CW01466635

Neuroanatomical Terminology

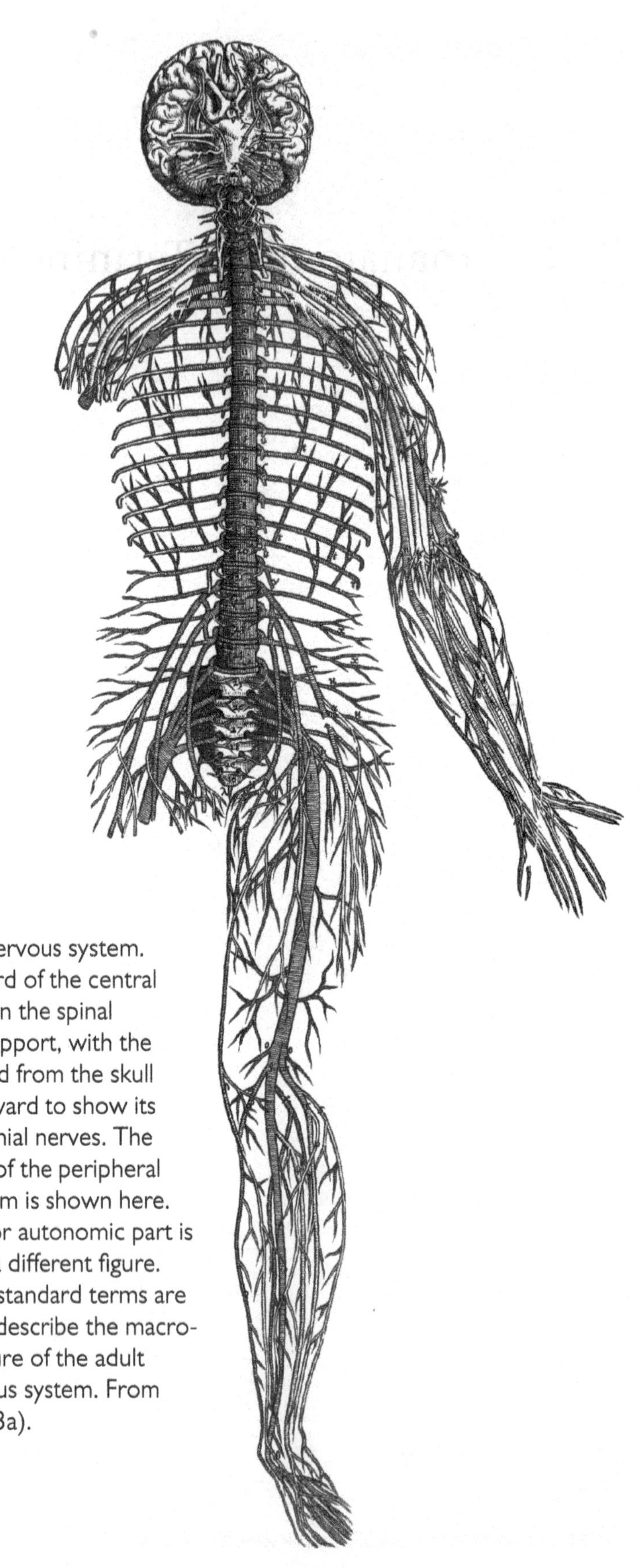

The human nervous system. The spinal cord of the central part remains in the spinal column for support, with the brain removed from the skull and tilted upward to show its base with cranial nerves. The somatic part of the peripheral nervous system is shown here. The visceral or autonomic part is illustrated in a different figure. About 1,300 standard terms are used now to describe the macroscopic structure of the adult human nervous system. From Vesalius (1543a).

Neuroanatomical **Terminology**

A LEXICON OF CLASSICAL ORIGINS AND HISTORICAL FOUNDATIONS

LARRY W. SWANSON, PhD

University Professor and
Appleman Professor of Biological Sciences
University of Southern California
Los Angeles

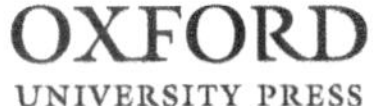

OXFORD
UNIVERSITY PRESS

Oxford University Press is a department of the University of Oxford.
It furthers the University's objective of excellence in research, scholarship,
and education by publishing worldwide.

Oxford New York
Auckland Cape Town Dar es Salaam Hong Kong Karachi
Kuala Lumpur Madrid Melbourne Mexico City Nairobi
New Delhi Shanghai Taipei Toronto

With offices in
Argentina Austria Brazil Chile Czech Republic France Greece
Guatemala Hungary Italy Japan Poland Portugal Singapore
South Korea Switzerland Thailand Turkey Ukraine Vietnam

Published in the United States of America by
Oxford University Press
198 Madison Avenue, New York, NY 10016

Library of Congress Cataloging-in-Publication
Swanson, Larry W., author.
Neuroanatomical terminology: a lexicon of classical origins and historical foundations / Larry W. Swanson.
p. ; cm.
Includes bibliographical references and index.
ISBN 978-0-19-534062-4 (alk. paper)
I. Title.
[DNLM: 1. Nervous System—anatomy & histology—Terminology—English.
2. Diagnostic Imaging. 3. Neuroanatomy—history. WL 15]
QM451
611'.8—dc23
2013042245

9 8 7 6 5 4 3 2 1
Printed in the United States of America
on acid-free paper

Table of Contents

List of Figures

Preface

Work on this book coincided with the explosive creation of the Internet and the rather more difficult birth of neuroinformatics toward the end of the 20th century. Without the former it probably could not have been finished in its present form during my lifetime, and without the latter it probably would not have been started at all.

The early stimulus for this research was a 1989 Committee on a National Neural Circuitry Database hosted by the Institute of Medicine (IOM) of the United States National Academies (Pechura & Martin, 1991). It helped pave the way for a decade of substantial National Institutes of Health (NIH) funding of the Human Brain Project (HBP) starting in 1995 (see De Schutter, 2005). During HBP conferences in San Diego, I met regularly and informally with three participants—Douglas Bowden, Steven Koslow, and Arthur Toga—to discuss broad strategies. We eventually agreed that the chaotic state of neuroanatomical nomenclature was perhaps the single greatest impediment to developing useful neuroinformatics tools for all aspects of neuroscience. Bowden went on to implement *NeuroNames* (Bowden & Dubach, 2003), which deals with contemporary sources of terminology, and I decided to take an historical approach, following the development of neuroanatomical terminology from the beginning. This approach was orders of magnitude more difficult than I had expected, and the initial results are presented here and in our broader Foundational Model of Connectivity (Swanson & Bota, 2011; Brown & Swanson, 2013).

Neuroinformatics is based on constructing databases and knowledge management systems for the nervous system (Koslow & Huerta, 1997). To construct tables for databases and to use inference engines in knowledge management systems it is necessary to create internally consistent defined vocabularies along with sets of rules for establishing relationships between concepts and terms. In contrast, neuroanatomy—now sometimes called *structural neuroscience* or *connectomics*—is thousands of years old and its terminology remains frustratingly disorganized, unlike mathematics, physics, and chemistry, where standardized nomenclatures have long been essential for progress.

I was originally drawn into this morass in the 1970s by the tradition of citing historical precedence in my own experimental neuroanatomical research papers on axonal connections between parts of the mammalian brain. It was accepted practice to determine which available terminologies for brain parts fitted the data best, and if none were adequate it was sometimes necessary to define new parts or different borders in relation to the older views (for example, Swanson, 1976). In the *Discussion* section the earlier literature could then be viewed and interpreted in relation to the internally consistent structural nomenclature adopted and defined for the experimental results.

As the body of this work grew and expanded to include the entire central nervous system (for example, Swanson & Hartman, 1975; Swanson & McKellar, 1979), the need for a systematic atlas became apparent, and the first edition of *Brain Maps: Structure of the Rat Brain* (Swanson, 1992, 1993) eventually appeared. This work contained a traditional atlas, with a set of photomicrographs of transverse histological sections through the rat brain accompanied by a set of corresponding interpretative maps (in print and the first atlas in digital format). But perhaps more importantly it contained the first systematic, hierarchically organized Nomenclature Tables of brain parts (gray matter regions and white matter tracts) to appear in modern times, with documentation from the primary literature. This required assessing the rather extensive contemporary literature and choosing an internally consistent parceling and accompanying nomenclature that appeared to be not only best documented in terms of experimental evidence, but also most appropriate in terms of historical precedence. These Nomenclature Tables are now in their third edition (Swanson, 2004).

The experience gained by this systematic exercise was taken to another level by our translation (Swanson & Swanson, 1995) of Santiago Ramón y Cajal's masterpiece, the *Histologie du Système Nerveux de l'Homme et des Vertébrés* (Cajal, 1909–1911). This monumental work of just over 680,000 words and 1,025 original illustrations not only documented Cajal's own contributions to neuroanatomy—especially in the arenas of neuron types and connections—but also formed a critical review of most contributions to the field in the second half of the 19th century. Thus, it became necessary for us to understand clearly the state of neuroanatomical terminology at the end of the 19th century, which was presented in the translation's *Index*.

The third level of structural neuroscience nomenclature analysis presented here emerged from the needs of a new field—neuroinformatics—mentioned above. We went on to create an online Brain Architecture Knowledge Management System (Google: *BAMS*) that was based initially on our atlas, nomenclature, and experimental circuit data in the rat (Bota et al., 2003). However, the need for a comprehensive neuroanatomical nomenclature for all parts of the nervous system (central and peripheral), and in all animals, remained and led to the formulation of a Foundational Model of Connectivity (Swanson & Bota, 2010) and the work presented here. The ultimate goal is to create a language that can be used to describe clearly, accurately, and unambiguously the wiring or schematic diagram of the nervous system and that can be refined with a set of rules to accommodate new data and conceptual frameworks (see Brown & Swanson, 2013).

A revolution in scholarly research methodology took place literally during the course of this investigation. I began in 1998 the traditional, time-honored way: reading books in a library and taking notes. Shortly thereafter, catalogs of most of the world's most important libraries came online, massive union catalogs like WorldCat and Karlsruher Virtueller Katalog (KVK) were created, and librarians could be contacted easily by email for more detailed information about individual holdings. The vast majority of Western literature from the 15th century on was digitized and made available by keyword searches online, often in text searchable format. And word processing software made note taking, file searching, and text organization much more convenient and efficient than ever before. Today there is no excuse but laziness for not examining the earlier literature on any topic, including the history of neuroscience, which goes back to the Smith Papyrus of about 1700 BC.

Aside from my personal library, the most useful by far has been the Louise M. Darling Biomedical Library at the University of California, Los Angeles, and the exceptionally knowledgeable and helpful staff in the History and Special Collections for the Sciences Division, including especially Katherine Donahue, Russell Johnson, and Teresa Johnson. Marie-Françoise Chesselet, Chair of the Neurobiology Department at UCLA at the time, also made the research go much more smoothly by arranging a Visiting Scholar appointment for me. The second most useful resource was the incomparable collection and staff at the U.S. National Library of Medicine in Bethesda, Maryland. Here I want especially to thank those in the History of Medicine Division who helped the most: Stephen Greenberg, Crystal Smith, Anne Rothfeld, and Karen Pitts. Other valuable resources in California included the Huntington Library and its Dibner Senior Curator Daniel Lewis, the William Andrews Clark Library of UCLA and its then Head Librarian Bruce Whiteman, the Arts Library of UCLA, the Charles E. Young Research Library of UCLA, and the Lane Medical Library of Stanford and its Historical Curator Drew Bourn. In New York City I especially thank Arlene Shaner at the superb New York Academy of Medicine Library, and Stephen Novak and Jennifer McGillan at the Archives and Special Collections of the Augustus C. Long Health Sciences Library of Columbia University. Exceptionally rare material was also examined at the Francis A. Countway Library of Medicine of Harvard University and the Bancroft Library and Marian Koshland Biosciences and Natural Resources Library of the University of California, Berkeley. This research was supported in part by NIH Grant R01NS050792.

Readers will understand that no undertaking like this by one individual in a limited time frame can be regarded as anything but a preliminary guide to the vast, multilingual literature and part of a never ending revision of nomenclature tables.

AUGUST 15, 2013
LOS ANGELES

Quotations

"He who can properly define and divide is to be considered a god."

Plato (quoted in Mackay, 1977, p. 119)

"For in order that nothing I say be misunderstood and that precision and clarity be everywhere present, it is most essential that the meaning of every term be accurately defined."

Galen (*On the Doctrines of Hippocrates and Plato*; De Lacy, 1980, p. 361)

"Truth is the daughter of Time and not of authority."

Leonardo da Vinci (quoted in Garrison, 1929, p. 14)

"I cannot set bounds to my astonishment at my own stupidity and excessive trust in the writings of Galen and other anatomists. I was so besotted by Galen that I had never undertaken to demonstrate a human head without the head of a lamb or ox at my public dissections; I was so keen not to gain the reputation of having been unable to find the plexus [rete mirable (Herophilus, c335–c280 BC)] whose name was familiar to everyone that I imposed upon my audience by demonstrating from a sheep's head something I had never found in a human one."

Andreas Vesalius (1543a; Richardson & Carman translation, 2002, p. xvii)

"I implore his Majesty the Emperor [Charles V] to punish severely, as he deserves, this monster born and reared in his own home, this most pernicious exemplar of ignorance, ingratitude, arrogance, and impiety; and to suppress him completely, lest he poison the rest of Europe with his pestilential breath. With his deadly spume, he has already infected certain Frenchmen, Germans, and Italians, but they, I believe, are ignorant of anatomy and of the other branches of medicine..."

Jacques Dubois (1551; from *A Repudiation of the Calumnies of a Certain Madman [Vesalius] Concerning Hippocratic and Galenic Anatomy by Jacobus Sylvius, the Royal Interpreter of Things Medical at Paris*; see Cushing translation, 1943, p. xxx)

"Among the parts of an animated Body, which are subject to Anatomical disquisition, none is presumed to be easier or better known than the brain; yet in the meantime, there is none less or more imperfectly understood."

Thomas Willis (1664; Pordage translation, 1681, p. 55)

"To examine each part [of the brain] thoroughly requires so much time and such application of mind that it would be necessary to give up all other labors and all other considerations on that particular task."

Nicolaus Steno (1669; see translation, 1965, p. 141)

"When a committee is made up of five or six people, one of them is reading, another is delivering his opinion, two are gossiping together, one is asleep, and one is diverting himself by leafing through one of the Dictionaries on the table."

Antoine Furetière (1688. A member of *l'Académie française*, founded in 1635 to produce a dictionary of the French language; quoted in Hitching, 2005, p. 51)

"Dictionaries are like watches. The worst is better than none, and the best cannot be expected to go quite true."

Samuel Johnson (shortly before his death in 1784, quoted in Hitching, 2005, p. 179)

"We shall provisionally adopt the more rational language which C. Chaussier has substituted for the whimsical and ridiculous names employed by the ancients to denote the different parts of the encephalic organ. But, it must be confessed, that zootomy will never be in possession of a nomenclature completely satisfactory, and susceptible of being generally adopted, until intelligent anatomists employ themselves, as the modern chemists [Antoine Lavoisier in particular] have done, to reform the language of their science; and until, after adopting a method of nomenclature, they shall have given to the different parts names suited not only to the organs of man, but also to the similar or analogous parts in animals, so as to connect by language two branches of natural history, which ought never to be separated."

Jean Burdin (1803 translation, Vol. 1, pp. 156–157)

"Anatomy may be likened to a harvest field. First come the reapers who, entering on untrodden ground, cut down great store of corn from all sides of them. These were the earliest anatomists of modern Europe, such as Vesalius, Fallopius, Malpighi, and Harvey. Then come the gleaners, all gather up ears enough from the bare ridges to make a few loaves of bread. Such were the anatomists of the last century—Winslow, Vicq d'Azyr, Camper, Hunter, and the two Monroes. Last of all come the geese, who still contrive to pick up a few grains scattered here and there among the stubble, and waddle home in the evening, poor things, cackling with joy because of their success. Gentlemen, we are the geese."

John Barclay (1758–1826; from a warning to his students, as quoted in Sinclair and Robb-Smith, 1950, p. 74)

"It is not a little remarkable that what is definitely known regarding the special functions of the nervous system has been ascertained within the last thirty years."

British and Foreign Medical Review (1840, Vol. 9, p. 98)

"The best workman uses the best tools. Terms are the tools of the teacher; and only an inferior hand persists in toiling with a clumsy instrument when a better one lies within his reach. But 'he has been used to the other.' No doubt; and some

extra practice is necessary to acquire the knack of applying the new tool. But in this acquisition a small capital of trouble will have been invested with a sure return of large profits. A single substantive term is a better instrument of thought than a paraphrase. But the substitution of such terms for definitions is still more advantageous when they are susceptible of becoming adjectives by inflection..."

Richard Owen (1866, p. xiii–xiv)

"Faced with an anatomical fact proven beyond doubt, any physiological result that stands in contradiction to it loses all its meaning... So, first anatomy and then physiology; but if first physiology, then not without anatomy"

Bernard von Gudden (quoted in Brodmann, 1909; Garey translation, 1994, p. 267)

"'A well-chosen word can save an enormous amount of thought,' because to name is to classify, to establish ideal affiliations—analogous relationships—between little-known phenomena, and to identify the general idea or principle wherein they lie latent, like the tree within its seed."

Santiago Ramón y Cajal (1999, p. 54)

"The terminology of the brain is in great confusion. Most of the more obvious parts were named before their functions were known, and the same part often receiving many different names, and sometimes the same name being applied to very different parts."

C. Judson Herrick (1915, p. 115)

"It is almost unbelievable how many people are unable to copy a name correctly, and once a mistake gets into print or into an official document it is difficult to eradicate."

Henry E. Sigerist (1960, p. 292)

"Regardless of how terms are defined by lexicographers or committees of experts, terms cannot be used outside a theory. That is true even when terms are contingent—'given so-and-so, that is a neuron'—or hedged with observational restrictions—'that is an object at this time and place which has observable properties a, b, ... n.' The principal reason for the frequent disputes over terminology is not so much about whether a new term muddles Greek with Latin. It is really about whether the term is biased toward their theory rather than ours."

Marcus Jacobson (1993, p. 16)

"Without the belief in some principle of organization of the nervous system there can be no science of the nervous system."

Marcus Jacobson (1993, p. 23)

Chapter I

LEXICON OF NERVOUS SYSTEM PARTS

Understanding how any system works requires four things: a general understanding of what the system does, a parts list, an account of how each part works, and knowledge of how the parts are interconnected to function as a whole. For the ***nervous system (Monro, 1783)*** in particular, there is a basic understanding of its role as a biological computer in controlling and coordinating both the internal physiological state of the body and behavioral interactions of the body with the external environment. However, a fundamental block to understanding mechanisms underlying this integration is the lack of a comprehensive, systematic, and widely accepted parts list for the ***nervous system (Monro, 1783)***.

A standard parts list is important for at least three main reasons. First, effective scientific communication requires an accurate, clearly defined vocabulary of technical terms. Second, a global parts list allows global analysis at the systems level. What is the internal configuration of each part and how does it work, how are the parts interconnected to function as a whole, and how does activity in one part or node influence activity in other parts or nodes of the network? And third, knowledge management systems that use inference engines with associated databases require unambiguous, systematic defined vocabularies of terms and relationships between terms.

Connectomes are one way to organize information about the wiring diagram of the ***nervous system (Monro, 1783)***. As originally conceived, a connectome is a global table of connections between ***nervous system (Monro, 1783)*** parts—a "from–to" lookup table or matrix (Sporns et al., 2005). Obviously, a comprehensive, internally consistent set of defined terms for parts that are connected is required for such a connectome (Bota et al., 2003; Bota & Swanson, 2010).

Foundational Model of Connectivity

Because the ***nervous system (Monro, 1783)*** is a biological computer, the "wiring" or schematic diagram of its structural connectivity provides one obligatory foundational model for understanding functional localization and mechanisms at all levels of organization from molecules to behavior and cognition. To facilitate accurate and clear scientific communication, global analysis of neural networks, and network modeling in knowledge management systems, a Foundational Model of Connectivity was formulated (Swanson & Bota, 2010). It is a high-level, downwardly extendible conceptual framework that applies to all animals with a ***nervous system (Monro, 1783)***, invertebrates and vertebrates alike, at all levels of analysis or resolution.

Any system or network has nodes and connections between nodes (see next section). This book has two major, interrelated parts: a Lexicon of defined terms and a set of 10 Nomenclature Tables. Fundamentally, they deal with the identity and location of nodes and connections within the ***nervous system (Monro, 1783)*** and are developed within the framework of the Foundational Model of Connectivity.

Location or position within the ***nervous system (Monro, 1783)***, and within the body as a whole, is described for any and all animals with a standard set of terms defined in the Foundational Model of Connectivity (Figure 1). This is a common approach in comparative anatomy, but for historical reasons it has been a major problem in human anatomy, where an idiosyncratic and deeply rooted set of positional terms is commonly used, especially in medical contexts. Nevertheless, the Foundational Model of Connectivity terms for positional information are used here as much as is practical for describing human ***nervous system (Monro, 1783)*** parts in the Lexicon (Figure 2).

Macrolevel, Mesolevel, and Microlevel of Analysis

An important feature of the Foundational Model of Connectivity is the precise definition for the ***nervous system (Monro, 1783)*** of three nested levels of analysis, resolution, granularity, and description (Swanson & Bota, 2010; Brown & Swanson, 2013). This approach (Figure 3) provides a strategy for attacking the well-known complexity of the ***nervous system (Monro, 1783)***, either from the top down (simple to complex) or bottom up (complex to simple).

The macrolevel of ***nervous system (Monro, 1783)*** connectivity is the simplest and lowest resolution. It deals with parceling ***gray matter (Meckel, 1817)*** and ***white matter (Meckel, 1817)*** into distinct ***gray matter regions (Swanson & Bota, 2010)*** and ***white matter tracts (Bell & Bell, 1826)***, respectively. At the macrolevel, ***nervous system (Monro, 1783)*** circuitry is described as ***gray matter region (Swanson & Bota, 2010)*** macronodes with ***white matter tract (Bell & Bell, 1826)*** input and output macroconnections. Before the microscope was used effectively for studying ***nervous system (Monro, 1783)*** connectivity organization in the mid 1830s, and the cell theory was introduced (Schleiden, 1838; Schwann, 1839), macrolevel examination was done with the naked eye, occasionally aided by a hand lens. Since then it has been examined predominantly with histological methods in animals and, more recently, with imaging techniques like MRI in living humans.

The mesolevel of ***nervous system (Monro, 1783)*** connectivity deals with neuron types (Bota & Swanson, 2007).

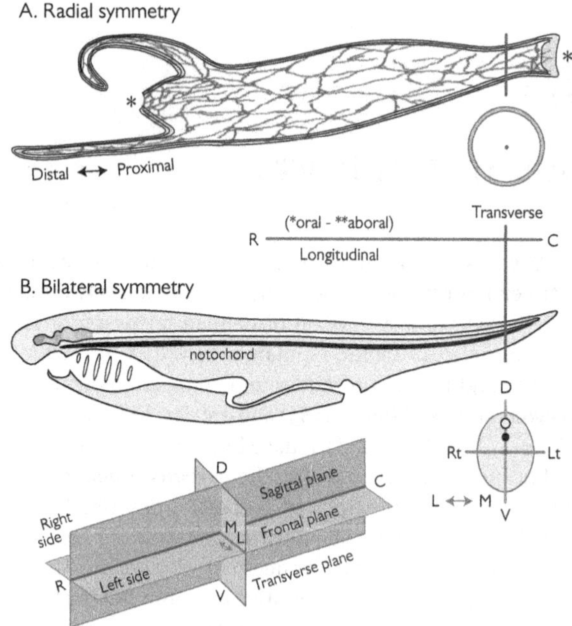

FIGURE 1. Describing position and symmetry in all animals with a ***nervous system (Monro, 1783)***. The basic assumption is that the body of all animals, whether radially or bilaterally symmetrical, has a longitudinal axis and one or two transverse axes, with the former having rostral and caudal ends. (A) Radially symmetrical animals like the hydra illustrated here have a ***nerve net (>1840)*** and two orthogonal axes, longitudinal (rostrocaudal or oral-aboral) and transverse. They also have two orthogonal planes of section, longitudinal or transverse. Relative position along body extensions, in this case tentacles, is indicated (distal or proximal to its attachment to the body). In bilaterally symmetrical animals, proximal and distal are used for extensions like fins, wings, limbs, or noses. (B) Bilaterally symmetrical invertebrates and vertebrates have three cardinal axes and three corresponding planes of section, as well as right and left halves or sides. An idealized chordate body plan is shown here. The ***central nervous system (Carus, 1814)*** lies dorsal to the notochord that in turn lies dorsal to the digestive system. A key principle in comparative schemes for indicating positional information is use of terms referring to the body itself, rather than to relationships of the body to the environment, which can change dramatically depending on behavior. Especially egregious offenders include horizontal (parallel to the horizon), superior (toward the sky, or heavens), and inferior (toward the earth). *Abbreviations*: C, caudal; D, dorsal; L, lateral; Lt, left; M, medial; R, rostral; Rt, right; V, ventral. *Reproduced with permission from Swanson & Bota (2010).*

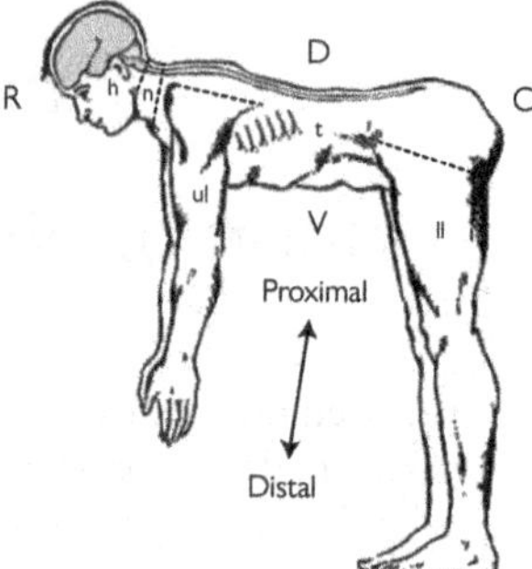

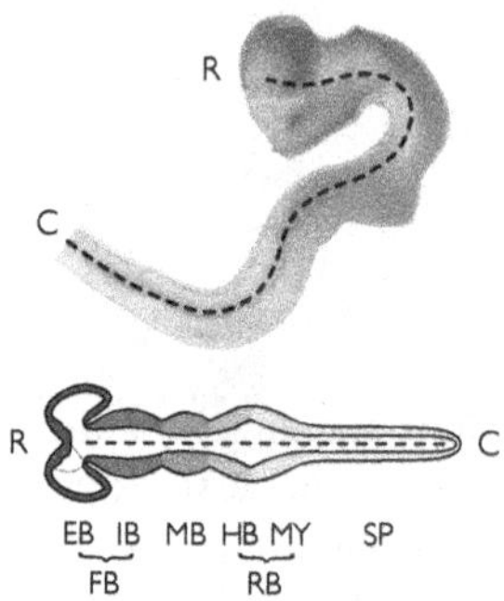

FIGURE 2. Describing position and symmetry in the developing and adult human. This problem is especially difficult because of dramatic changes in the longitudinal axis of the developing embryo, and of the adult body, which is vertical and bipedal with the palms facing forward in the standard human anatomical position. (A) Adult human in the comparative anatomical position where comparison with other bilaterally symmetrical animals (Figure 1B) is easy, and position along extensions like limbs is also easily described (compare with tentacle in Figure 1B). The body's longitudinal axis is indicated with a dashed line and has rostral (*R*) and caudal (*C*) ends. (B) ***Neural tube (Baer, 1837)*** of a one-month human embryo, with the longitudinal axis indicated by a dashed line. The ***endbrain (Kuhlenbeck, 1927)*** (*EB*) is at the rostral end and the ***spinal cord (Galen, c162–c166)*** (SP) is at the caudal end. The top part of the figure shows the right half of the ***neural tube (Baer, 1837)***, and the bottom half is a conceptualized straightened ***neural tube (Baer, 1837)*** in frontal (horizontal) section with topographic divisions listed in Appendix 2. *Other abbreviations*: *D*, dorsal; *FB*, ***forebrain (Goette, 1873)***; *HB*, ***hindbrain (Baer, 1837)***; *IB*, ***interbrain (Baer, 1837)***; *MB*, ***midbrain (Baer, 1837)***; *MY*, ***medulla (Winslow, 1733)*** or ***afterbrain (Baer, 1837)***; *RB*, ***rhombicbrain (His, 1893b)***; *V*, ventral. *Reproduced with permission from Swanson & Bota (2010).*

In essence, each ***gray matter region (Swanson & Bota, 2010)*** is defined by a unique set of neuron types. At the mesolevel, ***nervous system (Monro, 1783)*** connectivity is described as neuron type mesonodes within particular macronodes that have input and output mesoconnections following specific routes though ***white matter tracts (Bell & Bell, 1826)***.

The microlevel of ***nervous system (Monro, 1783)*** connectivity deals with individual neurons of a neuron type. At the microlevel, individual neurons form individual micronodes and the connection pattern of individual neurons at the level of axon branching patterns, and the distribution and size of individual synapses is accounted for.

In general, the macrolevel and mesolevel of ***nervous system (Monro, 1783)*** organization are genetically determined, discounting injury and disease. They are still commonly treated qualitatively, although differences between individuals are often measured. In contrast, the effects of experience—which include factors like learning, pharmacological agents, and stress—are measured at the microlevel. Microlevel features are commonly treated quantitatively and change rather quickly, and often more or less continuously, in the individual.

Goals and Scope of the Book

The general goal of this book was to provide a comprehensive, systematic defined vocabulary for describing the ***nervous system (Monro, 1783)*** in general and the human ***nervous system (Monro, 1783)*** in particular. This was approached by developing two major interrelated features. The first is the Lexicon. It provides for each ***standard term*** in the defined vocabulary a literature citation for the first use of the term; a textual definition including method used to describe the part, age, species, and sex to which the definition applies; a citation for the discovery of the part; and a list of other terms including alternate spellings, translations, synonyms, and those that partly correspond. The second feature is the comprehensive and systematic set of Nomenclature Tables based on the ***standard terms*** (see Chapter 3 and Appendices).

Based on these goals, an historical approach was taken starting at the beginning of surviving written documentation from the Middle Kingdom of Ancient Egypt about 3,700 years ago. As research on the goals progressed, it became apparent that the scope of the project would have to be limited. By the end of the 18th century the number of terms was clearly increasing exponentially (see Chapter 2 and Figure 6).

The scope of this book was thus limited in three ways. First, it was limited to the macrolevel of description (Figure 3), which is the easiest. Second, a comprehensive defined vocabulary for the ***nervous system (Monro, 1783)***

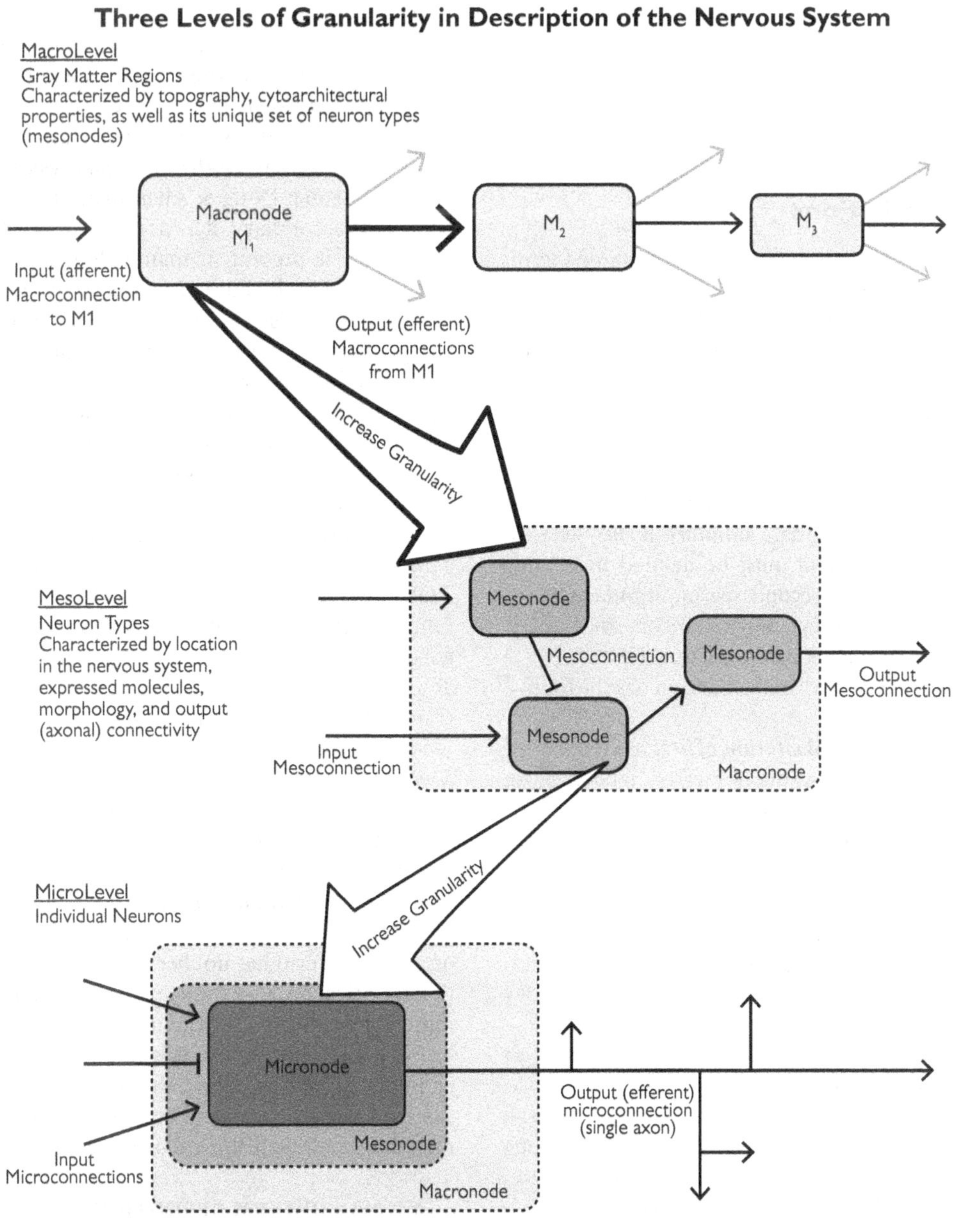

FIGURE 3. Levels of analysis for ***nervous system (Monro, 1783)*** connectivity. Because ***nervous system (Monro, 1783)*** circuitry is so complex, dividing it into three well-defined and nested levels helps clarify analysis strategies and provides a conceptual framework for clearer understanding of organizing principles. The origins of neural connections can be regarded as macronodes or ***gray matter regions (Swanson & Bota, 2010)***, mesonodes or neuron types, and micronodes or individual neurons. Individual ***gray matter regions (Swanson & Bota, 2010)*** are distinguished by a unique set of neuron types, and individual neuron types are distinguished by a unique set of individual neurons. *Reproduced with permission from Brown & Swanson (2013).*

was limited to human, where documented analysis at the macrolevel is by far most complete and where it is particularly relevant now for in vivo MRI imaging. And third, thorough historical documentation was limited to the Classic Era of neuroanatomy, which can be defined as ending with the introduction of the cell theory to biology (Schleiden, 1838; Schwann, 1839) and the rapid rise of histological analysis thereafter. Historical documentation of ***standard terms*** beyond 1840, symbolized as (>1840) when the original source was not established, was strictly limited to the best textbooks and to terms used relatively recently that may be confusing or ambiguous.

Following earlier attempts (Swanson, 1992, 1998, 2004; Swanson & Bota, 2010), the Nomenclature Tables (Appendices) present the higher levels of the hierarchies and are easily extendible in the future to lower levels containing documented finer subdivisions.

Terms and Definitions

The Lexicon is a defined vocabulary of 1,381 ***standard terms*** and 10,928 other, *nonstandard terms*. The use of ***standard terms*** is highly advantageous in a work like this for two reasons. First, the number of complete definitions required is proportional to the number of all terms, whereas without ***standard terms*** the number of complete definitions is proportional to the square of all terms (Dashti et al., 1997). In the former case *nonstandard terms* are defined in relation to ***standard terms*** (for example, synonyms need no definition, only a pointer to the appropriate ***standard term***), whereas in the latter case every term must be defined in relation to every other term. The second reason ***standard terms*** are advantageous is that they are used to construct clearly defined, internally consistent Nomenclature Tables.

A full ***standard term*** entry in the Lexicon has the following components:

Standard term name and citation of first use. Following recent international trends, the preferred language for ***standard terms*** is English (*Terminologia Anatomica*, 1998; Nieuwenhuys et al., 2008), with American English spelling. Anatomical literature has not been published in Latin since the 19th century, and very few experimental neuroscientists today are fluent in, or even acquainted with, Latin. In practice, this makes the use of existing Latin terminology meaningless and the creation of meaningful new terminology based on emerging research quite problematic.

Choosing ***standard terms*** from all those available, or even from new ones created specifically for this purpose, was particularly difficult. However, it is important to recall that human anatomy, including neuroanatomy, has a long and strong tradition—it has been taught continuously in medical schools for 2,500 years, since Classical Greece—and that macrolevel human anatomical terminology has been standardized by a succession of national and international committees since 1895 (see *Terminologia Anatomica*, 1998, pp. 157–162). Three main factors guided the choice of ***standard terms***. First, they followed, as closely as current evidence indicates, the standard nomenclature provided in *Nomina Anatomica* (1983) and *Terminologia Anatomica* (1998). The two sources are rather similar, although the latter includes Latin and English equivalents. They are strongest for ***peripheral nervous system (Meckel, 1817)*** anatomy and weakest for ***forebrain (Goette, 1873)*** anatomy. Creating a new rational neuroanatomical nomenclature, like Carl Linnaeus (1758) did for biological taxonomy or Antoine Lavoisier and colleagues (Guyton de Morveau et al., 1787) did for chemistry in the 18th century, is an undertaking for the future.

Second, possible choices were made with the long-term goal of creating a nomenclature common to mammals, with specialized terms for smaller subdivisions applicable to particular species. The choices made here were guided by the Foundational Model of Connectivity (Swanson & Bota, 2010) and the strategy taken in our nomenclature for the adult rodent ***central nervous system (Carus, 1814)*** (Swanson, 2004; Dong & Allen Institute for Brain Science, 2008). As a corollary, it is accepted procedure that when a structure is present in mammals including human, the term applied to the human is applied to the same structure in other forms (see Romer, 1962, p. 13). Other generally accepted procedures include the fact that any nomenclature should be logical, practical, and clear, and that for ***nerves (Herophilus, c335–c280 BC)*** in particular, terms should when possible correspond to accompanying bones, arteries, and/or veins, or to corresponding innervated structures like muscles and glands.

And third, the choices were made to construct and complete in a systematic way the 10 Nomenclature Tables presented in Chapter 3 and the Appendices. Since Linnaeus (1758), perhaps the single most important criterion for the acceptance of standard names in plant and animal taxonomy is historical precedence or priority (International Commission on Zoological Nomenclature, 1999, pp. 2, 24): if a species has been described and named adequately, it is not acceptable to use a new name. This principle has not yet been applied to structural neuroscience.

Following the ***standard term*** name is a citation to the first use of this specific term, as far as could be determined. Its format is ***standard term (Author, date)***, or ***standard term (>1840)*** when it was introduced after 1840 and the origin of the term has not been traced yet. The use of a citation is critical because the same term can have different definitions that must be distinguished, as is easy to see in the *List of All Defined Terms*. It is important to note that these citations are not eponyms, the use of which current practice discourages because they are sometimes used without regard to accurate historical precedence.

Standard Term Definition

All ***standard terms*** have a textual definition describing what they are in relation to other ***standard terms*** in the Lexicon. Other regular features of a definition include the species (for example, human or silkworm) or taxon (for example, vertebrate or mammal), age and sex to which the

standard term applies, and the method used to identify the structure indicated by the term (for example, macroscopic dissection, referred to as macrodissection). These features are important to include because the same term may have different (or the same) meaning in different species, in the embryo and adult, and in males, females, and hermaphrodites (see Bota & Swanson, 2010). Finally, each definition provides a citation to the first delineation of the structure indicated by the ***standard term***.

Some definitions include historical information about identification of the structure indicated by the ***standard term***. This was done when identification was unusually problematic, and is more complete for more important structures.

Alternate spellings

Alternate spellings of particularly important ***standard terms***, like ***brain (Smith Papyrus, c1700 BC)***, are given when of special interest or to clarify ambiguities. Variations between British English and American English spelling, or in hyphenation use, are not systematically given. Many ***standard terms*** can be either singular or plural, though only one is given; for example, ***nerves (Herophilus, c335–c280 BC)***, which is given, can obviously be used as ***nerve (Herophilus, c335–c280 BC)***. Alternate spellings are listed chronologically based on a citation to their first use as far as could be determined.

Translations

Full accounts of translations of standard and other terms into languages other than English are not provided and are relatively easy to access now on the Internet. One exception is the original term for ***standard terms*** when not in English. They are regularly given and are much more frequent in Latin than in German, French, Greek, and Italian. They are listed chronologically based on a citation to their first use as far as could be determined.

Earlier references

Earlier synonyms are terms used for a part before the ***standard term*** was first introduced. In addition, a part might have been delineated before receiving its first name, whether standard or an earlier synonym. Three separately listed possibilities were found, not necessarily in this order: (1) described, not named or illustrated; (2) illustrated, not named or described; and (3) illustrated and described, not named. All four types are defined with respect to ***standard terms*** and/or *nonstandard terms*, and are listed chronologically based on a citation to their first use as far as could be determined.

Later synonyms

They are terms used for a part after the ***standard term*** was introduced. They are listed chronologically based on a citation to their first use as far as could be determined.

Synonyms are the largest category of term in the Lexicon and the easiest to deal with conceptually, once it is admitted that exact synonymy is almost always impossible to determine unless explicitly stated by authors using them. Some authors used synonyms to the point of absurdity. Thomas Willis was one of the greatest abusers in this regard; for example: "The chamfered or streaked bodies, or the tops of the oblong marrow, are two lentiform processes..." uses 4 synonyms (chamfered bodies, streaked bodies, tops of oblong marrow, lentiform processes) in referring to another synonym, the (right and left) *corpus striatum (Willis, 1664)*; see Pordage translation (1681, p. 63). Other authors preferred long descriptive terms to simple terms. For example, compare *mental branch of maxillary branch of inferior maxillary branch of fifth pair of nerves (Bock, 1817)* to the earlier ***mental nerve (Cheselden, 1726)***. And finally, some distinctive parts lend themselves particularly to those inclined to create synonyms. The apparent favorite is ***mammillary body (Ludwig, 1779)***. Its entry in the Lexicon lists 45 earlier synonyms and 14 later synonyms. In contrast, the entry for ***retina (Herophilus, c335–c280 BC)*** lists only one earlier synonym and four later synonyms, the most recent being *coat of eye (Geminus, 1553)*.

Partly corresponds

These terms result from using a comprehensive defined vocabulary and are the hardest to deal with. Simply put, partly corresponding terms are not synonymous with any ***standard term*** in the defined vocabulary. However, in a hierarchically arranged nomenclature like that used here (Chapter 3 and Appendices) all terms related to the ***nervous system (Monro, 1783)*** can be defined with reference to one or more ***standard terms*** because ***nervous system (Monro, 1783)*** is at the top of the hierarchy—it is the universe or domain of discourse.

There are at least three major types of partly corresponding terms that have not been formally separated here. One type of partly corresponding term corresponds to two or more ***standard terms***. Examples include *midbrain (Burdin, 1803)*, which corresponds to ***tectum (Baer, 1837)*** and ***pons (Haller, 1747)*** considered together, and *lentiform nucleus (Burdach, 1822)*, which corresponds to ***globus pallidus (Burdach, 1822)*** and ***putamen (Burdach, 1822)*** considered together. Another type involves only part of one or more ***standard terms***—a part not recognized today and thus now considered a misinterpretation. An example is *cerebral part of oculomotor nerve (Arnold, 1834)*, which corresponds to the proximal segment of the ***oculomotor nerve (Estienne, 1545)*** before piercing the ***dura (Galen, c177)*** to enter the ***cavernous sinus (Winslow, 1733)***. And the third major type of partly corresponding term involves part of a ***standard term*** at the lowest level of the hierarchy that is not yet recognized as a legitimate ***standard term*** in the next lower level of the hierarchy but should or will be added. In summary, partly corresponding terms indicate misinterpretations as well as places where new ***standard terms*** can be added to new, lower levels of the hierarchy.

Methodology

The basic approach was to start at the beginning of recorded literature dealing with the structure of the ***nervous***

system (Monro, 1783), and systematically progress through history. Fortunately, virtually every relevant document through the beginning of the 16th century has been translated into English and is readily available in scholarly editions. For relevant information printed in Europe from the late 15th century to 1840, when the modern, microscopic era of structural neuroscience began, every attempt was made to examine an original copy, although fact checking has become much easier recently with the availability of printed material online. The goal was to provide for this period as complete an inventory as possible, without scholarly bias, of classical neuroanatomical terminology. This goal can, of course, never be achieved completely, as experience has taught for previous dictionaries of all kinds. Instead, methods and protocols were established with results limited by the author's knowledge, patience, and available time. The accuracy of information within the Lexicon was confirmed when possible by internal evidence within particular citations and by frequent reference to earlier work in later publications. For practical reasons, systematic examination was confined to the technical anatomical literature, so terms for ***nervous system (Monro, 1783)*** parts that have been used mostly in works on surgery, pathology, and the like may be missing. In addition, the etymology of terms is not treated systematically and pronunciation concerns are ignored, unlike many dictionaries.

In practice, systematic work on the historical origins of terms proceeded in parallel with construction of the 10 modern Nomenclature Tables presented in the Appendices. The two processes informed each other in a very synergistic way.

Chapter 2

Historical Trends

Localization of function is the single most important general principle emerging from the long history of clinical and scientific work in neuroscience (Sherrington, 1906; Neuburger, 1981; Clarke & Jacyna, 1987; Finger, 1994; Clarke & O'Malley, 1996), and is one reason clear communication about the parts of the ***nervous system (Monro, 1783)*** and their location is so critical. It is far beyond the scope of the present work to explore in detail the historical foundations of the results documented in the Lexicon, but some obvious trends in the Classical Era of neuroanatomy, defined as ending with the introduction of the cell theory at the end of the 1830s, are worth pointing out here.

Pattern of Discovery in the Classical Era

It is most interesting to begin with the discovery of ***nervous system (Monro, 1783)*** parts, whether or not, or what, they were named. For the present day macrolevel account of ***nervous system (Monro, 1783)*** parts in the Lexicon and Appendices, 1,381 ***standard terms*** are used, and of these, 1,162 (84%) corresponding parts were discovered by 1840. Almost all of the remaining 16% of parts with ***standard terms*** discovered since 1840 (>1840) are below the resolution of clear identification with current human in vivo imaging (MRI) methods, so it is clear that virtually everything in the ***nervous system (Monro, 1783)*** that can be identified with current human MRI technology was discovered by 1840.

Discovery in the Classical Era of neuroanatomy was not steady and progressive. Instead, it falls into four distinct periods separated by centuries of stagnation or even regression (Figure 4). Knowledge of the Egyptian Period is based on a single surviving papyrus with the only known original observations about ***nervous system (Monro, 1783)*** structure. The Edwin Smith Surgical Papyrus was written about 3,700 years ago by physicians dealing in living human patients with battle wounds, some so severe that the ***meninges (Smith Papyrus, c1700 BC)***, ***brain (Smith Papyrus, c1700 BC)***, and *cerebral convolutions (Smith Papyrus, c1700 BC)* were exposed to view. These were objective clinical observations accompanied by diagnoses and prognoses.

No new ***nervous system (Monro, 1783)*** structures were recorded over the next 1,200 years until the Greek Period of classical neuroanatomy, which coincided with Classical Greece in the 4th and 5th centuries BC. It was here that scientific observation of animal structure and function began: first with Alcmaeon and Anaxagoras, then with Hippocrates and Aristotle, and finally with Herophilus and Erasistratus, who also dissected human cadavers in Alexandria. Most notably, this group was responsible for clearly distinguishing major features including the ***nerves (Herophilus, c335–280 BC)***, ***retina (Herophilus, c335–c280 BC)***, ***ventricles (Hippocrates)***, *spinal medulla (Hippocrates)*, and ***cerebellum (Aristotle)***.

Following the work of Herophilus and Erasistratus, nothing original was added for over 300 years, until the Roman Period of classical neuroanatomy around the peak of the Roman Empire in the 2nd century. Galen was the towering figure of the period and a very large corpus of his vast writings has survived. He acknowledged a group of influential predecessor anatomists, including especially the respected Marinus of Pergamon, and had no successor. Galen, who was of Greek ethnicity and wrote in Greek, was far and away the greatest neuroanatomist of the Classical Era in terms of originality, breadth, and depth of discoveries. He discovered over two and a half times as many parts now referred to with ***standard terms*** as Andreas Vesalius, the next greatest discoverer (Figure 5).

Almost nothing was discovered in the ***nervous system (Monro, 1783)*** for 1,300 years after Galen's death, with two notable exceptions. First was the revival of Galen's writings, along with the practice of animal dissection, at the oldest western European medical school, in Salerno, during the late 11th to early 12th century. Four short anatomical texts used with the anatomical dissection of pigs have survived from that time (see Corner, 1927). One of them, associated with *Anatomia Magistri Nicolai physici*, first clearly identified the ***olfactory bulb (Weitbrecht, 1751)*** and ***cauda equina (Anatomia Magistri Nicolai, 12th century)***. The second exception occurred during the earliest stirrings of the Renaissance and was associated with the revival of human cadaver dissection, initially for autopsy purposes, at the medical school in Bologna. Mondino dei Luzzi was the author, and his book *Anathomia* (1316) was the first to mention the personal practice of human dissection since the work of Herophilus and Erasistratus 1,600 years earlier. He was the first to identify at least 5 parts of the ***nervous system (Monro, 1783)*** including the ***mammillary body (Ludwig, 1779)***.

The fruits of the Renaissance came surprisingly late to medicine and the life sciences. Almost 400 years passed after Mondino's *Anathomia* before the first few discoveries associated with the Renaissance Period of classical neuroanatomy in the 1490s, and its first great work didn't appear until 1543. That book, of course, was the *Fabrica* of Vesalius, and it stands second only to Galen's writing in terms of

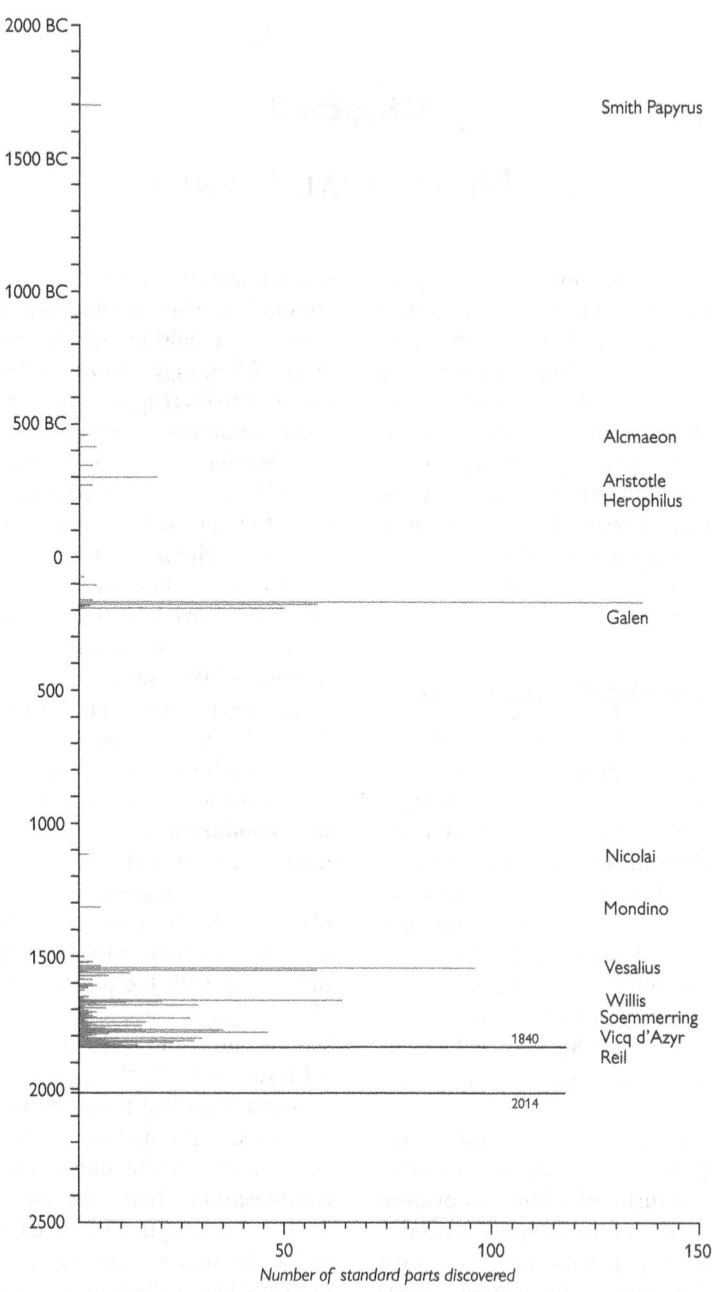

FIGURE 4. Patterns of discovery in the Classical Era. This histogram shows the year-by-year number of basic ***nervous system (Monro, 1783)*** parts discovered and documented in writing or illustration from c1700 BC to 1840. These are the parts given ***standard terms*** in the Lexicon and ten Nomenclature Tables of the Appendices. Authors responsible for significant peaks are listed on the right. The Modern Era of neuroanatomy between 1840 and the present is indicated between two horizontal lines. See text for discussion.

macrolevel ***nervous system (Monro, 1783)*** parts discovered (Figure 5). For our purposes, the Renaissance Period of classical neuroanatomy lasted about 350 years until the Modern Era of neuroanatomy began around 1840. During this period there were a number of great neuroanatomists (Figure 5), and the discovery of ***nervous system (Monro, 1783)*** parts designated with ***standard terms*** basically increased exponentially (Figures 4, 6).

Vesalius inspired a brilliant group of investigators, including most notably Bartolomeo Eustachi (1552), Gabriele Falloppio (1561), Volcher Coiter (1572), and Costanzo Varoli (1573). Then there was something of a lull until the conceptually brilliant work of Willis (1664, 1672), who actually made his most enduring anatomical discoveries in the ***peripheral nervous system (Meckel, 1817)***, which he called the *nervous system (Willis, 1664)*. Willis in turn inspired

Most discoveries in Classical Era

1.	Galen	c164-c192	250
2.	Vesalius	1543, 1555	97
3.	Willis	1664, 1672	67
4.	Vicq d'Azyr	1784, 1786	60
5.	Eustachi	1552	58
6.	Soemmerring	1778, 1791	36
7.	Vieussens	1684	29
8.	Reil	1807-1812	35
9.	Meckel	1817	28
10.	Winslow	1733	27

FIGURE 5 Most prolific discoverers of ***nervous system (Monro, 1783)*** parts in the Classical Era. The ten anatomists responsible for discovering the greatest number of parts before 1840 and the introduction of histological methods. Between c1700 BC and 1840, these ten people were responsible for discovering 59% (687/1,162) of the parts now constituting ***standard terms*** in the Lexicon. For other eminent authors see Figures 4, 6, and 7, and the text.

the work of Nicolas Steno (1669), Marcello Malpighi (1666, 1673), and Raymond Vieussens (1684) before another lull, broken by the superb general work of Jacob Winslow (1733) and Albrecht von Haller (1762) and the more specialized thesis of Samuel Thomas Soemmerring (1778). After the landmark atlas and commentary of Félix Vicq d'Azyr (1786) there was a rather steady increase of discoveries until the end of this period around 1840, most notably by Johann Christian Reil, Johann Friedrich Meckel the Younger, and Karl Friedrich Burdach.

Standard Terms, Synonyms, and Partly Corresponding Terms

The interpretation and definition of terms for parts of the ***nervous system (Monro, 1783)*** are, of course, retrospective—based on current evidence and informed by historical precedent. In general, the introduction of a ***standard term*** lags behind discovery of the corresponding part. For example, whereas Galen discovered at least 250 parts that now have ***standard terms***, only about 13 of the terms he used survive as current ***standard terms***. Similarly, Vesalius discovered almost 100 parts that now have ***standard terms***, and only about 10 of the terms he used survive as ***standard terms***. Unfortunately, there are no set rules for establishing neuroanatomical terms although reasonable best-practice guidelines have emerged over the years and have had some influence (see Chapter 1).

As of 1840, some 1,162 of the currently recognized 1,381 parts now assigned ***standard terms*** had been discovered (see preceding section), but only 386 (33%) of the 1,162 parts recognized in the Lexicon had received their currently assigned ***standard term*** (Figure 6). Burdach (1819, 1822), Meckel (1817), and Friedrich Arnold (1828, 1834, 1838a,b) contributed the most to standard terminology in the Classical Era of neuroanatomy (Figure 7). From Figures 5 and 7 it is clear that Galen (c164–c192), Vesalius (1543a), Winslow (1733), and Meckel (1817) were the greatest contributors during the Classical Era of neuroanatomy with respect to both original discoveries and contributions to standard terminology.

The discovery of structures corresponding to current ***standard terms*** was dealt with in the preceding section. Synonyms for ***standard terms*** constitute the largest category of terms in the Lexicon (Figure 6) and are the easiest to deal with—they correspond as far as can be reasonably determined to the ***standard term***. Synonyms have existed since the beginning, in the Edwin Smith Surgical Papyrus (c1700 BC), and for the ***nervous system (Monro, 1783)*** alone numbered at least 5,712 by 1840 not counting large numbers of alternate spellings and corresponding forms in other languages. This is a ratio of just over 4 (4.1) synonyms coined by 1840 for each ***standard term*** in the Lexicon. Their number obviously rose exponentially during the Renaissance Period of classical neuroanatomy (Figure 6), but the trend since then is impossible to pinpoint accurately because of changing interests, most notably the rise of histological approaches, and because of official nomenclature committees working for standardization since the 1890s (see Chapter 1).

The number of partly corresponding terms (see Chapter 1) also increased exponentially during the Renaissance Period at the end of the Classical Era of neuroanatomy (Figure 6), but not as fast as the number of synonyms. Thus, the ratio of partly corresponding terms in 1840 to current ***standard terms*** in the Lexicon was just under 3:1 (2.8:1; 3,933/1,381).

To summarize the research done here: at the end of the Classical Era of neuroanatomy in 1840, the vast majority of ***nervous system (Monro, 1783)*** parts having ***standard terms*** in the Lexicon had been discovered (1,162 of 1,381), although only 386 (33%) had received their current ***standard term***. In addition, at least 5,712 synonyms (not counting alternate spellings and equivalent forms in other languages) had been coined, and at least 3,922 partly corresponding terms had been delineated. This amounted to just over 10,000 terms for 1,162 ***nervous system (Monro, 1783)*** parts. For the sake of the complete Nomenclature Tables in the Appendices, just over 2,300 terms introduced after 1840 were added to the Lexicon and indicated as (>1840) if the citation to its first use was not determined; see Chapter 3. The number of parts discovered, ***standard terms***, partly corresponding terms, and synonyms all increased exponentially during the Classical Era of neuroanatomy. As pointed out in Chapter 1, by 1840 virtually every ***nervous system (Monro, 1783)*** part with a ***standard term*** that can be unambiguously identified with current human in vivo MRI technology had at least been delineated by 1840.

Methodological Innovations in the Classical Era

Methods used to study and delineate the ***nervous system (Monro, 1783)*** during the Classical Era seem crude

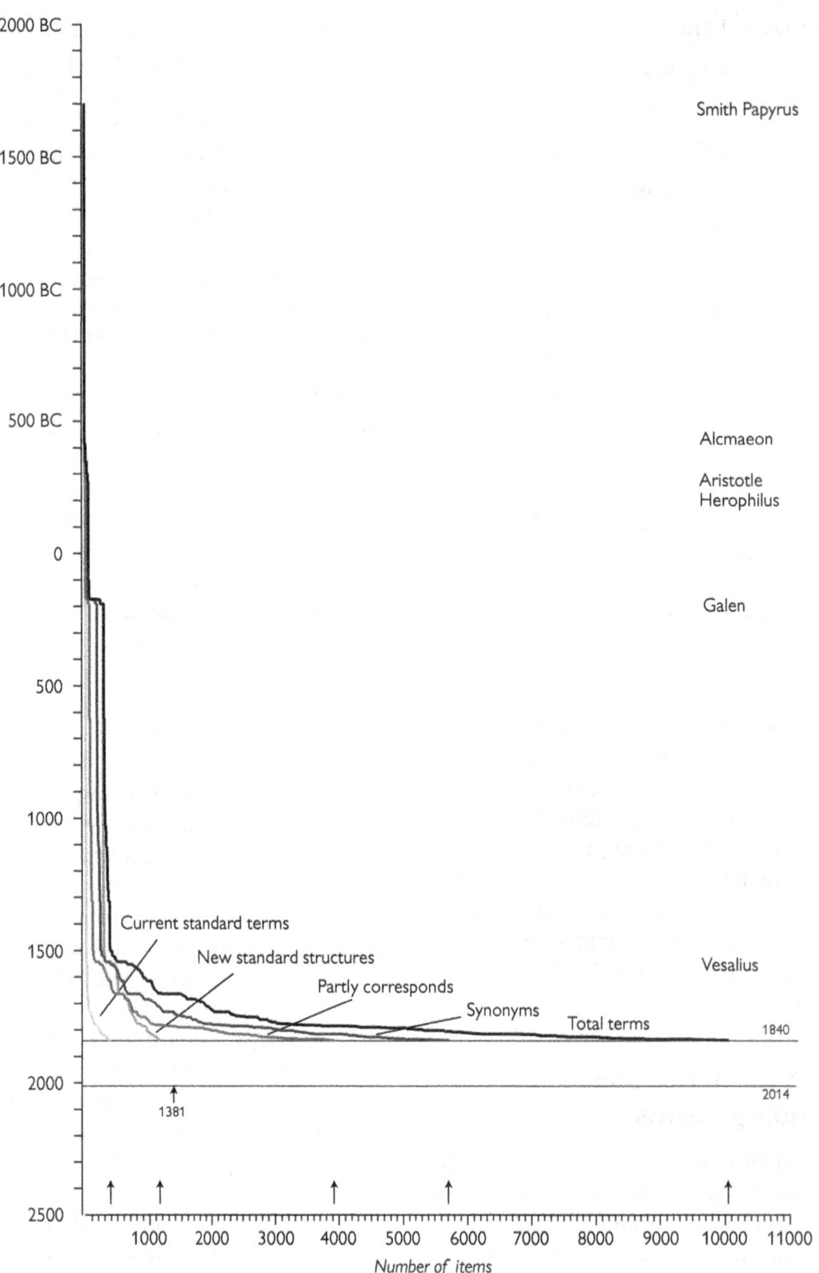

FIGURE 6. Cumulative timecourse for all parts delineated in the Classical Era. The five graphs begin in c1700 BC and end in 1840. They show an exponential rise in the number of new standard structures discovered each year in the ***nervous system (Monro, 1783)***, as well as the number of new ***standard terms*** given to standard structures, new synonyms, and new partly corresponding terms. The number of current ***standard terms*** (1,381) is shown below the horizontal line indicating 2014. The total number of items as of 1840 for each graph is indicated by an upward arrow just above the horizontal axis (Number of items). Some especially important changes along the graphs are associated with particular authors or sources, listed at right. See text for discussion.

today—essentially the gross anatomical dissection of human and other animal brains, viewed with the naked eye and occasionally magnified slightly with a hand lens in the Renaissance Period. As unbelievable as it may seem to modern scientists, the first major innovation since the scientific study of anatomy began in Classical Greece was the introduction of illustration to systematic description in the Renaissance Period. Plato, Aristotle, Galen, and Vesalius's teacher in Paris, Jacques Dubois, generally shunned illustration as too crude and misleading to represent what can actually be seen during dissection, and their predecessors Pythagoras and Socrates even refused to write down their thoughts, considering the written word too crude for conveying them accurately (see Singer & Rabin, 1946;

Singer, 1999). The first surviving records of anatomical research were written by Hippocrates (or his followers) and Aristotle.

While there were examples of crude, stylized drawings of the ***brain (Smith Papyrus, c1700 BC)*** in a few manuscripts (Clarke & Dewhurst, 1996), and printing with moveable type was introduced by Johannes Gutenberg in the mid 1450s, the first illustration of the ***brain (Smith Papyrus, c1700 BC)*** in a printed book did not appear until 1490, in an edition of Albertus Magnus's *Philosophia Pauperum* (Figure 8). It was a highly stylized, Medieval style drawing to illustrate the Three-cell Doctrine of ***nervous system (Monro, 1783)*** function (see Manzoni, 1998). Remarkably, the first naturalistic drawings of the ***brain (Smith Papyrus, c1700 BC)*** were not printed until 1517, and they were small, crude, and unlabeled (Figure 9). Six years later the first great realistic drawings of the ***brain (Smith Papyrus, c1700 BC)*** appeared in the second edition of Jacopo Berengario da Carpi's *Isagogae Breves* (1523) and they showed (Figure 10) what was considered its most important part, the ***ventricles (Hippocrates)***—compare with Figure 8, printed 33 years earlier.

Vesalius published a revolutionary series of brilliant drawings to illustrate the dissection of the entire ***nervous system (Monro, 1783)***, including what amounts to a modern atlas of the human ***brain (Smith Papyrus, c1700 BC)***; see Frontispiece and Figure 11. The ***brain (Smith Papyrus, c1700 BC)*** was revealed in a series of 15 drawings that included a sequence of frontal (horizontal) slices, the selective lifting of certain parts, and the selective removal of others (see Singer, 1952; Richardson & Carman, 2009). The result is a three-dimensional demonstration that would be useful today for autopsy purposes and for showing the

Most standard terms in Classical Era

1.	Burdach	1819, 1822	25
2.	Meckel	1817	20
3.	Arnold	1828, 1834, 1838a,b	20
4.	Winslow	1733	18
5.	Haller	1762	16
6.	Baer	1837	14
7.	Galen	c164-c192	13
8.	Cruveilhier	1836	11
9.	Vesalius	1543a	10
10.	Haase	1781	9
	Walter	1783	9

FIGURE 7. Most influential providers of standard terminology in the Classical Era of neuroanatomy. The anatomists responsible for providing the greatest number of ***standard terms*** in the Lexicon. These eleven people were responsible for providing 43% (165/382) of the ***standard terms*** coined between c1700 BC and 1840.

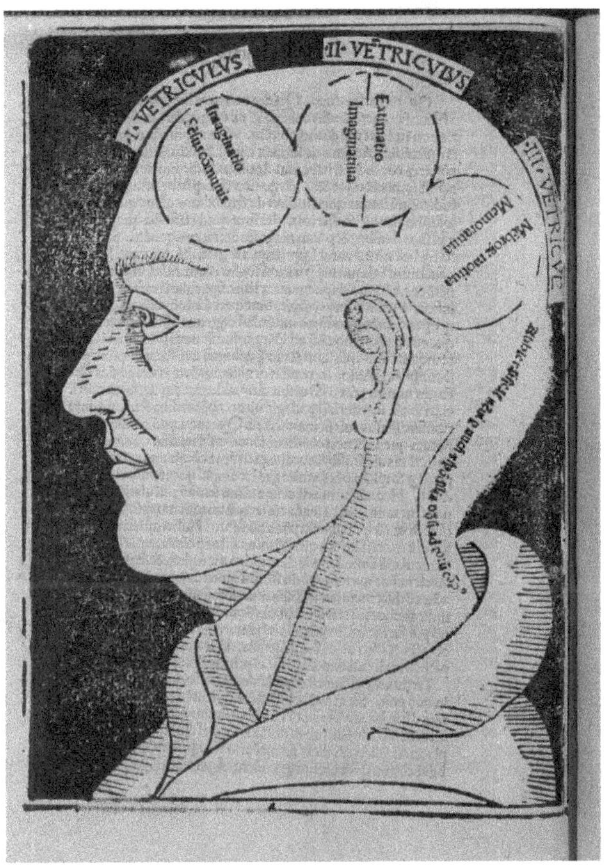

FIGURE 8. First printed illustration of the ***brain (Smith Papyrus, c1700 BC)***. This beautiful Renaissance drawing appeared in an early printed edition of the *Philosophia Pauperum* by Albertus Magnus (c1200–1280). It illustrates in highly schematic Medieval style the Three-cell Doctrine of ***nervous system (Monro, 1783)*** function projected on the side of the head. This theoretical framework attributed cognition to sequential processing of psychic pneuma brought to the ***ventricles (Hippocrates)***—and more specifically, the rostral end (front) of the ***lateral ventricles (Vesalius, 1543a)***—by the sensory ***nerves (Herophilus, c335–c280 BC)*** of the head. As shown, the ***lateral ventricles (Vesalius, 1543a)*** (*I ventriculus*, 1st ventricle or cell) subserve initially the common sense (*Sensus communis*), brought about by mingling of all sensory inputs, and then basic imagination (*Imaginatio*), which flows into the ***third ventricle (Galen, c173)*** (*II ventriculus*, 2nd ventricle or cell) through an unlabeled hole, the ***interventricular foramen (>1840)***, where creative imagination only found in humans (*Imaginativa*) and level of thought shared by all animals (*Ex[s]timatio*) reside. The next stage occurs after passing through another unlabeled hole indicating the ***cerebral aqueduct (>1840)*** and entering the ***fourth ventricle (Galen, c192)*** (*III ventriculus*, 3rd ventricle or cell), where memories (*Memorativa*) are formed and the power moving the limbs (*Membrorum motiva*) resides, before passing downward through the nerves of the neck and all the vertebrae to the whole body (as written on the neck). *Photograph courtesy of the National Library of Medicine.*

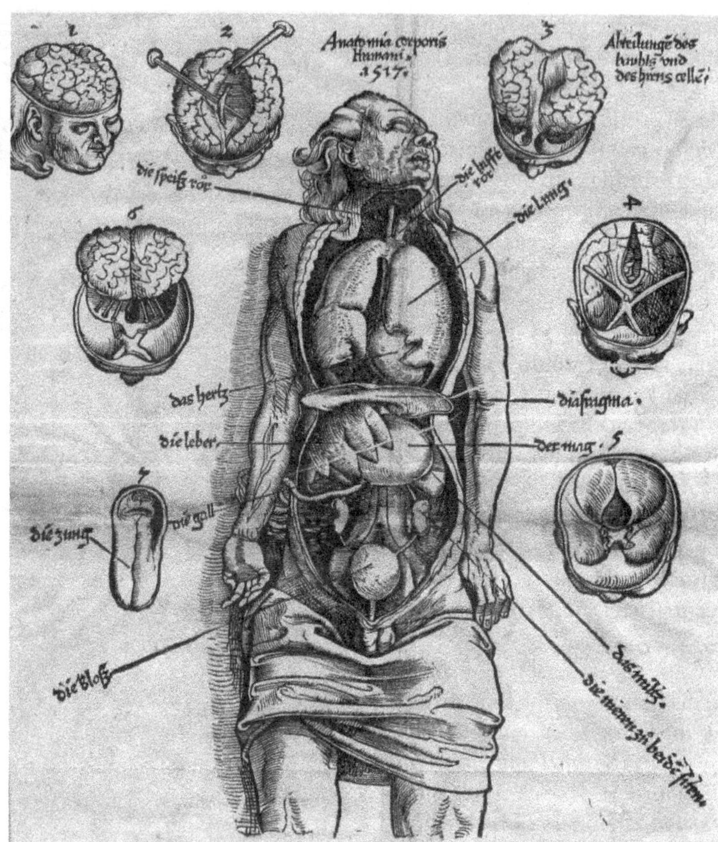

FIGURE 9. First printed naturalistic illustrations of the ***brain (Smith Papyrus, c1700 BC)***. The results of an actual dissection of an adult human cadaver are shown, with the viscera in the middle and a series of drawings around the periphery depicting the basic sequence of dissecting the head and ***brain (Smith Papyrus, c1700 BC)***, described since antiquity by Galen (c177) and Mondino (1316). It was probably drawn by Hans Wechtlin under supervision of the physician/anatomist Wendelin Hock von Brackenau and was first printed in 1517 as an independent fugitive sheet by Johann Schott in Strasbourg, who then included it in a book he published the same year: Hans von Gersdorff's *Feldbuch der Wundtartzney*.

basic structural organization of the human ***brain (Smith Papyrus, c1700 BC)***. The drawings themselves were done by Titian's studio and were not surpassed for well over 200 years, until the work of Soemmerring (1778) and Vicq d'Azyr (1786).

There were two other key methodological innovations during the Renaissance Period of classical neuroanatomy: tract tracing and fixation of nervous tissue. Willis (1664) proposed the revolutionary hypothesis that *gray substance (Vesalius, 1543a)* parts generate psychic pneuma ("neural information" in current terminology) whereas *tracts (Willis, 1664)* of *white matter (Vesalius, 1543a)* transmit it to other *gray substance (Vesalius, 1543a)* parts or to muscle. Willis (1664) speculated wildly about the overall organization of *tracts (Willis, 1664)* between various *gray substance (Vesalius, 1543a)* parts and was immediately criticized severely for doing so by Malpighi (1666) and Steno (1669). They both recommended carefully scraping away overlying *gray substance (Vesalius, 1543a)* to reveal more clearly the location and orientation of *tracts (Willis, 1664)*. This was soon done in a limited way by Willis (1672) for the *corpus striatum (Willis, 1664)* (Figure 12), and was illustrated quite remarkably for the ***corticospinal tract (>1840)*** a few years later by Vieussens (1684). The greatest practitioner of this approach in the Classical Era of neuroanatomy was Reil (1807–1812), who had the great advantage of using fixed human ***brain (Smith Papyrus, c1700 BC)*** tissue.

Fixation was a significant advance during the Renaissance Period of classical neuroanatomy because fresh nervous tissue is so soft, thus becoming rather distorted and decomposing quickly after removal from the body. The use of alcohol ("spirits of wine") to harden biological material and prevent putrification was suggested to the Royal Society in the 1660s by William Croone and Robert Boyle, and its use then became rather commonplace among anatomists (see Cole, 1944, pp. 445–448). However, its explicitly documented use in delineating parts of the ***nervous system (Monro, 1783)*** was essentially unknown until the magnificent ***brain (Smith Papyrus, c1700 BC)*** atlas of Vicq d'Azyr was published in 1786. It was an atlas in the broad tradition

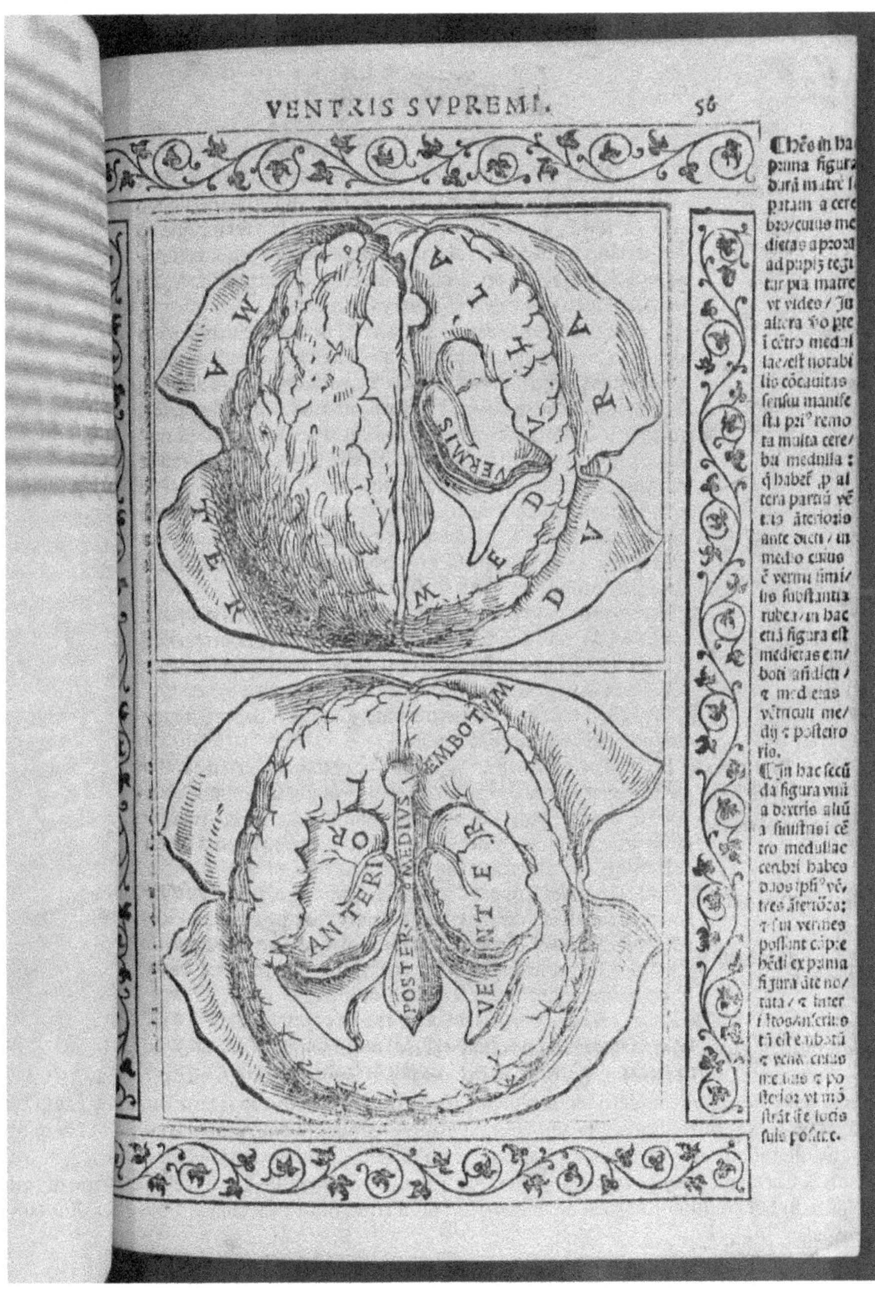

FIGURE 10. First printed naturalistic drawings of the ***brain (Smith Papyrus, c1700 BC)*** with labeled parts and description. It is from the 1523 book, *Isagogae Brevis* by Jacopo Berengario da Carpi, and shows the actual disposition of the ***ventricles (Hippocrates)*** in contrast to the schematic interpretation shown in Figure 8. The *dura mater (Haly Abbas or Ali ibn' ul-Abbas, d. 994)* of a fresh human cadaver was cut and reflected to show the ***brain (Smith Papyrus, c177 BC)*** from above, with rostral toward the top of each drawing, in four stages of dissection. In the upper left the *pia mater (Haly Abbas or Ali ibn' ul-Abbas, d. 994)* remains intact on the surface of the ***cerebral cortex (>1840)***. In the upper right a frontal (horizontal) slice of ***brain (Smith Papyrus, c177 BC)*** tissue, called *medulla (Berengario da Carpi, 1521)*, was removed to show the *venter anterior (Berengario da Carpi, 1521)* or ***lateral ventricle (Vesalius, 1543a)*** with its *vermis (Avicenna or Ibn Sina, c1030)* or ***choroid plexus of lateral ventricle (Vicq d'Azyr, 1784)***. In the bottom drawing the dorsal part (top) of the ***brain (Smith Papyrus, c1700 BC)*** was removed on both sides, clearly revealing near the median plane the *venter medius (Berengario da Carpi, 1521)* or ***third ventricle (Galen, c173)*** and *venter posterior (Berengario da Carpi, 1521)* or ***fourth ventricle (Galen, c192)***, as well as the *embotum (Berengario da Carpi, 1521)* or *infundibulum (Galen, c173)*. At this time, ***brain (Smith Papyrus, c1700 BC)*** function was commonly thought to reside in the ***ventricles (Hippocrates)***, with the *medulla (Berengario da Carpi, 1521)* playing only a supportive role. The ***posterior horn of lateral ventricle (Haller, 1747)*** is clearly illustrated (at *V* of VENTER in lower right). *Photographed courtesy of the Louise M. Darling Biomedical Library, University of California, Los Angeles.*

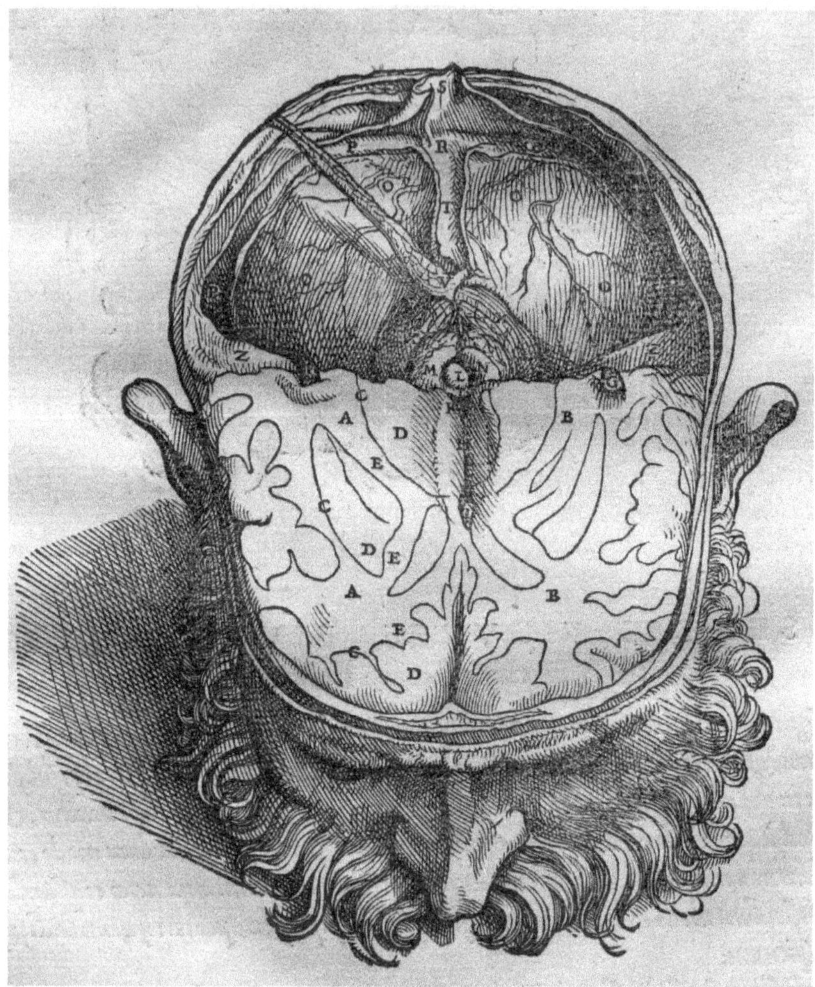

FIGURE 11. Part of adult human ***brain (Smith Papyrus, c1700 BC)*** series of drawings published by Andreas Vesalius (1543a). At this stage of dissection, the dorsal part (top) of the ***forebrain (Goette, 1873)*** was removed by a frontal (horizontal) slice, and the caudal (back) half was also removed to reveal the underlying ***cerebellar tentorium (Winslow, 1733)*** indicated by *O,O,O*. The great cerebral vein (of Galen), indicated by *V*, was moved caudally and laterally from the median plane for clarity (left side of figure). The many remaining features can be identified easily by consulting recent textbooks like Nieuwenhuys et al. (2008); also see Singer (1952, pp. 100–101), Richardson & Carman (2009, pp. 138–140). Vesalius (1543a) ridiculed the Three-cell Doctrine of ***brain (Smith Papyrus, c1700 BC)*** function (Figure 8) but could not suggest an alternative, preferring not to speculate. From Vesalius (1555), where the 1543 woodblocks were also used.

of Vesalius because it relied on slicing to expose various features (Figure 13); but a significant part of its success was due to hardening or fixing the tissue in alcohol, supplemented with hydrochloric acid (Vicq d'Azyr, 1786, Pl. 23 on p. 74; also see Burdach, 1822, p. 243). The other great work near the end of the Classical Era of neuroanatomy that relied to a significant degree on alcohol-fixed ***brain (Smith Papyrus, c1700 BC)*** tissue was that of Reil mentioned above. In fact, to separate ***gray matter (Meckel, 1817)*** and ***white matter (Meckel, 1817)***, he first hardened the tissue in alcohol alone (Reil, 1807–1808a, p. 18), alcohol and potash (Reil, 1809b, p. 139), or oil of turpentine followed by alcohol (Reil, 1812a, p. 96), and followed this treatment with maceration and gentle scraping. The best features of the approaches taken by Vicq d'Azyr and Reil were combined in the wonderful atlas of Arnold (1838b); see Figure 14.

The only other significant technical advance during the Classical Era of neuroanatomy was the occasional placement of ***nervous system (Monro, 1783)*** tissue between two thin sheets of glass for observation. For example, Georg Procháska (1779) ground parts of ***nerves (Herophilus, c335–c280 BC)*** between glass plates and concluded that their fundamental structure consists of tiny globules (see Garrison & McHenry, 1969), based on artifacts produced by the microscope he used (see next section). In contrast, Jules Baillarger

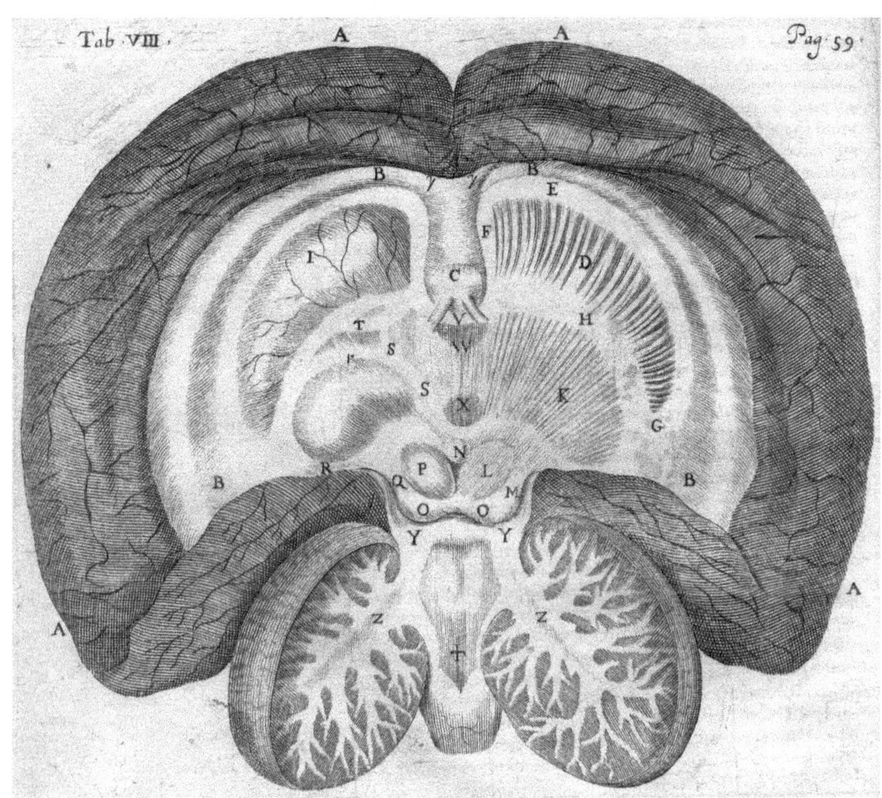

FIGURE 12. First illustration of physical *tract (Willis, 1664)* tracing by the scraping method. By carefully removing the somewhat softer overlying *gray substance (Vesalius, 1543a)*, Thomas Willis (1672) demonstrated the general location and orientation of segments of the adult human ***corticospinal tract (>1840)*** within the *corpus striatum (Willis, 1664)* or ***cerebral nuclei (Swanson, 2000a)*** indicated by D, ***interbrain (Baer, 1837)*** indicated by K, and ***tectum (Baer, 1837)*** indicated by L,O. He mistakenly thought the *tract (Willis, 1664)* did not extend to the ***cerebral cortex (>1840)***. Raymond Vieussens (1684) used the same method to clearly demonstrate continuity throughout the length of the *tract (Willis, 1664)*, from rostrally with the ***cerebral cortex (>1840)*** to caudally with the ***spinal cord (Galen, c162–c166)***. The ***brain (Smith Papyrus, c1700 BC)*** was cut down the median plane from dorsally, and then opened like a book to show the right and left sides with some medial parts of the ***cerebral nuclei (Swanson, 2000a)*** and ***interbrain (Baer, 1837)*** scraped away on the right side. *From Willis's Opera Omnia (1681).*

(1840) did brilliant work on lamination patterns in the ***cerebral cortex (>1840)*** by examining thin slices between glass plates with transmitted light, probably with magnifying glasses (see translation in von Bonin, 1960).

The Modern Era

The Modern Era of neuroanatomy is defined by effective use of the microscope for examining neural tissue and interpretation of the results in light of the cell theory of Matthias Jakob Schleiden (1838) and Theodor Schwann (1839). It is the histological era of structural neuroscience, beginning in the 1830s and defined for practical purposes as 1840. With the notable exception of work by Anton van Leeuwenhoek (1684, 1722) on ***nerves (Herophilus, c335–c280 BC)*** and the ***retina (Herophilus, c335–c280 BC)***, essentially everything observed in neural tissue under the microscope before the 1830s was artifactual—the universal fundamental unit seemed to be tiny spherules or globules—because of uncorrected optics (see Polyak, 1941; Clarke & Jacyna, 1987, pp. 58–62). This all changed with the development of achromatic microscope lenses, mainly by Giovanni Battista Amici and Joseph Jackson Lister (see Clarke & Jacyna, 1987, p. 60), and then serial sectioning of frozen ***central nervous system (Carus, 1814)*** tissue, first done brilliantly by hand (Stilling & Wallach, 1842; see Schiller, 1969) and later in the 1870s by microtome, the development of selective staining methods for neurons and neuron connections, and so on (see Clarke & Jacyna, 1987; Shepherd, 1991; Clarke & O'Malley, 1996). These developments stimulated a new vocabulary at the mesolevel and microlevel of analysis, and a shift from heavy emphasis on human anatomy, which is particularly amenable to macrodissection because of the relatively large size, to an emphasis on smaller animal anatomy, which is more practical at the histological level of analysis.

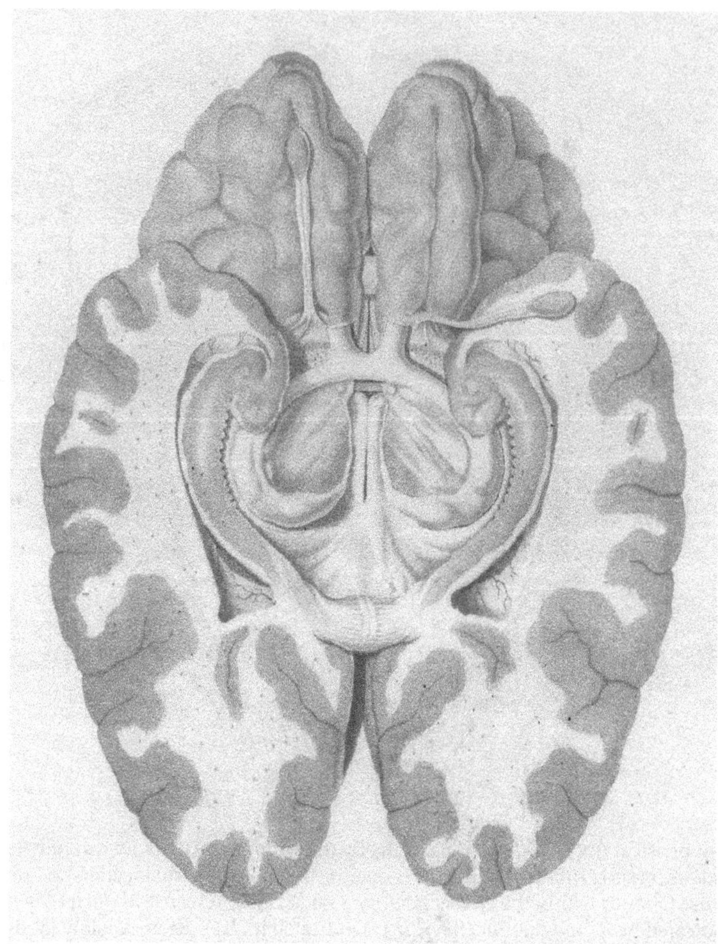

FIGURE 13. The most accurate and beautiful ***brain (Smith Papyrus, c1700 BC)*** atlas from the Classical Era of neuroanatomy. In this Plate, Félix Vicq d'Azyr (1786) showed the adult human ***brain (Smith Papyrus, c1700 BC)***, presumably hardened in alcohol, as viewed from the base (ventrally). Ventral parts of the right and left ***frontal region (Vicq d'Azyr, 1786)*** are seen toward the top of the figure, rostral to the ***optic chiasm (Galen, c173)*** near the median plane. On the left side of the ***brain (Smith Papyrus, c1700 BC)***, the ***olfactory peduncle (Solly, 1836)*** and ***olfactory bulb (Weitbrecht, 1751)*** were moved laterally to expose the ***olfactory sulcus (Quain, 1834)***, and the *insular threshold (Schwalbe, 1881)* is also clearly revealed near the proximal end of the ***olfactory peduncle (Solly, 1836)***. Ventral (basal or bottom) parts of the ***temporal region (>1840)*** and ***occipital region (Vesalius, 1543a)*** were sliced off to reveal the right and left *hippocampus (Aranzi, 1587)*, appearing like two seahorses facing each other from the ***inferior horn of lateral ventricle (Bell, 1802)*** on either side. Blood vessels, including those cut transversely in the ***cerebral cortex white matter (>1840)***, are colored red in the original Plate. Many other features, labeled on a corresponding outline drawing in the atlas, can be identified readily from modern textbooks like Nieuwenhuys et al. (2008).

History of Terminology Analysis

There is no need here to consider in depth such an arcane topic. It is, however, worth commenting on some of the more important contributions beginning, of course, with Aristotle, whose seminal generalization was that definitions should state what a term means, not what it doesn't mean, and should only use terms found elsewhere in the Lexicon (see Hitchings, 2005, p. 88 ff.). Ironically, he was also the first to introduce fundamental and lasting confusion into the neuroanatomical literature by using the same term, encephalon, in two very different ways. One was for the entire ***brain (Smith Papyrus, c1700 BC)*** and the other was for the *large brain (Aristotle)*, essentially the ***cerebrum (Obersteiner & Hill, 1900)*** and ***brainstem (Schwalbe, 1881)*** considered together—as opposed to the *small brain (Aristotle)* or its synonyms *parencephalon (Aristotle)* and ***cerebellum (Aristotle)***. Galen was the first to subject this and other ambiguities in neuroanatomical nomenclature to critical analysis (see, for example, Clarke & O'Malley, 1996, p. 630) and this tradition was continued in the 16th century by Berengario da Carpi (1521) and Vesalius (1543a,b),

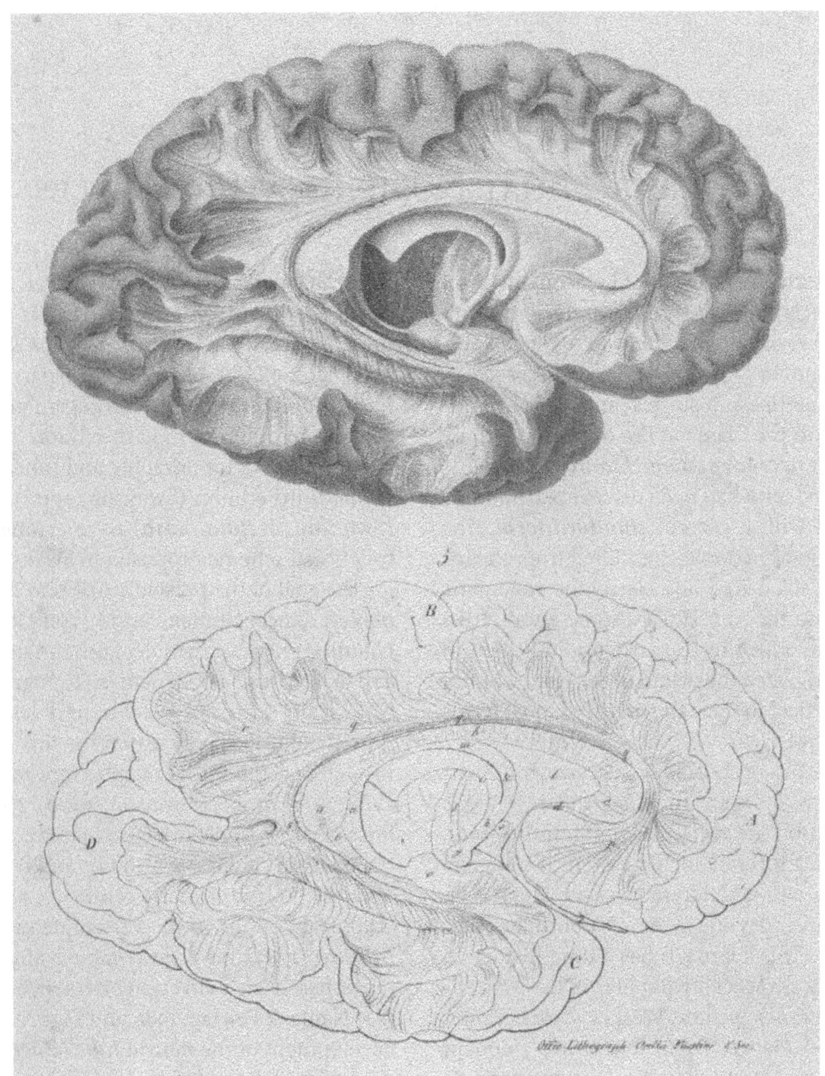

FIGURE 14. State of the art adult human *tract (Willis, 1664)* tracing in the 1830s. Friedrich Arnold (1838b) demonstrated the general location and orientation of ***white matter tracts (Bell & Bell, 1826)*** by selectively removing overlying ***gray matter (Meckel, 1817)*** with a process pioneered by Reil (1807–1812) and involving maceration and gentle scraping of alcohol-fixed tissue. This is Figure 5 of Plate 10, beautifully displaying many features including the ***cingulum (Burdach, 1822)*** (q), ***arcuate fibers (Arnold, 1838b)*** (unlabeled), ***fimbria (Honegger, 1890)*** (n), ***anterior commissure (Lieutaud, 1742)*** (e), ***postcommissural fornix (Loo, 1931)*** (h), ***mammillothalamic tract (Kölliker, 1896)*** (f), and ***zonal layer of thalamus (Burdach, 1822)*** (i). Plate 10 has four additional illustrations showing various stages of the dissection and is printed on two pages, one for drawings of the dissections (for example, Figure 5, top part of this figure) and one with matching outline drawings that are labeled (for example, Figure 5, bottom part of this figure). *Photographs courtesy of the National Library of Medicine.*

as analyzed in great detail by Singer and Rabin (1946) for anatomy in general.

Other authors who paid special attention to the origins and organization of neuroanatomical nomenclature included Caspar Bauhin (1605), Steno (1669), Haller (1762), Soemmerring (1778), Vicq d'Azyr (1786), and by far the most detailed of them all, Burdach (1819–1826). In the Modern Era of neuroanatomy, Jakob Henle (1871) and Wilhelm His (1895) had the most profound influence on macrolevel terminology, whereas the most detailed historical analysis was recently provided by Alfred Meyer (1971), who focused on the ***forebrain (Goette, 1873)***.

Chapter 3

Hierarchical Nomenclature Tables

This book has two interrelated parts, the Lexicon and a set of hierarchical Nomenclature Tables with ***standard terms*** to describe the entire ***nervous system (Monro, 1783)*** in all animals but especially human (Appendices). As discussed in Chapters 1 and 2, the complete historical analysis of terminology was restricted to the Classical Era of neuroanatomy when 1,162 of the 1,381 ***nervous system (Monro, 1783)*** parts with a current ***standard term*** had been discovered, but only 386 had been named with a current ***standard term***. The Lexicon contains just over 10,000 terms culled from the literature to 1840. To create, define, and clarify the systematic Nomenclature Tables in the Appendices, some 2,300 terms coined after 1840 were added to the Lexicon, indicated in the Lexicon by (>1840), when the origin of the term was not traced. It was not practical to trace the origin of most terms appearing after 1840 (see Figure 6).

It is well known that it "is absolutely necessary in scientific systematics to have a system in which different levels of generality or inclusion are recognized" (Simpson, 1961, p. 12), and that the best form of such a system is a hierarchy with a sequence of sets at different levels in which each set except the lowest includes one or more subordinate sets (Simpson, 1961, p. 13). This approach has a long history in human anatomy, and was especially popular in the 16th century, where good examples include Wecker (1562), Coiter (1564, 1566, 1672), and Platter (1583). It was less frequent thereafter, though one superb example is a hierarchical table (Bellingeri, 1818) of the complete branching pattern of the human ***trigeminal nerve (Winslow, 1733)***, the most complex of all the ***nerves (Herophilus, c335–c280)***. In the Modern Era the tables of anatomical parts in the *Basel Nomina Anatomica* (His, 1895) and its successors have been very useful but are not systematically hierarchical. The latest versions, the *Nomina Anatomica* (1983) and *Terminologia Anatomica* (1998), are better for the ***peripheral nervous system (Meckel, 1817)*** than the ***central nervous system (Carus, 1814)***, and are especially confusing for the ***forebrain (Goette, 1873)***.

The strategy of arranging a set of ***standard terms*** in hierarchical Nomenclature Tables allows every *nonstandard term*, now and in the future, to be synonymous or to partly correspond with one particular ***standard term*** at one particular level of the hierarchy. The highest level of the hierarchy is ***nervous system (Monro, 1783)***, which is the universe or domain of discourse for the neuroanatomical nomenclature ontology (Gruber, 1993; Gomez-Perez et al., 2003). These Nomenclature Tables are a modification and expansion of those appearing in the three editions of *Brain Maps* (Swanson, 1992, 1998, 2004). The latter provided complete hierarchical tables for ***gray matter regions (Swanson & Bota, 2010)*** and ***white matter tracts (Bell & Bell, 1826)*** of the adult male rat ***central nervous system (Carus, 1814)***, and incomplete tables for other parts of the ***nervous system (Monro, 1783)***. The arrangements within the hierarchies were different in each edition, based essentially on a combination of topographic and functional considerations. In the third edition (Swanson, 2004), ***gray matter regions (Swanson & Bota, 2010)*** were arranged according to the functional scheme proposed in Swanson (2003).

The goal of the present work is to provide a complete set of hierarchical Nomenclature Tables for the ***nervous system (Monro, 1783)*** as a whole, at the macrolevel of description and based just on structural topographic criteria, which historically are more stable and less theory-based than functional criteria. Research for this book began seriously in 1998 and the initial results were published in an article, *What is the brain?* (Swanson, 2000). Here some of the main lines of controversy in neuroanatomical nomenclature were traced from classical Antiquity, and it was documented that over the course of many centuries, 10 basic parts or topographical regions of the vertebrate ***central nervous system (Monro, 1783)*** have now gained almost universal acceptance based on converging evidence from adult structure (see Nauta & Feirtag, 1986 and Figure 15 lower left side) and development of the ***neural tube (Baer, 1837)*** (Appendix 2).

A global Foundational Model of Connectivity with a defined vocabulary for the ***nervous system (Monro, 1783)*** of all animals was developed several years ago (Swanson & Bota, 2010). It contains a standard set of terms for describing position or location in all animals with a ***nervous system (Monro, 1783)***, and the top levels of a general hierarchy of ***standard terms*** for ***nervous system (Monro, 1783)*** parts at the macrolevel, mesolevel, and microlevel of analysis (Figure 15). The 10 Nomenclature Tables in the Appendices are based on the Foundational Model of Connectivity hierarchy of parts, and provide a set of ***standard terms*** (on the order of 1,300) at or greater than the resolution needed for describing the human ***nervous system (Monro, 1783)*** at the macrolevel observable with MRI imaging.

The Nomenclature Tables in the Appendices are thematically grouped as follows. Appendix 1 is a basic parts list for the adult ***nervous system (Monro, 1783)*** in all animals, invertebrates and vertebrates alike, and is based on the Foundational Model of Connectivity (Figure 15). As such, the remaining 9 Appendices are consonant with it. Appendix 2 is a basic parts list for the early development of the vertebrate ***nervous system (Monro, 1783)***. It is fundamentally important that the basic parts of the vertebrate

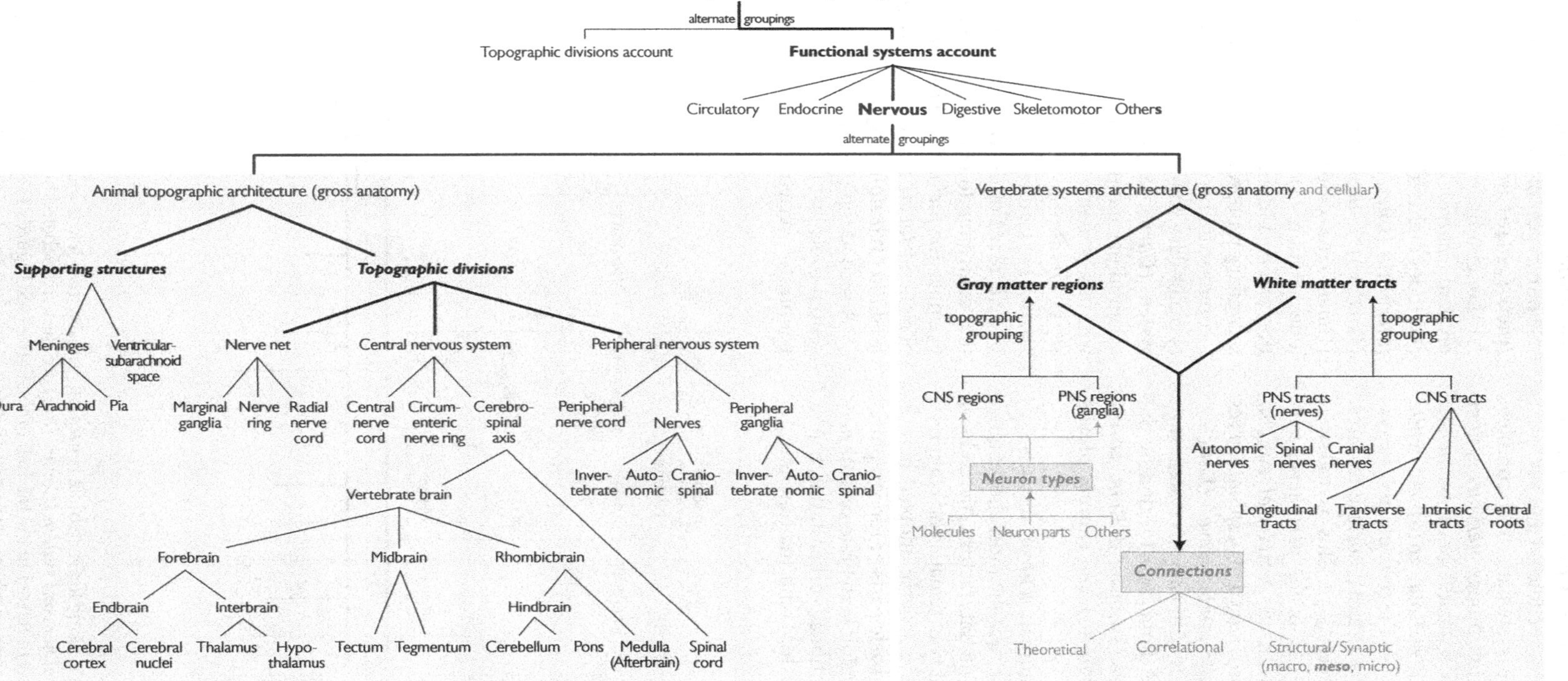

FIGURE 15. Hierarchical nomenclature scheme of the Foundational Model of Connectivity. The ***standard terms*** here apply to all animals with a ***nervous system (Monro, 1783)***. The organization of the ten Appendices is determined by this hierarchy. *Adapted slightly with permission from Swanson & Bota (2010).*

neural tube (Baer, 1837) are the same as the basic parts of the adult vertebrate ***central nervous system (Carus, 1814)*** shown in Figure 15 (lower left side) and Appendices 1 and 3–5.

Appendices 3–10 provide a systematic and complete macrolevel parts list for the adult human ***nervous system (Monro, 1783)***, separated into 8 tables for convenience. ***Gray matter regions (Swanson & Bota, 2010)*** and ***white matter tracts (Bell & Bell, 1826)*** of the ***central nervous system (Monro, 1783)***, followed by external surface features, are dealt with first (Appendices 3–5). This is followed by an account in Appendices 6–9 of the ***peripheral nervous system (Meckel, 1817)*** with its ***peripheral ganglia (>1840)***, ***cranial nerves (Soemmerring, 1791)***, ***spinal nerves (Camper, 1760–1762)***, and ***autonomic nerves (Langley, 1898)***. Finally, Appendix 10 deals with ***nervous system supporting structures (Swanson & Bota, 2010)*** including the ***ventricular-subarachnoid space (Swanson & Bota, 2010)***, ***meninges (Smith Papyrus, c1700 BC)***, and ***choroid plexus (Galen, c177)***.

A comprehensive table of human ***central nervous system white matter tracts (>1840)*** was the most challenging. As discussed in Appendix 4, no satisfactory hierarchical table of these features exists that is systematic and complete. The parceling and nomenclature scheme adopted here is based on two principles: the 10 basic parts or topographical regions of the developing and adult vertebrate ***central nervous system (Monro, 1783)*** mentioned earlier in the chapter (see Figure 2B, Figure 15 lower left), and the fundamental longitudinal-transverse organization of ***central nervous system white matter tracts (>1840)*** discussed in Appendix 4.

Four types of ***central nervous system white matter tracts (>1840)*** were defined for Appendix 4 (Figure 16). (1) Longitudinal tracts extend between rostrocaudally ordered ***central nervous system (Carus, 1814)*** secondary topographic divisions: ***endbrain (Kuhlenbeck, 1927)***, ***interbrain (Baer, 1837)***, ***midbrain (Baer, 1837)***, ***hindbrain (Baer, 1837)***, ***medulla (Winslow, 1733)***, and ***spinal cord (Galen, c162–c166)***. They can be unilateral or crossed with a decussation. (2) Transverse tracts are of two kinds. First, they can be a branch of a longitudinal tract to a primary or secondary topographic division. Or, second, they can form a commissure between the right and left sides of a primary or secondary topographic division of the ***central nervous system (Carus, 1814)***. (3) Intrinsic tracts are distinct from longitudinal and transverse tracts because they stay entirely within a primary topographic division: ***forebrain (Goette, 1873)***, ***midbrain (Baer, 1837)***, or ***rhombicbrain (His, 1893b)***. (4) Central roots are the ***white matter tracts (Bell & Bell, 1826)*** of the ***central nervous system (Carus, 1814)*** that contribute to ***craniospinal nerves (Herrick, 1915)***. For example, the ***facial nerve central root (>1840)*** becomes the peripheral ***facial nerve root (>1840)*** at the surface of the ***medulla (Winslow, 1733)***.

A second topic with critical implications is related to the central roots just mentioned. It deals conveniently with the naming of vertebrate ***spinal nerve (Camper, 1760–1762)***

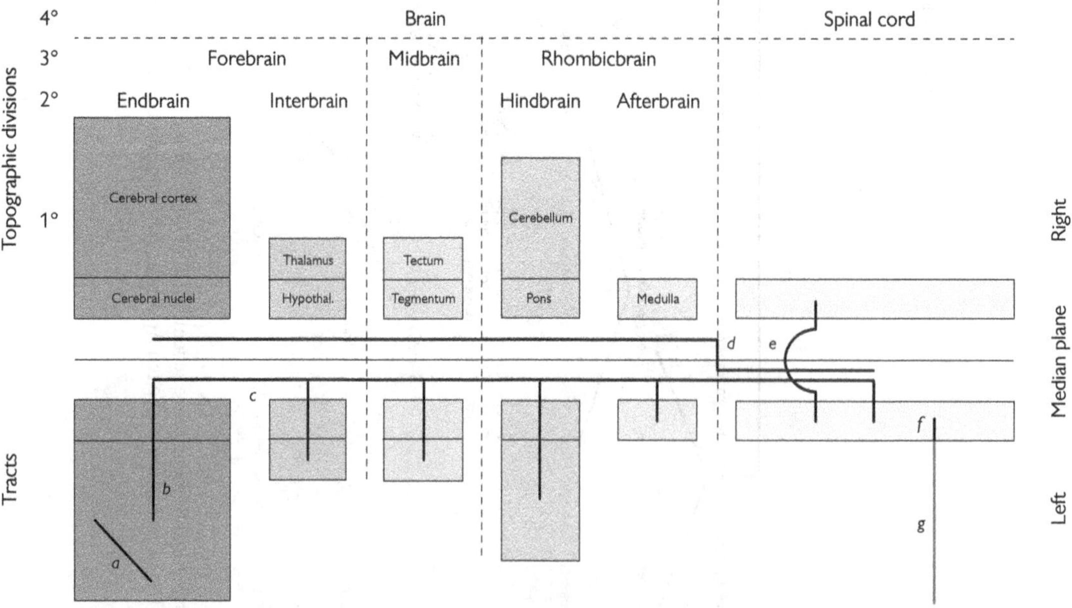

FIGURE 16. Parceling and naming scheme for vertebrate ***central nervous system white matter tracts (>1840)***. The ten primary topographic divisions of the ***central nervous system (Carus, 1814)*** are shown as labeled boxes and their grouping into secondary, tertiary, and quaternary divisions is indicated in the top half of the figure (see Figure 1 lower left and Appendix 1), above the line indicating the median plane. The naming scheme for *tracts (Willis, 1664)* is indicated in the bottom half of the figure and discussed in the text. Overall, there are longitudinal tracts, transverse tracts, intrinsic tracts, and central roots. *Abbreviations*: *a*, intrinsic tract; *b*, transverse tract that is branch of longitudinal tract; *c*, longitudinal tract; *d*, decussation of longitudinal tract; *e*, transverse tract that is a commissure; *f*, central root of a ***nerve (Herophilus, c335–c280 BC)***; *g*, ***nerve (Herophilus, c335–c280 BC)***.

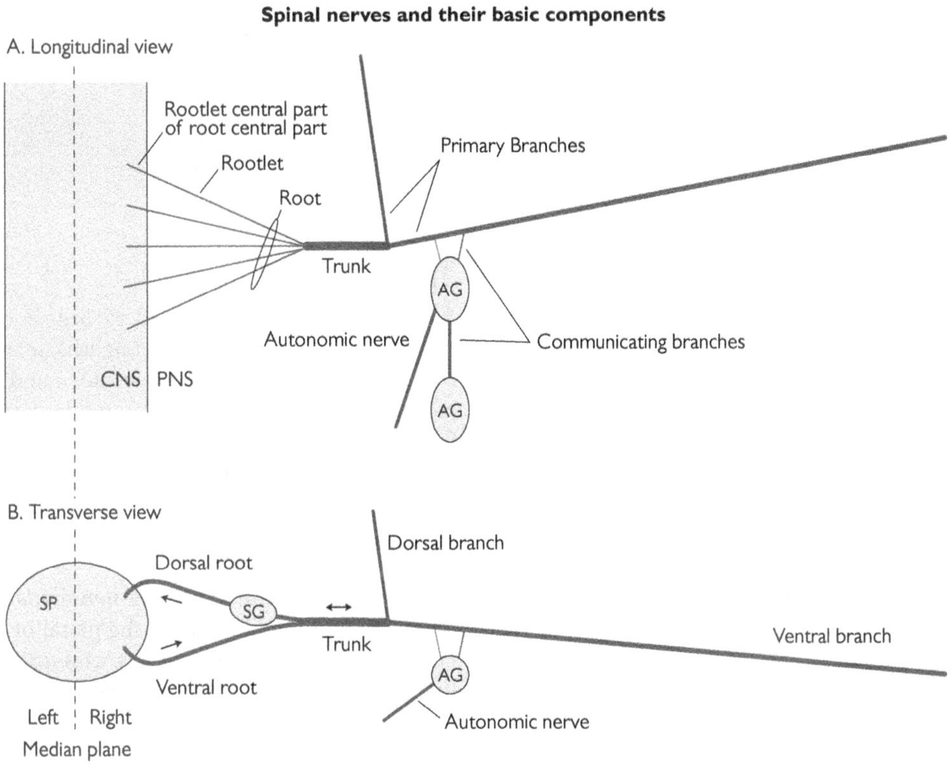

Spinal nerves and their basic components

FIGURE 17. Basic parts of ***spinal nerves (Camper, 1760–1762)***. In a hierarchy with topographic grouping (Figure 15, Appendix 1), ***spinal nerves (Camper, 1760–1762)*** are part of the ***peripheral nervous system (Meckel, 1817)***. In general, they have a ***ventral root (>1840)*** formed by a set of smaller ***ventral rootlets (>1840)***, and a ***dorsal root (Spurzheim, 1826)*** formed by a set of smaller ***dorsal rootlets (>1840)***. The proximal ends of these roots (and corresponding rootlets) meet the surface of the ***spinal cord (Galen, c162– c166)***, whereas the distal ends join to form a single mixed ***spinal nerve trunk (Frotscher, 1788)*** coursing a short distance before dividing into two ***spinal nerve primary branches (>1840)***: a typically larger ***spinal nerve ventral branch (>1840)***, and a typically smaller ***spinal nerve dorsal branch (Meckel, 1817)***. Each ***dorsal root (Spurzheim, 1840)*** has a ***spinal nerve ganglion (Burdach, 1819)*** associated with it, and each ***spinal nerve ventral branch (>1840)*** typically has one or more ***communicating branches of spinal nerve (Wutzer, 1817)*** with an ***autonomic ganglion (Langley, 1900)***, in particular with a ***sympathetic trunk ganglion (Winslow, 1733)***. In general, ***autonomic nerves (Langley, 1898)*** arise from ***autonomic ganglia (Langley, 1900)***. ***Nerves (Herophilus, c335–c280 BC)*** may branch a number of times, finally ending in terminal branches (not shown). In a hierarchy with topographic grouping (Figure 15, Appendix 1), ***dorsal root central parts (>1840)*** and ***ventral root central parts (>1840)***, with their corresponding ***ventral rootlet central parts (>1840)***, are part of the ***central nervous system (Carus, 1814)***; see text for details. *Abbreviations*: *AG*, ***autonomic ganglion (Langley, 1900)***; *CNS*, ***central nervous system (Carus, 1814)***; *PNS*, ***peripheral nervous system (Meckel, 1817)***; *SG*, ***spinal nerve ganglion (Burdach, 1819)***; *SP*, ***spinal cord (Galen, c162-c166)***.

parts. This might seem like a straightforward realm of neuroanatomical nomenclature but is complicated by two issues, one profound and one relatively trivial. The latter is that every textbook seems to use a slightly different set of terms for them. The ***standard terms*** adopted here are illustrated and explained in Figure 17. The profound issue is the fundamentally different way ***nervous system (Monro, 1783)*** structural organization may be described in different hierarchical arrangements, say structural versus functional.

For example, in a functional hierarchy, a motor component of a ***spinal nerve (Camper, 1760–1762)*** may be described as starting in neurons of the ***ventral horn (>1840)***, with axons passing through the ***ventral root central part (>1840)*** to enter the ***ventral root (>1840)*** peripheral part (illustrated clearly in Figure 5C of Swanson & Bota, 2010). In contrast, when a topographic hierarchy with ***central nervous system (Carus, 1814)*** and ***peripheral nervous system (Meckel, 1817)*** is used (Figures 15, 17; Appendix 1), ***spinal nerves (Camper, 1760-1762)*** are under the ***peripheral nervous system (Meckel, 1817)*** whereas ***ventral root central parts (>1840)*** are under the ***central nervous system (Carus, 1814)***. This example illustrates the critical need to distinguish clearly between topographic and functional descriptions of ***nervous system (Monro, 1783)*** structure, and is shown effectively in Swanson & Bota (2010, their Figure 5A–C).

Chapter 4

Notes on Using the Lexicon

Standard terms (main entries)

Articles in the Lexicon are a defined vocabulary used for the 10 Nomenclature Tables in the Appendices. They are followed by a citation to their first use (Author, date), or if their first use occurred after 1840 and was not determined here, followed by (>1840). The textual definition generally includes method used to identify, age (embryonic, infant, adult, and so on), species, sex (where relevant), and citation to discovery, whether or not the part was named and whether or not the ***standard term*** was used. Here and in general usage ***standard terms*** are bolded and italicized.

Nonstandard terms (subentries)

Following the definition, articles in the Lexicon contain chronological lists of related *nonstandard terms* when they are known. *Nonstandard terms* include alternate spellings of ***standard terms***, forms of ***standard terms*** in languages other than English (translations), synonyms introduced before a ***standard term*** was introduced, synonyms introduced after a ***standard term*** was introduced, and partly corresponding terms. Here and in general usage *nonstandard terms* are italicized. They include a citation to their first use (Author, date), or if their first use occurred after 1840 and was not determined here, followed by (>1840). They are generally defined with reference to a ***standard term*** or another *nonstandard term* like a synonym. Where appropriate, information about method used to identify, age, species, and sex is included.

Partly corresponding terms

Nonstandard terms that are not synonyms. A *partly corresponding term* refers to a zone of a ***reference term*** and thus does not fit exactly anywhere within the Nomenclature Table hierarchies in the Appendices. Above the lowest level of a hierarchy, *partly corresponding terms* are considered misinterpretations by definition. At the lowest level of a hierarchy, partly corresponding terms may be either misinterpretations or unrecognized ***standard terms***.

List of all defined terms

All ***standard terms*** and *nonstandard terms* are given alphabetically in the List of All Defined Terms. The List is used to find a particular *nonstandard term* in a particular ***standard term*** article of the Lexicon.

Spelling

American English is preferred to British English. In old Latin (and to some extent old English), *u* and *v*, as well as *i* and *j*, are typically interchangeable; *u* and *i*, respectively, are used where appropriate for modern spelling. In old German, *s* and *f* are interchanged in a regular way; *s* is used where appropriate for modern spelling.

Singular versus plural

In general, ***standard terms*** and *nonstandard terms* in the Lexicon can be used in either the plural or singular form. For example, ***nerves (Herophilus, c335–c280)***, an article in the Lexicon, can be used as ***standard term*** singular form, ***nerve (Herophilus, c335–c280)***.

Terms not in the Lexicon

There are many reasons a term is not found in the Lexicon. (1) No effort was made to document every minor spelling variation, including the use of hyphenation. (2) English ***standard terms*** are preferred, with original Latin form of ***standard term*** given if used. No effort was made systematically to provide alternate forms of ***standard terms*** and *nonstandard terms* in languages other than English. (3) Except for ***standard terms***, and common current synonyms for them, most terms introduced since 1840 are not included (see Figure 6). (4) Some terms have synonyms resulting from alternate word order; no attempt was made to document every such synonym, although many examples are provided. (5) In general, terms are culled from the anatomical literature, thus excluding specialized terms used in surgery, pathology, and related disciplines. (6) No dictionary or lexicon can be complete or completely accurate.

Defining terms not found in the Lexicon with respect to ***standard terms*** and *nonstandard terms* in the Lexicon, and thus the Nomenclature Tables in the Appendices, is much easier now than ever before. The place to start is with a combination of the best dictionaries and online search engines.

Eponyms

Citations (Author, date) following ***standard terms*** and *nonstandard terms* are not eponyms. Instead they refer to the first usage of the corresponding term as best determined thus far. Eponyms are included in Lexicon articles as *nonstandard terms*, with a citation to their first use.

Methods

During the Classical Era of neuroanatomy (c1700 BC–1840) almost all observations were macroscopic, made with the naked eye or sometimes a simple hand lens using gross dissection, often shortened in the Lexicon to "macro-dissection." During the Modern Era of neuroanatomy (1841–present) methodology obviously became much more complex and continues to evolve rapidly.

Etymology and pronunciation

These aspects of language nomenclature are not covered.

Standard Terms

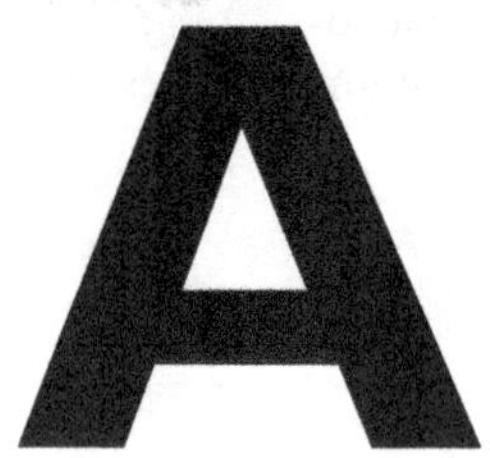

abducens nerve (Heister, 1717)

As described for macrodissected adult human, a ***cranial nerve (Soemmerring, 1791)*** attached to the ***medullopontine sulcus (>1840)***, between the rostral end of the ***pyramid (Willis, 1664)*** and caudal end of the ***pons (Haller, 1747)***, distal to the ***abducens nerve central root (>1840)***. Normally its action is through the lateral rectus extraocular muscle to rotate the eye laterally (abduction), although in nonhuman mammal it also supplies the retractor bulbi muscle; see Williams & Warwick (1980, pp. 1068-1069). Heister used the term for the *sixth pair of nerves arising within skull (Willis, 1664)* in macrodissected adult human; pp. 78, 94. Vicq d'Azyr (1786; Pl. XVII, Fig. I-51) reviewed the early history of exactly where it emerges from the surface of the ***brainstem (Schwalbe, 1881)***. Burdach (1822, p. 313) mentioned without citation that Riolan used the term *abducens*, and Schiller (1969, p. 78) wrote that Riolan (1610) used the term *abducens*; however, the source has not yet been traced; it does not appear to be in Riolan (1618). It was first clearly described as the *fourth pair of nerves from brain (Falloppio, 1561)*.

ALTERNATE SPELLINGS:

1. *abducent nerve (Heister, 1752)*
   Alternate spelling of ***abducens nerve (Heister, 1717)***; p. 230. Also see *Terminologia Anatomica* (1998, p. 135).

EARLIER REFERENCES:

Described, not named or illustrated:

1. ***[abducens nerve (Heister, 1717)] (Galen c173)***
   It has been suggested that Galen observed it in macrodissected adult mammal (see May translation, 1968, pp. 442, 444), but this is doubtful; see Duckworth translation (1962, p. 188), May (1968, p. 452), Savage-Smith (1971).

Earlier synonyms:

1. *fourth pair of nerves from brain (Falloppio, 1561)*
   Falloppio is credited with first clear description of ***abducens nerves (Heister, 1717)***, in macrodissected adult human; f. 147. Also see Zinn (1755, p. 200), Haller (1762, p. 222), Hierons & Meyer (1962, p. 289).
2. *seventh pair of nerves from brain (Bartholin, 1641)*
   Synonym for macrodissected adult human ***abducens nerves (Heister, 1717)***; see translation (1662, p. 325).
3. *sixth pair of nerves arising within skull (Willis, 1664)*
   Willis was first to use current number for ***abducens nerves (Heister, 1717)***; see Pordage translation (1681, p. 143) and Burdach (1822, p. 313), although Willis thought it contributes to origin of ***sympathetic trunk (Winslow, 1733)***; see Pordage translation (1681, p. 144).
4. *nervus timidus (Bidloo, 1685)*
   Synonym for macrodissected adult human ***abducens nerve (Heister, 1717)***, according to Burdach (1822, p. 313).

LATER SYNONYMS:

1. *nervi motores externi (Winslow, 1733)*
   Synonym listed for macrodissected adult human ***abducens nerves (Heister, 1717)***; Section VI, p. 59.
2. *nervi oculares externi (Winslow, 1733)*
   Synonym listed for macrodissected adult human ***abducens nerves (Heister, 1717)***; Section VI, p. 59; for singular form, *nervus ocularis externus*, see Burdach (1822, p. 313).
3. *nervi musculares externi (Winslow, 1733)*
   Synonym listed for macrodissected adult human ***abducens nerves (Heister, 1717)***; Section VI, p. 59.
4. *nervi oculo-musculares externi (Winslow, 1733)*
   Synonym listed for macrodissected adult human ***abducens nerves (Heister, 1717)***; Section VI, p. 59; for singular form, *nervus oculo-muscularis externus*, see Burdach (1822, p. 85). Burdin (see translation, 1803, Vol. 1, p. 144) used *exterior oculo-muscular pair of nerves*.
5. *nervi motores oculorum externi (Winslow, 1733)*
   Synonym listed for macrodissected adult human ***abducens nerves (Heister, 1717)***; Section X, p. 48. Alternately,

Andersch (1797) used singular, *nervus motorius externus oculi*; see Burdach (1822, p. 313).

6. *nervi opthalmici externi (Winslow, 1733)*
Synonym listed for macrodissected adult human ***abducens nerves (Heister, 1717)***; Section X, p. 48.
7. *tenth pair of nerves (Malacarne, 1791)*
Synonym for macrodissected adult human ***abducens nerves (Heister, 1717)***; in Latin, *par decimum* (see Burdach, 1822, p. 313).
8. *sixth pair of cranial nerves (Soemmerring, 1791)*
Synonym for macrodissected adult human ***abducens nerves (Heister, 1717)***; see ***cranial nerves (Soemmerring, 1791)***.
9. *sixth pair of cerebral nerves (Soemmerring, 1791)*
Synonym for *sixth pair of cranial nerves (Soemmerring, 1791)*; in the original Latin, *par sextum nervorum cerebri*, p. 125.
10. *par oculos abducens nervorum cerebri (Soemmerring, 1798)*
Synonym for *sixth pair of cerebral nerves (Soemmerring, 1798)*; p. 125.
11. *exterior oculo-muscular pair of nerves (Burdin, 1803)*
Synonym for macrodissected adult human ***abducens nerves (Heister, 1717)***; see translation (1803, Vol. 1, p. 178).
12. *abductor nerve of eye (Gordon, 1815)*
Synonym for macrodissected adult human ***abducens nerve (Heister, 1717)***; Gordon's original mixed Latin and English term (plural) was "*Abductores Oculorum* Nerves" (p. 113). Gall & Spurzheim (1810, p. 74) used the French, *nerf abducteur de l'oeil*, and Spurzheim (1826, p. 231 note 10) used the abbreviated *abductor nerve*.
13. *nervus oculomuscularis posterior (Meckel, 1817)*
Synonym for macrodissected adult human ***abducens nerve (Heister, 1717)***; p. 705, also see translation (1832, Vol. 3, p. 57).
14. *scornful nerve (Burdach, 1822)*
Synonym listed for macrodissected adult ***abducens nerve (Heister, 1717)***; in the original Latin, *nervus indignatorius*, p. 313. Apparently Casseri and Riolan used the term *indignatorius musculus* for the lateral rectus muscle; see Nysten (1814, p. 646).
15. *abducent oculo-muscular nerve (Swan, 1830)*
Synonym for macrodissected adult human ***abducens nerve (Heister, 1717)***; p. 18.

PARTLY CORRESPONDS:

1. *cerebral part of sixth pair (Arnold, 1834)*
Macrodissected adult human proximal segment of ***abducens nerve (Heister, 1717)*** before entering ***cavernous sinus (Winslow, 1733)***; in the original Latin, *par sextum, pars cerebralis*, p. 11.
2. *cerebral part of abducens nerve (Arnold, 1834)*
Synonym for *cerebral part of sixth pair (Arnold, 1834)*; in the original Latin, *nervus abducens, pars cerebralis*, p. 11.
3. *cerebral part of scornful nerve (Arnold, 1834)*
Synonym for *cerebral part of sixth pair (Arnold, 1834)*; in the original Latin, *nervus indignatorius, pars cerebralis*, p. 11.

abducens nerve central root (>1840)

As described for macrodissected adult human, and mammal generally with histological methods for ***axons (Kölliker, 1896)***, the central root *nerve fibers (Ehrenberg, 1833)* of the ***abducens nucleus (>1840)*** form bundles coursing ventrally to the ventral surface of the ***medulla (Winslow, 1733)*** at its junction with the ***pons (Haller, 1747)***; see Carpenter (1976, p. 349 and Figs. 12.1, 12.6), Nieuwenhuys et al. (2008, Figs. 6.25-30, 6.26-24). The bundles are ***abducens nerve central rootlets (>1840)*** together forming the ***abducens nerve central root (>1840)*** that on leaving the ***medulla (Winslow, 1733)*** becomes the peripheral ***abducens nerve root (>1840)***. It was discovered by Mayo; see ***[abducens nerve central root (>1840)] (Mayo, 1827)***.

EARLIER REFERENCES:

Illustrated and described, not named:

1. ***[abducens nerve central root (>1840)] (Mayo, 1827)***
Traced from rostral and ventral surface of macrodissected adult human ***medulla (Winslow, 1733)*** to back (dorsal) part of ***gray matter (Meckel, 1817)*** of ***pons (Haller, 1747)*** without, of course, recognizing ***abducens nucleus (>1840)*** in caudal ***tegmentum (Swanson, 2000b)***; Plate VII, Figure 2-*VI*.

Earlier synonyms:

1. *real origin of external ocular motor nerve (Cruveilhier, 1836)*
Synonym for macrodissected adult human ***abducens nerve central root (>1840)***. Cruveilhier noted without providing citations that Gall traced it along border of ***pyramid (Willis, 1664)*** and Herbert Mayo traced it through ***pons (Haller, 1747)*** to region below ***fourth ventricle (Galen, c192)***; in the original French, *origine réelle*, p. 896. Grainger (1837, p. 40) also traced it deep into macrodissected adult human ***pons (Haller, 1747)***.

abducens nerve central rootlets (>1840)

As described in macrodissected adult human, and mammal generally with histological methods for ***axons (Kölliker, 1896)***, the central root *nerve fibers (Ehrenberg, 1833)* of the ***abducens nucleus (>1840)*** form bundles coursing ventrally to the ventral surface of the ***medulla (Winslow, 1733)*** at its junction with the ***pons (Haller, 1747)***; see Carpenter (1976, p. 349 and Figs. 12.1, 12.6), Nieuwenhuys et al. (2008, Figs. 6.25-30, 6.26-24). The bundles are ***abducens nerve central rootlets (>1840)*** together forming the ***abducens nerve central root (>1840)***. On leaving the ventral surface of the ***medulla (Winslow, 1733)*** the ***abducens nerve central rootlets (>1840)*** become peripheral ***abducens nerve rootlets (>1840)***. They were not known by 1840.

abducens nerve root (>1840)

As described for macrodissected adult human, the ***abducens nerve (Heister, 1717)*** is attached to the side of the ***medulla (Winslow, 1733)*** just caudal to the ***pons (Haller, 1747)***, roughly in line with the ***hypoglossal nerve (Winslow, 1733)***; see Obersteiner & Hill (1900, Fig. 10), Crosby et al. (1962, p. 115). The ***abducens nerve root (>1840)*** consists of a variable number of ***abducens nerve rootlets (>1840)***. Meckel (1817) described the usual situation as 2 distinct roots, medial and lateral, with the latter about 2 times larger than the former and each made up of smaller filaments [rootlets]; see translation (1832, Vol. 3, p. 57). It was first observed by Du Verney; see ***[abducens nerve root (>1840)] (Du Verney, 1683).***

EARLIER REFERENCES:

Illustrated, not named or described:

1. ***[abducens nerve root (>1840)] (Du Verney, 1683)***
   Because Du Verney illustrated the ***abducens nerve rootlets (>1840)***, he illustrated the root for macrodissected adult human; Plate 1, Figure 1-*N*.

Earlier synonyms:

1. *external motor nerve roots (Günther, 1786)*
   Synonym for macrodissected adult human ***abducens nerve root (>1840)***. Günther described the usual situation as 2 distinct roots (p. 54), described in more detail by Meckel (1817) as internal [medial] and external [lateral], with the latter about 4 times larger than the former and each made up of smaller filaments [rootlets]. Meckel also described a right–left variation on how the 2 roots merge, which is always seen only on the left; see translation (1832, Vol. 3, p. 57).

abducens nerve rootlets (>1840)

As described for macrodissected adult human, the variable number of small *nerve fiber (Ehrenberg, 1833)* bundles between the surface of the ***medulla (Winslow, 1733)*** and the ***abducens nerve trunk (>1840)***, together constituting the ***abducens nerve root (>1840)***; see Gehuchten (1906, Fig. 5). They were discovered by Du Verney; see ***[abducens nerve rootlets (>1840)] (Du Verney, 1683).***

EARLIER REFERENCES:

Illustrated, not named or described:

1. ***[abducens nerve rootlets (>1840)] (Du Verney, 1683)***
   Illustrated for macrodissected adult human; Plate 1, Figure 1-*N*. Also see Bell & Bell (1829, p. 505).

Earlier synonyms:

1. *roots of external motor nerve of eyes (Malacarne, 1791)*
   Synonym mentioned in passing for macrodissected adult human ***abducens nerve rootlets (>1840)***; p. 227.
2. *external motor nerve filaments (Meckel, 1817)*
   Synonym for macrodissected adult human ***abducens nerve rootlets (>1840)***; see translation (1832, Vol. 3, p. 57).
3. *apparent origin of external ocular motor nerve (Cruveilhier, 1836)*
   Synonym for macrodissected adult human ***abducens nerve rootlets (>1840)***; in the original French, *origine apparente*, p. 896.

PARTLY CORRESPONDS:

1. *internal root of external ocular motor nerve (Cruveilhier, 1836)*
   Smaller of 2 macrodissected adult human ***abducens nerve rootlets (>1840)*** emerging from ***pons (Haller, 1747)***; in the original French, *racine interne*, p. 896.
2. *external root of external ocular motor nerve (Cruveilhier, 1836)*
   Larger of 2 macrodissected adult human ***abducens nerve rootlets (>1840)*** emerging just dorsal to rostral end of ***pyramid (Willis, 1664)***; in the original French, *racine externe*, p. 896.

abducens nerve trunk (>1840)

As described for macrodissected adult mammal, segment of the ***abducens nerve (Heister, 1717)*** between the ***abducens nerve root (>1840)*** proximally and the distal branching of the ***nerve (Herophilus, c335–c280 BC)*** to the lateral rectus and (when present) retractor bulbi muscles. It was probably first delineated by Willis; see ***[abducens nerve trunk (>1840)] (Willis, 1664).***

EARLIER REFERENCES:

Illustrated, not named or described:

1. ***[abducens nerve trunk (>1840)] (Willis, 1664)***
   Illustrated for macrodissected adult mammal; see Pordage translation (1681, p. 145, Fig. 2-C).

Earlier synonyms:

1. *sixth pair of nerves trunk (Vieussens, 1684)*
   Synonym for macrodissected adult human ***abducens nerve trunk (>1840)***; in the original Latin, *truncus nervi sexti paris*, Table 23-*D*.
2. *external motor nerve trunk (Günther, 1786)*
   Synonym for macrodissected adult human ***abducens nerve trunk (>1840)***; p. 54.

PARTLY CORRESPONDS:

1. *primary branch of sixth pair (Portal, 1803a)*
   Portal claimed it is not uncommon in macrodissected adult human to find such a branch of ***abducens nerve trunk (>1840)*** to ***nerve of pterygoid canal (>1840)***; in the original French, *le rameau primitif*, p. 158.
2. *secondary branch of sixth pair (Portal, 1803a)*
   Portal claimed it is not uncommon in macrodissected adult human to find such a branch of ***abducens nerve trunk (>1840)*** to 1st ***cervical spinal ganglion (>1840)***; in the original French, *le rameau secondaire*, p. 158.
3. *cavernous part of sixth pair (Arnold, 1834)*
   Macrodissected adult human segment of ***abducens nerve trunk (>1840)*** within ***cavernous sinus (Winslow, 1733)***; in the original Latin, *par sextum, pars cavernosa*, p. 11.
4. *cavernous part of abducens nerve (Arnold, 1834)*
   Synonym for *cavernous part of sixth pair (Arnold, 1834)*; in the original Latin, *nervus abducens, pars cavernosa*, p. 11.
5. *cavernous part of scornful nerve (Arnold, 1834)*
   Synonym for *cavernous part of sixth pair (Arnold, 1834)*; in the original Latin, *nervus indignatorius, pars cavernosa*, p. 11.
6. *orbital part of sixth pair (Arnold, 1834)*
   Macrodissected adult human segment of ***abducens nerve trunk (>1840)*** distal to ***cavernous sinus (Winslow, 1733)***, before it branches to enter lateral rectus muscle; in the original Latin, *par sextum, pars orbitalis*, p. 11.
7. *orbital part of abducens nerve (Arnold, 1834)*
   Synonym for *orbital part of sixth pair (Arnold, 1834)*; in the original Latin, *nervus abducens, pars orbitalis*, p. 11.

8. *orbital part of scornful nerve (Arnold, 1834)*
   Synonym for *orbital part of sixth pair (Arnold, 1834)*; in the original Latin, *nervus indignatorius, pars orbitalis*, p. 11.

abducens nucleus (>1840)

As described for mammal with cellular architecture and connections, the small ***gray matter region (Swanson & Bota, 2010)*** lying in the caudal dorsomedial ***pontine reticular nucleus (>1840)***, just ventral to the ventromedial tip of the ***pontine central gray (>1840)***, and generating the ***abducens nerve central root (>1840)*** continuing peripherally as the ***abducens nerve (Heister, 1717)*** to the lateral rectus muscle of the eye; see Nieuwenhuys et al. (2008, p. 203 and Fig. 6.26-*8*). It was first delineated by Desmoulins and Rolando; see ***[abducens nucleus (>1840)] (Desmoulins, 1825)***.

EARLIER REFERENCES:

Illustrated, not named or described:

1. ***[abducens nucleus (>1840)] (Desmoulins, 1825)***
   Clearly indicated in transverse section of macrodissected adult beef; Plate XIII, Figure 12, drawn by Rolando.

accessory cuneate nucleus (>1840)

As described for macrodissected adult human and for adult mammal in general with cellular architecture and connections, the ***gray matter region (Swanson & Bota, 2010)*** of the ***dorsal column nuclei (>1840)*** lying lateral to the rostral end of the ***cuneate nucleus (>1840)*** and receiving a massive input from the ***cuneate fascicle (Müller, 1834)***; histologically it contains larger ***neurons (Waldeyer, 1891)*** than the ***cuneate nucleus (>1840)***; see Williams & Warwick (1980, p. 902), *Terminologia Anatomica* (1998, p. 110), Nieuwenhuys et al. (2008, p. 194 and Figs. 6.22, 6.23, where it is called *lateral cuneate nucleus*). It was first recognized by Burdach; see ***[accessory cuneate nucleus (>1840)] (Burdach, 1822)***.

EARLIER REFERENCES:

Described, not named or illustrated:

1. ***[accessory cuneate nucleus (>1840)] (Burdach, 1822)***
   Described for macrodissected adult human; p. 36, see Dejerine & Dejerine-Klumpke (1901, p. 573).

accessory nerve (Vieussens, 1684)

As described for macrodissected adult human, a ***cranial nerve (Soemmerring, 1791)*** with a ***cranial root of accessory nerve (>1840)*** and a ***spinal root of accessory nerve (>1840)***. The ***cranial root of accessory nerve rootlets (>1840)*** and the ***spinal root of accessory nerve rootlets (>1040)*** caudal to it extend along a continuous longitudinal line on the outer surface of the ***medulla (Winslow, 1733)*** and ***spinal cord (Galen, c162-c166)***, caudal to the ***vagus nerve rootlets (>1840)***. The ***spinal root of accessory nerve rootlets (>1840)*** converge to form the long, rostrally directed (ascending) ***spinal root of accessory nerve trunk (>1840)***, and the ***cranial root of accessory nerve rootlets (>1840)*** converge to form the short ***cranial root of accessory nerve trunks (>1840)***. The ***spinal root of accessory nerve trunk (>1840)*** and ***cranial root of accessory nerve trunks (>1840)*** converge in the region of the jugular foramen to form the single short ***accessory nerve trunk (Wrisberg, 1786)***, in turn splitting to form the ***internal branch of accessory nerve trunk (Meckel, 1817)*** and ***external branch of accessory nerve (Meckel, 1817)***. The ***cranial root of accessory nerve (>1840)*** and ***spinal root of accessory nerve (>1840)*** are now described as essentially distinct parts anatomically as well as functionally; see Durward (1951, Fig. 908), Williams & Warwick (1980, pp. 1081–1083 and Fig. 7.189), *Terminologia Anatomica* (1998, p. 137). For Vieussens's use in macrodissected adult human see p. 179; also see *spinal accessory nerve (Willis, 1664)* and *accessory nerve of Willis (Vieussens, 1684)*. Ridley used the precise term, *accessory nerve*, in English (Fig. VIII-*P*). Meckel (1817; see translation, 1832, Vol. 3, p. 6) noted, without citation, that Portal and others considered the ***accessory nerve (Vieussens, 1684)*** an intermediate class of ***craniospinal nerve (Herrick, 1915)*** because it arises largely from the ***spinal cord (Galen, c162–c166)*** but exits from the cranium. It was known to Herophilus; see ***[accessory nerve (Vieussens, 1684)] (Herophilus, c335–c280 BC)***.

TRANSLATIONS:

1. *nervus accessorius (Vieussens, 1684)*
   Original Latin form of ***accessory nerve (Vieussens, 1684)***; p. 179, where it is plural. Also see Burdach (1822, p. 82) and Lobstein's thesis (1760).

EARLIER REFERENCES:

Described, not named or illustrated:

1. ***[accessory nerve (Vieussens, 1684)] (Herophilus, c335–c280 BC)***
   Herophilus, the founder of human anatomy, is credited with discovering but not naming ***glossopharyngeal nerve (Huber, 1744)***, ***vagus nerve (Galen, c192)***, and ***accessory nerve (Vieussens, 1684)***, which were apparently distinguished but considered together; see Solmsen (1961), von Staden (1969), Longrigg (1993), Clarke & O'Malley (1996, p. 261), *third division of nerve of sixth pair (Galen, c192)*. He dissected adult mammals and human cadavers.

Earlier synonyms:

1. *third division of nerve of sixth pair (Galen, c192)*
   Synonym for ***accessory nerve (Vieussens, 1684)***; see Duckworth translation (1962, p. 248). Galen carefully described this ***nerve (Herophilus, c335–c280 BC)***, which he included in the *sixth pair of nerves from brain (Galen, c192)*; see Duckworth translation (1962, pp. 202, 235), May translation (1968, pp. 696–697) Most if not all of his neuroanatomy was done on macrodissected adult beef, pig, and/or macaque but not human. Vesalius (1543a) mentioned it briefly for macrodissected adult human; see Richardson & Carman translation (2002, p. 195). The first modern, accurate description of the ***accessory nerve (Vieussens, 1684)*** was by Coiter in 1572; see Meyer (1971, p. 12 note 6).

Ridley (1695, p. 151) stated without citation that Guidi (1611) "painted and described" it.

2. *spinal accessory nerve (Willis, 1664)*
Synonym for macrodissected adult human ***accessory nerve (Vieussens, 1684)***; see Pordage translation (1681, Tab. IX legend). It was part of the *eighth pair of nerves arising within skull (Willis, 1664)*. Willis identified it consistently "not only in Man and four-footed Beasts, but also in Fowls and Fishes; and in these it seems to be destinated instead of Arms, and for the moving of their wings and fins" (Pordage translation, 1681, p. 173).
3. *accessory nerve of wandring pair (Willis, 1664)*
Synonym for ***accessory nerve (Vieussens, 1684)*** in macrodissected adult human and other vertebrates; see Pordage translation (1681, pp. 58, 146, 173, Tabs. 5-*N*, 6-*L*).
4. *spinal accessory nerve of wandring pair (Willis, 1664)*
Synonym for macrodissected adult human and other vertebrate ***accessory nerve (Vieussens, 1684)***, which Willis wrote arises entirely from the ***spinal cord (Galen, c162–c166)***, beginning caudally in human at levels six or seven of ***cervical part of spinal cord (>1840)***; see Pordage translation (1681, pp. 173–174). For Latin form, *nervus spinalis ad par vagum accessorius*, see Haase (1781, p. 114).
5. *accessory nerve of Willis (Vieussens 1684)*
Eponym for macrodissected adult human *spinal accessory nerve (Willis, 1664)*; in the original Latin (plural), *nervi accessorii Willisii*, p. 179.

LATER SYNONYMS:

1. *spinal nerve (Collins, 1685)*
Synonym for ***accessory nerve (Vieussens, 1684)***; p. 1052. Also see Vicq d'Azyr (1786, pp. 49, 54).
2. *nervus spinalis (Winslow, 1733)*
Latin form of *spinal nerve (Collins, 1685)*; Section X, p. 48.
3. *nervus accessorius octavi paris (Winslow, 1733)*
Synonym for macrodissected adult human ***accessory nerve (Vieussens, 1684)***; Section X, p. 48.
4. *recurrent spinal nerve (Albinus, 1744)*
Synonym for macrodissected adult human ***accessory nerve (Vieussens, 1684)***; in the original Latin, *nervus spinalis recurrens*; Table 18, Figures 1 & 3-ζ,η,θ,ι and Table 19-*f*. Also see Burdach (1822, p. 309).
5. *intermediate nerve (Huber, 1744)*
Synonym for macrodissected adult human ***accessory nerve (Vieussens, 1684)***; in the original Latin, *nervus intermedius*, p. 10. Also see Schreger (1803, p. 346).
6. *superior recurrent nerve of eighth pair (Neubauer, 1772)*
Synonym for macrodissected adult human ***accessory nerve (Vieussens, 1684)***; in Latin, *recurrens octavi paris superior*, according to Burdach (1822, p. 309).
7. *accessory nerves to eighth pair of Lobstein (Frotscher, 1788)*
Eponym for macrodissected adult human ***accessory nerves (Vieussens, 1684)***; in the original Latin, *nervi ad par octavum accessorii Lobsteinii*, p. 101, referring to Lobstein (1760). However, see *nervus accessorius octavi paris (Winslow, 1733)*.
8. *recurrent nerves of Willis (Frotscher, 1788)*
Eponym for macrodissected adult human ***accessory nerves (Vieussens, 1684)***; in the original Latin, *nervi recurrentes Willisii*, p. 101, without providing citation to Willis.
9. *accessory nerve to vagal pair (Frotscher, 1788)*
Synonym for macrodissected adult human ***accessory nerve (Vieussens, 1684)***; in the original Latin, *nervo ad par vagum accessorii*, p. 101.
10. *recurrent spinal nerve of Willis (Coopmans, 1789)*
Eponym for macrodissected adult human ***accessory nerve (Vieussens, 1684)***; in the original Latin, *spinalis recurrens Willisii*, p. 100, without providing citation to Willis.
11. *fifteenth pair (Malacarne, 1791)*
Synonym for macrodissected adult human right and left ***accessory nerves (Vieussens, 1684)***; see Burdach (1822, p. 309), who gave the Latin, *par decimum quintum*. The 15th of 17 pairs of *cerebral nerves (Malacarne, 1791)*.
12. *par accessorius ad sympathicum medium (Malacarne, 1791)*
Synonym for macrodissected adult human ***accessory nerves (Vieussens, 1684)***; according to Burdach (1822, p. 309).
13. *par vagum accessorius (Soemmerring, 1791)*
Synonym for macrodissected adult human ***accessory nerves (Vieussens, 1684)***, listed as 11th of 12 ***cranial nerves (Soemmerring, 1791)***; p. 254. Burdach (1822, p. 309) quoted without citation Soemmerring as using the term, *par undecimum, accessorius ad vocalem, Baynerve*.
14. *eleventh pair of cranial nerves (Soemmerring, 1791)*
Synonym for macrodissected adult human ***accessory nerves (Vieussens, 1684)***; see ***cranial nerves (Soemmerring, 1791)***.
15. *eleventh pair of cerebral nerves (Soemmerring, 1791)*
Synonym for *eleventh pair of cranial nerves (Soemmerring, 1791)*; see p. 103 and ***cranial nerves (Soemmerring, 1791)***. For original Latin form, *par undecimum nervorum cerebri*, see Soemmerring (1798, p. 125).
16. *adcessory pair of cerebral nerves (Soemmerring, 1798)*
Synonym for macrodissected adult human ***accessory nerves (Vieussens, 1684)***; in the original Latin, *par adcessorium nervorum cerebri*, p. 125.
17. *third division of eighth pair of nerves (Bell, 1803b)*
Synonym for macrodissected adult human ***accessory nerve (Vieussens, 1684)***; p. 159.
18. *nerfs spino-crânio-trapèziens (Portal, 1803b)*
Synonym for macrodissected adult human ***accessory nerves (Vieussens, 1684)***; Vol. 4, p. 217.
19. *trachelo-dorsal pair of nerves (Burdin, 1803)*
Synonym for macrodissected adult human ***accessory nerves (Vieussens, 1684)***; see translation (Vol. 1, p. 144).
20. *twelfth pair of encephalic nerves (Burdin, 1803)*
Synonym for macrodissected adult human ***accessory nerves (Vieussens, 1684)***; see translation (Vol. 1, p. 185).
21. *superior respiratory nerve of trunk (Bell, 1821)*
Synonym for macrodissected adult mammalian ***accessory nerve (Vieussens, 1684)***; p. 406. "To an anatomist it

is as plainly set forth as if it were written in our mother tongue, this is *the superior respiratory nerve of the trunk*." (Bell, 1822, p. 294; italics his).

22. *superior external respiratory nerve (Bell & Bell, 1826)*
Synonym for macrodissected adult human ***accessory nerve (Vieussens, 1684)***; Vol. 2, p. 400.
23. *ascending spinal nerve (Swan, 1830)*
Synonym for macrodissected adult human ***accessory nerve (Vieussens, 1684)***; p. 24.
24. *accessory nerve of Weber (Bischoff, 1832)*
Eponym for ***accessory nerve (Vieussens, 1684)*** as identified by Weber (1827, pp. 321-323) in macrodissected adult fish; in the original Latin, *nervus accessorius Weberi*, Table VI, Figures 1–3.

PARTLY CORRESPONDS:

1. *roots of accessory nerve of Willis (Malacarne, 1791)*
Alluded to for macrodissected adult human ***accessory nerve (Vieussens, 1684)*** without distinguishing ***cranial root of accessory nerve rootlets (>1840)*** from ***spinal root of accessory nerve rootlets (>1840)***; p. 227.
2. *anastomosis of third cervical nerve with recurrent nerve of Willis (Peipers, 1793)*
Macrodissected adult human short and long ***communicating branches (Winslow, 1733)*** between third ***cervical nerve (Galen, c173)*** and ***accessory nerve (Vieussens, 1784)***; in the original Latin, *anastomosis tertii cervicalium cum recurrente Willisii*, p. 33.
3. *spinal and cerebral part of eleventh pair (Arnold, 1834)*
Essentially synonym for macrodissected adult human **spinal root of accessory nerve (>1840)** and ***cranial root of accessory nerve (>1840)*** considered together; in the original Latin, *par undecimum, pars spinalis et cerebralis*, p. 14.
4. *spinal and cerebral part of accessory nerve of Willis (Arnold, 1834)*
Synonym for *spinal and cerebral part of eleventh pair (Arnold, 1834)*; in the original Latin, *nervus accessorius Willisii, pars spinalis et cerebralis*, p. 14.
5. *cervical part of eleventh pair (Arnold, 1834)*
Essentially macrodissected adult human ***accessory nerve trunk (Wrisberg, 1786)*** and its two major branches; in the original Latin, *par undecimum, pars cervicalis*, p. 14.
6. *cervical part of accessory nerve of Willis (Arnold, 1834)*
Synonym for *cervical part of eleventh pair (Arnold, 1834)*; in the original Latin, *nervus accessorius Willisii, pars cervicalis*, p. 14.

accessory nerve trunk (Wrisberg, 1786)

As described for macrodissected adult human, it lies distal to the site where the ***spinal root of accessory nerve trunk (>1840)*** and ***cranial root of accessory nerve trunks (>1840)*** merge in the region of the jugular foramen, and proximal to the site where it divides into ***internal branch of accessory nerve trunk (Meckel, 1817)*** and ***external branch of accessory nerve trunk (Meckel, 1817)***; see Durward (1951, p. 1043), Williams & Warwick (1980, pp. 10881–1083 and Fig. 7.189). For Wrisberg's use in macrodissected adult human, see Wrisberg reprint (1800, p. 429); in the original Latin, *truncus accessorii*. Bellingeri (1823; Tab. III, Fig. 5-*g*) illustrated it beautifully for macrodissected adult beef. It was perhaps first clearly delineated by Eustachi; see ***[accessory nerve trunk (Wrisberg, 1786)] (Eustachi, 1552)***.

EARLIER REFERENCES:

Illustrated, not named or described:

1. ***[accessory nerve trunk (Wrisberg, 1786)] (Eustachi, 1552)***
Illustrated for macrodissected adult human; see *trunk of recurrent spinal nerve (Albinus, 1744)*.

Earlier synonyms:

1. *trunk of recurrent spinal nerve (Albinus, 1744)*
Synonym for macrodissected adult human ***accessory nerve trunk (Wrisberg, 1786)***; in the original Latin, *truncus nervorum spinalium recurrentium*, Table 18, Figure 2-*f*.

PARTLY CORRESPONDS:

1. *anastomotic branch of accessory nerve of Willis with vagus nerve (Günther, 1786)*
Macrodissected adult human ***communicating branch (Winslow, 1733)*** between ***accessory nerve trunk (Wrisberg, 1786)*** and ***vagus nerve (Galen, c192)***; in the original Latin, *r. anastomaticos cum n. vago*, p. 90.
2. *anastomotic branch of accessory nerve of Willis with glossopharyngeal nerve (Günther, 1786)*
Macrodissected adult human ***communicating branch (Winslow, 1733)*** between ***accessory nerve trunk (Wrisberg, 1786)*** and ***glossopharyngeal nerve (Huber, 1744)***; in the original Latin, *r. anastomaticos cum n. glossopharyngeo*, p. 90.
3. *anastomotic branch of accessory nerve of Willis with ninth nerve (Günther, 1786)*
Macrodissected adult human ***communicating branch (Winslow, 1733)*** between ***accessory nerve trunk (Wrisberg, 1786)*** and ***hypoglossal nerve (Winslow, 1733)***; in the original Latin, *r. anastomaticos cum n. nono*, p. 90.

accessory obturator nerve (Schmidt, 1794)

As described for macrodissected adult human, it is observed in only about one in three individuals, arising from the third, or third and fourth ***lumbar nerves (Diemerbroeck, 1672)*** between the roots of the ***obturator nerve (Cheselden, 1726)*** and ***femoral nerve (Haller, 1762)***, and associated with although separable from the ***obturator nerve (Cheselden, 1726)***. It usually ends in three branches; one replaces the branch from the ***femoral nerve (Haller, 1762)*** to the pectineus muscle, a second goes to the hip joint, and a third communicates with the ***obturator nerve (Cheselden, 1726)***; see Durward (1951, p. 1098), *Terminologia Anatomica* (1998, p. 140). For Schmidt's use of this shorthand form of *accessory internal crural nerve (Schmidt, 1794)* see p. 82, where it is clearly described for the first time.

EARLIER REFERENCES:

Earlier synonyms:

1. *accessory internal crural nerve (Schmidt, 1794)*
   Synonym for macrodissected adult human ***accessory obturator nerve (Schmidt, 1794)***; in the original Latin, *accessorius nervi cruralis interioris*, pp. 81–83.
2. *accessory nerve of internal crural nerve (Schmidt, 1794)*
   Synonym for ***accessory obturator nerve (Schmidt, 1794)***; in the original Latin, *nervus accessorius nervi cruralis interioris*, Table II-76.

LATER SYNONYMS:

1. *accessory nerve of obturator nerve (Cloquet, 1828)*
   Synonym for macrodissected adult human ***accessory obturator nerve (Schmidt, 1794)***; in the original French, *nerf accessoire au nerf obturateur*, Plate CLXXII, Figure 1-90.
2. *nerve of coxofemoral joint (Cruveilhier, 1836)*
   Synonym for macrodissected adult human ***accessory obturator nerve (Schmidt, 1794)***; in the original French, *nerf de l'articulation coxo-fémorale*, p. 840.

accessory olfactory bulb (>1840)

As described for embryonic human primarily with histological methods, a small differentiation of the dorsal ***olfactory bulb (Weitbrecht, 1751)*** receiving the ***vomeronasal nerve (>1840)***. It regresses and is not present in adult human; see Crosby et al. (1962, p. 416). In macrosmatic adult mammal the small ***accessory olfactory bulb (>1840)*** forms a set of stacked layers with the ***vomeronasal nerve layer of accessory olfactory bulb (>1840)*** on the outside and forming the bulk of the ***vomeronasal nerve central root (>1840)***, which extends deeper to end in the glomeruli of the subjacent ***glomerular layer of accessory olfactory bulb (>1840)***; see Shipley et al. (1996), Swanson (2004, Atlas Level 3). The ***main olfactory bulb (>1840)*** and ***accessory olfactory bulb (>1840)*** were not distinguished by 1840.

accessory phrenic nerve (>1840)

As described for macrodissected adult human it not uncommonly arises from the ***subclavian nerve (>1840)***, sometimes with other filaments from the fifth and/or sixth ***cervical nerves (Galen, c173)***, and descends for variable distances before joining the main ***phrenic nerve (Galen, c173)*** in the lower neck or upper thorax; see Durward (1951, pp. 1065–1066, 1070), *Terminologia Anatomica* (1998, p. 137). It was perhaps first mentioned specifically by Meckel; see ***[accessory phrenic nerve (>1840)] (Meckel, 1817)***.

EARLIER REFERENCES:

Described, not named or illustrated:

1. ***[accessory phrenic nerve (>1840)] (Meckel, 1817)***
   Mentioned without naming for macrodissected adult human; see translation (1832, Vol. 3, p. 30).

accumbens nucleus (Ziehen, 1897–1901)

As described for macrodissected adult human, and with cellular architecture and connections for all mammals, a rostroventral differentiation of the ***striatum (Swanson, 2000a)*** between ***caudoputamen (Heimer & Wilson, 1975)*** dorsally and ***olfactory tubercle (Calleja, 1893)*** ventrally; see Nieuwenhuys et al. (2008, p. 436). There are no good histological criteria for determining a precise border between ***accumbens nucleus (Ziehen, 1897–1901)*** and ***caudoputamen (Heimer & Wilson, 1975)***. For Ziehen's use in macrodissection and histology of monotreme and marsupial, see p. 718. Not clearly described by 1840.

TRANSLATIONS:

1. *nucleus accumbens (Ziehen, 1897–1901)*
   Original Latin form of ***accumbens nucleus (Ziehen, 1897–1901)***; p. 718.

adenohypophysis (Rioch et al., 1940)

As described for adult mammal, a component of the ***pituitary gland (>1840)*** developing from Rathke's pouch with an ***anterior lobe of pituitary gland (>1840)*** derived from the rostral wall of the pouch, and an ***intermediate lobe of pituitary gland (>1840)*** derived from the caudal wall; see Simmons et al. (1990). It is thus non-neural tissue, and in English is *glandular pituitary*. By contrast, the other component of the ***pituitary gland (>1840)***, the ***neurohypophysis (Rioch et al., 1940)***, develops as a ventral and median, ventrally directed extension of the ***hypothalamus (Kuhlenbeck, 1927)*** and is thus neural tissue. For use by Rioch et al. in mammal see Table 2. It was perhaps first distinguished by Riolan; see ***[adenohypophysis (Rioch et al., 1940)] (Riolan, 1610)***.

EARLIER REFERENCES:

Described, not named or illustrated:

1. ***[adenohypophysis (Rioch et al., 1940)] (Riolan, 1610)***
   First identified vaguely in macrodissected adult human; see ***anterior lobe of pituitary gland (Haller, 1762)***.

Earlier synonyms:

1. *glandular lobe of hypophysis (Tilney, 1936)*
   Synonym for ***adenohypophysis (Rioch et al., 1940)***; p. 425. Tilney divided it into tuberal, infundibular [***intermediate lobe of pituitary gland (>1840)***], and distal parts; p. 425.

adrenal plexus (>1840)

As described for macrodissected adult human, it is formed by branches from the ***celiac ganglion (Walter, 1783)***, ***celiac plexus (Winslow, 1733)***, and ***greater splanchnic nerve (Walter, 1783)*** supplying the adrenal gland. Functionally the branches contain preganglionic sympathetic ***axons (Kölliker, 1896)*** synapsing with the gland's chromaffin cells, homologous to postganglionic ***neurons (Waldeyer, 1891)***; see Mitchell (1953, Fig. 104), Williams & Warwick (1980, p. 1134). It was known to Pietro da Cortona; see ***[adrenal plexus (>1840)] (Pietro da Cortona, c1618)***.

EARLIER REFERENCES:

Illustrated, not named or described:

1. ***[adrenal plexus (>1840)] (Pietro da Cortona, c1618)***
   Clearly illustrated in Table 8-Z for macrodissected adult human; see Haller (1762, p. 265-note *g*).

Described, not named or illustrated:

1. ***[adrenal plexus (>1840)] (Winslow, 1733)***
Mentioned for macrodissected adult human; Section VI, no. 406, p. 98.

Earlier synonyms:

1. *suprarenal plexus (Haase, 1781)*
Synonym for macrodissected adult human ***adrenal plexus (>1840)***; in the original Latin, *plexum(s) suprarenalis*, p. 125.
2. *capsular plexus (Wrisberg, 1808)*
Probably synonym for macrodissected adult human ***adrenal plexus (>1840)***, associated with *capsulis atrabilariis*, or *capsulam suprarenalem*; in the original Latin, *plexum capsularem*, p. 17.
3. *plexus of suprarenal capsule (Cruveilhier, 1836)*
Synonym for macrodissected adult human ***adrenal plexus (>1840)***; in the original French (plural), *plexus des capsules surrénales*, p. 1016.

PARTLY CORRESPONDS:

1. *suprarenal nerves (Cloquet, 1828)*
For macrodissected adult human, larger components of ***adrenal plexus (>1840)*** as it extends from ***celiac ganglion (Walter, 1783)*** and ***celiac plexus (Winslow, 1733)***; in the original French, *N. surrénaux*, Plate CLXXVI-*109*.

afterbrain (Baer, 1837)

Equally acceptable synonym for macrodissected embryonic and adult vertebrate ***medulla (Winslow, 1733)***; in the original German, *Nachhirn*, p. 107. Just 3 years earlier Bell (1834, p. 477) wrote, "After these dissections, it is impossible for us to consider the medulla oblongata as the mere commencement of the spinal marrow: it has a peculiar structure and distinct functions." Also see ***afterbrain vesicle (Baer, 1837)***.

TRANSLATIONS:

1. *Nachhirn (Baer, 1837)*
Original German form of ***afterbrain (Baer, 1837)***; p. 107.
2. *metencephalon (Sharpey et al., 1867)*
Original Latin form of ***afterbrain (Baer, 1837)***; p. 577.

afterbrain vesicle (Baer, 1837)

For macrodissected vertebrate embryos, the caudal division of the ***primary hindbrain vesicle (Baer, 1837)*** developing into the adult ***afterbrain (Baer, 1837)*** or equally acceptable synonym ***medulla (Winslow, 1733)***; the rostral division is the ***hindbrain vesicle (Baer, 1837)***. For Baer's use, see p. 107; it was clearly differentiated early on by Malpighi; see ***[afterbrain vesicle (Baer, 1837)] (Malpighi, 1673)***.

EARLIER REFERENCES:

Illustrated and described, not named:

1. ***[afterbrain vesicle (Baer, 1837)] (Malpighi, 1673)***
Clearly illustrated for chick embryo on third day of incubation; see Figure XVIII.

Earlier synonyms:

1. *medulla oblongata vesicle (Serres, 1824–1826)*
Synonym for ***afterbrain vesicle (Baer, 1837)*** in macrodissected chick embryo on third day of incubation; in the original French, *vésicule de la moelle allongée*; Plate I, Figure 3-5. Used later in the book for all vertebrates.

agranular retrosplenial area (>1840)

As described with cellular architecture in adult human, the dorsal, outer part of the ***retrosplenial region (>1840)***; Brodmann called it the *agranular retrolimbic area (Brodmann, 1909)*. It was not identified by 1840.

EARLIER REFERENCES:

Earlier synonyms:

1. *area retrolimbica agranularis (Brodmann, 1909)*
Original Latin form of *agranular retrolimbic area (Brodmann, 1909)*; p. 149.
2. *agranular retrolimbic area (Brodmann, 1909)*
Synonym for adult human ***agranular retrosplenial area (>1840)***; see p. 149.
3. *area 30 (Brodmann, 1909)*
Synonym for *agranular retrolimbic area (Brodmann, 1909)*; in the original German, *Feld 30*, see p. 149, Figure 86.

alar plate (>1840)

As described for developing vertebrate, right or left wall of the ***neural tube (Baer, 1837)*** between the ***roof plate (>1840)*** dorsally and ***limiting sulcus (>1840)*** ventrally; see Alvarez-Bolado & Swanson (1996, p. 13 ff.), Nieuwenhuys et al. (2008, p. 9). It was not clearly described by 1840.

alveus (Burdach, 1822)

As described in macrodissected adult human, and mammal generally with histological methods for ***axons (Kölliker, 1896)***, the components of the ***fimbria (Honegger, 1890)*** in direct contact with, and constituting the ***cerebral cortex white matter (>1840)*** of, ***Ammon's horn (Vicq d'Azyr, 1786)*** and the ***subiculum (>1840)***. It has two limbs, one on either side of the ***fimbria (Honegger, 1890)***, the longer extending toward the ***subiculum (>1840)*** and facing the ***inferior horn of lateral ventricle (Bell, 1802)*** and the shorter extending toward the ***dentate gyrus (>1840)***; see Swanson (2004, Atlas Levels 27–43). It was perhaps first clearly delineated as the *fibrous envelope of cornu ammonis (Meckel, 1817)*.

EARLIER REFERENCES:

Earlier synonyms:

1. *fibrous envelope of cornu ammonis (Meckel, 1817)*
Synonym for macrodissected adult human ***alveus (Burdach, 1822)***; see translation (1832, Vol. 2, p. 451).
2. *white envelope of pes hippocampi (Meckel, 1817)*
Synonym for macrodissected adult human ***alveus (Burdach, 1822)***; see translation (1832, Vol. 2, p. 451).
3. *medullary layer of cornu Ammonis (Meckel, 1817)*
Synonym for macrodissected adult human ***alveus (Burdach, 1822)***; see translation (1832, Vol. 2, p. 465).

PARTLY CORRESPONDS:

1. *external appendix of fimbria (Volkmann, 1831)*
Part of macrodissected adult mammalian ***alveus (Burdach, 1822)*** extending away from ***fimbria***

(Honegger, 1890) and toward ***subiculum (>1840)***, adjacent to ***inferior horn of lateral ventricle (Bell, 1802)***; in the original Latin, *appendicem fimbriae externum*, pp. 52–53, Table XVIIII, Figure 5-*h**. Dejerine & Dejerine-Klumpke (1901, p. 294) called it "intraventricular alveus", and Cajal (1911) called it "white matter layer on the side adjacent to the ventricle" (Swanson & Swanson translation, 1995, p. 604).

2. *internal appendix of fimbria (Volkmann, 1831)*
   Part of macrodissected adult mammalian ***alveus (Burdach, 1822)*** extending away from ***fimbria (Honegger, 1890)*** and toward ***dentate gyrus (>1840)***; in the original Latin, *appendicem fimbriae internum*, pp. 52–53, Table XVIIII, Figure 5-*h***. Dejerine & Dejerine-Klumpke (1901, pp. 294–295) called it "extraventricular alveus", and Blackstad (1956, pp. 420, 440) called it "deep root" of ***alveus (Burdach, 1822)***.

ambient gyrus (>1840)

As described for macrodissected adult human, a topographic subdivision of the ***olfactory region (>1840)*** between ***olfactory peduncle (Solly, 1836)*** rostrally and ***semilunar gyrus (>1840)*** caudally, and corresponding to the *limen insulae (>1840)*. Based on cellular architecture and connections, it basically corresponds to the ***piriform area (Smith, 1919)*** in mammal generally; see Nauta & Haymaker (1969, pp. 150–151, Fig. 4.10-*GA*), Nieuwenhuys et al. (2008, Fig. 5.6-*13*). It was perhaps first clearly distinguished as the *threshold of Sylvian fissure (Reil, 1809b)*.

TRANSLATIONS:

1. *gyrus ambiens (>1840)*
   Latin form of ***ambient gyrus (>1840)***; see Nauta & Haymaker (1969, p. 150).

EARLIER REFERENCES:

Earlier synonyms:

1. *threshold of Sylvian fissure (Reil, 1809b)*
   Synonym for macrodissected adult human *insular threshold (Schwalbe, 1881)*, indicating location of histologically defined ***piriform area (Smith, 1919)***; see Mayo translation (1823, p. 52).
2. *limen fissura Sylvii (Reil, 1809b)*
   Latin form of *threshold of Sylvian fissure (Reil, 1809b)*.

LATER SYNONYMS:

1. *insular threshold (Schwalbe, 1881)*
   Synonym for macrodissected adult human ***ambient gyrus (>1840)***; in the original German, *Inselschwelle*; see Nauta & Haymaker (1969, p. 156, Fig. 4.10), *Nomina Anatomica* (1983, p. A71), *Terminologia Anatomica* (1998, p. 125).
2. *limen insulae (>1840)*
   Current Latin form of *insular threshold (Schwalbe, 1881)*; see *Terminologia Anatomica* (1998, p. 125).
3. *lateral olfactory gyrus (>1840a)*
   According to some authors, synonym for macrodissected adult human ***ambient gyrus (>1840)***; see Nauta & Haymaker (1969, pp. 151, 156), Carpenter (1976, p. 525). For alternate view see *lateral olfactory gyrus (>1840b)*.

PARTLY CORRESPONDS:

1. *pyriform (Collins, 1685)*
   Term for differentiated region of ***endbrain (Kuhlenbeck, 1927)*** out of which extends ***olfactory peduncle (Solly, 1836)*** in skate, a cartilaginous fish: "In a Skate [the smelling nerves] arise out of the Apices of the *Pyriform* [called *pyramidal processes* in the legend to Table 61, Figure 1-*a* and Figure 2-*a*] being the First [rostralmost] Processes, and make their progress obliquely crossways, toward the inward Orbite of the Eyes, and then perforate the Skull, and afterward arrive the Organs of Smelling, and thence creeping all along, make a round ridge [bulb] on the Surfaces of them." (p. 1043). Thus, in very vague way *piriform (Collins, 1685)* may correspond to all or part of histologically defined ***piriform area (Smith, 1919)*** or macrodissected adult human ***ambient gyrus (>1840)***, though it is probably not possible to define correspondence more accurately.
2. *pyramidal process (Collins, 1685)*
   Synonym for *pyriform (Collins, 1685)*; see Table 61, Figure 1-*a* and Figure 2-*a*.
3. *lateral olfactory gyrus (>1840b)*
   According to some authors, corresponds in adult human to parts of ***piriform area (Smith, 1919)*** in direct proximity to ***lateral olfactory tract (>1840)***, with ***ambient gyrus (>1840)*** by this definition constituting rest of ***piriform area (Smith, 1919)*** more laterally; see Williams & Warwick (1980, p. 995). For alternate view see *lateral olfactory gyrus (>1840a)*.

ambiguus nucleus (>1840)

As described for adult mammal based on cellular architecture and connections, a thin longitudinal ***gray matter region (Swanson & Bota, 2010)*** in ventral and caudal parts of the ***medulla (Winslow, 1733)***, lying caudal to the ***facial nucleus (>1840)*** and generating motor components of the ***vagus nerve central roots (>1840)*** and continuing peripherally in the peripheral ***vagus nerve root (>1840)***. It has 2 spatially segregated functional components, one supplying striated muscles of the pharynx and larynx and the other supplying parts of the viscera, especially the heart, via the parasympathetic system; see Cheng & Powley (2000), Nieuwenhuys et al. (2008, pp. 194, 867 and Figs. 6.22–6.24). It was not identified by 1840.

amiculum of olive (>1840)

As described for macrodissected adult human, the dense band of myelinated axons surrounding the ***principal olivary nucleus (>1840)*** of the ***inferior olivary complex (>1840)***, formed at least partly by the caudal end of the ***medullary central tegmental tract (Bechterew, 1889)***; see Carpenter (1976, p. 299), *Terminologia Anatomica* (1998, p. 109), Williams & Warwick (1980, p. 904), Nieuwenhuys et al. (2008, p. 196 and Figs. 6.22-6.24). In English literally, *fleece of olive*. It was perhaps first clearly described as the *central nucleus of olivary eminence (Chaussier, 1807)*.

TRANSLATIONS:

1. *amiculum olivare (>1840)*
   Latin form of ***amiculum of olive (>1840)***; see *Terminologia Anatomica* (1998, p. 109).

EARLIER REFERENCES:

Earlier synonyms:

1. *central nucleus of olivary eminence (Chaussier, 1807)*
   For macrodissected adult human, the interlaced *white substance (Vesalius, 1543a)* surrounding the *dentate body of olivary eminence (Vicq d'Azyr, 1786)*, essentially the ***amiculum of olive (>1840)***; in the original French, *noyau central*, p. 123.
2. *dentate body of olives (Desmoulins, 1825)*
   In macrodissected adult human, the pleated capsule of fibrous matter associated with the ***inferior olivary complex (>1840)***, essentially the ***amiculum of olive (>1840)***; in the original French, *corps dentelé des olives*, Plate XIII, Figure 2-*d* and Figure 9-*d*.
3. *pleated capsule of olivary eminence (Cloquet, 1828)*
   Synonym for macrodissected adult human ***amiculum of olive (>1840)***; in the original French, *capsule plissée de l'éminence olivaire*, Plate CXLV, Figure 7-3.

PARTLY CORRESPONDS:

1. *funiculus siliquae externus (Burdach, 1822)*
   For macrodissected adult human the dorsal part of the ***amiculum of olive (>1840)***; Table III-*g*.
2. *tectum of white substance at anterior end of olivary nucleus (Arnold, 1838b)*
   For macrodissected adult human, the rostral part of the ***amiculum of olive (>1840)***; in the original Latin, *extremitas anterior nucleorum olivarum, substantia alba tecta*, Table II, Figure 10-*d*. See Carpenter (1976, p. 299).

Ammon's horn (Vicq d'Azyr, 1784)

As described for macrodissected adult human, one of two major parts of the ***hippocampal region (Swanson et al., 1987)***, the other being the medially adjacent ***dentate gyrus (>1840)***. As described with cellular architecture and connections in mammal, three longitudinal regions or areas of ***cerebral cortex gray matter (>1840)—field CA3 (Lorente de Nó, 1934)***, ***field CA2 (Lorente de Nó, 1934)***, and ***field CA1 (Lorente de Nó, 1934)***— arranged topologically and developmentally from medial to lateral. "CA" is abbreviation for *cornu ammonis*, the Latin form of Ammon's horn; see Brodmann (1906, p. 398 and Figs. 127, 128, 137, 156–162, 176–179, 191–194). Amun (Ammon in Greek) was one of the principal gods in Egyptian mythology, and as a symbol of virility was depicted as a ram with its typical curved horns—famously at Karnak, with its avenue of ram-headed sphinxes. Vicq d'Azyr distinguished clearly for the first time between ***dentate gyrus (>1840)*** and ***Ammon's horn (Vicq d'Azyr, 1784)*** in macrodissected adult human; in the original French, *corne d'Ammon*; pp. 518–520; also see Vicq d'Azyr, 1786, Plate XV:*20–23*, and Plate VIII, Figure 1-*25*,*26*. It is unclear whether he included any of the ***subiculum (>1840)***; compare his 1786 Plate XXVI, Figures 7 and 8 with Duvernoy (1988, Figs. 23, 91A, 92A). In addition, Vicq d'Azyr (1786) sometimes used the term more generally in the sense of *hippocampus (Aranzi, 1587)*, for example, Plate XXVI, Figures 4 and 6; also see *hippocampus proper (Vicq, d'Azyr, 1786)*. Vicq d'Azyr (1784, p. 520) emphasized that it is a special *cerebral convolution (Smith Papyrus, 1700 BC)*. Wenzel & Wenzel (1812, p. 151) also suggested that ***Ammon's horn (Vicq d'Azyr, 1784)*** is an infolding of the ***cerebral cortex (>1840)***, which was confirmed by Tiedemann (1816; see translation, 1826, p. 281). It is synonymous with *hippocampus (Vicq d'Azyr, 1784)* and is distinguished from *hippocampal gyrus (>1840)* or ***parahippocampal gyrus (>1840)***.

LATER SYNONYMS:

1. *hippocampus (Vicq d'Azyr, 1784)*
   Synonym for ***Ammon's horn (Vicq d'Azyr, 1784)***; p. 518.
2. *hippocampus major (Vicq d'Azyr, 1786)*
   Synonym for ***Ammon's horn (Vicq d'Azyr, 1784)***; in the original French, *grand hypocampe*, see Plate XV:*20–23*. In addition, Vicq d'Azyr sometimes used the term more generally in the sense of *hippocampus (Aranzi, 1587)*, for example, Plate XXVI, Figures 4 and 6; also see *hippocampus proper (Vicq, d'Azyr, 1786)*.
3. *hippocampus proper (Vicq d'Azyr, 1786)*
   Synonym for ***Ammon's horn (Vicq d'Azyr, 1784)***; in the original French, *hypocampe proprement dit*, see Plate XV:20–23.
4. *gerollte Wulst (Soemmerring, 1788)*
   German synonym for macrodissected adult human ***Ammon's horn (Vicq d'Azyr, 1784)***; see Burdach (1822, p. 372), Meyer (1971, p. 123). In English it refers to a rolled-in convolution.
5. *Kolben (Reil, 1809b)*
   Reil's term in German for macrodissected adult human ***Ammon's horn (Vicq d'Azyr, 1784)***, which he distinguished from ***dentate gyrus (>1840)***; see Mayo translation (1823, Pl. XIII-*G*,*H*), Meyer (1971, p. 127). In English, it refers to a club-shaped structure or bulb; a German synonym is *Wulst*.
6. *processus cerebri lateralis (Wenzel & Wenzel, 1812)*
   Apparently synonym for macrodissected adult human ***Ammon's horn (Vicq d'Azyr, 1784)***; pp. 134, 203.
7. *cylindrical protuberance (Cruveilhier, 1836)*
   Synonym listed for macrodissected adult human ***Ammon's horn (Vicq d'Azyr, 1784)***; in the original French, *protubérance cylindrïode*, p. 694.

PARTLY CORRESPONDS:

1. *lamina conjunctiva (Burdach, 1822)*
   Appears to indicate combined *stratum lacunosum-moleculare* and *stratum radiatum* of macrodissected adult human ***Ammon's horn (Vicq d'Azyr, 1784)***; p. 157. It is continuous with ***lamina medullaris (Burdach, 1822)***.

angular gyrus (>1840)

As described for macrodissected adult human, the caudal (posterior) topographic subdivision of the ***inferior parietal lobule (>1840)*** surrounding the caudal and dorsal end of the ***superior temporal sulcus (>1840)***;

see Williams & Warwick (1980, p. 986, Fig. 7.111A). It was clearly delineated by Rolando; see ***[angular gyrus (>1840)] (Rolando, 1831)***.

EARLIER REFERENCES:

Illustrated, not named or described:

1. ***[angular gyrus (>1840)] (Rolando, 1831)***
Very clearly illustrated for macrodissected adult human; Figure 1-29 indicates rostral limb of ***angular gyrus (>1840)***.

Earlier synonyms:

1. *area angularis (Brodmann, 1909)*
Original Latin form of *angular area (Brodmann, 1909)*; p. 140.
2. *angular area (Brodmann, 1909)*
Based on cellular architecture in adult human, corresponds roughly to ***angular gyrus (>1840)***; see Garey translation (1994, p. 119 and Fig. 85).
3. *area 39 (Brodmann, 1909)*
Synonym for adult human *angular area (Brodmann, 1909)*; in the original German, *Feld 39*, p. 140.

anococcygeal nerves (>1840)

As described for macrodissected adult human, they arise from the ***coccygeal plexus (>1840)*** and distribute to the coccygeus and adjacent parts of the levator ani muscles and to the skin and fascia near the coccyx and dorsal to (behind) the anus, medial to branches of the ***perforating cutaneous nerve (>1840)***; see Durward (1951, p. 1112 and Fig. 945), Williams & Warwick (1980, p. 1116 and Fig. 7.213), *Terminologia Anatomica* (1998, p. 140). They were known to Vieussens; see ***[anococcygeal nerves (>1840)] (Vieussens, 1684)***.

EARLIER REFERENCES:

Illustrated and described, not named:

1. ***[anococcygeal nerves (>1840)] (Vieussens, 1684)***
Vieussens provided a rudimentary description and illustration for macrodissected adult human; see Table 29-*18*. Fisher (1791, p. 23) described and illustrated them fairly accurately for macrodissected adult human.

Earlier synonyms:

1. *last branch of intercostal nerve (Günther, 1786)*
Synonym for macrodissected adult human ***anococcygeal nerves (>1840)***; in the original Latin, *r. ultimi intercostalis*, p. 96.

ansa cervicalis (>1840)

As described for macrodissected adult human, a complex part of the ***cervical plexus (Molinetti, 1675)*** with a ***superior root of ansa cervicalis (>1840)*** and ***inferior root of ansa cervicalis (>1840)*** joining to form a distal loop, the ansa cervicalis proper, with branches to the sternohyoid, sternothyroid, and omohyoid muscles; see Durward (1951, Figs. 909, 919), Hamilton (1976, Fig. 816), Williams & Warwick (1980, Figs. 7.193, 197), *Nomina Anatomica* (1983, p. A76 note *157*), *Terminologia Anatomica* (1998, p. 137). It was known at least partly to Galen; see ***[ansa cervicalis (>1840)] (Galen, c173)***.

EARLIER REFERENCES:

Described, not named or illustrated:

1. ***[ansa cervicalis (>1840)] (Galen, c173)***
Galen identified at least part of this loop in describing innervation of sternohyoid muscle from macrodissected adult beef, pig, and/or macaque but not human; see May translation (1968, p. 690) and Duckworth translation (1962, p. 204). Vesalius (1543a) described branches of *sixth pair of cerebral nerves (Vesalius, 1543a)* to sternohyoid and sternothyroid muscles in macrodissected adult human; see Richardson & Carman translation (2002, p. 195). Winslow (1733, Sect. VI, p. 75) clearly described the entire loop for macrodissected adult human. Asch (1750, see Figs. 4, 5) described and illustrated its major features in macrodissected adult human.

Earlier synonyms:

1. *ansam communicationis nervorum cervicalium cum nono pari cerebri nervorum (Neubauer, 1772)*
Macrodissected adult human ***ansa cervicalis (>1840)*** very clearly illustrated and described; Table 1-*156,245*.
2. *long arch of neck (Andersch & Soemmerring, 1792)*
Synonym for macrodissected adult human ***ansa cervicalis (>1840)***; in the original Latin, *arcus longus colli*, p. 161.
3. *arch of hyoidiam nerves (Burdin, 1803)*
Roughly synonymous with macrodissected adult human ***ansa cervicalis (>1840)***; see translation (1803, Vol. 1, p. 184).
4. *ansa formed by descending branch of hypoglossal nerve and third cervical nerve (Langenbeck, 1826–1830)*
Synonym for macrodissected adult human ***ansa cervicalis (>1840)***; in the original Latin, *ansa, quam formant ramus descendens nervi hypoglossi et nervus cervicalis tertius*, Fascicle III, Table XVII-*12*.

PARTLY CORRESPONDS:

1. *crooked nerve (Willis, 1664)*
Probably refers to at least part of macrodissected adult human ***ansa cervicalis (>1840)***; in the original Latin, *nervo incurvato;* see Pordage translation (1681, Tab. IX-*T*).
2. *ansa carotidi communi (Neubauer, 1772)*
Apparently segment of macrodissected adult human ***ansa cervicalis (>1840)*** adjacent to common carotid artery; Table 2-*156*.
3. *nerve to coracohyoid muscle (Andersch & Soemmerring, 1792)*
Branch of macrodissected adult human ***ansa cervicalis (>1840)*** to sternohyoid muscle; in the original Latin, *nervus musculi coracohyoidei*, p. 159.
4. *nerve to sternothyroid muscle (Andersch & Soemmerring, 1792)*
Branch of macrodissected adult human ***ansa cervicalis (>1840)*** to sternohyoid muscle; in the original Latin, *nervus musculi sternothyreoidei*, p. 159.
5. *middle plexus of neck (Andersch & Soemmerring, 1792)*
Relatively simple network of macrodissected adult human ***communicating branches (Winslow, 1733)*** at end of ***ansa***

cervicalis (>1840) generating ***nerves (Herophilus, c335–c280 BC)*** to sternohyoid and sternothyroid muscles; in the original Latin, *medius plexus colli*, p. 161.

6. *costohyoid nerve (Scarpa, 1794)*
   Branch of macrodissected adult human ***ansa cervicalis (>1840)*** to omohyoid muscle; in the original Latin, *nervus costo-hyoideus*, Table I-*28,29*.
7. *superficial cervical plexus (Bell & Bell, 1826)*
   Probably synonym for *middle plexus of neck (Andersch & Soemmerring, 1792)*; Vol. 2, pp. 587–588.
8. *branch of hypoglossal nerve descending branch to sternohyoid muscle (Arnold, 1834)*
   In macrodissected adult human, branch of ***ansa cervicalis (>1840)*** to sternohyoid muscle; in the original Latin, *nervus hypoglossus, ramus descendens, ramus musculi sternohyoidei*, p. 15.
9. *branch of hypoglossal nerve descending branch to omohyoid muscle (Arnold, 1834)*
   In macrodissected adult human, branch of ***ansa cervicalis (>1840)*** to superior belly of omohyoid muscle; in the original Latin, *nervus hypoglossus, ramus descendens, ramus musculi omohyoidei*, p. 15.
10. *branch of hypoglossal nerve descending branch to sternothyroid muscle (Arnold, 1834)*
    Synonym for macrodissected adult human *nerve to sternothyroid muscle (Andersch & Soemmerring, 1792)*; in the original Latin, *nervus hypoglossus, ramus descendens, ramus musculi sternothyroidei*, p. 15.
11. *cardiac branch of hypoglossal nerve descending branch (Arnold, 1834)*
    In macrodissected adult human, branch of ***ansa cervicalis (>1840)***, presumably to ***cardiac plexus (Keill, 1698)***; in the original Latin, *nervus hypoglossus, ramus descendens, ramus cardiacus*, p. 15.

ansa subclavia (Neubauer, 1772)

As defined for macrodissected adult human, two or more ***communicating branches of sympathetic trunk (>1840)*** between ***middle cervical ganglion (Haller, 1762)*** and ***inferior cervical ganglion (Vieussens, 1684)***, forming a loop around the subclavian artery; see Mitchell (1953, p. 223 and Fig. 104) and Williams & Warwick (1980, p. 1128). Neubauer should probably be given credit for naming it, "*ansa* circa arteriam *subclaviam*..." (his italics, p. 138), and distinguishing superficial and deep branches (Tab. 3, Fig. 3-*13,14*), in macrodissected adult human. It was clearly noted more than a century earlier by Willis; see ***[ansa subclavia (Neubauer, 1772)] (Willis, 1664)***.

TRANSLATIONS:

1. *subclavian ansa (>1840)*
   English form of ***ansa subclavia (Neubauer, 1772)***; see Mitchell (1953, p. 225). Another form is subclavian loop; see *Dorland's* (2004, p. 1067).

EARLIER REFERENCES:

Illustrated and described, not named:

1. ***[ansa subclavia (Neubauer, 1772)] (Willis, 1664)***
   Clearly illustrated and described for macrodissected adult human; see Pordage translation (1681, p. 158 and Tab. 9-Ξ), Mitchell (1953, p. 3).

Earlier synonyms:

1. *ansa of intercostal nerve (Krüger, 1758)*
   Synonym for macrodissected adult human ***ansa subclavia (Neubauer, 1772)***; in the original Latin, *nervi intercostalis ansa*, Table 2-*42*.

LATER SYNONYMS:

1. *ansularam subclavias (Camper, 1760–1762)*
   In a sentence describing macrodissected adult human, Camper wrote, "De ansularum usu nihil, ne conjecturâ quidem, detegere possumus, id constanter videmus, non modo corca subclavias..." (p. 10), clearly referring to ***ansa subclavia (Neubauer, 1772)***.
2. *ansa Vieussenii (Camper, 1760–1762)*
   Eponym for macrodissected adult human ***ansa subclavia (Neubauer, 1772)***, although Willis illustrated it clearly before Vieussens; Table 1, Figure 1-*5,7,10,9*. See ***[ansa subclavia (Neubauer, 1772)] (Willis, 1664)***.
3. *ansa magna circa subclaviam arteriam (Haller, 1772)*
   Synonym for macrodissected adult human ***ansa subclavia (Neubauer, 1772)***; p. 9-*94*.
4. *laquei subclavici (Andersch & Soemmerring, 1792)*
   Apparently synonym for macrodissected adult human right and left ***ansa subclavia (Neubauer, 1772)***; p. 175.
5. *laqueus ordinarius arteriae subclaviae (Andersch & Soemmerring, 1792)*
   Synonym for *laquei subclavici (Andersch & Soemmerring, 1792)*; pp. 189, 190.
6. *laqueus subclavicus (Andersch, 1797)*
   Singular form of *laquei subclavici (Andersch & Soemmerring, 1792)*; Vol. 2, p. 165.

ansiform lobule (Bolk, 1906)

As described for macrodissected adult human, the part of the ***cerebellar hemisphere (Willis, 1664)*** between ***simple lobule (Jansen & Brodal, 1954)*** and ***gracile lobule (>1840)***, lateral to the ***folium vermis (1840)*** of the ***cerebellar vermis (Meckel, 1817)***. It is subdivided into ***ansiform lobule crus 1 (Bock, 1906)***, adjacent to the ***simple lobule (Jansen & Brodal, 1954)***, and ***ansiform lobule 2 (Bock, 1906)***, adjacent to the ***gracile lobule (>1840)***; see Angevine et al. (1961, Fig. 24), Larsell & Jansen (1972, Fig. 118), Carpenter (1976, Fig. 14.1). It was not recognized as such by 1840.

EARLIER REFERENCES:

Earlier synonyms:

1. *semilunar lobules (>1840)*
   Synonym for macrodissected adult human ***ansiform lobule (Bolk, 1906)***; see His (1895, p. 83), *Terminologia Anatomica* (1998, p. 119).

ansiform lobule crus 1 (Bolk, 1906)

As described for macrodissected adult human, the part of the ***ansiform lobule (Bolk, 1906)*** of the ***cerebellar hemisphere (Willis, 1664)*** between ***simple lobule (Jansen & Brodal, 1954)*** and ***ansiform lobule crus 2***

(Bolk, 1906); see Angevine et al. (1961, Fig. 24), Larsell & Jansen (1972, Fig. 118), Carpenter (1976, Fig. 14.1). It was perhaps first clearly delineated as the *superior posterior lobe (Malacarne, 1776)*.

EARLIER REFERENCES:

Earlier synonyms:

1. *superior posterior lobe (Malacarne, 1776)*
   Synonym for macrodissected adult human ***ansiform lobule crus 1 (Bolk, 1906)***, p. 31; see Larsell (1967, p. 43). A Latin form is *lobus superior posterior*; see Burdach (1822, p. 294).
2. *posterior lobule of cerebellum (Chaussier, 1807)*
   According to Burdach (1822, p. 294), synonym for macrodissected adult human *superior posterior lobe (Malacarne, 1776)*; in the original French, *lobules postérieurs*, p. 91. Burdach gave the Latin form, *lobulus posterior*. Also see *superior lobule of cerebellum (Chaussier, 1807)*.
3. *superior semilunar lobe (Meckel, 1817)*
   Synonym for macrodissected adult human *superior posterior lobe (Malacarne, 1776)*, p. 465; also see translation (1832, Vol. 2, p. 428). For Latin form, *lobus superior semilunaris;* see Burdach (1822, p. 294).

PARTLY CORRESPONDS:

1. *superior external lobule (Vicq d'Azyr, 1784)*
   Apparently roughly corresponds to *superior posterior lobe (Malacarne, 1776)*, but without *deep lobule of superior fissure of Vicq d'Azyr (Dejerine & Dejerine-Klumpke, 1901)*; in the original French, *lobule supérieur et externe*, pp. 569, 571. Also see Vicq d'Azyr (1784, p. 89, Fig. 1). For Latin form, *lobulus cerebelli superior externus*, see Burdach (1822, p. 294).
2. *deep lobule of superior fissure of Vicq d'Azyr (Dejerine & Dejerine-Klumpke, 1901)*
   According to Dejerine & Dejerine-Klumpke (Fig. 339, *lobule profunde du sillon supérieur*), in current terms a region corresponding in macrodissected adult human to anterior sublobule of ***ansiform lobule crus I (Bolk, 1906)***, adjacent to ***posterior superior fissure (>1840)***; see Larsell & Jansen (1972, p. 51). It is probably referred to, though not with this exact name, in Vicq d'Azyr (1784, p. 569).

ansiform lobule crus 2 (Bolk, 1906)

As described for macrodissected adult human, the part of the ***ansiform lobule (Bolk, 1906)*** of the ***cerebellar hemisphere (Willis, 1664)*** between ***ansiform lobule crus 1 (Bolk, 1906)*** and ***gracile lobule (>1840)***; see Angevine et al. (1961, Fig. 24), Larsell & Jansen (1972, Fig. 118), Carpenter (1976, Fig. 14.1). It was perhaps first clearly delineated as the *inferior posterior lobe (Malacarne, 1776)*.

EARLIER REFERENCES:

Earlier synonyms:

1. *inferior posterior lobe (Malacarne, 1776)*
   Synonym for macrodissected adult human ***ansiform lobule crus 2 (Bolk, 1906)***. p. 42. Clarke & O'Malley (1996, p. 645) translated it *posteroinferior lobe*, whereas Larsell (1967, p. 4) translated it *superior inferior lobule*.

ansoparamedian fissure (>1840)

As described for macrodissected adult human, the groove between ***ansiform lobule crus 2 (Bolk, 1906)*** and ***gracile lobule (>1840)*** of the ***cerebellar hemisphere (Willis, 1664)***; see Angevine et al. (1961, p. 16 and Fig. 24), *Terminologia Anatomica* (1998, p. 119). It was perhaps first clearly identified by Malacarne; see ***[ansoparamedian fissure (>1840)] (Malacarne, 1776)***.

EARLIER REFERENCES:

Described, not named or illustrated:

1. *[ansoparamedian fissure (>1840)] (Malacarne, 1776)*
   Malacarne first distinguished clearly macrodissected adult human ***ansiform lobule crus 2 (Bolk, 1906)*** and ***gracile lobule (>1840)***. Thus he first identified, without naming, ***ansoparamedian fissure (>1840)***.

Earlier synonyms:

1. *semilunar fissure (Dejerine & Dejerine-Klumpke, 1901)*
   Synonym for macrodissected adult human ***ansoparamedian fissure (>1840)***; p. 465, Figure 344. Also see Angevine et al. (1961, p. 16) and *inferior cerebellar fissure (Vic d'Azyr, 1784)*.

anterior ampullary nerve (>1840)

As described for macrodissected adult human, commonly a terminal branch of the ***rostral part of vestibular nerve (>1840)*** to the ampulla of the anterior (superior) semicircular canal; see Durward (1951, Fig. 904), *Terminologia Anatomica* (1998, p. 136). It was probably first accurately described as the *branch of major anterior vestibular nerve to ampulla of anterior semicircular canal (Langenbeck, 1826–1830)*.

EARLIER REFERENCES:

Earlier synonyms:

1. *branch of major anterior vestibular nerve to ampulla of anterior semicircular canal (Langenbeck, 1826–1830)*
   Synonym for macrodissected adult human ***anterior ampullary nerve (>1840)***; in the original Latin, *ramus nervi vestibuli anterior—major—ad ampullam canalis semicircularis anterior*, Fascicle III, Table XXIX-7.
2. *branch of anterior vestibular nerve to ampulla of anterior membranous semicircular canal (Langenbeck, 1826–1830)*
   Synonym for macrodissected adult human ***anterior ampullary nerve (>1840)***; in the original Latin, *ramus nervi vestibuli anterior ad ampullam canalis semicircularis membranacei anterioris*; Fascicle III, Table XXIX, Figure IX-6.

anterior auricular nerves (>1840)

As described for macrodissected adult human, they are usually two branches of the ***auriculotemporal nerve (Haller, 1762)*** supplying skin of the tragus and sometimes a small part of the adjacent helix; see Williams & Warwick (1980, p. 1066), *Terminologia Anatomica* (1998, p. 134). They were known to Falloppio; see ***[anterior auricular nerves (>1840)] (Falloppio, 1561)***.

EARLIER REFERENCES:

Described, not named or illustrated:

1. ***[anterior auricular nerves (>1840)] (Falloppio, 1561)***
   According to Haller (1762, p. 220 note *o*), Falloppio alluded to them for macrodissected adult human on p. 145.

Illustrated and described, not named:

1. ***[anterior auricular nerves (>1840)] (Du Verney, 1683)***
   Mentioned and partly illustrated for macrodissected adult human; Plate 13-*I*.

Earlier synonyms:

1. *posterior branch of superficial temporal branch of third branch of fifth pair (Meckel, 1748)*
   Synonym for macrodissected adult human ***anterior auricular nerves (>1840)***; in the original Latin, *ramus temporalis superficialis tertii rami Quinti paris ramus auricularis*, pp. 102–103.
2. *auricular branch of superficial temporal branch of third branch of fifth pair (Meckel, 1748)*
   Synonym for macrodissected adult human ***anterior auricular nerves (>1840)***; in the original Latin, *ramus temporalis superficialis tertii rami Quinti paris ramus posterior*, pp. 102–103.
3. *auricular nerves (Haase, 1781)*
   Synonym for macrodissected adult human ***anterior auricular nerves (>1840)***; in the original Latin, *nervi auriculares*, see Index sections 144–146. Haase described anterior and posterior terminal branches; p. 76.
4. *minor posterior branches of auricular nerve (Soemmerring, 1791)*
   Synonym for macrodissected adult human ***anterior auricular nerves (>1840)***; p. 216. For original Latin form, *ramum posteriorem minorem*, see Soemmerring (1798, p. 237).
5. *first auricular branch of superficial temporal nerve (Bock, 1817)*
   Apparently synonym for macrodissected adult human ***anterior auricular nerves (>1840)***; in the original Latin, *ramus auricularis primus*, p. 50.
6. *superior auricular fascicle of cutaneous temporal surculus of inferior maxillary branch (Bellingeri, 1818)*
   Synonym for macrodissected adult human ***anterior auricular nerves (>1840)***; in the original Latin, *fasciculus auricularis superior*, see Table I.
7. *anterior auricular branches of superficial temporal nerve (Arnold, 1834)*
   Synonym for macrodissected adult human ***anterior auricular nerves (>1840)***; in the original Latin, *nervus temporalis superficialis, rami auriculares anteriores*, p. 11.
8. *anterior auricular branches of anterior auricular nerve (Arnold, 1834)*
   Synonym for macrodissected adult human ***anterior auricular nerves (>1840)***; in the original Latin, *nervus auricularis anterior, rami auriculares anteriores*, p. 11.
9. *external auricular branches of superficial temporal nerve (Todd, 1836–1839)*
   Synonym for macrodissected adult human ***anterior auricular nerves (>1840)***; p. 294.
10. *inferior branch of auriculotemporal nerve (Cruveilhier, 1836)*
    Synonym for macrodissected adult human ***anterior auricular nerves (>1840)***; in the original French, *branche inférieure*, p. 933.
11. *descending branch of auriculotemporal nerve (Cruveilhier, 1836)*
    Synonym for macrodissected adult human ***anterior auricular nerves (>1840)***; in the original French, *branche descendante*, p. 933.
12. *auricular branch of auriculotemporal nerve (Cruveilhier, 1836)*
    Synonym for macrodissected adult human ***anterior auricular nerves (>1840)***; in the original French, *branche auriculaire*, p. 933.

anterior branch of great auricular nerve (Bock, 1827)

As described for macrodissected adult human, it innervates skin of the face over the parotid gland and communicates in the substance of the gland with the ***cervical branch of facial nerve (>1840)***; see Williams & Warwick (1980, p. 1092) and Schwalbe (1881, Fig. 468-6,7). For Bock's use in macrodissected adult human see Table III-4. It was known to Galen; see ***[anterior branch of great auricular nerve (Bock, 1827)] (Galen, c192)***.

TRANSLATIONS:

1. *ramus anterior nervi auricularis magni (Bock, 1827)*
   Original Latin form of ***anterior branch of great auricular nerve (Bock, 1827)***; Table III-4.

EARLIER REFERENCES:

Described, not named or illustrated:

1. ***[anterior branch of great auricular nerve (Bock, 1827)] (Galen, c192)***
   Mentioned for macrodissected adult beef, pig, and/or macaque but not human; see Duckworth translation (1962, p. 225).

Illustrated, not named or described:

1. ***[anterior branch of great auricular nerve (Bock, 1827)] (Eustachi, 1552)***
   Clearly illustrated for macrodissected adult human; see Albinus edition (1761, Tab. 21/2-*h*). Du Verney probably illustrated its origin for macrodissected adult human (1683, Pl. 14-4,7).

Earlier synonyms:

1. *anterior branch of auricular nerve of third pair of cervical nerves (Meckel, 1753)*
   Synonym for macrodissected adult human ***anterior branch of great auricular nerve (Bock, 1827)***; p. 99.
2. *anterior branch of principal auricular nerve (Bang, 1770)*
   Synonym for macrodissected adult human ***anterior branch of great auricular nerve (Bock, 1827)***; in the

original Latin, *anterior ramus nervus auricularis principalis*, Figure I-*30,31*.

3. *anterior branch of greater posterior auricular nerve (Bang, 1770)*
   Synonym for macrodissected adult human ***anterior branch of great auricular nerve (Bock, 1827)***; in the original Latin, *anterior ramus nervus auricularis magnus posterior*, Figure I-*30,31*.
4. *lesser posterior auricular nerve (Neubauer, 1772)*
   Small component of macrodissected adult human *posterior auricular nerve (Neubauer, 1772)*, presumably ***anterior branch of great auricular nerve (Bock, 1827)***; in the original Latin, *parvum nervum auricularem posteriorem*, Table 1-*182*; also see Schwalbe (1881, Fig. 468-*6,7*).
5. *anterior twig of great cervical auricular nerve (Soemmerring, 1791)*
   Synonym for macrodissected adult human ***anterior branch of great auricular nerve (Bock, 1827)***; p. 269.
6. *anterior branches of auricular branch of cervical plexus (Cloquet, 1816)*
   Synonym for macrodissected adult human ***anterior branch of great auricular nerve (Bock, 1827)***; p. 640.

LATER SYNONYMS:

1. *facial branch of great auricular nerve (Arnold, 1834)*
   Synonym for macrodissected adult human ***anterior branch of great auricular nerve (Bock, 1827)***; in the original Latin, *nervus auricularis magnus ramus facialis*, Table IX-*43,44*.
2. *facial branchlets of auricular nerve (Cruveilhier, 1836)*
   Synonym for macrodissected adult human ***anterior branch of great auricular nerve (Bock, 1827)***; in the original French, *filets faciaux*, p. 783.
3. *parotid branchlets of auricular nerve (Cruveilhier, 1836)*
   Synonym for *facial branchlets of auricular nerve (Cruveilhier, 1836)*; in the original French, *filets parotidiens*, p. 783.

PARTLY CORRESPONDS:

1. *lateral cutaneous nerve of face of anterior branch of great auricular nerve (Meckel, 1753)*
   Dorsal (posterior) branch of macrodissected adult human ***anterior branch of great auricular nerve (Bock, 1827)***; in the original French, *le nerf cutané lateral du visage*, Table 1-*264* (also see p. 99).

anterior branch of lateral cerebral sulcus (>1840)

As described for macrodissected adult human, the rostral extension of the ***lateral cerebral sulcus (>1840)*** lying between ***straight gyrus (Valentin, 1841)*** ventrally and ***triangular part of inferior frontal gyrus (>1840)*** dorsally; see Williams & Warwick (1980, p. 984, Fig. 7.111A), *Terminologia Anatomica* (1998, p. 125). It was probably first alluded to accurately as the *anterior fissure (Burdach, 1822)*.

EARLIER REFERENCES:

Earlier synonyms:

1. *anterior fissure (Burdach, 1822)*
   May correspond to macrodissected adult human ***anterior branch of lateral cerebral sulcus (>1840)***. According to Foster (1892, p. 1597), it is a vaguely indicated adult human cerebral fissure corresponding to *presylvian fissure of Wilder*, which was then defined as *anterior limb* of ***lateral cerebral fissure (>1840)***, forming frontal boundary of *operculum (Burdach, 1822)*; see Foster, (1892, p. 1601). Meckel (1817) may have mentioned it earlier; see translation (1832, Vol. 2, p. 442). If it corresponds to ***anterior branch of lateral cerebral sulcus (>1840)***, it probably corresponds to rostrally directed part of *cruciform sulcus (Rolando, 1831)*, Figure 1-*8*. However, *anterior fissure (Burdach, 1822)* may correspond instead to ***ascending branch lateral cerebral sulcus (>1840)***; see Nieuwenhuys et al. (2008, Fig. 3.2-*27*). Meyer (1971, p. 130) suggested that *anterior fissure (Burdach, 1822)* may instead correspond to ***precentral sulcus (>1840)***, but this seems doubtful. Vicq d'Azyr (1784, pp. 505–506, and accompanying plate) may have alluded to *anterior fissure (Burdach, 1822)*. Burdach gave the German form, *Vorderspalte*; p. 166 and Table V-*9*.

anterior branch of lateral cutaneous branch of intercostal nerves (>1840)

As described for macrodissected adult human, the ventrally (anteriorly) directed branch of the ***lateral cutaneous branch of intercostal nerves (>1840)***; see Durward (1951, Fig. 935), Williams & Warwick (1980, p. 1103). It was probably first clearly described as *anterior branch of lateral cutaneous nerve of intercostal nerve (Bock, 1827)*.

EARLIER REFERENCES:

Earlier synonyms:

1. *anterior branch of lateral cutaneous nerve of intercostal nerve (Bock, 1827)*
   Synonym for ***anterior branch of lateral cutaneous branch of intercostal nerves (>1840)***; in the original Latin, *ram. anterior nervi cutanei lateralis intercostalis*, Table III-*27*.
2. *anterior filament of perforating branch of intercostal branches of dorsal nerves (Cruveilhier, 1836)*
   Synonym for macrodissected adult human ***anterior branch of lateral cutaneous branch of intercostal nerves (>1840)***; in the original French, *filet antérieur*, p. 825.

PARTLY CORRESPONDS:

1. *cutaneous branches of lateral pectoral nerve (Bock, 1827)*
   Apparently ***anterior branch of lateral cutaneous branch of intercostal nerve (>1840)*** of 2nd ***lateral cutaneous branch of intercostal nerve (>1840)***; in the original Latin, *rami cutanei nervi lateralis pectoris*, Table II-*80*.
2. *anterior branch of lateral pectoral nerve (Bock, 1827)*
   Synonym for macrodissected adult human ***anterior branch of lateral cutaneous branch of intercostal nerve (>1840)*** of 3rd–7th ***lateral cutaneous branches of intercostal nerves (>1840)***; in the original Latin, *ram. anterior nervi [cutanei] lateralis pectoris cutanei*, see Table II:*81–89*.
3. *anterior branch of lateral abdominal cutaneous nerve (Bock, 1827)*

Synonym for macrodissected adult human ***anterior branch of lateral cutaneous branch of intercostal nerve (>1840)*** of 8th–11th ***lateral cutaneous branches of intercostal nerves (>1840)***; in the original Latin, *ram. anterior nervi cutanei abdominis lateralis*, see Table II-92.

4. *anterior branch of lateral pectoral cutaneous nerve of intercostal nerve (Bock, 1827)*
   Synonym for macrodissected adult human ***anterior branch of lateral cutaneous branch of intercostal nerve (>1840)*** of 3rd–7th ***lateral cutaneous branch of intercostal nerves (>1840)***; in the original Latin, *ram. anterior nervi cutanei lateralis pectoris intercostalis*, see Table III-29.
5. *cutaneous nerves of intercostal nerve (Bock, 1827)*
   Synonym for macrodissected adult human ***anterior branch of lateral cutaneous branch of intercostal nerve (>1840)***, here for 11th ***lateral cutaneous branch of intercostal nerve (>1840)***; in the original Latin, *nervi cutanei intercostalis undecimi*, Table IV-56.
6. *inferior intercosto-humeral nerve (Knox, 1832)*
   In macrodissected adult human, apparently ***anterior branch of lateral cutaneous branch of intercostal nerve (>1840)*** of 4th ***lateral cutaneous branch of intercostal nerve (>1840)***, to skin overlying serratus anterior muscle; Plate XIX-27.

anterior branch of mandibular nerve (>1840)

As described for macrodissected adult human, the smaller of the two major divisions of the ***mandibular nerve (>1840)*** giving off one sensory ***nerve (Herophilus, c335–c280 BC)***, the ***buccal nerve (Meckel, 1748)***, and three substantial motor ***nerves (Herophilus, c335–c280 BC)***: the ***masseteric nerve (Meckel, 1748)***, ***deep temporal nerves (Haase, 1781)***, and ***lateral pterygoid nerve (>1840)***; see Durward (1951, pp. 1026–1029, Fig. 899) and Williams & Warwick (1980, p. 1066), who called it a trunk instead of branch—Hamilton called it a division (1976, p. 624). It was known to Vesalius; see *tendril-like offshoot of thicker root of third pair (Vesalius, 1543a)*.

EARLIER REFERENCES:

Earlier synonyms:

1. *tendril-like offshoot of thicker root of third pair (Vesalius, 1543a)*
   Roughly synonymous with macrodissected adult human ***anterior branch of mandibular nerve (>1840)***; see Richardson & Carman translation (2002, p. 189).
2. *first branch of fourth conjugation of nerves of brain (Crooke, 1615)*
   Roughly synonymous with macrodissected adult human ***anterior branch of mandibular nerve (>1840)***; p. 486. Crooke's description is a translation of Bauhin (1605).
3. *anterior branch of third branch of fifth cerebral pair (Albinus, 1744)*
   Synonym for macrodissected adult human ***anterior branch of mandibular nerve (>1840)***; in the original Latin, *ramus anterior tertii rami nervi quinti paris cerebri*, Table 18, Figures 1,3,4,5-*K*.
4. *superior branch of inferior maxillary nerve (Schaarschmidt, 1750)*
   Synonym for macrodissected adult human ***anterior branch of mandibular nerve (>1840)***; pp. 26–27.
5. *anterior branch of trunk of maxillary nerve (Le Cat, 1768)*
   Synonym for macrodissected adult human ***anterior branch of mandibular nerve (>1840)***; Plate VII, Figure 1-5.
6. *minor branches of inferior maxillary nerve (Loder, 1778)*
   Synonym for macrodissected adult human ***anterior branch of mandibular nerve (>1840)***; in the original Latin, *ramos minores*, p. 17.
7. *superior fascicle of inferior maxillary nerve (Günther, 1786)*
   Synonym for macrodissected adult human ***anterior branch of mandibular nerve (>1840)***; in the original Latin, *fasciculum superiorem*, p. 49.
8. *minor fascicle of inferior maxillary nerve (Günther, 1786)*
   Synonym for macrodissected adult human ***anterior branch of mandibular nerve (>1840)***; in the original Latin, *fasciculum minorem*, p. 49.
9. *upper anterior branch of inferior maxillary nerve (Meckel, 1817)*
   Synonym for macrodissected adult human ***anterior branch of mandibular nerve (>1840)***; see translation (1832, Vol. 3, p. 71).
10. *muscular branch of inferior maxillary nerve (Jacobson, 1818)*
    Essentially synonym for macrodissected adult mammalian ***anterior branch of mandibular nerve (>1840)***; in the original Latin, *nervus maxillaris inferior ramus muscularis*, p. 18.
11. *superior primary branch of inferior maxillary nerve (Quain, 1832)*
    Synonym for macrodissected adult human ***anterior branch of mandibular nerve (>1840)***; p. 675.
12. *muscular division of inferior maxillary nerve (Quain & Wilson, 1839)*
    Synonym for macrodissected adult human ***anterior branch of mandibular nerve (>1840)***; Plate XIII, Figure 2-*x*.

PARTLY CORRESPONDS:

1. *external branches of inferior maxillary nerve (Cruveilhier, 1836)*
   Macrodissected adult human ***deep temporal nerves (Haase, 1781)***, ***masseteric nerve (Meckel, 1748)***, and ***buccal nerve (Meckel, 1748)*** considered together; in the original French, *branches externes*, p. 930.

anterior branch of medial cutaneous nerve of forearm (>1840)

As described for macrodissected adult human, it is larger than the ***posterior branch of medial cutaneous nerve of forearm (>1840)*** and descends on the front of the medial side of the forearm, supplying skin as far as the wrist and communicating with the ***palmar branch of ulnar nerve (Soemmerring, 1791)***; see Williams & Warwick (1980, p. 1097 and Fig. 7.201, branch to the left), *Terminologia Anatomica* (1998, p. 138). It was first distinguished clearly by Eustachi; see ***[anterior branch of medial cutaneous nerve of forearm (>1840)] (Eustachi, 1552)***.

EARLIER REFERENCES:

Illustrated, not named or described:

1. *[anterior branch of medial cutaneous nerve of forearm (>1840)] (Eustachi, 1552)*
   Illustrated for macrodissected adult human; see Albinus edition (1761, Tab. 21/2-*16* upper branch).

Described, not named or illustrated:

1. *[anterior branch of medial cutaneous nerve of forearm (>1840)] (Winslow, 1733)*
   Described for macrodissected adult human; Section VI, no. 240, p. 83.

Earlier synonyms:

1. *palmar cutaneous nerve (Klint, 1784)*
   Synonym for macrodissected adult human ***anterior branch of medial cutaneous nerve of forearm (>1840)***; in the original Latin, *nervus cutaneus palmaris*, p. 65. Klint ascribed the term to Wrisberg without citation, presumably from his lectures.
2. *palmar cutaneous nerve of Wrisberg (Frotscher, 1788)*
   Eponym for macrodissected adult human *palmar cutaneous nerve (Klint, 1784)*; in the original Latin, *nervum cutaneum palmarem Wrisbergii*, p. 92, where Frotscher referred to Klint (1784, § XXIX), [p. 65].
3. *external branch of cutaneous nerve (Fyfe, 1800)*
   Synonym for macrodissected adult human ***anterior branch of medial cutaneous nerve of forearm (>1840)***; Vol. 2, p. 308.
4. *ramus magis palmaris nervi (Loder, 1803)*
   Synonym for macrodissected adult human ***anterior branch of medial cutaneous nerve of forearm (>1840)***; Table CLXXVIII-*144*.
5. *anterior branch of internal cutaneous nerve (Loder, 1803)*
   Synonym for macrodissected adult human ***anterior branch of medial cutaneous nerve of forearm (>1840)***; in the original Latin, *nervi cutanei interni ramus anterior*, Table CLXXVIII, Figure 2-*13*.
6. *middle cutaneous branch of internal cutaneous nerve (Caldani, 1813, 1814)*
   Synonym for macrodissected adult human ***anterior branch of medial cutaneous nerve of forearm (>1840)***; in the original Latin, *ramus medius cutaneus a nervo cutaneo interno*, Table CCLVIII, Figure 1-*29*.
7. *middle cutaneous nerve (Caldani, 1813, 1814)*
   Synonym for *middle cutaneous branch of internal cutaneous nerve (Caldani, 1813, 1814)*; in the original Latin, *nervus cutaneum medium*, Table CCLVIII, Figure 1-*30*.
8. *palmar branch of medial cutaneous nerve (Bock, 1827)*
   Synonym for macrodissected adult human ***anterior branch of medial cutaneous nerve of forearm (>1840)***; in the original Latin, *nervus cutaneus medius ramus palmaris*, Table II-*29,33*.
9. *palmar branch of major internal cutaneous nerve (Bock, 1827)*
   Synonym for macrodissected adult human ***anterior branch of medial cutaneous nerve of forearm (>1840)***; in the original Latin, *nervus cutaneus internus major ramus palmaris*, Table II-*29,33*.

PARTLY CORRESPONDS:

1. *branches of middle cutaneous nerve joining volar cutaneous branch of median nerve (Caldani, 1813, 1814)*
   For macrodissected adult human, two branches of ***anterior branch of medial cutaneous nerve of forearm (>1840)*** joining ***palmar branch of median nerve (Bock, 1827)***; in the original Latin, *rami nervi cutanei medii conjuncti cum ramus cutaneus volaris nervi mediani*, Table CCLVIII, Figure 1-*35*.
2. *palmar cutaneous branch of middle cutaneous branch of internal cutaneous nerve (Caldani, 1813, 1814)*
   For macrodissected adult human, extension of ***anterior branch of medial cutaneous nerve of forearm (>1840)*** to proximal part of palm; in the original Latin, *ramus cutaneus palmaris a ramo medio cutaneo derivatus*, Table CCLVIII, Figure 1-*39*.
3. *cutaneous palmar branch of middle cutaneous branch from internal cutaneous nerve (Knox, 1832)*
   Synonym for macrodissected adult human *palmar cutaneous branch of middle cutaneous branch of internal cutaneous nerve (Caldani, 1813, 1814)*; Table XX-*14*.

anterior branch of obturator nerve (Haase, 1781; Martin, 1781)

As described for macrodissected adult human, it has a ***cutaneous branch of obturator nerve (>1840)*** contributing to the ***subsartorial plexus (>1840)*** and ***muscular branches of anterior branch of obturator nerve (>1840)*** supplying the adductor longus, gracilis, usually the adductor brevis, and often the pectineus muscles; see Durward (1951, pp. 1092–1094), Williams & Warwick (1998, p. 1108). For Haase's use in macrodissected adult human, see p. 106; for Martin's, see p. 231. It was probably first identified as the *higher part of third deep nerve of thigh (Galen, c177)*.

TRANSLATIONS:

1. *nervus obturatorius ramus anterior (Haase, 1781)*
   Original Latin form of ***anterior branch of obturator nerve (Haase, 1781; Martin, 1781)***; p. 106.

EARLIER REFERENCES:

Earlier synonyms:

1. *higher part of third deep nerve of thigh (Galen, c177)*
   Probably corresponds to ***anterior branch of obturator nerve (Haase, 1781; Martin, 1781)***, with branch to gracilis muscle that Galen described for macrodissected adult beef, pig, and/or macaque but not human; see Singer translation (1999, p. 85). Eustachi (1552; see Albinus edition, 1761, Tab. 19/2-*2*) and Vieussens (1684, Tab. 28-*73,74*) probably illustrated part of it for macrodissected adult human.

LATER SYNONYMS:

1. *superior branch of obturator nerve (Günther, 1786)*
   Synonym for macrodissected adult human ***anterior branch of obturator nerve (Haase, 1781; Martin, 1781)***; in the original Latin, *r. superiorem*, p. 82.
2. *superficial branch of obturator nerve (Meckel, 1817)*
   Synonym for macrodissected adult human ***anterior branch of obturator nerve (Haase, 1781; Martin, 1781)***; see translation (1832, Vol. 3, p. 16).

anterior cerebellar notch (Chaussier, 1807)

As described for macrodissected adult human, the wide and shallow depression on the surface of the ***cerebellum (Aristotle)*** in the median plane. It is formed near the ***central lobule (Burdach, 1822)*** and is occupied by the ***inferior colliculi (Haller, 1762)*** and ***superior cerebellar peduncles (Procháska, 1800)***; see Carpenter (1976, Fig. 2.23, labeled *anterior incisure*), *Dorland's* (2003, pp. 920, 1280). For Chaussier's use in macrodissected adult human see pp. 78–79. It was first delineated as the *cliff (Malacarne, 1776)*.

TRANSLATIONS:

1. *échancrure antérieure (du cervelet) (Chaussier, 1807)*
   Original French form of ***anterior cerebellar notch (Chaussier, 1807)***; pp. 78–79.
2. *incisura anterior cerebelli (Burdach, 1822)*
   Latin form of macrodissected adult human ***anterior cerebellar notch (Chaussier, 1807)***; p. 49.
3. *incisura cerebelli anterior (Burdach, 1822)*
   Current Latin form of *incisura anterior cerebelli (Burdach, 1822)*; see *Dorland's* (2003, p. 920).

EARLIER REFERENCES:

Earlier synonyms:

1. *cliff (Malacarne, 1776)*
   Synonym for macrodissected adult human ***anterior cerebellar notch (Chaussier, 1807)***; see Clarke & O'Malley translation (1996, p. 643).
2. *anterior cerebellar fissure (Reil, 1807–1808a)*
   Synonym for macrodissected adult human ***anterior cerebellar notch (Chaussier, 1807)***; see Mayo translation (1823, Tab. I, Fig. I-*e,h*).
3. *semilunar cerebellar fissure (Reil, 1807–1808a)*
   Synonym for macrodissected adult human ***anterior cerebellar notch (Chaussier, 1807)***; see Mayo translation (1823, Tab. I, Fig. I-*e,h*).

LATER SYNONYMS:

1. *anterior semilunar notch (Tiedemann, 1816)*
   Synonym for macrodissected fetal human *semilunar cerebellar fissure (Reil, 1807–1808a)*; see translation (1826, p. 63).
2. *semilunar notch (Ranson, 1920)*
   Synonym for macrodissected adult human *anterior semilunar notch (Tiedemann, 1816)*; p. 197.

anterior cerebral artery plexus (Chaussier, 1789)

As described for macrodissected adult human, an extension of the ***internal carotid plexus (>1840)*** along the anterior cerebral artery and its branches; see Mitchell (1953, pp. 219–220). For Chaussier's observations and use of name in macrodissected human, see *Table synoptic du nerf tri-splanchnique*.

anterior cingulate region (>1840)

As described with cellular architecture for adult human, a subdivision of the ***cingulate region (>1840)*** between ***infralimbic area (Rose & Woolsey, 1948)*** rostrally and ***posterior cingulate region (>1840)*** caudally, and further divided into ***dorsal anterior cingulate area (Brodmann, 1909)***, or *area 32 (Brodmann, 1909)* and ***ventral anterior cingulate area (Brodmann, 1909)***, or *area 24 (Brodmann, 1909)*. See Nieuwenhuys et al. (2008, Fig. 12.13). It was not described by 1840.

anterior commissure (Lieutaud, 1742)

As described in macrodissected adult human and mammal generally with histological methods for ***axons (Kölliker, 1896)***, a part of the ***cerebral cortex white matter (>1840)*** crossing the median plane in the ***terminal lamina (Burdach, 1822)*** associated with the rostral and dorsal end of the ***hypothalamus (Kuhlenbeck, 1927)*** and having two major components, ***olfactory limb of anterior commissure (>1840)*** and ***temporal limb of anterior commissure (>1840)***; see Williams & Warwick (1980, p. 997), Nieuwenhuys et al. (2008, p. 596). For Lieutaud's use in macrodissected adult human, see p. 392. It was known to Eustachi; see ***[anterior commissure (Lieutaud, 1742)] (Eustachi, 1552)***.

EARLIER REFERENCES:

Illustrated, not named or described:

1. ***[anterior commissure (Lieutaud, 1742)] (Eustachi, 1552)***
   Illustrated crossing just rostral to macrodissected adult human ***postcommissural fornix (Loo, 1931)*** in plates not published until 1714, and without text. In his edition of the plates, Albinus (1744, p. 97) called ***anterior commissure (Lieutaud, 1742)*** the *portio transversa* of what corresponds to ***postcommissural fornix (Loo, 1931)***. Also see *transverse medullary process (Willis, 1664)*.
2. ***[anterior commissure (Lieutaud, 1742)] (Steno, 1669)***
   First accurate published illustration, shown crossing median plane in first published midsagittal view of ***brain (Smith Papyrus, c1700 BC)***, for macrodissected adult human; Plates I, II. Also see *transverse medullary process (Willis, 1664)*.

Earlier synonyms:

1. *transverse cord (Riolan, 1649)*
   First mention in writing of ***anterior commissure (Lieutaud, 1742)*** for macrodissected adult human; see Burdach (1822, p. 361), Bell (1802, p. 43), Meyer (1971, p. 14). Riolan wrote, "being spread out like a beam it [*septum lucidum (Galen, c177)*] bears up the Vaulted Arch of the Ventricles [***fornix (Vesalius, 1543a)***], the fore most [rostral] bifurcation cleaves

unto a little transverse cord, which resembles the Optick Nerve in thickness and in Color." (see translation, 1657, pp. 126–127). In the original Latin, *funiculus transversus.*

2. *processus transversus corpora striata conjugens (Bartholin, 1686)*
Synonym for macrodissected adult human ***anterior commissure (Lieutaud, 1742)***; p. 479, see Haller (1762, p. 56), Bartholin (1673, p. 479).

LATER SYNONYMS:

1. *portio transversa, qua radices fornicis conjunctae sunt (Albinus, 1744)*
Synonym for macrodissected adult human ***anterior commissure (Lieutaud, 1742)***; Table 17, Figure 6-*I*. Also see Burdach (1822, p. 361).
2. *anterior cerebral commissure (Tarin, 1753)*
Synonym for macrodissected adult human ***anterior commissure (Lieutaud, 1742)***; in the original Latin, *commissura anterior cerebri*, p. 24. Gordon (1815, p. 100) used English form, *anterior commissure of brain*, for macrodissected adult human.
3. *chorda Willisii (Santorini, 1775)*
Eponym for macrodissected adult human ***anterior commissure (Lieutaud, 1742)***; p. 39, see Burdach (1822, p. 361).
4. *junction of anterior convolutions of middle lobe (Gall & Spurzheim, 1810)*
Synonym for macrodissected adult human ***anterior commissure (Lieutaud, 1742)***; in the original French, *réunion des circonvolutions antérieures du lobe moyen*, Table VI-*61*. Burdach (1822, p. 361) gave the Latin, *reunio gyrorum anteriorum lobi medii.*
5. *commissure of hemispheres (Carus, 1814)*
Synonym for macrodissected adult human ***anterior commissure (Lieutaud, 1742)***; in the original German, *Commissur der Hemisphären*, p. 199.
6. *commissure of olfactory nerve ganglia (Carus, 1814)*
Synonym for macrodissected adult fish ***anterior commissure (Lieutaud, 1742)***; in the original German, *Commissur der Riechnervenganglien*, Table 2-*v*.
7. *commissure of olfactory ganglion (Schönlein, 1816)*
According to Burdach (1822, p. 361), synonym for macrodissected adult human ***anterior commissure (Lieutaud, 1742)***; in the original German, *Commissur der Riechganglien.*
8. *great commissure (Meckel, 1817)*
According to Burdach (1822, p. 361), synonym for macrodissected adult human ***anterior commissure (Lieutaud, 1742)***; in the original German, *grosse Commissur*; in Latin, *commissura magna*; Vol. 3, p. 519; also see translation (1832, Vol. 2, p. 457). Meckel pointed out that in adult human it is slightly thicker than the ***optic nerve (Vicq d'Azyr, 1786)***; also see *transverse cord (Riolan, 1649).*
9. *commissura magna (Meckel, 1817)*
Latin form of *great commissure (Meckel, 1817).*
10. *anterior junction of middle lobe (Knox, 1832)*
Synonym for macrodissected adult human ***anterior commissure (Lieutaud, 1742)***; Supplemental Plate IV-*29*.
11. *anterior commissure of middle lobe (Knox, 1832)*
Synonym for macrodissected adult human ***anterior commissure (Lieutaud, 1742)***; Supplemental Plate V-*9.a*.
12. *commissure of anterior cerebral ganglia (Combe et al., 1838)*
Synonym for macrodissected adult human ***anterior commissure (Lieutaud, 1742)***; p. xxix.
13. *commissure of corpus striatum (Combe et al., 1838)*
Synonym for macrodissected adult human ***anterior commissure (Lieutaud, 1742)***; p. xxix.
14. *cord (Gerdy, 1838)*
Synonym for macrodissected adult human ***anterior commissure (Lieutaud, 1742)***; in the original French, *le cordon*, p. 260.
15. *rostral commissure (>1840)*
Synonym for macrodissected adult human ***anterior commissure (Lieutaud, 1742)***; see *Nomina Anatomica* (1983, p. A72); in the original Latin, *commissura rostralis.*

PARTLY CORRESPONDS:

1. *commissura (Willis, 1664)*
Willis used Latin term *commissura* (p. 159) for "joining together" (Pordage translation, 1681, p. 103) across median plane of *transverse medullary process (Willis, 1664, p. 61)* or ***terminal stria (Wenzel & Wenzel, 1812)***, although what he actually described as *commissura* was almost certainly segment of ***anterior commissure (Lieutaud, 1742)*** in median plane.
2. *commissura crassioris nervi aemula (Vieussens, 1684)*
Corresponds to segment of macrodissected adult human ***anterior commissure (Lieutaud, 1742)*** near median plane; Table VIII-*b*. Also see Bell (1802, p. 24), Meyer (1971, p. 20).
3. *corpus medullare crassiorem nervum referens (Vieussens, 1684)*
Synonym for *commissura crassioris nervi aemula (Vieussens, 1684)*; see Meyer (1971, p. 16).
4. *tractus medullaris transversus et nonnihil obliquus (Vieussens, 1684)*
Corresponds to lateral regions of macrodissected adult human ***anterior commissure (Lieutaud, 1742)***; see Meyer (1971, p. 16).
5. *anterior commissure central part (Reil, 1809c)*
Corresponds to segment of macrodissected adult human ***anterior commissure (Lieutaud, 1742)*** near median plane, defined by interval between right and left ***postcommissural fornix (Loo, 1931)***; see Mayo translation (1823, Tab. XI-*o*, p. 108).

anterior cutaneous branch of iliohypogastric nerve (>1840)

As described for macrodissected adult human, it supplies small branches to the internal oblique and transversus muscles and then innervates abdominal skin above (rostral to) the pubis; see Williams & Warwick (1980, p. 1106 and Fig. 7.206), *Terminologia Anatomica* (1998, p. 139). It is sometimes considered a ***lumbar plexus ventral division (Paterson, 1887)***; see Durward (1951, Fig. 937),

Carpenter (1976, p. 181 and Fig. 7.19). It was first clearly delineated by Eustachi; see ***[anterior cutaneous branch of iliohypogastric nerve (>1840)] (Eustachi, 1552)***.

EARLIER REFERENCES:

Illustrated, not named or described:

1. ***[anterior cutaneous branch of iliohypogastric nerve (>1840)] (Eustachi, 1552)***
   Clearly illustrated for macrodissected adult human; see Albinus edition (1761, Tab. 21/2-*x,y,ζ*).

Described, not named or illustrated:

1. ***[anterior cutaneous branch of iliohypogastric nerve (>1840)] (Meckel, 1817)***
   Vaguely described without naming for macrodissected adult human; see translation (1832, Vol. 3, p. 14).

Earlier synonyms:

1. *internal branch of iliohypogastric nerve (Bock, 1827)*
   Synonym for macrodissected adult human ***anterior cutaneous branch of iliohypogastric nerve (>1840)***; in the original Latin, *Ram. internus nervi ileo-hypogastrici*, Table I, Figure 2-58,59.
2. *anterior branch of external cutaneous branch of lumbar plexus (Quain, 1828)*
   Synonym for macrodissected adult human ***anterior cutaneous branch of iliohypogastric nerve (>1840)***; p. 285.
3. *abdominal branch proper of greater abdominal branch of lumbar plexus (Cruveilhier, 1836)*
   Synonym for macrodissected adult human ***anterior cutaneous branch of iliohypogastric nerve (>1840)***; in the original French, *rameau abdominal proprement dit*, p. 834.

anterior cutaneous branch of intercostal nerves (>1840)

As described for macrodissected adult human, the terminal branches of the ***intercostal nerves (Vesalius, 1543a)*** that may be divided into thoracic and abdominal endings arising from the rostral (upper) and caudal (lower) ***intercostal nerves (Vesalius, 1543a)*** respectively; see Williams & Warwick (1980, pp. 1103–1105), *Nomina Anatomica* (1983, p. A77), *Terminologia Anatomica* (1998, p. 139). The feature was known to Galen; see ***[anterior cutaneous branch of intercostal nerves (>1840)] (Galen, c192)***.

EARLIER REFERENCES:

Described, not named or illustrated:

1. ***[anterior cutaneous branch of intercostal nerves (>1840)] (Galen, c192)***
   Described for macrodissected adult beef, pig, and/or macaque but not human; see Duckworth translation (1962, p. 259).

Illustrated and described, not named:

1. ***[anterior cutaneous branch of intercostal nerves (>1840)] (Vesalius, 1543a)***
   Described for macrodissected adult human without naming them as such; see Richardson & Carman translation (2002, p. 206). They were beautifully illustrated for macrodissected adult human by Eustachi (1552); see Albinus edition (1761, Tab. 21).

Earlier synonyms:

1. *cutaneous nerve of anterior thoracic nerves (Günther, 1786)*
   Synonym for macrodissected adult human ***anterior cutaneous branch of intercostal nerves (>1840)***; p. 72.
2. *anterior subcutaneous branch of intercostal branch of thoracic nerve (Bock, 1827)*
   Synonym for macrodissected adult human ***anterior cutaneous branch of intercostal nerve (>1840)***; in the original Latin, *ram. subcutaneus anterior*, Table I, Figure 2-52.
3. *internal branch of dorsal nerve (Swan, 1830)*
   Synonym for macrodissected adult human ***anterior cutaneous branch of intercostal nerve (>1840)***; Plate XVII.
4. *anterior perforating filaments of intercostal branch of intercostal branches of dorsal nerves (Cruveilhier, 1836)*
   Synonym for macrodissected adult human ***anterior cutaneous branch of intercostal nerves (>1840)***; in the original French, *filets perforans antérieurs*, p. 824.
5. *anterior perforating branches of dorsal nerves (Cruveilhier, 1836)*
   Synonym for macrodissected adult human ***anterior cutaneous branch of intercostal nerves (>1840)***; in the original French, *rameaux perforans antérieurs*, p. 830.
6. *anterior cutaneous branches of dorsal nerves (Cruveilhier, 1836)*
   Synonym for *anterior perforating branches of dorsal nerves (Cruveilhier, 1836)*; in the original French, *rameaux cutanés antérieurs*, p. 830.

PARTLY CORRESPONDS:

1. *pectoral anterior subcutaneous branch of intercostal branch of thoracic nerve (Bock, 1827)*
   As described for macrodissected adult human, ***anterior cutaneous branch of intercostal nerve (>1840)*** of 2nd ***intercostal nerve (Vesalius, 1543a)***; in the original Latin, *ram. subcutaneus anterior pectoris*, Table I, Figure 2-48.
2. *pectoral anterior cutaneous branch of intercostal nerves (Bock, 1827)*
   Synonym for *pectoral anterior subcutaneous branch of intercostal branch of thoracic nerve (Bock, 1827)*; in the original Latin, *nerv. cutaneus anterior pectoris*; Table II-90.
3. *internal subcutaneous branch of third subcostal nerve (Bock, 1827)*
   As illustrated for macrodissected adult human, lateral branch of ***anterior cutaneous branch of intercostal nerve (>1840)*** of 3rd ***intercostal nerve (Vesalius, 1543a)***; in the original Latin, *ram. subcutaneus internus nervi subcostalis tertii*; Table V, Figure 1-50.

anterior cutaneous branches of femoral nerve (Quain & Wilson, 1839)

As described for macrodissected adult human, they innervate skin on the dorsal side (front) of the thigh as far distally as the knee, where they end in the ***patellar plexus (>1840)***; see Williams & Warwick (1980, p. 1109, called *intermediate cutaneous nerve of thigh*). For Quain & Wilson's use in macrodissected adult human see Plate XXIII-*B,a*. They were first described as the *second cutaneous nerve at beginning of thigh (Galen, c177)*.

EARLIER REFERENCES:

Earlier synonyms:

1. *second cutaneous nerve at beginning of thigh (Galen, c177)*
   Synonym for ***anterior cutaneous branches of femoral nerve (Quain & Wilson, 1839)*** in macrodissected adult beef, pig, and/or macaque but not human; see Singer translation (1999, p. 83). They were clearly illustrated for macrodissected adult human by Eustachi (1552); see Albinus edition (1761, Tab. 21-*P*).
2. *most anterior branch of crural nerve forming cutaneous nerves (Winslow, 1733)*
   Synonym for macrodissected adult human ***anterior cutaneous branches of femoral nerve (Quain & Wilson, 1839)***; Section VI, p. 91.
3. *minor superior cutaneous branch of anterior femoral nerve (Soemmerring, 1798)*
   Synonym for macrodissected adult human ***anterior cutaneous branches of femoral nerve (Quain & Wilson, 1839)***; p. 318, also see Soemmerring (1791, p. 300).
4. *middle anterior femoral cutaneous nerve (Bock, 1827)*
   Synonym for macrodissected adult human ***anterior cutaneous branches of femoral nerve (Quain & Wilson, 1839)***; in the original Latin, *Nerv. cutaneus femoris anterior medius*, Table I, Figure 2-79. Bock also described external and internal branches of it, and used the Latin form, *nerv. cutaneus anterior medius femoris*, Table II-*111*.
5. *anterior cutaneous nerve (Cloquet, 1828)*
   Probably synonym for macrodissected adult human ***anterior cutaneous branches of femoral nerve (Quain & Wilson, 1839)***; in the original French, *nerf cutané antérieur*, Plate CLXXI, Figure 1-*44*.
6. *superior cutaneous perforant branch of crural musculocutaneous nerve (Cruveilhier, 1836)*
   Probably synonym for macrodissected adult human ***anterior cutaneous branches of femoral nerve (Quain & Wilson, 1839)***; in the original French, *perforante cutanée supérieure*, p. 842.
7. *anterior cutaneous branches of crural nerve (Quain & Wilson, 1839)*
   Synonym for macrodissected adult human ***anterior cutaneous branches of femoral nerve (Quain & Wilson, 1839)***; Plate XXIII-*B,a*.

PARTLY CORRESPONDS:

1. *middle cutaneous nerve of crural nerve (Styx, 1782)*
   Main macrodissected adult human ***anterior cutaneous branch of femoral nerve (Quain & Wilson, 1839)***; in the original Latin, *nervus cutaneus medius*, p. 8.
2. *anterior cutaneous nerve of crural nerve (Styx, 1782)*
   Minor macrodissected adult human ***anterior cutaneous branch of femoral nerve (Quain & Wilson, 1839)***; in the original Latin, *nervus cutaneus anterior*, p. 8.
3. *anterior cutaneous nerve (Styx, 1782)*
   Synonym for *anterior cutaneous nerve of crural nerve (Styx, 1782)*; in the original Latin, *nervus cutaneus anterior*, p. 8. Also see Schmidt (1794, p. 60).
4. *middle cutaneous nerve (Fyfe, 1800)*
   Synonym for macrodissected adult human *middle cutaneous nerve of crural nerve (Styx, 1782)*; Vol. 2, p. 327.
5. *anterior cutaneous branch of crural nerve (Fyfe, 1800)*
   Synonym for macrodissected adult human *anterior cutaneous nerve of crural nerve (Styx, 1782)*; Vol. 2, p. 328.
6. *middle cutaneous nerve of thigh (Bell, 1803a)*
   Lateral branch of macrodissected adult human ***anterior cutaneous branches of femoral nerve (Quain & Wilson, 1839)***; Plate VII-2.
7. *anterior cutaneous nerve of thigh (Bell, 1803a)*
   Medial branch of macrodissected adult human ***anterior cutaneous branches of femoral nerve (Quain & Wilson, 1839)***; Plate VII-3.
8. *anterior cutaneous nerve (Bell, 1803b)*
   Synonym for *anterior cutaneous nerve of thigh (Bell, 1803a)*; p. 197.
9. *short saphenous nerve (Quain & Wilson, 1839)*
   As illustrated for macrodissected adult human, ***anterior cutaneous branch of femoral nerve (Quain & Wilson, 1839)*** coursing just lateral to ***saphenous nerve (Haase, 1781)*** and ending proximal to knee; Plate XXIII-*e*. In some cadavers it might correspond to *lesser saphenous nerve (Fisher, 1791)*.
10. *middle cutaneous nerves of anterior crural nerve (Quain & Wilson, 1839)*
    Anterior cutaneous branches of femoral nerve (Quain & Wilson, 1839) on ventral (anterior) part of thigh; Plate XXIV-*a*; also see Plate XXIII-*B,a*.

anterior deep temporal nerve (Arnold, 1834)

As described for adult human, it is usually a component of the ***deep temporal nerves (Haase, 1781)*** although it is not uncommonly given off from the ***buccal nerve (Meckel, 1748)***. It courses rostrally (ascends) over the upper head of the lateral pterygoid muscle and supplies rostral (anterior) regions of the temporalis muscle; see Williams & Warwick (1980, p. 1066), Kwak et al. (2003, p. 394), and Henle's (1871, Fig. 243-*tpr*[2]) beautiful illustration. For Arnold's use in macrodissected adult human, see p. 10. It was perhaps first clearly delineated as the *internal deep temporal branch of third branch of fifth pair (Meckel, 1748)*.

TRANSLATIONS:

1. *nervus temporalis profundus anterior (Arnold, 1834)*
   Original Latin form of ***anterior deep temporal nerve (Arnold, 1834)***; p. 10.

EARLIER REFERENCES:

Earlier synonyms:

1. *internal deep temporal branch of third branch of fifth pair (Meckel, 1748)*

Synonym for macrodissected adult human ***anterior deep temporal nerve (Arnold, 1834)***; in the original Latin, *ramus temporalis profundus interior tertii rami quinti paris*, p. 82. Haase described anterior and posterior branches in macrodissected adult human (1781, p. 70).

2. *internal deep temporal nerve (Mayer, 1794)*
   Synonym for macrodissected adult human ***anterior deep temporal nerve (Arnold, 1834)***; in the original Latin, *nervus profundus temporalis internus*; Part 5, Table VIII-65 (p. 60).
3. *anterior deep temporal branch of inferior maxillary nerve (Todd, 1836–1839)*
   Synonym for macrodissected adult human ***anterior deep temporal nerve (>1840)***; p. 291. Also see Quain (1837, p. 764).
4. *internal deep temporal branch of inferior maxillary nerve (Todd, 1836–1839)*
   Synonym for macrodissected adult human ***anterior deep temporal nerve (>1840)***; p. 291.

anterior esophageal plexus (Haller, 1762)

As described for macrodissected adult human, a caudal (descending) extension of the ***esophageal plexus (Haller, 1762)*** derived predominantly, though by no means exclusively, from the left ***vagus nerve trunk (Wrisberg, 1786; Günther, 1786)***. It is concentrated around caudal (lower) thoracic parts of the ventral (anterior) esophagus; it receives sympathetic ***axons (Kölliker, 1896);*** and some parts of it condense into the ***anterior vagal trunk (Wrisberg, 1780)*** extending caudally (descending) into the abdomen, whereas other parts penetrate directly into the esophageal part of the ***enteric plexuses (Hill, 1927)***; see Mitchell (1953, pp. 184–185), Williams & Warwick (1980, p. 1079). For Haller's use in macrodissected adult human, see p. 235. It was known to Galen; see ***[anterior esophageal plexus (Haller, 1762)] (Galen, c173)***.

TRANSLATIONS:

1. *plexus oesophageus anterior (Haller, 1762)*
   Original Latin form of ***anterior esophageal plexus (Haller, 1762)***; p. 235.
2. *plexum gulae priorem (Soemmerring, 1798)*
   Latin form of *plexus oesophageus anterior (Haller, 1762)*; p. 269.
3. *plexus nervorum gulae prior (Soemmerring, 1798)*
   Latin form of *plexus oesophageus anterior (Haller, 1762)*; p. 269.
4. *anterior plexus gulae (Bell, 1803b)*
   Mixed English-Latin form of *plexus gulae priorem (Soemmerring, 1798)*; p. 158.

EARLIER REFERENCES:

Described, not named or illustrated:

1. ***[anterior esophageal plexus (Haller, 1762)] (Galen, c173)***
   Described briefly as part of entwined ***vagus nerves (Galen, c192)*** around distal (lower) part of esophagus in macrodissected adult beef, pig, and/or macaque but not human; see May translation (1968, pp. 290, 449), Duckworth translation (1962, p. 220). Winslow (1733, Sect. VI, p. 73) described it rather clearly for macrodissected adult human.

Illustrated, not named or described:

1. ***[anterior esophageal plexus (Haller, 1762)] (Pietro da Cortona, c1618)***
   Illustrated rather nicely for macrodissected adult human; see 1741 edition, Table 5, Figure 1. Also see Haller (1762, p. 235 note *r*).

anterior ethmoidal nerve (>1840)

As described for macrodissected adult human, the continuation of the ***nasociliary nerve (Meckel, 1817; Wutzer, 1817)*** distal to the origin of the ***infratrochlear nerve (Schaarschmidt, 1750)***. It supplies the ***nasal branches of anterior ethmoidal nerve (>1840)***; see Williams & Warwick (1980, p. 1061 and Figs. 7.171, 174), *Nomina Anatomica* (1983, p. A74), *Terminologia Anatomica* (1998, p. 134). It was first delineated as the *third offshoot of thinner root of third pair (Vesalius, 1543a)*.

EARLIER REFERENCES:

Earlier synonyms:

1. *third offshoot of thinner root of third pair (Vesalius, 1543a)*
   Synonym for ***anterior ethmoidal nerve (>1840)*** partly described and illustrated for macrodissected adult human; see Richardson & Carman translation (2002, p. 188).
2. *third branch of third conjugation of nerves of brain (Crooke, 1615)*
   Synonym for macrodissected adult human ***anterior ethmoidal nerve (>1840)***; p. 486. Crooke's description is a translation of Bauhin (1605).
3. *internal nasal nerve (Willis, 1664)*
   Synonym for mammalian ***anterior ethmoidal nerve (>1840)***; in the original Latin, *nervus nasalis internus;* see Meckel (1832, Vol. 3, p. 63).
4. *surculus secundus crassioris ac interioris propaginis K (Vieussens, 1684)*
   Roughly synonymous with macrodissected adult human ***anterior ethmoidal nerve (>1840)***; p. 171, Table 22-*m*.
5. *ethmoidal nerve (Günther, 1786)*
   Synonym for macrodissected adult human ***anterior ethmoidal nerve (>1840)***; in the original Latin, *nervis ethmoidalis*, p. 44.
6. *anterior trunk of ethmoidal nerve (Meckel, 1817)*
   Synonym for macrodissected adult human ***anterior ethmoidal nerve (>1840)***; see translation (1832, Vol. 3, p. 64).
7. *inferior nerve (Jacobson, 1818)*
   Synonym for macrodissected adult mammalian ***anterior ethmoidal nerve (>1840)***; in the original Latin, *nervus inferior*, p. 16.
8. *ethmoidal fascicle of nasal surculus (Bellingeri, 1818)*
   Synonym for macrodissected adult mammalian ***anterior ethmoidal nerve (>1840)***; in the original Latin, *fasciculus et[h]moidalis*, see Table I.

9. *ethmoidal branch of nasociliary nerve (Arnold, 1834)*
Synonym for macrodissected adult human ***anterior ethmoidal nerve (>1840)***; in the original Latin, *nervus nasociliaris, ramus ethmoidalis*, p. 8.
10. *ethmoidal branch of nasal nerve (Arnold, 1834)*
Synonym for macrodissected adult human ***anterior ethmoidal nerve (>1840)***; in the original Latin, *nervus nasalis, ramus ethmoidalis*, p. 8.
11. *internal nasal branch of nasal nerve (Cruveilhier, 1836)*
Synonym for macrodissected adult human ***anterior ethmoidal nerve (>1840)***; in the original French, *rameau nasal interne*, p. 915.
12. *internal nasal branch of nasal branch of ophthalmic nerve (Quain, 1837)*
Synonym for macrodissected adult human ***anterior ethmoidal nerve (>1840)***; pp. 761–762.
13. *internal nasal branch of nasociliary nerve (>1840)*
Synonym for macrodissected adult ***anterior ethmoidal nerve (>1840)***; see Durward (1951, p. 1019 and Fig. 893). Also see *internal nasal nerve (Willis, 1664)*.

anterior horn of lateral ventricle (Bell, 1803b)

As described for macrodissected adult human, the part of the ***lateral ventricle (Vesalius, 1543a)*** rostral to the transverse level of the ***interventricular foramen (>1840)***; see Millen & Woollam (1962, pp. 33–44, Figs. 13, 16) and Carpenter & Sutin (1983, pp. 41–45, Fig. 2.20). For Bell's use in macrodissected adult human, see p. 81; it was first referred to as the *front cavities (Galen, c177)*.

EARLIER REFERENCES:

Earlier synonyms:

1. *front cavities (Galen, c177)*
In *On Anatomical Procedures*, Galen referred to *septum (Galen, c177)* separating *front cavities (Galen, c177)*—clear allusion to right and left ***anterior horn of lateral ventricle (Bell, 1803b)***; see Singer translation (1999, pp. 227, 231). Galen referred to them variously as *front cavities (Galen, c177)* or *foremost ventricles (Galen, c177)* and recognized that they generate ***[olfactory ventricles (>1840)] (Galen, c173)*** in adult ox; see May translation (1968, p. 401 note 44). Later he wrote, "Betake yourself to the part where each of the two ventricles, stretching towards the front, is narrowed." (Duckworth translation, 1962, pp. 4, 186). And again, in *On Anatomical Procedures* he referred to rostral end of *foremost ventricle (Galen, c177)* as resembling a hollow horn; see Duckworth translation (1962, p. 3).
2. *foremost ventricles (Galen, c177)*
Alternate translation of *front cavities (Galen, c177)*; see Wiberg (1914, p. 19). Geminus (1553, f. BII) provided the singular in English, *formoste ventricle*.
3. *first ventricle (Geminus, 1553)*
Synonym for macrodissected adult human *foremost ventricle (Galen, c177)*; originally spelled *fyrst ventricle*, f. BII.
4. *foremost figure of brain (Geminus, 1553)*
Synonym for macrodissected adult human *foremost ventricle (Galen, c177)*; originally spelled *formost figure of brayne*, f. BII.

LATER SYNONYMS:

1. *anterior sinus of lateral ventricle (Bell, 1803b)*
Synonym for macrodissected adult human ***anterior horn of lateral ventricle (Bell, 1803b)***; p. 81.

anterior hypothalamic nucleus (>1840)

Based primarily on cellular architecture and connections in mammal, the component of the ***medial hypothalamic zone (Nauta & Haymaker, 1969)*** between ***medial preoptic nucleus (>1840)*** rostrally and ***ventromedial hypothalamic nucleus (>1840)*** caudally; see Swanson (1998, Table B, p. 206). It was not described by 1840.

anterior intercavernous sinus (>1840)

As described for macrodissected adult human, a component of the ***circulatory system***; the rostral transverse segment of the ***circular sinus (Ridley, 1695)***, rostral to the ***infundibulum (Rioch et al., 1940)*** and continuous with the rostral end of the right and left ***cavernous sinus (Winslow, 1733)***; see Williams & Warwick (1980, p. 748 and Figs. 6.126, 127B), *Terminologia Anatomica* (1998, p. 94). It was perhaps first clearly delineated as the *anterior clinoid sinus (Vicq d'Azyr, 1786)*.

EARLIER REFERENCES:

Earlier synonyms:

1. *sinus clinoïdeus anterior (Vicq d'Azyr, 1786)*
Synonym for macrodissected adult human ***anterior intercavernous sinus (>1840)***; p. 72; see Burdach (1822, p. 400).
2. *anterior clinoid sinus (Vicq d'Azyr, 1786)*
English form of *sinus clinoïdeus anterior (Vicq d'Azyr, 1786)*.

anterior interosseous nerve (Quain, 1832)

As described for macrodissected adult human, a branch of the ***median nerve (Du Verney, 1697)*** supplying the flexor pollicis longus, flexor digitorum profundus, and pronator quadratus muscles before ending in the distal radio-ulnar, radio-carpal, and carpal joints; see Williams & Warwick (1980, p. 1098), *Terminologia Anatomica* (1998, p. 138). For Quain's use in macrodissected adult human, see p. 688. It was known to Galen; see ***[anterior interosseous nerve (Quain, 1832)] (Galen, c177)***.

TRANSLATIONS:

1. *nervus inter-osseus anticus (Quain, 1832)*
Original Latin form of ***anterior interosseous nerve (Quain, 1832)***; p. 688.
2. *nervus interosseus antebrachii anterior (>1840)*
Current Latin form of ***anterior interosseous nerve (Quain, 1832)*** [of forearm]; see *Terminologia Anatomica* (1998, p. 138).

EARLIER REFERENCES:

Described, not named or illustrated:

1. ***[anterior interosseous nerve (Quain, 1832)] (Galen, c177)***

Alluded to in macrodissected adult beef, pig, and/or macaque but not human; see Singer translation (1999, p. 71). Vesalius (1543a) alluded to it as ***nerve (Herophilus, c335–c280 BC)*** branches to flexor digitorum profundus and pronator quadratus muscles in macrodissected adult human; see Richardson & Carman translation (2002, pp. 243–244).

Earlier synonyms:

1. *deep median nerve (Günther, 1786)*
   Synonym for macrodissected adult human ***anterior interosseous nerve (Quain, 1832)***; in the original Latin, *nervus medianum profundum*, p. 74.
2. *internal interosseous nerve (Günther, 1786)*
   Synonym for macrodissected adult human ***anterior interosseous nerve (Quain, 1832)***; in the original Latin, *nervus interosseum internum*, p. 74.
3. *anterior interosseous deep nerve (Mayer, 1794)*
   Synonym for macrodissected adult human ***anterior interosseous nerve (Quain, 1832)***; in the original Latin, *nervus profundus interosseus anterior*; Part 5, Table 5, Figure 1-*14* (p. 22).
4. *interosseal branch of median nerve (Cloquet, 1816)*
   Synonym for macrodissected adult human ***anterior interosseous nerve (Quain, 1832)***; in the original French, *rameau inter-osseux*, p. 648.
5. *deep branch of median nerve (Bock, 1827)*
   Synonym for macrodissected adult human ***anterior interosseous nerve (Quain, 1832)***; in the original Latin, *ram. profundus*, Table I, Figure 2-*26*. Langenbeck (1826–1830, Fasc. III, Tab. XIV-5) also used this term for macrodissected adult human, but Fascicle III was published in 1830.
6. *interosseous nerve (Quain, 1828)*
   Synonym for macrodissected adult human ***anterior interosseous nerve (Quain, 1832)***; p. 423.

PARTLY CORRESPONDS:

1. *long cutaneous branch of internal interosseous nerve (Caldani, 1813, 1814)*
   In macrodissected adult human, branch of ***anterior interosseous nerve (Quain, 1832)*** extending distally toward medial edge of wrist; in the original Latin, *ramus cutaneus longus*, Table CCLIX, Figure 2-*8*.

anterior labial nerves (>1840)

As described for macrodissected adult human female, branches of the ***ilio-inguinal nerve (>1840)*** to skin of the ventral (anterior) labial region of the labia majora and adjacent part of the thigh; see Durward (1951, p. 1092 and Fig. 918), *Terminologia Anatomica* (1998, p. 139). They were known to Winslow; see ***[anterior labial nerves (>1840)] (Winslow, 1733)***.

EARLIER REFERENCES:

Described, not named or illustrated:

1. ***[anterior labial nerves (>1840)] (Winslow, 1733)***
   Mentioned for macrodissected adult human female; Section VI, no. 274, p. 86. Also see Quain (1828, p. 284).

anterior limb of internal capsule (>1840)

As described for macrodissected adult human, typically in frontal (horizontal) section, the rostral ***internal capsule (Burdach, 1822)*** segment lying between ***caudate nucleus (Arnold, 1838b)*** rostromedially and *lentiform nucleus (Burdach, 1822)* caudolaterally; see Crosby et al. (1962, p. 394, Fig. 272). It was first delineated by Vesalius; see ***[anterior limb of internal capsule (>1840)] (Vesalius, 1543a)***.

EARLIER REFERENCES:

Illustrated, not named or described:

1. ***[anterior limb of internal capsule (>1840)] (Vesalius, 1543a)***
   Clearly illustrated in frontal (horizontal) section of macrodissected adult human; see Singer translation (1952, Fig. 7).

Earlier synonyms:

1. *bundle of striated bodies (Spurzheim, 1826)*
   Roughly synonymous with macrodissected adult human ***anterior limb of internal capsule (>1840)***; p. 230 note *P*.
2. *meditulli albi pars anterior (Arnold, 1838b)*
   Roughly synonymous with macrodissected adult human ***anterior limb of internal capsule (>1840)***; Table IV, Figure 4-*β*.

anterior lobe of pituitary gland (Haller, 1762)

As described for adult mammal, the part of the ***adenohypophysis (Rioch et al., 1940)*** derived developmentally from the rostral wall of Rathke's pouch and having up to 5 classical endocrine cell types, corticotropes, thyrotropes, gonadotropes, somatotropes, and lactotropes. It is typically divided somewhat arbitrarily into a ***distal part of anterior lobe (>1840)*** and ***tuberal part of anterior lobe (>1840)***; see Daniel & Pritchard (1975). For Haller's use in macrodissected adult human, see p. 59; in the original Latin, *lobus anterior*. It was perhaps first distinguished by Riolan; see ***[anterior lobe of pituitary gland (Haller, 1762)] (Riolan, 1610)***.

EARLIER REFERENCES:

Described, not named or illustrated:

1. ***[anterior lobe of pituitary gland (Haller, 1762)] (Riolan, 1610)***
   Burdach (1822, p. 330) credited Riolan (p. 160) with distinguishing two parts of macrodissected adult human *pituitary gland (Galen, c192)*. Willis (1664) also described two distinct lobes of macrodissected adult human *pituitary gland (Galen, c192)*, one of which [***anterior lobe of pituitary gland (Haller, 1762)***] is reddish, located on either side, and interwoven with blood vessels; see Pordage translation (1681, p. 104), Willis (1672, Tab. VI-*F*). None of these workers could have distinguished the regressed ***intermediate lobe of pituitary gland (>1840)*** in macrodissected adult human; they observed the ***adenohypophysis (Rioch et al., 1940)*** as a whole and generally.

Earlier synonyms:

1. *glandula pituitaria potior (Santorini, 1724)*
   Synonym for macrodissected adult human ***[anterior lobe of pituitary gland (Haller, 1762)] (Riolan, 1610)***; p. 70.

LATER SYNONYMS:

1. *anterior lobule of pituitary gland (Arnold, 1834)*
   Synonym for macrodissected adult human ***anterior lobe of pituitary gland (Haller, 1762)***; English form of the original Latin, *glandula pituitaria lobulus anterior*, Table III:*A-mm*.
2. *hypophysis cerebri lobulus anterior (Arnold, 1834)*
   Synonym for macrodissected adult human ***anterior lobe of pituitary gland (Haller, 1762)***; Table III:*A-mm*.

anterior nerve of lesser curvature (>1840)

As described for macrodissected adult human, it frequently presents as the largest of the ***gastric branches of anterior vagal trunk (>1840)***, coursing along the ventral (anterior) surface of the lesser curvature of the stomach between the layers of the lesser omentum; see Mitchell (1953, p. 185), *Terminologia Anatomica* (1998, p. 136). It was clearly illustrated by Eustachi; see ***[anterior nerve of lesser curvature (>1840)] (Eustachi, 1552)***.

EARLIER REFERENCES:

Illustrated, not named or described:

1. ***[anterior nerve of lesser curvature (>1840)] (Eustachi, 1552)***
   Clearly illustrated for macrodissected adult human; see Albinus edition (1744, Tab. 18, Fig. 2-*Ψ*).

Earlier synonyms:

1. *left gastro-epiploic nerve (Albinus, 1744)*
   Synonym for macrodissected adult human ***anterior nerve of lesser curvature (>1840)***; in the original Latin, *nervus gastro-epiploïcus sinister*; Table 18, Figure 2-*Ψ*.
2. *greater anterior gastric nerve (>1840)*
   Synonym for macrodissected adult human ***anterior nerve of lesser curvature (>1840)***; see Mitchell (1953, p. 185).
3. *principal anterior nerve of lesser curve (>1840)*
   Synonym for macrodissected adult human ***anterior nerve of lesser curvature (>1840)***; see Mitchell (1953, p. 185).

anterior olfactory nucleus (Herrick, 1910)

As described with cellular architecture and connections in mammal, a component of the ***olfactory region (>1840)*** between ***olfactory bulb (Weitbrecht, 1751)*** rostrally and ***piriform area (>1840)*** caudally. For topographic macroarchitecture it is the ***cerebral cortex gray matter (>1840)*** region of the ***olfactory peduncle (Solly, 1836)***. The term is a misnomer because it is an area of the ***cerebral cortex gray matter (>1840)***; see Haberly & Price (1978). For Herrick's use based on histology in amphibia and reptile, see p. 497. It was first glimpsed by Rolfinck; see ***[anterior olfactory nucleus (Herrick, 1910)] (Rolfinck, 1656)***, although the ***olfactory peduncle (Solly, 1836)*** had been separately identified at least since *olfactory nerve (Bartholin, 1611)*.

EARLIER REFERENCES:

Described, not named or illustrated:

1. ***[anterior olfactory nucleus (Herrick, 1910)] (Rolfinck, 1656)***
   In describing macrodissected adult human ***olfactory peduncle (Solly, 1836)***, Rolfinck identified gray and white stripes (Meyer 1971, p. 76), the ***anterior olfactory nucleus (Herrick, 1910)*** and accompanying segment of ***lateral olfactory tract (>1840)*** respectively; see *nervos odoratorios (Rolfinck, 1656)*.

Earlier synonyms:

1. *olfactory peduncle (Brodmann, 1909)*
   Synonym for mammalian ***anterior olfactory nucleus (Herrick, 1910)***; see Table 7 on p. 247.

anterior orbital gyrus (>1840)

As described for macrodissected adult human, the rostral topographic subdivision of the ***orbital gyri (>1940)***, separated from the others by the ***orbital sulci (>1840)***; see Williams & Warwick (1980, Fig. 7.116). It was first clearly delineated by Soemmerring; see ***[anterior orbital gyrus (>1840)] (Soemmerring, 1778)***.

EARLIER REFERENCES:

Illustrated, not named or described:

1. ***[anterior orbital gyrus (>1840)] (Soemmerring, 1778)***
   Illustrated for macrodissected adult human; Table II.

anterior paracentral gyrus (>1840)

As described for macrodissected adult human, a caudal topographic subdivision of the ***frontal region (Vicq d'Azyr, 1786)*** on the medial surface of the *cerebral hemisphere (Tiedemann, 1816)*, medial to the ***precentral gyrus (>1840)***, rostral to the ***central sulcus (Huschke, 1854)*** and caudal to the ***paracentral sulcus (>1840)***. It forms the rostral half of the *paracentral lobule (>1840)*; see Williams & Warwick (1980, Fig. 7.114A), *Terminologia Anatomica* (1998, p. 126), *Dorland's* (2003, p. 806). It was first clearly delineated by Soemmerring; see ***[anterior paracentral gyrus (>1840)] (Soemmerring, 1778)***.

EARLIER REFERENCES:

Illustrated, not named or described:

1. ***[anterior paracentral gyrus (>1840)] (Soemmerring, 1778)***
   Clearly illustrated for macrodissected adult human; Table III.

anterior parolfactory sulcus (>1840)

As described for macrodissected adult human, a dorsoventral (vertical) groove between the ventral end of the ***medial frontal gyrus (>1840)*** rostrally and the ***parolfactory gyrus (>1840)*** of the ***cingulate region (Brodmann, 1909)*** caudally; see Nauta & Haymaker (1969, Fig. 4.11), *Terminologia Anatomica* (1998, p. 126). It was first clearly distinguished by Soemmerring; see ***[anterior parolfactory sulcus (>1840)] (Soemmerring, 1778)***.

EARLIER REFERENCES:

Illustrated, not named or described:

1. ***[anterior parolfactory sulcus (>1840)] (Soemmerring, 1778)***
   Clearly illustrated for macrodissected adult human; Table III.

anterior pulmonary plexus (Haller, 1762)

As described for macrodissected adult human, a region of the ***pulmonary plexus (Winslow, 1733)*** arising from branches of the ***superior cervical cardiac branches of vagus nerve (>1840)*** and cervical levels of the ***sympathetic trunk (Winslow, 1733)***, as well as direct branches from both sources. It lies on the ventral (anterior) aspect of bronchial and vascular structures in the hila of the lungs and is much smaller than the ***posterior pulmonary plexus (Haller, 1672)***; see Mitchell (1953, Fig. 105), Williams & Warwick (1980, p. 1133). For Haller's use in macrodissected adult human, see p. 235; he was probably the first to distinguish it clearly.

ALTERNATE SPELLINGS:

1. *anterior pulmonic plexus (Bell & Bell, 1816)*
   Alternate spelling of macrodissected adult human ***anterior pulmonary plexus (Haller, 1762)***; p. 507.

TRANSLATIONS:

1. *anterioris plexus pulmonis (Haller, 1762)*
   Original Latin form of ***anterior pulmonary plexus (Haller, 1762)***; p. 235.
2. *plexum pulmonalem anteriorem (Haase, 1781)*
   Early Latin form of ***anterior pulmonary plexus (Haller, 1762)***; p. 87.

LATER SYNONYMS:

1. *anterior pulmonary plexus of eighth nerve (Scarpa, 1794)*
   Synonym for macrodissected adult human ***anterior pulmonary plexus (Haller, 1762)***; in the original Latin, *plexu pulmonali anteriore octavi nervi*, Table III-*51*.
2. *priori plexui nervorum pulmonum (Soemmerring, 1798)*
   Alternate form of macrodissected adult human *plexum pulmonalem anteriorem (Haase, 1781)*; p. 268.
3. *smaller anterior pulmonary plexus of pneumogastric (Knox, 1832)*
   Synonym for macrodissected adult human ***anterior pulmonary plexus (Haller, 1762)***; Plate III-*106*, in Knox's translation of Scarpa (1794).

PARTLY CORRESPONDS:

1. *plexum pulmonalem anteriorem minorem octavi (Scarpa, 1794)*
   Small component of macrodissected adult human ***anterior pulmonary plexus (Haller, 1762)*** associated particularly with ***vagus nerve (Galen, c192)***; Table III: *31–33*.

anterior renal ganglion (Tiedemann, 1822)

As described for macrodissected adult human, usually the second largest, but quite inconsistent, of the ***renal ganglia (Walther, 1735)***; see Mitchell (1953, p. 289). For Tiedemann's discovery and use in macrodissected adult human female see Table I-2.

TRANSLATIONS:

1. *ganglion renale anterius (Tiedemann, 1822)*
   Original Latin form of ***anterior renal ganglion (Tiedemann, 1822)***; Table I-2,*44*.

anterior scrotal nerves (>1840)

As described for macrodissected adult human male, branches of the ***ilio-inguinal nerve (>1840)*** to skin of the ventral (anterior) scrotal region; see Durward (1951, p. 1092 and Fig. 918), *Terminologia Anatomica* (1998, p. 139). They were known to Winslow; see ***[anterior scrotal nerves (>1840)] (Winslow, 1733)***.

EARLIER REFERENCES:

Described, not named or illustrated:

1. ***[anterior scrotal nerves (>1840)] (Winslow, 1733)***
   Mentioned for macrodissected adult human male; Section VI, no. 274, p. 86. Also see Quain (1828, p. 284).

anterior superior dental nerve (Haller, 1762)

As described for macrodissected adult human, a branch of the ***infraorbital nerve (Schaarschmidt, 1750)*** to the upper incisor and canine teeth, participating in the ***superior dental plexus (>1840)*** and giving off the ***nasal branch of anterior superior dental nerve (>1840)***; see Durward (1951, p. 1025) and Williams & Warwick (1980, p. 1064), both using the term. For Haller's use in macrodissected adult human, see p. 215. It was apparently discovered by Falloppio; see ***[anterior superior dental nerve (Haller, 1762)] (Falloppio, 1561)***.

TRANSLATIONS:

1. *nervus dentalis anterior superior (Haller, 1762)*
   Original Latin form of ***anterior superior dental nerve (Haller, 1762)***; p. 215.

EARLIER REFERENCES:

Described, not named or illustrated:

1. ***[anterior superior dental nerve (Haller, 1762)] (Falloppio, 1561)***
   According to Haller (1762, p. 215 note *f*), Falloppio mentioned it for macrodissected adult human (1561, pp. 143–144). Winslow clearly mentioned it for macrodissected adult human (1733, Sect. VI, p. 65).

Earlier synonyms:

1. *anterior dental branch of infraorbital nerve (Meckel, 1748)*
   Synonym for macrodissected adult human ***anterior superior dental nerve (Haller, 1762)***; in the original Latin, *nervus infraorbitalis... ramus dentalis anterior*, Figure 1-*61,b*.
2. *anterior dental branch of superior maxillary branch (Meckel, 1748)*
   Synonym for *anterior dental branch of infraorbital nerve (Meckel, 1748)*; p. 68.
3. *anterior dental nerve (Meckel, 1748)*
   Synonym for *anterior dental branch of infraorbital nerve (Meckel, 1748)*; in the original Latin, *nervi dentalis anterioris (maxillae superioris)* or *dentalis nervus anterior*, p. 114.

4. *anterior alveolar nerves of superior maxillary nerve (Schaarschmidt, 1750)*
   Synonym for macrodissected adult human ***anterior superior dental nerve (Haller, 1762)***; in the original Latin, *nervi alveolares anteriores maxillae superioris*, p. 24.

LATER SYNONYMS:

1. *anterior alveolar nerves (Soemmerring, 1798)*
   Synonym for macrodissected adult human ***anterior superior dental nerve (Haller, 1762)***; in the original Latin, *nervi alveolares priores*, p. 228.
2. *anterior dentar nerves (Meckel, 1817)*
   Synonym for macrodissected adult human ***anterior superior dental nerve (Haller, 1762)***; in the original Latin, *nervi dentales anteriores*, see translation (1832, Vol. 3, p. 69).
3. *third dental nerve of second trunk of fifth nerve (Swan, 1830)*
   Synonym for macrodissected adult human ***anterior superior dental nerve (Haller, 1762)***; Plate XII, Figure 5-4.
4. *anterior dental branch of superior maxillary nerve (Quain, 1832)*
   Synonym for macrodissected adult human ***anterior superior dental nerve (Haller, 1762)***; p. 675.
5. *greater anterior alveolar nerve (Arnold, 1834)*
   Synonym for macrodissected adult human ***anterior superior dental nerve (Haller, 1762)***; in the original Latin, *nervus alveolaris anterior major*, p. 9.
6. *greater anterior dental nerve (Arnold, 1834)*
   Synonym for macrodissected adult human ***anterior superior dental nerve (Haller, 1762)***; in the original Latin, *nervus dentalis anterior major*, p. 9.
7. *anterior alveolo-dental nerve (Cruveilhier, 1836)*
   Synonym for macrodissected adult human ***anterior superior dental nerve (Haller, 1762)***; in the original French, *nerf alvéolo-dentaire antérieur*, p. 927.
8. *anterior superior alveolar nerve (Henle, 1871)*
   Synonym for macrodissected adult human ***anterior superior dental nerve (Haller, 1762)***; in the original Latin, *nervus alveolaris superior anterior*, p. 370.

PARTLY CORRESPONDS:

1. *maxillary fasciculi of infraorbital surculus (Bellingeri, 1818)*
   Two branches of macrodissected adult human ***anterior superior dental nerve (Haller, 1762)*** to maxillary sinus and anterior teeth; in the original Latin, *fasciculi maxillares (duo)*, see Table I.
2. *dental branches of greater anterior alveolar nerve (Arnold, 1834)*
   Branches of macrodissected adult human ***anterior superior dental nerve (Haller, 1762)*** to teeth; in the original Latin, *nervus alveolaris anterior major, rami dentales*, p. 9.
3. *dental branches of greater anterior dental nerve (Arnold, 1834)*
   Branches of macrodissected adult human ***anterior superior dental nerve (Haller, 1762)*** to teeth; in the original Latin, *nervus dentalis anterior major, rami dentales*, p. 9.
4. *descending filaments of anterior alveolo-dental nerve (Cruveilhier, 1836)*
   Branches of macrodissected adult human ***anterior superior dental nerve (Haller, 1762)*** to teeth; in the original French, *filets descendans*, p. 928.

anterior thalamic nuclei (>1840)

As described for macrodissected adult human, and based on cellular architecture and connections in mammal, a rostromedial and dorsal component of the ***dorsal part of thalamus (Herrick, 1910)***. Its major ***gray matter regions (Swanson & Bota, 2010)*** include ***anteromedial thalamic nucleus (>1840)***, ***anterodorsal thalamic nucleus (>1840)***, ***anteroventral thalamic nucleus (>1840)***, and ***lateral dorsal thalamic nucleus (>1840)***; see Swanson (2004, Table B, p. 171), Nieuwenhuys et al. (2008, pp. 263–264). Their main projections to the ***cerebral cortex (>1840)*** involve the caudal half of the ***cingulate region (>1840)*** and the ***hippocampal formation (>1840)***. Some authors include the ***lateral dorsal thalamic nucleus (>1840)*** in the ***lateral thalamic nuclei (>1840)*** instead. They were first clearly identified as *subrotunda corpora alba (Vieussens, 1684)*.

EARLIER REFERENCES:

Earlier synonyms:

1. *subrotunda corpora alba (Vieussens, 1684)*
   Clearly illustrated ***anterior thalamic nuclei (>1840)*** for macrodissected adult human; Tables VII-*c*, VIII. See Meyer (1971, p. 14).
2. *small eminence at superior and anterior part of optic thalamus (Pourfour du Petit, 1710)*
   Synonym for macrodissected adult human ***anterior thalamic nuclei (>1840)***; in the original French, *la petite éminence que est à la partie superieure, & anterieure des Couches optiques*, p. 13. Used in first description of ***mammillothalamic tract (>1840)***.
3. *eminentiae thalamorum subrotundae (Tarin, 1750)*
   Synonym for macrodissected adult human ***anterior thalamic nuclei (>1840)***; Table I, Figure 2-*V*.
4. *round tubercles of optic thalamus (Tarin, 1750)*
   Synonym for macrodissected adult human *subrotunda corpora alba (Vieussens, 1684)*; in the original French, *tubercules arrondis de couches des nerfs optiques*, p. 25.
5. *tubercula subrotunda Vieussenii (Tarin, 1750)*
   Eponym for macrodissected adult human *subrotunda corpora alba (Vieussens, 1684)*; p. 25.
6. *corpus eminens oblongum album (Santorini, 1775)*
   Synonym for macrodissected adult human *subrotunda corpora alba (Vieussens, 1684)*; p. 39.
7. *anterior tubercle of optic thalamus (Vicq d'Azyr, 1786)*
   Synonym for macrodissected adult human ***anterior thalamic nuclei (>1840)***; Plate VIII, Figure II-*18*; Plate IX-*21*.
8. *anterior internal tubercle of optic thalamus (Vicq d'Azyr, 1786)*
   Synonym for *anterior tubercle of optic thalamus (Vicq d'Azyr, 1786)*; Plate XXV, Figure II-*c*.

9. *corpus geniculatum externum (Ramsay, 1813)*
   Mistakenly applied to macrodissected adult human *anterior tubercle of optic thalamus (Vicq d'Azyr, 1786)*; p. 45.
10. *anterior thalamic tubercle (Gordon, 1815)*
   Synonym for macrodissected adult human *anterior tubercle of optic thalamus (Vicq d'Azyr, 1786)*; in the original Latin, *tuberculum thalami anticum*, p. 100. See Burdach (1822, pp. 117, 341), who gave Latin form, *tuberculum thalami anterius*.
11. *superior gray nucleus (Burdach, 1822)*
   Synonym for ***anterior thalamic nuclei (>1840)*** observed with hand lens in alcohol-hardened slabs of macrodissected adult human material; in the original Latin, *nucleus cinereus superior*, p.122. See Jones (1985, p. 11), also see Meyer (1971, p. 31).
12. *anterior geniculate tubercle (Rolando, 1831)*
   Synonym for macrodissected adult human ***anterior thalamic nuclei (>1840)***; in the original Latin, *tuberculum geniculatum anterius*, Figure 10-24.
13. *anterior superior nucleus of thalamus of optic nerve (Arnold, 1838b)*
   Synonym for macrodissected adult human *superior gray nucleus (Burdach, 1822)*; in the original Latin, *nucleus anterior superior thalami nervi optici*, Table IV, Figure 5-*m*.
14. *superior nucleus of colliculus of optic nerve (Arnold, 1838b)*
   Synonym for macrodissected adult human *superior gray nucleus (Burdach, 1822)*; in the original Latin, *nucleus superior colliculi nervi optici*, Table VIII, Figure 2-*k*.

anterior vagal trunk (Wrisberg, 1780)

As described for macrodissected adult human, it has contributions from the right and left ***vagus nerve trunk (Wrisberg, 1786; Günther, 1876)***, though predominantly from the left, and extends caudally from the distal part of the ***anterior esophageal plexus (Haller, 1762)***; see Williams & Warwick (1980, p. 1079). For Wrisberg's formulation of the term in macrodissected adult human, see reprint in Wrisberg (1800, pp. 257, 259). It was perhaps first known as the *left stomach nerve (Crooke, 1615)*, from Crooke's rough translation of Bauhin (1605).

EARLIER REFERENCES:

Earlier synonyms:

1. *left stomach nerve (Crooke, 1615)*
   Roughly synonymous with macrodissected adult human ***anterior vagal trunk (Wrisberg, 1780)***; originally spelled *left stomacke (or stomack) nerve*, and in Latin *nervus stomachichus sinistrum*, p. 365. Crooke's text here was basically a translation of Bauhin (1605).
2. *superior stomachical branch of wandring pair (Willis, 1664)*
   Probably corresponds to macrodissected adult human and other common large mammal, ***anterior vagal trunk (Wrisberg, 1780)***; see Pordage translation (1681, p. 156 and Fig. 11-C).
3. *upper stomachical branch of wandring pair (Willis, 1664)*
   Synonymous with *superior stomachical branch of wandring pair (Willis, 1664)*; see Pordage translation (1681, p. 156 and Fig. 11-C).
4. *external trunk of vagus nerve (Drake, 1707)*
   Probably corresponds to *superior stomachical branch of wandring pair (Willis, 1664)* or, alternately, *inferior stomachical branch of wandring pair (Willis, 1664)*; p. 517.
5. *anterior rope of eighth pair (Winslow, 1733)*
   Synonym for macrodissected adult human ***anterior vagal trunk (Wrisberg, 1780)***; Section VI, p. 73.
6. *anterior stomachic nerve (Winslow, 1733)*
   Synonym for macrodissected adult human ***anterior vagal trunk (Wrisberg, 1780)***; Section VI, p. 73.

LATER SYNONYMS:

1. *anterior trunk of eighth pair of nerves (Wrisberg, 1780)*
   Synonym for ***anterior vagal trunk (Wrisberg, 1780)***; see Wrisberg reprint (1800, p. 257).
2. *lateral left vagus nerve (Haase, 1781)*
   Synonym for macrodissected adult human ***anterior vagal trunk (Wrisberg, 1780)***; in the original Latin, *nervus vagus sinistri lateris*, p. 88.
3. *anterior trunk of gastric and hepatic nerve (Walter, 1783)*
   Synonym for macrodissected adult human ***anterior vagal trunk (Wrisberg, 1780)***; in the original Latin, *truncus anterior nervorum ventriculi et hepatis*, Table III-456.
4. *anterior trunk of gastric and hepatic plexus (Walter, 1783)*
   Synonym for macrodissected adult human ***anterior vagal trunk (Wrisberg, 1780)***; in the original Latin, *truncus anterior plexus ventriculi et hepatis*, Table III-456.
5. *esophageal cord of left side (Cloquet, 1816)*
   Synonym for macrodissected adult human ***anterior vagal trunk (Wrisberg, 1780)***; in the original French, *cordon oesophagien du côté gauche*, p. 625.
6. *left cord of pneumogastric nerve (Meckel, 1817)*
   Synonym for macrodissected adult human ***anterior vagal trunk (Wrisberg, 1780)***; see translation (1832, Vol. 3, p. 49).

aorticorenal ganglion (>1840)

As described for macrodissected adult human, a small ***prevertebral ganglion (Quain, 1832)*** just caudal and lateral to the ***celiac ganglion (Walter, 1783)***; see Mitchell (1953, p. 273 and Fig. 104), *Terminologia Anatomica* (1998, p.143). It was probably first identified as the *renal infolding (Willis, 1664)*.

EARLIER REFERENCES:

Earlier synonyms:

1. *renal infolding (Willis, 1664)*
   Probably corresponds to ***aorticorenal ganglion (>1840)*** in macrodissected adult human and quadruped; in the original Latin, *plexum renalem*, Table IX-*I*; see Pordage translation (1681) for English form.
2. *renal mesenteric infolding (Willis, 1664)*
   Synonym for *renal infolding (Willis, 1664)*; in the original Latin, *plexum mesentericus renalem*, Table XI; see Pordage translation (1681) for English form.

arachnoid (Blasius, 1666)

Middle layer of the ***meninges (Smith Papyrus, c1700 BC)***, and outer layer of the ***pia-arachnoid (>1840)***, adjacent to the outermost ***dura (Galen, c177)***, separated in adults only by the potential *subdural space*. The ***arachnoid (Blasius, 1666)*** is divided into a thick outer ***arachnoid membrane (Meckel, 1817)*** adjacent to the ***dura (Galen, c177)*** and delicate intermediate ***arachnoid trabeculae (>1840)*** extending through the ***subarachnoid space (Magendie, 1827)*** to the thin vascular inner ***epipial layer (Key & Retzius, 1875)*** of the ***arachnoid (Blasius, 1666)***, lying on the outer surface of the ***pia (Galen, c192)***; see Millen & Woollam (1962). Blasius is usually credited with discovering and naming the macrodissected adult human **arachnoid (Blasius, 1666)**, presenting the vague appearance of a complex spider web; see Millen & Woollam (1962, p. 22). Also see Ridley (1695, p. 16) and Burdach (1822, pp. 24, 274), who used the full Latin term, *meninx arachnoidea*. However, it is impossible to know exactly which components Blasius actually observed, other than the ***arachnoid membrane (Meckel, 1817)***. Galen may have alluded to it much earlier, see ***[arachnoid (Blasius, 1666)] (Galen, c173)***, and Casseri clearly illustrated it; see ***[arachnoid (Blasius, 1666)] (Casseri, 1627)***.

EARLIER REFERENCES:

Described, not named or illustrated:

1. ***[arachnoid (Blasius, 1666)] (Galen, c173)***
 In *On the Usefulness of the Parts*, Galen may allude to it in region of ***pineal gland (Galen, c192)***; see May translation (1968, p. 421). In *On Anatomical Procedures*, he alluded to "empty space" between ***dura (Galen, c177)*** and ***pia (Galen, c192)***, and described how to manipulate its volume experimentally; see Singer translation (1999, p. 230). He macrodissected adult beef, pig, and/or macaque, not humans explicitly. Bell (1803b, p. 21) credited without citation Varoli for clearly describing it around the ***medulla (Winslow, 1733)***.

Illustrated, not named or described:

1. ***[arachnoid (Blasius, 1666)] (Casseri, 1627)***
 Illustrated well for macrodissected adult human, in plates published posthumously; see Mettler (1947, p. 66).

LATER SYNONYMS:

1. *tunica telae arachnoidis similiis (Molinetti, 1669)*
 Synonym for macrodissected adult human ***arachnoid (Blasius, 1666)***, p. 201, according to Haller (1762, p. 84) and Schreger (1803, p. 315).
2. *tertium involucrum (Vieussens, 1684)*
 Synonym for macrodissected adult human ***arachnoid (Blasius, 1666)***; p. 143, see Haller (1762, p. 84).
3. *meninx media (Bidloo, 1685)*
 Synonym for macrodissected adult human ***arachnoid (Blasius, 1666)***, according to Burdach (1822, p. 274).
4. *arachnoid membrane (Günther, 1786)*
 Synonym for macrodissected adult human ***arachnoid (Blasius, 1666)***; in the original Latin, *arachnoidea membrana*, p. 7.
5. *tunica arachnoidea (Bell, 1803b)*
 Synonym for macrodissected adult human ***arachnoid (Blasius, 1666)***; p. 21.
6. *membrana media cerebri (Wenzel & Wenzel, 1812)*
 Synonym for macrodissected adult human ***arachnoid (Blasius, 1666)***; p. 6, see Burdach (1822, p. 274).
7. *membrana mucosa (Meckel, 1817)*
 Synonym for macrodissected adult human ***arachnoid (Blasius, 1666)***; Vol. 3, p. 551. See Burdach (1822, p. 274) and Meckel translation (1832, Vol. 2, p. 475).

arachnoid granulations (>1840)

As described for macrodissected adult human, extensions of the ***arachnoid (Blasius, 1666)*** through the dural wall of venous sinuses (especially the superior sagittal sinus) by way of which ***cerebrospinal fluid (Magendie, 1827)*** from the ***subarachnoid space (Magendie, 1827)*** is reabsorbed into the venous blood; typically, the smaller *arachnoid villi* are included in this definition; see Millen & Woollam (1962, pp. 116–122). They were first mentioned clearly by Vesalius; see ***[arachnoid granulations (>1840)] (Vesalius, 1543a)***.

EARLIER REFERENCES:

Described, not named or illustrated:

1. ***[arachnoid granulations (>1840)] (Vesalius, 1543a)***
 Described briefly for macrodissected adult human; see Singer translation (1952, p. 11, Fig. 1-*K*).

Earlier synonyms:

1. *glandulis conglobatis durae meningis (Pacchioni, 1705)*
 Original description of macrodissected adult human ***arachnoid granulations (>1840)***; see title-page; also see Millen & Woollam (1962, p. 24).
2. *glands of Pacchioni (Fantoni, 1738)*
 Eponym for macrodissected adult human ***arachnoid granulations (>1840)***; in the original Latin, *Pacchioni glandulae*, p. 31. For English form see Meckel (1832, Vol. 2, p. 471).
3. *glandulae durae matris (Mayer, 1794)*
 Synonym for macrodissected adult human ***arachnoid granulations (>1840)***, illustrating both external and internal varieties; Part V, Table I, Figure 2-*C*,*a*.
4. *cerebral granulations (Bichat et al., 1801-1803)*
 Synonym for macrodissected adult human ***arachnoid granulations (>1840)***; in the original French, *granulationes cerebrales*; Vol. III, p. 59; see Meckel (1832, Vol. 2, p. 471) and Burdach (1822, p. 277).

arachnoid membrane (Meckel, 1817)

As described for macrodissected adult human, the major, condensed layer of ***arachnoid (Blasius, 1666)*** lying just subjacent to ***dura (Galen, c192)*** and generating delicate inwardly projecting ***arachnoid trabeculae (>1840)*** ending in the ***epipial layer (>1840)*** of ***arachnoid (Blasius, 1666)***; see Millen & Woollam (1962, p. 103 ff.). For Meckel's description in macrodissected adult human, see translation (1832, pp. 475–478). It was illustrated as early as ***[arachnoid membrane (Meckel, 1817)] (Casseri, 1627)***.

EARLIER REFERENCES:

Illustrated, not named or described:

1. ***[arachnoid membrane (Meckel, 1817)] (Casseri, 1627)*** Well illustrated for macrodissected adult human, in plates published posthumously; see Mettler (1947, p. 66).

Described, not named or illustrated:

1. ***[arachnoid membrane (Meckel, 1817)] (Blasius, 1666)*** It was undoubtedly the major, if not only, component of the ***arachnoid (Blasius, 1666)*** described.

arachnoid trabeculae (>1840)

Delicate fibrous threads passing through the ***subarachnoid space (Magendie, 1827)*** and connecting the inner surface of the ***arachnoid membrane (Meckel, 1817)*** with the ***epipial layer (>1840)*** of the ***arachnoid (Blasius, 1666)*** and immediately underlying ***pia (Galen, c192)***; see Millen & Woollam (1962, p. 103 ff.).

EARLIER REFERENCES:

Described, not named or illustrated:

1. ***[arachnoid trabeculae (>1840)] (Meckel, 1817)*** Clearly described for macrodissected adult human; see translation (1832, pp. 475–478).

arbor vitae (Winslow, 1733)

As described for macrodissected adult mammal, the deep ***central nervous system white matter tract (>1840)*** of the ***cerebellar cortex (Willis, 1664)*** distal to the three ***cerebellar peduncles (Ridley, 1695)*** and lateral to the ***cerebellar commissure (>1840)***; see Crosby et al. (1962, Fig. 153), *Dorland's* (2003, p. 122), Nieuwenhuys et al. (2008, p. 700). For Winslow's use in macrodissected adult human, see Section X, p. 40. It was first outlined by Dryander; see ***[arbor vitae (Winslow, 1733)] (Dryander, 1536)***.

EARLIER REFERENCES:

Illustrated, not named or described:

1. ***[arbor vitae (Winslow, 1733)] (Dryander, 1536)*** In *The Anatomy of the Human Head*, Dryander clearly if crudely illustrated in Figure 8 deep *white substance (Vesalius, 1543a)* of macrodissected adult human ***cerebellum (Aristotle)***, along with deep *white substance (Vesalius, 1543a)* of ***cerebral cortex (>1840)*** in Figure 6; see Lind translation (1975, pp. 301–302).

Described, not named or illustrated:

1. ***[arbor vitae (Winslow, 1733)] (Cortesi, 1625)*** According to Malpighi (1666), Cortesi described *white substance (Vesalius, 1543a)* of macrodissected adult human ***cerebellum (Aristotle)*** as resembling a branchy tree; see Meyer (1967, p. 189).

Earlier synonyms:

1. *middle marrow of cerebellum (Willis, 1664)* Synonym for macrodissected adult human ***arbor vitae (Winslow, 1733)***; see Pordage translation (1681, p. 124, Fig. VIII-*T*).
2. *meditullium (Willis, 1664)* Latin synonym for *middle marrow of cerebellum (Willis, 1664)*; Chapter 3, see Burdach (1822, p. 44). In general, *meditullium* refers to middle of anything; see Foster (1892, p. 2260). Collins (1685, pp. 1029, 1031) used the term specifically for ***arbor vitae (Winslow, 1733)***.
3. *ramificatio cerebelli ad forman arboris (Willis, 1664)* Synonym for *middle marrow of cerebellum (Willis, 1664)*; Chapter 3, see Burdach (1822, p. 291).
4. *tractus medullares cerebelli (Vieussens, 1684)* Synonym for macrodissected adult human ***arbor vitae (Winslow, 1733)***; Table XIII-*O,P*.
5. *central marrow of cerebellar hemisphere (Vieussens, 1684)* Synonym for macrodissected adult human ***arbor vitae (Winslow, 1733)***; in the original Latin, *centrum medullare hemisphaeriorum cerebelli*, p. 78, see (Burdach 1822, p. 289). Vicq d'Azyr (1784, p. 576) referred to it in French as *centre médullaire du Cervelet*.
6. *corpus callosum of cerebellum (Ridley, 1695)* Synonym for macrodissected adult human ***arbor vitae (Winslow, 1733)***; p. 136.
7. *root of peduncle (Pourfour du Petit, 1710)* Synonym for macrodissected adult human ***arbor vitae (Winslow, 1733)***; in the original French, *la racine du Peduncle*, p. 13. Pourfour de Petit referred to *white substance (Vesalius, 1543a)* emerging from *folia (Malacarne, 1776)* to join *root of peduncle (Pourfour du Petit, 1710)* as *branches of peduncular root*; in the original French, *les branches de la racine du Peduncle*, p. 13.
8. *arbusculis medullaribus (Heister, 1717)* Synonym for macrodissected adult human ***arbor vitae (Winslow, 1733)***; p. 211.

LATER SYNONYMS:

1. *cerebellar nucleus (Malacarne, 1776)* Synonym for macrodissected adult human ***arbor vitae (Winslow, 1733)***; p. 65, see Larsell (1967, p. 4).
2. *crus cerebelli (Monro, 1783)* Synonym for macrodissected adult human ***arbor vitae (Winslow, 1733)***; Table VII-*I*.
3. *central nucleus of peduncles (Chaussier, 1807)* Synonym for macrodissected adult human ***arbor vitae (Winslow, 1733)***; p. 98.
4. *central medullary nucleus (Reil, 1807–1808a)* Synonym for macrodissected adult human ***arbor vitae (Winslow, 1733)***, describing how *medullary stems* emerge from it and branch into lobes, lobules, and laminae or *folia (Malacarne, 1776)*; see Mayo translation (1822, p. 19).
5. *medullary nucleus (Reil, 1807–1808b)* Shortened form of *central medullary nucleus (Reil, 1807– 1808a)*; see Mayo translation (1822, p. 56).
6. *medullary nucleus of hemisphere (Reil, 1807–1808a)* Corresponds to *medullary nucleus (Reil, 1807–1808b)*; see Mayo translation (1823, p. 24).
7. *nucleus of cerebellum (Reil, 1809b)* Variation on *central medullary nucleus (Reil, 1807–1808a)*; see Mayo translation (1823, pp. 48, 53).
8. *nucleus of hemisphere (Reil, 1812c)* Variation on *central medullary nucleus (Reil, 1807–1808a)*.
9. *central mass of cerebellum (Gordon, 1815)*

Synonym for macrodissected adult human ***arbor vitae (Winslow, 1733)***; p. 143. Burdach (1822, p. 289) gave the Latin, *massa centralis cerebelli.*

10. *foliatus arbori (Tiedemann, 1821)*
Synonym for macrodissected adult monkey ***arbor vitae (Winslow, 1733)***; Table I, Figure 7-*l*.

11. *frondosae arbori (Tiedemann, 1821)*
Synonym for macrodissected adult monkey ***arbor vitae (Winslow, 1733)***; Table I, Figure 7-*l*.

12. *central white nucleus of cerebellum (Cruveilhier, 1836)*
Basically synonym for macrodissected adult human ***arbor vitae (Winslow, 1733)***; in the original French, *noyau blanc central*, p. 631.

PARTLY CORRESPONDS:

1. *trunk of arbor vitae (Langenbeck, 1826–1830)*
Central condensed part of macrodissected adult human ***arbor vitae (Winslow, 1733)***; in the original Latin, *truncus arbor vitae*, Fascicle I, Table XV-*s*.
2. *nucleus of cerebellum (Arnold, 1838a)*
Synonym for macrodissected adult human *trunk of arbor vitae (Langenbeck, 1826–1830)*; p. 35.
3. *trunk of cerebellum (Arnold, 1838a)*
Synonym for *nucleus of cerebellum (Arnold, 1838a)*; in the original Latin, *truncus*, p. 35.
4. *meditullium of cerebellar hemisphere (Arnold, 1838a)*
Synonym for *nucleus of cerebellum (Arnold, 1838a)*; p. 35. Also see Arnold (1838b, Tab. IV, Fig. 4-*s*), in Latin, *meditullium cerebelli haemisphaerii.*
5. *arbor medullaris (Arnold, 1838a)*
Part of macrodissected adult human ***arbor vitae (Winslow, 1733)*** extending into ***cerebellar cortex (Willis, 1664)*** from *trunk of cerebellum (Arnold, 1838a)*; p. 35.
6. *medullary body of cerebellar hemisphere (Arnold, 1838b)*
Synonym for *nucleus of cerebellum (Arnold, 1838a)*; in the original Latin, *corpus medullare hemisphaerii cerebelli*, Table IV, Figure 4-*p*.
7. *medullary body of cerebellum (Arnold, 1838b)*
Synonym for *nucleus of cerebellum (Arnold, 1838a)*; in the original Latin, *corpus medullare cerebelli*, Table VI, Figure 3-*n*.

arcuate fibers (Arnold, 1838b)

As described for macrodissected adult human, roughly *U*-shaped bundles of short ***association fibers of cerebral cortex (>1840)*** between nearby *cerebral gyri (Vesalius, 1543a)*; see Williams & Warwick (1980, pp. 1029–1030), where they are referred to as *short arcuate fibers* and *short association fibers*. Also see *Nomina Anatomica* (1983, p. A72), *Terminologia Anatomica* (1998, p. 131). For Arnold's use in macrodissected adult human, see Table X, Figures 1-*z*, 2-*t*.

TRANSLATIONS:

1. *fibrae arcuatae (Arnold, 1838b)*
Original Latin form of ***arcuate fibers (Arnold, 1838b)***; Table X, Figure 1-*z*.
2. *fibrae arcuatae cerebri (>1840)*
Currently accepted Latin form of ***arcuate fibers (Arnold, 1838b)***; see *Terminologia Anatomica* (1998, p. 131).

arcuate nucleus of medulla (>1840)

As described for macrodissected adult human, and based on cellular architecture and connections as well, narrow bands of ***gray matter (Meckel, 1817)*** on superficial parts of the ***pyramid (Willis, 1664)*** often regarded as caudally displaced extensions of the ***pontine nuclei (Jacobsohn, 1909)***, although their ***axons (Kölliker, 1896)***, unlike those from the ***pontine nuclei (Jacobsohn, 1909)***, contribute to the ***ventral external arcuate fibers (>1840)*** and enter the ***inferior cerebellar peduncle (Günther, 1786)***; see Williams & Warwick (1980, pp. 904–905), Nieuwenhuys et al. (2008, Figs. 6.22-*16*, 6.24-*14*). It was perhaps first clearly delineated by Gordon; see ***[arcuate nucleus of medulla (>1840)] (Gordon, 1815)***.

EARLIER REFERENCES:

Described, not named or illustrated:

1. ***[arcuate nucleus of medulla (>1840)] (Gordon, 1815)***
Clearly described for macrodissected adult human; p. 184.

area postrema (>1840)

As described for mammal, a tiny unpaired ***central nervous system gray matter region (>1840)*** lying dorsally in the median plane of the ***medulla (Winslow, 1733)***, just at the level of the ***obex (Burdach, 1822)***. As described for macrodissected adult human, it lies just medial to the ***funiculus separans (>1840)*** with its dorsal surface visible at the caudal tip of the ***floor of fourth ventricle (Reil, 1807–1808a)***. It is a circumventricular organ lacking a blood-brain barrier; see Williams & Warwick (1980, pp. 934–935). It was not described clearly by 1840.

articular branch of deep fibular nerve (>1840)

As described for macrodissected adult human, a thin branch of the ***deep fibular nerve (Fyfe, 1800)*** to the ankle joint; see Williams & Warwick (1980, p. 1115). It was perhaps first clearly identified as *branches of anterior tibial nerve to joints of foot (Quain & Wilson, 1839)*.

EARLIER REFERENCES:

Earlier synonyms:

1. *branches of anterior tibial nerve to joints of foot (Quain & Wilson, 1839)*
Synonym for macrodissected adult human ***articular branch of deep fibular nerve (>1840)***; Plate XXIV, Figure 2-*C,c*.
2. *branches of interosseous nerve to joints of foot (Quain & Wilson, 1839)*
Synonym for macrodissected adult human ***articular branch of deep fibular nerve (>1840)***; Plate XXIV, Figure 2-*C,c*.

articular branch of nerve to popliteus (>1840)

As described for macrodissected adult human, a branch of the ***nerve to popliteus (>1840)*** to the superior tibio-fibular joint; see Durward (1951, pp. 1109–1110), Williams & Warwick (1980, p. 1113). It was probably first pointed out by Jördens; see ***[articular branch of nerve to popliteus (>1840)] (Jördens, 1788).***

EARLIER REFERENCES:

Described, not named or illustrated:

1. ***[articular branch of nerve to popliteus (>1840)] (Jördens, 1788)***
   Mentioned for macrodissected adult human as arising from *first nerve to popliteus from tibial nerve trunk (Jördens, 1788)*; p. 9, § XIX.

articular branch of nerve to quadratus femoris (>1840)

As described for macrodissected adult human, a branch of the ***nerve to quadratus femoris (>1840)*** to the hip joint; see Durward (1951, p. 1100), Williams & Warwick (1980, p. 1111). It was perhaps first clearly delineated by Swan; see ***[articular branch of nerve to quadratus femoris (>1840)] (Swan, 1830).***

EARLIER REFERENCES:

Described, not named or illustrated:

1. ***[articular branch of nerve to quadratus femoris (>1840)] (Swan, 1830)***
   Clearly described for macrodissected adult human; p. 36.

Earlier synonyms:

1. *internal branches of nerve of quadratus femoris and gemellus inferior (Cruveilhier, 1836)*
   Synonym for macrodissected adult human ***articular branch of nerve to quadratus femoris (>1840)***; in the original French, *rameaux internes*, p. 859.
2. *articular branches of nerve of quadratus femoris and gemellus inferior (Cruveilhier, 1836)*
   Synonym for *internal branches of nerve of quadratus femoris and gemellus inferior (Cruveilhier, 1836)*; in the original French, *rameaux articulaires*, p. 859.

articular branch of posterior branch of obturator nerve (>1840)

As described for macrodissected adult human, a branch of the ***posterior branch of obturator nerve (Haase, 1781; Martin, 1781)*** to the dorsal (posterior) part of the knee joint; see Durward (1951, p. 1094), *Terminologia Anatomica* (1998, p. 140). It was first clearly described as the *articular nerve of knee (Cruveilhier, 1836, p. 840).*

EARLIER REFERENCES:

Earlier synonyms:

1. *articular nerve of knee (Cruveilhier, 1836, p. 840)*
   Synonym for macrodissected adult human ***articular branch of posterior branch of obturator nerve (>1840)***; in the original French, *nerf articulaire du genou*, p. 840.

articular branch of tibial nerve to ankle joint (>1840)

As described for macrodissected adult human, a branch of the ***tibial nerve (Haas, 1781)*** trunk to the ankle joint; see Williams & Warwick (1980, p. 1112). It was perhaps first clearly delineated by Swan; see ***[articular branch of tibial nerve to ankle joint (>1840)] (Swan, 1830).***

EARLIER REFERENCES:

Described, not named or illustrated:

1. ***[articular branch of tibial nerve to ankle joint (>1840)] (Swan, 1830)***
   Described for macrodissected adult human as branches from *posterior tibial nerve (Haller, 1762)* to deeper parts of ankle joint; p. 36.

articular branches of auriculotemporal nerve (>1840)

As described for macrodissected adult human, one or two small branches of the ***auriculotemporal nerve (Haller, 1762)*** to caudal (posterior) parts of the temporomandibular joint; see Williams & Warwick (1980, p. 1067). They were known to Galen; see ***[articular branches of auriculotemporal nerve (1840)] (Galen, c192).***

EARLIER REFERENCES:

Described, not named or illustrated:

1. ***[articular branches of auriculotemporal nerve (1840)] (Galen, c192)***
   Mentioned for macrodissected adult beef, pig, and/or macaque but not human; see Duckworth translation (1962, p. 193). They were described for macrodissected adult human by Swan (1830, Pl. XIV, Fig. 2-6) and Cruveilhier (1836, p. 933).

Earlier synonyms:

1. *articular fascicles of cutaneous temporal surculus of inferior maxillary branch (Bellingeri, 1818)*
   Synonym for two macrodissected adult human ***articular branches of auriculotemporal nerve (>1840)***; in the original Latin, *(duo) fasciculi articulares*, see Table I.

articular branches of common fibular nerve (>1840)

As described for macrodissected adult human, 1–3 commonly arise from the ***sciatic nerve (Keill, 1698)*** segment of the ***common fibular nerve (>1840)*** and supply the knee joint; see Durward (1951, p. 1106), Williams & Warwick (1980, p. 1115). They were perhaps first clearly described as the *superior popliteal nerve (Günther, 1786).*

EARLIER REFERENCES:

Earlier synonyms:

1. *superior popliteal nerve (Günther, 1786)*
   May correspond to macrodissected adult human ***articular branches of common fibular nerve (>1840)***; in the original Latin, *nervus popliteus superior*, p. 87. Also see ***articular branch of tibial nerve to knee joint (>1840).*** Burdin (1803; see translation, 1803, Vol. 1, p. 205) specifically mentioned such a branch for macrodissected adult human.
2. *inferior posterior cutaneous nerve (Meckel, 1817)*
   May correspond to macrodissected adult human ***articular branches of common fibular nerve (>1840)***; see translation (1832, Vol. 3, pp. 17–18).
3. *articular branch of external popliteal nerve (Bock, 1827)*
   Synonym for macrodissected adult human ***articular branches of common fibular nerve (>1840)***; in the

original Latin, *ram. articularis nerv. poplitaeus externus*, Table IV-*88*.

4. *articular branches of sciatic nerve (Cruveilhier, 1836)*
For macrodissected adult human probably ***articular branches of common fibular nerve (>1840)***; Cruveilhier mentioned three such branches (p. 860) but then only described one (p. 861) from *sciatic nerve trunk (Günther, 1786)*, the *articular nerve of knee (Cruveilhier, 1836)*; in the original French, *rameaux articulaires du nerf sciatique*.
5. *articular nerve of knee (Cruveilhier, 1836, p. 861)*
For macrodissected adult human, an *articular branch of sciatic nerve (Cruveilhier, 1836)*; in the original French, *nerf articulaire du genou*, p. 861.

articular branches of radial nerve (>1840)

As described for macrodissected adult human, branches from the trunk of the ***radial nerve (Du Verney, 1697)*** distributing to the elbow joint; see Williams & Warwick (1980, p. 1101). They were perhaps first clearly described as a *branch of musculo-spiral nerve distributed to joint (Quain & Wilson, 1839)*.

EARLIER REFERENCES:

Earlier synonyms:

1. *branch of musculo-spiral nerve distributed to joint (Quain & Wilson, 1839)*
Synonym for macrodissected adult human ***articular branches of radial nerve (>1840)***; Plate XIX, Figure 2-*a*.

articular branches of tibial nerve (>1840)

As described for macrodissected adult human, there are commonly 2–3 branches to the knee joint and one to the ankle joint from the trunk of the ***tibial nerve (Haas, 1781)***; see Durward (1951, p. 1109), Williams & Warwick (1980, p. 1112). At least some were first clearly delineated by Winslow; see ***[articular branches of tibial nerve (>1840)] (Winslow, 1733)***.

EARLIER REFERENCES:

Described, not named or illustrated:

1. ***[articular branches of tibial nerve (>1840)] (Winslow, 1733)***
Winslow mentioned branches to knee joint in macrodissected adult human; Section VI, no. 328, p. 91.

Earlier synonyms:

1. *internal articular branch of internal popliteal nerve (Bock, 1827)*
Synonym for macrodissected adult human ***articular branches of tibial nerve (>1840)***; in the original Latin, *ram. articularis internus nerv. poplitaeus internus*, Table IV-*93,94*.

articular branches of tibial nerve to knee joint (>1840)

As described for macrodissected adult human there are commonly 2–3 branches; see Durward (1951, p. 1109), Williams & Warwick (1980, p. 1112). They were perhaps first delineated by Winslow; see ***[articular branches of tibial nerve to knee joint (>1840)] (Winslow, 1733)***.

EARLIER REFERENCES:

Described, not named or illustrated:

1. ***[articular branches of tibial nerve to knee joint (>1840)] (Winslow, 1733)***
Mentioned for macrodissected adult human; Section VI, no. 328, p. 91.

Earlier synonyms:

1. *posterior articular nerve of knee (Cruveilhier, 1836)*
Synonym for macrodissected adult human ***articular branch of tibial nerve to knee joint (>1840)***; in the original French, *nerf articulaire postérieur du genou*, p. 870.

ascending branch of lateral cerebral sulcus (>1840)

As described for macrodissected adult human, the rostral and dorsal branch of the ***lateral cerebral sulcus (>1840)*** between ***triangular part of inferior frontal gyrus (>1840)*** rostrally and ***opercular part of inferior frontal gyrus (>1840)*** caudally; see Williams & Warwick (1980, p. 984, Fig. 7.111A), *Terminologia Anatomica* (1998, p. 124). It was first delineated as the *anterior vertical branch of Sylvian fissure (Vicq d'Azyr, 1784)*.

EARLIER REFERENCES:

Earlier synonyms:

1. *anterior vertical branch of Sylvian fissure (Vicq d'Azyr, 1784)*
Synonym for macrodissected adult human ***ascending branch of lateral cerebral sulcus (>1840)***; p. 506. It probably corresponds to dorsally directed part of ***cruciform sulcus (Rolando, 1831)***; Figure 1-*8*.

ascending superficial branches of cervical plexus (Quain, 1828)

As described for macrodissected adult human, branches of the second and third cervical ***spinal nerve ventral branches (>1840)*** generating the ***lesser occipital nerve (Andersch & Soemmerring, 1791)***, ***great auricular nerve (Haase, 1781)***, and ***transverse nerve of neck (>1840)***; see Durward (1951, p. 1061 and Fig. 919), Williams & Warwick (1980, p. 1092). For Quain's use in macrodissected adult human, see p. 489. They were known to Galen; see ***[ascending superficial branches of cervical plexus (Quain, 1828)] (Galen, c173)***.

EARLIER REFERENCES:

Described, not named or illustrated:

1. ***[ascending superficial branches of cervical plexus (Quain, 1828)] (Galen, c173)***
Galen described all three major branches in adult large mammals (beef, pig, and/or macaque) but not human; see May translation (1968, pp. 597–598, 698) and Duckworth translation (1962, pp. 225–226, 234–235, 238).

Earlier synonyms:

1. *cephalic part of trachelo-cutanean plexus (Burdin, 1803)*
Synonym for macrodissected adult human *cephalic part of tracheosubcutaneous nerves (Chaussier, 1809)*; see translation (1803, Vol. 1, p. 188).

2. *cephalic part of tracheosubcutaneous nerves (Chaussier, 1809)*
   Synonym for macrodissected adult human ***ascending superficial branches of cervical plexus (Quain, 1828)***.

PARTLY CORRESPONDS:

1. *lateral cutaneous nerve of face of first pair of cervical nerves (Meckel, 1753)*
   An inconsistent ***ascending superficial branch of cervical plexus (Quain, 1828)*** in macrodissected adult human ending near parotid gland and nearby parts of masseter muscle; Table 1-Φ (also see p. 101).

association fibers of cerebral cortex (>1840)

As described for macrodissected adult human, and mammal generally with histological methods, ***axons (Kölliker, 1896)*** connecting different areas of the ***cerebral cortex gray matter (>1840)*** on the same side (right or left) and generally taking a route through the underlying ***cerebral cortex white matter (>1840)***. For topographic description they are divided into short ***association fibers of cerebral cortex (>1840)***, or ***arcuate fibers (Arnold, 1838b)***, and long ***association fibers of cerebral cortex (>1840)*** including the ***uncinate fascicle (Reil, 1809b)***, ***inferior longitudinal fascicle (Burdach, 1822)***, ***external capsule (Burdach, 1822)***, ***superior longitudinal fascicle (>1840)***, and ***cingulum (Burdach, 1822)***; see Crosby et al. (1962, pp. 402–409 and Fig. 284), Williams & Warwick (1980, pp. 1029–1030, Fig. 7.148). They were perhaps first clearly distinguished by Reil; see ***[association fibers of cerebral cortex (>1840)] (Reil, 1809b)***.

EARLIER REFERENCES:

Illustrated and described, not named:

1. ***[association fibers of cerebral cortex (>1840)] (Reil, 1809b)***
   As described for macrodissected adult human, "it consists but of fasciculi which pass from the centre of any convolution to others more remote." (Mayo translation, 1823, p. 71). And "this structure is probably general, and is probably intended…for the common purpose of associating together in action the convolutions of the great divisions of either hemisphere" (Mayo translation, 1823, p. 81).

atrial plexuses (>1840)

As described for macrodissected adult human, derivatives of the right and left continuations of the ***cardiac plexus (Keill, 1698)*** extending along the pulmonary arteries to the right and left atria of the heart and overlapping with nerve fibers of the ***coronary plexuses (Meckel, 1817)***; see Williams & Warwick (1980, p. 1132). They were perhaps first clearly identified by Willis; see ***[atrial plexuses (>1840)] (Willis, 1664)***.

EARLIER REFERENCES:

Described, not named or illustrated:

1. ***[atrial plexuses (>1840)] (Willis, 1664)***
   Willis described for macrodissected adult human many "nerve fibers" going to "the Vessels hanging to the Heart, and to its little Ears [atria] and Pericardium" (Pordage translation, 1681, p. 147).

Earlier synonyms:

1. *auricular plexus (Swan, 1830)*
   Essentially synonym for macrodissected adult human ***atrial plexuses (>1840)***; pp. 6–7.

PARTLY CORRESPONDS:

1. *nerve to right auricle of heart (Andersch & Soemmerring, 1792)*
   In macrodissected adult human, associated with *anterior branch of right trunk of nerve of right pulmonary branches (Andersch & Soemmerring, 1792)* and contributes to right ***atrial plexus (>1840)***; in the original Latin, *nervus dextrae auriculae cordis, nervum auriculae dextrae cordis*, pp. 196–197.
2. *nerve to left auricle of heart (Andersch, 1797)*
   In macrodissected adult human, extends from *nerve layers of septum of heart (Andersch, 1797)* and contributes to left ***atrial plexus (>1840)***; in the original Latin, *nervus auriculae sinistrae cordis*, Vol. 2, pp. 78, 102.
3. *deep auricular branch of nerve to left auricle (Andersch, 1797)*
   Terminal branch of *nerve to left auricle of heart (Andersch, 1797)*; in the original Latin, *ramo auriculari profundo*, Vol. 2, p. 103.
4. *superficial auricular branches of nerve to left auricle (Andersch, 1797)*
   Terminal branches of *nerve to left auricle of heart (Andersch, 1797)*; in the original Latin, *ramos auricularos superficialos*, Vol. 2, p. 103.

atrium of lateral ventricle (>1840)

The part of the macrodissected adult human ***lateral ventricle (Vesalius, 1543a)*** between the ***body of lateral ventricle (Bell, 1803b)***, ***posterior horn of lateral ventricle (Haller, 1747)***, and ***inferior horn of lateral ventricle (Bell, 1802)***; see Williams & Warwick (1980, p. 1029), *Dorland's* (2003, p. 1949). If no ***posterior horn of lateral ventricle (Haller, 1747)*** is present, the ***body of lateral ventricle (Bell, 1803b)*** borders the ***inferior horn of lateral ventricle (Bell, 1802)*** at the level of the ***splenium of corpus callosum (Burdach, 1822)***; see Millen & Woollam (1962, pp. 33–44, Figs. 13, 16), *Terminologia Anatomica* (1998, p. 127). It was illustrated by Berengario da Carpi; see ***[atrium of lateral ventricle (>1840)] (Berengario da Carpi, 1523)***.

EARLIER REFERENCES:

Illustrated, not named or described:

1. ***[atrium of lateral ventricle (>1840)] (Berengario da Carpi, 1523)***
   First indicated and illustrated in macrodissected adult human; f. 56, top.

Described, not named or illustrated:

1. ***[atrium of lateral ventricle (>1840)] (Gordon, 1815)***
   Clearly described for macrodissected adult human; p. 107.

auditory radiation (>1840)

As described for macrodissected adult human, a topographic division of the ***cerebral cortex white matter (>1840)*** between ***sublentiform part of internal capsule (>1840)***, specifically its ***posterior thalamic radiation (>1840)*** component, and ***cerebral cortex gray matter (>1840)***. A major component is the projection from ***medial geniculate complex (>1840)*** to auditory areas centered in the ***transverse temporal gyri (Heschl, 1878)*** and adjacent parts of the ***superior temporal gyrus (>1840)***; see Mettler (1948, p. 409 and Figs. 96, 97), Crosby et al. (1962, pp. 275, 467 and Fig. 272), Carpenter (1976, Fig. 15.18), Nieuwenhuys et al. (1962, pp. 737, 742–744 and Fig. 18.1A-3). It was not clearly delineated by 1840.

auditory tubercle (>1840)

As described for macrodissected adult human, an eminence on the ***floor of fourth ventricle (Reil, 1807a–1808)***, associated with the ***lateral recess of fourth ventricle (>1840)*** and indicating the surface of the ***cochlear nuclei (>1840)***; see Williams & Warwick (1980, p. 934). It was distinguished by Procháska; see ***[auditory tubercle (>1840)] (Procháska, 1779)***.

EARLIER REFERENCES:

Described, not named or illustrated:

1. ***[auditory tubercle (>1840)] (Procháska, 1779)***
   Undoubtedly corresponds to surface of macrodissected adult human *gray band (Procháska, 1779)*; pp. 389–391.

Earlier synonyms:

1. *eminentias transversales ventriculi quarti (Procháska, 1800)*
   Synonym for at least part of macrodissected adult human right and left ***auditory tubercle (>1840)***; Vol. 1, p. 387 ff. See Burdach (1822, p. 311).

PARTLY CORRESPONDS:

1. *gray colliculus (Wenzel & Wenzel, 1812)*
   Apparently part of macrodissected adult human ***auditory tubercle (>1840)***; in the original Latin, *colliculus cinereus*, Table XI, Figure 4-*c*.

auricular branch of posterior auricular nerve (Arnold, 1834)

As described for macrodissected adult human, a secondary branch of the ***facial nerve trunk (>1840)*** supplying the posterior auricular muscle and intrinsic muscles on the cranial surface of the auricle and lying rostral (anterior) to the ***occipital branch of posterior auricular nerve (Arnold, 1834)***; see Hamilton (1976, Fig. 798), Williams & Warwick (1980, p. 1072). For Arnold's use in macrodissected adult human, see p. 12. It was known to Galen; see ***[auricular branch of posterior auricular nerve (Arnold, 1834)] (Galen, c173)***.

TRANSLATIONS:

1. *nervus auricularis posterior ramus auricularis (Arnold, 1834)*
   Original Latin form of ***auricular branch of posterior auricular nerve (Arnold, 1834)***; p. 12.

EARLIER REFERENCES:

Described, not named or illustrated:

1. ***[auricular branch of posterior auricular nerve (Arnold, 1834)] (Galen, c173)***
   Mentioned for macrodissected adult beef, pig, and/or macaque but not human; see May translation (1968, p. 686).

Illustrated, not named or described:

1. ***[auricular branch of posterior auricular nerve (Arnold, 1834)] (Du Verney, 1683)***
   Clearly illustrated for macrodissected adult human; Plate 12, Figure 3-*D*.

Earlier synonyms:

1. *auricular branch of external deep branch of hard nerve (Meckel, 1753)*
   Synonym for macrodissected adult human ***auricular branch of posterior auricular nerve (Arnold, 1834)***; in the original French, *le rameau postérieur profond auriculaire*, p. 75. Also see *occipital branch of external deep branch of hard nerve (Meckel, 1753)*.
2. *anterior auricular branch of hard nerve (Bang, 1770)*
   Synonym for macrodissected adult human ***auricular branch of posterior auricular nerve (Arnold, 1834)***; in the original Latin, *auriculari nervi duri anteriori*, Figure I-34.
3. *anterior branch of external deep branch of hard nerve (Haase, 1781)*
   Synonym for macrodissected adult human ***auricular branch of posterior auricular nerve (Arnold, 1834)***; p. 81.
4. *auricular branch proper of external deep branch of hard nerve (Günther, 1786)*
   Synonym for macrodissected adult human ***auricular branch of posterior auricular nerve (Arnold, 1834)***; in the original Latin, *auricularem proprium*, p. 57.
5. *anterior branch of auricular portion of hard part of acoustic nerve (Frotscher, 1788)*
   Synonym for macrodissected adult human ***auricular branch of posterior auricular nerve (Arnold, 1834)***; in the original Latin, *auriculari portionis durae nervi acustici anteriori*, see p. 87 of 1795 reprint.
6. *anterior branch of posterior auricular nerve (Meckel, 1817)*
   Synonym for macrodissected adult human ***auricular branch of posterior auricular nerve (Arnold, 1834)***; see translation (1832, Vol. 3, p. 54).
7. *auricular surculus of external deep branch of portio major and minor of facial nerve (Bellingeri, 1818)*
   Synonym for macrodissected adult human ***auricular branch of posterior auricular nerve (Arnold, 1834)***; in the original Latin, *surculus auricularis*, see Table II.
8. *nervus auricularis posterior rami musculorum retrahentium (Arnold,1834)*
   Synonym for macrodissected adult human ***auricular branch of posterior auricular nerve (Arnold, 1834)***; Table IX:VII-22. *Musculorum retrahentium* is posterior auricular muscle, also known as retractor muscle of ear; see Todd (1836–1839, Vol. 2, p. 552).

9. *ascending filament of posterior auricular branch of facial nerve (Cruveilhier, 1836)*
   Synonym for macrodissected adult human ***auricular branch of posterior auricular nerve (Arnold, 1834)***; in the original French, *filet ascendant*, p. 943.
10. *auricular filament of posterior auricular branch of facial nerve (Cruveilhier, 1836)*
   Synonym for *ascending filament of posterior auricular branch of facial nerve Cruveilhier, 1836)*; in the original French, *filet auriculaire*, p. 943.

auricular branch of vagus nerve (Arnold, 1834)

As described for macrodissected adult human, a proximal branch of the ***vagus nerve trunk (Wrisberg, 1786; Günther, 1786)*** appearing to arise from the ***proximal vagal ganglion (>1840)*** and soon joined by the ***communicating branch of glossopharyngeal nerve with auricular branch of vagus nerve (>1840)***. In the region of the facial canal, it is joined by the ***communicating branch of intermediofacial nerve with vagus nerve (>1840)*** before passing through the tympanomastoid fissure and dividing into two branches, one joining the ***posterior auricular nerve (Meckel, 1753)*** and the other distributing to skin on part of the cranial surface of the auricle and posterior wall and floor of the external auditory meatus and adjoining part of the outer surface of the tympanic membrane; see Mettler (1948, Fig. 61), Durward (1951, Fig. 907-*Aur.*), Williams & Warwick (1980, p. 1079). For Arnold's discovery and use in macrodissected adult human, see pp. 12, 13.

TRANSLATIONS:

1. *ramo auriculare nervi vagi (Arnold, 1834)*
   Original Latin form of ***auricular branch of vagus nerve (Arnold, 1834)***; pp. 12, 13.

LATER SYNONYMS:

1. *auricular branch of pneumogastric nerve (Cruveilhier, 1836)*
   Synonym for macrodissected adult human ***auricular branch of vagus nerve (Arnold, 1834)***; in the original French, *rameau auriculaire du pneumo-gastrique*, p. 942.
2. *Arnold's nerve (>1840)*
   Eponym for ***auricular branch of vagus nerve (Arnold, 1834)***; see Lekakis (2003, p. 28).

PARTLY CORRESPONDS:

1. *branchlet of auricular branch of vagus nerve to external auditory meatus (Arnold, 1834)*
   Macrodissected adult human branch of ***auricular branch of vagus nerve (Arnold, 1834)*** to external auditory meatus; in the original Latin, *ramus auricularis nervi vagi, ramuli meatus auditorii externi*, p. 14.

auriculotemporal nerve (Haller, 1762)

As described for macrodissected adult human, it generally arises from the ***posterior branch of mandibular nerve (>1840)*** as two roots encircling the middle meningeal artery and joining to form a trunk eventually dividing into ***superficial temporal branches of auriculotemporal nerve (>1840)***; see Hamilton (1976, Fig. 798), Williams & Warwick (1980, p. 1066), and Henle (1871, Fig. 243-*at*), who illustrated it beautifully. For Haller's original use in macrodissected adult human, see p. 219. It was known to Galen; see ***[auriculotemporal nerve (Haller, 1762)] (Galen, c173)***.

TRANSLATIONS:

1. *nervos temporales auricularem (Haller, 1762)*
   Original Latin form of ***auriculotemporal nerve (Haller, 1762)***; p. 219.
2. *nervus auriculo-temporalis (Henle, 1871)*
   Latin form of ***auriculotemporal nerve (Haller, 1762)***; p. 396.

EARLIER REFERENCES:

Described, not named or illustrated:

1. ***[auriculotemporal nerve (Haller, 1762)] (Galen, c173)***
   Described for macrodissected adult beef, pig, and/or macaque but not human; see May translation (1968, p. 444 note 38), Duckworth translation (1962, pp. 193, 196, 235). Winslow provided a rough description for macrodissected adult human, referring to 1st and 2nd branches of *inferior maxillary nerve (Heister, 1717)*; Section VI, pp. 65–66.

Illustrated and described, not named:

1. ***[auriculotemporal nerve (Haller, 1762)] (Du Verney, 1683)***
   Clearly illustrated for macrodissected adult human; Plate 13-*G*, also see Vieussens (1684, p. 173 and Tab. 22-9).

Earlier synonyms:

1. *superficial temporal branch of third branch of fifth pair (Meckel, 1748)*
   Synonym for macrodissected adult human ***auriculotemporal nerve (Haller, 1762)***; in the original Latin, *ramus temporalis superficialis tertii rami Quinti paris*, Figure 1-*81* and p. 97.
2. *superficial temporal nerve (Meckel, 1748)*
   Synonym for macrodissected adult human ***auriculotemporal nerve (Haller, 1762)***; in the original Latin, *nervus temporalis superficialis*, p. 98.
3. *posterior subcutaneous temporal nerve of third branch of fifth pair (Meckel, 1753)*
   Synonym for macrodissected adult human ***auriculotemporal nerve (Haller, 1762)***; in the original French, *le nerf sous-cutané postérieur des temples du troisième rameau du nerf de la cinquième paire*, pp. 58, 67.
4. *auricular branch of third trunk of fifth pair (Haller, 1762)*
   Synonym for macrodissected adult human ***auriculotemporal nerve (Haller, 1762)***, p. 229.

LATER SYNONYMS:

1. *posterior branch of inferior maxillary nerve (Le Cat, 1768)*
   Synonym for macrodissected adult human ***auriculotemporal nerve (Haller, 1762)***; Plate VII, Figure 1-*1*.
2. *external temporal branch of inferior maxillary nerve (Le Cat, 1768)*
   Synonym for macrodissected adult human ***auriculotemporal nerve (Haller, 1762)***; Plate VII, Figure 1-*1*.
3. *superficial temporal branch of inferior maxillary nerve (Le Cat, 1768)*

Synonym for macrodissected adult human ***auriculotemporal nerve (Haller, 1762)***; Plate VIII, Figure 1-Φ.

4. *external temporal nerve (Le Cat, 1768)*
   Synonym for macrodissected adult human ***auriculotemporal nerve (Haller, 1762)***; Plate VII, Figure 2-*1*.
5. *auricular nerve (Günther, 1786)*
   Synonym for macrodissected adult human ***auriculotemporal nerve (Haller, 1762)***; in the original Latin, *nervus auricularis*, p. 53.
6. *posterior superficial temporal nerve (Mayer, 1794)*
   Synonym for macrodissected adult human ***auriculotemporal nerve (Haller, 1762)***; in the original Latin, *nervus temporalis superficialis posterior*; Part 5, Table VII-*XI* (p. 53).
7. *cutaneous temporal nerve (Burdin, 1803)*
   Synonym for macrodissected adult human ***auriculotemporal nerve (Haller, 1762)***; see translation (1803, Vol. 1, p. 176).
8. *anterior auricular nerve (Bock, 1817)*
   Synonym for macrodissected adult human *superficial temporal nerve (Meckel, 1748)*; in the original Latin, *nervus auricularis anterior*, p. 47.
9. *cutaneous temporal surculus of inferior maxillary branch (Bellingeri, 1818)*
   Synonym for macrodissected adult human ***auriculotemporal nerve (Haller, 1762)***; in the original Latin, *surculus temporalis cutaneous*, see Table I.
10. *glandulocutaneous nerve (Jacobson, 1818)*
   Basically macrodissected adult mammalian ***auriculotemporal nerve (Haller, 1762)***; in the original Latin, *nervus maxillaris inferior ramus glandulo-cutaneus*, p. 18.
11. *superficial temporal nerve of third trunk of fifth (Swan, 1830)*
   Synonym for *superficial temporal branch of third branch of fifth pair (Meckel, 1748)*; Plate XIII-*13*.
12. *auricular branch of inferior maxillary nerve (Quain, 1832)*
   Synonym for macrodissected adult human ***auriculotemporal nerve (Haller, 1762)***; p. 676.
13. *ramus meatus auditorii externii Meckel (Quain, 1832)*
   Eponym for macrodissected adult human ***auriculotemporal nerve (Haller, 1762)***; p. 676. Quain provided no citation to Meckel's work.

PARTLY CORRESPONDS:

1. *lesser auricular nerves (Günther, 1786)*
   Macrodissected adult human ***anterior auricular nerves (>1840)*** and ***external acoustic meatus nerves (Meckel, 1817)*** considered together; in the original Latin, *auriculares minores*, p. 53.
2. *second auricular branch of superficial temporal nerve (Bock, 1817)*
   Apparently, trunk of macrodissected adult human ***auriculotemporal nerve (Haller, 1762)*** distal to where the ***anterior auricular nerves (>1840)*** branch off; in the original Latin, *ramus auricularis secundus*, p. 50.

autonomic ganglia (Langley, 1900)

As described for vertebrates, macrodissected ***ganglia (Galen, c173)*** in the ***peripheral nervous system (Meckel, 1817)*** that are distinguished from ***craniospinal ganglia (>1840)*** and for description are divided into sequentially more distal ***paravertebral ganglia (Durward, 1951)***, ***prevertebral ganglia (Quain, 1832)***, and ***terminal ganglia (Gaskell, 1886)***; see Crosby et al. (1962, p. 521). They are often embedded in ***prevertebral plexuses (Quain, 1837)*** and ***terminal plexuses (Swanson & Bota, 2010)***; also see ***autonomic nerves (Langley, 1898)***. Based on cellular architecture and connections, they are considered ***peripheral nervous system gray matter regions (Swanson & Bota, 2010)***. For Langley's use see pp. 677–678. Galen provided the first evidence for their existence; see ***[autonomic ganglia (Langley, 1900)] (Galen c173, c177, c192)***.

EARLIER REFERENCES:

Described, not named or illustrated:

1. ***[autonomic ganglia (Langley, 1900)] (Galen c173, c177, c192)***
   Galen described without naming three pairs of ***autonomic ganglia (Langley, 1900)***: the ***superior cervical ganglion (Vieussens, 1684)*** (see Duckworth translation, 1962, pp. 217–218; May translation, 1968, pp. 695–696; Savage-Smith 1971, p. 179), *cervicothoracic ganglion (>1840)* (see Duckworth translation, 1962, pp. 217–218; Savage-Smith, 1971, p. 179), and perhaps ***celiac ganglion (Walter, 1783)*** (see Savage-Smith 1971, p. 179). This is where he introduced the term ***ganglia (Galen, c173)***, which he described as having the consistency of ***nerve (Herophilus, c335–c280 BC)*** and lying on small ***nerves (Herophilus, c335–c280 BC)*** conducting over a long path; previous usage referred to a ganglion as an encapsulated tumor on a tendon or aponeurosis; see May translation (1968, p. 695).
2. ***[autonomic ganglia (Langley, 1900] (Willis, 1664)***
   Willis referred to a variety of them as *ganglioform infoldings (Willis 1664)* or *knots (Crooke, 1615)* that serve as animal spirit storehouses; see Pordage translation (1681, p. 165). His comprehensive description of the ***autonomic ganglia (Langley, 1900)*** and their connections was the first of its kind; see Sheehan (1936, p. 1088).

Earlier synonyms:

1. *vegetative system ganglia (Wutzer, 1817)*
   Basically equivalent to ***autonomic ganglia (Langley, 1900)***; in the original Latin, *ganglia systematis vegetativi*, pp. 52, 97.
2. *automatic system ganglia (Wutzer, 1817)*
   Basically equivalent to ***autonomic ganglia (Langley, 1900)***; in the original Latin, *ganglia systematis automaticum*, p. 52.
3. *ganglia of sympathetic nervous system (Wutzer, 1817)*
   Synonym for *vegetative system ganglia (Wutzer, 1817)*; in the original Latin, *ganglia systematis nervi sympathici (vegetativi)*, p. 97.

PARTLY CORRESPONDS:

1. *esophageal small ganglion (Walter, 1783)*
   Walter described at least two small ***ganglia (Galen, c173)*** associated with the macrodissected adult human

esophageal plexus (1762); in the original Latin, *gangliolum oesophageum*, Table III-*441,482*.

2. *esophageal ganglion (Cloquet, 1828)*
   Synonym for macrodissected adult human *esophageal small ganglion (Walter, 1783)*; in the original French, *ganglion oesophagien*, Plate CLXXVII-*203,208*.

autonomic nerves (Langley, 1898)

In macrodissected adult vertebrate, they consist of ***white matter (Meckel, 1817)***, and their origin—along with the anastomotic networks of ***communicating branches (Winslow, 1733)*** associated with them, *autonomic plexuses (Strong & Elwyn, 1943)*—appears to be from ***autonomic ganglia (Langley, 1900)*** in the ***peripheral nervous system (Meckel, 1817)***, not from the ***craniospinal nerves (Herrick, 1915)***. They are a component of what current usage (see *Nomina Anatomica*, 1983, p. A78) refers to as the *autonomic part of peripheral nervous system*. "The peripheral autonomous nervous system appears to be a direct survival of that diffuse type of nervous system which is found in the lowest animals which possess nerves at all, such as some jelly-fishes and worms" (Herrick, 1915, p. 227). ***Autonomic nerves (Langley, 1898)*** and ***autonomic ganglia (Langley, 1900)*** are distinguished macroscopically, although the latter are often embedded within *autonomic plexuses (Strong & Elwyn, 1943)*. For Langley's use, see p. 241); at least some were identified long ago: see *nerves to spongy flesh (Galen, c192)*.

EARLIER REFERENCES:

Earlier synonyms:

1. *sympathetic nerves (Sharpey et al., 1867)*
   Generally synonymous with macrodissected adult human ***autonomic nerves (Langley, 1898)***, p. cxxiii.

PARTLY CORRESPONDS:

1. *nerves to spongy flesh (Galen, c192)*
   Refers partly to ***autonomic nerves (Langley, 1898)*** supplying glands, in macrodissected adult beef, pig, and/or macaque, but not human; see Duckworth translation (1962, p. 111).
2. *inferior gastric nerves (Wrisberg, 1800)*
   As described for macrodissected adult human, probably associated with the *inferior gastric plexus (Portal, 1803a)* along the greater curvature of the stomach; in the original Latin, *nervos gastricos inferiores*, pp. 563, 568.
3. *superior gastric plexus (Portal, 1803a)*
   As described for macrodissected adult human, probably equivalent to ***right gastric plexus (>1840)*** and ***left gastric plexus (>1840)*** considered together; in the original French, *plexus gastrique supérieur*, p. 193. Also see *superior coronary plexus of stomach (Meckel, 1817)*.
4. *small coronary plexus (Portal, 1803a)*
   Synonym for macrodissected adult human *superior gastric plexus (Portal, 1803a)*; in the original French, *petit plexus coronaire*, p. 193.
5. *inferior gastric plexus (Portal, 1803a)*
   As described for macrodissected adult human, probably equivalent to ***right gastroepiploic plexus (Wrisberg, 1800)*** and ***left gastroepiploic plexus (Wrisberg, 1800)*** considered together; in the original French, *plexus gastrique inférieur*, p. 194.
6. *solar plexus (Cloquet, 1816)*
   For macrodissected adult human, all ***prevertebral plexuses (Quain, 1832)*** and ***terminal plexuses (Swanson & Bota, 2010)*** in the abdomen, ending with the ***inferior mesenteric plexus (Rau, 1720)***; in the original French, *plexus solaire*, pp. 703–709.
7. *superior coronary plexus of stomach (Meckel, 1817)*
   Synonym for macrodissected adult human *superior gastric plexus (Portal, 1803a)*; see translation (1832, Vol. 3, p. 86).
8. *inferior coronary plexus (Meckel, 1817)*
   Synonym for macrodissected adult human *inferior gastric plexus (Portal, 1803a)*; in the original Latin, *plexus coronarius stomachicus inferior*; see translation (1832, Vol. 3, p. 86).
9. *solar plexus (Cruveilhier, 1836)*
   For macrodissected adult human, essentially synonymous with *solar plexus (Cloquet, 1816)* and ***superior mesenteric plexus (Rau, 1720)*** considered together; in the original French, *plexus solaire*, pp. 1013, 1018.
10. *epigastric plexus (Cruveilhier, 1836)*
    Synonym for *solar plexus (Cruveilhier, 1836)*; in the original French, *plexus épigastrique*, p. 1013; see Mitchell (1953, p. 272).
11. *epigastric nervous center (Cruveilhier, 1836)*
    Synonym for *epigastric plexus (Cruveilhier, 1836)*; in the original French, *centre nerveux épigastrique*, p. 1014.
12. *visceral plexuses (Cruveilhier, 1836)*
    For macrodissected adult human, the four great visceral plexuses include the ***pharyngeal plexus (Neubauer, 1772)***, ***cardiac plexus (Keill, 1698)***, *solar plexus (Cruveilhier, 1836)*, ***superior hypogastric plexus (Tiedemann, 1822)***, and ***inferior hypogastric plexus (Tiedemann, 1822)*** considered together; in the original French, *plexus viscéraux*, p. 1032.
13. *autonomic plexuses (Strong & Elwyn, 1943)*
    Anastomotic networks of ***autonomic nerve (Langley, 1898)*** branches, and in macrodissected adult human distinguished from ***autonomic ganglia (Langley, 1900)*** that may be embedded within them; Figure 148.

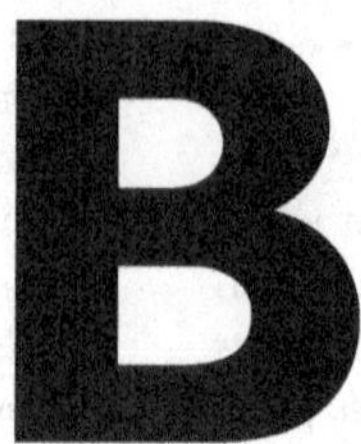

basal plate (>1840)

As described for developing vertebrate, right or left wall of the ***neural tube (Baer, 1837)*** between the ***floor plate (>1840)*** ventrally and ***limiting sulcus (>1840)*** dorsally; see Alvarez-Bolado & Swanson (1996, p. 13 ff.), Nieuwenhuys et al. (2008, p. 9). It was not clearly described by 1840.

basilar sulcus of pons (Gordon, 1815)

As described for macrodissected adult human, the longitudinal depression on the ventral surface of the ***pons (Haller, 1747)*** and its ***middle cerebellar peduncle (Rolando, 1819)*** in the median plane and usually lodging the basilar artery; see *Terminologia Anatomica* (1998, p. 112), Nieuwenhuys et al. (2008, Fig. 3.12-32). For Gordon's use in macrodissected adult human, see p. 112. It was first clearly delineated by Casseri; see ***[basilar sulcus of pons (Gordon, 1815)] (Casseri, 1609).***

TRANSLATIONS:

1. *sulcus pontis basilaris (>1840)*
   Latin form of ***basilar sulcus of pons (Gordon, 1815)***; see Foster (1894, p. 2874). Burdach (1822, p. 299) simply gave *sulcus basilaris*; see *Terminologia Anatomica* (1998, p. 112).

EARLIER REFERENCES:

Illustrated, not named or described:

1. ***[basilar sulcus of pons (Gordon, 1815)] (Casseri, 1609)***
   Clearly illustrated for macrodissected adult human; Table VII, *Organi olfactus*, Figure II, between right and left *B*.

Earlier synonyms:

1. *sinus protuberantiae annularis (Santorini, 1775)*
   Synonym for macrodissected adult human ***basilar sulcus of pons (Gordon, 1815)***; p. 15.
2. *medial longitudinal sulcus of annular protuberance (Vicq d'Azyr, 1786)*
   Synonym for macrodissected adult human ***basilar sulcus of pons (Gordon, 1815)***; in the original French, *sillon longitudinal et moyen de la protubérance annulaire*, Plate XVIII-23.
3. *basilar furrow of pons (Gordon, 1815)*
   Original English form of ***basilar sulcus of pons (Gordon, 1815)***; p. 112.

LATER SYNONYMS:

1. *longitudinal groove on base of pons for basilar artery (Tiedemann, 1826)*
   Synonym for macrodissected fetal human ***basilar sulcus of pons (Gordon, 1815)***; p. 77. For original description in German, see Tiedemann (1816, p. 50).

basolateral amygdalar complex (>1840)

Based on histology and connections in mammal, a major ventral part of the ***cortical subplate (>1840)*** including the ***lateral amygdalar nucleus (>1840), basolateral amygdalar nucleus (>1840), basomedial amygdalar nucleus (>1840)***, and ***posterior amygdalar nucleus (Canteras et al., 1992)***; see Johnston (1923, p. 456 ff., who referred to basal and lateral nuclei of amygdala or amygdaloid nuclei), Nieuwenhuys et al. (2008, Fig. 5.6-36), Price et al. (1987, who referred to *basolateral nuclei of amygdaloid complex*), Swanson & Petrovich (1998), Swanson (2004). It was first clearly delineated by Steno; see ***[basolateral amygdalar complex (>1840)] (Steno, 1669).***

EARLIER REFERENCES:

Illustrated, not named or described:

1. ***[basolateral amygdalar complex (>1840)] (Steno, 1669)***
   First clearly illustrated in transverse section through macrodissected adult human; Plate III.

Earlier synonyms:

1. *amygdalar nucleus (Burdach, 1822)*
   First description and illustration of macrodissected adult human ***basolateral amygdalar complex (>1840)***; in the original German, *den Mandelkern*, p. 173, Table III-*δ*. For modern comparison see Nieuwenhuys et al. (2008, Fig. 5.6-36).

2. *nucleus amygdalae (Burdach, 1822)*
   Original Latin form of *amygdalar nucleus (Burdach, 1822)*; p. 173, Table III-δ.
3. *amygdala (Arnold, 1838a)*
   Synonym for macrodissected adult human *amygdalar nucleus (Burdach, 1822)*; p. 68.

bed nuclei of terminal stria (Gurdjian, 1925)

As described for macrodissected adult human, and with cellular architecture and connections for all mammals, a dorsomedial component of the ***pallidum (Swanson, 2000a)*** surrounding the ***anterior commissure (Lieutaud, 1742)*** as it nears the median plane and characterized by a massive input from the ***terminal stria (Wenzel & Wenzel, 1812)***; see Swanson (2004, Tab. B). For Gurdjian's use in histological material from rat, see pp. 140, 152, 160. He used the singular, partly Latin, *bed nucleus of stria terminalis*. There are many ways of subdividing the ***bed nuclei of terminal stria (Gurdjian, 1925)***; see Swanson (2004, Tab. B), Bota & Swanson (2010). It was probably first identified vaguely as the *gray layer of taenia striata (Vicq d'Azyr, 1786)*.

TRANSLATIONS:

1. *bed nucleus of stria terminalis (Gurdjian, 1925)*
   Alternate form of ***bed nuclei of terminal stria (Gurdjian, 1925)***; pp. 140, 152, 160.
2. *bed nuclei of stria terminalis (Swanson et al., 1987)*
   Alternate form of ***bed nuclei of terminal stria (Gurdjian, 1925)*** for adult rat; p. 135, also see Ju & Swanson (1989, p. 587).

EARLIER REFERENCES:

Earlier synonyms:

1. *gray layer of taenia striata (Vicq d'Azyr, 1786)*
   Layer of *gray substance (Vesalius, 1543a)* around rostral (anterior) end of macrodissected adult human *taenia striata (Vicq d'Azyr 1786)*, or ***terminal stria (Wenzel & Wenzel, 1812)***, probably vague reference to ***bed nuclei of terminal stria (Gurdjian, 1925)***. Vicq d'Azyr also wrote that Tarin (1750) mentioned a semitransparent differentiation of horn-like color in this region of macrodissected adult human; Plates V-*o*, VI-32/33.
2. *horny layer of taenia striata (Vicq d'Azyr, 1786)*
   Synonym for *gray layer of taenia striata (Vicq d'Azyr, 1786)*; see Plates V-*o*, VI-32/33.
3. *tubercle of semicircular commissure (Serres, 1824–1826)*
   Gray substance (Vesalius, 1543a) mass in macrodissected adult human and monkey, probably corresponding to *gray layer of taenia striata (Vicq d'Azyr, 1786)*; in the original French, *tubercle de la commissure demi-circulaire, ou de la lame cornée*, Vol. 2, p. 464.

biventral lobule (>1840)

As described for macrodissected adult human, the part of the ***cerebellar hemisphere (Willis, 1664)*** between ***gracile lobule (>1840)*** and ***tonsil (Malacarne, 1776)***, and lateral to the ***pyramis (Malacarne, 1776)*** of the ***cerebellar vermis (Meckel, 1817)***; see Angevine et al. (1961, Fig. 24), Larsell & Jansen (1972, Figure 118), Carpenter (1976, Fig. 14.1), Williams & Warwick (1980, Fig. 7.74), *Terminologia Anatomica* (1998, p. 119), Nieuwenhuys et al. (2008, Fig. 20.2). On comparative anatomical grounds, Larsell & Jansen (1972, Fig. 118) called it the *ventral parafloccular lobule*. It was first described as the *biventral lobe (Malacarne, 1776)*.

EARLIER REFERENCES:

Earlier synonyms:

1. *biventral lobe (Malacarne, 1776)*
   Synonym for macrodissected adult human ***biventral lobule (>1840)***; p. 50, see Larsell & Jansen (1972, p. 52), Clarke & O'Malley (1996, p. 645).
2. *lateral lobule of inferior vermiform process (Vicq d'Azyr, 1784)*
   Synonym for macrodissected adult human ***biventral lobule (>1840)***; in the original French (plural), *lobules latérales du processus vermiforme inférieur*, p. 568.
3. *monticule of inferior vermiform process (Vicq d'Azyr, 1784)*
   Synonym for macrodissected adult human ***biventral lobule (>1840)***; in the original French (plural), *monticules du processus vermiforme inférieur*, p. 568. Vicq d'Azyr wrote that Haller (1762, p. 72) described this region well and used the singular term *colliculus*.
4. *lateral expansion of large part of inferior vermis (Vicq d'Azyr, 1784)*
   Synonym for macrodissected adult human ***biventral lobule (>1840)***; in the original French (plural), *expansions latérales de la grosse portion du vermis inferior*, p. 573 and Vicq d'Azyr (1786, Pl. XXX, Fig. 3-*16,17*).
5. *wing of large part of inferior vermis (Vicq d'Azyr, 1784)*
   Synonym for macrodissected adult human ***biventral lobule (>1840)***; in the original French (plural), *alies [alae in Latin] de la grosse portion du vermis inferior*, p. 573 and Vicq d'Azyr (1786, Pl. XXX, Fig. 3-*16,17*).
6. *inferior anterior lobe (Meckel, 1817)*
   Synonym for macrodissected adult human ***biventral lobule (>1840)***; p. 466, see (Burdach 1822, p. 295).
7. *cuneiform lobe (Meckel, 1817)*
   Synonym for macrodissected adult human ***biventral lobule (>1840)***; p. 466. Burdach (1822, p. 295) gave the Latin form, *lobus cuneiformis*.
8. *internal inferior lobe (Meckel, 1817)*
   Synonym for macrodissected adult human ***biventral lobule (>1840)***; see translation (1832, Vol. 2, p. 429).
9. *digastric lobe (Meckel, 1817)*
   Synonym for macrodissected adult human ***biventral lobule (>1840)***; see translation (1832, Vol. 2, p. 429)—*digastric* is a translation of the Latin *biventer*.

body of caudate nucleus (>1840)

As defined arbitrarily for macrodissected adult human, the middle segment of the ***caudate nucleus (Arnold, 1838b)*** between ***head of caudate nucleus (>1840)*** rostrodorsally and ***tail of caudate nucleus (Arnold, 1838b)*** caudoventrally; see Carpenter (1976, p. 497, Fig. 17.4). It was clearly illustrated by Vieussens; see ***[body of caudate nucleus (>1840)] (Vieussens, 1684).***

EARLIER REFERENCES:

Illustrated and described, not named:

1. ***[body of caudate nucleus (>1840)] (Vieussens, 1684)*** Clearly illustrated for macrodissected adult human; part of *striata corpora superna anteriora (Vieussens, 1684)* just to left of *F* in Table XIII, left side.

body of corpus callosum (Arnold, 1838a)

As described for macrodissected adult human, the main central part of the ***corpus callosum (Galen, c177)***, between ***genu of corpus callosum (Reil, 1809b)*** rostrally and ***splenium of corpus callosum (Burdach, 1822)*** caudally; see Mettler (1948, p. 100, Fig. 68). For Arnold's use in macrodissected adult human, see p. 76 (and p. 75). It was first clearly illustrated by Steno; see ***[body of corpus callosum (Arnold, 1838a)] (Steno, 1669).***

TRANSLATIONS:

1. *corpus corporis callosi (Arnold, 1838a)* Original Latin form of ***body of corpus callosum (Arnold, 1838a)***; p. 76.

EARLIER REFERENCES:

Illustrated, not named or described:

1. ***[body of corpus callosum (Arnold, 1838a)] (Steno, 1669)*** First clear indication of its shape, illustrated in midsagittal view of macrodissected adult human ***brain (Smith Papyrus, c1700 BC)***; Plate I.

Earlier synonyms:

1. *trunk of corpus callosum (Burdach, 1822)* Synonym for macrodissected adult human ***body of corpus callosum (Arnold, 1838a)***; in the original Latin, *truncus corporis callosi*, p. 141.
2. *middle part of corpus callosum (Spurzheim, 1826)* Synonym for macrodissected adult human ***body of corpus callosum (Arnold, 1838a)***; p. 231-*μ*.
3. *superior part of corpus callosum (Rolando, 1831)* Synonym for macrodissected adult human ***body of corpus callosum (Arnold, 1838a)***; in the original Italian, *parte superiore del corpo calloso*, Figure 2-*f*.

LATER SYNONYMS:

1. *body of great commissure (Arnold, 1838b)* Synonym for macrodissected adult human ***body of corpus callosum (Arnold, 1838a)***; in the original Latin, *corpus commissurae maximae*, Table VII, Fig. 2-*k*.

body of lateral ventricle (Bell, 1803b)

As described for macrodissected adult human, the part of the ***lateral ventricle (Vesalius, 1543a)*** between the level of the ***interventricular foramen (>1840)*** rostrally and the caudal end of the ***splenium of corpus callosum (Burdach, 1822)*** caudally; thus, it lies between ***anterior horn of lateral ventricle (Bell, 1803b)*** rostrally and ***atrium of lateral ventricle (>1840)*** caudally; see Millen & Woollam (1962, pp. 33–44, Figs. 13, 16), Carpenter & Sutin (1983, pp. 41–45, Fig. 2.20). If no ***posterior horn of lateral ventricle (Haller, 1747)*** is present, as in many other mammals, the ***body of lateral ventricle (Bell, 1803b)*** borders the ***inferior horn of lateral ventricle (Bell, 1802)*** at the level of the ***splenium of corpus callosum (Burdach, 1822)***; see Millen & Woollam (1962, pp. 33–44, Figs. 13, 16), *Terminologia Anatomica* (1998, p. 127). For Bell's use in macrodissected adult human, see p. 81. It was known generally to Galen; see ***[body of lateral ventricle (Bell, 1803b)] (Galen, c173).***

EARLIER REFERENCES:

Described, not named or illustrated:

1. ***[body of lateral ventricle (Bell, 1803b)] (Galen, c173)*** In *On the Usefulness of the Parts*, Galen referred to the part of the ***lateral ventricle (Vesalius, 1543a)*** adjacent to the *fornix (Galen, c177)*, roughly the ***body of lateral ventricle (Bell, 1803b)***; see May translation (1968, p. 416). He macrodissected adult beef, pig, and/or macaque but not human explicitly.

Earlier synonyms:

1. *hind recess of ventricle (Vesalius, 1543a)* Roughly synonymous with macrodissected adult human ***body of lateral ventricle (Bell, 1803b)***; see Singer translation (1952, p. 98 and Fig. 6).

LATER SYNONYMS:

1. *middle part of lateral ventricle (Meckel, 1817)* Synonym for *central part of lateral ventricle (Meckel, 1817)*; see translation (1832, Vol. 2, p. 463).
2. *central part of lateral ventricle (Meckel, 1817)* Synonym for macrodissected adult human ***body of lateral ventricle (Bell, 1803b)***; see translation (1832, Vol. 2, p. 463) and *Terminologia Anatomica* (1998, p. 127).

brachial plexus (Camper, 1760)

As described for macrodissected adult human, it is derived mainly from the ***spinal nerve ventral branches (>1840)*** of the 5th–8th ***cervical nerves (Galen, c173)*** and first ***thoracic nerve (Diemerbroeck, 1672)***; see Williams & Warwick (1980, Fig. 7.200). Variable contributions from the fourth ***cervical nerve (Galen, c173)*** and second ***thoracic nerve (Diemerbroeck, 1672)*** are also present in prefixed and postfixed patterns, respectively; see Kerr (1918, p. 298 ff.), Williams & Warwick (1980, p. 1094). As described by Schwalbe (1881, p. 915; also see Durward, 1951, Fig. 923) the adult human ***brachial plexus (Camper, 1760)*** is joined to the ***spinal cord (Galen, c162–c166)*** by ***brachial plexus roots (Schwalbe, 1881)*** and is then formed sequentially by ***brachial plexus trunks (Schwalbe, 1881), brachial plexus divisions (Paterson, 1887)***, and ***brachial plexus cords (Schwalbe, 1881)***, followed by the distal branches or *brachial nerves (Vesalius, 1543a)*. Kerr used the same plan with somewhat different terminology: trunks, branches, and fascicles, followed by the nerves (1928, p. 307 ff.). For Camper's use in macrodissected adult human, see p. 9; it was first described clearly as the *plexus of nerve pairs (Galen, c192)*.

TRANSLATIONS:

1. *plexus brachialis (Camper, 1760)* Original Latin form of ***brachial plexus (Camper, 1760)***; p. 9.

EARLIER REFERENCES:

Earlier synonyms:

1. *plexus of nerve pairs (Galen, c192)*
Synonym for ***brachial plexus (Camper, 1760)*** in macrodissected adult beef, pig, and/or macaque but not human; see Duckworth translation (1962, p. 244). Galen sensibly discussed differences between different types of animal, as well as between animals within a type; see Duckworth translation (1962, pp. 243–256) and May translation (1968, pp. 598–599). He wrote, "I have told previously about the nerves going to the arms, how they arise and are interwoven. I have also said that Nature creates such minglings of nerves for the sake of safety, and hence she takes care to do so particularly among those nerves that are unsupported or that must follow a long path." (May translation, 1968, p. 704). He also referred to the "long nerves which, beyond the plexus, extend to all these regions [of the arm]" (Duckworth translation, 1962, p. 243).
2. *plexus of nerves that enter arm (Vesalius, 1543a)*
Vesalius provided outstanding illustrations and detailed description of macrodissected adult human ***brachial plexus (Camper, 1760)***; Richardson & Carman translation (2002, p. 237 ff.). Eustachi (1552) also illustrated it beautifully for macrodissected adult human with a clear right-left asymmetry; see Albinus edition (1761, Tab. 18, Fig. 2-28).
3. *plexus in neck (Vesalius, 1543a)*
Synonym for macrodissected adult human ***brachial plexus (Camper, 1760)***; see Richardson & Carman translation (2002, p. 257).
4. *net-resembling fold under clavicle (Diemerbroeck, 1689)*
Synonym for macrodissected adult human ***brachial plexus (Camper, 1760)***; p. 561.
5. *axillary plexus (Salmon, 1714)*
Synonym for macrodissected adult human ***brachial plexus (Camper, 1760)***; p. 125.
6. *great plexus (Winslow, 1733)*
Synonym for macrodissected adult human ***brachial plexus (Camper, 1760)***; Section VI, p. 80.
7. *cervicobrachial plexus (Portal, 1803b)*
Synonym for macrodissected adult human ***brachial plexus (Camper, 1760)***; in the original French, *plexus cervico-brachial*, Vol. 4, p. 239.

PARTLY CORRESPONDS:

1. *brachial nerve (Vesalius, 1543a)*
In macrodissected adult human, general term for a ***nerve (Herophilus, c335–c280 BC)*** of the arm after emerging distally from the ***brachial plexus (Camper, 1760)***; in the original Latin, *nervorum brachii*; see Richardson & Carman (2002, p. 237). Galen clearly described them for macrodissected adult beef, pig, and/or macaque but not human, referring to the "long nerves which, beyond the [brachial] plexus, extend to all these regions [of the arm]" (Duckworth translation, 1962, p. 243).
2. *nerves to arm (Vesalius, 1543a)*
Set of *brachial nerves (Vesalius, 1543a)* for macrodissected adult human; in the original Latin, *nervi in brachium*; see Richardson & Carman translation (2002, p. 238).
3. *nerves to hand (Bauhin, 1605)*
Synonym for macrodissected adult human *nerves to arm (Vesalius, 1543a)*; see Crooke translation (1615, p. 900 ff.).
4. *subclavian nerves (Cheselden, 1713)*
In an obscure unillustrated section (p. 143) it is stated that macrodissected adult human *subclavian nerves (Cheselden, 1713)* arise from 5th cervical to 1st thoracic ***spinal nerves (Camper, 1760–1762)*** and have three branches—*inferior cubital nerve (Cheselden, 1713)*, *superior cubital nerve (Cheselden, 1713)*, and *nervus perforans (Cheselden, 1713)*— which possibly correspond to ***ulnar nerve (Cheselden, 1726)***, ***median nerve (Du Verney, 1697)***, and ***muscular branches of musculocutaneous nerve (Günther, 1786)***, respectively. Also see similar description in Cheselden (1722, p. 209).
5. *axillary nerve (Cheselden, 1713)*
Synonym for macrodissected adult human *subclavian nerves (Cheselden, 1713)*; p. 143, also see similar passage in Cheselden (1722, p. 209).
6. *axillary nerves (Salmon, 1714)*
Synonym for macrodissected adult human *nerves to arm (Vesalius, 1543a)*; p. 129.
7. *external thoracic nerves (Monro, 1783)*
Appears in macrodissected adult human to indicate as a group the ***long thoracic nerve (Quain & Wilson, 1839)***, ***upper subscapular nerve (>1840)***, ***thoracodorsal nerve (>1840)***, and ***lower subscapular nerve (>1840)***; see Table 16- 27, and also Table 15-21.
8. *scapular nerves (Günther, 1786)*
Macrodissected adult human ***lower subscapular nerve (>1840)*** and ***suprascapular nerve (Bang, 1770)*** considered together; in the original Latin, *nervi scapulares*, p. 73.
9. *posterior thoracic nerves (Günther, 1786)*
Macrodissected adult human ***long thoracic nerve (Quain & Wilson, 1839)*** and ***thoracodorsal nerve (>1840)*** considered together; in the original Latin, *nervi thoracici posteriores*, p. 73.
10. *anterior brachial plexus (Günther, 1786)*
For macrodissected adult human, included ***musculocutaneous nerve (Du Verney, 1697)***, ***median nerve (Du Verney, 1697)***, ***ulnar nerve (Cheselden, 1726)***, ***medial cutaneous nerve of forearm (>1840)***, and ***medial cutaneous nerve of arm (>1840)*** considered together; in the original Latin, *plexus brachialis anterior*, p. 73.
11. *superior brachial plexus (Günther, 1786)*
Synonym for *anterior brachial plexus (Günther, 1786)*; in the original Latin, *plexus brachialis superior*, p. 73.
12. *major brachial plexus (Günther, 1786)*
Synonym for *anterior brachial plexus (Günther, 1786)*; in the original Latin, *plexus brachialis major*, p. 73.
13. *thoracic nerves (Soemmerring, 1791)*
Probably synonymous with macrodissected adult human *external thoracic nerves (Monro, 1783)*; in the original Latin, *nervi thoracici*, p. 279.

14. *nervi extremitatis superioris (Meckel, 1817)*
Synonym for macrodissected adult human *brachial nerves (Vesalius, 1543a)*; see translation (1832, Vol. 3, p. 22).
15. *thoracic nerves (Quain, 1828)*
For macrodissected adult human, apparently three ***nerves (Herophilus, c335–c280 BC)*** considered together: ***long thoracic nerve (Quain & Wilson, 1839)***, ***medial pectoral nerve (>1840)***, and ***lateral pectoral nerve (>1840)***; pp. 417–418.
16. *anastomosis between fourth and fifth cervical nerve (Cloquet, 1828)*
In macrodissected adult human, ***communicating branch (Winslow, 1733)*** between fourth and fifth cervical ***brachial plexus roots (Schwalbe, 1881)***; in the original French, *anastomose entre le quatrième et le cinquième nerf cervical*, Plate CLX, Figure 2-56. See Durward (1951, Fig. 924), Williams & Warwick (1980, Fig. 7.200).

brachial plexus cords (Schwalbe, 1881)

As described for the macrodissected adult human ***brachial plexus (Camper, 1760)***, three ***brachial plexus ventral divisions (Paterson, 1887)*** and three ***brachial plexus dorsal divisions (Paterson, 1887)*** usually recombine distally to form three ***brachial plexus cords (Schwalbe, 1881)***: the ***brachial plexus lateral cord (Paterson, 1887)***, ***brachial plexus dorsal cord (Paterson, 1887)***, and ***brachial plexus medial cord (Schwalbe, 1881)***, which in turn generate the *brachial nerves (Vesalius, 1543a)*. Schwalbe (1881, p. 915) referred to three cords: external, posterior, and medial; Paterson (1887, p. 621) referred to [lateral and medial] ventral and dorsal cords; Kerr (1918, pp. 309–312) referred to lateral, posterior, and medial fasciculi; and Durward (1951, Fig. 923) referred to lateral, posterior, and medial cords. For Schwalbe's use in macrodissected adult human, see p. 915 where *cords* in the original German was *Stränge*. They were known to Galen; see ***[brachial plexus cords (Schwalbe, 1881)] (Galen, c192)***.

EARLIER REFERENCES:

Described, not named or illustrated:

1. ***[brachial plexus cords (Schwalbe, 1881)] (Galen, c192)***
Described for macrodissected adult beef, pig, and/or macaque but not human; see Duckworth translation (1962, pp. 247–248, 251–253). Meckel (1817) also vaguely described them for macrodissected adult human; see translation (1832, Vol. 3, pp. 23–24).

Illustrated, not named or described:

1. ***[brachial plexus cords (Schwalbe, 1881)] (Vesalius, 1543a)***
Vesalius indicated the ***brachial plexus lateral cord (Schwalbe, 1881)*** and ***brachial plexus dorsal cord (Paterson, 1887)*** in his illustrations, which are difficult to interpret because he only showed one of the usual six ***brachial plexus divisions (Paterson, 1887)***; see Richardson & Carman translation (2002, p. 237). Eustachi (1552) illustrated the three cords much more clearly, including three variations; see Albinus edition (1761, Tabs. 18, 19).

PARTLY CORRESPONDS:

1. *thoracic nerves of axillary plexus (Bell, 1803b)*
Included macrodissected adult ***thoracodorsal nerve (>1840)***, ***lateral pectoral nerve (>1840)***, and ***medial pectoral nerve (>1840)***, and related cutaneous ***nerves (Herophilus, c335–c280 BC)***; pp. 188–189.
2. *communicating arch between dorsal branches of radial and cubital nerves (Loder, 1803)*
Synonym for macrodissected adult human *dorsal arch of hand (Meckel, 1817)*; in the original Latin, *arcus communicans inter ramum dorsalem nervi radialis et ramum dorsalem nervi cubitalis*; Table CLXXVIII, Figure 2-74.
3. *volar plexus (Caldani, 1813, 1814)*
Macrodissected adult human network of ***communicating branches (Winslow, 1733)*** between ***lateral cutaneous nerve of forearm (>1840)*** and ***palmar branch of median nerve (Bock, 1827)*** in palm of hand; in the original Latin, *plexus volaris*, Table CCLIX, Figure 1-24.
4. *nervous ungual arch of thumb (Caldani, 1813, 1814)*
Macrodissected adult human network of ***communicating branches (Winslow, 1733)*** at tip of thumb from corresponding ***dorsal digital nerves of radial nerve (>1840)*** and ***proper palmar digital nerves of median nerve (>1840)***; in the original Latin, *arcus unguicularis nervosus pollicis*, Table CCLIX, Figure 2-14.
5. *nervous ungual arch of index finger (Caldani, 1813, 1814)*
Macrodissected adult human network of ***communicating branches (Winslow, 1733)*** at tip of index finger from corresponding ***dorsal digital nerves of radial nerve (>1840)*** and ***proper palmar digital nerves of median nerve (>1840)***; in the original Latin, *arcus unguicularis nervosus indicis*, Table CCLIX, Figure 2-21.
6. *anterior thoracic nerves (Meckel, 1817)*
Probably included macrodissected adult human ***medial pectoral nerve (>1840)*** and ***lateral pectoral nerve (>1840)***; see translation (1832, Vol. 3, p. 24).
7. *dorsal arch of hand (Meckel, 1817)*
Described for macrodissected adult human as consisting of terminal ramifications of ***superficial branch of radial nerve (Martin, 1781)*** communicating with terminal branches of ***ulnar nerve (Cheselden, 1726)*** and ***communicating branch of radial nerve with ulnar nerve (>1840)***; see translation (1832, Vol. 3, p. 26).
8. *dorsal digital nerves (Bock, 1827)*
Macrodissected adult human dorsal digital ***nerves (Herophilus, c335–c280 BC)*** of hand, including ***dorsal digital nerves of radial nerve (>1840)*** and ***dorsal digital nerves of ulnar nerve (>1840)***; in the original Latin, *nervi digitales dorsales*, Table IV-42.
9. *thoracic branches of brachial plexus (Cruveilhier, 1836)*
Synonym for macrodissected adult human ***lateral pectoral nerve (>1840)*** and ***medial pectoral nerve (>1840)*** considered together; in the original French, *branches thoraciques du plexus brachial*, p. 794.
10. *branch of communication of posterior branch of internal cutaneous nerve with radial cutaneous nerve (Quain & Wilson, 1839)*

Macrodissected adult human ***communicating branch (Winslow, 1733)*** between ***posterior branch of medial cutaneous nerve of forearm (>1840)*** and ***posterior cutaneous nerve of forearm (>1840)***; Plate XIX, Figure 1-*c*.

brachial plexus divisions (Paterson, 1887)

As described for the macrodissected adult human ***brachial plexus (Camper, 1760)***, three ***brachial plexus trunks (Schwalbe, 1881)*** each generate distally a ventral and a dorsal division, thus forming three ***brachial plexus ventral divisions (Paterson, 1887)*** and three ***brachial plexus dorsal divisions (Paterson, 1887)***—which then recombine to form three ***brachial plexus cords (Schwalbe, 1881)***, in the most usual pattern; see Kerr (1918, p. 307 ff.), Durward (1951, p. 1115 and Fig. 923), Williams & Warwick (1980, p. 1095). For Patterson's use in macrodissected adult human, see p. 621. They were known to Galen; see ***[brachial plexus divisions (Paterson, 1887)] (Galen, c192)***.

EARLIER REFERENCES:

Described, not named or illustrated:

1. ***[brachial plexus divisions (Paterson, 1887)] (Galen, c192)***
   Galen described but did not name systematically all six divisions for macrodissected adult beef, pig, and/or macaque but not human, and even referred to those from the ***brachial plexus upper trunk (>1840)*** and ***brachial plexus middle trunk (>1840)*** as *divisions*; see Duckworth translation (1962, pp. 245, 247–248, 252–253). Meckel (1817) described all six divisions for macrodissected adult human although they were not named systematically; see translation (1832, Vol. 3, p. 23).

Illustrated and described, not named:

1. ***[brachial plexus divisions (Paterson, 1887)] (Vesalius, 1543a)***
   Vesalius did a poor job with them, illustrating only dorsal division of ***brachial plexus lower trunk (>1840)***; see Richardson & Carman translation (2002, p. 237, part *M* of the figure).

Illustrated, not named or described:

1. ***[brachial plexus divisions (Paterson, 1887)] (Eustachi, 1552)***
   Eustachi did a much better job than Vesalius (1543a) in illustrating all six for macrodissected adult human, including three different variations; see Albinus edition (1761, Tabs. 18, 19).

Earlier synonyms:

1. *primary divisions of axillary plexus (Quain, 1828)*
   For macrodissected adult human, Quain accurately described all six ***brachial plexus divisions (Paterson, 1887)***; pp. 415–416.
2. *primary divisions of brachial plexus (Quain, 1828)*
   For macrodissected adult human, Quain accurately described all six ***brachial plexus divisions (Paterson, 1887)***; pp. 415–416.

brachial plexus dorsal cord (Paterson, 1887)

As described for macrodissected adult human, it arises from the three upper ***brachial plexus dorsal divisions (Paterson, 1887)*** and in turn generates the ***radial nerve (Du Verney, 1697)*** and ***axillary nerve (Winslow, 1733)***; it supplies extensor muscles. See Durward (1951, Figs. 923, 924), Williams & Warwick (1980, p. 1095). For Paterson's use in macrodissected adult human, see p. 621. It was known to Galen; see ***[brachial plexus dorsal cord (Paterson, 1887)] (Galen, c192)***.

EARLIER REFERENCES:

Described, not named or illustrated:

1. ***[brachial plexus dorsal cord (Paterson, 1887)] (Galen, c192)***
   Referred to for macrodissected adult beef, pig, and/or macaque but not human; see Duckworth translation (1962, p. 247). Meckel (1817) vaguely described it for macrodissected adult human in terms of a small trunk; see translation (1832, Vol. 3, p. 23).

Illustrated, not named or described:

1. ***[brachial plexus dorsal cord (Paterson, 1887)] (Vesalius, 1543a)***
   Vesalius illustrated it clearly for macrodissected adult human, although his view of ***brachial plexus (Camper, 1760)*** is difficult to interpret because he only showed one of the usual six ***brachial plexus divisions (Paterson, 1887)***; see Richardson & Carman translation (2002, p. 237, part *D* of the figure).

Earlier synonyms:

1. *large cord formed by great part of fourth and fifth cervicals (Monro, 1783)*
   Based on little description and good for the time illustration, probably indicates macrodissected adult human ***brachial plexus dorsal cord (Peterson, 1887)***, primarily because it generates the ***radial nerve (Du Verney, 1697)*** and ***axillary nerve (Winslow, 1733)***; Table 16-*16*. Monro followed *cervical nerves (Vesalius, 1543a)*.

PARTLY CORRESPONDS:

1. *scapular nerve (Du Verney, 1697)*
   According to Camper (1760, p. 9), Du Verney originated this term for macrodissected adult human, probably corresponding to Camper's description of ***upper subscapular nerve (>1840)*** and ***lower subscapular nerve (>1840)*** considered together; also see *scapular nerve (Monro, 1732)* and Winslow (1733, Sect. VI, pp. 79–81).
2. *posterior brachial plexus (Günther, 1786)*
   Main part of macrodissected adult human ***brachial plexus dorsal cord (Paterson, 1887)*** with ***radial nerve (Du Verney, 1697)*** and ***axillary nerve (Winslow, 1733)*** considered together; in the original Latin, *plexus brachialis posterior*, p. 78.
3. *inferior brachial plexus (Günther, 1786)*
   Synonym for *posterior brachial plexus (Günther, 1786)*; in the original Latin, *plexus brachialis inferior*, p. 78.
4. *minor brachial plexus (Günther, 1786)*
   Synonym for *posterior brachial plexus (Günther, 1786)*; in the original Latin, *plexus brachialis minor*, p. 78.

5. *infrascapular nerve (Mayer, 1794)*
   Probably synonym for macrodissected adult human *scapular nerve (Du Verney, 1697)*; in the original Latin, *nervus infrascapularis*; Part 5, Table V, Figure 1-*G*.
6. *subscapular nerve (Mayer, 1794)*
   Probably synonym for macrodissected adult human *scapular nerve (Du Verney, 1697)*; in the original Latin, *nervus infrascapularis*; Part 5, Table V, Figure 1-*G*.
7. *subscapular nerves (Bell, 1803a)*
   Synonym for macrodissected adult human *scapular nerve (Du Verney, 1697)*; Plate V-7.
8. *sub-scapulary nerves (Burdin, 1803)*
   Probably corresponds to ***upper subscapular nerve (>1840), thoracodorsal nerve (>1840)***, and ***lower subscapular nerve (>1840)*** considered together; see translation (1803, Vol. 3, p. 191).
9. *middle subscapular nerve (Bock, 1827)*
   Probably synonym for macrodissected adult human *scapular nerve (Du Verney, 1697)*; in the original Latin, *nervus subscapularis medius*; Table II-23. Also see *inferior subscapular nerve (Bock, 1827)*.
10. *sub-scapular nerves (Quain, 1832)*
   Synonym for macrodissected adult human *sub-scapulary nerves (Burdin, 1803)*; p. 682.

brachial plexus dorsal divisions (Paterson, 1887)

As described for the macrodissected adult human ***brachial plexus (Camper, 1760)***, the three ***brachial plexus trunks (Schwalbe, 1881)*** each generate a ventral and a dorsal division, thus forming three ***brachial plexus ventral divisions (Paterson, 1887)*** and three ***brachial plexus dorsal divisions (Paterson, 1887)***—which then recombine to form three ***brachial plexus cords (Schwalbe, 1881)***, in the most common pattern. Thus, there are upper, middle, and lower dorsal divisions. The dorsal divisions supply extensor muscles; see Kerr (1918, p. 307 ff.), Durward (1951, p. 1115 and Fig. 923), Williams & Warwick (1980, p. 1095). For Paterson's use in macrodissected adult human, see p. 621. They were known to Galen; see ***[brachial plexus dorsal divisions (Paterson, 1887)] (Galen, c192)***.

EARLIER REFERENCES:

Described, not named or illustrated:

1. ***[brachial plexus dorsal divisions (Paterson, 1887)] (Galen, c192)***
   Galen described but did not name all three dorsal divisions for macrodissected adult beef, pig, and/or macaque but not human—even referring to those from ***brachial plexus upper trunk (>1840)*** and ***brachial plexus middle trunk (>1840)*** as *divisions*; see Duckworth translation (1962, pp. 245, 247–248, 252–253). Meckel (1817) described for macrodissected adult human the three ***brachial plexus dorsal divisions (Paterson, 1887)*** without systematically naming them; see translation (1832, Vol. 3, p. 23).

Illustrated, not named or described:

1. ***[brachial plexus dorsal divisions (Paterson, 1887)] (Vesalius, 1543a)***
   Vesalius only illustrated (but did not name) dorsal division of ***brachial plexus lower trunk (>1840)*** for macrodissected adult human; see Richardson and Carman translation (2002, p. 237, part *E* in the figure).
2. ***[brachial plexus dorsal divisions (Paterson, 1887)] (Eustachi, 1552)***
   Eustachi illustrated all three for macrodissected adult human, including variations; see Albinus edition (1761, Tabs. 18, 19).

Earlier synonyms:

1. *posterior set of primary divisions of brachial plexus (Quain, 1828)*
   For macrodissected adult human, three ***brachial plexus dorsal divisions (Paterson, 1887)***; p. 415.

brachial plexus lateral cord (Schwalbe, 1881)

As described for macrodissected adult human, it arises distally from the two rostral ***brachial plexus ventral divisions (Paterson, 1887)*** and in turn generates the ***lateral pectoral nerve (>1840), musculocutaneous nerve (Du Verney, 1697)***, and ***lateral root of median nerve (>1840)***. It and the ***brachial plexus medial cord (Schwalbe, 1887)*** form two ventral ***brachial plexus cords (Schwalbe, 1881)*** supplying flexor muscles; see Paterson (1887, p. 621), Durward (1951, Figs. 923, 924), Williams & Warwick (1980, p. 1095). For Schwalbe's use in macrodissected adult human see p. 915, where *lateral cord* in the original German was *lateraler Strang*. It was known to Galen; see ***[brachial plexus lateral cord (Schwalbe, 1887)] (Galen, c192)***.

EARLIER REFERENCES:

Described, not named or illustrated:

1. ***[brachial plexus lateral cord (Schwalbe, 1887)] (Galen, c192)***
   Galen described clearly its formation in macrodissected adult beef, pig, and/or macaque but not human; see Duckworth translation (1962, p. 248). Meckel (1817) vaguely described it for macrodissected adult human in terms of a more or less complicated ***brachial plexus (Camper, 1760)***; see translation (1832, Vol. 3, p. 23) and Durward (1951, Fig. 924).

Illustrated, not named or described:

1. ***[brachial plexus lateral cord (Schwalbe, 1887)] (Vesalius, 1543a)***
   Vesalius indicated it in illustrations of macrodissected adult human, which are difficult to interpret because he only showed one of the usual six ***brachial plexus divisions (Paterson, 1887)***; see Richardson & Carman translation (2002, p. 237). Eustachi (1552) illustrated it much more clearly for macrodissected adult human, including three variations; see Albinus edition (1761, Tabs. 18, 19).

Earlier synonyms:

1. *large cord formed by all five undermost cervical nerves (Monro, 1783)*
   May indicate macrodissected adult human ***brachial plexus lateral cord (Schwalbe, 1887)*** because

it generates ***musculocutaneous nerve (Du Verney, 1697)***; Table 16–22.

brachial plexus lower trunk (>1840)

As described for macrodissected adult human, it is formed by the distal merging of the caudal two (8th cervical and 1st thoracic) ***brachial plexus roots (Schwalbe, 1881)***; see Durward (1951, Fig. 923). It was known to Galen; see ***[brachial plexus lower trunk (>1840)] (Galen, c192)***.

EARLIER REFERENCES:

Described, not named or illustrated:

1. ***[brachial plexus lower trunk (>1840)] (Galen, c192)***
Clearly described for macrodissected adult beef, pig, and/or macaque but not human; see Duckworth translation (1962, pp. 251–252), "This nerve [1st ***thoracic nerve (Diemerbroeck, 1672)***] blends and unites with that other one [8th ***cervical nerve (Galen, c173)***]. The unified nerve [***brachial plexus lower trunk (>1840)***] which is formed from both these two, after it has gone forward a little way, divides again, and unites with those ones which are higher than it and which originate from the sixth pair [***brachial plexus dorsal cord (Paterson, 1887)***]..." Vesalius (1543a) illustrated it for macrodissected adult human; see Richardson & Carman translation (2002, p. 237).

Earlier synonyms:

1. *common trunk formed by union of eighth cervical and first dorsal nerve (Meckel, 1817)*
Refers at least partly to macrodissected adult human ***brachial plexus lower trunk (>1840)***; see translation (1832, Vol. 3, p. 23).

brachial plexus medial cord (Schwalbe, 1881)

As described for macrodissected adult human, a continuation of the lower ***brachial plexus ventral division (Paterson, 1887)*** distally generating the ***medial pectoral nerve (>1840), medial cutaneous nerve of arm (>1840), medial cutaneous nerve of forearm (>1840), ulnar nerve (Cheselden, 1726)***, and ***medial root of median nerve (>1840)***. It and the ***brachial plexus lateral cord (Schwalbe, 1887)*** form two ventral cords supplying flexor muscles; see Paterson (1887, p. 621), Durward (1951, Figs. 923, 924), Williams & Warwick (1980, p. 1095). For Schwalbe's use in macrodissected adult human see p. 915, where *medial cord* in the original German was *medialer Strang*. It was first delineated clearly by Eustachi; see ***[brachial plexus medial cord (Schwalbe, 1881)] (Eustachi, 1552)***.

EARLIER REFERENCES:

Illustrated, not named or described:

1. ***[brachial plexus medial cord (Schwalbe, 1881)] (Eustachi, 1552)***
Illustrated for macrodissected adult human, including three variations; see Albinus edition (1761, Tabs. 18, 19).

Described, not named or illustrated:

1. ***[brachial plexus medial cord (Schwalbe, 1881)] (Meckel, 1817)***
Vaguely described for macrodissected adult human as part of a common trunk; see translation (1832, Vol. 3, p. 23).

PARTLY CORRESPONDS:

1. *sixth nerve entering arm (Vesalius, 1543a)*
For macrodissected adult human, ***medial cutaneous nerve of arm (>1840)*** and ***medial cutaneous nerve of forearm (>1840)*** considered together; see Richardson & Carman translation (2002, p. 246) and *subcutaneous nerve (Vesling, 1647)*.
2. *sixth sinew pertaining to arm (Geminus, 1553)*
Synonym for macrodissected adult human *sixth nerve entering arm (Vesalius, 1543a)*; originally spelled *syxte synowe pertayninge to arme*, see *The table of the figures of synowes*.
3. *sixth nerve of hand (Bauhin, 1605)*
Synonym for macrodissected adult human *sixth nerve entering arm (Vesalius, 1543a)*; see Crooke translation (1615, p. 903).
4. *subcutaneous nerve (Vesling, 1647)*
Synonym for macrodissected adult human *sixth nerve entering arm (Vesalius, 1543a)*; see Table 3 of Chapter 14, Figure V-*H*.
5. *internal cutaneous nerve (Schaarschmidt, 1750)*
Apparently, synonym for macrodissected adult human *sixth nerve entering arm (Vesalius, 1543a)*; in the original Latin, *nervus cutaneus internus*, p. 70.
6. *chiasma Camperi (Günther, 1786)*
Branches of macrodissected adult human ***brachial plexus (Camper, 1760)*** relating ***median nerve (Du Verney, 1697)*** and ***ulnar nerve (Cheselden, 1726)***, but not generally recognized today; p. 74. For contemporary illustrations see Camper (1760, Table I, Figure I), Mayer (1794, Part 5, Table V, Figure 2, and p. 28), Loder (1803, Table CLXXVIII-49).
7. *chiasm of Camper (Günther, 1786)*
English form of *chiasma Camperi (Günther, 1786)*.
8. *superficial volar arch (Mayer, 1794)*
communicating branch (Winslow, 1733) between ***superficial branch of ulnar nerve (Fyfe, 1800)*** and a ***common palmar digital nerve of median nerve (>1840)***; in the original Latin, *arcus superficialis volaris*, Part 5, Table III, Figure 1-5. Also see *superficial palmar arch (Meckel, 1817)*.
9. *chiasm (Loder, 1803)*
Shortened form of *chiasm of Camper (Günther, 1786)*; in the original Latin, *chiasma*, Table CLXXVII-*144*.
10. *great anastomotic branch between median and cubital nerves (Loder, 1803)*
Synonym for macrodissected adult human *superficial volar arch (Mayer, 1794)*; in the original Latin, *ramus anastomoticus magnus inter nervuum medianum et cubitalem*, Table CLXXX, Figure 1-*84*.
11. *volar neural arch of hand (Loder, 1803)*
Synonym for macrodissected adult human *superficial volar arch (Mayer, 1794)*; in the original Latin, *arcum nervosum volarem manus*, Table CLXXX, Figure 1-*84*.

12. *cubito-cutaneous nerve (Burdin, 1803)*
Synonym for macrodissected adult human *sixth nerve entering arm (Vesalius, 1543a)*; see Vol. 1, p. 192. Also see Cloquet (1816, p. 644) and Meckel (1832, Vol. 3, p. 29), neither of whom provided citations but refer to Chaussier, the source of Burdin's terminology.
13. *anastomotic nerve with second common digital branch of median nerve and ulnar volar nerve of fourth finger (Caldani, 1813, 1814)*
For macrodissected adult human, ***communicating branch (Winslow, 1733)*** between most lateral ***common palmar digital nerve of median nerve (>1840)*** and *ulnar volar nerve of fourth finger (Caldani, 1813, 1814)*; in the original Latin, *nervus anastomoticus cum ramo secundo [sic] digitali nervi mediani et cum nervus ulnaris volaris quarti digiti*, Table CCLIX, Figure 2-30.
14. *internal cutaneous nerve of arm (Cloquet, 1816)*
Synonym for macrodissected adult human *sixth nerve entering arm (Vesalius, 1543a)*; in the original French, *nerf brachial cutané interne*, p. 644.
15. *superficial palmar arch (Meckel, 1817)*
Described for macrodissected adult human hand as resulting from union of filament from ***superficial branch of ulnar nerve (Fyfe, 1800)*** with *cubito-palmar nerve of third finger (Meckel, 1817)*; see translation (1832, Vol. 3, p. 28) and Durward (1951, Fig. 931).

brachial plexus middle trunk (>1840)

As described for macrodissected adult human, arbitrarily defined as roughly the distal half of the seventh cervical ***brachial plexus root (Schwalbe, 1881)*** to complement the ***brachial plexus upper trunk (>1840)*** and ***brachial plexus lower trunk (>1840)***. It divides to form the ***brachial plexus ventral division (Paterson, 1887)*** and ***brachial plexus dorsal division (Paterson, 1887)***; see Durward (1951, Fig. 923). It was clearly delineated by Vesalius; see ***[brachial plexus middle trunk (>1840)] (Vesalius, 1543a)***.

EARLIER REFERENCES:

Illustrated and described, not named:

1. ***[brachial plexus middle trunk (>1840)] (Vesalius, 1543a)***
Vesalius clearly illustrated and described it for macrodissected adult human, pointing out that the configuration of ***brachial plexus (Camper, 1760)*** is quite variable between cadavers; see Richardson & Carman translation (2002, p. 237).

brachial plexus roots (Schwalbe, 1881)

As described for macrodissected adult human, the ***spinal nerve ventral branches (>1840)*** for the 5th–8th ***cervical nerves (Galen, c173)*** and the first ***thoracic nerve (Diemerbroeck, 1672)*** considered together, proximal to the ***brachial plexus trunks (Schwalbe, 1881)***; *roots* in the original German was *Wurzelin* (Fig. 471). For modern descriptions see Durward (1951, p. 1068 and Fig. 923), Williams & Warwick (1950, p. 1096). They were first described by Galen; see *root of nerves (Galen, c173)*.

EARLIER REFERENCES:

Earlier synonyms:

1. *root of nerves (Galen, c173)*
In this context Galen described ***brachial plexus roots (Schwalbe, 1881)*** of macrodissected adult beef, pig, and/or macaque but not human; see May translation (1968, p. 598). Vesalius (1543a) used the same basic terminology for macrodissected adult human; see Richardson & Carman translation (2002, p. 237).
2. *brachial nerves (Camper, 1760)*
Synonym for macrodissected adult human ***brachial plexus roots (Schwalbe, 1881)***; in the original Latin, *nervi brachiales*; p. 9 and Table 1, Figure 1:*a–e*.
3. *anterior branches of superior dorsal and four inferior cervical nerves (Meckel, 1817)*
Synonym for macrodissected adult human ***brachial plexus roots (Schwalbe, 1881)***; see translation (1832, Vol. 3, p. 23).

brachial plexus trunks (Schwalbe, 1881)

As described for the macrodissected adult human ***brachial plexus (Camper, 1760)***, the five ***brachial plexus roots (Schwalbe, 1881)*** merge distally into three trunks, each in turn dividing into ventral (lateral and medial) and dorsal ***brachial plexus divisions (Paterson, 1887)***; p. 915. Schwalbe (p. 915) referred to superior, middle, and inferior trunks, Kerr (1928, pp. 307–309) referred to cephalic, intermediate, and caudal trunks, and Durward (1951, Fig. 923) referred to upper, middle, and lower trunks. They were known to Galen; see ***[brachial plexus trunks (Schwalbe, 1881)] (Galen, c192)***.

EARLIER REFERENCES:

Described, not named or illustrated:

1. ***[brachial plexus trunks (Schwalbe, 1881)] (Galen, c192)***
Clearly described for macrodissected adult beef, pig, and/or macaque but not human; see Duckworth translation (1961, pp. 245–252).

Illustrated and described, not named:

1. ***[brachial plexus trunks (Schwalbe, 1881)] (Vesalius, 1543a)***
Illustrated for macrodissected adult human, although description not as clear as Galen's; see Richardson & Carman translation (2002, p. 237).

PARTLY CORRESPONDS:

1. *common trunks of great plexus (Winslow, 1733)*
Winslow referred to macrodissected adult human ***brachial plexus upper trunk (>1840)*** and ***brachial plexus lower trunk (>1840)*** individually as common trunks of corresponding ***brachial plexus roots (Schwalbe, 1881)***; Section VI, p. 80. He also referred to "the single Trunk of the 6th [7th ***cervical nerve (Galen, c173)***] Pair" (Sect. VI, p. 84), thus calling all three "trunks".
2. *common trunks of brachial plexus (Meckel, 1817)*
Meckel referred to macrodissected adult human ***brachial plexus upper trunk (>1840)*** and ***brachial plexus lower trunk (>1840)*** individually as common trunks of

corresponding ***brachial plexus roots (Schwalbe, 1881)***; see translation (1832, Vol. 3, p. 23).

brachial plexus upper trunk (>1840)

As described for macrodissected adult human, formed by merging of the rostral two (5th and 6th cervical) ***brachial plexus roots (Schwalbe, 1881)***; see Durward (1951, Fig. 923). It was known to Galen, see ***[brachial plexus upper trunk (>1840)] (Galen, c192)***.

EARLIER REFERENCES:

Described, not named or illustrated:

1. ***[brachial plexus upper trunk (>1840)] (Galen, c192)***
   Mentioned for macrodissected adult beef, pig, and/or macaque but not human: "...the one [***nerve (Herophilus, c335–c280 BC)***, that is, ***brachial plexus upper trunk (>1840)***] which originates from the junction of the two nerves which we mentioned [the 5th and 6th ***cervical nerves (Galen, c173)***]..." (Duckworth translation, 1962, p. 245). He described its three distal branches very accurately (Duckworth translation, 1962, pp. 245–251), just as illustrated by Williams & Warwick (1980, Fig. 7.200). Vesalius (1543a) illustrated ***brachial plexus upper trunk (>1840)***, but not its three distal branches, for macrodissected adult human; see Richardson & Carman translation (2002, p. 237).

Earlier synonyms:

1. *trunk formed by fourth and fifth subcervicals (Monro, 1783)*
   Synonym for macrodissected adult human ***brachial plexus upper trunk (>1840)***; Monro's numbering of cervical ***spinal nerve ventral branches (>1840)*** was one less than currently used, following *cervical nerves (Vesalius, 1543a)*, and he noted that this trunk also receives a small thread from third *subcervical nerve (Monro, 1783)*; Table 15-*10*. It was referred to as "large cord" in the next Table (16-*16*).
2. *common trunk formed by union of fifth and sixth cervical nerves (Meckel, 1817)*
   Synonym for macrodissected adult human ***brachial plexus upper trunk (>1840)***; see translation (1832, Vol. 3, p. 23).
3. *trunk formed by union of fifth and sixth cervical nerves (Meckel, 1817)*
   Synonym for macrodissected adult human ***brachial plexus upper trunk (>1840)***; see translation (1832, Vol. 3, p. 23).

brachial plexus ventral divisions (Paterson, 1887)

As described for the macrodissected adult human ***brachial plexus (Camper, 1760)***, the three ***brachial plexus trunks (Schwalbe, 1881)*** each generate a ventral and a dorsal division, thus forming three ***brachial plexus ventral divisions (Paterson, 1887)*** and three ***brachial plexus dorsal divisions (Paterson, 1887)***—which then recombine to form three ***brachial plexus cords (Schwalbe, 1881)***, in the most common pattern. Thus, there are upper, middle, and lower ventral divisions, which supply flexor muscles; see Kerr (1918, p. 307 ff.), Durward (1951, p. 1115 and Fig. 923), Williams & Warwick (1980, p. 1095). For Paterson's use in macrodissected adult human, see p. 621. They were known to Galen; see ***[brachial plexus ventral divisions (Paterson, 1887)] (Galen, c192)***.

EARLIER REFERENCES:

Described, not named or illustrated:

1. ***[brachial plexus ventral divisions (Paterson, 1887)] (Galen, c192)***
   Galen described but did not name all three ventral divisions for macrodissected adult beef, pig, and/or macaque but not human—even referring to those from ***brachial plexus upper trunk (>1840)*** and ***brachial plexus middle trunk (>1840)*** as *divisions*; see Duckworth translation (1962, pp. 245, 247–248, 252–253). Meckel (1817) described all three for macrodissected adult human, and referred to those from ***brachial plexus middle trunk (>1840)*** and ***brachial plexus lower trunk (>1840)*** as *anterior branches*, whereas he referred to that from ***brachial plexus upper trunk (>1840)*** as inferior ***nerve (Herophilus, c335–c280 BC)*** arising from *trunk formed by union of fifth and sixth cervical nerves (Meckel, 1817)*; see translation (1832, Vol. 3, p. 23).

Earlier synonyms:

1. *anterior set of primary divisions of brachial plexus (Quain, 1828)*
   For macrodissected adult human, three ***brachial plexus ventral divisions (Paterson, 1887)***; p. 415.

brachium of inferior colliculus (>1840)

As described for macrodissected adult human, and mammal generally with histological methods for ***axons (Kölliker, 1896)***, a short longitudinal ***central nervous system white matter tract (>1840)*** between ***inferior colliculus (Haller, 1762)*** caudally and ***medial geniculate complex (>1840)*** rostrally, on the dorsolateral surface of the ***tegmentum (Swanson, 2000b)*** just superficial to the ***nucleus of brachium of inferior colliculus (>1840)***; see Carpenter (1976, Fig. 2.19), Swanson (2004, Atlas Levels 40–44), Nieuwenhuys et al. (2008, Fig. 3.10-6). It was known to Willis; see ***[brachium of inferior colliculus (>1840)] (Willis, 1664)***.

EARLIER REFERENCES:

Illustrated and described, not named:

1. ***[brachium of inferior colliculus (>1840)] (Willis, 1664)***
   Discovered but not named for macrodissected adult human and sheep; see Pordage translation (1681, Tabs. IV-*N*, VIII-*I*), Meyer (1971, p. 17).

Earlier synonyms:

1. *processus versus principia nervorum opticorum (Santorini, 1775)*
   Synonym for macrodissected adult human ***brachium of inferior colliculus (>1840)***; p. 33, see Burdach (1822, p. 336).
2. *lateral ridge of lower corpus bigeminum (Gordon, 1815)*
   Synonym for macrodissected adult human ***brachium of inferior colliculus (>1840)***; p. 94.

3. *brachium of inferior quadrigeminal body (Burdach, 1822)* Synonym for macrodissected adult human ***brachium of inferior colliculus (>1840)***; the original Latin (plural), *brachia corporum quadrigeminorum inferiorum*, p. 113.
4. *posterior brachium of quadrigeminal body (Arnold, 1838a)* Synonym for macrodissected adult human ***brachium of inferior colliculus (>1840)***; the original Latin (plural), *brachia corporum quadrigeminorum post.*, p. 57.

brachium of superior colliculus (>1840)

As described in macrodissected adult human, and mammal generally with histological methods for ***axons (Kölliker, 1896)***, the caudal extension of the ***optic tract (Vicq d'Azyr, 1784)***, between ***dorsal lateral geniculate nucleus (>1840)*** rostrally and ***superior colliculus (Haller, 1762)*** caudally; see Williams & Warwick (1980, pp. 935, 977), Nieuwenhuys et al. (2008, Fig. 3.10-4). For topographic description it has ***thalamic brachium of superior colliculus (>1840)*** and ***pretectal brachium of superior colliculus (>1840)*** segments. It was first clearly delineated by Willis; see *appendix of nates (Willis, 1664)*.

EARLIER REFERENCES:

Earlier synonyms:

1. *appendix of nates (Willis, 1664)* Probably corresponds to ***brachium of superior colliculus (>1840)***, although it might refer to ***superior cerebellar peduncle (Prochâska, 1800)***, or possibly to both; see Pordage translation (1681, p. 65). However, the ***brachium of superior colliculus (>1840)*** itself was described and illustrated for macrodissected adult human and sheep; see Pordage translation (1681, p. 64, Tabs. IV-*N*, VIII-*I*). Also see Meyer (1971, p. 17).
2. *fibrous protuberance (Diemerbroeck, 1689)* Apparently corresponds to macrodissected adult human ***brachium of superior colliculus (>1840)***; Diemerbroeck wrote that optic (visual) nerve, and only *optic nerve (Galen, c173)*, proceeds from it; pp. 400–401.
3. *lateral ridge of upper corpus bigeminum (Gordon, 1815)* Synonym for macrodissected adult human ***brachium of superior colliculus (>1840)***; p. 93, see Burdach (1822, pp. 336–337) for early history.
4. *anterior brachium of quadrigeminal body (Arnold, 1838a)* Synonym for macrodissected adult human ***brachium of superior colliculus (>1840)***; the original Latin (plural), *brachia corp. quad. ant.*, p. 57.

brain (Smith Papyrus, c1700 BC)

A general term for the rostral topographic division of the ***central nervous system (Carus, 1814)***. ***Invertebrate brain (>1840)*** and ***vertebrate brain (Cuvier, 1800)*** are distinguished and treated separately because the evolutionary relationship between the two is not clear and because whereas there is a common basic plan for the ***vertebrate brain (Cuvier, 1800)*** based on development, there are multiple basic plans for the ***invertebrate brain (>1840)*** and many invertebrates have nothing resembling a ***brain (Smith Papyrus, c1700 BC)***. The terms listed below relate directly to the general term ***brain (Smith Papyrus, c1700 BC)***. For these definitions see Swanson & Bota (2010). A term equivalent to "brain" (the hieroglyph for *ais*) was used for the soft tissue ("marrow" in English) contents of the adult human skull (or more accurately the cranium) by the ancient Egyptians, who removed it with a hook through the nostrils as well as a hole in the cribriform plate of the ethmoid bone, and discarded it as unimportant before mummification; see direct quote of Herodotus (c480–c425 BC) in Longrigg (1998, p. 84) and Nunn (2002, p. 43). The best-known and oldest surviving use of the term is in the Edwin Smith Surgical Papyrus, a c1700 BC copy of a manuscript composed c3000 BC; see Breasted (1930), Nunn (2002, pp. 50–51), Allen (2005, p. 75). Thirteen cases of skull fracture accompanying war injuries were discussed. The term "brain" has been said to be unknown in any other language or treatise in this age, the third millennium BC (Breasted 1930, p. 12), although Walker (1998, p. 19) mentioned without reference that the first specific Egyptian reference to the ***brain (Smith Papyrus, c1700 BC)*** is found in a manuscript dating from about 4200 BC. In *On the Sacred Disease*, Hippocrates (c415 BC) stated that in humans, as in all other animals, a thin membrane divides the *encephalon (Homer, c9th century BC)* down the middle into two parts—the ***brain (Smith Papyrus, c1700 BC)*** " is double"; see Adams translation (1972, p. 351). According to Galen (see May translation, 1968, p. 417), Praxagoras (fl. c320–c300 BC) and Philotimus (a pupil of Praxagoras) and their followers believed that the ***brain (Smith Papyrus, c1700 BC)*** is an outgrowth of the ***spinal cord (Galen, c162–c166)***. This idea was revived in modern times by Bartholin (see 1662, p. 136) and Malpighi, who compared the ***spinal cord (Galen, c162–c166)*** and ***brain (Smith Papyrus, c1700 BC)*** to a cabbage plant, where sap is carried from the roots [***nerves (Herophilus, c335–c280 BC)***], up the stalk [***spinal cord (Galen, c162–c166)***] to the head [***brain (Smith Papyrus, c1700 BC)***]; see Collins (1685, pp. 1070–1072), Tiedemann (1826, p. 149 ff.), Meckel (1832, Vol. 2, p. 466), and Meyer (1967). The ***brain (Smith Papyrus, c1700 BC)*** was not illustrated realistically in print until 1517; see Gersdorff (1517), Clarke & O'Malley (1996, p. 384). The term *brain* came to have two different meanings; see *whole brain (Aristotle)* and *anterior part of brain (Aristotle)*.

ALTERNATE SPELLINGS:

1. *braegen (Anglo-Saxon)* Alternate form of ***brain (Smith Papyrus, c1700 BC)***; see Gordh & Headrick (2001, p. 138).
2. *braine (archaic English)* Alternate form of ***brain (Smith Papyrus, c1700 BC)*** in English until the 17th century; see Vicary (1548, p. 30), *Oxford English Dictionary* (Online).
3. *brane (archaic English)* Alternate form of ***brain (Smith Papyrus, c1700 BC)*** in English until the 17th century; see *Oxford English Dictionary* (Online).

4. *braynes (archaic English)*
Alternate form of ***brain (Smith Papyrus, c1700 BC)*** in English until the 17th century; see Brunschwig (1525, p. [5]), *Oxford English Dictionary* (Online).
5. *brayn (archaic English)*
Alternate form of ***brain (Smith Papyrus, c1700 BC)*** in English until the 17th century; see Brunschwig (1525, p. [8]), *Oxford English Dictionary* (Online).
6. *brayne (archaic English)*
Alternate form of ***brain (Smith Papyrus, c1700 BC)*** in English until the 17th century; see Brunschwig (1525, p. [8]), *Oxford English Dictionary* (Online).
7. *breine (archaic English)*
Alternate form of ***brain (Smith Papyrus, c1700 BC)*** in English until the 17th century; see *Oxford English Dictionary* (Online).

TRANSLATIONS:

1. *ais (Smith Papyrus, c1700 BC)*
English form of Egyptian hieroglyph for ***brain (Smith Papyrus, c1700 BC)***; see Rocca (2003, p. 21), Nunn (2002, pp. 50–51, 217).
2. *encephalos (Homer, c9th century BC)*
Greek word for ***brain (Smith Papyrus, c1700 BC)***, used in the *Iliad* to describe combat injuries near Troy; see Longrigg (1998, p. 168), Rocca (2003, p. 21). It was used in this sense for macrodissected adult human by Gibson (1684, pp. 349–351).
3. *enkephalos (Homer, c9th century BC)*
Alternate form of *encephalos (Homer, c9th century BC)*.
4. *encephalon (Homer, c9th century BC)*
Neuter form of Greek word *encephalos* (*enkephalos*); now standard usage in English, see *Oxford English Dictionary* (Online) and Rocca (2003, p. xvii). It was used seven times in the *Iliad* and three times in the *Odyssey*; see Skinner (1949, p. 132). Willis (1664) used the term for macrodissected adult humans and other mammals in the sense of *encephalon (Homer, c9th century BC)* and *whole brain (Aristotle)*, that is, for his *cerebrum (Willis, 1664)*, *oblong marrow (Willis, 1664)*, and ***cerebellum (Aristotle)***, considered together; see Pordage translation (1681, pp. 78, 81).
5. *enkephalon (Homer, c9th century BC)*
Alternate form of *encephalon (Homer, c9th century BC)*.
6. *cerebrum (Celsus, c30)*
Latin form of *encephalon (Homer, c9th century BC)*; Celsus published the first scientific work in Latin; see Singer (1959), May translation (1968, p. 394). In *On the Usefulness of the Parts*, Galen wrote, "To appreciate more clearly and plainly the significance of what I have said, call the encephalon by its Roman name, which was not taken from its position or from any other accident but is indicative of the very essence of it, and you will see clearly that there is nothing to prevent your saying that in man the *cerebrum* (for that is what the Romans call it) is in the head, and that in crabs it is in the breast." (May translation, 1968, pp. 394–395).
7. *encephalon (Galen, c173, c177)*
In *On the Usefulness of the Parts*, Galen wrote that the Greek term *encephalon* simply means "something in the head" and is derived from its location in the body; see May translation (1968, p. 393). In *On Anatomical Procedures*, Galen wrote or implied that he used the term *enkephalon* to indicate the *anterior brain (Aristotle)* and the *posterior brain (Aristotle)* considered together; see Wiberg translation (1914, p. 21), Singer translation (1999, p. 229).
8. *enkephalon (Galen, c177)*
Variant form of *encephalon (Galen, c177)*.

LATER SYNONYMS:

1. *marrow of skull (Smith Papyrus, c1700 BC)*
An alternate translation, term, or synonym for ***brain (Smith Papyrus, c1700 BC)***; see Breasted (1930, p. 167).

brain sand (Soemmerring & Lisignolo, 1785)

Small calcified bodies found primarily in the aging human ***pineal gland (Galen, c192)***, but also in the *pituitary gland (Galen, c192)* and ***choroid plexus (Galen, c177)***; see Crosby et al. (1962, p. 271), *Dorland's* (2003, p. 1654). Also see Soemmerring & Noethig (1786), Vicq d'Azyr (1786, Pl. XXVII, Fig. VII-*10*), Meckel (1817; see translation, 1832, Vol. 2, p. 439), Burdach (1822, p. 332). It was first observed by Galen; see ***[brain sand (Soemmerring & Lisignolo, 1785)] (Galen, c192)***.

TRANSLATIONS:

1. *acervulo cerebri (Soemmerring & Lisignolo, 1785)*
Original Latin form of ***brain sand (Soemmerring & Lisignolo, 1785)***; see title-page.

EARLIER REFERENCES:

Described, not named or illustrated:

1. ***[brain sand (Soemmerring & Lisignolo, 1785)] (Galen, c192)***
Observed in macrodissected adult ***pineal gland (Galen, c192)*** of horse, ox, and similar large mammals; see Duckworth translation (1962, p. 2) and Burdach (1822, p. 332).

Earlier synonyms:

1. *gravel (Winslow, 1733)*
Synonym for macrodissected adult human ***brain sand (Soemmerring & Lisignolo, 1785)***; Section X, p. 37.

LATER SYNONYMS:

1. *acervulus (Soemmerring & Lisignolo, 1785)*
Simply shortened form of *acervulo cerebri (Soemmerring & Lisignolo, 1785)* for macrodissected adult human; p. 13.
2. *acervulus of pineal gland (Bock, 1824)*
Synonym for macrodissected adult human *acervulus (Soemmerring & Lisignolo, 1785)*; in the original Latin, *acervulus glandulae pinealis*, p. 155.

brain vesicles (Malpighi, 1673)

The rostral topographic division of the vertebrate ***neural tube (Baer, 1837)***, which is followed by the caudal division, the ***spinal cord part of neural tube (>1840)***. Malpighi recognized three vesicles in the chick embryo at 40 hours of incubation, and then five vesicles in the 3-day chick embryo; Table II, Figure XI-C and Table III, Figure XVIII. Baer (1837, pp. 106–107) generalized this description for all vertebrates, calling the *five vesicles (Baer, 1837)*, or ***secondary brain vesicles (>1840)***, the morphological units from which the ***vertebrate brain (Cuvier, 1800)*** is built (p. 107) and lined up one after another sequentially, though curved ventrally (downward) at the rostral (front) end very early on (p. 108). Coiter observed them long ago; see *transparent globules (Coiter, 1572)*.

TRANSLATIONS:

1. *cerebri vesiculae (Malpighi, 1673)*
   Original Latin for ***brain vesicles (Malpighi, 1673)***; see p. 16.

EARLIER REFERENCES:

Earlier synonyms:

1. *transparent globules (Coiter, 1572)*
   Synonym for ***brain vesicles (Malpighi, 1673)***; Coiter described three of them in the 9-day macrodissected chick embryo, although their precise identification is unclear; in the original Latin, *tres globulos transparentes*, see translation (1969, p. 34).

LATER SYNONYMS:

1. *brain cells (Baer, 1837)*
   Probably synonym for ***brain vesicles (Malpighi, 1673)***; in the original German, *Hirnzellen*, p. 106. Also see Baer (1828, p. 29).
2. *cerebral cells (Baer, 1837)*
   Synonym for ***brain vesicles (Malpighi, 1837)***; in the original Latin, *cellulae cerebrales*, p. 106.
3. *head cells (Baer, 1837)*
   Synonym for ***brain vesicles (Malpighi, 1837)***; in the original German, *Hauptblase*, p. 107.

brainstem (Schwalbe, 1881)

A topographic division of the ***vertebrate brain (Cuvier, 1800)*** that is a combination of the ***interbrain (Baer, 1837)***, ***midbrain (Baer, 1837)***, ***pons (Haller, 1747)***, and ***medulla (Winslow, 1733)***; see Swanson & Bota (2010). Perhaps the first hint of it was *base of brain (Rufus of Ephesus, fl. c90–120)*. For Schwalbe's use in macrodissected adult human, see p. 396.The term was used more recently in this sense by Mettler (1948, Fig. 119), Carpenter & Sutin (1983, p. 27), Nauta & Feirtag (1986, Fig. 69), and Brodal (1992, p. 285).

TRANSLATIONS:

1. *Hirnstamm (Schwalbe, 1881)*
   Original German form of ***brainstem (Schwalbe, 1881)***; p. 396.

EARLIER REFERENCES:

Earlier synonyms:

1. *base of brain (Rufus of Ephesus, fl. c90–120)*
   In *On the Names of the Parts of the Human Body*, he wrote that the inner and posterior surface of the adult *encephalon (Homer, c9th century BC)*, or ***brain (Smith Papyrus, c1700 BC)***, is called the *base*, and that the *parencephalon (Aristotle)*, or ***cerebellum (Aristotle)***, is an extension of it. In his *Anatomy of the Parts of the Body*, he wrote that the *spinal marrow (Hippocrates)*, or ***spinal cord (Galen, c162–c166)***, is not a special substance but an extension of the ***brain (Smith Papyrus, c1700 BC)***—obviously the *base of brain (Rufus of Ephesus, fl. c90–120)*; see Clarke & O'Malley (1996, pp. 13–14). This may be the first vague reference in writing to the ***brainstem (Schwalbe, 1881)***, although it is not possible to know its exact extent; also see Todd (1983, p. 86) and *base of brain (Galen, c173)*. The English word *base* in Greek and Latin is *basis*.
2. *base of brain (Galen, c173)*
   In *On the Usefulness of the Parts*, Galen wrote that all *pairs of nerves from brain (Galen, c192)*—his first was the *optic nerve (Galen, c173)*—come off the base of the macrodissected ***brain (Smith Papyrus, c1700 BC)***, so his use of the term is roughly equivalent to ***brainstem (Schwalbe, 1881)*** in macrodissected adult mammal excluding human; see May translation (1968, pp. 417, 446).
3. *base of encephalon (Galen, c173)*
   Synonym for *base of brain (Galen, c173)*.
4. *entire base of brain (Galen, c173)*
   Synonym for *base of brain (Galen, c173)*. In *On the Usefulness of the Parts*, Galen at one point (May translation, 1968, p. 719) referred to the entire *base of brain (Galen, c173)*, in distinction to part of it associated with the ***cerebellum (Aristotle)***—that is, the *base of cerebellum (Galen, c173)*, which corresponds roughly to ***pons (Haller, 1747)*** and ***medulla (Winslow, 1733)***, considered together. The *entire base of brain* was usually referred to by Galen simply as the *base of brain (Galen, c173)*.
5. *entire base of encephalon (Galen, c173)*
   Alternate translation of *entire base of brain (Galen, c173)*.
6. *foundation of brain (Brunschwig, 1525)*
   The exact meaning of the term is unclear, but it was probably used in the sense of *base of brain (Galen, c173)*; the original text reads, "foundation of the braynes out of which the senewes [***nerves (Herophilus, c335–c280 BC)***] take their begynnynge" (p. [5]).

PARTLY CORRESPONDS:

1. *middle belly of brain (William of Saliceto, 1275)*
   An informed guess is macrodissected adult human ***interbrain (Baer, 1837)*** and ***midbrain (Baer, 1837)*** surrounding the ***lateral ventricle (Vesalius, 1543a)*** and ***cerebral aqueduct (>1840)*** respectively; see Rosenman translation (1998, p. 181).
2. *mid part of brain (Mondino, 1316)*
   Vaguely defined term probably refers roughly to macrodissected adult human ***interbrain (Baer, 1837)*** and ***midbrain (Baer, 1837)*** considered together. In his *Anathomia*, Mondino referred to the part of the ***brain (Smith Papyrus, c1700 BC)*** associated with the *great fore ventricle (Mondino, 1316)*, the right and left ***lateral ventricle (Vesalius, 1543a)*** together, in contrast to the part associated with the *middle ventricle (Galen, c173)*, or ***third ventricle (Galen, c173)***. One relevant passage reads: "Through this lacuna [***hypothalamic part of third ventricle (Swanson, 2004)*** and *infundibulum (Rufus of Ephesus, fl. c90–120)*; also see *lacuna cerebri (Mondino, 1316)*] the mid part of the brain is purged of superfluous matter. The fore part of the brain is purged of superfluous matter through the *colatoria narium* [cribriform plate]" (see Singer translation, 1925, p. 92). Further on he wrote, "Now raise the next following, to wit the mid part of the brain. Thou wilt see a second pair of nerves

[*second pair of nerves arising from brain (Galen, c173)*, the ***oculomotor nerve (Estienne, 1545)***], fine and hard, which go to the eyes to give them voluntary motion" (see Singer translation, 1925, p. 93). However, the situation is unclear because elsewhere, Mondino wrote, "But thou wilt ask why the mid ventricle did not have a mid brain separate, as the other ventricles had? It must be answered that the reason was that this ventricle is, as it were, the way and passage between these other two and so ought not to separated from them as regards the brain" (see Singer translation, 1925, p. 93). Possibly something was been lost in translation at some stage.

3. *anterior spinal marrow (Varoli, 1573)*
Varoli distinguished in macrodissected adult human an *anterior* part (within the cranium) of the *spinal marrow (Hippocrates)*, which roughly includes the ***midbrain (Baer, 1837)***, **pons (Haller, 1747)**, and ***medulla (Winslow, 1733)*** considered together; see Varoli (1573, Fig. II: *1-3* on f. 19), Clarke & O'Malley (1996, pp. 635, 821–822), and *cerebrum oblongatum (Colombo, 1559)*. Garrison & McHenry (1969, p. 43) claimed that Varoli dealt with the ***cerebral peduncle (Tarin, 1753)***, which is doubtful, and Clarke & O'Malley (1996, p. 634) claimed that he suggested four tracts (in the anterior spinal marrow)—two posterior (dorsal) ones related to the ***cerebellum (Aristotle)*** and two anterior (ventral) ones related to sensation, which is likely. Also see *base of brain (Varoli, 1573)*.
4. *primary origin of spinal marrow (Varoli, 1573)*
Synonym for *anterior spinal marrow (Varoli, 1573)*; see Clarke & O'Malley (1996, p. 822).
5. *other part of spinal marrow (Varoli, 1573)*
Synonym for *anterior spinal marrow (Varoli, 1573)*; see Clarke & O'Malley (1996, p. 822).
6. *medulla cauda (Bartholin, 1651)*
Latin form of *tail of marrow (Bartholin, 1662)*; p. 317.
7. *long part of marrow (Bartholin, 1662)*
At one point (p. 133) Bartholin used this term to indicate the macrodissected adult human ***midbrain (Baer, 1837)***, ***pons (Haller, 1747)***, and ***medulla (Winslow, 1733)*** considered together; in the original Latin, *medulla oblongata* (1651, p. 317). See *medulla oblongata (Bartholin, 1651)*. It is a synonym for *anterior spinal marrow (Varoli, 1573)*.
8. *tail of marrow (Bartholin, 1662)*
Synonym for *long part of marrow (Bartholin, 1662)*; p. 137.
9. *roots from brainlet (Bartholin, 1662)*
That component of the macrodissected adult human *part within skull of medulla oblongata (Bartholin, 1662)* associated directly with the ***cerebellum (Aristotle)***, thus including parts of the ***midbrain (Baer, 1837)***, especially the ***inferior colliculus (Haller, 1762)***, the ***pons (Haller, 1747)***, and the ***medulla (Winslow, 1733)*** derived from at least the ***superior cerebellar peduncle (Procháska, 1800)*** (p. 141) and ***inferior cerebellar peduncle (Günther, 1786)*** (Tab. IV, Fig. 1-C, p. 136). They are smaller than the *roots from brain (Bartholin, 1662)*; also see *trunk of spinal marrow (Bartholin, 1662)*.
10. *basis of oblong marrow (Willis, 1664)*
Vaguely defined term apparently includes roughly ***interbrain (Baer, 1837)*** and ***tegmentum (Swanson, 2000)*** considered together; see Pordage translation (1681, pp. 66–67).
11. *base of oblong marrow (Willis, 1664)*
Full English translation of *basis of oblong marrow (Willis, 1664)*.
12. *pedestal of oblong marrow (Willis, 1664)*
Synonym for *basis of oblong marrow (Willis, 1664)*; see Pordage translation (1681, p. 66).
13. *neck of medulla spinalis (Collins, 1685)*
Apparently a synonym for the *anterior spinal marrow (Varoli, 1573)*; p. 1070; also see *medulla vero cerebri oblongata (Bauhin, 1605)*.
14. *long process of medulla spinalis (Collins, 1685)*
Synonym for *neck of medulla spinalis (Collins, 1685)*; p. 1070.
15. *caudex of medulla oblongata (Collins, 1685)*
Apparently referred approximately to ***midbrain (Baer, 1837)***, **pons (Haller, 1747)**, and ***medulla (Winslow, 1733)*** considered together; pp. 1008, 1015. Described more clearly shortly thereafter by Ridley; see *caudex medullaris (Ridley, 1695)*. Collins did indicate specifically the ***pons (Haller, 1747)*** in an illustration; see p. 1017 and Table 48-*L*.
16. *caudex (Collins, 1685)*
Abbreviated form of *caudex of medulla oblongata (Collins, 1685)*; p. 1017.
17. *long pith (Diemerbroeck, 1689)*
Term used by the English for *long part of marrow (Bartholin, 1662)*; pp. 402–405.
18. *long pith of brain (Diemerbroeck, 1689)*
More complete form of *long pith (Diemerbroeck, 1689)* and complemented by *pith of spine (Diemerbroeck, 1689)*; p. 557.
19. *caudex medullaris (Ridley, 1695)*
Term referring approximately to macrodissected adult human ***tectum (Baer, 1837)***, **pons (Haller, 1747)**, and ***medulla (Winslow, 1733)*** considered together; p. 9. The *caudex medullaris* begins "where the *Crura Medulla Oblongata* come together in one body, constituting the *Caudex Medullae Oblongatae*" (p. 145). Dorsally the ***tectum (Baer, 1837)*** is part of the *caudex medullaris* (p. 9) whereas ventrally what he referred to as *thalami nervorum opticorum* was said to extend to or over the "forward and upper part of the Annular Process", roughly the ***pons (Haller, 1747)***; p. 145. In this ambiguous description, the rostral border of the *caudex medullaris* probably cuts diagonally from rostrodorsal, rostral to the ***tectum (Baer, 1837)***, to caudoventral at the rostral border of the commissure of the ***middle cerebellar peduncle (Rolando, 1819)***, the ***transverse pontine fibers (>1840)***. *Caudex* is an older Latin form of *codex*, the trunk of a tree.
20. *pons Varolii (Cowper, 1698)*
Cowper illustrated and described this "cerebellar matter" in macrodissected adult human as extending

rostrally as far as the caudal end of the ***mammillary body (Ludwig, 1779)***, which he called *white protuberances*; Table IX, Figure 1-Y.

21. *optic thalamus (Pourfour du Petit, 1710)*
Pourfour du Petit's use of the term (*couche optique* in French) for macrodissected adult human clearly included the ***interbrain (Baer, 1837)*** and ***midbrain (Baer, 1837)***, excluding the ***cerebral peduncle (Tarin, 1753)***. He referred to the *optic thalamus (Pourfour du Petit, 1710)* as a *superior part of medullary crura* and the ***cerebral peduncle (Tarin, 1753)*** as an *inferior part of medullary crura*; p. 14; unpublished translation of L. Kruger and L.W. Swanson.
22. *superior part of medullary crura (Pourfour du Petit, 1710)*
Synonymous with or includes (distinction unclear) the *optic thalamus (Pourfour du Petit, 1710)*; also see *inferior part of medullary crura (Pourfour du Petit, 1710)*.
23. *cerebral peduncle (Winslow, 1733)*
Winslow's definition for macrodissected adult human is quite vague and appears to include very roughly the ***tegmentum (Swanson, 2000b)*** and ***pons (Haller, 1747)*** exclusive of the ***cerebellar peduncles (Ridley, 1695)***. At one point he wrote that, "The great Branches of the Medulla Oblongata [a synonym for his cerebral peduncles] are two very considerable medullary Fasciculi, the anterior [rostral] Extremities of which are separated, and the posterior united, so that taken both together, they represent a *Roman V*. These fasciculi are flat, much broader before than behind; their Substance being composed of several longitudinal and distinctly prominent medullary Fibres. Their anterior Extremities seem to be lost at the lower part of the Corpora Striata; and it is for that reason that they are looked upon as the Pedunculi of the Cerebrum." (Sect. X, p. 41). But then he wrote, "We must observe in general concerning the Eminences of the Medulla Oblongata, that those which are medullary on their Outsides or Surfaces, are interiourly either intirely Cortical, or partly Cortical, and partly Medullary, or formed by a singular Mixture of these two Substances, which still remains to be unfolded, as well as many other particularities observable in examining the internal Structure of the Brain." (Sect. X, p. 43).
24. *large branch of medulla oblongata (Winslow, 1733)*
Synonym for *cerebral peduncle (Winslow, 1733)*; Section X, p. 41.
25. *great branch of medulla oblongata (Winslow, 1733)*
Synonym for *cerebral peduncle (Winslow, 1733)*; Section X, p. 41.
26. *anterior branch of medulla oblongata (Winslow, 1733)*
Synonym for *cerebral peduncle (Winslow, 1733)*; Section X, p. 41.
27. *crus anteriora medulla oblongata (Winslow, 1733)*
Synonym for *cerebral peduncle (Winslow, 1733)*; Section X, p. 41.
28. *femora medulla oblongata (Winslow, 1733)*
Synonym for *cerebral peduncle (Winslow, 1733)*; Section X, p. 41.
29. *crus cerebri (Haller, 1747)*
Haller's definition for macrodissected adult human included the fibrous ***cerebral peduncle (Tarin, 1753)*** and accompanying, though undefined and unillustrated, *gray substance (Vesalius, 1543a)* of the ***midbrain (Baer, 1837)*** and ***pons (Haller, 1747)***, exclusive of the ***tectum (Baer, 1837)***; p. 184. "The whole medulla of the brain is, in its lower part or basis, collected together into two very thick compressed columns, distinguished in their surface by a line running according to their length; and these have internally a cortical substance. These, which are the crura of the brain, meeting together downward, are covered by the subjacent crura of the cerebellum, and are inserted by apparent strata of fibres into the pyramidal bodies of the medulla oblongata; and with the other deeper fibres, which separate the inner transverse fibres that come from the cerebellum from the preceding, meet together with the medulla cerebelli to make up the beginning of the medulla oblongata."(see translation, 1754, pp. 294–295).
30. *basis of medulla of brain (Haller, 1754b)*
English form of *crus cerebri (Haller, 1747)*; pp. 294–295.
31. *crura of brain (Haller, 1754b)*
Refers in English to right and left *crus cerebri (Haller, 1747)*; pp. 294–295.
32. *processus cerebri ad pontem Varolii (Haase, 1781)*
Its meaning for macrodissected adult human is quite vague but probably is similar to *crus cerebri (Haller, 1747)*; p. 25.
33. *processus ad medullam oblongatam (Haase, 1781)*
Synonym for *processus cerebri ad pontem Varolii (Haase, 1781)*; p. 25.
34. *medulla oblongata (Vicq d'Azyr, 1786)*
Apparently used for macrodissected adult human ***medulla (Winslow, 1733)***, ***pons (Haller, 1747)*** without the ***pontine nuclei (Jacobsohn, 1909)*** and ***middle cerebellar peduncles (Rolando, 1819)***, and ***tegmentum (Swanson, 2000b)*** without the ***cerebral peduncles (Tarin, 1753)***, all considered together; Plate XXV, Figures I–II:*41/42*. Reil (1809c) used the term in essentially the same sense for macrodissected adult human; see Mayo translation (1823, p. 85).
35. *annular protuberance and its prolongations (Bichat, 1801)*
Corresponds roughly to macrodissected adult human ***pons (Haller, 1747)***, with the ***midbrain (Baer, 1837)*** rostrally and the ***medulla (Winslow, 1733)*** caudally; see translation (1822, Vol. 1, pp. 172–173).
36. *cerebral protuberance (Bichat et al., 1801–1803)*
Appears to correspond very roughly to macrodissected adult human ***midbrain (Baer, 1837)*** and ***pons (Haller, 1747)*** considered together, along with certain fiber tract prolongations to the ***forebrain (Goette, 1873)*** and ***cerebellum (Aristotle)***; in the original French, *protubérance cérébral*; pp. 107, 206. Also see Meckel (1832, Vol. 2, pp. 418–418).
37. *midbrain (Burdin, 1803)*
Apparently roughly corresponds to macrodissected adult human ***tectum (Baer, 1837)*** and ***pons (Haller,***

1747) considered together; in the original French, *mésocéphale*. Also see translation (1803, Vol. 1, pp. 165–166), where the Latin form, *mesencephalon*, is used. Also see Meckel (1832, Vol. 2, pp. 418–419), Todd (1845, pp. 157–159, 180 ff.).

38. *cerebral protuberance (Cloquet, 1816)*
Corresponds to macrodissected adult human ***tectum (Baer, 1837)*** and ***pons (Haller, 1747)*** considered together; in the original French, *protubérance cérébrale*, pp. 536–539.
39. *mesocephalon (Burdach, 1822)*
Latin translation provided for *midbrain (Burdin, 1803)*; p. 298, where it was also spelled *mesencephalon*. Meckel spelled it *mesocephalum*, see translation (1832, Vol. 2, p. 418).
40. *pyramidal bundle (Rolando, 1825a)*
In macrodissected adult human the ***cerebral peduncle (Tarin, 1753)*** and ***longitudinal pontine fibers (Arnold, 1838b)*** considered together; in the original French, *faisceaux pyramidaux*, Table 1, Figure 1-*p.e.* and Table III, Figure 1-*p*.
41. *pyramidal fascicle (Rolando, 1825a)*
Alternate translation for *pyramidal bundle (Rolando, 1825a)*.
42. *anterior pyramid (Rolando, 1825a)*
Rolando tended to use it in macrodissected adult mammals to include the ***longitudinal pontine fibers (Arnold, 1838b)*** and ***pyramid (Willis, 1664)*** considered together; the original French (plural), *pyramides antérieures*; see Table III, Figure 1-*p* and Table IV, Figure 1-*p*.
43. *annular protuberance (Cloquet, 1828)*
Synonym for macrodissected adult human *cerebral protuberance (Cloquet, 1816)*; in the original French, *protubérance annulaire*, p. 383.
44. *nodus encephali (Quain, 1828)*
Synonym for *cerebral protuberance (Cloquet, 1816)*; p. 623.
45. *node of brain (Cruveilhier, 1836)*
The macrodissected adult human ***midbrain (Baer, 1837)***, ***pons (Haller, 1747)***, and probably ***medulla (Winslow, 1733)*** considered together; in the original French, *noeud de l'encéphale*, p. 528.
46. *reinforcing fascicle of bulb (Cruveilhier, 1836)*
For macrodissected adult human a large and vaguely defined column—which Cruveilhier referred to as a nucleus (*noyau*)—of mixed ***central nervous system white matter tracts (>1840)*** and ***central nervous system gray matter regions (>1840)***—starting between the right and left ***inferior olivary complex (>1840)***, filling most of the rest of the ***medulla (Winslow, 1733)***, and extending rostrally through the ***midbrain (Baer, 1837)*** and caudally in and around the ***inferior cerebellar peduncle (Günther, 1786)***; in the original French, *fasceau de renforcement du bulb*, p. 596.
47. *unnamed fascicle of bulb (Cruveilhier, 1836)*
Synonym for *reinforcing fascicle of bulb (Cruveilhier, 1836)*; in the original French, *faisceau innominé*, p. 596. Todd (1845, pp. 177–178, 186, Figs. 20, 28-*i*) referred in Latin to right and left *fasciculi innominata* and called them the *olivary* or *central columns*.
48. *isthmus of brain (Cruveilhier, 1836)*
Synonym for *node of brain (Cruveilhier, 1836)*; in the original French, *isthme de l'encéphale*, p. 602. Cruveilhier wrote that he was following *isthmus (Ridley, 1695)*, although the latter was probably more restricted, essentially, to the ***midbrain (Baer, 1837)***.

branch of oculomotor nerve to ciliary ganglion (>1840)

As described for macrodissected adult human, a branch (or up to three smaller branches) of the ***oculomotor nerve (Estienne, 1545)*** usually arising from the ***nerve to inferior oblique (>1840)***. It carries preganglionic parasympathetic ***axons (Kölliker, 1896)*** from the ***Edinger-Westphal nucleus (>1840)*** of the ***midbrain (Baer, 1837)*** to the ***ciliary ganglion (Loder, 1778)***; see Williams & Warwick (1980, p. 1058), *Terminologia Anatomica* (1998, p. 133). It was perhaps first clearly distinguished by Pourfour du Petit; see ***[branch of oculomotor nerve to ciliary ganglion (>1840)] (Pourfour du Petit, 1729)***.

EARLIER REFERENCES:

Described, not named or illustrated:

1. ***[branch of oculomotor nerve to ciliary ganglion (>1840)] (Pourfour du Petit, 1729)***
Clearly described for macrodissected adult human; p. 10. For an account of early work, see Haller (1743, p. 45 note 39).

Earlier synonyms:

1. *short branch of oculomotor nerve (Winslow, 1733)*
Synonym for macrodissected adult human ***branch of oculomotor nerve to ciliary ganglion (>1840)***. Winslow specifically referred to small short branch of *third pair of nerves from medulla oblongata (Winslow, 1733)* forming a small *lenticular ganglion (Winslow, 1733)*; Section VI, p. 62. Beautifully illustrated for macrodissected adult human by Zinn (1755, Tab. VI, Fig. 1-*y*).
2. *short root of ophthalmic ganglion (Zinn, 1755)*
Synonym for macrodissected adult human ***branch of oculomotor nerve to ciliary ganglion (>1840)***; in the original Latin, *radix brevior ganglii ophthalmici*, Table VI, Figure 1-*z*.
3. *short root of ciliary ganglion (Langenbeck, 1826-1830)*
Synonym for macrodissected adult human ***branch of oculomotor nerve to ciliary ganglion (>1840)***; in the original Latin, *radix brevis ganglii ciliaris*, Fascicle III, Table XVI-*r*.
4. *short root of lenticular ganglion (Todd, 1836–1839)*
Synonym for macrodissected adult human ***branch of oculomotor nerve to ciliary ganglion (>1840)***; p. 281.
5. *branch of ophthalmic ganglion to inferior division of third nerve (Quain & Wilson, 1839)*
Synonym for macrodissected adult human ***branch of oculomotor nerve to ciliary ganglion (>1840)***; Plate XIII, Figure 2-*h*.

6. *ciliary ganglion branch of communication to inferior branch of third nerve (Quain & Wilson, 1839)*
   Synonym for macrodissected adult human ***branch of oculomotor nerve to ciliary ganglion (>1840)***; Plate XXVII-*E*,7.
7. *lenticular ganglion branch of communication to inferior branch of third nerve (Quain & Wilson, 1839)*
   Synonym for macrodissected adult human ***branch of oculomotor nerve to ciliary ganglion (>1840)***; Plate XXVII-*E*,7.

LATER SYNONYMS:

1. *parasympathetic root of ciliary ganglion (>1840)*
   Synonym for macrodissected adult human ***branch of oculomotor nerve to ciliary ganglion (>1840)***; see *Terminologia Anatomica* (1998, p. 133).
2. *oculomotor root of ciliary ganglion (>1840)*
   Synonym for macrodissected adult human ***branch of oculomotor nerve to ciliary ganglion (>1840)***; see *Terminologia Anatomica* (1998, p. 133).

buccal branch of facial nerve (>1840)

As described for macrodissected adult human, a terminal branch (or sometimes branches) of the ***facial nerve trunk (>1840)*** extending rostrally (forward) to the angle of the mouth and supplying muscles converging on the mouth, including the buccinator; see Durward (1951, p. 1032 and Fig. 902). Williams & Warwick (1980, p. 1072) referred to the lower ***zygomatic branches of facial nerve (>1840)*** as an upper buccal branch of facial nerve. It was first alluded to by Galen; see ***[buccal branch of facial nerve (>1840)] (Galen, c173)***.

EARLIER REFERENCES:

Described, not named or illustrated:

1. ***[buccal branch of facial nerve (>1840)] (Galen, c173)***
   Alluded to for macrodissected adult beef, pig, and/or macaque but not human; see May translation (1968, pp. 455, 539), Duckworth translation (1962, pp. 194, 196), and Meckel (1748, p. 2 notes *d,e*).

Illustrated and described, not named:

1. ***[buccal branch of facial nerve (>1840)] (Vesalius, 1543a)***
   Mentioned and illustrated for macrodissected adult human; see Richardson & Carman translation (2002, p. 193).

Earlier synonyms:

1. *buccal nerve of inferior branch of hard nerve (Meckel, 1753)*
   Corresponds roughly to macrodissected adult human ***buccal branch of facial nerve (>1840)***; in the original French, *le nerf buccal de le rameau inférieur du dur*, Table 1-*221*.
2. *buccal branch of inferior branch of hard nerve (Meckel, 1753)*
   Synonym for *buccal nerve of inferior branch of hard nerve (Meckel, 1753)*; in the original French, basically *le rameau buccal de la rameau inférieur du dur*, p. 93.
3. *buccal branch of portio dura of auditory nerve (Albinus, 1761)*
   Synonym for macrodissected adult human ***buccal branch of facial nerve (>1840)***; original Latin description was *nervorum auditoriorum portio dura, ramus ad buccinatorem*, Table 21/2-*f*.
4. *buccal branch of portio dura of seventh cerebral nerve (Albinus, 1761)*
   Synonym for macrodissected adult human ***buccal branch of facial nerve (>1840)***; original Latin description was *septimi paris nervorum cerebri portio dura, ramus ad buccinatorem*, Table 21/2-*f*.
5. *facial branches of superior branch of hard part of seventh pair (Haller, 1762)*
   Synonym for macrodissected adult human ***buccal branch of facial nerve (>1840)***; pp. 229–230.
6. *infraorbital branch of superior branch of anterior branch of hard nerve (Loder, 1778)*
   Synonym for macrodissected adult human ***buccal branch of facial nerve (>1840)***; in the original Latin, *ramum infraorbitalem*, p. 26 (called *supraorbitalis* in error on p. 27).
7. *buccal branches of lower facial branches of descending branch of superficial branch of hard nerve (Günther, 1786)*
   Synonym for macrodissected adult human ***buccal branch of facial nerve (>1840)***; p. 59.
8. *inferior facial branch of hard nerve (Peipers, 1793)*
   Synonym for macrodissected adult human ***buccal branch of facial nerve (>1840)***; in the original Latin, *ramus facialis inferior duri*, p. 35.
9. *buccal branch of hard nerves (Mayer, 1794)*
   Synonym for macrodissected adult human *buccal branch of inferior branch of hard nerve (Meckel, 1753)*; in the original Latin, *ramus buccalis nervi duri*; Part 5, Table VII-*150* (p. 51).
10. *inferior nerve (Soemmerring, 1798)*
    Probably synonym for macrodissected adult human ***buccal branch of facial nerve (>1840)***; in the original Latin, *nervus inferior*, p. 253.
11. *descending nerve (Soemmerring, 1798)*
    Probably synonym for macrodissected adult human ***buccal branch of facial nerve (>1840)***; in the original Latin, *nervus descendens*, p. 253.
12. *labial branches of facial nerve (Burdin, 1803)*
    Probably synonym for macrodissected adult human ***buccal branch of facial nerve (>1840)***; see translation (1803, Vol. 1, p. 180).
13. *buccal nerves (Meckel, 1817)*
    Synonym for macrodissected adult human ***buccal branch of facial nerve (>1840)***. Meckel recognized three branches: central or middle, with ascending and anterior twigs, and superior; see translation (1832, Vol. 3, p. 56).
14. *anterior branches of facial nerve (Meckel, 1817)*
    Synonym for ***buccal branch of facial nerve (>1840)***; see translation (1832, Vol. 3, p. 56).
15. *buccal surculus of inferior branch of portio major and minor of facial nerve (Bellingeri, 1818)*

Synonym for macrodissected adult human ***buccal branches of facial nerve (>1840)***; in the original Latin, *surculus buccalis*, see Table II.

16. *buccal surculus of cervico-facial branch of portio major and minor of facial nerve (Bellingeri, 1818)*
 Synonym for macrodissected adult human ***buccal branches of facial nerve (>1840)***; in the original Latin, *surculus buccalis*, see Table II.
17. *inferior facial branch of facial nerve (Cloquet, 1828)*
 Synonym for macrodissected adult human ***buccal branch of facial nerve (>1840)***; in the original French, *rameau facial inférieur*, Plate CLVII-*71*.
18. *inferior facial branch of portio dura (Knox, 1832)*
 Rough synonym for ***buccal branch of facial nerve (>1840)***; Plate II-*108*.
19. *buccal branches of superior branch of facial nerve (Arnold, 1834)*
 Synonym for ***buccal branch of facial nerve (>1840)***; in the original Latin, *ramus superior nervi facialis rami buccales*, p. 12.
20. *buccal branches of cervicofacial branch of facial nerve (Cruveilhier, 1836)*
 Synonym for ***buccal branch of facial nerve (>1840)***; in the original French, *rameaux buccaux*, pp. 946–947.

PARTLY CORRESPONDS:

1. *superior branch of buccal nerve (Meckel, 1753)*
 Dorsal (superior) branch of *buccal nerve of inferior branch of hard nerve (Meckel, 1753)*; p. 93, also see *inferior branch of buccal nerve (Meckel, 1753)*.
2. *inferior branch of buccal nerve (Meckel, 1753)*
 Ventral (inferior) branch of *buccal nerve of inferior branch of hard nerve (Meckel, 1753)*; in the original French, *la branche inférieure du buccal*, Table 1-*224*.
3. *internal maxillary plexus (Le Cat, 1768)*
 A ***plexus (Galen, c192)*** involving ***communicating branches (Winslow, 1733)*** of macrodissected adult human ***buccal branch of facial nerve (>1840)***; Plate VIII, Figure 1-*x*.
4. *buccal plexus (Le Cat, 1768)*
 A ***plexus (Galen, c192)*** involving ***communicating branches (Winslow, 1733)*** of macrodissected adult human ***buccal branch of facial nerve (>1840)***; Plate VIII, Figure 1-*x*.
5. *nervus anterior facialis infimus (Soemmerring, 1791)*
 Probably synonymous with macrodissected adult human *inferior branch of buccal nerve (Meckel, 1753)*; in the original Latin, *nervus anterior facialis infimus*, p. 238.
6. *facial communicating branch (Mayer, 1794)*
 Communicating branch (Winslow, 1733) associated with macrodissected adult human ***buccal branch of facial nerve (>1840)***; in the original Latin, *ramus communicans faciei*; Part 5, Table VII-*153* (p. 51).
7. *superior fascicle of buccal surculus of inferior branch of portio major and minor of facial nerve (Bellingeri, 1818)*
 Dorsal branch of macrodissected adult human ***buccal branch of facial nerve (>1840)***; in the original Latin, *fasciculus superior*, see Table II.
8. *superior fascicle of buccal surculus of cervico-facial branch of portio major and minor of facial nerve (Bellingeri, 1818)*
 Dorsal branch of macrodissected adult human ***buccal branch of facial nerve (>1840)***; in the original Latin, *fasciculus superior*, see Table II.
9. *middle fascicle of buccal surculus of inferior branch of portio major and minor of facial nerve (Bellingeri, 1818)*
 Intermediate branch of macrodissected adult human ***buccal branch of facial nerve (>1840)***; in the original Latin, *fasciculus medius*, see Table II.
10. *middle fascicle of buccal surculus of cervico-facial branch of portio major and minor of facial nerve (Bellingeri, 1818)*
 Intermediate branch of macrodissected adult human ***buccal branch of facial nerve (>1840)***; in the original Latin, *fasciculus medius*, see Table II.
11. *inferior fascicle of buccal surculus of inferior branch of portio major and minor of facial nerve (Bellingeri, 1818)*
 Ventral branch of macrodissected adult human ***buccal branch of facial nerve (>1840)***; in the original Latin, *fasciculus inferior*, see Table II.
12. *inferior fascicle of buccal surculus of cervico-facial branch of portio major and minor of facial nerve (Bellingeri, 1818)*
 Ventral branch of macrodissected adult human ***buccal branch of facial nerve (>1840)***; in the original Latin, *fasciculus inferior*, see Table II.

buccal nerve (Meckel, 1748)

As described for macrodissected adult human, a branch of the ***anterior branch of mandibular nerve (>1840)*** uniting with ***buccal branches of facial nerve (>1840)*** and supplying a branch to the lateral pterygoid muscle before innervating skin over the rostral (anterior) part of the buccinator muscle and mucous membrane lining its inner surface and the caudal (posterior) part of the buccal surface of the gum; see Williams & Warwick (1980, p. 1066). For Meckel's use in macrodissected adult human see pp. 82, 83; also see Meckel (1753, p. 64, Table 1-*101*). It was known to Galen; see ***[buccal nerve (Meckel, 1748)] (Galen, c173)***.

TRANSLATIONS:

1. *nervus buccinatorius (Schaarschmidt, 1750)*
 Early Latin form of ***buccal nerve (Meckel, 1748)***; p. 27.

EARLIER REFERENCES:

Described, not named or illustrated:

1. ***[buccal nerve (Meckel, 1748)] (Galen, c173)***
 Alluded to for macrodissected adult beef, pig, and/or macaque but not human; see May translation (1968, pp. 449–450) and Meckel (1748, p. 2 note *d*).
2. ***[buccal nerve (Meckel, 1748)] (Vesalius, 1543a)***
 Vesalius mentioned its muscular and cutaneous branches for macrodissected adult human; see Richardson & Carman translation (2002, p. 189). Du Verney clearly illustrated its origin (1683, Pl. 13-3).

LATER SYNONYMS:

1. *great buccal nerve (Meckel, 1753)*
 Synonym for macrodissected adult human ***buccal nerve (Meckel, 1748)***; Table 1-*232*.

2. *buccinator nerve (Meckel, 1753)*
Synonym for macrodissected adult human ***buccal nerve (Meckel, 1748)***; in the original French, *le nerf buccal, ou buccinatoire*, p. 64. For English use see Meckel (1832, Vol. 3, p. 72), where *buccal nerve* was also given.
3. *buccal branch of third branch of fifth pair (Loder, 1778)*
Synonym for macrodissected adult human ***buccal nerve (Meckel, 1748)***; in the original Latin, *ramus buccinatorius*, p. 18.
4. *bucco-labian nerve (Burdin, 1803)*
Synonym for macrodissected adult human ***buccal nerve (Meckel, 1748)***; in the original French, *bucco-labial.* Also see translation (1803, Vol. 1, p. 176).
5. *buccal surculus of ganglioform plexus with inferior maxillary branch (Bellingeri, 1818)*
Synonym for macrodissected adult human ***buccal nerve (Meckel, 1748)***; in the original Latin, *surculus buccinatorius*, see Table 1.
6. *buccolabial branch of fifth nerve (Bell, 1829)*
Apparently, synonym for macrodissected adult human *bucco-labian nerve (Burdin, 1803)*; in the original Latin, *ramus buccinalis labialis*; p. 323, Plate VIII, Figure 1-*E*.
7. *fourth trunk of fifth nerve (Swan, 1830)*
Synonym for macrodissected adult human ***buccal nerve (Meckel, 1748)***; Plate XIV, Figure 5-5.
8. *buccal branch of superior primary branch of inferior maxillary nerve (Quain, 1832)*
Synonym for macrodissected adult human ***buccal nerve (Meckel, 1748)***; p. 675.
9. *buccal branch of inferior maxillary nerve (Quain & Wilson, 1839)*
Synonym for macrodissected adult human ***buccal nerve (Meckel, 1748)***; Plate XIII, Figure 2-*b**.

PARTLY CORRESPONDS:

1. *muscular fascicles of buccal surculus of ganglioform plexus with inferior maxillary branch (Bellingeri, 1818)*
Macrodissected adult human branches of ***buccal nerve (Meckel, 1748)*** to pterygoid and temporal muscles; in the original Latin, *fasciculi musculares*, see Table 1.
2. *glandular fascicles of buccal surculus of ganglioform plexus with inferior maxillary branch (Bellingeri, 1818)*
Macrodissected adult human branches of ***buccal nerve (Meckel, 1748)*** to parotid duct and buccal mucous membrane; in the original Latin, *fasciculi glandulares*, see Table 1.
3. *buccal fascicle of buccal surculus of ganglioform plexus with inferior maxillary branch (Bellingeri, 1818)*
Macrodissected adult human branch of ***buccal nerve (Meckel, 1748)*** to buccinator muscle; in the original Latin, *fasciculus buccalis*, see Table 1.
4. *bucco-labial fascicle of buccal surculus of ganglioform plexus with inferior maxillary branch (Bellingeri, 1818)*
Macrodissected adult human branch of ***buccal nerve (Meckel, 1748)*** to "*m. buccinatorem, caninem, et triangularem*" (Tab. 1); in the original Latin, *fasciculus bucco-labialis.*
5. *ascending branches of buccal nerve (Cruveilhier, 1836)*
Branches of macrodissected adult human ***buccal nerve (Meckel, 1748)*** extending dorsally (ascending) to region of cheek; in the original French, *rameaux ascendans*, p. 931.
6. *middle branches of buccal nerve (Cruveilhier, 1836)*
Rostrally directed (horizontal) branches of macrodissected adult human ***buccal nerve (Meckel, 1748)*** to region lateral to lips; in the original French, *rameaux moyens*, p. 931.
7. *descending branches of buccal nerve (Cruveilhier, 1836)*
Branches of macrodissected adult human ***buccal nerve (Meckel, 1748)*** extending ventrally (descending) to region ventrolateral to lips; in the original French, *rameaux descendans*, p. 931.

bulb of posterior horn (>1840)

As described for macrodissected adult human, a bulge in the dorsal (upper) part of the medial wall of the ***posterior horn of lateral ventricle (Haller, 1747)*** formed by passage of the ***occipital forceps (>1840)***; see Williams & Warwick (1980, p. 1029 and Fig. 7.146). Not clearly described by 1840.

TRANSLATIONS:

1. *bulbus cornus posterioris (>1840)*
Latin form of ***bulb of posterior horn (>1840)***; see *Terminologia Anatomica* (1998, p. 127).

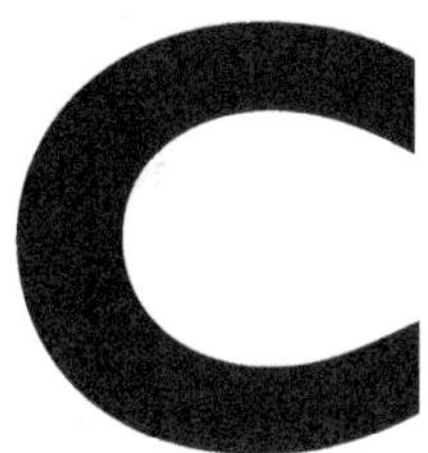

calcarine spur (Morand, 1748)

As described for macrodissected adult human, an elevation in the ventral (lower) part of the medial wall of the ***posterior horn of lateral ventricle (Haller, 1747)*** corresponding to the infolded ***occipital region (Vesalius, 1543a)*** associated with the rostral (anterior) part of the ***calcarine sulcus (>1840)***; see Williams & Warwick (1980, p. 1029, Fig. 7.146), *Terminologia Anatomica* (1998, p. 128), *Dorland's* (2003, p. 1746). It was probably first reported as the *pes hippocampi (Bergen, 1734)*, and Morand noted that it (sometimes) resembles a cock's spur; in French *l'ergot (Morand, 1748)*, and in Latin *calcar avis (Arnold, 1838a)*: "In this cavity one sees clearly an outgrowth or protuberance of the medulla [***cerebral cortex white matter (>1840)***], which I shall call *l'ergot* because it resembles perfectly the part of the claw of birds so named, in its outline, shape, and size, with this difference, that without presenting its entire thickness, it shows it only in relief." (p. 316; translated in Lewis, 1923, p. 226).

TRANSLATIONS:

1. *ergot (Morand, 1748)*
   Original French form, *l'ergot*, of ***calcarine spur (Morand, 1748)***; p. 316.
2. *calcar avis (Arnold, 1838a)*
   Latin form of ***calcarine spur (Morand, 1748)***; p. 88. See Meyer (1971, p. 21).

EARLIER REFERENCES:

Earlier synonyms:

1. *pes hippocampi (Bergen, 1734)*
   Probably refers to macrodissected adult human ***calcarine spur (Morand, 1748)***; see Tarin (1750, Tab. XIII, Fig. 3-*f*).

LATER SYNONYMS:

1. *eminentia minor (Günz, 1750)*
   Synonym for macrodissected adult human ***calcarine spur (Morand, 1748)***; see Haller (1762; p. 45, note *c* of Vol. IV, 1757).
2. *unguis (Haller, 1754a)*
   Synonym (meaning claw or nail) for macrodissected adult human ***calcarine spur (Morand, 1748)***; see Vicq d'Azyr (1786, pp. 7, 15), Lewis (1923, p. 227).
3. *colliculus (Haller, 1754a)*
   Synonym for macrodissected adult human ***calcarine spur (Morand, 1748)***; see Vicq d'Azyr (1786, pp. 7, 15).
4. *pes hippopotami minor (Mayer, 1779)*
   Mayer identified macrodissected adult human ***calcarine spur (Morand, 1748)*** as "small foot of the hippopotamus" (Tab. III-*r*; the German, *kleiner fuss des Seepferdes*, was used with Latin in parentheses) along with a number of clear digitations (Tab. III-*s*). The "small foot of the hippopotamus" comes off *leg of vault (Vesling, 1647)* and is in contrast to "large foot of the hippopotamus", the *pes hippopotami major (Mayer, 1779)*.
5. *small foot of hippopotamus (Mayer, 1779)*
   English form of *pes hippopotami minor (Mayer, 1779)*.
6. *pedis minoris hippocampi (Haase, 1781)*
   Haase "corrected" the term just introduced as *pes hippopotami minor (Mayer, 1779)*; p. 19. Also see Haller (1762, p. 34).
7. *small foot of seahorse (Haase, 1781)*
   English form of *pedis minoris hippocampi (Haase, 1781)*.
8. *digiti pedis minoris hippocampi (Haase, 1781)*
   Refinement in description of *pedis minoris hippocampi (Haase, 1781)*; p. 19.
9. *digits of small foot of seahorse (Haase, 1781)*
   English form of *digiti pedis minoris hippocampi (Haase, 1781)*. Also see *pes hippopotami minor (Mayer, 1779)*.
10. *hippocampus minor (Vicq d'Azyr, 1786)*
   Synonym for macrodissected adult human ***calcarine spur (Morand, 1748)***; in the original French, *petit hypocampe*, see Plate V-*x*, p. 9; Plate XXI, Figure I-29. Also see Meyer (1971, p. 21).
11. *second hippocampus (Vicq d'Azyr, 1786)*
   Synonym for macrodissected adult human ***calcarine spur (Morand, 1748)***; Plate V-*x*.

12. *colliculus caveae posterioris ventriculi lateralis (Vicq d'Azyr, 1786)*
Synonym for macrodissected adult human ***calcarine spur (Morand, 1748)***; pp. 7, 9 note *1*.
13. *ocrea (Günther, 1786)*
Synonym for macrodissected adult human ***calcarine spur (Morand, 1748)***; in English, a *greave*; p. 11.
14. *unciform eminence (Chaussier, 1807)*
Synonym for macrodissected adult human ***calcarine spur (Morand, 1748)***; p. 68, given by Burdach (1822, p. 376) in Latin as *eminentia unciformis*.
15. *hintre oder kleine Wulst (Tiedemann, 1816)*
Synonym for macrodissected adult human ***calcarine spur (Morand, 1748)***; p. 53, see Burdach (1822, p. 376).
16. *lesser hippocampus (Bell & Bell, 1816)*
Synonym for macrodissected adult human ***calcarine spur (Morand, 1748)***; Vol. 2, p. 447.
17. *digital eminence (Meckel, 1817)*
Synonym for macrodissected adult human ***calcarine spur (Morand, 1748)***; in the original Latin, *eminentia digitata*, see translation (1832, Vol. 2, p. 463) and Meyer (1971, p. 21).
18. *convolutions of digital cavity (Cruveilhier, 1836)*
Synonym for macrodissected adult human ***calcarine spur (Morand, 1748)***; in the original French, *circonvolutions de la cavité digitale*, p. 663.
19. *ergot de Morand (Cruveilhier, 1836)*
French eponym for macrodissected adult human ***calcarine spur (Morand, 1748)***; p. 697.

calcarine sulcus (>1840)

As described for macrodissected adult human, the deep and convoluted groove in the medial surface of the ***occipital region (Vesalius, 1543a)*** between ***lingual gyrus (>1840)*** ventrally and ***cuneus (Burdach, 1822)*** dorsally; see Williams & Warwick (1980, Fig. 7.114A), Nieuwenhuys et al. (2008, Figs. 5.17-*4*, 5.22-*10*). It was perhaps first delineated accurately by Soemmerring; see ***[calcarine sulcus (>1840)] (Soemmerring, 1778)***.

EARLIER REFERENCES:

Illustrated, not named or described:

1. ***[calcarine sulcus (>1840)] (Soemmerring, 1778)***
Accurately illustrated for macrodissected adult human in midsagittal view; Table III. Burdach reported that Malacarne (1780, Pt. II, p. 10) described without naming it, and Vicq d'Azyr (1786, Tab. III) also illustrated it.

Earlier synonyms:

1. *posterior cerebral fissure (Reil, 1809b)*
Synonym for macrodissected adult human ***calcarine sulcus (>1840)*** described as second only to *Sylvian fissure (Vicq d'Azyr, 1784)* in magnitude. Reil also noted one of its indentations produces a prominence in ***posterior horn of lateral ventricle (Haller, 1747)***, the ***calcarine spur (Morand, 1748)***; see Mayo translation (1823, p. 73). Burdach (1822, pp. 166, 387) reported that Reil used the German term, *kleine hintre Grube* (p. 185), and gave the Latin form, *fissura posterior*.
2. *sulcus under cuneus (Burdach, 1822)*
Synonym for macrodissected adult human ***calcarine sulcus (>1840)***; in the original German, *die Furche unter dem Zwickel*, p. 412. Also see Meyer (1971, p. 130).

cardiac branches of recurrent laryngeal nerve (>1840)

As described for macrodissected adult human, on the right side these small branches of the ***recurrent laryngeal nerve (Albinus, 1744)*** course to the ***cardiac plexus (Keill, 1698)***, whereas on the left side one relatively large branch typically arises near the origin of the left subclavian artery and courses past the left side of the aortic arch to the ***cardiac plexus (Keill, 1698)***; see Mitchell (1953, pp. 181–182), Williams & Warwick (1980, p. 1081). They were first identified by Eustachi; see ***[cardiac branches of recurrent laryngeal nerve (>1840)] (Eustachi, 1552)***.

EARLIER REFERENCES:

Illustrated, not named or described:

1. ***[cardiac branches of recurrent laryngeal nerve (>1840)] (Eustachi, 1552)***
Illustrated branch of macrodissected adult human ***recurrent laryngeal nerve (Albinus, 1744)*** joining ***thoracic cardiac branches of vagus nerve (>1840)***; see Albinus edition (1761, Tab. 18, Fig. 2-*s*, p. 105).

Described, not named or illustrated:

1. ***[cardiac branches of recurrent laryngeal nerve (>1840)] (Falloppio, 1561)***
Described for macrodissected adult human and attributed original observation to others without citation; see Diemerbroeck (1689, p. 418).

Illustrated and described, not named:

1. ***[cardiac branches of recurrent laryngeal nerve (>1840)] (Willis, 1664)***
Described and illustrated for right ***recurrent laryngeal nerve (>1840)*** in macrodissected adult human and other common large mammals; see Pordage translation (1681, p. 147 and Tab. 9-*n*). Vieussens provided considerably more detailed description for macrodissected adult human, including branches directly to left atrium and ventricle of heart; Table 23-*z,3,4*.

Earlier synonyms:

1. *descending branches of recurrent nerves (Scarpa, 1794)*
Roughly synonymous with macrodissected adult human ***cardiac branches of recurrent laryngeal nerve (>1840)***; in the original Latin, *recurrentis nervi rami descendentes*, Table III:*12,13,30–34*.
2. *filaments to cardiac nerves from pneumogastric nerve (Meckel, 1817)*
Synonym for macrodissected adult human ***cardiac branches of recurrent laryngeal nerve (>1840)***; see translation (1832, Vol. 3, p. 48).
3. *cardiac filaments of recurrent nerve (Cruveilhier, 1836)*
Synonym for macrodissected adult human ***cardiac branches of recurrent laryngeal nerve (>1840)***; in the original French, *filets cardiaques*, p. 963.

PARTLY CORRESPONDS:

1. *first cardiac branch of recurrent nerves (Mayer, 1794)*
First of two macrodissected adult human ***cardiac branches of recurrent laryngeal nerve (>1840)***; in the original Latin, *ramus cardiacus primus nervi recurrentis*; Part 6, Table II, Figure 1-*73* (p. 12).
2. *second cardiac branch of recurrent nerves (Mayer, 1794)*
Second of two macrodissected adult human ***cardiac branches of recurrent laryngeal nerve (>1840)***; in the original Latin, *ramus cardiacus secundus nervi recurrentis*; Part 6, Table II, Figure 1-*75* (p. 12).

cardiac ganglion (Neubauer, 1772; Haller, 1772)

As described for macrodissected adult human, the largest of a group of small ***terminal ganglia (Gaskell, 1886)*** embedded in superficial parts of the ***cardiac plexus (Keill, 1698)***; see Mitchell (1953, p. 252) and Williams & Warwick (1980, p. 1132) for human, and Al et al. (2007) for rat and mouse. For Neubauer's use in macrodissected adult human, see pp. 144-4, 154–157, and Table 2, Figure 1-*227*; for Haller's use, see p. 7, note *20*. Scarpa (1794, Tab. III-*114,115*) and Lobstein (1823, p. 19) clearly used the term in the modern sense for macrodissected adult human. It was first clearly indicated as the *cardiac infolding (Willis, 1664)*.

EARLIER REFERENCES:

Earlier synonyms:

1. *cardiac infolding (Willis, 1664)*
From illustrations, Willis clearly delineated ***cardiac ganglion (Neubauer, 1772; Haller, 1772)*** in macrodissected adult human and other large mammals, although the original Latin term is *plexum cardiacum*; see Pordage translation (p. 147; Tab. IX-*l*,*Δ*; and Tab. X).

LATER SYNONYMS:

1. *ganglion cervicale imum (Neubauer, 1772)*
Synonym for ***cardiac ganglion (Neubauer, 1772; Haller, 1772)***; p. 154.
2. *ganglion parvum cervicale imum (Neubauer, 1772)*
Synonym for ***cardiac ganglion (Neubauer, 1772; Haller, 1772)***; Table 2, Figure 1-*227*.
3. *cardiac ganglion of Wrisberg (Scarpa, 1794)*
Eponym for ***cardiac ganglion (Neubauer, 1772; Haller, 1772)***; in the original Latin, *ganglion cardiacum Wrisbergh*, Table IV-32. Wrisberg's description was from 1786 in the *Sylloge commentationum anatomicarum. II. Nervis arterias venasque comitantibus*.
4. *ganglion of cardiac nerves (Soemmerring, 1798)*
Probably synonym for ***cardiac ganglion (Neubauer, 1772; Haller, 1772)***; in the original Latin, *ganglion nervorum cordis*, p. 346.
5. *ganglion molle and pellucidum of Scarpa (Bell, 1803b)*
Eponym for macrodissected adult human *cardiac ganglion of Wrisberg (Scarpa, 1794)*; p. 175.
6. *cardiac ganglion of sympathetic (Knox, 1832)*
Synonym for macrodissected adult human ***cardiac ganglion (Neubauer, 1772; Haller, 1772)***; Plate III-*107*.
7. *soft and pellucid ganglion of deep cardiac nerve (Knox, 1832)*
Synonym for *ganglion molle and pellucidum of Scarpa (Bell, 1803b)*; Plate III-*154* in Knox's translation of Scarpa (1794).

PARTLY CORRESPONDS:

1. *lesser cardiac infolding (Willis, 1664)*
Willis divided *cardiac infolding (Willis, 1664)* into lesser and greater parts, with the former supplying right and anterior regions of the heart; see Pordage translation (1681, pp. 148, 151).
2. *greater cardiac infolding (Willis, 1664)*
Willis divided *cardiac infolding (Willis, 1664)* into lesser and greater parts, with the latter supplying left and posterior regions of the heart; see Pordage translation (1681, pp. 148, 151).
3. *olivary ganglion (Cloquet, 1828)*
Essentially, differentiation of macrodissected adult human ***cardiac ganglion (Neubauer, 1772; Haller, 1772)*** associated with ***coronary plexuses (Meckel, 1817)***; in the original French, *ganglion olivaire*, Plate CLXII-*83*.

cardiac plexus (Keill, 1698)

As described for macrodissected adult human, a ***terminal plexus (Swanson & Bota, 2010)*** formed by the various ***nerves (Herophilus, c335–c280 BC)*** associated with the heart and parasympathetic ***cardiac ganglion (Neubauer, 1772; Haller, 1772)***. It lies around the great vessels at the base of the heart and shows considerable variation between individuals. It is commonly divided now into arbitrary superficial and deep, or anterior (ventral) and posterior (dorsal) parts, and its main extensions are the ***preaortic plexus (Arnulf, 1939)***, ***coronary plexuses (Meckel, 1817)***, and ***atrial plexuses (>1840)***; see Durward (1951, pp. 1138–1140), Mitchell (1953, pp. 250–253), Williams & Warwick (1980, p. 1132). For Keill's use in macrodissected adult human, see pp. 293, 295. Falloppio is usually credited with discovering it; see ***[cardiac plexus (Keill, 1698)] (Falloppio, 1561)***.

TRANSLATIONS:

1. *plexus cardiacus (Keill, 1698)*
Original Latin form of ***cardiac plexus (Keill, 1698)***; p. 293.
2. *cordis plexum (Haase, 1781)*
Latin form of ***cardiac plexus (Keill, 1698)***, p. 119. Haase recognized superficial (*superficialem*) and deep (*profundum*) parts in macrodissected adult human.

EARLIER REFERENCES:

Described, not named or illustrated:

1. ***[cardiac plexus (Keill, 1698)] (Falloppio, 1561)***
Falloppio provided a detailed description of five, or less commonly four, ***nerves (Herophilus, c335–c280 BC)*** to this "infolding" in macrodissected adult human, and according to Johnstone (1795, p. 13) his account was much more accurate than Willis's and stood the test of time; see Diemerbroeck translation (1689, p. 418). In his excellent historical overview, Senac (1749, Vol. 1, p. 116) credited Falloppio with discovering the ***cardiac plexus (Keill, 1698)***.

Illustrated, not named or described:

1. ***[cardiac plexus (Keill, 1698)] (Willis, 1664)***
   Willis certainly illustrated it for macrodissected adult human, including a *cardiac infolding (Willis, 1664)*, even if he did not describe it as such; Table 9. He also referred to some "nerve fibers" distributed to anterior, and others to posterior, regions of the heart; Table 9-*o,s,τ*.

LATER SYNONYMS:

1. *great cardiac plexus (Neubauer, 1772)*
   Synonym for macrodissected adult human ***cardiac plexus (Keill, 1698)***; in the original Latin, *plexum cardiacum magnum*, p. 129.
2. *cardiac ganglion of Wrisberg (Quain, 1828)*
   Eponym for macrodissected adult human ***cardiac plexus (Keill, 1698)***; in the original Latin, *ganglion cardiacum*, Wrisberg, p. 667.
3. *aortic plexus (Quain, 1837, p. 814)*
   Alternate term Quain gave, in quotes, for macrodissected adult human ***cardiac plexus (Keill, 1698)***; p. 814.

PARTLY CORRESPONDS:

1. *nerveus plexus cardiacus superior (Vieussens, 1684)*
   Roughly equivalent to all but caudal (lower or inferior) end of ***cardiac plexus (Keill, 1698)***; Vieussens's description and illustration of it in macrodissected adult human was considerably better than that of ***[cardiac plexus (Keill, 1698)] (Willis, 1664)***; Table 23-43.
2. *nerveum plexum cardiacum superiorem (Vieussens, 1684)*
   Alternate form of *nerveus plexus cardiacus superior (Vieussens, 1684)*; Table 23-*8*.
3. *nerveo plexui cardiaco superiorem (Vieussens, 1684)*
   Alternate form of *nerveus plexus cardiacus superior (Vieussens, 1684)*; Table 23-*y*.
4. *nerveum plexum cardiacum inferiorem (Vieussens, 1684)*
   Roughly equivalent to caudal (lower) end of ***cardiac plexus (Keill, 1698)*** in macrodissected adult human; Table 23-*51*.
5. *lesser cardiack plex of par vagum (Collins, 1685)*
   Probably synonymous with *nerveum plexum cardiacum inferiorem (Vieussens, 1684)*; Collins described it as transmitting fibers to the forepart of the right chamber of the heart in macrodissected adult human; p. 1051.
6. *superior cardiac plexus (Drake, 1707)*
   Synonym for macrodissected adult human *nerveus plexus cardiacus superior (Vieussens, 1684)*; in the original Latin, *plexus cardiacus superior*, p. 517.
7. *great anterior plexus of heart (Senac, 1749)*
   Senac's description and illustration for macrodissected adult human were vague, but it lies dorsal to (behind) the aorta and probably corresponds roughly with *deep part of great cardiac plexus (Scarpa, 1794)*; in the original French, *grand plexus antérieur*, pp. 493–494 and Plate 5, Figure 3.
8. *great posterior plexus of heart (Senac, 1749)*
   Senac's description and illustration for macrodissected adult human were vague, but it probably corresponds roughly with *posterior plexus of heart (Haller, 1772)*; in the original French, *grand plexus postérieur*, pp. 493–494, and Plate 5, Figure 5.
9. *posterior plexus of heart (Haller, 1772)*
   Larger or superficial part of macrodissected adult human ***cardiac plexus (Keill, 1698)***; in the original Latin, *plexum cordis posteriorem*, p. 11-*[9]4*.
10. *superficial plexus of heart (Haller, 1772)*
    As described for macrodissected adult human, probably synonym for *superficial cardiac plexus (Lobstein, 1823)*; in the original Latin, *plexus superficiales cordis*, p. 12.
11. *magno nervo cardiaco (Wrisberg, 1786)*
    Synonym for macrodissected adult human *principal cardiac nerve (Lobstein, 1823)*; p. 29, see Lobstein (1831, p. 19). An English form is *large cardiac nerve*.
12. *novo nervo cardiaco (Wrisberg, 1786)*
    Synonym for macrodissected adult human *principal cardiac nerve (Lobstein, 1823)*; p. 29, see Lobstein (1831, p. 19). An English form is *new cardiac nerve*.
13. *communicating branches of superficial aortic nerves with anterior aortic plexus (Andersch & Soemmerring, 1792)*
    In macrodissected adult human, ***communicating branches (Winslow, 1733)*** of *superficial aortic nerves (Andersch & Soemmerring, 1792)* with *anterior aortic plexus (Andersch & Soemmerring, 1792)*; in the original Latin, *nervi cardiaci superficialis communicatorii rami plexus aortici anterioris*, p. 192.
14. *superficial cardiac plexus (Mayer, 1794)*
    Somewhat artificial division of macrodissected adult human ***cardiac plexus (Keill, 1698)***; in the original Latin, *plexus cardiacus superficialis*; Part 6, Table II, Figure 1-*38* (p. 11). Lobstein (see 1831, p. 21) described it as arising from three branches of ***superior cardiac nerve (Neubauer, 1772)*** encircling aorta and brachiocephalic artery and compared it to *deep seated cardiac plexus (Lobstein, 1823)*. According to Lobstein, left ***superior cardiac nerve (Neubauer, 1772)*** can arise from ***superior thoracic ganglion (Lieutaud, 1742)***; see translation (1831, p. 21).
15. *deep cardiac plexus (Mayer, 1794)*
    Somewhat artificial division of macrodissected adult human ***cardiac plexus (Keill, 1698)***; in the original Latin, *plexus cardiacus profundus*; Part 6, Table II, Figure 1-*38* (p. 11). Also see *deep seated cardiac plexus (Lobstein, 1823)*.
16. *great deep cardiac plexus (Scarpa, 1794)*
    Deeper ventral (anterior) parts of macrodissected adult human ***cardiac plexus (Keill, 1698)***; in the original Latin, *plexum cardiacum magnum profundum*, Table IV-22. English form from Knox (1832, Pl. IV-*31*).
17. *superficial nerve of heart (Andersch, 1797)*
    In macrodissected adult human, branch of *superficial cardiac nerve (Andersch & Soemmerring, 1792)*; in the original Latin, *nervum superficialem cordis*, Vol. 2, p. 50.
18. *inferior oblique nerve of ductus arteriosus (Andersch, 1797)*
    In macrodissected human, derived from left *external cardiac nerve (Andersch & Soemmerring, 1792)* and essentially component of ***cardiac plexus (Keill, 1698)***; in the original Latin, *nervum obliquum inferiorem ductus arteriosi*, Vol. 2, p. 31.
19. *anterior deep nerve of ductus arteriosus (Andersch, 1797)*

In macrodissected adult human, branch of *superficial branch of superficial cardiac nerve (Andersch, 1797)* and essentially component of ***cardiac plexus (Keill, 1698)***; in the original Latin, *nervum profundum anteriorem ductus arteriosi*, Vol. 2, p. 89.

20. *lateral deep nerve of ductus arteriosus (Andersch, 1797)*
In macrodissected adult human, derived from *superficial branch of superficial cardiac nerve (Andersch, 1797)* and essentially component of ***cardiac plexus (Keill, 1698)***; in the original Latin, *nervum profundum lateralem ductus arteriosi*, Vol. 2, p. 90.
21. *posterior superficial nerve of ductus arteriosus (Andersch, 1797)*
In macrodissected adult human, derived from *superficial branch of superficial cardiac nerve (Andersch, 1797)* and essentially component of ***cardiac plexus (Keill, 1698)***; in the original Latin, *ductus arteriosi nervo superficiali posteriori*, Vol. 2, p. 90.
22. *lateral superficial nerves of ductus arteriosus (Andersch, 1797)*
In macrodissected adult human, derived from *superficial branch of superficial cardiac nerve (Andersch, 1797)* and essentially component of ***cardiac plexus (Keill, 1698)***; in the original Latin, *nervi superficialis lateralis ductus arteriosi*, Vol. 2, p. 90.
23. *communicating branch of anterior aortic plexus (Andersch, 1797)*
Relatively small macrodissected adult human ***communicating branch (Winslow, 1733)*** between *superficial branches of superficial cardiac nerve (Andersch, 1797)* and *anterior aortic plexus (Andersch, 1797)*; in the original Latin, *ramus communicatorius plexus aortici anterioris*, Vol. 2, pp. 91–93.
24. *communicating nerves of anterior aortic plexus (Andersch, 1797)*
Relatively large macrodissected adult human ***communicating branches (Winslow, 1733)*** between *superficial branches of superficial cardiac nerve (Andersch, 1797)* and *anterior aortic plexus (Andersch, 1797)*; in the original Latin, *nervi communicatorii plexus aortici anterioris*, Vol. 2, p. 92.
25. *anterior aortic plexus (Andersch, 1797)*
Apparently part or extension of macrodissected adult human ***cardiac plexus (Keill, 1698)*** around ventral (anterior) parts of aorta in thorax, including descending aorta; in the original Latin, *plexum aorticum anteriorem*, Vol. 2, p. 92.
26. *interarterial superficial plexus (Andersch, 1797)*
Part or extension of macrodissected adult human ***cardiac plexus (Keill, 1698)*** under aortic arch; in the original Latin, *plexum superficialem inter arteriosum*, Vol. 2, p. 95.
27. *posterior lateral nerve of ductus arteriosus (Andersch, 1797)*
In macrodissected adult human, derived from *superficial branch of superficial cardiac nerve (Andersch, 1797)* and essentially component of ***cardiac plexus (Keill, 1698)***; in the original Latin, *nervum posteriorem ductus arteriosi*, Vol. 2, p. 98.
28. *highest superficial nerve of anterior ventricle of heart (Andersch, 1797)*
In macrodissected adult human, derived from *superficial nerve of heart (Andersch, 1797)* and essentially component of ***cardiac plexus (Keill, 1698)*** related to right ventricle; in the original Latin, *nervus superficialis supremus ventriculi anterioris cordis*, Vol. 2, p. 104.
29. *middle superficial branch of anterior ventricle of heart (Andersch, 1797)*
In macrodissected adult human, derived from *superficial nerve of heart (Andersch, 1797)* and essentially component of ***cardiac plexus (Keill, 1698)*** related to right ventricle; in the original Latin, *ramus superficialis medius ventriculi anterioris cordis*, Vol. 2, p. 106.
30. *lowest superficial branch of anterior ventricle of heart (Andersch, 1797)*
In macrodissected adult human, derived from *superficial nerve of heart (Andersch, 1797)* and essentially component of ***cardiac plexus (Keill, 1698)*** related to right ventricle; in the original Latin, *ramum superficialem infimum ventriculi anterioris cordis*, Vol. 2, p. 107.
31. *trunk of great deep cardiac nerve of left side (Fyfe, 1800)*
For macrodissected adult human, appears to correspond roughly to, or to generate, *anterior branch of cardiac ganglion (Lobstein, 1823)*, *middle branch of cardiac ganglion (Lobstein, 1823)*, and *posterior branch of cardiac ganglion (Lobstein, 1823)*; Vol. 2, p. 319.
32. *inferior cardiac plexus (Cuvier, 1800)*
Synonym for macrodissected adult human *nerveus plexus cardiacus inferiorem (Vieussens, 1684)*; in the original French, *plexus cardiaque inférieur*, Vol. 2, p. 232.
33. *anterior cardiac plexus (Burdin, 1803)*
For macrodissected adult human, part of ***cardiac plexus (Keill, 1698)*** associated specifically with right ventricle and left atrium; see translation (1803, Vol. 1, p. 210).
34. *posterior cardiac plexus (Burdin, 1803)*
For macrodissected adult human, part of ***cardiac plexus (Keill, 1698)*** associated specifically with left ventricle and right atrium; see translation (1803, Vol. 1, p. 211).
35. *deep seated cardiac plexus (Lobstein, 1823)*
Somewhat artificial division of macrodissected adult human ***cardiac plexus (Keill, 1698)***. Lobstein described its composition in detail—stating that each branch has triple origin from ***superior cardiac nerve (Neubauer, 1772)***, ***inferior cardiac nerve (Cloquet, 1816)***, and ***inferior cervical cardiac branches of recurrent laryngeal nerve (>1840)***—and contrasted it to *superficial cardiac plexus (Lobstein, 1823)*. He also described major differences between contributions from right and left ***nerves (Herophilus, c335–c280 BC)*** just listed; see translation (1831, pp. 18–23).
36. *great cardiac plexus (Lobstein, 1823)*
Synonym for *deep seated cardiac plexus (Lobstein, 1823)*; see translation (1831, p. 18).
37. *interior and anterior cardiac nerves (Lobstein, 1823)*
Branches in macrodissected adult human ***cardiac plexus (Keill, 1698)*** derived chiefly from ***superior cardiac nerve (Neubauer, 1772)***; see translation (1831, p. 18).

38. *middle cardiac nerves (Lobstein, 1823)*
   Branches in macrodissected adult human ***cardiac plexus (Keill, 1698)*** derived principally from ***inferior cardiac nerve (Cloquet, 1816)***; see translation (1831, p. 18).
39. *exterior and posterior cardiac nerves (Lobstein, 1823)*
   Branches in macrodissected adult human ***cardiac plexus (Keill, 1698)*** derived chiefly but not exclusively from ***inferior cervical cardiac branches of recurrent laryngeal nerve (>1840)***; see translation (1831, p. 18).
40. *middle nerves of cardiac plexus (Lobstein, 1823)*
   Synonym for *middle cardiac nerves (Lobstein, 1823)*; see translation (1831, p. 18).
41. *deep seated nerves of heart (Lobstein, 1823)*
   Two most conspicuous branches of *middle nerves of cardiac plexus (Lobstein, 1823)*—the ***inferior cardiac nerve (Cloquet, 1816)***—one being *principal cardiac nerve (Lobstein, 1823)* and the other *collateral branch of principal cardiac nerve (Lobstein, 1823)*; see translation (1831, pp. 18–19).
42. *cardiac nerves near heart (Lobstein, 1823)*
   The *interior and anterior cardiac nerves (Lobstein, 1823)*, *middle cardiac nerves (Lobstein, 1823)*, and *exterior and posterior cardiac nerves (Lobstein, 1823)*, considered together; see translation (1831, pp. 19–23).
43. *principal cardiac nerve (Lobstein, 1823)*
   As described for macrodissected adult human, branch of ***cardiac plexus (Keill, 1698)*** leading directly into ***cardiac ganglion (Neubauer, 1772, Haller, 1772)***; see translation (1831, p. 19).
44. *anterior branch of cardiac ganglion (Lobstein, 1823)*
   As described in detail for macrodissected adult human, branch of ***cardiac ganglion (Neubauer, 1772, Haller, 1772)*** going on to form much of ***right coronary plexus (Scarpa, 1794)***; see translation (1831, p. 19).
45. *middle branch of cardiac ganglion (Lobstein, 1823)*
   As described in detail for macrodissected adult human, continuation of *principal cardiac nerve (Lobstein, 1823)* past ***cardiac ganglion (Neubauer, 1772, Haller, 1772)*** going on to form, among other differentiations, ***left coronary plexus (Scarpa, 1794)***; see translation (1831, pp. 19–20).
46. *posterior branch of cardiac ganglion (Lobstein, 1823)*
   As described in detail for macrodissected adult human, component of ***cardiac plexus (Keill, 1698)*** related primarily to pulmonary artery; see translation (1831, p. 20).
47. *collateral branch of principal cardiac nerve (Lobstein, 1823)*
   As described in detail for macrodissected adult human, component of *deep seated nerves of heart (Lobstein, 1823)* not leading into ***cardiac ganglion (Neubauer, 1772, Haller, 1772)***; see translation description of its distribution (1831, p. 20).
48. *right lateral cardiac plexus (Swan, 1830)*
   In macrodissected adult human, Swan divided ***cardiac ganglion (Neubauer, 1772, Haller, 1772)*** into *right lateral cardiac plexus (Swan, 1830)* and *left lateral cardiac plexus (Swan, 1830)*; pp. 5–6.
49. *left lateral cardiac plexus (Swan, 1830)*
   In macrodissected adult human, Swan divided ***cardiac ganglion (Neubauer, 1772, Haller, 1772)*** into *right lateral cardiac plexus (Swan, 1830)* and *left lateral cardiac plexus (Swan, 1830)*; pp. 5–6.
50. *ventricular plexus (Swan, 1830)*
   For macrodissected adult human, basically combination of ***preaortic plexus (Arnulf, 1939)*** and ***coronary plexuses (Meckel, 1817)***; p. 6.
51. *superficial layer of cardiac nerves (Cruveilhier, 1836)*
   Synonym for macrodissected adult human *superficial cardiac plexus (Mayer, 1794)*, described as occupying anterior (ventral) surface of aortic arch, especially on right, and passing to anterior coronary artery; in the original French, *plan nerveux superficiel*, p. 1005.
52. *middle layer of cardiac nerves (Cruveilhier, 1836)*
   Essentially, synonym for macrodissected adult human *middle cardiac nerves (Lobstein, 1823)* described as having two parts: one between trachea and aortic arch above right pulmonary artery, and the other smaller one between right pulmonary artery and aortic arch; in the original French, *plan nerveux moyen*, p. 1005.
53. *deep layer of cardiac nerves (Cruveilhier, 1836)*
   Essentially, synonym for macrodissected adult human *deep seated cardiac nerves (Lobstein, 1823)* described as lying between right pulmonary artery and bifurcation of trachea; in the original French, *plan nerveux profond*, p. 1005.
54. *anterior auricular branches of deep cardiac plexus (Cruveilhier, 1836)*
   For macrodissected adult human, numerous extensions of *great deep cardiac plexus (Scarpa, 1794)*, which Cruveilhier defined as composed of *middle layer of cardiac nerves (Cruveilhier, 1836)* and *deep layer of cardiac nerves (Cruveilhier, 1836)* considered together; in the original French, *rameaux cardiaques antérieur*, p. 1006.

caroticotympanic nerves (>1840)

As described for macrodissected adult human, extensions—usually described as ***superior caroticotympanic nerve (>1840)*** and ***inferior caroticotympanic nerve (>1840)***—of the ***internal carotid plexus (>1840)*** passing through the wall of the carotid canal to the ***tympanic plexus (>1840)***; see Durward (1951, Figs. 901, 905), Williams & Warwick (1980, p. 1200, Fig. 7.184). Jacobson is usually credited with their discovery; see ***[caroticotympanic nerves (>1840)] (Jacobson, 1818)***.

EARLIER REFERENCES:

Described, not named or illustrated:

1. ***[caroticotympanic nerves (>1840)] (Jacobson, 1818)***
   Clearly described for macrodissected adult human; see Lobstein (1831, p. 36).

Earlier synonyms:

1. *anastomosis of Jacobson's nerve with sympathetic nerve (Langenbeck, 1826–1830)*
   For macrodissected adult human, at least one of the ***caroticotympanic nerves (>1840)***; in the original Latin, *anastomosis nervi Jacobsonii cum nervo sympathico*, Fascicle III, Table XVII-*d*.
2. *branch of Jacobson's nerve to sympathetic nerve (Langenbeck, 1826–1830)*

Synonym for *anastomosis of Jacobson's nerve with sympathetic nerve (Langenbeck, 1826–1830)*; in the original Latin, *ramus nervi Jacobsonii ad nervum sympathicum*, Fascicle III, Table XXV-*x*.

3. *connection of carotid nerve with tympanic nerve (Arnold, 1834)*
   Probably synonym for macrodissected adult human ***caroticotympanic nerves (>1840)***; in the original Latin, *conjunctio nervus caroticus ramus externus cum nervo tympanico*, p. 18.
4. *anastomotic filament of external branch of carotid branch of superior cervical ganglion with branch of Jacobson (Cruveilhier, 1836)*
   Synonym for macrodissected adult human ***caroticotympanic nerves (>1840)***; in the original French, *filet anastomotique avec le rameau de Jacobson*, p. 986.
5. *lesser superficial petrosal nerve (Quain & Wilson, 1839)*
   Synonym for macrodissected adult human ***caroticotympanic nerves (>1840)***; in the original Latin, *nervus petrosus superficialis minor*, Plate XXVII-*t*.

carotid branch of vagus nerve (>1840)

In somewhat over half of macrodissected adult humans, one or more branches of the ***vagus nerve trunk (Wrisberg, 1786; Günther, 1786)*** join the ***carotid branches of glossopharyngeal nerve (Todd, 1836–1839)*** and/or *intercarotid plexus (Luschka, 1862)* to innervate the carotid body and/or carotid sinus; see Funke (1904), Fuse (1950), Boyd (1937, p. 395), Mitchell (1953, p. 174), ***carotid branches of glossopharyngeal nerve (Todd, 1836-1839)***. It was discovered by Willis; see ***[carotid branch of vagus nerve (>1840)] (Willis, 1664)***.

EARLIER REFERENCES:

Described, not named or illustrated:

1. ***[carotid branch of vagus nerve (>1840)] (Willis, 1664)***
   Described for macrodissected adult human; see Pordage translation (1861, p. 147).

Earlier synonyms:

1. *posterior carotid artery nerve (Andersch & Soemmerring, 1792)*
   Probably macrodissected adult human ***carotid branch of vagus nerve (>1840)***; in the original Latin, *nervus arteriae carotidis posterioris*, p. 133. Nicely illustrated by Loder (1803, Tab. CLXXVII-*66*).

carotid branches of glossopharyngeal nerve (Todd, 1836–1839)

As described for macrodissected adult human, branches of the ***glossopharyngeal nerve trunk (Wrisberg, 1786; Günther, 1786)*** varying in number and origin and innervating the carotid sinus and carotid body after contributing to the nearby junctional region of the ***internal carotid plexus (>1840)*** and ***external carotid plexus (>1840)***, sometimes called the *intercarotid plexus (Luschka, 1862)*; see Funke (1904), Boyd (1937, p. 393 ff.), Fuse (1950), Hamilton (1976, Fig. 807), ***carotid branch of vagus nerve (>1840)***. Common synonyms include *carotid sinus nerve (Hering, 1924)* and *carotid sinus branch of glossopharyngeal nerve (>1840)*, which are misleading. For Todd's use in macrodissected adult human, see p. 496. They were first noted by Haller; see ***[carotid branches of glossopharyngeal nerve (Todd, 1836–1839)] (Haller, 1762)***.

EARLIER REFERENCES:

Described, not named or illustrated:

1. ***[carotid branches of glossopharyngeal nerve (Todd, 1836–1839)] (Haller, 1762)***
   Described vaguely for macrodissected adult human; p. 232.

Earlier synonyms:

1. *second glossopharyngeal branch (Neubauer, 1772)*
   Synonym for macrodissected adult human ***carotid branches of glossopharyngeal nerve (Todd, 1836–1839)***; in the original Latin, *secundus ramus glossopharyngei*, Table 2-77. A number of such branches were clearly illustrated and described by Scarpa (1794, Tab. II).
2. *carotid filaments of glossopharyngeal nerve (Cruveilhier, 1836)*
   Synonym for macrodissected adult human ***carotid branches of glossopharyngeal nerve (Todd, 1836–1839)***; in the original French, *filets carotidiens*, p. 953.

LATER SYNONYMS:

1. *carotid sinus nerve (Hering, 1924)*
   Common synonym for ***carotid sinus branches of glossopharyngeal nerve (>1840)***; see Boyd (1937, pp. 386, 397) and ***carotid branch of vagus nerve (Todd, 1836– 1839)***. It is not, however, accurate.
2. *carotid sinus branch of glossopharyngeal nerve (>1840)*
   Convenient synonym for ***carotid branches of glossopharyngeal nerve (Todd, 1836–1839)***. It is not, however, accurate.
3. *nervus glossopharyngeus ramus sinus carotici (>1840)*
   Latin form of *carotid sinus branch of glossopharyngeal nerve (>1840)*; see *Terminologia Anatomica* (1998, p. 136).

carotid ganglion (Wutzer, 1817; Bock, 1817)

As described for adult human, one or more macroscopic sympathetic ***paravertebral ganglia (Durward, 1951)*** and scattered sympathetic ganglion cells, commonly associated with the ***internal carotid plexus (>1840)*** in the carotid canal and/or cavernous sinus; see Mitchell (1953, p. 215), Williams & Warwick (1980, p. 1127). For Wutzer's use in macrodissected adult human see p. 97; for Bock's use see p. 66. It was probably discovered by Willis; see ***[carotid ganglion (Wutzer, 1817; Bock, 1817)] (Willis, 1664)***.

TRANSLATIONS:

1. *ganglion caroticum (Bock, 1817)*
   Original Latin form of ***carotid ganglion (Wutzer, 1817; Bock, 1817)***; p. 66.

EARLIER REFERENCES:

Described, not named or illustrated:

1. ***[carotid ganglion (Wutzer, 1817; Bock, 1817)] (Willis, 1664)***
   Willis may have noted it, as quoted by Bell & Bell (1829, p. 503). Meckel (1748, p. 129 note *a*) also may have noted it in macrodissected adult human; in the

original Latin,...*intra canalem caroticum ganglia nervi intercostalis*, p. 129.

Earlier synonyms:

1. *cavernous ganglion (Laumonier, 1793)*
   Synonym for macrodissected adult human ***carotid ganglion (Wutzer, 1817; Bock, 1817)***; p. 262, see Lobstein (1831, p. 34).

LATER SYNONYMS:

1. *sympathetic carotid ganglion (Langenbeck, 1826–1830)*
   Synonym for macrodissected adult human ***carotid ganglion (Wutzer, 1817; Bock, 1817)***; in the original Latin, *ganglion caroticum Sympathici*, Fascicle III, Table XVI-4.
2. *ganglion of Laumonier (Lobstein, 1831)*
   Eponym for ***carotid ganglion (Wutzer, 1817; Bock, 1817)***, according to translator of Lobstein's 1823 book, Joseph Pancoast; see p. 34.
3. *Bock's ganglion (>1840)*
   Eponym for ***carotid ganglion (Wutzer, 1817; Bock, 1817)***; see *Dorland's* (2003, p. 752).

cauda equina (Anatomia Magistri Nicolai physici, early 12th century)

As described for macrodissected adult human, the set of ***spinal nerve roots (Tiedemann, 1816)*** arising from the caudal part of the ***spinal cord (Galen, c162–c166)*** and extending caudally (descending) around the ***terminal filament (Tiedemann, 1821)*** in the vertebral canal; see Hamilton (1976, Fig. 808), *Dorland's* (2003, p. 310). The first surviving written description of the ***spinal cord (Galen, c162–c166)*** as resembling a horse's tail may be in an early 12th-century manuscript ascribed to Anatomia Magistri Nicolai physici; see Corner (1927, p. 27). Du Laurens (1599) is usually credited with popularizing the term *cauda equina*; he recommended placing the tissue in water and dissociating the ***nerves (Herophilus, c335–c280 BC)***; see Crooke (1615, p. 483), Mettler (1947, p. 49), Singer (1957, p. 145), Hagelin (1989, p. 53).

EARLIER REFERENCES:

Illustrated and described, not named:

1. ***[cauda equina (Anatomia Magistri Nicolai physici, early 12th century)] (Vesalius, 1543a)***
   Described and crudely illustrated for macrodissected adult human: "In the lower half of the thorax it must become suitable for sending out hard nerves that mainly serve movement; so there it is no longer simple but is divided into innumerable offshoots. There its structure is like a large number of very thin threads stretched out straight together and bound by a membrane; and through each of the foramina through which the nerves travel one thread after another is sent out from the complex until just a single thread is left [***terminal filament (Tiedemann, 1821)***]." (Robertson & Carman translation, 2002, p. 222 and Fig. on p. 205). It was much better illustrated by Eustachi (1552); see Albinus edition (1761, Tab. 17, Fig. 2-*R*). Illustrations by Estienne (1546, p. 366) are totally inadequate.

LATER SYNONYMS:

1. *horse's tail (Anatomia Magistri Nicolai physici, early 12th century)*
   English form of ***cauda equina (Anatomia Magistri Nicolai physici, early 12th century)***, used for example by Crooke (1615, p. 483), spelled *Horse tayle*.
2. *willow switch (Anatomia Magistri Nicolai physici, early 12th century)*
   Alternate descriptor for ***cauda equina (Anatomia Magistri Nicolai physici, early 12th century)***; see Corner (1927, p. 73).
3. *bundle of lumbar and sacral nerves (Burdin, 1803)*
   Synonym for macrodissected adult human ***cauda equina (Anatomia Magistri Nicolai physici, early 12th century)***; see translation (1803, Vol. 1, p. 221).
4. *caudiform expansion (Tiedemann, 1816)*
   Synonym for ***cauda equina (Anatomia Magistri Nicolai physici, early 12th century)***, as observed in a 6-month human fetus; see translation (1826, p. 74).

caudal fovea (>1840)

As described for macrodissected adult human, a slight depression in the ***floor of fourth ventricle (Reil, 1807–1808a)*** at the rostral tip of the ***vagal triangle (>1840)***, along the ***limiting sulcus of fourth ventricle (>1840)***; see Crosby et al. (1962, Fig. 97), *Nomina Anatomica* (1983, p. A66). It was probably first described as the *posterior fovea (Arnold, 1838a)*.

EARLIER REFERENCES:

Earlier synonyms:

1. *posterior fovea (Arnold, 1838a)*
   Synonym for macrodissected adult human ***caudal fovea (>1840)***; in the original Latin (pleural), *foveae posteriores*, p. 23.

caudal medullary velum (>1840)

As described for macrodissected adult human, a right and left thin crescentric layer forming part of the caudal half of the ***roof of fourth ventricle (Vesalius, 1543a)***. On closer inspection each layer consists of a ***central nervous system white matter tract (>1840)*** surfaced internally with ventricular ***ependyma (>1840)*** and externally with ***pia (Galen, c192)***. Each ***caudal medullary velum (>1840)*** extends from the side of the ***nodule (Reil, 1807–1808a)***, with the convex peripheral margin continuous with the ***arbor vitae (Winslow, 1733)*** and with the sides of the ***pyramid (Malacarne, 1776)***, ***uvula (Malacarne, 1776)***, and ***nodule (Reil, 1807–1808a)***. Its rostral border is free and continues as the ***choroid membrane of fourth ventricle (>1840)*** and underlying ***choroid epithelium of fourth ventricle (>1840)***, to the ***choroid line of fourth ventricle (>1840)***. Its ventrolateral corner merges with the ***floccular peduncle (Burdach, 1822)***; see Williams & Warwick (1980, p. 914, Fig. 7.75), Nieuwenhuys et al. (2008, Fig. 3.8). Vesalius probably first noted it; see ***[caudal medullary velum (>1840)] (Vesalius, 1543a)***.

EARLIER REFERENCES:

Described, not named or illustrated:

1. ***[caudal medullary velum (>1840)] (Vesalius, 1543a)*** Vesalius apparently referred vaguely to it in macrodissected adult human; see Singer translation (1952, pp. 37, 50).

Earlier synonyms:

1. *valvulae semicirculares inferiores & posteriores (Tarin, 1750)* First clear illustration, and name for, ***caudal medullary velum (>1840)*** as described for macrodissected adult human; Table II, Figure 2-*n*; see Foster (1894, p. 2998). It may actually only refer to part of the ***caudal medullary vellum (>1840)***; see Gordon (1817, p. 50).
2. *semilunar valves (Malacarne, 1776)* Synonym for macrodissected adult human ***caudal medullary velum (>1840)***; in the original Latin, *valvulas semilunares*, p. 61; see Burdach (1822, p. 297). Clarke & O'Malley (1996, p. 645) associated them with the ***lateral recesses of fourth ventricle (>1840)***.
3. *semicircular valves of mammillary eminence of inferior vermis (Vicq d'Azyr, 1784)* More precise term for *valvulae semicirculares inferiores & posteriores (Tarin, 1750)*—the ***caudal medullary velum (>1840)***; p. 573 and Vicq d'Azyr (1786, p. 95; Pl. XXX, Fig. III-*12,13*); in the original French, *les lames semi-lunaires de l'éminence mammillaire du vermis inferior*. Also see *mammillary process of inferior vermis (Vicq d'Azyr, 1786)*.
4. *lateral pedicles of laminated tubercles (Chaussier, 1807)* Synonym for macrodissected adult human *semilunar valves (Malacarne, 1776)*; in the original French, *pédicules latéraux des tubercules lamineaux*, p. 103.
5. *posterior medullary velum (Reil 1807–1808a)* Synonym for macrodissected adult human ***caudal medullary velum (>1840)***; in the original German, *hintere Marksegel*, see Mayo translation (1822, pp. 25, 47 ff.). Burdach (1822, p. 297) pointed out that Meckel (1817, p. 467) used the Latin term, *velum medullare posterius*.
6. *posterior valve (Burdach, 1822)* Synonym for macrodissected adult human ***caudal medullary vellum (>1840)***; in the original German, *hintre Klappe*, p. 50.
7. *inferior medullary velum (Arnold, 1838b)* Synonym for macrodissected adult human ***caudal medullary vellum (>1840)***; in the original Latin (plural), *vela medullaria inferiora*, Plate III, Figure 5-*k*.

PARTLY CORRESPONDS:

1. *wings of inferior vermiform process (Gordon, 1815)* Synonym for lateral parts of macrodissected adult human ***caudal medullary velum (>1840)***; p. 115; also see Gordon (1817, p. 50) who pointed out that Reil had clearly described and illustrated lateral parts of ***caudal medullary vellum (>1840)***. Thus, Gordon described it as having a middle part and two lateral parts (1817, p. 53). Burdach (1822, p. 297) gave the Latin form, *alas processus vermiformis inferioris*.
2. *alae of inferior vermiform process (Gordon, 1815)* Synonym for *wings of inferior vermiform process (Gordon, 1815)*; p. 115.

caudal part of vestibular nerve (>1840)

As described for macrodissected adult human, a branch of the ***vestibulocochlear nerve trunk (>1840)*** generating the ***posterior ampullary nerve (>1840)***, ***saccular nerve (>1840)***, and ***cochlear communicating branch of vestibular nerve (>1840)***; see *Nomina Anatomica* (1983, p. A75). It was first described as the *superior and posterior fascicle of soft nerve (Cotugno, 1760)* and is commonly known as the *inferior part of vestibular nerve (>1840)*.

EARLIER REFERENCES:

Earlier synonyms:

1. *superior and posterior fascicle of soft nerve (Cotugno, 1760)* Synonym for macrodissected adult human ***caudal part of vestibular nerve (>1840)***; in the original Latin, *fasciculus superior, & posterior*, p. 409, Table II-*g3*.
2. *posterior fascicle of soft nerve (Cotugno, 1760)* Synonym for *superior and posterior fascicle of soft nerve (Cotugno, 1760)*; p. 409.
3. *outer branch of portio mollis (Monro, 1783)* Synonym for macrodissected adult human ***caudal part of vestibular nerve (>1840)***; Table 30, Figure 4-*K*.
4. *middle posterior branch of auditory nerve proper (Günther, 1786)* Synonym for macrodissected adult human ***caudal part of vestibular nerve (>1840)***; in the original Latin, *nervus auditorius proprius ramus posterior medius*, p. 61.
5. *anterior fascicles of acoustic nerve (Scarpa, 1789)* Roughly corresponds to macrodissected adult human ***caudal part of vestibular nerve (>1840)***; Table 8, Figure 2-*f*.
6. *posterior branch of auditory nerve (Soemmerring, 1791)* Basically, macrodissected adult human ***caudal part of vestibular nerve (>1840)***; p. 225, and Soemmerring (1798, p. 258); also see Meckel (1832, Vol. 3, p. 52). It is also the smaller branch; see Soemmerring (1806, Tab. III, Fig. 9-α).
7. *anterior fasciculus of acustic nerve (Bell, 1803b)* Synonym for macrodissected adult human *anterior fascicles of acoustic nerve (Scarpa, 1789)*; Plate X, Figure 2-*f*.
8. *posterior branch of acoustic nerve (Cloquet, 1828)* Synonym for macrodissected adult human ***caudal part of vestibular nerve (>1840)***; in the original French, *branche postérieure du nerf acoustique*, Table CXXX, Figure 9-*19*.
9. *inferior part of vestibular nerve (>1840)* Synonym for macrodissected adult human ***caudal part of vestibular nerve (>1840)***; see *Terminologia Anatomica* (1998, p. 136).

caudate nucleus (Arnold, 1838b)

As described for macrodissected adult human, one of two distinct components of the ***caudoputamen (Heimer***

& Wilson, 1975) forming much of the lateral wall of the ***lateral ventricle (Vesalius, 1543a)***. It is separated from the other component, the ***putamen (Burdach, 1822)***, by the ***anterior limb of internal capsule (>1840)*** and is commonly described as having ***head of caudate nucleus (>1840)***, ***body of caudate nucleus (>1840)***, and ***tail of caudate nucleus (Arnold, 1838b)***; see Carpenter (1976, p. 497, Fig. 17.4). For Arnold's use in macrodissected adult human, see Table IV, Figure 4-ζ, also see Meyer (1971, p. 16). It was clearly illustrated by Vesalius; see ***[caudate nucleus (Arnold, 1838b)] (Vesalius, 1543a)***.

TRANSLATIONS:

1. *nucleus caudatus (Arnold, 1838b)*
   Original Latin form of ***caudate nucleus (Arnold, 1838b)***; Table IV, Figure 4-ζ.

EARLIER REFERENCES:

Illustrated, not named or described:

1. ***[caudate nucleus (Arnold, 1838b)] (Vesalius, 1543a)***
   Very clearly illustrated without comment for macrodissected adult human, both grossly and in section; see Singer translation (1952, Figs. 4–8).

Earlier synonyms:

1. *tailed structure (Avicenna, c1030)*
   According to Garrison & McHenry (1969, p. 24), Avicenna referred to a tailed structure later named ***caudate nucleus (Arnold, 1838b)***. See *cauda corporis striati (Malacarne, 1780)*.
2. *striata corpora superna anteriora (Vieussens, 1684)*
   In first parceling of *striated body (Willis, 1664)*, Vieussens distinguished and provided this synonym for macrodissected adult human ***caudate nucleus (Arnold, 1838b)***, according to Meyer (1971, p. 13); Tables IX-*E*, X-*C*. According to Chaussier (1807, p. 62 note *1*), it refers to *striated body (Willis, 1664)* as a whole.
3. *processus anteriores medullae oblongatae (Vieussens, 1684)*
   According to Burdach (1822, p. 348), synonym for macrodissected adult human *corpora striata superna anteriora (Vieussens, 1684)*.
4. *internal superior part of striated body (Pourfour du Petit, 1710)*
   Roughly synonymous with macrodissected adult human ***caudate nucleus (Arnold, 1838b)***; in the original French, *les corps cannelez internes &/ou superieurs*, pp. 7, 14; also see *corpus striatum (Willis, 1664)*. It is probably similar or equivalent to *corpora striata superna anteriora (Vieussens, 1684)*.
5. *cauda corporis striati (Malacarne, 1780)*
   Malacarne noted that *cauda* [tail] of macrodissected adult human *corpus striatum (Willis, 1664)* accompanies ***terminal stria (Wenzel & Wenzel, 1812)*** along ***inferior horn of lateral ventricle (Bell, 1802)***, a vague reference to ***caudate nucleus (Arnold, 1838b)***; Part 2, p. 56. See Burdach (1822, pp. 124, 349), Meyer (1971, p. 16). Arnold (1838b; Tab. I, Fig. 2-*μ*) used the form, *cauda corpora striatorum*.
6. *corpus striatum superior and internal part (Vicq d'Azyr, 1786)*
   Synonym for macrodissected adult human ***caudate nucleus (Arnold, 1838b)***; Plate IX, p. 27.
7. *inner portion of corpus striatum (Vicq d'Azyr, 1786)*
   Synonym Vicq d'Azyr used (p. 27) for macrodissected adult human ***caudate nucleus (Arnold, 1838b)***, according to Burdach (1822, p. 348), who gave the Latin, *portiones internae corporum striatorum*. Reil (1809b) also used this term and described a tail-like prolongation; see Mayo translation (1823, pp. 56, 62).
8. *pyriform eminences (Burdin, 1803)*
   Synonym for right and left ***caudate nucleus (Arnold, 1838b)***, referring to its appearance viewed from ***lateral ventricle (Vesalius, 1543a)***; see translation (1803, Vol. 1, p. 159), also see Burdach (1822, p. 348).
9. *colliculi nervorum ethmoidalium (Chaussier, 1807)*
   Synonym for macrodissected adult human right and left ***caudate nucleus (Arnold, 1838b)***; p. 63, according to Burdach (1822, p. 348).
10. *inner portion of cerebral ganglion (Reil, 1809b)*
    Synonym for macrodissected adult human ***caudate nucleus (Arnold, 1838b)***; in the original German, *innere Portion*, p. 144; see Meyer (1971, p. 29).
11. *internal part of superior great cerebral ganglion (Gall & Spurzheim, 1810)*
    Synonym for macrodissected adult human ***caudate nucleus (Arnold, 1838b)***; in the original French, *partie interne du grand ganglion cérébral supérieur*, Plate V-*l*.
12. *colliculus striatus (Wenzel & Wenzel, 1812)*
    Synonym for macrodissected adult human ***caudate nucleus (Arnold, 1838b)***; p. 262, Table III, Figure 1-*a*, according to Burdach (1822, p. 348).
13. *corpora striata antica inferiora (Meckel, 1817)*
    Synonym for macrodissected adult human right and left ***caudate nucleus (Arnold, 1838b)***; p. 513, according to Burdach (1822, p. 348).
14. *pyriformes prominentiae (Rolando, 1819)*
    Synonym for macrodissected adult human *eminentiae pyriformes (Burdin, 1803)*; Part 2, p. 9.

PARTLY CORRESPONDS:

1. *base of anterior ventricle both right and left (Manfredi, 1490)*
   Manfredi wrote that the very substance of the ***brain (Smith Papyrus, c1700 BC)*** forms the base of the *anterior ventricle (Galen, c173)*, seemingly referring to medial wall of macrodissected adult human ***caudate nucleus (Arnold, 1838b)***; see Singer translation (1917, p. 109). Also see *base of fore ventricle (Mondino, 1316)*.
2. *eminentiae similes coxis humanis (Berengario da Carpi, 1521)*
   Probably synonym for macrodissected adult human *base of anterior ventricle both right and left (Manfredi, 1490)*; f. 437, also see Burdach (1822, p. 347).
3. *anchae (Massa, 1536)*
   Fairly clearly referred to medial wall of macrodissected adult human ***caudate nucleus (Arnold, 1838b)***: "In [the ***lateral ventricles (Vesalius, 1543a)***] there are certain

elevated and more whitish substances called nates or anchae by modern anatomists, for they are humped, whitish, and elevated like human buttocks in the right and left cavities, or in the ventricle." (Lind translation, 1975, p. 237). They have nothing to do either with *buttocks (Galen, c177)*, as Massa himself pointed out (see Lind translation, 1975, p. 237), or apparently with *buttocks (Berengario da Carpi, 1522)*. Modern anatomists Massa referred to may base their terminology on *anchae (Mondino, 1316)*, although this is not clear, as contrasted with *buttocks (Galen, c177)*; see Lind translation (1975, p. 237).

4. *buttocks (Massa, 1536)*
   Synonym for *anchae (Massa, 1536)*; see Lind translation (1975, p. 237).
5. *nates (Massa, 1536)*
   Synonym for *anchae (Massa, 1536)*; see Lind translation (1975, p. 237).
6. *cone of striate body (Willis, 1672)*
   Roughly macrodissected adult human ***body of caudate nucleus (>1840)*** and ***tail of caudate nucleus (Arnold, 1838b)*** considered together; see Pordage translation (1683, p. 44, Tab. VIII-G). Also see *striated body (Willis, 1664)*.
7. *cauda of inner portion of corpus striatum (Reil, 1809b)*
   Roughly synonymous with macrodissected adult human *cone of striate body (Willis, 1672)*; see Mayo translation (1823, p. 65). Also see Carpenter (1976, p. 497, Fig. 17.4).
8. *body of caudate nucleus (Arnold, 1838b)*
   Macrodissected adult human ***head of caudate nucleus (>1840)*** and ***body of caudate nucleus (>1840)*** considered together; in the original Latin (plural), *corpus nuclei caudati*, Table IV, Figure 5-*r* and Table V, Figure 4-*η*. See Carpenter (1976, p. 497, Fig. 17.4), Nieuwenhuys et al. (2008, Fig. 5.31).

caudoputamen (Heimer & Wilson, 1975)

As described for macrodissected adult human the ***caudate nucleus (Arnold, 1838b)*** and ***putamen (Burdach, 1822)*** considered together and separated by the ***anterior limb of internal capsule (>1840)***; see Nieuwenhuys et al. (2008, pp. 429–435, called *caudate-putamen complex*). For mammals in general, based on cellular architecture and connections, the largest and dorsomedial component of the ***striatum (Swanson, 2000a)***; dorsal to ***accumbens nucleus (Ziehen, 1897–1901)***, ***medial amygdalar nucleus (Johnston, 1923)***, and ***central amygdalar nucleus (Johnston, 1923)***, and lateral to ***lateral septal complex (Risold & Swanson, 1997)***. For Heimer & Wilson's use in rat, see Figure 1-*CP*. It was not delineated as such by 1840.

cavernous nerves of clitoris (>1840)

As described for macrodissected adult human female, they extend from certain terminal branches of the ***vaginal nerves (Walter, 1783)*** to supply erectile tissue of the clitoris; see *Terminologia Anatomica* (1998, p. 143), *Dorland's* (2003, p. 1237). They were not clearly described by 1840.

cavernous nerves of penis (>1840)

As described for macrodissected adult human male, they extend from the ***prostatic plexus (1840)*** to supply erectile tissue of the penis; see *Terminologia Anatomica* (1998, p. 143), *Dorland's* (2003, p. 1237). They were not clearly described by 1840.

cavernous sinus (Winslow, 1733)

As described for macrodissected adult human, a component of the ***circulatory system***; a right and left irregularly shaped sinus of the ***dura (Galen, c177)*** lying on either side of the body of the sphenoid bone; see Williams & Warwick (1980, pp. 746–747, Figs. 6.126, 127A,B), *Dorland's* (2003, p. 1706). For Winslow's use in macrodissected adult human, see Section VI, p. 62. It was probably first identified as the *receptacula sellae equinae lateribus apposita (Vieussens, 1684)*.

TRANSLATIONS:

1. *sinus cavernosus (Winslow, 1733)*
   Original Latin form of ***cavernous sinus (Winslow, 1733)***; Section VI, p. 62.

EARLIER REFERENCES:

Earlier synonyms:

1. *receptacula sellae equinae lateribus apposita (Vieussens, 1684)*
   Description of, or synonym for, macrodissected adult human ***cavernous sinus (Winslow, 1733)***; p. 7, see Burdach (1822, p. 400). The *receptacle* was used in a translation by Best (1969, p. 161) of a passage from Morgagni (1719). A history of its early description was provided by Haller (1743, pp. 40–41 note *16*).

LATER SYNONYMS:

1. *sinus sphenoïdales (Malacarne, 1780)*
   Synonym for macrodissected adult human ***cavernous sinus (Winslow, 1733)***, according to Burdach (1822, p. 400), without a specific citation.
2. *sinus polymorphi (Schreger, 1803)*
   Synonym listed for macrodissected adult human ***cavernous sinus (Winslow, 1733)***; Burdach (1822, p. 400); in referring to it he also mentioned Ortelob without providing a citation.

celiac branches of anterior vagal trunk (>1840)

In macrodissected adult human, commonly 3–4 closely applied branches of the ***anterior vagal trunk (Wrisberg, 1780)*** arising near the cardiac orifice of the stomach and running along the left gastric artery, frequently uniting with the ***celiac branches of posterior vagal trunk (>1840)*** and entering and distributing within the ***celiac plexus (Winslow, 1733)***; see Mitchell (1953, p. 187 and Fig. 80), *Nomina Anatomica* (1983, p. A76). They were perhaps first clearly identified as the *anastomotic branch of anterior gastric plexus with branch of semilunar ganglion (Günther, 1786)*.

EARLIER REFERENCES:

Earlier synonyms:

1. *anastomotic branch of anterior gastric plexus with branch of semilunar ganglion (Günther, 1786)*

Essentially, synonym for macrodissected adult human ***celiac branches of anterior vagal trunk (>1840)***; in the original Latin, *r. anastomotici cum ganglii semilunaris ramis*, p. 66.

celiac branches of posterior vagal trunk (>1840)

As described for macrodissected adult human, 3–4 closely applied bundles from the ***posterior vagal trunk (Wrisberg, 1780)*** extending caudally (down) near the left gastric artery to enter and distribute within the ***celiac plexus (Winslow, 1733)***; see Mitchell (1953, p. 187 and Fig. 80), Williams & Warwick (1980, p. 1081), *Terminologia Anatomica* (1998, p. 137). They were probably first known to Willis; see ***[celiac branch of posterior vagal trunk (>1840)] (Willis, 1664)***.

EARLIER REFERENCES:

Illustrated and described, not named:

1. ***[celiac branch of posterior vagal trunk (>1840)] (Willis, 1664)***
   Probably mentioned and illustrated for macrodissected adult human and other common large mammals; see Pordage translation (1681, p. 158 and Fig. 11-η).

Earlier synonyms:

1. *fascia communicans memorabilis (Wrisberg, 1800)*
   Essentially synonymous with macrodissected adult human ***celiac branch of posterior vagal trunk (>1840)***; XV, p. 11.
2. *great abdomino-cephalic anastomotic branch (Lobstein, 1823)*
   Synonym for macrodissected adult human *fascia communicans memorabilis (Wrisberg, 1800)*; see translation (1831, p. 98).
3. *fascia communicans of Wrisberg (Lobstein, 1823)*
   Eponym for macrodissected adult human *fascia communicans memorabilis (Wrisberg, 1800)*; see translation (1831, Pl. III, Fig. 3-*d*).

celiac ganglion (Walter, 1783)

As described for macrodissected adult human, the largest and most constant ***prevertebral ganglion (Quain, 1832)*** of the ***celiac plexus (Winslow, 1733)***; see Mitchell (1953, p. 273), Williams & Warwick (1980, p. 1133). For Walter's use in macrodissected adult human, see Tables II:*1–10* and III:*244–258*; he described and named at least 12 "subganglia" whose number and size vary, p. 13. Mayer (1794; Part 6, Tab. VI:*a-m*, pp. 41-42; Tab. VII:*a-m*, p. 49; Tab. VIII:*a-n*, pp. 57–58) clearly described and illustrated either 11 or 12 for macrodissected adult human. It was probably discovered by Galen; see ***[celiac ganglion (Walter, 1783)] (Galen c173)***.

TRANSLATIONS:

1. *ganglion celiacum (Walter, 1783)*
   Original Latin form of ***celiac ganglion (Walter, 1783)***; see p. 13, Tables II:*1–10* and III:*244–258*.

EARLIER REFERENCES:

Described, not named or illustrated:

1. ***[celiac ganglion (Walter, 1783)] (Galen c173)***
   Probably described without naming for macrodissected adult beef, pig, and/or macaque but not human; see May translation (1968, pp. 695–696, 711), Duckworth translation (1962, pp. 217–218), Savage-Smith (1971, p. 179).

Earlier synonyms:

1. *chief mesenteric infolding (Willis, 1664)*
   From illustration almost certainly refers to macrodissected adult human and quadruped ***celiac ganglion (Walter, 1783)***; in the original Latin, *plexus mesentericus lateris primus*; see Pordage translation, p. 158 and Table XI-*H*.
2. *mesenteric infolding (Willis, 1664)*
   Synonym for *chief mesenteric infolding (Willis, 1664)* in macrodissected adult human and other common large mammals; see Pordage translation (1681, Tab. XI-*H*). Willis wrote it is infolding or ***ganglion (Galen, c173)*** for stomach and spleen on left (rostral or higher) side and infolding or ***ganglion (Galen, c173)*** for liver on right (caudal or lower) side; see Pordage translation (1681, pp. 166 and 168, respectively).
3. *superior mesenteric infolding (Willis, 1664)*
   Synonym for *chief mesenteric infolding (Willis, 1664)* in macrodissected adult human and other common large mammals; see Pordage translation (1681, Tab. XI-♂).
4. *plexus ganglioformis semilunaris nervi intercostalis (Vieussens, 1684)*
   Synonym for macrodissected adult human *chief mesenteric infolding (Willis, 1664)*; Table 23-57. A literal translation is "*semilunar ganglionic infolding of intercostal nerve.*"
5. *semilunar ganglion (Winslow, 1733)*
   Synonym for macrodissected adult human ***celiac ganglion (Walter, 1783)***; in the original Latin, *ganglion semilunaris*, Section VI, p. 98.
6. *semilunar plexus (Winslow, 1733)*
   Synonym for *semilunar ganglion (Winslow, 1733)*; in the original Latin, *plexus semilunaris*, Section VI, p. 98.
7. *great semilunar ganglion (Haller, 1762)*
   Synonym for macrodissected adult human *semilunar ganglion (Winslow, 1733)*; in the original Latin, *ganglion magnum semilunare*, p. 261. Johnstone (1765, p. 180) soon translated as *great semi-lunar ganglion*.
8. *great abdominal ganglion (Wrisberg, 1780)*
   Synonym for macrodissected adult human ***celiac ganglion (Walter, 1783)***; in the original Latin, *ganglion magnum abdominis*, see Wrisberg reprint (1800, p. 275).

LATER SYNONYMS:

1. *great celiac ganglion (Günther, 1786)*
   Günther's preferred term for macrodissected adult human ***celiac ganglion (Walter, 1783)***; in the original Latin, *ganglion magnum coeliacum*, p. 94.
2. *solar ganglion (Günther, 1786)*
   Synonym listed for macrodissected adult human ***celiac ganglion (Walter, 1783)***; in the original Latin, *ganglion solare*, p. 94.

3. *transverse ganglion (Günther, 1786)*
   Synonym listed for macrodissected adult human ***celiac ganglion (Walter, 1783)***; in the original Latin, *ganglion transversale*, p. 94.
4. *abdominal ganglion (Günther, 1786)*
   Synonym listed for macrodissected adult human ***celiac ganglion (Walter, 1783)***; in the original Latin, *ganglion abdominale*, p. 94.
5. *splanchnic ganglion (Günther, 1786)*
   Synonym listed for macrodissected adult human ***celiac ganglion (Walter, 1783)***; in the original Latin, *ganglion splanchnicum*, p. 94.
6. *great harmonic ganglion (Andersch, 1797)*
   Synonym for macrodissected adult human ***celiac ganglion (Walter, 1783)***; in the original Latin, *magnum ganglium harmonicum*, Vol. 2, p. 185.
7. *suprarenal ganglion (Meckel, 1817)*
   Synonym listed for macrodissected adult human ***celiac ganglion (Walter, 1783)***; see translation (1832, Vol. 3, p. 85).
8. *semilunar abdominal ganglion (Wrisberg, 1808)*
   Synonym for macrodissected adult human ***celiac ganglion (Walter, 1783)***; in the original Latin, *semilunare abdominis ganglion*, p. 17.
9. *ganglioso-abdominal centre (Lobstein, 1832)*
   Apparently synonym for macrodissected adult human ***celiac ganglion (Walter, 1783)***; see translation (1831, p. 101).

PARTLY CORRESPONDS:

1. *stomachical and splenetick infolding (Willis, 1664)*
   Synonym for macrodissected adult human left ***celiac ganglion (Walter, 1783)***, which Willis described as higher (more rostral) than right ***celiac ganglion (Walter, 1783)***; see Pordage translation (1681, p. 166).
2. *hepatick infolding (Willis, 1664)*
   Synonym for macrodissected adult human right ***celiac ganglion (Walter, 1783)***, which Willis described as lower (more caudal) than left ***celiac ganglion (Walter, 1783)***; see Pordage translation (1681, p. 168).
3. *hepatic plexus (Keill, 1698)*
   Synonym for macrodissected adult human *hepatick infolding (Willis, 1664)*; in the original Latin, *plexus hepaticus*, pp. 58, 293.
4. *splenic plexus (Keill, 1698)*
   Synonym for macrodissected adult human *stomachical and splenetick infolding (Willis, 1664)*; in the original Latin, *plexus splenicus*, pp. 65, 293.
5. *coeliac ganglia (Fyfe, 1800)*
   Fyfe wrote that macrodissected adult human *semilunar ganglion (Winslow, 1733)* is composed of many smaller ***ganglia (Galen, c173)***, termed *coeliac*; Vol. 2, p. 322.
6. *solar ganglia (Cruveilhier, 1836)*
   All macrodissected adult human ***ganglia (Galen, c173)*** in ***celiac plexus (Winslow, 1733)***; in the original French, *ganglions solaires*, p. 1014.

celiac plexus (Winslow, 1733)

As described for macrodissected adult human, the largest of the great ***prevertebral plexuses (Quain, 1832)***, lying near the last thoracic vertebra and upper part of the first lumbar vertebra, surrounding the celiac artery and root of the superior mesenteric artery; see Mitchell (1953, p. 272 ff.), Williams & Warwick (1980, p. 1133). Winslow used it for macrodissected adult human in Section VI, nos. 404–405. It was known by Galen; see ***[celiac plexus (Winslow, 1733)] (Galen, c173)***.

TRANSLATIONS:

1. *plexus caeliacus (Winslow, 1733)*
   Original Latin form of ***celiac plexus (Winslow, 1733)***; Section VI, p. 98.
2. *plexu coeliaco (Haller, 1762)*
   Latin form of ***celiac plexus (Winslow, 1733)***; p. 263.
3. *plexum coeliacum (Haase, 1781)*
   Latin form of ***celiac plexus (Winslow, 1733)***; p. 124.

EARLIER REFERENCES:

Described, not named or illustrated:

1. ***[celiac plexus (Winslow, 1733)] (Galen, c173)***
   Galen described briefly the general region of the ***celiac plexus (Winslow, 1733)***; see May translation (1968, pp. 695, 711), Savage-Smith (1971, p. 184). He dissected a variety of adult mammals but not explicitly human cadavers. According to Riolan (see translation, 1657, p. 67), this "intertexture of Nerves" was also described by Falloppio (1561).

Illustrated and described, not named:

1. ***[celiac plexus (Winslow, 1733)] (Willis, 1664)***
   Illustrated and described for macrodissected adult human and other common large mammals; see Pordage translation (1681, pp. 158–159 and Tab. XI). The most realistic early depiction in macrodissected adult human was by Lancisi (1728, Tab. 7-*o*).

Earlier synonyms:

1. *semilunar plexus (Palfijn, 1726)*
   Synonym for roughly the macrodissected adult human ***celiac plexus (Winslow, 1733)***; in the original French, *plexus semilunaire*, Part 2, pp. 334, 335.

LATER SYNONYMS:

1. *middle plexus of semilunar ganglia (Winslow, 1733)*
   Synonym for ***celiac plexus (Winslow, 1733)***; Section VI, p. 98.
2. *semilunar ganglioform plexus (Tarin, 1753)*
   Synonym for macrodissected adult human ***celiac plexus (Winslow, 1733)***; in the original Latin, *plexus ganglioformes semilunares*, p. 72.
3. *celiac plexus proper (Günther, 1786)*
   Synonym for macrodissected adult human ***celiac plexus (Winslow, 1733)***; in the original Latin, *plexus coeliacus proprius*, p. 95: associated with the celiac artery.
4. *median plexus (Chaussier, 1789)*
   Synonym listed for macrodissected adult human ***celiac plexus (Winslow, 1733)***; *Table synoptique du nerf tri-splanchnique.*
5. *opisto-gastric plexus (Chaussier, 1789)*
   Synonym listed for macrodissected adult human ***celiac plexus (Winslow, 1733)***; *Table synoptique du nerf tri-splanchnique.*

6. *transverse plexus (Chaussier, 1789)*
Synonym listed for macrodissected adult human ***celiac plexus (Winslow, 1733)***; *Table synoptique du nerf tri-splanchnique.*
7. *common plexus (Chaussier, 1789)*
Synonym listed for macrodissected adult human ***celiac plexus (Winslow, 1733)***; *Table synoptique du nerf tri-splanchnique.*
8. *plexus communis (Meckel, 1817)*
Synonym listed for macrodissected adult human ***celiac plexus (Winslow, 1733)***; see translation (1832, Vol. 3, p. 85).
9. *abdominal plexus (Meckel, 1817)*
Synonym listed for macrodissected adult human ***celiac plexus (Winslow, 1733)***; see translation (1832, Vol. 3, p. 85).

central amygdalar nucleus (Johnston, 1923)

As described for macrodissected adult human, and with cellular architecture and connections for all mammals, a caudal differentiation of the ***striatum (Swanson, 2000a)*** between ***caudoputamen (Heimer & Wilson, 1975)*** dorsally and ***medial amygdalar nucleus (Johnston, 1923)*** ventrally and medially; see Price et al. (1987). For Johnston's use in mammal, based on phylogeny and histology, see pp. 339, 398, 410, 456, where it is spelled *central amygdaloid nucleus*; current spelling was introduced by Swanson & Petrovich (1998, p. 324). Not clearly described by 1840.

central canal (Bellingeri, 1823)

As described for macrodissected adult human, the narrow caudal segment of the ***ventricles (Hippocrates)***, itself divided for topographic description into **central canal of *medulla* (>1840)** extending from the caudal end of the ***fourth ventricle (Galen, c192)*** through the caudal half of the ***medulla (Winslow, 1733)***, followed caudally by ***central canal of spinal cord (>1840)***; see Williams & Warwick (1980, pp. 869, 932). This distinction of rostral and caudal segments was not made before 1840. For Bellingeri's use in macrodissected adult beef see p. 19, where he referred to the *central canal of spinal medulla*; in the original Latin, *canalem centralem medullae spinalis*. Galen observed at least its rostral part; see ***[central canal (Bellingeri, 1823)] (Galen, c162–c166)***.

EARLIER REFERENCES:

Described, not named or illustrated:

1. ***[central canal (Bellingeri, 1823)] (Galen, c162–c166)***
In *On the Doctrines of Hippocrates and Plato*, *On the Usefulness of the Parts*, and *On Anatomical Procedures*, Galen noted that ***fourth ventricle (Galen, c192)*** narrows down and extends into region of ***spinal cord (Galen, c162–c166)*** associated with first cervical vertebra, but could trace it no farther caudally; see De Lacy translation (1980, pp. 447, 453), May translation (1968, p. 416), Duckworth translation (1962, p. 14). He macrodissected a variety of common large mammals, but not human.
2. ***[central canal (Bellingeri, 1823)] (Fernel, 1542)***
Sherrington (1946, p. 63) claimed that Fernel first noted that ***spinal cord (Galen, c162–c166)*** is hollow, "medulla spinalis cava est", although his description is vague, for example, in not stating whether it is hollow along its entire length. This presumably referred to human.
3. ***[central canal (Bellingeri, 1823)] (Estienne, 1545)***
Estienne claimed it extends the length of the macrodissected adult human ***spinal cord (Galen, c162–c166)***; Liber III, p. 337; see Craigie (1910–1911). However, whether this was actually observed before careful microscopic analysis in the 19th century is doubtful; see Todd (1845, p. 92 ff.). For example, the outstanding anatomist Coiter (1572, translation pp. 113–115) stated that the hole in the human ***spinal cord (Galen, c162–c166)*** reported by some anatomists is a dissection artifact.

Earlier synonyms:

1. *canal of Charles Estienne (Günther, 1786)*
Eponym for macrodissected adult human ***central canal (Bellingeri, 1823)***; in the original Latin, *canalis Caroli Stephani*, p. 33.
2. *ventricle of spinal marrow (Carus, 1814)*
Synonym for ***central canal (Bellingeri, 1823)*** in macrodissected adult vertebrate; in the original German, *Spaltung des Rückenmarks*, e.g., p. 171.
3. *canal of spinal marrow (Carus, 1814)*
Synonym for ***central canal (Bellingeri, 1823)*** in macrodissected adult vertebrate; in the original German, *Kanal des Rückenmarks*, e.g., pp. 129 (fish), 171 (amphibian), 191–192 (bird, where it is *Rückenmark-Kanals*), and mammal (p. 215) including human (pp. 260, 264). Spurzheim (1826, p. 52) used the English *canal of spinal cord*.
4. *medullary canal (Bojanus, 1819–1821)*
Synonym for macrodissected adult turtle ***central canal (Bellingeri, 1823)***; in the original Latin, *canalis medullaris*, Figures 95–100:*m*.
5. *small foramen (Bellingeri, 1823)*
In macrodissected adult beef, synonym for ***central canal (Bellingeri, 1823)*** in first level of ***cervical part of spinal cord (>1840)***; in the original Latin, *parvum foramen*, Table I, Figure 11-*l*. It was not observed in second level of ***cervical part of spinal cord (>1840)***; Table I, Figure 12. But it was observed at junction of ***thoracic part of spinal cord (>1840)*** and ***lumbar part of spinal cord (>1840)***, and at junction of ***lumbar part of spinal cord (>1840)*** and ***sacral part of spinal cord (>1840)***; Table 1, Figure 16-*l* and Table 1, Figure 18-*l*, respectively.
6. *canal of spinal cord (Spurzheim, 1826)*
Synonym for *canal of spinal marrow (Carus, 1814)*; p. 51.

PARTLY CORRESPONDS:

1. *rhomboid sinus (Jacobaeus, 1675)*
Dilation of macrodissected adult bird (parrot specifically) ***central canal (Bellingeri, 1823)*** in ***lumbar part of spinal cord (>1840)***; in the original Latin, *sinus*

rhomboidalis, p. 317 and figure thereon. Nicolai (1812, pp. 156–162) gave a detailed history of it.

central canal of medulla (>1840)

As described for macrodissected adult human, the short rostral segment of the ***central canal (Bellingeri, 1823)*** lying within the caudal half of the ***medulla (Winslow, 1733)***—as opposed to the long caudal segment, the ***central canal of spinal cord (>1840)***; see Williams & Warwick (1980, pp. 869, 932). Its presence was indicated long ago; see ***[central canal of medulla (>1840)] (Galen, c162–c166)***.

EARLIER REFERENCES:

Described, not named or illustrated:

1. ***[central canal of medulla (>1840)] (Galen, c162–c166)***
   Identified in macrodissected common large mammal but not human; see ***[central canal (Bellingeri, 1823)] (Galen, c162–c166)***.

Earlier synonyms:

1. *canal of medulla oblongata (Arnold, 1838b)*
   Specific identification of macrodissected adult human ***central canal of medulla (>1840)***; in the original Latin, *canalis medullae oblongatae*, Table II, Figure 13-*g*.

central canal of spinal cord (>1840)

As defined for macrodissected adult human, the long caudal segment of the ***central canal (Bellingeri, 1823)*** lying within the ***spinal cord (Galen, c162–c166)***—as opposed to the short rostral segment, the ***central canal of medulla (>1840)***; see Williams & Warwick (1980, pp. 869, 932). Its presence was first indicated by Galen; see ***[central canal of spinal cord (>1840)] (Galen, c162–c166)***.

EARLIER REFERENCES:

Described, not named or illustrated:

1. ***[central canal of spinal cord (>1840)] (Galen, c162–c166)***
   Galen identified it in macrodissected common large mammal but not human; see ***[central canal (Bellingeri, 1823)] (Galen, c162–c166)***.

Earlier synonyms:

1. *spinal canal (Tiedemann, 1816)*
   Synonym for ***central canal of spinal cord (>1840)*** observed in developing human fetus; see translation (1826, p. 20).

central ganglia (>1840)

Any ***ganglion (Galen, c173)*** of an invertebrate ***central nerve cord (Serres, 1824–1826)***; see Bullock & Horridge (1965, p. 52). First described as *globules (Malpighi, 1669)* in silkworm.

EARLIER REFERENCES:

Earlier synonyms:

1. *globules (Malpighi, 1669)*
   Synonym for silkworm ***central ganglia (>1840)*** viewed with a microscope; in the original Latin, *globuli*, pp. 45–46, Table VI. Described as lying along the *spinal medulla (Malpighi, 1669)* and composed of *cortical substance (Willis, 1664)*.
2. *nodules (Malpighi, 1669)*
   Synonym for *globules (Malpighi, 1669)*; in the original Latin, *noduli*, p. 47.
3. *ganglion (Swammerdam, c1675)*
   Synonym for *globule (Malpighi, 1669)*, viewed with a microscope; see Swammerdam (1737–1738); e.g., Tabs. VI, Figure I-*e* and XLI, Figure VII-*c*.
4. *knots (Swammerdam, c1675)*
   Synonym for *globules (Malpighi, 1669)*, viewed with a microscope; see translation (1758, e.g., Tab. XLI, Fig. VII-*c* in fly).
5. *swellings (Swammerdam, c1675)*
   Synonym for *globules (Malpighi, 1669)*, viewed with a microscope; see translation (1758, e.g., Tab. XLI, Fig. VII-*c* in fly).
6. *nodes (Gall & Spurzheim, 1810)*
   Synonym for *globules (Malpighi, 1669)*, viewed with a microscope; in the original French, *noeuds*, p. 38.
7. *nerve knots (Carus, 1814)*
   Synonym for *knots (Swammerdam, c1675)*, as in worms; in the original German, *Nervenknotten*, p. 85.

central lobule (Burdach, 1822)

As described for macrodissected adult human, the part of the ***cerebellar vermis (Meckel, 1817)*** between ***lingula (Malacarne, 1776)*** ventrally and caudally, and ***culmen (Henle, 1871)*** dorsally; see Angevine et al. (1961, Fig. 24), Larsell & Jansen (1972, Fig. 118), Carpenter (1976, Figs. 2.25, 2.26, 14.1), Nieuwenhuys et al. (2008, Fig. 3.8-26). For Burdach's use in macrodissected adult human, see p. 57. It was first clearly delineated as the *central lobe (Malacarne, 1776)*.

EARLIER REFERENCES:

Earlier synonyms:

1. *central lobe (Malacarne, 1776)*
   Synonym for macrodissected adult human ***central lobule (Burdach, 1822)***; see Larsell (1967, p. 3), Clarke & O'Malley (1996, p. 646). For Latin form, *lobus centralis*, see Burdach (1822, p. 294).

PARTLY CORRESPONDS:

1. *middle projection of central lobe (Malacarne, 1776)*
   As described for macrodissected adult human, zone near median plane of ***central lobule (Burdach, 1822)*** in line with ***lingula (Malacarne, 1776)*** and ***culmen (Henle, 1871)*** on either side; see Clarke & O'Malley (1996, p. 646). It is flanked by *wing of central lobule (Reil, 1807–1808a)*; see Williams & Warwick (1980, Fig. 7.74-*ala*), *Terminologia Anatomica* (1998, p. 119).
2. *lateral trunks of central lobule (Malacarne, 1776)*
   Synonym for macrodissected adult human *wing of central lobule (Reil, 1807–1808a)*; see Clarke & O'Malley (1996, p. 646).
3. *wing of central lobule (Reil, 1807–1808a)*
   Macrodissected adult human lateral zone of ***central lobule (Burdach, 1822)***, lateral to *middle projection of central*

lobe (Malacarne, 1776); see Mayo translation (1822, Tab. III, Figs. II-*a*, III-*a*). Also see Williams & Warwick (1980, Fig. 7.74-*ala*), *Terminologia Anatomica* (1998, p. 119).

4. *ala lobulus centralis (Reil, 1807–1808a)*
   Latin form of *wing of central lobule (Reil, 1807–1808a)*; plural, *alae lobuli centralis*, see Burdach (1822, p. 57).
5. *superior vermiform process (Gordon, 1815)*
   Probably macrodissected adult human ***central lobule (Burdach, 1822)***; p. 109.

central longitudinal communicating branch (>1840)

The segment of an invertebrate ***central nerve cord (Serres, 1824–1826)*** between two ***central ganglia (>1840)***; see Bullock & Horridge (1965, p. 52), Swanson & Bota (2010). As a topographic division, a ***communicating branch (Winslow, 1733)***. It was identified long ago by Malpighi; see ***[central longitudinal communicating branch (>1840)] (Malpighi, 1669)***.

EARLIER REFERENCES:

Illustrated and described, not named:

1. ***[central longitudinal communicating branch (>1840)] (Malpighi, 1669)***
   Viewed microscopically in silkworm; p. 47 and Table VI, Figure 2-*N*.

Earlier synonyms:

1. *conduit of spinal medulla (Lyonnet, 1762)*
   Synonym for ***central longitudinal communicating branch (>1840)*** in macrodissected caterpillar viewed under the microscope; in the original French (plural), *conduits de la moélle épinière*, p. 98.
2. *interganglionic cord (Serres, 1824-1826)*
   Synonym for ***central longitudinal communicating branch (>1840)*** in macrodissected insects viewed under the microscope; in the original French (plural), *cordons inter-ganglionnaires*, p. 35.
3. *longitudinal cord (Newport, 1832)*
   Synonym for ***central longitudinal communicating branch (>1840)*** in macrodissected hawkmoth, *Sphinx ligustri*; p. 384.
4. *communicating cord (Leuret, 1839)*
   Synonym for ***central longitudinal communicating branch (>1840)*** in macrodissected invertebrates; in the original French (plural), *cordons de communication*, p. 22.

central nerve cord (Serres, 1824–1826)

A ***nerve cord (Serres, 1824–1826)*** in the invertebrate ***central nervous system (Carus, 1814)***. For bilateral invertebrates, the ***central nervous system (Carus, 1814)*** generally consists of one or more ***central nerve cords (Serres, 1824–1826)***, with ***central transverse communicating branches (>1840)***—commonly referred to as commissures—typically interconnecting ***central ganglia (>1840)*** between ***central nerve cords (Serres, 1824–1826)*** (e.g., a right and a left) and forming a ladder-like, or orthogon (see Reisinger, 1925, 1972), arrangement with rostral and caudal ends. The most rostral of the ***central ganglia (>1840)*** is commonly called the ***invertebrate brain (>1840)*** or *cerebral ganglion (>1840)*. In annelids and arthropods the ***invertebrate brain (>1840)*** generally lies dorsal to the digestive system and is called the ***supraesophageal ganglion (Grant, 1834a)***, whereas the rest of the ***central nerve cord (Serres, 1824–1826)*** lies ventral to the digestive system and consists of ***circumesophageal connectives (>1840)*** and ***ventral cord (Anderson, 1837)***. See Bullock & Horridge (1965). For Serres's use of the term in molluscs see Vol. 2, p. 13. A complete ***central nerve cord (Serres, 1824–1826)*** was described earlier as a *nerve cord (Cuvier, 1800)*.

TRANSLATIONS:

1. *cordon nerveux central (Serres, 1824–1826)*
   Original French form of ***central nerve cord (Serres, 1824–1826)***; Vol. 2, p. 13.

EARLIER REFERENCES:

Earlier synonyms:

1. *medullary cord (Cuvier, 1800)*
   Synonym for octopus ***central nerve cord (Serres, 1824–1826)***; in the original French, *cordon médullaire*, Vol. 2, pp. 299, 317.
2. *longitudinal cord (Cuvier, 1800)*
   Synonym for leech ***central nerve cord (Serres, 1824–1826)***; in the original French, *cordon longitudinal*, Vol. 2, p. 355.
3. *nerve cord (Cuvier, 1800)*
   Synonym for ***central nerve cord (Serres, 1824–1826)*** for invertebrates generally; in the original French, *cordon nerveux*, e.g., Vol. 2, pp. 309, 318.
4. *trunk (Cuvier, 1800)*
   Synonym for ***central nerve cord (Serres, 1824–1826)***; in the original French, *tronc*, e.g., Vol. 2, p. 303 for a gastropod.
5. *main nerve cord of body (Carus, 1814)*
   Synonym for ***central nerve cord (Serres, 1824–1826)***; in the original German, *Hauptnervenstrang des Körpers*, p. 90.
6. *gangliated cord (Newport, 1834)*
   Synonym for macrodissected invertebrate ***central nerve cord (Serres, 1824–1826)***; pp. 402, 406.

central nerve cord trunk (>1840)

A ***central nervous system white matter tract (>1840)*** for an invertebrate ***central nerve cord (Serres, 1824–1826)***, with ***central ganglia (>1840)*** distributed along its length; see Swanson & Bota (2010). Not clearly described by 1840.

central nervous system (Carus, 1814)

In animals with bilateral symmetry, an obvious topographic division of the ***nervous system (Monro, 1783)*** in the longitudinal plane, lying in or near the median plane. For invertebrates this longitudinal division consists of one or more ***central nerve cords (>1840)***, whereas for vertebrates it consists of a single, hollow, and dorsal ***cerebrospinal axis (Meckel, 1817)***. In adult Echinoderms, which are radially symmetrical, a presumptive ***central***

nervous system (Carus, 1814) is formed by a ***circumoral nerve ring (>1840)*** with associated ***radial nerve cords (>1840)***, but there is no dominant ***ganglion (Galen, c173)*** that could be considered an ***invertebrate brain (>1840)***; see Bullock & Horridge (1965, pp. 9–14), Heinzeller & Welsch (2001, p. 41), Swanson & Bota (2010). When a ***central nervous system (Carus, 1814)*** is present, its obligate companion topographic division is a ***peripheral nervous system (Meckel, 1817)***. For systems architecture the ***central nervous system (Carus, 1814)*** consists of ***central nervous system gray matter regions (>1840)*** and ***central nervous system white matter tracts (>1840)***. Carus apparently first mentioned the term for both invertebrates and vertebrates; note on p. 76. However, the feature itself was noted in Classical Antiquity, ***[central nervous system (Carus, 1814)] (Herophilus, c335–c280 BC)***. For vertebrates, it is used interchangeably with ***cerebrospinal axis (Meckel, 1817)***.

TRANSLATIONS:

1. *centralen Nervensystems (Carus, 1814)*
   Original German for ***central nervous system (Carus, 1814)***; note on p. 76.

EARLIER REFERENCES:

Described, not named or illustrated:

1. ***[central nervous system (Carus, 1814)] (Herophilus, c335–c280 BC)***
   The founder of human anatomy recognized the ***brain (Smith Papyrus, c1700 BC)*** as the center of the ***nervous system (Monro, 1783)***; see von Staden (1989, p. 159).

Earlier synonyms:

1. *encephalon (Galen, c173)*
   In *On the Usefulness of the Parts*, Galen referred to the part of the *encephalon (Galen, c173)* within the vertebrae, implying that the ***spinal cord (Galen, c162–c166)*** is part of the ***brain (Smith Papyrus, c1700 BC)***, see May translation (1968, p. 570), and he also indicated that the *encephalon (Galen, c173)* is the source of all the ***nerves (Herophilus, c335–c280 BC)***; see May translation (1968, pp. 681–683). So in some places Galen appeared to use the term *encephalon* to mean the ***central nervous system (Carus, 1814)*** for large adult mammals but not humans specifically.
2. *brain (Piccolomini, 1586, definition 1)*
   Piccolomini appeared to used the term *cerebrum* or its English equivalent *brain* in three different ways: as *cerebrum proper (Piccolomini, 1586)* or the ***cerebral cortex gray matter (>1840)***; as the contents of the cranium or the ***brain (Smith Papyrus, c1700 BC)***; or as here, the equivalent of the ***central nervous system (Carus, 1814)***; see Bauhin (1605, p. 580 ff.) and Crooke's (rough) translation of Bauhin, "Wherefore the kernel or Marrow is the middle and white body of the braine, of which there are two parts; one contayned within the skull, the other falling out of it and lingthned downe to the great hole of the *occiput* and ending in the spine of the back." (1615, p. 459). Overall, Piccolomini apparently divided the ***central nervous system (Carus, 1814)*** into three main parts: *cerebrum (Piccolomini, 1586), or* ***cerebral cortex gray matter (>1840)***; ***cerebellum (Aristotle)***; and *medulla (Piccolomini, 1586)* with intracranial and spinal parts, the ***cerebrospinal trunk (>1840)*** and ***cerebral nuclei (Swanson, 2000)*** considered together; also see Bauhin (1605, pp. 624–625), Crooke (1615, pp. 479, 483), *encephalon (Galen, c173)*, and *medulla (Piccolomini, 1586)*. Spurzheim (1826, p. 30) discussed recent use of the term *brain* or *encephalon* for the ***central nervous system (Carus, 1814)***.
3. *brain and its appendix (Willis, 1664)*
   Synonym for macrodissected mammalian ***central nervous system (Carus, 1814)***. For Willis it had three major components: the *brain (Willis, 1664)* or ***cerebral cortex gray matter (>1840)***, the ***cerebellum (Aristotle)***, and the *medullary trunk (Willis, 1664)*—with the latter two forming the *appendix of brain (Willis, 1664)*; see Pordage translation (1681, p. 125).
4. *cerebrum broadly (Günther, 1786)*
   For macrodissected adult human, the *encephalon (Galen, c173)*; that is, the ***spinal cord (Galen, c162–c166)*** and ***brain (Smith Papyrus, c1700 BC)***; in the original Latin, *cerebrum sensu latissimo*, p. 1.
5. *middle part of nervous system (Cuvier, 1800)*
   Essentially the crustacean ***central nervous system (Carus, 1814)***; in the original French, *partie moyenne du système nerveux*, Vol. 2, p. 317.
6. *cerebral system (Burdin, 1803)*
   Synonym for ***central nervous system (Carus, 1814)*** in all animals, as opposed to *nervous system (Willis, 1664)* or ***peripheral nervous system (Meckel, 1817)***; see translation (1803, Vol. 1, pp. 141, 150).

LATER SYNONYMS:

1. *ganglion system (Carus, 1814)*
   Basically the macrodissected adult invertebrate ***central nervous system (Carus, 1814)***; in the original German, *Gangliensystem*, note on p. 74.
2. *central masses of nervous system (Carus, 1814)*
   Apparently the macrodissected adult invertebrate ***central nervous system (Carus, 1814)***; in the original German, *Centralmassen des Nervensystems*, p. 62.
3. *central mass (Gordon, 1815)*
   Synonym for macrodissected adult human ***central nervous system (Carus, 1814)***; p. 78.
4. *internal nervous system (Meckel, 1817)*
   Synonym for macrodissected adult human ***central nervous system (Carus, 1814)***; see translation (1832, Vol. 1, p. 152).
5. *central part of nervous system (Carus, 1818)*
   Synonym for macrodissected adult invertebrate ***central nervous system (Carus, 1814)***; in the original German, *Centraltheile des Nervensystems*, Table VI, Figure 1, p. 13.
6. *cerebrospinal system (Desmoulins, 1825)*
   Synonym for macrodissected adult vertebrate ***central nervous system (Carus, 1814)***; in the original French, *système cérébro-spinal*, Atlas Volume p. 3.

7. *cerebrospinal nervous system (Cloquet, 1828)*
   Synonym for macrodissected vertebrate ***central nervous system (Carus, 1814)***; in the original French, *système nerveux cérébo-spinal*, Plate CXXXII, Figure 1.
8. *cerebro-spinal mass (Quain, 1832)*
   Synonym for macrodissected adult human ***central nervous system (Carus, 1814)***; p. 634.
9. *spino-cerebral axis (Grant, 1834a)*
   Synonym for macrodissected vertebrate ***central nervous system (Carus, 1814)***; p. 481.
10. *cerebrospinal nervous center (Cruveilhier, 1836)*
   Synonym for macrodissected adult human ***central nervous system (Carus, 1814)***; in the original French, *centre nerveux céphalo-rachidien*, p. 527.

PARTLY CORRESPONDS:

1. *medulla (Piccolomini, 1586)*
   Basically, Piccolomini divided the macrodissected adult human ***central nervous system (Carus, 1814)*** into two main parts, *medulla (Piccolomini, 1586)* and *cerebrum (Piccolomini, 1586)*, the latter consisting of the *gray substance (Vesalius, 1543a)* of the ***cerebral cortex (>1840)*** and ***cerebellum (Aristotle)***. Explaining Piccolomini on the former division, Bauhin wrote, "Wherefore the kernel or Marrow [*medulla (Piccolomini, 1586)*] is the middle and white body of the braine, of which there are two parts; one contayned within the skull, the other falling out of it and lengthned downe to the great hole of the occiput and ending in the spine of the back." (p. 580, see Crooke translation,1615, p. 459). This corresponds roughly to the ***cerebral cortex white matter (>1840)***, ***cerebral nuclei (Swanson, 2000a)***, and ***cerebrospinal trunk (>1840)*** all considered together; that is, the ***central nervous system (Carus, 1814)*** without ***cerebral cortex gray matter (>1840)*** and ***cerebellum (Aristotle)***. In Piccolomini's view, the ***lateral ventricles (Vesalius, 1543a)*** are sculpted out of the ***corpus callosum (Galen, c177)***, which is also part of the *medulla (Piccolomini, 1586)*; p. 259, also see Crooke (1615, p. 459). He then divided the *medulla* or *marrow* into a *medulla globosa (Piccolomini, 1586)* and a *medulla oblongata (Piccolomini, 1586)*, with the latter subdivided into *intracranial medulla oblongata*—apparently the ***medulla (Winslow, 1733)***—and *spinal medulla oblongata*, the ***spinal cord (Galen, c162–c166)***; see corresponding entries; and Bauhin (1605, pp. 625–628), Crooke (1615, p. 479). This arrangement was illustrated in Piccolomini's pioneering though schematic sagittal drawing of the ***brain (Smith Papyrus, c1700 BC)***; p. 265; also see Clarke and Dewhurst (1996, Fig. 88:*D–F*).
2. *cerebral medulla (Piccolomini, 1586)*
   Synonym for *medulla (Piccolomini, 1586)*; in Latin, *medulla cerebri* or *cerebri medulla*, p. 259. Piccolomini referred to the "cerebrum [***cerebral cortex gray matter (>1840)***] *and its* medulla" (emphasis added). See Clarke and O'Malley (1996, p. 387), Bauhin (1605, p. 580), Crooke (1615, p. 459), and *cerebrum (Piccolomini, 1586)*.
3. *medulla vero (Bauhin, 1605)*
   More precise way of referring to macrodissected adult human *medulla (Piccolomini, 1586)*; p. 625, the "true marrow."
4. *totam cerebri medullam oblongatum (Bauhin, 1605)*
   Synonym for *medulla (Piccolomini, 1586)*; p. 625, see Crooke translation (1615, p. 479).
5. *medulla spinalis (Bauhin, 1605, p. 625)*
   Can be synonym for macrodissected adult human *medulla (Piccolomini, 1586)*; see *medulla spinalis (Bauhin, 1605, p. 628)*.
6. *spinal marrow (Bauhin, 1605)*
   English form of *medulla spinalis (Bauhin, 1605, p. 625)*.
7. *kernel (Crooke, 1615)*
   Synonym for *marrow (Crooke, 1615)*; p. 429.
8. *marrow (Crooke, 1615)*
   English form of *medulla (Piccolomini, 1586)*; pp. 458–459. Also see *spinal marrow (Hippocrates)*, *brain marrow (Piccolomini, 1586)*, and *spinal marrow in general (Bauhin, 1605)*.
9. *brain marrow (Crooke, 1615)*
   Translation of *cerebral medulla (Piccolomini, 1586)*; pp. 458–459, also see *cerebrum (Piccolomini, 1586)*.
10. *true marrow (Crooke, 1615)*
   Translation of *medulla vero (Bauhin, 1605)*, a more precise way of referring to *marrow (Crooke, 1615)*; p. 479.
11. *whole marrow of brain lengthened out (Crooke, 1615)*
   English form of *totam cerebri medullam oblongatum (Bauhin, 1605)*; p. 479.
12. *medulla oblongata (Bartholin, 1651)*
   Bartholin used this term—in English either *long part of marrow* or *lengthened marrow*—in two ways without distinguishing systematically between them. (A) Typically (pp. 317, 323, 451–455; in English, Bartholin, 1662, pp. 133, 137, 322–323), he referred to the *marrow* or *marrow in general* as the *lengthened marrow* or *medulla oblongata*—synonymous with *medulla (Piccolomini, 1586)*, or later, *totam cerebri medullam oblongatum (Bauhin, 1605)*. He then divided *medulla (Piccolomini, 1586)* into a *part within skull of medulla oblongata (Bartholin, 1651)*—the ***cerebral nuclei (Swanson, 2000a)*** and ***brainstem (Schwalbe, 1881)***—and a *part within backbone of medulla oblongata (Bartholin, 1662)*, the ***spinal cord (Galen, c162–c166)***. He noted that all ***nerves (Herophilus, c335–c280 BC)*** arise from the *medulla oblongata (Bartholin, 1651)*, counting 10 from the *part within skull of medulla oblongata (Bartholin, 1651)* and 30 from the *part within backbone of medulla oblongata (Bartholin, 1662)*; pp. 327, 451–455; translation (1662, pp. 138, 322–323). (B) He also wrote (p. 317; translation, 1662, p. 133) that the *marrow* consists of a *round part of marrow (Bartholin, 1662)* or *head of marrow (Bartholin, 1662)*, roughly the ***cerebral cortex white matter (>1840)***, ***cerebral nuclei (Swanson, 2000a)***, and ***interbrain (Baer, 1837)*** considered together, and a *long part of marrow (medulla oblongata)*, which he also called the *tail of marrow*, roughly the ***midbrain (Baer, 1837)***, ***pons (Haller, 1747)***, and ***medulla***

(Winslow, 1733), considered together. This is ambiguous because at least the first two of the *pairs of nerves from brain (Bartholin, 1611)*, the *olfactory sense instruments (Galen, c173)* and *optic nerves (Galen, c173)*, arise from the *round part of marrow (Bartholin, 1662)*, unless he included (without explanation or illustration) ventral regions of the ***cerebral nuclei (Swanson, 2000a)*** and ***interbrain (Baer, 1837)*** in *medulla oblongata (Bartholin, 1651)* rather than *round part of marrow (Bartholin, 1662)*.

13. *medulla elongata (Bartholin, 1651)*
Synonym for *medulla oblongata (Bartholin, 1651)*; p. 327.
14. *nervi glandulae pinealis (Wharton, 1656)*
Wharton wrote that two nerves, corresponding to right and left ***medullary stria (Wenzel & Wenzel, 1812)***, ***habenular commissure (>1840)***, and ***pineal stalk (Burdach, 1822)*** considered together, are distributed only to the ***pineal gland (Galen, c192)*** in macrodissected adult human. He mistakenly thought that the ***pineal stalk (Burdach, 1822)*** consists of two ***central nervous system white matter tracts (>1840)***; see translation p. 150 and Meyer (1971, p. 16). This mistake was clarified by Diemerbroeck (1689, p. 401).
15. *elongated marrow (Bartholin, 1662)*
English form of *medulla elongata (Bartholin, 1651)*; *lengthened marrow* is another possible translation.
16. *spinal marrow (Bartholin, 1662)*
Synonym for *medulla oblongata (Bartholin, 1662)*; see citations there.
17. *funiculi nervei (Le Boë, 1663)*
According to one interpretation, synonym for *nervi glandulae pinealis (Wharton, 1656)*; see Meyer (1971, p. 16). Wharton (1656, p. 150) wrote that Le Boë's term (not published until 1663) was *nerveos funiculos*. However, according to Collins (1685, pp. 1020–1021), the *nerveos funiculos* of Le Boë actually referred to the *pathetic nerve (Willis, 1664)* or ***trochlear nerve (Molinetti, 1669)***.
18. *nerve cords (Le Boë, 1663)*
English form of *funiculi nervei (Le Boë, 1663)*; see Wharton (1656, translation p. 150).
19. *pith (Willis, 1664)*
Probably synonym for *medullary trunk (Willis, 1664)*; see Pordage translation (1681, p. 60), also see Gibson (1684, p. 349).
20. *oblong stock (Willis, 1664)*
Synonym for *medullary trunk (Willis, 1664)*; see Pordage translation (1681, pp. 62, 64).
21. *whole nervous stock (Willis, 1664)*
Synonym for *medullary trunk (Willis, 1664)*; see Pordage translation (1681, pp. 89, 192).
22. *nervous stock (Willis, 1664)*
Abbreviated form of *whole nervous stock (Willis, 1664)*.
23. *medullary rope (Willis, 1664)*
Probably synonym for *medullary trunk (Willis 1664)*; see Pordage translation (1681, pp. 90, 124).
24. *medullary cord (Willis, 1664)*
Alternate translation of *medullary rope (Willis, 1664)*.
25. *appendix of brain (Willis, 1664)*
Probably synonym for *medullary trunk (Willis, 1664)*; see Pordage translation (1681, pp. 100, 125).
26. *medullary trunk (Willis, 1664)*
For Willis, the whole *medullary trunk* includes *oblong marrow (Willis, 1664)* and ***spinal cord (Galen, c162–c166)*** and generates all the ***craniospinal nerves (Herrick, 1915)***; see Pordage translation (1681, pp. 101, 124, 127). Thus the ***cerebral cortex (>1840)***, ***cerebellum (Aristotle)***, and ***nerves (Herophilus, c335–c280 BC)*** are attached to the *medullary trunk (Willis, 1664)*, going back to *medulla (Piccolomini, 1586)*.
27. *caudici medullari (Willis, 1664)*
Grammatical variation on *caudex medullaris (Willis, 1664)*; p. 155.
28. *caudex medullaris (Willis, 1664)*
Original Latin form of *medullary trunk (Willis, 1664)*; p. 231. *Caudex* is an old form of *codex*, or trunk.
29. *marrowy appendix (Willis, 1664)*
Synonym for *medullary trunk (Willis, 1664)*; see Pordage translation (1681, p. 125).
30. *medullary appendix (Willis, 1664)*
Synonym for *medullary trunk (Willis, 1664)*; see Pordage translation (1681, p. 125).
31. *genus nervosum (Willis, 1667)*
Latin form of *nervous stock (Willis, 1664)*; that is, the *medullary trunk (Willis, 1664)*. For English form see title of Pordage translation (1681).
32. *cerebral ring around esophagus (Burdin, 1803)*
For macrodissected gastropods, the complex ring formed by the ***central nervous system (Carus, 1814)*** around the esophagus region; see translation (1803, Vol. 1, p. 142). Also see Bullock & Horridge (1965, Vol. 2, Figs. 23.2, 23.3).
33. *spinal prolongation of brain (Chaussier, 1807)*
Synonym for macrodissected adult human ***medulla (Winslow, 1733)*** and ***spinal cord (Galen, c162–c166)*** considered together; in the original French, *prolongement rachidien de l'encéphale*, pp. 114, 194.
34. *summus corporis humani nervus (Chaussier, 1807)*
Synonym for macrodissected adult human ***medulla (Winslow, 1733)*** and ***spinal cord (Galen, c162–c166)*** considered together, the *spinal prolongation of brain (Chaussier, 1807)*; p. 115 in note 1. Also see *spinal bulb (Chaussier, 1807)*.
35. *axis of nervous system (Reil, 1809c)*
In a key formulation based on his examination of the adult human, Reil wrote, "Grey matter ascends uninterruptedly in the axis of the nervous system, chord-like below, a chain of ganglions above, the tubercula quadrigemina, the thalami, the corpora striata." (see Mayo translation, 1823, p. 86). *Axis of nervous system (Reil, 1809c)* corresponds to ***cerebrospinal trunk (1840)*** and ***cerebral nuclei (Swanson, 2000)*** considered together, going all the way back to *medulla Piccolomini (1586)*.
36. *nerve ring around esophagus (Carus, 1814)*
As described, a ring formed around the esophagus by the ***invertebrate brain (>1840)***, ***circumesophageal***

connectives (>1840), and most rostral ***ventral ganglia (>1840)*** of worms, molluscs, and all the other invertebrates examined by Carus and, as he noted, a characteristic difference with vertebrates; in the original German, *Nervenring um die Speiseröhre*, pp. 85, 121.

37. *marrow collar (Carus, 1814)*
The characteristic ring of ***central ganglia (>1840)*** and associated commissures, or ***central transverse communicating branches (>1840)***, and connectives, or ***central longitudinal communicating branches (>1840)*** near the rostral end of the ***central nerve cord (>1840)*** of macrodissected adult gastropods and cephalopods viewed under the microscope; in the original German, *Markhalsband*, p. 87. See Bullock & Horridge (1965, Figs. 23.3, 25.1).
38. *marrow ring (Carus, 1814)*
Synonym for *marrow collar (Carus, 1814)*; in the original German, *Markringes*, p. 88.
39. *brain ring (Treviranus, 1817)*
Synonym for *nerve ring around esophagus (Carus, 1814)* in macrodissected millipedes viewed under the microscope; in the original German, *Hirnring*; see Treviranus & Treviranus, Vol. 2 (1817), p. 32 and Table VII, Figure 2.
40. *nerve ring around mouth (Carus, 1818)*
Synonym for *nerve ring around esophagus (Carus, 1814)*, here for macrodissected bivalve viewed under microscope; in the original German, *Nervenring um den Mund*, Table II, Figure X-*b*. Carus also indicated a *ganglion of these nerve rings*; Table II, Figure X-*c*.
41. *nerve collar (Carus, 1818)*
Synonym for *nerve ring around esophagus (Carus, 1814)* in macrodissected adult *Aplysia* viewed under the microscope; in the original Latin, *Nervenhalsband*, Table III, Figure VII-*m*. See Bullock & Horridge (1965, Fig. 23.32).
42. *nervous ring of invertebrata (Müller, 1834)*
Synonym for *nerve ring around esophagus (Carus, 1814)*; see translation (1838, p. 592).
43. *oesophageal ring (Müller, 1834)*
Synonym for *nerve ring around esophagus (Carus, 1814)*; see translation (1838, p. 593).
44. *ganglionated circle around oesophagus (Grant, 1834a)*
Synonym for *nerve ring around esophagus (Carus, 1814)*; p. 485.
45. *ganglionated oesophageal ring (Grant, 1834a)*
Synonym for *nerve ring around esophagus (Carus, 1814)*; p. 485.
46. *spinal cord (Quain, 1837)*
For macrodissected adult human, the ***spinal cord (Galen, c162–c166)*** and ***medulla (Winslow, 1733)*** considered together; pp. 717–718.
47. *ganglionic chain (Leuret, 1839)*
The macrodissected adult ***central nervous system (Carus, 1814)*** of "articulated" invertebrate animals; in the original French, *chaîne ganglionaire*, e.g., p. 70.

central nervous system gray matter regions (>1840)

Gray matter regions (Swanson & Bota, 2010) are divided topographically into two parts, ***central nervous system gray matter regions (>1840)*** and ***peripheral nervous system gray matter regions (>1840)***. ***Central nervous system gray matter regions (>1840)*** are differentiations of ***gray matter (Meckel, 1817)*** now based essentially on cellular architecture and connections. The first clear differentiations, based on macrodissected adult human observations, were by Vesalius; see *cerebral lobe (Vesalius, 1543a)*, ***[cerebellar cortex (Willis, 1664)] (Vesalius, 1543a)***.

EARLIER REFERENCES:

Described, not named or illustrated:

1. ***[central nervous system gray matter regions (>1840)] (Rufus of Ephesus, fl. c90–c120)***
In the *Anatomy of the Parts of the Body*, Rufus wrote that the substance of the ***brain (Smith Papyrus, c1700 BC)*** is ash gray in color and that the *spinal marrow (Hippocrates)*, or ***spinal cord (Galen, c162–c166)***, is an extension of the ***brain (Smith Papyrus, c1700 BC)***; see Clarke & O'Malley (1996, p. 14). There is, however, no hint of a differentiation between ***central nervous system gray matter regions (>1840)*** and ***central nervous system white matter tracts (>1840)***. The conjecture that Galen made this distinction in the ***cerebrum (Obersteiner & Hill, 1900)*** is not strong; see May (1968, p. 398 note 41). In *On Anatomical Procedures*, Galen may have written that, "the component parts of the brain itself are a complex of veins and arteries, bound together by the pia mater..." (see Singer translation, 1999, p. 232). However, this translation is open to alternate interpretation not related to the substance of the ***brain (Smith Papyrus, c1700 BC)***; see Wiberg translation (1914, p. 24).
2. ***[central nervous system gray matter regions (>1840)] (Dryander, 1536)***
In *The Anatomy of the Human Head*, Dryander clearly if crudely illustrated it in a section through the macrodissected adult human ***cerebral cortex (>1840)*** on the right and left sides; Figure 6. The figure also shows crude *cerebral convolutions (Smith Papyrus, c1700 BC)* with *gray substance (Vesalius, 1543a)* superficial to *white substance (Vesalius, 1543a)*, although this arrangement was not written about in the text; see Lind translation (1975, p. 301).
3. ***[central nervous system gray matter regions (>1840)] (Vesalius, 1543a)***
For macrodissected adult human, Vesalius referred to *ash-gray substance (Vesalius, 1543a)* of ***cerebellum (Aristotle)*** checkered with *white substance (Vesalius, 1543a)*, see Singer translation (1952, p. 28), and clearly illustrated and described boundaries between them; see Singer translation (1952, pp. 94–95, Fig. 4). Vesalius also clearly distinguished between *ash-gray substance (Vesalius, 1543a)* and *white substance (Vesalius, 1543a)* in *cerebral lobe (Vesalius, 1543)*, especially in *cerebral convolutions (Smith Papyrus, c1700 BC)*; see Singer translation (1952, p. 28). The first clear distinction between ***central nervous system gray matter regions***

(>1840) and ***central nervous system white matter tracts (>1840)*** in the ***spinal cord (Galen, c162–c166)*** was made by Coiter (1572, see translation pp. 113–114). Willis (1672) pointed out that ***cerebral nuclei (Swanson, 2000a)*** as well as ***tectum (Baer, 1837)*** have *gray substance (Vesalius, 1543a)* intermixed with *white substance (Vesalius, 1543a)*; see Pordage translation (1683, p. 26). Malpighi (1665) wrote that ***brainstem (Schwalbe, 1881)*** is characterized by *white substance (Vesalius, 1543a)* peripherally and *gray substance (Vesalius, 1543a)* more centrally; see Meyer (1967, p. 189).

4. ***[central nervous system gray matter regions (>1840)] (Piccolomini, 1586)***
   Piccolomini is generally credited with first clear description in macrodissected adult human of difference between ***central nervous system gray matter regions (>1840)*** and ***central nervous system white matter tracts (>1840)***. For him, the former are softer, grayish, glandular, and concentrated in ***cerebral cortex gray matter (>1840)*** whereas the latter are more compact, white, and fibrous or medullary; see Ridley (1695, pp. 87–88), Clarke & O'Malley (1996, p. 387), and *cerebrum (Piccolomini, 1586)*.
5. ***[central nervous system gray matter regions (>1840)] (Reil, 1809c)***
   In a key formulation, Reil wrote, "Grey matter ascends uninterruptedly in the axis of the nervous system, chord-like below, a chain of ganglions above, the tubercula quadrigemina, the thalami, the corpora striata." (see Mayo translation, 1823, p. 86).

Earlier synonyms:

1. *ashy orange substance of brain (Vesalius, 1543a)*
   Synonym for macrodissected adult human *gray substance (Vesalius, 1543a)*; see Richardson & Carman translation (2009, p. 132).
2. *brown substance of brain (Vesalius, 1543a)*
   Synonym for macrodissected adult human *gray substance (Vesalius, 1543a)*; see Richardson & Carman translation (2009, p. 139). According to Gordon (1817, pp. 28–29), this is the most accurate description of its color in fresh tissue.
3. *discolored substance of brain (Vesalius, 1543a)*
   Synonym for macrodissected adult human *gray substance (Vesalius, 1543a)*; see Richardson & Carman translation (2009, p. 139).
4. *gray substance (Vesalius, 1543a)*
   Vesalius clearly distinguished in macrodissected adult human between ***central nervous system gray matter regions (>1840)*** and ***central nervous system white matter tracts (>1840)***, "The substance of the brain is not all white, but near the convolutions [*cerebral gyri (Vesalius, 1543a)*] it is yellowish or gray for a distance equal to the depth from the surface of the convolution. As the depth of the convolution, so is the depth of ash-gray matter, thus doubling the substance of that colour in the convolution. Any part of the brain which is not thus [ash] coloured is white and shining" (see Singer translation, 1952, pp. 28, 100). Schiller (1967, p. 516) elaborated on how the original Latin should or might be translated; also see ***[central nervous system gray matter regions (>1840)] (Rufus of Ephesus, fl. c90–c120)***.
5. *ash-gray substance (Vesalius, 1543a)*
   Synonym for macrodissected adult human *gray substance (Vesalius, 1543a)*; see Singer translation (1952, pp. 28, 100), Schiller (1967, p. 516).
6. *yellowish substance (Vesalius, 1543a)*
   Synonym for macrodissected adult human *gray substance (Vesalius, 1543a)*; see Singer translation (1952, pp. 28, 100). Geminus (1553) referred in English to "substaunce of the brayne... as it were yelowe, and somewhat moore lyke the colour of ashes" (see *The tables of the brayne*, Fig. 4-*D*).
7. *spongy substance (Paré, 1550)*
   Apparently synonym for macrodissected adult human *gray substance (Vesalius, 1543a)*; in the original French, *la substance spongieuse*, see Salomon & Trouilloud translation (2003, pp. 206, 207).
8. *ashen part (Valverde de Amusco, 1556)*
   Synonym for macrodissected adult human *gray substance (Vesalius, 1543a)*, in the original Spanish, *la parte... cenicienta*; Libro V, Figure VII-*D*.
9. *cineritious part (Valverde de Amusco, 1560)*
   Latin form of *cineritium*, of *ashen part (Valverde de Amusco, 1556)*; p. 242, see Schiller (1967, p. 517).
10. *bluish-white body (Piccolomini, 1586)*
    Synonym for macrodissected adult human *gray substance (Vesalius, 1543a)*; in the original Latin, *corpus in albo livescens*, p. 252. See Schiller (1967, p. 517).
11. *cortical substance (Willis, 1664)*
    Willis often referred thus to *gray substance (Vesalius, 1543a)*, or ***central nervous system gray matter regions (>1840)***; see Pordage translation (1681, p. 59) and Pordage translation (1683, p. 26).
12. *cortex (Malpighi, 1665)*
    Synonym for ***central nervous system gray matter regions (>1840)*** in general; see *Opera Omnia* (1686, Vol. 2, p. 115), and Meyer (1967, p. 186).
13. *cineritia substantia (Malpighi, 1665)*
    Slight variation on, and synonym for, *cineritious part (Valverde de Amusco, 1560)*; see *Opera Omnia* (1686, Vol. 2, p. 115) and quote in Adelmann (1966, p. 260).
14. *limbus (Molinetti, 1669)*
    Synonym for macrodissected adult human ***central nervous system gray matter regions (>1840)***; p. 81, according to Burdach (1822, p. 250).
15. *substantia glandulosa (Vieussens, 1684)*
    Synonym for macrodissected adult human ***central nervous system gray matter regions (>1840)***; p. 56, see Burdach (1822, p. 250).
16. *substantia vitrea (Leeuwenhoek, 1685)*
    Synonym for ***central nervous system gray matter regions (>1840)***; p. 883, according to Burdach (1822, p. 250).

17. *cineritious substance (Ridley, 1695)*
Simply English translation of macrodissected adult human *cineritia substantia (Malpighi, 1665)*; p. 120.
18. *ash-colored substance (Winslow, 1733)*
Variation on *gray substance (Vesalius, 1543a)*; see Section X, p. 44. Vicq d'Azyr (1784, p. 600) provided the French, *la substance cendrée*, p. 600; Clarke & O'Malley (1996, p. 269) translated it *ashen-colored substance*.
19. *cineritious matter (Monro, 1783)*
Slight variation on, and synonym for, macrodissected adult human *cineritious part (Valverde de Amusco, 1560)*, but probably the first actual use of the word *matter* rather than *substance* referring to ***central nervous system gray matter regions (>1840)***; p. 22.
20. *ash-coloured matter (Bell, 1803b)*
Synonym for macrodissected adult human ***central nervous system gray matter regions (>1840)***; p. 27.
21. *pulpy substance (Gall & Spurzheim, 1809)*
Synonym for macrodissected adult human ***central nervous system gray matter regions (>1840)***; in the original French, *substance pulpeuse*, e.g., p. 65.
22. *gelatinous substance (Gall & Spurzheim, 1809)*
Synonym for macrodissected adult human ***central nervous system gray matter regions (>1840)***; in the original French, *substance gélatineuse*, e.g., pp. 65, 168.
23. *gelatinous gray substance (Gall & Spurzheim, 1810)*
Synonym for macrodissected adult human ***central nervous system gray matter regions (>1840)***; in the original French, *substance gélatineuse grise*, p. 54.
24. *ganglion substance (Carus, 1814)*
Synonym for macrodissected adult vertebrate ***central nervous system gray matter regions (>1840)***; in the original German, *Gangliensubstanz*, e.g., pp. 76–77, 215. Carus attributed the concept to Gall.
25. *cerebral matter (Tiedemann, 1816)*
Synonym for macrodissected developing human ***central nervous system gray matter regions (>1840)***; see translation (1826, pp. 159–161), where it was also translated *cerebral substance* and contrasted with *medullary substance (Colombo, 1559)*.
26. *central nervous system gray matter (Meckel, 1817)*
Synonym for ***central nervous system gray matter regions (>1840)***. Meckel was the first to use this particular terminology, for macrodissected adult human, distinguishing it from *central nervous system white matter (Meckel, 1817)* and in fact stating explicitly that ***nervous system (Monro, 1783)*** as a whole may be divided into gray and white matter parts; see translation (1832, Vol. 2, pp. 152–154).
27. *substantia succosa (Langenbeck, 1826–1830)*
Synonym for macrodissected adult human ***central nervous system gray matter regions (>1840)***; Fascicle I, Table XVIII-*i*.

PARTLY CORRESPONDS:

1. *nucleus cinereus (Ludwig, 1779)*
A differentiable ***central nervous system gray matter region (>1840)***. Ludwig applied it to a part of the *thalami nervorum opticorum (Riolan, 1618)* of a bird (probably goose) as observed in an oblique sagittal cut; Figure 2-*b*, p. 36. See *nucleus (Vicq d'Azyr, 1784)*.
2. *gray nucleus (Ludwig, 1779)*
English form of *nucleus cinereus (Ludwig, 1779)*.
3. *nucleus (Vicq d'Azyr, 1784)*
Term applied to a yellowish layer of *gray substance (Vesalius, 1543a)* in the macrodissected adult human ***inferior olivary complex (>1840)***; p. 588. Vicq d'Azyr noted that the layer is analogous to *cortical substance (Willis, 1664)*, and that there is an analogous layer in ***dentate nucleus (>1840)*** of ***cerebellum (Aristotle)***. Stilling gave universal meaning to the term *nucleus (Vicq d'Azyr, 1784)* for a recognizable ***central nervous system gray matter region (>1840)***; see Schiller (1969), Jacobson (1993, p. 13), *nucleus cinereus (Ludwig, 1779)*.
4. *ganglion (Reil, 1809c)*
A differentiable mass of *gray substance (Vesalius, 1543a)* in macrodissected adult human ***central nervous system (Monro, 1783)***; in other words, an instance of a differentiable ***central nervous system gray matter region (>1840)***. See *nucleus (Vicq d'Azyr, 1784)*.
5. *brain ganglia (Gall & Spurzheim, 1810)*
Differentiations of ***central nervous system gray matter regions (>1840)*** in macrodissected adult human; according to Burdach (1822, p. 251), who gave the Latin as *ganglia encephali*, and the German as *Hirnganglien* (p. 7).
6. *Ganglionmasse (Carus, 1814)*
German synonym for a differentiable ***central nervous system gray matter region (>1840)*** in macrodissected adult human; p. 66, also see Burdach (1822, p. 250).
7. *collicular ganglia (Burdach, 1822)*
As described for macrodissected adult human, *brain ganglia (Gall & Spurzheim, 1810)* forming protrusions on surface of ***brain (Smith Surgical Papyrus, c1700 BC)***; in the original German, *gangliöse Hügel*, and in the original Latin, *colliculi gangliosi* (p. 7).
8. *nuclear ganglia (Burdach, 1822)*
As described for macrodissected adult human, *brain ganglia (Gall & Spurzheim, 1810)* lying within substance of ***brain (Smith Papyrus, c1700 BC)*** rather than on surface; in the original German, *gangliöse Kerne*, and in the original Latin, *nuclei gangliosi* (p. 7).

central nervous system surface features (>1840)

A physical differentiation described on the outer surface of the ***central nervous system (Carus, 1814)***. The first example has long been known; see ***[central nervous system surface features (>1840)] (Smith Papyrus, c1700 BC)***.

EARLIER REFERENCES:

Described, not named or illustrated:

1. ***[central nervous system surface features (>1840)] (Smith Papyrus, c1700 BC)***
First recorded example was *cerebral convolutions (Smith Papyrus, c1700 BC)*, described by surgeon for live adult human wounded in battle.

PARTLY CORRESPONDS:

1. *roof of Sylvian fissure (Reil, 1809b)*
   Corresponds to macrodissected adult human ***frontal operculum (>1840)*** and ***parietal operculum (>1840)*** considered together; in the original German, *dach der Sylvischen Grube*, p. 196, see Mayo translation (1823, p. 78).
2. *operculum (Burdach, 1822)*
   Synonym for macrodissected adult human *roof of Sylvian fissure (Reil, 1809b)*; in the original German, *der Klappdeckel*; p. 167 and Tables III-5, IV-8, III-12,13, VI-χ.
3. *operculum (Arnold, 1838a)*
   Modern definition of macrodissected adult human *operculum of insula (>1840)*, the ***frontal operculum (>1840)***, ***parietal operculum (>1840)***, and ***temporal operculum (>1840)***, considered together; p. 52. Also see *Dorland's* (2003, p. 1316).
4. *opercula of insula (>1840)*
   Synonym for macrodissected adult human *operculum (Arnold, 1838)*; see *Dorland's* (2003, p. 1316).

central nervous system white matter tracts (>1840)

White matter tracts (Bell & Bell, 1826) are divided topographically into two parts, ***central nervous system white matter tracts (>1840)*** and ***peripheral nervous system white matter tracts (>1840). Central nervous system white matter tracts (>1840)*** are differentiations of ***white matter (Meckel, 1817)*** now based essentially on histologically defined connections. The first clear differentiations, based on macrodissected adult human observations in the ***cerebral cortex (>1840)*** and ***cerebellum (Aristotle)***, were by Vesalius; see ***[central nervous system white matter tracts (>1840)] (Vesalius, 1543a)***.

EARLIER REFERENCES:

Illustrated, not named or described:

1. ***[central nervous system white matter tracts (>1840)] (Dryander, 1536)***
   In *The Anatomy of the Human Head*, Dryander clearly if crudely illustrated one instance of a ***central nervous system white matter tract (>1840)] (Dryander, 1536)*** in a section through the macrodissected adult human ***cerebral cortex (>1840)*** on the right and left sides; Figure 6. The figure shows crude *cerebral convolutions (Smith Papyrus, c1700 BC)*, with *gray substance (Vesalius, 1543a)* superficial to *white substance (Vesalius, 1543a)*, although this arrangement is not mentioned in the text; see Lind translation (1975, p. 301). Vesalius made the first distinction between different tracts; see ***[central nervous system white matter tracts (>1840)] (Vesalius, 1543a)***.
2. ***[central nervous system white matter tracts (>1840)] (Vesalius, 1543a)***
   For macrodissected adult human, Vesalius referred to gray (ash-gray) color of ***cerebellum (Aristotle)*** checkered with white lines, that is, *white substance (Vesalius, 1543a)*; see Singer translation (1952, p. 28). He also clearly distinguished between *ash-gray substance (Vesalius, 1543a)* in *cerebral lobe (Vesalius, 1543a)*, especially in *cerebral convolutions (Smith Papyrus, c1700 BC)*; see Singer translation (1952, p. 28). Later he wrote that deeper substance of *cerebral lobe (Vesalius, 1543a)* is "firmer and white" (see Singer translation, 1952, p. 31). Coiter made the first clear distinction between *gray substance (Vesalius, 1843a)* and *white substance (Vesalius, 1543a)* in ***spinal cord (Galen, c162–c166)***; see ***[central nervous system white matter tracts (>1840)] (Coiter, 1572)***.
3. ***[central nervous system white matter tracts (>1840)] (Coiter, 1572)***
   In perhaps the first indication of the fibrous nature of the ***brain (Smith Papyrus, c1700 BC)***, Coiter described in ***medullary substance (Colombo, 1559)*** hair-like fibers continuing into all *pairs of nerves from brain (Galen, c192)*; see translation p. 113. Bichat (Bichat et al., 1801–1803, Vol. 3, p. 96) was perhaps the last great anatomist to deny the fibrous nature of the ***brain (Smith Papyrus, c1700 BC)***; see Meckel (1832, Vol. 1, p. 162).
4. ***[central nervous system white matter tracts (>1840)] (Piccolomini, 1586)***
   Piccolomini is generally credited with the first clear description of a difference between ***central nervous system gray matter regions (>1840)*** and ***central nervous system white matter tracts (>1840)***. For him, the former are softer, grayish, glandular, and concentrated in ***cerebral cortex gray matter (>1840)***, whereas the latter is more compact, white, and fibrous or medullary; see Ridley (1695, pp. 87–88), Clarke & O'Malley (1996, p. 387), and *cerebrum (Piccolomini, 1586)*.

Earlier synonyms:

1. *white cerebral substance (Vesalius, 1543a)*
   Synonym for macrodissected adult human ***central nervous system white matter tracts (>1840)***; see Richardson & Carman translation (2009, p. 139).
2. *white substance (Vesalius, 1543a)*
   Vesalius clearly distinguished, for macrodissected adult human, between ***central nervous system white matter tracts (>1840)*** and ***central nervous system gray matter regions (>1840)***, "The substance of the brain is not all white, but near the convolutions [*cerebral gyri (Vesalius, 1543a)*] it is yellowish or gray for a distance equal to the depth from the surface of the convolution. As the depth of the convolution, so is the depth of ash-gray matter, thus doubling the substance of that colour in the convolution. Any part of the brain which is not thus [ash] coloured is white and shining" (see Singer translation, 1952, p. 28).
3. *medullary substance (Colombo, 1559)*
   Synonym for macrodissected adult human ***central nervous system white matter tracts (>1840)***. As quoted by Wharton (1656, translation p. 12), Colombo wrote, "under this thin membrane [***pia (Galen, c192)***] of the brain is concealed a white, soft substance, which is also described as medullary, although it differs a great deal from the substance marrow found in the hollow bones."

4. *corpus candicum (Bauhin, 1605)*
Synonym for macrodissected adult human *white substance (Vesalius, 1543a)*; p. 580, see Burdach (1822, p. 249).
5. *medullary part (Willis, 1664)*
Synonym for macrodissected adult mammalian ***central nervous system white matter tracts (>1840)***; see Pordage translation (1681, p. 93).
6. *marrowy substance (Willis, 1664)*
Synonym for macrodissected adult mammalian *medullary substance (Colombo, 1559)*; see Pordage translation (1681, pp. 60, 93, 101, 110).
7. *corpus callosum (Malpighi, 1665)*
Synonym for, occasionally at least, ***central nervous system white matter tracts (>1840)***; see Gordon translation (1817, p. 17), Meyer translation (1976, p. 186).
8. *callosal substance (Steno, 1669)*
Steno wrote that there is little reason to distinguish ***corpus callosum (Galen, c177)*** from the rest of the brain's *white substance (Vesalius, 1543a)*, or *medulla (Piccolomini, 1573)*, in macrodissected adult human; see translation p. 138. Thus, Steno suggested the term *callosal substance* for ***central nervous system white matter tracts (>1840)***; see Burdach (1822, p. 249).
9. *medullary matter (Monro, 1783)*
Slight variation on, and synonym for, macrodissected adult human *medullary substance (Colombo, 1559)*, but probably still the first actual use of the word *matter* rather than *substance* referring to the ***central nervous system white matter tracts (>1840)***; p. 22.
10. *white medullary matter (Bell, 1803b)*
Synonym for macrodissected adult human ***central nervous system white matter tracts (Swanson & Bota, 2010)***; p. 28.
11. *white matter (Bell, 1803b)*
Synonym for macrodissected adult human ***central nervous system white matter tracts (>1840)***; p. 107.
12. *central nerve mass (Carus, 1814)*
Probably synonym for macrodissected adult human ***central nervous system white matter tracts (>1840)***; in the original German, *centraler Nervenmasse*, p. 296.
13. *central nervous system white matter (Meckel, 1817)*
First use of this particular terminology, distinguishing it from *central nervous system gray matter (Meckel, 1817)* and in fact stating that the ***nervous system (Monro, 1783)*** as a whole may be divided into ***gray matter (Meckel, 1817)*** and ***white matter (Meckel, 1817)*** parts; see translation (1832, Vol. 2, pp. 152–154).
14. *fibrous substance of central organs of nervous system (Grainger, 1837)*
Synonym for macrodissected adult human ***central nervous system white matter tracts (>1840)***; p. 17.
15. *fibrous matter of central organs of nervous system (Grainger, 1837)*
Synonym for macrodissected adult human ***central nervous system white matter tracts (>1840)***; p. 17.

PARTLY CORRESPONDS:

1. *medullary capsule (Reil, 1809b)*
Term Reil used for a set of ***central nervous system white matter tracts (>1840)***: ***internal capsule (Burdach, 1822)***, ***external capsule (Burdach, 1822)***, and probably ***extreme capsule (>1840)*** in macrodissected adult human ***endbrain (Kuhlenbeck, 1927)***; see Mayo translation (1823, p. 52), Gordon (1817, p. 101 ff.), Meyer (1971, p. 29). Also see *inner wall of capsule (Reil, 1809b)* and *outer wall of capsule (Reil, 1809b)*.
2. *capsule (Reil, 1809b)*
Short form of *medullary capsule (Reil, 1809b)*; see Mayo translation (1823, pp. 69, 81).
3. *external part of medullary capsule (Reil, 1809b)*
Synonym for *outer wall of capsule (Reil, 1809b)*, including "that surface, which supports the convolutions of the island [*insula (Reil, 1809b)*]." (see Mayo translation, 1823, p. 52; Dejerine & Dejerine-Klumpke, 1895, p. 336).
4. *external capsule (Reil, 1809b)*
Synonym for *outer wall of capsule (Reil, 1809b)*; in the original German, *äussre Capsel*, p. 144; also see Burdach (1822, p. 351).
5. *corona radiata (Reil, 1809b)*
As described for macrodissected adult human, includes ***internal capsule (Burdach, 1822)***, its dorsal intersection with *oval center (Vieussens, 1684)*, and the latter's radiations into middle of *cerebral gyri (Vesalius, 1543a)*— radiations Reil called *medullary plates (Reil, 1809b)*— all three considered together. "The fibres derived from the crus cerebri, which diverge at the upper margin of the thalamus towards the circumference of either hemisphere, form the fibrous cone [*Stabkranz*]." (pp. 145, 157–166; see Mayo translation, 1823, p. 53). Thus, Reil considered *corona radiata (Reil, 1809b)* a "longitudinal" component of ***central nervous system white matter tracts (>1840)*** in contrast to "transverse" component associated with ***corpus callosum (Galen, c177)***. For detailed description see Dejerine & Dejerine-Klumpke (1901, pp. 1–19); also see Henle (1871, Fig. 72), Schwalbe (1881, Fig. 417), Crosby et al. (1962, pp. 395–396), Carpenter (1976, Fig. 2.8), Williams & Warwick (1980 p. 1030 and Fig. 7.150A).
6. *fibrous cone (Reil, 1809b)*
English form of original German form *Stabkranz*, for *corona radiata (Reil, 1809b)*; see Mayo translation (1823, p. 53).
7. *cerebral peduncle system (Reil, 1809b)*
As described for macrodissected adult human, the longitudinal (vertical) part of *nucleus of cerebrum (Reil, 1809b)*, the transverse (horizontal) part being *corpus callosum system (Reil, 1809b)*; in the original German, *Hirnschenkelsystem*; pp. 147–171, also see Mayo translation (1823, p. 53 ff.). Basically, *cerebral peduncle system (Reil, 1809b)* consisted, from rostral to caudal, of *corona radiata (Reil, 1809b)*, ***internal capsule (Burdach, 1822)***, ***cerebral peduncle (Tarin, 1753)***, ***longitudinal pontine fibers (Arnold, 1838b)***, and ***pyramid (Willis, 1664)*** on both sides of the ***brain (Smith Papyrus, c1700 BC)***. Reil wrote that rostral to the ***pyramids (Willis, 1664)*** this

fiber radiation, the *cerebral peduncle system (Reil, 1809b)* continually enlarges and diverges, especially rostral to the ***pons (Haller, 1747)***.

8. *Hirnschenkelsystem (Reil, 1809b)*
Original German form of *cerebral peduncle system (Reil, 1809b)*; pp. 147–171.
9. *vertical portion of nucleus of cerebrum (Reil, 1809b)*
Synonym for *cerebral peduncle system (Reil, 1809b)*; see Mayo translation (1823, p. 54).
10. *lemniscus (Reil, 1809b)*
Reil's description of the *fillet* (in English) or *Schleife* (in the original German; as well as *Schleifenbahn*) in macrodissected adult human included ***lateral lemniscus (Bechterew, 1885b)*** and ***medial lemniscus (>1840)***, and probably other nearby ***central nervous system white matter tracts (>1840)*** as well; see Mayo translation (1823, pp. 55 ff., 94 ff.), Burdach (1822, p. 323), Meyer (1971, pp. 29–30).
11. *fillet (Reil, 1809b)*
English form of *lemniscus (Reil, 1809b)*; see Mayo translation (1823, pp. 55 ff., 94 ff.).
12. *outer wall of capsule (Reil, 1809b)*
Term included both ***external capsule (Burdach, 1822)*** and ***extreme capsule (>1840)*** of macrodissected adult human; see Mayo translation (1823, pp. 80–81, Tab. X-*g*), and Dejerine & Dejerine-Klumpke (1895, p. 369).
13. *vertical layers (Reil, 1809c)*
Synonym for macrodissected adult human *stratum horizontale (Burdach, 1822)*; in the original German, *senkrechte Schichten*, p. 493.
14. *returning or converging nervous system (Gall & Spurzheim, 1809)*
Synonym for *apparatus of union (Gall & Spurzheim, 1810)*; in the original French, *système nerveux, rentrant ou convergent* (p. 153) or *systèmes nerveux rentrans ou convergens du cervelet et du cerveau* (p. 160).
15. *apparatus of union (Gall & Spurzheim, 1810)*
As described for macrodissected adult human and other mammals, basically all transverse components of ***central nervous system white matter tracts (>1840)*** connecting same structure on right and left sides—the commissural systems; in the original French, *appareils de réunion ou de jonction*, see pp. 182, 201; also see Gordon (1817, pp. 32 ff., 126 ff.), Spurzheim (1826, p. 179). Gall & Spurzheim thought of it as a system of convergence and as one of their two orders of cerebral fibers (basically transverse and longitudinal), the other being *apparatus of formation (Gall & Spurzheim, 1810)*.
16. *apparatus of formation (Gall & Spurzheim, 1810)*
As described for macrodissected adult human and other animals, basically all known (at the time) components of ***central nervous system white matter tracts (>1840)*** coursing longitudinally, similar to, though more comprehensive than, *cerebral peduncle system (Reil, 1809b)*; in the original French, *appareils de formation ou de renforcement*, pp. 185–186, 201, 221; also see Gordon (1817, p. 61 ff.). Gall & Spurzheim thought of it as a rostrally directed (ascending) system of divergence with two sets of bundles, the first going to ***frontal region (Vicq d'Azyr, 1786)*** and ***temporal region (>1840)*** and the second going to ***parietal region (>1840)*** and ***occipital region (Vesalius, 1543a)*** of ***cerebral cortex gray matter (>1840)***. It is one of their two orders of cerebral fibers (basically transverse and longitudinal), the other being *apparatus of union (Gall & Spurzheim, 1810)*.
17. *fascicle from olivary ganglion (Gall & Spurzheim, 1810)*
Probably macrodissected adult human *lemniscus (Reil, 1809b)*; pp. 192, 198 and Plate V-*a*; also see Meyer (1971, p. 30), Crosby et al. (1962, pp. 256–257). Gall & Spurzheim viewed it in their extremely vague description as a rostrally directed ***central nervous system white matter tract (>1840)***.
18. *radiation to ceiling of great ventricles (Carus, 1814)*
Apparently macrodissected adult human ***internal capsule (Burdach, 1822)*** and *corona radiata (Reil, 1809b)* considered together; in the original German, *Radiation der Decke der Grossen Hirnhöhlen*, p. 223.
19. *nucleus (Rosenthal, 1815)*
Rosenthal divided macrodissected adult human ***brain (Smith Papyrus, c1700 BC)*** into *mantle (Rosenthal, 1815)* and *nucleus (Rosenthal, 1815)*; in the original German, *Kern*, pp. 7, 11. The former is major part of ***cerebral cortex gray matter (>1840)*** and the latter constitutes major ***central nervous system white matter tracts (>1840)*** of ***brain (Smith Papyrus, c1700 BC)*** including ***cerebral cortex white matter (>1840)***, ***internal capsule (Burdach, 1822)***, ***cerebral peduncle (Tarin, 1753)***, and so on. Burdach (1822, pp. 10, 13) used the term for macrodissected adult human.
20. *middle bundle (Rosenthal, 1815)*
Probably corresponds roughly to macrodissected adult human *lemniscus (Reil, 1809b)*, which Rosenthal described as stretching between ***inferior olivary complex (>1840)*** and ***tectum (Baer, 1837)***; in the original German, *mittleres Bündel*, p. 24; see Burdach (1822, p. 281).
21. *olivary bundle (Rosenthal, 1815)*
Synonym for *middle bundle (Rosenthal, 1815)*; p. 24 and Table II; see Burdach (1822, p. 281). Serres (1824–1826, Pl. XVI, Fig. 288-2) used the French, *cordon olivaire*, and described extensions to dorsal (posterior) part of ***interbrain (Baer, 1837)***, ***inferior cerebellar peduncle (Günther, 1786)***, and ***pyramid (Willis, 1664)***, see Plate XVI, Figure 289.
22. *middle fasciculus of medulla oblongata (Rosenthal, 1815)*
Synonym for *olivary fasciculus (Tiedemann, 1816)*; pp. 24–27, see Tiedemann (1826, p. 49) and Meckel (1832, pp. 424, 467).
23. *olivary fasciculus (Tiedemann, 1816)*
According to Tiedemann, corresponds to *lemniscus (Reil, 1809b)* along with apparent extension in ***medulla (Winslow, 1733)*** of ***lateral funiculus (Burdach, 1822)*** to caudal end of ***olive (Tiedemann, 1821)***, which might be part of ***ventrolateral fascicle (>1840)***; see translation

(1826, p. 146). In Tiedemann's view, based on macroscopic dissection of alcohol-hardened human fetus, outer matter of ***spinal cord (Galen, c162–c166)*** differentiates into three fasciculi at level of ***medulla (Winslow, 1733)***: pyramidal (ventral), olivary (middle), and restiform (dorsal). The *olivary fasciculus (Tiedemann, 1816)* forms earlier than *olivary body (Vieussens, 1684)* in development and extends rostrally (ascends) through ***pons (Haller, 1747)***, distributing fibers to both sides of ***tectum (Baer, 1837)*** and then to ***interbrain (Baer, 1827)***; see translation (1826; pp. 62, 76, 90, 100, and 142 ff.). Tiedemann's work was an elaboration of Rosenthal (1815, pp. 24–27); see *middle fasciculus of medulla oblongata (Rosenthal, 1815)*. Arnold (1838a, p. 31; 1838b, Tab. II, Fig. 6-*b*; Tab. IX, Fig. 1-*i*) illustrated it clearly for macrodissected adult human and used *fasciculus olivaris*.

24. *circle of Reil (Gordon, 1817)*
Synonym for macrodissected adult human *corona radiata (Reil, 1809b)*; p. 100.

25. *stem system (Burdach, 1822)*
Essentially macrodissected adult human *apparatus of formation (Gall & Spurzheim, 1810)*; in the original German, *Stammsystem*, p. 10 ff.

26. *systema caudiceum (Burdach, 1822)*
Original Latin form of *Stammsystem* or *stem system (Burdach, 1822)*; p. 10.

27. *radiatio caudicea (Burdach, 1822)*
Synonym for macrodissected adult human *corona radiata (Reil, 1809b)*; Burdach also used the German, *Stammstrahlung*, p. 11.

28. *fibres of union (Spurzheim, 1826)*
Synonym for *apparatus of union (Gall & Spurzheim, 1810)*; p. 178.

29. *converging bundles (Spurzheim, 1826)*
Synonym for *apparatus of union (Gall & Spurzheim, 1810)*; p. 178.

30. *converging fibres (Spurzheim, 1826)*
Synonym for *apparatus of union (Gall & Spurzheim, 1810)*; p. 179.

31. *diverging fibres (Spurzheim, 1826)*
Synonym for *apparatus of formation (Gall & Spurzheim, 1810)*; p. 179.

32. *instruments of communication (Spurzheim, 1826)*
Synonym for *apparatus of formation (Gall & Spurzheim, 1810)*; p. 188.

33. *instruments of union (Spurzheim, 1826)*
Synonym for *apparatus of union (Gall & Spurzheim, 1810)*; p. 192.

34. *fillet of medulla oblongata (Mayo, 1827)*
Synonym for macrodissected adult human *lemniscus (Reil, 1809b)*; see Plate II, Figure 4-*i* and Pl. 4-ζ.

35. *respiratory tract (Quain, 1832)*
As described for macrodissected adult human, longitudinal "narrow line" or ***central nervous system white matter tract (>1840)*** between *olive (Tiedemann, 1821)* and *restiform body (Günther, 1786)*, or *inferior cerebellar peduncle (Günther, 1786)*, of ***medulla (Winslow, 1733)*** continuing down ***spinal cord (Galen, c162–c166)*** as ***lateral funiculus (Burdach, 1822)***; in the original Latin, *tractus respiratorius*, p. 637. Essentially the ***lateral funiculus (Burdach, 1822)*** and ***medullary ventrolateral fascicle (>1840)***.

36. *posterior column descending from hemisphere (Bell, 1834)*
As described for macrodissected adult human, difficult to describe with current terminology but includes, at least in part, ***thalamic radiations (Reil, 1809b)***, ***medial lemniscus (>1840)***, and ***medial lemniscus decussation (>1840)***, while more caudally Bell had it extending through ***lateral funiculus (Burdach, 1822)*** and forming ***dorsal roots (Spurzheim, 1826)***; pp. 473–476 and Plate XX, Figure 2. "Some authors describe these roots as derived from the cineritious [gray] matter. This is quite at variance with my dissections. The cineritious matter is not of a consistence or structure into which nerves can be traced" (Bell, 1835, p. 256). Also see *anterior column descending from hemisphere (Bell, 1834)*.

37. *posterior tract (Bell, 1834)*
Synonym for *posterior column descending from hemisphere (Bell, 1834)*; p. 475.

38. *sensible tract (Bell, 1834)*
Synonym for *posterior column descending from hemisphere (Bell, 1834)*; Plate XXI-*E*.

39. *tract of corpus olivare (Bell, 1834)*
For macrodissected adult human, Bell described it as extending rostrally (ascending) to *corpora quadrigemina (Wenzel & Wenzel, 1812)* and *crus cerebri (Vicq d'Azyr, 1784)* and descending to ***dorsal funiculus (>1840)*** and ***ventral funiculus (>1840)***; pp. 476–477. Also see *anterior column descending from hemisphere (Bell, 1834)*.

40. *cerebral part of second pair (Arnold, 1834)*
For macrodissected adult human, it included ***optic tract (Vicq d'Azyr, 1784)*** and ***brachium of superior colliculus (Haller, 1762)***, although Arnold described it as extending from ***inferior colliculus (Haller, 1762)***; in the original Latin, *par secundum, pars cerebralis*, p. 6.

41. *cerebral part of optic nerve (Arnold, 1834)*
Synonym for *cerebral part of second pair (Arnold, 1834)*; in the original Latin, *nervus opticus, pars cerebralis*, p. 6.

42. *pineal commissure (Solly, 1836)*
Apparently macrodissected adult mammalian ***habenular commissure (>1840)*** and right and left ***medullary stria (Wenzel & Wenzel, 1812)*** considered together; pp. 90, 178.

43. *grand soleil (Cruveilhier, 1836)*
French synonym for macrodissected adult human *corona radiata (Reil, 1809b)*; p. 716.

44. *éventail de Vieussens (Cruveilhier, 1836)*
Eponym in French for macrodissected adult human *corona radiata (Reil, 1809b)*; p. 716.

45. *real origin of trigeminal nerve (Cruveilhier, 1836)*
Considered together, *great root of trigeminal nerve (Cruveilhier, 1836)* and *small root of trigeminal nerve (Cruveilhier, 1836)*; in the original French, *origine réelle*, p. 894.

46. *cerebral medullary radiation (Arnold, 1838a)*
Synonym for macrodissected adult human *corona radiata (Reil, 1809b)*; in the original Latin, *radiatio medullaris cerebri*, p. 71.

central sulcus (Huschke, 1854)

As described for macrodissected adult human, the groove between ***precentral gyrus (>1840)*** rostrally and ***postcentral gyrus (>1840)*** caudally; see Williams & Warwick (1980, Fig. 7.111A). For Huschke's use in macrodissected adult carnivore and human, see p. 134 and Cunningham (1892, p. 162). It was first clearly distinguished by Vicq d'Azyr; see ***[central sulcus (Huschke, 1854)] (Vicq d'Azyr, 1786)***.

TRANSLATIONS:

1. *Centralfurche (Huschke, 1854)*
Original German form of ***central sulcus (Huschke, 1854)***; p. 134.

EARLIER REFERENCES:

Illustrated, not named or described:

1. ***[central sulcus (Huschke, 1854)] (Vicq d'Azyr, 1786)***
Clearly illustrated for macrodissected adult human; Plate III. See Rasmussen (1947, p. 15), Meyer (1971, p. 124).

Earlier synonyms:

1. *fissure of Rolando (Leuret, 1839)*
Eponym for macrodissected adult baboon ***central sulcus (Huschke, 1854)***; in the original French, *sillon de Rolando*, p. 398 and Plate XV, Figures 2, 4-*S.R.* Cunningham (1892, pp. 161–162) related how Leuret mistakenly attributed it to Rolando (in human) based on a defective edition of Vicq d'Azyr (1805) citing a detailed account by Broca (1876, p. 824). Also see Meyer (1971, p. 126).

PARTLY CORRESPONDS:

1. *cruciate sulcus (Leuret, 1839)*
A groove in rostral and medial parts of ***cerebral cortex gray matter (>1840)*** of some mammals like cat, sometimes thought to be homologous with ***central sulcus (Huschke, 1854)*** of human. Leuret described it in fox, cat, and seal, for example; in the original French, *sillon crucial*, pp. 376, 379, 392. Also see *Oxford English Dictionary* (Online).

central sulcus of insula (>1840)

As described for macrodissected human, the diagonal groove between ***short gyri of insula (Gall & Spurzheim, 1810)*** rostrally and ***long gyrus of insula (Valentin, 1841)*** caudally; see Williams & Warwick (1980, p. 988, Fig. 7113A), *Terminologia Anatomica* (1998, p. 125). It was perhaps first clearly delineated by Rolando; see ***[central sulcus of insula (>1840)] (Rolando, 1831)***.

EARLIER REFERENCES:

Illustrated, not named or described:

1. ***[central sulcus of insula (>1840)] (Rolando, 1831)***
Clearly illustrated for macrodissected adult human; Figure 3, within 3.

central tegmental tract (Bechterew, 1889)

As described in macrodissected adult human, and mammal generally with histological methods for ***axons (Kölliker, 1896)***, a diffusely organized longitudinal ***central nervous system white matter tract (>1840)*** extending roughly between ***red nucleus (Burdach, 1822)*** rostrally and ***inferior olivary complex (>1840)*** caudally. Rostrally, it is first visible in parts of the ***midbrain reticular nucleus (>1840)*** dorsomedial to the ***red nucleus (Burdach, 1822)*** and then extends caudally through dorsolateral parts of the ***pontine reticular nucleus (>1840)*** before shifting more medially and ventrally in the ***medulla (Winslow, 1733)*** to surround the ***inferior olivary complex (>1840)***; see Riley (1943, pp. 693–694), Crosby et al. (1962, pp. 256-257), Nieuwenhuys et al. (2008, Figs. 6.24–33). For topographic description, it has ***tegmental central tegmental tract (>1840), pontine central tegmental tract (>1840)***, and ***medullary central tegmental tract (>1840)*** segments, with the part of the latter surrounding the ***inferior olivary complex (>1840)*** called ***amiculum of olive (>1840)***. A main component is the *rubro-olivary projection*; see Nieuwenhuys et al. (2008, p. 208). It was not clearly delineated by 1840, although Rolando may have described part of it; see *anterolateral cord of oblong medulla (Rolando, 1825a)*.

central transverse communicating branch (>1840)

For invertebrates, a ***communicating branch (Winslow, 1733)*** between two corresponding ***central ganglia (>1840)*** on different ***central nerve cords (>1840)***, like the rungs of a ladder; see Swanson & Bota (2010, Thesaurus). A common synonym is *commissure*. Perhaps the first description was a *transverse filament (Serres, 1824–1826)*.

EARLIER REFERENCES:

Earlier synonyms:

1. *transverse filament (Serres, 1824–1826)*
Synonym for ***central transverse communicating branch (>1840)***; in the original French (plural), *filets transverses*, p. 21.

cerebellar commissure (>1840)

As described in macrodissected adult human, and mammal generally with histological methods for ***axons (Kölliker, 1896)***, a transverse ***central nervous system white matter tract (>1840)*** between right and left ***arbor vitae (Winslow, 1733)*** of the ***cerebellum (Aristotle)***; see Nieuwenhuys et al. (2008, p. 200 and Fig. 6.27). It was clearly illustrated by Steno; see ***[cerebellar commissure (>1840)] Steno (1669)***.

EARLIER REFERENCES:

Illustrated, not named or described:

1. ***[cerebellar commissure (>1840)] (Steno, 1669)***
Clearly illustrated in midsagittal view of macrodissected adult human; Plate I, bottom. For transverse view see Vicq d'Azyr (1786, Pl. XXIX, Fig. 2-24).

cerebellar cortex (Willis, 1664)

As described for vertebrate with gross dissection, cellular architecture, and connections, the remarkably uniform

gray matter region (Swanson & Bota, 2010) forming the outer layer of the ***cerebellum (Aristotle)***, superficial to the ***white matter (Meckel, 1817)*** of the ***cerebellar cortex (Willis, 1664)***, the ***arbor vitae (Winslow, 1733)***. The basic division of ***cerebellar cortex (Willis, 1664)***—into ***cerebellar vermis (Meckel, 1817)*** subdivisions and ***cerebellar hemisphere (Willis, 1664)*** lobules—adopted here follows the extensive comparative analysis of Larsell; see Larsell & Jansen (1972, Fig. 118), Angevine et al. (1961, p. 7, Fig. 24), Carpenter (1976, Fig. 14.1). For Willis's use in macrodissected adult human and other large mammals see Pordage translation (1681, pp. 67, 68). Reil (1807–1808b; see Mayo translation, 1822, p. 78) identified and physically separated two layers in the adult human ***cerebellar cortex (Willis, 1664)***: an outer gray layer, and an inner dirty yellowish layer. It was first delineated by Vesalius; see ***[cerebellar cortex (Willis, 1664)] (Vesalius, 1543a)***.

EARLIER REFERENCES:

Illustrated and described, not named:

1. ***[cerebellar cortex (Willis, 1664)] (Vesalius, 1543a)***
   Vesalius referred to gray (ashy) color of ***cerebellum (Aristotle)*** checkered with white lines [*white substance (Vesalius, 1543a)*]; see Singer translation (1952, p. 28). He also clearly illustrated and described boundaries between *gray substance (Vesalius, 1543a)* or *yellowish substance (Vesalius, 1543a)*, and *white substance (Vesalius, 1543a)* in Figure 4; see Singer translation (1952, pp. 94–95).

LATER SYNONYMS:

1. *cerebellar bark (Willis, 1664)*
   Synonym for ***cerebellar cortex (Willis, 1664)***; see Pordage translation (1681, p. 67).

PARTLY CORRESPONDS:

1. *folds (Erasistratus, c310–c250 BC, definition 2)*
   According to Galen, synonym for macrodissected adult presumably human *folia (Malacarne, 1776)*; see May translation (1968, p. 414), De Lacy (1980, pp. 441, 443), Clarke & O'Malley (1996, p. 630).
2. *convolutions (Erasistratus, c310-c250 BC)*
   According to Galen, synonym for macrodissected adult presumably human *folia (Malacarne, 1776)*; see May translation (1968, p. 414), De Lacy (1980, pp. 441, 443), Clarke & O'Malley (1996, p. 630).
3. *very small bodies (Galen, c173)*
   Synonym for macrodissected adult beef, pig, and/or macaque but not human *folia (Malacarne, 1776)*; see May translation (1968, p. 418).
4. *links in a chain (Haly Abbas or Ali ibn' ul-Abbas, d. 994)*
   Synonym for macrodissected adult presumably human *folia (Malacarne, 1776)*; see Wiberg translation (1914, p. 85).
5. *gyri (Vesalius, 1543a)*
   Synonym for macrodissected adult human *folia (Malacarne, 1776)*, noting they are not separate and discontinuous but instead form a single body, the ***cerebellar cortex (Willis, 1664)***; see Singer translation (1952, p. 26).
6. *circles (Hall, 1565)*
   Synonym for macrodissected adult human *folia (Malacarne, 1776)*; p. 36.
7. *globes (Bartholin, 1662)*
   Synonym for macrodissected adult human *folia (Malacarne, 1776)*; Table IV, Figure 1-*A*, p. 136.
8. *circumvolutions (Bartholin, 1662)*
   Synonym for macrodissected adult human *folia (Malacarne, 1776)*; p. 138.
9. *turnings (Bartholin, 1662)*
   Synonym for macrodissected adult human *folia (Malacarne, 1776)*; p. 138.
10. *windings (Bartholin, 1662)*
    Synonym for macrodissected adult human *folia (Malacarne, 1776)*; p. 138.
11. *lappets (Willis, 1664)*
    Synonym for macrodissected adult human *folia (Malacarne, 1776)*; see Pordage translation (1681, pp. 60, 67).
12. *lamellae (Willis, 1664)*
    Synonym for macrodissected adult human *folia (Malacarne, 1776)*; in the original Latin, *lamellis*, Ch. 3, translated by Pordage as *lappets (Willis, 1664)*. In his book published 21 years later, Collins (1685, pp. 995, 1029) examined and illustrated the ***brain (Smith Papyrus, c1700 BC)*** of many species of fish, birds, and mammals. He wrote, "The Antient and modern Anatomists have taken notice of some sort, of these Processes [*lamellae (Willis, 1664)*] on the Surface of the *Cerebellum*, but have not made (that I can read) any inspection into their more inward Recesses, how they are seated in Depth in Ranks and Files one under another in admirable order; and as far as I can apprehend, not any Anatomists have *mentioned* the lateral Provinces, only in general notices, of Circles and Episphaeres, and have not pried into their more retired parts, how they are parted from each other, taking no cognizance of their inward arrangements of Processes, lodged below one another..." (p. 1032).
13. *plates (Perrault, 1688)*
    Synonym for *folia (Malacarne, 1776)* in birds and terrestrial animals, and in particular here, the ostrich; p. 237.
14. *circilli (Tyson, 1699)*
    Synonym for macrodissected infant chimpanzee *folia (Malacarne, 1776)*; p. 56. It is probably derived from Willis's description, "...its folds are disposed in a certain orderly series; for the exterior frame of it seems to consist of thin lappets, or little rings or circles, being contiguous and infolded, also going about through the whole compass with a parallel site or situation." (Pordage translation, 1681, p. 67). See *circles (Hall, 1565)*, *lamellae (Willis, 1664)*.
15. *strata (Winslow, 1733)*
    Synonym for macrodissected adult human *folia (Malacarne, 1776)*; Section X, p. 39.
16. *laminated leaflets (Malacarne, 1776)*
    Synonym for macrodissected adult human *folia (Malacarne, 1776)*; see Clarke & O'Malley (1996, p. 644).
17. *folia (Malacarne, 1776)*

Term for convolutions of macrodissected adult human ***cerebellar cortex (Willis, 1664)***; see Soemmerring (1778, p. 62).

18. *yellowish substance between gray and white matter of cerebellum (Soemmerring, 1778)*
This material, which Soemmerring barely made out in several macrodissected adult human cadavers, may correspond to ***Purkinje cell layer (>1840)***; p. 63. Also see Vicq d'Azyr (1784, p. 576).
19. *annuli (Günther, 1786)*
Synonym for macrodissected adult human *folia (Malacarne, 1776)*; p. 17.
20. *concentric arcs (Günther, 1786)*
Synonym for macrodissected adult human *folia (Malacarne, 1776)*; in the original Latin, *arcus concentrici*, p. 17.
21. *substantia flavescens (Günther, 1786)*
Synonym for macrodissected adult human *yellowish substance between gray and white matter of cerebellum (Soemmerring, 1778)*; p. 18.

cerebellar falx (Günther, 1786)

As described for macrodissected adult human, the shallow longitudinal fold of ***dura (Galen, c177)*** in the median plane between the ***cerebellar hemispheres (Willis, 1664)***. It "is a small sickle-shaped fold, similar to the falx cerebri, which separates the posterior extremities of the cerebellar hemispheres. It is attached to the occipital bone from the occipital crest to the foramen magnum and its layers enclose the occipital sinus." (Millen & Woollam, 1962, p. 128). Also see *Terminologia Anatomica* (1998, p. 104). For Günther's use in macrodissected adult human, see p. 2. Perhaps the first clear description was *septum cerebelli (Winslow, 1733)*.

TRANSLATIONS:

1. *falx cerebelli (Günther, 1786)*
Original Latin form of ***cerebellar falx (Günther, 1786)***; p. 2; see *Terminologia Anatomica* (1998, p. 104).
2. *falx of cerebellum (Bell, 1803b; Burdin, 1803)*
English form of *falx cerebelli (Günther, 1786)*; Bell, p. 16; Burdin, see translation, 1803, Vol. 1, p. 153.

EARLIER REFERENCES:

Earlier synonyms:

1. *septum cerebelli (Winslow, 1733)*
Synonym for macrodissected adult human ***cerebellar falx (Günther, 1786)***; Section X, p. 25.
2. *small occipital septum (Winslow, 1733)*
Synonym for macrodissected adult human ***cerebellar falx (Günther, 1786)***; Section X, p. 26. In Latin, Winslow used *septum occiptalis minus*. Schreger (1803, p. 315) gave the Latin, *septum parvum occipitale*.
3. *occipital septum (Winslow, 1733)*
Synonym for macrodissected adult human ***cerebellar falx (Günther, 1786)***; Section X, pp. 26, 39.
5. *occipital falx (Malacarne, 1776)*
Synonym for macrodissected adult human ***cerebellar falx (Günther, 1786)***; p. 18, see Clarke & O'Malley (1996, p. 643).
6. *falx minor (Mayer, 1779)*
Synonym for macrodissected adult human ***cerebellar falx (Günther, 1786)***; Vol. 6, p. 23; see Burdach (1822, p. 319), who also preferred this term. Chaussier (1807, p. 24) used the French, *la petite faulx*, in English the *small falx*.
6. *processus falciformis cerebelli (Mayer, 1783-1794)*
Synonym for macrodissected adult human ***cerebellar falx (Günther, 1786)***; Vol. 6, p. 23; see Burdach (1822, p. 319).

LATER SYNONYMS:

1. *processus falciformis inferior (Schreger, 1803)*
Synonym for macrodissected adult human ***cerebellar falx (Günther, 1786)***; p. 315.
2. *median septum of cerebellum (Burdin, 1803)*
Synonym for macrodissected adult human ***cerebellar falx (Günther, 1786)***; see translation (1803, Vol. 1, p. 153). Burdach (1822, p. 319) also preferred this term.
3. *longitudinal septum of cerebellum (Chaussier, 1807)*
Synonym for macrodissected adult human ***cerebellar falx (Günther, 1786)***; in the original French, *septum longitudinal du cervelet*, p. 24.
4. *processus falciformis minor (Arnold, 1834)*
Synonym for macrodissected adult human ***cerebellar falx (Günther, 1786)***; Table II:*BB-ff*.

cerebellar fissures (>1840)

The transversely oriented grooves of various depths subdividing the macrodissected adult vertebrate ***cerebellar cortex (Willis, 1664)*** into lobes, lobules, and *folia (Malacarne, 1776)* (leaflets); see Williams & Warwick (1980, p. 912), *Terminologia Anatomica* (1998, p. 118), Nieuwenhuys et al. (2008, pp. 70, 808). Contrast with ***cerebral sulci (Vesalius, 1543a)***. They were first described as *grooves (Vesalius, 1543a)*.

EARLIER REFERENCES:

Earlier synonyms:

1. *grooves (Vesalius, 1543a)*
Synonym for macrodissected adult human ***cerebellar fissures (>1840)***; see Singer translation (1952, p. 26). Galen was undoubtedly familiar with them but his description was vague, "[The ***cerebellum (Aristotle)***] is composed not of large convolutions [*cerebral convolutions (Smith Papyrus, c1700 BC)*] separated by the thin membrane [***pia (Galen, c192)***] like the encephalon but of many very small bodies differently arranged from those in the encephalon." (May translation, 1962, p. 418).
2. *sulci (Heister, 1717)*
Synonym for macrodissected adult human ***cerebellar fissures (>1840)***; p. 78.
3. *furrows (Heister, 1722)*
English form of *sulci (Heister, 1717)*; p. 204.

cerebellar hemisphere (Willis, 1664)

As described for macrodissected adult mammal, the right or left part of the ***cerebellar cortex (Willis, 1664)*** lateral to the unpaired ***cerebellar vermis (Meckel, 1817)*** in the middle; see Angevine et al. (1961, Fig. 24), Larsell & Jansen (1972, Fig. 118), Carpenter (1976, Figs. 2.23–26, 14.1), Nieuwenhuys et al. (2008, Figs. 3.11, 3.13). For Willis's use in macrodissected adult human and other large mammals see Pordage translation (1681, p. 68, Tab. IV-*L*). It was first crudely delineated and illustrated by Dryander; see ***[cerebellar hemisphere (Willis, 1664)] (Dryander, 1536)***. It was clearly described on right and left as *globes (Vesalius, 1543a)*.

EARLIER REFERENCES:

Illustrated, not named or described:

1. *[cerebellar hemisphere (Willis, 1664)] (Dryander, 1536)*
   First illustrated in *Anatomy of the Human Head* for macrodissected adult human; see Figure 7 in Lind translation (1975, p. 301).

Earlier synonyms:

1. *globes (Vesalius, 1543a)*
   Vesalius wrote that ***cerebellum (Aristotle)*** is built in three parts, right, left, and middle [***cerebellar vermis (Meckel, 1817)***], and that the former "are as *globes* [***cerebellar hemispheres (Willis, 1664)***] pressed together, and in the space between there rests the third part." (Singer translation, 1952, p. 26).

LATER SYNONYMS:

1. *cerebellar eminence (Molinetti, 1669)*
   Synonym for macrodissected adult human ***cerebellar hemisphere (Willis, 1664)***; in the original Latin (plural), *eminentiae cerebelli*, p. 89.
2. *hemiglobi cerebelli (Molinetti, 1669)*
   Synonym for macrodissected adult human ***cerebellar hemispheres (Willis, 1664)***; p. 89.
3. *cerebellar lobe (Winslow, 1733)*
   Synonym for macrodissected adult human ***cerebellar hemisphere (Willis, 1664)***; Section X, p. 39.
4. *major cerebellar lobes (Günther, 1786)*
   Synonym for macrodissected adult human ***cerebellar hemispheres (Willis, 1664)***; in the original Latin, *lobi majores cerebelli*, p. 17.
5. *lateral part of cerebellum (Meckel, 1817)*
   Synonym for macrodissected adult human ***cerebellar hemisphere (Willis, 1664)***, objecting that Willis's term was very improper; see translation (1832, Vol. 2, p. 428).

PARTLY CORRESPONDS:

1. *lesser circuits of cerebellum (Collins, 1685)*
   Collins divided macrodissected adult human ***cerebellar hemisphere (Willis, 1664)*** into three lesser circuits, stories, or apartments [*lobes of cerebellar hemispheres (Malacarne, 1776)*], "The *Cerebellum* consisteth of Two great Provinces (T. 50 F.1 bbbb) seated on each side of the middle protuberance [***cerebellar vermis (Meckel, 1817)***], and each of these Provinces, may be divided into Three lesser Circuits, or Stories, the greatest of them (T. 50 F.1 eeee) is next the termination [typo?], and the middle (T. 50 F.1 dddd) is smaller then the Posterior, and the greater then the Anterior, or hightst Apartiment (T. 50 F.1 cccc).
   These several stories of each lateral Fabrick, (T. 50 F.1 bbbb) may be distinguished by their various protuberancies; the Posterior being the most depressed, and the Anterior most prominent, and the middle of a middle nature, more protuberant than the Posterior, and more depressed than the Anterior. ¶ And although the denomination speaketh a diminution, in reference to its slender bulk, yet it may in some sort challenge to its self preheminence above the Brain, in relation to the curious Fabrick of its *Cortex*; that of the Brain being framed of diverse *Anfractus* or Maeanders; but this of the *Cerebellum* is beautified with an innumerable company of Processes, embelished with variety of fine Models of different shapes and sizes, some resembling in a manner Triangles, others Quadrangles of unequal sides, Ovals, and others, are Orbicular, or Pyramidal." (pp. 1030–1031). Or again, "The Cerebellum of a Cat is composed of Five Apartiments, one in the middle, and another in the termination, and Four lateral, Two on each side of the middle Apartiment...The inward lateral Apartiments (T. 53 F.2 bb) are endued with a kind of Semi-lunary Figure, and are endued with many oblong transverse Processes, more short then those of the middle Apartiment, and somewhat akin to them in Figure." (p. 1096). The descriptions and illustrations are probably too vague to correlate with current ***cerebellar hemisphere (Willis, 1664)*** nomenclature, although its roots are obvious here.
2. *lesser stories of cerebellum (Collins, 1685)*
   Synonym for *lesser circuits of cerebellum (Collins, 1685)*; p. 1030.
3. *lesser apartments of cerebellum (Collins, 1685)*
   Synonym for *lesser circuits of cerebellum (Collins, 1685)*; p. 1030.
4. *lobes of cerebellum (Pourfour du Petit, 1710)*
   In outlining the substance of future (never published) work on the human ***brain (Smith Papyrus, c1700 BC)***, Pourfour du Petit made the intriguing but unelaborated statement, "I divide the superior part [of ***cerebellum (Aristotle)***] into four lobes. The inferior part has five paired lobes and one single unpaired lobe. I subdivided all of these lobes into leaves and grooves." (p. 13; L. Kruger & L.W. Swanson, unpublished translation). The passage is too vague to correlate with current ***cerebellar hemisphere (Willis, 1664)*** nomenclature.
5. *lobules of cerebellum (Heister, 1717)*
   Malacarne (1776; see Clarke & O'Malley, 1996, p. 644) pointed out that Heister used *lobuli* or *lobules* for smaller divisions of ***cerebellar hemisphere (Willis, 1664)***; p. 211. Heister also wrote that they had not been described adequately, and provided a nice illustration for macrodissected adult human; see translation (1721, p. 205 and Tab. IV, Fig. 16).
6. *cerebellar protuberances (Winslow, 1733)*
   Winslow divided macrodissected adult human ***cerebellar hemisphere (Willis, 1664)*** into three protuberances: anterior, middle or lateral, and posterior; Section X, p. 39. His description was brief and unillustrated, and impossible to correlate with current nomenclature but follows *lesser circuits of cerebellum (Collins, 1685)*; also see *cerebellar lobe (Winslow, 1733)*.

7. *lateral vermiform process (Winslow, 1733)*
Although Winslow's description is very brief and vague, probably refers roughly to macrodissected adult human *tubercula lateralia anteriora inferiora cerebelli (Tarin, 1750)*; Section X, p. 39. Burdach (1822, p. 296) gave the Latin form, *processus vermiformes laterales*. Ruysch also used the term; see *Thesaurus V* (no. 52, p. 13), dated 1744 and included in *Opera Omnia* (1737).
8. *tubercula lateralia anteriora inferiora cerebelli (Tarin, 1750)*
Appears to indicate roughly macrodissected adult human ***ansiform lobule crus 2 (>1840)***, ***gracile lobule (>1840)***, and ***biventral lobule (>1840)***, considered together (Tab. II, Fig. 2-*r,r*). Vicq d'Azyr (1786, Pl. XVIII-*50*) and Burdach (1822, p. 295) indicated inaccurately that Tarin used it for ***tonsil (Malacarne, 1776)***.
9. *lobules of cerebellum (Haller, 1762)*
Haller noted three of them, based on three *cerebellar protuberances (Winslow, 1733)*; in the original Latin, *lobulos*, p. 71.
10. *colliculus on side of inferior vermiform eminence (Haller, 1762)*
Although Haller's description is brief, it probably refers roughly to *tubercula lateralia anteriora inferiora cerebelli (Tarin, 1750)*; pp. 71–72 (including footnote *p*).
11. *lobes of cerebellar hemispheres (Malacarne, 1776)*
Indicates largest divisions of macrodissected adult human ***cerebellar hemisphere (Willis, 1664)***; see Clarke & O'Malley (1996, p. 644).
12. *superior anterior lobe (Malacarne, 1776)*
Macrodissected adult human *anterior quadrangular lobule (>1840)* and ***simple lobule (Jansen & Brodal, 1954)*** considered together; p. 26. Burdach (1822, pp. 57, 294) gave the Latin, *lobus superior anterior*.
13. *quadrilateral lobe (Malacarne, 1776)*
Synonym for *superior anterior lobe (Malacarne, 1776)*; p. 26.
14. *partis anterioris superioris cerebelli portio quaedam sulcis notata (Soemmerring, 1778)*
Corresponds roughly to macrodissected adult human ***ansiform lobule crus 2 (Bolk, 1906)***, ***gracile lobule (>1840)***, and ***biventral lobule (>1840)***, considered together; according to Vicq d'Azyr (1786, Pl. XVIII-*51*).
15. *tubercula anteriora inferiora Tarini (Haase, 1781)*
Eponym for macrodissected adult human *tubercula lateralia anteriora inferiora cerebelli (Tarin, 1750)*; p. 26.
16. *superior internal lobule (Vicq d'Azyr, 1784)*
Roughly synonymous with macrodissected adult human *superior anterior lobe (Malacarne, 1776)*; p. 569 and Vicq d'Azyr (1786, p. 89). Burdach (1822, p. 294) gave the Latin, *lobulus cerebelli superior internus*.
17. *inferior anterior tubercle of Tarin (Günther, 1786)*
Eponym for macrodissected adult human *tubercula lateralia anteriora inferiora cerebelli (Tarin, 1750)*; in the original Latin, *tubercula anteriora inferiora Tarini*, p. 18.
18. *monticuli of cerebellum (Fyfe, 1800)*
Synonym for macrodissected adult human *lobules of cerebellum (Heister, 1717)*; Vol. 2, p. 23.
19. *fascicles of cerebellum (Chaussier, 1807)*
Synonym for macrodissected adult human *lobes of cerebellar hemispheres (Malacarne, 1776)*; in the original French, *fascicules du cervelet*, p. 86.
20. *superior lobule of cerebellum (Chaussier, 1807)*
Chaussier divided each macrodissected adult human ***cerebellar hemisphere (Willis, 1664)*** into topographically named *superior lobule of cerebellum (Chaussier, 1807)*, *posterior lobule of cerebellum (Chaussier, 1807)*, and *inferior lobule of cerebellum (Chaussier, 1807)*; see Plates 1, 4. The *superior lobule of cerebellum (Chaussier, 1807)* has five smaller lobules; in the original French, *lobule supérieurs du cervelet*, pp. 89–91. It probably refers to parts of ***cerebellar hemisphere (Willis, 1664)*** dorsal to ***ansiform lobule crus 1 (Bolk, 1906)***; see *posterior lobule of cerebellum (Chaussier, 1807)*.
21. *inferior lobule of cerebellum (Chaussier, 1807)*
Chaussier divided each macrodissected adult human ***cerebellar hemisphere (Willis, 1664)*** into topographically named *superior lobule of cerebellum (Chaussier, 1807)*, *posterior lobule of cerebellum (Chaussier, 1807)*, and *inferior lobule of cerebellum (Chaussier, 1807)*; see Plates 1, 4. The *inferior lobule of cerebellum (Chaussier, 1807)* has four smaller lobules lateral to ***cerebellar vermis (>1840)***; in the original French, *lobule inférieurs du cervelet*, pp. 89–91. It probably refers to parts of ***cerebellar hemisphere (Willis, 1664)*** ventral to ***ansiform lobule crus 1 (Bolk)***; see *posterior lobule of cerebellum (Chaussier, 1807)*.
22. *square lobe (Reil, 1807-1808a)*
English form of *quadrilateral lobe (Malacarne, 1776)*; see Mayo translation (1822, p. 22), Burdach (1822, p. 294). Reil observed that here, *white substance (Vesalius, 1543a)* stems of ***arbor vitae (Winslow, 1733)*** are many and simple in macrodissected adult human; see Mayo translation (1822, Tab. V, Fig. I:*1-13*).
23. *anterior lobes of cerebellum (Gordon, 1815)*
While Gordon's description of macrodissected adult human is not entirely clear today, it may refer to parts of ***cerebellar hemisphere (Willis, 1664)*** rostral (anterior) to ***preculminate fissure (>1840)***; p. 108. See Larsell & Jansen (1972, Fig. 118) and *mons cerebelli (Gordon, 1815)*.
24. *posterior lobes of cerebellum (Gordon, 1815)*
While Gordon's description of macrodissected adult human is not entirely clear today, it may refer to parts of ***cerebellar hemisphere (Willis, 1664)*** between ***preculminate fissure (>1840)*** and ***horizontal cerebellar fissure (Malacarne, 1776)***; p. 108. See Larsell & Jansen (1972, Fig. 118) and *mons cerebelli (Gordon, 1815)*. However, also see Burdach (1822, p. 294).
25. *inferior lobe (Gordon, 1815)*
Apparently corresponds to macrodissected adult human ***ansiform lobule crus 2 (Bolk, 1906)*** and ***gracile lobule (>1840)*** considered together; p. 118, also see Burdach (1822, p. 295).
26. *quadrangular lobe (Meckel, 1817)*
Synonym for macrodissected adult human *quadrilateral lobe (Malacarne, 1776)*; in the original Latin, *lobus*

quadrangularis, p. 464. See Burdach (1822, p. 294), Larsell (1972, p. 43).

27. *inferior semilunar lobe (Meckel, 1817)*
Refers to macrodissected adult human *inferior posterior lobe (Malacarne, 1776)* and *gracile lobe (Malacarne, 1776)* considered together; see translation (1832, Vol. 2, p. 429).

28. *inferior posterior lobe (Burdach, 1822)*
Apparently corresponds to macrodissected adult human ***ansiform lobule crus 2 (Bolk, 1906)*** and ***gracile lobule (>1840)*** considered together; pp. 60, 295.

cerebellar nuclei (>1840)

As described for mammal with gross dissection, and with cellular architecture and connections, three incompletely separated ***gray matter regions (Swanson & Bota, 2010)*** buried within the ***arbor vitae (Winslow, 1733)*** except ventrally, where they approach the ***vestibular nuclei (>1840)***. The three commonly accepted parts, from medial to lateral, are the ***fastigial nucleus (>1840)***, the ***interposed nucleus (>1840)*** that may by subdivided in some species like human into a more medial ***emboliform nucleus (>1840)*** and a more lateral ***globose nucleus (>1840)***, and the ***dentate nucleus (>1840)***; see Nieuwenhuys et al. (pp. 200, 820 and Fig. 5.18). They were first identified generally by Willis; see ***[cerebellar nuclei (>1840)] (Willis, 1672)***.

EARLIER REFERENCES:

Illustrated, not named or described:

1. ***[cerebellar nuclei (>1840)] (Willis, 1672)***
Clearly illustrated without comment in macrodissected adult human; Table VIII, under *Z*.

cerebellar peduncles (Ridley, 1695)

As described in macrodissected adult human, and mammal generally with histological methods for ***axons (Kölliker, 1896)***, three ***central nervous system white matter tracts (>1840)*** extending from the ventral end of the ***arbor vitae (Winslow, 1733)*** as the rostrally directed ***superior cerebellar peduncle (Procháska, 1800)***, ventrally directed ***middle cerebellar peduncle (Rolando, 1819)***, and caudally directed ***inferior cerebellar peduncle (Günther, 1786)***; see Williams & Warwick (1980, pp. 915–918), Nieuwenhuys et al. (2008, Fig. 20.1). For Ridley's use in macrodissected adult human, see p. 135; also see *cerebellar peduncle (Willis, 1664)*. They were first referred to as the *round attachment (Vesalius, 1543a)* and *tracts connecting cerebellum with medulla (Vesalius, 1543a)*.

EARLIER REFERENCES:

Earlier synonyms:

1. *round attachment (Vesalius, 1543a)*
Vesalius described and illustrated in this way parts of macrodissected adult human ***cerebellar peduncles (Ridley, 1695)*** between ***cerebellum (Aristotle)*** dorsally and ***pons (Haller, 1747)*** and ***medulla (Winslow, 1733)*** ventrally; see Singer translation (1952, p. 27 and Figs. 10-*I,K*, 11-*G*).
2. *tracts connecting cerebellum with medulla (Vesalius, 1543a)*
Singer's translation (1952, p. 106) of passage describing macrodissected adult human *round attachment (Vesalius, 1543a)*.
3. *cerebellar peduncle (Willis, 1664)*
Willis introduced the term *cerebellar peduncle* for the three *white substance (Vesalius, 1543a)* extensions (anterior, middle, and posterior) relating ***cerebellum (Aristotle)*** to *oblong medulla (Willis, 1664)* in macrodissected adult human and other large mammals—the ***cerebellar peduncles (Ridley, 1695)*** together; see Pordage translation (1681, pp. 68, 113, Tab. VII-*Q,P,R*). Also see Meyer (1971, p. 12).
4. *cerebellar trunk (Willis, 1664)*
Synonym for *cerebellar peduncle (Willis, 1664)*; see Pordage translation (1681, p. 68).
5. *little foot of cerebellum (Willis, 1664)*
English form of Latin-based *cerebellar peduncle (Willis, 1664)*; see Pordage translation (1681, p. 110).
6. *cerebellar pedestal (Willis, 1664)*
Synonym for *cerebellar peduncle (Willis, 1664)*; see Pordage translation (1681, p. 110).
7. *hinder roots of oblongata medulla (Ridley, 1695)*
According to Ridley, term the ancients [16th century] used for ***cerebellar peduncles (Ridley, 1695)***; p. 135.
8. *cerebellar stalks (Ridley, 1695)*
Synonym for ***cerebellar peduncles (Ridley, 1695)***; p. 136.

LATER SYNONYMS:

1. *cerebellar roots (Lieutaud, 1742)*
Synonym for macrodissected adult human ***cerebellar peduncles (Ridley, 1695)***; in the original French, *racines du cervelet* (p. 398), in Latin, *radices cerebelli* (see Burdach, 1822, p. 288).
2. *cerebellar crura (Haller, 1747)*
Synonym for macrodissected adult human ***cerebellar peduncles (Ridley, 1695)***; in the original Latin, *crura cerebelli*, see Mihles translation (1754b, p. 295).
3. *crus cerebri posteriora (Tarin, 1750)*
Synonym for macrodissected adult human ***cerebellar peduncles (Ridley, 1695)***; Table I, Figure 4-S.
4. *small branches of oblong medulla (Tarin, 1753)*
Synonym for macrodissected adult human ***cerebellar peduncles (Ridley, 1695)***; in the original French, *les petites Branches de la moëlle allongée*, p. 25.
5. *crura minora medullae oblongatae (Haller, 1762)*
Synonym for macrodissected adult human *cerebellar crura (Haller, 1762)*; p. 72.
6. *cerebellar brachia (Malacarne, 1776)*
Synonym for macrodissected adult human ***cerebellar peduncles (Ridley, 1695)***; Article XII. For Latin form, *brachia cerebelli*, see Burdach (1822, pp. 42, 287).
7. *cerebellar processes (Günther, 1786)*
Synonym for macrodissected adult human ***cerebellar peduncles (Ridley, 1695)***; in the original Latin, *processus cerebelli*, p. 19.

8. *common trunk of cerebellar peduncle (Chaussier, 1807)*
Synonym for macrodissected adult human ***cerebellar peduncles (Ridley, 1695)***; in the original French, *tronc commun des pédoncules du cervelet*, p. 96.
9. *prolongations of cerebellum (Meckel, 1817)*
Synonym for macrodissected adult human ***cerebellar peduncles (Ridley, 1695)***; see translation (1832, Vol. 2, p. 434).
10. *medullary processes of cerebellum (Arnold, 1838a)*
Synonym for macrodissected adult human ***cerebellar peduncles (Ridley, 1695)***; in the original Latin, *processus medullares*, p. 33.

cerebellar tentorium (Winslow, 1733)

As described for macrodissected adult human, a reduplication of the inner meningeal layer of ***dura (Galen, c177)*** separating the ventral surface of the ***occipital region (Vesalius, 1543a)*** of the ***cerebral cortex (>1840)*** from the dorsal surface of the ***cerebellum (Aristotle)***. It lies within the outer or caudal part of the ***transverse cerebral fissure (>1840)*** and contains peripherally the right and left *transverse sinus*; see Millen & Woollam (1962, pp. 127–128, Figs. 87, 88). For Winslow's use in macrodissected adult human see Section X, p. 25. It was clearly described by Galen; see ***[cerebellar tentorium (Winslow, 1733)] (Galen, c173)***.

TRANSLATIONS:

1. *tent of cerebellum (Winslow, 1733)*
Original English form of ***cerebellar tentorium (Winslow, 1733)***; Section X, p. 25.
2. *tentorium cerebelli (Winslow, 1733)*
Latin form of ***cerebellar tentorium (Winslow, 1733)***; see *Terminologia Anatomica* (1998, p. 104).

EARLIER REFERENCES:

Described, not named or illustrated:

1. ***[cerebellar tentorium (Winslow, 1733)] (Galen, c173)***
Clearly described for macrodissected adult common large mammals but not human; see May translation (1968, p. 398).

Earlier synonyms:

1. *processus durae matris secundus (Vieussens, 1684)*
Synonym for macrodissected adult human ***cerebellar tentorium (Winslow, 1733)***; p. 14, see Burdach (1822, p. 319).
2. *processus durae matris posticus (Vieussens, 1684)*
Synonym for macrodissected adult human ***cerebellar tentorium (Winslow, 1733)***; p. 14, see Burdach (1822, p. 319).
3. *processus durae matris transversus (Slevogt, 1690)*
Synonym for macrodissected adult human ***cerebellar tentorium (Winslow, 1733)***; reprinted in Haller (1747–1751, Vol. 2, p. 820), see Burdach (1822, p. 319).
4. *falx transversalis (Ruysch, 1702)*
Synonym for macrodissected adult human ***cerebellar tentorium (Winslow, 1733)***; Vol. 2, p. 19, see Burdach (1822, p. 319).

LATER SYNONYMS:

1. *transverse septum (Winslow, 1733)*
Synonym for ***cerebellar tentorium (Winslow, 1733)***; Section X, pp. 26, 56.
2. *floor of cerebrum (Winslow, 1733)*
Synonym for ***cerebellar tentorium (Winslow, 1733)***; Section X, p. 25.
3. *diaphragm of brain (Winslow, 1733)*
Synonym for ***cerebellar tentorium (Winslow, 1733)***; Section X, p. 25.
4. *septum occipitale majus (Winslow, 1733)*
Synonym for ***cerebellar tentorium (Winslow, 1733)***; Section X, p. 26; English forms include *large occipital septum* and *great occipital septum*.
5. *processus transversus durae matris (Haller, 1762)*
Synonym for macrodissected adult human ***cerebellar tentorium (Winslow, 1733)***; Section X, p. 98.
6. *transverse cerebral septum (Günther, 1786)*
Synonym for macrodissected adult human ***cerebellar tentorium (Winslow, 1733)***; in the original Latin, *septum cerebri transversum*, p. 2.
7. *septum encephali (Soemmerring, 1791)*
Synonym for macrodissected adult human ***cerebellar tentorium (Winslow, 1733)***; p. 5.
8. *lateral process of dura mater (Fyfe, 1800)*
Synonym for macrodissected adult human ***cerebellar tentorium (Winslow, 1733)***; p. 12.
9. *tentorium (Bell, 1803b)*
Synonym for macrodissected adult human ***cerebellar tentorium (Winslow, 1733)***; p. 16.
10. *tentorium of cerebellum (Burdin, 1803)*
Synonym for macrodissected adult human ***cerebellar tentorium (Winslow, 1733)***; see translation (1803, Vol. 1, p. 153).

cerebellar vermis (Meckel, 1817)

As described for macrodissected adult mammal, the unpaired middle part of the ***cerebellar cortex (Willis, 1664)*** medial to the right and left ***cerebellar hemisphere (Willis, 1664)***; see Angevine et al. (1961, Fig. 24), Larsell & Jansen (1972, Fig. 118), Carpenter (1976, Figs. 2.25, 2.26, 14.1), Nieuwenhuys et al. (2008, Figs. 3.11, 3.13). For Meckel's use in macrodissected adult human, see translation (1832, Vol. 2, p. 430). Galen first described it as the *vermiform epiphysis (Galen, c173)*.

EARLIER REFERENCES:

Earlier synonyms:

1. *vermiform epiphysis (Galen, c173)*
In *On the Usefulness of the Parts* and *On Anatomical Procedures*, Galen described and basically named the ***cerebellar vermis (Meckel, 1817)***, which has a series of transverse folds, and thus resembles a worm that grows on wood; see May translation (1968, p. 419), *wormlike epifysis (Galen, c177)*, and *worm (Galen, c173)*. Galen dissected a variety of mammals including beef, pig, and/or macaque but not explicitly human. Vesalius (1543a) provided an excellent critique of earlier views on their function as well as illustrations; see Singer translation (1952, p. 70 and Figs.

8, 9, 11), Richardson & Carman translation (2009, pp. 208–210).

2. *worm (Galen, c173)*
   Synonym for *vermiform epiphysis (Galen, c173)*; see May translation (1968, p. 420), Singer translation (1999, p. 237). The term *worm* may also refer to ***choroid plexus of fourth ventricle (Vieussens, 1684)***, although this is doubtful; see Clarke & O'Malley (1996, p. 712), Singer (1999, p. 236). Geminus spelled it *worme* in English (1553, *The tables of the brayne*, Fig. 9-C).
3. *wormlike epifysis (Galen, c177)*
   Alternate form of *vermiform epiphysis (Galen, c173)*; see Wiberg translation (1914, p. 29).
4. *vermiform process (Galen, c177)*
   Translation Singer (1999, pp. 236–237) provided for *vermiform epiphysis (Galen, c173)*.
5. *vermiform excrescence (Galen, c177)*
   Translation Clarke & O'Malley (1996, p. 712) provided for *vermiform epiphysis (Galen, c173)*.
6. *grapes (Albertus Magnus, 13th century)*
   Albertus Magnus reported that some people refer to *vermiform epiphysis (Galen, c173)* by this name; see Kitchell & Resnick translation (1999, p. 248).
7. *uvae (Albertus Magnus, 13th century)*
   Latin form of *grapes (Albertus Magnus, 13th century)*; see Kitchell & Resnick translation (1999, p. 248).
8. *vermis (Galen, 1531)*
   Singer (1952, p. 81 note 69) pointed out that the specific Latin term *vermis*, for *worm (Galen, c173)* or ***cerebellar vermis (Meckel, 1817)***, was first used in Günther's 1531 translation of Galen's *De Anatomicis Administrationibus*, which was originally in Greek.
9. *silkworm (Vesalius, 1543a)*
   Synonym for *vermis (Galen, 1531)* of macrodissected adult human ***cerebellum (Aristotle)*** as appearing something like a silkworm chrysalis or even more a pupa; see Singer translation (1952, p. 70).
10. *middle part of cerebellum (Vesalius, 1543a)*
    Synonym for macrodissected adult human ***cerebellar vermis (Meckel, 1817)***; see Singer translation (1952, p. 26; Fig. 11, p. 107).
11. *scolicoides (Hall, 1565)*
    Synonym for macrodissected adult human ***cerebellar vermis (Meckel, 1817)***; p. 39. As Riolan (1657, p. 123) explained, "a certain portion of the Brain more firm than ordinary which represents the taile of a River-Crab when the shel is peeled off". Hall spelled it *scolecoeides*.
12. *cauda cerebelli (Molinetti, 1669)*
    Synonym for macrodissected adult human ***cerebellar vermis (Meckel, 1817)***; p. 89.
13. *vermiform eminence of cerebellum (Tarin, 1753)*
    Synonym for macrodissected adult human ***cerebellar vermis (Meckel, 1817)***; in the original French, *les eminences vermiculaires du cervelet*, and in the original Latin, *eminentiae vermiculares cerebelli*, p. 25. Like Galen, Tarin recognized anterior and posterior ends.
14. *raphe (Malacarne, 1776)*
    Synonym for macrodissected adult human ***cerebellar vermis (Meckel, 1817)***; p. 18, see Burdach (1822, p. 292).
15. *intermediate lobe (Mayer, 1779)*
    Synonym for macrodissected adult human ***cerebellar vermis (Meckel, 1817)***; in the original Latin, *lobus intermedius*, p. 18.
16. *minor cerebellar lobes (Günther, 1786)*
    Synonym for macrodissected adult human ***cerebellar vermis (Meckel, 1817)***; in the original Latin, *lobi minori (duo) cerebelli*, p. 17.
17. *middle protuberance of cerebellum (Chaussier, 1807)*
    Synonym for macrodissected adult human ***cerebellar vermis (Meckel, 1817)***; in the original French, *protubérance médiane du cervelet*, p. 83. Burdach (1822, p. 292) gave the Latin, *protuberantia media*.
18. *general commissure of cerebellum (Reil, 1807–1808a)*
    Synonym for macrodissected adult human ***cerebellar vermis (Meckel, 1817)***; in the original German, *Totalcommissur des kleinen Hirns*, p. 8. See Mayo translation for English form (1822, p. 20). Reil referred to depression between *general commissure of cerebellum (Reil, 1807–1808a)* and *cerebellar hemisphere (Willis, 1664)* as *isthmus* on right and left (Mayo, 1822, Tab. III, Fig. III-*b*).
19. *primitive part of cerebellum (Gall & Spurzheim, 1810)*
    Synonym for macrodissected adult human ***cerebellar vermis (Meckel, 1817)***; in the original Latin, *pars primitiva cerebelli*, p. 252. See Gordon (1817, p. 47).
20. *fundamental part of cerebellum (Gall & Spurzheim, 1810)*
    Synonym for macrodissected adult human ***cerebellar vermis (Meckel, 1817)***; in the original Latin, *pars fundamentalis cerebelli*, p. 252.
21. *corpus vermiforme (Bell & Bell, 1816)*
    Synonym for macrodissected adult human ***cerebellar vermis (Meckel, 1817)***; Vol. 2, p. 436.
22. *central part of cerebellum (Meckel, 1817)*
    Synonym for macrodissected adult human ***cerebellar vermis (Meckel, 1817)***; see translation (1832, Vol. 2, p. 430).
23. *median lobe of cerebellum (Serres, 1824–1826)*
    Synonym for macrodissected adult vertebrate ***cerebellar vermis (Meckel, 1817)***; in the original French, *lobe médian du cervelet*; see Figure 99-2, Figure 140-B,C, Figure 269-2. Cruveilhier (1836, p. 620) attributed without citation the term to Malacarne.

PARTLY CORRESPONDS:

1. *anterior end of worm (Galen, c173)*
   Corresponds roughly to macrodissected adult *inferior vermis (>1840)* in beef, pig, and/or macaque but not human; see May translation (1962, pp. 419–420), Clarke & O'Malley (1996, p. 712), Singer translation (1999, pp. 236–237). Also see *vermiform epiphysis (Galen, c173)*.
2. *posterior end of worm (Galen, c173)*
   Corresponds roughly to macrodissected adult *superior vermis (>1840)* in beef, pig, and/or macaque but not

human; see May translation (1968, pp. 419–420), Clarke & O'Malley (1996, p. 712), Singer translation (1999, pp. 236–237). Also see *vermiform epiphysis (Galen, c173)*.

3. *anterior worm (Massa, 1536)*
Vague reference to macrodissected adult human *inferior vermis (>1840)*; see Lind translation (1975, p. 239).
4. *superior worm (Massa, 1536)*
Vague reference to macrodissected adult human *superior vermis (>1840)*; see Lind translation (1975, p. 239).
5. *superior vermis (Massa, 1536)*
Latinized form of *superior worm (Massa, 1536)*, foreshadowing more precise *superior vermis (>1840)*.
6. *posterior worm (Massa, 1536)*
Vague reference to macrodissected adult human *superior vermis (>1840)*; see Lind translation (1975, p. 239).
7. *front part of middle part of cerebellum (Vesalius, 1543a)*
Roughly synonymous with macrodissected adult human *superior vermis (>1840)*; see Singer translation (1952, Fig. 11-*D*, p. 107).
8. *hind part of middle part of cerebellum (Vesalius, 1543a)*
Roughly synonymous with macrodissected adult human *inferior vermis (>1840)*; see Singer translation (1952, Figs. 9-*E* on p. 105, 11-*d* on p. 107).
9. *posterior vermiform process (Vieussens, 1684)*
Roughly synonymous with macrodissected adult human *superior vermis (>1840)*; in the original Latin, *processus vermiformis posterior*, see Soemmerring (1778, p. 173).
10. *anterior vermiform process (Vieussens, 1684)*
Roughly synonymous with macrodissected adult human *inferior vermis (>1840)*; in the original Latin, *processus vermiformis anterior*, pp. 65, 74. See Burdach (1822, p. 293).
11. *anterior vermicular eminences of cerebellum (Palfijn, 1726)*
Roughly synonymous with macrodissected adult human *inferior vermis (>1840)*; in the original French, *éminences vermiculaires anterieures du cervelet*, Part 2, pp. 28, 34.
12. *superior vermiform appendix (Winslow, 1733)*
Roughly synonymous with macrodissected adult human *superior vermis (>1840)*; Section X, p. 39.
13. *anterior vermiform appendix (Winslow, 1733)*
Roughly synonymous with macrodissected adult human *inferior vermis (>1840)*; Section X, p. 39.
14. *inferior vermiform appendix (Winslow, 1733)*
Roughly synonymous with macrodissected adult human *inferior vermis (>1840)*; Section X, p. 39.
15. *posterior vermiform appendix (Winslow, 1733)*
Roughly synonymous with macrodissected adult human *superior vermis (>1840)*; Section X, p. 39.
16. *superior process of vermis (Haller, 1762)*
Roughly synonymous with macrodissected adult human *superior vermis (>1840)*; in the original Latin, *processus superior vermis*, p. 71.
17. *inferior process of vermis (Haller, 1762)*
Roughly synonymous with macrodissected adult human *inferior vermis (>1840)*; in the original Latin, *processus inferior vermis*, p. 71.
18. *sutures of cerebellum (Malacarne, 1776)*
Roughly synonymous with macrodissected adult human *superior vermis (>1840)*; see Clarke & O'Malley (1996, p. 644).
19. *curvatura perpendicularis communis (Malacarne, 1776)*
Roughly synonymous with macrodissected adult human *inferior vermis (>1840)*, or at least its surface; p. 18. See Vicq d'Azyr (1786, Pl. XXVIII, Fig. 1-*15*).
20. *mammillary eminence of inferior vermis (Vicq d'Azyr, 1784)*
Macrodissected adult human ***nodule (Reil, 1807–1808a)*** and ***uvula (Malacarne, 1776)*** considered together; in the original French, *l'eminence mammillaire du vermis inferior*, p. 573. Also see Vicq d'Azyr (1786, Pl. XXX, Fig. 2-*12,13*) and Gordon (1815, p. 115).
21. *échancrure perpendiculaire posterieure moyenne (Vicq d'Azyr, 1786)*
French form of macrodissected adult human *curvatura perpencucularis communis (Malacarne, 1776)*; Plate XXVIII, Figure 1-*15*.
22. *inferior intermediate cerebellar lobule (Mayer, 1794)*
Synonym for macrodissected adult human *inferior process of vermis (Haller, 1762)*; in the original Latin, *lobulus intermedius cerebelli inferior*; Part 5, Table III, Figure 2-*P*.
23. *median protuberance of cerebellum (Burdin, 1803)*
Synonym for macrodissected adult human *superior vermis (>1840)*; see translation (1803, Vol. 1, p. 164).
24. *superior vermicular eminence (Burdin, 1803)*
Synonym for *median protuberance of cerebellum (Burdin, 1803)*; see translation (1803, Vol. 1, p. 164).
25. *median lobule (Burdin, 1803)*
Synonym for macrodissected adult human *inferior vermicular eminence of cerebellum (Burdin, 1803)*; see translation (1803, Vol. 1, p. 165).
26. *inferior vermicular eminence of cerebellum (Burdin, 1803)*
Synonym for macrodissected adult human *inferior process of vermis (Haller, 1762)*; see translation (1803, Vol. 1, p. 165).
27. *superior worm of cerebellum (Chaussier, 1807)*
Synonym for macrodissected adult human *superior process of vermis (Haller, 1762)*; in the original French, *ver supérieur du cervelet*, p. 83.
28. *inferior worm of cerebellum (Chaussier, 1807)*
Synonym for macrodissected adult human *inferior process of vermis (Haller, 1762)*; in the original French, *ver inférieur du cervelet*, p. 84.
29. *hinter oder beutelförminger Ausschnitt (Reil, 1807–1808a)*
German form of macrodissected adult human *curvatura perpendicularis communis (Malacarne, 1776)*; p. 8, see Burdach (1822, p. 293).
30. *superior vermiform process (Reil, 1807–1808a)*
Synonym for macrodissected adult human *superior vermis (>1840)*; see Mayo translation (1822, p. 20).
31. *single commissure of cerebellum (Reil, 1807–1808a)*
Synonym for macrodissected adult human *monticulus cerebelli (Meckel, 1817)*; see Mayo translation (1822, p. 23).
32. *inferior vermiform process (Reil, 1807–1808a)*

Synonym for macrodissected adult human *inferior vermis (>1840)*; see Mayo translation (1822, p. 20).

33. *semilunar fossa (Gordon, 1815)*
Macrodissected adult human transverse depression at anterior part of *superior vermis (>1840)*; p. 108, see definition in Foster (1892, p. 1635).
34. *mons cerebelli (Gordon, 1815)*
Synonym for macrodissected adult human *monticulus cerebelli (Meckel, 1817)*; p. 108, see Burdach (1822, p. 294). Also see *single commissure of cerebellum (Reil, 1807–1808a)*.
35. *monticulus cerebelli (Meckel, 1817)*
General region of macrodissected adult human ***culmen (Henle, 1871)*** and ***declive (>1840)*** considered together; p. 469 and translation (1832, pp. 430–431). Also see Burdach (1822, p. 294), Larsell & Jansen (1972, p. 42). First recognized as *single commissure of cerebellum (Reil, 1807–1808a)*.
36. *anterior vermiform process proper (Meckel, 1817)*
Basically, macrodissected adult human ***lingula (Malacarne, 1776)*** and ***central lobule (Burdach, 1822)*** considered together; see translation (1832, Vol. 2, p. 431).
37. *superior cerebellar vermis (Tiedemann, 1821)*
Synonym for macrodissected adult lion *superior vermis (>1840)*; in the original Latin, *vermis cerebelli superior*, Table III, Figure 6-*b*.
38. *inferior cerebellar vermis (Tiedemann, 1821)*
Synonym for macrodissected adult lion *inferior vermis (>1840)*; in the original Latin, *vermis cerebelli inferior*, Table III, Figure 6-*f*.
39. *superior cerebellar commissure (Tiedemann, 1821)*
Synonym for *superior cerebellar vermis (Tiedemann, 1821)*; in the original Latin, *commissura cerebelli superior*, see Table V, Figure 1-*g*.
40. *culmen (Burdach, 1822)*
Synonym for macrodissected adult human *monticulus cerebelli (Meckel, 1817)*; in the original German, *Gipfel des Bergs*, pp. 58, 294.
41. *posterior lobule of median lobe of cerebellum (Serres, 1824–1826)*
Macrodissected adult horse segment of ***cerebellar vermis (Burdach, 1822)*** interposed between *median lobule of median lobe of cerebellum (Serres, 1824–1826)* and *anterior lobule of median lobe of cerebellum (Serres, 1824–1826)*; in the original French, *lobule postérieur du lobe médian du cervelet*, Plate XV, Figure 274-C.
42. *median lobule of median lobe of cerebellum (Serres, 1824–1826)*
Roughly synonymous with macrodissected adult horse *median lobule (Burdin, 1803)*; in the original French, *lobule médian du lobe médian du cervelet*, Plate XV, Figure 274-*B*.
43. *anterior lobule of median lobe of cerebellum (Serres, 1824–1826)*
Macrodissected adult horse segment of ***cerebellar vermis (Burdach, 1822)*** superior (dorsal) to *posterior lobule of median lobe of cerebellum (Serres, 1824–1826)* and roughly synonymous with *superior vermiform process (Reil, 1807–1808a)*; in the original French, *lobule antérieur du lobe médian du cervelet*, Plate XV, Figure 274-*E*.
44. *laminated pyramid (Cruveilhier, 1836)*
Synonym for macrodissected adult human *inferior vermis (>1840)* attributed without citation to Malacarne; in the original French, *pyramide lamineuse*, p. 620.
45. *inferior vermis (>1840)*
According to Williams & Warwick (1980, p. 912), macrodissected adult human ***tuber vermis (>1840)***, ***pyramis (Malacarne, 1776)***, ***uvula (Malacarne, 1776)***, and ***nodule (Reil, 1807–1808a)*** of ***cerebellar vermis (Burdach, 1822)***, considered together. Separated from ***superior vermal regions (>1840)*** by ***horizontal cerebellar fissure (Malacarne, 1776)***.
46. *superior vermis (>1840)*
According to Williams & Warwick (1980, p. 912), macrodissected adult human ***lingula (Malacarne, 1776)***, ***central lobule (Burdach, 1822)***, ***culmen (Henle, 1871)***, ***declive (>1840)***, and ***folium vermis (>1840)*** of ***cerebellar vermis (Burdach, 1822)***, considered together. Separated from ***inferior vermal regions (>1840)*** by ***horizontal cerebellar fissure (Malacarne, 1776)***.

cerebellopontine angle (>1840)

As described for macrodissected adult human, the outer surface at the intersection of the ***pons (Haller, 1747)***, ***medulla (Winslow, 1733)***, and ***cerebellum (Aristotle)***, characterized as the site where the ***intermediofacial nerve (Strong & Elwyn, 1943)*** and ***vestibulocochlear nerve (>1840)*** emerge; see Carpenter (1976, p. 41 and Fig. 11.19), *Terminologia Anatomica* (1998, p. 112). It lies just dorsal to the ***medullopontine sulcus (>1840)***. It was not distinguished as such by 1840.

EARLIER REFERENCES:

Earlier synonyms:

1. *cerebellopontine trigone (>1840)*
Synonym for macrodissected adult human ***cerebellopontine angle (>1840)***; see *Nomina Anatomica* (1983, p. A66).

cerebellum (Aristotle)

The dorsal topographic division of the vertebrate ***hindbrain (Baer, 1837)*** connected to the ventral division—the ***pons (Haller, 1747)***—by the ***middle cerebellar peduncle (Rolando, 1819)***; see Swanson & Bota (2010). Mainly in *The Account of Animals* and *On the Parts of Animals*, Aristotle provided the first description with any detail of ***nervous system (Monro, 1783)*** structure; Ogle (1958, 652a 25 ff.), Thompson (1962, 494b 25 ff.), Clarke & O'Malley (1996, pp. 7 ff.). It included a distinction between *large brain (Aristotle)* rostrally in the cranium and *small brain (Aristotle)*, the *parencephalon (Aristotle)* or ***cerebellum (Aristotle)***, caudally in the cranium; Thompson (1962, 494b 30). It is unclear whether Aristotle included all or part of the ***brainstem (Schwalbe, 1881)*** in his definition of the ***cerebellum (Aristotle)***. In one passage he wrote that two of the three sets of ducts from the eye go to the ***cerebellum (Aristotle)***, see Thompson translation (1962 495a 10), but in another he wrote that the sense organs have no continuity with the ***brain (Smith Papyrus, c1700 BC)***; see Ogle translation (1958, 652b 5). Although the identity of the two pairs of ducts to the "cerebellum" is not entirely clear, the middle-sized pair is said to cross, and may refer to the *optic nerves (Galen, c173)*; Polyak (1957, p. 75). Thus, the first passage vaguely suggests that Aristotle's "cerebellum" included the ***brainstem (Schwalbe, 1881)***—because the ***optic chiasm (Galen, c173)*** attaches to the base of its rostral segment, the ***interbrain (Baer, 1837)***; for comparison, see ***cerebellum (Galen, c173)***. Aristotle based his statements on dissection of many animal species, but not on human material. Herophilus (335–280 BC) first observed the ***cerebellum (Aristotle)*** in macrodissected adult human; see von Staden (1989). Berengario da Carpi (1522) clearly used ***cerebellum (Aristotle)*** in the modern sense, stating that the ***fourth ventricle (Galen, c192)*** lies between the ***cerebellum (Aristotle)*** and the *large brain (Aristotle)*; see Lind translation (1959, p. 144). Vesalius first clearly distinguished between the *gray substance (Vesalius, 1543a)* and *white substance (Vesalius, 1543a)*, or ***cerebellar cortex (Willis, 1664)*** and ***arbor vitae (Winslow, 1733)***, of the ***cerebellum (Aristotle)***; see ***[central nervous system gray matter regions (>1840] (Vesalius, 1543a)***. For *lobes* in general, see ***cerebellar hemisphere (Willis, 1664)***.

TRANSLATIONS:

1. *parencephalis (Aristotle)*
   Aristotle's original Greek term for ***cerebellum (Aristotle)***; see Longrigg (1993, p. 212), Clarke & O'Malley (1996, pp. 629–630). Its literal translation is "beside the encephalon" (see May translation, 1968, p. 414 note 64).
2. *parenkephalis (Aristotle)*
   Alternate form of *parencephalis (Aristotle)*.
3. *parencephalon (Aristotle)*
   Alternate form of *parencephalis (Aristotle)*.
4. *epencranis (Erasistratus, c310–c250 BC)*
   According to Galen, this term for ***cerebellum (Aristotle)*** was from Erasistratus, who also first recorded that its structure is more complex than the *large brain (Aristotle)*, essentially the ***cerebrum (Obersteiner & Hill, 1900)***; see May translation (1968, p. 414). Also spelled *epenkranis*.
5. *encranis (Galen, c173)*
   In *On the Usefulness of the Parts*, Galen noted that some men refer to the *parencephalis (Aristotle)*, the ***cerebellum (Aristotle)***, as *encranis* or *encranion (Galen, c173)*. He also wrote that Herophilus used the terms *encephalon* and *parencephalon* for the *anterior brain (Aristotle)* and *posterior brain (Aristotle)*, respectively, because the anterior part had already [by Aristotle] appropriated the name of the whole (encephalon); see May translation (1968, p. 414), von Staden (1989, p. 197), Clarke & O'Malley (1996, p. 630). Also spelled *enkranis*.
6. *encranion (Galen, c173)*
   Alternate form of *encranis (Galen, c173)*. Also spelled *enkranion*.
7. *encranon (Galen, c173)*
   Alternate form of *encranion (Galen, c173)*; Clarke & O'Malley (1996, p. 630). Also spelled *enkranon*.
8. *encranium (Galen, c173)*
   In *On the Usefulness of the Parts*, Galen noted that some anatomists refer to the *parencephalis (Aristotle)*, the ***cerebellum (Aristotle)***, as the *encranium*; see May translation (1968, p. 398) and *encranis (Galen, c173)*. Also spelled *enkranium*.
9. *little brain (Geminus, 1553)*
   English form of ***cerebellum (Aristotle)***, actually spelled *lytle brayne*; see *The table of the figure of synowes*. Hall (1565, p. 36) spelled it *lyttle brayne*.
10. *lesser brain (Geminus, 1553)*
    Synonym for macrodissected adult human *little brain (Geminus, 1553)*; originally spelled *lesser brayne*, see *The tables of the brayne*, Figure 7.
11. *petty brain (Riolan, 1657)*
    English form of ***cerebellum (Aristotle)*** in Culpeper's version of Riolan; p. 119.
12. *brainlet (Bartholin, 1662)*
    English form of ***cerebellum (Aristotle)*** in Culpeper's version of Bartholin; pp. 133, 138.
13. *cerebel (Willis, 1664)*
    English form of ***cerebellum (Aristotle)***; see Pordage translation (1681, p. 57 ff.). Willis (1664, pp. 76–77) noted it has a very similar appearance in humans and other mammals, birds, and fish.

LATER SYNONYMS:

1. *posterior brain (Aristotle)*
   Synonym for ***cerebellum (Aristotle)***; see Thompson translation (1962, 494b 30), also see Ogle translation (1958, 652a 25 ff.), Thompson translation (1962, 494b 25 ff.), Clarke & O'Malley (1996, pp. 7 ff.). Galen (c173) adopted Aristotle's distinction; see May translation (1968, p. 417), von Staden (1989, p. 197), Clarke & O'Malley (1996, p. 630), and *cerebellum (Galen, c173)*. Burdach (1822, p. 287) noted that Mondino (1316) referred to the ***cerebellum (Aristotle)***, in Latin, as the *pars posterior cerebri*.
2. *posterior part of brain (Aristotle)*
   Alternate form of *posterior brain (Aristotle)*.
3. *small brain (Aristotle)*
   Synonym for *posterior brain (Aristotle)*; see Thompson translation (1962, 494b 30), also see Ogle translation (1958, 652a 25 ff.), Thompson translation (1962, 494b 25 ff.), Clarke & O'Malley (1996, pp. 7 ff.). Thus, Soemmerring (1778, p. 41) listed the Latin, *cerebrum parvum*, as a synonym for ***cerebellum (Aristotle)***.
4. *back part of brain (Galen, c177)*
   Posterior brain (Aristotle) in Galen's *On Anatomical Procedures* has also been translated as *back part of brain*; see Singer (1999, pp. 227, 229) and *cerebellum (Galen, c173)*.
5. *hind brain (Galen, c192)*
   Posterior brain (Aristotle) in Galen's *On Anatomical Procedures* has also been translated *hind brain* and

hind-brain; see Duckworth (1962, p. 18) and *cerebellum (Galen, c173)*. It was spelled *hynder brayne* in English by Geminus (1553, see *The tables of the brayne*, Fig. 9-*B,C,D*).

6. *occipital brain (Galen, c192)*
   Synonym for ***cerebellum (Aristotle)***; see Duckworth translation (1962, p. 18) and *cerebellum (Galen, c173)*.
7. *poop of brain (Zerbi, 1502)*
   Synonym for macrodissected adult human ***cerebellum (Aristotle)***; in the original Latin, *puppis cerebri*, f. 115. Also see Burdach (1822, p. 287) and *poop (Constantine the African, c1017–1087)*.
8. *hinder cell of brain (Geminus, 1553)*
   Synonym for macrodissected adult human ***cerebellum (Aristotle)***; original spelling was *hynder celle of brayne*, see *The table of the figures of sinowes*, 7th Figure part *D*.
9. *paregeophalida (Bartisch, 1583)*
   Bartisch stated it is the term for ***cerebellum (Aristotle)*** in Greek; see Blanchard (1996, p. 5).
10. *after-brain (Crooke, 1615)*
   Synonym for macrodissected adult human ***cerebellum (Aristotle)*** in Crooke's translation of Bauhin (1605, p. 575), "The forepart [of the ***brain (Smith Papyrus, c1700 BC)***, "Braine"] because it is the greater and most principall (for in it the Animall spirites are especially laboured) retaineth the name of the whole, and is properly called *Cerebrum* or [Greek]. The hinder part is much lesser, and is called by a diminutive word, *Cerebellum* we call it the After-braine." (p. 456). In Latin, Bauhin used anterior and posterior for forepart and hinder part, respectively.
11. *back-ward brain (Crooke, 1615)*
   Synonym for macrodissected adult human ***cerebellum (Aristotle)***; p. 432, see *back part of brain (Galen, c177)*.
12. *appendix of cerebrum (Soemmerring, 1778)*
   Listed as synonym for ***cerebellum (Aristotle)***; in the original Latin, *appendix ad cerebrum*, p. 61.
13. *unpaired spinal marrow ganglion (Carus, 1814)*
   Synonym for macrodissected vertebrate ***cerebellum (Aristotle)***; e.g., Table 2-ε.
14. *triangular leaflet (Solly, 1836)*
   Synonym for macrodissected adult fish (Whiting, Cod) ***cerebellum (Aristotle)***; p. 75.
15. *third cerebral mass (Anderson, 1837)*
   Synonym for macrodissected vertebrate ***cerebellum (Aristotle)***; pp. 16, 20.

PARTLY CORRESPONDS:

1. *superior surface of cerebellum (Malacarne, 1776)*
   For macrodissected adult human, Malacarne defined a *superior surface of cerebellum* and an *inferior surface of cerebellum (Malacarne, 1776)*, separated or distinguished by the *horizontal cerebellar fissure (Malacarne, 1776)*; p. 18, see translation in Clarke & O'Malley (1996, p. 643). This terminology was adopted by the *Basel Nomina Anatomica* (His, 1895, pp. 82, 83).
2. *inferior surface of cerebellum (Malacarne, 1776)*
   For macrodissected adult human, Malacarne defined an *inferior surface of cerebellum* and a *superior surface of cerebellum (Malacarne, 1776)*, separated or distinguished by the *horizontal cerebellar fissure (Malacarne, 1776)*; p. 18, see translation in Clarke & O'Malley (1996, p. 643). This terminology was adopted by the *Basel Nomina Anatomica* (His, 1895, pp. 82, 83). Vicq d'Azyr (1784, p. 567) distinguished two regions of the inferior surface.
3. *posterior surface of cerebellum (Vicq d'Azyr, 1784)*
   Synonym for macrodissected adult human *superior surface of cerebellum (Malacarne, 1776)*. Vicq d'Azyr referred to a single posterior surface and right and left anterior surfaces; pp. 568, 570.
4. *occipital surface of cerebellum (Vicq d'Azyr, 1784)*
   Synonym for macrodissected adult human *superior surface of cerebellum (Malacarne, 1776)*; pp. 568, 570.
5. *anterior surface of cerebellum (Vicq d'Azyr, 1784)*
   Synonym for macrodissected adult human *inferior surface of cerebellum (Malacarne, 1776)*. Vicq d'Azyr referred to a single posterior surface and right and left anterior surfaces; pp. 568, 570.
6. *temporal surface of cerebellum (Vicq d'Azyr, 1784)*
   Synonym for macrodissected adult human *inferior surface of cerebellum (Malacarne, 1776)*; p. 570.
7. *cone of cerebellum (Ramsay, 1813)*
   Apparently synonymous with macrodissected adult human *superior surface of cerebellum (Malacarne, 1776)*; p. 44. It was distinguished from the *inferior lobes of cerebellum (Ramsay, 1813)*.
8. *inferior lobes of cerebellum (Ramsay, 1813)*
   Apparently synonymous with macrodissected adult human *inferior surface of cerebellum (Malacarne, 1776)*; it was distinguished from the *cone of cerebellum (Ramsay, 1813)*; p. 44 (note 1).
9. *body of cerebellum (Meckel, 1817)*
   Meckel divided macrodissected adult human ***cerebellum (Aristotle)*** into arms or *crura (Haller, 1747)* and *body*, with the latter having right and left *lateral parts of cerebellum (Meckel, 1817)* and a *central part of cerebellum (Meckel, 1817)*; see translation (1832, Vol. 2, p. 427). He preferred *lateral part* to *cerebellar hemisphere (Willis, 1664)*, which he considered inaccurate, and central part to *vermis (Galen, 1531)*. Arnold (1838a, p. 33) gave the Latin, *corpus*. It is a standard term in *Nomina Anatomica* (1983, p. A67) and *Terminologia Anatomica* (1998, p. 118).
10. *corpus cerebelli (Meckel, 1817)*
   Latin form of *body of cerebellum (Meckel, 1817)*.

cerebral aqueduct (>1840)

The narrow passage between ***third ventricle (Galen, c173)*** and ***fourth ventricle (Galen, c192)***; see His (1895, p. 83), Millen & Woollam (1962, pp. 47–51). It was clearly distinguished by Vesalius; see *hind passage of third ventricle (Vesalius, 1543a)*.

TRANSLATIONS:

1. *aqueductus cerebri (>1840)*
   Latin form of ***cerebral aqueduct (>1840)***, see His (1895, p. 83).

EARLIER REFERENCES:

Earlier synonyms:

1. *hind passage of third ventricle (Vesalius, 1543a)*
Synonym for macrodissected adult human ***cerebral aqueduct (>1840)***; Singer translation (1952, p. 36). Later (1555), to clarify things, Vesalius wrote that it is "an important part of the third ventricle itself", as opposed to a part of the ***fourth ventricle (Galen, c192)***; Singer translation (1952, p. 36). That it corresponds to ***cerebral aqueduct (>1840)***—a channel *through* the ***tectum (Baer, 1837)***—is illustrated unambiguously in Figures 7, 8, and 10 of Book 7 (Singer translation, 1952, p. 52 and Figs. 7-*K*, 8-*K*, and 10), and its dissection by a longitudinal cut through the ***tectum (Baer, 1837)*** is described (Singer translation, 1952, pp. 68–69, 102). Also see *passage or canal extending from middle to posterior ventricle (Galen, c173, c177)*.
2. *posterior channel of third ventricle (Vesalius, 1543a)*
Alternate form of *hind passage of third ventricle (Vesalius, 1543a)*; see Richardson & Carman translation (2009, p. 196).
3. *passage from third to fourth ventricle (Vesalius, 1543a)*
Synonym for *hind passage of third ventricle (Vesalius, 1543a)*; see Singer translation (1952, p. 102). Burdach (1822, p. 377) quoted Vesalius as using the Latin term *meatus ex tertio ventriculo in quartum ventriculum pertinens* (1543a, p. 546).
4. *channel stretching from third to fourth ventricle (Vesalius, 1543a)*
Alternate form of *posterior channel of third ventricle (Vesalius, 1543a)*; see Richardson & Carman translation (2009, p. 141).
5. *aqueduct (Aranzi, 1587)*
Synonym for macrodissected adult human ***cerebral aqueduct (>1840)***; p. 549, see Clarke & O'Malley (1996, p. 721).
6. *posterior hole of third ventricle (Bauhin, 1605)*
Synonym for macrodissected adult human ***cerebral aqueduct (>1840)***; pp. 594–595, as translated by Crooke (1615, pp. 462–465).
7. *great hole of third ventricle (Bauhin, 1605)*
Synonym for macrodissected adult human ***cerebral aqueduct (>1840)***; pp. 594–595, as translated by Crooke (1615, pp. 462–465).
8. *canal connecting posterior ventricle with third ventricle (Spiegel, 1627)*
Synonym for macrodissected adult human ***cerebral aqueduct (>1840)***; p. 318, see Burdach (1822, p. 377), who provided the Latin form, *canalis, qui posteriorem ventriculum cum tertio conjungit.*
9. *chink (Bartholin, 1662)*
Synonym for macrodissected adult human ***cerebral aqueduct (>1840)***; p. 138 and Table V-*G*.
10. *anus (Bartholin, 1662)*
Synonym for macrodissected adult human ***cerebral aqueduct (>1840)***; p. 141.
11. *canal (Le Böe, 1663)*
Synonym for macrodissected adult human ***cerebral aqueduct (>1840)***; p. 49, see Burdach (1822, p. 377) and Schulte & Endtz (1977, p. 9).
12. *narrow den (Willis, 1664)*
Synonym for macrodissected adult mammalian ***cerebral aqueduct (>1840)***; see Pordage translation (1681, p. 107). Willis indicated that some consider it part of ***fourth ventricle (Galen, c192)***, others a passageway leading into it; see Pordage translation (1681, p. 65).
13. *straight den (Willis, 1664)*
Synonym for macrodissected adult human ***cerebral aqueduct (>1840)***; see Pordage translation (1681, p. 123).
14. *ventricle lying under orbicular protuberances (Willis, 1664)*
Synonym for macrodissected adult human ***cerebral aqueduct (>1840)***; see Pordage translation (1681, Figs. III-*N*, IV-*G*), also see Burdach (1822, p. 377). *Orbicular protuberances (Willis, 1664)* refers to ***tectum (Baer, 1837)***.
15. *fourth ventricle (Willis, 1664)*
Willis noted that some anatomists (mistakenly) refer to ***cerebral aqueduct (>1840)*** as *fourth ventricle*; see Pordage translation (1681, p. 107); also see Burdach (1822, p. 377).
16. *aqua emissarium (Vieussens, 1684)*
Synonym for macrodissected adult human ***cerebral aqueduct (>1840)***; p. 143, Table XI-*I*.
17. *Sylvius's aqueduct (Heister, 1721)*
Eponym for macrodissected adult human ***cerebral aqueduct (>1840)***; p. 203. Franz de Le Boë (Franciscus Sylvius in Latin) in 1663 used essentially the same description as Aranzi; see Baker (1909, p. 224), Millen & Woollam (1962, pp. 16–18), and *hind passage of third ventricle (Vesalius, 1543a)*.

12. *middle canal (Winslow, 1733)*
Synonym for macrodissected adult human ***cerebral aqueduct (>1840)***; Section X, p. 37.

18. *common canal (Winslow, 1733)*
Synonym for macrodissected adult human ***cerebral aqueduct (>1840)***; Section X, p. 40.
19. *canal of quadrigeminal eminences (Günz, 1750)*
Synonym for macrodissected adult human ***cerebral aqueduct (>1840)***; in the original Latin, *canalis eminentiae quadrigeminae*, p. 11, according to Schreger (1803, p. 321).
20. *incile (Haller, 1762)*
Synonym for macrodissected adult human ***cerebral aqueduct (>1840)***; p. 66.
21. *alveus Sylvii (Haller, 1762)*
Eponym for macrodissected adult human ***cerebral aqueduct (>1840)***; p. 68, see Schreger (1803, p. 321).
22. *iter ad quartum ventriculum (Monro, 1783)*
Synonym for macrodissected adult human ***cerebral aqueduct (>1840)***; Table II-*b*.
23. *iter à tertium ad quartum ventriculum (Monro, 1783)*

Synonym for macrodissected adult human ***cerebral aqueduct (>1840)***; Table VI-*I*.

24. *canal of quadrigeminal tubercles (Vicq d'Azyr, 1786)*
Synonym for macrodissected adult human ***cerebral aqueduct (>1840)***; p. 92. Meckel (1817; see translation, 1832, Vol. 2, p. 461) used the Latin form *canalis eminentiae quadrigeminae*, whereas Burdach (1822, p. 377) used *canalis tuberculorum quadrigeminorum*.

25. *intermediate canal of ventricles (Burdin, 1803)*
Synonym for macrodissected adult human ***cerebral aqueduct (>1840)***; see translation (1803, Vol. 1, p. 163).

26. *canalis sub corporibus quadrigeminis (Wenzel & Wenzel, 1812)*
Apparently a variation (Tab. X, Fig. 4) on, or synonym for, *ventricle lying under orbicular protuberances (Willis, 1664)*; they described four grooves in ***cerebral aqueduct (>1840)***, dorsal and ventral median, and right and left lateral (pp. 166–167), see Meckel (1817; and translation, 1832, Vol. 2, p. 461).

27. *middle cerebral canal (Tiedemann, 1821)*
Synonym for macrodissected adult lion ***cerebral aqueduct (>1840)***; in the original Latin, *canalis cerebri medius*, Table III, Figure 4-*l*.

28. *water pipe (Burdach, 1822)*
Synonym for macrodissected adult human ***cerebral aqueduct (>1840)***; in the original German, *Wasserleitung*, p. 159.

29. *ventricle of Sylvius (Müller, 1834)*
Eponym for ***cerebral aqueduct (>1840)*** in embryonic bird; see translation (1838, p. 810).

30. *aqueduct of quadrigeminal tubercles (Cruveilhier, 1836)*
Synonym for macrodissected adult human ***cerebral aqueduct (>1840)***; in the original French, *aqueduc des tubercules quadrijumeaux*, p. 685.

PARTLY CORRESPONDS:

1. *passage or canal extending from middle to posterior ventricle (Galen, c173, c177)*
Galen clearly described a connection between ***third ventricle (Galen, c173)*** and ***fourth ventricle (Galen, c192)***; see May translation (1968, pp. 416–423), Singer translation (1999, pp. 236–237). However, it is not likely that it corresponds to ***cerebral aqueduct (>1840)***, although some critics believe it does; see Woollam (1958, p. 17), Millen & Woollam (1962, Fig. 4), Clarke & O'Malley (1996, p. 712), Singer (1999, p. 236), Rocca (2003, p. 151 ff.). The best evidence that it does correspond to ***cerebral aqueduct (>1840)*** are two similar statements in *On Anatomical Procedures*, "One [duct] leads back to the cerebellum. If through this you introduce a probe you will find that it ends in the ventricle behind." (see Woollam, 1957, p. 17; for the similar quote, see Duckworth, 1962, pp. 1–2). However, other scholars including Wiberg (1914, pp. 98–101), Millen & Woollam (1962, p. 16), and May (1968, pp. 420–423) argue rather convincingly that Galen was actually describing a larger passage—between ***tectum (Baer, 1837)*** ventrally, and ***cerebellar vermis (Meckel, 1817)*** dorsally—whose floor is dorsal surface of ***tectum (Baer, 1837)*** and whose roof is ***arachnoid (Blasius, 1666)*** membrane, a region that would be much easier to see macroscopically and pass probes through. This interpretation has been questioned because of Galen's statements in *On the Usefulness of the Parts* that ***pineal gland (Galen, c192)*** is not part of and lies outside ***brain (Smith Papyrus, c1700 BC)***—and thus cannot regulate flow of pneuma from ***third ventricle (Galen, c173)*** to ***fourth ventricle (Galen, c192)***; Vesalius (1543a) as translated in Singer (1952, p. 45), May (1968, p. 419). However, in ox (which Galen dissected) the ***pineal gland (Galen, c192)*** is oriented essentially vertically, away from Galen's passage and dorsal surface of ***tectum (Baer, 1837)***; see Millen and Woollam (1962, Fig. 4). Historically, the interpretation that his passage lies between ***tectum (Baer, 1837)*** and ***cerebellum (Aristotle)*** seems to have been widely adopted: for example, by Haly Abbas (Wiberg, 1914, p. 86), Constantine the African (Manzoni, 1998, pp. 122–123), Albertus Magnus (Kitchell & Resnick, 1999, p. 249), Mondino (Singer, 1925, pp. 92–93), and Jacques Dubois (Jacobus Sylvius), Vesalius's teacher in Paris (Millen & Woollam, 1962, p. 160). Vesalius did describe a passage through substance of ***brain (Smith Papyrus, c1700 BC)*** (Singer translation,1952, pp. 36–37), and could not understand Galen's description of this general region, especially how ***cerebellar vermis (Meckel, 1817)*** could regulate opening of passage into ***fourth ventricle (Galen, c192)*** (Singer translation,1952, pp. 48–50; Meyer, 1971, p. 7 note 3), although there is a fairly clear description in later books of *On Anatomical Procedures* (Duckworth translation, 1962, p. 1), which was not available to Vesalius. Also see ***pineal recess (>1840)***.

2. *plumula (Arnold, 1838a)*
For macrodissected adult human, Arnold described angled striations in dorsal walls of ***cerebral aqueduct (>1840)***; p. 62, also see Arnold (1838b, Tab. IV, Fig. 2-*u*).

3. *pectunculi (Arnold, 1838a)*
For macrodissected adult human, Arnold described angled striations in lateral walls of ***cerebral aqueduct (>1840)***; p. 62, also see Arnold (1838b, Tab. IV, Fig. 2-*v*).

cerebral cortex (>1840)

The dorsal topographic division of the vertebrate ***endbrain (Kuhlenbeck, 1927)*** with a basically radial, laminated architecture; the ventral topographic division is the ***cerebral nuclei (Swanson, 2000a)***. The ***cerebral cortex (>1840)*** is divided into superficial ***cerebral cortex gray matter (>1840)*** and deep ***cerebral cortex white matter (>1840)***. See Swanson & Bota (2010) for these definitions, and Swanson (2004, Tab. B) for complete list of component ***gray matter regions (Swanson & Bota, 1010)*** in rat. The feature was recognized essentially as synonymous with *cerebral hemisphere (Willis, 1664)* by Herrick (1910, p. 491), "...the division of the cerebral hemisphere of Amphibia (and of higher animals) into dorsal or pallial [***cerebral cortex (>1840)***] and basal or subpallial [***cerebral nuclei (Swanson, 2000a)***] parts is primary and has its morphological basis in the configuration of the primitive neural tube antecedent to the evagination of the hemispheres [***endbrain (Kuhlenbeck, 1927)*** or ***cerebrum (Obersteiner & Hill, 1900)***]."

EARLIER REFERENCES:

Earlier synonyms:

1. *cerebral hemisphere (Willis, 1664)*
Synonym for macrodissected adult human ***cerebral cortex (>1840)***. Willis was the first to write that the *cerebrum (Willis, 1664)* is divided into two *hemispheres*; see Pordage translation (1681, pp. 60, 61, 91, Tab. I-*A*), also see Burdach (1822, p. 382), Meyer (1971, p. 122). His definition of *cerebrum (Willis, 1664)* included two *cerebral hemispheres (Willis, 1664)*—the right and left ***cerebral cortex (>1840)***—and the right and left ***lateral ventricle (Vesalius, 1543a)***, all four considered together. Willis (1664) also referred to anterior and posterior *cerebral lobes (Willis, 1664)* of the *cerebral hemisphere (Willis, 1664)*; see Pordage translation (1681, p. 91 and Fig. I-*A*). They are divided by the middle cerebral artery, so the *anterior cerebral lobe (Willis, 1664)* corresponds roughly to the ***frontal region (Haller, 1754)***, and his *posterior cerebral lobe (Willis, 1664)* corresponds roughly to the ***temporal region (>1840)***, ***parietal region (>1840)***, and ***occipital region (Vesalius, 1543a)*** considered together. As stated succinctly by Cheselden (1713, p. 134), the cerebrum's "upper side is divided into Two Hemispheres, and its lower side into Four Lobes, Two called anterior and Two posterior, which latter are much the largest." Also see *cerebral prominences (Varoli, 1573)*. Burdach (1822, pp. 382–386) gave a detailed history of early ideas about the composition of the *cerebral hemisphere (Willis, 1664)*.
2. *hemisphere (Willis, 1664)*
Synonym for *cerebral hemisphere (Willis, 1664)*; see Pordage translation (1681, pp. 60, 61).
3. *great lobe of brain (Winslow, 1733)*
Synonym for macrodissected adult human *cerebral hemisphere (Willis, 1664)*; Section X, pp. 25, 36.
4. *brain hemisphere (Tarin, 1753)*
Synonym listed for macrodissected adult human *cerebral hemisphere (Willis, 1664)*; in the original French (plural), *les Hémispheres du cerveau*, p. 22.
5. *quarter of oblong sphere of brain (Tarin, 1753)*
Synonym listed for macrodissected adult human *cerebral hemisphere (Willis, 1664)*; in the original French (plural), *les quarts de sphere oblongus du cerveau*, p. 22.
6. *cerebrum (Ramsay, 1813)*
In referring to macrodissected adult human, Ramsay wrote, "The cerebrum is composed of the two superior hemispheres, corpus callosum, and the inferior lobes." (p. 62). It is probably roughly synonymous with ***cerebral cortex (>1840)*** or *covering organs (Burdach, 1822)*.
7. *covering organs (Burdach, 1822)*
Apparently synonym for ***cerebral cortex (>1840)***; in the original German, *Belegungsorgane*, p. 12 ff. Also see Meyer (1971, p. 128 note 10). This term appears to be similar to *cerebrum (Ramsay, 1813)*.
8. *first cerebral mass (Anderson, 1837)*
Apparently synonymous with ***cerebral cortex (>1840)*** for vertebrates; pp. 16, 17 and p. 19, where Anderson wrote that it partly covers the ***corpus striatum (Willis, 1664)*** in the human embryo during the middle of the third month.
9. *lateral lobes of cerebrum (Gerdy, 1838)*
Apparently roughly synonymous with macrodissected adult human *cerebral hemispheres (Willis, 1664)*; in the original French, *lobes latéraux*, pp. 258–259.
10. *cerebral lobes (Gerdy, 1838)*
Synonym for *lateral lobes of cerebrum (Gerdy, 1838)*; in the original French, *lobes cérébraux*, p. 260.

PARTLY CORRESPONDS:

1. *organ of smell (Hippocrates)*
Vague reference to *outgrowth of brain to nose (Galen, c173)* in *Places in Man*; see Potter (1995, pp. 21–23), "The nature [structure and function] of the body is the beginning point of medical reasoning. Now first, the meningeal membrane is perforated at the point through which we hear, for the emptiness all around the ear only hears sounds and shouts, whereas what goes through the membrane into the brain is perceived distinctly. This is the only perforation through the membrane that covers the brain. In the region of the nostrils there is no perforation, but a kind of porousness, like a sponge [cribriform plate]; for this reason a person hears over a greater distance than he is able to smell, since odours are thoroughly broken up on their way to the organ of smell." Spelled *organes of smellynge* by Hall (1565, p. 45); also see Bauhin (1605, p. 870) and Crooke's translation (1615, p. 617).
2. *paired outgrowths from brain (Galen, c173)*
In *On the Usefulness of the Parts*, Galen described them as extending toward the nostrils, along with the ***[olfactory ventricle (>1840)] (Galen, c173)***, and attributed the sense of smell to them. He thought odors go through the cribriform plate, to the outgrowths, now called the right and left ***olfactory bulb (Weitbrecht, 1751)*** and ***olfactory peduncle (Solly, 1836)*** considered together. He did not regard the paired outgrowths as ***nerves (Herophilus, c335–c280 BC)***, but rather as "processes" of the ***brain (Smith Papyrus, c1700 BC)*** itself; the *optic nerves (Galen, c173)* were numbered the *first pair of nerves from brain (Galen c173)* because they exit the cranium; see May translation (1968, pp. 391, 401, 540), Meyer (1971, p. 75). Thus, Galen did not identify the ***olfactory nerve (Winslow, 1733)*** proper.
3. *olfactory sense instrument (Galen, c173)*
Synonym for *paired outgrowths from brain (Galen, c173)*; see May translation (1968, p. 407). They were referred to in English as *instruments of smelling* by Geminus (1553, see *The table of the figure of synowes*).
4. *olfactory instrument (Galen, c173)*
Apparently, synonym for *paired outgrowths from brain (Galen, c173)*. In *On the Usefulness of the Parts*, Galen

wrote, "...in the lower parts of them [the two ***anterior horns of lateral ventricles Bell, 1803b)***] toward the nose are both the olfactory instrument and a conduit, so to speak, for the discharge of the residues." (see May translation, 1968, p. 413).

5. *outgrowth of brain to nose (Galen, c173)*
Synonym for *paired outgrowths from brain (Galen, c173)*; see May translation (1968, pp. 438–439).

6. *two long hook-like processes from brain (Galen, c192)*
Later description (in later chapters of *On Anatomical Procedures*) of *paired outgrowths from brain (Galen, c173)*; see Duckworth translation (1962, pp. 186, 195). Galen also wrote that they resemble hollow horns; see Duckworth (1962, p. 3).

7. *primum nervorum par (Theophilos Protospatharios, fl. 610–641)*
Theophilos Protospatharios referred to the *paired outgrowths from brain (Galen, c173)* as first *pair of nerves from brain (Theophilos Protospatharios (fl. 610–641)*; see 1540 edition, f. 40v; and Meyer (1971, p. 75). It was the first real break on this topic with Galen, who referred to them as *paired outgrowths from brain (Galen, c173)*.

8. *first pair of nerves (Theophilos Protospatharios, fl. 610–641)*
English form of *primum nervorum par (Theophilos Protospatharios, fl. 610–641)*.

9. *nipple (Haly Abbas or Ali ibn' ul-Abbas, d. 994)*
Fairly obvious reference (singular) to *paired outgrowths from brain (Galen, c173)* in *The Complete Book of Medical Art, called the Royal Book*; see Wiberg translation (1914, p. 32).

10. *nerve to caruncle of nose (Anatomia Magistri Nicolai physici, early 12th century)*
The work refers to macrodissected adult human "nerves", presumably the ***olfactory peduncles (Solly, 1836)***, to the caruncles of the nose, which are spongy and formed like paps, that is, the ***olfactory bulbs (Weitbrecht, 1751)***; see Corner translation (1927, p. 72). Pap is slang for nipple; see *nipple (Haly Abbas or Ali ibn' ul-Abbas, d. 994)*; also see *caruncle (Anatomia Magistri Nicolai physici, early 12th century)* and *pap (Anatomia Magistri Nicolai physici, early 12th century)*.

11. *olfactory projection from brain (William of Saliceto, 1275)*
Synonym for macrodissected adult human *outgrowth of brain to nose (Galen, c173)*; see Rosenman translation (1998, p. 184). William attributed other sensory functions of nose to branches of ***trigeminal nerve (Winslow, 1733)***; p. 184.

12. *carunculae (Mondino, 1316)*
Synonym for macrodissected adult human *paired outgrowths from brain (Galen, c173)*; see Singer (1925, p. 93), Singer & Rabin (1945, p. 32), Meyer (1971, p. 75), O'Malley & Saunders (1982, p. 342). Also spelled *carunculi*. In Latin, a *caruncula* is a small fleshy eminence.

13. *carunculae similes capitibus mammillarum (Mondino, 1316)*
Meyer (1971, p. 75; see Soemmerring, 1778, p. 71) cited this complete term for Mondino's reference to *carunculae (Mondino, 1316)*. Meyer (1971, p. 75) wrote that Arabian followers of Galen invented the term *addimenta cerebri mammillaria* for *paired outgrowths from brain (Galen, c173)*; he based this statement on Burdach (1822, p. 394) and neither author provided citations.

14. *mammillary processes (Guy de Chauliac, 1363)*
Synonym for macrodissected adult human *paired outgrowths from brain (Galen, c173)* in Guy de Chauliac's surgical manual, presumably referring to macrodissected adult human extensions serving olfaction; see Rosenman translation (2005, p. 147).

15. *third pair of nerves from brain (Benedetti, 1502)*
Synonym for *mammillary carunculae (Benedetti, 1502)*; see Lind translation (1975, pp. 117–118).

16. *mammillary carunculae (Benedetti, 1502)*
Obvious synonym for macrodissected adult human *carunculae similes capitibus mammillarum (Mondino, 1316)*; see Lind translation (1975, p. 118). *Mammillary* is also spelled *mamillary*. Benedetti idiosyncratically considered this to be the third of the *pairs of nerves arising from brain (Benedetti, 1502)*.

17. *tubercula papillaria (Benedetti, 1502)*
Synonym for *paired outgrowths from brain (Galen, c173)*; see Lind translation (1975, p. 118).

18. *tubercles (Benedetti, 1502)*
Synonym for *tubercula papillaria (Benedetti, 1502)*; see Lind translation (1975, p. 118).

19. *caruncular nerves (Leonardo da Vinci, c1504–1506)*
In describing one of his magnificent unpublished drawings of the base of the skull, Leonardo used this term based on *carunculae (Mondino, 1316)*, which in turn was based on *paired outgrowths from brain (Galen, c173)*; see O'Malley & Saunders (1982, p. 342).

20. *mamillares cerebri (Brunschwig, 1525)*
Synonym for macrodissected adult human *paired outgrowths from brain (Galen, c173)*; p. 9.

21. *processus cerebri ad nares (Günther, 1536)*
Günther's Latin synonym for *paired outgrowths from brain (Galen, c173)*; see Soemmerring (1778, p. 73), Vicq d'Azyr (1786, p. 48).

22. *olfactory organ (Vesalius, 1543a)*
Synonym for macrodissected adult human *paired outgrowths from brain (Galen, c173)*; see Singer (1952, p. 10)—also translated *organ of smell*; see Singer (1952, p. 108).

23. *olfactory lobe (Vesalius, 1543a)*
Synonym for macrodissected adult human *paired outgrowths from brain (Galen, c173)*; see Singer translation (1952, p. 56).

24. *papillary process (Vesalius, 1543a)*
Synonym for macrodissected adult human *paired outgrowths from brain (Galen, c173)*; see Richardson & Carman translation (2002, p. 181). Obviously a variation on *nipple (Haly Abbas or Ali ibn' ul-Abbas, d. 994)*.

25. *monticulus (Vesalius, 1555)*
Meaning is unclear from vague unillustrated description on p. 786 for macrodissected adult human; see Singer

translation (1952, p. 35). Vicq d'Azyr (1786, p. 50, Pl. XVII-14,19) claimed Vesalius used it for ***temporal pole (Broca, 1878a)*** of ***temporal region (>1840)***; Burdach indicated it referred to the *uncus (Vicq d'Azyr, 1786)*, which seems most likely; and Singer (1952, p. 35) equated it with ***thalamus (His, 1893a)***.

26. *hillock (Vesalius, 1555)*
English form of *monticulus (Vesalius, 1555)*, see Schiller (1967, p. 527).

27. *Hügel (Vesalius, 1555)*
German form of *monticulus (Vesalius, 1555)*, see Schiller (1967, p. 527).

28. *instrument of smelling (Geminus, 1553)*
Synonym for macrodissected adult human *organ of smell (Hippocrates)*; originally spelled *instrument of smellynge*, see *The tables of the brayne*, Figure 12-C.

29. *nervos olfactibiles (Hall, 1565)*
Hall wrote that some men (misguidedly) call *paired outgrowths from brain (Galen, c173)* "olfactory nerves" (p. 45)—and regard them as *third pair of nerves from brain (Benedetti, 1502)*.

30. *productiones procerae (Coiter, 1572)*
Without providing a citation, Burdach (1822, p. 394) claimed this was a term Coiter used for *olfactory organs (Vesalius, 1543a)*; see translation (1572, p. LXXVI, note *21*).

31. *ductus instrumenti olfactus (Varoli, 1573)*
Synonym for macrodissected adult human *paired outgrowths from brain (Galen, c173)*; see Soemmerring (1778, p. 73). Also see *ductus nervei olfactus (Varoli, 1573)*.

32. *ductus nervei olfactus (Varoli, 1573)*
Synonym for macrodissected adult human *paired outgrowths from brain (Galen, c173)*; see Soemmerring (1778, p. 73). Meyer (1971, p. 77) suggested the term refers in part to ***lateral olfactory tract (>1840)***, although Varoli claimed somehow to trace this feature back as far as ***pons (Haller, 1747)*** or ***medulla (Winslow 1733)***.

33. *nerves of smelling (Piccolomini, 1586)*
Synonym for macrodissected adult human *paired outgrowths from brain (Galen, c173)*; see Bauhin (1605, p. 645), Crooke (1615, p. 485). Piccolomini referred to them as *second pair of nerves from brain (Piccolomini, 1586)*; see Soemmerring (1778, p. 73).

34. *nervi odoratorii (Piccolomini, 1586)*
Original Latin form of *nerves of smelling (Piccolomini, 1586)*; see Bauhin (1605, p. 645).

35. *second pair of nerves from brain (Piccolomini, 1586)*
Synonym for *nerves of smelling (Piccolomini, 1586)*; p. 262.

36. *tubercula mammillarum papillis simillima (du Laurens, 1599)*
Synonym for macrodissected adult human *paired outgrowths from brain (Galen, c173)*; pp. 407–408; see Soemmerring (1778, p. 73). Crooke translated it as *the processes which are like to the nipples of a womans paps* (1615, p. 527).

37. *processus mammarum ritu protuberantes (du Laurens, 1599)*
Synonym for macrodissected adult human *paired outgrowths from brain (Galen, c173)*; see Soemmerring (1778, p. 73).

38. *cerebri processus anteriores (Bauhin, 1605)*
Synonym for macrodissected adult human *paired outgrowths from brain (Galen, c173)*; p. 690.

39. *vaccinae papillae (Casseri, 1609)*
Synonym for macrodissected adult human *paired outgrowths from brain (Galen, c173)*; see Figure 4-*I* and Meyer (1971, p. 75). Singular in Latin is *vaccinis papillis*; see Soemmerring (1778, p. 89).

40. *processus medullares (Casseri, 1609)*
Synonym for macrodissected adult human *paired outgrowths from brain (Galen, c173)*; see Soemmerring (1778, p. 74).

41. *anterior processes of brain (Crooke, 1615)*
English form of *cerebri processus anteriores (Bauhin, 1605)*.

42. *processuum mammillarium principia (Bauhin, 1620)*
Synonym for macrodissected adult human *paired outgrowths from brain (Galen, c173)*; see Soemmerring (1778, p. 74).

43. *portiones mammillares (Cortesi, 1625)*
Synonym for macrodissected adult human *paired outgrowths from brain (Galen, c173)*; Figure 3-*F* on p. 21; also see Soemmerring (1778, p. 74).

44. *eighth pair of nerves from brain (Spiegel, 1627)*
Synonym for macrodissected adult human *paired outgrowths from brain (Galen, c173)*; pp. 210, 329; Casseri (1627, Lib. VII-*8*, Lib. X, Tab. X-*F*), Vicq d'Azyr (1786, p. 48). In Latin, *octavum par cerebri*; see Soemmerring (1778, p. 74).

45. *cerebral sphere (Willis, 1664)*
Right and left *cerebral hemisphere (Willis, 1664)* considered together; see Pordage translation (1681, p. 61).

46. *mole (Willis, 1664)*
Willis wrote that the *cerebral hemisphere (Willis, 1664)* in birds and fish has this appearance; see Pordage translation (1681, pp. 76–77).

47. *mammillary process (Willis, 1672, Tab. VI)*
At times Willis was inconsistent and included *olfactory nerve (Bartholin, 1611)*, which corresponds to ***olfactory peduncle (Solly, 1836)***, with *mammillary process (Willis, 1664)* to constitute *paired outgrowth from brain (Galen, c173)*; for example, Pordage translation (1681, Tab. VI-*A*).

48. *halves of cerebrum (Diemerbroeck, 1672)*
Apparently, synonym for macrodissected adult human right and left *cerebral hemisphere (Willis, 1664)*, according to Burdach (1822, pp. 382–383).

49. *combinationem primam (Molinetti, 1675)*
Synonym for macrodissected adult human *paired outgrowths from brain (Galen, c173)*; p. 188; see Soemmerring (1778, p. 75).

50. *nervi mamillares (Molinetti, 1675)*
Synonym for macrodissected adult human *paired outgrowths from brain (Galen, c173)*; p. 188.

51. *corporum striatorum propaginis (Rau, 1720)*
Synonym for macrodissected adult *paired outgrowths from brain (Galen, c173)*; p. 108.

52. *head of hippocampus (Duvernoy, 1735)*
Probably corresponds roughly to macrodissected adult human *uncus (Vicq d'Azyr, 1786)*. Duvernoy first illustrated it, though fancifully; p. 134, and C in the Figure; also see Lewis (1923, p. 224). For detailed modern interpretation of this region see Duvernoy (1988, p. 31 ff.).
53. *mammelon (Morand, 1748)*
Vaguely refers to general region of macrodissected adult human *uncus (Vicq d'Azyr, 1786)*, p. 318; see Burdach (1822, p. 375).
54. *olfactory nerve (Soemmerring, 1778)*
Synonym for macrodissected adult human *paired outgrowths from brain (Galen, c173)*; p. 69 ff. In the original Latin, *nervo olfactorio* (p. 68), *nervus olfactorius* (p. 179).
55. *fimbria medullaria transparente (Malacarne, 1780)*
May refer to part or all of macrodissected adult human *longitudinal cords (Lancisi, 1713)*, see Burdach (1822, pp. 369–370); the ***cingulum (Burdach, 1822)***, also see Meyer (1971, p. 29); and the ***indusium griseum (Valentin, 1841)***, all considered together. See Malacarne (1780, Part II, p. 25).
56. *pes hippocampi (Malacarne, 1780)*
By "foot of the hippocampus" Malacarne meant ventral (anterior or rostral), largest end of macrodissected adult human *hippocampus (Aranzi, 1587)*, toward tip of ***inferior horn of lateral ventricle (Bell, 1802)*** and including *uncus (Vicq d'Azyr, 1786)*; Part II, p. 66, see Burdach (1822, p. 375).
57. *great toe of pes hippocampi (Malacarne,1780)*
Synonym, at least roughly, for macrodissected adult human *uncus (Vicq d'Azyr, 1786)*—the "great toe of the foot of the hippocampus" (p. 67). Also see Burdach (1822, p. 375), Meyer (1971, p. 22).
58. *great toe of foot of hippocampus (Malacarne, 1780)*
Full English form of *great toe of pes hippocampi (Malacarne, 1780)*.
59. *fifth toe of pes hippocampi (Malacarne, 1780)*
Synonym, at least roughly, for macrodissected adult human *uncus (Vicq d'Azyr, 1786)*—the "fifth toe of the foot of the hippocampus" (p. 67). Also see Burdach (1822, p. 375), Meyer (1971, p. 22).
60. *fifth toe of foot of hippocampus (Malacarne, 1780)*
Full English form of *fifth toe of pes hippocampi (Malacarne, 1780)*.
61. *inner toe of pes hippocampi (Malacarne, 1780)*
Synonym, at least roughly, for macrodissected adult human *uncus (Vicq d'Azyr, 1786)*—the "great toe of the foot of the hippocampus" (p. 67). Also see Burdach (1822, p. 375) and Meyer (1971, p. 22).
62. *inner toe of foot of hippocampus (Malacarne, 1780)*
Full English form of *inner toe of pes hippocampi (Malacarne, 1780)*.
63. *uncus (Vicq d'Azyr, 1786)*
Hook-shaped topographic division of macrodissected adult human ***cerebral cortex (>1840)*** including rostroventral parts of ***temporal region (>1840)*** and adjacent parts of ***olfactory region (>1840)***. The best modern account of *uncus* morphology, going back to Giacomini (1884) and Retzius (1896), is in Duvernoy (1988, p. 31 ff., Figs. 17, 18). There is an *anterior segment* with ***gyrus ambiens (>1840)*** or ***piriform area (>1840)*** and the ***gyrus semilunaris (>1840)*** or ***cortical amygdalar nucleus (>1840)***; and a *posterior segment* with *uncinate gyrus (>1840)*, which includes primarily parts of ***subiculum (>1840)*** and ***field CA1 (Lorente de Nó, 1934)***, *band of Giacomini (>1840)*, which is part of ***dentate gyrus (>1840)***, and *intralimbic gyrus (>1840)*, which is basically part of ***field CA3 (Lorente de Nó, 1934)***. *Uncus* is a Latin form of the French term *crochet* introduced by Vicq d'Azyr (1786, Pl. XVI-*14,15*). Burdach (1822, p. 158) probably introduced the Latin form; see Meyer (1971, p. 22). The German form of uncus (*Haken*) was introduced by Reil (1809b; see Meyer 1971, p. 22).
64. *ethmoidal nerve (Chaussier, 1807)*
Synonym for macrodissected adult human *paired outgrowths from brain (Galen, c173)*; p. 195 and Plate 2-*1*. Burdach (1822, p. 392) gave the Latin, *nervus ethmöidalis*.
65. *innern gespaltnen Hügel (Reil, 1812b)*
German synonym for macrodissected adult human *uncus (Vicq d'Azyr, 1786)*; p. 110, also see Burdach (1822, p. 375).
66. *inner lobule of middle lobe (Gordon, 1815)*
Synonym for macrodissected adult human *uncus (Vicq d'Azyr, 1786)*; pp. 85, 105. Also see Burdach (1822, pp. 375, 389).
67. *eminence (Meckel, 1817)*
Synonym for macrodissected adult human *eminence of inferior lobe (Burdach, 1822)*, according to Burdach (1822, p. 389); in the original German, *der Vorsprung*, p. 457.
68. *cornu ammonis (Burdach, 1822)*
Burdach gave a more precise definition, in this Latin form, for macrodissected adult human *Ammon's horn (Garengeot, 1728)*—to include ***alveus (Burdach, 1822)*** and its *taenia (Burdach, 1822)*, *fascia dentata (Döllinger, 1814)*, and *subiculum cornu ammonis (Burdach, 1822)*; pp. 154–158. He also provided a detailed history of the nomenclature; pp. 372–376.
69. *eminence of inferior lobe (Burdach, 1822)*
Probably synonymous with macrodissected adult human *uncus (Vicq d'Azyr, 1786)*; in the original German, *der Vorsprung*; pp. 174, 389 and Tables VII-*η*, VIII-*5*. Also see Nauta & Haymaker (1969, Fig. 4-*10*), Nieuwenhuys et al. (2008, Figs. 3.3,3.6), and *eminence (Meckel, 1817)*.
70. *prominentia lobus inferior (Burdach, 1822)*
Original Latin form of *eminence of inferior lobe (Burdach, 1822)*; p. 174.
71. *uncus of fornicate gyrus (Arnold, 1838a)*
Synonym for macrodissected adult human *uncus (Vicq d'Azyr, 1786)*; in the original Latin, *uncus gyri fornicati*, Table VII, Figure 3-*f*, see Meyer (1971, p. 22).

cerebral cortex gray matter (>1840)

As described in adult vertebrate, ***gray matter (Meckel, 1817)*** forming the superficial component of the ***cerebral***

cortex (>1840) and distinguished from the deep component, ***cerebral cortex white matter (>1840)***. The ***cerebral cortex gray matter (>1840)*** is further parceled into ***gray matter regions (Swanson & Bota, 2010)*** based on cellular architecture and connections. For these precise definitions, see Swanson & Bota (2010). It was first delineated in broad outline as the *cerebral lobe (Vesalius, 1543a)* by Vesalius, who also referred to the *cerebrum applied to frontal bone (Vesalius, 1543a)*—roughly the ***frontal region (Vicq d'Azyr, 1786)***. In the classical prehistology era dealing with the macrodissected adult human *cerebral lobe (Vesalius, 1543a)*, Varoli distinguished an *anterior cerebral prominence (Varoli, 1573)*, a *middle cerebral prominence (Varoli, 1573)* or *middle and inferior cerebral prominence (Varoli, 1573)*, and a *posterior cerebral prominence (Varoli, 1573)* lying under corresponding bones of the skull, a scheme basically followed by Bauhin (1605, Table XVII:*A-C*, p. 671) and Crooke (1615, Table XXIIII:*A-C*, p. 492). Winslow defined this parceling more carefully in relation to the ***lateral cerebral sulcus (>1840)*** and called them *anterior lobe of cerebrum (Winslow, 1733)*, *middle lobe of cerebrum (Winslow, 1733)*, and *posterior lobe of cerebrum (Winslow, 1733)*. In contrast, Willis (1664) preferred just *anterior cerebral lobe (Willis, 1664)* and *posterior cerebral lobe (Willis, 1664)*, separated by the trunk of the middle cerebral artery, a scheme followed by Haller (1747; see 1754a translation, p. 288). They were referred to, respectively, by Gibson as *fore lobe of brain (Gibson, 1682)* and *hinder lobe of brain (Gibson, 1682)*, and by Cowper as *foremost lobe of brain (Cowper, 1698)* and *hindmost lobe of brain (Cowper, 1698)*. At about the same time as Willis, Bartholin (1662, p. 134) chose rather to distinguish upper and lower parts of the *brain (Piccolomini, 1586, definition 2)* in relation to the ***lateral cerebral sulcus (>1840)***. In more modern approaches, Chaussier instead referred to *frontal cerebral lobule (Chaussier, 1807)*, *temporal cerebral lobule (Chaussier, 1807)*, *parietal cerebral lobule (Chaussier, 1807)*, and *occipital cerebral lobule (Chaussier, 1807)*, named for the bones overlying them (see Carpenter, 1976, p. 22); and Burdach recognized five major lobes in macrodissected adult human: *stem lobe (Burdach, 1822)* or ***insular region (Brodmann, 1909)***, *anterior lobe (Burdach, 1822)* or ***frontal region (Vicq d'Azyr, 1786)***, *superior lobe (Burdach, 1822)* or ***parietal region (>1840)***, *inferior lobe (Burdach, 1822)* or ***temporal region (>1840)***, and *posterior lobe (Burdach, 1822)* or ***occipital region (Vesalius, 1543a)***. Vicq d'Azyr (1784, p. 512) pointed out that the pattern of human *cerebral gyri (Vesalius, 1543a)* is much more variable than in other mammals, where it is also considerably more symmetrical; also see Wenzel & Wenzel (1811, p. 23). Based on cellular architecture rather than macrodissection, Brodmann (1909) used *regions* and *areas* rather than *lobes* and *gyri* because his terms applied to all mammals, whether gyrencephalic or lissencephalic, and even in humans cellular architecture does not necessarily respect cortical folding patterns.

EARLIER REFERENCES:

Earlier synonyms:

1. *cerebral lobe (Vesalius, 1543a)*
   Vesalius referred in macrodissected adult human to a right and a left *cerebral lobe (Vesalius, 1543a)* or *lobe of brain (Vesalius, 1543a)*; see Singer translation (1952, pp. 21, 27). From Figure 6 and its legend it is clear that ***cerebral cortex white matter (>1840)***, ***cerebral nuclei (Swanson, 2000a)***, ***thalamus (His, 1893a)***, and ***midbrain (Baer, 1837)*** are in the unpaired *base of cerebrum (Vesalius, 1543a)*; see Singer translation (1952, p. 100 and Fig. 7), Richardson & Carman translation (2009, p. 180). Thus, *cerebral lobe (Vesalius, 1543a)* corresponds to right or left ***cerebral cortex gray matter (>1840)***. As late as 1807, Chaussier (p. 36) used essentially the same term. Before Vesalius, Dryander (1536) briefly mentioned cerebral lobe but it is impossible to know what features he included in the term; see Lind translation (1975, p. 300, Fig. 4-C).
2. *lobe of brain (Vesalius, 1543a)*
   Alternate translation of *cerebral lobe (Vesalius, 1543a)*.
3. *partes cerebri divisae (Varoli, 1573)*
   Probably roughly synonymous with macrodissected adult human right and left *cerebral lobe (Vesalius, 1543a)*; f. 6, also see *base of brain (Varoli, 1573)* and Burdach (1822, p. 382).
4. *cerebral prominences (Varoli, 1573)*
   Varoli divided macrodissected adult human *cerebral lobe (Vesalius, 1543a)*, roughly ***cerebral cortex gray matter (>1840)***, into three *cerebral prominences* (in the original Latin, *cerebri prominentiae*) as viewed from base of ***brain (Smith Papyrus, c1700 BC)*** and related to adjacent cranial bones: anterior, middle, and posterior. *Anterior cerebral prominence (Varoli, 1573)* lies in anterior cranial fossa and corresponds roughly to ***frontal region (Vicq d'Azyr, 1786)***; *middle cerebral prominence (Varoli, 1573)* lies in middle cranial fossa and corresponds roughly to ***temporal region (>1840)***; and *posterior cerebral prominence (Varoli, 1573)* corresponds roughly to ***occipital region (Vesalius, 1543a)*** and most or all of ***parietal region (>1840)*** considered together. See Varoli (1573, pp. 5–6, and Fig. I on f. 17v), Meyer (1971, p. 122), Clarke & O'Malley (1996, p. 822), *base of brain (Varoli, 1573)*.
5. *cerebrum (Piccolomini, 1586)*
   Synonym for macrodissected adult human *cerebral lobe (Vesalius, 1543a)* and *cerebrum proper (Piccolomini, 1586)*. Piccolomini also alluded to "certain lines" in *cerebrum (Piccolomini, 1586)*, possibly first vague hints of ***cerebral cortex gray matter (>1840)*** lamination. "I call the cerebrum that whole ashen-colored body, darkening from white, which very closely encompasses the medulla. The medulla is the whole of the white and more solid body which is concealed within the ashen-colored one. Thus the cerebrum differs and is distinguished from the medulla by color, because the cerebrum

is ashen-colored but the medulla white; in consistency, because the cerebrum is softer and medulla a little harder and more compact; in location, because the medulla is in the middle of the cerebrum which wholly covers it over; also the ashen-colored body is distinguished from the white by certain lines. The cerebrum commences everywhere by convolutions and extends as far as the corpus callosum and that middle white part. The medulla commences at the corpus callosum and is, I say, that whole, internal, middle, and white body which is lengthened out and slips forth into the spine of the back. Not only are the cerebrum and its medulla distinguished and separated from one another by the above indications, but also by the efficiency of one's dissection. For occasionally, working with slow deliberation and dexterity, I have separated the cerebrum from the corpus callosum and the whole middle, white part called the medulla." (Clarke & O'Malley translation, 1996, pp. 387–388; also see Clark & Dewhurst, 1996, Fig. 88).

6. *brain (Piccolomini, 1586, definition 2)*
English form of *cerebrum (Piccolomini, 1586)*; see Crooke translation (1615, pp. 458–459, 475). Also see *brain proper (Piccolomini, 1586).*
7. *cerebrum proper (Piccolomini, 1586)*
Synonym for *cerebrum (Piccolomini, 1586)*; see Bauhin (1605, p. 580), Crooke (1615, pp. 431, 456 ff.).
8. *brain proper (Piccolomini, 1586)*
English form of *cerebrum proper (Piccolomini, 1586)*; see Crooke translation (1615, pp. 431, 456 ff.).
9. *corpus cineritium (Piccolomini, 1586)*
Synonym for *cerebrum (Piccolomini, 1586)*; p. 252, see Bauhin (1605, p. 580), Clarke & O'Malley translation (1996, p. 387).
10. *cerebrum cineritium (Piccolomini, 1586)*
Synonym for *corpus cineritium (Piccolomini, 1586)*; p. 252.
11. *cerebral cortex (Bauhin, 1605)*
Bauhin was first to use term "cortex" in referring to macrodissected adult human ***cerebral cortex gray matter (>1840)***; p. 580, see Meyer (1971, p. 121). Crooke (1615) translated Bauhin's passage, "The substance therefore of the Braine is by *Archangelus* [Piccolomini] divided into the Braine and the Marrow. The Braine he calleth that Ash-colored part which compasseth the rest, whereby he meaneth the marrow: we will say it may be divided into the Shell and the Kernell." (pp. 458–459). Also see *cerebrum (Piccolomini, 1586).*
12. *brain shell (Crooke, 1615)*
Synonym for macrodissected adult human *cerebral cortex (Bauhin, 1605)*; it was actually spelled *Braine Shel*, pp. 458–459.
13. *brain bark (Crooke, 1615)*
Synonym for macrodissected adult human *cerebral cortex (Bauhin, 1605)*; it was actually spelled *Braine Barke*; pp. 458–459.
14. *forepart of whole brain (Crooke, 1615)*
Synonym for macrodissected adult human *cerebrum (Piccolomini, 1586)* in Crooke's translation (p. 456) of Bauhin (1605, p. 575), "The forepart [of the whole brain, 'Braine'] because it is the greater and most principall (for in it the Animall spirites are especially laboured) retaineth the name of the whole, and is properly called *Cerebrum* or [Greek]. The hinder part is much lesser, and is called by a diminitive word, *Cerebellum* we call it the After-braine." In Latin, Bauhin used anterior and posterior for forepart and hinder part, respectively. Also see *whole brain (Aristotle).*
15. *brain prominences (Crooke, 1615)*
Synonym for macrodissected adult human *cerebral prominences (Varoli, 1573)*; p. 497.
16. *brain itself (Bartholin, 1662)*
Synonym for macrodissected adult human *cerebral cortex (Bauhin, 1605)* as distinguished from *whole brain (Aristotle)*; p. 133.
17. *brain strictly so called (Bartholin, 1662)*
Synonym for *brain itself (Bartholin, 1662)*; p. 133.
18. *brain properly so-called (Bartholin, 1662)*
Synonym for *brain itself (Bartholin, 1662)*; p. 135.
19. *brain proper (Bartholin, 1662)*
Shorter form of *brain properly so-called (Bartholin, 1662).*
20. *forepart of brain commonly so called (Bartholin, 1662)*
Synonym for macrodissected adult human *forepart of whole brain (Crooke, 1615)*; p. 137, see *brain properly so-called (Bartholin, 1662).*
21. *external part of brain (Bartholin, 1662)*
Synonym for *brain itself (Bartholin, 1662)*; also referred to as external *substance* of brain, which is ash colored or yellowish white—some think is due to presence of veins; p. 133.
22. *process of marrow (Bartholin, 1662)*
Synonym for *brain itself (Bartholin, 1662)*. Bartholin revived ancient idea of Praxagoras and Philotimus (according to Galen; see May translation, 1968, p. 417) that ***brain (Smith Papyrus, c1700 BC)*** is outgrowth of ***spinal cord (Galen, c162–c166)***; pp. 136–137. He strengthened the argument with the comparative observation that in fish *medullary substance (Colombo, 1559)* is prominent but *brain bark (Crooke, 1615)* is very small; p. 136. Compare with *process of brain (Coiter, 1572).*
23. *bark as it were (Bartholin, 1662)*
Synonym for *brain bark (Crooke, 1615)*; p. 133.
24. *rind (Bartholin, 1662)*
Synonym for *brain bark (Crooke, 1615)*; spelled in the archaic way, *rinde*, p. 135.
25. *cerebral lobes (Willis, 1664)*
Willis was first to apply the term *lobes* to localized regions of macrodissected adult human ***cerebral cortex gray matter (>1840)*** and *lobes* considered together constitute ***cerebral cortex gray matter (>1840)*** as a whole. He divided each *cerebral hemisphere (Willis,

1664) into two *cerebral lobes, anterior cerebral lobe (Willis, 1664)* and *posterior cerebral lobe (1664)*; see Pordage translation (1681, p. 91 and Fig. I-*A*). As stated succinctly by Cheselden (1713, p. 134), the cerebrum's "upper side is divided into Two Hemispheres, and its lower side into Four Lobes, Two called anterior and Two posterior, which latter are much the largest." It is unclear whether Willis understood *cerebral lobes* to consist just of ***cerebral cortex gray matter (>1840)***, or whether he also included ***cerebral cortex white matter (>1840)***; however, see *cerebral lobe (Vesalius, 1543a)* and *cerebral prominence (Varoli, 1573)*, which both restricted term to ***cerebral cortex gray matter (>1840)***.

26. *enkar (Salmon, 1714)*
According to Salmon, Greek term for *brain proper (Piccolomini, 1586)*; p. 392. For Latin form, *encar*, see Foster (1892, p. 1439).
27. *enkaros (Salmon, 1714)*
Another form of *enkar (Salmon, 1714)*; p. 392.
28. *cortical substance (Carus, 1814)*
Synonym for macrodissected developing and adult human ***cerebral cortex gray matter (>1840)***; in the original German, *Rindensubstanz*, p. 294.
29. *hemispherical ganglia (Solly, 1836)*
Synonym for macrodissected adult human ***cerebral cortex gray matter (>1840)***; p. 167.
30. *cortical layer of cerebral convolution (Baillarger, 1840)*
Synonym for macrodissected adult human ***cerebral cortex gray matter (>1840)***; see von Bonin translation (1960, p. 22). Baillarger recognized six layers, three white alternating with three gray; see p. 24.
31. *outer gray substance of brain (Baillarger, 1840)*
Synonym for macrodissected adult human ***cerebral cortex gray matter (>1840)***; see von Bonin translation (1960, pp. 22, 23).
32. *gray cortical substance of convolutions of brain (Baillarger, 1840)*
Synonym for macrodissected adult human ***cerebral cortex gray matter (>1840)***; see von Bonin translation (1960, p. 24).
33. *pallium (>1840)*
Synonym for ***cerebral cortex gray matter (>1840)***; see Nauta & Feirtag (1986, p. 45) and *pallium (Burdach, 1822)*.
34. *cortical mantle (>1840)*
Synonym for ***cerebral cortex gray matter (>1840)***; see Nauta & Feirtag (1986, p. 45) and *mantle (Rosenthal, 1815)*.

PARTLY CORRESPONDS:

1. *cerebral convolutions (Smith Papyrus, c1700 BC)*
Synonym for *cerebral gyri (Vesalius, 1543a)* as seen by surgeons in living humans after battle injury. Outer surface of ***brain (Smith Papyrus, c1700 BC)*** was said to be *convoluted*, like *corrugations* forming on molten copper—floating slag forming on molten copper and removed by coppersmith before pouring metal into mold; see Breasted translation (1930, pp. 65, 167–168, 173), also see Allen (2005, pp. 75–76).
2. *corrugations (Smith Papyrus, c1700 BC)*
Synonym for *cerebral convolutions (Smith Papyrus, c1700 BC)*; see Breasted translation (1930, pp. 65, 167–168, 173), also see Allen (2005, pp. 75–76).
3. *small intestines (Erasistratus, c310–c250 BC)*
Synonym for macrodissected adult human *cerebral gyri (Vesalius, 1543a)*. As quoted by Galen, Erasistratus described outer surface of ***brain (Smith Papyrus, c1700 BC)*** as being "similar to the jejunum [small intestine] and has many folds [or coils]." (De Lacy translation, 1980, p. 441). Soemmerring (1778, p. 31) listed the Latin form *intestinula*.
4. *folds (Erasistratus, c310-c250 BC, definition 1)*
Synonym for *small intestines (Erasistratus, c310–c250 BC)*; see De Lacy translation (1980, p. 441). Berengario da Carpi (1523) noted that many cerebral *folds (Erasistratus, c310–c250 BC)* are hidden and revealed by dissection; see Lind translation (1959, p. 142).
5. *varicosities (Rufus of Ephesus, fl. c90–c120)*
Synonym for macrodissected adult human *cerebral gyri (Vesalius, 1543a)*; see Clarke & O'Malley translation (1996, p. 13). Soemmerring (1778, p. 31) listed the Latin term *varicosam cerebri partem*.
6. *anfractus (Zerbi, 1502)*
Synonym for macrodissected adult human *cerebral gyri (Vesalius, 1543a)*; p. 113. See Huard & Imbault-Huart (1980, p. 178), Soemmerring (1778, p. 33), and *anfractuosity* in Foster (1894, p. 262).
7. *cerebral gyri (Vesalius, 1543a)*
Tortuous convolutions on surface of macrodissected adult human ***cerebral cortex gray matter (>1840)***, separated by ***cerebral sulci (Vesalius, 1543a)***; see Singer translation (1952, p. 24), *Nomina Anatomica* (2003, p. 124), *Dorland's* (2003, pp. 805–806). Vesalius noted "the brain of man presents nothing peculiar [in its structure] and such convolutions [*cerebral gyri (Vesalius, 1543a)*] appear also in brains of asses, horses, oxen, and other creatures which I have so far examined. Yet perhaps it may be claimed as distinctive [of man] that Nature has in him wrought the winding sulci deeper, that thereby the substance of his brain may be the richer." (Singer translation, 1952, p. 24). Burdach (1822, p. 258) attributed the term *cerebral gyri* to Willis (1664, Ch. 10, p. 49), although Vesalius used *gyrus*, in Latin. They were first identified as *cerebral convolutions (Smith Papyrus, c1700 BC)*. Richardson & Carman (2009, p. 188) listed the following Latin terms they translated in Vesalius (1543a) as "convolutions": *circumactus, revolutiones, anfractus, inflexus*, and *involutiones*.
8. *cerebral gyrus (Vesalius, 1543a)*
Singular of *cerebral gyri (Vesalius, 1543a)*.
9. *clouds (Vesalius, 1543a)*
Synonym for macrodissected adult human *cerebral gyri (Vesalius, 1543a)*; see Singer translation (1952, p. 24).
10. *windings (Vesalius, 1543a)*
Synonym for macrodissected adult human *cerebral gyri (Vesalius, 1543a)*; see Singer translation (1952, p. 92). In the original Latin, *involutiones, revolutiones, implexus* (p. 542 ff.); see Burdach (1822, p. 258), Meyer (1971, p. 123).

11. *bendings (Vesalius, 1543a)*
Synonym for macrodissected adult human *cerebral gyri (Vesalius, 1543a)*; see Singer translation (1952, p. 92).
12. *coils (Vesalius, 1543a)*
Synonym for macrodissected adult human *cerebral gyri (Vesalius, 1543a)*; see Richardson & Carman translation (2002, p. 179).
13. *involutiones (Vesalius, 1543a)*
Synonym for macrodissected adult human *cerebral gyri (Vesalius, 1543a)*; see Richardson & Carman translation (2002, p. 188).
14. *revolutiones (Vesalius, 1543a)*
Synonym for macrodissected adult human *cerebral gyri (Vesalius, 1543a)*; see Richardson & Carman translation (2002, p. 188).
15. *implexus (Vesalius, 1543a)*
Synonym for macrodissected adult human *cerebral gyri (Vesalius, 1543a)*; see Burdach (1822, p. 258), Meyer (1971, p. 123).
16. *inflexus (Vesalius, 1543a)*
Synonym for macrodissected adult human *cerebral gyri (Vesalius, 1543a)*; see Richardson & Carman translation (2002, p. 188).
17. *compassings (Geminus, 1553)*
Synonym for macrodissected adult human *cerebral gyri (Vesalius, 1543a)*; originally spelled *compassynges*, see *The tables of the brayne*, Figure 3.
18. *turnings (Geminus, 1553)*
Synonym for macrodissected adult human *cerebral gyri (Vesalius, 1543a)*; originally spelled *turnynges*, see *The tables of the brayne*, Figure 3.
19. *foldings together of brain (Geminus, 1553)*
Synonym for *folds (Erasistratus, c310–c250 BC)*; originally spelled *foldynges together of the brayne*, see *The tables of the brayne*, Figure 3.
20. *posterior cerebral prominence (Varoli, 1573)*
Macrodissected adult human zone of ***cerebral cortex gray matter (>1840)*** lying caudal to middle cranial fossa, corresponding roughly to ***occipital region (Vesalius, 1543a)***, along with much or all (indeterminate extent) of ***parietal region (>1840)***; pp. 5–6, and Figure I on f. 17v. See Meyer (1971, p. 122), Clarke & O'Malley (1996, p. 822).
21. *spirae (Piccolomini, 1586)*
Synonym for macrodissected adult human *cerebral gyri (Vesalius, 1543a)*; p. 247, see Huard & Imbault-Huart (1980, p. 178). Soemmerring (1778, p. 31) listed the Latin term *spiras*.
22. *varicose part of cerebrum (du Laurens, 1600)*
According to Bauhin (1605, p. 578), the shallower macrodissected adult human *cerebral gyri (Vesalius, 1543a)*; in the original Latin, *pars varicosa cerebri*, see Crooke translation (1615, p. 456).
23. *orbicular circumvolutions (Bauhin, 1605)*
Synonym for macrodissected adult human *cerebral gyri (Vesalius, 1543a)*; p. 575, see Crooke translation (1615, p. 456).
24. *breaches (Crooke, 1615)*
Synonym for macrodissected adult human *cerebral gyri (Vesalius, 1543a)*; p. 458 and Table IX, Figure 3-*CC*.
25. *backward prominence of brain (Crooke, 1615)*
Synonym for macrodissected adult human *posterior cerebral prominence (Varoli, 1573)*; pp. 497–498.
26. *hindpart of brain (Crooke, 1615)*
Synonym for macrodissected adult human *posterior cerebral prominence (Varoli, 1573)*; p. 497.
27. *posterior cerebral lobe (Willis, 1664)*
Corresponds roughly to macrodissected adult human ***temporal region (>1840)***, ***occipital region (Vesalius, 1543a)***, and ***parietal region (>1840)*** considered together; see Pordage translation (1681, p. 91, Tab. I-*A*). Also see Haller (1762, pp. 14–15), Meyer (1971, p. 122), *cerebral lobes (Willis, 1664)*. Willis wrote that *anterior cerebral lobe (Willis, 1664)* and *posterior cerebral lobe (Willis, 1664)* have basically the same function (memory), with duplication being a safety factor, "So the Brain, like a Castle, divided into many Towers or places of Defense, is thereby made the stronger and harder to be taken." (Willis, 1664; see Pordage translation, 1681, p. 91). As stated succinctly about *cerebrum (Piccolomini, 1586)* by Cheselden (1713, p. 134), "[its] upper side is divided into Two Hemispheres, and its lower side into Four Lobes, Two called anterior and Two posterior, which latter are much the largest."
28. *plicae (Willis, 1664)*
Synonym for macrodissected adult human *cerebral gyri (Vesalius, 1543a)*; see Meyer (1971, p. 123). Soemmerring (1778, p. 31) listed the Latin form, *plicaturas*.
29. *corpora vorticosa (Malpighi, 1665)*
Synonym for macrodissected adult human *cerebral gyri (Vesalius, 1543a)*; see Burdach (1822, p. 258).
30. *hinder lobe of brain (Gibson, 1682)*
Synonym for macrodissected adult human *posterior cerebral lobe (Willis, 1664)*; Table XII-*A*.
31. *gyres (Collins, 1685)*
Alternate spelling, in English, of *cerebral gyri (Vesalius, 1543a)*; p. 1070 and Table XLVII, Figure 1-*eee*.
32. *intestine flexures of brain (Collins, 1685)*
Synonym for *cerebral gyri (Vesalius, 1543a)*; p. 998, also see *small intestines (Erasistratus, c310–c250 BC)*.
33. *anfractuosity (Perrault, 1688)*
English form of *anfractus (Zerbi, 1502)*, for *cerebral gyrus (Vesalius, 1543a)*, used for gazelle or antelope (p. 59), cat-a-mountain [mountain lion?] (p. 65), sea-lion (p. 72), lynx (p. 79), beaver (p. 90), chamois or gemp [wild goat] (p. 144–145), and monkey (p. 162). Exactly what was meant by the term *anfractuosity (Perrault, 1688)*, gyri and/or sulci, is not clear.
34. *hindmost lobe of brain (Cowper, 1698)*
Roughly synonymous with macrodissected adult human *posterior cerebral lobe (Willis, 1664)*, especially as viewed from base of ***brain (Smith Papyrus, c1700 BC)***; Tables VII, Figure 1-*A* and IX, Figure 1-*B,D*.
35. *anterior lobe of cerebrum (Winslow, 1733)*
Winslow defined *anterior lobe of cerebrum (Winslow, 1733)*, *middle lobe of cerebrum (Winslow, 1733)*, and *posterior*

lobe of cerebrum (Winslow, 1733) of macrodissected adult human ***cerebral cortex gray matter (>1840)*** in relation to ***lateral cerebral sulcus (>1840)***, with the first two dorsal and ventral, respectively, to the sulcus; Section X, p. 33. Thus, *anterior lobe of cerebrum (Winslow, 1733)* corresponds roughly to ***frontal region (Vicq d'Azyr, 1786)***, along with rostral half or so of ***parietal region (>1840)***.

36. *posterior lobe of cerebrum (Winslow, 1733)*
Roughly, *posterior cerebral prominence (Varoli, 1573)* of macrodissected adult human, although Winslow defined it more precisely with reference to ***lateral cerebral sulcus (>1840)***, so it roughly corresponds to ***occipital region (Vesalius, 1543a)*** and caudal half or so of ***parietal region (>1840)***—the *anterior lobe of cerebrum (Winslow, 1733)* and *middle lobe of cerebrum (Winslow, 1733)* lie dorsal and ventral to the sulcus, respectively; Section X, pp. 32, 33.

37. *circumgyrationes (Soemmerring, 1778)*
Latin synonym listed for macrodissected adult human *cerebral gyri (Vesalius, 1543a)*; p. 31.

38. *sphaericas prominentias (Soemmerring, 1778)*
Latin synonym listed for macrodissected adult human *cerebral gyri (Vesalius, 1543a)*; p. 31.

39. *maeandros (Soemmerring, 1778)*
Latin synonym listed for macrodissected adult human *cerebral gyri (Vesalius, 1543a)*; p. 31.

40. *flexus (Soemmerring, 1778)*
Latin synonym listed for macrodissected adult human *cerebral gyri (Vesalius, 1543a)*; p. 31.

41. *intestinorum simulacra (Soemmerring, 1778)*
Latin synonym listed for macrodissected adult human *cerebral gyri (Vesalius, 1543a)*; p. 31.

42. *involutiones intestiniformes (Soemmerring, 1778)*
Latin synonym listed for macrodissected adult human *cerebral gyri (Vesalius, 1543a)*; p. 31.

43. *processus enteroideos (Soemmerring, 1778)*
Latin synonym listed for macrodissected adult human *cerebral gyri (Vesalius, 1543a)*; p. 31, following *intestines (Erasistratus, c310–c250 BC)*. Meyer (1971, p. 123) attributed the term to Malacarne (1780).

44. *enteroid processes (Soemmerring, 1778)*
English form of *processus enteroideos (Soemmerring, 1778)*, referring to *cerebral gyri (Vesalius, 1543a)* as "gut-like prominences" (see Schiller translation, 1965, p. 326)—following *intestines (Erasistratus, c310–c250 BC)*.

45. *sinuosos cerebri flexus (Soemmerring, 1778)*
Latin synonym listed for macrodissected adult human *cerebral gyri (Vesalius, 1543a)*; p. 31.

46. *parietal region (Vicq d'Azyr, 1786)*
Roughly synonymous with macrodissected adult human ***parietal region (>1840)*** and ***temporal region (>1840)*** considered together; Plate III-*o*.

47. *Wulst (Soemmerring, 1788)*
German synonym for macrodissected adult human *cerebral gyrus (Vesalius, 1543a)*, in particular for some found more internally like ***Ammon's horn (Vicq d'Azyr, 1784)***, the *gerollte Wulst (Soemmerring, 1788)*; see p. 81 and Meyer (1971, p. 123, who gave English translation, *bulge*). Also see Soemmerring (1800, p. 27) as discussed by Burdach (1822, p. 258).

48. *bulge (Soemmerring, 1788)*
English form of *Wulst (Soemmerring, 1788)*; see Meyer (1971, p. 123).

49. *mantle (Rosenthal, 1815)*
English form of German, *der Mantel*; pp. 11–15. It referred roughly to macrodissected adult human ***cerebral cortex gray matter (>1840)*** but did not include certain features like ***hippocampal region (Swanson et al., 1987)***; see *pallium (Burdach, 1822)*, *pallium (>1840)*. Rosenthal also used the German, *die Schaale* (p. 7), now spelled *Schale*.

50. *ridge of anterior lobe near longitudinal fissure (Gordon, 1815)*
Synonym, as far as can be determined from Gordon's rather vague description, for continuous zone of macrodissected adult human ***cerebral cortex gray matter (>1840)*** including (a) rostral end of ***cingulate region (>1840)***; that is, zone ventral to ***frontal region (Vicq d'Azyr, 1786)***; (b) adjacent zones of ***frontal region (Vicq d'Azyr, 1786)*** including ***medial frontal gyrus (>1840)*** and caudally adjacent *paracentral lobule (>1840)*; (c) ***straight gyrus (Valentin, 1841)***; and (d) laterally adjacent ***medial orbital gyrus (>1840)***. It was described on p. 85; for helpful recent illustrations see Williams & Warwick (1980, Figs. 7.114A and 7.116).

51. *pallium (Burdach, 1822)*
Burdach's Latin synonym for macrodissected adult human *mantle (Rosenthal, 1815)*; p. 13. He divided it into five *lobes*, unlike the 2–3 parts of most previous authors: *stem lobe (Burdach, 1822)* or ***insular region (Brodmann, 1909)***, *anterior lobe (Burdach, 1822)* or ***frontal region (Vicq d'Azyr, 1786)***, *superior lobe (Burdach, 1822)* or ***parietal region (>1840)***, *inferior lobe (Burdach, 1822)* or ***temporal region (>1840)***, and *posterior lobe (Burdach, 1822)* or ***occipital region (Vesalius, 1543a)***. He did not, however, include certain other parts like ***hippocampal region (Swanson et al., 1987)***, so it is not strictly synonymous with ***cerebral cortex gray matter (>1840)***. He traced the origin of the term *der Mantel* or *Schale*, to Rosenthal (1815), pp. 7, 8, 11, 16, 47. It was also used in this general sense for human embryo by, for example, Herrick (1915, Figs. 46–50 and p. 216), Ranson (1920, pp. 32–33), Strong & Elwyn (1943, p. 17, Fig. 13).

52. *meditullium palii (Burdach, 1822)*
Synonym for *pallium (Burdach, 1822)*; in the original German, *Marklager*, p. 13; also see Foster (1892, p. 2260).

53. *torus marginalis (Burdach, 1822)*
Synonym for macrodissected adult human *cerebral gyrus (Vesalius, 1543a)*; p. 13, see Foster (1894, p. 2943).

54. *Randwülst (Burdach, 1822)*
Original German form of *torus marginalis (Burdach, 1822)*; p. 13.

55. *marginal bulge (Burdach, 1822)*
Translation Meyer (1971, p. 123) gave for *torus marginalis (Burdach, 1822)*, or *Randwülst (Burdach, 1822)*.

56. *cingulate gyrus (Burdach, 1822)*

Roughly corresponds to macrodissected adult human ***cingulate region (>1840)*** and adjacent parts of ***frontal region (Vicq d'Azyr, 1786)*** considered together. Burdach divided it into central cingulate gyrus, peripheral cingulate gyrus, and middle cingulate gyrus; in German, *Randwülst der Zwinge*, p. 150. Also see Dejerine & Dejerine-Klumpke (1895, p. 296), Meyer (1971, pp. 111, 123).

57. *superior lobes (Burdach, 1822)*
Burdach used this term (p. 171) in describing right or left macrodissected adult human ***parietal region (>1840)*** together with rostrally adjacent "motor areas" of ***frontal region (Vicq d'Azyr, 1786)***, roughly including *area 4 (Brodmann, 1909)*, *area 6 (Brodmann, 1909)*, and *area 8 (Brodmann, 1909)*—that is, roughly the zone lateral and then dorsal to ***insular region (Brodmann, 1909)***. Furthermore, he divided *superior lobes* into *outer part*, roughly equivalent to ***cerebral cortex gray matter (>1840)*** associated with ***frontal operculum (>1840)*** and ***parietal operculum (>1840)***, and inner part dorsally; p. 171. Burdach gave the Latin form, *lobi superiores*, and the German form, *die Oberlappen*.

58. *processes of longitudinal striae of Reil (Rolando, 1831)*
Apparently, macrodissected adult human medial zone of ***frontal region (Vicq d'Azyr, 1786)*** and ***parietal region (>1840)*** considered together, dorsal to ***cingulate region (>1840)*** and contributing to ***superior longitudinal fascicle (>1840)***; in the original Italian, *processi delle strie longitudinali di Reil*, Figures 2-*b*, 8-*b*.

59. *intermediate lobe (Arnold, 1838a)*
Macrodissected adult human ***cerebral cortex gray matter (>1840)*** associated with ***frontal operculum (>1840)***, ***parietal operculum (>1840)***, and ***temporal operculum (1840)*** considered together; in the original Latin, *lobus intermedius*, p. 52.

60. *hidden lobe (Arnold, 1838a)*
Synonym for *intermediate lobe (Arnold, 1838a)*; in the original Latin, *lobus opertus*, p. 52.

61. *retracted lobe (Arnold, 1838a)*
Synonym for *intermediate lobe (Arnold, 1838a)*; in the original Latin, *lobus retractus*, p. 52.

62. *first intermediate white layer of cortical layer (Baillarger, 1840)*
In mammalian ***cerebral cortex gray matter (>1840)***, corresponds to Baillarger's 2nd layer from inside out, now known as *inner layer of Baillarger*; see von Bonin translation (1960, p. 34). His 4th layer from inside out is now known as *outer layer of Baillarger*. He cut by hand thin slices of cortical tissue, placed them between two pieces of glass, and observed with transillumination, sometimes with a magnifying glass, or even a microscope.

63. *inner intermediate white layer of cortical layer (Baillarger, 1840)*
Synonym for *first intermediate white layer of cortical layer (Baillarger, 1840)*; see von Bonin translation (1960, p. 34).

64. *paracentral lobule (>1840)*
Macrodissected adult human zone lying between ***paracentral sulcus (>1840)*** and ***marginal sulcus (>1840)*** on medial face of ***cerebral cortex gray matter (>1840)***, consisting of ***anterior paracentral gyrus (>1840)*** and ***posterior paracentral gyrus (>1840)***; see Williams & Warwick (1980, Fig. 7.114A), *Terminologia Anatomica* (1998, p. 126). Soemmerring (1788, Tab. III) first accurately illustrated it for macrodissected adult human.

65. *area subcentralis (Brodmann, 1909)*
Original Latin form of *subcentral area (Brodmann, 1909)*; p. 133.

66. *subcentral area (Brodmann, 1909)*
Based on cellular architecture in adult human, zone of ***cerebral cortex gray matter (>1840)*** ventral to ventral tip of ***central sulcus (Huschke, 1854)*** and associated with caudal end of ***frontal operculum (>1840)*** and rostral end of ***parietal operculum (>1840)***; see Garey translation (1994, pp. 112–113 and Fig. 85).

67. *area 43 (Brodmann, 1909)*
Synonym for adult human *subcentral area (Brodmann, 1909)*; in the original German, *Feld 43*, p. 133.

cerebral cortex white matter (>1840)

As described for adult vertebrate with macrodissection and histological methods for ***axons (Kölliker, 1896)***, the ***white matter (Meckel, 1817)*** forming the deep component of the ***cerebral cortex (>1840)***, distinguished from the superficial component, ***cerebral cortex gray matter (>1840)***. For these precise definitions, see Swanson & Bota (2010). The ***cerebral cortex white matter (>1840)*** is subdivided topographically into ***central nervous system white matter tracts (>1840)*** such as ***anterior commissure (Lieutaud, 1742)***, ***corpus callosum (Galen, c177)***, ***radiation of corpus callosum (>1840)***, ***fimbria (Honegger, 1890)***, and ***association fibers of cerebral cortex (>1840)***. Overall, it contains projection, commissural, and association ***axons (Kölliker, 1896)***; see Dejerine & Dejerine-Klumpke (1895; Chs. 5, 6); Crosby et al. (1962, p. 394 ff.); Carpenter (1976, p. 29 ff.); Williams & Warwick (1980, p. 1029 ff.), Nieuwenhuys et al. (2008, p. 592). The first term for it defined in this inclusive way was probably *arbor vitae of brain (Cruveilhier, 1836)*.

EARLIER REFERENCES:

Earlier synonyms:

1. *arbor vitae of brain (Cruveilhier, 1836)*
Roughly synonymous with macrodissected adult human ***cerebral cortex white matter (>1840)***; in the original French, *arbre de vie du cerveau*, p. 705.
2. *central white substance (Baillarger, 1840)*
Roughly synonymous with macrodissected adult human ***cerebral cortex white matter (>1840)***; see translation, von Bonin (1960, p. 22 ff.).

PARTLY CORRESPONDS:

1. *psalidoeides (Vesalius, 1543a)*
Vesalius wrote that some (unnamed) Greeks used it for ***corpus callosum (Galen, c177)***, and that ancient Greeks also used it for *fornix (Galen, c177)*. Galen's use is at times ambiguous; see *psalidoeides (Galen, 177)*.

2. *arch (Vesalius, 1543a)*
English form of *psalidoeides (Vesalius, 1543a)*; see Singer translation (1952, p. 30).
3. *corpus callosum (Willis, 1664)*
Apparently corresponds to macrodissected adult large mammal (including human) ***cerebral cortex white matter (>1840)***—excluding ***white matter (Meckel, 1817)*** of the *gyri (Vesalius, 1543a)* called *medullary rays (Vieussens, 1684)*—comparing it to a chamber, vault, or arch; see Pordage translation (1681, pp. 60, 61, 93).
4. *chamber (Willis, 1664)*
Synonym for *corpus callosum (Willis, 1664)*; see Pordage translation (1681, p. 60).
5. *chambered body (Willis, 1664)*
Synonym for *corpus callosum (Willis, 1664)*; see Pordage translation (1681, p. 60).
6. *vault (Willis, 1664)*
Synonym for *corpus callosum (Willis, 1664)*; see Pordage translation (1681, p. 60).
7. *chamber of brain (Willis, 1664)*
Synonym for *corpus callosum (Willis, 1664)*; see Pordage translation (1681, p. 61). Also see *psalidoeides (Galen, 177)*.
8. *middle marrow of brain proper (Willis, 1664)*
Synonym for *corpus callosum (Willis, 1664)*; see Pordage translation (1681, p. 63).
9. *bottom of cerebral cortex (Willis, 1664)*
Synonym for *corpus callosum (Willis, 1664)*; see Pordage translation (1681, p. 91).
10. *middle of brain (Willis, 1664)*
Synonym for *corpus callosum (Willis, 1664)*; see Pordage translation (1681, p. 93).
11. *middle of cerebrum (Willis, 1664)*
Synonym for *corpus callosum (Willis, 1664)*; see Pordage translation (1681, p. 93).
12. *middle marrow of cerebrum (Willis, 1664)*
Synonym for *corpus callosum (Willis, 1664)*; see Pordage translation (1681, p. 93).
13. *base of cerebral cortex (Willis, 1664)*
Synonym for *corpus callosum (Willis, 1664)*; see Pordage translation (1681, p. 93).
14. *cerebri medulla (Malpighi, 1665)*
Essentially synonym for *corpus callosum (Willis, 1664)*; see Gordon (1817, p. 19).
15. *fornix vera (Vieussens, 1684)*
Synonym for macrodissected adult human *corpus callosum (Willis, 1664)*; p. 61. Also see Ridley (1695, p. 115), Burdach (1822, p. 363).
16. *camera anteriorum ventriculorum (Vieussens, 1684)*
Synonym for macrodissected adult human *corpus callosum (Willis, 1664)*; p. 59, see Burdach (1822, p. 363).
17. *oval center (Vieussens, 1684)*
Basically part of macrodissected adult human ***cerebral cortex white matter (>1840)*** lateral to ***corpus callosum (Galen, c177)*** and excluding *medullary rays (Vieussens, 1684)*; Table VI-*B*, also see Ridley (1695, p. 115), Bell (1802, p. 10). For detailed modern account see Dejerine & Dejerine-Klumpke (1901, pp. 1–19). There are varying interpretations of its full extent, but broad view adopted here is supported by Charpy (1889, Figs. 68, 108); also see *lateral centrum ovale (Vicq d'Azyr, 1786)*.
18. *ovale centrum (Vieussens, 1684)*
Original Latin form of *oval center (Vieussens, 1684)*; Table VI-*B*, also see Meyer (1971, p. 14). English form, *oval center*, used by Ridley (1695, p. 115).
19. *medullary rays (Vieussens, 1684)*
Essentially extensions of macrodissected adult human ***cerebral cortex white matter (>1840)*** into middle of *gyri (Vesalius, 1543a)*; Table VI-*a*.
20. *brawny body (Diemerbroeck, 1689)*
English form of macrodissected adult human *corpus callosum (Willis, 1664)*; p. 397.
21. *medullary part of brain (Ridley, 1695)*
Essentially synonym for macrodissected adult human *medullary rays (Vieussens, 1684)*; Figure 5.
22. *centrum ovale (Ridley, 1695)*
Alternate Latin form of *ovale centrum (Vieussens, 1684)*; p. 117.
23. *internal medullary circumvolution (Winslow, 1733)*
Synonym for macrodissected adult human *medullary rays (Vieussens, 1684)*; Section X, p. 33.
24. *white lamina (Winslow, 1733)*
Synonym for macrodissected adult human *medullary rays (Vieussens, 1684)*; Section X, p. 33.
25. *medullary lamina (Winslow, 1733)*
Synonym (singular) for macrodissected adult human *medullary rays (Vieussens, 1684)*; Section X, p. 34.
26. *medullary nucleus of cerebrum (Winslow, 1733)*
Essentially synonym for macrodissected adult human *oval center (Vieussens, 1684)*; Section X, p. 34.
27. *medullary arch (Winslow, 1733)*
Synonym for *medullary nucleus of cerebrum (Winslow, 1733)*; Section X, p. 34.
28. *medullary vault (Winslow, 1733)*
Synonym for *medullary nucleus of cerebrum (Winslow, 1733)*; Section X, p. 34.
29. *camera medullaris (Winslow, 1733)*
Latin form of *medullary vault (Winslow, 1733)*; see Burdach (1822, p. 385).
30. *nucleus of cerebrum (Winslow, 1733)*
Synonym for *medullary nucleus of cerebrum (Winslow, 1733)*; Section X, p. 34.
31. *cerebral nucleus (Winslow, 1733)*
Contracted form of *medullary nucleus of cerebrum (Winslow, 1733)*.
32. *great cerebral commissure (Lieutaud, 1742)*
Roughly synonymous with macrodissected adult human *corpus callosum (Willis, 1664)*; p. 390.
33. *commissura cerebri maxima (Lieutaud, 1742)*
Latin form of *great cerebral commissure (Lieutaud, 1742)*; see Soemmerring (1778).
34. *trabs medullaris (Haller, 1762)*
Synonym for macrodissected adult human *corpus callosum (Willis, 1664)*; p. 13, see Burdach (1822, p. 363).

35. *substantia medullaris (Santorini, 1775)*
Synonym for macrodissected adult human *ovale centrum (Vieussens, 1684)*; p. 38, according to Burdach (1822, p. 385).
36. *centrum semiovale Vieussenii (Mayer, 1779)*
Eponym for macrodissected adult human *ovale centrum (Vieussens, 1684)*; p. 6, see Burdach (1822, pp. 385–386).
37. *tegmentum ventriculorum (Mayer, 1779)*
Synonym for macrodissected adult human *ovale centrum (Vieussens, 1684)*; p. 6, see Günther (1786, p. 9), Burdach (1822, pp. 385–386).
38. *lateral oval center (Vicq d'Azyr, 1786)*
Corresponds to dorsal regions of macrodissected adult human *oval center (Vieussens, 1684)*; in the original French, *centre ovale latérale*, Plate IV, Figure 1-*a*.
39. *small oval center (Vicq d'Azyr, 1786)*
Synonym for *lateral oval center (Vicq d'Azyr, 1786)*; in the original French, *petit centre ovale*, Plate IV, Figure 1-*a*. Burdach (1822, p. 386) gave Latin form, *centrum ovale parvum*.
40. *medullary center of cerebrum (Vicq d'Azyr, 1786)*
Synonym for macrodissected adult human *oval center (Vieussens, 1684)* or *medullary nucleus of cerebrum (Winslow, 1733)*; in the original French, *centre ovale ou médullaire du cerveau*, Plate VI-6.
41. *superior striae of corpus striatum (Vicq d'Azyr, 1786)*
Topographic part of macrodissected adult human *corona radiata (Reil, 1809b)* lying between ***caudate nucleus (Arnold, 1838b)*** and ***claustrum (Burdach, 1822)***; Plate IX-26,27.
42. *superior oval center (Vicq d'Azyr, 1786)*
Synonym for *lateral oval center (Vicq d'Azyr, 1786)*; in the original French, *centre ovale supérieur*, Plate XXIV-30.
43. *commissura magna cerebri (Bell, 1802)*
Latin form of *great cerebral commissure (Lieutaud, 1742)*; p. 5 note 3.
44. *medullary plate (Reil, 1809b)*
Synonym for macrodissected adult human *medullary ray (Vieussens, 1684)*, all considered together forming the outer "tips" of *corona radiata (Reil, 1809b)*; and for deep ***white matter (Meckel, 1840)*** in *folia (Malacarne, 1776)* of ***cerebellar cortex Willis, 1664)***, which all together form "outer" part of ***arbor vitae (Winslow, 1733)***; see Mayo translation (1823, p. 53). German form is *Stabkraz*, see Burdach (1822, pp. 132, 352).
45. *corpus callosum system (Reil, 1809b)*
Macrodissected adult human transverse (horizontal) part of *nucleus of cerebrum (Reil, 1809b)*, longitudinal part being *cerebral peduncle system (Reil, 1809b)*; in the original German, *Balkensystem*, pp. 172–188, also see Mayo translation (p. 53 ff.). Basically, *corpus callosum system (Reil, 1809b)* is right and left ***cerebral cortex white matter (>1840)*** without *superior longitudinal fascicles (>1840)*.
46. *Balkensystem (Reil, 1809b)*
Original German form of *corpus callosum system (Reil, 1809b)*; pp. 172–188.
47. *horizontal portion of nucleus of cerebrum (Reil, 1809b)*
Synonym for *corpus callosum system (Reil, 1809b)*; see Mayo translation (1823, p. 66).
48. *magna reunio cerebri (Gall & Spurzheim, 1810)*
Synonym for macrodissected adult human *corpus callosum (Willis, 1664)*, according to Burdach (1822, p. 364).
49. *semilunar border (Reil, 1812c)*
Roughly segment of macrodissected adult human *corona radiata (Reil, 1809b)* corresponding to *oval center (Vieussens, 1684)*; see Mayo translation (1823, p. 122); in German, *halb-mond-förmiger Saum*.
50. *central white mass of convolutions (Gordon, 1815)*
Synonym for macrodissected adult human *oval center (Vieussens, 1684)*; p. 139. Burdach (1822, p. 386) gave Latin form, *corpus centrale gyrorum*.
51. *trabs cerebri (Bock, 1820)*
Synonym for macrodissected adult human *trabs medullaris (Haller, 1762)*; p. 259, see Burdach (1822, p. 364).
52. *maximus medullae orbis (Tiedemann, 1821)*
Synonym for macrodissected adult monkey *centrum semiovale Vieussenii (Mayer, 1779)*; Table II, Figure 1-*a*. In English, *great medullary circle*.
53. *great commissure of brain (Mayo, 1827)*
Synonym for macrodissected adult human *corpus callosum (Willis, 1664)*; Plate III-*g*.
54. *great commissure of cerebrum (Mayo, 1827)*
Synonym for macrodissected adult human *corpus callosum (Willis, 1664)*; Plate IV-*o*.
55. *medullary fascicle of crested process (Rolando, 1831)*
Apparently roughly synonymous with macrodissected adult human ***cingulum (Burdach 1822)*** and its ventral extension through medial ***temporal region (>1840)*** as far as *uncus (Vicq d'Azyr, 1786)*; in the original Italian, *fascio midollare del processo cristato*, pp. 125–126.
56. *great transverse commissure (Solly, 1836)*
Synonym for macrodissected adult human *corpus callosum (Willis, 1664)*; p. 88.
57. *transverse commissure (Solly, 1836)*
Synonym for macrodissected adult human *corpus callosum (Willis, 1664)*; p. 170.
58. *great transverse commissure of hemispheres (Combe et al., 1838)*
Synonym for macrodissected adult human *great transverse commissure (Solly, 1836)*; p. xxviii.
59. *body of corona radiata (Arnold, 1838a)*
Essentially, macrodissected adult human *oval center (Vieussens, 1684)*; in the original Latin, *corpus coronae radiatae*, p. 71.
60. *peripheral part of corona radiata (Arnold, 1838a)*
Synonym for macrodissected adult human *medullary plates (Reil, 1809b)*; in the original Latin, *pars peripherica*, p. 71.
61. *medullary cerebral radiation with cortex (Arnold, 1838b)*
Essentially synonymous with macrodissected adult human *oval center (Vieussens, 1684)*; in the original Latin, *radiatio cerebri medullaris cum cortice*, Table IV, Figure 4-*τ*.

cerebral falx (Vesalius, 1543a)

As described for macrodissected adult human, the longitudinal midsagittal folds of ***dura (Galen, c177)*** separating the right and left ***cerebral cortex (>1840)*** ventrally to the level of the ***corpus callosum (Galen, c177)*** and resembling a reaper's sickle or *falx*; see Millen & Woollam (1962, pp. 126–127), *Terminologia Anatomica* (1998, p. 104). Vesalius named and provided a beautiful description of it in macrodissected adult human; see Singer translation (1952, p. 11), also see Burdach (1822, pp. 399–400), who credited Mayer (1783–1794, Vol. 6, p. 18) with using the precise term, *falx cerebri*. Its existence has long been known; see ***[cerebral falx (Vesalius, 1543a)] (Hippocrates)***.

TRANSLATIONS:

1. *falx cerebri (Vesalius, 1543a)*
   Latin form of ***cerebral falx (Vesalius, 1543a)***; see *Terminologia Anatomica* (1998, p. 104).
2. *scythe (Diemerbroeck, 1689)*
   English form of *falx cerebri (Vesalius, 1543a)*; p. 385.
3. *falx of cerebrum (Meckel, 1832)*
   English form of *falx cerebri (Vesalius, 1543a)*; see Vol. 2, p. 480.

EARLIER REFERENCES:

Described, not named or illustrated:

1. ***[cerebral falx (Vesalius, 1543a)] (Hippocrates)***
   In *On the Sacred Disease*, Hippocrates noted that the ***brain (Smith Papyrus, c1700 BC)*** is divided through the middle into right and left sides by a thin membrane. This is probably the first reference to ***cerebral falx (Vesalius, 1543a)***, based most likely on macrodissected adult goat, although he claimed it is also true in human; see Adams translation (1972, p. 351), also see Millen & Woollam (1962, p. 19).
2. ***[cerebral falx (Vesalius, 1543a)] (Galen, c173)***
   Described for macrodissected adult beef, pig, and/or macaque but not specifically human; see May translation (1968, p. 437).

LATER SYNONYMS:

1. *falx durae matris (Vesalius, 1543a)*
   Synonym for macrodissected adult human ***cerebral falx (Vesalius, 1543a)***; see Schreger (1803, p. 314).
2. *processus durae matris longitudinalem (Slevogt, 1690)*
   Synonym for macrodissected adult human ***cerebral falx (Vesalius, 1543a)***; see reprinted thesis in Haller (1747–1751, Vol. 2, p. 820).
3. *septum sagittale (Winslow, 1733)*
   Synonym for macrodissected adult human ***cerebral falx (Vesalius, 1543a)***; Section X, p. 25.
4. *septum verticale (Winslow, 1733)*
   Synonym for macrodissected adult human ***cerebral falx (Vesalius, 1543a)***; Section X, p. 25.
5. *mediastinum cerebri (Winslow, 1733)*
   Synonym for macrodissected adult human ***cerebral falx (Vesalius, 1543a)***; Section X, p. 25.
6. *falx of dura mater (Winslow, 1733)*
   English form of macrodissected adult human *falx durae matris (Vesalius, 1543a)*; Section X, p. 26.
7. *great longitudinal septum (Winslow, 1733)*
   Synonym for macrodissected adult human ***cerebral falx (Vesalius, 1543a)***; Section X, p. 33.
8. *caudex (Pacchioni, 1741)*
   Synonym for macrodissected adult human ***cerebral falx (Vesalius, 1543a)***; p. 136.
9. *processus falciformis superior (Haller, 1762)*
   Synonym for macrodissected adult human ***cerebral falx (Vesalius, 1543a)***; Section X, pp. 96, 97.
10. *processus falciformis major (Haller, 1762)*
    Synonym for macrodissected adult human ***cerebral falx (Vesalius, 1543a)***; Section X, pp. 96, 97.
11. *processus falciformis (Mayer, 1783–1794)*
    Synonym for macrodissected adult human ***cerebral falx (Vesalius, 1543a)***; Vol. 6, p. 18.
12. *processus longitudinalis (Mayer, 1783–1794)*
    Synonym for macrodissected adult human ***cerebral falx (Vesalius, 1543a)***; Vol. 6, p. 18.
13. *superior longitudinal process (Fyfe, 1800)*
    Synonym for macrodissected adult human ***cerebral falx (Vesalius, 1543a)***; p. 12.
14. *septum cerebri (Fyfe, 1800)*
    Synonym for macrodissected adult human ***cerebral falx (Vesalius, 1543a)***; p. 12.
15. *falx (Fyfe, 1800)*
    Synonym for macrodissected adult human ***cerebral falx (Vesalius, 1543a)***; p. 12.
16. *median septum of brain (Burdin, 1803)*
    Synonym for macrodissected adult human ***cerebral falx (Vesalius, 1543a)***; see translation (1803, Vol. 1, p. 153).
17. *falx of brain (Burdin, 1803)*
    Synonym used in English for macrodissected adult human ***cerebral falx (Vesalius, 1543a)***; see translation (1803, Vol. 1, p. 153).
18. *falciform fold (Chaussier, 1807)*
    Synonym for macrodissected adult human ***cerebral falx (Vesalius, 1543a)***; in the original French, *repli falciforme*, p. 23.
19. *longitudinal fold of meninges (Chaussier, 1807)*
    Synonym for macrodissected adult human ***cerebral falx (Vesalius, 1543a)***; in the original French, *repli longitudinal de la méninge*, p. 23. For English form, *longitudinal fold of meninx*, see Meckel (1832, Vol. 2, p. 480).
20. *large falx (Chaussier, 1807)*
    Synonym for macrodissected adult human ***cerebral falx (Vesalius, 1543a)***; in the original French, *la grande faulx*, p. 193. For English form see Meckel (1832, Vol. 2, p. 480). It is also translated *great falx*.
21. *processus falciformis cerebri (Meckel, 1817)*
    Synonym for macrodissected adult human ***cerebral falx (Vesalius, 1543a)***; p. 560, see translation (1832, Vol. 2, p. 480).
22. *falx major (Meckel, 1817)*
    Latin form provided for *large falx (Chaussier, 1807)*; see translation (1832, Vol. 2, p. 480).

cerebral nuclei (Swanson, 2000a)

The ventral topographic division of the vertebrate ***endbrain (Kuhlenbeck, 1927)***; see Swanson & Bota (2010) for definition, and Swanson (2004, Tab. B) for complete list of component ***gray matter regions (Swanson & Bota, 1010)*** in rat. The dorsal topographic division of the vertebrate ***endbrain (Kuhlenbeck, 1927)*** is the ***cerebral cortex (>1840)***. For Swanson's original use in mammals, see p. 117. It was first clearly identified as the *striated body (Willis, 1664)*. "...the division of the cerebral hemisphere of Amphibia (and of higher animals) into dorsal or pallial [***cerebral cortex (>1840)***] and basal or subpallial [***cerebral nuclei (Swanson, 2000a)***] parts is primary and has its morphological basis in the configuration of the primitive neural tube antecedent to the evagination of the hemispheres." (Herrick, 1910, p. 491).

EARLIER REFERENCES:

Earlier synonyms:

1. *striated body (Willis, 1664)*
   Willis discovered in macrodissected adult human and other mammals the *corpus striatum (Willis, 1664)*, the most rostral or "top" segment of his *oblong medulla (Willis, 1664)*, corresponding roughly to the ***cerebral nuclei (Swanson, 2000a)***. He wrote that no other structures in the head have this appearance, and postulated that different medullary striations ascend to and descend from the *cerebral hemisphere (Willis, 1664)*; pp. 62–63, 101–102, Tab. VIII-*A*). He observed that *gray substance (Vesalius, 1543a)* and *white substance (Vesalius, 1543a)* are intermixed in the *striated body*; Willis (1672), see Pordage translation (1683, p. 26). The *striated body (Willis, 1664)* was actually mentioned earlier by Bartholin as the first segment of the *round trunk (Bartholin, 1662)* in macrodissected adult human, but he did not describe its unique internal structure.
2. *corpus striatum (Willis, 1664)*
   Latin form of *striated body (Willis, 1664)*.
3. *streaked body (Willis, 1664)*
   Another form of *striated body (Willis, 1664)*; see Pordage translation (1681, p. 62).
4. *chamfered body (Willis, 1664)*
   Synonym for *striated body (Willis, 1664)*; see Pordage translation (1681, pp. 61, 102).
5. *lentiform prominence (Willis, 1664)*
   Synonym for *striated body (Willis, 1664)*; see Pordage translation (1681, p. 63); plural in Latin, *prominentiae lentiformes*.
6. *lentiform process (Willis, 1664)*
   Synonym for *striated body (Willis, 1664)*; see Pordage translation (1681, p. 63).
7. *top of oblong marrow (Willis, 1664)*
   Synonym for *striated body (Willis, 1664)*; see Pordage translation (1681, p. 63).
8. *top of oblong marrow shank (Willis, 1664)*
   Synonym for *striated body (Willis, 1664)*; see Pordage translation (1681, pp. 62, 63).
9. *streaked membrane (Willis, 1664)*
   Apparently macrodissected adult bird equivalent of mammalian *streaked body (Willis, 1664)* or *striated body (Willis, 1664)*; see Pordage translation (1681, p. 75).
10. *first pair of tubercles (Steno, 1669)*
    Synonym for right and left macrodissected adult human *striated body (Willis, 1664)*; see Burdach (1822, p. 348).
11. *common sensory (Willis, 1672)*
    Functional synonym for *striated body (Willis, 1664)*; see Pordage translation (1683, p. 27). Willis thought this is where all of the sensory modalities converge, satisfying Aristotle's requirement for a *sensus communis* or "common sense", which in medieval times was placed in the ***lateral ventricle (Vesalius, 1543a)***; see Manzone (1998). A translation today would be *common sense*.
12. *corps canelez (Bourdon, 1683)*
    Synonym for macrodissected adult human *striated body (Willis, 1664)*; pp. 201, 400 and (in Atlas volume of 1678) Table 4, Figure 30-*e,i*. Also see *corps cannellez (Pourfour du Petit, 1710), channeled bodies (Poupart, 1712), corps canelés (Lieutaud, 1742)*, and "le *corps strié* ou *cannelé*" in Chaussier (1807, p. 62).
13. *little long mountain (Diemerbroeck, 1689)*
    Synonym for macrodissected adult human *striated body (Willis, 1664)*; plural in Latin, *insignes monticuli oblongi*, p. 400; also see Diemerbroeck (1672, p. 589).
14. *furrowed hillock (Diemerbroeck, 1689)*
    Synonym for macrodissected adult human *striated body (Willis, 1664)*; plural in Latin, *monticuli striati*, p. 420; also see Diemerbroeck (1672, p. 630).
15. *apex of medulla oblongata (Ridley, 1695)*
    Synonym for macrodissected adult human *top of oblong marrow (Willis, 1664)*; p. 115.
16. *processus lentiformes (Ridley, 1695)*
    Synonym for macrodissected adult human *lentiform prominence (Willis, 1664)*; p. 115.
17. *corps cannellez (Pourfour du Petit, 1710)*
    Synonym for *striated body (Willis, 1664)*; Letter 1, p. 3.
18. *channeled bodies (Poupart, 1712)*
    English form of *corpus striatum (Willis, 1664)*; p. 642.
19. *fibrous protuberance (Salmon, 1714)*
    Probably synonym for macrodissected adult human *striated body (Willis, 1664)*; p. 401.
20. *corps canelés (Lieutaud, 1742)*
    Apparently synonym in French for macrodissected adult human *striated body (Willis, 1664)*; p. 391, also see *corps cannelez (Pourfour du Petit, 1710)*.
21. *corpora striata interiora anteriora (Schreger, 1803)*
    Schreger claimed Vieussens (1684, Tab. XIV-*B*) used it for macrodissected adult human *striated body (Willis, 1664)*; p. 320.
22. *bed of ethmoidal nerve (Chaussier, 1807)*
    Synonym for macrodissected adult human *striated body (Willis, 1664)*; in the original French, *couche du nerf ethmoïdal*, p. 63. Also see Meckel (1832, Vol. 2, p. 454).
23. *colliculus nervi ethmoïdalis (Chaussier, 1807)*
    Latin form provided for *bed of ethmoidal nerve (Chaussier, 1807)*; p. 63.

24. *great cerebral ganglion (Reil, 1809b)*
Synonym for macrodissected adult human *striated body (Willis, 1664)*; in the original German, *grosse Hirnganglium*, p. 144; for English see Mayo translation (1823, p. 52).
25. *great striated cerebral ganglion (Reil, 1809b)*
Synonym for macrodissected adult human *striated body (Willis, 1664)*; in the original German, *das gestreifte grosse Hirnganglium*, p. 195, according to Meyer translation (1971, p. 29). Also see Schiller (1967, p. 528).
26. *anterior cerebral ganglion (Gall & Spurzheim, 1810)*
Synonym for macrodissected adult human *striated body (Willis, 1664)*; pp. 198–199.
27. *anterior and exterior cerebral ganglion (Gall & Spurzheim, 1810)*
Synonym for macrodissected adult human *striated body (Willis, 1664)*; pp. 198–199.
28. *great superior cerebral ganglion (Gall & Spurzheim, 1810)*
Synonym for macrodissected adult human *striated body (Willis, 1664)*; in the original French, *le grand ganglion supérieur*, p. 209. Also see Spurzheim (1826, p. 224).
29. *striated colliculus (Wenzel & Wenzel, 1812)*
Apparently synonym for macrodissected adult human *striated body (Willis, 1664)*; in the original Latin, *colliculus striatus*, see Table III, Figure 1-*a*; it refers at least to the ventricular surface of the *corpus striatum (Willis, 1664)*.
30. *anterior inner ganglia of optic tubercles (Carus, 1814)*
Synonym for ***cerebral nuclei (Swanson, 2000a)*** of macrodissected adult fish; in the original German, *vordern innern Ganglien des Sehhügels*, pp. 139, 155.
31. *ganglion of radiation to ceiling of great ventricles (Carus, 1814)*
Apparently synonym for macrodissected adult mammalian *corpus striatum (Willis, 1664)*; in the original German, *Ganglion für die Radiation der Decke der Grossen Hirnhöhlen*, p. 223.
32. *ganglia cerebri magna antica (Meckel, 1817)*
Listed as synonym for right and left macrodissected adult human *corpus striatum (Willis, 1664)*; see translation (1832, Vol. 2, p. 454), where Meckel went on to write, "The gray substance of the corpus striatum, seems then to be divided externally by a considerable layer of medullary substance, into an internal and upper half, and an external and lower" (p. 455). In English (singular), *great anterior cerebral ganglion*.
33. *anterior medullary nuclei of Reil (Tiedemann, 1821)*
Eponym for macrodissected adult monkey *striated body (Willis, 1664)*; in the original Latin, *nuclei medullares anteriores Reili*, Table II, Figure 2-*c*. Tiedemann did not provide a citation to Reil.
34. *ganglion of intellectual faculties (Spurzheim, 1826)*
Synonym for macrodissected adult *corpus striatum (Willis, 1664)*; p. 211.
35. *superior cerebral ganglion (Quain, 1828)*
Synonym for macrodissected adult mammalian ***cerebral nuclei (Swanson, 2000a)***; p. 625.
36. *greater and superior ganglion of brain (Knox, 1832)*
Knox's version in English of *great superior cerebral ganglion (Gall & Spurzheim, 1810)*; Supplemental Plate IV-*20,21*.
37. *ganglion of anterior columns (Solly, 1836)*
Synonym for macrodissected adult human ***cerebral nuclei (Swanson, 2000a)***; p. 175.
38. *ganglion of motory columns (Solly, 1836)*
Synonym for macrodissected adult human ***cerebral nuclei (Swanson, 2000a)***; p. 175.
39. *anterior ganglion of spinal cord (Solly, 1836)*
Synonym for macrodissected adult human ***cerebral nuclei (Swanson, 2000a)***; p. 179.
40. *motory ganglion of spinal cord (Solly, 1836)*
Synonym for macrodissected adult human ***cerebral nuclei (Swanson, 2000a)***; pp. 179, 185.
41. *anterior striated body (Solly, 1836)*
Synonym for macrodissected adult human ***cerebral nuclei (Swanson, 2000a)***; Figure 1-*F*, p. 180; also called *anterior corpus striatum* in Figure 1-*G*, p. 180.
42. *olfactory lobes (Cruveilhier, 1836)*
Synonym for macrodissected adult human ***cerebral nuclei (Swanson, 2000a)***, attributed without citation to Chaussier; in the original French, *lobes olfactifs*, p. 885.
43. *cendré supérieur (Gerdy, 1838)*
Synonym for macrodissected adult human ***cerebral nuclei (Swanson, 2000a)***; pp. 262, 263.
44. *striated eminence (Arnold, 1838a)*
Synonym for macrodissected adult human *striated body (Willis, 1664)*; in the original Latin (plural), *eminentiae striata*, p. 65.
45. *great anterior and superior cerebral ganglion (Arnold, 1838a)*
Synonym for macrodissected adult human *great superior cerebral ganglion (Gall & Spurzheim, 1810)* attributed without citation to Gall and Meckel; in the original Latin (plural), *ganglia cerebri magna superiora anteriora*, p. 65.

PARTLY CORRESPONDS:

1. *septum (Galen, c177)*
Term used in *On Anatomical Procedures* for the *diaphragm (Galen, c177)* separating the right and left ***lateral ventricle (Vesalius, 1543a)***, a set of ***gray matter regions (Swanson & Bota, 2010)*** and ***white matter tracts (Bell & Bell, 1826)*** that in the 20th century became known as the *septal region (Swanson & Cowan, 1979)*. Galen noted that its substance is like the rest of the ***brain (Smith Papyrus, c1700 BC)*** in macrodissected adult beef, pig, and/or macaque, but not human; see Singer translation (1999, pp. 231–232). According to Bauhin (1605, pp. 584–585; see Crooke translation, 1615, p. 460), he, Galen, Vesalius, and du Laurens regarded the *septum (Galen, c177)* as a stretched part of the ***brain (Smith Papyrus, c1700 BC)***, whereas Colombo and Piccolomini regarded it as ***pia (Galen, c192)***. Mayer (1783–1794, Vol. 6, p. 133) first clearly described ***gray matter regions (Swanson & Bota,***

2010) and ***white matter tracts (Bell & Bell, 1826)*** in the *septum (Galen, c177)*; see Burdach (1822, p. 353).

2. *septum lucidum (Galen, c177)*
   Synonym for *septum (Galen, c177)*; see Singer translation (1999, p. 234).
3. *septum pellucidum (Galen, c177)*
   Alternate form of *septum lucidum (Galen, c177)*. According to Burdach (1822, p. 352), Le Boë (1663) declared "*septum pellucidum, non lucidum*".
4. *diaphragma (Galen, c177)*
   Latin form of *septum (Galen, c177)*; see Singer translation (1999, pp. 231–232).
5. *diaphragm (Galen, c177)*
   English form of *diaphragma (Galen, c177)*.
6. *partition (Galen, c177)*
   Synonym for *septum (Galen, c177)*; see Singer translation (1999, pp. 231–232).
7. *membrane partitioning ventricles (Galen, c177)*
   Synonym for *septum (Galen, c177)*; see Singer translation (1999, pp. 231–232).
8. *speculum (Vesalius, 1543a)*
   Synonym for macrodissected adult human *septum (Galen, c177)*; see Singer translation (1952, pp. 65, 96). Burdach (1822, p. 352) attributed the term to Colombo (1559, p. 192).
9. *basal grayish substance of cerebrum (Vesalius, 1543a)*
   Vesalius clearly described deep *gray substance (Vesalius, 1543a)* distinguished by lines (or borders) from surrounding *white substance (Vesalius, 1543a)*; see Singer translation (1952, p. 100 and Fig. 7). It is in the unpaired *base of cerebrum (Vesalius, 1543a)*, not on the surface of the two *cerebral lobes (Vesalius, 1543a)*. Thus, it may refer roughly to the macrodissected adult human ***cerebral nuclei (Swanson, 2000a)***, or at least to regions of it near the ***corpus callosum (Galen, c177)***.
10. *hedge of right and left ventricles (Geminus, 1553)*
    Synonym for macrodissected adult human *septum (Galen, c177)*; see *The tables of the brayne*, Figure 5.
11. *enclosing of right and left ventricles (Geminus, 1553)*
    Synonym for macrodissected adult human *septum (Galen, c177)*; originally spelled *inclosynge of ryght and left ventricles*, see *The tables of the brayne*, Figure 5.
12. *locality where olfactory apparatus originates (Varoli, 1573)*
    Varoli clearly illustrated region of macrodissected adult human ***olfactory tubercle (Calleja, 1893)*** and ***diagonal band nucleus (>1840)***, known together as *anterior perforated substance (His, 1895)*; Figure I(8) on f. 17v, also see Polyak (1957, p. 98).
13. *corpus speculare (Piccolomini, 1586)*
    Synonym for macrodissected adult human *septum (Galen, c177)*; p. 252, see Burdach (1822, p. 352).
14. *speculum lucidum (du Laurens, 1600)*
    According to Burdach (1822, p. 352), synonym Du Laurens first used for macrodissected adult human *septum (Galen, c177)*; p. 528, also see Harvey (1961, p. 222).
15. *lapis specularis (du Laurens, 1600)*
    According to Burdach (1822, p. 352), synonym Du Laurens first used for the *septum (Galen, c177)*; also see Harvey (1961, p. 222).
16. *bright glass (du Laurens, 1600)*
    Translation of *lapis specularis (Du Laurens, 1600)*, the *septum (Galen, c177)*; see Crooke translation (1615, p. 431).
17. *looking glass (du Laurens, 1600)*
    Translation of *lapis specularis (Du Laurens, 1600)*, the *septum (Galen, c177)*; see Crooke translation (1615, p. 460).
18. *bright mirror (du Laurens, 1600)*
    Translation of *speculum lucidum (Du Laurens, 1600)*, the *septum (Galen, c177)*; see Riolan (1657, p. 122).
19. *partition-skin (Bartholin, 1662)*
    Synonym for macrodissected adult human *membrane partitioning ventricles (Galen, c177)*, or *septum (Galen, c177)*; p. 140.
20. *septum tenue (Bartholin, 1662)*
    Apparently synonym for macrodissected adult human *septum (Galen, c177)*; p. 142.
21. *corpora striata inferiora exteriora posteriora (Vieussens, 1684)*
    In the first parceling of the macrodissected adult human *striated body (Willis, 1664)*, Vieussens identified what roughly corresponds to the *lentiform nucleus (Burdach, 1822)*; p. 84, Table XIV-*B*. See Meyer (1971, p. 13).
22. *lucid enclosure (Diemerbroeck, 1689)*
    Synonym for macrodissected adult human *septum (Galen, c177)*; p. 397.
23. *lucid fence (Diemerbroeck, 1689)*
    Synonym for macrodissected adult human *septum (Galen, c177)*; p. 397.
24. *external inferior part of striated body (Pourfour du Petit, 1710)*
    Rough synonym for macrodissected adult human *lentiform nucleus (Burdach, 1822)*, although it may have included more ventral ***gray matter regions (Swanson & Bota, 2010)*** like the ***substantia innominata (Meynert, 1872)*** and ***olfactory tubercle (Calleja, 1893)***; in the original French, *les corps cannelez externes ou inferieurs*, pp. 3, 7, 14.It is probably roughly equivalent to *corpora striata inferiora exteriora et posteriora (Vieussens, 1684)*. See Arnold (1838b, Tab. VIII, Fig. 2-*n*), *pars externa et inferior corporis striati s. nucleus lenticularis*.
25. *tympanum (Duvernoy, 1735)*
    Synonym for macrodissected adult human *septum (Galen, c177)*; p. 133, see Burdach (1822, p. 353).
26. *pars cerebri subcinerea (Tarin, 1750)*
    Roughly synonymous with macrodissected adult human ***olfactory tubercle (Calleja, 1893)*** and ***diagonal band nucleus (>1840)***, known together as *anterior perforated substance (Vicq d'Azyr, 1784)*; Table I, Figure 4-*F*.
27. *pars crurum cerebri ante nervos opticos locata (Soemmerring, 1778)*
    Roughly synonymous with macrodissected adult human ***olfactory tubercle (Calleja, 1893)*** and ***diagonal band nucleus (>1840)***, known together as *anterior perforated substance (Vicq d'Azyr, 1784)*; p. 107, see Burdach (1822, p. 388).

28. *lamina septi medullaris triangularis intermedii interventriculos laterales (Soemmerring, 1778)*
Technical synonym Soemmerring preferred for macrodissected adult human *septum (Galen, c177)*; Table III-*g*.
29. *anterior perforated substance (Vicq d'Azyr, 1784)*
Synonym for roughly macrodissected adult human ***olfactory tubercle (Calleja, 1893)*** and ***diagonal band nucleus (>1840)*** considered together; p. 545. It had been alluded to earlier, at least briefly, by Varoli (1573, Fig. II-*8*) and Soemmerring (1778, see Meyer, 1971, p. 23). As defined today, it typically includes only the ***olfactory tubercle (Calleja, 1893)***; see Nauta & Haymaker (1969, pp. 151–153, 156–157).
30. *external part of corpus striatum (Vicq d'Azyr, 1786)*
Synonym for macrodissected adult human *corpora striata inferiora exteriora posteriora (Vieussens, 1684)*; p. 27, see Burdach (1822, p. 350).
31. *perforated white substance (Vicq d'Azyr, 1786)*
Synonym for *anterior perforated substance (Vicq d'Azyr, 1784)*; in the original French, *substance blanche perforée*; Plate XVII, Figures I-*27*, II-*6*; also see Meyer (1971, pp. 24, 85).
32. *perforated substance (Vicq d'Azyr, 1786)*
Synonym for *anterior perforated substance (Vicq d'Azyr, 1784)*; Plate XXI-*16*, see Meyer (1971, pp. 24, 85).
33. *middle cerebral septum (Günther, 1786)*
Synonym for macrodissected adult human *septum (Galen, c177)*; in the original Latin, *septum cerebri medium*, p. 11.
34. *median septum of ventricles (Burdin, 1803)*
Synonym for macrodissected adult human *septum (Galen, c177)*; see translation (1803, Vol. 1, p. 157). Also see Burdach (1822, p. 353), who wrote that Lindanus used the term *mediastinum, septum medium*; the reference has not been traced. Meckel (1817) gave Burdin's term in Latin as *septum median*; see translation (1832, Vol. 2, p. 449).
35. *transparent septum (Chaussier, 1807)*
Synonym listed for macrodissected adult human *septum (Galen, c177)*; in the original French, *cloîson transparente*, p. 53.
36. *outer portion of corpus striatum (Reil, 1809b)*
Synonym for macrodissected adult human *lentiform nucleus (Burdach, 1822)*, according to Mayo's translation (1823, p. 79). Also see Meyer (1971, p. 29) and *external part of corpus striatum (Vicq d'Azyr, 1786)*.
37. *outer portion of cerebral ganglion (Reil, 1809b)*
Synonym for *outer portion of corpus striatum (Reil, 1809b)*; in the original German, *äussere Portion*, p. 144. Also see Meyer (1971, p. 29).
38. *lamina cribrosa (Reil, 1809b)*
Approximate synonym for macrodissected adult human *anterior perforated substance (Vicq d'Azyr, 1784)*; p. 199. The German, *Siebplatte*, was used in Reil (1812a, p. 92). Also see Mayo translation (1823, pp. 80, 108–109); Burdach (1822, p. 169), who referred to Vicq d'Azyr (1786, Pl. XVII, Fig. 1-*16*); and Foster (1892, p. 2108).
39. *cribriform plate (Reil, 1809b)*
Translation of *lamina cribrosa (Reil, 1809b)* provided in Meckel (1832, Vol. 2, p. 441), where he noted "This cribriform plate is formed almost entirely of gray substance."
40. *external gray matter mass of great superior cerebral ganglion (Gall & Spurzheim, 1810)*
Synonym for macrodissected adult human *external part of corpus striatum (Vicq d'Azyr, 1786)*; in the original French, *amas externe de substance grise du grand ganglion cerebral supérieur*; p. 279, see Burdach (1822, p. 351).
41. *oblong flat surface (Gordon, 1815)*
Apparently, synonym for macrodissected adult human *anterior perforated substance (Vicq d'Azyr, 1784)*; pp. 87–88.
42. *anterior cribriform plate (Meckel, 1817)*
Synonym for macrodissected adult human *anterior perforated substance (Vicq d'Azyr, 1784)*; see translation (1832, Vol. 2, p. 442).
43. *anterior perforated plate (Meckel, 1817)*
Synonym for macrodissected adult human *anterior perforated substance (Vicq d'Azyr, 1784)*; see translation (1832, Vol. 3, p. 2).
44. *lentiform nucleus (Burdach, 1822)*
As described for macrodissected adult human, the ***globus pallidus (Burdach, 1822)***, a part of the ***pallidum (Swanson, 2000a)***, and the ***putamen (Burdach, 1822)***, a part of the ***striatum (Swanson, 2000a)***; see Williams & Warwick (1980, pp. 1032–1033). For Burdach's use in macrodissected adult human, see p. 127. It was probably first identified as the *corpora striata inferiora exteriora posteriora (Vieussens, 1684)*.
45. *nucleus lentiformis (Burdach, 1822)*
Original Latin form of *lentiform nucleus (Burdach, 1822)*; p. 127, where the plural *nuclei lentiformes* was used.
46. *lenticular nucleus (Burdach, 1822)*
Alternate accepted translation of *nucleus lentiformis (Burdach, 1822)*; see *Terminologia Anatomica* (1998, p. 130).
47. *olfactory field (Serres, 1824–1826)*
Essentially a synonym for the macrodissected adult mammalian *anterior perforated substance (Vicq d'Azyr, 1784)*; in the original French, *champ olfactif*, Pl. IX, Figure 203-*K* and elsewhere.
48. *hemispheric tubercle (Serres, 1824–1826)*
In macrodissected adult bird, possible equivalent of mammalian *corpus striatum (Willis, 1664)*; in the original French, *tubercule hémisphérique*; Vol. 2, pp. 441–442. There, Serres also equated it with Haller's *innominé* [unnamed] tubercle (no citation), which Malacarne called *Haller's tubercle* (again no citation). Serres critically reviewed the literature on the topic since Collins (1685).
49. *cribriform plate of brain (Mayo, 1827)*
Synonym for macrodissected adult human *cribriform plate (Reil, 1809b)*; Plate VII, Figure 1-*a*.
50. *perforated lamina (Rolando, 1831)*
Rough synonym for macrodissected adult human *anterior perforated substance (Vicq d'Azyr, 1784)*; in the original Italian, *lamina perforata*, Figure 8-*g*.

51. *internal striated body (Rolando, 1831)*
    For macrodissected adult human, Rolando here used terms *internal striated body (Rolando, 1831)* and *external striated body (Rolando, 1831)* to label parts of *striated body (Willis, 1664)* lying essentially medial and lateral to ***internal capsule (Burdach, 1822)***, respectively. The former includes but is not necessarily restricted to ***caudate nucleus (Arnold, 1838b)***; Figure 9-*b*. The latter includes but is not necessarily restricted to *lenticular nucleus (Burdach, 1822)*; pp. 124–125, Figure 9-*d*.
52. *external striated body (Rolando, 1831)*
    For macrodissected adult human, Rolando here used terms *internal striated body (Rolando, 1831)* and *external striated body (Rolando, 1831)* to label parts of *striated body (Willis, 1664)* lying essentially medial and lateral to ***internal capsule (Burdach, 1822)***, respectively. The former includes but is not necessarily restricted to ***caudate nucleus (Arnold, 1838b)***; Figure 9-*b*. The latter includes but is not necessarily restricted to *lenticular nucleus (Burdach, 1822)*; pp. 116–118, Figure 9-*d*.
53. *perforated lamina of Meckel (Rolando, 1831)*
    Presumably eponym for *perforated lamina (Rolando, 1831)*; in the original Italian, *lamina perforata di Mekel*; Figure 9-*o,p*.
54. *lateral perforated substance (Arnold, 1834)*
    Synonym for macrodissected adult human *anterior perforated substance (Vicq d'Azyr, 1784)*; in the original Latin, *substantia perforata lateralis*, Table I: *D-bb*.
55. *septum inter ventriculos (Quain, 1834)*
    Synonym for macrodissected adult human *septum (Galen, c177)*; p. 693.
56. *septum of lateral ventricles (Cruveilhier, 1836)*
    Synonym for macrodissected adult human *septum (Galen, c177)*; in the original French, *cloîson des ventricules latéraux*, p. 693.
57. *pyriform protuberance (Owen, 1837)*
    For macrodissected nonhuman mammals, like opossum and wombat, essentially synonym for *anterior perforated substance (Vicq d'Azyr, 1784)*; p. 95 and Plate V-8,9-1*b*.
58. *lateral anterior perforated substance (Arnold, 1838a)*
    Synonym for macrodissected adult human *anterior perforated substance (Vicq d'Azyr, 1784)*; in the original Latin, *substantia perforata antica lateralis*, p. 49.
59. *septal region (Swanson & Cowan, 1979)*
    As described for macrodissected adult human, and with cellular architecture and connections for all mammals, an arbitrary set of ***central nervous system gray matter regions (>1840)*** in the ***cerebral nuclei (Swanson, 2000a)***, including the ***lateral septal complex (Risold & Swanson, 1997)*** and ***triangular nucleus of septum (Cajal, 1901–1902)***, which are part of the ***striatum (Swanson, 2000a)***, and the ***medial septal complex (Swanson et al., 1987)*** and ***bed nuclei of stria terminalis (Gurdjian, 1925)***, which are part of the ***pallidum (Swanson, 2000a)***; see Swanson (2000a).

cerebral nuclei corticospinal tract (>1840)

As described for macrodissected adult human, the rostral topographic segment of the ***corticospinal tract (>1840)*** in the ***cerebral nuclei (Swanson, 2000a)*** between ***cerebral cortex white matter (>1840)*** rostrally and ***interbrain corticospinal tract (>1840)*** segment caudally. It courses through the ***anterior limb of internal capsule (>1840)***, where it is centered medially and laterally and tends to avoid intermediate parts; see Williams & Warwick (1980, Fig. 7.154). Its existence was clearly described by Malpighi; see ***[cerebral nuclei corticospinal tract (>1840)] (Malpighi, 1666)***.

EARLIER REFERENCES:

Described, not named or illustrated:

1. *[cerebral nuclei corticospinal tract (>1840)] (Malpighi, 1666)*
   Malpighi clearly described the origin of "nerve fibers" in ***cerebral cortex (>1840)*** coursing through ***cerebral nuclei (Swanson, 2000a)*** and ending in ***spinal cord (Galen, c162–c166)***; see Meyer (1967, p. 189). He dissected a variety of mammals, including human, although source of this observation is unclear.

Illustrated and described, not named:

1. *[cerebral nuclei corticospinal tract (>1840)] (Vieussens, 1684)*
   Clearly illustrated and described for macrodissected adult human with a scraping method; see Table XVI.

cerebral peduncle (Tarin, 1753)

As described for macrodissected adult human and other mammals, the segment of the ***corticospinal tract (>1840)*** in the ventral part (base) of the ***tegmentum (Swanson, 2000b)*** of the ***midbrain (Baer, 1837)***, between ***interbrain corticospinal tract (>1840)*** rostrally and ***longitudinal pontine fibers (Arnold, 1838b)*** caudally. Historically, its use is complex. In Latin, *peduncle* is the diminutive of *pes*, or *foot* in English, and generally refers to structures resembling a stalk or stem. Tarin (1753, p. 25) referred to cerebral peduncles (original Latin, *pedunculi cerebri*) in briefly describing a *white substance (Vesalius, 1543a)* bundle, listing *crus medulla oblongata (Collins, 1685)* as a synonym, and Soemmerring (1778, Tab. II-*K*) referred to *pedunculi cerebri* (plural) similarly. Gordon (1815, p. 89) defined it very clearly as a ***central nervous system white matter tract (>1840)*** without *gray substance (Vesalius, 1543a)* like the ***substantia nigra (Soemmerring, 1791)***—the *basis pedunculi (Arnold, 1838b)*. "This thick bundle of white fibers emerging from the base of the brain is called the foot of the crus cerebri, pes pedunculi, or crusta" (Edinger, 1890, p. 85). More recently it was used in this way by Crosby et al. (1962, pp. 261–262) and Nauta & Feirtag (1986, Fig. 83), but not in the *Basel Nomina Anatomica* (His, 1895) or those following it, like Mettler (1948), Carpenter (1976), and Williams & Warwick (1980), where it essentially corresponds to ***tegmentum (Swanson, 2000b)***. It was perhaps first clearly delineated as the *cerebelli anterior pars (Casseri, 1609)*.

EARLIER REFERENCES:

Earlier synonyms:

1. *cerebelli anterior pars (Casseri, 1609)*
   Very clearly illustrated synonym for macrodissected adult human ***cerebral peduncle (Tarin, 1753)***; pp. 123–124, Table VII, Figure 2-*C*.
2. *tractus medullaris ex media ovalis centri regione educti (Vieussens, 1684)*
   Very clearly illustrated synonym for macrodissected adult human ***cerebral peduncle (Tarin, 1753)***, and described as *Tractus medullaris è media ovalis centri regione educti, qui ad anticam spinalis medullae partem tendunt*; Tables IV-*N*, XIV-*I*.
3. *tractus medullaris striatis ex corporibus mediis emergentes (Vieussens, 1684)*
   Synonym for macrodissected adult human ***cerebral peduncle (Tarin, 1753)***; in full, *Tractus medullaris striatis è corporibus mediis emergentes, qui spinalem versus medullam tendendo*, Table V-*L*.
4. *crus medulla oblongata (Collins, 1685)*
   Synonym for macrodissected adult human ***cerebral peduncle (Tarin, 1753)***, vaguely referred to thus: "The *Crura Medullae oblongatae* [plural], composed of several *Fasciculi* of nervous Fibres, which continued, makes the *Striae* in the *Corpus Striata*" (Tab. XLVIII-*KK*). In Latin, *crus* means leg (between knee and ankle) or a structure resembling a leg. Also see *crus cerebri (Haller, 1747)*.
5. *medullary part of crus medulla oblongata (Ridley, 1695)*
   Vague though specific reference to macrodissected adult human ***cerebral peduncle (Tarin, 1753)***; the ***interbrain (Baer, 1837)*** "lies upon, and is continuous to the subjacent medullary [fibrous] part of the *Crura Medulla Oblongata*" (p. 195); see *crus of medulla oblongata (Willis, 1664)*, *caudex medullaris (Ridley, 1695)*, and *crus cerebri (Haller, 1747)*.
6. *cerebellar process (Ridley, 1695)*
   May refer to macrodissected adult human *medullary part of crus medulla oblongata (Ridley, 1695)*; see Soemmerring (1778, p. 107) as quoted by Burdach (1822, p. 320).
7. *inferior part of medullary crura (Pourfour du Petit, 1710)*
   Clear reference to macrodissected adult human ***cerebral peduncle (Tarin, 1753)***; p. 14. Contrasted with *superior part of medullary crura (Pourfour du Petit, 1710)*. Pourfour du Petit did not use the term *cerebral peduncle*; see Clarke & O'Malley (1996, p. 283).
8. *brachia medulla oblongata (Winslow, 1733)*
   Synonym for macrodissected adult human ***cerebral peduncles (Tarin, 1753)***; Section X, p. 41.
9. *crus cerebri anteriora (Tarin, 1750)*
   Apparently synonym for macrodissected adult human ***cerebral peduncle (Tarin, 1753)***; Table I, Figure 4-*G*. Also see Tarin (1753, p. 25, under *protuberantia mammillares Santorini*).

LATER SYNONYMS:

1. *large branch of oblong medulla (Tarin, 1753)*
   Synonym for macrodissected adult human ***cerebral peduncle (Tarin, 1753)***; in the original French (plural), *les grosses Branches de la moëlle allongée*, p. 25.
2. *crus oblongata cerebri (Camper & Albinus, 1767)*
   Apparently synonym for macrodissected adult human ***cerebral peduncle (Tarin, 1753)***; p. 14, Figure 2-*d,e*.
3. *cerebral medullary process (Soemmerring, 1778)*
   Apparently synonym for macrodissected adult human ***cerebral peduncle (Tarin, 1753)***; in the original Latin, *processus medullae cerebri*, p. 31, see Burdach (1822, p. 321). Term also used thus by Günther (1786, p. 15) and Wenzel & Wenzel (1812, p. 203; Tab. XIV, Fig. 4-*d*; Tab. XV, Fig. 5-*e*).
4. *crurum cerebri pars ante nervos opticos locata (Soemmerring, 1778)*
   Roughly synonymous with macrodissected adult human ***cerebral peduncle (Tarin, 1753)***; according to Vicq d'Azyr (1786, p. 55).
5. *columna medullaris centralis cerebri (Malacarne, 1780)*
   Apparently synonym for macrodissected adult human ***cerebral peduncle (Tarin, 1753)***; p. 61, see Burdach (1822, p. 321).
6. *medullary part of cerebral peduncle (Vicq d'Azyr, 1786)*
   Synonym for macrodissected adult human ***cerebral peduncle (Tarin, 1753)***; Plate XXI, Figure I-*40*.
7. *cerebral crus (Günther, 1786)*
   Synonym for macrodissected adult human ***cerebral peduncle (Tarin, 1753)***; in the original Latin (plural), *crura cerebri*, p. 15.
8. *processus ad pontem Varolii (Günther, 1786)*
   Synonym for macrodissected adult human ***cerebral peduncle (Tarin, 1753)***; in the original Latin, *processus ad pontem Varolii*, p. 15.
9. *cerebral process (Mayer, 1794)*
   Synonym for macrodissected adult human ***cerebral peduncle (Tarin, 1753)***; in the original Latin, *processus cerebri*; Part 5, Table III, Figure 1-*k*.
10. *crura medullarica (Mayer, 1794)*
    Apparently synonym for macrodissected adult human ***cerebral peduncles (Tarin, 1753)***; Vol. 6, p. 174, see Burdach (1822, p. 321).
11. *anterior prolongation of cerebral protuberance (Bichat et al., 1801–1803)*
    Apparently roughly synonymous with macrodissected adult human ***cerebral peduncle (Tarin, 1753)***; p. 114.
12. *cerebral prolongation of cerebral protuberance (Bichat et al., 1801–1803)*
    Synonym for *anterior prolongation of cerebral protuberance (Bichat et al., 1801–1803)*; p. 113.
13. *anterior branches of cerebrum (Chaussier, 1807)*
    Synonym listed for macrodissected adult human ***cerebral peduncles (Tarin, 1753)***; in the original French, *les branches antérieures du cerveau*, p. 43.
14. *anterior arms of cerebrum (Chaussier, 1807)*
    Synonym listed for macrodissected adult human ***cerebral peduncles (Tarin, 1753)***; in the original French, *les bras antérieures du cerveau*, p. 43.

15. *anterior legs of cerebrum (Chaussier, 1807)*
Synonym listed for macrodissected adult human ***cerebral peduncles (Tarin, 1753)***; in the original French, *les jambes antérieures du cerveau*, p. 43.
16. *brachia cerebri (Chaussier, 1807)*
Synonym listed for macrodissected adult human ***cerebral peduncles (Tarin, 1753)***; p. 43.
17. *femora cerebri (Chaussier, 1807)*
Synonym listed for macrodissected adult human ***cerebral peduncles (Tarin, 1753)***; p. 43.
18. *processus cerebri ad pontem varolii (Chaussier, 1807)*
Synonym listed for macrodissected adult human ***cerebral peduncle (Tarin, 1753)***; p. 43.
19. *processus cerebri ad medullam oblongatam (Chaussier, 1807)*
Synonym listed for macrodissected adult human ***cerebral peduncle (Tarin, 1753)***; p. 43.
20. *crus descendens cerebri (Chaussier, 1807)*
Synonym listed for macrodissected adult human ***cerebral peduncle (Tarin, 1753)***; p. 43.
21. *crust of crus cerebri (Reil, 1809b)*
Synonym for macrodissected adult human ***cerebral peduncle (Tarin, 1753)***, also synonymous with *basis pedunculi (Arnold, 1838b)*; see Mayo translation (1823, p. 56). The original German terms used by Reil (1809b, p. 150) were *Grundfläche* for *base*, and *Hirnschenkel* for *crus cerebri*.
22. *base of crus cerebri (Reil, 1809b)*
English form of German terms used by Reil (1809b, p. 150): *base* for *Grundfläche*, and *crus cerebri* for *Hirnschenkel*. See *crust of crus cerebri (Reil, 1809b)*, *base of cerebral peduncle (Meckel, 1817)*, and Schwalbe (1881, p. 450).
23. *basis crus cerebri (Reil, 1809b)*
Latin form of *base of crus cerebri (Reil, 1809b)*; also see Schwalbe (1881, p. 450).
24. *great fiber tract of hemisphere (Gall & Spurzheim, 1810)*
Synonym for macrodissected adult human ***cerebral peduncle (Tarin, 1753)***; in the original French (plural), *les grands faisceaux fibreux des hemisphères*, p. 195, see Burdach (1822, p. 321).
25. *crus of true olfactory nerve ganglia (Carus, 1814)*
Synonym for macrodissected adult fish ***cerebral peduncle (Tarin, 1753)***; in the original German, *Schenkel der wahren Riechnervenganglien*, Table 2-*ξ*.
26. *peduncle of brain proper (Gordon, 1815)*
Synonym for macrodissected adult human ***cerebral peduncle (Tarin, 1753)***; pp. 88, 132.
27. *anterior peduncles of cerebral protuberance (Cloquet, 1816)*
Synonym for macrodissected adult human ***cerebral peduncles (Tarin, 1753)***; in the original French, *pédoncules antérieurs de la protubérance cérébrale*, p. 532.
28. *base of cerebral peduncle (Meckel, 1817)*
Synonym for macrodissected adult human ***cerebral peduncle (Tarin, 1753)***; see translation (1832, Vol. 2, p. 467).
29. *hemispheric crus (Rolando, 1819)*
Synonym for macrodissected adult human ***cerebral peduncle (Tarin, 1753)***; in the original Latin (plural), *hemisphaeriorum crura*, Part 2, p. 4.
30. *peduncles of hemispheres (Rolando, 1825a)*
Synonym for macrodissected adult human ***cerebral peduncles (Tarin, 1753)***; in the original French, *péduncles des hémisphères*, Table I, Figure 1-*p.e.*
31. *peduncles of brain (Spurzheim, 1826)*
Synonym for macrodissected adult human ***cerebral peduncles (Tarin, 1753)***; p. 230 note *g*.
32. *superficial stratum of crus cerebri (Mayo, 1827)*
Synonym for macrodissected adult human ***cerebral peduncle (Tarin, 1753)***; Plate V-*b*.
33. *crura of brain (Swan, 1830)*
English form of *crura cerebri (Chaussier, 1807)*; Plate X, Figure 1-*G*. Swan also gave singular, *crus of brain*; Plate X, Figure 2-*B*.
34. *medullary processes of brain (Knox, 1832)*
English form (plural) of *cerebral medullary process (Soemmerring, 1778)*; Supplemental Plate IV-*16*.
35. *anterior peduncles (Cruveilhier, 1836)*
Synonym for macrodissected adult human ***cerebral peduncles (Tarin, 1753)***; in the original French, *pédoncules antérieurs*, p. 603.
36. *processus medullae oblongatae ad cerebrum (Cruveilhier, 1836)*
Synonym listed for macrodissected adult human ***cerebral peduncles (Tarin, 1753)***; p. 605.
37. *base of peduncle (Arnold, 1838b)*
Synonym for macrodissected adult human ***cerebral peduncle (Tarin, 1753)***; Plate III, Figure 1-*i*.
38. *basis pedunculi (Arnold, 1838b)*
Original Latin form of *base of peduncle (Arnold, 1838a)*; Plate III, Figure 1-*i*. See Ranson (1920, p. 158) for clarification and *base of cerebral peduncle (Meckel, 1817)*.

cerebral sulci (Vesalius, 1543a)

The grooves of various depths associated with the surface of the macrodissected adult vertebrate ***cerebral cortex gray matter (>1840)***; see Carpenter (1976, p. 22), Williams & Warwick (1980, pp. 982–984), *Terminologia Anatomica* (1998, p. 124). Contrast with ***cerebellar fissures (>1840)***. For Vesalius's use in macrodissected adult human and a variety of other mammals, including donkey, see Singer translation (1952, p. 24). They were written about very long ago; see ***[cerebral sulci (Vesalius, 1543a)] (Smith Papyrus, c1700 BC)***.

EARLIER REFERENCES:

Described, not named or illustrated:

1. ***[cerebral sulci (Vesalius, 1543a)] (Smith Papyrus, c1700 BC)***
By describing adult human *cerebral convolutions (Smith Papyrus, c1700 BC)*, ***cerebral sulci (Vesalius, 1543)*** in between were observed.

Earlier synonyms:

1. *grooves (Massa, 1536)*
Synonym for macrodissected adult human ***cerebral sulci (Vesalius, 1543a)***, described as *grooves (Massa, 1536)* or "sinuous depressions"; see Lind translation (1975, p. 237).

LATER SYNONYMS:

1. *recesses (Vesalius, 1543a)*
   Synonym for ***cerebral sulci (Vesalius, 1543a)***; see Singer translation (1952, p. 24).
2. *sinuses (Vesalius, 1543a)*
   Synonym for adult mammalian ***cerebral sulci (Vesalius, 1543a)***; see Richardson & Carman translation (2009, p. 183).
3. *circular ruts (Bauhin, 1605)*
   Synonym for macrodissected adult human ***cerebral sulci (Vesalius, 1543a)***; p. 575, see Crooke translation (1615, p. 456).
4. *chinks (Willis, 1664)*
   In this context a synonym for ***cerebral sulci (Vesalius, 1543a)***; see Pordage translation (1681, p. 60).
5. *streaks (Winslow, 1733)*
   Synonym for macrodissected adult human ***cerebral sulci (Vesalius, 1543a)***; Section X, p. 33.
6. *furrows (Winslow, 1733)*
   Synonym for macrodissected adult human ***cerebral sulci (Vesalius, 1543a)***; Section X, p. 33.
7. *fossulas (Soemmerring, 1778)*
   Latin synonym (diminutive of *fossa*) listed for macrodissected adult human ***cerebral sulci (Vesalius, 1543a)***; p. 31.
8. *anfractus (Vicq d'Azyr, 1786)*
   Synonym specifically for ***cerebral sulcus (Vesalius, 1543a)***; see dictionary on p. 57. Also see Haase (1781, p. 14), *Oxford English Dictionary* (Online).
9. *fossae (Gordon, 1815)*
   Synonym for macrodissected adult human ***cerebral sulci (Vesalius, 1543a)***; p. 86.

cerebrospinal axis (Meckel, 1817)

In popular usage, a gross anatomy topographic division corresponding to the vertebrate ***central nervous system (Carus, 1814)***, although in fact it applies more generally to the chordate ***central nervous system (Carus, 1814)***, a hollow tubular division of the ***nervous system (Monro, 1783)*** lying in the median plane, dorsal to the notochord, and flanked by a bilateral series of segmental muscles; see Nieuwenhuys (2002). Since Classical Antiquity at least six fundamentally different ways to divide the ***cerebrospinal axis (Meckel, 1817)*** have been used, although today there is rather broad consensus about a set of major topographic divisions arranged in a hierarchical parceling scheme that is based primarily on structural differentiation of the ***neural tube (Baer, 1837)*** culminating with adult macrostructure or gross anatomy; see Swanson (2000b), and Swanson & Bota (2010) for this precise definition. At the systems architecture level, the ***cerebrospinal axis (Meckel, 1817)*** consists of ***central nervous system gray matter regions (>1840)*** and ***central nervous system white matter tracts (>1840)***. For Meckel's use in macrodissected adult human, see translation (1832, Vol. 2, p. 410). It was known to Herophilus; see ***[cerebrospinal axis (Meckel, 1817)] (Herophilus, c335–c280 BC)***. It is used interchangeably with vertebrate ***central nervous system (Carus, 1814)***.

EARLIER REFERENCES:

Described, not named or illustrated:

1. ***[cerebrospinal axis (Meckel, 1817)] (Herophilus, c335–c280 BC)***
   Known in macrodissected adult human; see von Staden (1989, p. 159).

cerebrospinal fluid (Magendie, 1827)

In vertebrate, the watery fluid contained within the ***ventricles (Hippocrates)*** and ***subarachnoid space (Magendie, 1827)*** produced by the ***choroid plexuses (Galen, c177)*** and ***central nervous system (Carus, 1814)*** parenchyma and finally absorbed into the venous system; see Millen & Woollam (1962). Malpighi believed the ***ventricles (Hippocrates)*** were filled with air forcing the spirits into the substance of the ***brain (Smith Papyrus, c1700 BC)***; see Bell & Bell (1829, p. 415). For Magendie's use in macrodissected adult human and vertebrate generally, see p. 2. Cotunio (1764) is often credited with first clearly describing it; see Todd (1845, p. 39).

TRANSLATIONS:

1. *liquide céphalo-spinal (Magendie, 1827)*
   Original French form of ***cerebrospinal fluid (Magendie, 1827)***; p. 2.
2. *liquide céphalo-rachidien (Magendie, 1827)*
   Original French form of ***cerebrospinal fluid (Magendie, 1827)***; p. 2.

EARLIER REFERENCES:

Described, not named or illustrated:

1. ***[cerebrospinal fluid (Magendie, 1827)] (Smith Papyrus, c1700 BC)***
   The Edwin Smith Surgical Papyrus may refer to fluid surrounding ***brain (Smith Papyrus, c1700 BC)***, see Breasted (1930, pp. 171–172), that is, in ***subarachnoid space (Magendie, 1827)***. There is no clear reference to ***cerebrospinal fluid (Magendie, 1827)*** in Galen or other ancient writers, except for vague references to watery or moist humors; see Millen & Woollam (1962, p. 1), Clarke & O'Malley (1996, p. 721).
2. ***[cerebrospinal fluid (Magendie, 1827)] (Berengario da Carpi, 1521)***
   Vague reference made to it; see Clarke & O'Malley (1996, p. 721).
3. ***[cerebrospinal fluid (Magendie, 1827)] (de Laguna, 1535)***
   De Laguna wrote that ***lateral ventricles (Vesalius, 1543a)*** "seem to be pools of the clearest water..." (Lind translation, 1975, p. 289), and Massa (1536) provided a similar, even clearer, description; see Lind translation (1975, p. 237). Vesalius very clearly described fluid throughout ***ventricles (Hippocrates)*** and ***subarachnoid space (Magendie, 1827)***; see Richardson & Carman translation (2009, p. 197) for the former and Singer translation (1952, p. 17) for the latter.

PARTLY CORRESPONDS:

1. *ventricular fluid (Cruveilhier, 1836)*
   In macrodissected adult human, ***cerebrospinal fluid (Magendie, 1827)*** contained within ***ventricles***

(Hippocrates); in the original French, *liquide ventriculaire*, p. 701.

cerebrospinal trunk (>1840)

A topographic division of the vertebrate ***central nervous system (Carus, 1814)*** or ***cerebrospinal axis (Meckel, 1817)*** consisting of ***brainstem (Schwalbe, 1881)*** rostrally and ***spinal cord (Galen, c162–c166)*** caudally. In this grouping of basic parts, the vertebrate ***central nervous system (Carus, 1814)*** has three main topographic divisions: ***cerebrospinal trunk (>1840), cerebrum (Obersteiner & Hill, 1900)*** or ***endbrain (Kuhlenbeck, 1927)***, and ***cerebellum (Aristotle)***. For these definitions see Swanson & Bota (2010).

PARTLY CORRESPONDS:

1. *dorsal medulla (Vesalius, 1543a)*
Vesalius included ***pons (Haller, 1747), medulla (Winslow, 1733)*** [see *origin of dorsal medulla (Vesalius, 1543a)*] and ***spinal cord (Galen, c162–c166)*** in macrodissected adult human *dorsal medulla (Vesalius, 1543a)*, or *spinal marrow (Vesalius, 1543a)*, because of the large paired ***nerves (Herophilus, c335–c280 BC)*** arising from the whole structure. For Vesalius, ***cerebellum (Aristotle)*** arises from *spinal marrow (Vesalius, 1543a)*; see Singer translation (1952, pp. 21, 22, 27, 36, 46–47), Richardson & Carman translation (2002, pp. 205, 176–177). He wrote, "The spinal marrow may in fact be regarded as a second brain for all parts of the body below the head..." (Richardson & Carman translation, 2002, p. 221); and further on, "There is only one spinal marrow because the area of the brain from which it takes origin is single and simple." (Richardson & Carman translation, 2002, p. 222); also see *second brain (Galen c173)*.
2. *spinal marrow (Vesalius, 1543a)*
Synonym for *dorsal medulla (Vesalius, 1543a)*; see Richardson & Carman translation (2002, pp. 176–177), also see *spinal marrow proper (Vesalius, 1543a)*.
3. *marrow of back (Geminus, 1553)*
Translation of macrodissected adult human *spinal marrow (Vesalius, 1543a)*, in the original spelling, *marye of the backe*; see *The table of the figure of synowes*.
4. *cerebrum longum (Colombo, 1559)*
Synonym for *cerebrum oblongatum (Colombo, 1559)*; Book VIII, Ch. 4, p. 199; see Burdach (1819, p. 229).
5. *cerebrum oblongatum (Colombo, 1559)*
The macrodissected adult human *spinal marrow (Colombo, 1559)* is simply a long brain (*cerebrum oblongatum*) with a double beginning, the larger from the *cerebrum (Colombo, 1559)* and the smaller from the ***cerebellum (Aristotle)***, which actually is forked, with right and left parts. The English form, *long brain (Crooke, 1615)*, begins a little behind the *optic nerves (Galen, c173)* and so probably includes roughly ***midbrain (Baer, 1837), pons (Haller, 1747)***, and ***medulla (Winslow, 1733)***, as well as ***spinal cord (Galen, c162–c166)***; p. 187 ff. Colombo also countered Galen by stating that no ***nerves (Herophilus, c335–c280 BC)*** arise from ***cerebellum (Aristotle)***; see Bauhin (1605, p. 628) and Crooke (1615, pp. 480, 494). Also see *long brain (Benedetti, 1502), anterior spinal marrow (Varoli, 1573)*.
6. *spinal marrow (Colombo, 1559)*
He used the term, at least sometimes, synonymously with *cerebrum oblongatum (Colombo, 1559)*; in the original Latin, *spinalis medulla*, p. 187 ff. and Bannister (1578, f. 106v). Varoli (1573, Fig. 2-1,2,3 on f. 19) also used *spinal marrow* to include ***midbrain (Baer, 1837), pons (Haller, 1747), medulla (Winslow, 1733)***, and ***spinal cord (Galen, c162–c166)***. However, he did distinguish an *anterior spinal marrow (Varoli, 1573)*, which includes roughly ***midbrain (Baer, 1837), pons (Haller, 1747)***, and ***medulla (Winslow, 1733)***. He wrote that four roots—pairs of ***cerebral peduncles (Tarin, 1753)*** and ***cerebellar peduncles (Ridley, 1695)***—issue from the *cerebrum (Colombo, 1559)* and ***cerebellum (Aristotle)*** to make one notable *trunk (Varoli, 1573)* called the *spinal marrow (Varoli, 1573)* and issues ***nerves (Herophilus, c335–c280 BC)*** to all parts of the body, a view shared by du Laurens, who wrote that the *spinal marrow (Varoli, 1573)* is like a *stem (du Laurens, 1600)* arising from the four roots; Bauhin (1605, p. 628), Crooke (1615, pp. 480, 494). Bauhin (1605, p. 685), as translated by Crook (1615, p. 494), explained Varoli's view as follows: "Now the originall of the spinall marrow was to bee out of the middle part of the Braine, because through it as it were through a common water-course the spirits which are perfected in the middest of the Braine were to be derived into other Riverets and so into the whole body. Wherefore their beginning was to bee placed in the center of the Braine neere the Store-house or shop of the spirits, whence they might receive them as it were with a ful steame; like as Anatomy teacheth us, that the Arteries and the Veines do arise out of the middle of the Heart and the Liver [going back to Plato and Galen]." This view was stated more succinctly by Poupart (1712, p. 644) near the beginning of the 18th century: "The Cerebel and Brain [*cerebrum (Willis, 1664)*] are both plac'd and supported on the Medulla Oblongata [of *(Willis, 1664)*], or rather they are only principal Branches of this great Trunk, while the Nerves are the lesser ones." Varoli also believed that the ***inferior colliculi (Haller, 1762)*** contribute to the cerebellar roots, whereas the ***superior colliculi (Haller, 1762)*** contribute to the cerebral roots; see Crooke (1615, p. 499).
7. *caudex cerebri (Coiter, 1572)*
Synonym for *spinal marrow (Vesalius, 1543a), brain trunk (Coiter, 1572)*, or *brain stem (Coiter, 1572)*; see translation (1955, p. 112), also see Foster (1892, p. 875).
8. *brain stem (Coiter, 1572)*
English form of *caudex cerebri (Coiter, 1572)*; see translation (1955, p. 113).
9. *brain trunk (Coiter, 1572)*
Alternate English form of *brain stem (Coiter, 1572)*; see *Cassell's Concise Latin-English, English-Latin Dictionary* (1979).

10. *trunk (Varoli, 1573)*
Description of *spinal marrow (Varoli, 1573)*, roughly ***cerebrospinal trunk (>1840)***, without ***interbrain (Baer, 1837)***; in the original Latin, *truncorum spinalis medullae*; f. 6v, 7; see Bauhin (1605, p. 628) and Crooke (1615, pp. 480, 494).
11. *cerebrum elongatum (Bannister, 1578)*
Synonym for macrodissected adult human *cerebrum oblongatum (Colombo, 1559)*; f. 106v.
12. *medulla oblongata (Piccolomini, 1586)*
Shortened version of macrodissected adult human *medulla vero cerebri oblongata (Bauhin, 1605)*; ***medulla (Winslow, 1733)*** and ***spinal cord (Galen, c162–c166)*** considered together; p. 259. Illustrated in Piccolomini's schematic midsagittal drawing of the ***brain (Smith Papyrus, c1700 BC)***; p. 265, see Clarke and Dewhurst (1996, Fig. 88-*E,F*). He basically regarded ***spinal cord (Galen, c162–c166)*** as arising from *medulla globosa (Piccolomini, 1586)*; see Bauhin (1605, p. 628), Crooke (1615, p. 480). Also see *medulla (Piccolomini, 1586)*, *medulla globosa (Piccolomini, 1586)*, and *intracranial medulla oblongata (Piccolomini, 1586)*—the ***medulla (Winslow, 1733)***. *Oblongata* is Latin feminine of *oblongatus*, variously translated as "rather long" (*Stedman's Medical Dictionary*, 22nd Ed., 1972) or literally "prolonged" (*Oxford English Dictionary* Online).
13. *stem (du Laurens, 1600)*
Synonym for macrodissected adult human *trunk (Varoli, 1573)*; see Bauhin (1605, p. 628), Crooke (1615, p. 480).
14. *medulla vero cerebri oblongata (Bauhin, 1605)*
Basically, macrodissected adult human ***medulla (Winslow, 1733)*** and ***spinal cord (Galen, c162–c166)*** considered together. In explaining *medulla (Piccolomini, 1586)*, Bauhin wrote, "The marrow it selfe [*medulla vero (Bauhin, 1605)*, as opposed to ***cerebral cortex gray matter (>1840)***] may be said to be double—one Globous or round, the other Long. The Globous part [*medulla globosa (Bauhin, 1605)*] which is like the figure of the Scull, is of a great bulke and therein are ventricles excavated or hollowed. At this and continuall with it hangeth the other called *Cerebellum*...The Long Marrow of the Braine [*medulla vero cerebri oblongata (Bauhin 1605)*] which is like a Pith [*pith* used for *spinal marrow (Varoli, 1573)* since at least 1594, see *Oxford English Dictionary* (Online), and *pith (Crooke, 1615)*] or staff may bee divided into that part which is contained within the Scull [*medulla oblongata intracranium (Bauhin 1605)*], and that which is yssued out which properly is called the spinall marrow [*spinalis medullae proprie (Bauhin 1605)*]; although some there are that give this name [*spinal marrow, Spinalis medullae*] unto all the Long marrow of the Braine [e.g., see *long brain (Benedetti, 1502)*, *cerebrum oblongatum (Colombo, 1559)*, *medulla oblongata (Piccolomini, 1586)*] as well within the Scull as without..." (pp. 605–608; see Crooke translation, 1615, p. 479). This is one of the most difficult passages in the literature on neuroanatomical nomenclature. Eighty years later, Collins (1685, p. 1070) wrote, "...but Use being the great Master and Arbitrator of Language, I will take the freedom to keep the old appellative, as best understood; so that the *Medulla Spinalis*, or *Cerebrum elongatum* [*medulla vero cerebri oblongata (Bauhin, 1605)*] being a continuation of the *Medulla oblongata*, to its Origen is derived thence as being a Neck, or long Process of it; but as *Bauhinus* will have it [*anterior spinal marrow (Varoli, 1573)*], it is made up of Four orbicular Processes, the two greater proceed from the anterior part of the Brain, and the other lesser ones from the interior part of the *Cerebellum*, which are united in the *Medulla Spinalis*, contained within the Skull."
15. *medulla spinalis (Bauhin, 1605, p. 628)*
Macrodissected adult human ***medulla (Winslow, 1733)*** and ***spinal cord (Galen, c162–c166)*** considered together; p. 628. Another meaning is the *medulla (Piccolomini, 1586)*; as Bauhin explained (p. 625), "Now there is a double acceptation of the Spinall marrow, for in the larger signification it signifieth the whole marrow of the Brain lengthened out [*totam cerebri medullam oblongatam (Bauhin, 1605)*], one part whereof is yet contained in the Scull the other continuall with the former issueth at the great hole of the Nowle-bone [occipital bone] and desceendeth to the very end of the ridge. ¶ But in a strict and more proper acceptation it betokeneth that part of the marrow which without the skull is contayned in all the racke-bones or vertebrae of the spin or chine. Wherefore that it may bee free from all ambiguity, the history thereof is on this manner" (see Crooke translation, 1615, p. 479). Other people, Bauhin continued (p. 628), use the term *medulla spinalis* to mean the *medulla oblongata (Piccolomini, 1586)*; that is, ***medulla (Winslow, 1733)*** and ***spinal cord (Galen, c162–c166)*** considered together; see Crooke translation (1615, p. 479), where it is spelled *spinall marrow*. This latter basic usage was followed, for example, by Soemmerring (1778, p. 180; 1791, p. 56 ff.; 1798, p. 42) and Bell (1802, Pl. VII-*10*).
16. *dorsal marrow (Bauhin, 1605)*
Bauhin wrote that some people use it in referring to *medulla oblongata (Piccolomini, 1586)*; in the original Latin, *dorsalem medullam*, p. 628.
17. *long marrow of brain (Crooke, 1615)*
English form of *medulla vero cerebri oblongata (Bauhin, 1605)*, which more accurately could have been *true long marrow of brain* or *whole long marrow of brain*; p. 479.
18. *long marrow (Crooke, 1615)*
English form of *medulla oblongata (Piccolomini, 1586)*; p. 479.
19. *pith (Crooke, 1615)*
Synonym for macrodissected adult human *medulla oblongata (Piccolomini, 1586)* and *spinal marrow (Bauhin, 1605)*—***medulla (Winslow, 1733)*** and ***spinal cord (Galen, c162–c166)*** considered together; p. 479, also see Diemerbroeck (1689, p. 405).
20. *staff (Crooke, 1615)*
Synonym for *pith (Crooke, 1615)*; p. 479.
21. *spinal marrow (Crooke, 1615)*

Translation of *medulla spinalis (Bauhin, 1605)*, most commonly referring to ***medulla (Winslow, 1733)*** and ***spinal cord (Galen, c162–c166)*** considered together; p. 479.

22. *long brain (Crooke, 1615)*
English form of *cerebrum oblongatum (Colombo, 1559)*; p. 480.
23. *cerebrum elongatum (Collins, 1685)*
Apparently synonym for *medulla vero cerebri oblongata (Bauhin, 1605)*; p. 1070.
24. *spinal cord (Gordon, 1815)* Synonym for macrodissected adult human ***medulla (Winslow, 1733)*** and ***spinal cord (Galen, c162–c166)*** considered together; p. 79.
25. *central column of spinal cord (Gordon, 1815)*
Refers generally to ***central nervous system gray matter regions (>1840)*** of macrodissected adult human ***spinal cord (Galen, c162–c166)*** and caudal half of ***medulla (Winslow, 1733)***, consisting of *greyish-brown matter (Gordon, 1815)*; p. 183.
26. *vertebral marrow (Cloquet, 1816)*
Synonym for macrodissected adult human *spinal marrow (Crooke, 1615)*; in the original French, *moelle vertébrale*, p. 538.

cerebrum (Obersteiner & Hill, 1900)

Synonym for ***endbrain (Kuhlenbeck, 1927)***. Both terms are equally acceptable. Used in this sense by, for example, Williams & Warwick (1975, p. 805), *Nomina Anatomica* (1983, p. A70), Nauta & Feirtag (1986, p. 43), *Terminologia Anatomica* (1998, p. 124), Nieuwenhuys et al. (2008, p. 5, Fig. 1.2).

cervical branch of facial nerve (>1840)

As described for macrodissected adult human, the most ventral terminal branch of the ***facial nerve trunk (>1840)*** mainly innervating the platysma muscle; see Williams & Warwick (1980, p. 1072 and Fig. 7.186), *Terminologia Anatomica* (1998, p. 135). It was known to Galen; see ***[cervical branch of facial nerve (>1840)] (Galen, c173)***.

TRANSLATIONS:

1. *ramus colli nervi facialis (>1840)*
Current Latin form of ***cervical branch of facial nerve (>1840)***; see *Terminologia Anatomica* (1998, p. 135).

EARLIER REFERENCES:

Described, not named or illustrated:

1. ***[cervical branch of facial nerve (>1840)] (Galen, c173)***
Described for macrodissected adult beef, pig, and/or macaque but not human; see May translation (1962, pp. 700–701), Duckworth translation (1962, pp. 202, 225, 233, 237). Winslow (1733, Sect. VI, p. 70) briefly mentioned it for macrodissected adult human.

Illustrated, not named or described:

1. ***[cervical branch of facial nerve (>1840)] (Eustachi, 1552)***
Illustrated for macrodissected adult human; see Albinus edition (1761, Tab. 21, last branch below *f*).

Earlier synonyms:

1. *posterior subcutaneous branch of hard nerve (Meckel, 1753)*
Synonym for macrodissected adult human ***cervical branch of facial nerve (>1840)***; in the original French, *le rameau postérieur sous-cutané de l'inferior du nerf dur*, p. 92.
2. *posterior branch of inferior branch of hard nerve (Meckel, 1753)*
Synonym for *posterior subcutaneous branch of hard nerve (Meckel, 1753)*; in the original French, *le rameau postérieur de l'inferior du nerf dur*, p. 95.
3. *subcutaneous branch of neck of inferior branch of anterior branch of hard nerve (Loder, 1778)*
Synonym for macrodissected adult human ***cervical branch of facial nerve (>1840)***; in the original Latin, *subcutaneus colli*, p. 27.
4. *superior subcutaneous branch of neck of descending branch of superficial branch of hard nerve (Günther, 1786)*
Synonym for macrodissected adult human ***cervical branch of facial nerve (>1840)***; in the original Latin, *subcutaneum colli superiorem*, p. 60.
5. *sub-mentonniar branches of facial nerve (Burdin, 1803)*
Synonym for macrodissected adult human ***cervical branch of facial nerve (>1840)***; see translation (1803, Vol. 1, p. 180).
6. *submental branch of facial nerve (Burdin, 1803)*
English form of original French, *R. sous-mentonnier*; see *sub-mentonniar branches of facial nerve (Burdin, 1803)*.
7. *superior cutaneous submaxillary nerves (Meckel, 1817)*
Synonym for macrodissected adult human ***cervical branch of facial nerve (>1840)***; see translation (1832, Vol. 3, p. 57).
8. *subcutaneous branch of neck of hard nerve (Cloquet, 1828)*
Synonym for macrodissected adult human ***cervical branch of facial nerve (>1840)***; in the original French, *rameau sous-cutané du col*, Plate 157-74.
9. *subcutaneous cervical branch of portio dura (Knox, 1832)*
Apparently synonym for macrodissected adult human ***cervical branch of facial nerve (>1840)***; Plate III-g, in Knox's translation of Scarpa (1794).
10. *superior subcutaneous nerve of neck (Arnold, 1834)*
Synonym for macrodissected adult human ***cervical branch of facial nerve (>1840)***; in the original Latin, *nervus subcutaneus colli superior*, p. 12.
11. *cervical branches of cervicofacial branch of facial nerve (Cruveilhier, 1836)*
Synonym for macrodissected adult human ***cervical branch of facial nerve (>1840)***; in the original French, *rameaux cervicaux*, p. 947.

PARTLY CORRESPONDS:

1. *superior subcutaneous cervical nerves (Meckel, 1753)*
Branches of macrodissected adult human ***cervical branch of facial nerve (>1840)***, the *posterior subcutaneous branch of hard nerve (Meckel, 1753)*; in the original French, *les sous-cutanés supérieurs du col*, pp. 95–96. For Latin (*nervi subcutanei colli superiores*) and English forms see Meckel (1832, Vol. 3, p. 57). Meckel (1753) described three such ***nerves (Herophilus, c335–c280***

BC); pp. 95–96, Table 1:250–252. Also see Mayer (1794; Part 5, Tab. VII:*175–177*, p. 52), who called them anterior, middle, and posterior. Also see Bock (1827; Tab. V, Fig. 1-3).

2. *superior cutaneous cervical nerves (Meckel, 1753)*
   Synonym for *superior subcutaneous cervical nerves (Meckel, 1753)*; in the original French, *les cutanés supérieurs du col*, Table 1-246,262. Also see Bock (1827, Tab. III-6), *nerv. cutaneus colli superior*.
3. *superior cutaneous cervical branches of inferior branch of hard nerve (Meckel, 1753)*
   Synonym for *superior subcutaneous cervical nerves (Meckel, 1753)*; in the original French, *les cutanés supérieurs du col*, Table 1:250–252.
4. *submental nerve (Loder, 1778)*
   Branch of macrodissected adult human ***cervical branch of facial nerve (>1840)***; in the original Latin, *nervum submentalem*, p. 27.
5. *superior subcutaneous surculus of inferior branch of portio major and minor of facial nerve (Bellingeri, 1818)*
   Macrodissected adult human dorsal branch of ***cervical branch of facial nerve (>1840)***; in the original Latin, *surculus subcutaneus superior*, see Table II.
6. *superior subcutaneous surculus of cervico-facial branch of portio major and minor of facial nerve (Bellingeri, 1818)*
   Synonym for *superior subcutaneous surculus of inferior branch of portio major and minor of facial nerve (Bellingeri, 1818)*; in the original Latin, *surculus subcutaneus superior*, see Table II.
7. *middle subcutaneous surculus of inferior branch of portio major and minor of facial nerve (Bellingeri, 1818)*
   Macrodissected adult human intermediate branch of ***cervical branch of facial nerve (>1840)***; in the original Latin, *surculus subcutaneus medius*, see Table II.
8. *middle subcutaneous surculus of cervico-facial branch of portio major and minor of facial nerve (Bellingeri, 1818)*
   Synonym for *middle subcutaneous surculus of inferior branch of portio major and minor of facial nerve (Bellingeri, 1818)*; in the original Latin, *surculus subcutaneus medius*, see Table II.
9. *inferior subcutaneous surculus of inferior branch of portio major and minor of facial nerve (Bellingeri, 1818)*
   Macrodissected adult human ventral branch of ***cervical branch of facial nerve (>1840)***; in the original Latin, *surculus subcutaneus inferior*, see Table II.
10. *inferior subcutaneous surculus of cervico-facial branch of portio major and minor of facial nerve (Bellingeri, 1818)*
    Synonym for *inferior subcutaneous surculus of inferior branch of portio major and minor of facial nerve (Bellingeri, 1818)*; in the original Latin, *surculus subcutaneus inferior*, see Table II.
11. *twigs of superior subcutaneous nerve of neck to platysma muscle (Arnold, 1834)*
    Macrodissected adult human small branches of ***cervical branch of facial nerve (>1840)*** to platysma muscle; in the original Latin, *surculi nervus subcutaneus colli superior ad musculum platysmamyoiden*, Table IX:*VII-36*.

cervical enlargement (Arnold, 1838b)

As described for macrodissected adult human, the ***spinal cord differentiation (>1840)*** associated with attachment of the ***spinal nerves (Camper, 1760–1762)*** to the arms, most commonly from the 3rd ***cervical nerve (Galen, c173)*** to the 2nd ***thoracic nerve (Diemerbroeck, 1672)***; see Carpenter (1976, Fig. 9.1), *Terminologia Anatomica* (1998, p. 105), *Dorland's* (2003, p. 947). For Arnold's use in macrodissected adult human see Table I, Figure 2-*t*. It was first clearly distinguished by Estienne; see ***[cervical enlargement (Arnold, 1838b)] (Estienne, 1545)***.

TRANSLATIONS:

1. *intumescentia cervicalis (Arnold, 1838b)*
   Original Latin form of ***cervical enlargement (Arnold, 1838b)***; Table I, Figure 2-*t*.

EARLIER REFERENCES:

Illustrated, not named or described:

1. *[cervical enlargement (Arnold, 1838b)] (Estienne, 1545)*
   Very clearly illustrated for macrodissected adult human; p. 338. According to Diemerbroeck (1689, p. 406), Falloppio (1561) described it, and Willis (1664) certainly described it; for the latter see Pordage translation (1681, pp. 124–125).

Earlier synonyms:

1. *cervical prominence (Meckel, 1817)*
   Synonym for macrodissected adult human ***cervical enlargement (Arnold, 1838b)***; see translation (1832, Vol. 2, p. 411).
2. *superior enlargement (Serres, 1824–1826)*
   Synonym for macrodissected vertebrate ***cervical enlargement (Arnold, 1838b)***; in the original French, *renflement supérieur*, Plate I, Figure 21-3 and later. See Quain & Wilson (1839, Pl. 1, Fig. 2-*10*).
3. *middle swelling of spinal cord (Quain & Wilson, 1839)*
   Synonym for macrodissected adult human ***cervical enlargement (Arnold, 1838b)***; Plate I, Figure 2-*10*.
4. *brachial swelling of spinal cord (Quain & Wilson, 1839)*
   Synonym for *middle swelling of spinal cord (Quain & Wilson, 1839)*; Plate I, Figure 2-*10*.

cervical nerves (Galen, c173)

As described for macrodissected adult human, the eight pairs of ***spinal nerves (Camper, 1760–1762)*** associated with the ***cervical part of spinal cord (>1840)***; see Carpenter (1976, pp. 213–216). In *On the Usefulness of the Parts*, Galen described and named them for adult human; see May translation (1968, p. 599 for name, pp. 590–600, 699–700 for full description); also see Duckworth translation (1962, pp. 231–240) and Asch (1750, pp. 2–4). Galen dissected a wide range of mammals, but not human explicitly. There may be a vague reference to the first ***cervical nerve (Galen, c173)*** in the Hippocratic corpus; see Asch (1750, pp. 1–2). The classic description for macrodissected adult human was by Bang (1770).

LATER SYNONYMS:

1. *nerves from medulla of neck (Achillini, 1520)*
Synonym for macrodissected adult human ***cervical nerves (Galen, c173)***; see Lind translation (1975, p. 63).
2. *nerves of nape of neck (Berengario da Carpi, 1523)*
Synonym for macrodissected adult human ***cervical nerves (Galen, c173)***; see Lind translation (1959, p. 160).
3. *nerves of neck (Diemerbroeck, 1689)*
Synonym for macrodissected adult human ***cervical nerves (Galen, c173)***; p. 557.
4. *vertical nerves (Rau, 1720)*
Synonym for macrodissected adult human ***cervical nerves (Galen, c173)***; in the original Latin, *nervi verticales*, p. 112.
5. *nervi colli (Haase, 1781)*
Synonym for macrodissected adult human ***cervical nerves (Galen, c173)***; Index, section 79.
6. *trachelian pairs of nerves (Burdin, 1803)*
Synonym for macrodissected adult human ***cervical nerves (Galen, c173)***; see translation (1803, Vol. 1, pp. 190–195). Burdin referred to arm as *thoracic member*.
7. *tracheal nerves (Chaussier, 1809)*
Synonym for macrodissected adult human ***cervical nerves (Galen, c173)***; in the original French, *nerfs trachéliens*.

PARTLY CORRESPONDS:

1. *cervical nerves (William of Saliceto, 1275)*
William of Saliceto wrote that there are seven cervical vertebrae and seven corresponding *cervical nerves (William of Saliceto, 1275)*; see Rosenman translation (1998, p. 187). Vesalius (1543a) also counted seven pairs rather than the eight counted by Galen, and quite specifically called the ***nerve (Herophilus, c335–c280 BC)*** emerging between last cervical and first thoracic vertebrae the *first pair of thoracic nerves (Vesalius, 1543a)*; see Richardson & Carman translation (2002, p. 232).
2. *first pair of thoracic nerves (Vesalius, 1543a)*
The eighth pair of ***cervical nerves (Galen, c173)*** in macrodissected adult human; see Richardson & Carman translation (2002, p. 232).
3. *[cervical nerves] (Colombo, 1559)*
Colombo apparently counted only five pairs of macrodissected adult human ***cervical nerves (Galen, c173)***, rather than the eight Galen counted; see Crooke (1615, p. 895), ***cervical nerves (Galen, c173)***.
4. *first pair of sinews of hand (Colombo, 1559)*
Refers to sixth pair of macrodissected adult human ***cervical nerves (Galen, c173)***; according to Bauhin (1605), see Crooke translation (1615, p. 896).
5. *nerves from spinal marrow of neck (Crooke, 1615)*
Synonym in English for *cervical nerves (Vesalius, 1543a)*; pp. 488, 894, also spelled *necke*.
6. *tenth pair of nerves arising within skull (Willis, 1664)*
Willis's tenth and last *pair of nerves arising within skull (Willis, 1664)* apparently corresponds to parts of first and second ***cervical nerves (Galen, c173)***; see Pordage translation (1681, pp. 157, 178, Tab. 9-*H*).
7. *nerve of tenth pair (Willis, 1664)*
Synonym for *tenth pair of nerves arising within skull (Willis, 1664)*; see Pordage translation (1681, p. 178 and Tab. 9-*H*).
8. *cervical nerves (Winslow, 1733)*
Winslow counted for macrodissected adult human seven pairs rather than the eight ***cervical nerves (Galen, c173)***, beginning with the pair emerging between first and second cervical vertebrae; Section X, p. 76. Winslow called the first pair of ***cervical nerves (Galen, c173)*** the right and left ***suboccipital nerve (Winslow, 1733)***; also see *tenth pair of nerves arising within skull (Willis, 1664)*.
9. *intervertebral nerves of neck (Schaarschmidt, 1750)*
Synonym for macrodissected adult human *cervical nerves (Winslow, 1733)*; in the original Latin, *nervi intervertebrales colli*, p. 60.
10. *cerebrospinal nerve (Portal, 1803a)*
Synonym for macrodissected adult human *nerve of tenth pair (Willis, 1664)*; in the original French, *nerf cérébro-spinal, ou dixième paire de Willis*, p. 162.
11. *tenth pair of Willis (Portal, 1803a)*
Eponym for *tenth pair of nerves arising within skull (Willis, 1664)*; in the original French, *dixième paire de Willis*, p. 162.
12. *cerebrovertebral nerve (Portal, 1803a)*
Synonym for macrodissected adult human *nerve of tenth pair (Willis, 1664)*; in the original French, *nerf cérébro-vertébral*, p. 166.
13. *subatloidien nerve (Chaussier, 1809)*
The second macrodissected adult human ***cervical nerve (Galen, c173)***; in the original French, *nerf sous-atloïdien*.
14. *subaxoidien nerve (Chaussier, 1809)*
The third macrodissected adult human ***cervical nerve (Galen, c173)***; in the original French, *nerf sous-axoïdien*.
15. *tracheodiaphragmatic nerve (Chaussier, 1809)*
The fourth macrodissected adult human ***cervical nerve (Galen, c173)***; in the original French, *nerf trachélo-diaphragmatique*.
16. *superior division of fifth cervical nerve (Bell & Bell, 1816)*
According to Bell & Bell's description for macrodissected adult human, one of two main branches of fifth ***cervical nerve (Galen, c173)***; "it passes backwards to the muscles of the back and shoulder" and generates the ***long thoracic nerve (Quain & Wilson, 1839)***; Vol. 2, p. 515.
17. *inferior division of fifth cervical nerve (Bell & Bell, 1816)*
According to Bell & Bell's description for macrodissected adult human, one of two main branches of fifth ***cervical nerve (Galen, c173)***; it contributes to ***phrenic nerve (Galen, c173)*** and "communicates with the root of the sixth nerve, and sends muscular branches backward" (Vol. 2, p. 515).

cervical part of spinal cord (>1840)

As described for macrodissected adult vertebrate, the longitudinal ***spinal cord part (>1840)*** generating the *cervical nerves*; see Carpenter (1976, pp. 213–216). As described for macrodissected adult human, the longitudinal ***spinal cord part (>1840)*** generating the eight ***cervical nerves (Galen, c173)***; see *Nomina Anatomica* (1983, p. A64), *Terminologia Anatomica* (1998, p. 105). It was first described as *spinal medulla in neck (Galen, c173)*.

EARLIER REFERENCES:

Earlier synonyms:

1. *spinal medulla in neck (Galen, c173)*
   Synonym for ***cervical part of spinal cord (>1840)*** in macrodissected adult beef, pig, and/or macaque but not human; see May translation (1968, p. 597).
2. *cervical spinal medulla (Galen, c173)*
   In *On the Usefulness of the Parts*, Galen specifically referred thus to ***cervical part* of spinal cord (>1840)** for macrodissected adult beef, pig, and/or macaque but not human; see May translation (1968, p. 601).
3. *nape of neck (Berengario da Carpi, 1523)*
   Synonym for macrodissected adult human ***cervical part of spinal cord (>1840)***; see Lind translation (1959, p. 160).
4. *pith passing through vertebres of neck (Diemerbroeck, 1689)*
   Synonym for macrodissected adult human ***cervical part of spinal cord (>1840)***; p. 557.
5. *cervical portion of cord (Gordon, 1815)*
   Defined as that part of macrodissected adult human *spinal cord (Gordon, 1815)* lodged in cervical region of spinal canal; p. 157.
6. *cervical part of spinal medulla (Tiedemann, 1821)*
   Synonym for macrodissected adult monkey ***cervical part of spinal cord (>1840)*** with eight ***cervical nerves (Galen, c173)***; in the original Latin, *pars cervicalis medullae spinalis*, Table I, Figure 5-*e*.

cervical plexus (Molinetti, 1675)

As described for macrodissected adult human, formed by the ***spinal nerve ventral branches (>1840)*** of the 1st–4th ***cervical nerves (Galen, c173)*** with ***communicating loops of cervical plexus (>1840), communicating branches of cervical plexus (>1840)***, and branches distributing to certain neck muscles, the diaphragm, and parts of the skin associated with the head, neck, and chest; see Durward (1951, Fig. 919), Hamilton (1976, Fig. 816), Williams & Warwick (1980, Fig. 7.197). For Molinetti's use in macrodissected adult human, see p. 202. It was known to Galen, see ***[cervical plexus (Molinetti, 1675)] (Galen, c173)*** and was brilliantly illustrated in great detail for macrodissected adult human by Bang (1770, Fig. 1).

EARLIER REFERENCES:

Described, not named or illustrated:

1. ***[cervical plexus (Molinetti, 1675)] (Galen, c173)***
   Described without naming in macrodissected adult beef, pig, and/or macaque but not human explicitly; see May translation (1968, p. 598), Duckworth translation (1962, pp. 230, 249). He described at length the general features of ***plexuses (Galen, c192)***, which differ between classes of animals and between animals of the same type, as well as the functional uses of the ***plexuses (Galen, c192)***; see Duckworth translation (1962, pp. 230–231).

Illustrated and described, not named:

1. ***[cervical plexus (Molinetti, 1675)] (Vesalius, 1543a)***
   Described for macrodissected adult human, but account was much inferior to Galen's and illustration was very crude; see Richardson & Carman translation (2002, pp. 224–227). Vieussens (1684; Tabs. 23-*i*, 24-*f,g*) illustrated it relatively accurately for macrodissected adult human; also see Neubauer (1772, p. 56 ff. and Tab. 2).

PARTLY CORRESPONDS:

1. *middle branches of third cervical pair (Winslow, 1733)*
   Combination of some ***muscular branches of cervical plexus (Cruveilhier, 1836)*** and some ***descending superficial branches of cervical plexus (Quain, 1828)*** arising from fourth cervical ***spinal nerve ventral branch (>1840)*** of macrodissected adult human; Section VI, p. 79.
2. *exterior branch of fourth pair of cervical nerves (Neubauer, 1772)*
   Synonym for macrodissected adult human *middle branches of third cervical pair (Winslow, 1733)*; in the original Latin, *ramus exterior quartis paris*, Table 1-205; Neubauer also referred to it here as "anterior branch."
3. *sternothyrohyoid nerves (Andersch & Soemmerring, 1792)*
   Macrodissected adult human ***nerves (Herophilus, c335–c280 BC)*** associated with ***cervical plexus (Molinetti, 1675)*** and innervating at least some infrahyoid muscles; in the original Latin, *nervo sternothyreohyoideo*, p. 149.
4. *trachelo-cutaneous plexus (Burdin, 1803)*
   Synonym for *tracheosubcutaneous nerves (Chaussier, 1809)*; see translation (1803, Vol. 1, p. 187). Also spelled *trachelo-cutanean plexus* (1803 translation, Vol. 1, p. 187).
5. *trachelosubcutaneous nerves (Chaussier, 1809)*
   Basically, macrodissected adult human ***ascending superficial branches of cervical plexus (Quain, 1828)*** and ***descending superficial branches of cervical plexus (Quain, 1828)*** considered together; in the original French, *nerfs trachélo-sous-cutanés*.
6. *trachelosubcutaneous plexus (Cloquet, 1816)*
   Synonym for macrodissected adult human *tracheosubcutaneous nerves (Chaussier, 1809)*, attributed apparently in error to Chaussier; in the original French, *plexus trachélo-sous-cutané*, p. 636.
7. *third cervical nervous plexus (Meckel, 1817)*
   Macrodissected adult human part of ***cervical plexus (Molinetti, 1675)*** common to third and fourth cervical ***spinal nerve ventral branches (>1840)***; see translation (1832, Vol. 3, p. 31) and Williams & Warwick (1980, Fig. 7.197).
8. *first cervical nervous plexus (Meckel, 1817)*
   Macrodissected adult human part of ***cervical plexus (Molinetti, 1675)*** common to first and second cervical ***spinal nerve ventral branches (>1840)***; see translation (1832, Vol. 3, p. 33), and *ascending anastomotic nerve of second cervical nerve (Meckel, 1817)*.

9. *second cervical nervous plexus (Meckel, 1817)*
Macrodissected adult human part of ***cervical plexus (Molinetti, 1675)*** common to second and third cervical ***spinal nerve ventral branches (>1840)***; see translation (1832, Vol. 3, p. 33), *descending anastomotic nerve of second cervical nerve (Meckel, 1817)*, and Williams & Warwick (1980, Fig. 7.197).
10. *cutaneous branches of cervical plexus (Cruveilhier, 1836)*
Macrodissected adult human ***ascending superficial branches of cervical plexus (Quain, 1828)*** and ***descending superficial branches of cervical plexus (Quain, 1828)*** considered together, as opposed to ***muscular branches of cervical plexus (Cruveilhier, 1836)***; p. 781.

cervical spinal ganglia (>1840)

As described for macrodissected adult human, there is usually one ***spinal nerve ganglion (Burdach, 1819)*** for each ***dorsal root (Spurzheim, 1826)*** of the eight pairs of ***cervical nerves (Galen, c173)***, except that a ***spinal nerve ganglion (Burdach, 1819)*** may be absent from the first pair of ***cervical nerves (Galen, c173)***. They are numbered sequentially from rostral to caudal; see Williams & Warwick (1980, p. 1086). They were discovered by Coiter; see ***[cervical spinal ganglia (>1840)] (Coiter, 1572)***.

EARLIER REFERENCES:

Described, not named or illustrated:

1. ***[cervical spinal ganglia (>1840)] (Coiter, 1572)***
Coiter stated there is a *knot (Coiter, 1572)*, or ***spinal nerve ganglion (Burdach, 1819)***, for each *spinal nerve (Vesalius, 1543a)* in macrodissected adult human; see translation (1955, p. 115).

PARTLY CORRESPONDS:

1. *plexus ganglioformes nervorum cervicalium (Vieussens, 1684)*
Vieussens described and illustrated a ***cervical spinal ganglion (>1840)*** on ***dorsal root (>1840)*** of 2nd–7th ***cervical nerves (Galen, c173)*** for macrodissected adult human. He did not illustrate one for the first ***cervical nerve (Galen, c173)***, which sometimes occurs, and he followed Vesalius in having only seven *cervical nerves (Vesalius, 1543a)*; see Table 24-*a*.
2. *lateral small ganglion of neck (Andersch, 1797)*
Apparently variant form of macrodissected adult human fifth ***cervical spinal ganglion (>1840)***, which Andersch referred to as *small ganglion of fifth nerves of neck (Andersch, 1797)*; in the original Latin, *ganglioli lateralis colli*, Vol. 2, p. 142.
3. *small ganglion of fifth nerves of neck (Andersch, 1797)*
Apparently, macrodissected adult human fifth ***cervical spinal ganglion (>1840)***; in the original Latin, *gangliolum quinti nervi colli*, Vol. 2, p. 143.

cervical sympathetic ganglia (>1840)

As described for macrodissected adult human, commonly three major ***sympathetic trunk ganglia (Winslow, 1733)*** having ***gray communicating branches (>1840)*** with the ***cervical nerves (Galen, c173)***. They are the ***superior cervical ganglion (Vieussens, 1684)***, ***middle cervical ganglion (Haller, 1762)***, and ***inferior cervical ganglion (Vieussens, 1684)***; see Mitchell (1953, Ch. 15). They were perhaps first clearly delineated overall as the *cervical ganglia of intercostal nerve (Günther, 1786)*.

EARLIER REFERENCES:

Earlier synonyms:

1. *cervical ganglia of intercostal nerve (Günther, 1786)*
Synonym for macrodissected adult human ***cervical sympathetic ganglia (>1840)***; in the original Latin, *gangliorum n. intercostalis sunt in cervice tria*, p. 92.
2. *cervical ganglions of limiting cord (Meckel, 1817)*
Synonym for macrodissected adult human ***cervical sympathetic ganglia (>1840)***. Meckel described three for macrodissected adult human: ***superior cervical ganglion (Vieussens, 1684)***, ***middle cervical ganglion (Haller, 1762)***, and ***inferior cervical ganglion (Vieussens, 1684)***; see translation (1832, Vol. 3, pp. 88–96).

chorda tympani (Falloppio, 1561)

As described for macrodissected adult human, a ***communicating branch (Winslow, 1733)*** between ***intermediofacial nerve trunk (>1840)*** and ***lingual nerve (Vesalius, 1543a)***. It is secretomotor to the submandibular and sublingual salivary glands and supplies taste ***dendrites (His, 1889)*** to the rostral (anterior) two-thirds of the tongue; see Mitchell (1953, pp. 161–162 and Fig. 68), Williams & Warwick (1980, Fig. 7.177). According to Winslow, "This small Nerve is generally called Chorda Tympani, because in its passage through the Tympanum it has been compared to the Cord of a Drum." (1733, Sect. X, p. 111). For Falloppio's use in macrodissected adult human see pp. 28–29 and Haller (1762, Vol. 4, p. 226). For detailed accounts of early descriptions see Meckel (1748, p. 92 note *m*), Todd (1836–1839, p. 296). It was first depicted by Eustachi; see ***[chorda tympani (Falloppio, 1561)] (Eustachi, 1552)***.

TRANSLATIONS:

1. *cord of tympanum (Meckel, 1832)*
English form of ***chorda tympani (Falloppio, 1561)***; Vol. 3, p. 54.
2. *chord of tympanum (Swan, 1830)*
English form of ***chorda tympani (Falloppio, 1561)***; Plate XII, Figure 3-*21*.

EARLIER REFERENCES:

Illustrated, not named or described:

1. ***[chorda tympani (Falloppio, 1561)] (Eustachi, 1552)***
Clearly illustrated for macrodissected adult human; Table 18, Figures 1 and 3, see Albinus edition (1744, Tab. 18, Figs. 1,3-*T*). Du Verney (1683) clearly described and illustrated it for macrodissected adult human; see translation (1737, p. 53 and Pl. 12, Fig. 2; Pl. 13-*M*).

LATER SYNONYMS:

1. *recurrent acoustic nerve (Le Cat, 1768)*
Synonym for macrodissected adult human ***chorda tympani (Falloppio, 1561)***; p. 243 and Plate VII, Figure 4-*9*.

2. *recurrent lingual nerve (Le Cat, 1768)*
   Synonym for macrodissected adult human ***chorda tympani (Falloppio, 1561)***; p. 250; Plate VII, Figure 2-*d* and Plate IX, Figure 5-*1*.
3. *recurrent acoustico-laryngeal nerve (Le Cat, 1768)*
   Synonym for macrodissected adult human ***chorda tympani (Falloppio, 1561)***; p. 252; Plate VIII, Figure 1-*q* and Plate VIII, Figure 2-*h*.
4. *tympanic branch of facial nerve (Burdin, 1803)*
   Synonym for macrodissected adult human ***chorda tympani (Falloppio, 1561)***; see translation (1803, Vol. 1, p. 179).
5. *lingual branch of portio major and minor of facial nerve (Bellingeri, 1818)*
   Synonym for macrodissected adult human ***chorda tympani (Falloppio, 1561)***; in the original Latin, *ramus lingualis*, see Table II.
6. *chorda tympani nerve (Quain & Wilson, 1839)*
   Synonym for macrodissected adult human ***chorda tympani (Falloppio, 1561)***; Plate XV-*c*.

PARTLY CORRESPONDS:

1. *branch of chorda tympani to external malleus muscle (Langenbeck, 1826–1830)*
   Macrodissected adult human branch of ***chorda tympani (Falloppio, 1561)*** to laxator tympani (band of Meckel), now usually considered component of anterior ligament of malleus; in the original Latin, *ramus chordae tympani ad musculum mallei externum*, Fascicle III, Table 27-*e*.

choroid enlargement (>1840)

As described in macrodissected adult human, an oval swelling of the ***choroid plexus of lateral ventricle (Vicq d'Azyr, 1784)*** near the ***collateral triangle (>1840)***; p. 87. See Millen & Woollam (1962, p. 64 and Fig. 39), *Terminologia Anatomica* (1998, p. 127). It was perhaps first clearly defined as *button of choroid plexus of lateral ventricle (Vicq d'Azyr, 1784)*.

TRANSLATIONS:

1. *glomus choroideum (>1840)*
   Current Latin form of ***choroid enlargement (>1840)***; see *Terminologia Anatomica* (1998, p. 127). It was used by His (1895, p. 87) in the *Basel Nomina Anatomica*.

EARLIER REFERENCES:

Earlier synonyms:

1. *button of choroid plexus of lateral ventricle (Vicq d'Azyr, 1784)*
   Synonym for macrodissected adult human ***choroid enlargement (>1840)***; pp. 540–541; also see Meckel (1832, Vol. 2, p. 474).

choroid epithelium of fourth ventricle (>1840)

In developing vertebrate embryo, the simple ***ependymal roof plate (>1840)*** of the ***fourth ventricle (Galen, c192)*** is a free monolayer becoming covered by a double layer of ***pia (Galen, c192)***. In adult, the former is the ***choroid epithelium of fourth ventricle (>1840)*** and the latter is the ***choroid membrane of fourth ventricle (>1840)***. Accompanied by blood vessels, these layers invaginate into the lumen of the ***fourth ventricle (Galen, c192)*** to form the ***choroid plexus of fourth ventricle (Vieussens, 1684)***; see Millen & Woollam (1962, p. 66 ff.), Carpenter (1976, p. 132 ff.). It was not described by 1840.

choroid epithelium of lateral ventricle (>1840)

In developing vertebrate embryo, the simple ***ependymal roof plate (>1840)*** of the ***lateral ventricle (Vesalius, 1543a)*** is a free monolayer becoming covered by a layer of ***pia (Galen, c192)***. In adult, the former is the ***choroid epithelium of lateral ventricle (>1840)*** and the latter is the ***choroid membrane of lateral ventricle (>1840)***. Accompanied by blood vessels, both layers invaginate into the lumen of the ***lateral ventricle (Vesalius, 1543a)*** to form the ***choroid plexus of lateral ventricle (Vicq d'Azyr, 1784)***; see Millen & Woollam (1962, p. 66 ff.), Carpenter (1976, p. 132 ff.). In adult it is usually described as forming roughly the medial wall of the ***lateral ventricle (Vesalius, 1543a)***; embryologically it forms, to a first approximation, between the caudal end of the ***endbrain vesicle (Kuhlenbeck, 1927)*** and the rostral end of the thalamic or dorsal part of the ***interbrain vesicle (Baer, 1837)***; see Alvarez-Bolado & Swanson (1996, Figs. 9, 21, 22). It was not described by 1840.

choroid epithelium of third ventricle (>1840)

In developing vertebrate embryo, the simple ***ependymal roof plate (>1840)*** of the ***third ventricle (Galen, c173)*** is a free monolayer eventually covered by a double layer of ***pia (Galen, c192)***. In adult, the ***ependymal roof plate (>1840)*** is the ***choroid epithelium of third ventricle (>1840)*** and the associated ***pia (Galen, c192)*** is the ***choroid membrane of third ventricle (>1840)***. Accompanied by blood vessels, these layers invaginate into the lumen of the ***third ventricle (>Galen, c173)*** to form the ***choroid plexus of third ventricle (Vicq d'Azyr, 1784)***; see Millen & Woollam (1962, p. 66 ff.), Carpenter (1976, p. 132 ff.). It was not described by 1840.

choroid fissure (>1840)

As described for mammalian development, the earliest groove to appear on the lateral surface of the **endbrain (Kuhlenbeck, 1927)** in which the ***choroid plexus of lateral ventricle (Vicq d'Azyr, 1784)*** invaginates; see Millen & Woollam (1962, pp. 97–98 and Fig. 34), Carpenter (1976; pp. 65, 530 and Fig. 18.8), *Dorland's* (2003, p. 703). In macrodissected adult human, observed conventionally when ***choroid plexus of lateral ventricle (Vicq d'Azyr, 1784)*** is torn away and in this sense it is artifactual; see Williams & Warwick (1980, p. 1038). It was probably first clearly delineated as the *spiraglis (Malacarne, 1780)*.

ALTERNATE SPELLINGS:

1. *choroidal fissure of lateral ventricle (>1840)*
   Alternate form of ***choroid fissure (>1840)***; see *Terminologia Anatomica* (1998, p. 127).
2. *chorioid fissure (>1840)*

Alternate form of ***choroid fissure (>1840)***; see Mettler (1948, p. 148).

TRANSLATIONS:

1. *fissura choroidea (>1840)*
   Current Latin form of ***choroid fissure (>1840)***; see *Terminologia Anatomica* (1998, p. 127).

EARLIER REFERENCES:

Earlier synonyms:

1. *spiraglis (Malacarne, 1780)*
   Synonym for macrodissected adult human ***choroid fissure (>1840)***; p. 161, see Burdach (1822, p. 386).

choroid line of fourth ventricle (>1840)

As described for adult mammal, the line where the ***choroid epithelium of fourth ventricle (>1840)*** attaches to the lateral edge of the ***floor of fourth ventricle (Reil, 1807–1808a)*** along the ***inferior cerebellar peduncle (Günther, 1786)***; see Williams & Warwick (1980, p. 932). It was specifically noted by Burdach; see *taenia plexus choroidei ventriculi quarti (Burdach, 1822).*

TRANSLATIONS:

1. *tenia choroidea ventriculi quarti (>1840)*
   Latin form of ***choroid line of fourth ventricle (>1840)***; see *Dorland's* (2003, pp. 1851–1852). Also spelled *taenia choroidea ventriculi quarti.*

EARLIER REFERENCES:

Earlier synonyms:

1. *taenia plexus choroidei ventriculi quarti (Burdach, 1822)*
   Synonym for macrodissected adult human ***choroid line of fourth ventricle (>1840)***; p. 78, Table IV-*x*.
2. *ligula (Arnold, 1838b)*
   Synonym for macrodissected adult human ***choroid line of fourth ventricle (>1840)***; Table VIII, Figure 3-*h*.

choroid line of lateral ventricle (>1840)

As described for adult mammal, the line where the ***choroid epithelium of lateral ventricle (>1840)*** attaches to the ***dorsal part of thalamus (Herrick, 1919)*** at or near the ***terminal stria (Wenzel & Wenzel, 1812)***, associated with the ***lamina affixa (>1840)***; see Mettler (1948, p. 147), Crosby et al. (1962, p. 576). It was not clearly described by 1840.The other edge of the ***choroid epithelium of lateral ventricle (>1840)*** is formed by the ***fimbrial line of lateral ventricle (>1840).***

TRANSLATIONS:

1. *tenia choroidea ventriculi lateralis (>1840)*
   Latin form of ***choroid line of lateral ventricle (>1840)***; see *Dorland's* (2003, p. 1851). Also spelled *taenia choroidea.* Other synonyms include *tenia telae, tenia striae terminalis.* His (1895; see Eycleshymer translation, 1917, p. 161 ff.) used the term *taenia chorioidea.*

choroid line of third ventricle (>1840)

As described for adult mammal, the line where the ***choroid epithelium of third ventricle (>1840)*** attaches to the length of the ***thalamus (His, 1893a)***, specifically to the medial edge of the ***medullary stria (Wenzel & Wenzel, 1812)***; see Mettler (1948, p. 147), Crosby et al. (1962, p. 576 and Fig. 221), Williams & Warwick (1980, p. 954), where it is called *tenia thalami (>1840)*. It was not clearly described by 1840.

EARLIER REFERENCES:

Earlier synonyms:

1. *tenia of third ventricle (>1840)*
   Synonym for macrodissected adult human ***choroid line of third ventricle (>1840)***; see *Dorland's* (2003, p. 1852). Also spelled *taenia of third ventricle.*
2. *stria medullaris line (>1840)*
   Synonym for macrodissected adult human ***choroid line of third ventricle (>1840)***; see Mettler (1948, p. 147), Crosby et al. (1962, p. 576).
3. *tenia stria medullaris (>1840)*
   Latin form of *stria medullaris line (>1840).* Also spelled *taenia stria medullaris.*
4. *thalamic line (>1840)*
   Synonym for macrodissected adult human ***choroid line of third ventricle (>1840)***; see Mettler (1948, p. 147), Crosby et al. (1962, p. 576).
5. *tenia thalami (>1840)*
   Latin form of *thalamic line (>1840)*; see Williams & Warwick (1980, p. 954), *Terminologia Anatomica* (1998, p. 121), *Dorland's* (2003, p. 1852). Also spelled *taenia thalami.*

choroid membrane of fourth ventricle (>1840)

As described for adult human, a double layer or fold of ***pia (Galen, c192)*** in medial regions of the caudal half of the ***roof of fourth ventricle* (Vesalius, 1543a)**, overlying the ***choroid epithelium of fourth ventricle (>1840)*** between the more lateral ***caudal medullary velum (>1840)*** on the right and left sides. The dorsal layer of ***pia (Galen, c192)*** is associated with the ventral surface of the overlying ***cerebellar vermis (Meckel, 1817)***, whereas the ventral layer covers the ***choroid epithelium of fourth ventricle (>1840)***—and there are strands of ***arachnoid (Blasius, 1666)*** with accompanying blood vessels in between. Together with blood vessels, the ***choroid membrane of fourth ventricle (>1840)*** and underlying ***choroid epithelium of fourth ventricle (>1840)*** invaginate into the lumen of the ***fourth ventricle (Galen, c192)*** to form the right and left ***choroid plexus of fourth ventricle (Vieussens, 1684)***; see Mettler (1948, p. 98), Millen & Woollam (1962, p. 66 ff.), Carpenter (1976, p. 132 ff.), Williams & Warwick (1980, pp. 914, 932, Figs. 7.75, 87, 88). It was clearly described by Chaussier; see *choroid lamina of fourth ventricle (Chaussier, 1807).*

TRANSLATIONS:

1. *tela choroidea ventriculi quarti (>1840)*
   Current Latin form of ***choroid membrane of fourth ventricle (>1840)***; see *Dorland's* (2003, pp. 1860–1861).

EARLIER REFERENCES:

Earlier synonyms:

1. *choroid lamina of fourth ventricle (Chaussier, 1807)*
   Synonym for macrodissected adult human ***choroid membrane of fourth ventricle (>1840)***; in the

original French, *lame choroïdienne du quatrième ventricule*, p. 102.

2. *lamina chorioidea inferior (Burdach, 1822)*
   Synonym for macrodissected adult human ***choroid membrane of fourth ventricle (>1840)***; p. 77, Table VIII-*h*.
3. *ligula (Bergmann, 1831)*
   Synonym for macrodissected adult human ***choroid membrane of fourth ventricle (>1840)***; Table V-*n*.
4. *tela chorioidea (Arnold, 1838a)*
   Synonym for macrodissected adult human *choroid membrane of fourth ventricle (>1840)*; p. 23.

choroid membrane of lateral ventricle (>1840)

As described for human, a layer of ***pia (Galen, c192)*** lying just over the free medial layer of ***ependyma (>1840)*** of the ***lateral ventricle (Vesalius, 1543a)***, called developmentally the ***ependymal roof plate (>1840)*** and in adult the ***choroid epithelium of lateral ventricle (>1840). The choroid membrane of lateral ventricle (>1840)*** is a lateral extension of the deep or ventral layer of the ***choroid membrane of third ventricle (>1840)*** coursing through the ***interventricular foramen (>1840)*** to the ***lateral ventricle (Vesalius, 1543a)***; see Williams & Warwick (p. 1038), *Dorland's* (2003, p. 1861). Accompanied by blood vessels, the ***choroid membrane of lateral ventricle (>1840)***, along with the underlying ***choroid epithelium of lateral ventricle (>1840)***, is invaginated into the lumen of the ***lateral ventricle (Vesalius, 1543a)*** at the ***choroid fissure (>1840)*** to form the ***choroid plexus of lateral ventricle (Vicq d'Azyr, 1784)***. It was not clearly described by 1840.

TRANSLATIONS:

1. *tela choroidea ventriculi lateralis (>1840)*
   Current Latin form of ***choroid membrane of lateral ventricle (>1840)***; see *Dorland's* (2003, p. 1860).

choroid membrane of third ventricle (>1840)

As described for adult human, a double layer or fold of ***pia (Galen, c192)*** forming, along with the underlying ***choroid epithelium of third ventricle (>1840)***, the ***roof of third ventricle (>1840)*** and its invagination, the ***choroid plexus of third ventricle (Vicq d'Azyr, 1784)***. The dorsal layer of ***pia (Galen, c192)*** is associated with the ventral surface of the overlying ***fimbria (Honegger, 1890)***, whereas the ventral layer covers the ***choroid epithelium of third ventricle (>1840)***—and there are strands of ***arachnoid (Blasius, 1666)*** with accompanying blood vessels in between, all lying within the ***transverse cerebral fissure (>1840)***; see Millen & Woollam (1962, p. 99, Fig. 35), Williams & Warwick (1980, pp. 981, 1038; Fig. 7.157), *Dorland's* (2003, p. 1861). Its presence was first indicated by Galen; see ***[choroid membrane of third ventricle (>1840)] (Galen, c177)***.

TRANSLATIONS:

1. *tela choroidea ventriculi tertii (>1840)*
   Current Latin form of ***choroid membrane of third ventricle (>1849)***; see *Dorland's* (2003, p. 1860).

EARLIER REFERENCES:

Described, not named or illustrated:

1. ***[choroid membrane of third ventricle (>1840)] (Galen, c177)***
   In *On Anatomical Procedures*, Galen described at least its caudal regions; see Vicq d'Azyr (1786, p. 32), Singer translation (1999, p. 233), Wiberg translation (1914, pp. 25, 104). Galen macrodissected a broad range of common large mammals but did not explicitly mention human.

Illustrated, not named or described:

1. ***[choroid membrane of third ventricle (>1840)] (Steno, 1669)***
   Clearly illustrated, at least the more ventral part, for macrodissected adult human; Plates I, II.

Earlier synonyms:

1. *velum interpositum (Haller, 1754a)*
   Synonym for macrodissected adult human ***choroid membrane of third ventricle (>1840)***; Fascicle VII, Plate II-*N*; see Bell (1803b, pp. 50–51), Millen & Woollam (1962, p. 99, Fig. 35). The complete original Latin term was *veli sive plexus choroideis interpositi*; see Haller (1754a, p. 13). According to Burdach (1822, p. 398), certain authors beginning with Berengario da Carpi (1521) conflated the concepts of *velum interpositum (Haller, 1754a)* and ***choroid plexus of third ventricle (Vicq d'Azyr, 1784)***.
2. *velum triangulare (Haller, 1762)*
   Synonym for macrodissected adult human *velum interpositum (Haller, 1754a)*; p. 19, see Burdach (1822, p. 398).
3. *plexus choroideus tertius (Haase, 1781)*
   Synonym for macrodissected adult human *velum interpositum (Haller, 1754a)*; pp. 18, 22.See Burdach (1822, p. 398).
4. *plexus choroideus medius (Haase, 1781)*
   Synonym for macrodissected adult human *velum interpositum (Haller, 1754a)*; pp. 18, 22.See Burdach (1822, p. 398).
5. *plexus choroideus impar (Haase, 1781)*
   Synonym for macrodissected adult human *velum interpositum (Haller, 1754a)*; pp. 18, 22.See Burdach (1822, p. 398).
6. *tela choroïdea (Vicq d'Azyr, 1786)*
   Synonym for macrodissected adult human *velum interpositum (Haller, 1754a)*, more precisely defined than Haller in terms of constituent veins and arteries; in the original French, *la toile vasculare*; Plate VII, Figures 1–4, p. 20; Figure IV, p. 21. Also see Todd (1845, p. 28), Williams & Warwick (1980, p. 1038 and Fig. 7.159), Meckel (1832, Vol. 2, p. 474). Apparently, Cruveilhier (1836, p. 656) used the French, *toile choroïdienne*, a term he ascribed to Herophilus (p. 681).
7. *rete choroïdeum (Vicq d'Azyr, 1786)*
   Synonym for macrodissected adult human *tela choroïdea (Vicq d'Azyr, 1786)*; Plate VII, Figure I, p. 20.
8. *velum choroïdes (Vicq d'Azyr, 1786)*
   Synonym for macrodissected adult human *tela choroïdea (Vicq d'Azyr, 1786)*; p. 32.

9. *velum vasculosum (Bell, 1802)*
   Synonym for macrodissected adult human *velum interpositum (Haller, 1754a)*; Plate VI-*L*.
10. *velum of Haller (Bell, 1802)*
   Eponym for macrodissected adult human *velum interpositum (Haller, 1754a)*; Plate VIII, Figure II-*N*.
11. *vellum (Bell, 1803b)*
   Synonym for macrodissected adult human *velum interpositum (Haller, 1754a)*; p. 86.
12. *oblong passage (Gordon, 1815)*
   Synonym for macrodissected adult human *velum interpositum (Haller, 1754a)*; p. 92.
13. *choroid membrane (Gordon, 1815)*
   In macrodissected adult human, English form of *tela choroïdes (Vicq d'Azyr, 1786)*; p. 154, see Burdach (1822, p. 398).
14. *diaphragma interpositum (Bell & Bell, 1816)*
   Synonym for *velum vasculosum (Bell, 1802)*; Vol. 2, p. 448.
15. *Gefässblatt (Meckel, 1817)*
   German form of *tela choroïdea (Vicq d'Azyr, 1786)*; p. 548, according to Burdach (1822, p. 398).
16. *Gefässvorhang (Meckel, 1817)*
   German form of *tela choroïdea (Vicq d'Azyr, 1786)*; p. 548, according to Burdach (1822, p. 398).
17. *tela choroides superior (Burdach, 1822)*
   Synonym for macrodissected adult human *velum interpositum (Haller, 1754a)*; in the original German, *die obre Gefässplatte* or simply *die Gefässplatte*, pp. 184–185, 398.
18. *tela choroides (Burdach, 1822)*
   Synonym for *tela choroides superior (Burdach, 1822)*; in the original German, *Gefässplatte*, pp. 184–185, 398.
19. *velum cerebri vasculosum (Burdach, 1822)*
   Synonym for *tela choroides superior (Burdach, 1822)* Burdach attributed to Caldani without adequate citation; p. 398.

choroid plexus (Galen, c177)

General term for a hybrid structure formed by components of the ***nervous system (Monro, 1783)*** and ***vascular system*** producing ***cerebrospinal fluid (Magendie, 1827)*** entering the ***ventricles (Hippocrates)***. There are right and left strands of **choroid plexus of *lateral ventricle (Vicq d'Azyr, 1784)*** and ***choroid plexus of third ventricle (Vicq d'Azyr, 1784)***, which form continuous right and left strands passing through the ***interventricular foramen (>1840)***, and ***choroid plexus of fourth ventricle (Vieussens, 1684)***. Histologically, each strand is an invagination of the ***ependymal roof plate (>1840)*** associated developmentally with the corresponding ***ventricle (Hippocrates)***. In adult this layer of ***ependyma (>1840)*** is called the *choroid epithelium* and has ***cerebrospinal fluid (Magendie, 1827)*** on the inner side and a layer of highly vascularized ***arachnoid (Blasius, 1666)*** and ***pia (Galen, c192)*** on the outer side, along with *nerve fibers (Ehrenberg, 1833)*; see Millen & Woollam (1962, Ch. IV). The term was used in Galen's *On Anatomical Procedures* (see von Staden, 1989, p. 225; Singer translation, 1999, p. 231) for the macrodissected structure first identified as *choroid concatenations (Herophilus, c335–c280 BC)*.

ALTERNATE SPELLINGS:

1. *chorioid plexus (Galen, c177)*
   Alternate form of ***choroid plexus (Galen, c177)***.

TRANSLATIONS:

1. *plexus choroides (Galen, c177)*
   Latin form of ***choroid plexus (Galen, c177)***.
2. *plexus choroideus (Galen, c177)*
   Latin form of ***choroid plexus (Galen, c177)***.
3. *choroeidê plegmata (Galen, c177)*
   Greek form of ***choroid plexus (Galen, c177)***; see Singer translation (1999, p. 231).

EARLIER REFERENCES:

Earlier synonyms:

1. *choroid twisted clusters (Herophilus, c335–c280 BC)*
   According to Galen in *On Anatomical Procedure* (see von Staden, 1989, p. 225), those around Herophilus called macrodissected adult human ***choroid plexus (Galen, c177)*** "choroid twisted clusters" for similarity to membranes (*choria*) wrapped around fetus, membranes that are plexuses of veins and arteries held together by thin membranes.
2. *choroid concatenations (Herophilus, c335–c280 BC)*
   Singer's (1956, p. 321) translation of Herophilus's term for ***choroid plexus (Galen, c177)***.
3. *choroid coils (Herophilus, c335–c280 BC)*
   Longrigg's (1998, p. 87) translation of Herophilus's term for ***choroid plexus (Galen, c177)***.
4. *chorioid meninx (Herophilus, c335–c280 BC)*
   According to Rufus of Ephesus (c90–120), Herophilus used it for macrodissected adult human and animal ***choroid plexus (Galen, c177)***; see von Staden (1989, p. 225).
5. *choroid meninx (Herophilus, c335–c280 BC)*
   Alternate form of *chorioid meninx (Herophilus, c335–c280 BC)*.
6. *choroid membrane (Herophilus, c335–c280 BC)*
   English form of *choroid meninx (Herophilus, c335–c280 BC)*.
7. *chorioid tunic (Rufus of Ephesus, c90–120)*
   Synonym for ***choroid plexus (Galen, c177)***; see Millen & Woollam (1962, p. 5).
8. *choroid bodies (Galen, c173)*
   Synonym for ***choroid plexus (Galen, c177)*** used by Galen in *On the Usefulness of the Parts*; see May translation (1968, p. 392).
9. *chorioeidê sustremmata (Galen, c177)*
   Greek term Galen used in *On Anatomical Procedures* for the *choroid twisted clusters (Herophilus, c335–c280 BC)*; see Singer translation (1999, p. 231).

LATER SYNONYMS:

1. *secundines (Vesalius, 1543a)*
   Vesalius wrote that ***choroid plexus (Galen, c177)*** had been compared to membranes (*secundines* means

chorion) nourishing the fetus; see Singer translation (1952, p. 59 and Figs. 4–6).

2. *secundine plexus (Vesalius, 1543a)*
   More complete form of *secundines (Vesalius, 1543a)*; see Singer translation (1952, p. 98).
3. *plexus reteformis (Geminus, 1553)*
   Synonym for macrodissected adult human ***choroid plexus (Galen, c177)***, see *The tables of the brayne*, Figure 4-O.
4. *plexus reticulares (Colombo, 1559)*
   Apparently synonym for macrodissected adult human ***choroid plexus (Galen, c177)***; see Bauhin (1605, p. 596).
5. *plexus glandulosi (Varoli, 1573)*
   Varoli suggested that *glandular* is better description of ***choroid plexus (Galen, c177)*** than *net-like* (p. 8; see Crooke, 1615, p. 501). According to a description of Varoli's dissection method for human cadavers, "if you handle it [***choroid plexus (Galen, c177)***] nicely and mark it diligently you shall find that it is nothing else but a heape of broade and long membranes growing out of the *pia mater* of the braine, at the one side whereof through out their whole length hangeth a little thicke vessell full of excrementitious moysture, through which exceeding small vessels are derived..." (Crooke 1615 translation, p. 501, of Bauhin, 1605).
6. *plexus coriformes (Bauhin, 1605)*
   According to Bauhin, widely used term for macrodissected adult human ***choroid plexus (Galen, c177)***; p. 596; see Crooke translation, 1615, p. 464.
7. *plexus choreformes (Bauhin, 1605)*
   Crooke (1615, p. 464) translation of *plexus coriformes (Bauhin, 1605)*.
8. *plexus retiformis (Guidi, 1611)*
   Synonym for macrodissected adult human ***choroid plexus (Galen, c177)***; Table LXXVI, Figure VI-G.
9. *choroid fold (Diemerbroeck, 1689)*
   Synonym for macrodissected adult human ***choroid plexus (Galen, c177)***; p. 419.

PARTLY CORRESPONDS:

1. *red worm (Haly Abbas or Ali ibn' ul-Abbas, d. 994)*
   In *The Complete Book of Medical Art, called the Royal Book*, Haly Abbas referred to ***choroid plexus (Galen, c177)***, probably along with ***pineal gland (Galen, c192)***, as "red worm." It seems likely he referred to ***choroid plexus of lateral ventricle (Vicq d'Azyr, 1784)*** along with ***choroid plexus of third ventricle (Vicq d'Azyr, 1784)***; see, for example, Pagel (1958, p. 101), Manzoni (1998, p. 121). Unlike Galen, he wrote that two valves regulate flow of psychic pneuma through ***ventricles (Hippocrates)***, one (red worm) from ***lateral ventricle (Vesalius, 1543a)*** to ***third ventricle (Galen, c173)***, and the other, ***cerebellar vermis (Meckel, 1817)***—a view supported by Galen—from ***third ventricle (Galen, c173)*** to ***fourth ventricle (Galen, c192)***; see Manzoni (1998, p. 121).
2. *vermis (Avicenna or Ibn Sina, c1030)*
   Several sources claim that Avicenna first used the term *vermis* for ***choroid plexus of lateral ventricle (Vicq d'Azyr, 1784)***— for example, Lewy (1942, p. 2) and Garrison & McHenry (1969, p. 24)—although Haly Abbas had earlier used the term *red worm (Haly Abbas or Ali ibn' ul-Abbas, d. 994)*, with which it is probably synonymous. Use of the simple term *vermis* in this context is very clear in Mondino's *Anathomia*, where he described ***choroid plexus of lateral ventricle (Vicq d'Azyr, 1784)*** thus: "At the base of the lateral ventricles lies a red, sanguineous substance, called vermis...because it looks like an earthworm and because it behaves like it." (Lewy translation, 1942, p. 2). Alternately, part of the relevant passage has been translated, "At the side of each *ancha*, between the ventricles already mentioned, is a red blood-like substance made like a long or subterranean worm...This *worm* can lengthen itself by constriction...It is called *vermis* both for that it doth resemble a subterraneous worm in substance and shape and also by reason of this motion of contraction and extension" (Singer translation, 1925, p. 92). When lengthened, it supposedly blocked ***interventricular foramen (>1840)***, and thus formed at least part of ***choroid plexus of third ventricle (Vicq d'Azyr, 1784)***; Singer (1925, p. 92), Lewy (1942, p. 2). Albertus Magnus (see Lind, 1975, p. 58) claimed that a *caruncula (Albertus Magnus, 13th century)* of the little worm regulates flow of breath into ***lateral ventricles (Vesalius, 1543a)***, presumably via *paired outgrowths from encephalon (Galen, c173)*.
3. *worm (Mondino, 1316)*
   Synonym for macrodissected adult human *vermis (Avicenna or Ibn Sina, c1030)*; see *vermis (Avicenna or Ibn Sina, c1030)*, also see Burdach (1822, p. 398).
4. *vermiformis (Geminus, 1553)*
   Synonym for macrodissected adult human *vermis (Mondino, 1316)*; f. BII.

choroid plexus of fourth ventricle (Vieussens, 1684)

As described for macrodissected adult human, vascular infoldings of ***choroid membrane of fourth ventricle (>1840)***; on the right and left side there is a roughly *L*-shaped invagination, with one limb extending rostrally from the ***median aperture of fourth ventricle (>1840)*** and the other limb extending laterally (from the rostral end of the former) into the ***lateral recess of fourth ventricle (>1840)*** and then through the ***lateral aperture of fourth ventricle (>1840)*** into the ***subarachnoid space (Magendie, 1827)***; see Millen & Woollam (1962, Figs. 36, 37). For Vieussens's use in macrodissected adult human, see Table XII-*h,K*; also see Vicq d'Azyr (1786, p. 109), Burdach (1822, p. 317). It was first described clearly by Willis; see ***[choroid plexus of fourth ventricle (Vieussens, 1684)] (Willis, 1664)***.

TRANSLATIONS:

1. *plexus choroïdes quartus ventriculus (Vieussens, 1684)*
   Original Latin form of ***choroid plexus of fourth ventricle (Vieussens, 1684)***.
2. *plexus chorioïdei ventriculi quarti (Burdach, 1822)*
   Latin form of ***choroid plexus of fourth ventricle (Vieussens, 1684)***; p. 91.

3. *plexus choroideus ventriculi quarti (>1840)*
   Current Latin form of ***choroid plexus of fourth ventricle (Vieussens, 1684)***; see *Terminologia Anatomica* (1998, p. 105).

EARLIER REFERENCES:

Described, not named or illustrated:

1. ***[choroid plexus of fourth ventricle (Vieussens, 1684)] (Galen, c173, c177)***
   It has been claimed that Galen referred to it (Clarke & O'Malley, 1996, p. 712), but this does not seem likely from other interpretations; see Wiberg (1914, pp. 29–30), Singer (1999, pp. 236–237), and the observation of May (1968, p. 417) and Rocco (2003, pp. 135 note 100, 162 note 225). The two "worms" Galen referred to are almost certainly superior and inferior parts of ***cerebellar vermis (Meckel, 1817)***; see *veriform epiphysis (Galen, c173)*. In the *Epitome*, Vesalius (1543b) explicitly denied there is ***choroid plexus (Galen, c177)*** in ***fourth ventricle (Galen, c192)***; see Lind (1949, p. 68).
2. ***[choroid plexus of fourth ventricle (Vieussens, 1684)] (Willis, 1664)***
   Willis was the first (Millen & Woollam, 1962, p. 7; also see Burdach, 1822, p. 317) to describe it clearly, one strand on right side and one on left side, in macrodissected adult human and other common large mammals; see Pordage translation (1681, p. 67).

LATER SYNONYMS:

1. *fourth choroid plexus (Haller, 1754a)*
   Synonym for macrodissected adult human ***choroid plexus of fourth ventricle (Vieussens, 1684)***; in the original Latin, *plexus choroideus quartus*, Figure 3.
2. *fourth choroid plexus of Haller (Soemmerring, 1778)*
   Eponym for macrodissected adult human *fourth choroid plexus (Haller, 1754a)*; Table III-*z*.
3. *posterior choroid plexus (Desmoulins, 1825)*
   Synonym for macrodissected embryonic human ***choroid plexus of fourth ventricle (Vieussens, 1684)***; in the original French, *plexus choroïdes postérieurs*, p. 251.
4. *cerebellar choroid plexus (Desmoulins, 1825)*
   Synonym for macrodissected embryonic human ***choroid plexus of fourth ventricle (Vieussens, 1684)***; in the original French, *plexus choroïdes cérébelleux*, p. 251.
5. *choroides minor (Quain, 1828)*
   Synonym for macrodissected adult human ***choroid plexus of fourth ventricle (Vieussens, 1684)***; p. 622.
6. *choroid plexus minor (Quain, 1832)*
   Synonym for macrodissected adult human ***choroid plexus of fourth ventricle (Vieussens, 1684)***; p. 649.

PARTLY CORRESPONDS:

1. *lateral branches of choroid plexus of fourth ventricle (Vicq d'Azyr, 1784)*
   Vicq d'Azyr clearly described them (right and left) for macrodissected adult human; p. 586. They were clearly illustrated by Soemmerring (1778, Tab. II-*F*).
2. *wings of choroid plexus of fourth ventricle (Vicq d'Azyr, 1784)*
   Synonym for *lateral branches of choroid plexus of fourth ventricle (Vicq d'Azyr, 1784)*; p. 586.

choroid plexus of lateral ventricle (Vicq d'Azyr, 1784)

As described for macrodissected adult human, a vascular invagination along the ***choroid fissure (>1840)*** of the ***choroid membrane of lateral ventricle (>1840)*** and subjacent ***choroid epithelium of lateral ventricle (>1840)*** considered together. It is a rostral and then caudal extension through the ***interventricular foramen (>1840)*** of the ***choroid plexus of third ventricle (Vicq d'Azyr, 1784)***; see Millen & Woollam (1962, Figs. 34, 35), Williams & Warwick (1980, Figs. 7.157, 7.159). For Vicq d'Azyr's use in macrodissected adult human, see pp. 540–541.It was known long ago; see ***[choroid plexus of lateral ventricle (Vicq d'Azyr, 1784)] (Herophilus, c335–c280 BC)***.

EARLIER REFERENCES:

Described, not named or illustrated:

1. ***[choroid plexus of lateral ventricle (Vicq d'Azyr, 1784)] (Herophilus, c335–c280 BC)***
   Galen noted that Herophilus first observed it, probably in macrodissected adult human and other large mammals; see Wiberg (1914, p. 26), May translation (1968, p. 417), von Staden (1989, p. 225), Singer translation (1999, p. 231).

Earlier synonyms:

1. *plexus choriformis (Günther, 1531)*
   Synonym for ***choroid plexus of lateral ventricle (Vicq d'Azyr, 1784)***; see Singer & Rabin (1945, p. 14).
2. *secundine plexus of lateral ventricle (Vesalius, 1543a)*
   Vesalius specifically referred to and illustrated macrodissected adult human ***choroid plexus of lateral ventricle (Vicq d'Azyr, 1784)***, for which he also used this term; see Singer translation (1952, p. 98 and Fig. 6-*M*).
3. *retiform plexus (Varoli, 1573)*
   Synonym for macrodissected adult human ***choroid plexus of lateral ventricle (Vicq d'Azyr, 1784)***; see Clarke & O'Malley (1996, pp. 822–823).
4. *rete mirabile (du Laurens, 1599)*
   Synonym for macrodissected adult human ***choroid plexus of lateral ventricle (Vicq d'Azyr, 1784)***, "I like rather, saith my Author [du Laurens], to call the Plexus Choroides (which is manifest and obvious to every eye in the upper ventricles of the braine) Rete mirabile or the Wonderfull Net, as also some of the new Writers have done: for in it the vitall spirit is attenuated and the Animall getteth a certaine rudiment." (Crooke translation, 1615, p. 529; for original Latin see du Laurens, pp. 408–409).
5. *lateral choroid plexus (Haase, 1781)*
   Synonym for macrodissected adult human ***choroid plexus of lateral ventricle (Vicq d'Azyr, 1784)***; in the original Latin, *plexus choroideus lateralis*, p. 19.

LATER SYNONYMS:

1. *plexus of lateral ventricles (Bell, 1803b)*
   Synonym for macrodissected adult human ***choroid plexus of lateral ventricle (Vicq d'Azyr, 1784)***; p. 87.
2. *choroid plexus of brain (Cruveilhier, 1836)*

Synonym for macrodissected adult human ***choroid plexus of lateral ventricle (Vicq d'Azyr, 1784)***; in the original French (plural), *plexus choroïdes du cerveau*, p. 698.

PARTLY CORRESPONDS:

1. *caruncula (Albertus Magnus, 13th century)*
   In *De Animalibus*, Albertus Magnus described a *caruncula* (small fleshy eminence) of ***choroid plexus of lateral ventricle (Vicq d'Azyr, 1784)*** regulating flow of breath into ***lateral ventricle (Vesalius, 1543a)***; see Lind (1975, p. 58) and *vermis (Avicenna or Ibn Sina, c1030)*.
2. *reflected portion of choroid plexus (Cruveilhier, 1836)*
   In macrodissected adult human, segment of ***choroid plexus of lateral ventricle (Vicq d'Azyr, 1784)*** lying in ***inferior horn of lateral ventricle (Bell, 1802)***; in the original French, *portion réfléchie du plexus choroide*, p. 695.
3. *inferior portion of choroid plexus (Cruveilhier, 1836)*
   Synonym for *reflected portion of choroid plexus (Cruveilhier, 1836)*; in the original French, *portion inférieure du plexus choroide*, p. 695.

choroid plexus of third ventricle (Vicq d'Azyr, 1784)

As described for macrodissected adult human, right and left vascular infoldings along the length of the ***roof of third ventricle (>1840)***. Caudally the ends of the infoldings join across the median plane, whereas rostrally each extends through the ***interventricular foramen (>1840)*** and continues as the corresponding ***choroid plexus of lateral ventricle (Vicq d'Azyr, 1784)***; see Millen & Woollam (1962, Figs. 34, 35), Williams & Warwick (1980, Figs. 7.157, 7.159), Nieuwenhuys et al. (2008, Fig. 3.7-19). For Vicq d'Azyr's use in macrodissected adult human, see pp. 540–541. Also see Vicq d'Azyr (1786, p. 21), where in the original French he used *le plexus choroïdes du troisieme ventricule*; Burdach (1822, p. 398). It was observed long ago by Galen; see ***[choroid plexus of third ventricle (Vicq d'Azyr, 1784)] (Galen, c173)***.

EARLIER REFERENCES:

Described, not named or illustrated:

1. ***[choroid plexus of third ventricle (Vicq d'Azyr, 1784)] (Galen, c173)***
   Apparently described by Galen in macrodissected adult beef, pig, and/or macaque but not human. He described "veins" coursing rostrally (anteriorly) from region of ***pineal gland (Galen, c192)*** to pass through each *hole (Galen, c177)* or ***interventricular foramen (>1840)*** into right and left ***lateral ventricle (Vesalius, 1543a)***; see Wiberg translation (1914, p. 26), May translation (1968, p. 417), Singer translation (1999, p. 234), Rocca (2003, pp. 148–149, 221–222).
2. ***[choroid plexus of third ventricle (Vicq d'Azyr, 1784)] (Aranzi, 1587)***
   Aranzi very clearly described for macrodissected adult human that ***choroid plexus (Galen, c177)*** stretches rostrally from region of ***pineal gland (Galen, c192)*** along length of ***third ventricle (Galen, c173)*** to continue as ***choroid plexus of lateral ventricle (Vicq d'Azyr, 1784)***, in ***inferior horn of lateral ventricle (Bell, 1802)***, as described today; see Clarke & O'Malley (1996, p. 720).

Earlier synonyms:

1. *reticular broad expansion (Ridley, 1695)*
   Synonym for roughly macrodissected adult human ***choroid plexus of third ventricle (Vicq d'Azyr, 1784)***; p. 58. As suggested by Vicq d'Azyr (1786, p. 32), it may include more ***choroid membrane of third ventricle (>1840)*** than later understood. Burdach (1822, p. 398) gave the Latin form *reticularis expansio*.
2. *velum vasculosum (Haller, 1754a)*
   Synonym for macrodissected adult human ***choroid plexus of third ventricle (Vicq d'Azyr, 1784)***; Table 2.
3. *plexus choroidei medii pars, thalamus incumbens (Soemmerring, 1778)*
   Specific term for ***choroid plexus of third ventricle (Vicq d'Azyr, 1784)***; Table III-*l*.
4. *middle choroid plexus (Günther, 1786)*
   Synonym for macrodissected adult human ***choroid plexus of third ventricle (Vicq d'Azyr, 1784)***; in the original Latin, *plexus choroideus medius*, p. 13.
5. *third choroid plexus (Günther, 1786)*
   Synonym for macrodissected adult human ***choroid plexus of third ventricle (Vicq d'Azyr, 1784)***; in the original Latin, *plexus choroideus tertius*, p. 13.

LATER SYNONYMS:

1. *choroid plexus of pineal gland (Vicq d'Azyr, 1786)*
   Synonym for macrodissected adult human ***choroid plexus of third ventricle (Vicq d'Azyr, 1784)***; in the original French, *le plexus choroïdes de la glande pinéale*, p. 21.
2. *plexus of third ventricle (Bell, 1803b)*
   Synonym for macrodissected adult human ***choroid plexus of third ventricle (Vicq d'Azyr, 1784)***; p. 87.
3. *tela choroidea (Bock, 1824)*
   Synonym listed for macrodissected adult human ***choroid plexus of third ventricle (Vicq d'Azyr, 1784)***; p. 152.

ciliary ganglion (Loder, 1778)

As described for macrodissected adult human, a ***terminal ganglion (Gaskell, 1886)*** lying near the apex of the orbit, having three main roots—the ***branch of oculomotor nerve to ciliary ganglion (>1840)***, a branch of the ***internal carotid plexus (>1840)*** called the ***sympathetic root of ciliary ganglion (>1840)***, and a ***communicating branch of nasociliary nerve with ciliary ganglion (>1840)***—and generating the ***short ciliary nerves (>1840)*** distal to it; see Williams & Warwick (1980, p. 1058). It was nicely illustrated by Bock (1817; Tab. III, Fig. 4 and p. 12). For Loder's use in macrodissected adult human, see p. 11. It was discovered as the *infolding of third pair (Willis, 1664)*.

TRANSLATIONS:

1. *ganglion ciliare (Loder, 1778)*
   Original Latin form of ***ciliary ganglion (Loder, 1778)***; p. 11.

EARLIER REFERENCES:

Earlier synonyms:

1. *infolding of third pair (Willis, 1664)*

Synonym for macrodissected adult (presumably human) ***ciliary ganglion (Loder, 1778)***; see Pordage translation (1681, p. 145, legend for Fig. 2-*g*). Also see p. 140 and Figure 2 on p. 302, where it may be illustrated (but not indicated) just above and to right of *d*—having roots from ***oculomotor nerve (Estienne, 1545)*** and branch of ***trigeminal nerve (Winslow, 1733)***, and generating ***short ciliary nerves (>1840)***.

2. *round infolding (Willis, 1664, p. 285)*
Synonym for ***ciliary ganglion (Loder, 1778)*** in macrodissected adult human and other large mammals; in the original Latin, *plexus rotundi*, see Pordage translation (1681, p. 140) and Haller (1743, p. 46 note *30*).
3. *ophthalmic plexus (Keill, 1698)*
Synonym for macrodissected adult human ***ciliary ganglion (Loder, 1778)***; in the original Latin, *plexus ophthalmicus*, p. 290.
4. *ophthalmic ganglion (Pourfour du Petit, 1729)*
Synonym for macrodissected adult human ***ciliary ganglion (Loder, 1778)***; in the original French, *le ganglion ophthalmique*, p. 17. Loder (1778, p. 17) referred to *ophthalmic plexus* in quadruped.
5. *lenticular ganglion (Winslow, 1733)*
Synonym for macrodissected adult human ***ciliary ganglion (Loder, 1778)***; Section VI, p. 62; see Foster (1892, pp. 1674–1675). It was listed as *ganglion lenticulare* by Haase (1781, p. 58).

LATER SYNONYMS:

1. *Augennervenknötchens (Soemmerring, 1801)*
German synonym for macrodissected adult human ***ciliary ganglia (Loder, 1778)***; p. 45.
2. *Augenknöchtchen (Soemmerring, 1801)*
Shortened form (and singular) of *Augennervenknötchens (Soemmerring, 1801)*; Table III, Figure VI-*h*.
3. *orbitar ganglion (Burdin, 1803)*
Synonym for macrodissected adult human ***ciliary ganglion (Loder, 1778)***; see translation (1803, Vol. 1, p. 171).

PARTLY CORRESPONDS:

1. *filament from spheno-palatine ganglion to ciliary ganglion (Todd, 1836–1839)*
Todd noted it was not yet established in macrodissected adult human as a constant feature: ***communicating branch (Winslow, 1733)*** between ***pterygopalatine ganglion (>1840)*** and ***ciliary ganglion (Loder, 1778)***; pp. 281–282.

cingulate region (Brodmann, 1909)

As described for macrodissected adult human, the dorsal topographic subdivision of the ***limbic region (>1840)*** lying between ***olfactory region (>1840)*** rostrally and ***hippocampal formation (>Swanson & Cowan, 1977)*** caudally and ventrally. Its rostral end is formed by the ***parolfactory gyrus (>1840)*** and its caudal end by the ***isthmus of cingulate region (>1840)***. Based on cellular architecture and connections in human, it includes, from rostral to caudal, the ***infralimbic area (Rose & Woolsey, 1948)***, ***anterior cingulate region (>1840)***, ***posterior cingulate region (>1840)***, and ***retrosplenial region (>1840)***; see Nieuwenhuys et al. (2008, p. 617 ff., Figs. 12.3, 12.13). ***Cingulate region (Brodmann, 1909)*** is preferred to *cingulate gyrus (>1840)* because a distinct *cerebral gyrus (Vesalius, 1543a)* cannot always be distinguished in human and because the term *region* applies to all mammals, whether gyrencephalic or lissencephalic. For Brodmann's use, see pp. 129, 146–148 and Figure 84. It was first adequately delineated by Duvernoy; see ***[cingulate region (Brodmann, 1909] (Duvernoy, 1735)***.

TRANSLATIONS:

1. *regio cingularis (Brodmann, 1909)*
Original Latin form of ***cingulate region (Brodmann, 1909)***; p. 129.

EARLIER REFERENCES:

Illustrated, not named or described:

1. ***[cingulate region (Brodmann, 1909] (Duvernoy, 1735)***
Duvernoy probably gave first adequate illustration of it in macrodissected adult human; see Meyer (1971, pp. 111, 124), Mazzolini (1991, p. 104, Fig. 33). Soemmerring (1778, Tab. III) provided a very accurate illustration that could be used today, and Malacarne (1780, Vol. 2, p. 9) recognized it as a *cerebral gyrus (Vesalius, 1543a)* according to Meyer (1971, p. 111).

Earlier synonyms:

1. *convolution accompanying corpus callosum (Vicq d'Azyr, 1786)*
Vicq d'Azyr clearly illustrated its correspondence with macrodissected adult human ***cingulate region (Brodmann, 1909)***; Plate XXV, Figure I-*18,22,9,19,10,15*.
2. *long convolution (Reil, 1809b)*
Essentially synonym for macrodissected adult human ***cingulate region (Brodmann, 1909)***; in the original German, *Längenwindung*, see Mayo translation (1823, p. 67, Tab. IX-*o*), Meyer (1971, pp. 111, 126).

PARTLY CORRESPONDS:

1. *central cingulate gyrus (Burdach, 1822)*
Most of macrodissected adult human ***cingulate region (Brodmann, 1909)***; in the original German, *centrale Randwulst der Zwinge*, p. 150, Table VIII-*φ*. Most or all of *middle cingulate gyrus (Burdach, 1822)* would also be included in ***cingulate region (>1840)***.
2. *middle cingulate gyrus (Burdach, 1822)*
Refers approximately to rostral and dorsal strip of macrodissected adult human ***cingulate region (Brodmann, 1909)***; in the original German, *mittlere Randwulst der Zwinge*, p. 150, Table VIII-*ϰ*.

cingulate sulcus (>1840)

As described for macrodissected adult human, the long, irregular, curving groove on the medial surface of the ***cerebral cortex gray matter (>1840)*** separating ***cingulate region (Brodmann, 1909)*** from (rostral to caudal) ***medial frontal gyrus (>1840)***, ***anterior paracentral gyrus (>1840)***, and ***posterior paracentral gyrus (>1840)***. It has two dorsally directed branches, ***paracentral sulcus***

(>1840) and ***marginal sulcus (>1840)***; see Crosby et al. (1962, Fig. 234), Williams & Warwick (1980, Fig. 7.114). It was first clearly illustrated by Soemmerring; see ***[cingulate sulcus (>1840)] (Soemmerring, 1778)***.

EARLIER REFERENCES:

Illustrated, not named or described:

1. *[cingulate sulcus (>1840)] (Soemmerring, 1778)*
   Accurately illustrated for macrodissected adult human; Table III.

Earlier synonyms:

1. *callosomarginal sulcus (>1840)*
   Synonym for macrodissected adult human ***cingulate sulcus (>1840)***; see Crosby et al. (1962, p. 348), Carpenter (1976, p. 608).

cingulum (Burdach, 1822)

As described for macrodissected adult human, a longitudinal component of the ***association fibers of cerebral cortex (>1840)*** lying between ***corpus callosum (Galen, c177)*** ventrally and ***cingulate region (Brodmann, 1909)*** dorsally; see Crosby et al. (1962, pp. 404–405). For Burdach's use in macrodissected adult human, see p. 149; the Latin plural form is *cingula*. It was perhaps first distinguished as *tenia tecta (Reil, 1809b)* and was clearly identified as the *fillet of great commissure (Mayo, 1827)*.

EARLIER REFERENCES:

Earlier synonyms:

1. *tenia tecta (Reil, 1809b)*
   Latin form of term (in German, plural, *bedeckten Bänder*, p. 172 ff.) Reil used for longitudinal ***central nervous system white matter tract (>1840)*** dorsal to macrodissected adult human ***corpus callosum (Galen, c177)***; see Mayo translation (1823, pp. 52, 66–68). Although its exact identity is uncertain (Meyer 1971, p. 30 note 25), and he did not provide a clear illustration, *tenia tecta (Reil, 1809b)* probably corresponds broadly to ***cingulum (Burdach, 1822)***—he described pulling it up to remove ***cingulate region (Brodmann, 1909)***; see Mayo translation (1823, p. 72). He also noted that "The fornix on the under surface of the corpus callosum is to be compared with the covered bands of the upper. The use of these parts is apparently that of longitudinal commissures." (Mayo translation, 1823, p. 68; also see Burdach, 1822, p. 370). Furthermore, Reil specifically referred in a different context to *striae of Lancisi (Reil, 1812c)*; also see *external fornix (Arnold, 1838b)*.
2. *covered bands (Reil, 1809b)*
   Mayo's translation of German, *bedeckten Bänder* or (singular) *tenia tecta (Reil, 1809b)*.
3. *lateral longitudinal striae (Meckel, 1817)*
   Synonym (plural) for macrodissected adult human *tenia tecta (Reil, 1809b)*; see translation (1832, Vol. 2, p. 448).

LATER SYNONYMS:

1. *fillet of great commissure (Mayo, 1827)*
   Apparently synonym for macrodissected adult human ***cingulum (Burdach, 1822)***; Plate VI-X.
2. *peripheral part of fornix (Arnold, 1838b)*
   Synonym for macrodissected adult human ***cingulum (Burdach, 1822)***; in the original Latin, *pars fornicis peripherica*; Table X, Figure 5 legend.
3. *external fornix (Arnold, 1838b)*
   Synonym for *peripheral part of fornix (Arnold, 1838b)*; in the original Latin, *fornicis externi*, Table X, Figure 5 legend.
4. *peripheral fornix (Arnold, 1838b)*
   Synonym for *peripheral part of fornix (Arnold, 1838b)*; in the original Latin, *fornicis peripherici*, Table X, Figure 5 legend.

circular sinus (Ridley, 1695)

As described for macrodissected adult human, a component of the ***circulatory system***; the venous ring around the ***pituitary gland (>1840)*** formed laterally by the rostral ends of the right and left ***cavernous sinus (Winslow, 1733)***, rostrally by the ***anterior intercavernous sinus (>1840)***, and caudally by the ***posterior intercavernous sinus (>1840)***; see Williams & Warwick (1980, p. 748 and Figs. 6.126, 6.127B), *Dorland's* (2003, p. 1706). For Ridley's use in macrodissected adult human, see p. 44. It was perhaps first delineated as the *communicatio recentaculorum (Vieussens, 1684)*.

EARLIER REFERENCES:

Earlier synonyms:

1. *communicatio recentaculorum (Vieussens, 1684)*
   Vieussens was probably the first to observe and at least partly describe macrodissected adult human ***circular sinus (Ridley, 1695)***; p. 7. Also see Ridley (1695, p. 44) and Burdach (1822, p. 400). It was also described by Brunner (1688) in macrodissected adult human; see Burdach (1822, p. 400).

LATER SYNONYMS:

1. *sinus ovalis (Santorini, 1724)*
   Synonym for macrodissected adult human ***circular sinus (Ridley, 1695)***; p. 71, see Burdach (1822, p. 400).
2. *superior circular sinus (Winslow, 1733)*
   Synonym for macrodissected adult human ***circular sinus (Ridley, 1695)***; Section X, p. 28, see Burdach (1822, p. 400).
3. *sinus medius (Lieutaud, 1742)*
   Synonym for macrodissected adult human ***circular sinus (Ridley, 1695)***; p. 386.
4. *sinus circularis Ridleyi (Tarin, 1750)*
   Eponym for macrodissected adult human ***circular sinus (Ridley, 1695)***; p. 33.
5. *sinus ellipticus (Malacarne, 1780)*
   Synonym for macrodissected adult human ***circular sinus (Ridley, 1695)***, according to Burdach (1822, p. 400), without a specific citation.
6. *sinus clinoïdeus (Malacarne, 1780)*
   Synonym for macrodissected adult human ***circular sinus (Ridley, 1695)*** according to Burdach (1822, p. 400), without a specific citation.
7. *sinus coronoïdeus (Meckel, 1817)*

Synonym for macrodissected adult human ***circular sinus (Ridley, 1695)***; p. 333.

8. *sinus circularis sellae equinae (Burdach, 1822)*
Synonym for macrodissected adult human ***circular sinus (Ridley, 1695)***; p. 187.

circular sulcus (Schwalbe, 1881)

As described for macrodissected adult human, the groove separating ***insular region (Brodmann, 1909)*** from ***cerebral cortex gray matter (>1840)*** associated with the ***frontal operculum (>1840), parietal operculum (>1840)***, and ***temporal operculum (>1840)***. The ***circular sulcus (Schwalbe, 1881)*** is closed except for a short open segment facing the ***ambient gyrus (>1840)***, the *limen insulae (>1840)* or ***piriform area (Smith, 1919)*** of the ***olfactory region (>1840)***; see Williams & Warwick (1980, pp. 987–988 and Fig. 7.119), *Dorland's* (2003, p. 1786). For Schwalbe's use in macrodissected adult human, see p. 532. It was first delineated by Reil; see ***[circular sulcus (Schwalbe, 1881)] (Reil, 1809b)***.

EARLIER REFERENCES:

Illustrated and described, not named:

1. ***[circular sulcus (Schwalbe, 1881)] (Reil, 1809b)***
Described for macrodissected adult human; see Mayo translation (1823, p. 52). Reil wrote about how the "small, short, and covered convolutions [of the ***insular region (Brodmann, 1909)***] are surrounded by a groove." (Meyer translation, 1971, p. 127).

Earlier synonyms:

1. *superior sulcus (Burdach, 1822)*
Synonym for macrodissected adult human ***circular sulcus (Schwalbe, 1881)***; in the original Latin, *fissura superior*, and in the original German, *Oberspalte*, p. 166.

LATER SYNONYMS:

1. *circular sulcus of Reil (Schwalbe, 1881)*
Whole term (eponym) used for ***circular sulcus (Schwalbe, 1881)***; p. 532, see Foster (1894, p. 2873).

circumenteric nerve ring (>1840)

Regarded as the ***central nervous system (Carus, 1814)*** of nematodes and priapulids; see Bullock & Horridge (1965, pp. 605, 658), Swanson & Bota (2010). Not clearly described by 1840.

circumesophageal connective (>1840)

As described for annelids and arthropods, the segment of an invertebrate ***central nerve cord (Serres, 1824–1826)*** encircling the digestive system and connecting the ***supraesophageal ganglion (Grant, 1834a)*** or ***invertebrate brain (>1840)*** with the proximal (rostral) end of a ***ventral cord (Anderson, 1837)***, often formed by a *subesophageal ganglion (Straus Durckheim, 1828)*; see Bullock & Horridge (1965, pp. 662, 802–803). As a topographic division it is a ***central longitudinal communicating branch (>1840)***, and more generally a ***communicating branch (Winslow, 1733)***. It was described as long ago as *shank of oblong marrow (Willis, 1672)* in lobster.

EARLIER REFERENCES:

Earlier synonyms:

1. *shanks of oblong marrow (Willis, 1672)*
The two ***circumesophageal connectives (>1840)*** of the lobster he fancifully compared to roughly the mammalian ***pons (Haller, 1747)*** and ***medulla (Winslow, 1733)***; Table III, Figure 1-*D*; see Hanström, 1928, Figure 450.
2. *esophageal bridle (Lyonnet, 1762)*
Synonym for ***circumesophageal connective (>1840)*** in goat moth larva; in the original French, *bride de l'oesophage*, p. 579.
3. *cords of esophageal collar (Cuvier, 1800)*
Synonym for ***circumesophageal connectives (>1840)*** in a variety of invertebrates; in the original French, *cordons du collier de l'oesophage*, e.g., Vol. 2, p. 314.
4. *nerves of collar (Cuvier, 1800)*
Synonym for *cords of esophageal collar (Cuvier, 1800)* in annelid worms; in the original French, *nerfs du collier*, Vol. 2, p. 354.
5. *cerebral peduncle (Treviranus, 1817)*
Probably synonym for *shank of oblong marrow (Willis, 1672)*, described for macrodissected adult millipede (*Diplopoda*) viewed under the microscope; in the original German, *Hirnschenkel*; see Treviranus & Treviranus, 1816–1821, Vol. 2 (1817), p. 69, Table IX, Figure 3-*k*.
6. *esophageal ring (Serres, 1824–1826)*
Synonym for ***circumesophageal connective (>1840)*** in a variety of invertebrates; in the original French, *anneau oesophagien*, p. 16.

circumoral nerve ring (Tiedemann, 1815)

The ***nerve ring (>1840)*** in adult echinoderms where there is no convincing evidence the ***nervous system (Monro, 1783)***, which is a ***nerve net (>1840)***, is divided into ***central nervous system (Carus, 1814)*** and ***peripheral nervous system (Meckel, 1817)***; see Bullock & Horridge (1965, p. 1525), Cobb (1995, p. 411). There is also a ***circumoral nerve ring (>1840)*** with a ***ganglion (Galen, c173)*** in Phoronida; see Bullock & Horridge (1965, p. 641). For Tiedemann's use in adult starfish see p. 170; it was described a year earlier as simply a *nerve ring (Carus, 1814)*.

TRANSLATIONS:

1. *mundöffnung umgebenden Nervenringe (Tiedemann, 1815)*
Original German form of ***circumoral nerve ring (Tiedemann, 1815)***; p. 172; on p. 172, *mund umgebende nervenring* was used.

EARLIER REFERENCES:

Earlier synonyms:

1. *nerve ring (Carus, 1814)*
Synonym for ***circumoral nerve ring (>1840)*** in "animals with radial arms"; in the original German, *Nervenring*, p. 60.

LATER SYNONYMS:

1. *circular oral nervous chord (Grant, 1834a)*
Synonym for ***circumoral nerve ring (>1840)*** in starfish; p. 483.

2. *primary nervous ring (Anderson, 1837)*
Synonym for ***circumoral nerve ring (Tiedemann, 1815)***; p. 6. Anderson went on to claim finding modified forms of it in other animal classes, where he referred to it as *oral primary nervous ring*; see p. 32.

claustrum (Burdach, 1822)

As described for macrodissected adult human, an isolated mass of ***cerebral cortex gray matter (>1840)*** deep to the ***insular region (Brodmann, 1909)***, between ***extreme capsule (>1840)*** laterally and ***external capsule (Burdach, 1822)*** medially; see Nieuwenhuys et al. (2008, Figs. 5.4:*19–21* and p. 417). Based on cellular architecture and development, it has been interpreted to form a conspicuous part of the adult ***cortical subplate (>1840)***; see Swanson (2000, p. 130), Swanson (2004, Tabs. A note 5, B). For Burdach's use in macrodissected adult human, see p. 132. It was perhaps first clearly delineated by Vicq d'Azyr; see ***[claustrum (Burdach, 1822)] (Vicq d'Azyr, 1786)***.

EARLIER REFERENCES:

Illustrated and described, not named:

1. ***[claustrum (Burdach, 1822)] (Vicq d'Azyr, 1786)***
Clearly described and illustrated in frontal (horizontal) sections of macrodissected adult human; p. 27; Plates IX-*28*, X-*28*; also see Burdach (1822, p. 352).

Earlier synonyms:

1. *nucleus teniaformis (Reil, 1809b)*
According to Dejerine & Dejerine-Klumpke (1895, p. 369) without citation, Reil's term for macrodissected adult human ***claustrum (Burdach, 1822)***. Arnold (1838a, p. 68; 1838b, Tab. VII, Fig. 2-o) used it thus, spelled *nucleus taeniaeformis*.

LATER SYNONYMS:

1. *gray layer of insula (Rolando, 1831)*
Synonym for macrodissected adult human ***claustrum (Burdach, 1822)***; in the original Italian, *strato cinericcio dell' isola*, p. 113, Figure 4-*4*. Also see Henle (1871, p. 253).

coccygeal nerves (Camper, 1762)

As described for macrodissected adult human, the 1–3 (most commonly 1, sometimes 2, very rarely 3) pairs of ***spinal nerves (Camper, 1760–1762)*** associated with the ***coccygeal part of spinal cord (>1840)***; see Carpenter (1976, pp. 213–216). Camper appears to be the first to use this specific term for macrodissected adult human, applied to the single pair typically found exiting between the first and second coccygeal vertebrae; p. 8 and Table 1, Figure 2-*r,26*. Vesalius (1543a) denied the existence of ***coccygeal nerves (Camper, 1762)*** in macrodissected adult human; see Richardson & Carman translation (2002, pp. 208, 254). Vieussens (1684) suggested that the most caudal (lowest) ***spinal nerves (Camper, 1760–1762)*** in adult human may not always have visible ***ganglia (Galen, c173)*** associated with them; see Johnston (1767, p. 121). Benedetti may have been the first clearly to describe, but not name as such, a ***coccygeal nerve (Camper, 1762)*** in macrodissected adult human; see *sixth pair of sacral nerves (Benedetti, 1502)*.

TRANSLATIONS:

1. *nervi coccygei (Camper, 1762)*
Original Latin form of ***coccygeal nerves (Camper, 1762)***; p. 8.

EARLIER REFERENCES:

Earlier synonyms:

1. *sixth pair of sacral nerves (Benedetti, 1502)*
In macrodissected adult human, Benedetti counted six pairs of *sacral nerves (Benedetti, 1502)*, rather than five pairs of ***sacral nerves (Camper, 1760)*** and one pair of ***coccygeal nerves (Camper, 1762)***; see Lind translation (1975, pp. 130–133), also see *sacral nerves (Winslow, 1733)*.
2. *nerves of nape alhosos (Berengario da Carpi, 1523)*
Synonym for one pair of ***coccygeal nerves (Camper, 1762)*** counted in macrodissected adult human; see Lind translation (1959, p. 160). In 1536 Massa wrote, "The last bone of the spine is the tail bone [coccyx]; it is soft as if it were of cartilage and has one foramen in the middle from which one nerve only comes forth." (Lind translation, 1975, p. 251).
3. *three conjugations proceeding out of coccyx (Crooke, 1615)*
Refers to three pairs of ***coccygeal nerves (Camper, 1762)*** in macrodissected adult dog and monkey; p. 493. It was English translation of Bauhin (1605).

LATER SYNONYMS:

1. *sixth sacral nerve (Camper, 1762)*
Synonym for macrodissected adult human first ***coccygeal nerve (Camper, 1762)***; full term in the original Latin, *nervus sacer sextus seu coccygeus*, Plate I, Figure 2-*26*.
2. *caudal pairs of nerves (Burdin, 1803)*
Synonym for macrodissected adult mammalian ***coccygeal nerves (Camper, 1762)***; see translation (1803, Vol. 3, p. 150).

PARTLY CORRESPONDS:

1. *pairs of nerves associated with coccyx (Razi, c910)*
Razi counted three pairs of ***coccygeal nerves (Camper, 1762)*** in his account of human macroanatomy; see de Koning translation (1903, pp. 33–37, 487).
2. *nerves from medulla of alhosis (Achillini, 1520)*
Achillini's term for what was counted as three pairs of ***coccygeal nerves (Camper, 1762)*** in his description of human macroanatomy, although the observation must have been based ultimately on observations in macrodissected adult mammals other than human; see Lind (1975, p. 63). He implied that the term is derived from the first book of Razi's *Almansor*; see Lind translation (1975, p. 62).
3. *superior coccygeal nerve (Schlemm, 1834)*
For macrodissected adult human, Schlemm observed that occasionally there are two ***coccygeal nerves (Camper, 1762)***, rostral (superior) and caudal (inferior); in the original Latin, *nervus coccygeus superior*, Table 1, Figure 1-*4* and p. 5 ff.
4. *inferior coccygeal nerve (Schlemm, 1834)*
For macrodissected adult human, Schlemm observed that occasionally there are two ***coccygeal nerves***

(Camper, 1762), rostral (superior) and caudal (inferior); in the original Latin, *nervus coccygeus inferior*, Table 1, Figure 1-6 and p. 5 ff. Quain & Wilson (Pl. I-c) illustrated two for macrodissected adult human.

coccygeal part of spinal cord (>1840)

As described for macrodissected adult vertebrate, the longitudinal ***spinal cord part (>1840)*** generating the ***coccygeal nerves (Camper, 1762)***; see Carpenter (1976, pp. 213–216). As described for macrodissected adult human, the longitudinal ***spinal cord part (>1840)*** generating the 1–3 ***coccygeal nerves (Camper, 1762)***; see *Nomina Anatomica* (1983, p. A64), *Terminologia Anatomica* (1998, p. 105), Nieuwenhuys et al. (2008). It was perhaps first clearly indicated as the *medulla of alhosis (Achillini, 1520)*.

EARLIER REFERENCES:

Earlier synonyms:

1. *medulla of alhosis (Achillini, 1520)*
   Achillini used this synonym for ***coccygeal part of spinal cord (>1840)***, implying it was derived from the first book of Razi's *Almansor*; see Lind translation (1975, pp. 62–63).
2. *nape alhosis (Berengario da Carpi, 1523)*
   Synonym for macrodissected adult human ***coccygeal part of spinal cord (>1840)***; see Lind translation (1959, p. 160).

coccygeal plexus (>1840)

As described for macrodissected adult human, a plexiform cord resulting from the union of caudally directed (descending) branches of the fourth and fifth sacral and the coccygeal ***spinal nerve ventral branches (>1840)*** and generating the ***anococcygeal nerves (>1840)***; see Durward (1951, p. 1112), Williams & Warwick (1980, Fig. 7.213), *Terminologia Anatomica* (1998, p. 140). Perhaps the first specific reference to it was by Meckel; see ***[coccygeal plexus (>1840)] (Meckel, 1817)***.

EARLIER REFERENCES:

Described, not named or illustrated:

1. ***[coccygeal plexus (>1840)] (Meckel, 1817)***
   Vaguely described for macrodissected adult human; see translation (1832, Vol. 3, p. 15).

PARTLY CORRESPONDS:

1. *communicating branch between fourth and fifth sacral nerves (Bock, 1827)*
   Macrodissected adult human component of ***coccygeal plexus (>1840)*** formed by caudally directed (descending) branch of fourth sacral ***spinal nerve ventral branch (>1840)***; in the original Latin, *ram. communis nervi sacralis quarti et quinti*; Table VII, Figure 1-42. See Williams & Warwick (1980, Fig. 7.213).

coccygeal spinal ganglia (>1840)

As described for macrodissected adult human, there is one ***spinal nerve ganglion (Burdach, 1819)*** for each ***dorsal root (Spurzheim, 1826)*** of the one or more pairs of ***coccygeal nerves (Camper, 1762)***. They are numbered sequentially from rostral to caudal; see Williams & Warwick (1980, p. 1086). Other species may have a wide range of ***coccygeal nerves (Camper, 1762)*** and corresponding ***coccygeal spinal ganglia (>1840)***. They were probably first clearly delineated as *spinal ganglion of superior coccygeal nerve (Schlemm, 1834)*.

EARLIER REFERENCES:

Earlier synonyms:

1. *spinal ganglion of superior coccygeal nerve (Schlemm, 1834)*
   Schlemm described and illustrated that macrodissected adult humans often have one and occasionally two pairs of ***coccygeal nerves (Camper, 1762)***; in the latter case this term refers to ***coccygeal spinal ganglia (>1840)*** on the more rostral, or *superior coccygeal nerve (Schlemm, 1834)*; in the original Latin, *ganglion spinale nervus coccygeus superior*, Table 1, Figure 1-10.
2. *spinal ganglion of inferior coccygeal nerve (Schlemm, 1834)*
   Schlemm described and illustrated that macrodissected adult humans often have one and occasionally two ***coccygeal nerves (Camper, 1762)***; in the latter case this term refers to the ***coccygeal spinal ganglia (>1840)*** on the more caudal, or *inferior coccygeal nerve (Schlemm, 1834)*; in the original Latin, *ganglion spinale nervus coccygeus inferior*, Table 1, Figure 1-12.
3. *Schlemm's ganglion (Müller, 1837)*
   Eponym for macrodissected adult human ***coccygeal spinal ganglion (>1840)***; p. 290. Arnold (1835, p. 176; 1838a, p. 196) claimed without citations that Bichat and others had earlier clearly indicated its existence.
4. *ganglion of coccygeal nerve (Arnold, 1838b)*
   Synonym for macrodissected adult human ***coccygeal spinal ganglion (>1840)***; in the original Latin, *ganglion nervi coccygei*, Table II, Figure 1a-5.

coccygeal sympathetic ganglia (>1840)

As described for macrodissected adult human, ***sympathetic trunk ganglia (Winslow, 1733)*** having one or more ***gray communicating branches (>1840)*** between all ***coccygeal nerves (Camper, 1762)***. There is commonly one and occasionally two pairs of ***sacral sympathetic ganglia (>1840)***, numbered sequentially from rostral (superior) to caudal (inferior); see Mitchell (1953, Ch. 18), ***ganglion impar (Quain & Wilson, 1839)***. Other species may have considerably more pairs of ***coccygeal sympathetic ganglia (>1840)***. The first accurate account was probably given for the *coccygeal ganglion of intercostal nerve (Günther, 1786)*.

EARLIER REFERENCES:

Earlier synonyms:

1. *coccygeal ganglion of intercostal nerve (Günther, 1786)*
   Synonym for the one usual paired macrodissected adult human ***coccygeal sympathetic ganglion (>1840)***; in the original Latin, *ganglion coccygeum nervus intercostalis*, p. 96 (and p. 92).

2. *coccygeal ganglion (Mayer, 1794)*
   Synonym for macrodissected adult human *coccygeal ganglion of intercostal nerve (Günther, 1786)*; in the original Latin, *ganglion coccygeum*; Part 6, Table VI-*171* (p. 40).
3. *superior coccygeal ganglion (Bock, 1827)*
   Synonym for most rostral and largest macrodissected adult human ***coccygeal sympathetic ganglion (>1840)***; in the original Latin, *gangl. coccygeum superius*, Table VII, Figure 1-*62*.

cochlear communicating branch of vestibular nerve (>1840)

As described for macrodissected adult human, a ***communicating branch (Winslow, 1733)*** between ***caudal part of vestibular nerve (>1840)*** and ***cochlear ganglion (>1840)***; see Brödel (1946, Fig. 2, unlabeled), Mettler (1948, Fig. 58, labeled *vestibulocochlear ramus of Oort*, based on dissection by Brödel), *Terminologia Anatomica* (1998, p. 135). It was probably discovered by Scarpa; see ***[cochlear communicating branch of vestibular nerve (>1840)] (Scarpa, 1789)***.

EARLIER REFERENCES:

Illustrated and described, not named:

1. ***[cochlear communicating branch of vestibular nerve (>1840)] (Scarpa, 1789)***
   Probably described and illustrated for macrodissected adult human; Table 8, Figure 2.

Earlier synonyms:

1. *vestibulocochlear ramus (Oort, 1918)*
   Synonym for macrodissected adult mammalian ***cochlear communicating branch of vestibular nerve (>1840)***; also see Mettler (1948, Fig. 58).

cochlear ganglion (>1840)

As described for macrodissected adult human, the sensory ***cranial nerve ganglion (>1840)*** of the ***cochlear nerve (Cotugno, 1760)*** associated with the spiral canal of the modiolus; see Williams & Warwick (1980, p. 1213), *Terminologia Anatomica* (1998, p. 136). It was perhaps first mentioned by Cruveilhier; see ***[cochlear ganglion (>1840)] (Cruveilhier, 1836)***.

EARLIER REFERENCES:

Described, not named or illustrated:

1. ***[cochlear ganglion (>1840)] (Cruveilhier, 1836)***
   Cruveilhier wrote that macrodissected adult human ***cochlear nerve (Cotugno, 1760)*** "turns upon itself, as observed by Valsalva, and presents somewhat of a ganglionic appearance" (see translation, 1844, p. 842).

Earlier synonyms:

1. *spiral ganglion (>1840)*
   Synonym for macrodissected adult human ***cochlear ganglion (>1840)***; see Williams & Warwick (1980, p. 1213), *Terminologia Anatomica* (1998, p. 136).

cochlear nerve (Cotugno, 1760)

As described for macrodissected adult human, a component of the ***vestibulocochlear nerve (>1840)*** extending between the lateral surface of the ***medulla (Winslow, 1733)*** and the cochlear duct part of the membranous labyrinth. Its proximal part is associated with the ***vestibulocochlear nerve trunk (>1840)*** and its distal part, distal to the internal acoustic meatus, is free. This account is based on the work of Cannieu (1894), in turn built on Retzius (1884); see review in Streeter (1907, p. 154 ff.) and Durward (1951, Fig. 904). For Cotugno's use in macrodissected adult human see p. 408. It was probably first clearly identified by Du Verney; see ***[cochlear nerve (Cotugno, 1760)] (Du Verney, 1683)***.

EARLIER REFERENCES:

Described, not named or illustrated:

1. ***[cochlear nerve (Cotugno, 1760)] (Du Verney, 1683)***
   Du Verney distinguished in macrodissected adult human three branches of ***vestibulocochlear nerve (>1840)***: one to *cochlea*, one to *semicircular canals* and one to *vestibule*; the latter two arise from ***vestibular nerve (Cotugno, 1760)***; Section X, p. 110; also see translation (1737, pp. 49, 50).

Illustrated and described, not named:

1. ***[cochlear nerve (Cotugno, 1760)] (Valsalva, 1704)***
   Clearly illustrated for macrodissected adult human; Table 8, Figure 8-*e*.

Earlier synonyms:

1. *spirale intervallum nervi cochleae (Cotugno, 1760)*
   Whole Latin phrase related to ***cochlear nerve (Cotugno, 1760)***; p. 408.

LATER SYNONYMS:

1. *cochlear root of auditory nerve (>1840)*
   Can be synonym for ***cochlear nerve (Cotugno, 1760)*** as a whole; for example, see Cajal (1909–1911; and translation, 1995, Vol. 1, p. 616).

PARTLY CORRESPONDS:

1. *middle and anterior most inferior fascicle of soft nerve (Cotugno, 1760)*
   Free segment of macrodissected adult human ***cochlear nerve (Cotugno, 1760)*** distal to ***vestibulocochlear nerve trunk (>1840)***; in the original Latin, *fasciculus medius, & anterior omnium inferiorque*, Table II-*g2*.
2. *inner branch of portio mollis (Monro, 1783)*
   Synonym for macrodissected adult human *middle and anterior most inferior fascicle of soft nerve (Cotugno (1760)*; Table 30, Figure 4-*I*.
3. *inferior anterior branch of auditory nerve proper (Günther, 1786)*
   Synonym for macrodissected adult human *inner branch of portio mollis (Monro, 1783)*; in the original Latin, *ramus, anterior inferior*, p. 61.
4. *posterior fascicles of acoustic nerve trunk (Scarpa, 1789)*
   Apparently corresponds roughly to macrodissected adult human *middle and anterior most inferior fascicle of soft nerve (Cotugno (1760)*; Table 8, Figure 2-*n*.
5. *anterior branch of auditory nerve (Soemmerring, 1791)*
   Synonym for macrodissected adult human *inferior anterior branch of auditory nerve proper (Günther, 1786)*;

p. 225, also see Soemmerring (1798, p. 258). It is also the larger branch; see Soemmerring (1806, Tab. III, Fig. 9-*).

6. *posterior fasciculus of acustic nerve (Bell, 1803b)*
   Synonym for macrodissected adult human *posterior fascicles of acoustic nerve trunk (Scarpa, 1789)*; Plate X, Figure 2-*n*.
7. *anterior branch of acoustic nerve (Cloquet, 1828)*
   Synonym for macrodissected adult human *anterior branch of auditory nerve (Soemmerring, 1791)*; in the original French, *branche antérieure du nerf acoustique*, Table CXXX, Figure 9-*18*.
8. *cochlear nerve (Arnold, 1834)*
   Synonym for macrodissected adult human *anterior branch of auditory nerve (Soemmerring, 1791)*; in the original Latin, *nervus cochleae*, p. 12.
9. *cochlear root proper of auditory nerve (>1840)*
   Segment of ***cochlear nerve (Cotugno, 1760)*** between ***cochlear ganglion (>1840)*** and outer surface of ***medulla (Winslow, 1733)***; for example, see Cajal (1909–1911; and translation, 1995, Vol. 1, p. 634).
10. *cochlear root of vestibulocochlear nerve (>1840)*
   Synonym for *cochlear root proper of auditory nerve (>1840)*; see *Dorland's* (2003, p. 1566).

cochlear nerve central root (>1840)

As described for macrodissected adult human, and mammal generally with histological methods for ***axons (Kölliker, 1896)***, the short central continuation of the peripheral ***cochlear nerve (Cotugno, 1760)*** from the plane where it enters the ***medulla (Winslow, 1733)*** to its termination in the ***cochlear nuclei (>1840)***. For adult human, "The [cochlear] nerve enters the pons [***medulla (Winslow, 1733)***] just distal to the N. vestibuli (Plate II). The bundle [root] passes dorsalward a distance of 1/6 mm., growing gradually wider until it spreads out into a nucleus [ventral cochlear]." (Sabin, 1901, p. 82). It was probably first described as the *upper and external part of auditory nerve (Meckel, 1817)*.

EARLIER REFERENCES:

Earlier synonyms:

1. *upper and external part of auditory nerve (Meckel, 1817)*
   Probably synonym for macrodissected adult human ***cochlear nerve central root (>1840)***, although Meckel's description is difficult to follow; see translation (1832, Vol. 3, p. 52).

cochlear nuclei (>1840)

As described for macrodissected adult human, and for adult mammal in general with cellular architecture and connections, a ***gray matter region (Swanson & Bota, 2010)*** near the lateral surface of the rostral half of the ***medulla (Winslow, 1733)***, with two main divisions, ***dorsal cochlear nucleus (>1840)*** and ***ventral cochlear nucleus (>1840)***. The ***cochlear nerve (Cotugno, 1760)*** ends there, and they lie lateral to the ***vestibular nuclei (>1840)*** and ***spinal nucleus of trigeminal nerve (>1840)***; see Nieuwenhuys et al. (2008, pp. 194, 736 ff. and Fig. 6.24-*1,10*). They were probably first identified as the *gray band (Procháska, 1779)*.

EARLIER REFERENCES:

Earlier synonyms:

1. *gray band (Procháska, 1779)*
   Probably refers to at least main part of macrodissected adult human ***cochlear nuclei (>1840)***, and their relationship with *auditory nerve (Galen, c192)* was noted; pp. 387–391, see Meckel (1832, Vol. 2, p. 424), where it was noted that *gray bands (Proch   áska, 1779)* disappear in deaf people; the merit of having made profound researches on these striae belongs to Wenzel & Wenzel (1812).
2. *fasciola cinerea (Prochāska, 1779)*
   Original Latin form of *gray band (Procháska, 1779)*; see Meckel (1832, Vol. 2, p. 424).
3. *ganglion of acoustic nerve (Gall & Spurzheim, 1810)*
   Probably synonym for macrodissected adult human ***cochlear nuclei (>1840)***; p. 76, also see Gordon (1815, p. 180; 1817, p. 36) and Burdach (1822, p. 312). It was identified in macrodissected adult amphibian by Carus (1814, Tab. 3-π); in the original German, *Hörnervenganglion*.
4. *cinerea taenola (Wenzel & Wenzel, 1812)*
   Synonym for macrodissected adult human *gray band (Procháska, 1779)*; pp. 183–187, see Burdach (1822, p. 311), Foster (1894, p. 2901). According to Rolando (1825a, p. 36 & Tab. II, Fig. 3-*8*), Malacarne (1791, p. 66) referred to them as ribbons (*fiocchi*), and Gall & Spurzheim (1810, p. 183) referred to them as gray tubercles (*tubercules cendrés*).
5. *taenia grisea (Wenzel & Wenzel, 1812)*
   Synonym for *cinerea taenola (Wenzel & Wenzel, 1812)*; see *grey band of Wenzels (Tiedemann, 1816)*. They probably observed it in a 3-month human embryo; p. 321, see Gordon (1815, p. 192).
6. *brown ridge on peduncle of cord (Gordon, 1815)*
   Synonym for macrodissected adult human *gray band (Procháska, 1779)*; p. 192, also see pp. 180–181.
7. *ganglion of auditory nerve (Tiedemann, 1816)*
   Probably refers to ***cochlear nuclei (>1840)***, as observed here in 4-month and older human fetus; see translation (1826, pp. 47, 62), where Tiedemann noted Wenzel & Wenzel's reference (1812, p. 189) to *cinerea taenola (Wenzel & Wenzel, 1812)* in macrodissected adult human.
8. *grey band of Wenzels (Tiedemann, 1816)*
   Eponym for *cinerea taenola (Wenzel & Wenzel, 1812)*; see translation (1826, Pls. X, Fig. 2-*c*; XII-*d*).
9. *taenia cinerea foveae rhomboidalis (Burdach, 1822)*
   Synonym for macrodissected adult human *cinerea taenola (Wenzel & Wenzel, 1812)*; p. 84; see Foster (1894, p. 2900).

collateral branch of intercostal nerves (Davies et al., 1931)

As described for macrodissected adult human, each ***intercostal nerve (Vesalius, 1543a)*** generates a collateral branch following the caudal border of the space in the same intermuscular interval as the main trunk, which it may rejoin before distributing as a second ***anterior cutaneous branch of intercostal nerves (>1840)***; see Williams & Warwick (1980, p. 1103), *Terminologia Anatomica* (1998, p. 139). They were first clearly delineated by Vieussens; see ***[collateral branch of intercostal nerve (Davies et al., 1931)] (Vieussens, 1684)***.

EARLIER REFERENCES:

Illustrated and described, not named:

1. ***[collateral branch of intercostal nerve (Davies et al., 1931)] (Vieussens, 1684)***
   Described and illustrated clearly for macrodissected adult human; Table 27.

collateral eminence (Meckel, 1767)

As described for macrodissected adult human, the elevation in the floor of the ***inferior horn of lateral ventricle (Bell, 1802)*** caused by the ***collateral sulcus (>1840)***; see Mettler (1948, Fig. 101). "Sometimes, but rarely, we find a second eminence, which varies in length, at the side of and behind the cornu Ammonis [which is the first eminence] so that it seems divided into two parts situated one above the other. This eminence is termed the *collateral eminence* of Meckel (*eminentia collateralis Meckelii*), and seems to arise from suspended development." (Meckel translation, 1832, Vol. 2, p. 465). For Meckel's original use, see p. 91. It may first have been pointed out as the *tuber exterius (Günz, 1750)*.

TRANSLATIONS:

1. *protubérances collatérales (Meckel, 1767)*
   Original French form (plural) for ***collateral eminence (Meckel, 1767)***; p. 91.

EARLIER REFERENCES:

Earlier synonyms:

1. *tuber exterius (Günz, 1750)*
   Synonym for macrodissected adult human ***collateral eminence (Meckel, 1767)***; see Burdach (1822, p. 376).

LATER SYNONYMS:

1. *collateral cerebral eminence (Mayer, 1779)*
   Synonym for macrodissected adult human ***collateral eminence (Meckel, 1767)***; in the original Latin, *eminentia cerebri collateralis*, p. 8.
2. *gamberuolo (Malacarne, 1780)*
   Italian synonym for macrodissected adult human ***collateral eminence (Meckel, 1767)***; in English it refers to a greave—leg armor between the knee and ankle, p. 66.
3. *collateral cerebral eminence of Meckel (Günther, 1786)*
   Eponym for macrodissected adult human ***collateral eminence (Meckel, 1767)***; in the original Latin, *eminentia cerebri collateralis Meckelii*, p. 11.
4. *collateral eminence of Meckel (Meckel, 1817)*
   Eponym for macrodissected adult human ***collateral eminence (Meckel, 1767)***; see translation (1832, Vol. 2, p. 465).

collateral sulcus (>1840)

As described for macrodissected adult human, a longitudinal groove between ***lingual gyrus (>1840)*** and ***parahippocampal gyrus (>1840)*** medially, and ***medial occipitotemporal gyrus (>1840)*** laterally; see Williams & Warwick (1980, Fig. 7.114A), *Terminologia Anatomica (1998, p. 126)*. It was perhaps first clearly delineated by Soemmerring; see ***[collateral sulcus (>1840)] (Soemmerring, 1778)***.

EARLIER REFERENCES:

Illustrated, not named or described:

1. ***[collateral sulcus (>1840)] (Soemmerring, 1778)***
   Very clearly illustrated for macrodissected adult human; Tables I, II. Also see Vicq d'Azyr (1786, Pl. XVI).

collateral triangle (>1840)

As described for macrodissected adult human, a continuation of the ***collateral eminence (Meckel, 1767)*** triangular in shape and forming the floor of the ***atrium of lateral ventricle (>1840)***; see Williams & Warwick (1980, p. 1029). It was not clearly described by 1840.

TRANSLATIONS:

1. *trigonum collaterale (>1840)*
   Latin form of ***collateral triangle (>1840)***; see *Terminologia Anatomica* (1998, p. 127).
2. *collateral trigone (>1840)*
   English form of *trigonum collaterale (>1840)*; see *Terminologia Anatomica* (1998, p. 127).

common carotid plexus (Cloquet, 1816)

As described for macrodissected adult human, it arises from ventral (anterior) branches of the ***superior cervical ganglion (Vieussens, 1684)*** and/or the ***communicating branch of superior and middle cervical ganglia (Cruveilhier, 1836)*** and surrounds the common carotid artery; see Williams & Warwick (1980, p. 1128). Cloquet described it as arising from anterior branches of the ***communicating branch of superior and middle cervical ganglia (Cruveilhier, 1836)*** in macrodissected adult human; p. 692. It was probably alluded to long ago by Galen; see ***[common carotid plexus (Cloquet, 1816)] (Galen, c192)***.

TRANSLATIONS:

1. *plexus carotidien primitif (Cloquet, 1816)*
   Original French form of ***common carotid plexus (Cloquet, 1816)***; p. 692.

EARLIER REFERENCES:

Described, not named or illustrated:

1. ***[common carotid plexus (Cloquet, 1816)] (Galen, c192)***
   Galen probably alluded to it in macrodissected adult beef, pig, and/or macaque (but not human) although if so, misidentified its origin as ***vagus nerve (Galen, c192)***; see Duckworth translation (1962, p. 203).

common fibular nerve (>1840)

As described for macrodissected adult human, the smaller division of the ***sciatic nerve (Keill, 1698)***, arising from the fourth and fifth lumbar and first and second sacral ***sacral***

plexus dorsal divisions (Paterson, 1887) and generating the ***nerve to short head of biceps femoris (>1840), articular branches of common fibular nerve (>1840), lateral cutaneous nerve of calf (>1840), sural communicating branch of common fibular nerve (>1840), superficial fibular nerve (Fyfe, 1800)***, and ***deep fibular nerve (Fyfe, 1800)***; see Durward (1951, pp. 1104–1107, Figs. 946–948), Williams & Warwick (1980, pp. 1112–1115, Figs. 7.216, 217), *Terminologia Anatomica* (1998, p. 140). It corresponds to the ***radial nerve (Du Verney, 1697)*** of the upper limb; Durward (1951, p. 1106). It was known to Galen; see ***[common fibular nerve (>1840)] (Galen, c177)***.

TRANSLATIONS:

1. *nervus fibularis communis (>1840)*
   Current Latin form of ***common fibular nerve (>1840)***; see *Terminologia Anatomica* (1998, p. 140).

EARLIER REFERENCES:

Described, not named or illustrated:

1. ***[common fibular nerve (>1840)] (Galen, c177)***
   Described for macrodissected adult beef, pig, and/or macaque but not human; see Singer translation (1999, pp. 85–87).

Earlier synonyms:

1. *outer trunk of fourth nerve entering leg (Vesalius, 1543a)*
   Synonym for macrodissected adult human ***common fibular nerve (>1840)***; see Richardson & Carman translation (2002, pp. 259–260).
2. *lesser trunk of nerve of thigh (Vesalius, 1543a)*
   Synonym for *outer trunk of fourth nerve entering leg (Vesalius, 1543a)*; see Richardson & Carman translation (2002, p. 265).
3. *outer trunk or stock of fourth sinew going into leg (Geminus, 1553)*
   Synonym for *outer trunk of fourth nerve entering leg (Vesalius, 1543a)*; originally spelled *outter truncke or stocke of fourth synowe goynge into legge*, see *The table of the figures of sinowes*.
4. *less trunk of fourth sinew of thigh (Geminus, 1553)*
   Synonym for *outer trunk or stock of fourth sinew going into leg (Geminus, 1553)*; originally spelled *lesse truncke of fourth synowe of thigh*, see *The table of the figures of sinowes*, Figure 7.
5. *external branch of crural trunk (Diemerbroeck, 1672)*
   Synonym for macrodissected adult human ***common fibular nerve (>1840)***; pp. 875–876, translation (1689, p. 563).
6. *external branch of posterior crural nerve (Vieussens, 1684)*
   Synonym for macrodissected adult human ***common fibular nerve (>1840)***; in the original Latin, *nervus cruralis posticus, ramus exterior*, Table XXIX-Q.
7. *external branch of crural nerve proper (Salmon, 1713)*
   Synonym for macrodissected adult human ***common fibular nerve (>1840)***; p. 132.
8. *external sciatic nerve (Winslow, 1733)*
   Synonym for macrodissected adult human ***common fibular nerve (>1840)***; in the original Latin, *nervus sciaticus externus*, Section VI, p. 92.
9. *sciatico-peroneal nerve (Winslow, 1733)*
   Synonym for *external sciatic nerve (Winslow, 1733)*; in the original Latin, *nervus sciatico-peronaeus*, Section VI, p. 92.
10. *small sciatic ramus (Winslow, 1733)*
    Synonym for *external sciatic nerve (Winslow, 1733)*; Section VI, p. 92. Walter (1783) used the Latin, *ramus nervi ischiatici minor*, Table I-392.
11. *external popliteal nerve (Winslow, 1733)*
    Synonym for *external sciatic nerve (Winslow, 1733)*; in the original Latin, *nervus popliteus externus*, Section VI, p. 92.
12. *peroneal nerve (Schaarschmidt, 1750)*
    Synonym for macrodissected adult human ***common fibular nerve (>1840)***; in the original Latin, *nervus peroneus*, p. 89. See *Nomina Anatomica* (1983, p. A78).
13. *anterior tibial nerve (Haller, 1762)*
    Synonym for macrodissected adult human ***common fibular nerve (>1840)***; in the original Latin, *nervus tibialis anterior*, p. 251.
14. *external tibial nerve (Haller, 1762)*
    Synonym for macrodissected adult human ***common fibular nerve (>1840)***; in the original Latin, *nervus tibialis exterior*, p. 251.
15. *external popliteal sciatic nerve (Sabatier, 1775)*
    Synonym for macrodissected adult human ***common fibular nerve (>1840)***; in the original French, *nerf sciatique poplité externe*, pp. 744, 748.
16. *external branch of sciatic nerve trunk (Günther, 1786)*
    Synonym for macrodissected adult human ***common fibular nerve (>1840)***; in the original Latin, *r. exterior*, p. 86.
17. *minor branch of sciatic nerve trunk (Günther, 1786)*
    Synonym for macrodissected adult human ***common fibular nerve (>1840)***; in the original Latin, *r. minor*, p. 86.
18. *exterior sciatic nerve (Günther, 1786)*
    Synonym for macrodissected adult human ***common fibular nerve (>1840)***; in the original Latin, *ischiaticus exterior*, p. 88.
19. *minor sciatic nerve (Günther, 1786)*
    Synonym for macrodissected adult human ***common fibular nerve (>1840)***; in the original Latin, *ischiaticus minor*, p. 88.
20. *fibular nerve (Coopmans, 1789)*
    Synonym for macrodissected adult human ***common fibular nerve (>1840)***; p. 170; also see Bell (1803a, Pl. VII-10), *Nomina Anatomica* (1983, p. A78).
21. *peroniar nerve (Burdin, 1803)*
    Synonym for macrodissected adult human ***common fibular nerve (>1840)***; see translation (1803, Vol. 1, p. 205).
22. *peroneal branch of large sciatic nerve (Chaussier, 1809)*
    Synonym for macrodissected adult human ***common fibular nerve (>1840)***; in the original French, *branche péronière*.
23. *external division of great sciatic nerve (Quain, 1828)*

Synonym for macrodissected adult human ***common fibular nerve (>1840)***; p. 296.

24. *peroneal branch of great femoro-popliteal nerve (Quain, 1828)*
Synonym for macrodissected adult human ***common fibular nerve (>1840)*** attributed without citation to Chaussier; in the original French, *branche peronière du grand fémoro-poplité*, p. 296.

25. *peroneal branch of femoro-popliteal nerve (Quain, 1837)*
Synonym for macrodissected adult human ***common fibular nerve (>1840)***; in the original Latin, *ramus peroneus nervi femoro-poplitei*, p. 799.

26. *lateral popliteal nerve (>1840)*
Synonym for macrodissected adult human ***common fibular nerve (>1840)***, equivalent to *external popliteal nerve (Winslow, 1733)*; see Durward (1951, p. 1106), Williams & Warwick (1980, p. 1114).

27. *common peroneal nerve (>1840)*
Synonym for macrodissected adult human ***common fibular nerve (>1840)***; in Latin, *nervus peronaeus communis*, see His (1895, p. 92).

PARTLY CORRESPONDS:

1. *adductor longus femoris nerve (Jördens, 1788)*
Described for macrodissected adult human as typically arising from ***common fibular nerve (>1840)***, although often considered branch of ***obturator nerve (Cheselden, 1726)***; in the original Latin, *nervus* est *adductoris femoris longi*, p. 3.
2. *peroneal cutaneous nerve (Soemmerring, 1791)*
Probably macrodissected adult human ***lateral cutaneous nerve of calf (>1840)*** with ***sural communicating branch of common fibular nerve (>1840)***; in the original Latin, *cutaneus peroneus*, p. 311; also see Soemmerring (1798, p. 332).
3. *fibular nerve (Quain, 1828)*
For macrodissected adult human, name applied with justification to ***common fibular nerve (>1840)*** on reaching posterior surface of head of fibula; p. 297.
4. *peroneal nerve (Quain, 1828)*
Synonym for *fibular nerve (Quain, 1828)*; p. 297.
5. *collateral branches of external popliteal sciatic nerve (Cruveilhier, 1836)*
Macrodissected adult human branches of ***common fibular nerve (>1840)*** before it divides, including ***sural communicating branch of common fibular nerve (>1840)*** and ***lateral cutaneous nerve of calf (>1840)***; in the original French, *branches collatérales*, p. 862.

common palmar digital nerves of median nerve (>1840)

As described for macrodissected adult human, there are typically five such branches of the ***median nerve (Du Verney, 1697)*** in turn generating distally the ***proper palmar digital nerves of median nerve (>1840)***; see Williams & Warwick (1980, p. 1099), *Terminologia Anatomica* (1998, p. 138). They were known to Galen; see ***[common palmar digital nerves of median nerve (>1840)] (Galen, c177)***.

TRANSLATIONS:

1. *nervus medianus nervi digitales palmares communes (>1840)*
Current Latin form of ***common palmar digital nerves of median nerve (>1840)***; see *Terminologia Anatomica* (1998, p. 138).

EARLIER REFERENCES:

Described, not named or illustrated:

1. ***[common palmar digital nerves of median nerve (>1840)] (Galen, c177)***
Vaguely alluded to for macrodissected adult macaque but not human; see Singer translation (1999, p. 74). Vesalius (1543a) clearly described three for macrodissected adult human; see Richardson & Carman translation (2002, p. 244).

Earlier synonyms:

1. *bifid cutaneous digital branches of median nerve (Günther, 1786)*
Günther described three ***common palmar digital nerves of median nerve (>1840)*** for macrodissected adult human; in the original Latin (singular), *r. dig. cut. bifidus*, p. 75.
2. *common digital branches of median nerve (Loder, 1803)*
Synonym for macrodissected adult human *bifid cutaneous digital branches of median nerve (Günther, 1786)*; in the original Latin, *ramus digitalis communis* (*primus, secundus, tertius*), Table CLXXX, Figure 1-64,75,83.
3. *digital branches of median nerve (Cloquet, 1816)*
Cloquet carefully described for macrodissected adult human five individual ***common palmar digital nerves of median nerve (>1840)***; pp. 648–649, as illustrated by Williams & Warwick (1980, Fig. 7.204).

PARTLY CORRESPONDS:

1. *thumb branch of median nerve (Mayer, 1794)*
Macrodissected adult human ***common palmar digital nerve of median nerve (>1840)*** generating ***proper palmar digital nerves of median nerve (>1840)*** for thumb; in the original Latin, *ramus pollicaris*; Part 5, Table V, Figure 1-15 (p. 22).
2. *volar external musculo-cutaneous branch of hand (Mayer, 1794)*
Synonym for *thumb branch of median nerve (Mayer, 1794)*; in the original Latin, *ramus musculo-cutaneus externus volae manus*; Part 5, Table V, Figure 1-15 (p. 22).
3. *first common digital branch of median nerve (Caldani, 1813, 1814)*
Macrodissected adult human ***common palmar digital nerve of median nerve (>1840)*** generating ***proper palmar digital nerves of median nerve (>1840)*** to medial side of thumb and lateral side of index finger; in the original Latin, *ramus digitalis communis primus*, Table CCLIX, Figure 2-15.
4. *second common digital branch of median nerve (Caldani, 1813, 1814)*
Macrodissected adult human ***common palmar digital nerve of median nerve (>1840)*** generating ***proper palmar digital nerves of median nerve (>1840)*** to medial side of index finger and lateral side of middle finger; in

the original Latin, *ramus digitalis communis secundus*, Table CCLIX, Figure 2-22.

5. *third common digital branch of median nerve (Caldani, 1813, 1814)*
Macrodissected adult human ***common palmar digital nerve of median nerve (>1840)*** generating ***proper palmar digital nerves of median nerve (>1840)*** to medial side of middle finger and lateral side of ring finger; in the original Latin, *ramus digitalis communis tertius*, Table CCLIX, Figure 2-26.
6. *radial branch of median nerve (Bock, 1827)*
Macrodissected adult human lateral primary branch of ***common palmar digital nerves of median nerve (>1840)***; in the original Latin, *ram. radialis*, Table I, Figure 1-28.
7. *ulnar branch of median nerve (Bock, 1827)*
Macrodissected adult human medial primary branch of ***common palmar digital nerves of median nerve (>1840)***; in the original Latin, *ram. ulnaris*, Table I, Figure 1-29.
8. *external palmar branch of thumb of median nerve (Cloquet, 1828)*
Macrodissected adult human branch of ***common palmar digital nerves of median nerve (>1840)*** extending over thenar eminence; in the original French, *rameau palmaire externe du pouce*, Plate CLXIX, Figure 1-41.
9. *second terminal branch of median nerve (Cruveilhier, 1836)*
Synonym for macrodissected adult human *thumb branch of median nerve (Mayer, 1794)*; in the original French, *2e branche terminale du médian*, p. 807.
10. *median nerve external collateral branch of thumb (Cruveilhier, 1836)*
Synonym for *second terminal branch of median nerve (Cruveilhier, 1836)*; in the original French, *branche collatérale externe du pouce du médian*, p. 807.
11. *dorsal branch of median nerve external collateral branch of thumb (Cruveilhier, 1836)*
Macrodissected adult human dorsal terminal branch of *median nerve external collateral branch of thumb (Cruveilhier, 1836)*; in the original French, *rameau dorsal*, p. 807.
12. *unguinal branch of median nerve external collateral branch of thumb (Cruveilhier, 1836)*
Synonym for *dorsal branch of median nerve external collateral branch of thumb (Cruveilhier, 1836)*; in the original French, *rameau unguéal (proprement dit)*, p. 807.
13. *palmar branch of median nerve external collateral branch of thumb (Cruveilhier, 1836)*
Macrodissected adult human ventral terminal branch of *median nerve external collateral branch of thumb (Cruveilhier, 1836)*; in the original French, *rameau palmaire*, p. 807.
14. *third terminal branch of median nerve (Cruveilhier, 1836)*
Macrodissected adult human ***common palmar digital nerve of median nerve (>1840)*** extending along medial side of thumb; in the original French, *3e branche terminale du médian*, p. 807.
15. *median nerve internal collateral branch of thumb (Cruveilhier, 1836)*
Synonym for *third terminal branch of median nerve (Cruveilhier, 1836)*; in the original French, *branche collatérale interne du ponce du médian*, p. 807.
16. *fourth terminal branch of median nerve (Cruveilhier, 1836)*
Macrodissected adult human third ***common palmar digital nerve of median nerve (>1840)*** generating distally a *dorsal branch of fourth terminal branch of median nerve (Cruveilhier, 1836)* and a *ventral branch of fourth terminal branch of median nerve (Cruveilhier, 1836)*; in the original French, *4e branche terminale du médian*, p. 808.
17. *median nerve external collateral branch of index finger (Cruveilhier, 1836)*
Synonym for *fourth terminal branch of median nerve (Cruveilhier, 1836)*; in the original French, *branche collatérale externe de l'index du médian*, p. 808.
18. *fifth terminal branch of median nerve (Cruveilhier, 1836)*
Macrodissected adult human fourth ***common palmar digital nerve of median nerve (>1840)***; in the original French, *5e branche terminale du médian*, p. 808.
19. *median nerve common trunk for internal collateral branch of index finger and external collateral branch of middle finger (Cruveilhier, 1836)*
Synonym for *fifth terminal branch of median nerve (Cruveilhier, 1836)*; in the original French, *tronc commun des branches collatérale interne de l'index et collatérale externe du médius du médian*, p. 808.
20. *sixth terminal branch of median nerve (Cruveilhier, 1836)*
Macrodissected adult human fifth and last ***common palmar digital nerve of median nerve (>1840)***; in the original French, *sixième branche terminale du médian*, p. 808.
21. *median nerve common trunk for internal collateral branch of middle finger and external collateral branch of ring finger (Cruveilhier, 1836)*
Synonym for *fifth terminal branch of median nerve (Cruveilhier, 1836)*; in the original French, *tronc commun des branches collatérale interne du médius et collatérale externe de l'annulaire du médian*, p. 808.

common palmar digital nerves of ulnar nerve (>1840)

As described for macrodissected adult human, these branches of the ***superficial branch of ulnar nerve (Fyfe, 1800)*** in turn generate distally the ***proper palmar digital nerves of ulnar nerve (>1840)***; see Williams & Warwick (1980, pp. 1099–1100), *Terminologia Anatomica* (1998, p. 138). They were known to Galen; see ***[common palmar digital nerves of ulnar nerve (>1840)] (Galen, c177)***.

TRANSLATIONS:

1. *nervus ulnaris nervi digitales palmares communes (>1840)*
Current Latin form of ***common palmar digital nerves of ulnar nerve (>1840)***; see *Terminologia Anatomica* (1998, p. 138).

EARLIER REFERENCES:

Described, not named or illustrated:

1. ***[common palmar digital nerves of ulnar nerve (>1840)] (Galen, c177)***

Alluded to for macrodissected adult macaque but not human; see Singer translation (1999, p. 74). Vesalius (1543a) described three for macrodissected adult human; see Richardson & Carman translation (2002, p. 244).

Earlier synonyms:

1. *superficial volar branch of ulnar nerve (Bock, 1827)*
   Synonym for macrodissected adult human ***common palmar digital nerves of ulnar nerve (>1840)***; in the original Latin, *Ram. volaris sublimis*; Table I, Figure 2-*37*; Table II-*66*. Langenbeck (1826–1830; Fasc. III, XIV-*12*) used an equivalent term, *ramus sublimis rami volaris nervi ulnaris*, for macrodissected adult human but Fascicle III was published in 1830.

PARTLY CORRESPONDS:

1. *digital branch of cubital nerve (Cloquet, 1828)*
   Synonym for macrodissected adult human *external branch of superficial terminal branch of cubital nerve (Cruveilhier, 1836)*; in the original French, *rameau digital du nerf cubital*, Plate CLXIX, Figure 1-*72*.
2. *internal palmar branch furnished by cubital nerve (Cloquet, 1828)*
   Synonym for macrodissected adult human *internal branch of superficial terminal branch of cubital nerve (Cruveilhier, 1836)*; in the original French, *rameau palmaire interne fourni par le nerf cubital*, Plate CLXIX, Figure 1-*77*.
3. *internal branch of superficial terminal branch of cubital nerve (Cruveilhier, 1836)*
   Macrodissected adult human ***common palmar digital nerve of ulnar nerve (>1840)*** for ***proper palmar digital nerve of ulnar nerve (>1840)*** to medial side of little finger; in the original French, *rameau interne*, p. 813.
4. *external branch of superficial terminal branch of cubital nerve (Cruveilhier, 1836)*
   Macrodissected adult human ***common palmar digital nerve of ulnar nerve (>1840)*** for ***proper palmar digital nerves of ulnar nerve (>1840)*** to lateral side of little finger and medial side of ring finger; in the original French, *rameau interne*, p. 813.

common plantar digital nerves of lateral plantar nerve (>1840)

As described for macrodissected adult human, there are two branches (medial and lateral) of the ***lateral plantar nerve (>1840)*** in turn generating three ***proper plantar digital nerves of lateral plantar nerve (>1840)***; see Williams & Warwick (1980, p. 1114), *Terminologia Anatomica* (1998, p. 141), also see Durward (1951, Figs. 951, 952). They were known to Galen; see ***[common plantar digital nerves of lateral plantar nerve (>1840)] (Galen, c177)***.

EARLIER REFERENCES:

Described, not named or illustrated:

1. ***[common plantar digital nerves of lateral plantar nerve (>1840)] (Galen, c177)***
   Alluded to briefly in macrodissected adult macaque but not human; see Singer translation (1999, p. 87).

Illustrated, not named or described:

1. ***[common plantar digital nerves of lateral plantar nerve (>1840)] (Eustachi, 1552)***
   Illustrated for macrodissected adult human; see Albinus edition (1761, Tab. 20-25).

Illustrated and described, not named:

1. ***[common plantar digital nerves of lateral plantar nerve (>1840)] (Vieussens, 1684)***
   Accurately described and illustrated for macrodissected adult human; see Table 30-*T*, *V*.

Earlier synonyms:

1. *plantar nerves of external plantar nerve (Meckel, 1817)*
   Corresponds to both macrodissected adult human ***common plantar digital nerves of lateral plantar nerve (>1840)***; see translation (1832, Vol. 3, p. 21).
2. *digital branch of external plantar nerve (Quain & Wilson, 1839)*
   Synonym for macrodissected adult human ***common plantar digital nerve of lateral plantar nerve (>1840)***; Plate XXVI, Figure 1-*d*.

PARTLY CORRESPONDS:

1. *internal branch of external plantar nerve (Meckel, 1817)*
   Synonym for *fifth plantar nerve of toes (Meckel, 1817)*; see translation (1832, Vol. 3, p. 21).
2. *fifth plantar nerve of toes (Meckel, 1817)*
   Clearly described macrodissected adult human medial ***common plantar digital nerve of lateral plantar nerve (>1840)***; see translation (1832, Vol. 3, p. 21).
3. *external branch of external plantar nerve (Meckel, 1817)*
   Synonym for *sixth plantar nerve of toes (Meckel, 1817)*; see translation (1832, Vol. 3, p. 21).
4. *musculo-cutaneous nerve of external plantar nerve (Meckel, 1817)*
   Synonym for *sixth plantar nerve of toes (Meckel, 1817)*; see translation (1832, Vol. 3, p. 21).
5. *sixth plantar nerve of toes (Meckel, 1817)*
   Synonym for macrodissected adult human lateral ***common plantar digital nerve of lateral plantar nerve (>1840)***; see translation (1832, Vol. 3, p. 21).
6. *long external branch of external plantar nerve (Bock, 1827)*
   Synonym for macrodissected adult human *external branch of external plantar nerve (Meckel, 1817)*; in the original Latin, *ram. externus longus nervi plantaris externi*; Table VI, Figure 4-*20*.
7. *medial branch of external plantar nerve (Bock, 1827)*
   Synonym for macrodissected adult human *internal branch of external plantar nerve (Meckel, 1817)*; in the original Latin, *ram. medius nervi plantaris externi*; Table VI, Figure 4-*22*.
8. *external branch of superficial terminal branch of external plantar nerve (Cruveilhier, 1836)*
   Macrodissected adult human lateral ***common plantar digital nerve of lateral plantar nerve (>1840)***; in the original French, *rameau externe*, p. 875.
9. *internal branch of superficial terminal branch of external plantar nerve (Cruveilhier, 1836)*

Macrodissected adult human medial ***common plantar digital nerve of lateral plantar nerve (>1840)***; in the original French, *rameau interne*, p. 875.

10. *cutaneous nerves of external branch of superficial terminal branch of external plantar nerve (Cruveilhier, 1836)*
For macrodissected adult human, many cutaneous branches of *external branch of superficial terminal branch of external plantar nerve (Cruveilhier, 1836)*; in the original French, *nerfs cutanés*, p. 875.
11. *nerves of flexor digiti minimi brevis (Cruveilhier, 1836)*
Macrodissected adult human branches of *external branch of superficial terminal branch of external plantar nerve (Cruveilhier, 1836)* to flexor digiti minimi brevis of foot muscle; in the original French, *nerfs du court fléchisseur du petit orteil*, p. 875.
12. *nerves of interosseous muscles of fourth space (Cruveilhier, 1836)*
Macrodissected adult human branches of *external branch of superficial terminal branch of external plantar nerve (Cruveilhier, 1836)* to third and most lateral plantar interosseous muscle; in the original French, *nerfs des muscles interosseux du quatriéme espace*, p. 875.
13. *articular filaments of external branch of superficial terminal branch of external plantar nerve (Cruveilhier, 1836)*
Macrodissected adult human articular branchlets of *external branch of superficial terminal branch of external plantar nerve (Cruveilhier, 1836)*; in the original French, *filets articulaires*, p. 875.
14. *cutaneous nerves of internal branch of superficial terminal branch of external plantar nerve (Cruveilhier, 1836)*
For macrodissected adult human, many cutaneous branches of *internal branch of superficial terminal branch of external plantar nerve (Cruveilhier, 1836)*; in the original French, *nerfs cutanés*, p. 875.
15. *articular nerves of internal branch of superficial terminal branch of external plantar nerve (Cruveilhier, 1836)*
Macrodissected adult human articular branchlets of *internal branch of superficial terminal branch of external plantar nerve (Cruveilhier, 1836)*; in the original French, *nerfs articulaires*, p. 875.

common plantar digital nerves of medial plantar nerve (>1840)

As described for macrodissected adult human, these four major branches of the ***medial plantar nerve (>1840)*** in turn generate the ***proper plantar digital nerves of medial plantar nerve (>1840)***; see Williams & Warwick (1980, p. 1114), *Terminologia Anatomica* (1998, p. 141); also see Durward (1951, Figs. 951, 952). They were known to Galen; see ***[common plantar digital nerves of medial plantar nerve (>1840)] (Galen, c177)***.

EARLIER REFERENCES:

Described, not named or illustrated:

1. ***[common plantar digital nerves of medial plantar nerve (>1840)] (Galen, c177)***
Alluded to for macrodissected adult macaque but not human; see Singer translation (1999, p. 87). Vieussens beautifully described and illustrated them for macrodissected adult human; Table 30-*E,F,H,K*.

Earlier synonyms:

1. *digital branches of internal plantar branches of tibial nerve (Martin, 1781)*
Synonym for macrodissected adult human ***common plantar digital nerves of medial plantar nerve (>1840)***; in the original Latin, *nervus tibialis ramus plantaris interior rami digitales*, pp. 243–244 and Table XI.
2. *digital nerves of foot from internal plantar nerve (Soemmerring, 1798)*
Synonym for macrodissected adult human ***common plantar digital nerves of medial plantar nerve (>1840)***, where each of the four components was described accurately; in the original Latin, ex *nervo plantari interno* crassiori oriuntur *quatuor nervi digitorum pedis*, p. 331.
3. *plantar nerves of internal plantar nerve (Meckel, 1817)*
Synonym for macrodissected adult human *digital nerves of foot from internal plantar nerve (Soemmerring, 1798)*; see translation (1832, Vol. 3, p. 20).
4. *branches of internal plantar nerve (Bock, 1827)*
Synonym for macrodissected adult human ***common plantar digital nerves of medial plantar nerve (>1840)***; in the original Latin, *rami nervi plantaris interni*, Table VI, Figure 4-*11*.

PARTLY CORRESPONDS:

1. *bifid digital branches of internal plantar nerve (Günther, 1786)*
Günther described three of these ***common plantar digital nerves of medial plantar nerve (>1840)*** for macrodissected adult human; in the original Latin, *r. digitales bifidus*, p. 87.
2. *internal branch of internal plantar nerve (Jördens, 1788)*
Most medial of four major ***common plantar digital nerves of medial plantar nerve (>1840)*** in macrodissected adult human; in the original Latin, *ramus internus nervi plantaris interni*, p. 11 and Table III-*183**.
3. *internal lateral twig to abductor pollicis muscle from internal branch of internal plantar nerve (Jördens, 1788)*
Branch of *internal branch of internal plantar nerve (Jördens, 1788)* to abductor hallucis muscle in macrodissected adult human; in the original Latin, *surculus lateralis internus ad musculum abductorem pollicis*, p. 11 and Table III-*185*.
4. *external branch of internal plantar nerve (Jördens, 1788)*
Branch of macrodissected adult human ***medial plantar nerve (>1840)*** generating the three most lateral of the four major ***common plantar digital nerves of medial plantar nerve (>1840)***; in the original Latin, *ramus externus nervi plantaris interni*, p. 11 and Table III-*186*. According to Jördens's very detailed description, it divides into internal twig (Tab. III-*187*) and external twig

(Tab. III-*200*). The internal twig in turn generates internal minor twig (Tab. III-*188*) and external minor twig (Tab. III-*189*), with the former generating ***proper plantar digital nerves of medial plantar nerve (>1840)*** to lateral part of big toe and medial part of second toe, and the latter eventually generating such ***nerves (Herophilus, c335–c280 BC)*** to lateral part of second toe and medial part of third toe. The external (lateral) twig of *external branch of internal plantar nerve (Jördens, 1788)* (Tab. III-*200*) also generates two branches: an internal minor twig (Tab. III-*202*), in turn forming a common trunk (Tab. III-*203*) corresponding to the fourth and most lateral major ***common plantar digital nerve of medial plantar nerve (>1840)*** innervating lateral parts of third toe and medial parts of fourth toe; and a variable small external minor twig (Tab. III-*201*) generating ***common plantar digital nerves of medial plantar nerve (>1840)***, innervating lateral part of fourth toe and medial part of fifth toe when twig present. Furthermore, there is a communicating twig (Tab. III-*195*) between external minor twig (Tab. III-*189*) and internal minor twig (Tab. III-*202*). Other smaller cutaneous and articular branches are also described.

5. *metatarsal nerves (Fischer, 1791)*
   Fischer described four in macrodissected adult human, corresponding to the lateral three (of 4) major ***common plantar digital nerves of medial plantar nerve (>1840)*** and a minor, far lateral one. Two arise from each *tarsal nerve (Fischer, 1791)* and the largest, most medial one arises from *internal branch of internal plantar nerve (Fischer, 1791)*. The situation is complicated by the fact that both *metatarsal nerves (Fischer, 1791)* arising from internal (medial) *tarsal nerve (Fischer, 1791)* also generate an *interosseal twig of metatarsal nerves (Fischer, 1791)*, in turn generating two ***proper plantar digital nerves of medial plantar nerve (>1840)***. In the original Latin, *nervos metatarsicos*, pp. 36–37.
6. *interosseal twigs of metatarsal nerves (Fischer, 1791)*
   Part of macrodissected adult human hierarchy of ***common plantar digital nerves of medial plantar nerve (>1840)*** described by Fischer. In his dissection the internal (medial) *tarsal nerve (Fischer, 1791)* branched to produce an internal and an external *metatarsal nerve (Fischer, 1791)*, and each of the latter also branched, with one branch being an interosseal twig generating two ***proper plantar digital nerves of medial plantar nerve (>1840)***, from the lateral side of the big toe to the medial side of the third toe. The external (lateral) *tarsal nerve (Fischer, 1791)* branched to produce two *metatarsal nerves (Fischer, 1791)* directly generating four ***proper plantar digital nerves of medial plantar nerve (>1840)***, from the lateral side of the third toe to the medial side of the little toe. In the original Latin, *ramulum interosseum*, pp. 36–37.
7. *cutaneous plantar nervelet (Fischer, 1791)*
   Branch of external (lateral) *metatarsal nerve (Fischer, 1791)* derived from internal (medial) *tarsal nerve (Fischer, 1791)* and innervating parts of sole of foot nearest five toes; in the original Latin, *nervulus plantaris cutaneus*, p. 36.
8. *long branch of internal plantar nerve (Bock, 1827)*
   In macrodissected adult human, most medial (first) of ***common plantar digital nerves of medial plantar nerve (>1840)***; in the original Latin, *ram. longus internus plantaris*, Table VI, Figure 4-*6*.
9. *terminal branches of internal plantar nerve (Cruveilhier, 1836)*
   The lateral three macrodissected adult human ***common plantar digital nerves of medial plantar nerve (>1840)***, numbered from medial to lateral; in the original French, *rameaux terminaux du plantaire interne*, p. 873. In addition to their ***proper plantar digital nerves of medial plantar nerve (>1840)***, Cruveilhier described and even named other muscular, articular, and cutaneous branches for each of them; pp. 873–874.
10. *filament of first lumbrical of first terminal branch of internal plantar nerve (Cruveilhier, 1836)*
   Branchlet from first *terminal branch of internal plantar nerve (Cruveilhier, 1836)* to first lumbrical muscle of foot; in the original French, *filet du premier lombrical*, p. 873.
11. *articular filaments of first terminal branch of internal plantar nerve (Cruveilhier, 1836)*
   Branchlet from first *terminal branch of internal plantar nerve (Cruveilhier, 1836)* to metatarsopharyngeal joint of big toe; in the original French, *filets articulaires*, p. 873.
12. *cutaneous filaments of first terminal branch of internal plantar nerve (Cruveilhier, 1836)*
   Numerous cutaneous branchlets from first *terminal branch of internal plantar nerve (Cruveilhier, 1836)*; in the original French, *filets cutanés*, p. 873.

communicating branch (Winslow, 1733)

A topographic division of the ***nervous system (Monro, 1783)*** referring generally to a short segment of ***white matter (Meckel, 1817)*** between two ***central nerve cords (Serres, 1824–1826)***, two ***peripheral nerve cords (Swanson & Bota, 2010)***, two ***nerves (Herophilus, c335–c280 BC)***, two ***ganglia (Galen, c173)***, or any combination of two of them like a ***nerve (Herophilus, c335–c280 BC)*** and ***ganglion (Galen, c173)***. Galen (c180) referred less specifically to communications between ***nerves (Herophilus, c335–c280 BC)***; see translation by Goss (1966, p. 330). For Winslow's frequent use of the term *communicating branch* in describing macrodissected adult human ***nerves (Herophilus, c335–c280 BC)***, see Section VI.

TRANSLATIONS:

1. *ramus communicans (Winslow, 1733)*
   Latin form of ***communicating branch (Winslow, 1733)***; see Section VI.

communicating branch from internal carotid plexus to abducens nerve (>1840)

As described for adult human, it conveys postganglionic sympathetic ***axons (Kölliker, 1896)*** from ***superior***

cervical ganglion (Vieussens, 1684) to ***abducens nerve (Heister, 1717)***; see Mitchell (1953, p. 217). It was probably first mentioned by Achillini; see ***[communicating branch from internal carotid plexus to abducens nerve (>1840)] (Achillini, 1520)***.

EARLIER REFERENCES:

Described, not named or illustrated:

1. ***[communicating branch from internal carotid plexus to abducens nerve (>1840)] (Achillini, 1520)***
   In a rather confused statement, Achillini seemed to refer to it for macrodissected adult human; see Lind translation (1975, pp. 59–60) and Haller (1762, p. 223 note *q*). Morgagni (1719, Vol. 6, p. 30) also described it, according to Meckel (1817); see translation (1832, Vol. 3, p. 89). Walther (1733) described it even more clearly for macrodissected adult human; p. [6], see Neubauer (1772, p. 40 note 3).

Illustrated, not named or described:

1. ***[communicating branch from internal carotid plexus to abducens nerve (>1840)] (Eustachi, 1552)***
   Clearly illustrated for macrodissected adult human; see Albinus edition (1744, Tab. XVIII, Fig. 2). Later, Soemmerring (1778; Tab. III, Fig. VII-*β*) very clearly drew and labeled it for macrodissected adult human.

Earlier synonyms:

1. *ganglionnary nerve anastomosis with external motor nerve (Meckel, 1817)*
   Synonym for macrodissected adult human ***communicating branch from internal carotid plexus to abducens nerve (>1840)***; see translation (1832, Vol. 3, p. 89).
2. *ganglionnary nerve anastomosis with sixth pair (Meckel, 1817)*
   Synonym for macrodissected adult human ***communicating branch from internal carotid plexus to abducens nerve (>1840)***; see translation (1832, Vol. 3, p. 89).
3. *superior branch of sixth pair of nerves (Lobstein, 1823)*
   Synonym for macrodissected adult human ***communicating branch from internal carotid plexus to abducens nerve (>1840)***; see translation (1831, p. 10).
4. *abducens nerve branch to sympathetic (Langenbeck, 1826–1830)*
   Synonym for macrodissected adult human ***communicating branch from internal carotid plexus to abducens nerve (>1840)***; in the original Latin, *ramus nervi abducentis ad Sympathicum*, Fascicle III, Table XVI-*16*.
5. *communicating branches between abducens nerve and great sympathetic nerve (Langenbeck, 1826–1830)*
   Synonym for *abducens nerve branch to sympathetic (Langenbeck, 1826–1830)*; in the original Latin, *rami anastomotici inter nervum abducentem et nervum sympathicum magnum*; Fascicle III, Table XVII-*u*.
6. *connection of carotid nerve with abducens nerve (Arnold, 1834)*
   Synonym for macrodissected adult human ***communicating branch from internal carotid plexus to abducens nerve (>1840)***; in the original Latin, *conjunctio nervus caroticus ramus externus cum nervo abducente*, p. 18.
7. *anastomotic branches of carotid branch of superior cervical ganglion to sixth pair (Cruveilhier, 1836)*
   Synonym for macrodissected adult human ***communicating branch from internal carotid plexus to abducens nerve (>1840)***; in the original French, *branches anastomotiques avec la 6e paire*, p. 987.

PARTLY CORRESPONDS:

1. *first root of intercostal nerve (Bang, 1770)*
   As described for macrodissected adult human, first of two ascending branches from ***superior cervical ganglion (Vieussens, 1684)*** joining to form a single trunk, all three components constituting ***communicating branch from internal carotid plexus to abducens nerve (>1840)***; in the original Latin, *nervi intercostalis radicem primam*, Figure II-*b*.
2. *second root of intercostal nerve (Bang, 1770)*
   As described for macrodissected adult human, second of two ascending branches from ***superior cervical ganglion (Vieussens, 1684)*** joining to form a single trunk, all three components constituting the ***communicating branch from internal carotid plexus to abducens nerve (>1840)***; in the original Latin, *nervi intercostalis radicem secundum*, Figure II-*c*.
3. *communication of sympathetic with second division of fifth pair of nerves (Todd, 1836–1839)*
   In macrodissected adult human, Todd described it as extending from ***abducens nerve (Heister, 1717)*** to proximal end of ***maxillary nerve (Meckel, 1753)***, pointing out that it had been described previously by Laumonier (1793) and Munniks (1805) but denied by Arnold (1826a); p. 283. It partly corresponds to ***communicating branch from internal carotid plexus to abducens nerve (>1840)***.

communicating branch from internal carotid plexus to oculomotor nerve (>1840)

As described for adult human, it conveys postganglionic sympathetic ***axons (Kölliker, 1896)*** from ***superior cervical ganglion (Vieussens, 1684)*** to ***oculomotor nerve (Estienne, 1545)***, joining the latter at its point of division; see Williams & Warwick (1980, p. 1127). For its probable discovery see ***[communicating branch from internal carotid plexus to oculomotor nerve (>1840)] (Morgagni, 1719)***.

EARLIER REFERENCES:

Described, not named or illustrated:

1. ***[communicating branch from internal carotid plexus to oculomotor nerve (>1840)] (Morgagni, 1719)***
   Morgagni described it for macrodissected adult human, p. 105, according to Neubauer (1772, pp. 38–39); as did Munniks (1805, p. 25), according to Meckel (1817), see translation (1832, Vol. 3, p. 91).

Earlier synonyms:

1. *anastomotic branch between oculomotor nerve and anterior branch of sympathetic (Langenbeck, 1826–1830)*

Synonym for macrodissected adult human ***communicating branch from internal carotid plexus to oculomotor nerve (>1840)***; in the original Latin, *ramus anastomoticus inter nervum oculomotorium et ramus anteriorem Sympathici*; Fascicle III, Table XVI-*18*.

2. *sympathetic nerve branches to oculomotor nerve (Langenbeck, 1826–1830)*
   Synonym for *anastomotic branch between oculomotor nerve and anterior branch of sympathetic (Langenbeck, 1826–1830)*; in the original Latin, *rami nervi sympathici ad nervum oculomotorium*, Fascicle III, Table XVIII-*l*.
3. *communicating filaments of cavernous plexus with third nerve (Cruveilhier, 1836)*
   Synonym for macrodissected adult human ***communicating branch from internal carotid plexus to oculomotor nerve (>1840)***; in the original French, *filets de communication avec la 3^{e} paire*, p. 988.

communicating branch from internal carotid plexus to ophthalmic nerve (>1840)

As described for adult human, it conveys postganglionic sympathetic ***axons (Kölliker, 1896)*** from ***superior cervical ganglion (Vieussens, 1684)*** to ***ophthalmic nerve (Winslow, 1733)*** and/or its branch, the ***nasociliary nerve (Meckel, 1817; Wutzer, 1817)***, then extends to structures related to the eye by various and variable routes; see Mitchell (1953, pp. 157, 203–204, 217), Williams & Warwick (1980, p. 1127). According to Bell & Bell (1829, p. 490), it may accompany the ***abducens nerve (Heister, 1717)*** for some distance. It was described clearly by Pourfour du Petit; see ***[communicating branch from internal carotid plexus to ophthalmic nerve (>1840)] (Pourfour du Petit, 1729)***.

EARLIER REFERENCES:

Described, not named or illustrated:

1. ***[communicating branch from internal carotid plexus to ophthalmic nerve (>1840)] (Pourfour du Petit, 1729)***
   Described for macrodissected adult human; p. 4, reviewed by Meckel (1817; see translation, 1832, Vol. 3, p. 89).

Earlier synonyms:

1. *filaments of cavernous plexus joining first branch of fifth pair (Arnold, 1834)*
   Synonym for macrodissected adult human ***communicating branch from internal carotid plexus to ophthalmic nerve (>1840)***; in the original Latin, *filamenta (plexus cavernosus) se jungentia cum primo ramo quinti paris*, p. 18.
2. *communicating filaments of cavernous plexus with fifth pair (Cruveilhier, 1836)*
   Synonym for macrodissected adult human ***communicating branch from internal carotid plexus to ophthalmic nerve (>1840)***, including those to ***ophthalmic nerve (Winslow, 1733)*** and ***trigeminal ganglion (>1840)***; in the original French, *filets de communication avec la 5^{e} paire*, p. 988.

PARTLY CORRESPONDS:

1. *filaments of cavernous plexus joining Gasserian ganglion (Arnold, 1834)*
   In macrodissected adult human, branch of ***communicating branch from internal carotid plexus to ophthalmic nerve (>1840)*** to ***trigeminal ganglion (>1840)***; in the original Latin, *filamenta (plexus cavernosus) se jungentia cum primo ramo quinti paris*, p. 18.

communicating branch from internal carotid plexus to trochlear nerve (>1840)

As described for adult human, it conveys postganglionic sympathetic ***axons (Kölliker, 1896)*** from ***superior cervical ganglion (Vieussens, 1684)*** to ***trochlear nerve (Molinetti, 1669)***; see Durward (1951, p. 1134), Williams & Warwick (1980, p. 1127). It was definitely mentioned by Todd; see ***[communicating branch from internal carotid plexus to trochlear nerve (>1840)] (Todd, 1836–1839)***.

EARLIER REFERENCES:

Described, not named or illustrated:

1. ***[communicating branch from internal carotid plexus to trochlear nerve (>1840)] (Todd, 1836–1839)***
   Todd attributed its description for macrodissected adult human to Pauli (*Müller's Archiv*, 1834), although the article has not been located; p. 371.

communicating branch of digastric nerve with glossopharyngeal nerve (>1840)

As described for macrodissected adult human, a usual but not constant ***communicating branch (Winslow, 1733)*** between ***digastric nerve (Meckel, 1753)*** and ***glossopharyngeal nerve (Huber, 1744)***; see Williams & Warwick (1980, p. 1072), *Terminologia Anatomica* (1998, p. 135). It was probably first described as the *branch from wandring pair [to hard part of seventh pair of nerves arising within skull] (Willis, 1664)*.

EARLIER REFERENCES:

Earlier synonyms:

1. *branch from wandring pair [to hard part of seventh pair of nerves arising within skull] (Willis, 1664)*
   Synonym for macrodissected adult mammalian ***communicating branch of digastric branch of facial nerve with glossopharyngeal nerve (>1840)***; see Pordage translation (1681, p. 144). Also see Haller (1762, p. 228 note *n*).
2. *hard nerve anastomosis with eighth pair (Meckel, 1753)*
   Synonym for macrodissected adult human ***communicating branch of digastric branch of facial nerve with glossopharyngeal nerve (>1840)***; Table 1-*123*.
3. *ramus glossopharyngei cum nervo biventrico portionis durae anastomosin (Neubauer, 1772)*
   Synonym for macrodissected adult human ***communicating branch of digastric branch of facial nerve with glossopharyngeal nerve (>1840)***; Table 2-*76*.
4. *anastomotic branch of glossopharyngeal nerve with internal deep branch of hard nerve (Günther, 1786)*

Synonym for macrodissected adult human ***communicating branch of digastric branch of facial nerve with glossopharyngeal nerve (>1840)***; in the original Latin, *ramus anastomoticus cum r. profundo interno n. duri*, p. 62.

5. *ramus glosso-pharyngei ad nervum communicantem faciei (Scarpa, 1788)*
   Synonym for macrodissected adult human ***communicating branch of digastric branch of facial nerve with glossopharyngeal nerve (>1840)***; Table X, Figure 1-33.
6. *communication of facial nerve with digastric nerve (Scarpa, 1794)*
   Synonym for macrodissected adult human ***communicating branch of digastric branch of facial nerve with glossopharyngeal nerve (>1840)***; in the original Latin, *nervo digastrico communicantis faciei*, Table II-3.
7. *anastomosis of digastric branch of facial nerve with glossopharyngeal nerve (Meckel, 1817)*
   Synonym for macrodissected adult human ***communicating branch of digastric branch of facial nerve with glossopharyngeal nerve (>1840)***; see translation (1832, Vol. 3, pp. 54–55).
8. *glosso-pharyngeal anastomotic surculus of digastric branch (Bellingeri, 1818)*
   Synonym for macrodissected adult human ***communicating branch of digastric branch of facial nerve with glossopharyngeal nerve (>1840)***; in the original Latin, *surculus anastomoticus glosso-pharyng.*, see Table II.
9. *branch of digastric branch of facial joining glosso-pharyngeal nerve (Swan, 1830)*
   Synonym for macrodissected adult human ***communicating branch of digastric branch of facial nerve with glossopharyngeal nerve (>1840)***; Plate XVI, Figure 2-5.
10. *anastomotic filament of posterior mastoid branch of facial nerve with glossopharyngeal nerve (Cruveilhier, 1836)*
    Synonym for macrodissected adult human ***communicating branch of digastric branch of facial nerve with glossopharyngeal nerve (>1840)***; p. 943.
11. *anastomotic branch of glossopharyngeal nerve to facial nerve (Cruveilhier, 1836)*
    Synonym for *anastomotic filament of posterior mastoid branch of facial nerve with glossopharyngeal nerve (Cruveilhier, 1836)*; in the original French, *rameau anastomotique avec le nerf facial*, p. 953.
12. *branch of glossopharyngeal nerve for digastric and stylohyoid (Cruveilhier, 1836)*
    Synonym for *anastomotic filament of posterior mastoid branch of facial nerve with glossopharyngeal nerve (Cruveilhier, 1836)*; in the original French, *rameau du digastrique et du stylo-hyoïdien*, p. 953.
13. *communication of glosso-pharyngeal nerve with facial nerve (Quain & Wilson, 1839)*
    Synonym for macrodissected adult human ***communicating branch of digastric branch of facial nerve with glossopharyngeal nerve (>1840)***; Plate XV-*g*.

communicating branch of glossopharyngeal nerve with auricular branch of vagus nerve (>1840)

As described for macrodissected adult human, a ***communicating branch (Winslow, 1733)*** between the region of the ***distal glossopharyngeal ganglion (>1840)*** and proximal part of the ***auricular branch of vagus nerve (Arnold, 1834)***; see Mitchell (1953, p. 169), Williams & Warwick (1980, pp. 1075, 1079), *Terminologia Anatomica* (1998, p. 136). It was discovered by Andersch; see ***[communicating branch of glossopharyngeal nerve with auricular branch of vagus nerve (>1840)] (Andersch & Soemmerring, 1792)***.

EARLIER REFERENCES:

Described, not named or illustrated:

1. ***[communicating branch of glossopharyngeal nerve with auricular branch of vagus nerve (>1840)] (Andersch & Soemmerring, 1792)***
   Described for macrodissected adult human in Andersch's thesis (c1751–c1755) not available publicly until here; pp. 123–124. A footnote by Soemmerring on p. 124 noted that it was clearly illustrated by Scarpa (1788, see Tab. X). It was also clearly described for macrodissected adult human by Arnold (1834, p. 13:II.4).

communicating branch of glossopharyngeal nerve with meningeal branch of vagus nerve (>1840)

As described for macrodissected adult human, a small ***communicating branch (Winslow, 1733)*** between proximal part of ***glossopharyngeal nerve trunk (Wrisberg, 1786, Günther, 1786)*** and ***meningeal branch of vagus nerve (>1840)***; see Mitchell (1953, p. 174), *Nomina Anatomica* (1983, p. A75), *Terminologia Anatomica* (1998, p. 136). It was not identified by 1840.

communicating branch of intermediofacial nerve with tympanic plexus (>1840)

As described for macrodissected adult human, when present it arises from the region of the ***geniculate ganglion (Bischoff, 1832)*** and courses to the ***tympanic plexus (Müller, 1834)***, where it essentially merges with the ***lesser petrosal nerve (>1840)***; see Durward (1951, p. 1036 and Fig. 901), Mitchell (1953, p. 169), Williams & Warwick (1980, p. 1071 and Fig. 7.184, unlabeled just to left of *tympanic plexus*). Also see *communicating branch of otic ganglion with greater petrosal nerve (>1840)*. It was perhaps first alluded to by Drake; see ***[communicating branch of intermediofacial nerve with tympanic plexus (>1840)] (Drake, 1707)***.

EARLIER REFERENCES:

Described, not named or illustrated:

1. ***[communicating branch of intermediofacial nerve with tympanic plexus (>1840)] (Drake, 1707)***
   Probably alluded to for macrodissected adult human; p. 339, see Haller (1762, p. 227 note *a*). Winslow also reported it (1733, Sect. VI, no. 81, p. 68).

Earlier synonyms:

1. *nervus communicans faciei ramus anastomoticus (Günther, 1786)*

Synonym for macrodissected adult human *anastomotic branch of hard nerve (Günther, 1786)*; p. 56.

2. *anastomotic branch of hard nerve (Günther, 1786)*
   Probably synonym for macrodissected adult human ***communicating branch of intermediofacial nerve with tympanic plexus (>1840)***; in the original Latin, *nervus dura ramus anastomoticus*, p. 56.
3. *connection of facial nerve with tympanic nerve (Arnold, 1834)*
   Synonym for macrodissected adult human ***communicating branch of intermediofacial nerve with tympanic plexus (>1840)***; in the original Latin, *conjunctio nervus facialis cum nervo tympanico*, Table VII:*VII-48*. Also see Swan (1830, Pl. XII, Fig. 1-9).
4. *communicating branch of otic ganglion with greater petrosal nerve (>1840)*
   Synonym for macrodissected adult human ***communicating branch of intermediofacial nerve with tympanic plexus (>1840)*** when there is a variant arrangement such that ***communicating branch (Winslow, 1733)*** arises not from ***geniculate ganglion (Bischoff, 1832)*** but instead from ***greater petrosal nerve (>1840)***, or occasionally even from ***nerve of pterygoid canal (>1840)*** and directly joins ***lesser petrosal nerve (>1840)*** before it joins ***otic ganglion (Arnold, 1828)***, or even joins ***otic ganglion (Arnold, 1828)*** directly; see Brodal (1948, p. 233, Fig. 60), Mitchell (1953, p. 164).

communicating branch of intermediofacial nerve with vagus nerve (>1840)

As described for macrodissected adult human, a ***communicating branch (Winslow, 1733)*** between the ***intermediofacial nerve trunk (>1840)***, just before it leaves the stylomastoid foramen, and the ***auricular branch of vagus nerve (Arnold, 1834)***. It carries somatic sensation for the concha of the auricle, with the corresponding sensory ***neurons (Waldeyer, 1891)*** in the ***geniculate ganglion (Bischoff, 1832)***; see Durward (1951, Fig. 901), Williams & Warwick (1980, p. 1071 and Fig. 7.184). Its location defines the change of name between ***intermediofacial nerve trunk (>1840)*** and ***facial nerve trunk (>1840)***. It was discovered and named the *connection of petrous part of seventh pair with auricular branch of vagus nerve (Arnold, 1834)*.

EARLIER REFERENCES:

Earlier synonyms:

1. *connection of petrous part of seventh pair with auricular branch of vagus nerve (Arnold, 1834)*
   Synonym for macrodissected adult human ***communicating branch of intermediofacial nerve trunk with vagus nerve (>1840)***; in the original Latin, *par septimum pars petrosa conjunctio cum ramo auriculare nervi vagi*, pp. 11–12.
2. *connection of petrous part of facial nerve with auricular branch of vagus nerve (Arnold, 1834)*
   Synonym for macrodissected adult human ***communicating branch of intermediofacial nerve trunk with vagus nerve (>1840)***; in the original Latin, *nervus facialis pars petrosa conjunctio cum ramo auriculare nervi vagi*, pp. 11–12.
3. *connection of auricular branch of pneumogastric nerve with facial nerve (Arnold, 1834)*
   Apparently macrodissected adult human ***communicating branch of intermediofacial nerve trunk with vagus nerve (>1840)***; in the original Latin, *nervus pneumogastricus ramu auricularis conjunctio cum nervo faciali*, Table III-45,46 and p. 13.
4. *connection of auricular branch of vagus nerve with facial nerve (Arnold, 1834)*
   Apparently macrodissected adult human ***communicating branch of intermediofacial nerve trunk with vagus nerve (>1840)***; in the original Latin, *ramus auricularis nervi vagi conjunctiones cum nervo faciali*, Table V-43 and p. 13.
5. *anastomotic branch of ganglion of pneumogastric with facial nerve (Cruveilhier, 1836)*
   Synonym for macrodissected adult human *connection of auricular branch of pneumogastric nerve with facial nerve (Arnold, 1834)*; in the original French, *rameau anastomotique avec le nerf facial*, p. 955.
6. *branch of jugular fossa of pneumogastric nerve (Cruveilhier, 1836)*
   Synonym for macrodissected adult human *connection of auricular branch of pneumogastric nerve with facial nerve (Arnold, 1834)*; in the original French, *rameau de la fosse jugulaire*, p. 955.

communicating branch of lacrimal nerve with zygomatic nerve (>1840)

As described for macrodissected adult human, a ***communicating branch (Winslow, 1733)*** between the two named ***nerves (Herophilus, c335–c280 BC)***, branches of the ***ophthalmic nerve (Winslow, 1733)*** and ***maxillary nerve (Meckel, 1753)*** respectively; see Durward (1951, p. 892), Williams & Warwick (1980, Fig. 7.177), *Terminologia Anatomica* (1998, p. 133). It was first clearly described by Meckel; see ***[communicating branch of lacrimal nerve with zygomatic nerve (>1840)] (Meckel, 1748)***.

EARLIER REFERENCES:

Described, not named or illustrated:

1. ***[communicating branch of lacrimal nerve with zygomatic nerve (>1840)] (Meckel, 1748)***
   Clearly described for macrodissected adult human, although not named in terms of a communication between *lacrymal ramus of ophthalmic nerve (Winslow, 1733)* and *subcutaneous malar nerve (Meckel, 1748)*; p. 35.

Earlier synonyms:

1. *anastomosis of lacrimal nerve with subcutaneous malar nerve (Martin, 1781)*
   Synonym for macrodissected adult human ***communicating branch of lacrimal nerve with zygomatic nerve (>1840)***; Table II.
2. *spheno-maxillary fascicle of lacrimal surculus (Bellingeri, 1818)*

Synonym for macrodissected adult human ***communicating branch of lacrimal nerve with zygomatic nerve (>1840)***; in the original Latin, *fasciculus spheno-maxillaris*, see Table I.

3. *external branch of lacrimal nerve (Arnold, 1834)*
Synonym for macrodissected adult human ***communicating branch of lacrimal nerve with zygomatic nerve (>1840)***; in the original Latin, *nervus lacrymalis, ramus externus*, pp. 7–8.
4. *posterior branch of lachrymal nerve (Todd, 1836–1839)*
Synonym for macrodissected adult human ***communicating branch of lacrimal nerve with zygomatic nerve (>1840)***; p. 283.
5. *spheno-maxillary branch of lachrymal nerve (Todd, 1836–1839)*
Synonym for macrodissected adult human ***communicating branch of lacrimal nerve with zygomatic nerve (>1840)***; p. 283.
6. *temporal branch of lachrymal nerve (Todd, 1836–1839)*
Synonym for macrodissected adult human ***communicating branch of lacrimal nerve with zygomatic nerve (>1840)***; p. 283.

communicating branch of median nerve with ulnar nerve (Bock, 1827)

As described for macrodissected adult human, one or more branches frequently arise in the proximal (upper) forearm and pass distally and medially to join the ***ulnar nerve (Cheselden, 1726)***; see Williams & Warwick (1980, p. 1098), *Terminologia Anatomica* (1998, p. 138). For Bock's use in macrodissected adult human, see Table I, Figure 2-30. It was known to Galen; see ***[communicating branch of median nerve with ulnar nerve (Bock, 1827)] (Galen, c177)***.

TRANSLATIONS:

1. *Verbindungszweig (Ram. communicans) zwischen dem Median- und dem Ulnarnerven (Bock, 1827)*
Original German (Latin) form of ***communicating branch of median nerve with ulnar nerve (Bock, 1827)***; see Table I, Figure 2-30.

EARLIER REFERENCES:

Described, not named or illustrated:

1. ***[communicating branch of median nerve with ulnar nerve (Bock, 1827)] (Galen, c177)***
Mentioned for macrodissected adult beef, pig, and/or macaque but not human; see Singer translation (1999, p. 71).

Earlier synonyms:

1. *anastomotic nerve between median and cubital nerves (Caldani, 1813, 1814)*
Synonym for macrodissected adult human ***communicating branch of median nerve with ulnar nerve (Bock, 1827)***; in the original Latin, *nervus anastomoticus insignis inter medianum et cubitalem*, Table CCLIX, Figure 2-27.
2. *anastomotic branch of median and cubital nerves (Cloquet, 1828)*
Synonym for macrodissected adult human ***communicating branch of median nerve with ulnar nerve (Bock, 1827)***; in the original French, *rameau d'anastomose des N. médian et cubital*, Plate CLXIX, Figure 1-64.
3. *branch of median nerve communicating with ulnar (Swan, 1830)*
Synonym for macrodissected adult human ***communicating branch of median nerve with ulnar nerve (Bock, 1827)***; Plate XXII, Figure 2-7.
4. *communicating branch of ulnar nerve with median (Quain & Wilson, 1839)*
Synonym for macrodissected adult human ***communicating branch of median nerve with ulnar nerve (Bock, 1827)***; Plate XVIII, Figure 2-*p*.

communicating branch of nasociliary nerve with ciliary ganglion (>1840)

As described for adult human, sensory ***dendrites (His, 1889)*** from the eyeball reach the ***ciliary ganglion (Loder, 1778)*** in the ***short ciliary nerves (>1840)***, pass through the ganglion uninterrupted, and then course through the ***communicating branch of nasociliary nerve with ciliary ganglion (>1840)*** to the ***nasociliary nerve (Meckel, 1817; Wutzer, 1817)***; see Williams & Warwick (1980, p. 1058 and Fig. 7.176), *Terminologia Anatomica* (1998, p. 134). It was first clearly distinguished by Pourfour du Petit; see ***[communicating branch of nasociliary nerve with ciliary ganglion (>1840)] (Pourfour du Petit, 1729)***.

EARLIER REFERENCES:

Described, not named or illustrated:

1. ***[communicating branch of nasociliary nerve with ciliary ganglion (>1840)] (Pourfour du Petit, 1729)***
Pourfour du Petit clearly described it for macrodissected adult human (p. 10) as did Morgagni (in Valsalva, 1740, Vol. 2, p. 237). Meckel (1748, p. 37 note *r*) reviewed possible but doubtful earlier observations related to it.

Earlier synonyms:

1. *long root of ophthalmic ganglion (Meckel, 1748)*
Synonym for macrodissected adult human ***communicating branch of nasociliary nerve with ciliary ganglion (>1840)***; p. 37.
2. *long root of ciliary ganglion (Mayer, 1788)*
Synonym for macrodissected adult human ***communicating branch of nasociliary nerve with ciliary ganglion (>1840)***; in the original Latin, *radix longa ganglii ciliares*, Table 8, Figure 6-*1*.
3. *external branch of nasociliary nerve (Meckel, 1817)*
Synonym for macrodissected adult human ***communicating branch of nasociliary nerve with ciliary ganglion (>1840)***; see translation (1832, Vol. 3, p. 63).
4. *ciliary branch of nasociliary nerve (Meckel, 1817)*
Synonym for macrodissected adult human ***communicating branch of nasociliary nerve with ciliary ganglion (>1840)***; see translation (1832, Vol. 3, p. 63).
5. *ganglionic branch of nasociliary nerve (Meckel, 1817)*

Synonym for macrodissected adult human ***communicating branch of nasociliary nerve with ciliary ganglion (>1840)***; in the original Latin, *ramus ad ganglion*; see translation (1832, Vol. 3, p. 63).

6. *ciliary branch of nasal nerves (Wutzer, 1817)*
   Synonym for macrodissected adult human ***communicating branch of nasociliary nerve with ciliary ganglion (>1840)***; in the original Latin, *ramus ciliaris nervi nasalis*, Figure 3-*e*.
7. *ganglionic root of nasal surculus (Bellingeri, 1818)*
   Synonym for macrodissected adult human ***communicating branch of nasociliary nerve with ciliary ganglion (>1840)***; in the original Latin, *radix ganglii*, see Table I.
8. *lenticular branch of nasal nerve (Todd, 1836–1839)*
   Synonym for macrodissected adult human ***communicating branch of nasociliary nerve with ciliary ganglion (>1840)***; p. 281.
9. *long root of lenticular ganglion (Todd, 1836–1839)*
   Synonym for macrodissected adult human ***communicating branch of nasociliary nerve with ciliary ganglion (>1840)***; p. 281.
10. *branch of nasal nerve to ophthalmic ganglion (Quain & Wilson, 1839)*
    Synonym for macrodissected adult human ***communicating branch of nasociliary nerve with ciliary ganglion (>1840)***; Plate XIII, Figure 2-*f*.
11. *ciliary ganglion branch of communication to nasal nerve (Quain & Wilson, 1839)*
    Synonym for macrodissected adult human ***communicating branch of nasociliary nerve with ciliary ganglion (>1840)***; Plate XIII-*E*,*4*.
12. *lenticular ganglion branch of communication to nasal nerve (Quain & Wilson, 1839)*
    Synonym for macrodissected adult human ***communicating branch of nasociliary nerve with ciliary ganglion (>1840)***; Plate XIII-*E*,*4*.
13. *sensory root of ciliary ganglion (>1840)*
    Synonym for macrodissected adult human ***communicating branch of nasociliary nerve with ciliary ganglion (>1840)***; see *Terminologia Anatomica* (1998, p. 134).
14. *nasociliary root of ciliary ganglion (>1840)*
    Synonym for macrodissected adult human ***communicating branch of nasociliary nerve with ciliary ganglion (>1840)***; see *Terminologia Anatomica* (1998, p. 134).

communicating branch of otic ganglion with chorda tympani (>1840)

As described for macrodissected adult human, a small ***communicating branch (Winslow, 1733)*** between ***otic ganglion (Arnold, 1828)*** and ***chorda tympani (Falloppio, 1561)***; see Mitchell (1953, pp. 164, 175), and Brodal (1948, p. 233, Fig. 60), Durward (1951, p. 1037), Williams & Warwick (1980, p. 1076). It was discovered and described as the *nerve from otic ganglion to tensor tympani (Arnold, 1834)*.

EARLIER REFERENCES:

Earlier synonyms:

1. *nerve from otic ganglion to tensor tympani (Arnold, 1834)*
   Synonym for macrodissected adult human ***communicating branch of otic ganglion with chorda tympani (>1840)***; in the original Latin, *nervus tensoris tympani e ganglio otico*, Table V:V-27 and p. 10.
2. *nerve from auricular ganglion to tensor tympani (Arnold, 1834)*
   Synonym for macrodissected adult human ***communicating branch of otic ganglion with chorda tympani (>1840)***; in the original Latin, *nervus tensoris tympani e ganglio auriculare*, Table VII:V-28 and p. 10.

communicating branch of radial nerve with ulnar nerve (>1840)

As described for macrodissected adult human, it arises from the ***superficial branch of radial nerve (Martin, 1781)*** and communicates with the ***ulnar nerve (Cheselden, 1726)*** in the dorsum of the hand; see Williams & Warwick (1980, p. 1102 and Fig. 7.202), *Terminologia Anatomica* (1998, p. 139). It was first indicated by Eustachi; see ***[communicating branch of radial nerve with ulnar nerve (>1840)] (Eustachi, 1552)***.

EARLIER REFERENCES:

Illustrated, not named or described:

1. ***[communicating branch of radial nerve with ulnar nerve (>1840)] (Eustachi, 1552)***
   Clearly illustrated for macrodissected adult human; see Albinus edition (1761, Tab. 23-dorsal surface of right hand).

Earlier synonyms:

1. *anastomotic branch of radial nerve with cubital nerve (Klint, 1784)*
   Synonym for macrodissected adult human ***communicating branch of radial nerve with ulnar nerve (>1840)***; pp. 42–43.
2. *anastomotic arch of dorsal nerves of hand (Mayer, 1794)*
   Synonym for macrodissected adult human ***communicating branch of radial nerve with ulnar nerve (>1840)***; in the original Latin, *arcus anastomoticus nervosus dorsalis manus*; Part 5, Table VI-η (p. 35).
3. *branch of cubital nerve communicating with radial nerve (Cloquet, 1828)*
   Synonym for macrodissected adult human ***communicating branch of radial nerve with ulnar nerve (>1840)***; in the original French, *rameau du nerf cubital communiquant avec le nerf radial*, Plate CLXVII, Figure 2-*46*.
4. *communicating branch of dorsal branch of ulnar nerve with radial (Quain & Wilson, 1839)*
   Synonym for macrodissected adult human ***communicating branch of radial nerve with ulnar nerve (>1840)***; Plate XIX, Figure 1-*m*.

communicating branch of superior and middle cervical ganglia (Cruveilhier, 1836)

As described for macrodissected adult human, a ***communicating branch of sympathetic trunk (>1840)*** between ***superior cervical ganglion (Vieussens, 1684)*** and ***middle cervical ganglion (Haller, 1762)*** when present; see Mitchell (1953, p. 223). For Cruveilhier's use in macrodissected adult human, see p. 991. It was clearly identified by Willis; see ***[communicating branch of superior and middle cervical ganglia (Cruveilhier, 1836)] (Willis, 1664)***.

TRANSLATIONS:

1. *branche de communication du ganglion cervical supérieur au ganglion cervical moyen (Cruveilhier, 1836)*
   Original French form of ***communicating branch of superior and middle cervical ganglia (Cruveilhier, 1836)***; p. 991.

EARLIER REFERENCES:

Illustrated and described, not named:

1. ***[communicating branch of superior and middle cervical ganglia (Cruveilhier, 1836)] (Willis, 1664)***
   Described and illustrated for macrodissected adult human; see Pordage translation (1681, p. 157, Tab. IX).

Earlier synonyms:

1. *inferior branch of superior cervical ganglion (Cloquet, 1816)*
   Synonym for macrodissected adult human ***communicating branch of superior and middle cervical ganglia (>1840)***; in the original French, *filet inferior du ganglion cervical supérieur*, p. 690, where Cloquet referred to it as a *nerve cord (cordon nerveux)*. Meckel (1817) described branches from *inferior branch of superior cervical ganglion (Cloquet, 1816)* to ***vestibulocochlear nerve (>1840), glossopharyngeal nerve (Huber, 1744), vagus nerve (Galen, c192)***, and ***accessory nerve (Ridley, 1695)***; see translation (1832, Vol. 3, pp. 93–94).
2. *superior branch of middle cervical ganglion (Meckel, 1817)*
   Synonym for macrodissected adult human *inferior branch of superior cervical ganglion (Cloquet, 1816)*; see translation (1832, Vol. 3, p. 94).
3. *intermediate trunk between supreme and middle cervical ganglia (Arnold, 1834)*
   Synonym for macrodissected adult human ***communicating branch of superior and middle cervical ganglia (>1840)***; in the original Latin, *truncus intermedius inter ganglion cervicale supremum et medium*, p. 18.

communicating branch of superior laryngeal nerve with inferior laryngeal nerve (Langenbeck, 1826–1830)

As described for macrodissected adult human, a ***communicating branch (Winslow, 1733)*** or bridge between the caudally directed (descending) ***internal branch of superior laryngeal nerve (Fyfe, 1800)*** and the rostrally directed (ascending) ***inferior laryngeal nerve (>1840)*** branch of the ***recurrent laryngeal nerve (Albinus, 1744)***. It is also common to describe communication of the ***internal branch of superior laryngeal nerve (Fyfe, 1800)*** with the ***recurrent laryngeal nerve (Albinus, 1744)*** when its rostrally directed terminal branch is not called the ***inferior laryngeal nerve (>1840)***; see Durward (1951, p. 1040), Williams & Warwick (1980, p. 1080), *Terminologia Anatomica* (1998, p. 136). As detailed by Scarpa (1794, Tab. III), there also may be multiple ***communicating branches (Winslow, 1733)*** between ***recurrent laryngeal nerve (Albinus, 1744)*** and ***internal branch of superior laryngeal nerve (Fyfe, 1800)***. For Langenbeck's description of several such branches in macrodissected adult human, see Fascicle II, Table IX-79. It was beautifully illustrated by Swan (1830, Pl. XVI, Figs. 6, 7) and was discovered by Galen; see ***[communicating branch of superior laryngeal nerve with inferior laryngeal nerve (Langenbeck, 1826–1830)] (Galen, c173)***.

TRANSLATIONS:

1. *rami communicantes inter nervum laryngeum inferiorem et superiorem (Langenbeck, 1826–1830)*
   Original Latin form (plural) of ***communicating branch of superior laryngeal nerve with inferior laryngeal nerve (Langenbeck, 1826–1830)***; Fascicle II, Table IX-79.

EARLIER REFERENCES:

Described, not named or illustrated:

1. ***[communicating branch of superior laryngeal nerve with inferior laryngeal nerve (Langenbeck, 1826–1830)] (Galen, c173)***
   Clearly described for macrodissected adult "bears, dogs, oxen, and other animals of this kind" (see Scarpa, 1794, Tab. III).

Illustrated, not named or described:

1. ***[communicating branch of superior laryngeal nerve with inferior laryngeal nerve (Langenbeck, 1826–1830)] (Eustachi, 1552)***
   Illustrated for macrodissected adult human; see Albinus edition (1761, Tab. 18, Fig. 2-*n,o,p*).

Illustrated and described, not named:

1. ***[communicating branch of superior laryngeal nerve with inferior laryngeal nerve (Langenbeck, 1826–1830)] (Willis, 1664)***
   Described and illustrated for macrodissected adult human and other common large mammals; see Pordage translation (1681, p. 147, Tab. IX-*h*, Tab. X). Very clearly illustrated by Scarpa (1794); see Knox translation (1832, Pl. III-92).

Earlier synonyms:

1. *communicating branch of internal laryngeal nerve and recurrent nerve (Andersch & Soemmerring, 1792)*
   Synonym for macrodissected adult human ***communicating branch of superior laryngeal nerve with inferior laryngeal nerve (Langenbeck, 1826–1830)***; in the original Latin, *nervi laryngei interni et nervi recurrentis communicatorius ramus*, p. 129.

2. *communicating nerve betwixt internal laryngeal nerve and recurrent branch of par vagum (Bell & Bell, 1816)*
   Synonym for macrodissected adult human ***communicating branch of superior laryngeal nerve with inferior laryngeal nerve (Langenbeck, 1826–1830)***; p. 505.
3. *anastomotic branch of internal branch of superior laryngeal nerve with recurrent laryngeal nerve (Meckel, 1817)*
   Synonym for macrodissected adult human ***communicating branch of superior laryngeal nerve with inferior laryngeal nerve (Langenbeck, 1826–1830)***; see translation (1832, Vol. 3, p. 47).
4. *twig connecting inferior laryngeal nerve with superior laryngeal nerve (Arnold, 1834)*
   Synonym for macrodissected adult human ***communicating branch of superior laryngeal nerve with inferior laryngeal nerve (Langenbeck, 1826–1830)***; in the original Latin, *surculus coiens nervus laryngeus inferior cum nervo laryngeo superiore*, p. 14, Table V-57.
5. *anastomotic filament of superior laryngeal branches of pneumogastric nerve (Cruveilhier, 1836)*
   Synonym for macrodissected adult human ***communicating branch of superior laryngeal nerve with inferior laryngeal nerve (Langenbeck, 1826–1830)***; in the original French, *filet anastomotique*, p. 960.
6. *descending filament of superior laryngeal branches of pneumogastric nerve (Cruveilhier, 1836)*
   Synonym for *anastomotic filament of superior laryngeal branches of pneumogastric nerve (Cruveilhier, 1836)*; in the original French, *filet descendant*, p. 960.

LATER SYNONYMS:

1. *communicating branch of superior laryngeal nerve with recurrent laryngeal nerve (>1840)*
   Synonym for macrodissected adult human ***communicating branch of superior laryngeal nerve with inferior laryngeal nerve (Langenbeck, 1826–1830)***; see Durward (1951, p. 1040), Williams & Warwick (1980, p. 1080), *Terminologia Anatomica* (1998, p. 136).

PARTLY CORRESPONDS:

1. *laryngeal plexus (Soemmerring, 1791)*
   Probably related to macrodissected adult human ***communicating branch of superior laryngeal nerve with inferior laryngeal nerve (Langenbeck, 1826–1830)***; in the original Latin, *plexus laryngeus*, p. 317.
2. *descending branch of internal laryngeal nerve (Knox, 1832)*
   Apparently *superior laryngeal nerve (Loder, 1778)* component of macrodissected adult human ***communicating branch of superior laryngeal nerve with inferior laryngeal nerve (Langenbeck, 1826–1830)***; Plate III-*94,97,178*, in Knox's translation of Scarpa (1794).

communicating branch of tympanic plexus with greater petrosal nerve (>1840)

As described for macrodissected adult human, a ***communicating branch (Winslow, 1733)*** between ***tympanic plexus (Müller, 1834)*** and ***greater petrosal nerve (>1840)***; see Mitchell (1953, p. 169), Williams & Warwick (1980, pp. 1071, 1200). It was discovered by Jacobson; see ***[branch of tympanic plexus to greater petrosal nerve (>1840)] (Jacobson, 1818)***.

EARLIER REFERENCES:

Described, not named or illustrated:

1. ***[branch of tympanic plexus to greater petrosal nerve (>1840)] (Jacobson, 1818)***
   Described for macrodissected adult human; see Lobstein translation (1831, p. 36).

communicating branch of vagus nerve with glossopharyngeal nerve (>1840)

As described for macrodissected adult human, one or more typically extend between ***distal glossopharyngeal ganglion (>1840)*** and ***proximal vagal ganglion (>1840)***; see Durward (1951, Fig. 907, unlabeled), Mitchell (1953, p. 169), Williams & Warwick (1980, p. 1075), *Terminologia Anatomica* (1998, p. 136). It was probably first clearly described with the *communicating branchlets of tenth nerves of head (Andersch, 1797)*.

EARLIER REFERENCES:

Earlier synonyms:

1. *communicating branchlets of tenth nerves of head (Andersch, 1797)*
   Description of this feature in macrodissected adult human included ***communicating branch of vagus nerve with glossopharyngeal nerve (>1840)***; in the original Latin, *ramulum communicatorium decimi nervi capitis*, p. 7. Kilian (1822, pp. 87, 89, 91) described at least four such ***communicating branches (Winslow, 1733)*** in macrodissected adult human.

communicating branches of auriculotemporal nerve with facial nerve (>1840)

As described for macrodissected adult human, two ***communicating branches (Winslow, 1733)*** commonly extend from the ***auriculotemporal nerve (Haller, 1762)*** rostrally (forward) and laterally, deep to the neck of the mandible, to join branches of the ***facial nerve trunk (>1840)*** at the caudal (posterior) border of the masseter muscle in or near the parotid gland; see Durward (1951, p. 1028), Williams & Warwick (1980, p. 1066), *Terminologia Anatomica* (1998, p. 134). They were known to Eustachi; see ***[communicating branches of auriculotemporal nerve with facial nerve (>1840)] (Eustachi, 1552)***.

EARLIER REFERENCES:

Illustrated, not named or described:

1. ***[communicating branches of auriculotemporal nerve with facial nerve (>1840)] (Eustachi, 1552)***
   Illustrated for macrodissected adult human; see Albinus edition (1761, Tab. 18, Fig. 1-*V*, p. 102). So, apparently, did Valsalva (1704, Tab. 7, Fig. 3-*f*).

Described, not named or illustrated:

1. ***[communicating branches of auriculotemporal nerve with facial nerve (>1840)] (Winslow, 1733)***

Winslow probably mentioned two in macrodissected adult human as communications associated with second and third branches of *inferior maxillary nerve (Heister, 1717)*; Section VI, pp. 65–66.

Earlier synonyms:

1. *anastomotic branches of superficial temporal nerve with facial nerve (Meckel, 1817)*
   Synonym for macrodissected adult human ***communicating branches of auriculotemporal nerve with facial nerve (>1840)***; see translation (1832, Vol. 3, p. 73).
2. *anastomotic fascicles of cutaneous temporal surculus of inferior maxillary branch (Bellingeri, 1818)*
   Synonym for two macrodissected adult human ***communicating branches of auriculotemporal nerve with facial nerve (>1840)***; in the original Latin, *(duo) fasciculi anastomotici*, see Table I.
3. *communicating branches of superficial temporal nerve with facial nerve (Arnold, 1834)*
   Synonym for macrodissected adult human ***communicating branches of auriculotemporal nerve with facial nerve (>1840)***; in the original Latin, *nervus temporalis superficialis, rami communicantes cum nervo faciali*, p. 11.
4. *communicating branches of anterior auricular nerve with facial nerve (Arnold, 1834)*
   Synonym for macrodissected adult human ***communicating branches of auriculotemporal nerve with facial nerve (>1840)***; in the original Latin, *nervus auricularis anterior, rami communicantes cum nervo faciali*, p. 11.

communicating branches of cervical plexus (>1840)

As described for macrodissected adult human, ***communicating branches (Winslow, 1733)*** of the ***communicating loops of cervical plexus (>1840)*** with the ***vagus nerve (Galen, c192), accessory nerve (Vieussens, 1684), hypoglossal nerve (Winslow, 1733)***, and ***superior cervical ganglion (Vieussens, 1684)***, the latter of which are ***gray communicating branches (>1840)***; and a ***communicating branch (Winslow, 1733)*** between the fourth and fifth cervical ***spinal nerve ventral branches (>1840)***; see Durward (1951, Fig. 919), Williams & Warwick (1980, pp. 1092–1094, Fig. 7.193). At least one was known to Galen; see ***[communicating branches of cervical plexus (>1840)] (Galen, c192)***.

EARLIER REFERENCES:

Described, not named or illustrated:

1. ***[communicating branches of cervical plexus (>1840)] (Galen, c192)***
   Galen clearly described one with ***accessory nerve (Vieussens, 1684)*** in macrodissected adult large mammals, including macaque, but not human; see Duckworth translation (1962, p. 235). Galen wrote there, "the third pair of these [***cervical nerves (Galen, c173)***]...communicates in these anterior regions...with a branch [***accessory nerve (Vieussens, 1684)*** to trapezius muscle] from the sixth pair of nerves which arise from the brain."
2. ***[communicating branches of cervical plexus (>1840)] (Vieussens, 1684)***
   Vieussens clearly described and illustrated for macrodissected adult human a branch from rostral ***communicating loop of cervical plexus (>1840)*** to ***vagus nerve (Galen, c192)***—Tables 23-*K* descending branch, and 24-*e*—and a ***gray communicating branch (>1840)*** between ***superior cervical ganglion (Vieussens, 1684)*** and second cervical ***spinal nerve ventral branch (>1840)***—Table 23-*89*.
3. ***[communicating branches of cervical plexus (>1840)] (Asch, 1750)***
   Asch clearly described and illustrated all of them for macrodissected two-year-old infant and adult human, including those with ***hypoglossal nerve (Winslow, 1733)***, and generally referred to each as a communicating branch (*ramulum communicatorium*); see Figures 3–5 and pp. 42–43. Also see historical review in Haller (1762, pp. 238–239) and a detailed illustration in Neubauer (Tab. 3, Fig. 4) for macrodissected adult human.

PARTLY CORRESPONDS:

1. *communicating branch from anterior rami of first nerve of neck to inferior branches (Andersch & Soemmerring, 1792)*
   Probably macrodissected adult human ***communicating branch of ansa cervicalis (>1840)*** between first cervical ***spinal nerve ventral branch (>1840)*** and ***hypoglossal nerve (Winslow, 1733)*** leading to ***superior root of ansa cervicalis (>1840)***; in the original Latin, *ramus communicatorius a primi nervi colli anterioris rami inferiori ramo*, p. 145.
2. *communicating branch of anterior rami of first nerve of neck and inferior rami (Andersch, 1797)*
   Synonym for *communicating branch from anterior rami of first nerve of neck to inferior branches (Andersch & Soemmerring, 1792)*; in the original Latin, *ramum communicatorium primi nervi colli rami anterioris inferioris rami*, p. 64.

communicating branches of lingual nerve with hypoglossal nerve (>1840)

As described for macrodissected adult human, loops of communication between ***lingual nerve (Vesalius, 1543a)*** and small branches of the ***hypoglossal nerve (Winslow, 1733)***; see Williams & Warwick (1980, p. 1067), *Terminologia Anatomica* (1998, p. 135). They were probably first delineated by Falloppio; see ***[communicating branches of lingual nerve with hypoglossal nerve (>1840)] (Falloppio, 1561)***.

EARLIER REFERENCES:

Described, not named or illustrated:

1. ***[communicating branches of lingual nerve with hypoglossal nerve (>1840)] (Falloppio, 1561)***
   According to Scarpa (1794, Tab. I), Falloppio described them on p. 155. According to Haller (1762, p. 218 note

y), Vieussens (1684, p. 173) mentioned or alluded to them for macrodissected adult human, with reference to the *ninth pair of nerves arising within skull (Willis, 1664)*. Winslow (1733, Sect. VI, p. 67) clearly described several such ***communicating branches (Winslow, 1733)*** for macrodissected adult human. Monro (1783, Tab. 26*-*L*) described, "A small plexus formed by the joining of the fifth with the ninth pair."

Illustrated and described, not named:

1. ***[communicating branches of lingual nerve with hypoglossal nerve (>1840)] (Meckel, 1748)***
   Clearly described and illustrated for macrodissected adult human; p. 96 note *z* and Figure 1-*78,92*.

Earlier synonyms:

1. *anastomotic branch of ninth pair with branch of lingual nerve of fifth pair (Günther, 1786)*
   Synonym for macrodissected adult human ***communicating branch of lingual nerve with hypoglossal nerve (>1840)***; in the original Latin, *r. anastomotieus cum ramis nervi lingualis quinti paris*, p. 68.
2. *ascending communicating branch part of tenth nerves of head with superior lingual nerve (Andersch & Soemmerring, 1792)*
   Synonym for macrodissected adult human ***communicating branch of lingual nerve with hypoglossal nerve (>1840)***; in the original Latin, *decimi nervi capitis partis ascendentis ramus communicatorius nervi lingualis superioris*, p. 153.
3. *anastomosis of ninth nerve with lingual nerve of fifth pair (Scarpa, 1794)*
   Synonym for ***communicating branches of lingual nerve with hypoglossal nerve (>1840)***; in the original Latin, *anastomosis Noni cum Linguali nervo Paris Quinti*, Table I-39. Scarpa described a double anastomosis in macrodissected adult human.
4. *lingual nerve filaments anastomosing with hypoglossal nerve (Meckel, 1817)*
   Synonym for macrodissected adult human ***communicating branches of lingual nerve with hypoglossal nerve (>1840)***; see translation (1832, Vol. 3, p. 75).
5. *double anastomosis of great hypoglossal nerve with lingual branch of fifth pair (Knox, 1832)*
   Synonym for macrodissected adult human ***communicating branches of lingual nerve with hypoglossal nerve (>1840)***; Plate I-69.
6. *connection of lingual nerve with hypoglossal nerve (Arnold, 1834)*
   Synonym for macrodissected adult human ***communicating branches of lingual nerve with hypoglossal nerve (>1840)***; in the original Latin, *nervus lingualis, conjunctio cum nervo hypoglosso*, p. 11.
7. *connection of gustatory nerve with hypoglossal nerve (Arnold, 1834)*
   Synonym for macrodissected adult human ***communicating branches of lingual nerve with hypoglossal nerve (>1840)***; in the original Latin, *nervus gustatorius, conjunctio cum nervo hypoglosso*, p. 11.
8. *connection of lingual part of hypoglossal nerve with lingual nerve (Arnold, 1834)*
   Synonym for *connection of lingual nerve with hypoglossal nerve (Arnold, 1834)*; in the original Latin, *conjunctio nervus hypoglossus pars lingualis cum nervo linguali*, p. 15.
9. *branches of communication of ninth nerve with gustatory nerve (Quain & Wilson, 1839)*
   Synonym for macrodissected adult human ***communicating branches of lingual nerve with hypoglossal nerve (>1840)***; Plate XVI-*a*.
10. *branches of communication of lingual nerve with gustatory nerve (Quain & Wilson, 1839)*
    Synonym for macrodissected adult human ***communicating branches of lingual nerve with hypoglossal nerve (>1840)***; Plate XVI-*a*.

PARTLY CORRESPONDS:

1. *lingual muscular fascicle of lingual surculus with chorda tympani (Bellingeri, 1818)*
   As described for macrodissected adult human, ***communicating branch of lingual nerve with hypoglossal nerve (>1840)*** supplying posterior part of hyoglossus muscle, the "*musculum cerato-glossum*"; in the original Latin, *fasciculi musculares linguales*, see Table I.

communicating branches of lingual nerve with submandibular ganglion (>1840)

As described for macrodissected adult human, usually two or sometimes three ***communicating branches (Winslow, 1733)*** between ***lingual nerve (Vesalius, 1543a)*** and ***submandibular ganglion (>1840)***; typically the caudal (posterior) branch is the motor or parasympathetic root of the ***submandibular ganglion (>1840)*** with ***axons (Kölliker, 1896)*** from the ***superior salivatory nucleus (>1840)***, whereas the rostral (anterior) branch has ***axons (Kölliker, 1896)*** from the ***submandibular ganglion (>1840)*** joining the ***lingual nerve (Vesalius, 1543a)*** and extending to the sublingual and anterior lingual glands; see Williams & Warwick (1980, pp. 1067, 1072, and Figs. 7.177, 179) and His (1895, p. 89). They were perhaps first alluded to by Vieussens; see ***[communicating branches of lingual nerve with submandibular ganglion (>1840)] (Vieussens, 1684)***.

EARLIER REFERENCES:

Illustrated and described, not named:

1. ***[communicating branches of lingual nerve with submandibular ganglion (>1840)] (Vieussens, 1684)***
   Alluded to in macrodissected adult human as branches to maxillary (submandibular) gland; p. 173 and Tables 22-6 and 23-*g*.

Earlier synonyms:

1. *branchlets from lingual nerve to maxillary ganglion (Meckel, 1748)*
   Synonym for macrodissected adult human ***communicating branches of lingual nerve with submandibular ganglion (>1840)***; in the original Latin, *ramuli ex nervo linguali ad ganglion maxillare*, Figures 1-*72,73* and p. 94.

2. *filaments of lingual nerve to maxillary ganglion (Meckel, 1817)*
   Synonym for macrodissected adult human ***communicating branches of lingual nerve with submandibular ganglion (>1840)***; see translation (1832, Vol. 3, p. 75).
3. *ganglionic fascicles of lingual surculus with chorda tympani (Bellingeri, 1818)*
   Synonym for three macrodissected adult human ***communicating branches of lingual nerve with submandibular ganglion (>1840)***; in the original Latin, *(tres) fasciculi gangliosi*, see Table I.
4. *branches of lingual nerve to maxillary ganglion (Arnold, 1834)*
   Synonym for macrodissected adult human ***communicating branches of lingual nerve with submandibular ganglion (>1840)***; p. 10.
5. *branches of gustatory nerve to maxillary ganglion (Arnold, 1834)*
   Synonym for *branches of lingual nerve to maxillary ganglion (Arnold, 1834)*; p. 10.
6. *short root of glottic ganglion (Arnold, 1834)*
   Synonym for macrodissected adult human ***communicating branches of lingual nerve with submandibular ganglion (>1840)***; in the original Latin, *ganglion glotticum, radix brevis*, p. 10.
7. *short root of lingual ganglion (Arnold, 1834)*
   Synonym for macrodissected adult human ***communicating branches of lingual nerve with submandibular ganglion (>1840)***; in the original Latin, *ganglion linguale, radix brevis*, p. 10.
8. *short root of maxillary ganglion (Arnold, 1834)*
   Synonym for macrodissected adult human ***communicating branches of lingual nerve with submandibular ganglion (>1840)***; in the original Latin, *ganglion maxillare, radix brevis*, p. 10.
9. *short root of Meckel's ganglion (Arnold, 1834)*
   Synonym for macrodissected adult human ***communicating branches of lingual nerve with submandibular ganglion (>1840)***; in the original Latin, *ganglion Meckelii, radix brevis*, p. 10.
10. *connection of maxillary ganglion with lingual nerve (Arnold, 1834)*
   Synonym for macrodissected adult human ***communicating branches of lingual nerve with submandibular ganglion (>1840)***; in the original Latin, *conjunctio ganglion maxillare cum nervo linguali*, Table VII:*V-43*.
11. *nervous filament quitting gustatory nerve to communicate with submaxillary ganglion (Quain & Wilson, 1839)*
   Synonym for macrodissected adult human ***communicating branch of lingual nerve with submandibular ganglion (>1840)***; Plate XXVII-*s*.
12. *ganglionic branches to submandibular ganglion (>1840)*
   Synonym for macrodissected adult human ***communicating branches of lingual nerve with submandibular ganglion (>1840)***; see *Terminologia Anatomica* (1998, p. 135).
13. *sensory root of submandibular ganglion (>1840)*
   Synonym for macrodissected adult human ***communicating branches of lingual nerve with submandibular ganglion (>1840)***; see *Terminologia Anatomica* (1998, p. 135)—seems like an obvious error.

PARTLY CORRESPONDS:

1. *posterior branchlets from lingual nerve to maxillary ganglion (Meckel, 1748)*
   In macrodissected adult human there are usually two or three ***communicating branches of lingual nerve with submandibular ganglion (>1840)***, and this refers to the caudal (posterior) two of the three; in the original Latin, *ramuli posteriores ex nervo linguali ad ganglion maxillare*, see Figure 1-72 and Williams & Warwick (1980, Figs. 7.177–179).
2. *retrograde anterior branchlet from lingual nerve to maxillary ganglion (Meckel, 1748)*
   In macrodissected adult human there are usually two or three ***communicating branches of lingual nerve with submandibular ganglion (>1840)***, one of which is separated from the other(s) and lies more rostrally (anteriorly); in the original Latin, *ramulus anterior eiusdem* [referring to *posterior branchlets from lingual nerve to maxillary ganglion (Meckel, 1748)*] *ex linguali retrogradus*, see Figure 1-73 and Williams & Warwick (1980, Figs. 7.177–179).

communicating branches of otic ganglion with auriculotemporal nerve (>1840)

As described for adult human, ***communicating branches (Winslow, 1733)*** between ***otic ganglion (Arnold, 1828)*** and ***auriculotemporal nerve (Haller, 1762)*** carrying postganglionic parasympathetic ***axons (Kölliker, 1896)*** to the parotid gland; see Durward (1951, Fig. 899), Williams & Warwick (1980, p. 1076). First clearly described as *branchlet of otic ganglion to anterior auricular nerve (Arnold, 1834)*.

EARLIER REFERENCES:

Earlier synonyms:

1. *branchlet of otic ganglion to anterior auricular nerve (Arnold, 1834)*
   Synonym for macrodissected adult human ***communicating branches of otic ganglion with auriculotemporal nerve (>1840)***; in the original Latin, *ramulus ganglii otici ad nervum auricularem anteriorem*, Table VII:*V-31* (also see p. 10 for description).
2. *filaments of communication of otic ganglion with auricular nerve (Quain & Wilson, 1839)*
   Synonym for macrodissected adult human ***communicating branches of otic ganglion with auriculotemporal nerve (>1840)***; Plate XIII, Figure 1-*n*.

communicating branches of spinal nerves (Wutzer, 1817)

As described for macrodissected adult human, relatively short branches connecting ***spinal nerves***

(Camper, 1760–1762) with ***sympathetic cord (>1840).*** Each ***spinal nerve (Camper, 1760–1762)*** typically has one ***gray communicating branch (>1840)***, whereas the ***lumbar nerves (Diemerbroeck, 1672)*** and upper ***thoracic nerves (Diemerbroeck, 1672)***, as well as the middle ***sacral nerves (Camper, 1760)***, also have at least one ***white communicating branch (>1840)***; see Mitchell (1953, pp. 205–207). Their functional significance remained unclear until Gaskell's work in the 1880s; see Clarke & Jacyna (1987, p. 325). Scarpa (1779) demonstrated they are primarily associated with ***spinal nerve ventral branches (>1840)***. A ***gray communicating branch (>1840)*** typically joins a ***spinal nerve ventral branch (>1840)*** proximal to the point where the ***white communicating branch (>1840)*** leaves it, contrary to many schematic illustrations; see Williams & Warwick (1980, p. 1103). For Wutzer's use in macrodissected adult human, see p. 97; for translation see Lobstein (1831, p. 54), "communicating branches with the spinal nerves." For an early analysis of gray and white *nerve fibers (Ehrenberg, 1833)* associated with ***communicating branches of spinal nerves (Wutzer, 1817)***, see Müller (1838, p. 672 ff.). Their existence was first indicated by Galen; see ***[communicating branches of spinal nerves (Wutzer, 1817)] (Galen, c173).***

TRANSLATIONS:

1. *rami communicantis illi nervorum spinalium (Wutzer, 1817)*
   Original Latin form of ***communicating branches of spinal nerves (Wutzer, 1817)***; p. 97.
2. *rami communicantes nervorum spinalium (>1840)*
   Current Latin form of ***communicating branches of spinal nerves (Wutzer, 1817)***; see *Terminologia Anatomica* (1998, p. 141).

EARLIER REFERENCES:

Described, not named or illustrated:

1. ***[communicating branches of spinal nerves (Wutzer, 1817)] (Galen, c173)***
   In *On the Usefulness of the Parts* and *On Anatomy of Nerves*, Galen described thoraco-lumbar ***communicating branches (Winslow, 1733)***; see Goss (1966, pp. 333–334), May (1968, p. 695), Clarke & Jacyna (1987, p. 312); also see Duckworth (1962, pp. 218–219). Galen explicitly admitted macrodissecting adult beef, pig, macaque, and other common large mammals but not human cadavers, and suggested that these anastomotic branches were for support rather than exchange of nervous material; see Duckworth translation (1962, p. 220). Vesalius (1543a) described and illustrated ***communicating branches of spinal nerves (Wutzer, 1817)*** for ***thoracic nerves (Diemerbroeck, 1672)*** and rostral two ***lumbar nerves (Diemerbroeck, 1672)*** in macrodissected adult human; see Richardson & Carman translation (2002, pp. 195, 199, 234, 252). Vieussens (1684; Tab. 23-*89,91*) described and illustrated for macrodissected adult human all of them, except for a second one associated with ***lumbar nerves (Diemerbroeck, 1672)***; that is, he had two ***communicating branches of spinal nerves (Wutzer, 1817)*** for each ***thoracic nerve (Diemerbroeck, 1672)***, although he had their relationship with the ***sympathetic trunk (Winslow, 1733)*** wrong.

Earlier synonyms:

1. *vertebral branch (Willis, 1664)*
   Synonym for macrodissected adult human and other large mammalian ***communicating branch of spinal nerves (Wutzer, 1817)***; see Pordage translation (1681, p. 158 and Tab. 9-*11*).
2. *branches which communicate with great sympathetic nerve (Winslow, 1733)*
   Synonym for macrodissected adult human ***communicating branches of spinal nerves (Wutzer, 1817)***; Section VI, p. 85. They were called "communicating branches" in the English translation of Lobstein (1831, p. 16).
3. *ganglions communicate by short branches with vertebral nerves (Winslow, 1733)*
   Synonym for macrodissected adult human ***communicating branches of spinal nerves (Wutzer, 1817)***; Section VI, p. 96.
4. *rami communicanti cum intercostali (Martin, 1781)*
   Synonym for macrodissected adult human ***communicating branches of spinal nerves (Wutzer, 1817)***; Table X.
5. *anastomoseos cum sympathico (Martin, 1781)*
   Synonym for macrodissected adult human ***communicating branches of spinal nerves (Wutzer, 1817)***; p. 229.
6. *anastomotic root between ganglia and trunk of great sympathetic nerve (Walter, 1783)*
   Synonym for macrodissected adult human ***communicating branch of spinal nerves (Wutzer, 1817)***; in the original Latin, *radix anastomotica inter ganglion... atque nervi sympathici magni*, e.g., Table 1-*101*.
7. *communicating root between ganglia and trunk of great sympathetic nerve (Walter, 1783)*
   Synonym for macrodissected adult human ***communicating branch of spinal nerves (Wutzer, 1817)***; in the original Latin, *radix communicans...*, e.g., Table 1-*149*.
8. *spinal roots of great sympathetic nerve (Günther, 1786)*
   Synonym for macrodissected adult human ***communicating branches of spinal nerves (Wutzer, 1817)***; in the original Latin, *radicibus spinalibus nervus intercostalis magnus*, p. 92.
9. *branch of union with sympathetic (Bell & Bell, 1816)*
   Synonym for a macrodissected adult human ***communicating branch of spinal nerves (Wutzer, 1817)***; Vol. 2, p. 517.
10. *filaments of communication with anterior cords of spinal nerves (Meckel, 1817)*
    Synonym for macrodissected adult human ***communicating branches of spinal nerves (Wutzer, 1817)***; see translation (1832, Vol. 1, p. 179).
11. *anastomosing branches communicate with limiting ganglions of ganglionnary system (Meckel, 1817)*
    Synonym for macrodissected adult human ***communicating branches of spinal nerves (Wutzer, 1817)***; see translation (1832, Vol. 3, p. 8).

LATER SYNONYMS:

1. *communicating branches of sympathetic nerve (Lobstein, 1823)*
   Synonym for ***communicating branches of spinal nerves (Wutzer, 1817)***; see translation (1831, p. 44).
2. *exterior branches of sympathetic nerve (Lobstein, 1823)*
   Synonym for ***communicating branches of spinal nerves (Wutzer, 1817)***; see translation (1831, p. 44).
3. *ganglionic spinal branches (Cruveilhier, 1836)*
   Synonym for macrodissected adult human ***communicating branches of spinal nerves (Wutzer, 1817)***; in the original French, *branches spinales ganglionnaires*, p. 765.
4. *communicating branches of spinal pairs with ganglia of great sympathetic (Cruveilhier, 1836)*
   Synonym for macrodissected adult human ***communicating branches of spinal nerves (Wutzer, 1817)***; in the original French, *branches de communication des paires spinales avec les ganglions du grand sympathique*, p. 1008.

PARTLY CORRESPONDS:

1. *commixtion of intercostall nerves with descending branch of sixt conjugation of brain (Crooke, 1615)*
   Refers to ***communicating branches of spinal nerves (Wutzer, 1817)*** associated specifically with subset of macrodissected adult human ***intercostal nerves (Vesalius, 1543a)***; p. 492. Crooke's passage is translation of Bauhin (1605).
2. *roots of proper intercostal nerves (Monro, 1783)*
   Communicating branches of spinal nerves (Wutzer, 1817), illustrated for ***thoracic nerves (Diemerbroeck, 1672)*** of macrodissected adult ox; Table 23-G. Monro observed, "Some branches, as T, seem, by their direction, to go from the proper intercostal to the great sympathetic ganglion; others seem to come from the ganglion of the sympathetic to the proper intercostal nerve." (Tab. 23-*RS*).
3. *communicating branches to sympathetic (Bell, 1803b)*
   Synonym for macrodissected adult human ***communicating branches of spinal nerves (Wutzer, 1817)*** associated specifically with ***thoracic nerves (Diemerbroeck, 1672)***; p. 169. Bell also referred to them as *communicating nerves from spinal marrow*; p. 168.
4. *communicating branch between supreme cervical ganglion and second cervical nerve (Bischoff, 1832)*
   For macrodissected adult human, ***communicating branch of spinal nerves (Wutzer, 1817)*** between ***superior cervical ganglion (Vieussens, 1684)*** and second ***cervical nerve (Galen, c173)***; in the original Latin, *ramus communicans inter ganglion cervicale supremum et secundum nervum cervicalem*, Table 1, Figure 1-45.
5. *external branches of superior cervical ganglion (Cruveilhier, 1836)*
   For macrodissected adult human, ***communicating branches of spinal nerves (Wutzer, 1817)*** for first three, or sometimes four, ***cervical nerves (Galen, c173)***; in the original French, *rameaux externes*, p. 990.
6. *external branches of thoracic part of great sympathetic (Cruveilhier, 1836)*
   For macrodissected adult human, ***communicating branches of spinal nerves (Wutzer, 1817)*** for ***thoracic nerves (Diemerbroeck, 1672)***; in the original French, *rameaux externes*, p. 1008.
7. *spinal branches of thoracic part of great sympathetic (Cruveilhier, 1836)*
   Synonym for *external branches of thoracic part of great sympathetic (Cruveilhier, 1836)*; in the original French, *branches rachidiennes*, p. 1008.
8. *communicating branches between lumbar pairs and ganglia (Cruveilhier, 1836)*
   For macrodissected adult human, ***communicating branches of spinal nerves (Wutzer, 1817)*** for ***lumbar nerves (Diemerbroeck, 1672)***; *rameaux de communication entre les paires et les ganglions lombaires*, p. 1023.

communicating branches of sympathetic trunk (>1840)

Macroscopic segments of the ***sympathetic trunk (Winslow, 1733)*** between discrete ***sympathetic trunk ganglia (Winslow, 1733)***; see Mitchell (1953, pp. 207–209). They were clearly identified by Willis; see ***[communicating branches of sympathetic trunk (>1840)] (Willis, 1664)***.

EARLIER REFERENCES:

Illustrated, not named or described:

1. ***[communicating branches of sympathetic trunk (>1840)] (Willis, 1664)***
   Clearly illustrated in macrodissected adult human; Table IX, also see Pordage translation (1681, pp. 157–158).

Earlier synonyms:

1. *intercostal trunk (Neubauer, 1772)*
   Synonym for macrodissected adult human ***communicating branches of sympathetic trunk (>1840)***; for example, p. 99.
2. *anastomotic nerve of great sympathetic nerve (Walter, 1783)*
   Synonym for macrodissected adult human ***communicating branch of sympathetic trunk (>1840)***; for example, *nervus anastomoticus inter sextum et septimum ganglion thoracicum seu Truncus Nervi Sympathici magni*, Table I-42; also in the form *nervum anastomoticum*, Table 2-65.
3. *trunk of great sympathetic nerve (Walter, 1783, Tab. 2)*
   Synonym for macrodissected adult human ***communicating branch of sympathetic trunk (>1840)***; for example, *nervus anastomoticus inter sextum et septimum ganglion thoracicum seu Truncus Nervi Sympathici magni*, Table I-42; also in the form *nervum anastomoticum*, Table 2-65.
4. *anastomotic nerve of intercostal nerve (Walter, 1783)*
   Synonym for macrodissected adult human ***communicating branch of sympathetic trunk (>1840)***; for example, *truncus Nervi Intercostalis, seu anastomoticus nervus inter septimum et octavum ganglion*, Table 1-47.
5. *trunk nerve of intercostal nerve (Walter, 1783)*
   Synonym for macrodissected adult human ***communicating branch of sympathetic trunk (>1840)***;

for example, *truncus Nervi Intercostalis, seu anastomoticus nervus inter septimum et octavum ganglion*, Table 1-47.

6. *communicating nerve of great sympathetic nerve (Walter, 1783)*
Synonym for macrodissected adult human ***communicating branch of sympathetic trunk(>1840)***; for example, *truncus nervi sympathici magni...seu nervus communicans inter ganglion sacrale primum et ganglion lumbare quintum*, Table 1, Figure 2-3.
7. *communicating branch into forty-fourth (sympathetic) nerve of body (Andersch & Soemmerring, 1792)*
Synonym for macrodissected adult human ***communicating branch of sympathetic trunk (>1840)***; in the original Latin, *communicatorium ramum in quadragesunum quartum (sympathicum) nervum corporis*, p. 182.
8. *filaments of union of limiting ganglia (Meckel, 1817)*
Synonym for macrodissected adult human ***communicating branches of sympathetic trunk (>1840)***; see translation (1832, Vol. 3, pp. 97). Meckel also wrote, "[The limiting ganglions] anastomose by some longitudinal cords with each other" (1832, Vol. 3, p. 84).
9. *communicating branch of intercostal nerve (Lobstein, 1823)*
Synonym for macrodissected adult human ***communicating branch of sympathetic trunk (>1840)***; see translation (1831, p. 71). Quain (1828, see p. 669) used *branch of communication*.
10. *cords of connexion of sympathetic nerve (Quain, 1828)*
Synonym for macrodissected adult human ***communicating branch of sympathetic trunk (>1840)***; p. 668. Also see *communicating branch of intercostal nerve (Lobstein, 1823)*.
11. *anastomosing branch of great sympathetic (Knox, 1832)*
Synonym for macrodissected adult human ***communicating branch of sympathetic trunk (>1840)***; Plate XI-8, describing Table I, Figure 2 of Walter (1783).
12. *anastomosing nerve of sympathetic (Knox, 1832)*
Synonym for *anastomosing branch of great sympathetic (Knox, 1832)*; Plate XI-*146*.
13. *communicating nerve of sympathetic (Knox, 1832)*
Synonym for *anastomosing branch of great sympathetic (Knox, 1832)*; Plate XI-*150*.
14. *intermediate trunk (Arnold, 1834)*
Synonym for macrodissected adult human ***communicating branch of sympathetic trunk (>1840)***; in the original Latin, *truncus intermedius*, p. 18.
15. *cord of communication between ganglia (Quain & Wilson, 1839)*
Synonym for macrodissected adult human ***communicating branch of sympathetic trunk (>1840)***; Plate XXVII-*h**, and similar use elsewhere in Plate.

LATER SYNONYMS:

1. *interganglionic branches of sympathetic trunk (>1840)*
Currently sanctioned synonym for ***communicating branches of sympathetic trunk (>1840)***; see *Terminologia Anatomica* (1998, p. 141).

PARTLY CORRESPONDS:

1. *communicating branches of thoracic ganglia (Cloquet, 1816)*
For macrodissected adult human, ***communicating branches of sympathetic trunk (>1840)*** for ***thoracic sympathetic ganglia (>1840)***; in the original French, *filets de communication des ganglions thoraciques*, p. 701.
2. *communicating branches of lumbar ganglia (Cloquet, 1816)*
For macrodissected adult human, ***communicating branches of sympathetic trunk (>1840)*** for ***lumbar sympathetic ganglia (>1840)***; in the original French, *filets de communication des ganglions lombaires*, p. 710.

communicating loops of cervical plexus (>1840)

As described for macrodissected adult human there are four of them: one rostral (superior), two middle forming the double roots of the ***great auricular nerve (Haase, 1781)*** and ***transverse nerve of neck (>1840)***, and one caudal (inferior) between the 1st and 2nd, 2nd and 3rd, and 3rd and 4th cervical ***spinal nerve ventral branches (>1840)*** respectively; see Hamilton (1976, p. 642 and Fig. 816), Williams & Warwick (1980, p. 1091 for the term itself, and Fig. 7.197). They were described in outline by Galen; see ***[communicating loops of cervical plexus (>1840)] (Galen, c173)***.

EARLIER REFERENCES:

Described, not named or illustrated:

1. ***[communicating loops of cervical plexus (>1840)] (Galen, c173)***
Galen provided general description for macrodissected adult common large mammals but not human explicitly; see May translation (1968, p. 598), Duckworth translation (1962, pp. 230–238).

Illustrated and described, not named:

1. ***[communicating loops of cervical plexus (>1840)] (Vieussens, 1684)***
Accurately described and illustrated at least partly for macrodissected adult human; Table 24.

PARTLY CORRESPONDS:

1. *superior branch of second cervical nerve (Bell & Bell, 1816)*
Synonym for macrodissected adult human *first ansa cervicalis (Bock, 1827)*; Vol. 2, p. 513.
2. *ascending anastomotic nerve of second cervical nerve (Meckel, 1817)*
Macrodissected adult human rostral ***communicating loop of cervical plexus (>1840)*** associated with ***communicating branches of cervical plexus (>1840)*** to ***superior cervical ganglion (Vieussens, 1684)***, ***vagus nerve (Galen, c192)***, and ***hypoglossal nerve (Winslow, 1733)***; see translation (1832, Vol. 3, p. 33) and Durward (1951, Fig. 919). Component of *first cervical nervous plexus (Meckel, 1817)*.
3. *descending anastomotic nerve of second cervical nerve (Meckel, 1817)*
Macrodissected adult human rostral (descending) component of middle ***communicating loop of cervical plexus (>1840)*** generating ***great auricular nerve (Haase,***

1781); see translation (1832, Vol. 3, p. 33) and Williams & Warwick (1980, Fig. 7.197). Component of *second cervical nervous plexus (Meckel, 1817)*.

4. *anastomotic branch between anterior branches of cervical nerve two and cervical nerve three (Langenbeck, 1826–1830)*
   Synonym for macrodissected adult human *second ansa cervicalis (Bock, 1827)*; in the original Latin, *ramus anastomoticus inter ramum anteriorem nervi cervicalis secundi et nervum cervicalem tertium*, Fascicle III, Table XV-*n*.
5. *anastomotic branch between cervical nerves three and four (Langenbeck, 1826–1830)*
   Synonym for macrodissected adult human *third ansa cervicalis (Bock, 1827)*; in the original Latin, *ramus anastomoticus inter nervum cervicalem tertium et quartum*, Fascicle III, Table XV-*s*.
6. *first ansa cervicalis (Bock, 1827)*
   Macrodissected adult human rostral ***communicating loop of cervical plexus (>1840)***; in the original Latin, *ansa cervicalis prima*, Table V, Figure 2-*10*.
7. *second ansa cervicalis (Bock, 1827)*
   Macrodissected adult human middle ***communicating loop of cervical plexus (>1840)***; in the original Latin, *ansa cervicalis secunda*, Table V, Figure 2-*22*.
8. *third ansa cervicalis (Bock, 1827)*
   Macrodissected adult human caudal ***communicating loop of cervical plexus (>1840)***; in the original Latin, *ansa cervicalis tertia*, Table V, Figure 2-*30*.
9. *first anastomotic ansa of cervical nerves (Cloquet, 1828)*
   Synonym for macrodissected adult human *first ansa cervicalis (Bock, 1827)*; in the original French, *première anse anastomotique des nerfs cervicaux*, Plate CLVI, Figure 2-*49*.
10. *second anastomotic ansa of cervical nerves (Cloquet, 1828)*
    Synonym for macrodissected adult human *second ansa cervicalis (Bock, 1827)*; in the original French, *seconde anse anastomotique des nerfs cervicaux*, Plate CLVI, Figure 2-*54*.
11. *anastomosis between first and second cervical nerve (Cloquet, 1828)*
    Synonym for *first anastomotic ansa of cervical nerves (Cloquet, 1828)*; in the original French, *anastomose entre le premier et le second nerf cervical*, Plate CLIX-*89*.
12. *anastomosis of second and third cervical nerves (Cloquet, 1828)*
    Synonym for *second anastomotic ansa of cervical nerves (Cloquet, 1828)*; in the original French, *anastomose des second et troisième nerfs cervicaux*, Plate CLIX-*94*.
13. *anastomosis between third and fourth cervical nerve (Cloquet, 1828)*
    Synonym for macrodissected adult human *third ansa cervicalis (Bock, 1827)*; in the original French, *anastomose entre le troisième et le quatrième nerf cervical*, Plate CLX, Figure 2-*54*.
14. *union of second and third cervical nerves (Swan, 1830)*
    Synonym for macrodissected adult human *second ansa cervicalis (Bock, 1827)*; Plate XVII-*29*.
15. *union of first and second cervical nerves (Swan, 1830)*
    Synonym for macrodissected adult human *first ansa cervicalis (Bock, 1827)*; Plate XVII-*32*.
16. *arched anastomosis between first and second cervical nerves (Knox, 1832)*
    Synonym for macrodissected adult human *first ansa cervicalis (Bock, 1827)*; Plate II-*89*, in Knox's translation of Scarpa (1794).
17. *anastomotic branch of first cervical nerve with second cervical nerve (Arnold, 1834)*
    Macrodissected adult human first cervical ***spinal nerve ventral branch (>1840)*** component of *first ansa cervicalis (Bock, 1827)*; in the original Latin, *ramus anastomoticus nervus cervicalis primus cum nervo cervicali secundo*, pp. 15–16.
18. *ascending anastomotic branchlet of second cervical nerve with first cervical nerve (Arnold, 1834)*
    Macrodissected adult human second cervical ***spinal nerve ventral branch (>1840)*** component of *first ansa cervicalis (Bock, 1827)*; in the original Latin, *ramulus ascendens anastomoticus nervus cervicalis secundus cum nervo cervicali primo*, pp. 15–16.
19. *descending anastomotic branch of second cervical nerve with third cervical nerve (Arnold, 1834)*
    Macrodissected adult human second cervical ***spinal nerve ventral branch (>1840)*** component of *second ansa cervicalis (Bock, 1827)*; in the original Latin, *ramus descendens anastomoticus nervus cervicalis secundus cum nervo cervicali tertio*, pp. 15–16.
20. *ascending anastomotic branch of third cervical nerve (Arnold, 1834)*
    Macrodissected adult human third cervical ***spinal nerve ventral branch (>1840)*** component of *second ansa cervicalis (Bock, 1827)*; in the original Latin, *ramus anastomoticus ascendens nervus cervicalis tertius*, pp. 16–17.
21. *descending anastomotic branch of third cervical nerve (Arnold, 1834)*
    Macrodissected adult human third cervical ***spinal nerve ventral branch (>1840)*** component of *third ansa cervicalis (Bock, 1827)*; in the original Latin, *ramus anastomoticus descendens nervus cervicalis tertius*, pp. 16–17.
22. *ascending branch of fourth cervical nerve (Arnold, 1834)*
    Macrodissected adult human fourth cervical ***spinal nerve ventral branch (>1840)*** component of *third ansa cervicalis (Bock, 1827)*; in the original Latin, *ramus ascendens nervus cervicalis quartus*, p. 17.
23. *connection of third with fourth cervical nerves (Arnold, 1834)*
    Synonym for macrodissected adult human *third ansa cervicalis (Bock, 1827)*; in the original Latin, *conjunctio nervi cervicalis tertii cum quarto*, Table IX-*49*.

compact part of substantia nigra (>1840)

One of two major ***gray matter regions (Swanson & Bota, 2010)*** of mammalian ***substantia nigra (Soemmerring, 1791)***, lying generally dorsomedial to the ***reticular part of substantia nigra (>1840)*** and characterized in adult human by darkly pigmented ***neurons (Waldeyer, 1891)*** that in all mammals utilize dopamine as a neurotransmitter; see Nieuwenhuys et al. (2008, pp. 438–439). It was first illustrated clearly by Vicq d'Azyr; see ***[compact part of substantia nigra (>1840)] (Vicq d'Azyr, 1786)***.

EARLIER REFERENCES:

Illustrated, not named or described:

1. *[compact part of substantia nigra (>1840)] (Vicq d'Azyr, 1786)*
   Clearly illustrated for macrodissected adult human in cross section, where dark rays are shown radiating toward ***cerebral peduncle (Tarin, 1753)***. Vicq d'Azyr did not specifically describe the presence of a ***gray matter region (Swanson & Bota, 2010)*** between the rays, which would have identified unambiguously the ***reticular part of substantia nigra (>1840)***; Plate XXI, Figure 1-41.

coronary plexuses (Meckel, 1817)

As described for macrodissected adult human, there is a smaller ***right coronary plexus (Scarpa, 1794)*** and larger ***left coronary plexus (Scarpa, 1794)***; each is derived from the ***cardiac plexus (Keill, 1698)***, accompanies the corresponding coronary artery, and supplies the corresponding atrium and ventricle; see Williams & Warwick (1980, p. 1132). For Meckel's use in macrodissected adult human see translation (1832, Vol. 3, p. 96). They were noted by Willis; see ***[coronary plexuses (Meckel, 1817)] (Willis, 1664)***.

TRANSLATIONS:

1. *plexus coronarii (Meckel, 1817)*
   Original Latin form of ***coronary plexuses (Meckel, 1817)***; see translation (1832, Vol. 3, p. 96).

EARLIER REFERENCES:

Described, not named or illustrated:

1. ***[coronary plexuses (Meckel, 1817)] (Willis, 1664)***
   Willis described ***nerves (Herophilus, c335–c280 BC)*** to macrodissected adult human vessels of the heart; see Pordage translation (1681, p. 147).

Earlier synonyms:

1. *great double plexus of arteries of heart (Andersch, 1797)*
   Synonym for macrodissected adult human ***coronary plexuses (Meckel, 1817)***; in the original Latin, *plexum duarum magnarum arteriarum cordis*, Vol. 2, p. 44.
2. *nerve layers of septum of heart (Andersch, 1797)*
   Overview of Andersch's very detailed description of *great double plexus of arteries of heart (Andersch, 1797)*, the ***coronary plexuses (Meckel, 1817)***; in the original Latin, *strata nervosa septi cordis*, Vol. 2, p. 44. He described superficial, middle, and deep ***nerves (Herophilus, c335–c280 BC)*** associated with these layers.

PARTLY CORRESPONDS:

1. *middle nerve of nerve layers of septum of heart (Andersch, 1797)*
   One of three components of *nerve layers of septum of heart (Andersch, 1797)*; in the original Latin, *nervum medii strati nervorum septi cordis*, Vol. 2, pp. 48, 51.
2. *superficial nerve of nerve layers of septum of heart (Andersch, 1797)*
   One of three components of *nerve layers of septum of heart (Andersch, 1797)*; in the original Latin, *nervum superficialis strati nervorum septi cordis*, Vol. 2, pp. 48, 59–60.
3. *deep nerve of nerve layers of septum of heart (Andersch, 1797)*
   One of three components of *nerve layers of septum of heart (Andersch, 1797)*; in the original Latin, *nervus profundus strati nervorum septi cordis*, Vol. 2, pp. 52–53.
4. *superficial nerve of posterior ventricle of heart (Andersch, 1797)*
   Branch of *highest trunk of nerves of superficial layer of septum of heart (Andersch, 1797)* going to left ventricle; in the original Latin, *nervus superficialis ventriculi posterioris cordis*, Vol. 2, pp. 54, 60.
5. *highest trunk of nerves of superficial layer of septum of heart (Andersch, 1797)*
   One of three main branches of *superficial nerve of nerve layers of septum of heart (Andersch, 1797)*; in the original Latin, *truncus supremus nervi strati superficialis septi cordis*, Vol. 2, p. 60.
6. *middle trunk of superficial nerve of nerve layers of septum of heart (Andersch, 1797)*
   One of three main branches of *superficial nerve of nerve layers of septum of heart (Andersch, 1797)*; in the original Latin, *truncus medius*, Vol. 2, p. 60.
7. *lowest trunk of superficial nerve of nerve layers of septum of heart (Andersch, 1797)*
   One of three main branches of *superficial nerve of nerve layers of septum of heart (Andersch, 1797)*; in the original Latin, *truncus infimus*, Vol. 2, p. 60.
8. *lowest nerve of posterior ventricle of heart (Andersch, 1797)*
   Branch to macrodissected adult human left ventricle of *deep nerve of nerve layers of septum of heart (Andersch, 1797)*; in the original Latin, *nervus infimus ventriculi posterioris cordis*, Vol. 2, p. 67.
9. *superior circumflex nerves of arteries of heart (Andersch, 1797)*
   Components of macrodissected adult human ***coronary plexuses (Meckel, 1817)***; in the original Latin, *nervi circumflexi superioris arteriae septi cordis*, Vol. 2, p. 68.
10. *inferior circumflex nerve of arteries of heart (Andersch, 1797)*
    Components of macrodissected adult human ***coronary plexuses (Meckel, 1817)***; in the original Latin, *nervum circumflexum inferiorem arteriae septi cordis*, Vol. 2, p. 69.
11. *coronary nerve of posterior ventricle (Andersch, 1797)*
    Branch of *deep nerve of nerve layers of septum of heart (Andersch, 1797)* apparently related to left coronary artery and left ventricle; in the original Latin, *nervus coronarius ventriculi posterioris*, Vol. 2, p. 73.
12. *nerve between right auricle and ventricle of heart (Andersch, 1797)*
    Apparently, component of macrodissected adult human ***coronary plexuses (Meckel, 1817)*** associated with *superficial nerve of heart (Andersch, 1797)*; in the original

Latin, *nervum intermedium auriculae et ventriculi dextri cordis*, Vol. 2, p. 109.

corpus callosum (Galen, c177)

As described for adult human, the division of the ***cerebral cortex white matter (>1840)*** near the median plane, dorsal to the right and left ***anterior horn of lateral ventricle (Bell, 1803b)*** and ***body of lateral ventricle (Bell, 1803b)***, consisting predominantly of commissural (between right and left sides) ***axons (Kölliker, 1896)***, or *commissural fibers of cerebral cortex* to complement ***association fibers of cerebral cortex (>1840)*** that remain on the right or left side. It is subdivided for topographic description into four somewhat arbitrarily defined parts, from rostral to caudal: the ***rostrum of corpus callosum (Reil, 1809b), genu of corpus callosum (Reil, 1809b), body of corpus callosum (Arnold, 1838a)***, and ***splenium of corpus callosum (Burdach, 1822)***; see Cloquet (1828, Pl. CXXXVI), Mettler (1948, p. 100, Fig. 68). The ***corpus callosum (Galen, c177)*** is found in all mammals except monotremes and marsupials; see Nieuwenhuys et al. (2008, p. 596). Galen alluded to the longitudinal "callus-like body" in the median plane of the *cerebrum (Aristotle)* just superficial to the *fornix (Galen, c177)* and overlying the ***anterior horn of lateral ventricle (Bell, 1803b)*** and ***body of lateral ventricle (Bell, 1803b)***; see Singer translation (1999, p. 231). Clarke & O'Malley (1996, p. 577) suggested that Galen might also have included more lateral parts of the ***cerebral cortex white matter (>1840)*** in his understanding of ***corpus callosum (Galen, c177)***, but the factual basis of this conjecture is unclear. Vesalius clearly illustrated the ***corpus callosum (Galen, c177)*** and, although more lateral ***cerebral cortex white matter (>1840)*** was also clearly illustrated, it was not named; see Singer translation (1952, pp. 30–31). Jacques Dubois (Sylvius), the famous teacher of Vesalius, has been credited (Singer, 1957, p. 109) with introducing the exact Latin term *corpus callosum*, as has Vesalius himself (Burdach 1822, p. 363)—Galen wrote in Greek. According to Ridley (1695, p. 115), "The middle and uppermost part of this [cerebral] Medullary Substance, by the Ancients [was] always called Corpus Callosum". Winslow (1733) essentially defined the modern view of the ***corpus callosum (Galen, c177)*** as a region of the ***cerebral cortex white matter (>1840)*** near the median plane: "if we separate gently the two lateral Parts or Hemispheres of the Cerebrum, we see a longitudinal Portion of a white convex Body, which is named Corpus Callosum. It is a middle Portion of the medullary Substance, which under the inferior Sinus of the Falx, and also a little toward each side, is parted from the Mass of the Cerebrum... Both Extremities of this medullary Body terminate by a small Edge bent transversely downward [the ***genu of corpus callosum (Reil, 1809b)*** and ***splenium of corpus callosum (Burdach, 1822)***]... The Corpus Callosum becomes afterwards continuous on each side, with the medullary Substance, which through all the remaining part of its extent, is intirely united with the cortical Substance, and together with the Corpus Callosum forms a medullary Arch or Vault of an oblong or oval Figure. To perceive this, the whole cortical Substance, together with the medullary Laminae [***cerebral cortex white matter (>1840)*** within *gyri (Vesalius, 1543a), medullary rays (Vieussens, 1684)*] mixed with it, must be cautiously and dexterously cut off in the same Direction with the Convexity of the Cerebrum. After which we will observe a medullary Convexity much smaller than that which is common to the whole Cerebrum, but of the same form; so that it appears like a medullary Nucleus of the Cerebrum, especially when we consider it together with the medullary Substance of the inferior Part or Basis of the Cerebrum. And from thence *M. Vieussens* took occasion to name this Nucleus the Centrum Ovale." (Sect. X, p. 34). And, the ***fornix (Vesalius, 1543a)*** " is in reality nothing but the Corpus Callosum, the lower side of which is like a hollow Cieling with three Angles, one anterior and two posterior..." (Sect. X, p. 35). Reil was more precise in distinguishing it from the ***external capsule (Burdach, 1822)*** [see *outer wall of capsule (Reil, 1809b)*], which, he observed, converges with the ***internal capsule (Burdach, 1822)*** dorsally in a rather amorphous region [the *semilunar border (Reil, 1811c)*] just lateral to the roof of the ***lateral ventricle (Vesalius, 1543a)***; 1809b, see Mayo translation (1823, pp. 69–70). In light of this, Reil suggested for practical purposes that the ***corpus callosum (Galen, c177)*** proper extends from the median plane roughly as far laterally as it is covered by the *long convolution (Reil, 1809b)* or ***cingulate region (Brodmann, 1909)***; 1812c, see Mayo translation (1823, p. 121).

TRANSLATIONS:

1. *brawny body (Geminus, 1553)*
   Synonym for macrodissected adult human ***corpus callosum (Galen, c177)***; originally spelled *brawnye bodye*, see *The tables of the brayne*, Figure 3, where Geminus also seemed to call it the *wectye* or *wectie body*.
2. *hard body (Geminus, 1553)*
   Synonym for *brawny body (Geminus, 1554)*; originally spelled *harde bodye*, see *The tables of the brayne*, Figure 4.
3. *callous body (Haller, 1754b)*
   English form of macrodissected adult human ***corpus callosum (Galen, c177)***; p. 289.

LATER SYNONYMS:

1. *copula alba cerebri (Varoli, 1573)*
   Synonym for macrodissected adult human ***corpus callosum (Galen, c177)***; see Burdach (1822, p. 363). Arnold (1838a, p. 75) gave *copula cerebri alba*.
2. *corpus callosum medium (Haller, 1747)*
   Synonym for macrodissected adult human ***corpus callosum (Galen, c177)***; see Mihles translation (1754b, p. 291).
3. *mesolobe (Burdin, 1803)*
   Synonym for macrodissected adult human ***corpus callosum (Galen, c177)***, credited to Chaussier (unpublished by 1803); see translation (1803, Vol. 1, p. 156). Burdach (1822, p. 364) gave the Latin, *mesolobium*.

4. *great commissure (Bell & Bell, 1823)*
 Synonym for macrodissected adult human ***corpus callosum (Galen, c177)***; Vol. 2, pp. 370, 404.
5. *great superior commissure of cerebral hemispheres (Grant, 1834c)*
 Synonym for macrodissected adult human ***corpus callosum (Galen, c177)***; p. 552.
6. *commissure of hemispheres (Owen, 1837)*
 Synonym for macrodissected adult mammalian ***corpus callosum (Galen, c177)***; p. 95.
7. *superior cerebral commissure (Gerdy, 1838)*
 Synonym for macrodissected adult human ***corpus callosum (Galen, c177)***; in the original French, *commissure cérébrale supérieure*, p. 258.
8. *cerebral ceiling (Gerdy, 1838)*
 Synonym for macrodissected adult human ***corpus callosum (Galen, c177)***; in the original French, *plafond du cerveau*, pp. 258, 259.
9. *great cerebral commissure (Arnold, 1838a)*
 Synonym for macrodissected adult human ***corpus callosum (Galen, c177)***; in the original Latin, *commissura cerebri maxima*, p. 75.

PARTLY CORRESPONDS:

1. *striae medullares pectiniformes (Lancisi, 1718)*
 Synonym for macrodissected adult human *superior raphe of corpus callosum (Reil, 1809b)*, which Lancisi described and illustrated clearly; p. 316.
2. *raphe of corpus callosum (Winslow, 1733)*
 Synonym for macrodissected adult human *superior raphe of corpus callosum (Reil, 1809b)*. "This Raphe is made more perceivable by two small medullary Cords [***longitudinal striae (>1840)***] which accompany it on each side, and adhere closely to the transverse Fibres." (Sect. X, p. 34).
3. *striae transversa corporis callosi in medio decussatae (Tarin, 1753)*
 Crossing fibers of macrodissected adult human ***corpus callosum (Galen, c177)*** forming its substance; p. 23.
4. *transverse striae of Willis (Günther, 1786)*
 Eponym for macrodissected adult human *striae transversa corporis callosi in medio decussatae (Tarin, 1753)*; in the original Latin, *strias transversales Willisii*, p. 9.
5. *median line of mesolobe (Chaussier, 1807)*
 Synonym for macrodissected adult human *raphe of corpus callosum (Winslow, 1733)*; in the original French, *ligne médiane du mésolobe*, p. 47.
6. *superior raphe of corpus callosum (Reil, 1809b)*
 Refers to median depression on dorsal surface of macrodissected adult human ***corpus callosum (Galen, c177)***, between right and left sets of ***longitudinal striae (>1840)***; see Mayo translation (1823, p. 66), and Dejerine & Dejerine-Klumpke (1895, Fig. 199).
7. *inferior raphe of corpus callosum (Reil, 1809b)*
 Refers to median depression on ventral surface of macrodissected adult human ***corpus callosum (Galen, c177)***, with dorsal end of right and left *septum lucidum (Galen, c177)* attached on either side and extending to ***splenium of corpus callosum (Burdach, 1822)***; see Mayo translation (1823, p. 66). First clearly illustrated by Willis (1664, Fig. VII-*K*).
8. *raphe externa (Reil, 1809b)*
 Original form of *superior raphe of corpus callosum (Reil, 1809b)*; p. 172.
9. *raphe interna (Reil, 1809b)*
 Original form of *inferior raphe of corpus callosum (Reil, 1809b)*; p. 172.
10. *forceps of corpus callosum (Reil, 1809b)*
 Corresponds to macrodissected adult human ***frontal forceps (>1840)*** and ***occipital forceps (>1840)*** as a pair; see Mayo translation (1823, pp. 68–69), based on the German form *Zangen* (see Meyer, 1971, p. 29). Burdach (1822, p. 148) supplied the Latin form, *forcipes*, and Arnold (1838a, p. 77) used the Latin form, *forceps*.
11. *external suture of corpus callosum (Meckel, 1817)*
 Synonym for macrodissected adult human *raphe of corpus callosum (Winslow, 1733)*; see translation (1832, Vol. 2, p. 448).

cortical amygdalar area (>1840)

As defined with cellular architecture and connections in mammal, the main component of the ***cortical amygdalar complex >1840)***. For its recent use in adult rat, see Swanson (2004, Tab. B, p. 168); also see Canteras et al. (1992). Price (1973, pp. 94–95, Fig. 5) emphasized its inclusion within the ***cerebral cortex gray matter (>1840)***; for comparison see *cortical amygdalar nucleus (Johnston, 1923)*. It was not identified by 1840.

EARLIER REFERENCES:

Earlier synonyms:

1. *cortical amygdalar nucleus (Johnston, 1923)*
 Synonym for amniote ***cortical amygdalar area (Swanson, 2004)*** based on phylogeny and histology; see pp. 339, 410, 456, where it was spelled *cortical amygdaloid nucleus*; current spelling was introduced by Swanson & Petrovich (1998, p. 326).

cortical amygdalar complex (>1840)

As described with cellular architecture and connections in mammal, the caudal component of the ***olfactory region (>1840)*** between ***piriform area (Smith, 1919)*** rostrally and ***entorhinal area (Brodmann, 1909)*** caudally. In the rat, where it has been analyzed most carefully, it consists of the ***cortical amygdalar area (>1840)***, and several "periamygdalar areas" (see Krettek & Price, 1978, pp. 265–266) including ***postpiriform transition area (Canteras et al., 1992)***, ***piriform-amygdalar area (Canteras et al., 1992)***, and ***nucleus of lateral olfactory tract (>1840)***; see Canteras et al. (1992), Swanson (2004, Tab. B). In macrodissected adult human and some other primates, it corresponds to the ***semilunar gyrus (>1840)***; see Nauta & Haymaker (1969, pp. 151, 156). It was not identified by 1840.

cortical plate (>1840)

As described histologically with cellular architecture during mammalian development, the entire breadth of *cerebral cortex gray matter (>1840)* displays a layer, the *cortical plate (>1840)*, that may (isocortex) or may not (allocortex) be fitted into a basic six-layered scheme (Vogt & Vogt, 1919) numbered 1–6 from superficial to deep. The *olfactory region (>1840)* and *hippocampal formation (Swanson & Cowan, 1977)* are allocortex and the rest is isocortex, according to the scheme presented here; see Swanson (2004, Tab. A, note 4). Thus, the term *cortical plate (>1840)* has a specific histological meaning in development as well as in the adult, where it refers to the classic six layers of isocortex and three layers of allocortex; for this use in adult mammal, see Swanson (2000, p. 129). Contrast with *cortical subplate (>1840)* that, where present, lies deep to the *cortical plate (>1840)*. In macrodissected adult human, the major components of the *cortical plate (>1840)* and *cortical subplate (>1840)* are easily distinguished; see Nieuwenhuys et al. (2008, Fig. 5.6). It was first delineated by Burdach; see *[cortical plate (>1840)] (Burdach, 1822)*.

EARLIER REFERENCES:

Described, not named or illustrated:

1. *[cortical plate (>1840)] (Burdach, 1822)*
   Burdach described and illustrated the main features and topographic relationships of *cortical plate (Burdach, 1922)* and *cortical subplate (>1840)* in macrodissected adult human; see Table III-δ.

cortical subplate (>1840)

Based on cellular architecture in mammal, a layer of *cerebral cortex gray matter (>1840)* deep to most but not all of the *cortical plate (>1840)*, with some *neurons (Waldeyer, 1891)* scattered into the subjacent *cerebral cortex white matter (>1840)*. The most obvious components include, from ventral to dorsal, the *basolateral amygdalar complex (>1840), endopiriform nucleus (>1840)* deep to the *piriform area (>1840), claustrum (Burdach, 1822), and isocortex layer 6b (>1840)*; see Swanson (2000, p. 130), Swanson (2004, Tabs. A note 5, B), Torres-Reveron & Friedlander (2007), Judas et al. (2010). The *claustrum (Burdach, 1840)* and *basolateral amygdalar complex (>1840)* are easily observed in macrodissected adult human; see Nieuwenhuys et al. (2008, Fig. 5.6). It was first broadly delineated by Burdach; see *[cortical subplate (>1840)] (Burdach, 1822)*.

EARLIER REFERENCES:

Described, not named or illustrated:

1. *[cortical subplate (>1840)] (Burdach, 1822)*
   Burdach described and illustrated essential continuity between two largest components in macrodissected adult human, *claustrum (Burdach, 1822)* and *amygdalar nucleus (Burdach, 1822)*; pp. 132, 173, Table III-δ.

LATER SYNONYMS:

1. *claustral complex (Swanson, 2000a)*
   Synonym for adult mammalian *cortical subplate (>1840)*; p. 130.

corticospinal tract (>1840)

As described for adult human and other mammals with macrodissection and histological methods for *axon (Kölliker, 1896)* pathway tracing, a longitudinal *central nervous system white matter tract (>1840)* arising in the *cerebral cortex (>1840)* and ending in the *spinal cord (Galen, c162–c166)*, with a major branch to the *pontine nuclei (Jacobsohn, 1909)*, the *corticopontine fibers (>1840)*, and smaller branches to other parts of the *midbrain (Baer, 1837), pons (Haller, 1747)*, and *medulla (Winslow, 1733)*. It is first distinguished rostrally in medial and lateral (but not intermediate) parts of the *anterior limb of internal capsule (>1840)*, and then in roughly the lateral half of the *posterior limb of internal capsule (>1840)*; see Williams & Warwick (1980, Fig. 7.154). For ease of topographic description, two segments are recognized in these parts of the *internal capsule (Burdach, 1822)*—the *cerebral nuclei corticospinal tract (>1840)* and *interbrain corticospinal tract (>1840)*, respectively. The *corticospinal tract (>1840)* continues in the *midbrain (Baer, 1837)* as the *cerebral peduncle (Tarin, 1753)* and then as the *longitudinal pontine fibers (Arnold, 1838b)*, after giving off the *corticopontine fibers (>1840)*; see Carpenter (1976, Figs. 12.18, 12.23, and 13.1 with *crus cerebri* for *cerebral peduncle*). In the *medulla (Winslow, 1733)* it forms the *pyramid (Willis, 1664)*, which then forms the *pyramidal decussation (Reil, 1809c)* in the junctional region with the *spinal cord (Galen, c162–c166)*. In the *spinal cord (Galen, c162–c166)*, most *axons (Kölliker, 1896)* of the *corticospinal tract (>1840)* form the *crossed corticospinal tract (>1840)*, whereas a small minority continue on the same side as the *uncrossed corticospinal tract (>1840)*. The *spinothalamic tract (>1840)* is a topographically separate, rostrally directed, longitudinal *central nervous system white matter tract (>1840)* originating in the *spinal cord (Galen, c162–c166)* and extending all the way to the *cerebral cortex (>1840)* as the *spinocortical tract (>1840)*. The *corticospinal tract (>1840)* was first clearly identified by Malpighi; see *[corticospinal tract (>1840)] (Malpighi, 1666)*.

EARLIER REFERENCES:

Described, not named or illustrated:

1. *[corticospinal tract (>1840)] (Malpighi, 1666)*
   Malpighi clearly described the origin of "nerve fibers" in the *cerebral cortex (>1840)* coursing through the *cerebral nuclei (Swanson, 2000a)* and ending in the *spinal cord (Galen, c162–c166)*; see Meyer (1967, p. 189). He dissected a variety of mammals, including human, but the source of this observation is unclear. Willis (1664) thought these fibers arise in the *striated body (Willis, 1664)*, or *cerebral nuclei (Swanson, 2000a)*, not the *cerebral cortex (>1840)*; see Pordage translation (1681, pp. 62, 102).

Illustrated and described, not named:

1. *[corticospinal tract (>1840)] (Vieussens, 1684)*
   Clearly illustrated and described for macrodissected adult human with a scraping method; see Table XVI.

Earlier synonyms:

1. *anterior column descending from hemisphere (Bell, 1834)*
   Corresponds roughly to macrodissected adult human ***corticospinal tract (>1840)***; pp. 473–475. It was one of three great longitudinal columns Bell distinguished in ***central nervous system (Carus, 1814)***; also see *posterior column descending from hemisphere (Bell, 1834), tract of corpus olivare (Bell, 1834).*
2. *motor tract (Bell, 1834)*
   Synonym for *anterior column descending from hemisphere (Bell, 1834)*; p. 475.

cranial nerve ganglia (>1840)

As described for macrodissected adult vertebrate, sensory ***ganglia (Galen, c173)*** associated with ***cranial nerves (Soemmerring, 1791)*** contrasted with ***autonomic ganglia (Langley, 1900)*** associated with ***cranial nerves (Soemmerring, 1791)***. The first example discovered was *olive body (Falloppio, 1561)* or ***distal vagal ganglion (>1840)***.

EARLIER REFERENCES:

Earlier synonyms:

1. *cerebral system ganglia (Wutzer, 1817)*
   Roughly synonymous with macrodissected adult human ***cranial nerve ganglia (>1840)***; in the original Latin, *ganglia systematis cerebralis*, p. 52.

PARTLY CORRESPONDS:

1. *barley-shaped ganglioform enlargement of accessory nerve (Cruveilhier, 1836)*
   Term attributed without citation to Huber, related to macrodissected adult human ***cranial nerve ganglion (>1840)*** associated with ***accessory nerve (Vieussens, 1684)***; in the original Latin, *in ganglion vix hordeaceum intumescit nervus accessorius.*

cranial nerves (Soemmerring, 1791)

The rostral topographic division of the ***craniospinal nerves (Herrick, 1915)***, the caudal division being the ***spinal nerves (Camper, 1760–1762)***. The 12 ***cranial nerves (Soemmerring, 1791)*** exit the *cranium* (see *Dorland's*, 2003, p. 432) and traditionally are enumerated from rostral to caudal, followed by the ***spinal nerves (Camper, 1760–1762)***, also enumerated from rostral to caudal. Following today's terminology, the first (I) ***cranial nerve (Soemmerring, 1791)*** is the ***olfactory nerve (Winslow, 1733)***, the second (II) is the ***optic nerve (Vicq d'Azyr, 1786)***, the third (III) is the ***oculomotor nerve (Estienne, 1545)***, the fourth (IV) is the ***trochlear nerve (Molinetti, 1669)***, the fifth (V) is the ***trigeminal nerve (Winslow, 1733)***, the sixth (VI) is the ***abducens nerve (Heister, 1717)***, the seventh (VII) is the ***intermediofacial nerve (Strong & Elwyn, 1943)***, the eighth (VIII) is the ***vestibulocochlear nerve (>1840)***, the ninth is the ***glossopharyngeal nerve (Huber, 1744)***, the tenth (X) is the ***vagus nerve (Galen, c192)***, the eleventh (XI) is the ***accessory nerve (Vieussens, 1684)***, and the twelfth (XII) is the ***hypoglossal nerve (Winslow, 1733)***. This account does not formally account for the ***terminal nerve (>1840)*** and ***vomeronasal nerve (>1840)***, which are often described with the ***olfactory nerve (Winslow, 1733)***. For Soemmerring's account of the 12 ***cranial nerve (Soemmerring, 1791)*** pairs in macrodissected adult human, see sections 128, 203–272; also see Soemmerring (1798, p. 125). At least a third of the ***cranial nerves (Soemmerring, 1791)*** were postulated by Alcmaeon, and most of them were discovered by Herophilus; see ***[cranial nerves (Soemmerring, 1791)] (Alcmaeon, c490–c430 BC), [cranial nerves (Soemmerring, 1791)] (Herophilus, c335–c280 BC)***, and *ducts (Aristotle)*.

TRANSLATIONS:

1. *Schedelnerven (Soemmerring, 1791)*
   Original German form of ***cranial nerves (Soemmerring, 1791)***; pp. 103, 106. Currently it is usually spelled *Schädelnerven*.

EARLIER REFERENCES:

Described, not named or illustrated:

1. ***[cranial nerves (Soemmerring, 1791)] (Alcmaeon, c490–c430 BC)***
   In *De Sensu*, Aristotle's successor Theophrastus (c327–c287 BC), clearly stated that Alcmaeon postulated the existence of channels (alternate translations: *passages, ducts*) between most sense organs of the head (eyes, ears, nostrils, and probably tongue) and the ***brain (Smith Papyrus, c1700 BC)***. It has been claimed that Alcmaeon discovered the *optic nerve (Galen, c173)* by dissection, but this is far from certain. It can be said, however, that at least he postulated the existence of ***olfactory nerve (Winslow, 1733), optic nerve (Vicq d'Azyr, 1786), vestibulocochlear nerve (>1840)***, and ***hypoglossal nerve (Winslow, 1733)***; see Solmsen (1961, pp. 151–152), Lloyd (1975).
2. ***[cranial nerves (Soemmerring, 1791)] Anaxagoras of Athens, c488–c428 BC)***
   Anaxagoras may have asserted that ***brain (Smith Papyrus, c1700 BC)*** generates ***nerves (Herophilus, c335–c280 BC)***; see Rasmussen (1947, p. 1), von Staden (1989, p. 155).
3. ***[cranial nerves (Soemmerring, 1791)] (Herophilus, c335–c280 BC)***
   Herophilus, the founder of human anatomy, is credited with discovering ***nerves (Herophilus, c335–c280 BC)***, including most of the ***cranial nerves (Soemmerring, 1791)*** and ***spinal nerves (Camper, 1760–1762)*** in macrodissected adult human; see Solmsen (1961), von Staden (1989), Longrigg (1993), Clarke & O'Malley (1996, p. 261). He recognized *optic nerve (Galen, c173)*, ***oculomotor nerve (Estienne, 1545), trigeminal nerve sensory root (>1840), trigeminal nerve motor root (>1840)***, *facial nerve (Vicq d'Azyr, 1784)*, ***vestibulocochlear nerve (>1840), hypoglossal nerve (Winslow, 1733)***— and probably ***glossopharyngeal nerve (Huber, 1744), vagus nerve (Galen, c192)***, and ***accessory nerve (Vieussens, 1684)***, all three referred to together as *sixth pair of nerves from brain (Galen,*

c192); see von Staden 1989 (pp. 159–161). Herophilus macrodissected adult animals and human cadavers.

LATER SYNONYMS:

1. *cerebral nerves (Soemmerring, 1791)*
Synonym for macrodissected adult human ***cranial nerves (Soemmerring, 1791)***; in the original German, *Hirnnerven* (p. 103), in the original Latin, *nervorum cerebri* (Soemmerring, 1798, p. 125).
2. *cerebrine nerves (Hooper, 1797)*
Synonym for macrodissected adult human ***cranial nerves (Soemmerring, 1791)***; p. 93.
3. *cerebral nerves (Carus, 1814)*
Carus recognized for macrodissected adult human the 12 ***cranial nerves (Soemmerring, 1791)*** but grouped them idiosyncratically—Group I: olfactory nerve (I); Group II: visual nerves (II, III, IV, VI); Group III: auditory nerves (VIII, VII); Group IV: anterior intervertebral nerves of head (V, IX, XII); and Group V: posterior intervertebral nerves of head (X, XI); in the original German, *Hirnnerven*, see Table on p. 276.

PARTLY CORRESPONDS:

1. *ducts (Aristotle)*
In *The Account of Animals*, Aristotle apparently referred to perhaps three ***cranial nerves (Soemmerring, 1791)*** associated with the eye as *ducts* (in Greek, *poroi*; alternate translations: *passages, channels*); this was almost certainly based on observations in macrodissected adult mammal; see Lloyd (1975), von Staden (1989, p. 157). This conclusion is strengthened by his description in *On the Generation of Animals* of animal eye development, which may represent the first definite identification of a ***nerve (Herophilus, c335–c280 BC)***—the *optic nerve (Galen, c173)*—although Aristotle did not recognize it as a ***nerve (Herophilus, c335–c280 BC)*** proper, probably because of theoretical preconceptions related to his cardiocentric theory of body control; Platt (1958, pp.743–744), Solmsen (1961, pp. 169 ff., 193–194).
2. *[pairs of nerves from skull (Galen, c192)] (Marinus of Pergamum, fl. c50)*
Although this great anatomist's books have not survived, Galen fully acknowledged using his classification of seven *pairs of nerves from skull (Galen, c192)*; see May translation (1968, pp. 31–32, 438).
3. *outgrowths of brain (Galen, c173)*
Synonym for *pairs of nerves from skull (Galen, c192)*; see May translation (1968, pp. 438, 444).
4. *pairs of nerves from brain (Galen, c192)*
Synonym for *pairs of nerves from skull (Galen, c192)*. Goss (1966) translated it simply as *pairs of nerves from brain (Galen, c192)*, whereas Duckworth (1962, pp. 10, 181–222) translated it *pairs of nerves arising from brain*; also see May translation (1968, pp. 31–32, 438–454).
5. *pairs of nerves from skull (Galen, c192)*
Galen freely acknowledged using the classification scheme of Marinus, with seven *[pairs of nerves from skull (Galen, c192)] (Marinus of Pergamum, fl. c50)*; see Duckworth translation (1962, pp. 181–222), where *pairs of nerves springing from skull* was used. Galen's scheme remained in wide use until Willis introduced a new system of ten *pairs of nerves arising within skull (Willis, 1664)* and Soemmerring introduced his classification of *nervorum per ossa capitis egredientium (Soemmerring, 1778)*, still used today with some modification as the 12 pairs of ***cranial nerves (Soemmerring, 1791)***. Galen's account is thus: first pair, *optic nerve (Galen, c173)*, which includes the ***optic nerve (Vicq d'Azyr, 1786), optic chiasm (Galen, c173)***, and ***optic tract (Vicq d'Azyr 1784)*** considered together; second pair, probably just the ***oculomotor nerve (Estienne, 1545)***; third and fourth pairs, roughly the ***trigeminal nerve sensory root (>1840)*** and ***trigeminal nerve motor root (Bell, 1829)***, respectively; fifth pair, the ***intermediofacial nerve (Strong & Elwyn, 1943)*** and ***vestibulocochlear nerve (>1840)***, considered together; sixth pair, the ***glossopharyngeal nerve (Huber, 1744), vagus nerve (Galen, c192)***, and ***accessory nerve (Vieussens, 1684)*** considered together; and seventh pair, the ***hypoglossal nerve (Winslow, 1733)***; see Savage-Smith (1971). Thus, by Galen's time all of the traditional ***cranial nerves (Soemmerring, 1791)*** but the ***olfactory nerve (Winslow, 1733), trochlear nerve (Molinetti, 1669), abducens nerve (Heister, 1717)***, and ***intermediate nerve (>1840)*** had been clearly differentiated and identified. Galen also acknowledged that other anatomists begin an account of the *pairs of nerves from skull (Galen, c192)* with the *olfactory sense instrument (Galen, c173)* rather than *optic nerve (Galen, c173)*, "Whoever desires to enumerate simply the processes arising from the brain will say that the first pair of nerves springing from the brain goes to the two nasal cavities, and its course travels along the middle region of the skull. The second pair is that of the optic nerves, and in their course its two components travel one on each side of the nerves of the first pair. The third pair is that of the nerves which move the eyes. Nevertheless anyone who does not wish to reckon simply the processes, but the nervous processes and their points of origin, will count the optic nerves as the first pair, and as the second pair, that of the nerves moving the eye. For as we explained previously in our description of the eye, the eye is moved by means of the pair of the 'hard' nerves, but the things which it perceives with its gaze it apprehends by means of the pair of 'soft' nerves..." (Duckworth translation, 1962, p. 188). This clearly distinguishes between a sensory and a motor ***nerve (Herophilus, c335–c280 BC)*** that are functionally related. Also see *pairs of nerves from brain (Theophilos Protospatharios, fl. 610–641)*.
6. *conjugations of nerves from brain (Galen, c192)*
The Latin term *conjugatio* (archaic spelling: *coniugatio*) is traditionally used as a translation from the Greek of *pairs of nerves from brain (Galen, c192)*; see Galen (1528, Index, under *nervorum coni[j]ugationes*) and Foster (1892, p. 1121).
7. *conjugatio (Galen, c192)*
Shortened form of *conjugations of nerves from brain (Galen, c192)*.

8. *coniugatio (Galen, c192)*
Archaic spelling of *conjugatio (Galen, c192)*; see Benedetti (1502; Lind translation, 1975, p. 118) and Estienne (1545, p. 248).
9. *fifth pair of nerves from brain (Galen, c192)*
Included ***intermediofacial nerve (Strong & Elwyn, 1943)*** and ***vestibulocochlear nerve (>1840)*** considered together, for macrodissected adult beef, pig, and/or macaque but not human; see May translation (1968, p. 445), Savage-Smith (1971, p. 181 ff.), *pairs of nerves from brain (Galen, c192)*.
10. *sixth pair of nerves from brain (Galen, c192)*
Included three distinct components: ***glossopharyngeal nerve (Huber, 1744), vagus nerve (Galen, c192)***, and ***accessory nerve (Vieussens, 1684)***; see Duckworth translation (1962, pp. 197 ff.); also see May translation (1968, pp. 445 ff.), Savage-Smith (1971, pp. 183 ff.), and *pairs of nerves from brain (Galen, c192)*. In some of his writings Galen described ***sympathetic trunk (Winslow, 1733)*** as arising from, and thus being component of, *sixth pair of nerves from brain (Galen, c192)*; see *nerve extending along roots of ribs (Galen, c173)*. Galen dissected a variety of mammals, but not human cadavers explicitly.
11. *roots of sixth pair of nerves from brain (Galen, c192)*
Galen wrote that "In regard to the sixth pair of nerves, neither of its two units [right and left] consists of a single nerve springing from either side of the brain, but each of the two consists of three nerves which come off from three roots," thus alluding to ***glossopharyngeal nerve root (>1840), vagus nerve root (>1840)***, and ***cranial root of accessory nerve (>1840)***. He macrodissected adult beef, pig, and macaque but not human; see Duckworth translation (1962, pp. 197–198), May (1968, p. 445 note *41*).
12. *sixth pair of nerves from brain (Theophilos Protospatharios, fl. 610–641)*
Synonym for *fifth pair of nerves from brain (Galen, c192)*; see *pairs of nerves from brain (Theophilos Protospatharios, fl. 610–641)*.
13. *seventh pair of nerves from brain (Theophilos Protospatharios, fl. 610–641)*
Synonym for *sixth pair of nerves from brain (Galen, c192)*. Benedetti (1502) used essentially the same nomenclature as Theophilos; see Lind translation (1975, p. 117). Also see *pairs of nerves from brain (Theophilos Protospatharios, fl. 610–641)*.
14. *nerve outgrowths from skull (Vesalius, 1543a)*
Synonym for seven macrodissected adult human *pairs of nerves from skull (Galen, c192)*; see Richardson & Carman translation (2002, p. 176).
15. *cerebral nerves (Vesalius, 1543a)*
Synonym for seven macrodissected adult human *pairs of nerves from skull (Galen, c192)*, although Vesalius's description is considerably clearer than Galen's, especially for his third and fourth pairs, corresponding to ***trigeminal nerve sensory root (>1840)*** and ***trigeminal nerve motor root (Bell, 1829)***, respectively; see Richardson & Carman translation (2002, pp. 177–204).
16. *root of fifth pair of cerebral nerves (Vesalius, 1543a)*
Vague term referring to region of *fifth pair of nerves from brain (Galen, c192)* associated with its attachment to rostral end of ***medulla (Winslow, 1733)***; see Richardson & Carman translation (2002, p. 205, no. 6 in the figure).
17. *larger root of fifth pair of cerebral nerves (Vesalius, 1543a)*
Synonym for macrodissected adult human *fifth pair of nerves from brain (Galen, c192)*; see Richardson & Carman translation (2002, p. 265), Singer translation (1952, Fig. 14-*M*).
18. *root of sixth pair of cerebral nerves (Vesalius, 1543a)*
As illustrated for macrodissected adult human, ***glossopharyngeal nerve root (>1840)*** and ***vagus nerve root (>1840)*** considered together; see Richardson & Carman translation (2002, p. 205, no. 6 in the figure).
19. *little roots of sixth pair of cranial nerves (Vesalius, 1543a)*
Based on illustrations, probably refers to combination of macrodissected adult human ***glossopharyngeal nerve rootlets (>1840)*** and ***vagus nerve rootlets (>1840)***; see Singer translation (1952, Fig. 14-*N*).
20. *beginnings and twigs of sixth pair of cerebral nerves (Vesalius, 1543a)*
Probably refers to macrodissected adult human ***glossopharyngeal nerve rootlets (>1840), vagus nerve rootlets (>1840)***, and ***cranial root of accessory nerve rootlets (>1840)*** considered together; in the original Latin, *sexti paris nervorum cerebri principia ac surculi*, see Richardson & Carman (2009, p. 156). Eustachi (1552) illustrated them for macrodissected adult human; see Albinus edition (1761, Tab. 18, Figs. 1, 3, 4-ε and 2-*d*).
21. *fifth pair (Estienne, 1545)*
Synonym for macrodissected adult human *sixth pair of nerves from brain (Galen, c192)*; see Vicq d'Azyr (1786, p. 49).
22. *fifth pair of sinews of brain (Geminus, 1553)*
Synonym for macrodissected adult human *fifth pair of nerves from brain (Galen, c192)*; originally spelled, *fifte payre of sinowes of the brayne*, see *The table of the figures of sinowes*; or *fyft payre of synowes of the brayne*, see *The tables of the brayne*, Figure 9-*M*.
23. *root of fifth pair of sinews of brain (Geminus, 1553)*
Synonym for macrodissected adult human *root of fifth pair of cerebral nerves (Vesalius, 1543a)*; originally spelled, *roote of fifte payre of sinowes of the brayne*, see *The table of the figures of sinowes*.
24. *goodliest and safest root of fifth pair of sinews of brain (Geminus, 1553)*
Synonym for macrodissected adult human *larger root of fifth pair of cerebral nerves (Vesalius, 1543a)*; originally spelled *goodlyest and sayfest roote of fyft payre of sinowes of the brayne*, see *The table of the figures of sinowes*, Figure 7-*I,O*.
25. *greater root of fifth pair of sinews of brain (Geminus, 1553)*
Synonym for macrodissected adult human *larger root of fifth pair of cerebral nerves (Vesalius, 1543a)*; originally spelled *greater roote of the fyfte payre of synowes of the brayne*, see *The tables of the brayne*, Figure 14-*M,N*.

26. *sixth pair of sinews of brain (Geminus, 1553)*
Synonym for macrodissected adult human *sixth pair of nerves from brain (Galen, c192)*; the original spelling was, *syxte payre of synowes of the brayne*, see The table of the figure of synowes; or *sixte payre of synowes of the brayne*, see The tables of the brayne, Figure 9-N.
27. *root of sixth pair of sinews of brain (Geminus, 1553)*
Synonym for macrodissected adult human *root of sixth pair of cerebral nerves (Vesalius, 1543a)*; originally spelled, *roote of syxte payre of sinowes of brayne*, see The table of the figures of sinowes.
28. *pairs of sinews of brain (Geminus, 1553)*
Synonym for macrodissected adult human *pairs of nerves from brain (Galen, c192)*, or *cerebral nerves (Vesalius, 1543a)*, originally spelled *synowes of the braynes*, see The table of the figure of synowes.
29. *small branches of sixth pair of sinews of brain (Geminus, 1553)*
Synonym for macrodissected adult human *little roots of sixth pair of cranial nerves (Vesalius, 1543a)*; originally spelled *small braunches of fyrst payre of sinowes of brayne*, see The tables of the brayne, Figure 14-N.
30. *seven pair of sensitive sinews from brain (Geminus, 1553)*
Synonym for macrodissected adult human *pairs of nerves from brain (Galen, c192)*; originally spelled *seven payre of sensative synowes frome the brayne*, f. BII. Geminus qualified the term by writing that "all these Synowes have both selyinge [sensing] and movynge, althoughe in some more and in some lesse" (f. Bvi).
31. *pairs of nerves arising from brain (Colombo, 1559)*
Colombo counted nine pairs in macrodissected adult human, adding two to the seven *cranial nerves (Galen, c192)*. His eighth was *thinner root of fifth pair of nerves (Vesalius, 1543a)*, probably ***abducens nerve (Heister, 1717)***, and his ninth was *lesser root of third pair of nerves (Vesalius, 1543a)*, probably ***trochlear nerve (Molinetti, 1669)***; see p. 195 ff.
32. *pairs of nerves from brain (Falloppio, 1561)*
Falloppio enumerated eight pairs in macrodissected adult human, modified from *pairs of nerves from brain (Galen, c192)*, roughly as follows: first pair was *optic nerve (Galen, c173)*; second pair included ***oculomotor nerve (Estienne, 1545)***; third pair probably included ***trigeminal nerve sensory root (>1840)*** and ***trigeminal nerve motor root (Bell, 1829)*** considered together; fourth pair was ***abducens nerve (Heister, 1717)***; fifth pair included *facial nerve (Vicq d'Azyr, 1784)* and ***vestibulocochlear nerve (>1840)*** considered together; sixth pair included ***glossopharyngeal nerve (Huber, 1744)***, ***vagus nerve (Galen, c192)***, and ***accessory nerve (Vieussens, 1684)*** considered together; seventh pair included ***hypoglossal nerve (Winslow, 1733)***; and eighth pair was ***trochlear nerve (Molinetti, 1669)***; ff. 137–155. Also see Hierons & Meyer (1962, p. 289).
33. *posterior nerve of sixth conjugation of nerves of brain (Bauhin, 1605)*
Macrodissected adult human ***vagus nerve (Galen, c192)*** and ***accessory nerve (Vieussens, 1684)*** considered together; see Crooke translation (1615, p. 892). Bauhin also described here that it arises from ***brain (Smith Papyrus, c1700 BC)*** as some fibers (rootlets).
34. *outward branch of sixth pair of nerves (Crooke, 1615)*
Synonym for macrodissected adult human *posterior nerve of sixth conjugation of nerves of brain (Bauhin, 1605)*; p. 365.
35. *wandering conjugation (Crooke, 1615)*
Synonym for *sixth pair of nerves from brain (Galen, c192)*. According to Crooke's translation of Bauhin (1605), "because it runneth almost through all the bowels of the body it is therefore called Conjugatio vaga, the gadding or wandering conjugation [pair]." (p. 893).
36. *eighth pair of nerves from brain (Bartholin, 1641)*
Synonym for macrodissected adult human *fifth pair of nerves from brain (Galen, c192)*; see translation (1662, pp. 325–326).
37. *ninth pair of nerves from brain (Bartholin, 1641)*
Bartholin's enumeration of *sixth pair of nerves from brain (Galen, c192)*; see translation (1662, pp. 324–326), also see Huard & Imbault-Huart (1980, p. 29).
38. *ambulatorium (Vesling, 1647)*
Synonym for macrodissected adult human *sixth pair of nerves from brain (Galen, c192)*; see Soemmerring (1778, p. 165). Burdach (1822, p. 309) used the form *ambulatorius*.
39. *auditory nerve (Willis, 1664)*
Synonym for *seventh pair of nerves arising within skull (Willis, 1664)*; see Pordage translation (1681, p. 58).
40. *hearing nerve (Willis, 1664)*
Synonym for *auditory nerve (Willis, 1664)*; see Pordage translation (1681, p. 58).
41. *wandring pair (Willis, 1664)*
Synonym for macrodissected adult mammalian *wandering conjugation (Crooke, 1615)*; see Pordage translation (1681), p. 58. Modern spelling is *wandering pair*.
42. *seventh pair of nerves arising within skull (Willis, 1664)*
Synonym for macrodissected adult human *fifth pair of nerves from brain (Galen, c192)*; see Pordage translation (1681, p. 140 ff.), *pairs of nerves arising within skull (Willis, 1664)*.
43. *eighth pair of nerves arising within skull (Willis, 1664)*
Synonym for *sixth pair of nerves from brain (Galen, c192)*; see Pordage translation (1681, p. 146 ff.).
44. *wandring pair of nerves (Willis, 1664)*
Synonym for *eighth pair of nerves arising within skull (Willis, 1664)*; see Pordage translation (1681, pp. 58, 120, 146 ff.). Modern spelling is *wandering pair of nerves*.
45. *vagus nerve (Willis, 1664)*
Either member of *wandring pair of nerves (Willis, 1664)*.
46. *pari vago (Willis, 1664)*
Latin form of *wandring pair of nerves (Willis, 1664)*; in English the *vagal pair*.
47. *third branch of second division of fifth pair of nerves arising within skull (Willis, 1664)*
As described for macrodissected adult (presumably human), apparently included a nonsensical combination

of ***masseteric nerve (Meckel, 1748), superior labial branches of infraorbital nerve Meckel, 1748)***, and ***buccal branches of facial nerve (>1840)***; see Pordage translation (1681, pp. 144–145, Fig. 1-*E,e,f,g*).

48. *maxillary branch of second division of fifth pair of nerves arising within skull (Willis, 1664)*
Synonym for *third branch of second division of fifth pair of nerves arising within skull (Willis, 1664)*; see Pordage translation (1681, pp. 144–145, Fig. 1-*E,e,f,g*), where it was originally spelled *maxillar*.

49. *nerves proceeding from pith within skull (Diemerbroeck, 1689)*
Synonym for macrodissected adult human *pairs of nerves from skull (Galen, c192)*; p. 408.

50. *par vagum (Ridley, 1695)*
Form of *pari vago (Willis, 1664)*; p. 150.

51. *nervus sympatheticus medius (Winslow, 1733)*
Synonym for macrodissected adult human *vagus nerve (Willis, 1664)* or *sixth pair of nerves from brain (Galen, c192)*; in the original Latin (plural), *nervi sympathetici medii*, Section VI, p. 59.

52. *middle sympathetic nerve (Winslow, 1733)*
English form of *nervus sympatheticus medius (Winslow, 1733)*.

53. *par vagum minus (Winslow, 1733)*
Synonym for macrodissected adult human *pari vago (Willis, 1664)*; Section VI, p. 59.

54. *infraorbital plexus (Meckel, 1753)*
Network of ***communicating branches (Winslow, 1733)*** between ***infraorbital nerve (Schaarschmidt, 1750)*** and ***zygomatic branches of facial nerve (>1840)*** in region between orbit and upper lip of macrodissected adult human; in the original French, *le plexus sous-orbital (des nerfs)*, pp. 56, 90.

55. *ocular nerves (Zinn, 1755)*
All ***nerves (Herophilus, c335–c280 BC)*** taken together associated with the macrodissected adult human eye and its muscles, including *optic nerve (Galen, c173)*, ***oculomotor nerve (Estienne, 1545), trochlear nerve (Molinetti, 1669), short ciliary nerves (>1840)***, and ***abducens nerve (Heister, 1717)***; p. 183 ff.

56. *roots of intermediate sympathetic nerve (Malacarne, 1791)*
For macrodissected adult human, ***glossopharyngeal nerve rootlets (>1840)*** and ***vagus nerve rootlets (>1840)*** considered together; pp. 227, 238.

57. *intermediate sympathetic nerve (Malacarne, 1791)*
Corresponds to macrodissected adult human ***glossopharyngeal nerve (Huber, 1744)*** and ***vagus nerve (Galen, c192)*** considered together; p. 192.

58. *fourteenth pair of nerves (Malacarne, 1791)*
Synonym for *intermediate sympathetic nerve (Malacarne, 1791)*; p. 192.

59. *pairs of nerves of head (Andersch, 1797)*
Andersch's naming scheme for the 12 ***cranial nerves (Soemmerring, 1791)*** in macrodissected adult human was somewhat idiosyncratic: *primus nervus olfactorius, secundus visorius* [*visual nerve (Theophilos Protospatharios, fl. 610–641)*], *tertius motorius medius oculi* [***oculomotor nerve (Estienne, 1545)***], *quartus motorius internus oculi* [***trochlear nerve (Molinetti, 1669)***], *quintus consensorius medius capitis* [*nervi sympathetici medii (Wrisberg, 1777)*], *sextus motorius externus oculi* [*nervi oculo-musculares externi (Winslow, 1733)*], *septimus consensorius parvus capitis* [*small sympathetic nerve (Winslow, 1733)*], *octavus auditorius* [*eighth pair of nerves leaving skull (Soemmerring, 1778)*], *nonus sensorius linguae* [***glossopharyngeal nerve (Huber, 1744)***], *decimus consentiens magnus capitis* [*middle sympathetic nerve (Winslow, 1733)], undecimus motorius linguae* [*motor nerve for tongue (Galen, c173)*], *et duodecimus nervus motorius capitis*: p. 1. The first 11 correspond to *nervorum per ossa capitis egredientium (Soemmerring, 1778)*, though often with different synonyms.

60. *nerves from tuber annulare and its extensions (Bichat, 1801)*
In Bichat's scheme there were only two *cerebral nerves (Bichat, 1801)*: ***olfactory nerve (Winslow, 1733)*** and ***optic nerve (Vicq d'Azyr, 1786)***; he listed nine other ***cranial nerves (Soemmerring, 1791)*** as *nerves from tuber annulare and its elongations (Bichat, 1801)*, excluding ***accessory nerve (Vieussens, 1684)***, which he assigned to *nerves from spinal marrow (Bichat, 1801)*; see translation (1822, Vol. 1, pp. 172–173).

61. *nerves of cerebral protuberance (Bichat et al., 1801–1803)*
Corresponds to six pairs of ***cranial nerves (Soemmerring, 1791)***: ***oculomotor nerve (Estienne, 1545), trochlear nerve (Molinetti, 1669), trigeminal nerve (Winslow, 1733), abducens nerve (Heister, 1717), intermediofacial nerve (Strong & Elwyn, 1943)***, and ***vestibulocochlear nerve (>1840)***; Vol. 3, p. 156 ff.

62. *pairs of encephalic nerves (Burdin, 1803)*
For macrodissected adult human Burdin listed 12 in same order as *pairs of nerves of head (Andersch, 1797)*—see translation (1803, Vol. 1, pp. 167–185)—but used an almost completely novel nomenclature based on at the time unpublished teachings of Chaussier (see Vol. 1, p. 156). They were, in order, *ethmoidal pair of nerves (Burdin, 1803), ocular pair of nerves (Burdin, 1803), common oculo-muscular pair of nerves (Burdin, 1803), interior oculo-muscular pair of nerves (Burdin, 1803), trifacial pair of nerves (Burdin, 1803), exterior oculo-muscular pair of nerves (Burdin, 1803), facial nerves (Vicq d'Azyr, 1784), labyrinthic pair of nerves (Burdin, 1803), pharyngio-glossian pair of nerves (Burdin, 1803), pneumo-gastric pair of nerves (Burdin, 1803), hyo-glossian pair of nerves (Burdin, 1803)*, and *trachelo-dorsal pair of nerves (Burdin, 1803)*.

63. *cerebral nerves (Wenzel & Wenzel, 1812)*
For macrodissected adult human, ***cranial nerves (Soemmerring, 1791)*** were listed but not numbered; however, ***intermediofacial nerve (Strong & Elwyn, 1943)*** was listed eighth and ***vestibulocochlear nerve (>1840)*** was listed seventh; p. 205.

64. *cerebellar nerves (Gordon, 1815)*
Five pairs of *cerebral nerves (Gordon, 1815)* arising from *cerebellum (Haller, 1762)*: *internal oculo-muscular*

nerves (Chaussier, 1807), external oculo-muscular nerves (Winslow, 1733), ***trigeminal nerves (Winslow, 1733),*** *facial nerves (Vicq d'Azyr, 1786),* and *auditory nerves (Galen, c192)*; p. 202 ff.

65. *encephalic nerves (Meckel, 1817)*
Synonym for macrodissected adult human ***cranial nerves (Soemmerring, 1791)***, although Meckel had ***intermediofacial nerve (Strong & Elwyn, 1943)*** listed eighth and ***vestibulocochlear nerve (>1840)*** listed seventh, and he numbered the set from caudal to rostral, rather than rostral to caudal so ***olfactory nerve (Winslow, 1733)*** was twelfth; see translation (1822, Vol. 3, p. 36 ff.).

66. *cerebral nerves (Solly, 1836)*
For macrodissected adult human, Solly had 11 of the 12 ***cranial nerves (Soemmerring, 1791)***, logically leaving out ***accessory nerve (Vieussens, 1684)*** arising from ***spinal cord (Galen, c162–166). Hypoglossal nerve (Winslow, 1733)*** thus became eleventh *cerebral nerve (Solly, 1836)*; p. 237 ff.

67. *mental plexus (Cruveilhier, 1836)*
In macrodissected adult human, associated with lower lip and formed by ***communicating branches (Winslow, 1733)*** between ***inferior labial branches of mental nerve (Meckel, 1753)*** and branches of ***marginal mandibular branch of facial nerve (>1840)***; in the original French, *plexus mentonnier*, p. 936.

68. *posterior cranial pairs (Cruveilhier, 1836)*
For macrodissected adult human, and based on Cruveilhier's analysis of cranial bone organization, right and left ***glossopharyngeal nerves (Huber, 1744), vagus nerves (Galen, c192), accessory nerves (Vieussens, 1684)***, and ***hypoglossal nerves (Winslow, 1733)*** considered together—with the former two pairs forming mixed sensory and motor roots and the latter two forming just motor roots; in the original French, *paire crânienne postérieure*, p. 979.

69. *anterior cranial pairs (Cruveilhier, 1836)*
For macrodissected adult human, and based on Cruveilhier's analysis of cranial bone organization, right and left ***trigeminal nerves (Winslow, 1733), oculomotor nerves (Estienne, 1545), trochlear nerves (Molinetti, 1669), abducens nerves (Heister, 1717)***, and ***intermediofacial nerves (Strong & Elwyn, 1943)*** considered together; in the original French, *paire crânienne antérieure*, p. 979.

cranial root of accessory nerve (>1840)

As described for macrodissected adult human, commonly 4–8 short, thin ***cranial root of accessory nerve rootlets (>1840)*** converge to form the one or more commonly two ***cranial root of accessory nerve trunks (>1840)***, in turn converging near the jugular foramen with the ***spinal root of accessory nerve trunk (>1840)*** to form the ***accessory nerve trunk (Wrisberg, 1786)***. The ***cranial root of accessory nerve (1840)*** is best viewed as a branch of the ***vagus nerve (Galen, c192)*** distributing mainly in the ***pharyngeal branches of vagus nerve (Wrisberg, 1786)*** and ***pharyngeal branches of recurrent laryngeal nerve (>1840)***; see *medulla oblongata roots of accessory nerve (Meckel, 1817)* and Williams & Warwick (1980, pp. 1081–1082, Fig. 7.189). It may have been known to Galen; see ***[cranial root of accessory nerve (>1840)] (Galen, c192)***. Winslow clearly distinguished it; see ***[cranial root of accessory nerve (>1840)] (Winslow, 1733)***.

EARLIER REFERENCES:

Described, not named or illustrated:

1. ***[cranial root of accessory nerve (>1840)] (Galen, c192)***
Galen probably referred to it for macrodissected adult beef, pig, and/or macaque (but not human) because he described three *roots of sixth pair of nerves from brain (Galen, c192)*, although he did not elaborate on the third and most caudal root associated with the ***accessory nerve (Vieussens, 1684)*** and certainly did not distinguish between ***cranial root of accessory nerve (>1840)*** and ***spinal root of accessory nerve (>1840)***; see Duckworth translation (1962, pp. 197–198).
2. ***[cranial root of accessory nerve (>1840)] (Winslow, 1733)***
Clearly described for macrodissected adult human as "two Filaments from the posterior Portion of the Medulla" (Sect. VI, p. 74).

Illustrated and described, not named:

1. ***[cranial root of accessory nerve (>1840)] (Du Verney, 1683)***
Crudely illustrated for macrodissected adult human; Plate 11, Figure 1 lateral to Q. Lobstein (1760, Tab. V-*d*; also see Vicq d'Azyr, 1786, Pl. XVIII-69) clearly described and illustrated distinction between it and ***spinal root of accessory nerve (>1840)*** in macrodissected adult human.

Earlier synonyms:

1. *medulla oblongata roots of accessory nerve (Meckel, 1817)*
Synonym for macrodissected adult human ***cranial root of accessory nerve (>1840)***; see translation (1832, Vol. 3, p. 43), where he wrote, "The spinal roots also are usually single, while those arising from the medulla oblongata are generally composed of two short radicles united at an acute angle, each of which is formed by three or four filaments." The filaments are now called ***cranial root of accessory nerve rootlets (>1840)*** and the radicles ***cranial root of accessory nerve trunks (>1840)***, together forming the ***cranial root of accessory nerve (>1840)***; see Williams & Warwick (1980, p. 1082 and Fig. 7.189).
2. *cerebral part of accessory nerve (Arnold, 1838b)*
Synonym for macrodissected adult human ***spinal root of accessory nerve (>1840)***; in the original Latin, *pars cerebralis nervi accessorii*, Table I, Figure 2-8.

cranial root of accessory nerve rootlets (>1840)

As described for macrodissected adult human, 3–4 of them converge to form a ***cranial root of accessory nerve trunk (>1840)***. There are commonly two sets of ***cranial root of accessory nerve rootlets (>1840)*** and thus two

cranial root of accessory nerve trunks (>1840) merging near the jugular foramen with the ***spinal root of accessory nerve (>1840)*** to form the ***accessory nerve trunk (Wrisberg, 1786)***. The ***cranial root of accessory nerve rootlets (>1840)*** are attached in a longitudinal line to the outside of the ***medulla (Winslow, 1733)***, just caudal to the ***vagus nerve rootlets (>1840)***; see *medulla oblongata roots of accessory nerve (Meckel, 1817)* and Williams & Warwick (1980, p. 1082 and Fig. 7.189). They were perhaps first clearly delineated by Lobstein; see ***[cranial root of accessory nerve rootlets (>1840)] (Lobstein, 1760)***.

EARLIER REFERENCES:

Illustrated and described, not named:

1. ***[cranial root of accessory nerve rootlets (>1840)] (Lobstein, 1760)***
   Clearly illustrated for macrodissected adult human in Lobstein's classic thesis on the ***accessory nerve (Vieussens, 1684)***; Table V, Figure 1-*d*.

Earlier synonyms:

1. *cerebral roots of accessory nerve of Willis (Günther, 1786)*
   Günther described 3–4 ***cranial root of accessory nerve rootlets (>1840)*** for macrodissected adult human; in the original Latin, *radicibus cerebralibus*, p. 89.
2. *roots [of accessory nerve] from medulla oblongata (Frotscher, 1788)*
   Synonym for macrodissected adult human ***cranial root of accessory nerve rootlets (>1840)***; in the original Latin, *radicibus ex medulla oblongata*, p. 102. According to Frotscher there are commonly two of them. Also see *roots of accessory nerve from spinal medulla (Frotscher, 1788)*.
3. *accessory roots from medulla oblongata (Scarpa, 1788)*
   Synonym for macrodissected adult human ***cranial root of accessory nerve rootlets (>1840)***; in the original Latin, *radices accessorii ex medulla oblongata*, Table X, Figure 1-3.
4. *filaments of medulla oblongata roots of accessory nerve (Meckel, 1817)*
   Synonym for macrodissected adult human ***cranial root of accessory nerve rootlets (>1840)***, "The spinal roots also are usually single, while those arising from the medulla oblongata are generally composed of two short radicles united at an acute angle, each of which is formed by three or four filaments." (translation, 1832, Vol. 3, p. 43). The filaments are now referred to in English as *rootlets*.

cranial root of accessory nerve trunks (>1840)

As described for macrodissected adult human, a set of ***cranial root of accessory nerve rootlets (>1840)*** converges distally to form a ***cranial root of accessory nerve trunk (>1840)*** and commonly two sets of ***cranial root of accessory nerve rootlets (>1840)*** and ***cranial root of accessory nerve trunks (>1840)*** together constitute the ***cranial root of accessory nerve (>1840)***, which joins the ***spinal root of accessory nerve (>1840)*** to form the ***accessory nerve trunk (Wrisberg, 1786)***; see *medulla oblongata roots of accessory nerve (Meckel, 1817)* and Williams & Warwick (1980, p. 1082 and Fig. 7.189). They were perhaps first clearly delineated by Lobstein; see ***[cranial root of accessory nerve trunks (>1840)] (Lobstein, 1760)***.

EARLIER REFERENCES:

Illustrated and described, not named:

1. ***[cranial root of accessory nerve trunks (>1840)] (Lobstein, 1760)***
   Clearly illustrated for macrodissected adult human in Lobstein's classic thesis on ***accessory nerve (Vieussens, 1684)***; Table V, Figure 1-*d*. They were illustrated earlier, though inaccurately without ***cranial root of accessory nerve rootlets (>1840)***, by Du Verney (1683, Pl. 11, Fig. 1 lateral to Q). Also beautifully illustrated by Soemmerring (1778, Tab. II-γ).

Earlier synonyms:

1. *radicles of medulla oblongata roots of accessory nerve (Meckel, 1817)*
   Synonym for macrodissected adult human ***cranial root of accessory nerve trunks (>1840)***, "The spinal roots also are usually single, while those arising from the medulla oblongata are generally composed of two short radicles united at an acute angle, each of which is formed by three or four filaments." (translation, 1832, Vol. 3, p. 43). The radicles are now referred to in English as *trunks*.

craniospinal ganglia (>1840)

As described for macrodissected vertebrate, the ***cranial nerve ganglia (>1840)*** and ***spinal nerve ganglia (Burdach, 1819)*** considered together, all of which are sensory in function, and contrasted with ***autonomic ganglia (Langley, 1900)***. They were first identified in part as *knots (Coiter, 1572)*, the ***spinal nerve ganglia (Burdach, 1819)***.

EARLIER REFERENCES:

Earlier synonyms:

1. *ganglionated part of nervous system (Blainville, 1821)*
   For vertebrates in general, that part of the ***nervous system (Monro, 1783)*** directly related to ***craniospinal ganglia (>1840)*** dealing with special senses and general sensation and locomotion; in the original French, *ganglionaire*, p. 205.

craniospinal nerves (Herrick, 1915)

For macrodissected vertebrates the 12 pairs of ***cranial nerves (Soemmerring, 1791)*** exiting the *cranium* (see *Dorland's*, 2003, p. 432), and a variable number in different species of pairs of ***spinal nerves (Camper, 1760–1762)*** exiting the *spinal column* (see *Dorland's*, 2003, p. 394), considered together and distinguished from the ***autonomic nerves (Langley, 1898)***. Obersteiner and Hill (1900, p. 200) emphasized that most ***craniospinal nerves (Herrick, 1915)*** have a *central root* within the ***central nervous system (Carus, 1814)***, and a *peripheral root* in the ***peripheral nervous system (Meckel, 1817)***. The only clear exception is the neural connection between eye and ***brain (Smith Papyrus, c1700 BC)***, which is described in terms of ***optic nerve (Vicq d'Azyr, 1786)***, ***optic chiasm (Galen, c173)***, and multiple fiber systems proximal or central to the chiasm. Herrick wrote specifically of "cranial and spinal nerves" (p. 106). They were referred to long ago; see *nerves from brain and spinal cord (Galen, c192)*.

EARLIER REFERENCES:

Earlier synonyms:

1. *nerves from brain and spinal cord (Galen, c192)*
   Clear reference to macrodissected adult mammal, though not explicitly human, ***craniospinal nerves (Herrick, 1915)***; see Duckworth translation (1962, p. 181).
2. *nerves of animal life (Bichat, 1801)*
   Refers to ***craniospinal nerves (Herrick, 1915)***; distinguished from *nerves of organic life (Bichat, 1801)*. The macrodissected adult human *nerves of animal life (Bichat, 1801)* were divided here into two pairs of *cerebral nerves (Bichat, 1801)*, nine pairs of *nerves from tuber annulare and its elongations (Bichat, 1801)*, and 30–31 pairs of *nerves from spinal marrow (Bichat, 1801)*. *Cerebral nerves (Bichat, 1801)* included ***olfactory nerve (Winslow, 1733)*** and ***optic nerve (Vicq d'Azyr, 1786)***, and he assigned ***accessory nerve (Vieussens, 1684)*** to *nerves from spinal marrow (Bichat, 1801)*; see translation (1822, Vol. 1, pp. 172–173).
3. *nerves of animal life (Bichat et al., 1801–1803)*
   Description here differed from that in *nerves of animal life (Bichat, 1801)*. Here it included the two *cranial nerves (Bichat, 1801)*, six pairs of *nerves of cerebral protuberance (Bichat et al., 1801–1803)*, five pairs of *nerves of origin of vertebral medulla (Bichat et al., 1801–1803)*, and 29–30 *spinal nerves (Vesalius, 1543a)*; Vol. 3, p. 143 ff.
4. *nervous system of animal life (Bichat et al., 1801–1803)*
   Apparently synonym for *nerves of animal life (Bichat et al., 1801–1803)*; Vol. 3, p. 142. However, see *nervous system of animal life (Bichat, 1801)*.
5. *nerves of origin of vertebral medulla (Bichat et al., 1801–1803)*
   Included for macrodissected adult human ***glossopharyngeal nerve (Huber, 1744)***, ***vagus nerve (Galen, c192)***, ***accessory nerve (Vieussens, 1684)***, ***hypoglossal nerve (Winslow, 1733)***, and first ***cervical nerve (Galen, c173)***—the ***suboccipital nerve (Winslow, 1733)***; Vol. 3, p. 205 ff.
6. *cerebral system (Reil, 1807)*
   Probably corresponds at least roughly to macrodissected adult human *cerebral nervous system (Bichat et al., 1801–1803)*; in the original German, *cerebralsystem*, p. 189.
7. *cerebro-spinal nerves (Müller, 1834)*
   Generally refers to ***craniospinal nerves (Herrick, 1915)*** and distinguished from *organic nerves (Ackerman, 1813)*; see translation (1838, p. 789). Sharpey et al. (1867, p. 582) used this general term because they used ***cerebrospinal axis (Meckel, 1817)***, although they referred to ***cranial nerves (Soemmerring, 1791)*** and ***spinal nerves (Camper, 1760–1762)*** separately.
8. *cephalo-rachidian nerves (Cruveilhier, 1836)*
   Overall, macrodissected adult human ***cerebrospinal nerves (Herrick, 1915)***; in the original French, *nerfs céphalo-rachidiens*, p. 759.

PARTLY CORRESPONDS:

1. *communicating branch of ascending part of tenth nerves of head and superior lingual nerves (Andersch & Soemmerring, 1792)*
   In macrodissected adult human, ***communicating branch (Winslow, 1733)*** between ***superior root of ansa cervicalis (>1840)*** and ***lingual nerve (Vesalius, 1543a)***; in the original Latin, *decimi nervi capitis partis ascendentis ramus communicatorius nervi lingualis superioris*, p. 153. It was referred to as ascending part of *eleventh* nerve in Andersch (1797, p. 40).
2. *spinal nerves (Gordon, 1815)*
   Gordon listed 34 pairs arising from macrodissected adult human *spinal cord (Gordon, 1815)* and purposefully did not number them: ***glossopharyngeal nerves (Huber, 1744)***, *pneumogastric nerves (Chaussier, 1807)*, ***hypoglossal nerves (Winslow, 1733)***, ***accessory nerves (Vieussens, 1684)***, ***suboccipital nerves (Winslow, 1733)***, seven pairs of *cervical nerves (William of Saliceto, 1275)*, twelve pairs of *dorsal nerves (Winslow, 1733)*, five pairs of ***lumbar nerves (Diemerbroeck, 1672)***, and five pairs of ***sacral nerves (Camper, 1760)***; p. 203.
3. *encephalic nerves proper (Cloquet, 1816)*
   For macrodissected adult human, ***cranial nerves (Soemmerring, 1791)*** and ***suboccipital nerve (Winslow, 1733)*** considered together; in the original French, *nerfs encéphaliques en particulier*, p. 584 ff.
4. *symmetrical system of nerves (Bell, 1821)*
   For all macrodissected animals from leeches and worms to human, equivalent of ***spinal nerves (Camper, 1760–1762)*** and ***trigeminal nerve (Winslow, 1733)*** considered together, because all of them have both sensory and motor functions and two roots, one with an accompanying ***ganglion (Galen, c173)***; p. 404. Bell did not here assign specific functions to the two roots. Also see Bell & Bell (1829, p. 318 and Pl. IX, Fig. 3).
5. *original nerves (Bell, 1821)*
   Synonym for *symmetrical system of nerves (Bell, 1821)*; p. 404.
6. *superadded nerves (Bell, 1821)*
   Eleven of 12 ***cranial nerves (Soemmerring, 1791)***, without ***trigeminal nerve (Winslow, 1733)***; p. 404. Contrasted with the *original nerves (Bell, 1821)*.
7. *respiratory nerves (Bell, 1821)*
   For macrodissected adult mammal, included ***vagus nerve (Galen, c192)***, *facial nerve (Vicq d'Azry, 1784)*, ***accessory nerve (Vieussens, 1684)***, ***phrenic nerve (Galen, c173)***, and ***long thoracic nerve (Quain & Wilson, 1839)***; pp. 406–407.

8. *superadded system of nerves (Bell, 1822)*
   Synonym for *superadded nerves (Bell, 1821)* to which Bell attributed "our condition of mental superiority including respiration, language and the expression of sentiment" (p. 310). "The nerves treated of in these papers, are the instruments of expression, from the smile upon the infant's cheek to the last agony of life." (p. 309).
9. *irregular system of nerves (Bell & Bell, 1826)*
   As defined here, ***oculomotor nerve (Estienne, 1545), trochlear nerve (Molinetti, 1669), abducens nerve (Heister, 1717),*** *facial nerve (Vicq d'Azyr, 1784),* ***vestibulocochlear nerve (>1840), vagus nerve (Galen, c192), accessory nerve (Vieussens, 1684), hypoglossal nerve (Winslow, 1733), phrenic nerve (Galen, c173),*** and ***long thoracic nerve (Quain & Wilson, 1839)***; Vol. 2, p. 390.
10. *irregular nerves (Bell & Bell, 1829)*
   Synonym for *irregular system of nerves (Bell & Bell, 1829)*; p. 318.
11. *nerves originating from spinal marrow (Bichat, 1801)*
   For macrodissected adult human Bichat counted the traditional 30 or 31 pairs (8 cervical, 12 thoracic, 5 lumbar, and 5 or 6 sacral), see *spinal nerves (Benedetti, 1502)*, but also included the ***accessory nerve (Vieussens, 1684)***; see translation (1822, Vol. 1, pp. 172–173).

crossed corticospinal tract (>1840)

As described for adult human with experimental methods for pathway tracing, the contralateral caudal segment of the right or left ***corticospinal tract (>1840)***, caudal to the ***pyramidal decussation (>1840)*** and centered in intermediate regions of the left or right ***lateral funiculus (Burdach, 1822)*** respectively; see Williams & Warwick (1980, pp. 877–878 and Fig. 7.44), who called it *lateral corticospinal tract (>1840)*, and Nieuwenhuys et al. (2008, Fig. 6.1-20). Its size and location can vary greatly between individuals and species. For example, in adult rat it lies ventrally in the ***dorsal funiculus (>1840)***; see Craigie (1925, pp. 27–28). In adult mammal it is typically much larger than the ***uncrossed corticospinal tract (>1840)***. It was not clearly delineated by 1840.

EARLIER REFERENCES:

Earlier synonyms:

1. *lateral corticospinal tract (>1840)*
   Synonym for macrodissected adult human ***crossed corticospinal tract (>1840)***; see *Terminologia Anatomica* (1998, p. 107).

cruciform sulcus (>1840)

As described for macrodissected adult human, the two orthogonal grooves on the dorsal surface of the ***tectum (Baer, 1837)***: the ***transverse tectal sulcus (>1840)*** separating the ***superior colliculi (Haller, 1762)*** rostrally from the ***inferior colliculi (Haller, 1762)*** caudally, and the **longitudinal tectal sulcus (>1840)** separating the right ***superior colliculus (Haller, 1762)*** and ***inferior colliculus (Haller, 1762)*** from the left ***superior colliculus (Haller, 1762)*** and ***inferior colliculus (Haller, 1762)***; see Williams & Warwick (1980, p. 935). It was known to Galen; see ***[cruciform sulcus (>1840)] (Galen, c173)***.

EARLIER REFERENCES:

Described, not named or illustrated:

1. ***[cruciform sulcus (>1840)] (Galen, c173)***
   In describing ***superior colliculi (Haller, 1762)*** and ***inferior colliculi (Haller, 1762)*** of macrodissected adult beef, pig, and/or macaque but not human, Galen must have observed it; see *little buttocks (Galen, c173, definition 1)*.

Illustrated and described, not named:

1. ***[cruciform sulcus (>1840)] (Vesalius, 1543a)***
   Clearly described and illustrated for macrodissected adult human; see Singer translation (1952, p. 106, Fig. 10).

Earlier synonyms:

1. *crucial depression (Meckel, 1817)*
   Synonym for macrodissected adult human ***cruciform sulcus (>1840)***; see translation (1832, Vol. 2, p. 445).
2. *central sulcus separating four quadrigeminal tubercles (Cloquet, 1828)*
   Synonym for macrodissected adult human ***cruciform sulcus (>1840)***; in the original French, *sillon central qui sépare les quatre tubercules quadrijumeaux*, Plate CXXXVII, Figure 1-23.

culmen (Stroud, 1895)

As described for macrodissected adult human and other mammals, the part of the ***cerebellar cortex (Willis, 1664)*** lying between ***central lobule (Burdach, 1822)*** rostrally, and ***declive (>1840)*** and ***simple lobule (Jansen & Brodal, 1954)*** caudally. In macrodissected adult human, the ***paramedian fissure (>1840)*** extends at least partly into the ***culmen (Stroud, 1895)*** from the ***declive (>1840)***. The zone of the ***culmen (Stroud, 1895)*** near the median plane thus lies within the ***cerebellar vermis (Meckel, 1817)***, and at least part of the ***culmen (Stroud, 1895)*** adjacent to the ***simple lobule (Jansen & Brodal, 1954)*** lies more laterally within the ***cerebellar hemisphere (Willis, 1664)***, where it has received various names including *quadrangular lobule (>1840)* and *anterior quadrangular lobule (>1840)*; see Angevine et al. (1961, Figs. 1-24), Larsell & Jansen (1972, Fig. 118), Carpenter (1976, Figs. 2.25, 2.26, 14.1), Nieuwenhuys et al. (2008, Fig. 3.8-28). For Stroud's use in macrodissected adult human, see p. 102. It was not recognized as such by 1840.

PARTLY CORRESPONDS:

1. *anterior quadrangular lobule (>1840)*
   As described for macrodissected adult human, lateral zone of ***culmen (Stroud, 1895)***; see His (1895, p. 82), Carpenter (1976, Fig. 14.1), Nieuwenhuys et al. (2008, Fig. 20.2). For synonyms see Angevine et al. (1961, Figs. 1-24).
2. *quadrangular lobule (>1840)*
   As described for macrodissected adult human, lateral zone of ***culmen (Stroud, 1895)***; see *Nomina Anatomica*

(1955, p. 41, *lobulus quadrangulus*), Williams & Warwick (1980, p. 912 and Fig. 7.74). For synonyms see Angevine et al. (1961, Figs. 1–24).

cuneate fascicle (Müller, 1834)

As described for macrodissected adult human, a rostrally directed ***central nervous system white matter tract (>1840)*** in the ***dorsal funiculus (>1840)*** of the ***spinal cord (Galen, c162–c166)*** and caudal part of the ***medulla (Winslow, 1733)***. It receives contributions from and is found in the rostral (upper) ***thoracic part of spinal cord (>1840)*** and the ***cervical part of spinal cord (>1840)***, where it lies lateral to the ***gracile fascicle (Müller, 1834)*** and ***dorsolateral sulcus of spinal cord (>1840)***; see Williams & Warwick (1980, p. 881). For topographic description it has ***medullary cuneate fascicle (>1840)*** and ***spinal cuneate fascicle (>1840)*** segments, with the former separated from the ***medullary gracile fascicle (>1840)*** by the ***dorsolateral sulcus of medulla (>1840)***. For Müller's use in macrodissected adult human, see translation (1838, p. 827). It was first clearly delineated by Santorini; see ***[cuneate fascicle (Müller, 1834)] (Santorini, 1775)***.

TRANSLATIONS:

1. *fasciculus cuneatus (Müller, 1834)*
   Original Latin form of ***cuneate fascicle (Müller, 1834)***; see translation (1838, p. 827).

EARLIER REFERENCES:

Illustrated, not named or described:

1. ***[cuneate fascicle (Müller, 1834)] (Santorini, 1775)***
   Clearly illustrated for macrodissected adult human; Table III, Figure 2.

Earlier synonyms:

1. *outer bundle of posterior funiculus (Rosenthal, 1815)*
   Synonym for macrodissected adult human ***cuneate fascicle (Müller, 1834)***; in the original German, *äussres Bündel des hintern Strangs*, p. 29; see Burdach (1822, p. 285).
2. *external posterior cord of spinal marrow (Meckel, 1817)*
   Synonym for macrodissected adult human ***cuneate fascicle (Müller, 1834)***; see translation (1832, Vol. 2, p. 414).
3. *funiculus cuneatus (Burdach, 1822)*
   Synonym for macrodissected adult human ***cuneate fascicle (Müller, 1834)***; in the original German, *Keilstrang*, p. 36, Table IV-*s*.

cuneate nucleus (>1840)

As described for macrodissected adult human, and for adult mammal in general with cellular architecture and connections, the ***gray matter region (Swanson & Bota, 2010)*** of the ***dorsal column nuclei (>1840)*** lying between ***gracile nucleus (>1840)*** medially and ***accessory cuneate nucleus (>1840)*** rostrolaterally and receiving a massive input from the ***cuneate fascicle (Müller, 1834)***; histologically it contains smaller ***neurons (Waldeyer, 1891)*** than the ***accessory cuneate nucleus (>1840)***; see Williams & Warwick (1980, p. 901), *Terminologia Anatomica* (1998, p. 110), Nieuwenhuys et al. (2008, p. 194 and Figs. 6.21–23, called *medial cuneate nucleus*). It was first recognized by Burdach; see ***[cuneate nucleus (>1840)] (Burdach, 1822)***.

EARLIER REFERENCES:

Described, not named or illustrated:

1. ***[cuneate nucleus (>1840)] (Burdach, 1822)***
   Burdach described presence of ***gray matter (Meckel, 1817)*** associated with *funiculus cuneatus (Burdach, 1822)* in macrodissected adult human; p. 36.

cuneate tubercle (>1840)

As described for macrodissected adult human, the surface of the expanded rostral end of the ***cuneate fascicle (Müller, 1840)***, the ***medullary cuneate fascicle (>1840)*** lying dorsal to the ***cuneate nucleus (>1840)***; see Crosby et al. (1962, p. 114), *Terminologia Anatomica* (1998, p. 109), *Dorland's* (2003, p. 1961), Nieuwenhuys et al. (2008, Fig. 3.10-17). It was perhaps first clearly delineated as the *posterior olivary body (Ruysch, 1737)*.

EARLIER REFERENCES:

Earlier synonyms:

1. *posterior olivary body (Ruysch, 1737)*
   Probably synonym for macrodissected adult human *posterior olive (Huber, 1741)*; in the original Latin, *corpora olivaria posteriora*, see Epistle XII, p. 25, Table XIV, Figure 5. The description first appeared in a response Ruysch wrote in 1699 to a thesis written the same year by Ettmuller; it was printed in Ruysch's *Opera Omnia* (1737), where it was dated 1728.
2. *posterior olive (Huber 1741)*
   Synonym for macrodissected adult human ***cuneate tubercle (>1840)***; Figure 2-*N*.
3. *inferior olivary body (Günther, 1786)*
   Apparently synonym for macrodissected adult human *posterior olivary body (Ruysch, 1737)*; in the original Latin (plural), *corpora olivaria inferiora*, p. 23.

cuneus (Burdach, 1822)

As described for macrodissected adult human, a triangular topographic subdivision on the medial face of the ***occipital region (Vesalius, 1543a)*** lying between ***parieto-occipital sulcus (>1840)*** dorsally and ***calcarine sulcus (>1840)*** ventrally; see Williams & Warwick (1980, Fig. 7.114A). For Burdach's use in macrodissected adult human, see pp. 151, 175. It was perhaps first clearly delineated by Soemmerring; see ***[cuneus (Burdach, 1822)] (Soemmerring, 1778)***.

EARLIER REFERENCES:

Illustrated, not named or described:

1. ***[cuneus (Burdach, 1822)] (Soemmerring, 1778)***
   Clearly illustrated for macrodissected adult human; Table III.

cutaneous branch of obturator nerve (>1840)

As described for macrodissected adult human, a branch of the ***anterior branch of obturator nerve (Haase, 1781; Martin, 1781)*** contributing, when present, to the ***subsartorial plexus (>1840)*** in turn supplying skin on the medial surface of the thigh; see Durward (1951, Fig. 939), Williams & Warwick (1980, p. 1108 and Fig. 7.211), *Terminologia Anatomica* (1998, p. 140). It was known to Vesalius; see ***[cutaneous branch of obturator nerve (>1840)] (Vesalius, 1543a)***.

EARLIER REFERENCES:

Described, not named or illustrated:

1. ***[cutaneous branch of obturator nerve (>1840)] (Vesalius, 1543a)***
   Described for macrodissected adult human; see Richardson & Carman translation (2002, p. 258).

Earlier synonyms:

1. *external branch of anterior branch of obturator nerve (Cloquet, 1816)*
   Synonym for macrodissected adult human ***cutaneous branch of obturator nerve (>1840)***; p. 665.
2. *cutaneous filaments of obturator nerve (Quain & Wilson, 1839)*
   Synonym for macrodissected adult human ***cutaneous branch of obturator nerve (>1840)***; Plate XXIII-*m*.

cystic plexus (Wrisberg, 1808)

As described for macrodissected adult human, a tiny extension of the ***hepatic plexus (Rau, 1720)*** communicating with a cystic branch of the ***vagus nerve (Galen, c192)*** and innervating the gall bladder; see Mitchell (1953, p. 280), Williams & Warwick (1980, p. 1134). For Wrisberg's use in macrodissected adult human, see p. 16; it was first described as the *nerve conferred on bladder called container of bile (Galen, c173)*.

TRANSLATIONS:

1. *plexus cysticus (Wrisberg, 1808)*
   Original Latin form of ***cystic plexus (Wrisberg, 1808)***; p. 16.

EARLIER REFERENCES:

Earlier synonyms:

1. *nerve conferred on bladder called container of bile (Galen, c173)*
   Synonym for ***cystic plexus (Wrisberg, 1808)*** as described for macrodissected adult beef, pig, and/or macaque but not human; see May translation (1968, pp. 263 for name, and 262).
2. *twig to gall bladder (Vesalius, 1543a)*
   Synonym for macrodissected adult human ***cystic plexus (Wrisberg, 1808)***; see Richardson & Carman translation (2002, p. 200).
3. *cystic nerves (Walter, 1783)*
   Basically synonym for macrodissected adult human ***cystic plexus (Wrisberg, 1808)***; in the original Latin, *nervi cystici*, Table IV:*161–165*.

LATER SYNONYMS:

1. *middle hepatic plexus (Wrisberg, 1808)*
   Synonym for ***cystic plexus (Wrisberg, 1808)***; in the original Latin, *plexus hepaticus medius*, p. 16.

PARTLY CORRESPONDS:

1. *anterior cystic nerves (Mayer, 1794)*
   Components of macrodissected adult human ***cystic plexus (Wrisberg, 1808)*** ending around ventral (anterior) aspects of base of gall bladder; in the original Latin, *nervi cystici anteriores*; Part 6, Table IV-*54,55* (p. 28).
2. *inferior cystic nerves (Mayer, 1794)*
   Synonym for *anterior cystic nerves (Mayer, 1794)*; in the original Latin, *nervi cystici inferiores*; Part 6, Table IV-*54,55* (p. 28).
3. *deep cystic nerve (Mayer, 1794)*
   Component of macrodissected adult human ***cystic plexus (Wrisberg, 1808)*** ending around dorsal (posterior) aspects of base of gall bladder; in the original Latin, *nervus cysticus profundus*; Part 6, Table IV-*60* (p. 28).
4. *posterior cystic nerve (Mayer, 1794)*
   Synonym for *deep cystic nerve (Mayer, 1794)*; in the original Latin, *nervus cysticus posterior*; Part 6, Table IV-*60* (p. 28).

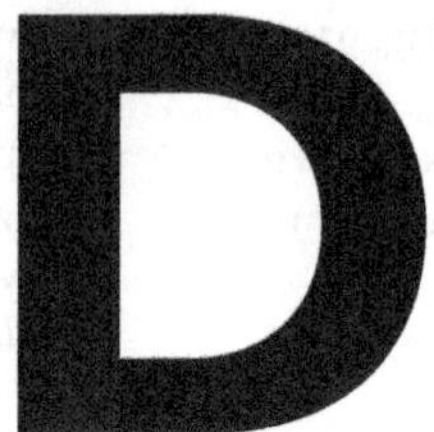

declive (>1840)

As described for macrodissected adult human, the part of the ***cerebellar vermis (Meckel, 1817)*** between ***culmen (Stroud, 1895)*** and ***folium vermis (>1840)***, medial to the right and left ***simple lobule (Jansen & Brodal, 1954)*** of the ***cerebellar hemisphere (Willis, 1664)***; see Larsell & Jansen (1972, Fig. 118), Angevine et al. (1961, Fig. 24), Carpenter (1976, Figs. 2.26, 14.1), Nieuwenhuys et al. (2008, Fig. 3.8-*30*). It was not recognized as such by 1840.

deep branch of lateral plantar nerve (>1840)

As described for macrodissected adult human, one of two terminal branches of the ***lateral plantar nerve (>1840)***, along with the ***superficial branch of lateral plantar nerve (>1840)***. It supplies the 2nd through 4th lumbrical, adductor hallucis, and all interossei (except sometimes those of the 4th space) muscles of the foot; see Durward (1951, p. 1112 and Figs. 951, 952), *Terminologia Anatomica* (1998, p. 141). It was perhaps first clearly delineated by Eustachi; see ***[deep branch of lateral plantar nerve (>1840)] (Eustachi, 1552)***.

EARLIER REFERENCES:

Illustrated, not named or described:

1. ***[deep branch of lateral plantar nerve (>1840)] (Eustachi, 1552)***
   Origin illustrated for macrodissected adult human; see Albinus edition (1761, Tab. 20-*21*).

Illustrated and described, not named:

1. ***[deep branch of lateral plantar nerve (>1840)] (Vieussens, 1684)***
   Accurately described and illustrated for macrodissected adult human; see Table 30-*R*.

Earlier synonyms:

1. *deep branch of external plantar branch of tibial nerve (Martin, 1781)*
   Synonym for macrodissected adult human ***deep branch of lateral plantar nerve*** (**>1840**); in the original Latin, *nervus tibialis ramus plantaris exterior ramus profundus*, p. 245.
2. *deep branch of external plantar nerve (Günther, 1786)*
   Synonym for macrodissected adult human ***deep branch of lateral plantar nerve (>1840)***; in the original Latin, *r. profundos*, p. 88.
3. *muscular branch of external plantar nerve (Günther, 1786)*
   Synonym for macrodissected adult human ***deep branch of lateral plantar nerve (>1840)***; in the original Latin, *r. musculares*, p. 88.
4. *internal branch of external plantar nerve (Jördens, 1788)*
   Synonym for macrodissected adult human ***deep branch of lateral plantar nerve (>1840)***; in the original Latin, *ramus internus nervi plantaris externi*, p. 12 and Table III-*213*.
5. *profound branch of exterior branch of tibial nerve (Burdin, 1803)*
   Synonym for macrodissected adult human ***deep branch of lateral plantar nerve (>1840)***; see translation (1803, Vol. 1, pp. 207–208).
6. *deep trunk of external plantar nerve (Meckel, 1817)*
   Synonym for macrodissected adult human ***deep branch of lateral plantar nerve (>1840)***; see translation (1832, Vol. 3, p. 21).
7. *muscular trunk of external plantar nerve (Meckel, 1817)*
   Synonym for macrodissected adult human ***deep branch of lateral plantar nerve (>1840)***; see translation (1832, Vol. 3, p. 21).
8. *middle branch of external plantar nerve (Meckel, 1817)*
   Synonym for macrodissected adult human ***deep branch of lateral plantar nerve (>1840)***; see translation (1832, Vol. 3, pp. 20–21).
9. *middle trunk of external plantar nerve (Meckel, 1817)*

Synonym for macrodissected adult human ***deep branch of lateral plantar nerve (>1840)***; see translation (1832, Vol. 3, p. 21).

10. *deep internal branch of external plantar nerve (Cloquet, 1828)*
    Synonym for macrodissected adult human ***deep branch of lateral plantar nerve (>1840)***; in the original French, *rameau interne profond du N. plantaire externe*, Plate CLXXIV, Figure 3-*16*.
11. *deep plantar nerve (Swan, 1830)*
    Synonym for macrodissected adult human ***deep branch of lateral plantar nerve (>1840)***; Plate XXV, Figure 3-*14*. Swan described its branches in detail.
12. *deep terminal branch of external plantar nerve (Cruveilhier, 1836)*
    Synonym for macrodissected adult human ***deep branch of lateral plantar nerve (>1840)***; in the original French, *branche terminale profonde*, p. 875.

PARTLY CORRESPONDS:

1. *superficial twig of deep branch of external plantar nerve (Jördens, 1788)*
   Described for macrodissected adult human as 1st root of *nerve to abductor digiti minimi and flexor brevis digiti minimi muscles (Jördens, 1788)*; in the original Latin, *ramulus ex ramus profundus nervi plantaris externi superficialis*, p. 12 and Table III-*214*. Thus, branch of ***deep branch of lateral plantar nerve (>1840)***.
2. *deep twig of deep branch of external plantar nerve (Jördens, 1788)*
   Branch of ***deep branch of lateral plantar nerve (>1840)*** described for macrodissected adult human as dividing into two muscular twigs; in the original Latin, *ramulus ex ramus profundus nervi plantaris externi profundus*, p. 12 and Table III-*215*.
3. *first twig of deep twig of deep branch of external plantar nerve to flexor digiti minimi brevis (Jördens, 1788)*
   Macrodissected adult human secondary branch of ***deep branch of lateral plantar nerve (>1840)*** to flexor digiti minimi brevis muscle of foot; in the original Latin, *surculus primus ramulus ex ramus profundus nervi plantaris externi profundus ad flexorem brevem digiti minimi*, p. 12 and Table III-*216*.
4. *second twig of deep twig of deep branch of external plantar nerve to abductor pollicis (Jördens, 1788)*
   Macrodissected adult human secondary branch of ***deep branch of lateral plantar nerve (>1840)*** to dorsal (posterior) part of abductor hallucis muscle; in the original Latin, *surculus secundus ramulus ex ramus profundus nervi plantaris externi profundus ad abductorem pollicis*, p. 12 and Table III-*217*.
5. *nerve to abductor pollicis muscle from deep branch of external plantar nerve (Fischer, 1791)*
   Branch of ***deep branch of lateral plantar nerve (>1840)*** to macrodissected adult human abductor hallucis muscle; in the original Latin, *nervus musculi abductoris pollicis*, p. 37.
6. *nerve to flexor digiti minimi brevis muscle from deep branch of external plantar nerve (Fischer, 1791)*
   Branch of ***deep branch of lateral plantar nerve (>1840)*** to macrodissected adult human flexor digiti minimi brevis muscle of foot; in the original Latin, *nervus musculi flexoris brevis digiti minimi*, p. 37.
7. *articular filaments of deep terminal branch of external plantar nerve (Cruveilhier, 1836)*
   Macrodissected adult human thin branches of *deep terminal branch of external plantar nerve (Cruveilhier, 1836)* to tarsometatarsal and intermetatarsal joints; in the original French, *filets articulaires*, p. 876.
8. *filament of third lumbrical of deep terminal branch of external plantar nerve (Cruveilhier, 1836)*
   Macrodissected adult human thin branch of *deep terminal branch of external plantar nerve (Cruveilhier, 1836)* to 3rd lumbrical muscle of foot; in the original French, *filet du troisième lombrical*, p. 876.
9. *filament of transverse abductor of deep terminal branch of external plantar nerve (Cruveilhier, 1836)*
   Macrodissected adult human thin branch of *deep terminal branch of external plantar nerve (Cruveilhier, 1836)* to transverse head of adductor hallucis muscle; in the original French, *filet de l'abducteur transverse*, p. 876.
10. *filaments of interosseous muscles of deep terminal branch of external plantar nerve (Cruveilhier, 1836)*
    Macrodissected adult human thin branches of *deep terminal branch of external plantar nerve (Cruveilhier, 1836)* to plantar interossei muscles; in the original French, *filets des muscles interosseux du troisième, du deuxième, et du premier espace*, p. 876.

deep branch of radial nerve (Martin, 1781)

As described for macrodissected adult human, one of two ***radial nerve (Du Verney, 1697)*** terminal branches continuing as the ***posterior interosseous nerve (Quain & Wilson, 1839)*** after crossing the supinator muscle; see Hamilton (1976, p. 651). For Martin's use in macrodissected adult human, see p. 200; beautifully illustrated by Loder (1803, Tab. CLXXX, Fig. 2). It was known to Galen; see ***[deep branch of radial nerve (Martin, 1781)] (Galen, c177)***.

TRANSLATIONS:

1. *nervus radialis ramus profundus (Martin, 1781)*
   Original Latin form of ***deep branch of radial nerve (Martin, 1781)***; p. 185.

EARLIER REFERENCES:

Described, not named or illustrated:

1. ***[deep branch of radial nerve (Martin, 1781)] (Galen, c177)***
   Galen described most of its muscular branches in macrodissected beef, pig, and/or macaque but not human; see Singer translation (1999, pp. 72–73).

Earlier synonyms:

1. *lower branch of fourth nerve entering arm (Vesalius, 1543a)*
   Synonym for ***deep branch of radial nerve (Martin, 1781)***; Vesalius described most of its muscular branches in macrodissected adult human; see Richardson & Carman translation (2002, pp. 242–243).
2. *internal branch of radial nerve (Haase, 1781)*

Synonym for macrodissected adult human ***deep branch of radial nerve (Martin, 1781)***; in the original Latin, *nervus radialis ramus internus*, pp. 101–102.

LATER SYNONYMS:

1. *deep branch of muscular spiral nerve (Monro, 1783)*
Synonym for macrodissected adult human ***deep branch of radial nerve (Martin, 1781)***; Table 26-*I*.
2. *posterior branch of radial nerve (Cloquet, 1816)*
Synonym for macrodissected adult human ***deep branch of radial nerve (Martin, 1781)***; p. 653.
3. *deep nerve of muscular spiral nerve (Bell & Bell, 1816)*
Synonym for macrodissected adult human ***deep branch of radial nerve (Martin, 1781)***; in the original Latin, *nervus profundus*, Vol. 2, p. 538.
4. *muscular branch of radial nerve (Meckel, 1817)*
Synonym for macrodissected adult human ***deep branch of radial nerve (Martin, 1781)***; see translation (1832, Vol. 3, pp. 25–26).
5. *external interosseous nerve of forearm (Bock, 1827)*
Synonym for macrodissected adult human ***deep branch of radial nerve (Martin, 1781)***; in the original Latin, *nerv. interosseus externus antibrachii*, Table IV-*31*.
6. *muscular branch of musculo-spiral nerve (Quain, 1832)*
Synonym for macrodissected adult human ***deep branch of radial nerve (Martin, 1781)***; p. 690.
7. *antibrachial deep branch of radial nerve (Cruveilhier, 1836)*
Synonym for macrodissected adult human ***deep branch of radial nerve (Martin, 1781)***; in the original French, *branche profonde anti-brachiale du radial*, p. 817.
8. *antibrachial muscular branch of radial nerve (Cruveilhier, 1836)*
Synonym for macrodissected adult human ***deep branch of radial nerve (Martin, 1781)***; in the original French, *branche musculaire anti-brachiale du radial*, p. 817.
9. *posterior branch of musculo-spiral nerve (Quain & Wilson, 1839)*
Synonym for macrodissected adult human ***deep branch of radial nerve (Martin, 1781)***; Plate XIX, Figure 2-*b*.

deep branch of ulnar nerve (Fyfe, 1800)

As described for macrodissected adult human, a terminal branch supplying the three short muscles of the little finger, the interossei and 3rd and 4th lumbricals, and the adductor pollicis, first palmar interosseous, and flexor pollicis brevis muscles; see Williams & Warwick (1980, p. 1100). For Fyfe's use in macrodissected adult human, see Vol. 2, p. 313. It was probably known to Vesalius; see ***[deep branch of ulnar nerve (Fyfe, 1800)] (Vesalius, 1543a)***.

EARLIER REFERENCES:

Described, not named or illustrated:

1. ***[deep branch of ulnar nerve (Fyfe, 1800)] (Vesalius, 1543a)***
Probably alluded to for macrodissected adult human in terms of some associated muscles; see Richardson & Carman translation (2002, p. 244).

Illustrated, not named or described:

1. ***[deep branch of ulnar nerve (Fyfe, 1800)] (Eustachi, 1552)***
Origin illustrated for macrodissected adult human; see Albinus edition (1761, Tab. 19-52, p. 116).

Earlier synonyms:

1. *internal branch of cubital nerve (Haase, 1781)*
Synonym for macrodissected adult human ***deep branch of ulnar nerve (Fyfe, 1800)***; in the original Latin, *nervus cubitalis ramus internus*, pp. 99–100. Haase described 3 branches, one *deep* and two *superficial*.
2. *ramus profundus volaris ramus volaris nervus cubitalis (Martin, 1781)*
Latin form of macrodissected adult human ***deep branch of ulnar nerve (Fyfe, 1800)***; p. 217.
3. *deep volar branch of ulnar nerve (Günther, 1786)*
Synonym for macrodissected adult human ***superficial branch of ulnar nerve (Fyfe, 1800)***; in the original Latin, *ramus profundum volarem*; p. 76.

LATER SYNONYMS:

1. *deep palmar nerve (Fyfe, 1800)*
Synonym for macrodissected adult human ***deep branch of ulnar nerve (Fyfe, 1800)***; Vol. 2, p. 313.
2. *deep branch of volar branch of cubital nerve (Loder, 1803)*
Synonym for macrodissected adult human ***deep branch of ulnar nerve (Fyfe, 1800)***; *ramus profundus rami volaris*, Table CLXXX, Figure 1-*94*.
3. *deep branch of cubital nerve (Caldani, 1813, 1814)*
Synonym for macrodissected adult human ***deep branch of ulnar nerve (Fyfe, 1800)***; in the original Latin, *ramus nervus cubitalis profundus*, Table CCLIX, Figure 2-*33*.
4. *deep twig of palmar branch of ulnar nerve (Meckel, 1817)*
Synonym for macrodissected adult human ***deep branch of ulnar nerve (Fyfe, 1800)***; see translation (1832, Vol. 3, p. 28) and *palmar branch of ulnar nerve (Meckel, 1817)*.
5. *muscular twig of palmar branch of ulnar nerve (Meckel, 1817)*
Synonym for macrodissected adult human ***deep branch of ulnar nerve (Fyfe, 1800)***; see translation (1832, Vol. 3, p. 28) and *palmar branch of ulnar nerve (Meckel, 1817)*.
6. *deep-seated palmar branch of ulnar nerve (Quain, 1828)*
Synonym for macrodissected adult human ***deep branch of ulnar nerve (Fyfe, 1800)***; p. 420.
7. *deep branch of palmar branch of cubital nerve (Cloquet, 1828)*
Synonym for macrodissected adult human ***deep branch of ulnar nerve (Fyfe, 1800)***; in the original French, *rameau profond*, Plate CLXIX, Figure 1-*70*.
8. *deep terminal branch of cubital nerve (Cruveilhier, 1836)*
Synonym for macrodissected adult human ***deep branch of ulnar nerve (Fyfe, 1800)***; in the original French, *branche terminale profonde*, p. 813.
9. *muscular branch of hand of cubital nerve (Cruveilhier, 1836)*
Synonym for *deep terminal branch of cubital nerve (Cruveilhier, 1836)*; in the original French, *branche musculaire*, pp. 813, 814. Branches described in detail.
10. *deep palmar branch of ulnar nerve (Quain & Wilson, 1839)*
Synonym for macrodissected adult human ***deep branch of ulnar nerve (Fyfe, 1800)***; Plate XVIII, Figure 2-*r*.

PARTLY CORRESPONDS:

1. *anastomotic branch of volar deep branch of ulnar nerve with superficial nerve (Günther, 1786)*
   Macrodissected adult human ***communicating branch (Winslow, 1733)*** between *volar deep branch of ulnar nerve (Günther, 1786)* and *volar superficial branch of ulnar nerve (Gunther, 1786)*; in the original Latin, *r. anastomoticum cum n. superficiali*, p. 76.
2. *muscular branch of volar deep branch of ulnar nerve (Günther, 1786)*
   Basically ***deep branch of ulnar nerve (Fyfe, 1800)*** trunk in macrodissected adult human; in the original Latin, *r. muscularem*, p. 76.
3. *branch of deep branch of ulnar nerve to adductor muscle of little finger and last lumbrical muscle (Swan, 1830)*
   Macrodissected adult human branch of ***deep branch of ulnar nerve (Fyfe, 1800)***, essentially to 3rd palmar interosseous muscle and 4th lumbrical muscle; Plate XXII-27.
4. *branches for three muscles of hypothenar eminence from deep terminal branch of cubital nerve (Cruveilhier, 1836)*
   For macrodissected adult human, three branches of ***deep branch of ulnar nerve (Fyfe, 1800)*** to the three hypothenar muscles; in the original French, *branches pour les trois muscles de l'éminence hypothénar*, p. 813.

deep fibular nerve (Fyfe, 1800)

As described for macrodissected adult human, a terminal branch of the ***common fibular nerve (>1840)*** generating ***muscular branches of deep fibular nerve (>1840)*** and ***digital branch of deep fibular nerve (>1840)***; see Durward (1951, p. 1107 and Figs. 948, 949; referred to as *anterior tibial nerve*), Hamilton (1976, Figs. 835, 836), and Williams & Warwick (1980, Fig. 7.212). For Fyfe's use in macrodissected adult human, see Vol. 2, p. 331. He divided it into three branches: dorsal, deep of foot, and superficial; see Bell (1803b, p. 209). It was known to Galen; see ***[deep fibular nerve (Fyfe, 1800)] (Galen, c173)***.

EARLIER REFERENCES:

Described, not named or illustrated:

1. ***[deep fibular nerve (Fyfe, 1800)] (Galen, c173)***
   Described for macrodissected adult beef, pig, and/or macaque but not human; see May translation (1968, p. 706).

Illustrated, not named or described:

1. ***[deep fibular nerve (Fyfe, 1800)] (Eustachi, 1552)***
   Clearly illustrated for macrodissected adult human; see Albinus edition (1761, Tab. 19/2-*15,16*). Vieussens (1684, Tab. 29-*81,94*) described and illustrated at least part of it for macrodissected adult human.

Earlier synonyms:

1. *superior anterior branch of small sciatic branch (Winslow, 1733)*
   Synonym for macrodissected adult human ***deep fibular nerve (Fyfe, 1800)***; Section VI, p. 93.
2. *deep branch of peroneal nerve (Haase, 1781)*
   Synonym for macrodissected adult human ***deep fibular nerve (Fyfe, 1800)***; in the original Latin, *ramus nervus peroneus profundus*, p. 113.
3. *deep peroneal nerve (Günther, 1781)*
   Synonym for macrodissected adult human ***deep fibular nerve (Fyfe, 1800)***; in the original Latin, *nervus peroneum profundum*, p. 88.
4. *muscular branch of peroneal nerve (Martin, 1781)*
   Synonym for macrodissected adult human ***deep fibular nerve (Fyfe, 1800)***; in the original Latin, *nervus peroneus ramus muscularis*, p. 248. Referred to in Table XI as *nervus muscularis*.
5. *deep muscular branch of peroneal nerve (Soemmerring, 1791)*
   Synonym for macrodissected adult human ***deep fibular nerve (Fyfe, 1800)***; p. 312; also see Soemmerring (1798, p. 333) where Soemmerring used the Latin, *nervus musculos adiens profundior*.
6. *interosseal nerve (Mayer, 1794)*
   Synonym for macrodissected adult human ***deep fibular nerve (Fyfe, 1800)***; in the original Latin, *nervus interosseus*; Part 5, Table V, Figure 1-*E* (p. 26). Quain (1837, p. 801) in English spelled it *inter-osseous nerve* for macrodissected adult human.

LATER SYNONYMS:

1. *deep peroneal nerve (Bell, 1803a)*
   Synonym for macrodissected adult human ***deep fibular nerve (Fyfe, 1800)***; in the original Latin, *nervi peronei profundae*, Table VIII-*16*.
2. *praetibio-super-plantaris nerve (Burdin, 1803)*
   Synonym for macrodissected adult human ***deep fibular nerve (Fyfe, 1800)***; see translation (1803, Vol. 1, p. 206).
3. *anterior tibial branch of external popliteal nerve (Cloquet, 1816)*
   Synonym for macrodissected adult human ***deep fibular nerve (Fyfe, 1800)***; in the original French, *branche tibiale antérieure*, p. 675.
4. *anterior tibial nerve (Meckel, 1817)*
   Synonym for macrodissected adult human ***deep fibular nerve (Fyfe, 1800)***; see translation (1832, Vol. 3, p. 18). Cloquet (1816, p. 675) attributed the term (dubiously) to Soemmerring without citation.
5. *deep seated branch of fibular nerve (Bell & Bell, 1829)*
   Synonym for macrodissected adult human ***deep fibular nerve (Fyfe, 1800)***; p. 590.
6. *deeper division of fibular nerve (Bell & Bell, 1829)*
   Synonym for macrodissected adult human ***deep fibular nerve (Fyfe, 1800)***; p. 590.
7. *interosseal branch of external popliteal sciatic nerve (Cruveilhier, 1836)*
   Synonym for macrodissected adult human ***deep fibular nerve (Fyfe, 1800)***; in the original French, *branche interosseuse*, p. 866.

PARTLY CORRESPONDS:

1. *internal branch of deep peroneal nerve (Fischer, 1791)*
   Fischer described for macrodissected adult human two terminal branches of ***deep fibular nerve (Fyfe, 1800)***,

internal and external. The internal branch in turn generates *common twig to extensor digitorum brevis muscle and superior interossei muscles (Fischer, 1791)* and *metatarsus pollicis nerve (Fischer, 1791)*. In the original Latin, *ramus internus nervi peronei profundi*, p. 33.

2. *interosseal nerve (Soemmerring, 1791)*
   Extension of *deep muscular branch of peroneal nerve (Soemmerring, 1791)*; in the original Latin, *nervus interosseus*, p. 312; also see Soemmerring (1798, p. 333).
3. *branch of peroneal nerve to anterior tibial artery (Swan, 1830)*
   Macrodissected adult human branch of ***deep fibular nerve (Fyfe, 1800)*** coursing along anterior tibial artery; Plate XXIII, Figure 4-6.

deep petrosal nerve (Meckel, 1817)

As described for macrodissected adult human, it extends from the ***internal carotid plexus (>1840)*** to the junction of the ***nerve of pterygoid canal (>1840)*** and ***greater petrosal nerve (>1840)***. It contains postganglionic sympathetic ***axons (Kölliker, 1896)*** from the ***superior cervical ganglion (Vieussens, 1684)*** and is thus a ***paravertebral nerve (>1840)***. As such, it played a central role in early descriptions of the ***sympathetic trunk (Winslow, 1733)*** as arising either from what is now recognized as the ***intermediofacial nerve trunk (>1840)*** or from the ***maxillary nerve (Meckel, 1753)***, or from both; see review by Meckel (1748, p. 53 note *q*), also see Mitchell (1953, p. 217 and Fig. 93), Williams & Warwick (1980, Fig. 7.184). For Meckel's (1817) use see translation (1832, Vol. 3, p. 67), where it is given as *deep petrous nerve* in contrast to *superficial petrous nerve (Meckel, 1817)*. It was clearly described by Meckel's grandfather—see *deep major branch of Vidian nerve (Meckel, 1748)*— although its existence was probably indicated by Willis; see ***[deep petrosal nerve (Meckel, 1817)] (Willis, 1664)***.

ALTERNATE SPELLINGS:

1. *deep petrous nerve (Meckel, 1832)*
   English form of ***deep petrosal nerve (Meckel, 1817)***; Vol. 3, p. 67.

EARLIER REFERENCES:

Earlier synonyms:

1. *deep major branch of Vidian nerve (Meckel, 1748)*
   Synonym for macrodissected adult human ***deep petrosal nerve (Meckel, 1817)***; in the original Latin, *ramus nervus Vidianus majorem profundum*, pp. 52, 53 and Figures 2, 5-*q*, 3, 6-*r*, and 4-*s*.
2. *root of intercostal nerve (Meckel, 1751)*
   Synonym for *deep major branch of Vidian nerve (Meckel, 1748)*; in the original French, *la racine du nerf intercostal*, Figure 1-*s*.
3. *third root of intercostal nerve (Bang, 1770)*
   In Bang's description of macrodissected adult human, deep ascending branch of ***superior cervical ganglion (Vieussens, 1684)*** probably corresponding to ***deep petrosal nerve (Meckel, 1817)***; in the original Latin, *(profundus) radicem nervi intercostalis tertiam*, Figure II-*n*.
4. *deep branch of Vidian nerve (Neubauer, 1772)*
   Shorter form of *deep major branch of Vidian nerve (Meckel, 1748)*; in the original Latin, *profundus ramus Vidiani nervi*, p. 29.
5. *deep Vidian nerve (Günther, 1786)*
   Synonym for *deep branch of Vidian nerve (Neubauer, 1772)*; in the original Latin, *Vidianum profundum*, p. 47.
6. *pterygoid nerve (Andersch & Soemmerring, 1792)*
   Synonym for macrodissected adult human ***deep petrosal nerve (Meckel, 1817)***; in the original Latin, *nervo pterygoideo*; pp. 163–165. Regarded as derived from ***trigeminal nerve (Winslow, 1733)***: *quinti nervi capitis*.
7. *second root of intercostal nerves (Mayer, 1794)*
   Synonym for macrodissected adult human ***deep petrosal nerve (Meckel, 1817)***; in the original Latin, *radix secunda nervi intercostalis*, Part 5, Table VIII, Figure 3-*q*. In an accompanying figure (Fig. 4-*s*) referred to as *third root of intercostal nerve (Bang, 1770)*, perhaps reflecting different arrangements in different cadavers.
8. *inferior branch of vidian nerve (Burdin, 1803)*
   Synonym for macrodissected adult human ***deep petrosal nerve (Meckel, 1817)***; see translation (1803, Vol. 1, p. 174).
9. *inferior branch of pterygoid nerve (Cloquet, 1816)*
   Synonym for macrodissected adult human ***deep petrosal nerve (Meckel, 1817)***; in the original French, *rameau inférieur du nerf ptérygoïdien*, p. 685.
10. *carotid branch of Vidian nerve (Cloquet, 1816)*
    Synonym for macrodissected adult human ***deep petrosal nerve (Meckel, 1817)***; in the original French, *rameau carotidien du nerf vidien*, p. 685. Todd (1836–1839, p. 288) referred to it in English as *carotidean branch of Vidian nerve*; he also noted that in macrodissected adult human it sometimes joins ***pterygopalatine ganglion (>1840)*** directly.
11. *carotid branch of pterygoid nerve (Cloquet, 1816)*
    Synonym for macrodissected adult human ***deep petrosal nerve (Meckel, 1817)***; in the original French, *rameau carotidien du nerf ptérygoïdien*, p. 685.

LATER SYNONYMS:

1. *inferior petrosal nerve (Meckel, 1817)*
   Synonym for ***deep petrosal nerve (Meckel, 1817)***; in the translation (1832, Vol. 3, p. 67) it was given as *inferior petrous nerve*.
2. *deep thread of Vidian fascicle (Bellingeri, 1818)*
   Synonym for macrodissected adult human ***deep petrosal nerve (Meckel, 1817)***; in the original Latin, *stamen profundus*, see Table I.
3. *intercostal thread of Vidian fascicle (Bellingeri, 1818)*
   Synonym for macrodissected adult human ***deep petrosal nerve (Meckel, 1817)***; in the original Latin, *stamen intercostalis*, see Table I.

4. *sympathetic branch of Vidian nerve (Arnold, 1834)*
 Synonym for macrodissected adult human ***deep petrosal nerve (Meckel, 1817)***; in the original Latin, *ramo sympathico nervi Vidiani*, p. 8.
5. *lesser deep petrosal nerve (Arnold, 1834)*
 Apparently synonym for macrodissected adult human ***deep petrosal nerve (Meckel, 1817)***; in the original Latin, *nervus petrosus profundus minor*, p. 13. Arnold described a connection from ***tympanic nerve (Arnold, 1834)*** to *lesser deep petrosal nerve (Arnold, 1834)*; p. 13, II3e. See Williams & Warwick (1980, Fig. 7.184), where it goes partly via ***internal carotid plexus (>1840)***.
6. *connection of carotid nerve with nasal ganglion (Arnold, 1834)*
 Synonym for macrodissected adult human ***deep petrosal nerve (Meckel, 1817)***; in the original Latin, *conjunctio nervus caroticus ramus externus cum ganglio nasali*, p. 18.
7. *anastomotic branch of external branch of carotid branch of superior cervical ganglion with sphenopalatine ganglion (Cruveilhier, 1836)*
 Synonym for macrodissected adult human *carotid branch of Vidian nerve (Cloquet, 1816)*; in the original French, *rameau anastomotique avec le ganglion sphéno-palatin*, p. 986.
8. *carotid branch of posterior branch of spheno-palatine ganglion (Quain & Wilson, 1839)*
 Synonym for macrodissected adult human ***deep petrosal nerve (Meckel, 1817)***; Plate XXVII-*o,p*.
9. *sympathetic root of sphenopalatine ganglion (>1840)*
 Synonym for ***deep petrosal nerve (Meckel, 1817)***; see Mitchell (1953, p. 217).

PARTLY CORRESPONDS:

1. ***[deep petrosal nerve (Meckel, 1817)] (Willis, 1664)***
 Willis indicated for macrodissected adult (presumably) human several communications between ***trigeminal nerve (Winslow, 1733)*** and ***sympathetic trunk (Winslow, 1733)***, which in a crude, inaccurate way may indicate existence of ***deep petrosal nerve (Meckel, 1817)***; see Figure 1-*b,b* on p. 302.

deep temporal nerves (Haase, 1781)

As described for macrodissected adult human, two or three branches of the ***anterior branch of mandibular nerve (>1840)*** supplying the temporal muscle; see Williams & Warwick (1980, p. 1066) and beautiful illustration by Henle (1871, Fig. 243). For Haase's use in macrodissected adult human see Index, sections 133–134, where he described external and internal ***nerves (Herophilus, c335–c280 BC)*** or branches. They were known to Galen; see ***[deep temporal nerves (Haase, 1781)] (Galen, c173)***.

TRANSLATIONS:

1. *nervus temporalis profundus (Haase, 1781)*
 Original Latin (singular) form of ***deep temporal nerves (Haase, 1781)***; see Index, sections 133–134.

EARLIER REFERENCES:

Described, not named or illustrated:

1. ***[deep temporal nerves (Haase, 1781)] (Galen, c173)***
 Described for macrodissected adult beef, pig, and/or macaque but not human; see May translation (1968, pp. 440–441, 451, 453, 507).

Illustrated and described, not named:

1. ***[deep temporal nerves (Haase, 1781)] (Vesalius, 1543a)***
 Mentioned and illustrated for macrodissected adult human; see Richardson & Carman translation (2002, p. 189). Du Verney clearly illustrated their origin for macrodissected adult human (1683, Pl. 13-*1*).

Earlier synonyms:

1. *deep temporal branches of third branch of fifth pair (Meckel, 1748)*
 Synonym for ***deep temporal nerves (Haase, 1781)***, described and illustrated with two major branches for macrodissected adult human; in the original Latin, *ramorum temporalium profundorum tertii rami quinti paris*, p. 82.
2. *temporal nerve (Schaarschmidt, 1750)*
 Synonym for macrodissected adult human ***deep temporal nerves (Haase, 1781)***; in the original Latin, *nervus temporalis*, p. 27.

LATER SYNONYMS:

1. *temporo-muscular nerves (Burdin, 1803)*
 Synonym for macrodissected adult human ***deep temporal nerves (Haase, 1781)***; see translation (1803, Vol. 1, p. 175).
2. *crotaphitic surculus of ganglioform plexus of inferior maxillary branch (Bellingeri, 1818)*
 Essentially synonym for macrodissected adult human ***deep temporal nerves (Haase, 1781)***; in the original Latin, *surculus crotaphiticus*, see Table I. Also see *nervus crotaphiticus-nervus buccinatorius (Palletta, 1784)*.
3. *deep temporal branches of inferior maxillary nerve (Todd, 1836–1839)*
 Synonym for macrodissected adult human ***deep temporal nerves (Haase, 1781)***; p. 291. Also see Quain (1837, p. 764) who provided Latin form, *r. temporales profundi*.

PARTLY CORRESPONDS:

1. *internal fascicle of crotaphitic surculus of ganglioform plexus of inferior maxillary branch (Bellingeri, 1818)*
 Essentially corresponds to macrodissected adult human ***middle deep temporal nerve (>1840)*** and ***anterior deep temporal nerve (Arnold, 1834)*** considered together; in the original Latin, *fasciculus internus*, see Table I.

deferential plexus (Cruveilhier, 1836)

As defined for macrodissected adult human male, an extension of the ***extrinsic vesical plexus (1840)*** to the deferent duct (ductus deferens, vas deferens); see Mitchell (1953, pp. 295–296), Williams & Warwick (1980, p. 1135), *Terminologia Anatomica* (1998, p. 143). For Cruveilhier's use in macrodissected adult human male, see p. 1027.

TRANSLATIONS:

1. *plexus déférentiel (Cruveilhier, 1836)*
 Original French form of ***deferential plexus (Cruveilhier, 1836)***; p. 1027.

dentate gyrus (>1840)

As described for macrodissected adult mammal and with cellular architecture, connections, and development, topologically the most medial component of the ***hippocampal region (>1840)***, lying adjacent to the more lateral ***Ammon's horn (Vicq d'Azyr, 1784)*** component; see Swanson et al. (1987), Williams & Warwick (1980, Fig. 7.121), Duvernoy (1988). The term was used early on by, for example, Honegger (1890, p. 266) and Ranson (1920, Fig. 209). It was first vaguely delineated as the *substantia cinerea (Tarin, 1750)*.

EARLIER REFERENCES:

Earlier synonyms:

1. *substantia cinerea (Tarin, 1750)*
   Tarin provided first vague description and illustration of ***dentate gyrus (>1840)*** in describing macrodissected adult human ***hippocampal region (>1840)***; Table II, Figure 6; see Meyer (1971, p. 22).
2. *internal dentate margin of Ammon's horn (Vicq d'Azyr, 1784)*
   Synonym for macrodissected adult human ***dentate gyrus (>1840)***; in the original French, *bord interne et dentelé de la corne d'Ammon*; see Vicq d'Azyr (1786, Pl. XV-37,39). Also see Burdach (1822, p. 374).
3. *internal margin of hippocampus major (Vicq d'Azyr, 1786)*
   Synonym for macrodissected adult human ***dentate gyrus (>1840)***; in the original French, *bord interne du grand hippocampe*, Plate XX-*a/d*. Also see Meyer (1971, p. 22).
4. *concave margin of hippocampus major (Vicq d'Azyr, 1786)*
   Synonym for macrodissected adult human ***dentate gyrus (>1840)***; in the original French, *bord concave du grand hippocampe*, Plate XX-*a/d*. Also Meyer (1971, p. 22).
5. *dentate margin of hippocampus major (Vicq d'Azyr, 1786)*
   Synonym for macrodissected adult human ***dentate gyrus (>1840)***; in the original French, *bord dentelé du grand hippocampe*, Plate XX-*a/d*. Also see Meyer (1971, p. 22).
6. *gadroonate margin of hippocampus major (Vicq d'Azyr, 1786)*
   Synonym for macrodissected adult human ***dentate gyrus (>1840)***; in the original French, *bord godronné du grand hippocampe*, Plate XX-*a/d*. Also see Meyer (1971, p. 22).
7. *crenate part of hippocampus major (Vicq d'Azyr, 1786)*
   Synonym for macrodissected adult human ***dentate gyrus (>1840)***; in the original French, *portion crenelée du grand hippocampe*, Plate XXV, Figure III-*m*.
8. *plaited margin of pedes hippocampi (Fyfe, 1800)*
   Synonym for macrodissected adult human ***dentate gyrus (>1840)***; Vol. 2, p. 20.
9. *serrated margin of pedes hippocampi (Fyfe, 1800)*
   Synonym for macrodissected adult human ***dentate gyrus (>1840)***; Vol. 2, p. 20.
10. *indented margin of pedes hippocampi (Fyfe, 1800)*
    Synonym for macrodissected adult human ***dentate gyrus (>1840)***; Vol. 2, p. 20.
11. *indented border (Reil, 1812c)*
    Synonym for macrodissected adult human ***dentate gyrus (>1840)***; Table XIII-*H*.
12. *fascia dentata (Döllinger, 1814)*
    Döllinger's German synonym, *gezähnte Leiste* (p. 10), for ***dentate gyrus (>1840)*** was translated into Latin (*fascia dentata*) by Meckel (1817; Vol. 3, p. 488); also see Burdach (1822, p. 374), Meyer (1971, p. 22).
13. *indented band (Gordon, 1815)*
    Synonym for macrodissected adult human ***dentate gyrus (>1840)***; p. 105, also see Burdach (1822, p. 374).
14. *taeniam cornu Ammonis cineream (Volkmann, 1831)*
    Essentially synonym for macrodissected adult mammalian ***dentate gyrus (>1840)***; p. 53, Table XVII, Figure 3-*b,b**and Table XVIII, Figure 5-*b*.

PARTLY CORRESPONDS:

1. *tail of fascia dentata (Arnold, 1838b)*
   Macrodissected adult human *band of Giacomini (>1840)*; in the original Latin, *cauda fascia dentata*, Table IV, Figure 1-δ. See Duvernoy (1988, p. 31).
2. *band of Giacomini (>1840)*
   Slight elevation on medial and ventral surface of macrodissected adult human *uncus (Vicq d'Azyr, 1786)*, indicating underlying ventral (anterior, temporal) end of ***dentate gyrus (>1840)***; see Duvernoy (1988, pp. 31–32, Figs. 11, 17, 18, 75B), Giacomini (1884).

dentate nucleus (>1840)

As described for adult human with gross dissection, and for adult mammal in general with cellular architecture and connections, the large lateral component of the ***cerebellar nuclei (>1840)***, lying lateral to the ***interposed nucleus (>1840)*** or when present its more lateral differentiation the ***globose nucleus (>1840)***; see Nieuwenhuys et al. (2008, pp. 200, 820 and Fig. 5.12-23). It was first described as the *rhomboid body (Vieussens, 1684)*.

EARLIER REFERENCES:

Earlier synonyms:

1. *rhomboid body (Vieussens, 1684)*
   Synonym for macrodissected adult human ***dentate nucleus (>1840)***; in the original Latin, *corpus rhomboïdeum*, p. 78, Table XIII-*d*. See Burdach (1822, p. 289).
2. *rhomboid substance (Vieussens, 1684)*
   Synonym for *rhomboid body (Vieussens, 1684)*; in the original Latin, *rhomboidaem substantiam*; p. 78.
3. *dentate body of cerebellum (Vicq d'Azyr, 1784)*
   Synonym for macrodissected adult human ***dentate nucleus (>1840)***; in the original French *le corps dentelé*, and in the original Latin *corpus dentatum cerebelli*, p. 580 and Vicq d'Azyr (1786, Pl. XXXI, Fig. III:20-23).
4. *serrated body of cerebellum (Vicq d'Azyr, 1784)*
   Synonym for macrodissected adult human ***dentate nucleus (>1840)***; in the original French *le corps festonné*,

and in the original Latin *corpus serratum cerebelli*, p. 580 and Vicq d'Azyr (1786, Pl. XXXI, Fig. III:*20-23*).

5. *corpus truncus medullaris (Günther, 1786)*
   Synonym for macrodissected adult human ***dentate nucleus (>1840)***; p. 18.
6. *nucleus (Soemmerring, 1791)*
   Refers to macrodissected adult human *dentate body of cerebellum (Vicq d'Azyr, 1786)*. Soemmerring also compared it with ***inferior olivary complex (>1840)***; in the original German, *Kern*, pp. 53–54, see Burdach (1822, p. 289).
7. *central nucleus (Chaussier, 1807)*
   Synonym for macrodissected adult human ***dentate nucleus (>1840)***; in the original Latin, *nucleus centralis*, p. 98, see Burdach (1822, p. 289).
8. *ciliary body (Reil, 1807-1808a)*
   Synonym for macrodissected adult human ***dentate nucleus (>1840)***; see Mayo translation (1822, Tab. V, Fig. I-*t*). Reil observed "The ciliary bodies lie strictly in the hemispheres of the cerebellum, whence it happens that they are wanting in animals which have diminutive hemispheres, or none at all." (1812c; see Mayo translation, 1823, p. 129). Arnold (1838a, p. 37) gave the Latin (plural), *corpora ciliaria*.
9. *cerebellar ganglion (Gall & Spurzheim, 1810)*
   Synonym for macrodissected adult human ***dentate nucleus (>1840)***; in the original Latin, *ganglion cerebelli*, p. 261, see Burdach (1822, p. 289). "…this ganglion is not situated in the middle of the cerebellum, but commences where this mass is connected with the medulla oblongata" (Spurzheim, 1826, p. 122—where it was also called *ganglion of cerebellum*, p. 230 note *s*). In his translation, Knox (1832, Suppl. Pl. IV-*g*) also called it *ganglion of cerebellum*.
10. *moriform body (Tiedemann, 1816)*
    Synonym for ***dentate nucleus (>1840)***, as possibly observed in 4-month human fetus; see translation (1826, p. 48).
11. *great medullary nucleus (Tiedemann, 1816)*
    Tiedemann ascribed this synonym for ***dentate nucleus (>1840)*** to Reil, without providing a citation; see translation (1826, p. 65).
12. *corpus fimbriatum (Meckel, 1817)*
    Synonym for macrodissected adult human ***dentate nucleus (>1840)***; Vol. 3, p. 475. Also see Burdach (1822, p. 290).
13. *dentate body of cerebellar peduncles (Desmoulins, 1825)*
    Synonym for macrodissected adult human ***dentate nucleus (>1840)***; in the original French, *corps dentelé des pédoncules du cervelet*, Plate XIII, Figure 3-*q*.
14. *ganglion of increase to cerebellum (Quain, 1832)*
    Synonym for macrodissected adult human ***dentate nucleus (1840)***; p. 649, also see Quain (1837, Fig. 154-*m*).
15. *cerebellar olive (Cruveilhier, 1836)*
    Synonym for macrodissected adult human ***dentate nucleus (1840)***; in the original French, *olive du cervelet*, p. 632.

denticulate ligament (Monro, 1783)

As described for macrodissected adult human, there is one on each side of the ***spinal cord (Galen, c162–c166)*** arising from a line midway between the origins of the ***dorsal roots (Spurzheim, 1826)*** and ***ventral roots (>1840)***. Each is a row of about 21 flattened lateral bands of collagenous tissue associated medially with the ***pia (Galen, c192)*** and/or ***epipial layer (Key & Retzius, 1875)*** and extending through the ***subarachnoid space (Magendie, 1827)*** with their lateral tips firmly attached to the ***arachnoid (Blasius, 1666)*** and overlying ***dura (Galen, c177)***; see Millen & Woollam (1962, p. 95), *Dorland's* (2003, p. 1039). For Monro's use in macrodissected adult human, see p. 29 and Table 10, Figure 1:*a-x*. He provided the first clear description of it.

TRANSLATIONS:

1. *ligamentum denticulatum (Monro, 1783)*
   Original Latin form of *denticulate ligament (Monro, 1783)*; p. 29.

LATER SYNONYMS:

1. *serrated membrane (Gordon, 1815)*
   Synonym for macrodissected adult human ***denticulate ligament (Monro, 1783)***; p. 185.

descending superficial branches of cervical plexus (Quain, 1828)

As described for macrodissected adult human, branches of the 3rd and 4th cervical ***spinal nerve ventral branches (>1840)*** generating the ***supraclavicular nerves (Meckel, 1817)***; see Durward (1951, p. 1061 and Fig. 919), Williams & Warwick (1980, p. 1092). For Quain's use in macrodissected adult human, see p. 490. They were known to Galen; see ***[descending superficial branches of cervical plexus (Quain, 1828)] (Galen, c173)***.

EARLIER REFERENCES:

Described, not named or illustrated:

1. ***[descending superficial branches of cervical plexus (Quain, 1828)] (Galen, c173)***
   Alluded to for macrodissected adult beef, pig, and/or macaque but not human; see May translation (1968, p. 598) and Duckworth translation (1962, p. 238).

Earlier synonyms:

1. *thoracic part of trachelo-cutanean plexus (Burdin, 1803)*
   Synonym for macrodissected adult human *thoracic part of tracheosubcutaneous nerves (Chaussier, 1809)*; see translation (1803, Vol. 1, p. 188).
2. *thoracic part of tracheosubcutaneous nerves (Chaussier, 1809)*
   Synonym for macrodissected adult human ***descending superficial branches of cervical plexus (Quain, 1828)***.
3. *descending external branches of cervical plexus (Cloquet, 1816)*

Synonym for macrodissected adult human ***descending superficial branches of cervical plexus (Quain, 1828)***; in the original French, *branches descendantes externes*, p. 638.

LATER SYNONYMS:

1. *descending branches of cervical plexus (Knox, 1832)*
   Synonym for macrodissected adult human ***descending superficial branches of cervical plexus (Quain, 1828)***; Supplemental Plate II-29.

diagonal band (Broca, 1879)

As described in macrodissected adult human, and mammal generally with histological methods for ***axons (Kölliker, 1896)***, a ***central nervous system white matter tract (>1840)*** diffusely dispersed through the ***medial septal complex (Swanson et al., 1987)*** with individual ***axons (Kölliker, 1896)*** coursing roughly parallel to the outer surface of the ***medial septal complex (Swanson et al., 1987)***. It lies between the ***medial forebrain bundle (Edinger, 1893)*** ventrally and caudally, and the ***precommissural fornix (Loo, 1931)*** and ***postcommissural fornix (Loo, 1931)*** dorsally. For Broca's use in mammal generally, see pp. 401, 428; also see Figures 5-*d*, 6-*d*. It was perhaps first clearly delineated by Lancisi; see ***[diagonal band (Broca, 1879)] Lancisi (1718)***.

EARLIER REFERENCES:

Illustrated and described, not named

1. ***[diagonal band (Broca, 1879)] (Lancisi, 1718)***
   Clearly described and illustrated for macrodissected adult human; for the right and left sides, *Nervuli longitudinales in partes inferiores thalamorum nervorum opticorum definentes*, thus a rostroventral extension, expansion, and differentiation of the *longitudinal nerve (Lancisi, 1718)*, p. 317, Figure 2-*d*. Soemmerring (1778, Fig. 1, region inside *b*, *θ*, *ξ*; Fig. 2, region indicated by *l*) seems clearly to have differentiated between it and ***olfactory tubercle (Calleja, 1893)***.

Earlier synonyms:

1. *lemniscus of lamina cribrosa (Reil, 1812a,b)*
   Synonym for macrodissected adult human ***diagonal band (Broca, 1879)***; see Mayo translation (1823, pp. 108–109, 114), "The septum [*septum (Galen, c177)*] contains, within its double layer of epithelium, fibres derived from the fillets of the lamina cribrosa, and from the upper surface of the fornix." (Mayo translation, 1823, p. 114). Also see *lamina cribrosa (Reil, 1809)*.
2. *septal arcuate fibers (Burdach, 1822)*
   Burdach described arching fibers of macrodissected adult human *septum (Galen, c177)* coursing dorsally (ascending) and then rostrocaudally (horizontally) to reach ***hippocampal region (Swanson et al., 1987)***; p. 135. Probably correspond to all or part of ***diagonal band (Broca, 1879)***; see Meyer (1971, pp. 100–101).

LATER SYNONYMS:

1. *diagonal band of quadrilateral space (Broca, 1879)*
   Synonym for ***diagonal band (Broca, 1879)***; p. 401.
2. *internal arcuate fibers of septum (Cajal, 1901–1902)*
   Roughly synonymous with ***diagonal band (Broca, 1879)*** described in Golgi material from young mouse and rat; in the original Spanish, *fibras arciformes internas*, see Figures 11-*E*, 19-*F*, p. 187. Also see *external arcuate fibers of septum (Cajal, 1901–1902)*.

diagonal sulcus (Beccari, 1911)

As described for macrodissected adult human, the shallow groove between the surface of the ***olfactory tubercle (Calleja, 1893)*** laterally and the ***diagonal band nucleus (>1840)*** of the ***medial septal complex (Swanson et al., 1987)*** medially. For Beccari's use in mammal generally see Figure 1-*d*, and for human specifically see Figure 2. It was probably first delineated clearly by Soemmerring; see ***[diagonal sulcus (Beccari, 1911)] (Soemmerring, 1778)***.

EARLIER REFERENCES:

Illustrated, not named or described:

1. ***[diagonal sulcus (Beccari, 1911)] (Soemmerring, 1778)***
   Clearly illustrated for macrodissected adult human; Table 1 above *b*,*ζ*; Table 2 between *H* and *I*).

digastric nerve (Meckel, 1753)

As described for macrodissected adult human, a branch of the ***facial nerve trunk (>1840)*** mainly supplying the posterior belly of digastric muscle; it often has other small branches and often arises from a common trunk with the ***stylohyoid nerve (Meckel, 1753)***; see Durward (1951, Figs. 901, 902), Williams & Warwick (1980, p. 1072), *internal deep nerve of hard nerve (Meckel, 1753)*. For Meckel's use in macrodissected adult human, see Table 1-*122*. It was probably first delineated by Willis; see ***[digastric nerve (Meckel, 1753)] (Willis, 1664)***.

TRANSLATIONS:

1. *nerf digastrique (Meckel, 1753)*
   Original French form of ***digastric nerve (Meckel, 1753)***; Table 1-*122*.
2. *nervus biventricus (Neubauer, 1772)*
   Latin form of ***digastric nerve (Meckel, 1753)***; Table 2-*73*.

EARLIER REFERENCES:

Illustrated and described, not named:

1. ***[digastric nerve (Meckel, 1753)] (Willis, 1664)***
   Probably mentioned and illustrated for macrodissected adult human; see Pordage translation (1681, p. 144 and Tab. IX-*1*). It was clearly referred to by Winslow (1733, Sect. VI, p. 68).

LATER SYNONYMS:

1. *posterior branch of internal deep nerve of hard nerve (Meckel, 1753)*
   Synonym for macrodissected adult human ***digastric nerve (Meckel, 1753)***; in the original French, *le rameau postérieur du nerf profond intérieur du nerf dur*, p. 73, Table 1:*120-122*.
2. *digastric branch of internal deep nerve of hard nerve (Meckel, 1753)*
   Synonym for macrodissected adult human ***digastric nerve (Meckel, 1753)***; in the original French, *le rameau biventrique du nerf profond intérieur*, p. 73.

3. *par septimum portionis durae ramus biventricus (Haase, 1781)*
   Latin synonym for macrodissected adult human ***digastric nerve (Meckel, 1753)***; see Index section 180. It roughly translates "digastric branch of hard part of seventh pair."
4. *digastric branch of hard part of acoustic nerve (Scarpa, 1794)*
   Synonym for macrodissected adult human ***digastric nerve (Meckel, 1753)***; in the original Latin, *portionis durae nervi acustici ramus digastricus*, Table III-*155*.
5. *digastric muscle nerve (Soemmerring, 1798)*
   Synonym for macrodissected adult human ***digastric nerve (Meckel, 1753)***; in the original Latin, *nervum musculi digastrici*, p. 248.
6. *sub-mastoidian branch of facial nerve (Burdin, 1803)*
   Apparently, synonym for macrodissected adult human ***digastric nerve (Meckel, 1753)***; see translation (1803, Vol. 3, p. 179). Quain (1828, p. 653) spelled it *submastoïd branch*.
7. *digastric branch of facial nerve (Meckel, 1817)*
   Synonym for macrodissected adult human ***digastric nerve (Meckel, 1753)***; see translation (1832, Vol. 3, p. 54).
8. *digastric branch of communicating nerve of face (Knox, 1832)*
   Synonym for macrodissected adult human ***digastric nerve (Meckel, 1753)***; Plate II-*41*.
9. *posterior mastoid branch of facial nerve (Cruveilhier, 1836)*
   Synonym for macrodissected adult human ***digastric nerve (Meckel, 1753)***; in the original French, *rameau mastoïdien postérieur*, p. 943.

PARTLY CORRESPONDS:

1. *anastomotic filament of digastric branch (Bellingeri, 1818)*
   Macrodissected adult human ***communicating branch (Winslow, 1733)*** of ***digastric nerve (Meckel, 1753)*** with ***stylohyoid nerve (Meckel, 1753)***; in the original Latin, *filamentum anastomoticum*, see Table II.
2. *digastric surculus proper of digastric branch (Bellingeri, 1818)*
   Macrodissected adult human branch of ***digastric nerve (Meckel, 1753)*** to digastric muscle; in the original Latin, *surculus digastrici proprii*, see Table II.
3. *laryngeal anastomotic surculus of digastric branch (Bellingeri, 1818)*
   Macrodissected adult human ***communicating branch (Winslow, 1733)*** of ***digastric nerve (Meckel, 1753)*** with ***superior laryngeal nerve (Loder, 1778)***; in the original Latin, *surculus anastomoticus laryngeus*, see Table II.

digital branch of deep fibular nerve (>1840)

As described for macrodissected adult human, a branch of the ***deep fibular nerve (Fyfe, 1800)***, in turn generating medial branches, the ***dorsal digital nerves of deep fibular nerve (>1840)***, and small lateral branches to associated muscles, especially the extensor digitorum brevis muscle and sometimes the dorsal interossei muscles of the foot and the tarsal, tarso-metatarsal, and metatarso-phalangeal joints; see Durward (1951, p. 1108, referred to as *collateral branches of anterior tibial nerve*), Hamilton (1976, p. 665 and Fig. 835, called *digital branch of deep peroneal nerve*), Williams & Warwick (1980, p. 1115, called *terminal branches of deep peroneal nerve*). It was perhaps first clearly delineated by Eustachi; see ***[digital branch of deep fibular nerve (>1840)] (Eustachi, 1552)***.

EARLIER REFERENCES:

Illustrated, not named or described:

1. ***[digital branch of deep fibular nerve (>1840)] (Eustachi, 1552)***
   Illustrated for macrodissected adult human; see Albinus edition (1761, Tab. 19/2-associated with *16*).

Earlier synonyms:

1. *metatarsus pollicis nerve (Fischer, 1791)*
   Synonym for macrodissected adult human ***digital branch of deep fibular nerve (>1840)***; in the original Latin, *nervus metatarsicus pollicis*, p. 33. It would now be called *metatarsus hallucis nerve*.
2. *internal dorsal branch of deep peroneal nerve (Fischer, 1791)*
   Synonym for macrodissected adult human ***digital branch of deep fibular nerve (>1840)***; in the original Latin, *ramus nervi peronei profundi dorsalis internus*, Table IV, Figure 1-*350*.
3. *superficial branch of deep peroneal nerve (Fischer, 1791)*
   Synonym for macrodissected adult human ***digital branch of deep fibular nerve (>1840)***; in the original Latin, *ramus nervi peronei profundi superficialis*, Table IV, Figure 1-*350*.
4. *superficial dorsal branch of foot of deeper seated branch of fibular nerve (Bell & Bell, 1816)*
   Term emerging from Bell & Bell's description of macrodissected adult human ***digital branch of deep fibular nerve (>1840)***; in the original Latin, *ramus dorsalis pedis superficialis*, Vol. 2, p. 551.
5. *dorsal branch of deep peroneal nerve (Bock, 1827)*
   Synonym for macrodissected adult human ***digital branch of deep fibular nerve (>1840)***; in the original Latin, *ram. dorsalis nervi peronei profundi*, Table II-*122*.
6. *superficial nerve of deep peroneal nerve (Knox, 1832)*
   Synonym for *superficial branch of deep peroneal nerve (Fischer, 1791)*; Plate XVII-*350*.

PARTLY CORRESPONDS:

1. *deep dorsal twig of foot of deep branch of peroneal nerve (Jördens, 1788)*
   Branch of macrodissected adult human ***digital branch of deep fibular nerve (>1840)*** to some dorsal interossei muscles of foot; in the original Latin, *ramulus dorsalis pedis profundus rami profundi nervi peronei*, pp. 4, 14.
2. *external dorsal twig of foot of deep branch of peroneal nerve (Jördens, 1788)*
   Synonym for *deep dorsal twig of foot of deep branch of peroneal nerve (Jördens, 1788)*; in the original Latin, *ramulus dorsalis pedis externus rami profundi nervi peronei*, pp. 4, 14.

3. *deep dorsal branch of foot (Bell, 1803b)*
   Lateral branch of macrodissected adult human ***digital branch of deep fibular nerve (>1840)***; in the original Latin, *ramus dorsalis, pedis profundus*, p. 209.
4. *superficial dorsal branch of foot (Bell, 1803b)*
   Medial branch of macrodissected adult human ***digital branch of deep fibular nerve (>1840)***; in the original Latin, *ramus dorsalis, pedis superficialis*, p. 209.
5. *internal and deep branch of back of foot of anterior tibial branch of external popliteal nerve (Cloquet, 1816)*
   Medial branch of macrodissected adult human ***digital branch of deep fibular nerve (>1840)***; in the original French, *rameau interne et profond du dos du pied*, p. 676.
6. *external and deep branch of back of foot of anterior tibial branch of external popliteal nerve (Cloquet, 1816)*
   Lateral branch of macrodissected adult human ***digital branch of deep fibular nerve (>1840)***; in the original French, *rameau externe et profond du dos du pied*, p. 676.
7. *external branch of deep peroneal nerve (Bock, 1827)*
   Lateral branch of macrodissected adult human ***digital branch of deep fibular nerve (>1840)***; in the original Latin, *Ram. externus nerv. profundus peroneus*; Table I, Figure 2-85,86.
8. *internal branch of deep peroneal nerve (Bock, 1827)*
   Medial branch of macrodissected adult human ***digital branch of deep fibular nerve (>1840)***; in the original Latin, *Ram. internus nerv. profundus peroneus*; Table I, Figure 2-85,87.
9. *internal dorsal branch of deep peroneal nerve (Cloquet, 1828)*
   Medial branch of macrodissected adult human ***digital branch of deep fibular nerve (>1840)*** supplying dorsal digital nerves to first two toes; in the original French, *rameau dorsal interne du N. péronier profond*, Plate CLXXIV, Figure 1-85.
10. *internal deep branch of dorsum of foot of anterior tibial branch of external peroneal sciatic nerve (Cruveilhier, 1836)*
    Major branch of macrodissected adult human ***digital branch of deep fibular nerve (>1840)*** generating ***dorsal digital nerves of deep fibular nerve (>1840)*** and branch to 1st interosseous space; in the original French, *rameau interne et profond du dos du pied*, p. 866.
11. *external deep branch of dorsum of foot of anterior tibial branch of external peroneal sciatic nerve (Cruveilhier, 1836)*
    Small branch of macrodissected adult human ***digital branch of deep fibular nerve (>1840)*** generating branches to extensor digitorum brevis muscle and dorsal interossei muscles of foot; in the original French, *rameau externe et profond du dos du pied*, p. 866.
12. *lateral terminal branch of deep peroneal nerve (>1840)*
    Synonym for macrodissected adult human *external branch of deep peroneal nerve (Bock, 1827)* and *external deep branch of dorsum of foot of anterior tibial branch of external peroneal sciatic nerve (Cruveilhier, 1836)*; that is, lateral terminal branches of ***digital branch of deep fibular nerve (>1840)***, see Williams & Warwick (1980, p. 1115).

distal glossopharyngeal ganglion (>1840)
As described for macrodissected adult human, the larger of two sensory ***cranial nerve ganglia (>1840)*** of the ***glossopharyngeal nerve (Huber, 1744)*** associated with the proximal part of the ***glossopharyngeal nerve trunk (Wrisberg, 1786; Günther, 1786)*** just distal to the ***proximal glossopharyngeal ganglion (>1840)*** in a notch in the lower border of the petrous part of the temporal bone; see Williams & Warwick (1980, p. 1075 and Fig. 7.189). It was probably first described as the *glossopharyngeal nerve ganglion (Huber, 1744)*.

EARLIER REFERENCES:

Earlier synonyms:

1. *glossopharyngeal nerve ganglion (Huber, 1744)*
   Probably synonym for macrodissected adult human ***distal glossopharyngeal ganglion (>1840)***; in the original Latin, *ganglio nervi glossopharyngei*, p. 12, see Neubauer (1772, p. 46). Its discovery has been attributed without citation or apparent justification to Winslow (1733); see Kilian (1822, p. 75), Rasmussen (1947, p. 14).
2. *petrosal ganglion (Wrisberg, 1786)*
   Synonym for macrodissected adult human ***distal glossopharyngeal ganglion (>1840)***; see Wrisberg reprint (1800, p. 416).
3. *petrosal ganglion of eighth nerve of head (Andersch & Soemmerring, 1792)*
   Synonym for ***distal glossopharyngeal ganglion (>1840)*** described for macrodissected adult human in Andersch's thesis finished c1751–c1755; it was not distributed then and was edited and reprinted by Soemmerring only in 1792. The simple term, *petrosal ganglion* (*ganglio petroso*), is used on p. 115. Also see *small ganglion of ninth nerves of head (Andersch, 1797)*.
4. *small ganglion of ninth nerves of head (Andersch, 1797)*
   Synonym for macrodissected adult human ***distal glossopharyngeal ganglion (>1840)*** in 1st unedited edition of Andersch's thesis work; in the original Latin, *gangliolum noni nervi capitis*, p. 6. Also see *petrosal ganglion of eighth nerve of head (Andersch & Soemmerring, 1792)*.
5. *petrosal small ganglion (Andersch, 1797)*
   Synonym for macrodissected adult human ***distal glossopharyngeal ganglion (>1840)***; in the original Latin (plural), *ganglioli petrosi*, p. 7.
6. *petrosal neuronode (Kilian, 1822)*
   Synonym for macrodissected adult human ***distal glossopharyngeal ganglion (>1840)***; in the original Latin, *neuronodus petrosus*, p. 76.
7. *inferior ganglion of glossopharyngeal nerve (Todd, 1836–1839)*
   Synonym for macrodissected adult human ***distal glossopharyngeal ganglion (>1840)***; p. 495.
8. *ganglion of Andersch (Todd, 1836–1839)*
   Eponym for macrodissected adult human ***distal glossopharyngeal ganglion (>1840)***; p. 495.

distal vagal ganglion (>1840)

As described for macrodissected adult human, the larger of two sensory ***cranial nerve ganglia (>1840)*** of the ***vagus nerve (Galen, c173)*** associated with the proximal part of the ***vagus nerve trunk (Wrisberg, 1786; Günther, 1786)*** just distal to the ***proximal vagal ganglion (>1840)***; see Williams & Warwick (1980, pp. 1076, 1078 and Fig. 7.189). It was probably discovered and described as the *olive body (Falloppio, 1561)*.

EARLIER REFERENCES:

Earlier synonyms:

1. *olive body (Falloppio, 1561)*
   Probably refers to macrodissected adult human ***distal vagal ganglion (>1840)***; in the original Latin, *corpus olivare*, p. 152. See Willis (1664; and Pordage translation, 1681, p. 146), Diemerbroeck (1689, p. 417), Schiller (1967, p. 533). According to Bauhin (1605), Falloppio noted that it is sometimes single and sometimes double, implying that he may have also observed the ***proximal vagal ganglion (>1840)***—although he may well have been referring to the ***superior cervical ganglion (Vieussens, 1684)***; see Crooke translation (1615, p. 893). Scarpa (1794) stated "there is nothing, I think, more certain than that Falloppius described in this place the superior cervical ganglion..." (Knox translation, 1832, Pl. II-74).
2. *plexus ganglioformis cervicalis nervi octavis paris (Vieussens, 1684)*
   Apparently, synonym for macrodissected adult human ***distal vagal ganglion (>1840)***; Table 23-*H*, see Johnston (1765, p. 182). However, involvement of the ***distal glossopharyngeal ganglion (>1840)*** is not clear.
3. *ganglioform plexus of par vagum (Collins, 1685)*
   Term appears in margin note for text where Collins wrote, "The *Caudex* [***vagus nerve trunk (Wrisberg, 1786; Günther, 1786)***] of the *Par Vagum* is amplified in an oblong Tumor, called the *Plexus ganglioformis*, now and then single and sometimes double" (p. 1050). He referred to *plexus ganglioformis cervicalis nervi octavis paris (Vieussens, 1684)*, or ***distal vagal ganglion (>1840)***, although involvement of ***distal glossopharyngeal ganglion (>1840)*** is not clear.
4. *contorted fold (Diemerbroeck, 1689)*
   Synonym for macrodissected adult human *olive body (Falloppio, 1561)*; p. 417.
5. *truncum octavi tumidulum (Pfeffinger, 1783)*
   Synonym for macrodissected adult human *olive body (Falloppio, 1561)*; Section II, §. XXX.
6. *octavi nervorum cerebri truncus gangliformis (Scarpa, 1794)*
   Synonym for macrodissected adult human *olive body (Falloppio, 1561)*; Table II-45.
7. *primary ganglion of vagus nerves (Wutzer, 1817)*
   Apparently, synonym for macrodissected adult human *olive body (Falloppio, 1561)*; in the original Latin, *ganglion primum nervi vagi*, Figure VII-*r*.
8. *ganglioform trunk of pneumogastric (Knox, 1832)*
   Synonym for *octavi nervorum cerebri truncus gangliformis (Scarpa, 1794)*; Plate II-74.
9. *secondary vagal ganglion (Bischoff, 1832)*
   Synonym for macrodissected kitten ***distal vagal ganglion (>1840)***; in the original Latin, *ganglion secundum Vagi*, Table II, Figure 1-*12*.
10. *vagus nerve ganglion (Arnold, 1834)*
   Synonym for macrodissected adult human ***distal vagal ganglion (>1840)***; in the original Latin, *ganglion nervi vagi*, p. 13.
11. *ganglion of pneumogastric (Cruveilhier, 1836)*
   Synonym for macrodissected adult human ***distal vagal ganglion (>1840)***; in the original French, *ganglion du pneumo-gastrique*, p. 955.
12. *nodose ganglion (>1840)*
   Synonym for macrodissected adult human ***distal vagal ganglion (>1840)***; see Williams & Warwick (1980, p. 1078).

dorsal anterior cingulate area (Brodmann, 1909)

As described with cellular architecture for adult human, the dorsal part of the ***anterior cingulate region (>1840)***; p. 148. It was not identified by 1840.

TRANSLATIONS:

1. *area cingularis anterior dorsalis (Brodmann, 1909)*
   Original Latin form of ***dorsal anterior cingulate area (Brodmann, 1909)***; p. 148.

EARLIER REFERENCES:

Earlier synonyms:

1. *area 32 (Brodmann, 1909)*
   Synonym for adult human ***dorsal anterior cingulate area (Brodmann, 1909)***; in the original German, *Feld 32*, see p. 148.

dorsal branch of ulnar nerve (Günther, 1786)

As described for macrodissected adult human, it arises about 5 cm proximal to the wrist and eventually divides into 2–3 ***dorsal digital nerves of ulnar nerve (>1840)***; see Williams & Warwick (1980, p. 1100). For Günther's use in macrodissected adult human, see p. 76. It was known to Vesalius; see ***[dorsal branch of ulnar nerve (Günther, 1786)] (Vesalius, 1543a)***.

TRANSLATIONS:

1. *nervus ulnaris ramus dorsalis (Günther, 1786)*
   Original Latin form of ***dorsal branch of ulnar nerve (Günther, 1786)***; p. 76.

EARLIER REFERENCES:

Described, not named or illustrated:

1. ***[dorsal branch of ulnar nerve (Günther, 1786)] (Vesalius, 1543a)***
   Illustrated and clearly described for macrodissected adult human; see Richardson & Carman translation (2002, pp. 244–245).

Earlier synonyms:

1. *dorsal branch of cubital nerve (Martin, 1781)*

Synonym for macrodissected adult human ***dorsal branch of ulnar nerve (Günther, 1786)***; in the original Latin, *ramus dorsalis nervus cubitalis*, p. 217.

LATER SYNONYMS:

1. *anterior branch of cubital nerve (Frotscher, 1788)*
   Synonym for macrodissected adult human *dorsal branch of cubital nerve (Martin, 1781)*; p. 92 of 1795 reprint.
2. *dorsal nerve (Fyfe, 1800)*
   Synonym for macrodissected adult human ***dorsal branch of ulnar nerve (Günther, 1786)***; Vol. 2, p. 313.
3. *dorsal branch of cubital nerve (Loder, 1803)*
   Synonym for macrodissected adult human ***dorsal branch of ulnar nerve (Günther, 1786)***; in the original Latin, *nervi cubitalis ramus dorsalis*, Table CLXXVIII, Figure 2-75.
4. *minor branch of cubital nerve trunk (Loder, 1803)*
   Synonym for *dorsal branch of cubital nerve (Loder, 1803)*; Table CLXXX, Figure 1-92.
5. *dorsal branch of hand of ulnar nerve (Bock, 1827)*
   Synonym for macrodissected adult human ***dorsal branch of ulnar nerve (Günther, 1786)***; in the original Latin, *ram. dorsalis ulnaris manus*, Table IV-26.
6. *cubital nerve internal dorsal branch of hand (Cruveilhier, 1836)*
   Synonym for macrodissected adult human ***dorsal branch of ulnar nerve (Günther, 1786)***; in the original French, *branche dorsale interne de la main*, p. 812.
7. *cutaneous dorsal branch of cubital nerve (Cruveilhier, 1836)*
   Synonym for macrodissected adult human ***dorsal branch of ulnar nerve (Günther, 1786)***; in the original French, *branche dórsale cutanée*, p. 814.

PARTLY CORRESPONDS:

1. *dorsal nerve of hand (Klint, 1784)*
   Largest branch of macrodissected adult human ***dorsal branch of ulnar nerve (Günther, 1786)*** generating the two ***dorsal digital nerves of ulnar nerve (>1840)***; in the original Latin, *(verus) nervus dorsalis manus*, p. 45. Klint distinguished two smaller branches.
2. *communicating branchlet of dorsal branch of cubital nerve with middle cutaneous nerve (Caldani, 1813, 1814)*
   Macrodissected adult human small ***communicating branch (Winslow, 1733)*** between ***dorsal branch of ulnar nerve (Günther, 1786)*** and ***anterior branch of medial cutaneous nerve of forearm (>1840)***; in the original Latin, *ramulus communicans cum ramo medio nervi cutanei*; Table CCLX, Figure 2-2.
3. *common trunk of dorsal branch of cubital nerve for ulnar dorsal nerve of ring finger, radial dorsal nerve of auricular finger, and radial dorsal nerve of ring finger (Caldani, 1813, 1814)*
   Macrodissected adult human complex branching of ***dorsal branch of ulnar nerve (Günther, 1786)*** generating three ***dorsal digital nerves of ulnar nerve (>1840)*** to medial side of ring finger, lateral side of little finger, and lateral side of ring finger, respectively; Table CCLX, Figure 2-3.

dorsal column nuclei (>1840)

As described for macrodissected adult human, and for adult mammal in general with cellular architecture and connections, a set of ***gray matter regions (Swanson & Bota, 2010)*** lying in the caudal dorsolateral ***medulla (Winslow, 1733)***, dorsomedial to the ***spinal nucleus of trigeminal nerve (>1840)*** and receiving massive inputs from ***gracile fascicle (Müller, 1834)*** and ***cuneate fascicle (Müller, 1834)***. The main parts are ***gracile nucleus (>1840)***, ***cuneate nucleus (>1840)***, and ***accessory cuneate nucleus (>1840)***, from medial to lateral; see Williams & Warwick, 1980, p. 901), Nieuwenhuys et al. (2008, p. 194 and Figs. 6.21-23). They were first noted by Burdach; see ***[dorsal column nuclei (>1840)] (Burdach, 1822)***.

EARLIER REFERENCES:

Described, not named or illustrated:

1. ***[dorsal column nuclei (>1840)] (Burdach, 1822)***
   Burdach noted ***gray matter (Meckel, 1817)*** in region of macrodissected adult human ***[gracile nucleus (>1840)] (Burdach, 1822)*** and ***[cuneate nucleus (>1840)] (Burdach, 1822)***.

dorsal digital nerves of deep fibular nerve (>1840)

As described for macrodissected adult human, they innervate the lateral side of the big toe, along with a ***dorsal digital nerve of medial dorsal cutaneous nerve (>1840)***, and the medial side of the second toe, also with a ***dorsal digital nerve of medial dorsal cutaneous nerve (>1840)***; see Durward (p. 1108 and Fig. 949; referred to as *anterior tibial nerve*), *Terminologia Anatomica* (1998, p. 140). They were perhaps first delineated by Eustachi; see ***[dorsal digital nerves of deep fibular nerve (>1840)] (Eustachi, 1552)***.

EARLIER REFERENCES:

Illustrated, not named or described:

1. ***[dorsal digital nerves of deep fibular nerve (>1840)] (Eustachi, 1552)***
   Illustrated for macrodissected adult human; see Albinus edition (1761, Table 19/2, at the end of *16*).

Earlier synonyms:

1. *internal anterior branches of muscular branch of peroneal nerve (Martin, 1781)*
   Synonym for macrodissected adult human ***dorsal digital nerves of deep fibular nerve (>1840)***; in the original Latin, *nervus peroneus ramus muscularis ramus anterior internus*, p. 248.
2. *inferior anterior branches of muscular nerve (Martin, 1781)*
   Synonym for macrodissected adult human ***dorsal digital nerves of deep fibular nerve (>1840)***; in the original Latin, *nervus muscularis ramus anterior inferior*, Table XI.
3. *dorsal digital nerves of deep branch of peroneal nerve (Langenbeck, 1826–1830)*
   Synonym for macrodissected adult human ***dorsal digital nerves of deep fibular nerve (>1840)***; in the original Latin, *nervi digitales dorsales, ramus profundus nervi peronei*; Fascicle III, Table VII, Figure 2.

PARTLY CORRESPONDS:

1. *superficial dorsal twig of foot of deep branch of peroneal nerve (Jördens, 1788)*
   Dorsal digital nerve of deep fibular nerve (>1840) splitting into internal (medial) twig to big toe and external (lateral) twig to second toe; in the original Latin, *ramulus dorsalis pedis superficialis rami profundi nervi peronei*, pp. 4, 14.
2. *internal twig from superficial dorsal twig of foot of deep branch of peroneal nerve (Jördens, 1788)*
   Branch of *superficial dorsal twig of foot of deep branch of peroneal nerve (Jördens, 1788)* to big toe; in the original Latin, *ramulus internus ex ramulus dorsalis pedis superficialis rami profundi nervi peronei*, pp. 4, 14. Jördens described here three smaller branches of this branch.
3. *external twig from superficial dorsal twig of foot of deep branch of peroneal nerve (Jördens, 1788)*
   Branch of *superficial dorsal twig of foot of deep branch of peroneal nerve (Jördens, 1788)* to second toe; in the original Latin, *ramulus externus ex ramulus dorsalis pedis superficialis rami profundi nervi peronei*, pp. 4, 14. Jördens described here three smaller branches of this branch.
4. *external dorsal digital nerve of big toe from metatarsus pollicis nerve (Fischer, 1791)*
   Dorsal digital nerve of digital branch of deep fibular nerve (>1840) contribution to lateral side of macrodissected adult human big toe; in the original Latin, *nervus dorsalis digitalis pollicis externus*; p. 32. See Durward (1951, Fig. 949).
5. *internal dorsal digital nerve of second toe from metatarsus pollicis nerve (Fischer, 1791)*
   Dorsal digital nerve of medial dorsal cutaneous nerve (>1840) contribution to medial side of macrodissected adult human second toe; in the original Latin, *nervus dorsalis digitalis digiti secundi internus*; p. 32. See Durward (1951, Fig. 949).
6. *external dorsal nerve of big toe (Mayer, 1794)*
   Dorsal digital nerve of digital branch of deep fibular nerve (>1840) contribution to lateral side of macrodissected adult human big toe; in the original Latin, *nervus dorsalis externus pollicis*; Part 5, Table V, Figure 1-25 (p. 26); also referred to as *nervus dorsalis externus pollicis pedis;* Part 5, Table V, Figure 1-27 (p. 27).
7. *internal dorsal nerve of first small toe (Mayer, 1794)*
   Dorsal digital nerve of digital branch of deep fibular nerve (>1840) contribution to medial side of macrodissected adult human second toe; in the original Latin, *nervus dorsalis internus digiti primi minoris*; Part 5, Table V, Figure 1-26 (p. 26).
8. *external dorsal nerve of first small toe (Mayer, 1794)*
   Dorsal digital nerve of digital branch of deep fibular nerve (>1840) contribution to lateral side of macrodissected adult human second toe; in the original Latin, *nervus dorsalis externus digiti primi minoris*; Part 5, Table V, Figure 1-27 (p. 26).
9. *deep dorsal external collateral nerve of big toe (Cruveilhier, 1836)*
   For macrodissected adult human, ***dorsal digital nerve of digital branch of deep fibular nerve (>1840)*** contribution to lateral side of big toe; in the original French, *nerf collatéral externe dorsal profond du gros orteil*, p. 866.
10. *dorsal internal collateral nerve of second toe (Cruveilhier, 1836)*
    For macrodissected adult human, ***dorsal digital nerve of digital branch of deep fibular nerve (>1840)*** contribution to medial side of second toe; in the original French, *nerf collatéral interne dorsal du second*, p. 866.

dorsal digital nerves of intermediate dorsal cutaneous nerve (>1840)

As described for macrodissected adult human, there is commonly one for the lateral side of the third toe, one each for the medial and lateral sides of the fourth toe, and one for the medial side of the fifth (little) toe, also receiving a contribution from the ***sural nerve (Pietro da Cortona, 1741)***; see Durward (1951, p. 1108 and Fig. 949; referred to as *lateral branch of musculo-cutaneous nerve*), *Terminologia Anatomica* (1998, p. 140). They were perhaps first clearly delineated by Eustachi; see ***[dorsal digital nerves of intermediate dorsal cutaneous nerve (>1840)] (Eustachi, 1552)***.

EARLIER REFERENCES:

Illustrated, not named or described:

1. ***[dorsal digital nerves of intermediate dorsal cutaneous nerve (>1840)] (Eustachi, 1552)***
   Illustrated for macrodissected adult human; see Albinus edition (1761, Tab. 21-3).

Illustrated and described, not named:

1. ***[dorsal digital nerves of intermediate dorsal cutaneous nerve (>1840)] (Vieussens, 1684)***
   Vieussens described and illustrated for macrodissected adult human at least medial component to third and fourth toes, including at its origins with ***dorsal digital nerves of medial dorsal cutaneous nerve (>1840)*** a "ganglioform plexus" that Durward (1951, p. 1108) called a "ganglioform enlargement"; that is, a *pseudoganglion (>1840)*; Table 29:*85,88-91*.

Earlier synonyms:

1. *metatarsal nerves (Soemmerring, 1798)*
   Synonym for macrodissected adult human ***dorsal digital nerves of intermediate dorsal cutaneous nerve (>1840)***, which Soemmerring described; in the original Latin, *nervos metatarsicos*, p. 332.

PARTLY CORRESPONDS:

1. *dorsal external twig of third digit (Jördens, 1788)*
   Dorsal digital nerve of intermediate dorsal cutaneous nerve (>1840) to lateral part of third toe in macrodissected adult human; in the original Latin, *ramulus externus digiti tertii dorsalis*, p. 7, Table I-*104*.
2. *dorsal internal twig of fourth digit (Jördens, 1788)*
   Dorsal digital nerve of intermediate dorsal cutaneous nerve (>1840) to medial part of fourth toe in macrodissected adult human; in the original Latin, *ramulus internus digiti quarti dorsalis*, p. 7, Table I-*105*.

3. *dorsal external twig of fourth digit (Jördens, 1788)* ***Dorsal digital nerve of intermediate dorsal cutaneous nerve (>1840)*** to lateral part of fourth toe in macrodissected adult human; in the original Latin, *ramulus externus digiti quarti dorsalis*, p. 8, Table I-*107*.
4. *dorsal internal twig of fifth digit (Jördens, 1788)* ***Dorsal digital nerve of intermediate dorsal cutaneous nerve (>1840)*** to medial part of fifth (little) toe in macrodissected adult human; in the original Latin, *ramulus internus digiti quinti dorsalis*, p. 8, Table I-*108*.
5. *external dorsal digital nerve of third toe from external branch of superficial peroneal nerve (Fischer, 1791)* ***Dorsal digital nerve of intermediate dorsal cutaneous nerve (>1840)*** to lateral side of macrodissected adult human third toe; in the original Latin, *nervum dorsalem digitalem digiti tertii externum*, p. 32.
6. *internal dorsal digital nerve of fourth toe from external branch of superficial peroneal nerve (Fischer, 1791)* ***Dorsal digital nerve of intermediate dorsal cutaneous nerve (>1840)*** to medial side of macrodissected adult human fourth toe; in the original Latin, *nervum dorsalem digitalem digiti tertii internum*, p. 32.
7. *external dorsal digital nerve of fourth toe from external branch of superficial peroneal nerve (Fischer, 1791)* ***Dorsal digital nerve of intermediate dorsal cutaneous nerve (>1840)*** to lateral side of macrodissected adult human fourth toe; in the original Latin, *nervus dorsalis digitalis digiti quarti externus*, p. 32.
8. *internal dorsal digital nerve of fifth toe from external branch of superficial peroneal nerve (Fischer, 1791)* ***Dorsal digital nerve of intermediate dorsal cutaneous nerve (>1840)*** to medial side of macrodissected adult human fifth (little) toe; in the original Latin, *nervum dorsalem digitalem digiti quinti internum*, p. 32.
9. *internal dorsal nerve of second small toe (Mayer, 1794)* ***Dorsal digital nerve of intermediate dorsal cutaneous nerve (>1840)*** to medial side of macrodissected adult human third toe; in the original Latin, *nervus dorsalis internus digiti secundi minoris*; Part 5, Table V, Figure 1-32 (p. 26).
10. *external dorsal nerve of second small toe (Mayer, 1794)* ***Dorsal digital nerve of intermediate dorsal cutaneous nerve (>1840)*** to lateral side of macrodissected adult human third toe; in the original Latin, *nervus dorsalis externus digiti secundi minoris*; Part 5, Table V, Figure 1-33 (p. 26).
11. *internal dorsal nerve of third small toe (Mayer, 1794)* ***Dorsal digital nerve of intermediate dorsal cutaneous nerve (>1840)*** to medial side of macrodissected adult human fourth toe; in the original Latin, *nervus dorsalis internus digiti tertii minoris*; Part 5, Table V, Figure 1-34 (p. 26).
12. *external dorsal nerve of third small toe (Mayer, 1794)* ***Dorsal digital nerve of intermediate dorsal cutaneous nerve (>1840)*** to lateral side of macrodissected adult human fourth toe; in the original Latin, *nervus dorsalis externus digiti tertii minoris*; Part 5, Table V, Figure 1-35 (p. 26).
13. *internal dorsal nerve of fourth small toe (Mayer, 1794)* ***Dorsal digital nerve of intermediate dorsal cutaneous nerve (>1840)*** to medial side of macrodissected adult human fifth (little) toe; in the original Latin, *nervus dorsalis internus digiti quarti minoris*; Part 5, Table V, Figure 1-36 (p. 26).
14. *external dorsal nerve of fourth small toe (Mayer, 1794)* ***Dorsal digital nerve of intermediate dorsal cutaneous nerve (>1840)*** to lateral side of macrodissected adult human fifth (little) toe; in the original Latin, *nervus dorsalis externus digiti quarti minoris*; Part 5, Table V, Figure 1-37 (p. 26).
15. *internal dorsal nerve of smallest toe (Mayer, 1794)* ***Dorsal digital nerve of intermediate dorsal cutaneous nerve (>1840)*** to medial side of macrodissected adult human fifth (little) toe; in the original Latin, *nervus dorsalis internus digiti minimi*; Part 5, Table V, Figure 1-34 (p. 28).
16. *external dorsal nerve of smallest toe (Mayer, 1794)* ***Dorsal digital nerve of intermediate dorsal cutaneous nerve (>1840)*** to lateral side of macrodissected adult human fifth (little) toe; in the original Latin, *nervus dorsalis externus digiti minimi*; Part 5, Table V, Figure 1-36 (p. 28).
17. *tibial nerve of little toe (Meckel, 1817)* ***Dorsal digital nerve of intermediate dorsal cutaneous nerve (>1840)*** to medial side of macrodissected adult human fifth (little) toe; see translation (1832, Vol. 3, p. 18).
18. *dorsal nerves of fourth toe (Meckel, 1817)* Medial and lateral ***dorsal digital nerves of intermediate dorsal cutaneous nerve (>1840)*** of macrodissected adult human fourth toe; see translation (1832, Vol. 3, p. 18).
19. *peroneal nerve of third toe (Meckel, 1817)* ***Dorsal digital nerve of intermediate dorsal cutaneous nerve (>1840)*** to lateral side of macrodissected adult human third toe; see translation (1832, Vol. 3, p. 18).
20. *external dorsal collateral nerve of third toe (Cruveilhier, 1836)* ***Dorsal digital nerve of intermediate dorsal cutaneous nerve (>1840)*** to lateral side of macrodissected adult human third toe; in the original French, *collatéral dorsaux, externe du 3e*, p. 866.
21. *internal dorsal collateral nerve of fourth toe (Cruveilhier, 1836)* ***Dorsal digital nerve of intermediate dorsal cutaneous nerve (>1840)*** to medial side of macrodissected adult human fourth toe; in the original French, *interne du 4e*, p. 866.

dorsal digital nerves of lateral dorsal cutaneous nerve (>1840)

As described for macrodissected adult human there is commonly one for the lateral side of the little toe, and they become decreasingly common for the lateral and medial sides of the fourth toe and the lateral side of the third toe; see Durward (p. 1108 and Fig. 949). They were perhaps first clearly delineated and named individually, but not named as a group, by Fischer (1791, p. 34).

PARTLY CORRESPONDS:

1. *external dorsal digital nerve of third toe from internal metatarsal branch of inframalleolar nerve (Fischer, 1791)*
   Dorsal digital nerves of lateral dorsal cutaneous nerve (>1840) contribution to lateral side of macrodissected adult human third toe; in the original Latin, *nervus dorsalis digitalis digiti tertii externus*, p. 34. See Durward (1951, Fig. 949).
2. *internal dorsal digital nerve of fourth toe from internal metatarsal branch of inframalleolar nerve (Fischer, 1791)*
   Dorsal digital nerves of lateral dorsal cutaneous nerve (>1840) contribution to medial side of macrodissected adult human fourth toe; in the original Latin, *nervus dorsalis digitalis digiti quarti internus*, p. 34. See Durward (1951, Fig. 949).
3. *external dorsal digital nerve of fourth toe from internal metatarsal branch of inframalleolar nerve (Fischer, 1791)*
   Dorsal digital nerves of lateral dorsal cutaneous nerve (>1840) contribution to lateral side of macrodissected adult human fourth toe; in the original Latin, *nervus dorsalis digitalis digiti quarti externus*, p. 34. See Durward (1951, Fig. 949).
4. *internal dorsal digital nerve of little toe from internal metatarsal branch of inframalleolar nerve (Fischer, 1791)*
   Dorsal digital nerves of lateral dorsal cutaneous nerve (>1840) contribution to medial side of macrodissected adult human little toe; in the original Latin, *nervus dorsalis digitalis digiti minimi internus*, p. 34. See Durward (1951, Fig. 949).
5. *external dorsal digital nerve of fifth toe from external metatarsal branch of inframalleolar nerve (Fischer, 1791)*
   Dorsal digital nerve of lateral dorsal cutaneous nerve (>1840) contribution to lateral side of macrodissected adult human little toe; in the original Latin, *nervus dorsalis digitalis digiti minimi externus*, p. 34. See Durward (1951, Fig. 949).
6. *external dorsal nerve of little toe (Bock, 1827)*
   Dorsal digital nerves of lateral dorsal cutaneous nerve (>1840) contribution to lateral side of macrodissected adult human little toe; in the original Latin, *nerv. dorsalis externus digiti minimi*; Table VI, Figure 3-*16*.
7. *external dorsal nerve of third toe (Bock, 1827)*
   Dorsal digital nerves of lateral dorsal cutaneous nerve (>1840) contribution to lateral side of macrodissected adult human third toe; in the original Latin, *nerv. dorsalis externus digiti tertii*; Table VI, Figure 3-*18*.
8. *internal dorsal nerve of fourth toe (Bock, 1827)*
   Dorsal digital nerves of lateral dorsal cutaneous nerve (>1840) contribution to medial side of macrodissected adult human fourth toe; in the original Latin, *nerv. dorsalis internus digiti quarti*; Table VI, Figure 3-*19*.
9. *external dorsal nerve of fourth toe (Bock, 1827)*
   Dorsal digital nerves of lateral dorsal cutaneous nerve (>1840) contribution to medial side of macrodissected adult human fourth toe; in the original Latin, *nerv. dorsalis externus digiti quarti*; Table VI, Figure 3-*19*.
10. *internal dorsal nerve of little toe (Bock, 1827)*
    Dorsal digital nerves of lateral dorsal cutaneous nerve (>1840) contribution to medial side of macrodissected adult human little toe; in the original Latin, *nerv. dorsalis internus digiti minimi*; Table VI, Figure 3-*20*.
11. *internal dorsal collateral nerve of little toe (Cruveilhier, 1836)*
    Dorsal digital nerves of lateral dorsal cutaneous nerve (>1840) contribution to medial side of macrodissected adult human little toe; in the original French, *collatéral interne dorsal du petit orteil*, p. 869.
12. *external dorsal collateral nerve of fifth metatarsal (Cruveilhier, 1836)*
    Dorsal digital nerves of lateral dorsal cutaneous nerve (>1840) contribution to lateral side of macrodissected adult human little toe; in the original French, *nerf collatéral externe [dorsal] du cinquième metatarsien*, p. 869.
13. *external dorsal collateral nerve of fourth toe (Cruveilhier, 1836)*
    Dorsal digital nerves of lateral dorsal cutaneous nerve (>1840) contribution to lateral side of macrodissected adult human fourth toe; in the original French, *collateral externe dorsal du quatrième*, p. 869.

dorsal digital nerves of medial dorsal cutaneous nerve (>1840)

As described for macrodissected adult human, there is commonly one for the medial side of the big toe, one for the lateral side of the big toe that is also contributed to by the ***deep fibular nerve (Fyfe, 1800)***, one for the medial side of the second toe that is also contributed to by the ***deep fibular nerve (>1840)***, one for the lateral side of the second toe, and one for the medial side of the third toe; see Durward (p. 1108 and Fig. 949, referred to as *medial branch of musculo-cutaneous nerve*). They were perhaps first clearly delineated by Eustachi; see ***[dorsal digital nerves of medial dorsal cutaneous nerve (>1840)] (Eustachi, 1552)***.

EARLIER REFERENCES:

Illustrated, not named or described:

1. ***[dorsal digital nerves of medial dorsal cutaneous nerve (>1840)] (Eustachi, 1552)***
   Illustrated for macrodissected adult human; see Albinus edition (1761, Tab. 21-*4*).

Illustrated and described, not named:

1. ***[dorsal digital nerves of medial dorsal cutaneous nerve (>1840)] (Vieussens, 1684)***
   Described and illustrated for macrodissected adult human (Tab. 29-*92,95-101*) along with a "ganglioform plexus" that Durward (1951, p. 1108) called a "ganglioform enlargement"; that is, a *pseudoganglion (>1840)*; Table 29-*85*.

Earlier synonyms:

1. *dorsal nerves of two external toes and peroneal nerve of third (Meckel, 1817)*
   Synonym (possibly mistranslated or described in error) for macrodissected adult human ***dorsal digital nerves of medial dorsal cutaneous nerve (>1840)***; see translation (1832, Vol. 3, p. 18).

PARTLY CORRESPONDS:

1. *internal dorsal twig of big toe (Jördens, 1788)*
   Dorsal digital nerve of medial dorsal cutaneous nerve (>1840) to medial side of macrodissected adult human big toe; in the original Latin, *ramulus dorsalis pollicis internus*; see p. 6 and Table I-*92*.
2. *dorsal external twig of second digit (Jördens, 1788)*
   Dorsal digital nerve of medial dorsal cutaneous nerve (>1840) to lateral side of second toe in macrodissected adult human; in the original Latin, *ramulus externus digiti secundi dorsalis*; see p. 7 and Table I-*100*.
3. *dorsal internal twig of third digit (Jördens, 1788)*
   Dorsal digital nerve of medial dorsal cutaneous nerve (>1840) to medial side of third toe in macrodissected adult human; in the original Latin, *ramulus internus digiti tertii dorsalis*; see p. 7 and Table I-*100*.
4. *internal dorsal digital nerve of big toe (Fischer, 1791)*
   Dorsal digital nerve of medial dorsal cutaneous nerve (>1840) to medial side of macrodissected adult human big toe; in the original Latin, *nervus dorsalis digitalis pollicis internus*, p. 32.
5. *external dorsal digital nerve of big toe from external metatarsal twig (Fischer, 1791)*
   Dorsal digital nerve of medial dorsal cutaneous nerve (>1840) contribution to lateral side of macrodissected adult human big toe; in the original Latin, *nervus dorsalis digitalis pollicis externus*, p. 32. See Durward (1951, Fig. 949).
6. *internal dorsal digital nerve of second toe from external metatarsal twig (Fischer, 1791)*
   Dorsal digital nerve of medial dorsal cutaneous nerve (>1840) contribution to medial side of macrodissected adult human second toe; in the original Latin, *nervus dorsalis digitalis digiti secundi internus*, p. 32. See Durward (1951, Fig. 949).
7. *external dorsal digital nerve of second toe (Fischer, 1791)*
   Dorsal digital nerve of medial dorsal cutaneous nerve (>1840) to lateral side of macrodissected adult human second toe; in the original Latin, *nervus dorsalis digitalis digiti secundi externus*, p. 32. Fischer had it arising from *external branch of superficial peroneal nerve (Fischer, 1791)* in his dissections.
8. *internal dorsal digital nerve of third toe (Fischer, 1791)*
   Dorsal digital nerve of medial dorsal cutaneous nerve (>1840) to medial side of macrodissected adult human third toe; in the original Latin, *nervum dorsalem digitalem digiti tertii internum*, p. 32. Fischer had it arising from *external branch of superficial peroneal nerve (Fischer, 1791)* in his dissections.
9. *internal dorsal nerve of big toe (Mayer, 1794, p. 27)*
   Dorsal digital nerve of medial dorsal cutaneous nerve (>1840) to medial side of macrodissected adult human big toe; in the original Latin, *nervus dorsalis internus pollicis pedis*; Part 5, Table V, Figure 1-*29* (p. 27).
10. *tibial dorsal nerve of big toe (Bock, 1827)*
    Synonym for macrodissected adult human *internal dorsal nerve of big toe (Mayer, 1794, p. 27)*; in the original Latin, *nerv. dorsalis tibialis halucis*; Table VI, Figure 3-*6*.
11. *external dorsal nerve of big toe (Bock, 1827)*
    Dorsal digital nerve of medial dorsal cutaneous nerve (>1840) contribution to lateral side of macrodissected adult human big toe; in the original Latin, *nerv. dorsalis externus halucis*; Table VI, Figure 3-*11*.
12. *internal dorsal nerve of second toe (Bock, 1827)*
    Dorsal digital nerve of medial dorsal cutaneous nerve (>1840) contribution to medial side of macrodissected adult human second toe; in the original Latin, *nerv. dorsalis internus digiti secundi*; Table VI, Figure 3-*11*.
13. *external dorsal nerve of second toe (Bock, 1827)*
    Dorsal digital nerve of medial dorsal cutaneous nerve (>1840) contribution to lateral side of macrodissected adult human second toe; in the original Latin, *nerv. dorsalis externus digiti secundi*; Table VI, Figure 3-*12*.
14. *internal dorsal nerve of third toe (Bock, 1827)*
    Dorsal digital nerve of medial dorsal cutaneous nerve (>1840) contribution to medial side of macrodissected adult human third toe; in the original Latin, *nerv. dorsalis internus digiti tertii*; Table VI, Figure 3-*12*.
15. *lateral branch of internal dorsal branch of superficial peroneal nerve (Cloquet, 1828)*
    Dorsal digital nerve of medial dorsal cutaneous nerve (>1840) to medial side of macrodissected adult human big toe; in the original French, *rameau latéral du rameau dorsal interne du N. péronier superficiel*; Plate CLXXIII, Figure 1-*76* (and *74*). It should be called "medial branch of internal dorsal branch of superficial peroneal nerve."
16. *metatarsal branch of internal dorsal branch of superficial peroneal nerve (Cloquet, 1828)*
    Synonym for *lateral branch of internal dorsal branch of superficial peroneal nerve (Cloquet, 1828)*; in the original French, *rameau métatarsien*; Plate CLXXIII, Figure 1-*76*.
17. *internal metatarsal nerve (Knox, 1832)*
    Proximal segments of macrodissected adult human ***dorsal digital nerves of medial dorsal cutaneous nerve (>1840)*** before entering fingers; Plate XVII-*296*.
18. *internal dorsal collateral nerve of big toe (Cruveilhier, 1836)*
    Dorsal digital nerve of medial dorsal cutaneous nerve (>1840) to medial side of macrodissected adult human big toe; in the original French, *nerf collatéral interne dorsal du gros orteil*, p. 865.
19. *external dorsal collateral nerve of big toe (Cruveilhier, 1836)*
    Dorsal digital nerve of medial dorsal cutaneous nerve (>1840) to lateral side of macrodissected adult human big toe; in the original French, *collatéral dorsal externe du gros orteil*, p. 865.
20. *internal dorsal collateral nerve of second toe (Cruveilhier, 1836)*
    Dorsal digital nerve of medial dorsal cutaneous nerve (>1840) to medial side of macrodissected adult human second toe; in the original French, *collatéral interne du second*, p. 865.
21. *external dorsal collateral nerve of second toe (Cruveilhier, 1836)*
    Dorsal digital nerve of medial dorsal cutaneous nerve (>1840) to lateral side of macrodissected adult human

second toe; in the original French, *collatéral externe du deuxiéme*, p. 865.

22. *internal dorsal collateral nerve of third toe (Cruveilhier, 1836)* ***Dorsal digital nerve of medial dorsal cutaneous nerve (>1840)*** to medial side of macrodissected adult human third toe; in the original French, *collatéral interne du troisième*, p. 865.

dorsal digital nerves of radial nerve (>1840)

As described for macrodissected adult human, 4 or 5 terminal branches of the ***superficial branch of radial nerve (Martin, 1781)*** to dorsal regions of fingers; see Durward (1951, p. 1083), Hamilton (1976, Fig. 823), Williams & Warwick (1980, pp. 1101–1102), *Nomina Anatomica* (1983, p. A77). They were known to Vesalius; see ***[dorsal digital nerves of radial nerve (>1840)] (Vesalius, 1543a)***.

EARLIER REFERENCES:

Described, not named or illustrated:

1. ***[dorsal digital nerves of radial nerve (>1840)] (Vesalius, 1543a)***
   Five described for macrodissected adult human but not named as a group; see Richardson & Carman translation (2002, p. 242).

Earlier synonyms:

1. *dorsal branches of superficial branch of radial nerve (Martin, 1781)*
   Synonym for macrodissected adult human ***dorsal digital nerves of radial nerve (>1840)***; in the original Latin, *nervus radialis ramus superficialis rami dorsales*, pp. 220–221.
2. *dorsal cutaneous branches of dorsal superficial branch of radial nerve (Günther, 1786)*
   Günther described three ***dorsal digital nerves of radial nerve (>1840)*** for macrodissected adult human; in the original Latin (singular), *ramus cutaneus dorsalis*, p. 79.
3. *dorsal branch of superficial branch of spiral nerve (Fyfe, 1800)*
   Synonym for macrodissected adult human ***dorsal digital nerves of radial nerve (>1840)***; Vol. 2, p. 310.
4. *dorsal digital nerves of dorsal branch of radial nerve (Langenbeck, 1826–1830)*
   Synonym for macrodissected adult human ***dorsal digital nerves of radial nerve (>1840)***; in the original Latin, *nervi digitales dorsales ex ramo dorsali nervi radialis*; Fascicle III, Table XIII, Figure 2-*18*.

PARTLY CORRESPONDS:

1. *[dorsal cutaneous nerves of thumb (Meckel, 1817)] (Vesalius, 1543a)*
   Described without naming as branches of ***superficial branch of radial nerve (Martin, 1781)*** in macrodissected adult human; see Richardson & Carman translation (2002, p. 242).
2. *[radio-dorsal nerve of index finger (Meckel, 1817)] (Vesalius, 1543a)*
   Described without naming as branch of ***superficial branch of radial nerve (Martin, 1781)*** in macrodissected adult human to lateral part of index finger; see Richardson & Carman translation (2002, p. 242).
3. *[cubito-dorsal nerve of index finger (Meckel, 1817)] (Vesalius, 1543a)*
   Described without naming as branch of ***superficial branch of radial nerve (Martin, 1781)*** in macrodissected adult human to medial part of index finger; see Richardson & Carman translation (2002, p. 242).
4. *[radio-dorsal nerve of middle finger (Meckel, 1817)] (Vesalius, 1543a)*
   Described without naming as branch of ***superficial branch of radial nerve (Martin, 1781)*** in macrodissected adult human to lateral part of middle finger; see Richardson & Carman translation (2002, p. 242).
5. *[cubito-dorsal nerve of middle finger (Meckel, 1817)] (Vesalius, 1543a)*
   Described without naming as branch of branch of ***dorsal branch of ulnar nerve (Günther, 1786)*** in macrodissected adult human to medial part of middle finger; see Richardson & Carman translation (2002, p. 245). He also noted that occasionally this ***nerve (Herophilus, c335–c280 BC)*** is a branch of the ***radial nerve (Du Verney, 1697)***, in which case there is no branch from ***dorsal branch of ulnar nerve (Günther, 1786)***; see Richardson & Carman translation (2002, p. 245).
6. *external dorsal nerve of thumb (Mayer, 1794)*
   Macrodissected adult human ***dorsal digital nerve of radial nerve (>1840)*** described as extending from *volar branch of radial nerve (Mayer, 1794)* to lateral and dorsal region of thumb; in the original Latin, *nervus dorsalis externus pollicis*; Part 5, Table VI-*14* (p. 35).
7. *internal dorsal nerve of thumb (Mayer, 1794)*
   Macrodissected adult human ***dorsal digital nerve of radial nerve (>1840)*** described as extending from medial branch of ***superficial branch of radial nerve (Martin, 1781)*** to medial and dorsal region of thumb; in the original Latin, *nervus dorsalis internus pollicis*; Part 5, Table VI-*15* (p. 35).
8. *external dorsal nerve of index finger (Mayer, 1794)*
   Macrodissected adult human ***dorsal digital nerve of radial nerve (>1840)*** described as extending from medial branch of ***superficial branch of radial nerve (Martin, 1781)*** to lateral and dorsal region of index (2nd) finger; in the original Latin, *nervus dorsalis externus indicis*; Part 5, Table VI-*17* (p. 35).
9. *internal dorsal nerve of index finger (Mayer, 1794)*
   Macrodissected adult human ***dorsal digital nerve of radial nerve (>1840)*** described as extending from medial branch of ***superficial branch of radial nerve (Martin, 1781)*** to medial and dorsal region of index (2nd) finger; in the original Latin, *nervus dorsalis internus indicis*; Part 5, Table VI-*19* (p. 35).
10. *external dorsal nerve of middle finger (Mayer, 1794)*
   Macrodissected adult human ***dorsal digital nerve of radial nerve (>1840)*** described as extending from medial branch of ***superficial branch of radial nerve (Martin, 1781)*** to lateral and dorsal region of middle

(3rd) finger; in the original Latin, *nervus dorsalis externus digiti medii*; Part 5, Table VI-20 (p. 35).

11. *ulnar dorsal nerve of thumb (Loder, 1803)*
Synonym for macrodissected adult human *internal dorsal nerve of thumb (Mayer, 1794)*; in the original Latin, *nervus dorsalis ulnaris pollicis*, Table CLXXIX, Figure 1-17.

12. *radial dorsal nerve of thumb (Loder, 1803)*
Synonym for macrodissected adult human *external dorsal nerve of thumb (Mayer, 1794)*; in the original Latin, *nervus dorsalis radialis pollicis*, Table CLXXIX, Figure 1-28.

13. *radial dorsal nerve of index finger (Loder, 1803)*
Synonym for macrodissected adult human *external dorsal nerve of index finger (Mayer, 1794)*; in the original Latin, *nervus dorsalis radialis indicis*, Table CLXXVIII, Figure 2-66.

14. *ulnar dorsal nerve of index finger (Loder, 1803)*
Synonym for macrodissected adult human *internal dorsal nerve of index finger (Mayer, 1794)*; in the original Latin, *nervus dorsalis ulnaris indicis*, Table CLXXVIII, Figure 2-69.

15. *radial dorsal nerve of middle finger (Loder, 1803)*
Synonym for macrodissected adult human *external dorsal nerve of middle finger (Mayer, 1794)*; in the original Latin, *nervus dorsalis radialis digiti medii*, Table CLXXVIII, Figure 2-70.

16. *ulnar dorsal nerve of middle finger (Loder, 1803)*
Macrodissected adult human ***dorsal digital nerve of radial nerve (>1840)*** described as extending from *divided branch of dorsal branch of radial nerve (Loder, 1803)* to medial and dorsal region of middle (3rd) finger; in the original Latin, *nervus dorsalis ulnaris digiti medii*, Table CLXXVIII, Figure 2-72.

17. *radial dorsal nerve of ring finger (Loder, 1803)*
Macrodissected adult human ***dorsal digital nerve of radial nerve (>1840)*** described as extending from *divided branch of dorsal branch of radial nerve (Loder, 1803)* to lateral and dorsal region of ring (4th) finger; in the original Latin, *nervus dorsalis radialis digiti annularis*, Table CLXXVIII, Figure 2-73.

18. *anastomoses between ulnar and radial dorsal nerves of thumb (Caldani, 1813, 1814)*
Macrodissected adult human ***communicating branches (Winslow, 1733)*** between *ulnar dorsal nerve of thumb (Loder, 1803)* and *radial dorsal nerve of thumb (Loder, 1803)*; in the original Latin, *anastomoses inter nervos pollicis dorsales ulnarem et radialem*, Table CCLVIII, Figure 2-19.

19. *dorsal cutaneous nerves of thumb (Meckel, 1817)*
Described as two small branches in macrodissected adult human arising from anterior branch of ***superficial branch of radial nerve (Martin, 1781)*** and descending on thumb's dorsal side along radial and ulnar edges to its anterior extremity, furnishing filaments to its dorsal face and anastomosing with palmar nerves of thumb; in the original Latin, *nervi cutanei pollicis dorsales*, see translation (1832, Vol. 3, p. 25). They are ***dorsal digital nerves of radial nerve (>1840)*** to medial and lateral sides of thumb. See *[dorsal cutaneous nerves of thumb (Meckel, 1817)] (Vesalius, 1543a)*.

20. *radio-dorsal nerve of index finger (Meckel, 1817)*
Described for macrodissected adult human as arising from anterior ramuscule (branchlet) of posterior branch of ***superficial branch of radial nerve (Martin, 1781)*** and going to radial (lateral) side of index finger; in the original Latin, *nervus dorsalis radialis indicis*, see translation (1832, Vol. 3, p. 25). It is a ***dorsal digital nerve of radial nerve (>1840)*** to lateral side of index finger. See *[radio-dorsal nerve of index finger (Meckel, 1817)] (Vesalius, 1543a)*.

21. *cubito-dorsal nerve of index finger (Meckel, 1817)*
Described for macrodissected adult human as arising from first of two filaments of posterior ramuscule (branchlet) of posterior branch of ***superficial branch of radial nerve (Martin, 1781)*** and going to medial and dorsal part of index finger; see translation (1832, Vol. 3, p. 25). It is a ***dorsal digital nerve of radial nerve (>1840)*** to medial side of index finger. See *[cubito-dorsal nerve of index finger (Meckel, 1817)] (Vesalius, 1543a)*.

22. *radio-dorsal nerve of middle finger (Meckel, 1817)*
Described for macrodissected adult human as arising from first of two filaments (small branches) of posterior ramuscule (branchlet) of posterior branch of ***superficial branch of radial nerve (Martin, 1781)*** to lateral and dorsal part of middle finger; see translation (1832, Vol. 3, p. 25). It is a ***dorsal digital nerve of radial nerve (>1840)*** to lateral side of middle finger. See *[radio-dorsal nerve of middle finger (Meckel, 1817)] (Vesalius, 1543a)*.

23. *cubito-dorsal nerve of middle finger (Meckel, 1817)*
Described for macrodissected adult human as arising from second of two filaments (small branches) of posterior ramuscule (branchlet) of posterior branch of ***superficial branch of radial nerve (Martin, 1781)*** to medial and dorsal part of middle finger; see translation (1832, Vol. 3, p. 25). It is a ***dorsal digital nerve of radial nerve (>1840)*** to medial side of middle finger. See *[cubito-dorsal nerve of middle finger (Meckel, 1817)] (Vesalius, 1543a)*.

24. *external branch of dorsal radial nerve (Bock, 1824)*
Basically, synonym for macrodissected adult human *external dorsal nerve of thumb (Mayer, 1794)*; in the original Latin, *ram. externus Nervi radialis dorsalis*, Table XV, Figure 13-3.

25. *dorsal nerves of thumb (Bock, 1827)*
For macrodissected adult human, medial and lateral ***dorsal digital nerve of radial nerve (>1840)*** for thumb; in the original Latin, *nervi dorsales pollicis*, Table III-24.

26. *dorsal nerves of index finger (Bock, 1827)*
Macrodissected adult human medial and lateral ***dorsal digital nerves of radial nerve (>1840)*** for index finger; in the original Latin, *nervi dorsales indicis*, Table III-25.

27. *internal dorsal branch of thumb of anterior branch of radial nerve (Cloquet, 1828)*

Macrodissected adult human ***dorsal digital nerve of radial nerve (>1840)*** for medial side of thumb; in the original French, *rameau dorsal interne du pouce*, Plate CLXVII, Figure 2-*31*.

28. *external dorsal branch of thumb of anterior branch of radial nerve (Cloquet, 1828)*
Macrodissected adult human ***dorsal digital nerve of radial nerve (>1840)*** for lateral side of thumb; in the original French, *rameau dorsal externe du pouce*, Plate CLXVII, Figure 2-*32*.

29. *internal dorsal branch of thumb of palmar branch of radial nerve (Coquet, 1828)*
Synonym for *internal dorsal branch of thumb of anterior branch of radial nerve (Cloquet, 1828)*; in the original French, *rameau dorsal interne du pouce du rameau palmaire du n. radial*, Plate CLXVIII, Figure 1-*16*.

30. *external branch of superficial branch of radial nerve (Cruveilhier, 1836)*
Macrodissected adult human proximal part in wrist of ***dorsal digital nerve of radial nerve (>1840)*** extending to lateral side of thumb; in the original French, *rameau externe*, p. 818.

31. *dorsal external collateral nerve of thumb (Cruveilhier, 1836)*
Macrodissected adult human distal part of ***dorsal digital nerve of radial nerve (>1840)*** for lateral side of thumb; in the original French, *nerf collatéral externe dorsal du pouce*, p. 818.

32. *internal branch of superficial branch of radial nerve (Cruveilhier, 1836)*
Macrodissected adult human large medial branch of ***superficial branch of radial nerve (Martin, 1781)*** generating three secondary branches: *internal dorsal collateral branch of thumb of radial nerve (Cruveilhier, 1836)*, *external dorsal collateral branch of index finger of radial nerve (Cruveilhier, 1836)*, and *internal dorsal collateral branch of index finger of radial nerve (Cruveilhier, 1836)*; in the original French, *rameau interne*, p. 818.

33. *internal dorsal collateral branch of thumb of radial nerve (Cruveilhier, 1836)*
Macrodissected adult human ***dorsal digital nerve of radial nerve (>1840)*** for medial side of thumb; in the original French, *rameau collatéral dorsal interne du pouce*, p. 819.

34. *external dorsal collateral branch of index finger of radial nerve (Cruveilhier, 1836)*
Macrodissected adult human ***dorsal digital nerve of radial nerve (>1840)*** for lateral side of index finger; in the original French, *rameau collatéral dorsal externe de l'index*, p. 819.

35. *internal dorsal collateral branch of index finger of radial nerve (Cruveilhier, 1836)*
Macrodissected adult human ***dorsal digital nerve of radial nerve (>1840)*** for medial side of index finger; in the original French, *rameau collatéral dorsal interne de l'index*, p. 819.

36. *posterior collateral branch to thumb of radial nerve (Quain & Wilson, 1839)*
Macrodissected adult human ***dorsal digital nerve of radial nerve (>1840)*** for lateral side of thumb; Plate XIX, Figure 1-*h*.

dorsal digital nerves of ulnar nerve (>1840)

As described for macrodissected adult human, two or three of them arise from the ***dorsal branch of ulnar nerve (Günther, 1786)***, the first supplying the dorsal and medial side of the little finger, the second the adjacent dorsal sides of the little and ring fingers and, when present, the third supplying the adjoining dorsal sides of the ring and middle fingers; see Hamilton (1976, Fig. 823), Williams & Warwick (1980, p. 1100), *Nomina Anatomica* (1983, p. A77). They were known to Vesalius; see ***[dorsal digital nerves of ulnar nerve (>1840)] (Vesalius, 1543a)***.

EARLIER REFERENCES:

Described, not named or illustrated:

1. ***[dorsal digital nerves of ulnar nerve (>1840)] (Vesalius, 1543a)***
Vesalius described and named five in macrodissected adult human without naming the group; see Richardson & Carman translation (2002, p. 245).

Earlier synonyms:

1. *dorsal digital branches of dorsal branch of ulnar nerve (Günther, 1786)*
Günther described two ***dorsal digital nerves of ulnar nerve (>1840)*** for macrodissected adult human; in the original Latin (singular), *r. dig. dors.*, p. 76.
2. *dorsal digital nerves of dorsal branch of ulnar nerve (Langenbeck, 1826–1830)*
Synonym for macrodissected adult human ***dorsal digital nerves of ulnar nerve (>1840)***; in the original Latin, *nervi digitales dorsales, ex ramo dorsali nervi ulnaris*; Fascicle III, Table XIII, Figure 1-*21*.
3. *dorsal collateral branches of digital nerves of ulnar nerve (Quain & Wilson, 1839)*
Synonym for macrodissected adult human ***dorsal digital nerves of ulnar nerve (>1840)***; Plate XIX, Figure 2-*g*.

PARTLY CORRESPONDS:

1. *[radio-dorsal nerve of fourth finger (Meckel, 1817)] (Vesalius, 1543a)*
Described as branch of branch of ***dorsal branch of ulnar nerve (Günther, 1786)*** to lateral side of fourth finger in macrodissected adult human; see Richardson & Carman translation (2002, p. 245). Vesalius also noted that occasionally this ***nerve (Herophilus, c335–c280 BC)*** is a branch of the ***radial nerve (Du Verney, 1697)***, in which case there is no branch from ***dorsal branch of ulnar nerve (Günther, 1786)***; see Richardson & Carman translation (2002, p. 245).
2. *[cubito-dorsal nerve of fourth finger (Meckel, 1817)] (Vesalius, 1543a)*
Described as branch of branch of ***dorsal branch of ulnar nerve (Günther, 1786)*** to medial side of fourth finger in macrodissected adult human; see Richardson & Carman translation (2002, p. 245).

3. *[radio-dorsal nerve of fifth finger (Meckel, 1817)] (Vesalius, 1543a)*
Described as branch of branch of ***dorsal branch of ulnar nerve (Günther, 1786)*** to lateral side of little finger in macrodissected adult human; see Richardson & Carman translation (2002, p. 245).
4. *[cubito-dorsal nerve of fifth finger (Meckel, 1817)] (Vesalius, 1543a)*
Described as branch of branch of ***dorsal branch of ulnar nerve (Günther, 1786)*** to medial side of little finger in macrodissected adult human; see Richardson & Carman translation (2002, p. 245).
5. *internal dorsal nerve of auricular finger (Mayer, 1794)*
Macrodissected adult human ***dorsal digital nerve of ulnar nerve (>1840)*** described as extending from ***dorsal branch of ulnar nerve (Günther, 1786)*** to medial and dorsal region of fifth (little or auricular) finger; in the original Latin, *nervus dorsalis internus digiti auricularis*; Part 5, Table VI-27 (p. 35).
6. *external dorsal nerve of little finger (Mayer, 1794)*
Macrodissected adult human ***dorsal digital nerve of ulnar nerve (>1840)*** described as extending from ***dorsal branch of ulnar nerve (Günther, 1786)*** to lateral and dorsal region of fifth (little) finger; in the original Latin, *nervus dorsalis externus digiti minimi*; Part 5, Table VI-29 (p. 35).
7. *internal dorsal nerve of ring finger (Mayer, 1794)*
Macrodissected adult human ***dorsal digital nerve of ulnar nerve (>1840)*** described as extending from ***dorsal branch of ulnar nerve (Günther, 1786)*** to medial and dorsal region of fourth finger; in the original Latin, *nervus dorsalis internus digiti annularis*; Part 5, Table VI-30 (p. 35).
8. *external dorsal nerve of ring finger (Mayer, 1794)*
Macrodissected adult human ***dorsal digital nerve of ulnar nerve (>1840)*** described as extending from ***dorsal branch of ulnar nerve (Günther, 1786)*** to lateral and dorsal region of fourth finger; in the original Latin, *nervus dorsalis externus digiti annularis*; Part 5, Table VI-32 (p. 35).
9. *internal dorsal nerve of middle finger (Mayer, 1794)*
Macrodissected adult human ***dorsal digital nerve of ulnar nerve (>1840)*** described as extending from ***dorsal branch of ulnar nerve (Günther, 1786)*** to medial and dorsal region of third finger; in the original Latin, *nervus dorsalis internus digiti medii*; Part 5, Table VI-33 (p. 36).
10. *ulnar dorsal nerve of ring finger (Loder, 1803)*
Synonym for macrodissected adult human *internal dorsal nerve of ring finger (Mayer, 1794)*; in the original Latin, *nervus dorsalis ulnaris digiti annularis*, Table CLXXVIII, Figure 2-79.
11. *radial dorsal nerve of auricular finger (Loder, 1803)*
Synonym for macrodissected adult human *external dorsal nerve of auricular finger (Mayer, 1794)*; in the original Latin, *nervus dorsalis ulnaris digiti auricularis*, Table CLXXVIII, Figure 2-80.
12. *ulnar dorsal nerve of auricular finger (Loder, 1803)*
Synonym for macrodissected adult human *internal dorsal nerve of auricular finger (Mayer, 1794)*; in the original Latin, *nervus dorsalis ulnaris digiti auricularis*, Table CLXXVIII, Figure 2-81.
13. *ulnar nerve of little finger of cubital nerve (Caldani, 1813, 1814)*
Synonym for macrodissected adult human *ulnar dorsal nerve of auricular finger (Loder, 1803)*; in the original Latin, *nervus ulnaris digiti minimi a nervo cubitali*, Table CCLX, Figure 2-8.
14. *radio-dorsal nerve of fourth finger (Meckel, 1817)*
Described as arising from second filament of anterior twig of ***dorsal branch of ulnar nerve (Günther, 1786)*** supplying lateral side of ring finger in macrodissected adult human; see translation (1832, Vol. 3, p. 28). See *[radio-dorsal nerve of fourth finger (Meckel, 1817)] (Vesalius, 1543a)*.
15. *cubito-dorsal nerve of fourth finger (Meckel, 1817)*
Described as arising from first filament of anterior twig of ***dorsal branch of ulnar nerve (Günther, 1786)*** supplying medial side of ring finger in macrodissected adult human; see translation (1832, Vol. 3, p. 28). See *[cubito-dorsal nerve of fourth finger (Meckel, 1817)] (Vesalius, 1543a)*.
16. *radio-dorsal nerve of fifth finger (Meckel, 1817)*
Described as arising from first filament of anterior twig of ***dorsal branch of ulnar nerve (Günther, 1786)*** supplying lateral side of little finger in macrodissected adult human; see translation (1832, Vol. 3, p. 28). See *[radio-dorsal nerve of fifth finger (Meckel, 1817)] (Vesalius, 1543a)*.
17. *cubito-dorsal nerve of fifth finger (Meckel, 1817)*
Described as arising from posterior twig of ***dorsal branch of ulnar nerve (Günther, 1786)*** supplying medial side of little finger in macrodissected adult human; see translation (1832, Vol. 3, p. 28). See *[cubito-dorsal nerve of fifth finger (Meckel, 1817)] (Vesalius, 1543a)*.
18. *dorsal ulnar nerve of ring-finger (Knox, 1832)*
Synonym for macrodissected adult human *ulnar dorsal nerve of ring finger (Loder, 1803)*; Plate XXII, Figure 2-4,7.
19. *nerve for radial side of little finger (Knox, 1832)*
Synonym for macrodissected adult human *radial dorsal nerve of auricular finger (Loder, 1803)*; Plate XXII, Figure 2-6.
20. *internal dorsal branch of cubital nerve internal dorsal branch of hand (Cruveilhier, 1836)*
In macrodissected adult human, tiny proximal segment in wrist of ***dorsal digital nerve of ulnar nerve (>1840)*** to medial side of little finger; in the original French, *rameau dorsal interne*, p. 812.
21. *internal dorsal collateral branch of cubital nerve internal dorsal branch of hand (Cruveilhier, 1836)*
Macrodissected adult human distal segment of ***dorsal digital nerve of ulnar nerve (>1840)*** to medial side of little finger; in the original French, *collatéral dorsal interne*, p. 812.
22. *external dorsal branch of cubital nerve internal dorsal branch of hand (Cruveilhier, 1836)*
Macrodissected adult human proximal segment of ***dorsal digital nerve of ulnar nerve (>1840)*** generating two

secondary *external dorsal collateral branches of cubital nerve internal dorsal branch of hand (Cruveilhier, 1836)*, each in turn generating two tertiary branches to adjacent fingers; in the original French, *rameau dorsal externe*, p. 812.

23. *anastomotic filament of external dorsal branch of cubital nerve internal dorsal branch of hand (Cruveilhier, 1836)*
Macrodissected adult human ***communicating branch (Winslow, 1733)*** between *external dorsal branch of cubital nerve internal dorsal branch of hand (Cruveilhier, 1836)* and its counterpart from ***radial nerve (Du Verney, 1697)***; in the original French, *filet anastomotique*, p. 812.

24. *dorsal collateral branches of cubital nerve internal dorsal branch of hand (Cruveilhier, 1836)*
In macrodissected adult human, two secondary branches of *external dorsal branch of cubital nerve internal dorsal branch of hand (Cruveilhier, 1836)*, each generating two tertiary branches to adjacent fingers; in the original French, *rameaux collatéraux dorsaux*, p. 812.

25. *external collateral branch of little finger of dorsal collateral branches of cubital nerve internal dorsal branch of hand (Cruveilhier, 1836)*
Macrodissected adult human ***dorsal digital nerve of ulnar nerve (>1840)*** along lateral side of little finger; in the original French, *collatéral externe du petit doigt*, p. 812.

26. *internal collateral branch of ring finger of dorsal collateral branches of cubital nerve internal dorsal branch of hand (Cruveilhier, 1836)*
Macrodissected adult human ***dorsal digital nerve of ulnar nerve (>1840)*** along medial side of ring finger; in the original French, *collatéral interne de l'annulaire*, p. 812.

27. *external collateral branch of ring finger of dorsal collateral branches of cubital nerve internal dorsal branch of hand (Cruveilhier, 1836)*
Macrodissected adult human ***dorsal digital nerve of ulnar nerve (>1840)*** along lateral side of ring finger; in the original French, *collatéral externe de l'annulaire*, p. 812.

28. *internal collateral branch of middle finger of dorsal collateral branches of cubital nerve internal dorsal branch of hand (Cruveilhier, 1836)*
Macrodissected adult human ***dorsal digital nerve of ulnar nerve (>1840)*** along medial side of middle finger; in the original French, *collatéral interne du médius*, p. 812.

dorsal fornix (Sprague & Meyer, 1950)

As described in macrodissected adult human, and mammal generally with histological methods for ***axons (Kölliker, 1896)***, a longitudinal differentiation of the ***fimbria (Honegger, 1890)*** lying just ventral to the ***corpus callosum (Galen, c177)*** in the median plane. In eutherian mammals where ***Ammon's horn (Vicq d'Azyr, 1784)*** extends rostrodorsally just ventral to the ***corpus callosum (Galen, c177)***, the caudal end of the ***dorsal fornix (Sprague & Meyer, 1950)*** lies between ***corpus callosum (Galen, c177)*** dorsally and ***field CA1 (Lorente de Nó, 1934)*** ventrally, and the rostral end lies at the level of the rostral tip of the ***ventral hippocampal commissure (Craigie, 1925)*** and caudal tip of the ***lateral septal complex (Risold & Swanson, 1997)***; see Swanson (2004, Atlas Levels 21–33). For Sprague & Meyer's use in adult rabbit with experimental degeneration and normal histological methods for ***axons (Kölliker, 1896)***, see p. 355. It was probably first clearly delineated by Carus; see ***[dorsal fornix (Sprague & Meyer, 1950)] (Carus, 1814)***.

EARLIER REFERENCES:

Described, not named or illustrated:

1. ***[dorsal fornix (Sprague & Meyer, 1950)] (Carus, 1814)***
According to Honegger (1890, p. 228), Carus first described it for macrodissected adult human, p. 226. Honegger (1890, p. 247) also noted Stieda (1869 p. 87, Tab. III, Fig. 61-c') referred to it as a *Markschicht der Rinde* in mouse (also see Kölliker, 1896, p. 787).

Earlier synonyms:

1. *arcuate fascicle of septum pellucidum (Ganser, 1882)*
Synonym for ***dorsal fornix (Sprague & Meyer, 1950)*** in adult mole with histological methods for ***axons (Kölliker, 1896)***; in the original Latin, *fasciculus arcuatus septi pellucidi*; in the original German, *Bogenbündel der Scheidewand*, p. 640, Figures 17–20.
2. *olfactory fascicle of trigone (Dejerine & Dejerine-Klumpke, 1901)*
Largely corresponds to macrodissected adult human ***dorsal fornix (Sprague & Meyer, 1950)***; in the original French, *faisceau olfactif du trigone*, pp. 264, 283; Figures 252-*Fol*, 262-*Fol*.
3. *olfactory fascicle of Ammon's horn of Zuckerkandl (Dejerine & Dejerine-Klumpke, 1901)*
Eponym for *olfactory fascicle of trigone (Dejerine & Dejerine-Klumpke, 1901)*; in the original French, *faisceaux olfactif de la corne d'Ammon de Zuckerkandl*, p. 283.
4. *olfactory fasciculus of fornix (Tilney & Riley, 1923)*
Synonym for macrodissected adult human *olfactory fascicle of trigone (Dejerine & Dejerine-Klumpke, 1901)*; Figure 506-*Fol*.

dorsal funiculus (>1840)

As described for macrodissected adult human and other mammal, the dorsal topographic division of the ***funiculi of spinal cord (Burdach, 1822)***, between the ***dorsal median septum (>1840)*** in the median plane and the ***dorsolateral tract (>1840)*** of the ***lateral funiculus (Burdach, 1822)*** laterally. See Carpenter (1976, pp. 214–216 and Fig. 9.2), called *posterior funiculus (Rosenthal, 1815)*; Williams & Warwick (1980, p. 868 and Fig. 7.36), called *posterior funiculus (Rosenthal, 1815)*; *Terminologia Anatomica* (1998, p. 107); Nieuwenhuys et al. (2008, Fig. 6.1-3). It was first identified in illustration by Blasius; see ***[dorsal funiculus (>1840)] (Blasius, 1666)***.

EARLIER REFERENCES:

Illustrated, not named or described:

1. ***[dorsal funiculus (>1840)] (Blasius, 1666)***
   Clearly illustrated for macrodissected adult human; Figures 10, 11, 18.

Earlier synonyms:

1. *posterior cord (Vicq d'Azyr, 1784)*
   Synonym for macrodissected adult human ***dorsal funiculus (>1840)***; pp. 602–603, see Clarke & O'Malley translation (1996, p. 270) and *medullary columns (Vicq d'Azyr, 1784)*.
2. *posterior funiculus (Rosenthal, 1815)*
   Synonym for macrodissected adult human ***dorsal funiculus (>1840)***; in the original German, *hintern Strang(s)*, p. 29; see Burdach (1822, pp. 31, 35–36). Blasius (1674, p. 59) may have mentioned the posterior funiculus.
3. *posterior medullary cord (Meckel, 1817)*
   Synonym for macrodissected adult human ***dorsal funiculus (>1840)***; see translation (1832, Vol. 2, p. 413).
4. *posterior half of spinal marrow (Meckel, 1817)*
   Basically synonym for macrodissected adult human ***dorsal funiculus (>1840)***; see translation (1832, Vol. 2, p. 414).
5. *posterior column of spinal marrow (Bell, 1822)*
   Synonym for macrodissected adult human and other mammalian ***dorsal funiculus (>1840)***; p. 292. Bell (1835, pp. 257, 259) later thought from macrodissection that it comes from *restiform body (Günther, 1786)* and thus ***cerebellum (Aristotle)***; see *cerebellar fascicle (Bellingeri, 1823)*.
6. *posterior fascicle of spinal medulla (Bellingeri, 1823)*
   Synonym for macrodissected adult human and other mammalian ***dorsal funiculus (>1840)***; in the original Latin (plural), *fasciculi posteriores medullae spinalis*, Table 1, Figure 1-*e*.
7. *cerebellar fascicle (Bellingeri, 1823)*
   Synonym for macrodissected adult human and other mammalian ***dorsal funiculus (>1840)***; in the original Latin (plural), *fasciculi cerebellosi*, p. 10. See *posterior column of spinal marrow (Bell, 1822)*.
8. *abdominal cord of spinal medulla (Cloquet, 1828)*
   Synonym for macrodissected adult human *posterior cord (Vicq d'Azyr, 1784)*; in the original French (plural), *cordons abdominaux de la moelle épinière*, Plate CXLV, Figure 6-15.
9. *posterior part of white substance of spinal medulla (Arnold, 1838b)*
   Synonym for macrodissected adult human ***dorsal funiculus (>1840)***; in the original Latin (plural), *substantiae albae pars postica*, Plate II, Figure 16-*e*.

dorsal hippocampal commissure (Craigie, 1925)

As described in macrodissected adult human, and mammal generally with histological methods for ***axons (Kölliker, 1896)***, the caudal differentiation of the ***hippocampal commissures (Johnston, 1913)***, caudal to the ***intermediate hippocampal commissure (>1840)*** and containing commissural ***axons (Kölliker, 1896)*** from the ***retrohippocampal region (Swanson et al., 1987)***; see Swanson and Cowan (1977), Swanson et al. (1978). Gall and Spurzheim (1810, p. 205) first claimed that the adult human *lyre (Winslow, 1733)* contains commissural fibers, although they believed the fibers arose form caudal *gyri (Vesalius, 1543a)* of the ***temporal region (>1840)***; see Gordon (1817, p. 132). A clearer term would be *caudal hippocampal commissure*. For Craigie's use in adult rat with the Weigert myelin method see p. 103 and Plate XXVI. It was known to Vesalius; see ***[dorsal hippocampal commissure (Craigie, 1925)] (Vesalius, 1543a)***.

EARLIER REFERENCES:

Illustrated and described, not named:

1. ***[dorsal hippocampal commissure (Craigie, 1925)] (Vesalius, 1543a)***
   Vesalius clearly illustrated the region of this feature (see Figs. 5-*T* and 6-*A* in Singer translation, 1952), and wrote "that part of this body [of the ***fornix (Vesalius, 1543a)***] which springs from the right [lateral] ventricle is continuous with that from the left [***lateral ventricle (Vesalius, 1543a)***], and the two form one broad mass." (Singer translation, 1952, p. 41). There was, however, no hint of a distinction between ***fimbria (Honegger, 1890)*** and ***dorsal hippocampal commissure (Craigie, 1925)***.

Earlier synonyms:

1. *lyre (Winslow, 1733)*
   Synonym for macrodissected adult human ***dorsal hippocampal commissure (Craigie, 1925)***. Winslow defined it as lying between right and left *posterior pillar of fornix (Winslow, 1733)* just before coming together to form *anterior pillar of fornix (Winslow, 1733)*, and wrote that it was named by "the ancients" for its resemblance to a stringed musical instrument resembling somewhat a dulcimer (Sect. X, p. 35). Winslow did not state the source of this name, although *testudo (Achillini, 1520)*, synonymous with *fornix (Galen, c177)*, refers to something shaped like either an arch (*fornix*) or a lyre. Vicq d'Azyr concluded that "the ancients" used terms related to lyre in referring to the entire structure they regarded as the fornix (1786, pp. 31–32)—see ***[dorsal hippocampal commissure (Craigie, 1925)] (Vesalius, 1543a)***—and illustrated Winslow's conception of fornix very clearly (Pls. VII, VIII, and XV).
2. *psaloides (Winslow, 1733)*
   Term Winslow indicated "the ancients" applied to *lyre (Winslow, 1733)*, although he was probably the first to identify it as a distinct component of ***fornix (Vesalius, 1543a)***; Section X, p. 35. See discussion of this history in Meyer (1971, pp. 20–21). *Psaloides (Galen, 177)* referred to entire *fornix (Galen, c177)* as Galen observed it in macrodissected adult beef, pig, and/or monkey but not human.

3. *psalterium (Tarin, 1750)*
   Tarin is usually credited with providing the first illustration of ***dorsal hippocampal commissure (Craigie, 1925)*** as a distinct structure; Table I, Figure 1-*P*; see Meyer (1971, p. 21). Transverse shading between *C,B,C* in Figure IIII of Willis (1664) might be interpreted as resembling the *psalterium (Tarin, 1750)*, but he did not label it and did not mention anything of the sort in the text. Also see *lyre (Winslow, 1733)*.
4. *lamina medullaris triangularis (Günz, 1750)*
   Synonym for macrodissected adult human *lyre (Winslow, 1733)*, according to Schreger (1803, p. 319), Burdach (1822, p. 368).
5. *lyra Davidis (Mayer, 1779)*
   Mayer attached David eponymously to *lyre (Winslow, 1733)*, apparently referring to the anatomist Jean-Pierre David (1737–1784), although Winslow used the term before David was born; p. 10, see Burdach (1822, p. 368).
6. *corpus psalloideum (Mayer, 1779)*
   Synonym for *lyra Davidis (Mayer, 1779)*; p. 10, see Burdach (1822, p. 368).
7. *membrana medullaris inter crura posteriora fornicis (Haase, 1781)*
   Synonym for macrodissected adult human *lyre (Winslow, 1733)*; see Burdach (1822, p. 368).
8. *corpus psalloïdes (Vicq d'Azyr, 1786)*
   Synonym for macrodissected adult human *lyre (Winslow, 1733)*; Plate VII, Figure IV:3–6, p. 22. Vicq d'Azyr defined it (Pl. XXVI, Fig. III-*h*) as lying between dorsal (posterior or septal) end of right and left *posterior pillar of fornix (Vicq d'Azyr, 1786)*.
9. *dorsal commissure of Ammon's horn (Kölliker, 1896)*
   Synonym for adult human ***dorsal hippocampal commissure (Craigie, 1925)*** observed with histological methods for ***axons (Kölliker, 1896)***; in the original German, *dorsale Kommissur der Ammonshörner*, p. 776. Dejerine & Dejerine-Klumpke (1901, pp. 295–296) credited Ganser (1882, p. 659?) with first noting a dorsal part of *psalterium (Ganser, 1882)* in mole.

dorsal horn (>1840)

As described for macrodissected adult human, and for mammal in general with cellular architecture and connections, the ***gray matter region (Swanson & Bota, 2010)*** of the ***spinal cord (Galen, c162–166)*** lying dorsal to the ***intermediate spinal zone (>1840)*** and often divided, from ventral to dorsal, into base, neck, head, and apex; see *Terminologia Anatomica* (1998, p. 106). The base is formed by the ***basal nucleus of dorsal horn (Cajal, 1899–1904)*** medially and ***spinal reticular nucleus (>1840)*** laterally; the neck is formed by the ***nucleus proprius of spinal cord (>1840)***; the head is formed by the ***gelatinous substance of spinal cord (>1840)*** or *substantia gelatinosa of spinal cord (>1840)*; and the apex is formed by the ***marginal nucleus of spinal cord (>1840)***. For a good comparison of classical ***spinal cord (Galen, c162–166)*** parceling with the laminar scheme proposed by Rexed (1952), see Carpenter (1976, pp. 222–229); also see Cajal (1899-1904, Vol. 1, pp. 225–228), Swanson (1998–1999, pp. 212–213). The ***dorsal horn (>1840)*** was first distinguished by Blasius; see ***[dorsal horn (>1840)] (Blasius, 1666)***.

EARLIER REFERENCES:

Illustrated and described, not named:

1. ***[dorsal horn (>1840)] (Blasius, 1666)***
   Very clearly illustrated for macrodissected adult human, showing it is thinner than ***ventral horn (>1840)***; see Schulte & Endtz (1977, p. 13).

Earlier synonyms:

1. *cauda of spinal ash-colored substance (Winslow, 1733)*
   Roughly synonymous with macrodissected adult human ***dorsal horn (>1840)*** viewed in transverse section; Section X, p. 44.
2. *extremities of spinal ash-colored substance (Winslow, 1733)*
   Synonym for *cauda of spinal ash-colored substance (Winslow, 1733)*.
3. *posterior cineritious substance (Monro, 1783)*
   Monro roughly indicated difference in macrodissected adult human between ***dorsal horn (>1840)*** and ***ventral horn (>1840)***, although his account was vague: "...when either of these two cords [halves of ***spinal cord (Galen, c162–c166)***] is accurately examined it will be found to be subdivided by a slight furrow, into a small posterior cord and a large anterior cord. In the former, fasciculi of longitudinal fibres readily appear; in the latter, the disposition of the medullary fibres is much less evident...When we cut the spinal marrow transversely, the internal cineritious substance makes a cruciform appearance [***X***-shaped], or consists of four portions, one corresponding to each of the four cords of which I have observed it consists." (pp. 28–29). In contemporaneous work, Vicq d'Azyr (1784, pp. 600–601) divided lateral part of spinal *ash-colored substance (Winslow, 1733)* into anterior extremity, body or central part, and posterior extremity.
4. *posterior end of lateral part of spinal ash-colored substance (Vicq d'Azyr, 1784)*
   Roughly synonymous with macrodissected adult human ***dorsal horn (>1840)***; in the original French, *l'extrémité postérieure*, p. 601.
5. *posterior horn of cineritious substance (Günther, 1786)*
   Roughly synonymous with macrodissected adult human ***dorsal horn (>1840)***; in the original Latin (plural), *cornua postrorsum substantia cinerea*, p. 33.
6. *posterior crus of gray substance (Keuffel, 1810)*
   Roughly synonymous with macrodissected adult human ***dorsal horn (>1840)*** viewed in transverse section; in the original Latin (plural), *crura posteriora substantiae cinereae*, Figure 1-*l,m*.
7. *posterior gray column (Burdach, 1819)*
   Roughly synonymous with macrodissected adult human ***dorsal horn (>1840)***; in the original German, *hintern graue Strang*, p. 134. Also see Burdach (1822, p. 30).

8. *posterior horn (Rolando, 1825a)*
   Roughly synonymous with macrodissected calf ***dorsal horn (>1840)***; in the original French (plural), *cornes postérieures*, Table VII, Figure 1-*y*.
9. *posterior horn of medulla (Quain, 1828)*
   Roughly synonymous with macrodissected adult human ***dorsal horn (>1840)***; p. 609.
10. *posterior horn of spinal cord (Quain, 1828)*
   Roughly synonymous with macrodissected adult human ***dorsal horn (>1840)***; p. 720.
11. *posterior crus of spinal medulla (Arnold, 1838b)*
   Roughly synonymous with macrodissected adult human ***dorsal horn (>1840)***; in the original Latin (plural), *crura posteriora*, Table II, Figure 2-*e*.
12. *posterior gray fascicle (Wagner, 1839)*
   Roughly synonymous with macrodissected adult human ***dorsal horn (>1840)***; in the original Latin, *fasciculus cinereus posterior*, Table XXVII, Figure 10-7.

PARTLY CORRESPONDS:

1. *posterior gray substance (Rolando, 1824)*
   Corresponds to macrodissected adult human ***gelatinous substance of spinal cord (>1840)*** and ***marginal nucleus of spinal cord (>1840)*** considered together, as viewed in transverse section; in the original Italian, *sostanza cinericcia posteriori*, p. 59. Also see *posterior gray substance darker and almost gelatinous (Rolando, 1824)*.
2. *posterior gray substance darker and almost gelatinous (Rolando, 1824)*
   Synonym for *posterior gray substance (Rolando, 1824)*; in the original Italian, *sostanza cinericcia posterior quasi gelatinosa e più oscura*, Table III, Figure 3-*sp*.
3. *gelatinous substance of spinal medulla (Stilling & Wallach, 1842–1843)*
   Synonym for macrodissected adult human *posterior gray substance (Rolando, 1824)*; in the original German, *gelatinöse Substanz des Rückenmarkes*, Vol. 1, p. 9.

dorsal intermediate sulcus (>1840)

As described for macrodissected adult human, the groove on the dorsal surface of the ***medulla (Winslow, 1733)*** between ***gracile fascicle (Müller, 1834)*** medially and ***cuneate fascicle (Müller, 1834)*** laterally; see Nieuwenhuys et al. (2008, Fig. 3.10-22, called *posterior intermediate sulcus*). It was perhaps first clearly delineated by Santorini; see ***[dorsal intermediate sulcus (>1840)] (Santorini, 1775)***.

EARLIER REFERENCES:

Illustrated, not named or described:

1. ***[dorsal intermediate sulcus (>1840)] (Santorini, 1775)***
   Clearly illustrated for macrodissected adult human; Table III, Figure 2.

Earlier synonyms:

1. *collateral sulcus (Gall & Spurzheim, 1810)*
   Synonym for macrodissected adult human ***dorsal intermediate sulcus (>1840)***; in the original French, *sillon collateral*, p. 59. See Burdach (1822, p. 285).
2. *lateral fissure (Meckel, 1817)*
   Synonym for macrodissected adult human ***dorsal intermediate sulcus (>1840)***; see translation (1832, Vol. 2, p. 412), and Henle (1871, p. 41).
3. *posterior intermediate sulcus (Bellingeri, 1823)*
   Synonym for macrodissected adult human ***dorsal intermediate sulcus (>1840)***; in the original Latin (plural), *sulci intermedii posteriores*, Table I, Figure 2-*i*.
4. *sulci of posterior pyramids (Rolando, 1824)*
   Synonym for macrodissected adult human right and left ***dorsal intermediate sulcus (>1840)***; in the original Italian, *solchi delle piramidi posteriori*, p. 41 and Table I, Figure 1-*spp*.

dorsal intersegmental tract (>1840)

As described in macrodissected adult human, and mammal generally with histological methods for ***axons (Kölliker, 1896)***, a narrow ***central nervous system white matter tract (>1840)*** in the deepest part of the ***dorsal funiculus (>1840)***, predominantly but not exclusively formed by ***axons (Kölliker, 1896)*** connecting different ***gray matter regions (Swanson & Bota, 2010)*** within the ***spinal cord (Galen, c162-c166)***; see Mettler (1948, pp. 236–237), Crosby et al. (1962, p. 108), Williams & Warwick (1980, p. 882 and Figs. 7.43–44), called *posterior intersegmental tract (>1840)*, and *Dorland's* (2003, p. 678), under *fasciculus proprius posterior medullae spinalis*. It was not identified by 1840.

EARLIER REFERENCES:

Earlier synonyms:

1. *posterior fasciculus proprius (>1840)*
   Synonym for macrodissected adult human ***dorsal intersegmental tract (>1840)***; see *Terminologia Anatomica* (1998, p. 107).
2. *dorsal fasciculus proprius (>1840)*
   Synonym for macrodissected adult human ***dorsal intersegmental tract (>1840)***; see Williams & Warwick (1980, Fig. 7.44), *Terminologia Anatomica* (1998, p. 107).
3. *posterior intersegmental tract (>1840)*
   Synonym for macrodissected adult human ***dorsal intersegmental tract (>1840)***; see Williams & Warwick (1980, p. 882).

dorsal lateral geniculate nucleus (>1840)

As described for macrodissected adult human, and based on cellular architecture and connections in mammals generally, a ***gray matter region (Swanson & Bota, 2010)*** in the caudal and lateral end of the ***dorsal part of thalamus (Herrick, 1910)*** receiving a visual input directly from the ***retina (Herophilus, c335–c280 BC)*** and projecting to the ***primary visual area (>1840)*** or *area 17 (Brodmann, 1909)* of ***cerebral cortex gray matter (>1840)***; see Williams & Warwick (1980, p. 977), Jones (1985, Ch. 9). Also see ***ventral lateral geniculate nucleus (>1840)***. It was probably known to Galen; see ***[dorsal lateral geniculate nucleus (>1840)] (Galen, c192)***.

EARLIER REFERENCES:

Described, not named or illustrated:

1. ***[dorsal lateral geniculate nucleus (>1840)] (Galen, c192)*** In the later books of *On Anatomical Procedures*, apparently described for macrodissected adult beef, pig, and/or macaque but not human; see Duckworth translation (1962, p. 3), Woollam (1958, p. 15).

Illustrated and described, not named:

1. ***[dorsal lateral geniculate nucleus (>1840)] (Varoli, 1573)*** Clearly illustrated for macrodissected adult human; see Figure II-*e* on f. 19. Also see Polyak (1957, p. 98). Platter (1603, p. 122) first credited Varoli with the discovery.

Earlier synonyms:

1. *stringy protuberance (Diemerbroeck, 1689)* Apparently refers to macrodissected adult human ***dorsal lateral geniculate nucleus (>1840)***; p. 410.
2. *lateral geniculate body (Santorini, 1724)* Synonym for macrodissected adult human ***dorsal lateral geniculate nucleus (>1840)***; see Meyer (1971, p. 20).
3. *gibber inferius (Soemmerring, 1778)* Synonym for macrodissected adult human ***dorsal lateral geniculate nucleus (>1840)***; p. 108, according to Burdach (1822, p. 342).
4. *large round tubercle (Vicq d'Azyr, 1786)* Synonym for macrodissected adult human ***dorsal lateral geniculate nucleus (>1840)***, according to Burdach (1822, p. 342), who gave the Latin form, *tuberculum magnum rotundum*.
5. *outer corpus geniculatum (Gordon, 1815)* Synonym for macrodissected adult human ***dorsal lateral geniculate nucleus (>1840)***; p. 88.
6. *anterior tubercle of thalamus opticus (Gordon, 1815)* Synonym for macrodissected adult human ***dorsal lateral geniculate nucleus (>1840)***; p. 92.
7. *tuberculum thalami posticum inferius (Meckel, 1817)* Synonym for macrodissected adult human ***dorsal lateral geniculate nucleus (>1840)***; see translation (1832, Vol. 2, p. 453).
8. *tuberculum thalami posticum externus (Meckel, 1817)* Synonym for macrodissected adult human ***dorsal lateral geniculate nucleus (>1840)***; see translation (1832, Vol. 2, p. 453).
9. *tuberculum pedunculi cerebri (Treviranus, 1820)* Synonym for macrodissected adult human ***dorsal lateral geniculate nucleus (>1840)***; p. 20 according to Burdach (1822, p. 342).
10. *external geniculate body (Burdach, 1822)* Synonym for macrodissected adult human ***dorsal lateral geniculate nucleus (>1840)***; in the original Latin, *corpus geniculatum externum*, p. 118. Gordon (1815, p. 92) called it *external corpus geniculatum* in English.
11. *geniculate tubercle (Rolando, 1825a)* Synonym for macrodissected adult human ***dorsal lateral geniculate nucleus (>1840)***; in the original Latin, *tuberculum geniculatum*, and original French, *tubercule noueux*, Table V, Figure 1-*t.n*.
12. *posterior and external tubercle of optic bed (Meckel, 1832)* Translation of *tuberculum thalami posticum externus (Meckel, 1817)*; Vol. 3, p. 77.
13. *ganglioform intumescence at origin of optic nerve (Arnold, 1834)* Synonym for macrodissected adult human ***dorsal lateral geniculate nucleus (>1840)***; in the original Latin, *intumescentia ganglioformis in origine nervi optici*, p. 6.
14. *greater geniculate body (Solly, 1836)* Synonym for macrodissected adult human ***dorsal lateral geniculate nucleus (>1840)***; p. 245.
15. *anterior geniculate (Gerdy, 1838)* Synonym for macrodissected adult human ***dorsal lateral geniculate nucleus (>1840)***; in the original French, *genouillé antérieur*, p. 262.
16. *external geniculate tubercle (Arnold, 1838b)* Synonym for macrodissected adult human ***dorsal lateral geniculate nucleus (>1840)***; in the original Latin, *tuberculum geniculatum externum*, Table IV, Figure 3-ζ.

dorsal longitudinal fascicle (Schütz, 1891)

As described in adult human with histological methods for ***axons (Kölliker, 1896)***, a diffusely organized, longitudinal ***central nervous system white matter tract (>1840)*** stretching the length of the ***periaqueductal gray (>1840)*** and caudally adjacent ***pontine central gray (>1840)***. It is continuous rostrally with the ***periventricular bundle of hypothalamus (>1840)*** and ***periventricular bundle of thalamus (>1840)***, all three together often regarded as forming the periventricular system, with most ***axons (Kölliker, 1896)*** tending to orient longitudinally; see Crosby et al. (1962, pp. 318–320), Sutin (1966), Nauta & Haymaker (1969, pp. 172–173, 197–198 and Fig. 4.26), *Terminologia Anatomica* (1998, p. 116), Swanson (2004, p. 178 notes 125, 130). For topographic description it has ***tegmental dorsal longitudinal fascicle (Schütz, 1891)*** and ***pontine dorsal longitudinal fascicle (Schütz, 1891)*** segments. The rostral end of the ***midbrain dorsal longitudinal fascicle (Schütz, 1891)*** joins the caudal end of the ***hypothalamic medial forebrain bundle (>1840)*** as well as the caudal ends of the ***periventricular bundle of hypothalamus (>1840)*** and ***periventricular bundle of thalamus (>1840)***. For Schütz's use in normal histological material see pp. 531, 576 and Table XI, Figure 1-*dl*. It was not identified by 1840.

TRANSLATIONS:

1. *dorsales Längsbündel (Schütz, 1891)* Original German form of ***dorsal longitudinal fascicle (Schütz, 1891)***; see pp. 531, 576 and Table XI, Figure 1-*dl*.

LATER SYNONYMS:

1. *posterior longitudinal fasciculus (>1840)* Synonym for macrodissected adult human ***dorsal longitudinal fascicle (Schütz, 1891)***; see *Terminologia Anatomica* (1998, p. 116).

dorsal median septum (>1840)

As described for macrodissected adult human, the longitudinal division between right and left ***gracile fascicle (Müller, 1834)*** of the ***spinal cord (Galen, c162–c166)***, deep to the shallow ***dorsal median sulcus of spinal cord (>1840)*** on the dorsal surface in the median plane; see Williams & Warwick (1980, p. 865 and Fig. 7.36, called *posterior median septum*), *Nomina Anatomica* (1983, p. A64), *Terminologia Anatomica* (1998, p. 105). It was probably first mentioned by Mondino; see ***[dorsal median sulcus (>1840] (Mondino, 1316)***.

EARLIER REFERENCES:

Described, not named or illustrated:

1. *[dorsal median septum (>1840)] (Mondino, 1316)*
   Mentioned for macrodissected adult human; see Singer translation (1925, Vol. 1, p. 97). It presumably included ***dorsal median sulcus of spinal cord (>1840)***. Coiter (1572; see translation p. 113) clearly described it for macrodissected adult human, including observation that it is "covered by a thin membrane", presumably of ***pia (Galen, c192)***.

Earlier synonyms:

1. *major posterior fissure (Blasius, 1666)*
   Synonym for macrodissected adult human ***dorsal median septum (>1840)***; Figure X-*e*, also see Haller (1762, p. 82). It presumably included ***dorsal median sulcus of spinal cord (>1840)***.
2. *posterior partition (Pourfour du Petit, 1710)*
   Synonym for macrodissected adult human ***dorsal median septum (>1840)***; in the original French, *la division postérieure*, Letter 1, p. 15, see translation in Clarke & O'Malley (1996, p. 265). It presumably included ***dorsal median sulcus of spinal cord (>1840)***.
3. *posterior median fissure (Morgagni, 1719)*
   Synonym for macrodissected adult human ***dorsal median septum (>1840)***; p. 18, see Haller (1762, p. 82).
4. *posterior fissure (Vic d'Azyr, 1784)*
   Synonym for macrodissected adult human ***dorsal median septum (>1840)***; in the original French, *le sillon postérieur*, p. 599 ff.; see translation in Clarke & O'Malley (1996, p. 270). It presumably included ***dorsal median sulcus of spinal cord (>1840)***.
5. *posterior longitudinal groove (Tiedemann, 1816)*
   Synonym for macrodissected fetal human ***dorsal median septum (>1840)***; see translation (1826, p. 30).
6. *posterior median sulcus (Bellingeri, 1823)*
   Synonym for macrodissected adult mammalian, including human, ***dorsal median septum (>1840)***; in the original Latin, *sulcus medius posterior*, Table I, Figure 1-*b*.

dorsal median sulcus of medulla (>1840)

As described for macrodissected adult human, a dorsal longitudinal groove in the median plane of the caudal half of the ***medulla (Winslow, 1733)*** between ***obex (Burdach, 1822)*** rostrally and ***dorsal median sulcus of spinal cord (>1840)*** caudally; see Crosby et al. (1962, Fig. 97), Williams & Warwick (1980, p. 897), *Terminologia Anatomica* (1998, p. 109). It was first delineated by Vesalius; see ***[dorsal median sulcus of medulla (>1840)] (Vesalius, 1543a)***.

EARLIER REFERENCES:

Illustrated, not named or described:

1. ***[dorsal median sulcus of medulla (>1840)] (Vesalius, 1543a)***
   Clearly illustrated for macrodissected adult human; see Singer translation (1952, Fig. 10, above *P*).

Earlier synonyms:

1. *posterior median fissure (Gordon, 1815)*
   Synonym here for macrodissected adult human ***dorsal median sulcus of medulla (>1840)***; p. 178.
2. *posterior median sulcus of medulla oblongata (Quain, 1832)*
   Synonym for macrodissected adult human ***dorsal median sulcus of medulla (>1840)***; p. 636. See *Terminologia Anatomica* (1998, p. 109).
3. *posterior longitudinal fissure (Arnold, 1838b)*
   Synonym for macrodissected adult human ***dorsal median fissure of medulla (>1840)***; in the original Latin, *fissura longitudinalis posterior*, Table II, Figure 13-*b*.

dorsal median sulcus of spinal cord (>1840)

As described for macrodissected adult human, the shallow dorsal groove between right and left ***dorsal funiculus (>1840)*** in the median plane. It extends deeply (ventrally) all the way to the ***spinal central gray (>1840)*** as the ***dorsal median septum (>1840)*** and also extends rostrally as the ***dorsal median sulcus of medulla (>1840)***; see Williams & Warwick (1980, p. 865 and Fig. 7.36, called *posterior median sulcus*), *Nomina Anatomica* (1983, p. A64), *Terminologia Anatomica* (1998, p. 105). It was probably first mentioned by Mondino; see ***[dorsal median sulcus of spinal cord (>1840] (Mondino, 1316)***.

EARLIER REFERENCES:

Described, not named or illustrated:

1. ***[dorsal median sulcus of spinal cord (>1840] (Mondino, 1316)***
   Mentioned for macrodissected adult human; see Singer translation (1925, Vol. 1, p. 97).

Illustrated and described, not named:

1. ***[dorsal median sulcus of spinal cord (>1840)] Blasius (1666)***
   Clearly illustrated for macrodissected adult human; Figure XIII-*b*.

Earlier synonyms:

1. *superior medullary sulcus (Bojanus, 1819–1821)*
   Synonym for macrodissected adult turtle ***dorsal median sulcus of spinal cord (>1840)***; in the original Latin, *sulcus medullae superior*, Figure 83-*k*.
2. *superior sulcus of spinal medulla (Bojanus, 1819–1821)*
   Synonym for macrodissected adult turtle ***dorsal median sulcus of spinal cord (>1840)***; in the original Latin, *sulcus medullae spinalis superior*, Figures 95–100:*k*.

3. *posterior median sulcus of spinal medulla (Rolando, 1824)*
   Synonym for macrodissected adult human ***dorsal median sulcus of spinal cord (>1840)***; in the original Italian, *solco mediano posteriore*, p. 38.
4. *dorsal median fissure of spinal cord (Spurzheim, 1826)*
   Synonym for macrodissected adult human ***dorsal median sulcus of spinal cord (>1840)***; from description on p. 65.
5. *posterior median furrow of spinal marrow (Mayo, 1827)*
   Synonym for macrodissected adult human ***dorsal median sulcus of spinal cord (>1840)***; Plate I, Figure 1-*b*.
6. *posterior longitudinal sulcus (Arnold, 1838a)*
   Synonym for macrodissected adult human ***dorsal median sulcus of spinal cord (>1840)***; in the original Latin, *sulcus longitudinalis posterior*, p. 12.

dorsal midbrain sulcus (>1840)

As described for macrodissected adult human and other vertebrates, a longitudinal groove on the dorsolateral surface of the ***midbrain (Baer, 1837)*** between ***tectum (Baer, 1837)*** dorsally and ***tegmentum (Swanson, 2000b)*** ventrally; see Crosby et al. (1962, p. 221, called *dorsolateral fissure*), Williams & Warwick (1980, p. 935). During development it is often regarded as the ***midbrain vesicle (Baer, 1837)*** equivalent of the ***limiting sulcus (>1840)***, and has been called the *lateral tectal sulcus (Palmgren, 1921)* or *midbrain sulcus (Alvarez-Bolado & Swanson, 1996)*; see Alvarez-Bolado & Swanson (1996, p. 14). It was perhaps first clearly delineated by Vesalius; see ***[dorsal midbrain sulcus (>1840)] (Vesalius, 1543a)***.

EARLIER REFERENCES:

Illustrated, not named or described:

1. ***[dorsal midbrain sulcus (>1840)] (Vesalius, 1543a)***
   Illustrated but not described for macrodissected adult human; see Singer (1952, Figs. 8, 10).

Earlier synonyms:

1. *dorsolateral fissure (>1840)*
   Synonym for macrodissected adult human ***dorsal midbrain sulcus (>1840)***; see Crosby et al. (1962, p. 221).

dorsal motor nucleus of vagus nerve (>1840)

As described for adult mammal based on cellular architecture and connections, a thin longitudinal ***gray matter region (Swanson & Bota, 2010)*** in dorsomedial parts of the ***medulla (Winslow, 1733)***, lying between ***hypoglossal nucleus (>1840)*** medially and ***nucleus of solitary tract (>1840)*** laterally and generating motor components of the ***vagus nerve central root (>1840)*** continuing in the peripheral ***vagus nerve root (>1840)***. Functionally, it consists mostly of preganglionic parasympathetic ***neurons (Waldeyer, 1891)*** supplying many parts of the viscera; see Williams & Warwick (1980, pp. 1076, 1123 and Fig. 7.224), Nieuwenhuys et al. (2008, pp. 191, 194 and Figs. 6.22–23). It was not identified by 1840.

dorsal nerve of clitoris (>1840)

As described for macrodissected adult human female, a very small branch of the ***pudendal nerve (Camper, 1762)*** supplying erectile tissue of the crus and corpus cavernosum of the clitoris before passing onto its dorsal side to supply its distal two-thirds; see Durward (1951, p. 1102), Williams & Warwick (1980, p. 1116), *Terminologia Anatomica* (1998, p. 140). It was first clearly delineated as the *superior pudendal nerve in female (Camper, 1762)*.

EARLIER REFERENCES:

Earlier synonyms:

1. *superior pudendal nerve in female (Camper, 1762)*
   Synonym for macrodissected adult human female ***dorsal nerve of clitoris (>1840)***; p. 7. Haller also touched on it in the same year (1762, p. 253), without providing a name.
2. *clitoral pudendal nerve (Walter, 1783)*
   Synonym for macrodissected adult human female ***dorsal nerve of clitoris (>1840)***; in the original Latin, *nervus pudendalis clytorideus*, Table I-*512*.
3. *clitoral nerve (Walter, 1783)*
   Synonym for macrodissected adult human female ***dorsal nerve of clitoris (>1840)***; in the original Latin, *nervus clytorideius*, Table I-*521*. Walter also described its complex system of roots and branches; Table I:*513–530*.
4. *superior external pudendal nerve (Mayer, 1794)*
   Synonym for macrodissected adult human female ***dorsal nerve of clitoris (>1840)***; in the original Latin, *nervus pudendalis externus superior*; Part 6, Table VIII-*98* (p. 56).
5. *ischioclitoral nerve (Chaussier, 1809)*
   Synonym for macrodissected adult human female ***dorsal nerve of clitoris (>1840)***; in the original French, *nerf iskio-clitorien*. Also spelled *nerf ischio-clitorien*.
6. *nerf honteux chez la femme (Cloquet, 1816)*
   French synonym for macrodissected adult human female ***dorsal nerve of clitoris (>1840)***; p. 672.
7. *nerve of clitoris (Meckel, 1817)*
   Synonym for macrodissected adult human female ***dorsal nerve of clitoris (>1840)***; see translation (1832, Vol. 3, p. 15).
8. *superior pudic nerve (Knox, 1832)*
   Synonym for macrodissected adult human female ***dorsal nerve of clitoris (>1840)***; Plate XI-*128* in Knox's translation of Walter (1783, Tab. I, Fig. 2).
9. *clitoral branch of internal pudendal nerve (Cruveilhier, 1836)*
   Synonym for macrodissected adult human female ***dorsal nerve of clitoris (>1840)***; in the original French, *branche clitoridienne*, p. 855.

PARTLY CORRESPONDS:

1. *dorsal nerve of clitoris (Mayer, 1794)*
   Branch of macrodissected adult human ***dorsal nerve of clitoris (>1840)*** just to dorsal part of clitoris itself; in the original Latin, *nervus dorsalis clitoridis*; Part 6, Table VIII-*100* (p. 56).

dorsal nerve of penis (Camper, 1762)

As described for macrodissected adult human male, a branch of the ***pudendal nerve (Camper, 1762)*** providing a branch to the corpus cavernosum penis, supplying the distal two-thirds of the penis and ending in the glans penis; see Durward (1951, p. 1102), Williams & Warwick (1980, p. 1116, Fig. 6.94), *Terminologia Anatomica* (1998, p. 140). For Camper's use in macrodissected adult human male, see Table 1, Figure 1:*14–16*; also see ***dorsal nerve of clitoris (>1840)***. It was first described as the *nerve to penis (Galen, c192)*.

EARLIER REFERENCES:

Earlier synonyms:

1. *nerve to penis (Galen, c192)*
   Synonym for ***dorsal nerve of penis (Camper, 1762)*** in macrodissected adult beef, pig, and/or macaque but not human; see Duckworth translation (1962, pp. 132, 263), also see May translation (1968, p. 651) for Galen's first mention of it. Eustachi (1552) illustrated it for macrodissected adult human; see Albinus edition (1761, Table 21-*K*). Vieussens described and illustrated it for macrodissected adult human male (1684, Tab. 29:*21–24*).

LATER SYNONYMS:

1. *superior pudendal nerve in male (Camper, 1762)*
   Synonym for macrodissected adult human male ***dorsal nerve of penis (Camper, 1762)***; p. 7.
2. *superior nerve of penis (Soemmerring, 1791)*
   Synonym for macrodissected adult human male ***dorsal nerve of penis (Camper, 1762)***; in the original Latin, *nervi superioris penis*, p. 303, also see Soemmerring (1798, p. 322).
3. *penile nerves (Mayer, 1794)*
   Synonym for macrodissected adult human male ***dorsal nerve of penis (Camper, 1762)***; in the original Latin, *nervi penis*; Part 5, Table VI-2 (p. 36).
4. *superior external pudendal nerves (Mayer, 1794)*
   Synonym for macrodissected adult human male ***dorsal nerve of penis (Camper, 1762)***; in the original Latin, *nervi pudendales externi superiores*; Part 5, Table VI-2 (p. 36).
5. *external common pudendal nerve (Mayer, 1794)*
   Synonym for macrodissected adult human male ***dorsal nerve of penis (Camper, 1762)***; in the original Latin, *nervus pudendus communis externus*; Part 6, Table VI-*183* (p. 41).
6. *nerf honteux (Cloquet, 1816)*
   French synonym for macrodissected adult human male ***dorsal nerve of penis (Camper, 1762)***; p. 671.
7. *penile pudendal nerve (Bock, 1827)*
   Synonym for macrodissected adult human male ***dorsal nerve of penis (Camper, 1762)***; in the original Latin, *n. pudendus penis*, Table VI, Figure 1-*37*.
8. *superior branch of internal pudendal nerve (Cruveilhier, 1836)*
   Synonym for macrodissected adult human male ***dorsal nerve of penis (Camper, 1762)***; in the original French, *branche supérieure*, p. 853.
9. *deep branch of internal pudendal nerve (Cruveilhier, 1836)*
   Synonym for *superior branch of internal pudendal nerve (Cruveilhier, 1836)*; in the original French, *branche profonde*, p. 853.
10. *dorsal branch of penis of internal pudendal nerve (Cruveilhier, 1836)*
    Synonym for *superior branch of internal pudendal nerve (Cruveilhier, 1836)*; in the original French, *branche dorsale de la verge*, p. 853.
11. *penile branch of internal pudendal nerve (Cruveilhier, 1836)*
    Synonym for *superior branch of internal pudendal nerve (Cruveilhier, 1836)*; in the original French, *branche pénienne*, p. 853.

PARTLY CORRESPONDS:

1. *dorsal nerve of penis (Mayer, 1794)*
   Distal end of macrodissected adult human male ***dorsal nerve of penis (Camper, 1762)***, just within penis itself; in the original Latin, *nervus dorsalis penis*; Part 6, Table VI-*185* (p. 41).
2. *rameau inférieur du nerf honteux chez l'homme (Cloquet, 1816)*
   Branch of macrodissected adult human ***dorsal nerve of penis (Camper, 1762)*** to anal sphincter, scrotum, urethra, and adjacent regions; p. 671.
3. *rameau supérieur du nerf honteux chez l'homme (Cloquet, 1816)*
   Terminal branch of macrodissected adult human ***dorsal nerve of penis (Camper, 1762)*** to glans penis; p. 672.
4. *branches of dorsal nerve of penis to prepuce (Langenbeck, 1826–1830)*
   In macrodissected adult human male, branches of ***dorsal nerve of penis (Camper, 1762)*** to foreskin; in the original Latin, *rami nervi dorsalis penis ad praeputium*, Fascicle III, Table X-9.
5. *external branch of penile nerve (Bock, 1827)*
   Branch of macrodissected adult human ***dorsal nerve of penis (Camper, 1762)*** to lateral side of penis; in the original Latin, *ram. externus nervi penis*, Table VI, Figure 2-*6*.
6. *internal branch of penile nerve (Bock, 1827)*
   Branch of macrodissected adult human ***dorsal nerve of penis (Camper, 1762)*** to medial side of penis; in the original Latin, *ram. internus nervi penis*, Table VI, Figure 2-*7*.
7. *dorsal plexus of penis (Bock, 1827)*
   In macrodissected adult human, ***plexus (Galen, c192)*** on dorsal surface of penis formed by *external branch of penile nerve (Bock, 1827)* and *internal branch of penile nerve (Bock, 1827)*; in the original Latin, *plex. dorsalis penis*; Table VI, Figure 2-*8,9*; from a "Negro" cadaver.
8. *cutaneous branches of dorsal plexus of penis (Bock, 1827)*
   As described by the term, for macrodissected adult human; in the original Latin, *rami cutanei*, Table VI, Figure 2-*10*.
9. *internal branch of deep branch of internal pudendal nerve (Cruveilhier, 1836)*
   Deeper branch of *deep branch of internal pudendal nerve (Cruveilhier, 1836)* ending in glans penis; in the original French, *rameau interne*, p. 855.

10. *internal branch of dorsal branch of penis of internal pudendal nerve (Cruveilhier, 1836)*
    Deeper branch of *dorsal branch of penis of internal pudendal nerve (Cruveilhier, 1836)* ending in glans penis; in the original French, *rameau interne*, p. 855.
11. *glans branch of deep branch of internal pudendal nerve (Cruveilhier, 1836)*
    Deeper branch of *deep branch of internal pudendal nerve (Cruveilhier, 1836)* ending in glans penis; in the original French, *rameau du gland*, p. 855.
12. *glans branch of dorsal branch of penis of internal pudendal nerve (Cruveilhier, 1836)*
    Deeper branch of *dorsal branch of penis of internal pudendal nerve (Cruveilhier, 1836)* ending in glans penis; in the original French, *rameau du gland*, p. 855.
13. *external branch of deep branch of internal pudendal nerve (Cruveilhier, 1836)*
    Superficial branch of *deep branch of internal pudendal nerve (Cruveilhier, 1836)*; in the original French, *rameau externe*, p. 855.
14. *external branch of dorsal branch of penis of internal pudendal nerve (Cruveilhier, 1836)*
    Superficial branch of *dorsal branch of penis of internal pudendal nerve (Cruveilhier, 1836)*; in the original French, *rameau externe*, p. 855.
15. *cutaneous branch of deep branch of internal pudendal nerve (Cruveilhier, 1836)*
    Superficial branch of *deep branch of internal pudendal nerve (Cruveilhier, 1836)*; in the original French, *rameau cutané*, p. 855.
16. *cutaneous branch of dorsal branch of penis of internal pudendal nerve (Cruveilhier, 1836)*
    Superficial branch of *dorsal branch of penis of internal pudendal nerve (Cruveilhier, 1836)*; in the original French, *rameau cutané*, p. 855.

dorsal part of thalamus (Herrick, 1910)

As described for macrodissected adult human, and based on cellular architecture, connections, and development in vertebrate, the very large middle topographic subdivision of the ***thalamus (His, 1893a)*** lying between ***epithalamus (His, 1893b)*** dorsomedially and ***ventral part of thalamus (Herrick, 1910)*** ventrally and laterally. Based on cellular architecture and connections, it is further divided into ***midline thalamic nuclei (>1840), anterior thalamic nuclei (>1840), medial thalamic nuclei (>1840), intralaminar thalamic nuclei (>1840), ventral thalamic nuclei (>1840), lateral thalamic nuclei (>1840), posterior thalamic nuclei (>1840), dorsal lateral geniculate nucleus (>1840)***, and ***medial geniculate complex (>1840)***; see Carpenter (1976, pp. 441–443), Williams & Warwick (1980, p. 955), Jones (1985, p. 87 ff.), Swanson (1998, Tab. B, pp. 203–204), Nieuwenhuys et al. (2008, p. 253 ff.). For Herrick's use in vertebrate, see p. 498, as well as pp. 468–469, 492. It was first identified at least roughly as the *globular part of thalamus (Reil, 1809c)*.

TRANSLATIONS:

1. *pars dorsalis thalami (Herrick, 1910)*
   Original Latin form of ***dorsal part of thalamus (Herrick, 1910)***; see p. 498.

EARLIER REFERENCES:

Earlier synonyms:

1. *globular part of thalamus (Reil, 1809c)*
   Roughly synonymous with macrodissected adult human ***dorsal part of thalamus (Herrick, 1910)***, that part of ***interbrain (Baer, 1837)*** dorsal and medial to ***medial lemniscus (>1840)***; see Mayo translation (1823, Tab. XI-*x*).

PARTLY CORRESPONDS:

1. *lacunar (Vieussens, 1684)*
   Corresponds to parts of macrodissected adult human ***midline thalamic nuclei (>1840)*** and ***intralaminar thalamic nuclei (>1840)*** actually crossing the median plane in the ***interthalamic adhesion (>1840)***. Vieussens described it as containing a soft gray substance; p. 64; see Burdach (1822, p. 341), Meyer (1971, p. 16).
2. *gray transverse lamina of Morgagni (Tarin, 1753)*
   Eponym for macrodissected adult human *lacunar (Vieussens, 1684)*; in the original Latin, *lamina transversa cinerea Morgagni*, p. 24.
3. *soft commissure of optic thalamus (Vicq d'Azyr, 1784)*
   Synonym for macrodissected adult human *lacunar (Vieussens, 1684)*, which Vicq d'Azyr also noted consists of *gray substance (Vesalius, 1543a)*; in the original French, *la commissure molle des couches optiques*, p. 527. Also see Vicq d'Azyr (1786, Pl. VIII, Fig. I-3/4; p. 37; Pl. XXIII-*e*) and *nexus thalamorum nervorum opticorum (Santorini, 1775)*.
4. *commissura mollis (Vicq d'Azyr, 1784)*
   Latin form of *soft commissure of optic thalamus (Vicq d'Azyr, 1784)*; see Burdach (1822, p. 341).
5. *transversa cinerea thalamorum (Schreger, 1803)*
   Synonym for macrodissected adult human *soft commissure of optic thalamus (Vicq d'Azyr, 1784)*; p. 320, also see Burdach (1822, p. 341).
6. *external gray nucleus (Burdach, 1822)*
   Corresponds roughly to ***lateral thalamic nuclei (>1840)*** and probably at least part of ***ventral thalamic nuclei (>1840)***, described for slabs of macrodissected adult human ***thalamus (His, 1893a)*** hardened in alcohol and observed with a hand lens; in the original Latin, *nucleus cinereus externus*, p. 122; see Jones (1985, p. 11); also see Meyer (1971, p. 31).
7. *gray commissure of thalamus (Rolando, 1831)*
   Synonym for macrodissected adult human *soft commissure of optic thalamus (Vicq d'Azyr, 1784)*; in the original Italian, *commessura cinerea dei thalami*, Figure 10–26.
8. *external nucleus of thalamus of optic nerve (Arnold, 1838b)*
   Synonym for macrodissected adult human *external gray nucleus (Burdach, 1822)*; in the original Latin, *nucleus externus thalami nervi optici*, Table IV, Figure 5-*l*.
9. *external nucleus of colliculus of optic nerve (Arnold, 1838b)*
   Synonym for macrodissected adult human *external gray nucleus (Burdach, 1822)*; in the original Latin, *nucleus externus colliculi nervi optici*, Table VIII, Figure 2-*i*.

dorsal posterior cingulate area (Brodmann, 1909)

As described with cellular architecture for adult human, the dorsal part of the ***posterior cingulate area (Brodmann, 1909)***; p. 147. It was not identified by 1840.

TRANSLATIONS:

1. *area cingularis posterior dorsalis (Brodmann, 1909)*
   Original Latin form of ***dorsal posterior cingulate area (Brodmann, 1909)***; p. 147.

EARLIER REFERENCES:

Earlier synonyms:

1. *area 31 (Brodmann, 1909)*
   Synonym for adult human ***dorsal posterior cingulate area (Brodmann, 1909)***; in the original German, *Feld 31*, see p. 147. Also see Nieuwenhuys et al. (2008, Fig. 12.13).

dorsal premammillary nucleus (>1840)

Based primarily on cellular architecture and connections in mammal, the small component of the ***medial hypothalamic zone (Nauta & Haymaker, 1969)*** surrounded by ***ventromedial hypothalamic nucleus (>1840)*** rostrally, ***ventral premammillary nucleus (>1840)*** ventrally, and ***mammillary body (Ludwig, 1779)*** caudally; see Swanson (1998, Tab. B, p. 206). It was not described by 1840.

dorsal root (Spurzheim, 1826)

As described for macrodissected adult human, a ***spinal nerve trunk (Frotscher, 1788)*** typically has associated with it two proximal fascicles, medial and lateral, each diverging into a more proximal bundle of ***dorsal rootlets (>1840)*** entering the ***spinal cord (Galen, c162–166)*** along the ***dorsolateral sulcus of spinal cord (>1840)*** as the ***dorsal root central part (>1840)***; see Durward (1951, p. 1052 and Fig. 915, not exactly corresponding to Fig. 913), Williams & Warwick (1980, p. 1086 and Fig. 7.195A, called there *dorsal nerve roots*), *Terminologia Anatomica* (1998, p. 133), Nieuwenhuys et al. (2008, Figs. 6.1-10). The medial and lateral filaments may be called primary dorsal roots, whereas the more proximal bundles associated with them may be called secondary dorsal roots. For Spurzheim's use in macrodissected adult vertebrate see p. 57. They were discovered by Coiter; see ***[dorsal root (Spurzheim, 1826)] (Coiter, 1572)***.

TRANSLATIONS:

1. *radix dorsalis (>1840)*
   Current Latin form of ***dorsal root (Spurzheim, 1826)***; part of full term, *radix dorsalis nervi spinalis*; see *Dorland's* (2003, p. 1565).

EARLIER REFERENCES:

Described, not named or illustrated:

1. ***[dorsal root (Spurzheim, 1826)] (Coiter, 1572)***
   Coiter clearly described ***dorsal root (Spurzheim, 1826)*** component of macrodissected adult human ***spinal nerves (Camper, 1760–1762)***. He referred to them as a row of *posterior medullar threads (Coiter, 1572), posterior medullar filaments (Coiter, 1572)*, or *posterior medullar fibers (Coiter, 1572)*, more or less of which combine to form a ***nerve (Herophilus, c335–c280 BC)*** of greater or lesser thickness, respectively, and provided evidence that the substance of the ***spinal cord (Galen, c162–c166)*** contributes to them; see translation pp. 115–117. The medullary threads are ***dorsal rootlets (>1840)*** together forming a ***dorsal root (Spurzheim, 1826)***. Rasmussen (1947) stated that Galen distinguished ***dorsal root (Spurzheim, 1826)*** and ***ventral root (>1840)***, but Rasmussen's source is unknown and his interpretation is not confirmed elsewhere; see Siegel (1970). More likely, Rasmussen's source confused ***dorsal root (Spurzheim, 1826)*** and ***ventral root (>1840)*** with ***spinal nerve dorsal branch (Meckel, 1817)*** and ***spinal nerve ventral branch (>1840)***, which Galen described extensively; see May (1968).

Earlier synonyms:

1. *posterior fasciculus (Winslow, 1733)*
   Synonym for macrodissected adult human ***dorsal root (Spurzheim, 1826)***; Section VI, p. 76; Section X, p. 45.
2. *posterior filaments (Huber, 1741)*
   Synonym for macrodissected adult human ***dorsal root (Spurzheim, 1826)***; pp. 2–5, see Clarke & O'Malley translation (1996, p. 267).
3. *posterior root (Asch, 1750)*
   Synonym for macrodissected 2-year old human infant ***dorsal root (Spurzheim, 1826)***, which Asch described as composed of filaments for ***cervical nerves (Galen, c173)***; in the original Latin, *radix postica*, p. 39 and Figure 1:*a–f*.
4. *posterior bundle (Monro, 1783)*
   English form of macrodissected adult human *posterior fasciculus (Winslow, 1733)*; Table 10, Figure 1-O.
5. *sensitive root (Bell, 1829)*
   Synonym for macrodissected adult human ***dorsal root (Spurzheim, 1826)***; Plate IX, Figure 2-A.
6. *ganglionic root (Cruveilhier, 1836)*
   Synonym for macrodissected adult human ***dorsal root (Spurzheim, 1826)***; in the original French (plural), *racines ganglionnaires*, p. 764.

dorsal root central part (>1840)

As described for macrodissected adult human, and mammal generally with histological methods for ***axons (Kölliker, 1896)***, the central extension of the peripheral ***dorsal root (Spurzheim, 1826)*** coursing through and to the ***dorsolateral tract (>1850), dorsal horn (>1840)*** and ***dorsal funiculus (>1840)***; see Nieuwenhuys et al. (2008, Figs. 6.1-10, unlabeled). Not clearly identified by 1840.

dorsal rootlets (>1840)

As described for macrodissected adult human, the set of individual filaments together constituting a ***dorsal root (Spurzheim, 1826)***; see Williams & Warwick (1980, p. 1086), *Terminologia Anatomica* (1998, p. 133). They were first distinguished by Eustachi; see ***[dorsal rootlets (>1840)] (Eustachi, 1552)***.

EARLIER REFERENCES:

Illustrated, not named or described:

1. ***[dorsal rootlets (>1840)] (Eustachi, 1552)***
   Eustachi clearly illustrated the whole series for macrodissected adult human; see Albinus edition (1761, Tab. 17, Fig. 2:*1-30*).

Earlier synonyms:

1. *posterior medullar threads (Coiter, 1572)*
   Synonym for macrodissected adult human ***dorsal rootlets (>1840)***; see translation, p. 115.
2. *posterior medullar filaments (Coiter, 1572)*
   Synonym for macrodissected adult human ***dorsal rootlets (>1840)***; see translation, p. 115.
3. *posterior medullar fibers (Coiter, 1572)*
   Synonym for macrodissected adult human ***dorsal rootlets (>1840)***; see translation, p. 115.
4. *nervi à parte spinalis medullae posteriore procedents (Blasius, 1666)*
   Synonym for macrodissected adult human ***dorsal rootlets (>1840)***; Figure X-*a*.
5. *posterior nervous filaments (Winslow, 1733)*
   Synonym for macrodissected adult human ***dorsal rootlets (>1840)***; Section VI, p. 76.
6. *posterior bundles of spinal nerves (Swan, 1830)*
   Synonym for macrodissected adult human ***dorsal rootlets (>1840)***; Plate X, Figure 6.

dorsal scapular nerve (Bock, 1827)

As described for macrodissected adult human, a branch of the 5th cervical ***brachial plexus root (Schwalbe, 1881)*** innervating primarily the rhomboid muscles, although it may innervate the levator scapulae muscle as well; see Williams & Warwick (1980, pp. 1095–1096). For Bock's use in macrodissected adult human see Table V, Figure 1-*41*. It was known to Galen; see ***[dorsal scapular nerve (Bock, 1827)] (Galen, c173)***.

TRANSLATIONS:

1. *nervus dorsalis scapulae (Bock, 1827)*
   Original Latin form of ***dorsal scapular nerve (Bock, 1827)***; see Table V, Figure 1-*41*.

EARLIER REFERENCES:

Described, not named or illustrated:

1. ***[dorsal scapular nerve (Bock, 1827)] (Galen, c173)***
   Clearly described in macrodissected adult beef, pig, and/or macaque but not human; see May translation (1968, p. 701). Vesalius (1543a) may have alluded to it in macrodissected adult human; see Richardson & Carman translation (2002, p. 228).

Illustrated, not named or described:

1. ***[dorsal scapular nerve (Bock, 1827)] (Eustachi, 1552)***
   Clearly illustrated for macrodissected adult human; see Albinus edition (1761, Tab. 20/2-*d*).

Earlier synonyms:

1. *suprascapular nerve (Haase, 1781)*
   Synonym for macrodissected adult human ***dorsal scapular nerve (Bock, 1827)***; in the original Latin, *nervus suprascapularis*, p. 96.

PARTLY CORRESPONDS:

1. *angular muscle branch of brachial plexus (Cruveilhier, 1836)*
   As currently described in typical macrodissected adult human, branch of ***dorsal scapular nerve (Bock, 1827)*** to levator scapulae muscle; in the original French, *branche du muscle angulaire du plexus brachial*, p. 792.
2. *rhomboid branch of brachial plexus (Cruveilhier, 1836)*
   As currently described in typical macrodissected adult human, branch of ***dorsal scapular nerve (Bock, 1827)*** to rhomboid muscles; in the original French, *branche du rhomboïde du plexus brachial*, p. 792.

dorsal spinocerebellar tract (>1840)

As described for macrodissected adult human, and mammal generally with histological methods for ***axons (Kölliker, 1896)***, a rostrally directed, uncrossed, longitudinal ***central nervous system white matter tract (>1840)*** arising from the ***dorsal thoracic nucleus (>1840)*** and extending rostrally through the dorsolateral ***lateral funiculus (Burdach, 1822)*** to enter the ***inferior cerebellar peduncle (Günther, 1786)***; see Williams & Warwick (1980, p. 879 and Fig. 7.43, called *posterior spinocerebellar tract*), *Terminologia Anatomica* (1998, p. 107). For topographic description it has ***spinal dorsal spinocerebellar tract (>1840)*** and ***medullary dorsal spinocerebellar tract (1840)*** segments. It was not delineated clearly by 1840.

EARLIER REFERENCES:

Earlier synonyms:

1. *posterior spinocerebellar tract (>1840)*
   Synonym for macrodissected adult human ***dorsal spinocerebellar tract (>1840)***; see *Terminologia Anatomica* (1998, p. 107).

dorsal tegmental decussation (>1840)

As described in macrodissected adult human, and mammal generally with histological methods for ***axons (Kölliker, 1896)***, a transverse ***central nervous system white matter tract (>1840)*** along the median plane of the ***tegmentum (Swanson, 2000b)*** where the right and left ***tegmental tectospinal tracts (>1840)*** decussate, between the ***rostral linear nucleus of raphe (>1840)*** dorsally and ***central linear nucleus of raphe (>1840)*** ventrally; see Williams & Warwick (1980, pp. 939, 942), Swanson (2004, Atlas Levels 40–42), Nieuwenhuys et al. (2008, pp. 206, 778–779 and Fig. 19.10, labeled *predorsal fascicle*). It was not known by 1840.

dorsal thoracic nucleus (>1840)

As described for macrodissected adult human, a thin longitudinal ***central nervous system gray matter region (>1840)*** in the dorsomedial ***intermediate spinal zone (>1840)***, most prominent from the 8th level of the ***cervical part of spinal cord (>1840)*** rostrally to the 3rd or 4th level of the ***lumbar part of spinal cord (>1841)*** caudally. Similar though not identical ***central nervous system gray matter regions (>1840)*** are found caudally in the

sacral part of spinal cord (>1841) and rostrally in the ***central cervical nucleus (>1840)***; see Carpenter (1976, p. 249, called *Clarke's column* or *dorsal nucleus*), Edgley & Grant (1991, p. 138 and Fig. 2), *Terminologia Anatomica* (1998, p. 106). It was first delineated as the thoracic part of the *posterior vesicular column (Clarke, 1851)*.

EARLIER REFERENCES:

Earlier synonyms:

1. *posterior vesicular column (Clarke, 1851)*
   Roughly synonymous with adult mammalian ***dorsal thoracic nucleus (>1840)*** observed in unstained histological sections, although Clarke described it along the length of the ***spinal cord (Galen, c162–c166)***; p. 611.
2. *Clarke's column (Kölliker, 1896)*
   Eponym for macrodissected adult human *posterior vesicular column (Clarke, 1851)*; in the original German, Clarke*'sche Säulen*, see p. 62 and Figure 373-*g*. Also see Carpenter (1976, p. 249), Edgley & Grant (1991, p. 130).
3. *Stilling's nucleus (>1840)*
   Eponym for macrodissected adult human *posterior vesicular column (Clarke, 1851)*; see Kölliker (1896, p. 62 and Fig. 373-*g*, in the original German, Stilling*'scher Kern*) and Stilling (1859).
4. *thoracic nucleus (>1840)*
   Synonym for macrodissected adult human ***dorsal thoracic nucleus (>1840)***; see Williams & Warwick (1980, p. 879).
5. *dorsal nucleus of spinal cord (>1840)*
   Synonym for macrodissected adult human ***dorsal thoracic nucleus (>1840)***; see Carpenter (1976, p. 249).
6. *posterior thoracic nucleus (>1840)*
   Synonym for macrodissected adult human ***dorsal thoracic nucleus (>1840)***; see *Terminologia Anatomica* (1998, p. 106).

dorsolateral sulcus of medulla (>1840)

As described for macrodissected adult human, the longitudinal groove on the surface of the ***medulla (Winslow, 1733)*** with its rostral end lying just dorsal to the ***olive (Tiedemann, 1821)*** and extending caudally as the ***dorsolateral sulcus of spinal cord (>1840)***. Along its length emerge the ***glossopharyngeal nerve rootlets (>1840), vagus nerve rootlets (>1840)***, and ***cranial root of accessory nerve rootlets (>1840)***, from rostral to caudal; see Williams & Warwick (1980, p. 898 and Fig 7.189), *Terminologia Anatomica* (1998, p. 108). It was first clearly delineated by Soemmerring; see ***[dorsolateral sulcus of medulla (>1840)] (Soemmerring, 1778)***.

EARLIER REFERENCES:

Described, not named or illustrated:

1. ***[dorsolateral sulcus of medulla (>1840)] (Soemmerring, 1778)***
   Definitively illustrated for macrodissected adult human; Table II, especially on right side of figure, where it is shaded in the outline plate.

Earlier synonyms:

1. *posterolateral sulcus of medulla (>1840)*
   Synonym for macrodissected adult human ***dorsolateral sulcus of medulla (>1840)***; see *Terminologia Anatomica* (1998, p. 108).

dorsolateral sulcus of spinal cord (>1840)

As described for macrodissected adult human, a longitudinal groove on the surface of the ***spinal cord (Galen, c162–c166)*** indicating the ***dorsal root (Spurzheim, 1826)*** entry zone and border between ***dorsal funiculus (>1840)*** and ***lateral funiculus (Burdach, 1822)***. It extends rostrally as the ***dorsolateral sulcus of medulla (>1840)***; see Williams & Warwick (1980, pp. 867, 898 and Fig. 7.189; called *anterolateral sulcus*), *Terminologia Anatomica* (1998, p. 108). It was first noted by Blasius; see ***[dorsolateral sulcus of spinal cord (>1840)] (Blasius, 1666)***.

EARLIER REFERENCES:

Illustrated, not named or described:

1. ***[dorsolateral sulcus of spinal cord (>1840)] (Blasius, 1666)***
   Indicated for macrodissected adult human in Figures 10, 11, 18.

Earlier synonyms:

1. *collateral sulcus (Chaussier, 1807)*
   Synonym for macrodissected adult human ***dorsolateral sulcus of spinal cord (>1840)***; in the original French (plural), *sillons collatéraux*, p. 135.
2. *posterior lateral sulcus of spinal medulla (Meckel, 1817)*
   Synonym for macrodissected adult human ***dorsolateral sulcus of spinal cord (>1840)***; see translation (1832, Vol. 2, p. 412).
3. *posterior collateral sulcus (Bellingeri, 1823)*
   Synonym for macrodissected adult human ***dorsolateral sulcus of spinal cord (>1840)***; in the original Latin (plural), *sulci collaterales posteriores*, Table 1, Figure 1-*c*.
4. *lateral dorsal channels (Spurzheim, 1826)*
   Synonym (plural) for macrodissected adult human ***dorsolateral sulcus of spinal cord (>1840)***; Plate 1, Figure 5-*α*.
5. *posterior lateral furrow of spinal marrow (Mayo, 1827)*
   Synonym for macrodissected adult human ***dorsolateral sulcus of spinal cord (>1840)***; Plate I, Figure 1-*d*.
6. *sulcus of posterior roots (Cruveilhier, 1836)*
   Synonym for macrodissected adult human ***dorsolateral sulcus of spinal cord (>1840)***; in the original French, *silions des racines postérieures*, p. 575.

dorsolateral tract (>1840)

As described in macrodissected adult human, and mammal generally with histological methods for ***axons (Kölliker, 1896)***, a longitudinal ***central nervous system white matter tract (>1840)*** extending the length of the ***spinal cord (Galen, c162–c166)*** between the dorsolateral end of the ***dorsal horn (>1840)*** and outer surface of the ***spinal cord (Galen, c162–c166)***, just lateral to the ***dorsal***

funiculus (>1840) and, when present, its ***cuneate fascicle (Müller, 1834)***; see Williams & Warwick (1980, Fig. 7.43), *Terminologia Anatomica* (1998, p. 107), Nieuwenhuys et al. (2008, Figs. 6.1-*18*, 6.9-*10*), called *dorsolateral fascicle (>1840)*. It was not described by 1840.

EARLIER REFERENCES:

Earlier synonyms:

1. *posterolateral tract (>1840)*
   Synonym for ***dorsolateral tract (>1840)***; see *Terminologia Anatomica* (1998, p. 107).
2. *Lissauer's tract (>1840)*
   Eponym for ***dorsolateral tract (>1840)***; see Crosby et al. (1962, p. 76) and Lissauer (1886).
3. *zone of Lissauer (>1840)*
   Eponym for ***dorsolateral tract (>1840)***; see Carpenter (1976, p. 286) and Lissauer (1886).
4. *dorsolateral fascicle (>1840)*
   Synonym for ***dorsolateral tract (>1840)***; see Mettler (1948, Fig. 172), Nieuwenhuys et al. (2008, Fig. 6.1-*18*).

dura (Galen, c177)

As described for macrodissected adult human, the outermost, toughest, and most fibrous layer of the ***meninges (Smith Papyrus, c1700 BC)***. The ***dura (Galen, c177)*** surrounding the ***brain (Smith Papyrus, c1700 BC)*** is now described as having two layers, outer *periosteal* and thinner inner *meningeal*, which alone descends as the single layer of ***dura (Galen, c177)*** surrounding the ***spinal cord (Galen, c162–c166)***; see Millen & Woollam (1962, pp. 123–126). For Galen's use in *On Anatomical Procedures*, see Wiberg translation (1914, p. 21). It was clearly distinguished in the Hippocratic Corpus; see *thick membrane (Hippocrates)*.

EARLIER REFERENCES:

Earlier synonyms:

1. *thick membrane (Hippocrates)*
   Referring rather vaguely to ***dura (Galen, c177)***, Hippocrates wrote in *Fleshes*, "...for the brain itself is moist, and the membrane around it is moist and thick" (Potter translation, 1995, p. 155; also see p. 139). In *Places in Man*, Hippocrates referred to two membranes (the plural in Greek is *meninges*) around ***brain (Smith Papyrus, c1700 BC)***, "Of the brain, there are two membranes; the fine one cannot be healed, when once it is injured." (Potter translation, 1995, p. 23). Galen used it much more decisively; for example, see May translation (1968, p. 410). His descriptions were not based on human dissection.
2. *stronger membrane (Aristotle)*
   In *The Account of Animals*, Aristotle described two membranes around ***brain (Smith Papyrus, c1700 BC)***, a stronger one nearer the skull [***dura (Galen, c177)***] and a finer one around the ***brain (Smith Papyrus, c1700 BC)*** itself [***pia (Galen, c192)***]; see Thompson translation (1962, p. 494b) and Clarke & O'Malley (1996, p. 8). He dissected a variety of animals, but not human.
3. *tunica prima (Rufus of Ephesus, c90–120)*
   Synonym for ***dura (Galen, c177)***; see Burdach (1822, p. 275).
4. *crassa (Galen, c173)*
   Latin term meaning thick, referring to *thick membrane (Hippocrates)*, or ***dura (Galen, c177)***; for example, see Vesalius (1543a; Singer translation, 1952, p. 8).
5. *hard membrane (Galen, c177)*
   Synonym for ***dura (Galen, c177)***; see Singer translation (1999, p. 226).
6. *dura meninx (Galen, c177)*
   Latin form of *hard membrane (Galen, c177)*; for example, see Meckel (1832, Vol. 2, p. 478).
7. *cuticular membrane (Galen, c177)*
   According to Singer's translation (1999, p. 226), synonym Galen mentioned for ***dura (Galen, c177)***. Wiberg (1914, p. 18) translated the same passage as "membranous" membrane, and Rocca (2003, p. 87) as "skin-like".
8. *cuticularis (Galen, c177)*
   Latin term for "skin-like", referring to *cuticular membrane (Galen, c177)* or ***dura (Galen, c177)***; for example, see Vesalius (1543a; Singer translation, 1952, p. 8).

LATER SYNONYMS:

1. *dura mater (Haly Abbas or Ali ibn' ul-Abbas, d. 994)*
   Haly Abbas apparently is responsible for adding the Arabic term *mater* (mother) to ***dura (Galen, c177)***; see Wiberg (1914, p. 86). The actual Latin term came from Stephen of Antioch's 1127 Latin translation of *Liber Regius*; Singer (1957, p. 81). In the Second Salernitan Demonstration (c1070–1100), *pia mater (Haly Abbas or Ali ibn' ul-Abbas, d. 994)* is described as protecting ***brain (Smith Papyrus, c1700 BC)*** "like a devoted mother" from harshness of *dura mater (Haly Abbas or Ali ibn' ul-Abbas, d. 994)*, whereas the latter protects ***brain (Smith Papyrus, c1700 BC)*** and *pia mater (Haly Abbas or Ali ibn' ul-Abbas, d. 994)* from harshness of cranium; see Corner (1927, p. 66). Singer's use of the term *dura mater* in his translation of Galen's *On Anatomical Procedures* (Singer, 1999, p. 230) is not literal. The same may well apply to Duckworth's translation (1962, p. 5) of the later books of *On Anatomical Procedures*; also see *matres (Stephen of Antioch, 1127)*.
2. *panniculus grossus (Averroes, 12th century)*
   Synonym for adult human ***dura (Galen, c177)***; see Burdach (1822, p. 275).
3. *outer dense membrane (William of Saliceto, 1275)*
   Synonym for adult human ***dura (Galen, c177)***; see Rosenman translation (1998, p. 182).
4. *outer meninge (William of Saliceto, 1275)*
   Synonym for adult human ***dura (Galen, c177)***; see Rosenman translation (1998, p. 182). Soemmerring (1798, p. 23) gave the Latin form, *meninx exterior*.
5. *outer miringe (William of Saliceto, 1275)*
   Synonym for adult human ***dura (Galen, c177)***; see Rosenman translation (1998, p. 182).
6. *grossa mininga (Zerbi, 1502)*
   Synonym for macrodissected adult human ***dura (Galen, c177)***; p. 111, also see Burdach (1822, p. 275) and *panniculus grossus (Averroes, 12th century)*.

7. *custodian of brain (Benedetti, 1502)*
   Synonym for macrodissected adult human ***dura (Galen, c177)***; in the original Latin, *custos cerebri*, p. 1234; see Lind translation (1975, p. 115).
8. *dura membrana (Geminus, 1553)*
   Latin synonym for macrodissected adult human ***dura (Galen, c177)***; see f. BII.
9. *hard pannicle (Geminus, 1553)*
   Variation directly in English of *hard membrane (Galen, c177)*; actually spelled *harde pannicle*, see *The tables of the brayne, fyrst fygure*. Also see *panniculus grossus (Averroes, 12th century)*.
10. *strong mother (Hall, 1565)*
   Direct translation in English of *dura mater (Haly Abbas or Ali ibn' ul-Abbas, d. 994)*; p. 41.
11. *tough veil (Hall, 1565)*
   Variation directly in English of *hard membrane (Galen, c177)*, actually spelled there *toughe veyle*, p. 41.
12. *crassa meninx (Hall, 1565)*
   Synonym for macrodissected adult human ***dura (Galen, c177)***; p. 41.
13. *hard mother (Diemerbroeck, 1689)*
   English form of *dura mater (Haly Abbas or Ali ibn' ul-Abbas, d. 994)*; p. 384.
14. *musculus triventer & quadritendineus (Pacchioni, 1741)*
   Synonym for macrodissected adult human ***dura (Galen, c177)***; p. 136.
15. *meninx exterior (Soemmerring, 1798)*
   Synonym for macrodissected adult human ***dura (Galen, c177)***; p. 23.
16. *meninx (Chaussier, 1807)*
   Synonym for macrodissected adult human ***dura (Galen, c177)***, distinguished from *meningine (Burdin, 1803)*, the ***pia (Galen, c192)*** and ***arachnoid (Blasius, 1666)*** considered together; Vol. 1, p. 153.
17. *meninx scléra (Chaussier, 1807)*
   Synonym listed for macrodissected adult human ***dura (Galen, c177)***; p. 20.
18. *meninx pachéia (Chaussier, 1807)*
   Synonym listed for macrodissected adult human ***dura (Galen, c177)***; p. 20.
19. *dura membrana cerebrum ambiens (Chaussier, 1807)*
   Synonym listed for macrodissected adult human ***dura (Galen, c177)***; p. 20.
20. *externa membrana cerebri (Wenzel & Wenzel, 1812)*
   Synonym for macrodissected adult human ***dura (Galen, c177)***; p. 6, see Burdach (1822, p. 275).
21. *meninx fibrosa (Burdach, 1822)*
   Synonym for macrodissected adult human ***dura (Galen, c177)***; p. 24.

PARTLY CORRESPONDS:

1. *hard cerebral membrane (Vesalius, 1543a)*
   Term for ***dura (Galen, c177)*** associated specifically with macrodissected adult human ***brain (Smith Papyrus, c1700 BC)***; in the original Latin, *durae cerebri membranae*, see Richardson & Carman translation (2009, p. 124).
2. *dura cerebri meninx (Wrisberg, 1777)*
   Term for ***dura (Galen, c177)*** associated specifically with macrodissected adult human ***brain (Smith Papyrus, c1700 BC)***; p. 14.

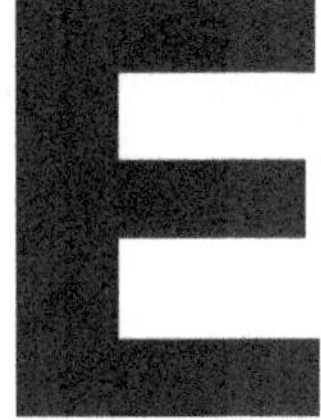

emissary veins (Santorini, 1724)

As described for macrodissected adult human, a component of the ***circulatory system***; small valveless veins passing through holes in the skull and connecting the dural venous sinuses with scalp veins or with deep veins below the base of the skull; see Carpenter (1976, p. 624 and Fig. 20.16), Williams & Warwick (1980, pp. 749–750), *Dorland's* (2003, p. 2022, under *vena emissaria*). According to Haase (1781, p. 9), Vicq d'Azyr (1784, p. 504), Bell (1803b, p. 67), and Chaussier (1807, p. xxiii) the term comes from Santorini (see pp. 74–76).

LATER SYNONYMS:

1. *venae emissariae Santorini (Bell & Bell, 1816)*
   Eponym for macrodissected adult human ***emissary veins (Santorini, 1724)***; Vol. 2, p. 431.

endbrain (Kuhlenbeck, 1927)

The paired right and left rostrodorsal topographic divisions of the vertebrate ***forebrain (Goette, 1873)***, connected to the single caudal division of the ***forebrain (Goette, 1873)***, the ***interbrain (Baer, 1837)***; see Swanson & Bota (2010). It is the topographic division of the ***central nervous system (Carus, 1814)*** developing from the neuroepithelium of, and coextensive with, the ***lateral ventricles (Vesalius, 1543a)***. It is divided into ***cerebral nuclei (Swanson, 2000a)*** ventrally and ***cerebral cortex (>1840)*** dorsally. The definition of Kuhlenbeck (1927, Chs. 3, 10) is based on vertebrate phylogeny, development, and histology; it was probably first recognized thus as the *fore part of brain (Mondino, 1316)*. This English translation (endbrain) of *telencephalon (Kuhlenbeck, 1927)* has been used routinely by, among others, Strong & Elwyn (1943, p. 11), Carpenter (1976, p. 60), Williams & Warwick (1975, Table of Content), Williams & Warwick (1980, p. 982), Nauta and Feirtag (1986, p. 39), and Nieuwenhuys et al. (2008, p. 9). An equally acceptable synonym is ***cerebrum (Obersteiner & Hill, 1900)***, and another common synonym is *cerebral hemispheres (Tiedemann, 1816)*.

TRANSLATIONS:

1. *Endhirn (Kuhlenbeck, 1927)*
   Original German form of ***endbrain (Kuhlenbeck, 1927)***; Chapter 3.
2. *telencephalon (Kuhlenbeck, 1927)*
   Original Latin form of ***endbrain (Kuhlenbeck, 1927)***; Chapter 2.

EARLIER REFERENCES:

Earlier synonyms:

1. *fore part of brain (Mondino, 1316)*
   Synonym for macrodissected adult human ***endbrain (Kuhlenbeck, 1927)***. In *Anathomia*, Mondino referred to part of ***brain (Smith Papyrus, c1700 BC)*** associated with ***lateral ventricles (Vesalius, 1543a)*** as opposed to part associated with ***third ventricle (Galen, c173)***. The most relevant passage reads: "Through this lacuna [***hypothalamic part of third ventricle (Swanson, 2004)*** and *infundibulum (Rufus of Ephesus, fl. c90–120)*, considered together] the mid part of the brain is purged of superfluous matter. The fore part of the brain is purged of superfluous matter through the *colatoria narium* [cribriform plate]." (Singer translation, 1925, Vol. 1, p. 92). In Latin, Burdach (1822, p. 319) gave Mondino's term as *pars anterior cerebri*.
2. *lobe of brain (Dryander, 1536)*
   In *The Anatomy of the Human Head*, Dryander illustrated and referred to right and left *lobes of brain*, a seemingly obvious though vague reference to macrodissected adult human ***endbrain (Kuhlenbeck, 1927)***; see Lind translation (1975, p. 300).
3. *body of brain (Steno, 1669)*
   Roughly synonymous with macrodissected adult human ***endbrain (Kuhlenbeck, 1927)***; see translation, p. 137.

4. *superior olfactory tubercle (Haller, 1768)*
Roughly synonymous with macrodissected adult fish ***endbrain (Kuhlenbeck, 1927)***; in the original Latin, *tuberculis olfactoriis superioribus*, pp. 199–200, 206, 214; also see Arsaky (1813, p. 35).
5. *olfactory tubercle (Arsaky, 1813)*
Synonym for macrodissected adult fish *superior olfactory tubercle (Haller, 1768)*; in the original Latin, *tuberculorum olfactoriorum*, pp. 29, 35.
6. *olfactory nerve ganglia (Carus, 1814)*
Roughly synonymous with macrodissected adult fish and amphibian ***endbrain (Kuhlenbeck, 1927)*** or *cerebral hemispheres (Tiedemann, 1816)*; in the original German, *Riechnerven-Ganglien*, Tables 2-*a*, 3-*a*.
7. *cerebral hemispheres (Tiedemann, 1816)*
Synonym for developing human ***endbrain (Kuhlenbeck, 1927)***. "The two anterior vesicles represent the two hemispheres of the brain; the two middle, the optic chambers; and the posterior, the cerebellum" (see translation, 1826, p. 15). The term has been used for macrodissected developing and adult human more recently by, for example, Strong & Elwyn (1943, pp. 13–16), Hamilton et al. (1952, pp. 263, 294–295), Crosby et al. (1962, p. 356), Williams & Warwick (1980, p. 982; also see p. 864), and Nauta & Feirtag (1986, p. 38).
8. *forebrain (Baer, 1837)*
Synonym for vertebrate embryonic and adult ***endbrain (Kuhlenbeck, 1927)***; in the original German, *Vorderhirn*, p. 107.

PARTLY CORRESPONDS:

1. *anterior belly of brain (William of Saliceto, 1275)*
Basically, macrodissected adult human ***endbrain (Kuhlenbeck, 1927)*** surrounding but not necessarily including ***lateral ventricle (Vesalius, 1543a)***, one on right and one on left; see Rosenman translation (1998, p. 181).
2. *brain (Willis, 1664)*
Willis's definition of *cerebrum (Willis, 1664)*—occasionally clarified with the more specific *cerebrum proper (Willis, 1664)* or *brain proper (Willis, 1664)*—included for macrodissected adult human and other common large mammals the right and left ***cerebral cortex (>1840)*** and ***lateral ventricle (Vesalius, 1543a)***, all four considered together; see Pordage translation (1681, pp. 57, 91 ff.). In contrast, he referred to *whole brain (Willis, 1664)*, or contents of cranium, as *encephalon (Homer, c9th century BC)*. This distinction was used by Samuel Johnson (1755) in his great dictionary, and the linguistic distinction remains common in English today. In birds and fish, Willis wrote that the *brain* lacks a *corpus callosum (Willis, 1664)*, and has an inverted appearance compared to mammals; see Pordage translation (1681, pp. 75–77).
3. *brain proper (Willis, 1664)*
Synonym for *brain (Willis, 1664)*; see Pordage translation (1681, pp. 60, 95).
4. *brain properly so called (Willis, 1664)*
Synonym for *brain (Willis, 1664)*; see Pordage translation (1681, pp. 60, 95).
5. *cerebrum (Willis, 1664)*
Latin form of *brain (Willis, 1664)*.
6. *cerebrum proper (Willis, 1664)*
Latin-based form of *brain proper (Willis, 1664)*.
7. *cerebrum properly so called (Willis, 1664)*
Latin-based form of *brain properly so called (Willis, 1664)*.
8. *whole brain (Willis, 1664)*
Synonym for *brain properly so called (Willis, 1664)*; see Pordage translation (1681, p. 91).
9. *double origination of olfactory nerve (Collins, 1685)*
Collins claimed for the first time to note, in macrodissected adult human, ***lateral olfactory tract (>1840)*** and *medial olfactory stria (>1840)*; Table XLVIII-*oooo*. Also see *olfactory nerve (Bartholin, 1651)* and ***[lateral olfactory tract (>1840)] (Casseri, 1609)***.
10. *brain in particular (Ridley, 1695)*
Synonym for macrodissected adult human *brain (Willis 1664)* or *cerebrum (Willis, 1664)*; pp. 113–115.
11. *peduncle of corpus callosum (Vicq d'Azyr, 1784)*
Difficult term in adult human neuroanatomy; see p. 546 and Vicq d'Azyr (1786, Pls. XXI-*13*; XXV-*31,s*). His (1895; see Eycleshymer translation, 1917, p. 166 ff.) gave perhaps the best analysis, claiming it is synonymous with *peduncle of septum (Burdach, 1822)* and *subcallosal gyrus (Zuckerkandl, 1887)*.
12. *peduncle of septum (Burdach, 1822)*
Synonym for macrodissected adult human *peduncle of corpus callosum (Vicq d'Azyr, 1784)* according to His (1895; see Eycleshymer translation, 1917, p. 166 ff.); in the original German, *Stiele der Scheidewand*; in Latin, *pedunculus septi*, p. 135. Burdach followed the description of Gall & Spurzheim (1810), who did not name the structure or refer to Vicq d'Azyr (1786, Pl. XIII-*63*), who clearly labeled the ***diagonal band (Broca, 1879)***. According to Foster's description (1894, p. 2538), the *septal peduncle (Burdach, 1822)* consists of a fiber bundle projecting downward from the anterior extremity of the septum lucidum (prolongations of their *laminae*) in front of the anterior commissure to enter the white substance of the frontal lobe near the base of the lenticular nucleus, which is how Zuckerkandl (1887, Fig. 38-*P.c.c.*) illustrated it.
13. *septal peduncle (Burdach, 1822)*
Alternate form of *peduncle of septum (Burdach, 1822)*.
14. *caelamina inter pedunculos corporis callosi (Burdach, 1822)*
Synonym for right and left *peduncle of corpus callosum (Vicq d'Azyr, 1784)*; see p. 366, where Burdach referred to Vicq d'Azyr (1786, p. 73).
15. *funiculi inter pedunculos corporis callosi (Burdach, 1822)*
Synonym for right and left *peduncle of corpus callosum (Vicq d'Azyr, 1784)*; p. 366.
16. *cerebral hemispheres (Serres, 1824-1826)*
For macrodissected bony fish, amphibians, reptiles, birds, and mammals (but not "lower" fish) Serres

distinguished *olfactory lobes (Serres, 1824–1826)* from *cerebral hemispheres (Serres, 1824–1826)* or, as he also called them, *cerebral lobes (Serres, 1824–1826)*. Thus, in these animals he divided ***endbrain (Kuhlenbeck, 1927)*** into two pairs of lobes, olfactory and cerebral, laying the groundwork for the concept of the *rhinencephalon (Turner, 1891)*. In the original French, *hémisphères cérébraux*, p. 208 ff.

17. *hemispheric lobes (Serres, 1824–1826)*
Synonym for *cerebral hemispheres (Serres, 1824-1826)*; in the original French, *lobes des hémisphères*, p. 209.
18. *cerebral lobes (Serres, 1824-1826)*
Synonym for *cerebral hemispheres (Serres, 1824-1826)*; in the original French, *lobes cérébraux*, p. 211.
19. *reflected portion of corpus callosum (Cruveilhier, 1836)*
Synonym for macrodissected adult human *peduncle of corpus callosum (Vicq d'Azyr, 1784)*; in the original French, *portion réfléchie du corps calleux*, p. 654.
20. *central end of olfactory nerve (Cruveilhier, 1836)*
Considered together, *apparent origin of olfactory nerve (Cruveilhier, 1836)* and *real origin of olfactory nerve (Cruveilhier, 1836)*; in the original French, *extrémité central du nerf olfactif*, pp. 883, 885.
21. *apparent origin of olfactory nerve (Cruveilhier, 1836)*
In macrodissected adult human, *gray root of olfactory nerve (Cruveilhier, 1836)* and white roots described by Vicq d'Azyr; in the original French, *origine apparente*, pp. 884–885.
22. *peduncle of septum lucidum (Arnold, 1838a)*
Synonym for macrodissected adult human *peduncle of septum (Burdach, 1822)*; in the original Latin, *pedunculus septi lucidi*, p. 50. Clearly illustrated by Arnold (1838b, Tab. VII, Fig. 1-*v*).
23. *supraoptic layer (Gerdy, 1838)*
Probably synonym for, or partly corresponds to, macrodissected adult human *peduncle of corpus callosum (Vicq d'Azyr, 1784)*; in the original French, *lame sus-optiques*, pp. 260–261. Supraoptic filaments (*filets sus-optiques*, p. 261) are associated with it.
24. *cerebral ganglia (Leuret, 1839)*
Macrodissected adult fish *cerebral hemispheres (Serres, 1824–1826)*; in the original French, *ganglions cérébraux*, p. 140.
25. *subcallosal gyrus (Zuckerkandl, 1887)*
According to His (1895; see Eycleshymer translation, 1917, p. 166 ff.), synonym for macrodissected adult human *peduncle of corpus callosum (Vicq d'Azyr, 1784)*. For Zuckerkandl's use, see pp. 15, 59 ff. and Figures 37-*G.s.*, 38-*P.c.c.*
26. *geniculate gyrus of Zuckerkandl (Dejerine & Dejerine-Klumpke, 1895)*
Eponym for *subcallosal gyrus (Zuckerkandl, 1887)*; in the original French, *circonvolution géniculée de Zuckerkandl*, Figure 211-*Cgn*.
27. *subcallosal area (>1840)*
As described for macrodissected adult human, sometimes described as outer surface of two adjacent parts, ***tenia tecta (Swanson, 1992)***, a component of ***cerebral cortex (>1840)***, and ***medial septal complex (Swanson et al., 1987)*** or *paraterminal gyrus (>1840)*, a component of ***cerebral nuclei (Swanson, 2000a)***. Bounded rostrally by ***posterior parolfactory sulcus (>1840)*** and caudally by ***terminal lamina (Burdach, 1822)***; see Nauta & Haymaker (1969, p. 158 and Figs. 4.1, 11, 27). Other authorities define it as corresponding to ***parolfactory gyrus (>1840)***; see Williams & Warwick (1980, p. 988), Nieuwenhuys et al. (2008, Fig. 3.6-7, p. 67).
28. *subcallosal gyrus (>1840)*
Synonym for macrodissected adult human *subcallosal area (>1840)* according to Nauta & Haymaker (1969, p. 158 and Figs. 4.1, 11, 27), Nieuwenhuys et al. (2008, Fig. 3.6-5).
29. *amygdalar region (>1840)*
As described for macrodissected adult human, and with cellular architecture and connections for all mammals, arbitrary set of ***central nervous system gray matter regions (>1840)*** in ***endbrain (Kuhlenbeck, 1927)***, including parts of ***cerebral cortex (>1840)*** and ***cerebral nuclei (Swanson, 2000a)***; see Swanson & Petrovich (1998) for a contemporary account of its components and their connections. It was first clearly illustrated in a transverse section through the macrodissected adult human by Steno (1669, Pl. III). Meckel (1817) probably alluded for the first time in writing to the adult human *amygdalar region (>1840)* in an extremely vague way. He noted that the region of the *eminence (Meckel, 1817)*, or *convolution of hippocampus major (Vicq d'Azyr, 1786)*, rostral to the *uncus (Vicq d'Azyr, 1786)*, terminates in a blunt extremity continuous with the ***terminal stria (Wenzel & Wenzel, 1812)***; see translation (1832, Vol. 2, p. 440). The first great modern account was by Johnston (1923); see Price et al. (1987).
30. *amygdala (>1840)*
See *amygdalar region (>1840)*.

endbrain vesicle (Kuhlenbeck, 1927)

For macrodissected vertebrate embryo, the paired rostral topographic division of the ***primary forebrain vesicle (Baer, 1837)*** developing into the adult ***endbrain (Kuhlenbeck, 1927)*** or ***cerebrum (Obersteiner & Hill, 1900)***, with ***cerebral nuclei (Swanson, 2000a)*** ventrally and ***cerebral cortex (>1840)*** dorsally; the caudal topographic division is the ***interbrain vesicle (Baer, 1837)***. For Kuhlenbeck's use, see p. 80. It was identified long ago in the chick embryo; see *vesicle represents brain (Harvey, 1651)*.

TRANSLATIONS:

1. *Endhirnblasen (Kuhlenbeck, 1927)*
Original German form of ***endbrain vesicle (Kuhlenbeck, 1927)***; p. 80.

EARLIER REFERENCES:

Earlier synonyms:

1. *vesicle represents brain (Harvey, 1651)*
Synonym for ***endbrain vesicle (Kuhlenbeck, 1927)*** of chick embryo at end of 5th day of incubation or beginning of 6th; see translation (1653, p. 111). It is too late in development to be the ***primary forebrain vesicle (Baer, 1837)***; see Malpighi (1673, Fig. XVIII).

2. *cerebral lobes vesicle (Serres, 1824–1826)*
   Synonym for ***endbrain vesicle (Kuhlenbeck, 1927)*** in macrodissected chick embryo on 3rd day of incubation; in the original French, *vésicule des lobes cérébraux*; e.g., Plate I, Figure 3-*8*. Used later in the book for all vertebrates.
3. *cerebral hemispheres vesicle (Serres, 1824–1826)*
   Synonym for *cerebral lobes vesicle (Serres, 1824–1826)*; in the original French, *vésicule des hémisphères cérébraux*, e.g., Plate I, Figure 4-9 and Plate II, Figure 45-5.
4. *forebrain vesicle (Baer, 1837)*
   Synonym for macrodissected embryonic vertebrate ***endbrain vesicle (Kuhlenbeck, 1927)***; p. 107.
5. *anterior cerebral cell (Wagner, 1839)*
   Synonym for macrodissected embryonic chick ***endbrain vesicle (Kuhlenbeck, 1927)***; in the original Latin, *cellula cerebri anterior hemisphaeria*, Table IV, Figure 5-*b*.

enteric plexuses (Hill, 1927)

As described for macrodissected adult human, they extend uninterrupted from the rostral (upper) end of the esophagus to the caudal (lower) end of the rectum. In general there are three concentric ***enteric plexuses (Hill, 1927)*** interconnected by *nerve fibers (Ehrenberg, 1833)*; from inner to outer they are the *mucosal plexus* at the level of the muscularis mucosae, the *submucosal plexus* (called *Meissner's plexus*) on the submucosal surface of the external muscle, and the *myenteric plexus* (called *Auerbach's plexus*) between the inner and outer layers of the external muscle. Differentiations of the ***enteric plexuses (Hill, 1927)*** are described for each segment of the digestive tract: esophagus, stomach, small intestine, large intestine, and rectum. See Mitchell (1953, pp. 50–59), Williams & Warwick (1980, p. 1316 ff.) They were not described by 1840.

entorhinal area (Brodmann, 1909)

As described for adult mammal with cellular architecture and connections, developmentally and topologically the most lateral component of the ***hippocampal formation (Swanson & Cowan, 1777)***, lateral to the ***parasubiculum (>1840)*** and most simply divided into medial and lateral parts; see Swanson et al. (1987). For Brodmann's use in mammal, see pp. 209–210, Table 7 on p. 247, and pp. 182, 188, 192, where he noted a *medial entorhinal area* and *lateral entorhinal area*, at least in the flying fox, kinkajou, rabbit, and ground squirrel. In macrodissected adult human, it is topologically the most lateral component of the ***parahippocampal gyrus (>1840)***; see Williams & Warwick (1980, Fig. 7.119-*EA*). It was not clearly described by 1840.

EARLIER REFERENCES:

Earlier synonyms:

1. *area 28 (Brodmann, 1909)*
   Synonym for macrodissected adult human ***entorhinal area (Brodmann, 1909)***; in the original German, *Feld 28*, see pp. 209–210.

PARTLY CORRESPONDS:

1. *dorsal entorhinal area (Brodmann, 1909)*
   Small differentiation of adult human ***entorhinal area (Brodmann, 1909)*** not observed by Brodmann in other mammals; see p. 149 and Figure 86.
2. *area 34 (Brodmann, 1909)*
   Synonym for *dorsal entorhinal area (Brodmann, 1909)*; in the original German, *Feld 34*, see p. 149 and Figure 86.

ependyma (>1840)

The thin, ciliated columnar epithelium lining the ***ventricles (Hippocrates)***. It is the adult remnant of the ventricular layer of the neuroepithelium, and is a type of ***glia (Virchow, 1846)***; see Williams & Warwick (1980, pp. 160, 835–837). It was not described by 1840.

ependymal roof plate (>1840)

In certain embryonic ***secondary brain vesicles (>1840)***, a more or less wide transverse expansion of the ***roof plate (>1840)*** to form a thin, free layer of ***ependyma (>1840)***, with the inner side facing the lumen of the ***ventricles (Hippocrates)*** and the outer side acquiring a layer of ***pia (Galen, c192)***. As development progresses, the ***ependymal roof plate (>1840)*** comes to form the ***choroid epithelium of lateral ventricle (>1840), choroid epithelium of third ventricle (>1840)***, and ***choroid epithelium of fourth ventricle (>1840)***; see Hamilton & Mossman (1972, pp. 463–465, 467–468, 471–472, 474–478, Figs. 437, 448–453). It was not clearly described by 1840.

epipial layer (Key & Retzius, 1875)

As described for macrodissected adult human, the thin layer of ***arachnoid (Blasius, 1666)*** consisting of highly vascular innermost condensations of ***arachnoid trabeculae (>1840)*** lying just outside the ***pia (Galen, c192)***; see Millen & Woollam (1962, pp. 90–94). It was well described by Vesalius; see ***[epipial layer (Key & Retzius, 1875)] (Vesalius, 1543a)***.

EARLIER REFERENCES:

Described, not named or illustrated:

1. *[epipial layer (Key & Retzius, 1875)] (Vesalius, 1543a)*
   Very clearly described for macrodissected adult human, "It [***pia (Galen, c192)***] is of equal thickness all over and everywhere presents the appearance of a very thin membrane covered with innumerable vessel ducts." (Richardson & Carman translation, 2009, p. 176).

epithalamic medullary stria (>1840)

As described in macrodissected adult human, and mammal generally with histological methods for ***axons (Kölliker, 1896)***, the dorsal segment of the ***medullary stria (Wenzel & Wenzel, 1812)*** extending near the median plane of the ***epithalamus (His, 1893b)*** between ***hypothalamic medullary stria (>1840)*** rostrally and ***habenular commissure (>1840)*** caudally. It was known to Vesalius; see ***[epithalamic medullary stria (>1840)] (Vesalius, 1543a)***.

EARLIER REFERENCES:

Described, not named or illustrated:

1. ***[epithalamic medullary stria (>1840)] (Vesalius, 1543a)***
Very clearly illustrated for macrodissected adult human; see Singer translation (1952, p. 107, Fig. 10).

PARTLY CORRESPONDS:

1. *tenia thalami (Wenzel & Wenzel, 1812)*
Synonym for part of macrodissected adult human ***medullary stria (Wenzel & Wenzel, 1812)*** specifically associated with ***habenular nuclei (>1840)*** according to Dejerine & Dejerine-Klumpke (1901); that is, all but the rostral end of the ***epithalamic medullary stria (>1840)***. According to Burdach (1822, p. 333), the term Wenzel & Wenzel used (in Latin) was *taenia medullosa juxta interiorem marginem colliculi optici* (see p. 86 ff.).

epithalamus (His, 1893b)

As described for macrodissected adult human, and based on cellular architecture and development in vertebrate, the most dorsal of the three topographic subdivisions of the ***thalamus (His, 1893a)*** lying dorsomedial to the ***dorsal part of thalamus (Herrick, 1910)***. Based on cellular architecture and connections it has two main parts, ***habenular nuclei (>1840)*** and ***pineal gland (Galen, c192)***; see Nieuwenhuys et al. (2008, p. 44 and Fig. 5.31). For His's use in macrodissected adult human, see pp. 178–179. It was not delineated as such by 1840.

esophageal branches of recurrent laryngeal nerve (Arnold, 1834)

As described for macrodissected adult human, they arise from the rostrally directed (ascending) limb of the ***recurrent laryngeal nerve (Albinus, 1744)*** and supply mucous membrane and muscle coat of the esophagus; see Williams & Warwick (1980, p. 1081), *Terminologia Anatomica* (1998, p. 136). For Arnold's use in macrodissected adult human, see p. 14. They were perhaps first clearly described by Loder; see ***[esophageal branches of recurrent laryngeal nerve (>1840)] (Loder, 1778)***.

TRANSLATIONS:

1. *rami oesophagei nervus recurrens laryngeus (Arnold, 1834)*
Original Latin form of ***esophageal branches of recurrent laryngeal nerve (Arnold, 1834)***; p. 14.

EARLIER REFERENCES:

Described, not named or illustrated:

1. ***[esophageal branches of recurrent laryngeal nerve (>1840)] (Loder, 1778)***
Described for macrodissected adult human; pp. 30–31.

Earlier synonyms:

1. *aesophagian branches of tracheal nerve (Burdin, 1803)*
Synonym for macrodissected adult human ***esophageal branches of recurrent laryngeal nerve (>1840)***; see translation (1803, Vol. 1, p. 183).

LATER SYNONYMS:

1. *esophageal branches of inferior laryngeal nerve (Arnold, 1834)*
Synonym for macrodissected adult human ***esophageal branches of recurrent laryngeal nerve (>1840)***; in the original Latin, *rami oesophagei nervus laryngeus inferior*, p. 14.
2. *esophageal branches of recurrent nerve (Cruveilhier, 1836)*
Synonym for macrodissected adult human ***esophageal branches of recurrent laryngeal nerve (>1840)***; in the original French, *rameaux oesophagiens*, p. 963.

PARTLY CORRESPONDS:

1. *small oesophageal plexus (Fyfe, 1800)*
Partly surrounds esophagus and arises from macrodissected adult human ***esophageal branches of recurrent laryngeal nerve (>1840)*** and from ***vagus nerve (Galen, c192)*** near origin of ***recurrent laryngeal nerve (Albinus, 1744)***; Vol. 2, p. 317. Also see *great oesophageal plexus (Fyfe, 1800)*.

esophageal branches of sympathetic trunk (>1840)

As described for macrodissected adult human, they commonly arise from the ***thoracic pulmonary nerves (>1840)*** and extend to the esophagus; see Mitchell (1953, pp. 238–239), Williams & Warwick (1980, p. 1131). They were first mentioned by Vieussens; see ***[esophageal branches of sympathetic trunk (>1840)] (Vieussens, 1684)***.

EARLIER REFERENCES:

Illustrated and described, not named:

1. ***[esophageal branches of sympathetic trunk (>1840)] (Vieussens, 1684)***
Alluded to for macrodissected adult human; Table 23-40.

Earlier synonyms:

1. *sympathetic branches to esophagus (Bischoff, 1832)*
For macrodissected adult human, Bischoff illustrated two ***esophageal branches of sympathetic trunk (>1840)***; in the original Latin, duo *rami Sympathici ad Oesophagum*, Table I, Figure 1-46,47.

esophageal plexus (Haller, 1762)

As described for macrodissected adult human, branches of the right and left ***vagus nerve trunk (Wrisberg, 1786; Günther, 1786)*** arising distal to (below) the ***pulmonary branches of vagus nerve (Cloquet, 1828)*** and forming a network around the outside of the esophagus. The ***esophageal plexus (Haller, 1762)*** is divided roughly into ***anterior esophageal plexus (Haller, 1762)*** and ***posterior esophageal plexus (Haller, 1762)*** before entering the abdomen through the esophageal hiatus of the diaphragm. Proximal branches of the ***esophageal plexus (Haller, 1762)*** include the ***upper esophageal branches of vagus nerve (Cloquet, 1828)*** and small branches of the thoracic ***sympathetic trunk (Winslow, 1733)*** and ***greater splanchnic nerve (Walter, 1783)***. Distal branches include sympathetic and parasympathetic ***axons (Kölliker, 1896)*** sinking into the esophageal wall to end in its component of the ***enteric plexuses (Hill, 1927)***; see Mitchell (1953, pp. 184–185 and Figs. 104, 110, 111, 119, 120), Williams & Warwick (1980, pp. 1079, 1081). A common synonym is *lower esophageal branches of vagus nerve (>1840)*. For Haller's use in macrodissected adult human, see p. 235.

It was discovered by Galen; see ***[esophageal plexus (Haller, 1762)] (Galen, c173)***.

TRANSLATIONS:

1. *plexus oesophageus (Haller, 1762)*
   Original Latin form of ***esophageal plexus (Haller, 1762)***; p. 235.
2. *plexum gulae (Soemmerring, 1798)*
   Latin form of ***esophageal plexus (Haller, 1762)***; p. 269. Also see Bell & Bell (1816, Vol. 2, p. 508) who used *plexus gulae*; see Mitchell (1953, p. 184).

EARLIER REFERENCES:

Described, not named or illustrated:

1. ***[esophageal plexus (Haller, 1762)] (Galen, c173)***
   Mentioned for macrodissected adult pig, beef, and/or monkey but not human; see May translation (1968, pp. 290, 449), Duckworth translation (1962, p. 220). Vesalius (1543a) barely alluded to it for macrodissected adult human (see Richardson & Carman translation, 2002, p. 199), but it was rather clearly described by Paré (1561, p. cxiii); see English translation (1634, p. 153). Vieussens (1684, p. 186) and Winslow (1733, Sect. VI, p. 71) described it very clearly for macrodissected adult human.

Illustrated, not named or described:

1. ***[esophageal plexus (Haller, 1762)] (Eustachi, 1552)***
   Illustrated for macrodissected adult human; see Albinus edition (1761, Tab. 18-*η*), Haller (1762, p. 235-*u*).

LATER SYNONYMS:

1. *plexum circa oesophagum (Ludwig, 1772)*
   Synonym for macrodissected adult human ***esophageal plexus (Haller, 1762)***; p. 8.
2. *great esophageal plexus of eighth pair (Scarpa, 1794)*
   Synonym for macrodissected adult human ***esophageal plexus (Haller, 1762)***; in the original Latin, *octavi magnus plexus oesophageus*, Table V:37-39.
3. *great oesophageal plexus (Fyfe, 1800)*
   English form of *great esophageal plexus of eighth pair (Scarpa, 1794)*; Vol. 2, p. 317. Also see *small oesophageal plexus (Fyfe, 1800)*.
4. *anterior and posterior plexus gulae (Bell & Bell, 1816)*
   Synonym for macrodissected adult human ***esophageal plexus (Haller, 1762)***; Vol. 2, p. 508.
5. *oesophageal branches of vagus nerve (Quain, 1832)*
   Synonym for macrodissected adult human ***esophageal plexus (Haller, 1762)***; p. 669.
6. *lower esophageal branches of vagus nerve (>1840)*
   Synonym for macrodissected adult human ***esophageal plexus (>1840)***; see Williams & Warwick (1980, p. 1081).

PARTLY CORRESPONDS:

1. *stomachical branches of wandring pair (Willis, 1664)*
   Corresponds roughly to ***anterior vagal trunk (Wrisberg, 1780)*** and ***posterior vagal trunk (Wrisberg, 1780)*** considered together in macrodissected adult human and other common large mammals; see Pordage translation (1681, p. 156 and Tab. 9-*T*).
2. *stomachical nerves (Willis, 1664)*
   Synonym for *stomachical branches of wandring pair (Willis, 1664)*; see Pordage translation (1681, p. 158 and Tab. 11-*D*).

external acoustic meatus nerves (Meckel, 1817)

As described for macrodissected adult human, they are usually two branches of the ***auriculotemporal nerve (Haller, 1762)*** supplying the external acoustic (auditory) meatus, with the dorsal (upper) ***nerve (Herophilus, c335–c280 BC)*** sending a tiny branch to the tympanic membrane; see Williams & Warwick (1980, p. 1066), *Terminologia Anatomica* (1998, p. 134). For Meckel's use in macrodissected adult human, see translation (1832, Vol. 3, p. 73); also see Bock (1817, p. 48). It was perhaps first mentioned by Rau; see ***[external acoustic meatus nerves (Meckel, 1817)] (Rau, 1694)***.

TRANSLATIONS:

1. *nervi meatus auditorii externi (Meckel, 1817)*
   Original Latin form of ***external acoustic meatus nerves (Meckel, 1817)***; see translation (1832, Vol. 3, p. 73).

EARLIER REFERENCES:

Described, not named or illustrated:

1. ***[external acoustic meatus nerves (Meckel, 1817)] (Rau, 1694)***
   Mentioned for macrodissected adult human; pp. 193–194, see Haller (1762, p. 220 note *r*). Meckel's illustrious grandfather (Meckel; 1748, pp. 99–100) clearly described them for macrodissected adult human.

Earlier synonyms:

1. *auricular fascicles proper of cutaneous temporal surculus of inferior maxillary branch (Bellingeri, 1818)*
   Synonym for macrodissected adult human ***external acoustic meatus nerves (Meckel, 1817)***; in the original Latin, *fasciculi auriculares proprii*, see Table I.
2. *external auditory meatus branch of superficial temporal nerve (Arnold, 1834)*
   Synonym for macrodissected adult human ***external acoustic meatus nerves (Meckel, 1817)***; in the original Latin, *nervus temporalis superficialis, ramus meatus auditorii externi*, p. 11.
3. *external auditory meatus branch of anterior auricular nerve (Arnold, 1834)*
   Synonym for macrodissected adult human ***external acoustic meatus nerves (Meckel, 1817)***; in the original Latin, *nervus auricularis anterior, ramus meatus auditorii externi*, p. 11.
4. *internal auricular branches of superficial temporal nerve (Todd, 1836–1839)*
   Synonym for macrodissected adult human ***external acoustic meatus nerves (Meckel, 1817)***; p. 293.

external branch of accessory nerve trunk (Meckel, 1817)

As described for macrodissected adult human, one of two major terminal branches of the ***accessory nerve trunk (Meckel, 1817)*** arising from the ***spinal root of accessory nerve (Meckel, 1817)*** and supplying mainly the sternocleidomastoid and trapezius muscles; see Williams & Warwick (1980, p. 1082). For Meckel's use in macrodissected adult human, see translation (1832, Vol. 3, pp. 44). It was known to Galen; see ***[external branch of accessory nerve trunk (>1840)] (Galen, c192)***.

EARLIER REFERENCES:

Described, not named or illustrated:

1. ***[external branch of accessory nerve trunk (>1840)] (Galen, c192)***
   Distribution to trapezius and sternocleidomastoid muscles clearly described for macrodissected adult beef, pig, and/or macaque but not human; see Duckworth translation (1962, p. 202).

Earlier synonyms:

1. *descending trunk of accessory spinal nerve (Willis, 1664)*
   Basically synonymous with macrodissected adult human ***external branch of accessory nerve trunk (Meckel, 1817)***; see Pordage translation (1681, Tab. 9-♃, ♀, ♂).
2. *external branch of accessory nerve (Scarpa, 1788)*
   Synonym for macrodissected adult human ***external branch of accessory nerve trunk (Meckel, 1817)***; in the original Latin, *accessorii ramus externus*, Table X, Figure 1-*6*.
3. *external branch of accessory vagal pair (Soemmerring, 1791)*
   Synonym for macrodissected adult human ***external branch of accessory nerve trunk (Meckel, 1817)***; p. 256, also see Soemmerring (1798, p. 276).
4. *greater external branch of accessory eighth nerve (Scarpa, 1794)*
   Basically, synonym for macrodissected adult human *external branch of accessory vagal pair (Soemmerring, 1791)*; see Table I:*47-51*.

LATER SYNONYMS:

1. *greater external branch of spinal accessory nerve (Knox, 1832)*
   Synonym for macrodissected adult human *greater external branch of accessory eighth nerve (Scarpa, 1794)*; Plate II-*60*.
2. *muscular branch of accessory nerve (Cruveilhier, 1836)*
   Synonym for macrodissected adult human ***external branch of accessory nerve trunk (Meckel, 1817)***; in the original French, *branche musculaire*, p. 970.
3. *muscular branch of spinal nerve (Cruveilhier, 1836)*
   Synonym for *muscular branch of accessory nerve (Cruveilhier, 1836)*; in the original French, *branche musculaire du nerf spinal*, pp. 970, 971.

PARTLY CORRESPONDS:

1. *anastomotic branches of external accessory nerve with second and third cervical nerves (Scarpa, 1788)*
   Macrodissected adult human ***communicating branches (Winslow, 1733)*** between ***external branch of accessory nerve trunk (Meckel, 1817)*** and 2nd and 3rd ***cervical nerves (Galen, c173)***; in the original Latin, *anastomosis rami externi accessorii cum secundo et tertio cervicalium*, Table X, Figure 1-*14,15*. Scarpa also described ***communicating branches (Winslow, 1733)*** between ***external branch of accessory nerve trunk (Meckel, 1817)*** and 4th and 5th ***cervical nerves (Galen, c173)***; Table X, Figure 1-*17*.
2. *connection of external branch of accessory nerve of Willis with third and second cervical nerves (Arnold, 1834)*
   Synonym for macrodissected adult human *anastomotic branches of external accessory nerve with second and third cervical nerves (Scarpa, 1788)*; in the original Latin, *conjunctio ramus externus nervus accessorius Willisii cum nervo cervicali tertio et secundo*; p. 14, Table VIII-*64*, Table IV-*18*.

external branch of superior laryngeal nerve (Fyfe, 1800)

As described for macrodissected adult human, it ends in the cricothyroid muscle after supplying branches to the ***pharyngeal plexus (Neubauer, 1772)*** and inferior pharyngeal constrictor muscle and communicating with the ***superior cardiac nerve (Neubauer, 1772)*** and ***superior cervical ganglion (Vieussens, 1684)***; see Williams & Warwick (1980, p. 1080), *Terminologia Anatomica* (1998, p. 136). For Fyfe's description in macrodissected adult human, see Vol. 2, p. 295. It was known to Galen; see ***[external branch of superior laryngeal nerve (Fyfe, 1800)] (Galen, c173)***.

EARLIER REFERENCES:

Described, not named or illustrated:

1. ***[external branch of superior laryngeal nerve (Fyfe, 1800)] (Galen, c173)***
   Described in macrodissected adult beef, pig, and/or macaque but not human; see May translation (1968, pp. 689–690), Duckworth translation (1962, pp. 76, 203–204). Vesalius (1543a) described it for macrodissected adult human; see Richardson & Carman translation (2002, p. 195).

Earlier synonyms:

1. *superficial branchlets of superior laryngeal nerve (Loder, 1778)*
   Synonym for macrodissected adult human ***external branch of superior laryngeal nerve (Fyfe, 1800)***; in the original Latin, *ramulum superficialem*, p. 85.
2. *external branch of laryngeal nerve (Haase, 1781)*
   Synonym for macrodissected adult human ***external branch of superior laryngeal nerve (Fyfe, 1800)***; in the original Latin, *nervus laryngeus ramus externus*, p. 85.
3. *outer laryngeal nerve (Günther, 1786)*
   Synonym for macrodissected adult human ***external branch of superior laryngeal nerve (Fyfe, 1800)***; in the original Latin, *nervus laryngeus exteriorem*, p. 63.
4. *external laryngeal nerve (Soemmerring, 1791)*
   Synonym for macrodissected adult human ***external branch of superior laryngeal nerve (Fyfe, 1800)***; in the original Latin, *nervus laryngeus externus*, p. 247.

LATER SYNONYMS:

1. *pharyngolaryngeal nerve (Bell, 1803b)*
   Synonym listed for macrodissected adult human ***external branch of superior laryngeal nerve (Fyfe, 1800)***; in the original Latin, *pharyngo-laryngeus*, p. 154. Knox (1832, Pl. II-*79*) hyphenated it in English, *pharyngo-laryngeal nerve*.

2. *external laryngeal branch of vocal nerve (Bock, 1817)*
Synonym for macrodissected adult human ***external branch of superior laryngeal nerve (Fyfe, 1800)***; in the original Latin (and German), *ramus laryngeus externus (des Stimmnerven)*, p. 68.
3. *external branch of descending laryngeal nerve (Swan, 1830)*
Synonym for macrodissected adult human ***external branch of superior laryngeal nerve (Fyfe, 1800)***; p. 756.
4. *external laryngeal branch of superior laryngeal branch of pneumogastric nerve (Cruveilhier, 1836)*
Synonym listed for macrodissected adult human ***external branch of superior laryngeal nerve (Fyfe, 1800)***; in the original French, *laryngé externe*, p. 959.

PARTLY CORRESPONDS:
1. *laryngeal plexus of soft nerves (Scarpa, 1794)*
Term attributed without citation to Haller (it could derive from a sentence in Haller, 1762, p. 233) referring to branches of macrodissected adult human ***external branch of superior laryngeal nerve (Fyfe, 1800)*** to inferior pharyngeal constrictor muscle, larynx, and thyroid gland; in the original Latin, *plexus laryngaei nervorum mollium*, Table III-*140*; see Knox translation (1832, Pl. III-*176*).
2. *branches of superior laryngeal nerve to arytenoid muscle (Langenbeck, 1826–1830)*
Macrodissected adult human branches of ***external branch of superior laryngeal nerve (Fyfe, 1800)*** to arytenoid muscle; in the original Latin, *rami laryngei superioris ad musculos arytaenoideos*; Fascicle III, Tables XVI-*9*, XVIII-*31*.
3. *branch of superior laryngeal nerve to cricothyroid muscle (Langenbeck, 1826–1830)*
Macrodissected adult human branch of ***external branch of superior laryngeal nerve (Fyfe, 1800)*** to cricothyroid muscle; in the original Latin, *ramus laryngei superioris ad musculos cricothyreoideum*, Fascicle III, Table XVIII-*32*.
4. *branch of superior laryngeal nerve to lateral cricoarytenoid muscle (Langenbeck, 1826–1830)*
Macrodissected adult human branch of ***external branch of superior laryngeal nerve (Fyfe, 1800)*** to lateral cricoarytenoid muscle; in the original Latin, *ramus laryngei superioris ad musculos cricoarytaenoideum lateralem*, Fascicle III, Table XVIII-*33*.

external capsule (Burdach, 1822)

As described for macrodissected adult human, a topographic division of the ***cerebral cortex white matter (>1840)*** between ***putamen (Burdach, 1822)*** medially and ***claustrum(Burdach, 1822)*** laterally; see Crosby et al. (1962, pp. 396–398 and Fig. 284). For Burdach's use in macrodissected adult human, see p. 130. It was delineated by Vesalius; see ***[external capsule (Burdach, 1822)] (Vesalius, 1543a)***.

TRANSLATIONS:
1. *capsula externa (Burdach, 1822)*
Original Latin form of ***external capsule (Burdach, 1822)***; p. 130.

EARLIER REFERENCES:

Illustrated, not named or described:
1. ***[external capsule (Burdach, 1822)] (Vesalius, 1543a)***
Very clearly illustrated for macrodissected adult human; see Singer translation (1952, Figs. 7 and 8).

Earlier synonyms:
1. *corporis striati limbus anterior (Willis, 1672)*
Roughly corresponds to ***external capsule (Burdach, 1822)*** in macrodissected adult sheep and human; in the original Latin (plural) a fuller description included, *corporus striati limbus anterior, corpori calloso conjunctus*; Tables V-*N* and VIII-*E*, also see Schiller (1967, p. 529).
2. *anterior limbus of striate body (Willis, 1672)*
English form (singular) of *corporus striati limbus anterior (Willis, 1672)*.
3. *foremost border of streaked body (Willis, 1672)*
English form of *anterior limbus of striate body (Willis, 1672)*; see Pordage translation (1683, Table VIII-*D,E*).
4. *exterior smaller medullary tract of anterior process of medulla oblongata (Vieussens, 1684)*
Probably corresponds at least partly to macrodissected adult human ***external capsule (Burdach, 1822)***; p. 66, see translations in Gordon (1817, p. 94), Clarke & O'Malley (1996, p. 587).

LATER SYNONYMS:
1. *medullary capsule of lentiform nucleus (Arnold, 1838b)*
Synonym for macrodissected adult human ***external capsule (Burdach, 1822)***; in the original Latin, *capsula medullaris nuclei lentiformis*, Table IV, Figure 4-*ι*.

external carotid plexus (>1840)

As described for macrodissected adult human, it begins as 4–6 filaments leaving the ventral (anterior) aspect of the ***superior cervical ganglion (Vieussens, 1684)*** and then forming a rich ***plexus (Galen, c192)*** around the external carotid artery and all its branches; see Mitchell (1953, pp. 220–221). "It has been often observed, that the branches of the carotid artery have a peculiar provision of nerves, and that these nerves are more numerous and minutely distributed than in any other part of the body. There are indeed no nerves in any part of the body which have so extensive and intricate connections with important vital nerves as the cutaneous nerves of the face and neck. This distribution of the nerves has been considered a provision for that power possessed by the imagination, or rather that uncontrollable connection which exists betwixt the feelings and the action of the vessels in blushing, and in the expression of the passions." (Bell & Bell, 1829, p. 561). It was perhaps first clearly described by Neubauer; see ***[external carotid plexus (>1840)] (Neubauer, 1772)***.

EARLIER REFERENCES:

Described, not named or illustrated:
1. ***[external carotid plexus (>1840)] (Neubauer, 1772)***
Neubauer mentioned at least one branch from ***superior cervical ganglion (Vieussens, 1684)*** to external

carotid artery of macrodissected adult human; see p. 8-*e*, Table 1-9. Cloquet (1816, p. 693) clearly described it and its extensions to all external carotid artery branches for macrodissected adult human. Scarpa (1794) described its appearance minutely in macrodissected adult human (see Knox translation, 1832, Pl. III-*115*) and Lobstein (1823) described its appearance under the microscope in adult human; see translation (1831, p. 43).

Earlier synonyms:

1. *soft nerves of anterior carotid artery (Andersch & Soemmerring, 1792)*
   Synonym for macrodissected adult human ***external carotid plexus (>1840)***; in the original Latin, *nervi mollis arteriae carotidis anterioris*, p. 166.
2. *external carotid soft nerve trunk (Arnold, 1834)*
   Synonym for macrodissected adult human ***external carotid plexus (>1840)***; in the original Latin, *truncus nervorum mollium carotidis externae*, p. 18.
3. *external carotid vascular nerve trunk (Arnold, 1834)*
   Synonym for macrodissected adult human ***external carotid plexus (>1840)***; in the original Latin, *truncus nervorum vasorum carotidis externae*, p. 18.
4. *soft nerve net accompanying trunk of external carotid artery (Arnold, 1834)*
   Synonym for macrodissected adult human ***external carotid plexus (>1840)***; in the original Latin, *retia nervorum mollium, truncum arteriae carotidis externae comitantia*, Table VII:*XX-113*.

PARTLY CORRESPONDS:

1. *transverse nerve of anterior carotid artery (Andersch & Soemmerring, 1792)*
   Mixing of ***communicating branches (Winslow, 1733)*** from ***glossopharyngeal nerve (Huber, 1744)*** and ***vagus nerve (Galen, c192)*** associated with macrodissected adult human ***external carotid plexus (>1840)***; in the original Latin, *nervum transversalem arteriae carotidis anterioris*, p. 167.
2. *reverse nerve of occipital artery (Andersch & Soemmerring, 1792)*
   Basically, extension of macrodissected adult human ***external carotid plexus (>1840)*** described as coursing along occipital artery and generating ascending branch along ***glossopharyngeal nerve (Huber, 1744)***; in the original Latin, *nervus reversivus arteriae occipitalis*, p. 167.
3. *reverse nerve of superior thyroid artery (Andersch & Soemmerring, 1792)*
   Basically, extension of macrodissected adult human ***external carotid plexus (>1840)*** described as coursing along superior thyroid artery; in the original Latin, *nervo reversivo arteriae thyreoidae superioris*, p. 168.
4. *soft nerve of labial artery (Andersch & Soemmerring, 1792)*
   Basically, extension of macrodissected adult human ***external carotid plexus (>1840)*** described as coursing along labial artery; in the original Latin, *nervum mollem arteriae labialis*, p. 170.
5. *labial soft nerves (Andersch & Soemmerring, 1792)*
   Synonym for *soft nerve of labial artery (Andersch & Soemmerring, 1792)*; in the original Latin, *nervi mollis labialis*, p. 171.
6. *labial artery nerves (Andersch & Soemmerring, 1792)*
   Synonym for *soft nerve of labial artery (Andersch & Soemmerring, 1792)*; in the original Latin, *nervi arteriae labialia*, p. 171.
7. *reverse soft nerve of occipital artery (Andersch, 1797)*
   Synonym for *reverse nerve of occipital artery (Andersch & Soemmerring, 1792)*; in the original Latin, *nervus mollis reversivus arteriae occipitalis*, p. 109.
8. *reverse soft nerve of superior thyroid artery (Andersch, 1797)*
   Synonym for *reverse nerve of superior thyroid artery (Andersch & Soemmerring, 1792)*; in the original Latin, *nervo molli reversivo arteriae thyreoideae superioris*, p. 110. Also see Arnold (1834, Tab. VII:*XX-110*).
9. *anastomotic filament of portio major and minor of facial nerve with intercostal branch (Bellingeri, 1818)*
   May correspond to macrodissected adult human *connection of soft nerves of external carotid vascular nerve trunk with facial nerve (Arnold, 1834)*; in the original Latin, *filamentum anastomoticum*, see Table II.
10. *carotid plexus of glossopharyngeal nerves (Kilian, 1822)*
   As described for macrodissected adult human, fixed with alcohol, very fine ***plexus (Galen, c192)*** associated at least initially with ***external carotid plexus (>1840)*** and derived from *main communicating branch of glossopharyngeal nerve (Kilian, 1822)*; in the original Latin, *plexus carotideus nervi glossopharyngei*, p. 90. Kilian used the term *nerve net* (*Nervennetz*, p. 90) to describe this feature, which undoubtedly contributes to the *intercarotid plexus (Boyd, 1937)*.
11. *connection of soft nerves of external carotid soft nerve trunk with facial nerve (Arnold, 1834)*
   For macrodissected adult human, ***communicating branch (Winslow, 1733)*** of ***external carotid plexus (>1840)*** with *facial nerve (Vic d'Azyr, 1784)*; in the original Latin, *conjunctio truncus nervorum mollium carotidis externae nervi molles cum nervo facialis*, p. 18.
12. *connection of soft nerves of external carotid vascular nerve trunk with facial nerve (Arnold, 1834)*
   For macrodissected adult human, ***communicating branch (Winslow, 1733)*** of ***external carotid plexus (>1840)*** with *facial nerve (Vic d'Azyr, 1784)*; in the original Latin, *conjunctio truncus nervorum vasorum carotidis externae nervi molles cum nervo facialis*, p. 18 (and Tab. VII:*XX-111*). It might correspond to inconsistent *external petrosal nerve (>1840)*, usually described as extending between *middle meningeal plexus (>1840)* and *genu of facial nerve (Langenbeck, 1826-1830)*; see Williams & Warwick (1980, p. 1071). Also see *anastomotic filament of portio major and minor of facial nerve (Bellingeri, 1818)*.
13. *soft nerves of temporal artery (Arnold, 1834)*
   In macrodissected adult human, extension of ***external carotid plexus (>1840)*** along superficial temporal

artery; in the original Latin, *nervi molles arteriae temporalis*, Table VII:*XX-114*.

14. *soft nerves of internal maxillary artery (Arnold, 1834)*
In macrodissected adult human, extension of ***external carotid plexus (>1840)*** along maxillary artery; in the original Latin, *nervi molles arteriae maxillaris internae*, Table VII:*XX-116*.

15. *soft nerves of facial artery (Arnold, 1834)*
In macrodissected adult human, extension of ***external carotid plexus (>1840)*** along facial artery; in the original Latin, *nervi molles arteriae facialis*, Table IX-*51*.

16. *soft nerves of occipital artery (Arnold, 1834)*
In macrodissected adult human, extension of ***external carotid plexus (>1840)*** along occipital artery; in the original Latin, *nervi molles arteriae occipitalis*, Table IX-*51*.

17. *thyroid plexus (Cruveilhier, 1836)*
Extension of macrodissected adult human ***external carotid plexus (>1840)*** coursing along superior thyroid artery into thyroid gland; in the original French, *plexus thyroïdien*, p. 992.

18. *lingual plexus (Cruveilhier, 1836)*
Extension of macrodissected adult human ***external carotid plexus (>1840)*** coursing along lingual artery into tongue where Cruveilhier described communication with ***lingual nerve (Vesalius, 1543a)*** and even ***hypoglossal nerve (Winslow, 1733)***; in the original French, *plexus lingual*, p. 992.

19. *facial plexus (Cruveilhier, 1836)*
Extension of macrodissected adult human ***external carotid plexus (>1840)*** coursing along facial artery with some branches entering submandibular gland, and according to some the ***submandibular ganglion (>1840)***—the ***sympathetic root of submandibular ganglion (>1840)***; in the original French, *plexus facial*, p. 992.

20. *occipital plexus (Cruveilhier, 1836)*
Extension of macrodissected adult human ***external carotid plexus (>1840)*** coursing along occipital artery; in the original French, *plexus occipital*, p. 993.

21. *auricular plexus (Cruveilhier, 1836)*
Extension of macrodissected adult human ***external carotid plexus (>1840)*** coursing along posterior auricular artery; in the original French, *plexus auriculaire*, p. 993.

external medullary lamina (>1840)

As described in macrodissected adult human, and mammal generally with histological methods for ***axons (Kölliker, 1896)***, a ***central nervous system white matter tract (>1840)*** between the medial edge of the ***reticular thalamic nucleus (>1840)*** and lateral edge of the ***dorsal part of thalamus (Herrick, 1910)***; see Williams & Warwick (1980, p. 955). It was perhaps first clearly delineated by Rolando; see ***[external medullary lamina (>1840)] (Rolando, 1825)***.

EARLIER REFERENCES:

Illustrated and described, not named:

1. ***[external medullary lamina (>1840)] (Rolando, 1825)***
Illustrated and described in transverse section of macrodissected adult beef; Table VIII, Figure 1-*y*.

external nasal branch of anterior ethmoidal nerve (>1840)

As described for macrodissected adult human, it supplies skin of the ala, apex, and vestibule of the nose; see Williams & Warwick (1980, p. 1061), *Terminologia Anatomica* (1998, p. 134). It was first delineated vaguely by Willis; see ***[external nasal branch of anterior ethmoidal nerve (>1840)] (Willis, 1664)***.

EARLIER REFERENCES:

Illustrated and described, not named:

1. ***[external nasal branch of anterior ethmoidal nerve (>1840)] (Willis, 1664)***
Vaguely illustrated and described for macrodissected adult mammal; see p. 302, Figure 1-*c*.

Earlier synonyms:

1. *superior nasal cutaneous branch of nasal nerve (Meckel, 1753)*
Roughly synonymous with macrodissected adult human ***external nasal branch of anterior ethmoidal nerve (>1840)***; in the original French, *le rameau cutané du nés supérieur du nerf nasal*, p. 40, Table 1-*28*.
2. *exterior branch of nasal nerve (Scarpa, 1785)*
Synonym for macrodissected adult human ***external nasal branch of anterior ethmoidal nerve (>1840)***; in the original Latin, *nervi nasalis ramus exterior*, Table I, Figure 1-*i*.
3. *external branch of nasal nerve (Scarpa, 1785)*
Synonym for macrodissected adult human ***external nasal branch of anterior ethmoidal nerve (>1840)***; in the original Latin, *nervi nasalis ramus externus*, Table II, Figure II-*p*. Scarpa described two branches of this branch, Table II, Figure II-*q,r*.
4. *external superior nasal nerves (Günther, 1786)*
Synonym for macrodissected adult human ***external nasal branch of anterior ethmoidal nerve (>1840)***; in the original Latin, *N. nasales superiores externi*, p. 44.
5. *dorsal superior nasal nerves (Günther, 1786)*
Synonym for macrodissected adult human ***external nasal branch of anterior ethmoidal nerve (>1840)***; in the original Latin, *N. nasales superiores dorsales*, p. 44.
6. *external nasal branch of ethmoidal branch of nasociliary nerve (Arnold, 1834)*
Synonym for macrodissected adult human ***external nasal branch of anterior ethmoidal nerve (>1840)***; in the original Latin, *nervus nasociliaris, ramus ethmoidalis, ramus externus narium*, p. 8.
7. *external nasal branch of ethmoidal branch of nasal nerve (Arnold, 1834)*
Synonym for macrodissected adult human ***external nasal branch of anterior ethmoidal nerve (>1840)***; in the original Latin, *nervus nasalis, ramus ethmoidalis, ramus externus narium*, p. 8.
8. *naso-lobar nerve (Todd, 1836–1839)*

Todd attributed without citation term to Chaussier, synonym for macrodissected adult human ***external nasal branch of anterior ethmoidal nerve (>1840)***; p. 282. Cruveilhier (1836, p. 916) also attributed term to Chaussier without citation, and referred to it as larger of two terminal branches of *nerve of external wall of nasal fossa (Cruveilhier, 1836)*.

9. *nerve of Cotunnius (Todd, 1836–1839, p. 282)*
   Eponym for macrodissected adult human ***external nasal branch of anterior ethmoidal nerve (>1840)***; p. 282.
10. *external filament of internal nasal branch of nasal nerve (Cruveilhier, 1836)*
   Synonym for macrodissected adult human ***external nasal branch of anterior ethmoidal nerve (>1840)***; in the original French, *filet externe*, p. 916.
11. *external filament of ethmoidal branch of nasal nerve (Cruveilhier, 1836)*
   Synonym for macrodissected adult human ***external nasal branch of anterior ethmoidal nerve (>1840)***; in the original French, *filet externe*, p. 916.
12. *nerve of external wall of nasal fossa (Cruveilhier, 1836)*
   Synonym for macrodissected adult human ***external nasal branch of anterior ethmoidal nerve (>1840)***; in the original French, *nerf de la paroi externe*, p. 916. Also see Cruveilhier (1844, p. 830).
13. *external nasal nerve (>1840)*
   Synonym for macrodissected adult human ***external nasal branch of anterior ethmoidal nerve (>1840)***; see *Terminologia Anatomica* (1998, p. 134).

external nasal branches of infraorbital nerve (>1840)

As described for macrodissected adult human they innervate skin on the side of the nose and communicate with the ***external nasal branch of anterior ethmoidal nerve (>1840)***; see Williams & Warwick (1980, p. 1064), *Terminologia Anatomica* (1998, p. 134). They were perhaps first mentioned by Winslow; see ***[external nasal branches of infraorbital nerve (>1840)] (Winslow, 1733)***.

EARLIER REFERENCES:

Described, not named or illustrated:

1. ***[external nasal branches of infraorbital nerve (>1840)] (Winslow, 1733)***
   Mentioned without naming for macrodissected adult human; Section VI, p. 65.

Earlier synonyms:

1. *superficial nasal branches of infraorbital nerve (Meckel, 1748)*
   Meckel described for macrodissected adult human superior and inferior branches that anastomose, constituting ***external nasal branches of infraorbital nerve (>1840)***; see Figure 1-*d,f,g,h*. Also see Todd (1836–1839, p. 289).
2. *superficial nasal nerves (Schaarschmidt, 1750)*
   Synonym for macrodissected adult human *superficial nasal branches of infraorbital nerve (Meckel, 1748)*; in the original Latin, *nervi nasales superficiales*, p. 25.
3. *cutaneous nerves of nose (Meckel, 1753)*
   Synonym for macrodissected adult human ***external nasal branches of infraorbital nerve (>1840)***. Meckel distinguished superior, middle, and inferior *cutaneous nerves of nose (Meckel, 1753)*; in the original French, *le nerf cutané du nés (supérieur, moyen, inférieur)*, p. 50, Table 1:35-41.
4. *superior superficial nasal branches of infraorbital nerve (Loder, 1778)*
   Synonym for macrodissected adult human ***external nasal branches of infraorbital nerve (>1840)***. Loder noted they also lie external and inferior; in the original Latin, *nasalis superficialis superior*, p. 50, Table 1:35-41.
5. *external inferior superficial nasal nerve (Meckel, 1817)*
   Synonym for macrodissected adult human ***external nasal branches of infraorbital nerve (>1840)***; see translation (1832, Vol. 3, p. 71).
6. *external inferior cutaneous nasal nerve (Meckel, 1817)*
   Synonym for macrodissected adult human ***external nasal branches of infraorbital nerve (>1840)***; see translation (1832, Vol. 3, p. 71).
7. *inferior nasal subcutaneous branch of infraorbital nerve (Bock, 1817)*
   Synonym for macrodissected adult human ***external nasal branches of infraorbital nerve (>1840)***; in the original Latin, *ramus subcutaneus nasi inferior*, p. 36.
8. *internal filaments of superior maxillary nerve (Cruveilhier, 1836)*
   Synonym for macrodissected adult human ***external nasal branches of infraorbital nerve (>1840)***; in the original French, *filets internes*, p. 928.
9. *nasal filaments of superior maxillary nerve (Cruveilhier, 1836)*
   Synonym for macrodissected adult human ***external nasal branches of infraorbital nerve (>1840)***; in the original French, *filets nasaux*, p. 928.

PARTLY CORRESPONDS:

1. *middle nasal cutaneous nerve (Mayer, 1794)*
   Macrodissected adult human ***external nasal branch of infraorbital nerve (>1840)*** to ventral (inferior) third of nose; in the original Latin, *nervus cutaneus nasi medius*; Part 5, Table VII-*26* (p. 44).
2. *inferior nasal cutaneous nerve (Mayer, 1794)*
   Macrodissected adult human ***external nasal branch of infraorbital nerve (>1840)*** to ventral (inferior) tip of nose; in the original Latin, *nervus cutaneus nasi inferior*; Part 5, Table VII-*28* (p. 44).
3. *superior nasal subcutaneous fascicle of infraorbital surculus (Bellingeri, 1818)*
   Macrodissected adult human branch of ***external nasal branch of infraorbital nerve (>1840)*** to muscles and

skin near root of nose; in the original Latin, *fasciculus subcutaneus nasi sup.*, see Table I.

4. *inferior nasal subcutaneous fasciculi of infraorbital surculus (Bellingeri, 1818)*
Macrodissected adult human branches of ***external nasal branch of infraorbital nerve (>1840)*** to lower eyelid, muscles and skin of nose, and upper lip; in the original Latin, *fasciculi subcutaneus nasi inf.*, see Table I.

extrinsic vesical plexus (>1840)

As described for macrodissected adult human, a ventral (anterior) extension of the ***inferior hypogastric plexus (Tiedemann, 1822)*** accompanying the vesical artery to the urinary bladder, along the way looping around the distal ends of the ureters. It is distinguished from the ***intrinsic vesical plexus (>1840)***, the terminal extension within the muscular wall of the bladder itself. In male the basal fiber bundles of the ***extrinsic vesical plexus (1840)*** are closely associated with the ***prostatic plexus (>1840)***, and in female with the ***uterovaginal plexus (>1840)***; see Mitchell (1953, pp. 303, 305 and Fig. 131), Williams & Warwick (1980, pp. 1135–1136). It was known to Vesalius; see ***[extrinsic vesical plexus (>1840)] (Vesalius, 1543a)***.

EARLIER REFERENCES:

Described, not named or illustrated:

1. ***[extrinsic vesical plexus (>1840)] (Vesalius, 1543a)***
Mentioned and vaguely illustrated for macrodissected adult human; see Robertson & Carman translation (2002, pp. 200, 255 and Fig. 2-ε,μ). Willis described for macrodissected adult human and other common large mammals a ***nerve (Herophilus, c335–c280 BC)*** broken into shoots distributing to right and left sides of bladder and its sphincter; see Pordage translation (1681, p. 172 and Tab. 11-*f*).

Earlier synonyms:

1. *urinary vesical branch of primary hypogastric plexus (Walter, 1783)*
Essentially, macrodissected adult human ***extrinsic vesical plexus (>1840)***; in the original Latin, *ramus vesicae urinariae primus plexus hypogastricus*, Table I-*438*.
2. *vesical nerves (Bock, 1827)*
Essentially, macrodissected adult human ***extrinsic vesical plexus (>1840)***; in the original Latin, *nervi vesicales*, Table VI, Figure 1-*28*.
3. *vesical branches of small plexus from first hypogastric plexus (Cloquet, 1828)*
Essentially, macrodissected adult human ***extrinsic vesical plexus (>1840)***; in the original French, *rameaux vésicaux*; Plate CLXXV-*227*.
4. *vesical plexus (Cruveilhier, 1836)*
Synonym for macrodissected adult human ***extrinsic vesical plexus (>1840)***; in the original French (plural), *plexus vésicaux*, p. 1026.

PARTLY CORRESPONDS:

1. *superior vesical nerves (Walter, 1783)*
Rostral (upper) component of ***extrinsic vesical plexus (>1840)*** for macrodissected adult human; in the original Latin, *nervi vesicales superiores*, Table I-*474*.
2. *ascending vesical plexus (Cruveilhier, 1836)*
Rostral (ascending) component of *vesical plexus (Cruveilhier, 1836)*; in the original French, *ascendans vésicaux*, p. 1026.
3. *horizontal vesical plexus (Cruveilhier, 1836)*
Transverse component of *vesical plexus (Cruveilhier, 1836)*; in the original French, *vésicaux horizontaux*, p. 1026.

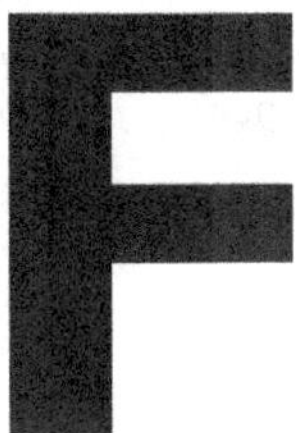

facial colliculus (>1840)

As described for macrodissected adult human, a convexity in the ***floor of fourth ventricle (Reil, 1807–1808a)*** produced by the underlying ***genu of facial nerve (>1840)*** and then ***abducens nucleus (>1840)***; see Williams & Warwick (1980, p. 33, Fig. 7.69) and *Terminologia Anatomica* (1998, p. 115). It was probably identified by Herophilus; see ***[facial colliculus (>1840)] (Herophilus, c335–c280 BC).***

EARLIER REFERENCES:

Described, not named or illustrated:

1. ***[facial colliculus (>1840)] (Herophilus, c335–c280 BC)***
   In *On Anatomical Procedures*, Galen (c177) told how Herophilus first described the caudal end of macrodissected adult human ***floor of fourth ventricle (Reil, 1807–1808a)*** as having the shape of a quill peculiar to Alexandria, where he taught, and where he dissected both animals and human cadavers. The ***facial colliculus (>1840)*** is probably an integral part of the description; see Singer (1999, pp. 237, 277).

Illustrated and described, not named:

1. ***[facial colliculus (>1840)] (Ridley, 1695)***
   Ridley clearly described and illustrated region of **medial eminence** (>1840) and ***facial colliculus (>1840)*** in macrodissected adult human; p. 198, Figure VII-*k*. Rolando (1825a; Tab. IX, Figs. 1, 2:*e.l*) clearly illustrated it in transverse section for macrodissected adult cattle.

facial ganglion (Lazorthes, 1949)

As described for macrodissected adult human, a ***paravertebral ganglion (Durward, 1951)*** often found in the ***external carotid plexus (>1840)*** near the origin of the facial artery; see Mitchell (1953, p. 220). For Lazorthes's use in macrodissected adult human, see p. 119. Not to be confused with ***geniculate ganglion (Bischoff, 1832)*** of the ***intermediofacial nerve trunk (>1840)***. Its relationship to the ***temporal ganglion (Andersch & Soemmerring, 1792)*** is unclear. It was probably first delineated as the *small ganglion (Neubauer, 1772)*.

EARLIER REFERENCES:

Earlier synonyms:

1. *small ganglion (Neubauer, 1772)*
   Described and beautifully illustrated small ***ganglion (Galen, c173)*** in ***external carotid plexus (>1840)*** of macrodissected adult human, in position of ***facial ganglion (Lazorthes, 1949)***; in the original Latin, *ganglio parvo* or *parvum ganglion*; Table 2-*144,148*.

facial nerve central root (>1840)

As described for macrodissected adult human, and mammal generally with histological methods for ***axons (Kölliker, 1896)***, the central root *nerve fibers (Ehrenberg, 1833)* of the ***facial nucleus (>1840)*** form a stout bundle becoming the peripheral ***facial nerve root (>1840)*** at the ventral surface of the ***medulla (Winslow, 1733)***. In its course through the ***medulla (Winslow, 1733)***, the ***facial nerve central root (>1840)*** takes a unique arching course with an initial ascending part extending dorsomedially; an internal, central, or medullary genu of facial nerve curving over the dorsal part (top) of the ***abducens nucleus (>1840)***; and a final descending part extending ventrolaterally to continue as the peripheral ***facial nerve root (>1840)***; see Mettler (1948, p. 301 and Figs. 208, 235), Williams & Warwick (1980, p. 910 and Fig. 7.69). It was known to Mayo, though not in its full course; see ***[facial nerve central root (>1840)] (Mayo, 1827)***.

EARLIER REFERENCES:

Illustrated and described, not named:

1. ***[facial nerve central root (>1840)] (Mayo, 1827)***

Mayo traced 2–3 large fascicles to dorsal part (back) of macrodissected adult human ***medulla (Winslow, 1733)***; Plate VII, Figure 2-*VII*.

Earlier synonyms:

1. *real origin of portio dura (Cruveilhier, 1836)*
   Synonym for macrodissected adult human ***facial nerve central root (>1840)***; in the original French, *origine réelle*, p. 897.

facial nerve root (>1840)

As described for macrodissected adult human, one of two ***intermediofacial nerve roots (>1840)***—the other being the ***intermediate nerve (>1840)***—stretching from the outer surface of the ***medulla (Winslow, 1733)*** to the region in the internal acoustic meatus where it joins the ***intermediate nerve (>1840)*** to form the ***intermediofacial nerve trunk (>1840)***; see Hamilton (1976, pp. 628–629), Williams & Warwick (1980, p. 1071 and Fig. 7.184). It is currently often referred to as the *motor root of facial nerve (>1840)*. It was probably first clearly distinguished by Soemmerring; see ***[facial nerve root (>1840)] (Soemmerring, 1778)***.

EARLIER REFERENCES:

Described, not named or illustrated:

1. ***[facial nerve root (>1840)] (Soemmerring, 1778)***
   Clearly differentiated without naming for macrodissected adult human; see p. 93. Also see ***intermediate nerve (>1840)***.

Earlier synonyms:

1. *roots of portio dura of acoustic nerve (Malacarne, 1791)*
   Synonym for macrodissected adult human ***facial nerve root (>1840)***; p. 227.
2. *internal and anterior root of facial nerve (Meckel, 1817)*
   Synonym for macrodissected adult human ***facial nerve root (>1840)***; see translation (1832, Vol. 3, p. 53).
3. *principal root of facial nerve (Meckel, 1817)*
   Synonym for macrodissected adult human ***facial nerve root (>1840)***; see translation (1832, Vol. 3, p. 53).
4. *apparent origin of portio dura (Cruveilhier, 1836)*
   Synonym for macrodissected adult human ***facial nerve root (>1840)***; in the original French, *origine apparente de la portion dure*, p. 897.
5. *motor part of facial nerve (Kölliker, 1896)*
   Synonym for macrodissected adult human ***facial nerve root (>1840)***; Vol. 2, p. 272.
6. *motor root of facial nerve (>1840)*
   Synonym for mammalian ***facial nerve root (>1840)***; see Cajal (1899–1904, Vol. 2, pt. 1, p. 171).

facial nerve trunk (>1840)

As described for macrodissected adult human, the segment of the ***intermediofacial nerve (Strong & Elwyn, 1943)*** between the distal end of the ***intermediofacial nerve trunk (>1840)***, indicated by a branch point for the ***communicating branch of intermediofacial nerve trunk with vagus nerve (>1840)***, and the proximal end of the ***parotid plexus (Meckel, 1817)***, where terminal branches of the ***facial nerve trunk (>1840)*** begin; see Durward (1951, Figs. 901, 902). It was not identified as such by 1840.

PARTLY CORRESPONDS:

1. *superior branch of portio dura (Du Verney, 1683)*
   As described for macrodissected adult human, ***facial nerve trunk (1840)*** can be described as dividing into superior (dorsal) and inferior (ventral) terminal branches (Hovelacque, 1927, p. 183); this is the former, see translation (1737, Pl. 12, Fig. 3-*F*). Also see *superior facial branch of hard nerve (Haller, 1762)*.
2. *inferior branch of portio dura (Du Verney, 1683)*
   As described for macrodissected adult human, ***facial nerve trunk (1840)*** can be described as dividing into superior (dorsal) and inferior (ventral) terminal branches (Hovelacque, 1927, p. 183); this is the latter, see translation (1737, Pl. 12, Fig. 3-*G*). Also see *inferior facial branch of hard nerve (Haller, 1762)*. Durward (1951, p. 1032 and Fig. 902) referred to it as *lower part of facial nerve (Vicq d'Azyr, 1784)*.
3. *superior branch of hard part of nerve of seventh pair (Bonhomme, 1748)*
   From brief description, corresponds to macrodissected adult human *superior branch of portio dura (Du Verney, 1683)*; p. 78.
4. *inferior branch of hard part of nerve of seventh pair (Bonhomme, 1748)*
   From brief description, corresponds to macrodissected adult human *inferior branch of portio dura (Du Verney, 1683)*; p. 78.
5. *internal deep nerve of hard nerve (Meckel, 1753)*
   Branch of ***facial nerve trunk (1840)*** dividing into ***digastric nerve (Meckel, 1753)*** and ***stylohyoid nerve (Meckel, 1753)*** for macrodissected adult human; in the original French, *rameau profond intérieur du nerf dur*, Table 1-*119*; also see Haase (1781, p. 80), Durward (1951, Fig. 902).
6. *internal muscular branch of hard nerve (Meckel, 1753)*
   Synonym for *internal deep nerve of hard nerve (Meckel, 1753)*; in the original French, *le rameau musculaire interne du nerf dur*, Table 1-*119*.
7. *superior branch of hard nerve (Meckel, 1753)*
   Essentially dorsal (ascending) terminal branch of macrodissected adult human ***facial nerve trunk (1840)*** generating ***temporal branches of facial nerve Swan, 1830)*** and ***zygomatic branches of facial nerve (>1840)*** considered together; in the original French, *rameau supérieur du nerf dur*, pp. 76, 122. Clearly illustrated in Durward (1951, Fig. 902).
8. *inferior branch of hard nerve (Meckel, 1753)*
   Essentially ventral (descending) terminal branch of macrodissected adult human ***facial nerve trunk (1840)*** generating ***buccal branch of facial nerve (>1840)***, ***marginal mandibular branch of facial nerve (>1840)***, and ***cervical branch of facial nerve (>1840)*** considered together; in the original French, *rameau inférieur du dur*, pp. 76, 90, 126. Clearly illustrated in Durward (1951, Fig. 902).

9. *ascending suprazygomatic branch of superior branch of hard nerve (Meckel, 1753)*
Synonym for *ascending branch of superior branch of hard nerve (Meckel, 1753)*; in the original French, *ascendant supra-zygomatique*, p. 77.
10. *temporal branch of superior branch of hard nerve (Meckel, 1753)*
Synonym for *ascending branch of superior branch of hard nerve (Meckel, 1753)*; p. 77.
11. *zygomatic branch of hard nerve (Meckel, 1753)*
Synonym for *ascending branch of superior branch of hard nerve (Meckel, 1753)*; p. 77.
12. *ascending branch of superior branch of hard nerve (Meckel, 1753)*
First branch in macrodissected adult human of *superior branch of hard nerve (Meckel, 1753)*, basically generating ***temporal branches of facial nerve (Swan, 1830)*** and upper set of ***zygomatic branches of facial nerve (>1840)*** considered together; in the original French, *rameau ascendant du supérieur du dur*, Table 1-*136*.
13. *great zygomatic branch of hard nerve (Meckel, 1753)*
Synonym for *ascending branch of superior branch of hard nerve (Meckel, 1753)*; in the original French, *rameau grand zygomatique du supérieur du dur*, Table 1-*136*.
14. *inferior facial branch of hard nerve (Meckel, 1753)*
Synonym for *inferior branch of hard nerve (Meckel, 1753)*; Table 1-*233, 242*.
15. *temporal branches of hard nerve (Meckel, 1753)*
Corresponds to macrodissected adult human ***temporal branches of facial nerve (Swan, 1830)*** and upper set of ***zygomatic branches of facial nerve (>1840)***; Table 1-*141* ff.
16. *superior facial branch of hard nerve (Haller, 1762)*
Synonym for macrodissected adult human *superior branch of portio dura (Du Verney, 1683)*, including ***temporal branches of facial nerve (Swan, 1830)***, ***zygomatic branches of facial nerve (>1840)***, and ***buccal branch of facial nerve (>1840)***; pp. 229–230.
17. *inferior facial branch of hard nerve (Haller, 1762)*
Synonym for macrodissected adult human *inferior branch of portio dura (Du Verney, 1683)*, including ***marginal mandibular branch of facial nerve (>1840)*** and ***cervical branch of facial nerve (>1840)***; pp. 230–231.
18. *temporal branch of superior facial branch of hard part of seventh nerve (Haller, 1762)*
Appears to correspond roughly to macrodissected adult human ***temporal branches of facial nerve (Swan, 1830)*** and ***zygomatic branches of facial nerve (>1840)*** considered together; p. 229.
19. *internal deep branch of hard part of seventh pair (Haase, 1781)*
Synonym for macrodissected adult human *internal deep nerve of hard nerve (Meckel, 1753)*; in the original Latin, *par septimum portionis durae ramus profundus inferior*, p. 80 and Index section 153.
20. *nervus communicans faciei ramos profundos (Günther, 1786)*
Synonym for *deep branch of hard nerve (Günther, 1786)*; p. 57.
21. *deep branch of hard nerve (Günther, 1786)*
Basically, segment of macrodissected adult human ***facial nerve trunk (1840)*** between stylomastoid foramen and ***parotid plexus (Meckel, 1817)***; in the original Latin, *ramos profundos*, p. 57.
22. *internal deep branch of hard nerve (Günther, 1786)*
Synonym for macrodissected adult human *internal deep nerve of hard nerve (Meckel, 1753)*; in the original Latin, *nervus durus ramum profundum internum*, p. 57.
23. *nervus communicans faciei ramos superficiales (Günther, 1786)*
Synonym for *superficial branch of hard nerve (Günther, 1786)*; p. 58.
24. *superficial branch of hard nerve (Günther, 1786)*
Basically entire component of macrodissected adult human ***facial nerve trunk (1840)*** distal to *deep branch of hard nerve (Günther, 1786)*; in the original Latin, *ramus superficiales*, p. 58.
25. *ascending branch of superficial branch of hard nerve (Günther, 1786)*
Synonym for macrodissected adult human *superior branch of hard nerve (Meckel, 1753)*; in the original Latin, *ramus ascendentem*, p. 58. Günther also referred to it as the superior or major branch.
26. *descending branch of superficial branch of hard nerve (Günther, 1786)*
Synonym for macrodissected adult human *inferior branch of hard nerve (Meckel, 1753)*; in the original Latin, *ramus descendentem*, p. 59. Günther also referred to it as the inferior or minor branch.
27. *lower facial branches of descending branch of superficial branch of hard nerve (Günther, 1786)*
Macrodissected adult human ***buccal branch of facial nerve (>1840)*** and ***marginal mandibular branch of facial nerve (>1840)*** considered together; in the original Latin, *facialem infimum*, p. 59.
28. *interior deep branch of hard nerve (Mayer, 1794)*
Synonym for macrodissected adult human *internal deep nerve of hard nerve (Meckel, 1753)*; in the original Latin, *ramus profundus interior nervi duri*; Part 5, Table VII-*84* (p. 47).
29. *deep muscular branch of hard nerve (Mayer, 1794)*
Synonym for macrodissected adult human *internal muscular branch of hard nerve (Meckel, 1753)*; in the original Latin, *ramus muscularis profundus nervi duri*; Part 5, Table VII-*84* (p. 47).
30. *superior superficial branch of hard nerve (Mayer, 1794)*
Synonym for macrodissected adult human *superior branch of hard nerve (Meckel, 1753)*; in the original Latin, *ramus superficialis superior nervi duri*; Part 5, Table VII- *V* (pp. 47–48).
31. *facial plexus (Mayer, 1794)*
Plexus (Galen, c192) of ***communicating branches (Winslow, 1733)*** associated mainly with ***zygomatic branches of facial nerve (>1840)*** and ***buccal branch of facial nerve (>1840)***; in the original Latin, *plexus facialis*; Part 5, Table VII-*141* (p. 50).
32. *ascending branch of hard nerve (Mayer, 1794)*

Synonym for macrodissected adult human *superior branch of hard nerve (Meckel, 1753)*; in the original Latin, *ramus ascendens nervi duri*; Part 5, Table VIII-*85* (p. 61).

33. *descending branch of hard nerve (Mayer, 1794)*
Synonym for macrodissected adult human *inferior branch of hard nerve (Meckel, 1753)*; in the original Latin, *ramus descendens nervi duri*; Part 5, Table VIII-*88* (p. 61).
34. *temporofacial branch of facial nerve (Meckel, 1817)*
Synonym for macrodissected adult human *superior branch of portio dura (Du Verney, 1683)* including ***temporal branches of facial nerve (Swan, 1830)*** and ***zygomatic branches of facial nerve (>1840)***; see Meckel (1832, Vol. 3, p. 55), who ascribed it without citation to Chaussier.
35. *ascending branches of facial nerve (Meckel, 1817)*
Synonym for *temporofacial branch of facial nerve (Chaussier, 1807)*; see translation (1832, Vol. 3, p. 55).
36. *descending branches of facial nerve (Meckel, 1817)*
Synonym for *cervicofacial branch of facial nerve (Chaussier, 1807)*; see translation (1832, Vol. 3, p. 56).
37. *cervicofacial branch of facial nerve (Meckel, 1817)*
Synonym for macrodissected adult human *inferior branch of portio dura (Du Verney, 1683)*, including ***buccal branch of facial nerve (>1840)***, ***marginal mandibular branch of facial nerve (>1840)***, and ***cervical branch of facial nerve (>1840)***; see Meckel (1832, Vol. 3, p. 56), who ascribed it without citation to Chaussier.
38. *superior branch of portio major and minor of facial nerve (Bellingeri, 1818)*
Synonym for macrodissected adult human *temporofacial branch of facial nerve (Meckel, 1817)*; in the original Latin, *ramus superior*, see Table II.
39. *inferior branch of portio major and minor of facial nerve (Bellingeri, 1818)*
Synonym for macrodissected adult human *cervicofacial branch of facial nerve (Meckel, 1817)*; in the original Latin, *ramus inferior*, see Table II.
40. *superior division of facial nerve (Swan, 1830)*
Synonym for macrodissected adult human *superior branch of portio dura (Du Verney, 1683)*; Plate XIII-*2*.
41. *inferior division of facial nerve (Swan, 1830)*
Synonym for macrodissected adult human *inferior branch of portio dura (Du Verney, 1683)*; Plate XIII-*9*.
42. *superior branch of facial nerve (Knox, 1832)*
Synonym for macrodissected adult human *superior branch of portio dura (Du Verney, 1683)*; Supplemental Plate II-*1*.
43. *stylohyoid and digastric nerve (Arnold, 1834)*
Synonym for macrodissected adult human *internal deep nerve of hard nerve (Meckel, 1753)*; in the original Latin, *nervus stylohyoideus et biventericus*, p. 12.
44. *inferior branch of facial nerve (Arnold, 1834)*
Synonym for macrodissected adult human *inferior branch of portio dura (Du Verney, 1683)*; in the original Latin, *ramus inferior nervi facialis*, p. 12.
45. *terminal branches of facial nerve (Cruveilhier, 1836)*
Two major branches of macrodissected adult human ***facial nerve trunk (1840)*** beginning in and extending distal to ***parotid plexus (Meckel, 1817)***, *temporofacial branch of facial nerve (Chaussier, 1807)*, and *cervicofacial branch of facial nerve (Chaussier, 1807)* considered together; in the original French, *rameaux terminales du nerf facial*, p. 943.

facial nucleus (>1840)

As described for adult mammal based on cellular architecture and connections, the ***gray matter region (Swanson & Bota, 2010)*** in rostral and ventral parts of the ***medulla (Winslow, 1733)***, lying ventromedial to the ***spinal nucleus of trigeminal nerve (>1840)*** and generating the dorsally and then ventrally arching ***facial nerve central root (>1840)***, continuing as the peripheral ***facial nerve root (>1840)***; see Nieuwenhuys et al. (2008, pp. 203, 865–867 and Figs. 6.25-*10*, 6.26-*11*). It was not identified by 1840.

fasciola cinerea (Arnold, 1838b)

As described for macrodissected adult human, and with cellular architecture in all mammals, a very thin extension of the ***hippocampal region (>1840)*** around the ***splenium of corpus callosum (Burdach, 1822)*** to the dorsomedial surface of the ***body of corpus callosum (Arnold, 1838a)***, where it extends rostrally as the ***indusium griseum (Valentin, 1841)***; see Williams & Warwick (1980, p. 998), who use *gyrus fasciolaris (>1840)*. For Arnold's use in macrodissected adult human, see Table VII, Figure 3-*i,k* and Table X, Figure 1-*o*. It was probably first identified by Reil; see ***[fasciola cinerea (Arnold, 1838b)] (Reil, 1809b)***.

EARLIER REFERENCES:

Described, not named or illustrated:

1. *[fasciola cinerea (Arnold, 1838b)] (Reil, 1809b)*
Reil described this small band of *gray matter (Meckel, 1817)*, *graue Substanz* in German, in macrodissected adult human; see Mayo translation (1823, p. 67), also see Meyer (1971, p. 94).

Earlier synonyms:

1. *fasciola dentata (Arnold, 1838a)*
Synonym for macrodissected adult human ***fasciola cinerea (Arnold, 1838b)***; p. 76.

LATER SYNONYMS:

1. *fascia dentata (Arnold, 1838b)*
Synonym for ***fasciola cinerea (Arnold, 1838b)***; Table VII, Figure 3-*i,k*.
2. *fasciola cinerea cinguli (>1840)*
Synonym for macrodissected adult human ***fasciola cinerea (Arnold, 1838b)***; see Foster (1892, p. 1548).
3. *fasciolar gyrus (>1840)*
Synonym for macrodissected adult human ***fasciola cinerea (Arnold, 1838b)***; in Latin, *gyrus fasciolaris*, see *Terminologia Anatomica* (1998, p. 126), *Dorland's* (2003, p. 806).
4. *splenial gyrus (>1840)*
Synonym for macrodissected adult human ***fasciola cinerea (Arnold, 1838b)***; see Williams & Warwick (1980, p. 998).
5. *area ectosplenialis (Brodmann, 1909)*
Original Latin form of *ectosplenial area (Brodmann, 1909)*; see p. 148.

6. *ectosplenial area (Brodmann, 1909)*
   As described with cellular architecture in adult human and lemur, the small, ventral, inner part of *retrosplenial region (Brodmann, 1909)*, deep to ***granular retrosplenial area (>1840)***, apparently corresponding to ***fasciola cinerea (Arnold, 1838b)***; in the original Latin, *area ectosplenialis*, see p. 148.
7. *area 26 (Brodmann, 1909)*
   Synonym for *ectosplenial area (Brodmann, 1909)*; in the original German, *Feld 26*, see p. 149, Figure 86.

fastigial nucleus (>1840)

As described with cellular architecture and connections in mammal, the medial component of the ***cerebellar nuclei (>1840)***, lying medial to the ***interposed nucleus (>1840)*** or when present its more medial differentiation the ***emboliform nucleus (>1840)***; see Nieuwenhuys et al. (2008, pp. 200, 820 and Fig. 5.12-*21*.). Not clearly described by 1840.

fastigium of fourth ventricle (Burdach, 1822)

As described for macrodissected adult human, the dorsal peak of the ***roof of fourth ventricle (Vesalius, 1543a)*** at the junction between ***rostral medullary vellum (>1840)*** and ***nodule (Reil, 1807–1808a)***; see *Terminologia Anatomica* (1998, p. 115), *Dorland's* (2003, p. 679). For Burdach's use and first clear description in macrodissected adult human, see p. 79.

TRANSLATIONS:

1. *fastigium ventriculi quarti (Burdach, 1822)*
   Original Latin form of ***fastigium of fourth ventricle (Burdach, 1822)***; p. 79.

femoral branch of genitofemoral nerve (>1840)

As described for macrodissected adult human, it supplies skin over the rostral (upper) part of the femoral triangle and communicates with the ***anterior cutaneous branches of femoral nerve (Quain & Wilson, 1839)***; see Williams & Warwick (1980, p. 1107 and Fig. 7.206), *Terminologia Anatomica* (1998, p. 140). It was perhaps first delineated by Eustachi; see ***[femoral branch of genitofemoral nerve (>1840)] (Eustachi, 1552)***.

EARLIER REFERENCES:

Illustrated, not named or described:

1. ***[femoral branch of genitofemoral nerve (>1840)] (Eustachi, 1552)***
   Clearly illustrated for macrodissected adult human; see Albinus edition (1761, Tab. 21-*H*).

Described, not named or illustrated:

1. ***[femoral branch of genitofemoral nerve (>1840)] (Winslow, 1733)***
   Mentioned for macrodissected adult human; Section VI, no. 276, p. 86.

Earlier synonyms:

1. *inguinal branch of singular nerve from second and third lumbar nerves (Monro & Coopmans, 1754)*
   Synonym for macrodissected adult human ***femoral branch of genitofemoral nerve (>1840)***; in the original Latin (plural), *ramos inguinis nervus singularis ex lumbalibus secundo & tertio*, p. 64 note *a*. The note was by Coopmans, expanding on his Latin translation of Monro's *The Anatomy of the Human Nerves.*
2. *external branch of external spermatic nerve (Walter, 1783)*
   Synonym for macrodissected adult human ***femoral branch of genitofemoral nerve (>1840)***; in the original Latin, *ramus externus nervi externi spermatici*, Table 1-*91*.
3. *external inguinal branch of eternal spermatic branch of first lumbar nerve (Günther, 1786)*
   Synonym for macrodissected adult human ***femoral branch of genitofemoral nerve (>1840)***; in the original Latin, *ramus inguinalem externum*, p. 81.
4. *external inguinal nerve (Fischer, 1791)*
   Synonym for macrodissected adult human ***femoral branch of genitofemoral nerve (>1840)***; p. 2.
5. *femoral anterior cutaneous nerve (Fischer, 1791)*
   Synonym for macrodissected adult human ***femoral branch of genitofemoral nerve (>1840)***; p. 2.
6. *spermatic nerve (Mayer, 1794)*
   Apparently synonym for macrodissected adult human *external inguinal nerve (Fischer, 1791)*; in the original Latin, *nervus spermaticus*; Part 5, Table V, Figure 1-*32*.
7. *lumboinguinal nerve (Schmidt, 1794)*
   Synonym for macrodissected adult human ***femoral branch of genitofemoral nerve (>1840)***; in the original Latin, *nervus lumbo-inguinalis*, p. 43, where there is a detailed history of its identification.
8. *external branch of genitocrural nerve (Meckel, 1817)*
   Synonym for macrodissected adult human ***femoral branch of genitofemoral nerve (>1840)***; see translation (1832, Vol. 3, pp. 13–14).
9. *external branch of external pudic nerve (Quain, 1828)*
   Synonym for macrodissected adult human ***femoral branch of genitofemoral nerve (>1840)***; p. 286.
10. *external branch of internal inguinal branch of lumbar plexus (Cruveilhier, 1836)*
    Synonym for macrodissected adult human ***femoral branch of genitofemoral nerve (>1840)***; in the original French, *rameau externe*, p. 837.
11. *cutaneous femoral branch of internal inguinal branch of lumbar plexus (Cruveilhier, 1836)*
    Synonym for macrodissected adult human ***femoral branch of genitofemoral nerve (>1840)***; in the original French, *rameau fémoral cutané*, p. 837.
12. *crural branch of external pudic nerve (Quain & Wilson, 1839)*
    Synonym for macrodissected adult human ***genital branch of genitofemoral nerve (>1840)***; also gave the Latin, *n. pudendus externus*, Plate XXI-*m,o*.
13. *crural branch of external spermatic nerve (Quain & Wilson, 1839)*
    Synonym for macrodissected adult human ***genital branch of genitofemoral nerve (>1840)***; also gave the Latin, *n. spermaticus externus*, Plate XXI-*m,o*.
14. *crural branch of genito-crural nerve (Quain & Wilson, 1839)*

Synonym for macrodissected adult human ***genital branch of genitofemoral nerve (>1840)***; also gave the Latin, *n. genito-cruralis*, Plate XXI-*m,o*.

PARTLY CORRESPONDS:

1. *nerve of crural artery proper (Schmidt, 1794)*
Branch of macrodissected adult human ***femoral branch of genitofemoral nerve (>1840)*** supplying twigs to femoral artery; in the original Latin, *nervus arteriae crurali proprius*, pp. 73–75, Table II-*K*, with branches to it.
2. *cutaneous branch of external spermatic nerve (Bock, 1827)*
Superficial branch of macrodissected adult human ***femoral branch of genitofemoral nerve (>1840)*** distinct from *lumboinguinal nerve (Schmidt, 1794)*; in the original Latin, *ram. cutaneus nervi spermatici externi*, Table II-*105*.
3. *external branch of lumboinguinal nerve (Bock, 1827)*
Superficial, dorsally (posteriorly) directed branch of macrodissected adult human ***femoral branch of genitofemoral nerve (>1840)*** distinct from *lumboinguinal nerve (Schmidt, 1794)*; in the original Latin, *ram. externus nervi lumbo-inguinalis*, Table III-*46*.
4. *internal branch of lumbo-inguinal nerve (Cloquet, 1828)*
Macrodissected adult human medial branch of ***femoral branch of genitofemoral nerve (>1840)***; in the original French, *rameau interne du nerf lombo-inguinal*, Plate CLXXII, Figure 1-*63*.

femoral nerve (Haller, 1762)

As described for macrodissected adult human, the largest branch of the ***lumbar plexus (Vesalius, 1543a)***. It arises from the ***lumbar plexus dorsal divisions (Paterson, 1887)*** of the 2nd–4th ***lumbar nerves (Diemerbroeck, 1672)*** and eventually generates ***muscular branches of femoral nerve (Quain & Wilson, 1839)***, ***anterior cutaneous branches of femoral nerve (Quain & Wilson, 1839)***, the ***medial cutaneous nerve of thigh (>1840)***, and the ***saphenous nerve (Haase, 1781)***; see Durward (1951, pp. 1094–1098), Williams & Warwick (1980, pp. 1108–1110). For Haller's use in macrodissected adult human, see p. 400; also see Haase (1781, p. 106). It was originally known as the *first deep nerve of thigh (Galen, c177)*.

EARLIER REFERENCES:

Earlier synonyms:

1. *first deep nerve of thigh (Galen, c177)*
Galen's term for ***femoral nerve (Haller, 1762)*** in macrodissected adult beef, pig, and/or macaque but not human; see Singer translation (1999, pp. 83–84); also see May translation (1968, p. 707), Duckworth translation (1962, pp. 262, 263). Eustachi provided the first relatively accurate illustration of its origin and course in macrodissected adult human; see Albinus edition (1761, Tab. 19/2-*ω,Γ,6*).
2. *anterior crural nerve (Vieussens, 1684)*
Synonym for macrodissected adult human ***femoral nerve (Haller, 1762)***; Table XXVIII-C. Vieussens noted it has 4 branches and illustrated accurately, for the first time in print, its origin from ***lumbar plexus (Vesalius, 1543a)***; in the original Latin, *nervus cruralis anticus*,Table XXVIII-*D*.
3. *anterior femoral nerve (Keill, 1698)*
Synonym for macrodissected adult human ***femoral nerve (Haller, 1762)***; in the original Latin, *nervus anterior femuris*, p. 300.
4. *crural nerve (Heister, 1717)*
Synonym for macrodissected adult human ***femoral nerve (Haller, 1762)***; in the original Latin, *nervus cruralis*, see translation (1721, p. 249).
5. *middle crural nerve (Lieutaud, 1742)*
Synonym for macrodissected adult human ***femoral nerve (Haller, 1762)***; in the original German, *mittlere Schenkelnerve*, Vol. 2, p. 178; see Fischer (1791, p. 6).
6. *great femoral nerve (Haller, 1762)*
Synonym for ***femoral nerve (Haller, 1762)***; in the original Latin, *nervus femoralis magnus* (p. 400) or *nervum femoralem magnum* (p. 249).

LATER SYNONYMS:

1. *lumbar trunk (Bell, 1803b)*
Synonym listed for macrodissected adult human ***femoral nerve (Haller, 1762)***; in the original Latin, *truncus lumborum*, p. 198.
2. *femoro-praetibial nerve (Burdin, 1803)*
Synonym for macrodissected adult human ***femoral nerve (Haller, 1762)***; in the original French, *nerf fémoro-prétibial*; see translation (1803, Vol. 1, p. 205).
3. *deep-seated branches of crural nerve (Quain, 1828)*
Apparently roughly synonymous with macrodissected adult human ***femoral nerve (Haller, 1762)***; p. 287.

PARTLY CORRESPONDS:

1. *second cutaneous nerve of thigh (Galen, c177)*
Probably synonymous with *small saphena nerve (Meckel, 1817)* for macrodissected adult beef, pig, and/or macaque but not human; see Singer translation (1999, p. 83), where attribution of modern equivalence is probably not accurate.
2. *second nerve entering leg (Vesalius, 1543a)*
Synonym for medial ***muscular branches of femoral nerve (Quain & Wilson, 1839)*** and ***saphenous nerve (Haase, 1781)*** considered together in macrodissected adult human; see Richardson & Carman translation (2002, p. 257). Vesalius's description of the ***femoral nerve (Haller, 1762)*** was confused.
3. *second nerve traveling to thigh (Vesalius, 1543a)*
Synonym for *second nerve entering leg (Vesalius, 1543a)*; see Richardson & Carman translation (2002, p. 265).
4. *second sinew of leg (Geminus, 1553)*
Synonym for macrodissected adult human *second nerve entering leg (Vesalius, 1543a)*; originally spelled *seconde synowe creapynge into legge*, see *The table of the figures of synowes*.
5. *second sinew going to thigh (Geminus, 1553)*
Synonym for *second sinew of leg (Geminus, 1553)*; originally spelled *seconde synowe goyng to thighe*, see *The table of the figures of sinowes*, Figure 7.
6. *great crural nerve trunk (Pietro da Cortona, 1741)*

Synonym for macrodissected adult human *crural nerve trunk (Styx, 1782)*; in the original Latin, *magnorum cruralium nervorum truncum*; Table III, Figure I-*o* and p. 7.

7. *crural nerve trunk (Styx, 1782)*
Unbranched proximal segment of macrodissected adult human ***femoral nerve (Haller, 1762)***, just distal to *crural nerve roots (Walter, 1783)*; p. 30.

8. *crural nerve roots (Walter, 1783)*
Walter described three roots of ***femoral nerve (Haller, 1762)*** arising from 2nd–4th ***lumbar plexus dorsal divisions (Paterson, 1887)*** associated with 2nd–4th ***lumbar nerves (Diemerbroeck, 1672)*** for macrodissected adult human; in the original Latin, *prima, secunda, tertia radix nervi cruralis*; Table III:*185–187*.

9. *second root of crural nerve (Günther, 1786)*
Part of macrodissected adult human *crural nerve roots (Walter, 1783)* formed by third and fourth ***lumbar nerves (Diemerbroeck, 1672)***; in the original Latin, *radicem alteram n. cruralis*, p. 81.

10. *cutaneous branches of crural nerve (Günther, 1786)*
Macrodissected adult human ***medial cutaneous nerve of thigh (>1840)*** and ***saphenous nerve (Haase, 1781)*** considered together; in the original Latin, *rami cutanei*, p. 83.

11. *inferior external femoral cutaneous nerve (Mayer, 1794)*
Mayer illustrated and described for macrodissected adult human a branch of ***femoral nerve (Haller, 1762)*** descending essentially unbranched to supply superficial lateral regions of calf and distinct from ***lateral cutaneous nerve of thigh (>1840)***; in the original Latin, *nervus cutaneus externus inferior femoris*; Part 5, Table V, Figure 1-9 (p. 25).

12. *inferior external cutaneous nerve of leg (Mayer, 1794)*
Synonym for *inferior external femoral cutaneous nerve (Mayer, 1794)*; in the original Latin, *nervus cutaneus externus inferior cruris*; Part 5, Table V, Figure 1-*10* (p. 27).

13. *small saphena nerve (Meckel, 1817)*
Meckel apparently regarded ***anterior cutaneous branches of femoral nerve (>1840)*** and ***medial cutaneous nerve of thigh (>1840)*** thus, as a single ***nerve (Herophilus, c335– c280 BC)***; in the original Latin, *nervus saphenus minor*, see translation (1832, Vol. 3, p. 16). Another translation is *lesser saphenous nerve*.

14. *superior saphena nerve (Meckel, 1817)*
Synonym for *small saphena nerve (Meckel, 1817)*; in the original Latin, *nervus saphenus superior*, see translation (1832, Vol. 3, p. 16).

15. *musculocutaneous trunk of crural nerve (Cloquet, 1828)*
Short trunk of *musculocutaneous nerve of crural nerve (Cloquet, 1828)*; in the original French, *tronc musculo-cutané du nerf crural*, Plate CLXXI, Figure 1-*38*.

16. *musculocutaneous nerve of crural nerve (Cloquet, 1828)*
Macrodissected adult human short branch of ***femoral nerve (Haller, 1762)*** supplying a number of ***muscular branches of femoral nerve (Quain & Wilson, 1839)***, including *nerve to pectineus muscle (>1840)* and ***medial cutaneous nerve of thigh (>1840)***; in the original French, *nerf musculo-cutané fourni par le nerf crural*, Plate CLXXIV, Figure 1-*36*.

17. *deep-seated branches of anterior crural nerve (Quain, 1832)*
Basically, macrodissected adult human ***muscular branches of femoral nerve (Quain & Wilson, 1839)*** and ***saphenous nerve (Haase, 1781)*** considered together; p. 697.

18. *superficial branches of anterior crural nerve (Quain, 1832)*
Synonym for macrodissected adult human *anterior cutaneous branches of anterior crural nerve (Quain, 1837)*; p. 697.

19. *terminal branches of crural nerve (Cruveilhier, 1836)*
For macrodissected adult human, Cruveilhier described: *crural musculocutaneous nerve (Cruveilhier, 1836)*, *small branch of sheath of femoral vessels of crural nerve (Cruveilhier, 1836)*, *nerve to rectus femoris muscle (Frotscher, 1788)*, *nerve of vastus externus (Cruveilhier, 1836)*, *nerves of vastus internus (Cruveilhier, 1836)*, and *internal saphenous nerve (Cloquet, 1816)*; in the original French, *rameaux terminaux du nerf crural*, pp. 841–842.

20. *crural musculocutaneous nerve (Cruveilhier, 1836)*
Macrodissected adult human *muscular branches of crural musculocutaneous nerve (Cruveilhier, 1836)*—to sartorius muscle—and *cutaneous branches of crural musculocutaneous nerve (Cruveilhier, 1836)*, considered together; in the original French, *nerf musculo-cutané crural*, p. 842.

21. *small branch of sheath of femoral vessels of crural nerve (Cruveilhier, 1836)*
The second of Cruveilhier's macrodissected adult human *terminal branches of crural nerve (Cruveilhier, 1836)*; in the original French, *petite branche de la gaine des vaisseaux fémoraux*, p. 841.

22. *anterior cutaneous branches of anterior crural nerve (Quain, 1837)*
Macrodissected adult human ***anterior cutaneous branches of femoral nerve (Quain & Wilson, 1839)*** and ***medial cutaneous nerve of thigh (>1840)*** considered together; p. 788.

23. *anterior cutaneous branches of femoral nerve (Quain, 1837)*
Synonym for macrodissected adult human *anterior cutaneous branches of anterior crural nerve (Quain, 1837)*; p. 788 (and p. 787).

field CA1 (Lorente de Nó, 1934)

As described with cellular architecture and connections in mammal, the topologically and developmentally lateral subdivision of ***Ammon's horn (Vicq d'Azyr, 1784)*** lying between ***field CA2 (Lorente de Nó, 1934)*** medially and ***subiculum (>1840)*** laterally; see Swanson et al. (1987), Nieuwenhuys et al. (2008, Fig. 12.5). It was not identified by 1840.

field CA2 (Lorente de Nó, 1934)

As described with cellular architecture and connections in mammal, the topologically and developmentally middle and narrowest subdivision of ***Ammon's horn (Vicq d'Azyr, 1784)*** lying between ***field CA3 (Lorente de Nó,***

1934) medially and ***field CA1 (Lorente de Nó, 1934)*** laterally; see Swanson et al. (1987), Nieuwenhuys et al. (2008, Fig. 12.5). It was not identified by 1840.

field CA3 (Lorente de Nó, 1934)

As described with cellular architecture and connections in mammal, the topologically and developmentally medial subdivision of ***Ammon's horn (Vicq d'Azyr, 1784)*** lying between the ***dentate gyrus (>1840)*** medially and ***field CA2 (Lorente de Nó, 1934)*** laterally; see Swanson et al. (1987), Nieuwenhuys et al. (2008, Fig. 12.5). It was not identified by 1840.

fimbria (Honegger, 1890)

As described for macrodissected adult mammal, the caudal division of the ***fornix (Vesalius, 1543a)*** with the rostral division divided into ***precommissural fornix (Loo, 1931)*** and ***postcommissural fornix (Loo, 1931)***. For topographic description, the ***fimbria (Honegger, 1890)*** of the ***fornix (Vesalius, 1543a)*** has two segments. The ventral (temporal, anterior) segment is distinguished by a clear differentiation along its entire length, the ***alveus (Burdach, 1822)*** and accompanying underlying ***hippocampal region (Swanson et al., 1987)***, and another differentiation along part of its length, the ***dorsal hippocampal commissure (Craigie, 1925)***. The dorsal (septal, posterior) segment begins ventrally at the dorsal (septal, posterior) end of the macroscopically visible ***hippocampal region (Swanson et al., 1987)*** and so is not directly associated with the ***alveus (Burdach, 1822)***; it lies ventral to the ***corpus callosum (Galen, c177)*** in all eutherian mammals and its major differentiation is the ***ventral hippocampal commissure (Craigie, 1925)***. There are two other differentiations of the ***fimbria (Honegger, 1890)*** as a whole; one is the ***dorsal fornix (Sprague & Meyer, 1950)*** extending near the median plane just ventral to the ***corpus callosum (Galen, c177)***, and the other consists of the ***longitudinal striae (>1840)*** extending around the ***splenium of corpus callosum (Burdach, 1822)*** and then coursing rostrally near the median plane, just dorsal to the ***corpus callosum (Galen, c177)*** and associated with the ***fasciola cinerea (Arnold, 1838b)*** and ***indusium griseum (Valentin, 1841)*** respectively. For Honegger's use in adult human and other mammals, based on macroscopic dissection and classical normal histological stains, see pp. 316–321. It was quickly adopted by Dejerine and Dejerine-Klumpke (1895, pp. 348–349; 1901, p. 294) for human; and by Johnston (1913, p. 399), Craigie (1925, Pl. XXI), and Gurdjian (1927, Fig. 27-*fi*) for rat. At least part of it was known to Vesalius; see ***[fimbria (Honegger, 1890)] (Vesalius, 1543a)***.

EARLIER REFERENCES:

Illustrated and described, not named:

1. ***[fimbria (Honegger, 1890)] (Vesalius, 1543a)***
   Vesalius apparently described and illustrated at least its dorsal end for macrodissected adult human, ascending along ***inferior horn of lateral ventricle (Bell, 1802)*** to join *body of fornix (Vesalius, 1543a)*; see Singer translation (1952, pp. 41–42, Fig. 6-*B,C*), and ***[hippocampal region (>1840)] Vesalius (1543a)***.

Earlier synonyms:

1. *posterior angles of cerebral trigone (Cloquet, 1816)*
   Basically, synonym for macrodissected adult human right and left ***fimbria (Honegger, 1890)***; in the original French, *angles postérieurs du trigóne cérébral*, p. 554.

PARTLY CORRESPONDS:

1. *oven of brain (Massa, 1536)*
   The text is brief and unclear, but Massa apparently divided macrodissected adult human *psalidoeides (Galen, 177)* or *fornix (Galen, c177)* into two parts: *oven of brain (Massa, 1536)*, also called *psalidoeides (Massa, 1536)*, and *extremities of septum (Massa, 1536)*; see Lind translation (1975, p. 237). *Oven of brain (Massa, 1536)* may correspond roughly to *body of fornix (Vesalius, 1543a)*, whereas *extremities of septum (Massa, 1536)* may correspond to segment of ***fimbria (Honegger, 1890)*** rostral to *body of fornix (Vesalius, 1543a)* along with ***septal postcommissural fornix (Loo, 1931)***. However, his description (or its translation) is confusing with respect to *corpus callosum (Galen, c177)*; see Lind translation (1975, p. 237); also see *psalidoeides (Galen, c177)*.
2. *psalidoeides (Massa, 1536)*
   Synonym for *oven of brain (Massa, 1536)*; see Lind translation (1975, p. 237).
3. *body of fornix (Vesalius, 1543a)*
   Vesalius originated the term for macrodissected adult human, "from the hind part of the lateral ventricles, where they turn down and forward [***inferior horn of lateral ventricle (Bell, 1802)***], there extends [this] body [of the ***fornix (Vesalius, 1543a)***] of like substance to the ventricles, except that it is somewhat whiter and harder. That part of this body which springs from the right ventricle is continuous with that from the left and the two form one broad mass [*body of fornix (Vesalius, 1543a)*]" (Singer translation, 1952, p. 41; also see pp. 96–97, Figs. 4–6). Basically, *body of fornix (Vesalius, 1543a)* is a triangular region of macrodissected adult human ***fimbria (Honegger, 1890)*** opposed to ventral surface of ***splenium of corpus callosum (Burdach, 1822)*** and containing ***dorsal hippocampal commissure (Craigie, 1925)***; that is, coextensive with macroscopically visible *lyre (Winslow, 1733)*.
4. *buttocks of brain (Vesalius, 1543a)*
   Vesalius wrote that many anatomists mistakenly identified what were later called *posterior pillars of fornix (Paré, 1564)* as *buttocks of brain*; see Richardson & Carman translation (2009, p. 202 and Fig. 5-*S,T* on p. 133).
5. *vaulted body (Paré, 1550)*
   Probably synonym for macrodissected adult human *body of fornix (Vesalius, 1543a)*; f. 56v.
6. *fornix (Colombo, 1559)*
   As implied from the text, synonym for macrodissected adult human *body of fornix (Vesalius, 1543a)*; p. 192.
7. *posterior crus of fornix (Colombo, 1559)*

Reference to it in macrodissected adult human was very brief, and presumably corresponds to *posterior pillar of fornix (Paré, 1564)*; p. 192. Paré had earlier referred briefly to *vaulted body with three legs (Paré, 1550)* without referring to or describing each leg/pillar separately, or actually naming them anterior and posterior.

8. *posterior pillar of fornix (Paré, 1564)*
Paré referred to right and left *posterior pillar of fornix* extending caudally and ventrally in macrodissected adult human from *vaulted body with three legs (Paré, 1550)* or *vaulted body with three pillars (Paré, 1561)*; see translation (1634, p. 168). His description was based on Vesalius but much briefer, and he used Vesalius's figures. Based on this, *posterior pillar of fornix (Paré, 1564)* probably corresponds to short segment of ***fimbria (Honegger, 1890)*** starting just caudal to *body of fornix (Vesalius, 1543a)* and perhaps extending caudally and ventrally over dorsal end of ***hippocampal region (Swanson et al., 1987)***, with its associated ***alveus (Burdach, 1822)***—an interpretation supported by Longet (1842, p. 541). It was illustrated very clearly in Eustachi's (1552) plates, not published until 1714 (and without text); see Albinus edition (1744, Plate XVII, Fig. V-*F*), labeled *crura fornicis*, following *crus of fornix (Riolan, 1618)*.
9. *psalloidique corpori (Aranzi, 1587)*
Derived from *psalloides (Galen, 177)* and apparently synonym for macrodissected adult human *body of fornix (Vesalius, 1543a)*; p. 45, see Lewis (1923, p. 217).
10. *psalloid body (Aranzi, 1587)*
English form of *psalloidique corpori (Aranzi, 1587)*; see Lewis (1923, p. 217).
11. *crus of fornix (Riolan, 1618)*
Probably synonym for macrodissected adult human *posterior crus of fornix (Vesling, 1647)*; p. 418, also see *leg of vault (Vesling, 1647)*.
12. *posterior column of fornix (Riolan, 1618)*
Probably synonym for macrodissected adult human *posterior pillar of fornix (Paré, 1564)*; in the original Latin (plural), *posteriores fornicis columnas*, p. 419.
13. *leg of vault (Vesling, 1647)*
English form of *crus of fornix (Riolan, 1618)*; see Culpeper translation (1653, 1st Tab., Ch. 14, Fig. 3-*b*).
14. *posterior crus of fornix (Vesling, 1647)*
Clearly illustrated and labeled synonym for macrodissected adult human *corpus fimbriatum (Winslow, 1733)*, distinguished from *hippocampus (Aranzi, 1587)* and apparently even ***alveus (Burdach, 1822)***; see Culpeper translation (1653, 2nd Tab., Ch. 14, Fig. 1-*G*). Vesling indicated *posterior crus of fornix (Vesling, 1647)* extends roughly length of ***inferior horn of lateral ventricle (Bell, 1802)***, unlike earlier workers except possibly Aranzi. Diemerbroeck (1689 translation, p. 399) wrote that these *hinder thighs of fornix* were called *pedes hippocampi* by Hippocrates and that Riolan, following Aranzi, considered them upward branches of *optic nerves (Galen, c173)*. Hippocrates certainly did not use this term, and Aranzi did not make this suggestion; see *hippocampus (Aranzi, 1587)* and *lateral column of fornix (Riolan, 1649)*.
15. *hinder leg of vault (Vesling, 1647)*
English form of *posterior crus of fornix (Vesling, 1647)*; see Culpeper translation (1653, 2nd Tab., Ch. 14, Fig. 1-*G*).
16. *lateral column of fornix (Riolan, 1649)*
Apparently synonym for macrodissected adult human *posterior crus of fornix (Vesling, 1647)*. According to Riolan, it is a product of the optic nerve [the ***optic tract (Vicq d'Azyr, 1784)***], and the columns on each side join in the ventricles [***body of lateral ventricle (Bell, 1803b)***] just as they do at their other ends in the ***optic chiasm (Galen, c173)***; see translation (1657, p. 123, and Tab. 17, Fig. 1-*G*; the figure was taken directly without attribution from Vesling, 1647). In the original Latin, the term is derived from the following paragraph with the marginal notation *Fornix*, "Supra anteriores ventriculos extensum est corpus trifidum, quod est corpus Psalloides, tribus columnis sussultum: quarum duae sunt laterales: revolutae circa illas eminentias, quas vocat Galenus, thalamos nervorum Opticorum." (1649, p. 247).
17. *thigh of fornix (Bartholin, 1662)*
Culpeper's translation for macrodissected adult human of *crus of fornix (Riolan, 1618)*; compare Bartholin (1662, Book III, Table IV, Fig. 3-*I*) with Bartholin (1651, same Table—the figure is directly from Vesling, 1647).
18. *hinder thigh of fornix (Bartholin, 1662)*
Variation on translation of *thigh of fornix (Bartholin, 1662)*, and thus *posterior crus of fornix (Vesling, 1647)*; Book III, Table V-*CC*.
19. *hind shank of fornix (Bartholin, 1662)*
Alternate form of *hinder thigh of fornix (Bartholin, 1662)*, the *crus of fornix (Riolan, 1618)*; p. 140.
20. *trunk of fornix (Willis, 1664)*
Corresponds to caudal half or so of *fornix itself (Willis, 1664)* in macrodissected adult sheep, dorsal and rostral to *arm of fornix (Willis, 1664)* and corresponding roughly to segment of ***fimbria (Honegger, 1890)*** containing ***hippocampal commissures (>1840)***; Figure VII-*B*.
21. *arm of fornix (Willis, 1664)*
Essentially synonym for *posterior crus of fornix (Vesling, 1647)*; illustrated in Figure VIII-*C* for both sides of macrodissected adult sheep, and described for macrodissected adult human in the text. In the original Latin (plural), *fornicis brachia* (Fig. VII-*C*), and see Pordage translation (1681, pp. 60–61, 94). As Drake (1707, pp. 642, 647) explained, they are named "because in Effect they embrace the Thighs [*crura*] of the *Medulla Oblongata* [roughly ***brainstem (Schwalbe, 1881)***]." Willis's account was very brief and did not deal with its ventral extension.
22. *brachium of fornix (Willis, 1664)*
Latin-based form of *arm of fornix (Willis, 1664)*; see Lewis (1923, p. 222).
23. *pes hippocampi (Diemerbroeck, 1672)*
Diemerbroeck claimed quite mistakenly that Hippocrates called the *posterior crus of fornix (Vesling, 1647)* the *pes hippocampi*; see translation (1689, p. 399).
24. *fascia (Molinetti, 1675)*

Synonym for macrodissected adult human *posterior crus of fornix (Vesling, 1647)*; p. 186, according to Burdach (1822, p. 374), who also wrote that Molinetti believed earlier authors had referred to it as "limbus."

25. *columnas posteriores veri fornicis (Vieussens, 1684)*
Probably synonym for macrodissected adult human right and left *brachium of fornix (Willis, 1664)*; Table VII-*a,b*. Also see *fimbriatae veri fornicis appendix (Vieussens, 1684)*.
26. *posterior column of true fornix (Vieussens, 1684)*
English form (singular) of *columnas posteriores veri fornicis (Vieussens, 1684)*.
27. *cornua fornicis (Lancisi, 1714)*
In his annotation of Eustachi's plates, published here for the first time though completed in 1552, Lancisi referred thus to right and left macrodissected adult human *posterior pillar of fornix (Paré, 1564)*; see Meyer (1971, p. 21).
28. *Ammon's horn (Noguez, 1726)*
Apparently synonym for macrodissected adult human *posterior pillar of fornix (Paré, 1564)*; p. 280. Noguez suggested it is ventral differentiation of *corpus callosum (Willis, 1664)*; see Meyer (1971, p. 21). This view was elaborated by Haller (1762); see Lewis (1923, pp. 226–227).
29. *posterior pillar of fornix (Winslow, 1733)*
In this clearly original account of ***fornix (Vesalius, 1543a)***, perhaps inspired by work of Pourfour du Petit (1710), Winslow described macrodissected adult human *posterior pillar of fornix (Winslow, 1733)* as extending from ventral end of ***inferior horn of lateral ventricle (Bell, 1802)*** to rostral end of *lyre (Winslow, 1733)*, roughly ***dorsal hippocampal commissure (Craigie, 1925)***. Thus, *posterior pillar of fornix (Winslow, 1733)* includes segment of ***fimbria (Honegger, 1890)*** from ventral pole of ***hippocampal region (Swanson et al., 1987)*** to rostral end of ***dorsal hippocampal commissure (Craigie, 1925)***, including ***alveus (Burdach, 1822)***: "The posterior Pillars are bent downward, and continued through the lower Portions of the Ventricles all the way to their Extremities, resembling a Ram's Horn, which is a name that has been given to them. They diminish gradually in thickness during this course [whereas the ***hippocampal region (Swanson et al., 1987)*** increases], and at their outsides they have each a small, thin, flat, collateral Border, to which the name of Corpora Fimbriata is owing" (Sect. X, p. 35). *Corpus fimbriatum (Winslow, 1733)* is a long ventral segment of *posterior pillar of fornix (Winslow, 1733)*, corresponding to *arm of fornix (Willis, 1664)*. This was the interpretation of Meckel (1817; see translation, 1832, Vol. 2, p. 451), who referred to its "center" as *body*; see *body of fornix (Monro, 1783)*.
30. *ram's horn (Winslow, 1733, p. 35)*
Synonym for macrodissected adult human *posterior pillar of fornix (Winslow, 1733)*; note that Winslow earlier (Sect. X, p. 34) used the term *ram's horn (Winslow, 1733, p. 34)* differently, for ***inferior horn of lateral ventricle (Bell, 1802)***.
31. *corpus fimbriatum (Winslow, 1733)*
Corresponds to long ventral segment of *posterior pillar of fornix (Winslow, 1733)*, caudal to shorter dorsal and rostral segment corresponding to *body of fornix (Vesalius, 1543a)* or *vaulted body (Paré, 1550)*—the *arm of fornix (Willis, 1664)*; Section X, p. 35.
32. *corpus fimbriatum Sylvii (Bergen, 1734)*
Eponym for macrodissected adult human *corpus fimbriatum (Winslow, 1733)*; see Burdach (1822, p. 374), referring to Frans de Le Boë (Sylvius).
33. *cornice of vault (Bonhomme, 1748)*
Synonym for macrodissected adult human *corpus fimbriatum (Winslow, 1733)*; in the original French, *la corniche de la voûte*, p. 51.
34. *fimbria (Günz, 1750)*
Burdach (1822, p. 374) credited Günz with using it instead of *corpus fimbriatum (Winslow, 1733)*.
35. *taenia cerebri (Haller, 1762)*
Synonym for macrodissected adult human *corpus fimbriatum (Winslow, 1733)*; p. 37, according to Haase (1781, p. 19). Also see Mayer (1779, p. 9).
36. *posterior crus of fornix (Haller, 1762)*
Probably synonym for macrodissected adult human *body of fornix (Vesalius, 1543a)* or *vaulted body (Paré, 1550)*, dorsal and rostral to *fimbria (Günz, 1750)*; p. 36.
37. *limbus Sylvii (Haller, 1762)*
Eponym for *corpus fimbriatum (Winslow, 1733)*; p. 37, according to Burdach (1822, p. 374), referring to Frans de Le Boë (Sylvius).
38. *silkworm (Malacarne, 1780)*
Synonym for macrodissected adult human *corpus fimbriatum (Winslow, 1733)*; the complete passage reads, "Aranzio is perhaps the first to have called 'bombicine appendixes' those semi-cylindrical, curved bodies that descend from the posterior pillars of the vault down through the Horns of Ammon; they are very white and soft, and on their inner side the fimbriate bodies—which I call the silkworms—hang" (Vol. 2, p. 64; unpublished translation from the Italian kindly provided by Frederick Mario Fales). In the original Italian, *Bachi*.
39. *taenia hippocampi (Vicq d'Azyr, 1786)*
Corresponds to ventral segment of macrodissected adult human ***fimbria (Honegger, 1890)***, coextensive with ***hippocampal region (Swanson et al., 1987)***. Vicq d'Azyr regarded it a caudal extension of *posterior column of medullary triangle (Vicq d'Azyr, 1786)*, ventral to ***splenium of corpus callosum (Burdach, 1822)***; see Plates XV:34–36 and XXV, Figure III-*k,i,h*; and Meyer (1971, p. 21). In the original French, *bandelette de l'hippocampe*; Plates XV:*34–36* and XXVIII, Figure II-*6*. Thus, *taenia hippocampi (Vicq d'Azyr, 1786)* is probably not synonymous with *corpus fimbriatum (Winslow, 1733)*, which probably extends more rostrally to caudal end of ***dorsal hippocampal commissure (Craigie, 1925)*** and thus includes the short *posterior and lateral part of vault with three pillars (Vicq d'Azyr, 1786)*. Note that Vicq d'Azyr associated *taenia hippocampi (Vicq d'Azyr, 1786)* with ***hippocampal region (Swanson et al., 1987)*** not ***fornix***

(Vesalius, 1543a). Also see *taenia (Burdach, 1822)*. Bell & Bell (1829, p. 421) spelled it *tenia hippocampi*.

40. *marginal body (Vicq d'Azyr, 1786)*
Vicq d'Azyr wrote that this term (in the original French, *corps bordé*), derived from *corpus fimbriatum (Winslow, 1733)*, is a poor one. He preferred *taenia hippocampi (Vicq d'Azyr, 1786)*; p. 87; Plate XXVIII, Figure II-6.

41. *bandelette du grand hippocampe (Vicq d'Azyr, 1786)*
French synonym for *taenia hippocampi (Vicq d'Azyr, 1786)*; also see *hippocampus major (Vicq d'Azyr, 1786)*.

42. *posterior pillar of vault with three pillars (Vicq d'Azyr, 1786)*
Synonym for *posterior column of medullary triangle (Vicq d'Azyr, 1786)*; in the original French both pillars were referred to as *piliers postérieurs de la voûte*; see Plates V-*s*, XV-49.

43. *posterior pillar of fornix (Vicq d'Azyr, 1786)*
Synonym for *posterior column of medullary triangle (Vicq d'Azyr, 1786)*; Plate VII, Figure VI-2.

44. *posterior column of medullary triangle (Vicq d'Azyr, 1786)*
Corresponds to *posterior crus of fornix (Haller, 1762)* and *crus of fornix (>1840a)* considered together; Plate XV-49, also see *medullary triangle (Vicq d'Azyr, 1786)*.

45. *posterior and lateral part of vault with three pillars (Vicq d'Azyr, 1786)*
Caudal segment of *posterior pillar of vault with three pillars (Vicq d'Azyr, 1786)*, corresponding to *crus of fornix (>1840a)*; see 23 in Plates IX–XI, and Plate XV-34.

46. *posterior and lateral part of medullary triangle (Vicq d'Azyr, 1786)*
Synonym for *posterior and lateral part of vault with three pillars (Vicq d'Azyr, 1786)*; 23 in Plates IX–XI.

47. *Saum des Wulstes (Soemmerring, 1791)*
German synonym for macrodissected adult human *taenia hippocampi (Vicq d'Azyr, 1786)*; pp. 32–36, also see Burdach (1822, p. 375).

48. *limbus of Ammon's horn (Soemmerring, 1791)*
English form of *Saum des Wulstes (Soemmerring, 1791)*; see p. 32.

49. *bordered or fringed bodies (Burdin, 1803)*
Synonym for macrodissected adult human *taenia hippocampi (Vicq d'Azyr, 1786)*; see translation (1803, Vol. 1, p. 160), also see Burdach (1822, p. 375).

50. *posterior peduncles of trigone (Chaussier, 1807)*
Synonym for macrodissected adult human *posterior pillars of vault with three pillars (Vicq d'Azyr, 1786)*; in the original French, *pédoncules postérieurs du trigône*, p. 56.

51. *posterior angles of cerebral trigone (Chaussier, 1807)*
Synonym for macrodissected adult human *posterior pillars of vault with three pillars (Vicq d'Azyr, 1786)*; in the original French, *les angles postérieurs du trigône cérébral*, p. 56.

52. *posterior columns of vault (Chaussier, 1807)*
Synonym listed for macrodissected adult human *posterior pillars of vault with three pillars (Vicq d'Azyr, 1786)*; in the original French, *les colonnes postérieurs de la voûte*, p. 56.

53. *posterior arches of vault (Chaussier, 1807)*
Synonym listed for macrodissected adult human *posterior pillars of vault with three pillars (Vicq d'Azyr, 1786)*; in the original French, *les arcs de la postérieurs voûte*, p. 56.

54. *fimbria hippocampi (Wenzel & Wenzel, 1812)*
Synonym for macrodissected adult human *taenia hippocampi (Vicq d'Azyr, 1786)*; p. 88.

55. *fimbria medullosa (Wenzel & Wenzel, 1812)*
Synonym for macrodissected adult human *taenia hippocampi (Vicq d'Azyr, 1786)*, p. 203. Burdach (1822, p. 375) quoted the term *fimbria medullaris hippocampi*, and wrote that it included epithelium and ***white matter (Meckel, 1817)***.

56. *posterior crus of fornix (Reil, 1812b)*
Synonym for macrodissected adult human *posterior pillar of fornix (Winslow, 1733)*; see Mayo translation (1823, pp. 115–116).

57. *band of fornix (Tiedemann, 1816)*
Synonym for *corpus fimbriatum (Winslow, 1733)*, as observed in macrodissected 4-month human fetus; see translation (1826, p. 54).

58. *markiger Saum (Bock, 1820)*
German synonym for macrodissected adult human *taenia hippocampi (Vicq d'Azyr, 1786)*; p. 267, according to Burdach (1822, p. 375). A rough translation is *white matter limbus*.

59. *body of fornix (Burdach, 1822)*
Part of macrodissected adult human ***fimbria (Honegger, 1890)*** rostral to *body of fornix (Vesalius, 1543a)*; in the original Latin, *corpus fornicis*, p. 138 and Table VII-*i*.

60. *crus of fornix (Burdach, 1822)*
Synonym for macrodissected adult human *posterior crus of fornix (Reil, 1812b)*; in the original Latin (plural), *crura fornicis*, pp. 139, 155–156 and Table. VII-*k*.

61. *taenia (Burdach, 1822)*
Synonym for macrodissected adult human *taenia hippocampi (Vicq d'Azyr, 1786)*; p. 156.

62. *vault proper (Longet, 1842)*
Synonym for macrodissected adult human *body of fornix (Burdach, 1822)*; in the original French, *voûte proprement dite*, p. 539.

63. *posterior pillar of vault (Longet, 1842)*
Synonym for macrodissected adult human *posterior crus of fornix (Reil, 1812b)*; in the original French (plural), *piliers postérieurs de la voûte*, p. 541.

64. *corpus fimbriatum (Longet, 1842)*
Synonym for macrodissected adult human *taenia (Burdach, 1822)*; p. 539 note *1*.

65. *fimbria of hippocampus (Henle, 1871)*
Synonym for macrodissected adult human *taenia (Burdach, 1822)*; in the original Latin, *fimbria (hippocampi)*, p. 168.

66. *fornix longus (Forel, 1872)*
As observed in small mammals with histological methods for ***axons (Kölliker, 1896)***, ***dorsal fornix (Sprague & Meyer, 1950)*** and ***longitudinal striae (>1840)*** considered together; p. 19 and Figure 5-8, see Honegger (1890,

p. 252), Smith (1898, p. 242 ff.). Also see *fornix superior (Kölliker, 1896)* and *dorsal fornix (Smith, 1898)*.

67. *posterior pillar of trigone (Dejerine & Dejerine-Klumpke, 1895)*
Synonym for macrodissected adult human *corpus fimbriatum (Winslow, 1733)*; in the original French (plural), *piliers postérieurs du trigone*, p. 348.
68. *posterior pillar proper of trigone (Dejerine & Dejerine-Klumpke, 1895)*
Synonym for macrodissected adult human *posterior pillar of fornix (Winslow, 1733)*; in the original French, *piliers postérieurs proprement dit du trigone*, pp. 273–277.
69. *fornix superior (Kölliker, 1896)*
Corresponds to macrodissected adult human ***dorsal fornix (Sprague & Meyer, 1950)*** and ***longitudinal striae (>1840)***—considered together the *fornix longus (Forel, 1876)*—as well as *perforating fibers of fornix longus (Kölliker, 1896)*; p. 787, see Smith (1898, p. 242 ff.) and Dejerine & Dejerine-Klumpke (1901, pp. 296–297).
70. *perforating fibers of fornix longus (Kölliker, 1896)*
Axons (Kölliker, 1896) penetrating ***corpus callosum (Galen, c177)*** more or less perpendicularly, first noted by Meynert (1872, Fig. 264); p. 787, also see Dejerine & Dejerine-Klumpke (1901, pp. 279–283).
71. *dorsal fornix (Smith, 1898)*
Essentially synonym for *fornix longus (Forel, 1876)* and *fornix superior (Kölliker, 1896)* considered together, "In order not further to prejudice Kölliker's term 'fornix superior,' I propose to use the designation 'fornix dorsalis' for all those uncrossed fibres of the fornix whose arrangement is disturbed by the development of a corpus callosum, and which arise from or end in the dorsal limb of the hippocampal arc. The fornix dorsalis thus includes the striae Lancisii and all the fibres connected with these striae, as well as the uncrossed fibres which arise from the subsplenial hippocampal flexure." (pp. 242–243).
72. *posterior column of fornix (Demeter et al., 1985)*
For adult monkey with macrodissection and histological methods showing ***axons (Kölliker, 1896)***, synonym for *crus of fornix (>1840a)*; p. 32.
73. *taenia fornicis (>1840)*
Synonym for macrodissected adult human *taenia (Burdach, 1822)*; see His (1895, p. 86).
74. *crus of fornix (>1840a)*
Very short segment of macrodissected adult human ***fimbria (Honegger, 1890)*** between caudal end of ***dorsal hippocampal commissure (Craigie, 1925)*** and dorsal (septal, posterior) end of macroscopically visible ***hippocampal region (Swanson et al., 1987)***, where ***alveus (Burdach, 1822)*** begins to form. See Herrick (1915, p. 330), and clear illustration in Ranson (1920, Fig. 203). It was first recognized by Vesalius, see quote in *body of fornix (Vesalius, 1543a)* and was later called *posterior and lateral part of vault with three pillars (Vicq d'Azyr, 1786)*.
75. *crus of fornix (>1840b)*
Macrodissected adult human *body of fornix (Burdach, 1822)* and *crus of fornix (Burdach, 1822)* considered together; see Larsell (1939, p. 270).
76. *body of fornix (>1840)*
Macrodissected adult human *body of fornix (Vesalius, 1543a)* and *body of fornix (Burdach, 1822)* considered together; see Ranson (1920, pp. 271–272).
77. *fimbria of fornix (>1840)*
Ventral segment of macrodissected adult human ***fimbria (Honegger, 1890)*** coextensive with ***hippocampal region (Swanson et al., 1987)***; see Mettler (1948, p. 15). Originally called *taenia hippocampi (Vicq d'Azyr, 1786)*.

fimbrial line of lateral ventricle (>1840)

As described for adult mammal, the line where the ***choroid epithelium of lateral ventricle (>1840)*** attaches to the length of the ***fimbria (Honegger, 1890)***; see Mettler (1948, p. 147), Crosby et al. (1962, p. 576). It was not clearly described by 1840. The other edge of the ***choroid epithelium of lateral ventricle (>1840)*** is formed by the ***choroid line of lateral ventricle (>1840)***.

TRANSLATIONS:

1. *tenia fimbriae ventriculi lateralis (>1840)*
Latin form of ***choroid line of lateral ventricle (>1840)***; see *Dorland's* (2003, pp. 1851). Also spelled *taenia choroidea*. Other synonyms include *tenia telae, tenia striae terminalis*. His (1895; see Eycleshymer translation, 1917, p. 161 ff.) used the term *taenia fornicis et fimbriae* and noted Reichert (1861) originated the term *taenia fornicis*.

fimbriodentate sulcus (>1840)

As described for macrodissected adult human, a shallow groove between the proximal end of the ***fimbria (Honegger, 1890)*** and ***field CA3 (Lorente de Nó, 1934)*** of ***Ammon's horn (Vicq d'Azyr, 1784)***, on the side of the ***fimbria (Honegger, 1890)*** facing the ***hippocampal sulcus (Gratiolet, 1854)***; see Mettler (1948, p. 151), Williams & Warwick (1980, Fig. 7.121D), *Terminologia Anatomica* (1998, p. 127). It was first clearly delineated by Vicq d'Azyr; see ***[fimbriodentate sulcus (>1840)] (Vicq d'Azyr, 1786)***.

EARLIER REFERENCES:

Illustrated, not named or described:

1. ***[fimbriodentate sulcus (>1840)] (Vicq d'Azyr, 1786)***
Clearly illustrated for macrodissected adult human in transverse section; Table XXVI, Figure 7, just to the right of 5.

floccular peduncle (Burdach, 1822)

As described for macrodissected adult human, a component of the ***arbor vitae (Winslow, 1733)*** connecting ***flocculus (Meckel, 1817)*** with ***nodule (Reil, 1807–1808a)*** and ***uvula (Malacarne, 1776)***, and with ***caudal medullary velum (>1840)***; see Larsell & Jansen (1972, p. 63), Williams & Warwick (1980, p. 913), *Nomina Anatomica* (1983, p. A67), *Terminologia Anatomica* (1998, p. 119), *Dorland's* (2003, p. 1390). For Burdach's use in macrodissected adult human, see p. 65. It was first known as the *medullary stem of laminated flakes (Malacarne, 1776)*.

TRANSLATIONS:

1. *pedunculus flocci (Burdach, 1822)*
   Original Latin form of ***floccular peduncle (Burdach, 1822)***; p. 65.

EARLIER REFERENCES:

Earlier synonyms:

1. *medullary stem of laminated flakes (Malacarne, 1776)*
   Synonym for macrodissected adult human ***floccular peduncle (Burdach, 1822)***; see Clarke & O'Malley translation (1996, p. 645).
2. *medullary cord of laminated flakes (Malacarne, 1776)*
   Synonym for *medullary stem of laminated flakes (Malacarne, 1776)*; see Clarke & O'Malley translation (1996, p. 645).
3. *principal root of flock (Reil, 1809c)*
   Synonym for macrodissected adult human *medullary stem of laminated flakes (Malacarne, 1776)*; see Mayo translation (1809c, p. 88). Nicely illustrated by Wenzel & Wenzel (1812, Tab. XI, Fig. 4-*g*).

flocculus (Meckel, 1817)

As described for macrodissected adult human, the part of the ***cerebellar hemisphere (Willis, 1664)*** adjacent to the ***tonsil (Malacarne, 1776)*** and its ***paraflocculus (Stroud, 1895)***, and lateral to the ***nodule (Reil, 1807–1808a)*** of the ***cerebellar vermis (Meckel, 1817)***; see Angevine et al. (1961, Figs. 2, 3, 5–8, 10, 11, 13, 15–24), Larsell & Jansen (1972, Fig. 118), Carpenter (1976, Fig. 14.1), Williams & Warwick (1980, Fig. 7.74), *Terminologia Anatomica* (1998, p. 119), Nieuwenhuys et al. (2008, Fig. 20.2). For Meckel's use in macrodissected adult human, see p. 467, and translation (1832, Vol. 2, p. 429). Also see Burdach (1822, p. 296). It was perhaps first clearly delineated by Salmon; see ***[flocculus (Meckel, 1817] (Salmon, 1714)***.

EARLIER REFERENCES:

Illustrated, not named or described:

1. ***[flocculus (Meckel, 1817] (Salmon, 1714)***
   Very clearly illustrated for macrodissected adult human; Table 20. Compare with Nieuwenhuys et al. (2008, Fig. 3.13).

Earlier synonyms:

1. *vermiformes (Winslow, 1733)*
   Probably alludes to right and left macrodissected adult human ***flocculus (Meckel, 1817)***, "two lateral Appendices, both turned outward." (Sect. X, p. 39).
2. *tubercula minima cerebelli (Tarin, 1750)*
   Synonym for macrodissected adult human ***flocculus (Meckel, 1817)***; see Burdach (1822, p. 296).
3. *laminated flakes (Malacarne, 1776)*
   Translation of term Malacarne used for macrodissected adult human ***flocculus (Meckel, 1817)***; in the original Italian, *fiocchi laminosi*, p. 24. See Larsell (1967, p. 4), Larsell & Jansen (1972, p. 62), Clarke & O'Malley (1996, p. 645).
4. *flossi laminosi (Malacarne, 1776)*
   Latin form of *laminated flakes (Malacarne, 1776)*; see Burdach (1822, p. 296).
5. *particulae segregatae cerebelli mediae (Soemmerring, 1778)*
   Synonym for macrodissected adult human ***flocculus (Meckel, 1817)***; p. 16, see Burdach (1822, p. 296).
6. *lobule of eighth pair (Vicq d'Azyr, 1784)*
   Synonym for *lobule of vagus nerve (Vicq d'Azyr, 1786)*; p. 570.
7. *lobule of vagus nerve (Vicq d'Azyr, 1786)*
   Synonym for macrodissected adult human ***flocculus (Meckel, 1817)***; p. 54, Plate XVII, Figure I-*71*. See Burdach (1822, p. 296), Henle (1871, p. 119).
8. *lobuli minima (Günther, 1786)*
   Synonym for macrodissected adult human *tubercula minima cerebelli (Tarin, 1750)*; p. 18.
9. *lobuli parvi cerebelli, que communiter septimo et octavo pari interjacent (Procháska, 1800)*
   Synonym for right and left macrodissected adult human ***flocculus (Meckel, 1817)***; Vol. 1, p. 355. See Burdach (1822, p. 296).
10. *lobular appendix (Chaussier, 1807)*
    Synonym for macrodissected adult human ***flocculus (Meckel, 1817)***; in the original French, *appendice lobulaire*, p. 94. Burdach (1822, p. 296) gave the Latin (plural), *appendices lobulares*.
11. *flock (Reil, 1807–1808a)*
    Synonym for macrodissected adult human ***flocculus (Meckel, 1817)***; in the original German, *Flocke*, or the plural *Flocken*; see Mayo translation (1822, p. 25). Also see Burdach (1822, p. 296).
12. *subpeduncular lobule (Gordon, 1815)*
    Synonym for macrodissected adult human ***flocculus (Meckel, 1817)***; in the original Latin (plural), *lobuli subpedunculares*, p. 117. Also see Burdach (1822, p. 296).

LATER SYNONYMS:

1. *lobe of pneumogastric nerve of Vicq d'Azyr (Meckel, 1817)*
   Eponym for macrodissected adult human *lobule of vagus nerve (Vicq d'Azyr, 1786)*; see translation (1832, Vol. 2, p. 429) and *pneumo-gastric nerve (Chaussier, 1807)*.

floor of fourth ventricle (Reil, 1807–1808a)

As described for macrodissected adult mammal, the ventral part or base of the ***fourth ventricle (Galen, c192)*** residing within the dorsal walls of the ***pons (Haller, 1747)*** and ***medulla (Winslow, 1733)***; see Williams & Warwick (1980, pp. 933–935). For Reil's use in macrodissected adult human, see Mayo translation (1822, Tab. 3, Fig. I-*m*). It was recognized long ago as the *calamus scriptorius (Herophilus, c335–c280 BC)*.

EARLIER REFERENCES:

Earlier synonyms:

1. *calamus scriptorius (Herophilus, c335–c280 BC)*
   In *On Anatomical Procedures*, Galen (c177) told how Herophilus first described macrodissected adult human ***floor of fourth ventricle Reil, 1807–1808a)*** as having the shape of a quill peculiar to Alexandria, where he taught and where he dissected both animals and human cadavers. The ***facial colliculus (>1840), obex (Burdach,***

1822), and ***median sulcus of fourth ventricle (>1840)*** are probably integral parts of the description; see Singer translation (1999, pp. 237, 277) and Vesalius (1543a; see Singer translation, 1952, p. 37 and Fig. 10).

2. *kalamos (Herophilus, c335–c280 BC)*
   Original Greek term for the Latin ***calamus scriptorius (Herophilus, c335–c280 BC)***, meaning "reed pen"; see Von Staden (1989, p. 158).
3. *cavity of medulla dorsalis forming part of fourth ventricle (Vesalius, 1543a)*
   Synonym for macrodissected adult human ***floor of fourth ventricle (Reil, 1807–1808a)***; see Singer translation (1952, p. 104).
4. *pointed part of scribe's quill (Vesalius, 1543a)*
   Synonym for macrodissected adult human ***floor of fourth ventricle (Reil, 1807–1808a)***; see Singer translation (1952, pp. 104, 106).
5. *point of a pen with which we write (Geminus, 1553)*
   Synonym for macrodissected adult human ***floor of fourth ventricle (Reil, 1807–1808a)***; originally spelled *poynte of a penne wherewith we wryte*, see *The tables of the brayne*, Figure 9-*I*.
6. *fourth ventricle (Molinetti, 1675)*
   Synonym for macrodissected adult human ***floor of fourth ventricle (Reil, 1807–1808a)***; according to Burdach (1822, p. 302).
7. *rhomboid ventricle (Albinus, 1744)*
   Synonym for macrodissected adult human ***floor of fourth ventricle (Reil, 1807–1808a)*** as illustrated by Eustachi; in the original Latin, *ventriculus rhomboidalis*, according to Burdach (1822, p. 302).
8. *scrobs ventriculi quarti (Santorini, 1775)*
   Synonym for macrodissected adult human ***floor of fourth ventricle (Reil, 1807–1808a)***; p. 24, according to Burdach (1822, p. 302).
9. *rhomboid cavity (Malacarne, 1776)*
   Synonym for macrodissected adult human ***floor of fourth ventricle (Reil, 1807–1808a)***; in Latin, *cavitas rhomboidalis*, according to Burdach (1822, p. 302).
10. *inferior floor of fourth ventricle (Vicq d'Azyr, 1786)*
   Roughly synonymous with macrodissected adult human ***floor of fourth ventricle (Reil, 1807–1808a)***; Plates XXIX, Figure III-6; XXX, -Figure I-6.

LATER SYNONYMS:

1. *lozenge-shaped field (Reil, 1809c)*
   Synonym for macrodissected adult human ***floor of fourth ventricle (Reil, 1807–1808a)***; see Mayo translation (1823, p. 86).
2. *lozenge (Reil, 1809c)*
   Synonym for *lozenge-shaped field (Reil, 1809c)*; see Mayo translation (1823, p. 87).
3. *rhomboid fossa (Burdach, 1822)*
   Synonym for macrodissected adult human ***floor of fourth ventricle (Reil, 1807–1808a)***; p. 74. It is a preferred term in *Nomina Anatomica* (1983) and *Terminologia Anatomica* (1998) but is not complementary to ***roof of fourth ventricle (Vesalius, 1543a)***.
4. *fourth ventricle fovea (Arnold, 1838a)*
   Synonym for macrodissected adult human *rhomboid fossa (Burdach, 1822)*; in the original Latin, *fovea ventriculi quarti*, p. 22.

PARTLY CORRESPONDS:

1. *eminentias perpendiculares (Prochâska, 1800)*
   For macrodissected adult human, probably included right and left ***hypoglossal triangle (>1840)*** and ***medial eminence (>1840)***; Vol. 1, p. 391; see Burdach (1822, p. 285). According to Arnold (1838a) the name was first used by Santorini ("C18, p. 90"), but it is not found in Santorini (1724, 1775).
2. *anterior face of cerebellar ventricle (Chaussier, 1807)*
   In macrodissected adult human, literally base of ***floor of fourth ventricle (Reil, 1807–1808a)***, because he also described right and left *lateral walls of cerebellar ventricle (Chaussier, 1807)* formed by ***cerebellar peduncles (Ridley, 1695)***, and *posterior face of cerebellar ventricle (Chaussier, 1807)*; in the original French, *la face antérieure de la ventricule du cervelet*, pp. 99–100.
3. *lateral faces of cerebellar ventricles (Chaussier, 1807)*
   Synonym for *lateral walls of cerebellar ventricle (Chaussier, 1807)*; in the original French, *les faces latérales de la ventricule du cervelet*, pp. 99–100.
4. *lateral walls of cerebellar ventricle (Chaussier, 1807)*
   In macrodissected adult human, lateral walls of ***floor of fourth ventricle (Reil, 1807–1808a)***, dorsal to *anterior face of cerebellar ventricle (Chaussier, 1807)* and ventral to *posterior face of cerebellum (Chaussier, 1807)*; in the original French, *les parois latérales de la ventricule du cervelet*; pp. 99–100.
5. *longitudinal eminences (Rolando, 1825a)*
   Probably synonym for macrodissected adult human and beef *eminentias perpendiculares (Prochâska, 1800)*; in the original French, *éminences longitudinales*; Plate IV, Figures 3, 4-*e.l.*
6. *corpora teretia (Arnold, 1838a)*
   Synonym for *eminentiae teretes (Arnold, 1838a)*; p. 18.
7. *eminentia teres (Arnold, 1838a)*
   Synonym for macrodissected adult human right and left ***medial eminence (>1840)*** and ***hypoglossal triangle (>1840)*** considered together, the *eminentias perpendiculares (Prochâska, 1800)*; p. 18. Also see Arnold, 1838b; Table II, Figure 10-g; Table IV, Figure 3-*i.*; and Table VIII, Figure 3-*l*.
8. *funiculus teres (Arnold, 1838a)*
   Synonym *eminentia teres (Arnold, 1838a)*; p. 20.
9. *fasciculus teres (Arnold, 1838b)*
   Synonym for *eminentia teres (Arnold, 1828a)*; Table VIII, Figure 3-*l*.

floor plate (>1840)

As described for the developing vertebrate ***neural tube (Baer, 1837)***, the thin ventral region in the median plane of ***spinal cord part of neural tube (>1840)*** and ***primary hindbrain vesicle (Baer, 1837)*** not generating neural tissue; see Kingsbury (1934) and Alvarez-Bolado &

Swanson (1996, p. 13 ff.) for classical histological view. It was identified early on as the *anterior plate of spinal marrow (Meckel, 1817)*.

EARLIER REFERENCES:

Earlier synonyms:

1. *anterior plate of spinal marrow (Meckel, 1817)*
   For macrodissected embryonic human, ***floor plate (>1840)*** of ***spinal cord part of neural tube (>1840)***; see translation (1832, Vol. 2, p. 484).

folium vermis (>1840)

As described for macrodissected adult human, the part of the ***cerebellar vermis (Meckel, 1817)*** between ***declive (>1840)*** and ***tuber vermis (>1840)***, medial to the right and left ***ansiform lobule crus I (Bolk, 1906)*** of the ***cerebellar hemisphere (Willis, 1664)***; see Angevine et al. (1961, Fig. 24), Larsell & Jansen (1972, Fig. 118), Carpenter (1976, Figs. 2.26, 14.1), Nieuwenhuys et al. (2008, Fig. 3.8-32). It was first clearly described as the *chorda laminosa transversalis (Malacarne, 1776)*.

EARLIER REFERENCES:

Earlier synonyms:

1. *chorda laminosa transversalis (Malacarne, 1776)*
   Synonym for macrodissected adult human ***folium vermis (>1840)***; see Larsell (1967, p. 3).
2. *commissura cerebelli (Malacarne, 1776)*
   Synonym for macrodissected adult human ***folium vermis (>1840)***; see Larsell (1972, p. 44).
3. *commissure of superior posterior lobes (Malacarne, 1776)*
   Synonym for macrodissected adult human ***folium vermis (>1840)***; see Meckel (1832, Vol. 2, p. 430), *commissura cerebelli (Malacarne, 1776)*, and *superior posterior lobe (Malacarne, 1776)*.
4. *short exposed commissure of cerebellum (Reil, 1807–1808a)*
   Synonym for macrodissected adult human ***folium vermis (>1840)***; see Mayo translation (1822, p. 23) and Burdach (1822, p. 295).
5. *folium cacuminis (Burdach, 1822)*
   Synonym for macrodissected adult human ***folium vermis (>1840)***; p. 60.

foramen cecum of medulla (>1840)

As described for macrodissected adult human, a tiny ventral, rostrally directed indentation of the ***medullo-pontine sulcus (>1840)*** in the median plane at the rostral end of the ***ventral median fissure of medulla (>1840)***; see Crosby et al. (1962, Fig. 98 unlabeled), *Terminologia Anatomica* (1998, p. 108, listed as *foramen cecum of medulla oblongata*), *Dorland's* (2003, p. 722). It was probably first delineated as the *alveus (Haller, 1762)*.

EARLIER REFERENCES:

Earlier synonyms:

1. *alveus (Haller, 1762)*
   Synonym for macrodissected adult human ***foramen cecum of medulla (>1840)***; p. 68. Haller indicated that Le Boë may have used the term earlier, although he was mistaken in this attribution according to Burdach (1822, p. 286).
2. *foramen coecum posterius (Soemmerring, 1778)*
   Synonym for macrodissected adult human ***foramen cecum of medulla (>1840)***; Table II, p. 178.
3. *foramen coecum (Vicq d'Azyr, 1784)*
   Synonym for macrodissected adult human ***foramen cecum of medulla (>1840)***; p. 587. Spelled *foramen caecum* by Bell & Bell (1829, p. 441).
4. *posterior foramen cecum of pons (Mayer, 1794)*
   Synonym for macrodissected adult human ***foramen cecum of medulla (>1840)***; in the original Latin, *foramen coecum posterius pontis*; Part 5, Table III, Figure 2-θ.
5. *inferior acoustic fovea (Bergmann, 1831)*
   Synonym for macrodissected adult human ***foramen cecum of medulla (>1840)***; in the original Latin, *fovea acustica inferior*, p. 69.

forebrain (Goette, 1873)

The most rostral of the three main topographic divisions of the ***vertebrate brain (Cuvier, 1800)*** lying rostral to the ***midbrain (Baer, 1837)***; the third main topographic division is the ***rhombicbrain (His, 1893b)*** lying most caudal. The adult vertebrate ***endbrain (Kuhlenbeck, 1927)*** and ***interbrain (Baer, 1837)*** considered together. For these precise definitions see Swanson & Bota (2010, Thesaurus); also see Carpenter (1976, p. 38), Nieuwenhuys et al. (2008, Fig 2.2). Goette (p. 400) used it thus for toad embryos and Kupffer (1885, p. 473) clearly used it thus for all vertebrates; see Wilder & Gage (1882, p. 405). It was relatively clearly identified early on as the *cerebrum (Colombo, 1559)*.

TRANSLATIONS:

1. *prosencephalon (Mihalkovics, 1877)*
   Latin form of ***forebrain (Goette, 1873)*** used for comparative vertebrate embryology; p. 22.

EARLIER REFERENCES:

Earlier synonyms:

1. *cerebrum (Colombo, 1559)*
   Essentially, macrodissected adult human ***forebrain (Goette, 1873)***, contrasted with *cerebrum oblongatum (Colombo, 1559)*; p. 187 ff., also see Bannister (1578, f. 106v). Varoli clearly followed this usage; see Clarke & O'Malley (1996, pp. 635, 881–882), *base of brain (Varoli, 1573)*, and *spinal marrow (Varoli, 1573)*.
2. *principal cavity (Ridley, 1695)*
   For obscure reasons Ridley assigned to the large or principal cavity a list of macrodissected adult human structures corresponding nicely to ***forebrain (Goette, 1873)***; p. 116.
3. *cerebrum proper (Chaussier, 1807)*
   Synonym for macrodissected adult human *cerebrum (Colombo, 1559)*; in the original French, *le Cerveau en particulier, le Cerveau proprement dit*, p. 35.
4. *brain proper (Chaussier, 1807)*
   Alternate translation of *cerebrum proper (Chaussier, 1807)*.

5. *hemispheric ganglia (Solly, 1836)*
   Synonym for macrodissected adult fish ***forebrain (Goette, 1873)***; pp. 73–74.

PARTLY CORRESPONDS:

1. *ganglia of cord (Solly, 1836)*
   For macrodissected adult human, ***cerebral nuclei (Swanson, 2000a)*** and ***interbrain (Baer, 1837)*** considered together; p. 179.
2. *central nucleus of brain (Cruveilhier, 1836)*
   For macrodissected adult human, ***cerebral nuclei (Swanson, 2000a)*** and ***interbrain (Baer, 1837)*** considered together; in the original French, *noyau central du cerveau*, p. 702.
3. *root of brain (Cruveilhier, 1836)*
   Synonym for *central nucleus of brain (Cruveilhier, 1836)*; in the original French, *racine du cerveau*, p. 702.
4. *telencephalon (His, 1893a)*
   Based on comparative embryology including human, composed of ***endbrain (Kuhlenbeck, 1927)*** and preoptic region (see Swanson, 1976, pp. 229–235) of ***hypothalamus (Kuhlenbeck, 1927)***; pp. 159–162.
5. *telencephalon (His, 1893b)*
   Based on comparative embryology including human, composed of ***endbrain (Kuhlenbeck, 1927)*** and preoptic, anterior, and tuberal regions (see Swanson, 1987, p. 2) of ***hypothalamus (Kuhlenbeck, 1927)***, an interpretation adopted by the *Basel Nomina Anatomica* (His, 1895, p. 158); pp. 173, 178, 179. See *hypothalamus (His, 1893b)*.

fornix (Vesalius, 1543a)

As described for adult mammal with macrodissection and experimental ***axon (Kölliker, 1896)*** pathway tracing methods, a heterogeneous ***central nervous system white matter tract (>1840)*** with two major divisions distinguished primarily at the level of the ***subfornical organ (>1840)*** and ***interventricular foramen (>1840)***. The first major division is the ***fimbria (Honegger, 1890)*** of the ***fornix (Vesalius, 1543a)***, the part of the transverse ***cerebral cortex white matter (>1840)*** associated with the ***hippocampal formation (Swanson & Cowan, 1977)***; the second major division has two subdivisions, the transverse ***precommissural fornix (Loo, 1931)*** and the longitudinal ***postcommissural fornix (Loo, 1931)***. The ***fimbria (Honegger, 1890)*** is divided arbitrarily into ventral (temporal, anterior) and dorsal (septal, posterior) segments in mammals with a ***corpus callosum (Galen, c177)***. The ventral segment is distinguished by a clear differentiation along its length, the ***alveus (Burdach, 1822)***, and another differentiation along part of its length, the ***dorsal hippocampal commissure (Craigie, 1925)***. The dorsal segment is not associated with the ***alveus (Burdach, 1822)*** and lies entirely ventral to the ***corpus callosum (Galen, c177)***; its major differentiation is the ***ventral hippocampal commissure (Craigie, 1925)***. There are two other differentiations of the ***fimbria (Honegger, 1890)*** as a whole; one is the ***dorsal fornix (Sprague & Meyer, 1950)*** extending near the median plane just ventral to the ***corpus callosum (Galen, c177)***, and the other consists of the ***longitudinal striae (>1840)*** extending around the ***splenium of corpus callosum (Burdach, 1822)*** and then coursing rostrally near the median plane, just dorsal to the ***corpus callosum (Galen, c177)*** and associated with the ***fasciola cinerea (Arnold, 1838b)*** and ***indusium griseum (Valentin, 1841)*** respectively. The ***postcommissural fornix (Loo, 1931)*** and ***precommissural fornix (Loo, 1931)*** are similar to the ***internal capsule (Burdach, 1822)*** and its branches for the ***hippocampal formation (Swanson & Cowan, 1977)***. As the right and left ***fimbria (Honegger, 1890)*** extend dorsally along the ***inferior horn of lateral ventricle (Bell, 1802)***, they converge and come to lie adjacent to one another at the median plane, meeting at various distances rostral and ventral or caudal and ventral to the ***splenium of corpus callosum (Burdach, 1822)*** in different species (see Johnston, 1913, Figs. 86–90). The rostral end of the ***ventral hippocampal commissure (Craigie, 1925)*** lies at about the level of the ***subfornical organ (>1840)*** and ***interventricular foramen (>1840)***, and here the dorsal segment of the adjacent right and left ***fimbria (Honegger, 1890)*** diverge again, extending rostrally and ventrally as the right and left ***precommissural fornix (Loo, 1931)*** and ***postcommissural fornix (Loo, 1931)***. Vesalius's (1543a) description was much more complete than *fornix (Galen, c 177)* and while vague, corresponds broadly to current usage. Vesalius wrote that the adult human ***fornix (Vesalius, 1543a)*** or *tortoise (Vesalius, 1543a)* is a single, triangular structure forming a link between the two sides of the *cerebrum (Vesalius, 1543a)* and is of the same substance as the ***corpus callosum (Galen, c177)***; see Singer translation (1952, pp. 41–42, Fig. 5:*S-V*). Unlike Galen, he apparently included the ***fimbria (Honegger, 1890)***, down into the ***inferior horn of lateral ventricle (Bell, 1802)***, with the ***fornix (Vesalius, 1543a)***, stating that it merges there with the substance of the ***brain (Smith Papyrus, c1700 BC)***, presumably the ***hippocampal region (Swanson et al., 1987)***; see Singer translation (1952, pp. 41–42, Fig. 6-*B,C*). Vesalius also noted that the rostral angle of the ***fornix (Vesalius, 1543a)*** enters and extends (in an undescribed way) through the substance of the ***brain (Smith Papyrus, c1700 BC)***, presumably the ***interbrain (Baer, 1837)***, at the level of the ***interventricular foramen (>1840)***; see Singer translation (1952, pp. 41–42).

TRANSLATIONS:

1. *cameratum (Vesalius, 1543a)*
   Simply, a revival of *camera (Galen, c177)*; Vesalius used it as alternate translation of ***fornix (Vesalius, 1543a)*** for macrodissected adult human; see Singer translation (1952, p. 3). In Latin, *camera* or *camara* means dome, vault, or vaulted body.
2. *camaratum (Vesalius, 1543a)*
   Alternate form of *cameratum (Vesalius, 1543a)*.
3. *zac (Vesalius, 1543a)*
   According to Vesalius, Arabic form (Latinized) of *fornix (Galen, c177)*. Only Arabist word Vesalius used in his

account of ***brain (Smith Papyrus, c1700 BC)***; see Singer translation (1952, p. 41 and note 59), also see ***fornix (Vesalius, 1543a)***.

4. *zachd (Vesalius, 1543a)*
Alternate form of *zac (Vesalius, 1543a)*; see Singer translation (1952, p. 41 and note 59).
5. *tortoise (Vesalius, 1543a)*
Alternate translation of ***fornix (Vesalius, 1543a)***; see Singer translation (1952, p. 41), also see *tortoise shell (Achillini, 1520)*. According to Burdach (1822, p. 374), Bergen (1734) believed Vesalius was referring specifically to *corpus fimbriatum (Winslow, 1733)*.
6. *vault (Geminus, 1553)*
Alternate translation for macrodissected adult human ***fornix (Vesalius, 1543a)***; originally spelled *vaute* and *vaulte*; see *The tables of the brayne*, Figures 3-*K* and 5-*S, T, V*. Also see Gerdy (1838, p. 260).
7. *chamber built after manner of arch (Geminus, 1553)*
Alternate form of ***fornix (Vesalius, 1543a)*** for macrodissected adult human; originally spelled *chamber buylded after the maner of an arche*, see *The tables of the brayne*, Figure 3-*K*.
8. *body made like vault (Geminus, 1553)*
Alternate translation of *vault (Geminus, 1553)*; originally spelled *bodye made like a vaulte*, see *The tables of the brayne*, Figure 5, where it is also referred to as a *bodye made like a furneves [furnace?]*.
9. *body like arch (Geminus, 1553)*
Alternate translation of *vault (Geminus, 1553)*; originally spelled *bodye like arche*, see *The tables of the brayne*, Figure 5-*X*.
10. *arch (Hall, 1565)*
Alternate English form of ***fornix (Vesalius, 1543a)*** for macrodissected adult human; p. 38. Also see *arch with three columns (Crooke, 1615)*.
11. *camarion (Hall, 1565)*
Alternate form of *cameratum (Vesalius, 1543a)*; p. 38.
12. *concameration (Tyson, 1699)*
English form of *cameratum (Vesalius, 1543a)*; p. 57.

LATER SYNONYMS:

1. *vaulted body with three legs (Paré, 1550)*
Synonym for macrodissected adult human ***fornix (Vesalius, 1543a)***, although here, in a very brief description, Paré did not actually designate the legs as anterior and posterior; in the original French, *vouste soustenue par trois pieds*, f. 56v. Term used in English by Bannister (1578, f. 100v). Colombo (1559, p. 192) referred to it in Latin, using *crura* for *legs*.
2. *corpus cameratum (Colombo, 1559)*
Obviously derived from *camera (Galen, c177)* referring to macrodissected adult human ***fornix (Vesalius, 1543a)*** or *cameratum (Vesalius, 1543a)*; see Bauhin (1605, p. 595; translation in Crooke, 1615, p. 463).
3. *vaulted body with three pillars (Paré, 1561)*
Synonym for macrodissected adult human *vaulted body with three legs (Paré, 1550)*; from passage that could also be translated *vault with three pillars*, *vault atop three pillars*, *arch with three pillars*, *fornix with three pillars*, or *psalloides with three pillars* or *stays*; see translation (1634, p. 168). It consists of right and left *posterior pillar of fornix (Paré, 1564)* extending caudally [down length of right and left ***inferior horn of lateral ventricle (Bell, 1802)***], and single *anterior pillar of fornix (Paré, 1564)* extending toward "the nose under the *Septum lucidum*".
4. *fornicem (Hall, 1565)*
Listed as vulgar synonym for macrodissected adult human ***fornix (Vesalius, 1543a)***; p. 38.
5. *corpus fornicatum (Hall, 1565)*
Listed as vulgar synonym for macrodissected adult human ***fornix (Vesalius, 1543a)***; p. 38.
6. *fornicate body (Hall, 1565)*
English form of *corpus fornicatum (Hall, 1565)*.
7. *cornix (Valverde de Amusco, 1589)*
Synonym in Latin translation of Valverde de Amusco's textbook, for macrodissected adult human ***fornix (Vesalius, 1543a)***; p. 243, see Burdach (1822, p. 357). For original passage in Spanish, see Valverde de Amusco (1556, f. 80v).
8. *arch with three columns (Crooke, 1615)*
For macrodissected adult human, Crooke wrote about "the Arch [***fornix (Vesalius, 1543a)***] of the braine called *Corpus cameratum* which is supported by three *Columnes* which like Atlas do sustaine the weight of the braine, so that the thirde ventricle which liethy under them is not obliterated." (p. 431). Also see *corpus cameratum (Colombo, 1559)* and *vaulted body with three pillars (Paré, 1561)*.
9. *corpus trifidum (Riolan, 1649)*
Riolan's reference to a "three-forked body" in macrodissected adult human goes back to ***fornix (Vesalius, 1543a)*** and *vaulted body with three pillars (Paré, 1561)*; p. 247. It was clearly illustrated by Vesling (1647); see Culpeper translation (1653, 2nd Tab., Ch. 14, Fig. 1).
10. *corpus psalloides (Riolan, 1649)*
Derived from *psalloidique corpori (Aranzi, 1587)*, going back ultimately to *psalloides (Galen, 177)*; p. 247. However, Riolan used it here in a more modern sense, as synonym for *corpus trifidum (Riolan, 1648)*.
11. *tripartite body (Riolan, 1657)*
Culpeper's translation of *corpus trifidum (Riolan, 1649)*; p. 123.
12. *Welch harp (Riolan, 1657)*
Synonym for macrodissected adult human ***fornix (Vesalius, 1543a)***; p. 123. Now spelled *Welsh harp*.
13. *arched roof of ventricles (Riolan, 1657)*
Synonym for macrodissected adult human ***fornix (Vesalius, 1543a)***; p. 126.
14. *harp fashioned body (Riolan, 1657)*
Synonym for macrodissected adult human ***fornix (Vesalius, 1543a)***; p. 127.
15. *vaulted arch of ventricles (Riolan, 1657)*
Synonym for macrodissected adult human ***fornix (Vesalius, 1543a)***; pp. 126–127. Willis (1664; see Pordage translation, 1681, p. 60) simply used *arched vault* for ***fornix (Vesalius, 1543a)***.

16. *vault of ventricles (Riolan, 1657)*
    Synonym for macrodissected adult human ***fornix (Vesalius, 1543a)***; p. 127.
17. *belly of lute (Bartholin, 1662)*
    Synonym for macrodissected adult human ***fornix (Vesalius, 1543a)***; p. 140.
18. *arched vault (Willis, 1664)*
    Variation on *vaulted arch of ventricles (Riolan, 1657)*; see Pordage translation (1681, p. 60).
19. *arched chamber (Willis, 1664)*
    Variation on *vaulted arch of ventricles (Riolan, 1657)*; see Pordage translation (1681, Tab. III-C).
20. *fornix callosus (Winslow, 1733)*
    Synonym for macrodissected adult human ***fornix (Vesalius, 1543a)***; Section X, p. 36. Winslow regarded it as part of ***corpus callosum (Galen, c177)***; Section X, p. 35.
21. *medullary triangle (Lieutaud, 1742)*
    Description of macrodissected adult human *vault with three pillars (Paré, 1564)*, going back to description of ***fornix (Vesalius, 1543a)***; p. 392.
22. *four-horned medullary tracts (Haller, 1747)*
    Synonym for macrodissected adult human ***fornix (Vesalius, 1543a)***; see Mihles translation (1754b, p. 291).
23. *medullary vault (Tarin, 1753)*
    Synonym for macrodissected adult human ***fornix (Vesalius, 1543a)***; in the original French, *la Voûte medullaire*, p. 102.
24. *cerebral trigone (Burdin, 1803)*
    Synonym for macrodissected adult human *vault with three pillars (Paré, 1564)*, or ***fornix (Vesalius, 1543a)***; see translation (1803, Vol. 1, p. 159).
25. *fornix trilaterus (Chaussier, 1807)*
    Synonym for macrodissected adult human ***fornix (Vesalius, 1543a)***, attributed without citation to [Stephen] Blancard by Chaussier; p. 54 note *1*.
26. *twin column of beam (Reil, 1809b)*
    Synonym for macrodissected adult human ***fornix (Vesalius, 1543a)***; in the original German, *Zwillingsbinde des Balkens*, see Mayo translation (1823, p. 52). Also see Cruveilhier (1836, p. 677) and Dejerine & Dejerine-Klumpke (1895, p. 344), who gave the French form, *bandelette géminée*.
27. *corpus communionis cerebri (Gall & Spurzheim, 1810)*
    Synonym for macrodissected adult human ***fornix (Vesalius, 1543a)***; see Burdach (1822, p. 358), Foster (1892, p. 1156).
28. *longitudinal commissure (Solly, 1836)*
    Synonym for macrodissected adult human ***fornix (Vesalius, 1543a)***; pp. 90, 183.
29. *inferior longitudinal commissure (Solly, 1836)*
    Synonym for macrodissected adult human ***fornix (Vesalius, 1543a)***; pp. 176, 183. Solly had it arising at one end from ***substantia nigra (Soemmerring, 1791)***; p. 185.
30. *hippocampal commissure (Owen, 1837)*
    Synonym for macrodissected adult mammalian ***fornix (Vesalius, 1543a)***; pp. 91, 92, 95 note *m*. Also see Leuret (1839, p. 412).
31. *internal fornix (Arnold, 1838b)*
    Synonym for macrodissected adult human ***fornix (Vesalius, 1543a)***; in the original Latin, *fornicis interni*, Table X, Figure 5 legend.

PARTLY CORRESPONDS:

1. *vaulted body (Galen, c173)*
   Synonym for *fornix (Galen, c177)*; see May translation (1968, pp. 392, 415–416).
2. *vault-shaped body (Galen, c173)*
   Synonym for *vaulted body (Galen, c173)*; see May translation (1968, p. 415).
3. *little vault (Galen, c173)*
   Synonym for *vaulted body (Galen, c173)*; see May translation (1968, p. 415).
4. *arch (Galen, c173)*
   Synonym for *vaulted body (Galen, c173)*; see May translation (1968, p. 415). The Latin word for *arch* is *fornix*; see Richardson & Carman (2009, p. 192).
5. *little arch (Galen, c173)*
   Synonym for *vaulted body (Galen, c173)*; see May translation (1968, p. 415).
6. *vault (Galen, c173)*
   Synonym for *vaulted body (Galen, c173)*; see May translation (1968, p. 416).
7. *arch-like body (Galen, c177)*
   Synonym for *vaulted body (Galen, c173)*; see Singer translation (1999, pp. 233–235).
8. *fornix (Galen, c177)*
   In *On Anatomical Procedures*, Galen described vaguely an arch-like body lying over ***third ventricle (Galen, c173)*** and under ***corpus callosum (Galen, c177)*** in macrodissected adult beef, pig, and macaque but not human. It is hard or callous like ***corpus callosum (Galen, c177)*** and begins rostrally near ***anterior commissure (Lieutaud, 1742)***; see Wiberg translation (1914, p. 26), Singer translation (1999, p. 234). *Fornix (Galen, c177)* thus apparently corresponds essentially to ***septal postcommissural fornix (>1840)*** and caudally continuous segment of ***fimbria (Honegger, 1890)*** ventral to ***corpus callosum (Galen, c177)***. The Latin word for *arch* is *fornix*; see Richardson & Carman (2009, p. 192).
9. *camera (Galen, c177)*
   Latin word meaning dome, vault, or vaulted body, mentioned by Galen in relation to *fornix (Galen, c177)*; see Singer translation (1999, p. 234). Vesalius (1543a) later referred to ***fornix (Vesalius, 1543a)*** as *cameratum (Vesalius, 1543a)*.
10. *psalidoeides (Galen, c177)*
    Greek word from which *arch-like body (Galen, 177)* is derived; see Singer translation (1999, p. 234). In the same passage, Galen noted that some people mistakenly call ***corpus callosum (Galen, c177)*** the *psalidoeides*. Massa (1536) probably used the term for *fornix (Galen, 177)*, although his description (or its translation) is confusing with respect to ***corpus callosum (Galen, c177)***; see Lind translation (1975, p. 237), also see *psalidoeides (Vesalius, 1543a)*.

11. *psaloides (Galen, c177)*
Alternate form of *psalidoeides (Galen, c177)*.
12. *psalloides (Galen, c177)*
Alternate form of *psalidoeides (Galen, c177)*.
13. *cupola (Galen, c192)*
Synonym for *fornix (Galen, c177)* in Duckworth translation (1962, p. 14).
14. *ajaz (Avicenna or Ibn Sina, c1030)*
In the *Canon*, Avicenna referred to *fornix (Galen, c177)* as *ajaz*, which in Arabic can mean "long-roofed chamber"; see Singer (1952, p. 80 note 59).
15. *tortoise shell (Achillini, 1520)*
Synonym for macrodissected adult human *fornix (Galen, c177)*; see Lind translation (1975, p. 58). According to Singer (1952, pp. 42–43, 80 note 58), when Vesalius (and presumably Achillini) used the term they had in mind a siege device known as *testudo*, a curved rectangular shield held by a group of heavily armed soldiers over their heads in a combined defensive maneuver.
16. *testudo (Achillini, 1520)*
Latin word for *tortoise shell (Achillini, 1520)*. *Testudo* also means a curved stringed instrument such as a lyre, as well as an arch or vault, and Vicq d'Azyr (1786, p. 31) quoted a Latin translation from Galen's *On the Usefulness of the Parts* (see May translation, 1968, p. 415) where "arches" is rendered "testudines."
17. *extremity of septum (Massa, 1536)*
May refer to rostral end of macrodissected adult human *fornix (Galen, c177)*; that is, segment of ***fimbria (Honegger, 1890)*** rostral to *body of fornix (Vesalius, 1543a)* along with ***septal postcommissural fornix (>1840)***; see f. 83 and Lind (1975, p. 237), who translated it *extremity of diaphragm*. Also see *oven of brain (Massa, 1536)*.
18. *extremitates septi (Massa, 1536)*
Latin form (plural) of *extremity of septum (Massa, 1536)*; f. 83. See Burdach (1822, p. 359) and Lind (1975, p. 237), who translated it (plural) *extremities of diaphragm*.
19. *leg of vaulted body (Paré, 1550)*
One of the legs of the *vaulted body with three legs (Paré, 1550)*; f. 56v.
20. *corpus psalloeides (Dubois, 1556)*
Probably synonym for *psalidoeides (Galen, c177)*; f. 91, see Burdach (1822, p. 357). Also spelled *corpus psalloides*; see Günther (1786, p. 12).
21. *anterior crus of fornix (Colombo, 1559)*
Colombo's reference to this macrodissected adult human structure was very brief, and presumably corresponds to *anterior pillar of fornix (Paré, 1564)*; p. 192. Paré referred earlier in French to *vaulted body with three legs (Paré, 1550)* but did not actually name the legs anterior and posterior.
22. *anterior pillar of fornix (Paré, 1564)*
From Paré's brief reference to this term it is impossible to know exactly what he meant; see translation (1634, p. 168). It might be safest to assume that Vesling (1647, Ch. 14, Tab. 2-*F*) illustrated what was commonly understood by the term in macrodissected adult human; see *anterior crus of fornix (Vesling, 1647)*. Also see *vaulted body with three pillars (Paré, 1561)*. Vesling's description was based directly on ***fornix (Vesalius, 1543a)***.
23. *anterior column of fornix (Riolan, 1618)*
Apparently synonym for macrodissected adult human *anterior pillar of fornix (Paré, 1564)*; in the original Latin, *anteriores fornicis columna*, p. 418.
24. *anterior crus of fornix (Vesling, 1647)*
In modern terms, it seems likely that what Vesling illustrated for macrodissected adult human *anterior crus of fornix (Vesling, 1647)* included segment of ***fimbria (Honegger, 1890)*** rostral to ***dorsal hippocampal commissure (Craigie, 1925)***, along with accompanying ***intermediate hippocampal commissure (>1840)*** and ***ventral hippocampal commissure (Craigie, 1925)***, ***septal postcommissural fornix (>1840)***, and probably initial, dorsal part of ***hypothalamic postcommissural fornix (>1840)***; Ch. 14, Table 2-*F*. Also see *anterior pillar of fornix (Paré, 1564)*.
25. *foremost leg of vault (Riolan, 1657)*
English form of *anterior crus of fornix (Colombo, 1559)*; second Table, Ch. 14, Figure 1-*F*. Haller (1762, p. 35) used the Latin (plural) form, *crura anteriora fornicis*.
26. *fornix itself (Willis, 1664)*
Roughly describes macrodissected adult human and sheep part of ***fornix (Vesalius, 1543a)*** between *root of fornix (Willis, 1664)* rostrally and *arm of fornix (Willis, 1664)* caudally. It is segment of ***fimbria (Honegger, 1890)*** coextensive with ***hippocampal commissures (>1840)*** and part or all of ***septal postcommissural fornix (>1840)***; see Pordage translation (1681, p. 61). Willis divided it into *trunk of fornix (Willis, 1664)* caudally and *base of fornix (Willis, 1664)* rostrally.
27. *vault itself (Willis, 1664)*
Synonym for *fornix itself (Willis, 1664)*, at least partly because Willis also used the simple term *vault (Willis, 1664)* for *corpus callosum (Willis, 1664)*; see Pordage translation (1681, p. 61). Also see *psalidoeides (Galen, 177)*, *oven of brain (Massa, 1536)*.
28. *fornix (Willis, 1664)*
In macrodissected adult sheep, and presumably human, it included a caudal *arm of fornix (Willis, 1664)*, an intermediate *fornix itself (Willis, 1664)*—subdivided into caudal *trunk of fornix (Willis, 1664)* and rostral *basis of fornix (Willis, 1664)*—and a rostral *root of fornix (Willis, 1644)*; see Pordage translation (1681, pp. 61, 93–94 and Tab. VII).
29. *fimbria fornicis (Vieussens, 1684)*
Essentially synonymous with *fornix itself (Willis, 1664)* for macrodissected adult human; p. 60, see Meyer (1971, p. 21).
30. *fimbria of fornix (Vieussens, 1684)*
English form of *fimbria fornicis (Vieussens, 1684)*.
31. *fimbriatae veri fornicis appendix (Vieussens, 1684)*
The "fimbrial appendix of true fornix" is a synonym (English singular for Latin plural) for *fimbria fornicis (Vieussens, 1684)*; see p. 61 and Tables VI-*D*, VII-*E*, VIII-*B*, IX-*C*, XI-*G*. Also see *fornix vera (Vieussens, 1684)*. Burdach (1822, pp. 59–61) gave Vieussens's

term somewhat incorrectly as *appendix fimbriata veri fornicis*.

32. *fimbrial appendix of true fornix (Vieussens, 1684)*
English form of *fimbriatae veri fornicis appendix (Vieussens, 1684)*.

33. *foremost thigh of arch (Diemerbroeck, 1689)*
Synonym for macrodissected adult human *foremost leg of vault (Riolan, 1657)*; p. 398.

34. *body of fornix (Ridley, 1695)*
A "broadish medullary Body" essentially corresponding to macrodissected adult human *fornix (Willis, 1664)*; pp. 117–118.

35. *fornix (Ridley, 1695)*
Synonym for *body of fornix (Ridley, 1695)*.

36. *posterior pillar of fornix (Pourfour du Petit, 1710)*
Very brief account of macrodissected adult human ***fornix (Vesalius, 1543a)*** vaguely described *posterior pillar of fornix (Pourfour du Petit, 1710)* as extending up from ***inferior horn of lateral ventricle (Bell, 1802)*** to run under ***corpus callosum (Galen, c177)*** and then turn down into *septum (Galen, c177)*, where it splits into right and left [*anterior*] *pillar of fornix (Pourfour du Petit, 1710)* extending to ***mammillary body (Ludwig, 1779)***; in the original French (plural), *piliers posterieurs de la voute*, p. 13. Also see *pillar of fornix (Pourfour du Petit, 1710)*. Thus, *posterior pillar of fornix (Pourfour du Petit, 1710)* consisted of ***fimbria (Honegger, 1890)*** and indeterminate part of rostrally adjacent ***septal postcommissural fornix (>1840)***.

37. *anterior pillar of fornix (Winslow, 1733)*
As described for macrodissected adult human ***fornix (Vesalius, 1543a)***, segment between *posterior pillar of fornix (Winslow, 1733)* caudally and *root of anterior pillar of fornix (Winslow, 1733)* rostrally; Section X, p. 35. In modern terms, segment of ***fornix (Vesalius, 1543a)*** containing ***intermediate hippocampal commissure (>1840)***, ***ventral hippocampal commissure (Craigie, 1925)***, and ***septal postcommissural fornix (>1840)***.

38. *anterior crus of fornix (Haller, 1762)*
Probably corresponds to macrodissected adult human *anterior pillar of fornix (Winslow, 1733)* and *root of anterior pillar of fornix (Winslow, 1733)* considered together; p. 36. Also see Honegger (1890, p. 216).

39. *body of fornix (Monro, 1783)*
Apparently synonymous with macrodissected adult human *fornix (Galen, c177)*; Table II-P. Burdach (1822, pp. 138, 357) also used the term thus; in Latin, *corpus fornicis*.

40. *anterior column of medullary triangle (Vicq d'Azyr, 1786)*
Synonym for macrodissected adult human *anterior pillar of fornix (Winslow, 1733)*; Plate XXV-38, and Plates VI and VIII. Also see *medullary triangle (Vicq d'Azyr, 1786)*.

41. *anterior column of vault with three pillars (Vicq d'Azyr, 1786)*
Synonym for *anterior column of medullary triangle (Vicq d'Azyr, 1786)*; Plate XIV, Figure III-7 and Plate XXV-38.

42. *tegmentum of third ventricle (Günther, 1786)*
Synonym for macrodissected adult human *fornix (Galen, c177)*; in the original Latin, *tertius ventriculus tegmentum*, p. 12.

43. *anterior peduncle of trigone (Chaussier, 1807)*
Apparently synonym for macrodissected adult human *anterior column of medullary triangle (Vicq d'Azyr, 1786)*; in the original French (plural), *pédoncules antérieur du trigone*, p. 55. Burdach (1822, p. 357) gave the Latin (plural), *pedunculi anteriores trigoni cerebralis*.

44. *body of fornix (Reil, 1812b)*
Synonym for macrodissected adult human *anterior column of medullary triangle (Vicq d'Azyr, 1786)*; see Mayo translation (1823, pp. 52, 115).

45. *anterior extremity of vault (Cloquet, 1816)*
Synonym for macrodissected adult human *anterior pillar of fornix (Paré, 1564)*; in the original French, *extrémité antérieure de la voûte*, p. 553.

46. *anterior pillar of longitudinal commissure (Solly, 1836)*
Synonym for macrodissected adult human *anterior pillar of fornix (Winslow, 1733)*; p. 182.

47. *fornix column (Herrick, 1915)*
Synonym for macrodissected adult human *anterior crus of fornix (Haller, 1762)*; see p. 330.

48. *anterior pillar of fornix (Herrick, 1915)*
Synonym for macrodissected adult human *anterior crus of fornix (Haller, 1762)*; see p. 330.

49. *fornix (Demeter et al., 1985)*
In adult monkey with macrodissection and histological methods for ***axons (Kölliker, 1896)***, *postcommissural fornix (Loo, 1931)* and *fimbria of hippocampus (Henle, 1871)* considered together, although definition is vague; p. 32 and Figures 4–8, 12.

fourth ventricle (Galen, c192)

The ***ventricle (Hippocrates)*** associated with the ***primary hindbrain vesicle (Baer, 1837)*** of the ***vertebrate neural tube (Baer, 1837)***, both during development and in adult; it lies between the ***cerebral aqueduct (>1840)*** rostrally and ***central canal (Bellingeri, 1823)*** caudally. It was clearly described long ago as *base of brain (Herophilus, c335–c280 BC)*, and Galen used the term in its modern sense in *On Anatomical Procedures* for macrodissected adult beef, pig, and/or macaque but not human; see Duckworth translation (1962, p. 19), Singer translation (1999, p. 235).

ALTERNATE SPELLINGS:

1. *fourth ventrycle (Geminus, 1553)*
Early English form of ***fourth ventricle (Galen, c192)***; see *The tables of the brayne*, Figure 9-*I*.

EARLIER REFERENCES:

Earlier synonyms:

1. *base of brain (Herophilus, c335–c280 BC)*
According to Galen in *De Historia Philosopha*, Herophilus referred thus to ***fourth ventricle (Galen, c192)***, which he is credited with discovering. The term may have also included ***cerebellum (Aristotle)***; see von Staden (1989, p. 247, 314). Herophilus suggested that this part of the ***brain (Smith Papyrus, c1700 BC)*** is the most important "command center" of the body, perhaps the earliest significant attempt

at ***brain (Smith Papyrus, c1700 BC)*** localization of function; see Pagel (1958, p. 97), von Staden (1989, pp. 247- 248), Gross (1998, p. 27).

2. *ventricle of cerebellum (Herophilus, c335–c280 BC)*
According to Galen in *On the Usefulness of the Parts* (c173), Herophilus also referred to ***fourth ventricle (Galen, c192)*** thus; see von Staden (1989, p. 247). Haller (1762, p. 76) referred to Oribasius on this matter.
3. *most principal ventricle (Herophilus, c335–c280 BC)*
According to Bauhin (1605, p. 603), synonym for ***fourth ventricle (Galen, c192)***; in Latin, *principalissimum*, see Crooke translation (1615, p. 469).
4. *noble ventricle (Herophilus, c335–c280 BC)*
According to Burdach (1822, p. 301), synonym for ***fourth ventricle (Galen, c192)***, which Herophilus considered the most important ***ventricle (Hippocrates)***. The most relevant documentation is in Galen (c173; see May translation, 1968, p. 415), also see Bartholin (1651, p. 326; 1662, pp. 137, 138).
5. *ventriculus nobilis (Herophilus, c335–c280 BC)*
Latin form of *noble ventricle (Herophilus, c335–c280 BC)*; see Burdach (1822, p. 301).
6. *posterior ventricle (Galen, c177)*
Synonym frequently used for ***fourth ventricle (Galen, c192)***, in, for example, *On Anatomical Procedures*; see von Staden (1989, p. 199).

LATER SYNONYMS:

1. *first ventricle (Galen, c192)*
In the later books of *On Anatomical Procedures*, Galen referred to *posterior ventricle (Galen, c177)* or ***fourth ventricle (Galen, c192)*** as such; see Duckworth translation (1962, p. 25). Tiedemann (1816) used the term more recently; see translation (1826, p. 178).
2. *hindmost ventricle (Avicenna, c1030)*
According to du Laurens (1599, p. 408), Avicenna referred thus to *posterior ventricle (Galen, 177)* or ***fourth ventricle (Galen, c192)***; p. 528, see Crooke translation (1615, p. 528). By extension, it would be Avicenna's *third ventricle*; see *cerebral ventricles (Galen, c192)* and *cells (Anatomia Magistri Nicolai physici, early 12th century)*. Hall (1565, p. 40) referred to it as *hindermost ventricle of cerebellum*.
3. *third ventricle (Avicenna, c1030)*
Synonym for *hindmost ventricle (Avicenna, c1030)*; also used by Geminus (1553, f. BII).
4. *cellula memorialis (Anatomia Magistri Nicolai physici, early 12th century; Guillaume de Conches, c1100–1154)*
According to the most popular version of the three cell theory of ***brain (Smith Papyrus, c1700 BC)*** function, the ***fourth ventricle (Galen, c192)*** is the "cell for memory" (see Corner, 1927, p. 71; Manzoni, 1998, p. 125).
5. *hind ventricle (Mondino, 1316)*
Synonym for macrodissected adult human ***fourth ventricle (Galen, c192)*** in *Anathomia*; see Singer translation (1925, pp. 91–93).
6. *sinus of cerebellum (Benedetti, 1502)*
Synonym for macrodissected adult human ***fourth ventricle (Galen, c192)***; see Lind translation (1975, p. 116).
7. *venter posterior (Berengario da Carpi, 1522)*
Alternate Latin form of macrodissected adult human *posterior ventricle (Galen, c177)*; f. 443. Also see Berengario da Carpi (1523, bottom figure on f. 56).
8. *rear ventricle (Berengario da Carpi, 1522)*
Synonym for macrodissected adult human ***fourth ventricle (Galen, c192)***; see Lind translation (1959, p. 144).
9. *posterior sinus (de Laguna, 1535)*
Synonym for macrodissected adult human ***fourth ventricle (Galen, c192)***; see Lind translation (1975, p. 287).
10. *ventriculus cerebello et medullae dorsali communis (Vesalius, 1543a)*
Synonym for macrodissected adult human ***fourth ventricle (Galen, c192)***; p. 530, as pointed out by Burdach (1822, p. 302).
11. *common cavity of cerebellum and dorsal marrow (Vesalius, 1543a)*
English form of *ventriculus cerebello et medullae dorsalis communis (Vesalius, 1543a)*; see Singer (1952, p. 100).
12. *ventricle common to medulla dorsalis and cerebellum (Vesalius, 1543a)*
Synonym for *common cavity of cerebellum and dorsal marrow (Vesalius, 1543a)*; see Singer translation (1952, p. 104).
13. *hollowness common to cerebellum and marrow of back (Geminus, 1553)*
Synonym for macrodissected adult human *common cavity of cerebellum and dorsal marrow (Vesalius, 1543a)*; originally spelled *holounes common to cerebellum and marie of the backe*, see *The tables of the brayne*, Figure 7-*K*.
14. *common ventricle of marrow of back and cerebellum (Geminus, 1553)*
Synonym for *hollowness common to cerebellum and marrow of back (Geminus, 1553)*; originally spelled *common ventricle of marye of the backe and of the cerebellum*, see *The tables of the brayne*, Figure 9-*I*.
15. *last ventricle (Hall, 1565)*
Synonym for macrodissected adult human ***fourth ventricle (Galen, c192)***; p. 38.
16. *cerebellar cistern (Aranzi, 1587)*
Synonym for macrodissected adult human ***fourth ventricle (Galen, c192)***; see Gall & Spurzheim (1810, p. 185), Clarke & O'Malley (1996, p. 720).
17. *cistern between cerebellum and spinal cord (Aranzi, 1587)*
Synonym for macrodissected adult human ***fourth ventricle (Galen, c192)***; see Diemerbroeck (1689, p. 404), Clarke & O'Malley translation (1996, p. 720).
18. *cisterna spirituum (Aranzi, 1587)*
Synonym for macrodissected adult human ***fourth ventricle (Galen, c192)***; see Ridley (1695, pp. 133–134).
19. *fourth sinus (du Laurens, 1600)*
Synonym for macrodissected adult human ***fourth ventricle (Galen, c192)***; in Latin, *sinus quartus*, see Bauhin (1605, p. 602).
20. *backward ventricle (Crooke, 1615)*
English form of *posterior ventricle (Galen, 177)*, that is, ***fourth ventricle (Galen, c192)***; p. 528. Crooke's translation was based on du Laurens (1599, p. 408).

21. *hinder braine-pan (Nemesius, 1636)*
English term used for ***fourth ventricle (Galen, c192)*** in this translation of Nemesius's 4th-century work, *On the Nature of Man*; p. 306.
22. *calamus scriptorius (Read, 1638)*
Apparently synonym for macrodissected adult human ***fourth ventricle (Galen, c192)*** as a whole; p. 421. Many years later Chaussier (1807, p. 100) noted that the term (*plume à écrive* in French) was still sometimes used in this sense.
23. *four bellies (Willis, 1664)*
Synonym for ***fourth ventricle (Galen, c192)***; see Pordage translation (1681, p. 67).
24. *ventriculum nobilem (Collins, 1685)*
Different form of *ventriculus nobilis (Herophilus, c335–c280 BC)*; p. 1019.
25. *rhomboidaea caveae (Haller, 1762)*
Synonym for macrodissected adult human ***fourth ventricle (Galen, c192)***; p. 76. In 1747 (see Mihles translation, 1754b, p. 296) Haller noted that ***fourth ventricle (Galen, c192)*** has rhomboid figure or shape.
26. *rhomboid cavity (Haller, 1762)*
English form of *rhomboidaea caveae (Haller, 1762)*.
27. *fifth ventricle (Wenzel & Wenzel, 1812)*
Synonym for macrodissected adult human ***fourth ventricle (Galen, c192)***; in Latin, *ventriculus quintus*, see Burdach (1822, p. 302).
28. *stylus scriptorius (Ramsay, 1813)*
Synonym listed for macrodissected adult human ***fourth ventricle (Galen, c192)***; p. 46.
29. *central fissure of cerebellum (Gordon, 1815)*
Apparently synonym for macrodissected adult human ***fourth ventricle (Galen, c192)***; pp. 113, 119, 186.
30. *spino-cerebellar ventricle (Gordon, 1815)*
Gordon suggested it as better synonym for macrodissected adult human ***fourth ventricle (Galen, c192)***; p. 187.

PARTLY CORRESPONDS:

1. *calamus scriptorius (Ridley, 1695)*
Extreme caudal end of macrodissected adult human ***fourth ventricle (Galen, c192)***; Figure VII-*n*.
2. *cistern of Aranzi (Tarin, 1753)*
Eponym for *ventricle of Aranzi (Mayer, 1779)*; in the original Latin, *cysterna Arantii*, p. 24.
3. *ventricle of Aranzi (Mayer 1779)*
Eponym for roughly caudal or medullary half of macrodissected adult human ***fourth ventricle (Galen, c192)*** associated with ***floor of fourth ventricle (Reil, 1807–1808a)***; in the original Latin, *ventriculus Arantii*, p. 22, according to Burdach (1822, p. 303). Foster (1894, p. 3013) defined it as "The small depression or cavity at the pointed extremity of the calamus scriptorius."
4. *fossette of fourth ventricle (Chaussier, 1807)*
Synonym for macrodissected adult human *rhomboidal sinus (Meckel, 1817)*; in the original French, *fossette du quatrième ventricule*, p. 125.
5. *foveola ventriculi quarti (Chaussier, 1807)*
Latin form of *fossette of fourth ventricle (Chaussier, 1807)*; see Meckel (1832, Vol. 2, p. 422).
6. *angular fossette of fourth ventricle (Chaussier, 1807)*
Synonym for *fossette of fourth ventricle (Chaussier, 1807)*; in the original French, *fossette angulaire du quatrième ventricule*, p. 194.
7. *triangular fossa (Gordon, 1815)*
Apparently synonym for macrodissected adult human *rhomboidal sinus (Meckel, 1817)*; pp. 120, 179–180. Meckel (1817) gave the Latin as *fossa triangularis*, see translation (1832, Vol. 2, p. 422).
8. *rhomboidal sinus (Meckel, 1817)*
For macrodissected adult human, caudal part of ***fourth ventricle (Galen, c192)***, caudal to ***lateral recess of fourth ventricle (>1840)*** and roughly coextensive with ***medulla (Winslow, 1733)***; see translation (1832, Vol. 2, pp. 422, 458, 460) and Burdach (1822, p. 303); in Latin, *sinus rhomboideus*. Also see *fourth ventricle (Meckel, 1817)*.
9. *sinus of medulla oblongata (Meckel, 1817)*
Synonym listed for macrodissected adult human *rhomboidal sinus (Meckel, 1817)*; see translation (1832, Vol. 2, p. 422).
10. *sinus bulbi rachidici (Meckel, 1817)*
Synonym listed for macrodissected adult human *rhomboidal sinus (Meckel, 1817)*; see translation (1832, Vol. 2, p. 422).
11. *ventricle of Aranzi (Meckel, 1817)*
Eponym listed for macrodissected adult human *rhomboidal sinus (Meckel, 1817)*; in Latin, *ventriculus Arantii*, see translation (1832, Vol. 2, p. 422).
12. *fossa of fourth ventricle (Meckel, 1817)*
Synonym listed for macrodissected adult human *rhomboidal sinus (Meckel, 1817)*; see translation (1832, Vol. 2, p. 422); variation on *foveola ventriculi quarti (Chaussier, 1807)*.
13. *fourth ventricle (Meckel, 1817)*
For macrodissected adult human, rostral half of ***fourth ventricle (Galen, c192)***, roughly associated with ***pons (Haller, 1747)***; see translation (1832, Vol. 2, p. 460), *ventricle of cerebellum (Meckel, 1817)*, and *rhomboidal sinus (Meckel, 1817)*.
14. *ventricle of cerebellum (Meckel, 1817)*
Synonym for *fourth ventricle (Meckel, 1817)*; see translation (1832, Vol. 2, p. 460).
15. *fifth ventricle (Meckel, 1817)*
Synonym for *fourth ventricle (Meckel, 1817)*; see translation (1832, Vol. 2, p. 460).

frenulum (Vieussens, 1684)

As described for macrodissected adult human, a rostral extension in the median plane of the ***rostral medullary vellum (>1840)*** between the adult human right and left ***inferior colliculus (Haller, 1762)***; see Mettler (1948, Fig. 106, *frenulum veli*), Crosby et al. (1962, Fig. 97). For Vieussens's use in macrodissected adult human, its first description, see Chapter 11, p. 73 and Tables VIII-*g*, IX-*f*; also see Burdach (1822, p. 336).

EARLIER REFERENCES:

Earlier synonyms:

1. *parvus ac brevis tractus medullaris (Vieussens, 1684)*
Synonym for ***frenulum (Vieussens, 1684)***; Tables VIII-*g*, IX-*f*.

LATER SYNONYMS:
1. *frenulum veli anterioris (Arnold, 1838a)*
   Synonym for macrodissected adult human ***frenulum (Vieussens, 1684)***; p. 41.

frontal forceps (>1840)

As described for macrodissected adult human, extension of the ***rostrum of corpus callosum (Reil, 1809b)*** into the region of the ***frontal pole (>1840)*** and thus a ***radiation of corpus callosum (Dejerine & Dejerine-Klumpke, 1895)*** in the ***cerebral cortex white matter (>1840)***; see Crosby et al. (1962, Fig. 277, called *anterior forceps*), *Nomina Anatomica* (1983, p. A71), *Terminologia Anatomica* (1998, p. 127), *Dorland's* (2003, p. 726). It was probably first clearly delineated as one of the two *forceps of corpus callosum (Reil, 1809b)* and first separately named the *lateral expansion of rostrum of corpus callosum (Reil, 1812c)*.

TRANSLATIONS:
1. *forceps frontalis (>1840)*
   Current Latin form of ***frontal forceps (>1840)***; see *Terminologia Anatomica* (1998, p. 127).

EARLIER REFERENCES:

Earlier synonyms:
1. *lateral expansion of rostrum of corpus callosum (Reil, 1812c)*
   Synonym for macrodissected adult human ***frontal forceps (>1840)***; see Mayo translation (1823, p. 120).
2. *forceps minor (Arnold, 1838a)*
   Synonym for macrodissected adult human *anterior forceps (Arnold, 1838a)*; p. 79.
3. *anterior forceps (Arnold, 1838a)*
   Synonym for macrodissected adult human ***frontal forceps (>1840)***; in the original Latin, *forceps anterior*, p. 79.

frontal nerve (Cheselden, 1726)

As described for macrodissected adult human, the largest branch of the ***ophthalmic nerve (Winslow, 1733)*** dividing into a smaller ***supratrochlear nerve (Schaarschmidt, 1750)*** and a larger ***supraorbital nerve (Meckel, 1753, p. 42)***; see Williams & Warwick (1980, p. 1059 and Fig. 7.186), Hamilton (1976, Fig. 791). For Cheselden's use in macrodissected adult human, see p. 262 (and p. 254); Alexander Monro *primus* wrote the chapter on the ***nerves (Herophilus, c335–c280 BC)*** in Cheselden. It was known to Galen; see ***[frontal nerve (Cheselden, 1726)] (Galen, c173)***.

TRANSLATIONS:
1. *nervus frontalis (Cheselden, 1726)*
   Original Latin form of ***frontal nerve (Cheselden, 1726)***; in full, *nervus frontalis quinti*, p. 262.
2. *frontalis nervus (Haase, 1781)*
   Latin form of ***frontal nerve (Cheselden, 1726)***; see Index, section 102.

EARLIER REFERENCES:

Described, not named or illustrated:
1. ***[frontal nerve (Cheselden, 1726)] (Galen, c173)***
   Described for macrodissected adult beef, pig, and/or macaque but not human; see May translation (1968, p. 455).

Illustrated, not named or described:
1. ***[frontal nerve (Cheselden, 1726)] (Eustachi, 1552)***
   Clearly illustrated for macrodissected adult human; see Albinus edition (1761, Tab. 18, Figs. 1, 3, 5-*y,A,B,Z*) and Meckel (1748, p. 31 note *z*).

Earlier synonyms:
1. *superior branch of first and superior branch of third pair (Marchetti, 1652)*
   Synonym for macrodissected adult human ***frontal nerve (Cheselden, 1726)***; p. 122.
2. *second–fourth shoots of uppermost branch of second division of fifth pair of nerves arising within skull (Willis, 1664)*
   Roughly synonymous with macrodissected adult, presumably human, ***frontal nerve (Cheselden, 1726)***; see Pordage translation (1681, p. 144, Fig. 1-*C,d,ee*).
3. *ramulus primus rami minoris superioris nervus quintae conjugationis (Vieussens, 1684)*
   Roughly synonymous with macrodissected adult human ***frontal nerve (Cheselden, 1726)***; p. 170 and Table 22-*d*.

LATER SYNONYMS:
1. *superior ramus of ophthalmic nerve (Winslow, 1733)*
   Synonym for macrodissected adult human ***frontal nerve (Cheselden, 1726)***; Section VI, p. 63 (and p. 59).
2. *frontal ramus of ophthalmic nerve (Winslow, 1733)*
   Synonym for macrodissected adult human ***frontal nerve (Cheselden, 1726)***; Section VI, p. 63 (and p. 59).
3. *superciliary nerve (Winslow, 1733)*
   Synonym for macrodissected adult human ***frontal nerve (Cheselden, 1726)***; in the original Latin, *nervus superciliaris*, Section VI, p. 63 (and p. 59). Burdin (1803 translation, Vol. 1, p. 170) spelled it *supercilian nerve*.
4. *frontal branch of first branch of fifth pair of nerves (Meckel, 1753)*
   Synonym for macrodissected adult human ***frontal nerve (Cheselden, 1726)***; in the original French, *le rameau frontal du premier rameau du nerf de la cinquième paire*, p. 40.
5. *ophthalmico-frontal branch of first branch of fifth pair of nerves (Meckel, 1753)*
   Synonym for macrodissected adult human ***frontal nerve (Cheselden, 1726)***; in the original French, *le rameau ophtalmico-frontal du premier rameau du nerf de la cinquième paire*, p. 40.
6. *first branch of superior palpebral nerve (Meckel, 1753)*
   Apparently synonym for macrodissected adult human ***frontal nerve (Cheselden, 1726)***; in the original French, *le premier rameau du nerf de la paupiere supérieure*, p. 40.
7. *ophthalmicofrontal nerve (Le Cat, 1768)*
   Synonym for macrodissected adult human ***frontal nerve (Cheselden, 1726)***; Plate VIII, Figure 1-*S*.
8. *palpebro-frontal nerve (Burdin, 1803)*
   Synonym for macrodissected adult human ***frontal nerve (Cheselden, 1726)***; see translation (1803, Vol. 1, p. 170).

9. *frontal branch of ophthalmic nerve (Knox, 1832)*
   Synonym for macrodissected adult human *frontal ramus of ophthalmic nerve (Winslow, 1733)*; Supplemental Plate I-3.
10. *superior branch of first division of fifth pair of nerves (Todd, 1836–1839)*
   Synonym for macrodissected adult human ***frontal nerve (Cheselden, 1726)***; p. 279.
11. *middle branch of first division of fifth pair of nerves (Todd, 1836–1839)*
   Synonym for macrodissected adult human ***frontal nerve (Cheselden, 1726)***; p. 279.

PARTLY CORRESPONDS:

1. *anastomotic branch of greater frontal nerve (Mayer, 1794)*
   Communicating branch (Winslow, 1733) of macrodissected adult human ***frontal nerve (Cheselden, 1726)*** with ***temporal branches of facial nerve (Swan, 1830)***; in the original Latin, *ramus anastomoticus nervi frontalis majoris*; Part 5, Table VII-3 (p. 43).
2. *ocular fat fascicle (Bellingeri, 1818)*
   Macrodissected adult human branch of ***frontal nerve (Cheselden, 1726)*** to retro-orbital fat pad; in the original Latin, *fasciculus pinguedineus oculi*, see Table I.
3. *frontonasal branch of frontal nerve (Cruveilhier, 1836)*
   Not infrequent third major branch from inner side of macrodissected adult human ***frontal nerve (Cheselden, 1726)*** ending in upper eyelid; in the original French, *rameau fronto-nasal*, p. 912.

frontal operculum (>1840)

As described for macrodissected adult human, the surface of the ***frontal region (Vicq d'Azyr, 1786)*** lining the dorsal wall of the ***lateral cerebral sulcus (>1840)*** up to the ***circular sulcus (Schwalbe, 1881)*** and involving the ***orbital part of inferior frontal gyrus (>1840), triangular part of inferior frontal gyrus (>1840), opercular part of inferior frontal gyrus (>1840)***, and ventral (lower) end of ***precentral gyrus (>1840)***; see Carpenter (1976, Fig. 2.3), *Terminologia Anatomica* (1998, p. 125), *Dorland's* (2003, p. 1316). It was perhaps first clearly described as the *roof of Sylvian fissure (Meckel, 1817)*.

EARLIER REFERENCES:

Earlier synonyms:

1. *roof of Sylvian fissure (Meckel, 1817)*
   Roughly synonymous with macrodissected adult human ***frontal operculum (>1840)***; see translation (1832, Vol. 2, p. 442).

frontal pole (>1840)

As described for macrodissected adult human, the rostral tip of the ***frontal region (Vicq d'Azyr, 1786)*** of the ***cerebral cortex gray matter (>1840)***; see Williams & Warwick (1980, p. 982), *Terminologia Anatomica* (1998, p. 125). Attention was first drawn to it as the *mamillary process (Vesalius, 1543a)*.

EARLIER REFERENCES:

Earlier synonyms:

1. *mamillary process (Vesalius, 1543a)*
   Vesalius wrote that what roughly corresponds to macrodissected adult human ***frontal pole (>1840)*** is usually called thus; see Richardson & Carman translation (2009, p. 247 and Figs. 12-*I*, 13-C). Vesalius also pointed out that some people believe it has olfactory function; see Richardson & Carman translation (2002, pp. 179, 267). Also see ***[olfactory ventricle (>1840)] (Galen, c173)*** and *organ of smelling (du Laurens, 1599)*. Haly Abbas had long before referred to underlying ***olfactory bulb (Weitbrecht, 1751)***, perhaps along with ***olfactory peduncle (Solly, 1836)***, as a *nipple (Haly Abbas or Ali ibn' ul-Abbas, d. 994)*. Singer (1952; p. 70 and Figs. 12-*I*, 13-C) loosely translated it *mammillary prominence*.
2. *mammillary prominence (Vesalius, 1543a)*
   Singer's (1952; p. 70 and Figs. 12-*I*, 13-C) loose translation of *processus mamillares (Vesalius, 1543a)*.
3. *processus mamillares (Vesalius, 1543a)*
   Latin form of *mamillary process (Vesalius, 1543a)*; Book 7, Figure 12-*I*. Also see Geminus (1553, *The tables of the brayne*, Fig. 12-*I*).
4. *mastoid process (Vesalius, 1543a)*
   Richardson and Carman (2002, p. 170) translated Vesalius's "*mamillarem*" as *mastoid* rather than *mamillary* for ***frontal pole (>1840)***.
5. *mastoid swelling (Vesalius, 1543a)*
   Synonym for *mastoid process (Vesalius, 1543a)*; see Richardson & Carman translation (2002, p. 181).
6. *mamillaris processus cerebri (Geminus, 1553)*
   Synonym for macrodissected adult human *processus mamillares (Vesalius, 1543a)*. Geminus wrote, "The knobbes of the brayne, which for the similitude and lykenes that they have with the teates, are called Mamillaris processus cerebri." (see *The tables of the brayne*, Fig. 13-C).
7. *teat (Crooke, 1615)*
   Translation of *processus mamillares (Vesalius, 1543a)*; p. 454 and Table 14, Fig. 19-CC. Also see the description in English of *mamillaris processus cerebri (Geminus, 1553)*.
8. *frontal horn (Cruveilhier, 1836)*
   Synonym for macrodissected adult human ***frontal pole (>1840)***; in the original French, *corne frontale*, p. 658.
9. *mammillary caruncle (Arnold, 1838b)*
   Synonym for macrodissected adult human ***frontal pole (>1840)***; in the original Latin, *caruncula mammillaris*, Plate III, Figure 1-η.

frontal region (Vicq d'Azyr, 1786)

As described for macrodissected adult human, a topographic division of the ***cerebral cortex gray matter (>1840)*** lying rostral to the ***parietal region (>1840)***. Its main parts are the ***orbital region (Rolando, 1831), inferior frontal gyrus (>1840), middle frontal gyrus (>1840), superior frontal gyrus (>1840), medial frontal gyrus (>1840)***, and ***precentral gyrus (>1840)***; for general modern overview, see Nieuwenhuys et al. (2008, p. 620 ff.). ***Frontal region (Vicq d'Azyr, 1786)*** is preferred to *frontal lobe (Rolando, 1831)* because an actual lobe cannot be distinguished and because the term *region* applies to all mammals, whether gyrencephalic or lissencephalic. For Vicq d'Azyr's use in macrodissected adult human see Plate III-*o* and Plate III-*f*, where he noted that its *cerebral gyri (Vesalius, 1543a)* are arranged roughly longitudinally. It was first alluded to vaguely as the *lowest brain substance (Dryander, 1536)*, and then more specifically as the *cerebrum applied to frontal bone (Vesalius, 1543a)*.

EARLIER REFERENCES:

Earlier synonyms:

1. *lowest brain substance (Dryander, 1536)*
   Dryander indicated roughly location of macrodissected adult human ***frontal region (Vicq d'Azyr, 1786)*** in Figure 8 and its legend (see Lind translation, 1975, p. 302), where he indicated it is lowest substance of *anterior part of brain (Berengario da Carpi, 1523)*. He also indicated position of ***temporal region (>1840)*** with term *lower substance of brain (Dryander, 1536)*, and indicated "posterior" in the cranium (Fig. 7; see Lind translation, 1975, p. 301). This crudely foreshadowed *anterior cerebral prominence (Varoli, 1573)*, *middle cerebral prominence (Varoli, 1573)*, and *posterior cerebral prominence (Varoli, 1573)*.
2. *cerebrum applied to frontal bone (Vesalius, 1543a)*
   Vesalius referred to "those parts of the cerebrum... applied to the frontal bone" (Singer translation, 1952, p. 34), description of what would later be named ***frontal region (Vicq d'Azyr, 1786)***.
3. *anterior cerebral prominence (Varoli, 1573)*
   Roughly synonymous with macrodissected adult human ***frontal region (Vicq d'Azyr, 1786)***, lying in anterior cranial fossa; see folios 5–6 and Figure I on f. 17v. Also see Meyer (1971, p. 122), Clarke & O'Malley (1996, p. 822).
4. *forward prominence of brain (Crooke, 1615)*
   Translation of *anterior cerebral prominence (Varoli, 1573)*; pp. 497–498.
5. *forepart of brain (Crooke, 1615)*
   Translation of *anterior cerebral prominence (Varoli, 1573)*; p. 497.
6. *prow of brain (Willis, 1664)*
   Roughly synonymous with macrodissected adult human ***frontal region (Vicq d'Azyr, 1786)***; see Pordage translation (1681, p. 57).
7. *anterior cerebral lobe (Willis, 1664)*
   Roughly synonymous with macrodissected adult human ***frontal region (Vicq d'Azyr, 1786)***; see Pordage translation (1681, p. 91, Tab. I-*A*), also see Meyer (1971, p. 122) and *cerebral lobes (Willis, 1664)*. Willis suggested *anterior cerebral lobe (Willis, 1664)* and *posterior cerebral lobe (Willis, 1664)* have basically the same function (memory), with duplication being a safety factor, "So the Brain, like a Castle, divided into many Towers or places of Defense, is thereby made the stronger and harder to be taken." (Pordage translation, 1681, p. 91).
8. *fore lobe of brain (Gibson, 1682)*
   Synonym for macrodissected adult human *anterior cerebral lobe (Willis, 1664)*; Table XII-*A*.
9. *former lobe of brain (Ridley, 1695)*
   Synonym for macrodissected adult human *anterior cerebral lobe (Willis, 1664)*; p. 142.
10. *foremost lobe of brain (Cowper, 1698)*
   Synonym for macrodissected adult human *fore lobe of brain (Ridley, 1695)*; Table IX, Figure 1-*C*.

LATER SYNONYMS:

1. *frontal cerebral lobule (Chaussier, 1807)*
   Synonym for macrodissected adult human ***frontal region (Vicq d'Azyr, 1786)***; p. 37, see Meyer (1971, p. 122).
2. *frontal lobe (Rolando, 1831)*
   Synonym for macrodissected adult human ***frontal region (Vicq d'Azyr, 1786)***; in the original text, *lobo frontale*, p. 114. Also see *frontal lobe (Arnold, 1838a)*.

PARTLY CORRESPONDS:

1. *anterior lobe (Burdach, 1822)*
   Burdach meant by this term roughly "prefrontal region" of macrodissected adult human ***frontal region (Vicq d'Azyr, 1786)***, corresponding approximately to *areas 9–12* and *44–47 (Brodmann, 1909)*; p. 169.
2. *frontal lobe (Arnold, 1838a)*
   Macrodissected adult human *frontal lobe (Rolando, 1831)* but specifically without ***cerebral cortex gray matter (>1840)*** associated with ***frontal operculum (>1840)***, included in *intermediate lobe (Arnold, 1838a)*; in the original Latin, *lobus frontalis*, pp. 51–52.
3. *area frontopolaris (Brodmann, 1909, p. 137)*
   Original Latin form of *frontopolar area (Brodmann, 1909, p. 137)*; p. 137.
4. *frontopolar area (Brodmann, 1909, p. 137)*
   Based on cellular architecture in adult human, most rostral zone of ***frontal region (Vicq d'Azyr, 1786)***, including parts of ***medial frontal gyrus (>1840)***, ***superior frontal gyrus (>1840)***, and ***middle frontal gyrus (>1840)***; see Garey translation (1994, p. 116 and Figs. 85, 86).
5. *area 10 (Brodmann, 1909)*
   Synonym for adult human *frontopolar area (Brodmann, 1909, p. 137)*; in the original German, *Feld 10*, p. 137.
6. *area frontalis granularis (Brodmann, 1909)*
   Original Latin form of *frontal granular area (Brodmann, 1909)*; p. 137.
7. *granular frontal area (Brodmann, 1909)*
   Based on cellular architecture in adult human, middle zone of ***frontal region (Vicq d'Azyr, 1786)*** between *frontopolar area (Brodmann, 1909, p. 137)* rostrally and *intermediate frontal area (Brodmann, 1909)* caudally and including parts of ***medial frontal gyrus (>1840)***, ***superior frontal gyrus (>1840)***, and ***middle frontal gyrus (>1840)***; see Garey translation (1994, p. 116 and Figs. 85, 86).
8. *area 9 (Brodmann, 1909)*
   Synonym for adult human *granular frontal area (Brodmann, 1909)*; in the original German, *Feld 9*, p. 137.
9. *area frontalis intermedia (Brodmann, 1909)*

Original Latin form of *intermediate frontal area (Brodmann, 1909)*; p. 137.

10. *intermediate frontal area (Brodmann, 1909)*
Based on cellular architecture in adult human, middle zone of ***frontal region (Vicq d'Azyr, 1786)*** between *granular frontal area (Brodmann, 1909)* rostrally and *agranular frontal area (Brodmann, 1909)* caudally and including parts of ***medial frontal gyrus (>1840)***, ***superior frontal gyrus (>1840)***, and ***middle frontal gyrus (>1840)***; see Garey translation (1994, p. 116 and Figs. 85, 86).

11. *area 8 (Brodmann, 1909)*
Synonym for adult human *intermediate frontal area (Brodmann, 1909)*; in the original German, *Feld 8*, p. 137.12. *area frontalis agranularis (Brodmann, 1909)*
Original Latin form of *agranular frontal area (Brodmann, 1909)*; p. 136.

13. *agranular frontal area (Brodmann, 1909)*
Based on cellular architecture in adult human, caudal zone of ***frontal region (Vicq d'Azyr, 1786)*** between *intermediate frontal area (Brodmann, 1909)* rostrally and *giant pyramidal area (Brodmann, 1909)* caudally, and including parts of ***anterior paracentral gyrus (>1840)***, ***superior frontal gyrus (>1840)***, ***middle frontal gyrus (>1840)***, and ***precentral gyrus (>1840)***, especially ventrally; see Garey translation (1994, p. 115 and Figs. 85, 86).

14. *area 6 (Brodmann, 1909)*
Synonym for adult human *agranular frontal area (Brodmann, 1909)*; in the original German, *Feld 6*, p. 136.

15. *area gigantopyramidalis (Brodmann, 1909)*
Original Latin form of *giant pyramidal area (Brodmann, 1909)*; pp. 134–136.

16. *giant pyramidal area (Brodmann, 1909)*
Based on cellular architecture in adult human, most caudal zone of ***frontal region (Vicq d'Azyr, 1786)*** between *agranular frontal area (Brodmann, 1909)* rostrally and *rostral postcentral area (Brodmann, 1909)* caudally, and including parts of ***anterior paracentral gyrus (>1840)*** and ***precentral gyrus (>1840)***, especially dorsally; see Garey translation (1994, pp. 113–114 and Figs. 85, 86).

17. *area 4 (Brodmann, 1909)*
Synonym for adult human *giant pyramidal area (Brodmann, 1909)*; in the original German, *Feld 4*, p. 134.

18. *area frontopolaris (Brodmann, 1909, p. 156)*
Original Latin form of *frontopolar area (Brodmann, 1909, p. 156)*; p. 156.

19. *frontopolar area (Brodmann, 1909, p. 156)*
Based on cellular architecture in adult monkey, flying fox, kinkajou, and rabbit, but not human rostroventral zone of *frontal region (Vicq d'Azyr, 1786)*; see Garey translation (1994, pp. 135, 142, 166 and Figs. 90, 91, 96, 97, 102, 103, 105–107).

20. *area 12 (Brodmann, 1909)*
Synonym for adult monkey, flying fox, kinkajou, and rabbit, but not human *frontopolar area (Brodmann, 1909, p. 156)*; in the original German, *Feld 12*, p. 156.

funiculi of spinal cord (Burdach, 1822)

As described for macrodissected adult human and other mammal, the "little cords" of ***white matter (Meckel, 1817)*** forming the periphery of the ***spinal cord (Galen, c162–c166)***, completely surrounding the *H*-shaped ***gray matter (Meckel, 1817)*** in the center and divided for topographic description into ***ventral funiculus (>1840)***, ***lateral funiculus (Burdach, 1822)***, and ***dorsal funiculus (>1840)***—the first two by the ***ventral root central parts (>1840)*** and the last two by the ***dorsal root central parts (>1840)***; see Carpenter (1976, pp. 214–216 and Fig. 9.2), (Williams & Warwick (1980, p. 868 and Fig. 7.36), *Terminologia Anatomica* (1998, pp. 105, 107). In general, the many named ***central nervous system white matter tracts (>1840)*** extending through the ***funiculi of spinal cord (Burdach, 1822)*** partly overlap and are not clearly distinguished; see Carpenter (1976, pp. 218, 238), Williams & Warwick (1908, pp. 874–875). For Burdach's use in macrodissected adult human, see pp. 30–31 (*Stränge* in the original German, *funiculi* in the original Latin). They were first clearly illustrated by Blasius; see ***[funiculi of spinal cord (Burdach, 1822)] (Blasius, 1666)***.

EARLIER REFERENCES:

Illustrated and described, not named:

1. ***[funiculi of spinal cord (Burdach, 1822)] (Blasius, 1666)***
Blasius first clearly illustrated this basic feature of macrodissected adult human ***spinal cord (Galen, c162–c166)***; Figure 18.

Earlier synonyms:

1. *medullary columns (Vicq d'Azyr, 1784)*
Synonym for macrodissected adult human ***funiculi of spinal cord (Burdach, 1822)***. Vicq d'Azyr wrote, "having been separated entirely the one from the other [right and left halves or cords of the ***spinal cord (Galen, c162–c166)***] and from the cortical substance [***gray matter (Meckel, 1817)***], these cords are somewhat flattened and resemble ribbons which run side by side, as seen from in front and from behind, forming the medullary columns [*funiculi*] as they are seen in the vertebral canal... instead of two cords in the spinal cord, there are four quite distinct, two of which are located posteriorly between the semilunar and convex portions of the cortical substance and divided by the posterior sulcus [referring to ***dorsal funiculi (>1840)***]; and two others situated laterally in the concavity of these same semilunar portions of the cortical substance, and divided anteriorly by the anterior sulcus [referring to ***ventral funiculus (>1840)*** and ***lateral funiculus (Burdach, 1822)***, considered together; the *anterolateral funiculus (>1840)*]." (pp. 602–603; see Clarke & O'Malley translation, 1996, p. 270).

LATER SYNONYMS:

1. *spinal funicular white substance (Arnold, 1838b)*
Synonym for macrodissected adult human ***funiculi of spinal cord (Burdach, 1822)***; in the original Latin, *substantia alba funiculi spinalis*, Table II, Figure 2-*a*.

PARTLY CORRESPONDS:

1. *lateral cord (Vicq d'Azyr, 1784)*
Synonym for macrodissected adult human *anterolateral funiculus (>1840)*; pp. 602–603, see Clarke & O'Malley

translation (1996, p. 270) and *medullary columns (Vicq d'Azyr, 1784)*.

2. *anterior funiculus (Rosenthal, 1815)*
   Synonym for macrodissected adult human *lateral cord (Vicq d'Azyr, 1784)*; in the original German, *vordern Strangs*, p. 27, according to Burdach (1822, p. 284).
3. *anterior cord (Rolando, 1824)*
   Synonym for macrodissected adult human *lateral cord (Vicq d'Azyr, 1784)*; in the original Italian (plural), *cordoni anteriori*, pp. 48–51 and Table I, Figure 1-*c.a.*
4. *anterior cords of spinal medulla (Rolando, 1825a)*
   Synonym for *anterior cords (Rolando, 1824)*; in the original French, *cordons antérieurs de la moelle épinière*, Table I, Figure 1-*c.a.*
5. *anterolateral cord of spinal medulla (Rolando, 1825a)*
   Synonym for *anterolateral funiculus (>1840)*; in the original French (plural), *cordons antéro-latéraux de la moelle épinière*, Table I, Figure 1-*c.a.*
6. *anterolateral funiculus (>1840)*
   Macrodissected adult human ***ventral funiculus (>1840)*** and ***lateral funiculus (Burdach, 1822)*** considered together; see Williams & Warwick (1980, p. 865), Nieuwenhuys et al. (2008, Fig. 6.1-7).

funiculus separans (>1840)

In the macrodissected adult human ***floor of fourth ventricle (Reil, 1807–1808a)***, a surface feature separating ***area postrema (>1840)*** from ***vagal triangle (>1840)***; see Crosby et al. (1962, p. 114), Williams & Warwick (1980, p. 934). It was not described clearly by 1840.

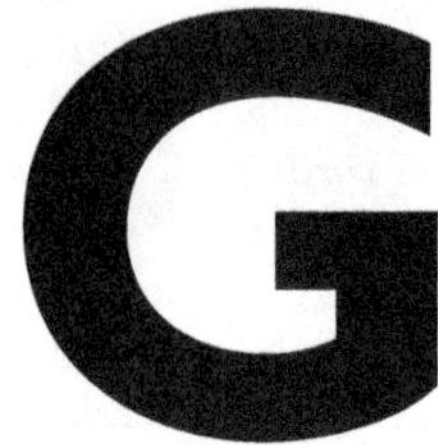

ganglia (Galen, c173)

A topographic division of the ***nervous system (Monro, 1783)*** forming a recognizable swelling in a ***nerve net (>1840)***, ***nerve (Herophilus, c335–c280 BC)***, or ***nerve cord (Serres, 1824–1826)***, as well as a recognizable ***gray matter region (Swanson & Bota, 2010)*** within the same features at a gross anatomical or cellular level. There are ***marginal ganglia (>1840)*** associated with some invertebrate ***nerve nets (>1840)***, ***central ganglia (>1840)*** associated with invertebrate ***central nerve cords (Serres, 1824–1826)***, and ***peripheral ganglia (>1840)*** in the invertebrate and vertebrate ***peripheral nervous system (Meckel, 1817)***. For vertebrates it has long been best practice to restrict the term *ganglion* (and terms derived from ganglion) to parts of the ***peripheral nervous system (Meckel, 1817)***. As Herrick wrote, "The term 'ganglion' is also sometimes used for nuclei or centers within the brain...but this usage is objectionable, for the use of the word ganglion in vertebrate neurology should be restricted to collections of neurons outside the central nervous system, such as the ganglia of the cranial and spinal nerves and the sympathetic [autonomic] ganglia." (1915, p. 108). A prime example is the unfortunate use of *basal ganglia (>1840)* for ***cerebral nuclei (Swanson, 2000a)***. For Galen's discovery in macrodissected adult mammal, but not human, see May translation (1968, pp. 695–696). Also see Swanson & Bota (2010, Thesaurus).

LATER SYNONYMS:

1. *neuronode (Kilian, 1822)*
   Synonym for ***ganglion (Galen, c173)***; in the original Latin, *neuronodus*, see pp. 75–76.

ganglion impar (Quain & Wilson, 1839)

As described for macrodissected adult human, the unpaired terminal ***sympathetic trunk ganglion (Winslow, 1733)*** of the right and left ***sympathetic trunks (Winslow, 1733)*** ventral to (in front of) the coccyx in the median plane. If present it represents a fused right and left ***coccygeal sympathetic ganglion (>1840)***; see Mitchell (1953, p. 207). For Quain & Wilson's use in macrodissected adult human, see Plate XXI-*d**. It was probably first described as the *round infolding (Willis, 1664, p. 348)*.

EARLIER REFERENCES:

Earlier synonyms:

1. *round infolding (Willis, 1664, p. 348)*
   Synonym for macrodissected adult human ***ganglion impar (Quain & Wilson, 1839)***; in the original Latin, *plexum rotundum*, Chapter XXV last paragraph (p. 348). For translation see Pordage (1681, p. 160).
2. *coccygeal ganglion (Walter, 1783)*
   Synonym for macrodissected adult human ***ganglion impar (Quain & Wilson, 1839)***; Table II, Figure 2-64.
3. *common coccygeal ganglion (Soemmerring, 1798)*
   Synonym for macrodissected adult human ***ganglion impar (Quain & Wilson, 1839)***; in the original Latin, *commune ganglion coccygeum*, p. 352.
4. *ganglion sine pare (Bell & Bell, 1826)*
   Synonym for macrodissected adult human ***ganglion impar (Quain & Wilson, 1839)***; Vol. 2, p. 607.
5. *lowest coccygeal ganglion (Bock, 1827)*
   Synonym for macrodissected adult human ***ganglion impar (Quain & Wilson, 1839)***; in the original Latin, *gangl. coccygeum infimum*; Table VII, Figure 1-63.
6. *azygos ganglion (Quain & Wilson, 1839)*
   Synonym for macrodissected adult human ***ganglion impar (Quain & Wilson, 1839)***; in the original Latin, *ganglion azygos*, Plate XXI-*d**. Also spelled *azygous ganglion*.
7. *terminal ganglion (Quain & Wilson, 1839)*
   Synonym for macrodissected adult human ***ganglion impar (Quain & Wilson, 1839)***; Plate XXVIII-*M*.
8. *ganglion of Walter (Hovelacque, 1927)*
   Eponym for macrodissected adult human ***ganglion impar (Quain & Wilson, 1839)***; p. 735.

gastric branches of anterior vagal trunk (>1840)

As described for macrodissected adult human, 4–10 join the ***left gastric plexus (>1840)*** on the ventral (anterior) aspect of the lesser curvature of the stomach, distributing like the ***gastric branches of posterior vagal trunk (>1840)*** but with a slightly wider distribution; see Mitchell (1953, pp. 185, 277–278, Figs. 77, 79). They were alluded to by Galen; see ***[gastric branches of anterior vagal trunk (>1840)] (Galen, c173)***.

EARLIER REFERENCES:

Described, not named or illustrated:

1. ***[gastric branches of anterior vagal trunk (>1840)] (Galen, c173)***
   Alluded to as forming a network most dense near the cardiac orifice in macrodissected adult beef, pig, and/or macaque but not human; see May translation (1968, p. 209).

Illustrated and described, not named:

1. ***[gastric branches of anterior vagal trunk (>1840)] (Vesalius, 1543a)***
   Dealt with rather crudely for macrodissected adult human; see Richardson & Carman translation (2002, p. 199).

Earlier synonyms:

1. *abdominal branches of lateral left vagus nerve (Haase, 1781)*
   Synonym for macrodissected adult human ***gastric branches of anterior vagal trunk (>1840)***; in the original Latin, *nervus vagus sinistri lateris abdominales ramos*, pp. 88–89.
2. *descending branches of anterior trunk of eighth pair of nerves (Walter, 1783)*
   Synonym for macrodissected adult human ***gastric branches of anterior vagal trunk (>1840)***; in the original Latin (singular), *ramos descendentes truncus anterior nervi octavi paris*, Table IV-*456*.
3. *gastric branches of anterior trunk of eighth pair of nerves (Walter, 1783)*
   Synonym for macrodissected adult human ***gastric branches of anterior vagal trunk (>1840)***; in the original Latin, *ramos stomachicos truncus anterior nervi octavi paris*, Table IV-*456*. Walter described at least five of them; Table IV-*108*.
4. *anterior gastric plexus (Günther, 1786)*
   Basically synonym for macrodissected adult human ***gastric branches of anterior vagal trunk (>1840)***; in the original Latin, *plexum gastricum anteriorem*, p. 66. Günther described *rami coeuntes* between it and *posterior gastric plexus (Günther, 1786)*; p. 66.
5. *descending branch of left vagus nerve (Mayer, 1794)*
   Synonym for macrodissected adult human ***gastric branch of left vagus nerve (Mayer, 1794)***; in the original Latin, *ramus descendens nervi vagi sinistri*; Part 6, Table IV-*1* (p. 25).
6. *gastric branch of left vagus nerve (Mayer, 1794)*
   Synonym for macrodissected adult human ***gastric branches of anterior vagal trunk (>1840)***, generating *cardiac branches of gastric branch of left vagus nerve (Mayer, 1794)*, *left anterior and superior gastric nerves (Mayer, 1794)*, and *middle anterior and superior gastric nerves (Mayer, 1794)*; in the original Latin, *ramus gastricus nervi vagi sinistri*; Part 6, Table IV-*1* (p. 25).
7. *left gastric nerves (Wrisberg, 1800)*
   Probably roughly synonymous with macrodissected adult human ***gastric branches of anterior vagal trunk (>1840)***; in the original Latin, *nervi gastrici sinistri*, p. 562.

PARTLY CORRESPONDS:

1. *nerve plexus to coronary arteries (Walter, 1783)*
   Branches of macrodissected adult human ***gastric branches of anterior vagal trunk (>1840)*** along left gastric artery; in the original Latin, *plexum nervosum arteriae coronariae*, Table II-*31*.
2. *cardiac nerves of anterior trunk of eighth pair of nerves (Walter, 1783)*
   Branches of macrodissected adult human ***gastric branches of anterior vagal trunk (>1840)*** to cardia region of stomach; in the original Latin, *nervi cardiaci truncus anterior nervi octavi paris*, Table IV:*1-3* (and Tab. III-*456*, not *256*).
3. *cardiac branches of descending branch of left vagus nerve (Mayer, 1794)*
   Three branches of *descending branch of left vagus nerves (Mayer, 1794)* to cardia region of stomach described for macrodissected adult human; in the original Latin, *rami cardiaci*; Part 6, Table IV-*2* (p. 25).
4. *left anterior and superior gastric nerves (Mayer, 1794)*
   Two branches of *descending branch of left vagus nerves (Mayer, 1794)* to fundus region of stomach described for macrodissected adult human; in the original Latin, *nervi gastrici superiores et anteriores sinistri*; Part 6, Table IV-*3* (p. 25).
5. *middle anterior and superior gastric nerves (Mayer, 1794)*
   Two main branches of *descending branch of left vagus nerves (Mayer, 1794)* to body region of stomach described for macrodissected adult human; in the original Latin, *nervi gastrici superiores et anteriores medii*; Part 6, Table IV-*4* (p. 25).
6. *anterior cardiac nerves (Mayer, 1794)*
   Synonym for macrodissected adult human *cardiac nerves of anterior trunk of eighth pair of nerves (Walter, 1783)*; in the original Latin, *nervi cardiaci anteriores*; Part 6, Table VI-*270* (p. 44).

gastric branches of posterior vagal trunk (>1840)

As described for macrodissected adult human, they join the ***left gastric plexus (>1840)*** on the dorsal (posterior) aspect of the lesser curvature of the stomach, distributed in a manner similar to the ***gastric branches of anterior vagal trunk (>1840)*** but with a slightly more restricted distribution; see Mitchell (1953, p. 187, Figs. 77, 79). They were alluded to by Galen; see ***[gastric branches of posterior vagal trunk (>1840)] (Galen, c173)***.

EARLIER REFERENCES:

Described, not named or illustrated:

1. ***[gastric branches of posterior vagal trunk (>1840)] (Galen, c173)***
   Alluded to as forming a network most dense near the cardiac oriface in macrodissected adult beef, pig, and/or macaque but not human; see May translation (1968, p. 209).

Illustrated and described, not named:

1. ***[gastric branches of posterior vagal trunk (>1840)] (Vesalius, 1543a)***
   Described in roughly the same way as ***[gastric branches of posterior vagal trunk (>1840] (Galen, c173)*** for macrodissected adult human; see Richardson & Carman translation (2002, p. 199).

Earlier synonyms:

1. *posterior gastric plexus (Loder, 1778)*
   Probably essentially synonymous with macrodissected adult human ***gastric branches of posterior vagal trunk (>1840)***; in the original Latin, *plexum gastricum posteriorem*, p. 32.
2. *posterior gastric nerves (Wrisberg, 1780)*
   Synonym for macrodissected adult human ***gastric branches of posterior vagal trunk (>1840)***; in the original Latin, *nervos gastricos posteriores*, see Wrisberg reprint (1800, p. 258).
3. *right gastric nerves (Wrisberg, 1780)*
   Synonym for macrodissected adult human ***gastric branches of posterior vagal trunk (>1840)***; in the original Latin, *nervi gastrici dextri*, see Wrisberg reprint (1800, p. 563).
4. *gastric branches of posterior trunk of gastric and hepatic plexus (Walter, 1783)*
   Synonym for macrodissected adult human ***gastric branches of posterior vagal trunk (>1840)***; in the original Latin (singular), *ramus gastricus truncus posterior plexus ventriculi et hepatis*, Table III:489–504.
5. *inferior branch of right vagus nerve (Mayer, 1794)*
   Synonym for macrodissected adult human ***gastric branches of posterior vagal trunk (>1840)***; in the original Latin, *ramus inferior nervi vagi dextri*; Part 6, Table IV-13 (p. 26).
6. *gastric branch of right vagus nerve (Mayer, 1794)*
   Synonym for macrodissected adult human ***gastric branches of posterior vagal trunk (>1840)***; in the original Latin, *ramus gastricus nervi vagi dextri*; Part 6, Table IV-13 (p. 26).

PARTLY CORRESPONDS:

1. *left posterior and superior gastric nerves (Mayer, 1794)*
   Three branches of *inferior branch of right vagus nerves (Mayer, 1794)* to fundus region of stomach for macrodissected adult human; in the original Latin, *nervi gastrici superiores et posteriores sinistri*; Part 6, Table IV-15 (p. 26).
2. *middle posterior and superior gastric nerves (Mayer, 1794)*
   Branches of *inferior branch of right vagus nerves (Mayer, 1794)* to body region of stomach for macrodissected adult human; in the original Latin, *nervi gastrici superiores et posteriores medii*; Part 6, Table IV-18 (p. 26).
3. *posterior cardiac nerves (Mayer, 1794)*
   Macrodissected adult human ***gastric branches of posterior vagal trunk (>1840)*** supplying dorsal (posterior) regions of cardiac region of stomach; in the original Latin, *nervi cardiaci posteriores*; Part 6, Table VI-225 (p. 43).

gastroduodenal plexus (>1840)

As described for macrodissected adult human, 2–3 filaments of the ***celiac plexus (Winslow 1733)*** surrounding the gastroduodenal artery and its main branches and supplying *nerve fibers (Ehrenberg, 1833)* to the duodenum, pancreas, stomach, and transverse colon; see Mitchell (1953, p. 280), Williams & Warwick (1980, p. 1134 called *plexus accompanying gastroduodenal artery*). It was known to Vesalius; see ***[gastroduodenal plexus (>1840)] (Vesalius, 1543a)***.

EARLIER REFERENCES:

Illustrated and described, not named:

1. ***[gastroduodenal plexus (>1840)] (Vesalius, 1543a)***
   Vesalius vaguely and poorly described and illustrated it for macrodissected adult human, referring to ***nerves (Herophilus, c335–c280 BC)*** supplying duodenum, stomach, and colon; see Richardson & Carman translation (2002, pp. 172-α, 200), Richardson & Carman translation (2007, legend to Fig. 4, p. 8).

PARTLY CORRESPONDS:

1. *duodenal nerves (Walter, 1783)*
   Walter described six of them for macrodissected adult human ***gastroduodenal plexus (>1840)***; in the original Latin, *nervi duodenales*, Table IV:117-120.
2. *superior duodenal nerves (Mayer, 1794)*
   Rostral (upper) components of macrodissected adult human *duodenal nerves (Walter, 1783)*; in the original Latin, *nervi duodenales superiores*; Part 6, Table IV-48 (p. 28).
3. *duodenal plexus (Wrisberg, 1800)*
   Duodenal component of macrodissected adult human ***gastroduodenal plexus (>1840)***; p. 568, also see Lobstein (1831 p. 40).

geniculate ganglion (Bischoff, 1832)

As described for macrodissected adult human, the sensory ***cranial nerve ganglion (>1840)*** of the ***intermediofacial nerve (Strong & Elwyn, 1943)***. It is associated with the ***intermediofacial nerve trunk (>1840)***, in the so-called *genu of facial nerve (Langenbeck, 1826–1830)* within the facial canal of the temporal bone. Its ***axons (Kölliker, 1896)*** extend proximally to reach the ***medulla (Winslow, 1733)*** through the ***intermediate nerve (>1840)***, whereas its ***dendrites (His, 1889)*** extend distally through the ***intermediofacial nerve trunk (>1840), chorda tympani (Falloppio, 1561)***, and then ***lingual nerve (Vesalius, 1543a)*** to the tongue; see Williams & Warwick (1980, p. 1071, Fig. 7.184). For Bischoff's use in macrodissected adult human, and first clear description, see p. 73. For early history see Haller (1762, p. 201 note *o*), Henle (1871, pp. 400–401).

LATER SYNONYMS:

1. *ganglioform intumescence of genu of facial nerve (Arnold,1834)* Synonym for macrodissected adult human **geniculate ganglion (Bischoff, 1832)**; in the original Latin, *intumescentia ganglioformis genu nervi facialis*, p. 11. See Henle (1871, p. 400).
2. *facial ganglion (>1840)* Synonym for macrodissected adult human **geniculate ganglion (Bischoff, 1832)**; see Williams & Warwick (1980, p. 1065).
3. *intermediate ganglion (>1840)* Most appropriate synonym for macrodissected adult human **geniculate ganglion (Bischoff, 1832)**.

genital branch of genitofemoral nerve (>1840)

As described for macrodissected adult human male it supplies the cremaster muscle and sends a few branchlets to skin of the scrotum, whereas in female it ends in skin of the mons pubis and labium majus; see Williams & Warwick (1980, p. 1107), *Terminologia Anatomica* (1998, p. 140). It was known to Galen; see ***[genital branch of genitofemoral nerve (>1840)] (Galen, c192)***.

EARLIER REFERENCES:

Described, not named or illustrated:

1. ***[genital branch of genitofemoral nerve (>1840)] (Galen, c192)*** Galen identified supply to cremaster muscle in macrodissected adult beef, pig, and/or macaque but not human male; see Duckworth translation (1962, p. 130) and *fourth cutaneous nerve of thigh (Galen, c177)*.

Illustrated and described, not named:

1. ***[genital branch of genitofemoral nerve (>1840)] (Vesalius, 1543a)*** Described and illustrated for macrodissected adult human; see Richardson & Carman translation (2002, p. 252).

Earlier synonyms:

1. *cremasteric branch of singular nerve from second and third lumbar nerves (Monro & Coopmans, 1754)* Synonym for macrodissected adult human **genital branch of genitofemoral nerve (>1840)**; in the original Latin (plural), *ramos inguinis nervus singularis ex lumbalibus secundo & tertio*, p. 64 note *a*. The note was by Coopmans, expanding on his Latin translation of Monro's *The Anatomy of the Human Nerves*.
2. *internal inguinal nerve (Martin, 1781)* Synonym for macrodissected adult human **genital branch of genitofemoral nerve (>1840)**; p. 228. See Schmidt (1794, p. 39).
3. *internal branch of external spermatic nerve (Walter, 1783)* Synonym for macrodissected adult human **genital branch of genitofemoral nerve (>1840)**; in the original Latin, *ramus internus nervi externi spermatici*, Table 1-*88*.
4. *internal inguinal branch of external spermatic branch of first lumbar nerve (Günther, 1786)* Synonym for macrodissected adult human **genital branch of genitofemoral nerve (>1840)**; in the original Latin, *ramus inguinalem internum*, p. 81.
5. *inferior branches of spermatic nerve (Fyfe, 1800)* Synonym for macrodissected adult human **genital branch of genitofemoral nerve (>1840)**; Vol. 2, p. 325.
6. *external branches of spermatic nerve (Fyfe, 1800)* Synonym for macrodissected adult human **genital branch of genitofemoral nerve (>1840)**; Vol. 2, p. 325.
7. *internal ramusculus of external pudic nerve (Quain, 1828)* Synonym for macrodissected adult human **genital branch of genitofemoral nerve (>1840)**; p. 285.
8. *internal branch of internal inguinal branch of lumbar plexus (Cruveilhier, 1836)* Synonym for macrodissected adult human **genital branch of genitofemoral nerve (>1840)**; in the original French, *rameau interne*, p. 837.
9. *scrotal branch of internal inguinal branch of lumbar plexus (Cruveilhier, 1836)* Synonym for macrodissected adult human **genital branch of genitofemoral nerve (>1840)**; in the original French, *rameau scrotal*, p. 837.
10. *spermatic branch of external pudic nerve (Quain & Wilson, 1839)* Synonym for macrodissected adult human **genital branch of genitofemoral nerve (>1840)**; also gave the Latin, *n. pudendus externus*, Plate XXI-*m,n*.
11. *spermatic branch of external spermatic nerve (Quain & Wilson, 1839)* Synonym for macrodissected adult human **genital branch of genitofemoral nerve (>1840)**; also gave the Latin, *n. spermaticus externus*, Plate XXI-*m,n*.
12. *spermatic branch of genito-crural nerve (Quain & Wilson, 1839)* Synonym for macrodissected adult human **genital branch of genitofemoral nerve (>1840)**; also gave the Latin, *n. genito-cruralis*, Plate XXI-*m,n*.

genitofemoral nerve (>1840)

As described for macrodissected adult human it arises as two independent roots or ***lumbar plexus ventral divisions (Paterson, 1887)***, associated with the first and second ***lumbar nerves (Diemerbroeck, 1672)***, and merges in the substance of the psoas major muscle before eventually dividing distally into ***genital branch of genitofemoral nerve (>1840)*** and ***femoral branch of genitofemoral nerve (>1840)***; see Durward (1951, p. 1092 and Fig. 937), Williams & Warwick (1980, p. 1107). It was first described as the *fourth cutaneous nerve of thigh (Galen, c177)*.

EARLIER REFERENCES:

Earlier synonyms:

1. *fourth cutaneous nerve of thigh (Galen, c177)* Synonym for **genitofemoral nerve (>1840)** in macrodissected adult beef, pig, and/or macaque but not human; see Singer translation (1999, p. 83). Eustachi clearly illustrated it for macrodissected adult human;

see Albinus edition (1761, Tab. 19-*Φ*), and Vieussens (1684, Tab. 28) described and illustrated at least parts of it for macrodissected adult human.

2. *inguinal nerve (Camper, 1762)*
Synonym for macrodissected adult human ***genitofemoral nerve (>1840)***; in the original Latin, *nervus inguinalis*, p. 7 and Table I, Figure 2-*27,28*. Also see Fischer (1791, p. 2).
3. *first of three anterior branches of first lumbar pair (Sabatier, 1775)*
Synonym for macrodissected adult human ***genitofemoral nerve (>1840)***; in the original French, *premiere des trois branches anterieures de la premiere paire lombaire*, pp. 717, 727, 728. See Schmidt (1794, p. 39), Schreger (1803, p. 352).
4. *external inguinal nerve (Martin, 1781)*
Synonym for macrodissected adult human *external spermatic nerve (Walter, 1783)*; in the original Latin, *nervus inguinalis externus*, p. 227.
5. *external spermatic nerve (Walter, 1783)*
Synonym for macrodissected adult human ***genitofemoral nerve (>1840)***; in the original Latin, *nervus spermaticus externus*, Table 1-*86*. For further discussion see Schmidt (1794, p. 39).
6. *external spermatic branch of first lumbar nerve (Günther, 1786)*
Synonym for macrodissected adult human ***genitofemoral nerve (>1840)***; in the original Latin, *primus lumbaris, r. spermaticus externus*, p. 81.
7. *super-pubian nerve (Burdin, 1803)*
Synonym for macrodissected adult human *suprapubic nerve (Chaussier, 1809)*; see translation (1803, Vol. 1, p. 199).
8. *suprapubic nerve (Chaussier, 1809)*
Probably synonym for macrodissected adult human ***genitofemoral nerve (>1840)***; in the original French, *nerf sus-pubien*.
9. *genitocrural branch of lumbar plexus (Cloquet, 1816)*
Probably synonym for macrodissected adult human ***genitofemoral nerve (>1840)***; in the original French, *branche génito-crurale*, p. 663. Cruveilhier (1836, p. 831) attributed the term to Bichat without citation.
10. *external pudic nerve (Meckel, 1817)*
Synonym listed for macrodissected adult human ***genitofemoral nerve (>1840)***; in the original Latin, *nervus pudendus externus*, see translation (1832, Vol. 3, p. 13).
11. *genitocrural nerve (Meckel, 1817)*
Synonym listed for macrodissected adult human ***genitofemoral nerve (>1840)***; in the original Latin, *nervus genito-curalis*, see translation (1832, Vol. 3, p. 13). Quain (1828, p. 285) attributed the term to Soemmerring without citation.
12. *internal inguinal branch of second lumbar pair (Cruveilhier, 1836)*
Synonym for macrodissected adult human *genitocrural branch of lumbar plexus (Cloquet, 1816)*; in the original French, *inguinale interne*, p. 831.
13. *internal inguinal branch of lumbar plexus (Cruveilhier, 1836)*
Synonym for *internal inguinal branch of second lumbar pair (Cruveilhier, 1836)*; in the original French, *branche inguinale interne*; p. 837.

PARTLY CORRESPONDS:

1. *anastomotic branch of first lumbar pair (Cruveilhier, 1836)*
For macrodissected adult human, probably rostral (upper) root of ***genitofemoral nerve (>1840)***; in the original French, *branche anastomotique*, p. 831.

genu of corpus callosum (Reil, 1809b)

As described for macrodissected adult human, the rostral curved end of the ***corpus callosum (Galen, c177)*** between ***rostrum of corpus callosum (Reil, 1809b)*** rostrally and ***body of corpus callosum (>1840)*** caudally; see Mettler (1948, p. 100, Fig. 68). Reil noted that for macrodissected adult human, "The corpus callosum is terminated by an anterior fold" (Mayo translation, 1823, p. 52). Burdach (1822, p. 146) provided the Latin form *genu corpus callosum*. It was first clearly delineated by Steno; see ***[genu of corpus callosum (Reil, 1809b)] (Steno, 1669)***.

TRANSLATIONS:

1. *Knie des Balkens (Reil, 1809b)*
Original German form of ***genu of corpus callosum (Reil, 1809b)***; see Mayo translation (1823, p. 52).
2. *anterior fold of corpus callosum (Reil, 1809b)*
English form of ***genu of corpus callosum (Reil, 1809b)***; see Mayo translation (1823, p. 52).
3. *knee of corpus callosum (Reil, 1809b)*
English form of ***genu of corpus callosum (Reil, 1809b)***; see Meckel (1832, Vol. 2, p. 448).

EARLIER REFERENCES:

Illustrated, not named or described:

1. ***[genu of corpus callosum (Reil, 1809b)] (Steno, 1669)***
First clear indication of its shape, illustrated in midsagittal view of macrodissected adult human ***brain (Smith Papyrus, c1700 BC)***; Plate I.

Described, not named or illustrated:

1. ***[genu of corpus callosum (Reil, 1809b)] (Winslow, 1733)***
Referring to macrodissected adult human ***genu of corpus callosum (Reil, 1809b)*** and ***splenium of corpus callosum (Burdach, 1822)*** Winslow wrote, "Both Extremities of this medullary Body [***corpus callosum (Galen, c177)***] terminate by a small Edge bent transversely downward." (Sect. X, p. 34).

Earlier synonyms:

1. *bourrelet antérieur du corps calleux (Vicq d'Azyr, 1786)*
Synonym for macrodissected adult human ***genu of corpus callosum (Reil, 1809b)***; Plate XX-*23*.

LATER SYNONYMS:

1. *commissure of anterior lobe (Spurzheim, 1826)*
Synonym for macrodissected adult human ***genu of corpus callosum (Reil, 1809b)***; p. 224.
2. *genu of great commissure (Arnold, 1838b)*

Synonym for macrodissected adult human ***genu of corpus callosum (Reil, 1809b)***; in the original Latin, *genu commissurae maximae*, Table VII, Figure 2-*i*.

genu of internal capsule (>1840)

As described for macrodissected adult human, typically in frontal (horizontal) section, the general topographic region occupying the angle between ***anterior limb of internal capsule (>1840)*** and ***posterior limb of internal capsule (>1840)***; see Crosby et al. (1962, p. 394, Fig. 272). It was first delineated by Vesalius; see ***[genu of internal capsule (>1840)] (Vesalius, 1543a)***.

EARLIER REFERENCES:

Illustrated, not named or described:

1. ***[genu of internal capsule (>1840)] (Vesalius, 1543a)*** Clearly illustrated in frontal (horizontal) section of macrodissected adult human; see Singer translation (1952, Fig. 7).

glandular branches of submandibular ganglion (>1840)

As described for macrodissected adult human, there are typically 5–6 ***nerve (Herophilus, c335–c280 BC)*** branches from the ***submandibular ganglion (>1840)*** to the submandibular gland and its duct and to the sublingual gland; see Williams & Warwick (1980, p. 1072 and Figs. 7.177, 179), *Nomina Anatomica* (1983, p. A75). They were discovered by Meckel; see ***[glandular branches of submandibular ganglion (>1840)] (Meckel, 1748)***.

EARLIER REFERENCES:

Illustrated and described, not named:

1. ***[glandular branches of submandibular ganglion (>1840)] (Meckel, 1748)*** Meckel clearly described and illustrated five or six such branches from ***submandibular ganglion (>1840)*** in macrodissected adult human; p. 95 and Figure 1-75.

PARTLY CORRESPONDS:

1. *branches of maxillary ganglion to submaxillary gland (Langenbeck, 1826–1830)* For macrodissected adult human, ***glandular branches of submandibular ganglion (>1840)*** specifically just to submandibular gland; in the original Latin, *ganglion maxillare, rami ad glandulam submaxillarem*; Fascicle II, Table I-5.
2. *branches of maxillary ganglion to sublingual gland (Langenbeck, 1826–1830)* For macrodissected adult human, ***glandular branches of submandibular ganglion (>1840)*** specifically just to sublingual gland; in the original Latin, *ganglion maxillare, rami ad glandulam sublingualem*; Fascicle II, Table I-6.

globus pallidus (Burdach, 1822)

As described for macrodissected adult human, the medial component of the *lentiform nucleus (Burdach, 1822)* in turn divided into ***medial globus pallidus (>1840)*** and ***lateral globus pallidus (>1840)***. It is separated from the lateral component of the *lentiform nucleus (Burdach, 1822)*, the ***putamen (Burdach, 1822)***, by the ***lateral medullary lamina (>1840)***. In mammal generally, it is differentiated by cellular architecture and connections as the large, intermediate component of the ***pallidum (Swanson, 2000a)***; see Nieuwenhuys et al. (2008, p. 437). For Burdach's use in macrodissected adult human, see p. 130. It was first illustrated by Vesalius; see ***[globus pallidus (Burdach, 1822)] (Vesalius, 1543a)***.

EARLIER REFERENCES:

Illustrated, not named or described:

1. ***[globus pallidus (Burdach, 1822)] (Vesalius, 1543a)*** Clearly illustrated in a frontal (horizontal) section through macrodissected adult human; see Singer translation (1952, Fig. 7).

glossopharyngeal nerve (Huber, 1744)

As described for macrodissected adult human, a ***cranial nerve (Soemmerring, 1791)*** with a proximal part, the ***glossopharyngeal nerve root (>1840)*** attached to the outer surface of the ***medulla (Winslow, 1733)*** in a longitudinal line just rostral to the ***vagus nerve root (>1840)***, and a distal part, the ***glossopharyngeal nerve trunk (Wrisberg, 1786; Günther, 1786)*** with a variety of branches; see Mettler (1948, Figs. 57, 59, 60), Durward (1951, Fig. 905), Hamilton (1976, Fig. 802), Williams & Warwick (1980, Fig. 7.189). For Huber's use (plural) in macrodissected adult human, see pp. 12, 17. It was probably discovered by Herophilus; see ***[glossopharyngeal nerve (Huber, 1744)] (Herophilus, c335–c280 BC)***.

TRANSLATIONS:

1. *nervi glossopharyngei (Huber, 1744)* Original Latin (plural) form of ***glossopharyngeal nerve (Huber, 1744)***; see pp. 12, 17.
2. *nervus glossopharyngeus (Haller, 1762)* Singular Latin form of ***glossopharyngeal nerve (Huber, 1744)***; it was sometimes hyphenated, as *nervus glosso-pharyngeus*.

EARLIER REFERENCES:

Described, not named or illustrated:

1. ***[glossopharyngeal nerve (Huber, 1744)] (Alcmaeon, c490–c430 BC)*** In *De Sensu*, Aristotle's successor Theophrastus (c327–c287 BC) wrote that Alcmaeon postulated the existence of a channel (alternate translations: *passage, duct*) between tongue and ***brain (Smith Papyrus, c1700 BC)*** for sensory experience, presumably taste; see Solmsen (1961, pp. 151–152), Lloyd (1975).
2. ***[glossopharyngeal nerve (Huber, 1744)] (Herophilus, c335–c280 BC)*** Herophilus, the founder of human anatomy, is credited with discovering but not naming the ***glossopharyngeal nerve (Huber, 1744)***, which he apparently considered together with the ***vagus nerve (Galen, c192)*** and ***accessory nerve (Vieussens, 1684)***; see Solmsen (1961), von Staden (1969), Longrigg (1993), Clarke & O'Malley (1996, p. 261). Herophilus dissected animals and human cadavers.

Earlier synonyms:

1. *special pharyngeal nerve (Galen, c192)*
Galen specifically described and named at least part of the macrodissected adult beef, pig, and/or macaque but not human ***glossopharyngeal nerve (Huber, 1744)***; see Duckworth translation (1962, pp. 201, 210). Earlier he also gave a very good description without naming in *On the Usefulness of the Parts*; see May translation (1968, p. 697). It was included in the *sixth pair of nerves from brain (Galen, c192)*; also see ***cranial nerves (Soemmerring, 1791)***. He also described the results of experimentally interrupting the *special pharyngeal nerve (Galen, c192)*; see Duckworth translation (1962, pp. 210–211).
2. *qui ad musculos linguae et faucium tendit (Falloppio, 1561)*
Roughly synonymous with macrodissected adult human ***glossopharyngeal nerve (Huber, 1744)***; see Vicq d'Azyr (1786, p. 49).
3. *anterior nerve of sixth conjugation of nerves of brain (Bauhin, 1605)*
Synonym for macrodissected adult human ***glossopharyngeal nerve (Huber, 1744)***; see Crooke translation (1615, pp. 365, 892).
4. *superior branch of eighth pair of nerves arising within skull (Willis, 1664)*
Roughly synonymous with macrodissected adult human ***glossopharyngeal nerve (Huber, 1744)***; see Vicq d'Azyr (1786, p. 49).
5. *anterior fibers of vagus nerve pair (Morgagni, 1719)*
Synonym for macrodissected adult human ***glossopharyngeal nerve (Huber, 1744)***; p. 14. Also see Burdach (1822, pp. 310–311), who used the Latin *fibras anteriores paris octavi*.
6. *small branch of eighth pair of nerves of medulla oblongata (Winslow, 1733)*
Roughly synonymous with macrodissected adult human ***glossopharyngeal nerve (Huber, 1744)***; Section X, p. 132. Vicq d'Azyr (1786, p. 49) claimed that Winslow used the term *lingual branch of eighth pair of nerves of medulla oblongata*, but the reference has not been found. According to Burdach (1822, p. 310), Willis first used this term, but Burdach did not provide a specific citation either.

LATER SYNONYMS:

1. *glossopharyngeal branch of eighth pair (Haller, 1762)*
Synonym for macrodissected adult human ***glossopharyngeal nerve (Huber, 1744)***; p. 231.
2. *lingual branch of eighth pair (Haller, 1762)*
Synonym for macrodissected adult human ***glossopharyngeal nerve (Huber, 1744)***; in the original Latin, *lingualis octavi paris ramus*, p. 232.
3. *glossopharyngeal eighth pair of nerves (Haller, 1772)*
Synonym for macrodissected adult human ***glossopharyngeal nerves (Huber, 1744)*** used in describing Andersch's unpublished plate from some 18 years earlier; in the original Latin, *nervus paris octavi glossopharyngeus*, p. 7, #1. Also see *glossopharyngeal branch of eighth pair (Haller, 1762)*.
4. *first spinal nerve (Soemmerring, 1778)*
Listed as synonym for macrodissected adult human ***glossopharyngeal nerve (Huber, 1744)***; in the original Latin, *nervus spinalis primus*, p. 180.
5. *first pair of nerves of medulla oblongata (Haller & Wrisberg, 1780)*
Wrisberg's synonym for macrodissected adult human ***glossopharyngeal nerves (Huber, 1744)***; see translation (Haller, Cullen, & Wrisberg, 1786, p. 208).
6. *minor and anterior part of eighth pair (Haase, 1781)*
Synonym for macrodissected adult human ***glossopharyngeal nerve (Huber, 1744)***; in the original Latin, *paris octavi portio minor et anterior*, p. 41.
7. *lingual nerve of eighth pair of nerves (Vicq d'Azyr, 1784)*
Synonym for macrodissected adult human ***glossopharyngeal nerve (Huber, 1744)***; pp. 593–594.
8. *par octavum sensorius linguae (Vicq d'Azyr, 1784)*
Vicq d'Azyr credited Andersch with using it for ***glossopharyngeal nerves (Huber, 1744)***; p. 593, as did Burdach (1822, p. 311). However, it is an amalgam of *eighth pair of nerves of head (Andersch & Soemmerring, 1792)* and *lingual sensory nerve (Andersch, 1797)*. Also see Haller (1772).
9. *ninth pair of cranial nerves (Soemmerring, 1791)*
Synonym for macrodissected adult human ***glossopharyngeal nerves (Huber, 1744)***; see ***cranial nerves (Soemmerring, 1791)***.
10. *ninth pair of cerebral nerves (Soemmerring, 1791)*
Synonym for *ninth pair of cranial nerves (Soemmerring, 1791)*; see p. 103 and *cerebral nerves (Soemmerring, 1791)*. In the original Latin, *par nonum nervorum cerebri*, Soemmerring (1798, p. 125).
11. *eighth pair of nerves of head (Andersch & Soemmerring, 1792)*
Synonym for macrodissected adult human ***glossopharyngeal nerves (Huber, 1744)***; in the original Latin, *octavus nervus capitis*, p. 114.
12. *ninth nerves of head (Andersch, 1797)*
Synonym for macrodissected adult human ***glossopharyngeal nerves (Huber, 1744)***; in the original Latin, *nono nervo capitis*, p. 1. Meckel (1817; see translation, 1832, Vol. 3, p. 38) credited Andersch with separating clearly for the first time ***glossopharyngeal nerve (Huber, 1744)***, ***vagus nerve (Galen, c192)***, and ***accessory nerve (Vieussens, 1684)***.
13. *lingual sensory nerve (Andersch, 1797)*
Synonym for macrodissected adult human ***glossopharyngeal nerve (Huber, 1744)***; in the original Latin, *nervo sensorio linguae*, p. 1.
14. *lateral lingual nerve (Fyfe, 1800)*
Synonym for macrodissected adult human ***glossopharyngeal nerve (Huber, 1744)***; in the original Latin, *lingualis lateralis*, p. 294.
15. *pharyngo-glossian pair of nerves (Burdin, 1803)*
Synonym for macrodissected adult human ***glossopharyngeal nerve (Huber, 1744)***; see translation (1803, Vol.

1, p. 144). Burdach (1822, p. 311) gave the Latin, *nervus pharyngoglossicus*.

16. *ninth pair of nerves leaving skull (Burdach, 1822)*
According to Burdach (p. 311), Soemmerring's 1778 enumeration of macrodissected adult human ***glossopharyngeal nerves (Huber, 1744)***, although Soemmerring did not use this term; in Latin, *par nonum*. See *nervorum per ossa capitis egredientium (Soemmerring, 1778)*.

17. *associate of eighth pair of nerves (Swan, 1830)*
Synonym for macrodissected adult human ***glossopharyngeal nerve (Huber, 1744)***; p. 22.

PARTLY CORRESPONDS:

1. *first branch of eighth pair (Winslow, 1733)*
Winslow indicated this name is given in macrodissected adult human to ***glossopharyngeal nerve (Huber, 1744)*** after leaving cranium and separating from ***vagus nerve (Galen, c192)***; Section VI, p. 70.

2. *anastomosis of glossopharyngeal nerve with pharyngeal nerves of eighth pair (Scarpa, 1788)*
Macrodissected adult human ***communicating branch (Winslow, 1733)*** between ***glossopharyngeal nerve (Huber, 1744)*** and ***pharyngeal branches of vagus nerve (Wrisberg, 1786)***; in the original Latin, *anastomosis glosso-pharyngei cum nervo pharyngeo octavi*, Table X, Figure 1-31.

5. *circulus tonsillaris (Andersch & Soemmerring, 1792)*
Plexus (Galen, c192) of branches of macrodissected adult human ***glossopharyngeal nerve (Huber, 1744)*** helping form *tonsillar plexus (Andersch & Soemmerring, 1792)*; pp. 118–119. Alternate form, *circuli tonsillaris*. See Scarpa (1794, Tab. II-20) for nice illustration.

4. *tonsillar plexus (Andersch & Soemmerring, 1792)*
Associated with palatine tonsil and formed by various branches of macrodissected adult human ***glossopharyngeal nerve (Huber, 1744)***; in the original Latin, *plexum tonsillarem*, p. 118. From it many ***lingual branches of glossopharyngeal nerve (Haller, 1762)*** proceed rostrally; see Scarpa (1794, Tab. II-20) for nice illustration.

5. *digastric branch of glossopharyngeal nerves (Kilian, 1822)*
Branch of macrodissected adult human ***glossopharyngeal nerve (Huber, 1744)*** to digastric muscle; in the original Latin, *ramus digastricus nervi glossopharyngei*, p. 89. Swann (1830, Pl. XVII, Figs. 2, 3) and Todd (1836–1839, p. 496) indicated a ***communicating branch (Winslow, 1733)*** with ***digastric nerve (Meckel, 1753)***.

6. *stylohyoid branch of glossopharyngeal nerves (Kilian, 1822)*
Branch of macrodissected adult human ***glossopharyngeal nerve (Huber, 1744)*** to stylohyoid muscle; in the original Latin, *ramus stylohyoideus nervi glossopharyngei*, p. 89.

7. *main communicating branch of glossopharyngeal nerve (Kilian, 1822)*
It generates on the order of ten branches and lies between *digastric branch of glossopharyngeal nerves (Kilian, 1822)* and *pharyngolingual branch of glossopharyngeal nerves (Kilian, 1822)* for macrodissected adult human; in the original Latin, *ramus communicans maximus nervi glossopharyngei*, pp. 90–91, [106].

8. *ascending branch of glossopharyngeal nerve to accessory nerve of Willis (Kilian, 1822)*
Branch from macrodissected adult human ***glossopharyngeal nerve (Huber, 1744)*** to ***accessory nerve (Vieussens, 1684)***; in the original Latin, *ramus ascendens ad nervus accessorium Willisii*, p. 91.

9. *branches of glossopharyngeal nerve to soft nerves (Kilian, 1822)*
Macrodissected adult human branches of ***glossopharyngeal nerve (Huber, 1744)*** to *soft nerves (Haller, 1762)*; in the original Latin, *ramusculi ad nervos molles*, pp. 91–92.

10. *cardiac branch of glossopharyngeal nerve (Kilian, 1822)*
Macrodissected adult human branches of ***glossopharyngeal nerve (Huber, 1744)*** to ***cardiac plexus (Keill, 1698)***, and associated with *pharyngocarotid plexus of vagus nerve (Kilian, 1822)*; in the original Latin, *ramus cardiacus*, pp. 92–93.

11. *bifid branch of main communicating branches of glossopharyngeal nerve (Kilian, 1822)*
Macrodissected adult human branch of ***glossopharyngeal nerve (Huber, 1744)*** to *pharyngocarotid plexus of vagus nerve (Kilian, 1822)*; in the original Latin, *ramus bifidus rami communicantis maximi nervi glossopharyngei*, p. 93.

12. *branch of glossopharyngeal nerve to nodular plexus of vagus nerve of Meckel (Kilian, 1822)*
Macrodissected adult human branch of ***glossopharyngeal nerve (Huber, 1744)*** to *nodular plexus of vagus nerves of Meckel (Kilian, 1822)*, that is, to region of ***vagus nerve (Galen, c192)*** generating ***pharyngeal branches of vagus nerve (Wrisberg, 1786)***; in the original Latin, *ramulus ad plexum nodulosum n. vagi Meck.*, pp. 94–95.

13. *superior lingual branch of glossopharyngeal nerve (Kilian, 1822)*
Substantial branch of macrodissected adult human ***glossopharyngeal nerve (Huber, 1744)*** generating ***stylopharyngeal branch of glossopharyngeal nerve (>1840)***, some ***tonsillar branches of glossopharyngeal nerve (Wrisberg, 1786)***, and some ***lingual branches of glossopharyngeal nerve (Haller, 1762)*** that supply vallate papillae and adjacent regions; in the original Latin, *ramus lingualis superior*, p. 102.

14. *inferior lingual branch of glossopharyngeal nerve (Kilian, 1822)*
Macrodissected adult human branch of ***glossopharyngeal nerve (Huber, 1744)***, supplying muscles it passes by and ending in hyoglossus muscle; in the original Latin, *ramus lingualis inferior*, p. 103.

15. *lingual muscle branch of glossopharyngeal nerve (Kilian, 1822)*
Synonym for *inferior lingual branch of glossopharyngeal nerve (Kilian, 1822)*; in the original Latin, *ramus muscularis linguae*, p. 105.

16. *circulus tonsillaris Anderschii (Cloquet, 1828)*
Eponym for macrodissected adult human *circulus tonsillaris (Andersch & Soemmerring, 1792)*; Plate CLIX-55.

17. *tonsillar circular plexus (Cloquet, 1828)*

Synonym for macrodissected adult human *tonsillar plexus (Andersch & Soemmerring, 1792)*; in the original French, *plexus circulaire tonsillaire*, Plate CLIX-55.

18. *smaller external lingual branch of glossopharyngeal (Knox, 1832)*
   Small branch of macrodissected adult human ***glossopharyngeal nerve (Huber, 1744)*** to *circuli tonsillaris (Andersch & Soemmerring, 1792)*; Plate II-53.
19. *pharyngeal and laryngeal part of ninth pair (Arnold, 1834)*
   Part of macrodissected adult human ***glossopharyngeal nerve (Huber, 1744)*** including and distal to origin of ***pharyngeal branches of glossopharyngeal nerve (Neubauer, 1772)***; in the original Latin, *par nonum, pars pharyngea et lingualis*, p. 13.
20. *pharyngeal and laryngeal part of glossopharyngeal nerve (Arnold, 1834)*
   Synonym for *pharyngeal and laryngeal part of ninth pair (Arnold, 1834)*; in the original Latin, *nervus glossopharyngeus, pars pharyngea et lingualis*, p. 13.

glossopharyngeal nerve central root (>1840)

As described for macrodissected adult human, and mammal generally with histological methods for ***axons (Kölliker, 1896)***, the central extension of the peripheral ***glossopharyngeal nerve root (>1840)*** coursing transversely through the ***medullary segment of spinal tract of trigeminal nerve (>1840)*** and medially adjacent ***spinal nucleus of trigeminal nerve (>1840)***, rostral to the **vagus nerve central root** (>1840), to parts of the ***inferior salivatory nucleus (>1840)***, ***ambiguus nucleus (>1840)***, ***spinal nucleus of trigeminal nerve (>1840)***, and ***nucleus of solitary tract (>1840)***. It is formed by smaller individual fascicles, the ***glossopharyngeal nerve central rootlets (>1840)***; see Villiger et al. (1951, Fig. 12), Carpenter (1976, pp. 312–313 and Figs. 11.16–18). Mayo perhaps first identified at least part of it; see ***[glossopharyngeal nerve central root (>1840)] (Mayo, 1827)***.

EARLIER REFERENCES:

Illustrated and described, not named:

1. ***[glossopharyngeal nerve central root (>1840)] (Mayo, 1827)***
   Traced at least part of it in macrodissected adult human to region of ***inferior cerebellar peduncle (Günther, 1786)***; Plate VII, Figure 2-*VIII*. Grainger (1837, p. 41) accurately traced at least part of it in macrodissected adult human to "the grey matter placed in the posterior part of the medulla oblongata."

glossopharyngeal nerve central rootlets (>1840)

As described in macrodissected adult human, and mammal generally with histological methods for ***axons (Kölliker, 1896)***, the central extensions of the peripheral ***glossopharyngeal nerve rootlets (>1840)***, together forming the ***glossopharyngeal nerve central root (>1840)***; see Villiger et al. (1951, Fig. 12), Carpenter (1976, pp. 312–313). They were not clearly identified by 1840.

glossopharyngeal nerve root (>1840)

As described for macrodissected adult human, the proximal part of the ***glossopharyngeal nerve (Huber, 1744)*** consisting of ***glossopharyngeal nerve rootlets (>1840)*** attached proximally to the outer surface of the ***medulla (Winslow, 1733)*** in a longitudinal line just rostral to the ***vagus nerve root (>1840)*** and continued distally as the ***glossopharyngeal nerve trunk (Wrisberg, 1786; Günther, 1786)***; see Williams & Warwick (1980, Fig. 7.189). It was known to Galen; see ***[glossopharyngeal nerve root (>1840)] (Galen, c192)***.

EARLIER REFERENCES:

Described, not named or illustrated:

1. ***[glossopharyngeal nerve root (>1840)] (Galen, c192)***
   Clearly referred to as one of three *roots of sixth pair of nerves arising from brain (Galen, c192)* in macrodissected adult beef, pig, and/or macaque but not human; see May translation (1968, p. 445 note *41*).

Earlier synonyms:

1. *cerebral part of ninth pair (Arnold, 1834)*
   Essentially synonymous with macrodissected adult human ***glossopharyngeal nerve root (>1840)***; in the original Latin, *par nonum pars cerebralis*, p. 13.
2. *cerebral part of glossopharyngeal nerve (Arnold, 1834)*
   Essentially synonymous with macrodissected adult human ***glossopharyngeal nerve root (>1840)***; in the original Latin, *nervus glossopharyngeus, pars cerebralis*, p. 13.

glossopharyngeal nerve rootlets (>1840)

As described for adult human, thin bundles of ***axons (Kölliker, 1896)*** between outer surface of ***medulla (Winslow, 1733)*** and ***glossopharyngeal nerve trunk (Wrisberg, 1786; Günther, 1786)***, together forming the ***glossopharyngeal nerve root (>1840)***; see ***vagus nerve rootlets (>1840)***. They were called rootlets by Durward (1951, p. 1035); also see *little roots of sixth pair of cranial nerves (Vesalius, 1543a)*. Williams & Warwick (1980, p. 1074) mentioned 3–6 of them for macrodissected adult human. They were perhaps first clearly distinguished as the *anterior nerve of sixth conjugation of nerves of brain fibers (Bauhin, 1605)*.

EARLIER REFERENCES:

Earlier synonyms:

1. *anterior nerve of sixth conjugation of nerves of brain fibers (Bauhin, 1605)*
   From description, clearly synonymous with macrodissected adult human ***glossopharyngeal nerve rootlets (>1840)***; see Crooke translation (1615, p. 892).
2. *anterior filaments of nerves of eighth pair (Winslow, 1733)*
   Winslow stated that in macrodissected adult human they are separated from the main body of (posterior) filaments by a thin septum, referring to ***glossopharyngeal nerve rootlets (>1840)*** and ***vagus nerve rootlets (>1840)*** respectively; Section VI, no. 106, p. 70.

3. *smaller nerve bundles of glossopharyngeal nerve (Wrisberg, 1786)*
For macrodissected adult human, Wrisberg described 4–6 ***glossopharyngeal nerve rootlets (>1840)***; in the original Latin, *minoribus fasciculis nerveis*, see Wrisberg reprint (1800, p. 415).
4. *glossopharyngeal nerve filaments (Meckel, 1817)*
Synonym for macrodissected adult human ***glossopharyngeal nerve rootlets (>1840)***; see translation (1832, Vol. 3, p. 50).
5. *glossopharyngeal roots (Bischoff, 1832)*
Synonym for macrodissected adult human ***glossopharyngeal nerve rootlets (>1840)***; in the original Latin, *radices glossopharyngei*, Table I, Figure 1-25.

glossopharyngeal nerve trunk (Wrisberg, 1786; Günther, 1786)

As described for macrodissected adult human, the condensed part of the ***glossopharyngeal nerve (Haller, 1762)*** distal to the ***glossopharyngeal nerve root (>1840)***. It forms proximally in the jugular foramen and extends distally to the origin of the ***pharyngeal branches of glossopharyngeal nerve (Neubauer, 1772)***, where the two terminal branches—***tonsillar branches of glossopharyngeal nerve (>1840)*** and ***lingual branches of glossopharyngeal nerve (Haller, 1762)***—form; see Durward (1951, pp. 1036– 1037), Mitchell (1953, p. 176), Hamilton (1976, Fig. 802). For Wrisberg's use in macrodissected adult human, see Wrisberg reprint (1800, p. 416). It was also mentioned for macrodissected adult human by Günther (1786, p. 61).

TRANSLATIONS:

1. *truncus nervi glossopharyngaei (Wrisberg, 1786)*
Original Latin form of ***glossopharyngeal nerve trunk (Wrisberg, 1786; Günther, 1786)***; see Wrisberg reprint (1800, p. 416).

PARTLY CORRESPONDS:

1. *first branch of glossopharyngeal nerve (Wrisberg, 1786)*
Synonym for *first communicating branch of glossopharyngeal nerve (Wrisberg, 1786)*; see Wrisberg reprint (1800, pp. 416–417).
2. *first communicating branch of glossopharyngeal nerve (Wrisberg, 1786)*
Macrodissected adult human ***communicating branch (Winslow, 1733)*** from ***glossopharyngeal nerve trunk (Wrisberg, 1786; Günther, 1786)*** to ***pharyngeal branches of vagus nerve (Wrisberg, 1786)***; see Wrisberg reprint (1800, pp. 416–417).
3. *third branch of glossopharyngeal nerve (Wrisberg, 1786)*
Synonym for *second communicating branch of glossopharyngeal nerve (Wrisberg, 1786)*; see Wrisberg reprint (1800, p. 418).
4. *second communicating branch of glossopharyngeal nerve (Wrisberg, 1786)*
Macrodissected adult human ***communicating branch (Winslow, 1733)*** from ***glossopharyngeal nerve trunk (Wrisberg, 1786; Günther, 1786)*** to ***pharyngeal branches of vagus nerve (Wrisberg, 1786)***; see Wrisberg reprint (1800, pp. 416–417).
5. *long root of otic ganglion (Arnold, 1834)*
Apparently, macrodissected adult human ***tympanic nerve (Arnold, 1834)***, ***tympanic plexus (Müller, 1834)***, and ***lesser petrosal nerve (>1840)*** considered together; in the original Latin, *ganglion oticum, radix longa*, p. 10.
6. *long root of auricular ganglion (Arnold, 1834)*
Synonym for *long root of otic ganglion (Arnold, 1834)*; in the original Latin, *ganglion auriculare, radix longa*, p. 10.
7. *petrous part of ninth pair (Arnold, 1834)*
Macrodissected adult human segment of ***glossopharyngeal nerve trunk (Wrisberg, 1786; Günther, 1786)*** in petrous part of temporal bone; in the original Latin, *par nonum, pars petrosa*, pp. 12–13.
8. *petrous part of glossopharyngeal nerve (Arnold, 1834)*
Synonym for *petrous part of ninth pair (Arnold, 1834)*; in the original Latin, *nervus glossopharyngeus, pars petrosa*, pp. 12–13.

gracile fascicle (Müller, 1834)

As described for macrodissected adult human, a rostrally directed ***central nervous system white matter tract (>1840)*** extending the length of the ***dorsal funiculus (>1840)*** of the ***spinal cord (Galen, c162–c166)*** and caudal part of the ***medulla (Winslow, 1733)***. It receives contributions from the caudal (lower) ***thoracic part of spinal cord (>1840)***, ***lumbar part of spinal cord (>1840)***, ***sacral part of spinal cord (>1840)***, and ***coccygeal part of spinal cord (>1840)***. At more rostral levels it lies between ***dorsal median sulcus of spinal cord (>1840)*** and ***dorsolateral sulcus of spinal cord (>1840)***, which partly separates it from the ***cuneate fascicle (Müller, 1834)*** laterally; see Williams & Warwick, 1980, p. 881 and Figure 7.35A. For topographic description it has ***medullary gracile fascicle (>1840)*** and ***spinal gracile fascicle (>1840)*** segments, with the former partly separated from the ***medullary cuneate fascicle (>1840)*** by the ***dorsolateral sulcus of medulla (>1840)***. For Müller's use in macrodissected adult human, see translation (1838, p. 827). It was first clearly delineated by Santorini; see ***[gracile fascicle (Müller, 1834)] (Santorini, 1775)***.

TRANSLATIONS:

1. *fasciculus gracilis (Müller, 1834)*
Original Latin form of ***gracile fascicle (Müller, 1834)***; see translation (1838, p. 827).

EARLIER REFERENCES:

Illustrated, not named or described:

1. ***[gracile fascicle (Müller, 1834)] (Santorini, 1775)***
Clearly illustrated for macrodissected adult human; Table III, Figure 2. See Burdach (1822, p. 285).

Earlier synonyms:

1. *gracile bundle (Reil, 1809c)*
Synonym for macrodissected adult human ***gracile fascicle (Müller, 1834)***; in the original German, *zarte Bündel*, p. 488; see Burdach (1822, p. 285). Tiedemann

(1816) clearly described it for 5-month human fetus; see translation (1826, p. 148).

2. *inner bundle of posterior funiculus (Rosenthal, 1815)*
Synonym for macrodissected adult human ***gracile fascicle (Müller, 1834)***; in the original German, *inneres Bündel des hintern Strangs*, p. 29, according to Burdach (1822, p. 285).
3. *internal posterior cord of spinal marrow (Meckel, 1817)*
Synonym for macrodissected adult human ***gracile fascicle (Müller, 1834)***; see translation (1832, Vol. 2, p. 414).
4. *funiculus gracilis (Burdach, 1822)*
Synonym for macrodissected adult human ***gracile fascicle (Müller, 1834)***; in the original German, *der zarte Strang*, p. 36, Table IV-*r*.
5. *posterior intermediate fascicles (Bellingeri, 1823)*
Synonym for macrodissected adult human ***gracile fascicle (Müller, 1834)***; in the original Latin (plural), *fasciculi intermedii posteriores*, Table 1, Figure 10-*l*.
6. *posterior median column (Cruveilhier, 1836)*
Synonym for macrodissected adult human ***gracile fascicle (Müller, 1834)***; in the original French (plural), *cordons médians postérieurs*, p. 588. See Henle (1871, p. 42).
7. *Goll's fasciculus (>1840)*
Eponym for macrodissected adult human ***gracile fascicle (Müller, 1834)***; see Henle (1871, p. 42), who attributed it without citation to Kölliker. Also see Goll (1860).

gracile lobule (>1840)

As described for macrodissected adult human, the part of the ***cerebellar hemisphere (Willis, 1664)*** between ***ansiform lobule crus 2 (Bock, 1906)*** and ***biventral lobule (>1840)***, and lateral to adjacent parts of ***tuber vermis (>1840)*** and ***pyramis (Malacarne, 1776)*** of the ***cerebellar vermis (Meckel, 1817)***; see Angevine et al. (1961, Fig. 24), Larsell & Jansen (1972, Fig. 118), Carpenter (1976, Fig. 14.1), Williams & Warwick (1980, Fig. 7.74), *Terminologia Anatomica* (1998, p. 119), Nieuwenhuys et al. (2008, Fig. 20.2). It was first recognized as the *gracile lobe (Malacarne, 1776)*.

EARLIER REFERENCES:

Earlier synonyms:

1. *gracile lobe (Malacarne, 1776)*
Malacarne called "slender" (in Italian, *lobo sottile*) one of his five major lobes of macrodissected adult human ***cerebellar hemisphere (Willis, 1664)***, the ***gracile lobule (>1840)***; p. 22, see Clarke & O'Malley (1996, p. 645).
2. *lobus subtilus (Malacarne, 1776)*
Latin form of ***gracile lobe (Malacarne, 1776)***; see Burdach (1822, p. 295).

gracile nucleus (>1840)

As described for macrodissected adult human, and for adult mammal in general with cellular architecture and connections, the ***gray matter region (Swanson & Bota, 2010)*** of the ***dorsal column nuclei (>1840)*** lying medial to the ***cuneate nucleus (>1840)*** and receiving a massive input from the ***gracile fascicle (Müller, 1834)***; see Williams & Warwick (1980, p. 901), *Terminologia Anatomica* (1998, p. 110), Nieuwenhuys et al. (2008, p. 194 and Figs. 6.21–22). It was first recognized by Burdach; see ***[gracile nucleus (>1840)] (Burdach, 1822)***.

EARLIER REFERENCES:

Described, not named or illustrated:

1. ***[gracile nucleus (>1840)] (Burdach, 1822)***
Burdach alluded to ***gray matter (Meckel, 1817)*** associated with ***funiculus gracilis (Burdach, 1822)*** in macrodissected adult human; p. 37.

Earlier synonyms:

1. *mamillary swelling of posterior median column (Cruveilhier, 1836)*
Synonym for macrodissected adult human ***gracile nucleus (>1840)***; in the original French, *renflemens mamelonnés des cordons médians postérieurs*, p. 588. See *posterior median column (Cruveilhier, 1836)*.

gracile tubercle (>1840)

As described for macrodissected adult human, the surface of the expanded rostral end of the ***gracile fascicle (Müller, 1834)***, the ***medullary gracile fascicle (>1840)***, lying dorsal to the ***gracile nucleus (>1840)***; see Crosby et al. (1962, p. 114), *Terminologia Anatomica* (1998, p. 109), *Dorland's* (2003, p. 1961), Nieuwenhuys et al. (2008, Fig. 3.10-*18*). It was probably first noticed by Aranzi; see ***[gracile tubercle (>1840)] (Aranzi, 1587)***.

EARLIER REFERENCES:

Described, not named or illustrated:

1. ***[gracile tubercle (>1840)] (Aranzi, 1587)***
Aranzi was the first to notice it in macrodissected adult human, according to Burdach (1822, p. 304).

Earlier synonyms:

1. *posterior pyramidal body (Ruysch, 1737)*
Synonym for macrodissected adult human ***gracile tubercle (>1840)***; in the original Latin (plural), *corpora pyramidalia postica*; p. 25, Table XIV, Figure 5. See Burdach (1822, p. 304). Huber (1741, Fig. 2-*M*) used the term for macrodissected adult human shortly thereafter.
2. *posterior pyramid (Haller, 1762)*
Synonym for macrodissected adult human *posterior pyramidal body (Ruysch, 1737)*; p. 80.
3. *pyramidal eminence (Malacarne, 1776)*
Synonym for macrodissected adult human ***gracile tubercle (>1840)***; in the original Italian, *le eminenze piramidali*, p. 81. Also see Clarke & O'Malley (1996, p. 645).
4. *clava (Burdach, 1822)*
Synonym for macrodissected adult human ***gracile tubercle (>1840)***; pp. 37, 75 and Table IV-*u*. See Crosby et al. (1962, p. 114).
5. *pyramidal columns (Rolando, 1824)*
Synonym for macrodissected adult human ***gracile tubercle (>1840)***; in the original Italian, *fasci piramidali*, p. 53.

6. *superior pyramid (Desmoulins, 1825)*
Apparently synonym for macrodissected adult mammalian *posterior pyramid (Haller, 1762)*; in the original French (plural), *pyramides supérieures*, p. 221.

granular retrosplenial area (>1840)

As described with cellular architecture in adult human, the ventral, inner part of the ***retrosplenial region (>1840)***, between ***agranular retrosplenial area (>1840)*** dorsally and caudally and ***fasciola cinerea (Arnold, 1838b)*** ventrally and rostrally. Brodmann called it the *granular retrolimbic area (Brodmann, 1909)*. It was not identified by 1840.

EARLIER REFERENCES:

Earlier synonyms:

1. *area retrolimbica granularis (Brodmann, 1909)*
Original Latin form of *granular retrolimbic area (Brodmann, 1909)*; p. 149.
2. *granular retrolimbic area (Brodmann, 1909)*
Synonym for adult human ***granular retrosplenial area (>1840)***; see p. 149.
3. *area 29 (Brodmann, 1909)*
Synonym for *agranular retrolimbic area (Brodmann, 1909)*; in the original German, *Feld 29*, see p. 149, Figure 86.

gray communicating branch (>1840)

As described for adult human, a ***communicating branch of spinal nerves Wutzer, 1817)***, with each of the ***spinal nerves (Camper, 1760–1762)*** typically having one; see Mitchell (1953, pp. 205–207). ***Gray communicating branches (>1840)*** typically carry postganglionic sympathetic ***axons (Kölliker, 1896)*** and autonomic sensory ***dendrites (His, 1889)***; see Mitchell (1953, p. 124), Williams & Warwick (1980, pp. 1136–1137). Most often the ***white communicating branch (>1840)*** lies just distal to the ***gray communicating branch (>1840)*** on the ***spinal nerve ventral branch (>1840)***; see Williams & Warwick (1980, pp. 1103, 1125). They were clearly identified by Meckel; see ***[gray communicating branch (>1840)] (Meckel, 1751)***.

TRANSLATIONS:

1. *ramus communicans griseus (>1840)*
Current Latin form of ***gray communicating branch (1840)***; see *Terminologia Anatomica* (1998, p. 141).

EARLIER REFERENCES:

Described, not named or illustrated:

1. ***[gray communicating branch (>1840)] (Meckel, 1751)***
Meckel distinguished between ***white communicating branch (>1840)*** and ***gray communicating branch (>1840)*** in macrodissected adult human. He wrote that some are white and others reddish [which they are in the fresh state]—later referred to as gray; see Clarke & Jacyna (1987, p. 325).

PARTLY CORRESPONDS:

1. *anastomotic branch of anterior branch of first cervical nerve with supreme cervical ganglion (Arnold, 1834)*
In macrodissected adult human, ***gray communicating branch (>1840)*** between ***superior cervical ganglion (Vieussens, 1684)*** and ***spinal nerve ventral branch (>1840)*** of first ***cervical nerve (Galen, c173)***; in the original Latin, *ramus anastomoticus nervus cervicalis primus ramus anterior cum ganglio cervicali superior*, p. 16.
2. *connection of anterior branch of second cervical nerve with supreme cervical ganglion (Arnold, 1834)*
In macrodissected adult human, ***gray communicating branch (>1840)*** between ***superior cervical ganglion (Vieussens, 1684)*** and ***spinal nerve ventral branch (>1840)*** of second ***cervical nerve (Galen, c173)***; in the original Latin, *conjunctio nervus cervicalis primus ramus anterior cum ganglio cervicali superior*, p. 16.
3. *anastomotic branch of anterior branch of third cervical nerve with supreme cervical ganglion (Arnold, 1834)*
In macrodissected adult human, ***gray communicating branch (>1840)*** between ***superior cervical ganglion (Vieussens, 1684)*** and ***spinal nerve ventral branch (>1840)*** of the third ***cervical nerve (Galen, c173)***; in the original Latin, *ramus anastomoticus nervus cervicalis tertius ramus anterior cum ganglio cervicali superior*, pp. 16–17.
4. *connection of great anterior branch of fourth cervical nerve with trunk of sympathetic nerve (Arnold, 1834)*
In macrodissected adult human, ***gray communicating branch (>1840)*** between ***communicating branch of superior and middle cervical ganglia (>1840)*** and ***spinal nerve ventral branch (>1840)*** of fourth ***cervical nerve (Galen, c173)***; in the original Latin, *conjunctio nervus cervicalis quartus ramus anterior major cum trunco nervi sympathici*, p. 17.

gray matter (Meckel, 1817)

Since the 16th century, the entire ***nervous system (Monro, 1783)*** has been divided more and more precisely into ***gray matter (Meckel, 1817)*** and ***white matter (Meckel, 1817)*** based on their appearance in freshly dissected material observed with the naked eye—a systems architecture approach. This began with Vesalius's (1543a) macrodissection observations on ***central nervous system gray matter regions (>1840)*** and on Morgagni's (1719) macrodissection observations on ***peripheral nervous system gray matter regions (>1840)***. Since the late 1830s this differentiation has also been made at the cellular level; see Purkinje (1838, Pl. between pp. 174–175, Figs. 16–19). Starting with the latter, it is now known that ***gray matter (Meckel, 1817)*** is the ***nervous system (Monro, 1783)*** compartment consisting of the ***cell bodies (Deiters, 1865)*** of ***neurons (Waldeyer, 1891)***; the cytoplasmic ***neuron extensions (>1840)—axons (Kölliker, 1896)***, ***dendrites (His, 1889)***, and ***amacrine extensions (>1840)***; and ***synapses (Foster & Sherrington, 1897)*** between the ***neuron extensions (>1840)***—as well as ***glia (Virchow, 1846)*** and parts of the *circulatory system (vascular cells)*. ***Neuropil (Waldeyer, 1891)*** refers to the ***gray matter (Meckel, 1817)*** compartment exclusive of *cell bodies* and *vascular cells* (blood vessels) and thus consists of the cytoplasmic extensions of ***neurons (Waldeyer, 1891)*** and ***glia (Virchow, 1846)***, including ***synapses (Foster***

& Sherrington, 1897). There is often a fuzzy border of variable and difficult-to-measure width between ***gray matter (Meckel, 1817)*** and ***white matter (Meckel, 1817)***. ***Gray matter (Meckel, 1817)*** is parceled into ***gray matter regions (Swanson & Bota, 2010)*** based now on regional differences in cellular architecture and connections. For early history, see Clarke & O'Malley (1996, Ch. 10); for modern histological interpretation, see Nauta & Feirtag (1986, p. 45 footnote), Peters et al. (1991), Swanson (2012, pp. 90–103). This definition is adapted from Swanson & Bota (2010, Thesaurus). The general term *gray matter* found anywhere in the ***nervous system (Monro, 1783)*** was probably first used by Meckel for macrodissected adult human; see translation (1832, Vol. 2, pp. 152–154, 166–167); also see Herrick (1915, p. 108). It was described earlier, however, as *nervous brown matter (Gordon, 1815)*.

EARLIER REFERENCES:

Earlier synonyms:

1. *nervous brown matter (Gordon, 1815)*
   Synonym for macrodissected adult human ***gray matter (Meckel, 1817)***; p. 120. Gordon described it as having a slightly different color in different places: *wood-brown matter (Gordon, 1815)* or *greyish-brown matter (Gordon, 1815)*; p. 120.
2. *cineritious matter (Bell & Bell, 1816)*
   Synonym for macrodissected adult human ***gray matter (Meckel, 1817)***; e.g., Vol. 2, pp. 374, 378.

LATER SYNONYMS:

1. *nervous system gray matter (Meckel, 1817)*
   Synonym for ***gray matter (Meckel, 1817)***. Meckel was the first to use this particular terminology, for macrodissected adult human, distinguishing it from *nervous system white matter (Meckel, 1817)*; see translation (1832, Vol. 2, pp. 152–154, 166–167).
2. *secondary substance (Wutzer, 1817)*
   Synonym for macrodissected adult human ***gray matter (Meckel, 1817)***; in the original Latin, *substantia secundaria*, p. 53, see Burdach (1819, p. 168; 1822, p. 250).
3. *nervous system gelatinous substance (Spurzheim, 1826)*
   Synonym for ***gray matter (Meckel, 1817)*** in all animals; p. 1.
4. *nervous system pulpy substance (Spurzheim, 1826)*
   Synonym for ***gray matter (Meckel, 1817)*** in all animals; p. 1.
5. *cineritious neurine (Solly, 1836)*
   Synonym for macrodissected ***gray matter (Meckel, 1817)*** in all animals; pp. 6, 119.
6. *nervous system grey substance (Grainger, 1837)*
   Synonym for ***gray matter (Meckel, 1817)*** in all animals; p. 120.

PARTLY CORRESPONDS:

1. *wood-brown matter Gordon, 1815)*
   One variety of *nervous brown matter (Gordon, 1815)*; p. 120.
2. *greyish-brown matter (Gordon, 1815)*
   One variety of *nervous brown matter (Gordon, 1815)*; p. 120.

gray matter regions (Swanson & Bota, 2010)

Recognizable volumes of ***gray matter (Meckel, 1817)*** in the ***nervous system (Monro, 1783)*** divided topographically into ***central nervous system gray matter regions (>1840)*** and ***peripheral nervous system gray matter regions (>1840)***. All ***gray matter regions (Swanson & Bota, 2010)*** are parceled at the histological level on the basis of a unique set of ***neuron types (Bota & Swanson, 2007)*** with unique spatial distributions and connections—a systems architecture approach. In general, ***gray matter regions (Swanson & Bota, 2010)*** are the sites of origin and termination of axonal connections, whereas the routes taken by connections are through ***white matter tracts (Bell & Bell, 1826)***. The entire ***gray matter (Meckel, 1817)*** is regionalized, and individual regions may contain ***white matter (Meckel, 1817)***, including ***axons-of-passage (Swanson & Bota, 1010)***, which are ***axons (Kölliker, 1896)*** passing through without forming ***synapses (Foster & Sherrington, 1897)***. The traditional way to view regionalization is with a Nissl stain, whose interpretation is based on connectional and histochemical methods identifying ***neuron types (Bota & Swanson, 2007)*** and their spatial distribution; see Brodal (1981, p. 4), Swanson (2004, p. 8). Examples of ***gray matter regions (Swanson & Bota, 2010)*** include areas of the ***cerebral cortex gray matter (>1840)***, nuclei of the ***thalamus (His, 1893a)***, and ***peripheral ganglia (>1840)***. As a complete set, ***gray matter regions (Swanson & Bota, 2010)*** can be arranged in various different ways, for example, *topographic arrangement of gray matter regions* and *subsystems arrangement of gray matter regions*. For this definition see Swanson & Bota (2010, Fig. 1 and Thesaurus). Vesalius first recognized multiple (2) ***gray matter regions (Swanson & Bota, 2010)*** based on macrodissection or gross anatomy; see *cerebral lobe (Vesalius, 1543a)*, ***[cerebellar cortex (Willis, 1664)] (Vesalius, 1543a)***. Purkinje (1838, Pl. between pp. 174–175, Figs. 16–19) clearly laid the groundwork for their histological identification.

great auricular nerve (Haase, 1781)

As described for macrodissected adult human, an ***ascending superficial branch of cervical plexus (Quain, 1828)*** commonly arising from the second and third cervical ***spinal nerve ventral branches (>1840)*** and innervating skin behind the auricle (pinna, external ear), on both sides of the auricle's lower part, and over the ventral (inferior) part of the masseter muscle and parotid gland; see Durward (1951, pp. 1062–1063). For Haase's use in macrodissected adult human, see p. 94. It was known to Galen; see ***[great auricular nerve (Haase, 1781)] (Galen, c173)***.

TRANSLATIONS:

1. *nervus auricularis maximus (Haase, 1781)*
   Original Latin form of ***great auricular nerve (Haase, 1781)***; p. 94.

EARLIER REFERENCES:

Described, not named or illustrated:

1. ***[great auricular nerve (Haase, 1781)] (Galen, c173)***
   Clearly described for macrodissected adult beef, pig, and/or macaque but not human; see May translation (1962, p. 698) and Duckworth translation (1962, pp. 225, 234–235).

Illustrated, not named or described:

1. ***[great auricular nerve (Haase, 1781)] (Eustachi, 1552)***

Illustrated for macrodissected adult human; Table 21/2-*h*.

Illustrated and described, not named:

1. ***[great auricular nerve (Haase, 1781)] (Du Verney, 1683)*** Clearly illustrated and described for macrodissected adult human; see Plate 14:5-7,*D,E*.

Earlier synonyms:

1. *auricular nerve (Meckel, 1753)* Synonym for macrodissected adult human ***great auricular nerve (Haase, 1781)***; in the original French, *le nerf auriculaire*, p. 97.
2. *greater posterior auricular nerve (Meckel, 1753)* Synonym for macrodissected adult human ***great auricular nerve (Haase, 1781)***; in the original French, *le grand nerf auriculaire postérieur*, Table 1-*Λ*; also see *lesser posterior auricular nerve (Meckel, 1753)*.
3. *auricular nerve of third cervical pair (Meckel, 1753)* Synonym for macrodissected adult human ***great auricular nerve (Haase, 1781)***; in the original French, *le nerf auriculaire de la troisième paire des cervicaux*, p. 99.
4. *principal auricular nerve (Bang, 1770)* Synonym for macrodissected adult human ***great auricular nerve (Haase, 1781)***; in the original Latin, *nervus auricularis principalis*, Figure I-30 (see 1791 reprint).
5. *posterior auricular nerve (Neubauer, 1772)* Apparently synonym for macrodissected adult human ***great auricular nerve (Haase, 1781)***; in the original Latin, *nervum auricularem posteriorem*, Table 1-*159,173*. Neubauer referred to greater and lesser components.

LATER SYNONYMS:

1. *zygomatico-auricular branch of cephalic part of trachelo-cutanean plexus (Burdin, 1803)* Synonym for *zygomatico-auricular branch of cephalic part of tracheosubcutaneous nerves (Chaussier, 1809)*; see translation (1803, Vol. 1, p. 188).
2. *zygomatico-auricular branch of cephalic part of tracheosubcutaneous nerves (Chaussier, 1809)* Synonym for macrodissected adult human ***great auricular nerve (Haase, 1781)***, according to Meckel (1832, Vol. 3, p. 32); in the original French, *branche zygomato-oriculaire*.
3. *auricular branch of cervical plexus (Cloquet, 1816)* Synonym for macrodissected adult human ***great auricular nerve (Haase, 1781)***; in the original French, *branche auriculaire*, p. 640.
4. *cervical auricular nerve (Meckel, 1817)* Synonym for macrodissected adult human ***great auricular nerve (Haase, 1781)***; in the original Latin, *nervus auricularis cervicalis*, see translation (1832, Vol. 3, p. 32).
5. *middle ascending superficial branch of cervical plexus (Quain, 1828)* Synonym for macrodissected adult human ***great auricular nerve (Haase, 1781)***; p. 489.
6. *middle branch of cervical plexus (Quain & Wilson, 1839)* Synonym for macrodissected adult human ***great auricular nerve (Haase, 1781)***; Plate XIV-*l*.

greater occipital nerve (Haase, 1781)

As described for macrodissected adult human, formed by the ***medial branch of spinal nerve dorsal branch (>1840)*** arising from the second ***cervical nerve (Galen, c173)*** and a small branch from the ***medial branch of spinal nerve dorsal branch (>1840)*** arising from the third ***cervical nerve (Galen, c173)***. It supplies skin of the scalp as far rostrally (forward) as the vertex of the skull, and the semispinalis capitis muscle; see Williams & Warwick (1980, p. 1089). For Haase's use in macrodissected adult human, see p. 94. It was known to Galen; see ***[greater occipital nerve (Haase, 1781)] (Galen, c173)***.

TRANSLATIONS:

1. *nervus occipitalis magnus (Haase, 1781)* Original Latin form of ***greater occipital nerve (Haase, 1781)***; p. 94.

EARLIER REFERENCES:

Described, not named or illustrated:

1. ***[greater occipital nerve (Haase, 1781)] (Galen, c173)*** Clearly described for macrodissected beef, pig, and/or macaque but not human; see May translation (1968, pp. 597, 698, 701) and Duckworth translation (1962, pp. 225–226).

Illustrated and described, not named:

1. ***[greater occipital nerve (Haase, 1781)] (Vesalius, 1543a)*** Described and illustrated for macrodissected adult human; see Richardson & Carman translation (2002, p. 225).

Earlier synonyms:

1. *great occipital nerve (Winslow, 1733)* Probably corresponds to macrodissected adult human ***greater occipital nerve (Haase, 1781)***; Section VI, no. 180, p. 78 (also see Sect. VI, no. 172, p. 77).

LATER SYNONYMS:

1. *posterior greater occipital nerve (Peipers, 1793)* Synonym for macrodissected adult human ***greater occipital nerve (Haase, 1781)***; in the original Latin, *nervus occipitalis maximus posterior*; p. 33.
2. *posterior occipital nerve (Quain & Wilson, 1839)* Synonym for macrodissected adult human ***greater occipital nerve (Haase, 1781)***; Plate XIV-*s*.

PARTLY CORRESPONDS:

1. *connection of greater occipital nerve with lesser occipital nerve (Arnold, 1834)* Macrodissected adult human ***communicating branch (Winslow, 1733)*** between ***greater occipital nerve (Haase, 1781)*** and ***lesser occipital nerve (Mayer, 1794)***; in the original Latin, *conjunctio nervus occipitalis major cum nervo occipitali minori*, Table IX-*40,41*.

greater palatine nerve (Cloquet, 1816)

As described for macrodissected adult human, it courses ventrally (descends) from the ***pterygopalatine ganglion (>1840)*** to supply the gums and the mucous membrane and glands of the hard palate, and it communicates rostrally (in front), below the hard palate, with terminal branches of the ***nasopalatine nerve (Scarpa, 1785)***; its major branches are the ***posterior inferior nasal nerves***

(Günther, 1786); see Williams & Warwick (1980, p. 1065 and Fig. 7.178). For Cloquet's use in macrodissected adult human see p. 684, where he described a multitude of external and internal branches. Vesalius may have been the first to recognize it; see ***[greater palatine nerve (Cloquet, 1816)] (Vesalius, 1543a)***.

ALTERNATE SPELLINGS:

1. *great palatine nerve (Meckel, 1832)*
   English form of *nervus palatini major (Meckel, 1817)*; see translation (1832, Vol. 3, p. 68).

TRANSLATIONS:

1. *grand nerf palatin (Cloquet, 1816)*
   Original French form of ***greater palatine nerve (Cloquet, 1816)***; p. 684.
2. *nervus palatini major (Meckel, 1817)*
   Latin form of ***greater palatine nerve (Cloquet, 1816)***; see translation (1832, Vol. 3, p. 68).

EARLIER REFERENCES:

Illustrated and described, not named:

1. ***[greater palatine nerve (Cloquet, 1816)] (Vesalius, 1543a)***
   Vesalius may have described and illustrated it for macrodissected adult human according to Meckel, who reviewed the vague earlier literature (1748, p. 62 note *s*); also see the more skeptical interpretation in Richardson & Carman (2002, p. 192, and *Z* in Fig. 2 on p. 169).

Earlier synonyms:

1. *anterior greater palatine nerve (Meckel, 1748)*
   Synonym for macrodissected adult human ***greater palatine nerve (Cloquet, 1816)***; in the original Latin, *nervi palatini major anterior*, p. 61. Mayer (1794; Part 5, Tab. VIII-ς) gave it as *nervus palatinus anterior major*.
2. *anterior palatine nerve (Meckel, 1748)*
   Synonym for *anterior greater palatine nerve (Meckel, 1748)*; in the original Latin, *palatinus anterior nervus*, p. 62.
3. *anterior branch of palatine nerve (Bang, 1770)*
   Synonym for macrodissected adult human ***greater palatine nerve (Cloquet, 1816)***; in the original Latin, *nervus palatinus ramus anterior*; Figure II-*h*.
4. *anterior greater branch of palatine nerve (Loder, 1778)*
   Synonym for macrodissected adult human ***greater palatine nerve (Cloquet, 1816)***; in the original Latin, *majorem anteriorem*, p. 14 (and p. 13).
5. *ethmoidal nerve (Burdin, 1803)*
   Synonym for macrodissected adult human ***greater palatine nerve (Cloquet, 1816)***; see translation (1803, Vol. 1, p. 175).
6. *spheno-palatine nerve (Burdin, 1803)*
   Synonym for *ethmoidal nerve (Burdin, 1803)*; see translation (1803, Vol. 1, p. 175).

LATER SYNONYMS:

1. *inferior palatine nerve (Cloquet, 1816)*
   Synonym for macrodissected adult human ***greater palatine nerve (Cloquet, 1816)*** attributed without citation to Chaussier; in the original French, *nerf palatin inférieur*, p. 684.
2. *anterior palatine fascicle of sphenopalatine ganglion (Bellingeri, 1818)*
   Synonym for macrodissected adult human ***greater palatine nerve (Cloquet, 1816)***; in the original Latin, *fascicle palatinus anterior*, see Table I.
3. *internal branches of spheno-palatine ganglion (Quain, 1828)*
   Synonym for macrodissected adult human ***greater palatine nerve (Cloquet, 1816)***; p. 666.
4. *spheno-palatine branches of spheno-palatine ganglion (Quain, 1828)*
   Synonym for macrodissected adult human ***greater palatine nerve (Cloquet, 1816)***; p. 666. A typographical error had it spelled *pheno-palatine*.
5. *principal palatine nerve (Swan, 1830)*
   Synonym for macrodissected adult human ***greater palatine nerve (Cloquet, 1816)***; Plate XIV, Figure 8-*8*.
6. *spheno-palatine branches of Meckel's ganglion (Quain & Wilson, 1839)*
   Synonym for *spheno-palatine branches of spheno-palatine ganglion (Quain, 1828)*; Plate XIII, Figure 2-*q*.

PARTLY CORRESPONDS:

1. *inferior nasal nerves (Schaarschmidt, 1750)*
   Branches of macrodissected adult human ***greater palatine nerve (Cloquet, 1816)*** to nasal septum; in the original Latin, *nervi nasales inferiores*, p. 22.
2. *exterior minor branch of major palatine nerve (Scarpa, 1785)*
   Branch of macrodissected adult human ***greater palatine nerve (Cloquet, 1816)*** to gingiva of molar and premolar regions; in the original Latin, *ramus minor exterior*, Table II, Figure II-*19*.
3. *palatine gland threads of anterior palatine fascicle (Bellingeri, 1818)*
   Branches of macrodissected adult human ***greater palatine nerve (Cloquet, 1816)*** to palatine glands; in the original Latin, *stamina palatinus glandularis*, see Table I.
4. *external palatine thread of anterior palatine fascicle (Bellingeri, 1818)*
   Synonym for macrodissected adult human *exterior minor branch of major palatine nerve (Scarpa, 1785)*; in the original Latin, *stamen palatinus externus*, see Table I.
5. *internal palatine thread of anterior palatine fascicle (Bellingeri, 1818)*
   Branch of macrodissected adult human ***greater palatine nerve (Cloquet, 1816)*** to palatine glands and mucosa; in the original Latin, *stamen palatinus internus*, see Table I.
6. *staphyline branch of anterior palatine nerve (Cruveilhier, 1836)*
   Branch of ***greater palatine nerve (Cloquet, 1816)*** to both sides of soft palate, supplied by superior and inferior branchlets; in the original French, *rameau staphylin*, pp. 921–922.

greater petrosal nerve (>1840)

As described for macrodissected adult human, a branch of the ***intermediofacial nerve trunk (>1840)*** leaving from the ***geniculate ganglion (Bischoff, 1832)*** and extending rostrally (forward) to meet the ***deep petrosal nerve (Meckel, 1817)***; the merged ***greater petrosal nerve (>1840)*** and ***deep petrosal nerve (Meckel, 1817)*** together form the ***nerve of pterygoid canal (>1840)*** ending in the ***pterygopalatine ganglion (>1840)***; see Williams & Warwick (1980, Figure 7.184). It was discovered by Vesalius; see ***[greater petrosal nerve (>1840)] (Vesalius, 1543a)***.

EARLIER REFERENCES:

Illustrated and described, not named:

1. *[greater petrosal nerve (>1840)] (Vesalius, 1543a)* According to Richardson & Carman (2002, p. 193), Vesalius (1543a) described and illustrated it for macrodissected adult human.

Earlier synonyms:

1. *superficial minor branch of Vidian nerve (Meckel, 1748)* Synonym for macrodissected adult human ***greater petrosal nerve (>1840)***; in the original Latin, *ramus nervus Vidianus minorem superficialem*, p. 52 and Figure 1-57,κ.
2. *petrosal nerve (Schaarschmidt, 1750)* Synonym for macrodissected adult human ***greater petrosal nerve (>1840)***; in the original Latin, *nervus petrosus*, p. 21.
3. *superficial branch of Vidian nerve (Scarpa, 1785)* Synonym for macrodissected adult human *greater petrosal nerve (>1840)*; in the original Latin, *nervi vidiani ramos superficialem*, Table II, Figure II-*11*.
4. *facial communicating nerve (Wrisberg, 1786)* Synonym for macrodissected adult human ***greater petrosal nerve (>1840)***; in the original Latin, *nervo communicante faciei*, see Wrisberg reprint (1800, p. 387 and also p. 374).
5. *superficial Vidian nerve (Günther, 1786)* For macrodissected adult human, shorter form of *superficial minor branch of Vidian nerve (Meckel, 1748)*; in the original Latin, *Vidianum superficialem*, p. 47.
6. *superior Vidian nerve (Günther, 1786)* Synonym for macrodissected adult human ***greater petrosal nerve (>1840)***; in the original Latin, *Vidianum superiorem*, p. 47.
7. *petrous nerve (Günther, 1786)* Synonym for macrodissected adult human ***greater petrosal nerve (>1840)***; in the original Latin, *petrosum*, p. 47.
8. *cranial branch of pterygoid branch of superior maxillary branch of trigeminal nerve (Bichat et al., 1801–1803)* Synonym for macrodissected adult human ***greater petrosal nerve (>1840)***; in the original French, *filet crânien*, Vol. 3, p. 179.
9. *superior branch of Vidian nerve (Burdin, 1803)* Synonym for macrodissected adult human ***greater petrosal nerve (>1840)***; see translation (1803, Vol. 1, p. 174). Also see Cloquet (1816, p. 685).
10. *pterygoid branch of facial nerve (Chaussier, 1809)* Synonym for macrodissected adult human ***greater petrosal nerve (>1840)***; in the original French, *filet ptérygoïdien*.
11. *superior branch of pterygoid nerve (Cloquet, 1816)* Probably macrodissected adult human ***greater petrosal nerve (>1840)***; in the original French, *rameau supérieur du nerf ptérygoïdien*, p. 685.
12. *superior petrous nerve (Meckel, 1817)* Synonym for macrodissected adult human ***greater petrosal nerve (>1840)***; see translation (1832, Vol. 3, p. 67).
13. *superficial petrous nerve (Meckel, 1817)* Synonym for macrodissected adult human ***greater petrosal nerve (>1840)***; in the original Latin, *nervus petrosus superficialis*, see translation (1832, Vol. 3, pp. 53, 67).
14. *anastomotic petrosal thread of Vidian fascicle with trunk of facial nerve (Bellingeri, 1818)* Synonym for macrodissected adult human ***greater petrosal nerve (>1840)***; in the original Latin, *stamen petrosus anastomoticus cum trunco nervi facialis*, see Table I.
15. *deep-seated Vidian nerve (Lobstein, 1823)* Synonym for ***greater petrosal nerve (>1840)***; see translation (1831, Pl. VI-*g*).
16. *cranial branch of Vidian nerve (Cloquet, 1828)* Synonym for macrodissected adult human ***greater petrosal nerve (>1840)***; in the original French, *filet crânien du nerf vidian*, Plate CXXIX, Figure 14-*19*.
17. *greater superficial petrosal nerve (Arnold, 1834)* Synonym for macrodissected adult human ***greater petrosal nerve (>1840)***; in the original Latin, *nervus petrosus superficialis major*, pp. 9, 11. It was used in the *Basel Nomina Anatomica*; His (1895, p. 88).
18. *superficial petrous branch of Vidian nerve (Todd, 1836–1839)* Synonym for macrodissected adult human ***greater petrosal nerve (>1840)***; p. 288.
19. *superior twig of Vidian nerve (Todd, 1836–1839)* Synonym for macrodissected adult human ***greater petrosal nerve (>1840)***; p. 371.
20. *nervus innominatus (Todd, 1836–1839)* Synonym for macrodissected adult human ***greater petrosal nerve (>1840)***; p. 371.
21. *petrous branch of posterior branch of spheno-palatine ganglion (Quain & Wilson, 1839)* Synonym for macrodissected adult human ***greater petrosal nerve (>1840)***; Plate XXVII-*o,q*.
22. *petrous branch of Vidian nerve (Quain & Wilson, 1839)* Synonym for macrodissected adult human ***greater petrosal nerve (>1840)***; Plate XXVII-*o,q*.
23. *parasympathetic root of pterygopalatine ganglion (>1840)* Synonym for macrodissected adult human ***greater petrosal nerve (>1840)***; it is inappropriate because the ***nerve (Herophilus, c335–c280 BC)*** has other

functional components; see Williams & Warwick (1980, p. 1071), *Terminologia Anatomica* (1998, p. 135).

PARTLY CORRESPONDS:

1. *branch of superficial branch of Vidian nerve to internal malleus muscle (Langenbeck, 1826–1830)*
   Macrodissected adult human branch of ***greater petrosal nerve (>1840)*** to tensor tympani muscle; in the original Latin, *ramus rami superficialis nervi Vidiani ad musculum mallei internum*, Fascicle III, Table XXVI-*l*.

greater splanchnic nerve (Walter, 1783)

As described for macrodissected adult human, it is almost always larger than the more caudal ***lesser splanchnic nerve (Haller, 1762)*** and ***least splanchnic nerve (>1840)***, and usually arises by 3–4 larger roots and an inconsistent number of smaller rootlets from the fifth or sixth to the ninth or tenth ***thoracic sympathetic ganglia (>1840)***. The right and left ***greater splanchnic nerves (Walter, 1783)*** extend caudally (descend) in the thorax—communicating with the ***esophageal plexus (Haller, 1762)*** and ***thoracic aortic plexus (>1840)***—enter the abdomen by piercing the homolateral diaphragmatic crus, and shortly thereafter end in the ***celiac plexus (Winslow, 1733)***, ***celiac ganglion (Walter, 1783)***, ***aorticorenal ganglion (>1840)***, and adrenal gland; see Mitchell (1953, pp. 240–243 and Fig. 104), Williams & Warwick (1980, p. 1131). For Walter's use in macrodissected adult human, see Table I-*214,215*. It probably first appeared in English in the translation of Lobstein (1831, pp. 24–25). It was probably known to Galen; see ***[greater splanchnic nerve (Walter, 1783)] (Galen, c177)***.

TRANSLATIONS:

1. *nervus splanchnicus major (Walter, 1783)*
   Original Latin form of ***greater splanchnic nerve (Walter, 1783)***; Table I-*214,215*.

EARLIER REFERENCES:

Described, not named or illustrated:

1. ***[greater splanchnic nerve (Walter, 1783)] (Galen, c177)***
   Probably mentioned in passing for macrodissected adult beef, pig, and/or macaque but not human; see Singer (1999, p. 142 note *115*).

Illustrated, not named or described:

1. ***[greater splanchnic nerve (Walter, 1783)] (Eustachi, 1552)***
   Illustrated for macrodissected adult human; see Albinus edition (1761, Table 18, Fig. 2-*ψ,ω*).

Earlier synonyms:

1. *mesenteric nerve (Willis, 1664)*
   Synonym for macrodissected adult human ***greater splanchnic nerve (Walter, 1783)***; in the original Latin, *nervus mesentericus* (Tab. XI-G); also see Pordage translation (1681, p. 158 and Tab. XI-G).
2. *mesenteric branch of intercostal nerve (Willis, 1664)*
   Synonym for *mesenteric nerve (Willis, 1664)*; see Pordage translation (1681, p. 158).
3. *supreme mesenteric branch (Willis, 1664)*
   Synonym for *mesenteric nerve (Willis, 1664)*, referring to branch of *intercostal nerve (Willis, 1564)*; see Pordage translation (1681, p. 166).
4. *superior mesenteric branch of intercostal trunk (Drake, 1707)*
   Variation on *supreme mesenteric branch (Willis, 1664)* for macrodissected adult human; p. 519.
5. *anterior intercostal nerve (Schaarschmidt, 1750)*
   Synonym for macrodissected adult human ***greater splanchnic nerve (Walter, 1783)***; in the original Latin, *nervus intercostalis anterior*, p. 52.
6. *superior splanchnic nerve (Haase, 1781)*
   Synonym for macrodissected adult human ***greater splanchnic nerve (Walter, 1783)***; in the original Latin, *nervus splanchnicus superior*, p. 126.

LATER SYNONYMS:

1. *principal splanchnic nerve (Walter, 1783)*
   Synonym for macrodissected adult human ***greater splanchnic nerve (Walter, 1783)***; in the original Latin, *nervus splanchnicus principalis*, Table III-*220*, or *nervum splanchnicum principem*, Table III-*221*.
2. *splanchnic nerve (Günther, 1786)*
   Günther's preferred term for macrodissected adult human ***greater splanchnic nerve (Walter, 1783)***; in the original Latin, *n. splanchnicum*, p. 94.
3. *collateral intercostal nerve (Günther, 1786)*
   Synonym for macrodissected adult human ***greater splanchnic nerve (Walter, 1783)***; in the original Latin, *n. intercostalem collateralem*, p. 94.
4. *great suprarenal nerve (Chaussier, 1789)*
   Synonym listed for macrodissected adult human ***greater splanchnic nerve (Walter, 1783)***; in the original French, *le grand surrenal*, in *Table synoptique du nerf tri-splanchnique*.
5. *collateral trunk (Chaussier, 1789)*
   Synonym listed for macrodissected adult human ***greater splanchnic nerve (Walter, 1783)***; in the original French, *tronc collatéral*, in *Table synoptique du nerf tri-splanchnique*.
6. *great splanchnic nerve (Knox, 1832)*
   Synonym for macrodissected adult human ***greater splanchnic nerve (Walter, 1783)***; Plate VIII-*4*.

PARTLY CORRESPONDS:

1. *splanchnic nerve trunk (Wrisberg, 1780)*
   Segment of ***greater splanchnic nerve (Walter, 1783)*** distal to point where *splanchnic nerve roots (Wrisberg, 1780)* from 6th–9th ***thoracic sympathetic ganglia (>1840)*** have joined in macrodissected adult human; in the original Latin, *splanchnici nervi truncus*; see Wrisberg (1800, p. 268).
2. *splanchnic nerve roots (Wrisberg, 1780)*
   Separate origins of ***greater splanchnic nerve (Walter, 1783)*** from 6th–9th ***thoracic sympathetic ganglia (>1840)*** before joining to form *splanchnic nerve trunk (Wrisberg, 1780)* in macrodissected adult human; in the original Latin, *splanchnici nervi radices*; see Wrisberg (1800, p. 268).

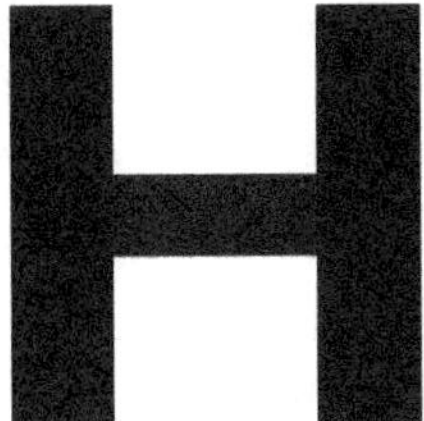

habenular commissure (>1840)

As described in macrodissected adult human, and mammal generally with histological methods for ***axons (Kölliker, 1896)***, a very short transverse ***central nervous system white matter tract (>1840)*** connecting the caudal ends of the right and left ***medullary stria (Wenzel & Wenzel, 1812)*** through the base of the dorsal lamella of the ***pineal stalk (Burdach, 1822)***; see Williams & Warwick (1980, pp. 962–963), Nieuwenhuys et al. (2008, pp. 52, 69). It was probably known to Vesalius; see ***[habenular commissure (>1840)] (Vesalius, 1555)***.

EARLIER REFERENCES:

Described, not named or illustrated:

1. ***[habenular commissure (>1840)] (Vesalius, 1555)***
   Vesalius described without naming a transverse ***central nervous system white matter tract (>1840)*** near the ***pineal gland (Galen, c192)*** in macrodissected adult human, almost certainly ***habenular commissure (>1840)*** rather than ***posterior commissure (Winslow, 1733)***; see Singer translation (1952, p. 36), also see *tractus medullaris transversus natibus antipositus (Vieussens, 1684)*.

Earlier synonyms:

1. *glandulae pinealis frena (Tarin, 1750)*
   Tarin very clearly illustrated crossing of right and left ***medullary stria (Wenzel & Wenzel, 1812)*** dorsal to and distinct from ***posterior commissure (Winslow, 1733)*** in macrodissected adult human, the ***habenular commissure (>1840)***. Whether he included ***pineal stalk (Burdach, 1822)*** is unclear; Table I, Figure 3-*K*; Table II, Figure 2-*f*. Also see *columna medullaris (Tarin, 1750)*.
2. *commissura taeniae (Haller, 1762)*
   Synonym for macrodissected adult human ***habenular commissure (>1840)*** as distinguished from ***medullary stria (Wenzel & Wenzel, 1812)***; see Meyer (1971, pp. 16, 107).
3. *transverse commissure of conarium (Cruveilhier, 1836)*
   Synonym for macrodissected adult human ***habenular commissure (>1840)***; in the original French, *commissure transversale*, p. 687.
4. *transverse commissure of pineal body (Cruveilhier, 1836)*
   Synonym for macrodissected adult human ***habenular commissure (>1840)***; in the original French, *commissure transversale*, p. 687.
5. *pineal commissure (Combe et al., 1838)*
   Presumably synonym for macrodissected adult human ***habenular commissure (>1840)***; p. xxviii.

habenular nuclei (>1840)

As described for macrodissected adult human, and for adult vertebrate in general with cellular architecture and connections, the ***gray matter region (Swanson & Bota, 2010)*** of the ***epithalamus (His, 1893b)*** lying medial to the ***medullary stria (Wenzel & Wenzel, 1812)***, and further divided into ***medial habenular nucleus (>1840)*** and ***lateral habenular nucleus (>1840)***; see Jones (1985, Ch. 15.2), Nieuwenhuys et al. (2008, Figs. 5.9, 5.31). Not clearly identified by 1840.

EARLIER REFERENCES:

Earlier synonyms:

1. *habenular ganglion (Meynert, 1872)*
   Synonym for macrodissected adult human ***habenular nuclei (>1840)***; in the original Latin, *ganglion habenulae*, p. 695 and Figure 271.

habenular sulcus (>1840)

As described for macrodissected adult human, a groove separating the ventrolateral edge of ***habenular trigone (>1840)*** of the ***epithalamus (His, 1893b)*** from the adjacent dorsomedial edge of the ***dorsal part of thalamus (Herrick, 1910)***; see Williams & Warwick (1980, pp. 955,

962), *Dorland's* (2003, p. 1786), Nieuwenhuys et al. (2008, Fig. 5.9, unlabeled between *23, 28*). In mammal generally it lies along the lateral margin of the ***medullary stria (Wenzel & Wenzel, 1812)*** and accompanying ***lateral habenular nucleus (>1840)***, indicating the surface border between ***epithalamus (His, 1893b)*** and ***dorsal part of thalamus (Herrick, 1910)***. Not described by 1840.

habenular triangle (>1840)

As described for macrodissected adult human, the surface between ***habenular sulcus (>1840)*** laterally and ***choroid line of third ventricle (>1840)*** medially, formed mostly by the surface of the ***medullary stria (Wenzel & Wenzel, 1812)***; see Williams & Warwick (1980, p. 955 and Fig. 7.97), Nieuwenhuys et al. (2008, Figs. 3.19-*14*, 5.9 surface of *28*). Not clearly described by 1840.

TRANSLATIONS:

1. *trigonum habenulare (>1840)*
   Current Latin form of ***habenular triangle (>1840)***; see *Terminologia Anatomica* (1998, p. 120), where the English form, *habenular trigone*, is given.

habenulo-interpeduncular tract (>1840)

As described in macrodissected adult human, and mammal generally with histological methods for ***axons (Kölliker, 1896)***, a ***central nervous system white matter tract (>1840)*** extending longitudinally from the caudal end of the ***habenular nuclei (>1840)*** of the ***epithalamus (His, 1893b)*** to the adjacent rostral end of the ***midbrain (Baer, 1837)*** before coursing ventrally (transversely) to end in the ***interpeduncular nucleus (>1840)***; see *Terminologia Anatomica* (1998, p. 121), Nieuwenhuys et al. (2008, Fig. 7.1). For topographic description, it has ***thalamic habenulo-interpeduncular tract (>1840)*** and ***tegmental habenulo-interpeduncular tract (>1840)*** segments. It was probably first identified as *sphincter of anus (Chaussier, 1807)*.

EARLIER REFERENCES:

Earlier synonyms:

1. *sphincter of anus (Chaussier, 1807)*
   Described in macrodissected adult human as very thin ***central nervous system white matter tracts (>1840)*** coursing on right and left side past region where ***third ventricle (Galen, c173)*** leads into ***cerebral aqueduct (>1840)***, the ***opening of cerebral aqueduct (>1840)*** sometimes called *anus (Bauhin, 1605)*. These ***central nervous system white matter tracts (>1840)*** are probably right and left ***habenulo-interpeduncular tracts (>1840)***, and Chaussier (1807, p. 71; in the original French, *sphincter de l'anus*) attributed without citation the description and name to "Fr. Petit," probably François Pourfour du Petit. There is reference to *white substance (Vesalius, 1543a)* sphincters on p. 13 of Letter 1 (Pourfour du Petit, 1710), but this passage hardly fits Chaussier's description.
2. *inferior peduncles of conarium (Cruveilhier, 1836)*
   Synonym for macrodissected adult human right and left ***habenulo-interpeduncular tract (>1840)***; in the original French, *pédoncules inférieurs*, p. 687.
3. *inferior peduncles of pineal body (Cruveilhier, 1836)*
   Synonym for macrodissected adult human right and left ***habenulo-interpeduncular tract (>1840)***; in the original French, *pédoncules inférieurs*, p. 687.
4. *tegmental bundle from ganglion of pineal peduncles (Meynert, 1871–1872)*
   Synonym for adult human and guinea pig ***habenulo-interpeduncular tract (>1840)*** observed histologically; Vol. II, pp. 737–738, Figure 241-*I*; see translation (1872, p. 695 and Fig. 264-*I*).
5. *fasciculus retroflexus (>1840)*
   Synonym for ***habenulo-interpeduncular tract (>1840)***; see *Terminologia Anatomica* (1998, p. 121).
6. *Meynert's bundle (>1840)*
   Eponym for ***habenulo-interpeduncular tract (>1840)***; see Meyer (1971, p. 46).

PARTLY CORRESPONDS:

1. *interpeduncular fascicle (Cruveilhier, 1836)*
   Apparently indicates segment of macrodissected adult human ***habenulo-interpeduncular tract (>1840)*** within ***interpeduncular nucleus (>1840)***; in the original French (plural), *faisceaux interpédonculaires*, p. 606.

head of caudate nucleus (>1840)

As defined arbitrarily for macrodissected adult human, the expanded rostrodorsal end of the ***caudate nucleus (Arnold, 1838b)*** lying rostral to the ***body of caudate nucleus (>1840)*** and the ***thalamus (His, 1893a)***, and bulging medially into the ***anterior horn of lateral ventricle (Bell, 1803b)***; see Carpenter (1976, p. 497, Fig. 17.4). It was clearly illustrated by Vesalius; see ***[head of caudate nucleus (>1840)] (Vesalius, 1543a)***.

EARLIER REFERENCES:

Illustrated, not named or described:

1. ***[head of caudate nucleus (>1840)] (Vesalius, 1543a)***
   Clearly illustrated for macrodissected adult human; see Singer translation (1952, Figs. 6-*D,E* and 7).

Earlier synonyms:

1. *head of striated body (Willis, 1664)*
   Roughly synonymous with ***head of caudate nucleus (>1840)***; see Pordage translation (1681, p. 63). Also see *striated body (Willis, 1664)*.
2. *basis of striate body (Willis, 1672)*
   Synonym for *head of striated body (Willis, 1664)*; see Pordage translation (1683, p. 44, Tab. VIII-*F*).
3. *base of striate body (Willis, 1672)*
   Alternate form of *basis of striate body (Willis, 1672)*.

hemispheric sulcus (Grönberg, 1902)

As described for the developing vertebrate ***neural tube (Baer, 1837)***, the surface groove between ***endbrain vesicle (Kuhlenbeck, 1927)*** and ***interbrain vesicle (Baer,***

1837); see Alvarez-Bolado & Swanson (1996, pp. 14, 22, 25 and embryonic days 11–17). It was first delineated by Malpighi; see ***[hemispheric sulcus (Grönberg, 1902)] (Malpighi, 1673)***.

EARLIER REFERENCES:

Illustrated, not named or described:

1. ***[hemispheric sulcus (Grönberg, 1902)] (Malpighi, 1673)***
   Illustrated clearly but not described for early chick embryo; see Table III.

hepatic branches of anterior vagal trunk (>1840)

As described for macrodissected adult human, usually 2–4 of them extend to the liver, often with branches to the common and cystic ducts, and to the gall bladder. They are complemented by 1–2 ***hepatic branches of posterior vagal trunk (>1840)***; see Mitchell (1953, p. 187), *Terminologia Anatomica* (1998, p. 136). They were known to Galen; see ***[hepatic branches of anterior vagal trunk (>1840)] (Galen, c173)***.

EARLIER REFERENCES:

Described, not named or illustrated:

1. ***[hepatic branches of anterior vagal trunk (>1840)] (Galen, c173)***
   Mentioned for macrodissected adult beef, pig, and/or macaque but not human; see May (1968, pp. 223, 228, 246). Vesalius (1543a) described and illustrated them for macrodissected adult human; see Richardson & Carman translation (2002, p. 172-*x,ß2**).

Earlier synonyms:

1. *left hepatic plexus (Wrisberg, 1780)*
   Synonym for macrodissected adult human ***hepatic branches of anterior vagal trunk (>1840)***; in the original Latin, *plexum hepaticum sinistrum*, see Wrisberg reprint (1800, p. 259).
2. *minor hepatic plexus (Wrisberg, 1780)*
   Synonym for macrodissected adult human ***hepatic branches of anterior vagal trunk (>1840)***; in the original Latin, *plexum hepaticum minorem*, see Wrisberg reprint (1800, p. 259).
3. *ascending branches of anterior trunk of eighth pair of nerves (Walter, 1783)*
   Synonym for macrodissected adult human ***hepatic branches of anterior vagal trunk (>1840)***; in the original Latin, *ramos adscendentes truncus anterior nervi octavi paris*, Table IV-*456*.
4. *hepatic branches of anterior trunk of eighth pair of nerves (Walter, 1783)*
   Synonym for macrodissected adult human ***hepatic branches of anterior vagal trunk (>1840)***; in the original Latin, *ramos hepaticos truncus anterior nervi octavi paris*, Table IV-*456*.
5. *ascending branch of left vagus nerve (Mayer, 1794)*
   Synonym for macrodissected adult human ***hepatic branches of anterior vagal trunk (>1840)***; in the original Latin, *ramus adscendens nervi vagi sinistri*; Part 6, Table IV-*5* (pp. 25–26).
6. *hepatic branch of left vagus nerve (Mayer, 1794)*
   Synonym for macrodissected adult human ***hepatic branches of anterior vagal trunk (>1840)***; in the original Latin, *ramus hepaticus nervi vagi sinistri*; Part 6, Table IV-*5* (p. 26).

hepatic branches of posterior vagal trunk (>1840)

As described for macrodissected adult human, 1–2 branches of the ***gastric branches of posterior vagal trunk (>1840)*** to the liver, supplementing the 2–4 ***hepatic branches of anterior vagal trunk (>1840)***; see Mitchell (1953, p. 187), Williams & Warwick (1980, p. 1081), *Nomina Anatomica* (1983, p. A76). At least one was known to Vesalius; see ***[hepatic branch of posterior vagal trunk (>1840)] (Vesalius, 1543a)***.

EARLIER REFERENCES:

Described, not named or illustrated:

1. ***[hepatic branch of posterior vagal trunk (>1840)] (Vesalius, 1543a)***
   Vesalius described and illustrated branch of right ***vagus nerve (Galen, c192)*** extending from stomach along portal vein to concave area of liver; see Richardson & Carman translation (2002, p. 199).

Earlier synonyms:

1. *hepatico-gastric branch of posterior trunk of gastric and hepatic plexus (Walter, 1783)*
   Essentially synonym for macrodissected adult human ***hepatic branch of posterior vagal trunk (>1840)***; in the original Latin, *ramus hepaticus-gastricus truncus posterior plexus ventriculi et hepatis*, Table III-*505*.
2. *superior branch of right vagus nerves (Mayer, 1794)*
   Synonym for macrodissected adult human ***hepatic branch of posterior vagal trunk (>1840)***; in the original Latin, *ramus superior nervi vagi dextri*; Part 6, Table IV-*12* (p. 26).

hepatic ganglia (Walter, 1783)

As described for macrodissected adult human, ***terminal ganglia (Gaskell, 1886)*** around the hepatic artery that are variable in size (though usually small) and number; see Foster (1892, p. 1674). For Walter's use in macrodissected adult human see Table IV:*183–188*.

TRANSLATIONS:

1. *ganglia hepatica (Walter, 1783)*
   Original Latin form of ***hepatic ganglia (Walter, 1783)***, Table IV:*183–188*.

hepatic plexus (Rau, 1720)

As described for macrodissected adult human, the largest ***terminal plexus (Swanson & Bota, 2010)*** extension of the ***celiac plexus (Winslow, 1733)***. It receives small branches from the right and left ***vagus nerves (Galen, c192)*** and the right ***phrenic nerve (Galen c173)***. The ***hepatic plexus (Rau, 1720)*** accompanies the portal vein (see Swan, 1830, p. 11) and all branches of the hepatic artery and is apparently confined to the region of blood vessels in the liver. Branches of the ***hepatic plexus (Rau,***

1720) extend as the ***cystic plexus (Wrisberg, 1808)*** to the gall bladder, the ***hepatic plexus branches to bile ducts (>1840)***, and ***right gastric plexus (>1840)*** to the pylorus, superior part of the duodenum, right part of the stomach and greater curvature, descending duodenum, and head of the pancreas; see Mitchell (1953, pp. 278–280), Williams & Warwick (1980, p. 1134). For Rau's use in macrodissected adult human, see p. 110. It was known at least in outline by Galen; see *nerve to liver (Galen, c173)*.

TRANSLATIONS:

1. *plexus hepaticus (Rau, 1720)*
   Original Latin form of ***hepatic plexus (Rau, 1720)***; p. 110.

EARLIER REFERENCES:

Earlier synonyms:

1. *nerve implanted in liver (Galen, c173)*
   Synonym for ***hepatic plexus (Rau, 1720)*** as mentioned for macrodissected adult beef, pig, and/or macaque but not human; see May translation (1968, pp. 223, 224 note 51, 246).
2. *nerve to liver (Galen, c173)*
   Synonym for ***hepatic plexus (Rau, 1720)*** as mentioned for macrodissected adult beef, pig, and/or macaque but not human; see May translation (1968, p. 228). Vesalius (1543a) also described and illustrated a *nerve to liver (Galen, c173)* in macrodissected adult human; see Richardson & Carman translation (2007, p. 8, legend to Fig. 4-*ß*) and Richardson & Carman translation (2002, pp. 199–200). More accurately, Willis (1664) described it for macrodissected adult human thus: the ***celiac ganglion (Walter, 1783)*** "sends forth from it self many little bundles of nervous Fibres; the greatest of which being carried towards the Liver, cloaths the Hepatick Artery as it were with a Net made of Fibres" (Pordage translation, 1681, p. 168 and Tab. 11-*a*).
3. *nerve conferred on liver (Galen, c173)*
   Synonym for ***hepatic plexus (Rau, 1720)*** as mentioned for macrodissected adult beef, pig, and/or macaque but not human; see May translation (1968, p. 263).
4. *nerve inserted into liver (Galen, c173)*
   Synonym for ***hepatic plexus (Rau, 1720)*** as mentioned for macrodissected adult beef, pig, and/or macaque but not human; see May translation (1968, p. 263).
5. *nerve branch to liver (Galen, c192)*
   Synonym for ***hepatic plexus (Rau, 1720)*** as mentioned for macrodissected adult beef, pig, and/or macaque but not human; see Duckworth translation (1962, p. 222).
6. *nerveum plexum hepaticum (Vieussens, 1684)*
   Synonym for ***hepatic plexus (Rau, 1720)***; Table 23-*21,59*. Walter (1783, Tab. IV-*83*) used the form *plexum nervosum hepaticum*. Palfijn (1726, Part 2, p. 346) gave the French, *plexus hépatique nerveux*.
7. *nerveus plexus hepaticum (Vieussens, 1684)*
   Alternate form of *nerveum plexum hepaticum (Vieussens, 1684)*; Table 23-*60*.

LATER SYNONYM:

1. *portal plexus (Wrisberg, 1800)*
   Synonym for macrodissected adult human ***hepatic plexus (Rau, 1720)***; in the original Latin, *plexus portarum*, p. 568.

PARTLY CORRESPONDS:

1. *hepatic nerves (Walter, 1783)*
   At least four were described as generating macrodissected adult human *hepatic plexus (Walter, 1783)*, so they are proximal part of ***hepatic plexus (Rau, 1720)*** extending from ***celiac plexus (Winslow, 1733)***; in the original Latin, *nervus hepaticus, quartus*; Tables II, IV-*58*.
2. *posterior hepatic nerves (Walter, 1783)*
   Appear to form part of ***hepatic plexus (Rau, 1720)*** associated with macrodissected adult human quadrate lobe; in the original Latin, *nervi hepatici posteriores*, Table IV:*169–182*.
3. *hepatic plexus (Walter, 1783)*
   Distal part of macrodissected adult human ***hepatic plexus (Rau, 1720)***, formed by the *hepatic nerves (Walter, 1783)*; in the original Latin, *plexum hepaticum* (Tab. II-*73*), *plexus hepaticus* (Tab. III after *285*), *plexu hepatico* (Tab. IV after *32*).
4. *hepaticogastric nerve (Walter, 1783)*
   Proximal part of macrodissected adult human ***hepatic plexus (Rau, 1720)*** arising from ***celiac ganglion (Walter, 1783)***; in the original Latin, *hepatico-gastricus nervus*, Table III-*274*.
5. *nerve plexus of hepatic artery (Walter, 1783)*
   Part of ***hepatic plexus (Rau, 1720)*** accompanying macrodissected adult human hepatic artery; in the original Latin, *plexus nervosus arteriam hepaticam*, Table IV-*54*.
6. *nerves disappearing in hepatic duct (Walter, 1783)*
   Self-explanatory component of macrodissected adult human ***hepatic plexus (Rau, 1720)***; in the original Latin, *nervi in ductu hepatico evanescentes*, Table IV-*167,168*.
7. *right major posterior hepatic plexus (Soemmerring, 1791)*
   Component of macrodissected adult human ***hepatic plexus (Rau, 1720)***; p. 251, and Soemmerring (1798, p. 270, referred to in Latin as *plexum iecoris posteriorem majorem dextrum*).
8. *hepaticogastric plexus (Mayer, 1794)*
   Proximal part of macrodissected adult human ***hepatic plexus (Rau, 1720)***; in the original Latin, *plexus hepatico-gastricus*, Part 6, Table IV-*9* (p. 26).
9. *anterior hepatic plexus (Mayer, 1794)*
   Topographic but artificial division of macrodissected adult human ***hepatic plexus (Rau, 1720)***; in the original Latin, *plexus hepaticus anterior*; Part 6, Table IV, p. 28.
10. *posterior hepatic plexus (Mayer, 1794)*
    Topographic but artificial division of macrodissected adult human ***hepatic plexus (Rau, 1720)***; in the original Latin, *plexus hepaticus posterior*; Part 6, Table IV, p. 28.
11. *right hepatic nerves (Mayer, 1794)*
    Extensions of macrodissected adult human ***hepatic plexus (Rau, 1720)*** to right regions of liver; in the original Latin, *nervi hepatici dextri*; Part 6, Table IV-*51* (p. 28).

12. *middle hepatic nerves (Mayer, 1794)*
   Extensions of macrodissected adult human ***hepatic plexus (Rau, 1720)*** to middle regions of liver; in the original Latin, *nervi hepatici medii*; Part 6, Table IV-52 (p. 28).
13. *left hepatic nerves (Mayer, 1794)*
   Extensions of macrodissected adult human ***hepatic plexus (Rau, 1720)*** to left regions of liver; in the original Latin, *nervi hepatici sinistri*; Part 6, Table IV-53 (p. 28).
14. *portal plexus (Wrisberg, 1808)*
   Macrodissected adult human right ***hepatic plexus (Rau, 1720)***; in the original Latin, *plexus portarum*, p. 16.
15. *umbilical plexuses (Wrisberg, 1808)*
   As described for macrodissected adult human, extension of left ***hepatic plexus (Rau, 1720)***; in the original Latin, *plexu umbilicali*, p. 16.
16. *remaining hepatic nerves (Wrisberg, 1808)*
   Synonym for *minor hepatic nerves (Wrisberg, 1808)*; in the original Latin, *nervi hepatis reliqui*, pp. 16, 26.
17. *minor hepatic nerves (Wrisberg, 1808)*
   Parts of macrodissected adult human ***hepatic plexus (Rau, 1720)***; in the original Latin, *nervi hepatis minores*, p. 16. Wrisberg provided a detailed history of ***nerves (Herophilus, c335–c280 BC)*** to the liver on pp. 26–27 note *f*.
18. *umbilical nervous plexuses (Wrisberg, 1808)*
   Apparently synonym for *umbilical plexuses (Wrisberg, 1808)*; in the original Latin, *plexus nervorum umbilicalis*, pp. 23–26. There Wrisberg provided detailed history of relevant observations.
19. *umbilical nerves (Wrisberg, 1808)*
   Larger differentiations of *umbilical nervous plexuses (Wrisberg, 1808)*; in the original Latin, *nervorum umbilicalium*, p. 24.

hepatic plexus branches to bile ducts (>1840)

As described for macrodissected adult human, the term is self-explanatory; see Williams & Warwick (1980, p. 1134). It was known to Willis; see ***[hepatic plexus branches to bile ducts (>1840)] (Willis, 1664)***.

EARLIER REFERENCES:

Described, not named or illustrated:

1. ***[hepatic plexus branches to bile ducts (>1840)] (Willis, 1664)***
   Described for macrodissected adult human and other common large mammals; see Pordage translation (1681, p. 158 and Tab. 11-*o*).

Earlier synonyms:

1. *nerves ending in cystic duct (Walter, 1783)*
   Synonym for macrodissected adult human ***hepatic plexus branches to bile ducts (>1840)***; in the original Latin, *nervi qui in ductu cystico consumuntur*, Table IV:156–159.

hindbrain (Baer, 1837)

The topographic division of the ***vertebrate brain (Cuvier, 1800)*** including the ***cerebellum (Aristotle)*** and ***pons (Haller, 1747)***, considered together. Used more recently in this sense by, for example, the *Basel Nomina Anatomica* (His; 1895, p. 162) and Obersteiner & Hill (1900, p. 46). It should not be confused with the ***primary hindbrain vesicle (Baer, 1837)*** of early ***neural tube (Baer, 1837)*** development, which divides into two smaller divisions: the ***hindbrain (Baer, 1837)*** rostrally, sometimes called *secondary hindbrain (Sharpey et al., 1867)*, and ***afterbrain (Baer, 1837)*** caudally, now more commonly known as the ***medulla (Winslow, 1733)***. For these precise definitions see Swanson & Bota (2010); for Baer's use in vertebrate see p. 107. It was recognized early on as the *cerebellar vesicle (Malpighi, 1675)*.

TRANSLATIONS:

1. *Hinterhirn (Baer, 1837)*
   Original German form of ***hindbrain (Baer, 1837)***. The original English translation was in Sharpey et al. (1867, p. 577).
2. *epencephalon (Sharpey et al., 1867)*
   Original Latin form of ***hindbrain (Baer, 1837)***; p. 577. The original English translation was in Sharpey et al. (1867, p. 577).

EARLIER REFERENCES:

Earlier synonyms:

1. *cerebellar vesicle (Malpighi, 1675)*
   Synonym for ***hindbrain (Baer, 1837)*** in chick embryo after 4 days of incubation; Table V, Figure XXXVI-*B*; see Adelmann (1966, p. 1005). Serres (1824–1826) used it for all vertebrates.
2. *cerebellum (Haller, 1762)*
   Synonym for macrodissected adult human ***hindbrain (Baer, 1837)***; p. 60. Soemmerring (1791, pp. 51–55) and Gordon (1815, pp. 79–80, 175) used it in the same way.

LATER SYNONYMS:

1. *secondary hindbrain (Sharpey et al., 1867)*
   Synonym for ***hindbrain (Baer, 1837)***; from explanation in footnote on p. 577.

PARTLY CORRESPONDS:

1. *cerebellum (Varoli, 1573)*
   For macrodissected adult human it included ***cerebellum (Aristotle)*** and ***middle cerebellar peduncle (Rolando, 1819)***—the *pons of cerebellum (Varoli, 1573)*—and because *auditory nerve (Hundt, 1501)* emerges from *pons of cerebellum (Varoli, 1573)*, Varoli suggested that hearing is a function of *cerebellum (Varoli, 1573)*; see Harvey (1961, p. 230, note 824), Clarke & O'Malley (1996, pp. 634–635, 831).

hindbrain vesicle (Baer, 1837)

For macrodissected vertebrate embryo, the rostral division of the ***primary hindbrain vesicle (Baer, 1837)*** developing into the adult ***hindbrain (Baer, 1837)***—the ***pons (Haller, 1747)*** ventrally and ***cerebellum (Aristotle)*** dorsally; the caudal division is the ***afterbrain vesicle (Baer, 1837)***. For Baer's use, see p. 107. It was clearly differentiated early on by Malpighi; see ***[hindbrain vesicle (Baer, 1837)] (Malpighi, 1673)***.

EARLIER REFERENCES:

Illustrated and described, not named:

1. ***[hindbrain vesicle (Baer, 1837)] (Malpighi, 1673)***
   Clearly illustrated for 3-day-old chick embryo; see Figure XVIII.

hippocampal commissures (Johnston, 1913)

As described in macrodissected adult human, and mammal generally with histological methods for ***axons (Kölliker, 1896)***, the ***cerebral cortex white matter (>1840)*** differentiations for the ***hippocampal region (Swanson et al., 1987)*** equivalent to and continuous with (though folded ventral to or under) the ***corpus callosum (Galen, c177)*** for much of the rest of the ***cerebral cortex gray matter (>1840)***. In his work on adult rat with the Marchi technique for myelin, Craigie (1925, p. 103, Pl. XXVI) defined three parts of the ***hippocampal commissures (>1840)***: a rostral ***ventral hippocampal commissure (Craigie, 1925)***, an intermediate *thin part of dorsal hippocampal commissure (Craigie, 1925)*, and a distinct caudal ***dorsal hippocampal commissure (Craigie, 1925)***, which is more deeply stained in Marchi preparations. Demeter et al. (1985, see Fig. 2-C) confirmed this description for adult macaque monkey with normal myelin stains and the autoradiographic pathway tracing method; they defined three overlapping components, from caudal to rostral: ***dorsal hippocampal commissure (Craigie, 1925)***, *hippocampal decussation (Demeter et al., 1985)* or *thin part of dorsal hippocampal commissure (Craigie, 1925)*, and ***ventral hippocampal commissure (Craigie, 1925)***. Their account was confirmed in all essential details for adult human by Gloor et al. (1993). As defined here, the ***hippocampal commissures (Johnston, 1913)*** consist of dorsal, intermediate, and ventral regions: ***dorsal hippocampal commissure (Craigie, 1925)***, ***intermediate hippocampal commissure (>1840)***, and ***ventral hippocampal commissure (Craigie, 1925)***; there is no clear boundary between them. Autoradiographic pathway tracing in rat indicates that ***axons (Kölliker, 1896)*** from the ***hippocampal region (Swanson et al., 1987)*** cross in the ***ventral hippocampal commissure (Craigie, 1925)***, ***axons (Kölliker, 1896)*** from the ***retrohippocampal region (Swanson et al., 1987)*** cross in the ***dorsal hippocampal commissure (Craigie, 1925)***, and smaller numbers of ***axons (Kölliker, 1896)*** from both regions cross in the ***intermediate hippocampal commissure (>1840)***; see Swanson and Cowan (1977), Swanson et al. (1978). For Johnston's clear overall description in mammals generally based on histological stains for ***axons (Kölliker, 1896)***, see p. 399. Their existence generally was known to Vesalius; see ***[dorsal hippocampal commissure] (Vesalius, 1543a)***.

EARLIER REFERENCES:

Earlier synonyms:

1. *fornix transversus (Forel, 1872)*
   Synonym for ***hippocampal commissures (Johnston, 1913)*** observed in a variety of mammals with normal histological stains; p. 46, see Dejerine & Dejerine-Klumpke (1901, p. 276). Forel noted it is equivalent to "*Lyra fornicis*" of human (p. 46).
2. *Ammon's horn commissure (Forel, 1872)*
   Synonym for *fornix transversus (Forel, 1872)*; see Figure 5 legend, and Kölliker (1896, pp. 776, 782).
3. *psalterium (Ganser, 1882)*
   Synonym for ***hippocampal commissures (Johnston, 1913)*** in histological sections of adult mole; in the original German, *Kommissurenfascern*, pp. 637–641, 656–569. Also see Dejerine & Dejerine-Klumpke (1901, p. 276) and Kölliker (1896, pp. 776, 787), who noted Ganser identified dorsal and ventral parts.
4. *fornix commissure (Smith, 1895)*
   Synonym for *fornix transversus (Forel, 1872)*, with dorsal and ventral limbs; pp. 185, 188, 200–201.

hippocampal formation (Swanson & Cowan, 1977)

As described for macrodissected adult human, the caudal and dorsal topographic subdivision of the ***limbic region (>1840)*** lying between ***olfactory region (>1840)*** rostrally and ***cingulate region (>1840)*** dorsally. It in turn has two major subdivisions, ***parahippocampal gyrus (>1840)*** and ***hippocampal region (Swanson et al., 1987)***. Based on cellular architecture and connections in mammal, the corresponding ***retrohippocampal region (Swanson et al., 1987)*** and ***hippocampal region (Swanson et al., 1987)***, respectively, are recognized. For general overviews see Swanson et al. (1987), Nieuwenhuys et al. (2008, p. 361 ff.). For Swanson & Cowan's use in adult rat based on cytoarchitecture and connections, see pp. 51–52. Blackstad (1956, p. 417, Fig. 2) called it the *hippocampal region* in rat. Based on development and topological relations, a more natural subdivision and nomenclature for macrodissected adult human would be ***parahippocampal gyrus (>1840)*** laterally, hippocampal gyrus for ***Ammon's horn (Vicq d'Azyr, 1784)*** in the middle, and ***dentate gyrus (>1840)*** medially. It was not recognized as such by 1840.

hippocampal region (Swanson et al., 1987)

As described with cellular architecture, connections, and development in mammal, the developmentally and topologically medial subdivision of the ***hippocampal formation (Swanson & Cowan, 1977)***, the lateral subdivision being the ***retrohippocampal region (Swanson et al., 1987)***. Major parts of the ***hippocampal region (Swanson et al., 1987)*** are ***dentate gyrus (>1840)*** medially and ***Ammon's horn (Vicq d'Azyr, 1784)*** laterally; minor parts extend around the caudal end, dorsal surface, and rostral end of the ***corpus callosum (Galen, c177)*** and include ***fasciola cinerea (Arnold, 1838b)***, ***indusium griseum (Valentin, 1841)***, and ***tenia tecta (Swanson, 1992)***, respectively. Meckel (1817) wrote that "These parts are then evidently similar to the corresponding halves of two adjacent circumvolutions, between which a medullary layer penetrates instead of the pia-mater alone, and which is covered internally only by a very thin medullary layer" (1832 translation,

Vol. 2, p. 466). For original use in rat by Swanson et al., see p. 126. For the classic description of its development in human, see Hines (1922). Credit for its discovery is usually given to Aranzi; see *hippocampus (Aranzi, 1587)*. However, it was probably described by Vesalius; see ***[hippocampal region (>1840)] (Vesalius, 1543a)***.

EARLIER REFERENCES:

Illustrated, not named or described:

1. *[hippocampal region (>1840)] (Vesalius, 1543a)*
In at least three places Vesalius possibly referred to it in macrodissected adult human, though none are unambiguous. First and most probable, he illustrated what may correspond to the dorsal (posterior or septal) end of the ***hippocampal region (Swanson et al., 1987)*** and wrote that it is the "Part of the 'tortoise' [***fornix (Vesalius, 1543a)***]…arising here from the substance of the cerebrum" (Singer translation, 1952, p. 98 and Fig. 6-*B,C*). This conclusion is strengthened by his description in the body of the text, "from the hind part of the lateral ventricles, where they turn down and forward [***inferior horn of lateral ventricle (Bell, 1802)***], there extends [this] body [of the ***fornix (Vesalius, 1543a)***] of like substance to the ventricles, except that it is somewhat whiter and harder" (Singer translation, 1952, p. 41). Second, he referred to rounded surfaces in the ***lateral ventricles (Vesalius, 1543a)***, although it is more likely they were the *anchae (Mondino, 1316)*, probably the ***caudate nucleus (Arnold, 1838b)***; see Singer translation (1952, p. 42). And third, in the 1555 edition of the *Fabrica*, Vesalius referred to an infolding in the ***inferior horn of lateral ventricle (Bell, 1802)***; see Singer translation (1952, p. 34).

PARTLY CORRESPONDS:

1. *hippocampus (Aranzi, 1587)*
Aranzi's brief, unillustrated description of this differentiation in macrodissected adult human ***cerebrum (Obersteiner & Hill, 1900)*** was ambiguous; see entire original passage, and translation, in Lewis (1922, p. 217). For the sake of discussion, two clearly different interpretations are possible. First, the term may refer to ***hippocampal region (Swanson et al., 1987)*** and adjacent ventral segment of ***fimbria (Honegger, 1890)*** with its ***alveus (Burdach, 1822)*** differentiation. This interpretation, adopted here, was clearly illustrated by Vesling (1647, 2nd Tab. for Ch. 14, Fig. 1-*H*: Sea-horse, or Silkworms of Arantius; see 1653 translation). Alternately, Aranzi may have referred to only ventral segment of ***fimbria (Honegger, 1890)*** with its ***alveus (Burdach, 1822)*** differentiation as hippocampus, without including *gray substance (Vesalius, 1543a)* of ***hippocampal region (Swanson et al., 1987)***; these two *white substance (Vesalius, 1543a)* differentiations are continuous dorsally with dorsal segment of ***fimbria (Honegger, 1890)***. Aranzi was the first to describe in any detail surface features of ***inferior horn of lateral ventricle (Bell, 1802)***, and the outline on the medial wall reminded him of a seahorse (see Clarke & O'Malley, 1996, p. 720)—the word *hippocampus* literally means horse-caterpillar in Latin (see Lewis, 1923, p. 218). The first definite illustration of ***hippocampal region (Swanson et al., 1987)*** surface is probably in Cortesi (1625, Fig. VI; also see Haller 1774, p. 355) for macrodissected adult human. Perhaps the first great illustration of ***gray matter (Meckel, 1817)*** of ***hippocampal region (Swanson et al., 1987)*** in relation to ***white matter (Meckel, 1817)*** was by Vicq d'Azyr (1786, Plate XX). Also see *posterior pillar of fornix (Paré, 1564)*.
2. *seahorse (Aranzi, 1587)*
English form of *hippocampus (Aranzi, 1587)*.
3. *vermis bombycinus (Aranzi, 1587)*
The *hippocampus (Aranzi, 1587)* reminded Aranzi of a white silkworm, as well as a seahorse; see Meyer (1971, p. 14), Clarke & O'Malley (1996, p. 720).
4. *silkworm (Aranzi, 1587)*
English form of *vermis bombycinus (Aranzi, 1587)*.
5. *white silkworm (Aranzi, 1587)*
English form of *vermis bombycinus (Aranzi, 1587)*.
6. *pes hippocampi (Riolan, 1618)*
Synonym for macrodissected adult human *hippocampus (Aranzi, 1587)*; p. 418, where plural is used, *pedes hippocampi (Riolan, 1618)*. Haller (1747; see Mihles translation, 1753, p. 292) noted it is "outwardly medullary, inwardly of a cortical substance"—***alveus (Burdach, 1822)*** and ***hippocampal region (Swanson et al., 1987)***, respectively.
7. *foot of seahorse (Riolan, 1618)*
English form of *pes hippocampi (Riolan, 1618)*. The consequences of this poor choice of terminology were incredible (see below).
8. *pedes hippocampi (Riolan, 1618)*
Plural of *pes hippocampi (Riolan, 1618)*, the term actually found in Riolan, p. 418. Variations found in Haller (1747) include *pedibus hippocampi* (p. 180) and *pedum hippocampi* (p. 182). Diemerbroeck made the fanciful statement, "The hinder Thighs *Hippocrates* calls *Pedes Hippocampi*" (1672; p. 585; see 1689 translation, p. 398).
9. *hyppocampum (Cortesi, 1625)*
Variant form of *hippocampus (Aranzi, 1587)* for macrodissected adult human; p. 26, Figure VI-*H*. Probably first definite illustration of ***hippocampal region (Swanson et al., 1987)*** surface.
10. *bombyx (Marchetti, 1652)*
Synonym for macrodissected adult human *hippocampus (Aranzi, 1587)*; p. 119, see Burdach (1822, p. 372) and *vermis bombycinus (Aranzi, 1587)*.
11. *thighs of arch (Diemerbroeck, 1689)*
Probably synonym for macrodissected adult human *pedes hippocampi (Riolan, 1618)*; p. 410, see Lewis (1923, p. 223).
12. *hippocampus Aurantius (Ridley, 1695)*
Eponym for macrodissected adult human *hippocampus (Aranzi, 1587)*; p. 118.
13. *bombycinus Aurantius (Ridley, 1695)*
Eponym for macrodissected adult human *hippocampus (Aranzi, 1587)*; p. 118, see *vermis bombycinus (Aranzi, 1587)*.

14. *Ammon's horn (Garengeot, 1728)*
Synonym for macrodissected adult human *hippocampus (Aranzi, 1587)* or *thigh of arch (Diemerbroeck, 1689)*; in the original French, *les jambes de la voute que nous avon dit ressembler aux cornes d'*Ammon (see p. 468 and Pl. XVIII-*E*).
15. *ram's horn (Duvernoy, 1735)*
Used (p. 135) to describe macrodissected adult human *hippocampus (Aranzi, 1587)*—not ***fimbria (Honegger, 1890)*** with its ***alveus (Burdach, 1822)***, as Winslow had done; see *ram's horn (Winslow, 1733, Sect. X, p. 35)*. On the *hippocampus (Aranzi, 1587)*, Duvernoy very clearly illustrated digitations or striations (grossly exaggerated) and noted it seems to resemble a ram's horn, although he did not distinguish in the figure between ***fimbria (Honegger, 1890)***, ***alveus (Burdach, 1822)***, and ***hippocampal region (Swanson et al., 1987)***; see Lewis (1923, p. 224).
16. *crus fornicis (Wreeden, 1741)*
Synonym for macrodissected adult human *hippocampus (Aranzi, 1587)*; p. 12 and Burdach (1822, p. 372).
17. *posterior pillar of vault (Lieutaud, 1742)*
Synonym for macrodissected adult human *hippocampus (Aranzi, 1587)*; p. 392 and Plate V, Figure 2-*e*.
18. *pedibus hippocampi (Haller, 1747)*
Original Latin form (plural) of *foot-stalk of hippocampus (Haller, 1747)*; p. 180.
19. *pedum hippocampi (Haller, 1747)*
Original Latin form (plural) of *foot-stalk of hippocampus (Haller, 1747)*; p. 180.
20. *foot-stalk of hippocampus (Haller, 1747)*
English form of *pes hippocampi (Riolan, 1618)* in Mihles's translation (1754b, p. 289, §360), referring to macrodissected adult human *hippocampus (Aranzi, 1587)*, "which [for right and left] are outwardly medullary [***alveus (Burdach, 1822)***] and inwardly of a cortical substance [***hippocampal region (Swanson et al., 1987)***]" (Mihles translation, 1754b, p. 202; also see Hill, 1893, p. 390). However, the translation, at least, is confusing because on p. 291 (§291), *crus* is translated "foot-stalk".
21. *corpus fimbriatum (Bonhomme, 1748)*
Given as synonym for *Ammon's horn (Garengeot, 1728)*; p. 51, see Burdach (1822, p. 372). Tarin apparently referred to right and left *corpus fimbriatum (Bonhomme, 1748)* in French as *les corps bordés* (1753, p. 25).
22. *cornu arietis (Günz, 1750)*
Apparently a convoluted eponym for macrodissected adult human *hippocampus (Aranzi, 1587)*; p. 6, as quoted by Hill (1893, p. 391). Also see *Ammon's horn (Garengeot, 1728)* and Meckel (1832, Vol. 2, p. 465).
23. *pedes hippocampi Arantii (Tarin, 1753)*
Eponym (plural) for macrodissected adult human *hippocampus (Aranzi, 1587)*; p. 25.
24. *digiti pedis hippocampi (Haller, 1762)*
Haller noted that macrodissected adult human *hippocampus (Aranzi, 1587)* displays series of 3–5 swellings, resembling "toes on the foot of the hippocampus", and pointed out they were illustrated by Morand (1744) and Tarin (1750); p. 34, also see *pedes hippocampi (Haller, 1747)*. Burdach (1822, pp. 372, 375) noted they were also described by Duvernoy (1735). For a modern description of these swellings see Duvernoy (1988).
25. *toes of hippocampus (Haller, 1762)*
English form of *digiti pedes hippocampi (Haller, 1762)*.
26. *pes hippopotami major (Mayer, 1779)*
Mayer introduced term "foot of the larger hippopotamus" for macrodissected adult human *hippocampus (Aranzi, 1587)* or *pes hippocampi (Riolan, 1618)*; Table V-*g*, in the original German legend, *grosse fusse des Seepferdes*; the Latin was given in Table III-*t*. Also see Burdach (1822, p. 372), Lewis (1923, p. 227), Meyer (1971, p. 21). He illustrated it coming off end of ***fimbria (Honegger, 1890)***, or *leg of vault (Riolan, 1657)*, with several vague digitations apparently reminding him of toes (Tab. V-*g*). It was complemented by "foot of the smaller hippopotamus", the *pes hippopotami minor (Mayer, 1779)*. Also see *ram's horn (Duvernoy, 1735)*.
27. *foot of larger hippopotamus (Mayer, 1779)*
English form of *pes hippopotami major (Mayer, 1779)*.
28. *digitationes pes hippopotami major (Mayer, 1779)*
Series of eminences between oblique grooves on surface of macrodissected adult human *hippocampus (Aranzi, 1587)* referred to by Mayer as "toes of the foot of the larger hippopotamus" (p. 8). Also see Haller (1762, p. 34), Burdach (1822, p. 375). As late as 1867 Meynert (see Tab. III, Fig. 3, p. 120) still referred to *pedis hyppopotami*.
29. *toes of foot of larger hippopotamus (Mayer, 1779)*
English form of *digitationes pes hippopotami major (Mayer, 1779)*.
30. *bombicine appendix (Malacarne, 1780)*
Term Malacarne attributed to Aranzi, synonym for macrodissected adult human *hippocampus (Aranzi, 1587)*; for English translation of passage in Vol. II, p. 64, see *silkworm (Malacarne, 1780)*.
31. *pede hippocampi majore (Haase, 1781)*
Haase "corrected" the term just introduced as *pes hippopotami major (Mayer, 1779)*; p. 36, also see Haller (1762, p. 34).
32. *foot of larger hippocampus (Haase, 1781)*
English form of *pede hippocampi majore (Haase, 1781)*.
33. *foot of larger seahorse (Haase, 1781)*
Full English form of *pede hippocampi majore (Haase, 1781)*.
34. *pedes major hippoocampi (Haase, 1781)*
Plural form of *pede hippocampi majore (Haase, 1781)*; p 19.
35. *pes hippopotami major & anterior (Günther, 1786)*
Synonym for macrodissected adult human *pes hippopotami major (Mayer, 1779)*; p. 11.
36. *digital processes of Ammon's horn (Günther, 1786)*
Synonym for macrodissected adult human *toes of foot of larger hippopotamus (Mayer, 1779)*; in the original Latin, *processus digitatus*, p. 11.
37. *cylindroid protuberance (Burdin, 1803)*
Synonym for macrodissected adult human *hippocampus (Aranzi, 1587)*; see translation (1803, Vol. 1, p. 160, where also called cylindric).

38. *anchor (Chaussier, 1807)*
Synonym listed for macrodissected adult human *hippocampus (Aranzi, 1587)*; in the original French, *une ancre*, p. 66.

39. *accessory foot of hippocampus (Cruveilhier, 1836)*
In macrodissected adult human a not uncommon differentiation of *pes hippocampi (Riolan, 1618)*; in the original French, *accessoire du pied d'hippocampe*, p. 695. Cruveilhier noted there, without citation, that it was regarded by Meckel as a product of arrested development.

40. *area praegenualis (Brodmann, 1909)*
Based on cellular architecture in adult human, ***tenia tecta (Swanson, 1992)*** and rostral part of ***indusium griseum (Valentin, 1841)***; p. 148.

41. *pregenual area (Brodmann, 1909)*
English form of *area praegenualis (Brodmann, 1909)*; see Garey translation (1994, p. 127).

42. *area 33 (Brodmann, 1909)*
Synonym for *pregenual area (Brodmann, 1909)*; in the original German, *Feld 33*, p. 148.

hippocampal sulcus (Gratiolet, 1854)

As described for macrodissected adult human and other mammal, the very deep groove invaginating the ***hippocampal formation (Swanson & Cowan, 1977)***, basically with the ***subicular complex (Swanson & Cowan, 1997)*** and ***field CA 1 (Lorente de Nó, 1934)*** on one side, and ***field CA3 (Lorente de Nó, 1934)*** and ***dentate gyrus (>1840)*** on the other side; see Williams & Warwick (1980, Fig. 7.121), *Nomina Anatomica* (1983, p. A71, given as *sulcus hippocampi or hippocampalis*), *Terminologia Anatomica* (1998, p. 126), Nieuwenhuys et al. (2008, Figs. 12.2, 12.5A). It is continuous dorsally and rostrally with the caudal end of the ***sulcus of corpus callosum (>1840)***; see Carpenter (1996, p. 27). For the classic account of its development in human, see Hines (1922). ***Hippocampal sulcus (Gratiolet, 1854)*** is preferred to *hippocampal fissure (Gratiolet, 1854)* for the sake of consistency with ***cerebral sulci (Vesalius, 1543a)***—as, for example, ***lateral cerebral sulcus (>1840)*** rather than *lateral fissure (>1840)*. For Gratiolet's use in macrodissected adult human and other primates, see Figure 3 (*B'-B"*) and Meyer (1971, p. 139). It was perhaps first clearly delineated by Vicq d'Azyr; see ***[hippocampal sulcus (Gratiolet, 1854)] (Vicq d'Azyr, 1786)***.

TRANSLATIONS:

1. *scissure des hippocampes (Gratiolet, 1854)*
Original French form of ***hippocampal sulcus (Gratiolet, 1854)***; see Figure 3 (*B'-B"*) and Meyer (1971, p. 139).

EARLIER REFERENCES:

Illustrated, not named or described:

1. ***[hippocampal sulcus (Gratiolet, 1854)] (Vicq d'Azyr, 1786)***
Illustrated clearly in cross section, without naming, labeling, or describing, for macrodissected adult human; Table XXVI, Figures 7, 8. Its longitudinal extent, as viewed from the surface, was nicely illustrated for macrodissected adult human by Burdach (1822, Tab. 7:*βx-γ*), see Meyer (1971, p. 130).

Earlier synonyms:

1. *fissure upon which hippocampus is folded (Owen, 1837)*
Synonym for macrodissected adult mammalian ***hippocampal sulcus (Gratiolet, 1854)***; p. 90.

LATER SYNONYMS:

1. *hippocampal fissure (Gratiolet, 1854)*
Common synonym for mammalian ***hippocampal sulcus (Gratiolet, 1854)***; see Carpenter (1976, p. 530 and Fig. 18.8), Swanson et al. (1987), Nieuwenhuys et al. (2008, p. 52). In the original French, *scissure des hippocampes*, with *scissure* translated either *fissure* or *sulcus*.

horizontal fissure (Malacarne, 1776)

As described for macrodissected adult human, the groove between ***ansiform lobule crus 1 (Bolk, 1906)*** and ***ansiform lobule crus 2 (Bolk, 1906)*** of the ***cerebellar cortex (Willis, 1664)*** continuing across the median plane between ***folium vermis (>1840)*** and ***tuber vermis (>1840)*** of the ***cerebellar vermis (Meckel, 1817)***; see Angevine et al. (1961, p. 17 and Figs. 1–3, 6, 11, 14, 17, 20–24), *Terminologia Anatomica* (1998, p. 119). For Malacarne's use in macrodissected adult human, see Clarke & O'Malley translation (1996, p. 643).

LATER SYNONYMS:

1. *common lateral cerebellar fissure (Malacarne, 1776)*
Synonym for macrodissected adult human ***horizontal fissure (Malacarne, 1776)***; see Clarke & O'Malley translation (1996, p. 643).

2. *great cerebellar fissure (Vicq d'Azyr, 1784)*
Synonym for macrodissected adult human ***horizontal fissure (Malacarne, 1776)***; in the original French, *grand sillon du cervelet*, p. 569 and Vicq d'Azyr (1786, Pl. XXXI, Fig. I:*26–28*). See Larsell & Jansen (1972, p. 51).

3. *lateral circumferential fissure (Vicq d'Azyr, 1784)*
Synonym for macrodissected adult human ***horizontal fissure (Malacarne, 1776)***; in the original French, *sillon latéral et circulaire*, pp. 569–570 and Vicq d'Azyr (1786, Pl. XXXI, Fig. I:*26–28*). See Larsell & Jansen (1972, p. 51).

4. *transverse sulcus (Chaussier, 1807)*
Synonym for macrodissected adult human ***horizontal fissure (Malacarne, 1776)***; in the original French, *sillon transversal*, p. 79.

5. *perpendicular fossa (Meckel, 1817)*
Synonym for macrodissected adult human ***horizontal fissure (Malacarne, 1776)***; see translation (1832, Vol. 2, p. 463).

6. *great horizontal sulcus (Arnold, 1834)*
Synonym for macrodissected adult human ***horizontal fissure (Malacarne, 1776)***; in the original Latin, *sulcus horizontalis magnus*, Table I:*C-p*.

hypogastric nerve (Walter, 1783)

As described for macrodissected adult human, the right and left "nerves" form through bifurcation of the unpaired ***superior hypogastric plexus (Tiedemann,***

1822) and extend caudally (descend) medial to the internal iliac arteries (older synonym, hypogastric arteries) to merge imperceptibly with the ***inferior hypogastric plexuses (Tiedemann, 1822)***. Each ***hypogastric nerve (Walter, 1783)*** may be single or consist of 2–3 interconnected *nerve fiber (Ehrenberg, 1833)* bundles forming a narrow elongated ***plexus (Galen, c192)***, and the two ***hypogastric nerves (Walter, 1783)*** are often bridged themselves by a delicate *middle hypogastric plexus (Mitchell, 1953)*; see Mitchell (1953, pp. 299–301 and Figs. 120, 131), *Terminologia Anatomica* (1998, p. 143), and *hypogastric plexus (Winslow, 1733)*. Thus, based on structure and position it is best regarded as an integral part of the ***prevertebral plexuses (Quain, 1832)*** and might be named more appropriately the *interhypogastric plexus*. It is the main source of sympathetic ***axons (Kölliker, 1896)*** to the ***inferior hypogastric plexus (Tiedemann, 1822)***; see Mitchell (1953, p. 301). For Walter's use in macrodissected adult human, see Table II-*175,176*. It was clearly distinguished by Willis; see ***[hypogastric nerve (Walter, 1783)] (Willis, 1664)***.

TRANSLATIONS:

1. *nervus hypogastricus (Walter, 1783)*
   Original Latin form of ***hypogastric nerve (Walter, 1783)***, see Table II-*175,176*.

EARLIER REFERENCES:

Illustrated and described, not named:

1. ***[hypogastric nerve (Walter, 1783)] (Willis, 1664)***
   Described and illustrated for macrodissected adult human and common quadrupeds; see Pordage translation (p. 159, Tab. XI-C).

LATER SYNONYMS:

1. *secondary plexiform cord of lumboaortic plexus (Cruveilhier, 1836)*
   Probably synonym for macrodissected adult human ***hypogastric nerve (Walter, 1783)***; in the original French (plural), *cordons plexiformes secondaires*, p. 1025.

hypoglossal nerve (Winslow, 1733)

As described for macrodissected adult human, the motor ***nerve (Herophilus, c335–c280 BC)*** of the tongue. It is a ***cranial nerve (Soemmerring, 1791)*** attached to the lateral surface of the ***medulla (Winslow, 1733)*** by the ***hypoglossal nerve root (>1840)***, which is continuous with the ***hypoglossal nerve central root (>1840)***. The ***hypoglossal nerve root (>1840)*** attachment is in a longitudinal line corresponding to the ***ventrolateral sulcus of medulla (>1840)***, just rostral to the cervical ***ventral roots (>1840)***. The ***hypoglossal nerve root (>1840)*** consists of a set of ***hypoglossal nerve rootlets (>1840)*** converging distally to form the ***hypoglossal nerve trunk (Günther, 1786)***, which in turn generates ***thyrohyoid branches of hypoglossal nerve (Meckel, 1817)*** and ***lingual branches of hypoglossal nerve (Cloquet, 1816)***; see Durward (1951, Fig. 909), Williams & Warwick (1980, p. 1083 and Fig. 7.189). For Winslow's use in macrodissected adult human, see Section VI, p. 60. It was discovered by Herophilus; see ***[hypoglossal nerve (Winslow, 1733)] (Herophilus, c335–c280 BC)***. The earlier literature was thoroughly reviewed by Boehmer (1777).

TRANSLATIONS:

1. *nervi hypoglossi (Winslow, 1733)*
   Original Latin form of ***hypoglossal nerves (Winslow, 1733)***; Section VI, p. 60.

EARLIER REFERENCES:

Described, not named or illustrated:

1. ***[hypoglossal nerve (Winslow, 1733)] (Herophilus, c335–c280 BC)***
   Herophilus, the founder of human anatomy, is credited with discovering the ***hypoglossal nerve (Winslow, 1733)***, which he apparently did not name. He dissected animals and adult human cadavers; see Solmsen (1961), von Staden (1969), Longrigg (1993), Clarke & O'Malley 1996, p. 261).
2. ***[hypoglossal nerve (Winslow, 1733)] (Erasistratus, c310–c250 BC)***
   In *The Doctrines of Hippocrates and Plato* (c162–166), Galen quoted from a book of Erasistratus (now lost) where "from the [human] brain nerves led to the tongue and the eyes." (see Longrigg, 1998, p. 93).

Earlier synonyms:

1. *motor nerve for tongue (Galen, c173)*
   Synonym in *On the Usefulness of the Parts* for macrodissected adult beef, pig, and/or macaque but not human ***hypoglossal nerve (Winslow, 1733)***; see May translation (1968, p. 450). Also see Duckworth translation (1962, pp. 200–201), Savage-Smith (1971, p. 188 ff.). Galen wrote, "If here you expose the tough [hard] nerve of the tongue—and there is one of these on each side of the tongue—and then tie a ligature round it, or sever it, then you deprive the whole tongue of mobility but not of sensibility. For it is the 'soft' nerve which passes by the bone of the mandible and goes to the tongue [the ***lingual nerve (Vesalius, 1543a)***] which, coming from the brain, conveys sense-impressions of taste [and does so] without distributing itself in a single muscle, or in the substance of the tongue..." (Duckworth translation, 1962, pp. 54, 200). Soemmerring (1778, p. 167) listed it in Latin as *nervum linguae motorium* vel *motorem*.
2. *seventh pair of nerves from brain (Galen, c192)*
   Synonym for *motor nerve for tongue (Galen, c173)*; see Duckworth translation (1962, pp. 200–201). Also see May translation (1968, p. 449), Savage-Smith (1971, p. 199 ff.).
3. *eighth pair of nerves from brain (Theophilos Protospatharios, fl. 610–641)*
   Synonym for *seventh pair of nerves from brain (Galen, c192)*; see *pairs of nerves from brain (Theophilos Protospatharios, fl. 610–641)*. Massa (1536) also used this designation for macrodissected adult human ***hypoglossal nerves (Winslow, 1733)***, see Lind translation (1975, p. 225), as did Piccolomini (1586, p. 262). Also see Burdach (1822, p. 308).

4. *seventh pair of sinews of brain (Geminus, 1553)*
Synonym for macrodissected adult human *seventh pair of nerves from brain (Galen, c192)*; originally spelled *seventh payre of synowes of brayne*, see *The table of the figures of synowes*.
5. *tenth pair of nerves from brain (Bartholin, 1641)*
Bartholin's enumeration of Galen's *seventh pair of nerves from brain (Galen, c192)*; for English version see Bartholin (1662, p. 326).
6. *ninth pair of nerves arising within skull (Willis, 1664)*
Synonym for *seventh pair of nerves from brain (Galen, c192)*; see Pordage translation (1681, pp. 58, 177). Willis, along with Ridley (1695), thought these ***nerves (Herophilus, c335–c280 BC)*** arise from ***inferior olivary complex (>1840)***; see Burdach (1822, p. 308).
7. *lingual motor pair (Diemerbroeck, 1672)*
Synonym for macrodissected adult human ***hypoglossal nerves (Winslow, 1733)***; in the original Latin, *par linguam movens*, p. 366. Heister (1717) gave the Latin form, *par linguae motorium*, see translation (1721, p. 247).
8. *eleventh pair (Bidloo, 1685)*
Synonym for macrodissected adult human *seventh pair of nerves from brain (Galen, c192)*; see Soemmerring (1778, p. 167), Vicq d'Azyr (1786, p. 49), Burdach (1822, p. 308).
9. *nervi indeterminati (Salmon, 1714)*
Synonym for macrodissected adult human ***hypoglossal nerve (Winslow, 1733)***, named because the author believed it was unclear whether it proceeds from within or from without the skull; p. 120.
10. *par linguale (Heister, 1717)*
Synonym for macrodissected adult human ***hypoglossal nerves (Winslow, 1733)***; see translation (1721, p. 247).
11. *par gustatorium (Heister, 1717)*
Heister noted that *par linguale (Heister, 1717)* was sometimes called *par gustatorium*; see translation (1721, p. 247).
12. *great sublingual nerve (Winslow, 1732)*
Synonym for macrodissected adult human ***hypoglossal nerve (Winslow, 1733)***; in the original Latin, *nervum sublingualis magnus*; Section III, p. 248, see Burdach (1822, p. 308).
13. *nervi gustatorii (Winslow, 1733)*
Synonym listed for ***hypoglossal nerves (Winslow, 1733)***; Section VI, p. 60, also see *par gustatorium (Heister, 1717)*. According to Burdach (1822, p. 308), Boerhaave used this term for a set of ***nerves (Herophilus, c335–c280 BC)*** but Burdach gave no citation.
14. *gustatory nerve (Winslow, 1733)*
English form (singular) of *nervi gustatorii (Winslow, 1733)*.
15. *nervi linguales (Winslow, 1733)*
Synonym listed for ***hypoglossal nerves (Winslow, 1733)***; Section VI, p. 60, also see *par linguale (Heister, 1717)*.
16. *lingual nerve (Winslow, 1733)*
English form (singular) of *nervi linguales (Winslow, 1733)*; see Vicq d'Azyr (1786, p. 49).
17. *nervi hypoglossi externi (Winslow, 1733)*
Synonym for ***hypoglossal nerves (Winslow, 1733)***; Section X, p. 48.
18. *nervi hypoglossi majores (Winslow, 1733)*
Synonym for ***hypoglossal nerves (Winslow, 1733)***; Section VI, p. 74; listed as *nervum hypoglossum magnum* (singular) by Soemmerring (1778, p. 166).

LATER SYNONYMS:

1. *middle lingual pair (Haller, 1762)*
Synonym for macrodissected adult human ***hypoglossal nerves (Winslow, 1733)***; in the original Latin, *par linguale medium*, p. 238, see Vicq d'Azyr (1786, p. 50).
2. *middle lingual nerve (Haller, 1762)*
Synonym for macrodissected adult human ***hypoglossal nerve (Winslow, 1733)***; in the original Latin, *nervus lingualis medius*, p. 238, see Burdach (1822, p. 308).
3. *third gustatory nerve (Soemmerring, 1778)*
Synonym for macrodissected adult human ***hypoglossal nerve (Winslow, 1733)***; in the original Latin, *nervum gustatorium tertium*, p. 167. According to Burdach (1822, p. 308), Boerhaave used this term earlier, but Burdach gave no citation.
4. *third spinal nerve (Soemmerring, 1778)*
Synonym for macrodissected adult human ***hypoglossal nerve (Winslow, 1733)***; in the original Latin, *nervus spinalis tertius*, p. 180.
5. *third pair of nerves of medulla oblongata (Haller & Wrisberg, 1780)*
Synonym for macrodissected adult human ***hypoglossal nerves (Winslow, 1733)***; see Haller, Cullen, & Wrisberg translation (1786, p. 208). Burdach (1822, p. 309) apparently wrongly ascribed the term to ***accessory nerve (Vieussens, 1684)***.
6. *ninth pair of cerebral nerves (Haase, 1781)*
Synonym for macrodissected adult human ***hypoglossal nerves (Winslow, 1733)***; pp. 42, 90.
7. *twelfth pair of cranial nerves (Soemmerring, 1791)*
Synonym for macrodissected adult human ***hypoglossal nerves (Winslow, 1733)***; see ***cranial nerves (Soemmerring, 1791)***.
8. *twelfth pair of cerebral nerves (Soemmerring, 1791)*
Synonym for *twelfth pair of cranial nerves (Soemmerring, 1791)*; see p. 103 and *cerebral nerves (Soemmerring, 1791)*. In the original Latin, *par duodecimum nervorum cerebri*, Soemmerring (1798, p. 125).
9. *sixteenth pair (Malacarne, 1791)*
Synonym for macrodissected adult human ***hypoglossal nerves (Winslow, 1733)***; in the original Latin, *par decimum sextum*, p. 193. The 16th of 17 *cerebral nerves (Malacarne, 1791)*.
10. *tenth nerve of head (Andersch & Soemmerring, 1792)*
Synonym for macrodissected adult human ***hypoglossal nerve (Winslow, 1733)***; in the original Latin, *decimus nervus capitis*, p. 124.

11. *tenth pair of nerves of head (Andersch & Soemmerring, 1792)*
Synonym for macrodissected adult human ***hypoglossal nerves (Winslow, 1733)***; in the original Latin, *decimi paris capitis nervorum*, p. 150.
12. *eleventh pair of nerves of head (Andersch, 1797)*
Synonym for macrodissected adult human ***hypoglossal nerves (Winslow, 1733)***; pp. 1, 54.
13. *eleventh nerves of head (Andersch, 1797)*
Synonym for macrodissected adult human ***hypoglossal nerves (Winslow, 1733)***; in the original Latin, *undecimo nervo capitis*, p. 54.
14. *great hypoglossal nerve (Cuvier, 1800)*
Synonym for macrodissected adult human ***hypoglossal nerve (Winslow, 1733)***; in the original French, *nerf grand hypoglosse*, simply a translation of the Latin (plural) *nervi hypoglossi majores (Winslow, 1733)*, Vol. 2, p. 147. Knox (1832, Pl. I-49) used the term in English itself.
15. *laryngeal nerve (Bell, 1802)*
Misnomer for macrodissected adult human *ninth pair of nerves arising within skull (Willis, 1664)*, synonym for ***hypoglossal nerve (Winslow, 1733)***; Plate XI-*10*.
16. *hyo-glossian pair of nerves (Burdin, 1803)*
Synonym for macrodissected adult human ***hypoglossal nerves (Winslow, 1733)***, his 11th pair; see translation (1803, Vol. 1, p. 144) and *eleventh pair of nerves of head (Andersch, 1797)*. For Latin form, *nervus hyoglossus*, see Burdach (1822, p. 308).
17. *myo-glossal nerve (Swan, 1830)*
Synonym for macrodissected adult human ***hypoglossal nerve (Winslow, 1733)***; p. 22.
18. *speaking nerve (Arnold, 1834)*
Synonym for macrodissected adult human ***hypoglossal nerve (Winslow, 1733)***; in the original Latin, *nervus loquens*, p. 15.

PARTLY CORRESPONDS:

1. *transverse arch of tenth pair of nerves of head (Andersch & Soemmerring, 1792)****Communicating branch (Winslow, 1733)*** of macrodissected adult human ***hypoglossal nerve (Winslow, 1733)*** associated in part with genioglossus muscles; in the original Latin, *arcum transversalem decimi paris capitis nervorum*, p. 150.
2. *communicating branches of [tenth nerves of head and] ninth nerves of head (Andersch & Soemmerring, 1792)*
Three macrodissected adult human ***communicating branches (Winslow, 1733)*** between ***hypoglossal nerve (Winslow, 1733)*** and ***vagus nerve (Galen, c192)*** were described; pp. 143–144.
3. *communicating branches of [eleventh nerves of head and] tenth nerves of head (Andersch, 1797)*
Synonym for *communicating branches of [tenth nerves of head and] ninth nerves of head (Andersch & Soemmerring, 1792)*; p. 62.
4. *transverse arch of eleventh pair of nerves of head (Andersch, 1797)*
Communicating branch (Winslow, 1733) of macrodissected adult human ***hypoglossal nerve (Winslow, 1733)*** associated in part with genioglossus muscles; in the original Latin, *arcum transversalem undecimi paris nervorum capitis*, p. 73.

hypoglossal nerve central root (>1840)

As described for macrodissected adult human, and mammal generally with histological methods for ***axons (Kölliker, 1896)***, the central root *nerve fibers (Ehrenberg, 1833)* of the ***hypoglossal nucleus (>1840)*** form bundles coursing ventrally through the ***medulla (Winslow, 1733)*** to its surface between ***pyramid (Willis, 1664)*** and ***inferior olivary complex (>1840)***; see Nieuwenhuys et al. (2008, Figs. 6.14, 6.23). The bundles are ***hypoglossal nerve central rootlets (>1840)***, together forming the ***hypoglossal nerve central root (>1840)*** that, on leaving the ventral surface of the ***medulla (Winslow, 1733)*** at the ***ventrolateral sulcus of medulla (>1840)***, becomes the peripheral ***hypoglossal nerve root (>1840)***. It was perhaps first delineated by Rolando; see ***[hypoglossal nerve central root (>1840)] (Rolando, 1825a)***.

EARLIER REFERENCES:

Illustrated, not named or described:

1. ***[hypoglossal nerve central root (>1840)] (Rolando, 1825a)***
Clearly illustrated in transverse section through macrodissected adult beef ***medulla (Winslow, 1733)***; Plate IX, Figure 7, running diagonally between *x* and *ca*.
2. ***[hypoglossal nerve central root (>1840)] (Desmoulins, 1825)***
Clearly illustrated in transverse section through macrodissected adult human ***medulla (Winslow, 1733)***; Plate XIII, Figure 12, which was drawn by Rolando; compare with Nieuwenhuys et al. (2008, Fig. 6.23).

Earlier synonyms:

1. *real origin of great hypoglossal nerve (Cruveilhier, 1836)*
Synonym for macrodissected adult human ***hypoglossal nerve central root (>1840)***; in the original French, *origine réelle*, p. 901.

hypoglossal nerve central rootlets (>1840)

As described in macrodissected adult human, and mammal generally with histological methods for ***axons (Kölliker, 1896)***, the central root *nerve fibers (Ehrenberg, 1833)* of the ***hypoglossal nucleus (>1840)*** form bundles coursing ventrally through the ***medulla (Winslow, 1733)*** to its surface at the ***ventrolateral sulcus of medulla (>1840)***; see Nieuwenhuys et al. (2008, Figs. 6.14, 6.23). The bundles are ***hypoglossal nerve central rootlets (>1840)*** together forming the ***hypoglossal nerve central root (>1840)***. On leaving the ventral surface of the ***medulla (Winslow, 1733)***, the ***hypoglossal nerve central rootlets (>1840)*** become peripheral ***hypoglossal nerve rootlets (>1840)***. They were known to Rolando; see ***[hypoglossal nerve central rootlets (>1840)] (Rolando, 1825a)***.

EARLIER REFERENCES:

Illustrated, not named or described:

1. ***[hypoglossal nerve central rootlets (>1840)] (Rolando, 1825a)***
   Two on right and on left side of macrodissected adult beef ***medulla (Winslow, 1733)*** clearly illustrated in transverse section; Plate IX, Figure 7, running diagonally between *x* and *ca*.
2. ***[hypoglossal nerve central rootlets (>1840)] (Desmoulins, 1825)***
   Two on right and on left side of macrodissected adult human ***medulla (Winslow, 1733)*** clearly illustrated in transverse section; Plate XIII, Figure 12, which was drawn by Rolando; compare with Nieuwenhuys et al. (2008, Fig. 6.23).

hypoglossal nerve root (>1840)

As described for macrodissected adult human, the aggregate of two bundles of ***hypoglossal nerve rootlets (>1840)*** perforating ***dura (Galen, c177)*** separately, opposite the hypoglossal canal in the occipital bone, and then converging to form the single ***hypoglossal nerve trunk (Günther, 1786)***. The ***hypoglossal nerve root (>1840)*** is attached to the ***ventrolateral sulcus of medulla (>1840)***, in line with and just rostral to the ***ventral root (>1840)*** of the first ***cervical nerve (Galen, c173)***; see Williams & Warwick (1980, Fig. 7.189). It was first clearly delineated as the *root of seventh pair of cerebral nerves (Vesalius, 1543a)*.

EARLIER REFERENCES:

Earlier synonyms:

1. *root of seventh pair of cerebral nerves (Vesalius, 1543a)*
   Synonym for macrodissected adult human ***hypoglossal nerve root (>1840)***, and constituent ***hypoglossal nerve rootlets (>1840)*** were also illustrated; see Richardson & Carman translation (2002, p. 205, no. 7 in the figure).
2. *root of seventh pair of sinews of brain (Geminus, 1553)*
   Synonym for macrodissected adult human *root of seventh pair of cerebral nerves (Vesalius, 1543a)*; originally spelled *roote of [seventh] payre of sinowes of brayne*, see *The table of the figures of sinowes*.
3. *cerebral part of twelfth pair (Arnold, 1834)*
   Essentially synonym for macrodissected adult human ***hypoglossal nerve root (>1840)***; in the original Latin, *par duodecimum, pars cerebralis*, p. 15.
4. *cerebral part of hypoglossal nerve (Arnold, 1834)*
   Synonym for *cerebral part of twelfth pair (Arnold, 1834)*; in the original Latin, *nervus hypoglossus, pars cerebralis*, p. 15.
5. *cerebral part of speaking nerve (Arnold, 1834)*
   Synonym for *cerebral part of twelfth pair (Arnold, 1834)*; in the original Latin, *nervus loquens, pars cerebralis*, p. 15.

hypoglossal nerve rootlets (>1840)

As described for macrodissected adult human, the set of some 10–15 filaments making up the ***hypoglossal nerve root (>1840)*** and commonly aggregating in 2 subsets. They emerge from the ***ventrolateral sulcus of medulla (>1840)***, in longitudinal line with and just rostral to the ***ventral rootlets (>1840)*** of the 1st ***cervical nerve (Galen, c173)***; see Williams & Warwick (1980, p. 1083 and Fig. 7.189). They were first clearly delineated as *little roots of seventh pair of cerebral nerves (Vesalius, 1543a)*.

EARLIER REFERENCES:

Earlier synonyms:

1. *little roots of seventh pair of cerebral nerves (Vesalius, 1543a)*
   Vesalius described and illustrated macrodissected adult human ***hypoglossal nerve rootlets (>1840)***; see Singer translation (1952, Fig. 14-O), Richardson & Carman translation (2002, fig. on p. 205, nerve 7). Elsewhere he wrote that the *seventh pair of nerves from brain (Galen, c192)* "begins as a number of separate twigs, which arise from the spinal marrow when this is on the point of leaving the skull [the ***medulla (Winslow, 1733)***]" (Richardson & Carman translation, 2002, p. 204). Also see Richardson & Carman translation (2009, p. 156), Haller (1762, p. 238 note *q*).
2. *roots of seventh conjugation (Bauhin, 1605)*
   Synonym for macrodissected adult human ***hypoglossal nerve rootlets (>1840)***; see Crooke translation (1615, pp. 487, 894).
3. *filaments of par linguale (Winslow, 1733)*
   Synonym for macrodissected adult human ***hypoglossal nerve rootlets (>1840)***; Section VI, p. 74.
4. *hypoglossal nerve fibers (Günther, 1786)*
   Description of macrodissected adult human ***hypoglossal nerve rootlets (>1840)*** referred to 4–8 fibers (Latin, *fibris*) coalescing in two major *fasciculi*; p. 67.
5. *roots of gustatory nerve (Malacarne, 1791)*
   Synonym mentioned without elaboration for macrodissected adult human ***hypoglossal nerve rootlets (>1840)***; pp. 227, 239.
6. *hypoglossal nerve fasciculi (Soemmerring, 1791)*
   Synonym for macrodissected adult human ***hypoglossal nerve rootlets (>1840)***; p. 259, also see Soemmerring (1798, p. 278). They were described in detail by Andersch & Soemmerring (1792, pp. 142–143).

hypoglossal nerve trunk (Günther, 1786)

As described for macrodissected adult human, the part of the ***hypoglossal nerve (Winslow, 1733)*** distal to the ***hypoglossal nerve root (>1840)*** and generating ***thyrohyoid branches of hypoglossal nerve (Meckel, 1817)*** and ***lingual branches of hypoglossal nerve (Cloquet, 1816)***; see Hamilton (1976, p. 636), Williams & Warwick (1980, p. 1083 and Figs. 7.189, 193). It was known to Vesalius; see ***[hypoglossal nerve trunk (Günther, 1786)] (Vesalius, 1543a)***.

EARLIER REFERENCES:

Described, not named or illustrated:

1. ***[hypoglossal nerve trunk (Günther, 1786)] (Vesalius, 1543a)***
   Alluded to for macrodissected adult human; see Richardson & Carman translation (2002, p. 204).

Earlier synonyms:

1. *trunk of par lingulae (Winslow, 1733)*
   Synonym for macrodissected adult human ***hypoglossal nerve trunk (Günther, 1786)***; Section VI, p. 75.
2. *trunk of ninth pair (Haase, 1781)*
   Synonym for macrodissected adult human ***hypoglossal nerve trunk (Günther, 1786)***; in the original Latin, *truncus noni paris*, p. 91.

LATER SYNONYMS:

1. *trunk of ninth cerebral nerve (Scarpa, 1794)*
   Synonym for macrodissected adult human ***hypoglossal nerve trunk (Günther, 1786)***; in the original Latin, *noni nervorum cerebri truncus*, Table I-32.
2. *trunk of great hypoglossal nerve (Knox, 1832)*
   Synonym for macrodissected adult human ***hypoglossal nerve trunk (Günther, 1786)***; Plate I-64.

PARTLY CORRESPONDS:

1. *condyloid part of twelfth pair (Arnold, 1834)*
   Proximal segment of macrodissected adult human ***hypoglossal nerve trunk (Günther, 1786)*** in hypoglossal canal; in the original Latin, *par duodecimum, pars condyloidea*, p. 15.
2. *condyloid part of hypoglossal nerve (Arnold, 1834)*
   Synonym for *condyloid part of twelfth pair (Arnold, 1834)*; in the original Latin, *nervus hypoglossus, pars condyloidea*, p. 15.
3. *condyloid part of speaking nerve (Arnold, 1834)*
   Synonym for *condyloid part of twelfth pair (Arnold, 1834)*; in the original Latin, *nervus loquens, pars condyloidea*, p. 15.
4. *connection of hypoglossal nerve with first cervical nerve (Arnold, 1834)*
   Macrodissected adult human ***communicating branch (Winslow, 1733)*** between ***hypoglossal nerve trunk (Günther, 1786)*** and first ***cervical nerve (Galen, c173)***; in the original Latin, *conjunctio nervus hypoglossus cum nervo cervicali primo*, p. 15. See Williams & Warwick (1980, Fig. 7.189).
5. *connection of hypoglossal nerve with ganglioform plexus of vagus nerve (Arnold, 1834)*
   Macrodissected adult human ***communicating branch (Winslow, 1733)*** between ***hypoglossal nerve trunk (Günther, 1786)*** and *ganglioform plexus of vagus nerve (Arnold, 1834)*, a *pseudoganglion (>1840)* on ***vagus nerve (Galen, c192)*** just proximal to origin of ***superior laryngeal nerve (Loder, 1778)***; in the original Latin, *conjunctio nervus hypoglossus cum plexu ganglioformi nervi vagi*, p. 15.
6. *cervical part of twelfth pair (Arnold, 1834)*
   Segment of macrodissected adult human ***hypoglossal nerve trunk (Günther, 1786)*** between *condyloid part of twelfth pair (Arnold, 1834)* and *lingual part of twelfth pair (Arnold, 1834)*; in the original Latin, *par duodecimum, pars cervicalis*, p. 15.
7. *cervical part of hypoglossal nerve (Arnold, 1834)*
   Synonym for *cervical part of twelfth pair (Arnold, 1834)*; in the original Latin, *nervus hypoglossus, pars cervicalis*, p. 15.
8. *cervical part of speaking nerve (Arnold, 1834)*
   Synonym for *cervical part of twelfth pair (Arnold, 1834)*; in the original Latin, *nervus loquens, pars cervicalis*, p. 15.

hypoglossal nucleus (>1840)

As described for macrodissected adult human, and for adult mammal in general with cellular architecture and connections, the cylindrical ***gray matter region (Swanson & Bota, 2010)*** extending longitudinally near the median plane of the caudal half of the ***medulla (Winslow, 1733)***, just ventral to the ***floor of fourth ventricle (Reil, 1807–1808a)*** and generating the ***hypoglossal nerve central root (>1840)*** continuing as the peripheral ***hypoglossal nerve root (>1840)*** to the muscles of the tongue; see Williams & Warwick (1980, p. 1083). It was first clearly delineated by Rolando; see ***[hypoglossal nucleus (>1840)] (Rolando, 1825a)***.

EARLIER REFERENCES:

Illustrated, not named or described:

1. ***[hypoglossal nucleus (>1840)] (Rolando, 1825a)***
   Clearly illustrated in transverse section of macrodissected adult cattle; Plate IX, Figure 7, small clear oval just ventral to (above in figure) the label abbreviation "*f.c.*"
2. ***[hypoglossal nucleus (>1840)] (Desmoulins, 1825)***
   Clearly illustrated in transverse section of macrodissected adult human; Plate XIII, Figure 12 (clear ovals below "*p*" on either side), which was drawn by Rolando; compare with Nieuwenhuys et al. (2008, Fig. 6.23).

hypoglossal triangle (>1840)

As described for macrodissected adult human, an elevation in the caudal half of the ***floor of fourth ventricle (Reil, 1807–1808a)*** between ***median sulcus of fourth ventricle (>1840)*** and ***vagal triangle (>1840)***, and caudal to ***medial eminence (>1840)***; see Williams & Warwick (1980, pp. 933–934, Fig. 7.89). It was described first by Willis; see ***[hypoglossal triangle (>1840] (Willis, 1664)***.

EARLIER REFERENCES:

Described, not named or illustrated:

1. ***[hypoglossal triangle (>1840)] (Willis, 1664)***
   Willis described in macrodissected adult human ***floor of fourth ventricle (Reil, 1807–1808a)*** a swelling indicating origin of ***hypoglossal nerve (Winslow, 1733)***; see Pordage translation (1681, p. 58).

Illustrated, not named or described:

1. ***[hypoglossal triangle (>1840)] (Vicq d'Azyr, 1786)***
   Clearly illustrated for macrodissected adult human; Plate XXX, Figure III, near 3.

Earlier synonyms:

1. *descending fibers of calamus scriptorius (Laurencet, 1825)*
   Synonym for macrodissected adult human ***hypoglossal triangle (>1840)***; in the original French, *fibres descendant du Calamus Scriptorius*, see legend to Figure XII-*IV* and Figure XIII.
2. *fasciculus teres (Wagner, 1839)*
   Clearly synonym for macrodissected adult human ***hypoglossal triangle (>1840)***; Table XXVII, Figure 6-*1*.

hypophysial plexus (>1840)

In adult mammal, a ramification in the ***pituitary gland (>1840)*** of sympathetic ***axons (Kölliker, 1896)*** derived from the ***internal carotid plexus (>1840)***, and ultimately the ***superior cervical ganglion (Vieussens, 1684)***; see Mitchell (1953, p. 217). It was probably first alluded to by Girardi; see ***[hypophysial plexus (>1840)] (Girardi, 1791)***.

EARLIER REFERENCES:

Described, not named or illustrated:

1. *[hypophysial plexus (>1840)] (Girardi, 1791)*
Described for macrodissected adult human; see reprint in Ludwig (1791–1795, Vol. 3, p. 85). Meckel (1832, Vol. 3, p. 91) noted that Cloquet (1816, Vol. 2, p. 687) reported fibers from ***sympathetic trunk (Winslow, 1733)*** to *infundibulum (Galen, c173)* in macrodissected adult human. Swan (1830, Pl. XII, Fig. 7-9) illustrated "A plexus formed on the internal carotid artery, and giving filaments to the pituitary gland."

Earlier synonyms:

1. *suprasphenoidal filament (Cloquet, 1816)*
Extension of macrodissected adult human ***internal carotid plexus (>1840)*** forming ***hypophysial plexus (>1840)***; in the original French, *filet sus-sphénoïdaux*, p. 689. Cloquet attributed without citation the term to Chaussier.

hypothalamic mammillotegmental tract (>1840)

As described in macrodissected adult human, and mammal generally with histological methods for ***axons (Kölliker, 1896)***, the rostral topographic segment of the ***mammillotegmental tract (>1840)*** in the ***hypothalamus (Kuhlenbeck, 1927)*** between ***principal mammillary tract (Kölliker, 1896)*** rostrally and ***midbrain mammillotegmental tract (>1840)*** segment caudally. It was first clearly delineated by Vicq d'Azyr; see ***[hypothalamic mammillotegmental tract (>1840)] (Vicq d'Azyr, 1786)***.

EARLIER REFERENCES:

Illustrated and described, not named:

1. *[hypothalamic mammillotegmental tract (>1840)] (Vicq d'Azyr, 1786)*
Described and illustrated clearly in macrodissected adult human, though without distinguishing ***principal mammillary tract (Kölliker, 1896)***; Plate XXV, Figure II-*41*.

hypothalamic mammillothalamic tract (>1840)

As described in macrodissected adult human, and mammal generally with histological methods for ***axons (Kölliker, 1896)***, the ventral topographic segment of the ***mammillothalamic tract (>1840)*** in the ***hypothalamus (Kuhlenbeck, 1927)*** between ***principal mammillary tract (Kölliker, 1896)*** ventrally and ***thalamic mammillothalamic tract (>1840)*** segment dorsally. It was probably first clearly observed by Pourfour du Petit; see ***[hypothalamic mammillothalamic tract (1840)] (Pourfour du Petit, 1710)***.

EARLIER REFERENCES:

Described, not named or illustrated:

1. *[hypothalamic mammillothalamic tract (1840)] (Pourfour du Petit, 1710)*
Delineated without separately naming for macrodissected adult human and without distinguishing ***principal mammillary tract (Kölliker, 1896)***; see ***[mammillothalamic tract (>1840)] (Pourfour du Petit, 1710)***.

hypothalamic medial forebrain bundle (>1840)

As described in macrodissected adult human, and vertebrate generally with histological methods for ***axons (Kölliker, 1896)***, the most rostral and largest topographic segment of the ***medial forebrain bundle (Edinger, 1893)***, rostral to the ***tegmental medial forebrain bundle (>1840)*** segment and centered in the ***lateral hypothalamic zone (Nauta & Haymaker, 1969)***. It is continuous rostrally with a number of components in the ***endbrain (Kuhlenbeck, 1927)***, including ***septal postcommissural fornix (>1840)***, ***diagonal band (Broca, 1879)***, ***lateral septal arcuate fibers (>1840)***, ***terminal stria (>1840)***, and ***peduncular loop (Gratiolet, 1857)***. A conspicuous dorsal branch is the ***hypothalamic medullary stria (>1840)***. Caudally, at the border between ***hypothalamus (Kuhlenbeck, 1927)*** and ***tegmentum (Swanson, 2000b)***, the rostral end of the ***dorsal longitudinal fascicle (Schütz, 1891)*** also meets the caudal end of the ***hypothalamic medial forebrain bundle (>1840)***. See Osborn (1888, p. 78), Saper et al. (1976), Swanson (2004, Tab. C, p. 178). It was first identified by Meckel; see ***[hypothalamic medial forebrain bundle (>1840)] (Meckel, 1817)***.

EARLIER REFERENCES:

Described, not named or illustrated:

1. *[hypothalamic medial forebrain bundle (>1840)] (Meckel, 1817)*
Clearly delineated in outline for macrodissected adult human; see ***[medial forebrain bundle (Edinger, 1893)] (Meckel, 1817)***.

hypothalamic medullary stria (>1840)

As described in adult mammal with histological methods for ***axons (Kölliker, 1896)***, a dorsally directed branch of the ***hypothalamic medial forebrain bundle (>1840)*** centered in the ***hypothalamus (Kuhlenbeck, 1927)*** and meeting the rostral end of the ***epithalamic medullary stria (>1840)***. It is most obvious at about the level of the ***anterior hypothalamic nucleus (>1840)***; see Nauta & Haymaker (1969, Fig. 4.23-*OH*), Kruger et al. (1995, Pl. 12). It was clearly illustrated by Kölliker as the *descending part of medullary stria (Kölliker, 1896)*. It was not identified by 1840.

EARLIER REFERENCES:

Earlier synonyms:

1. *descending part of medullary stria (Kölliker, 1896)*
Clearly illustrated synonym for ***hypothalamic medullary stria (>1840)*** in adult rabbit with histological stains

for ***axons (Kölliker, 1896)***; in the original German, *absteigender Theil der Stria medullaris (Kölliker, 1896)*, see Figure 618.

2. *lateral olfacto-habenular tract (Gurdjian, 1925)*
   Essentially synonym for ***hypothalamic medullary stria (>1840)*** in adult rat histological sections stained for ***axons (Kölliker, 1896)***; see p. 154. Gurdjian (1925, pp. 152–153) also described a diffusely organized *medial olfacto-habenular tract* arising from parts of the ***hypothalamus (Kuhlenbeck, 1927)*** medial to the ***hypothalamic medial forebrain bundle (>1840)*** and ascending medial to the *lateral olfacto-habenular tract (Gurdjian, 1925)*, partly through rostral and medial regions of the ***dorsal part of thalamus (Herrick, 1910)***.

hypothalamic optic tract (>1840)

As described for macrodissected adult mammal, the ventral topographic segment of the ***optic tract (Vicq d'Azyr, 1786)***, between ***optic chiasm (Galen, c173)*** ventrally and ***thalamic optic tract (>1840)*** segment dorsally. It was known to Galen, who did not name or delineate it separately; see ***[hypothalamic optic tract (>1840)] (Galen, c173)***.

EARLIER REFERENCES:

Described, not named or illustrated:

1. *[hypothalamic optic tract (>1840)] (Galen, c173)*
   Observed as part of *optic nerve (Galen, c173)* in macrodissected adult beef, pig, and/or macaque, but not described separately.

hypothalamic part of third ventricle (Swanson, 2004)

Part of ***third ventricle (Galen, c173)*** ventral to ***hypothalamic sulcus (>1840)***, in contrast to ***thalamic part of third ventricle (Swanson, 2004)*** dorsal to ***hypothalamic sulcus (>1840)***; p. 166. It may first have been referred to as *infundibulum (Rufus of Ephesus, fl. c90–120)*. It was first illustrated, schematically, by Hans Peyligk (1499); see Clarke and Dewhurst (1996, Fig. 46b).

EARLIER REFERENCES:

Earlier synonyms:

1. *infundibulum (Rufus of Ephesus, fl. c90–120)*
   Perhaps referred roughly to all or most of ***hypothalamic part of third ventricle (Swanson, 2004)***, according to Burdach (1822, p. 328).
2. *ditch (Rufus of Ephesus, fl. c90–120)*
   Synonym for *infundibulum (Rufus of Ephesus, fl. c90–120)*; English translation of Greek term Rufus of Ephesus used. See Meyer (1971, p. 7).
3. *hollow (Rufus of Ephesus, fl. c90–120)*
   Synonym for *ditch (Rufus of Ephesus, fl. c90–120)*; English translation of Greek term Rufus of Ephesus used. See Meyer (1971, p. 7).
4. *pyelos (Galen, c177)*
   Galen used this Greek term in association with *infundibulum (Rufus of Ephesus, fl. c90–120)*. It can be translated *trough (Galen, c177)*; see Singer (1999, p. 227)—or presumably *ditch (Rufus of Ephesus, fl. c90–120)*.
5. *trough (Galen, c177)*
   English form of *pyelos (Galen, c177)*; see Singer (1999, p. 227).
6. *pool (Galen, c192)*
   Apparently synonym for *trough (Galen, c177)*; see Duckworth translation (1962, pp. 4, 6, 7).
7. *cistern (Galen, c192)*
   Synonym for *pool (Galen, c192)*; see Duckworth translation (1962, p. 6, 7).
8. *lacuna cerebri (Mondino, 1316)*
   In *Anathomia*, Mondino appeared to apply it (and simply *lacuna*) to *trough (Galen, c177)*; see Singer translation (1925, p. 92). It was first illustrated schematically by Peyligk in 1499; see Clarke & Dewhurst (1996, Fig. 46a).
9. *lacuna (Mondino, 1316)*
   Synonym for *lacuna cerebri (Mondino, 1316)*; listed by Soemmerring (1778, p. 47) as *lacunam*.
10. *concavitas conchularis (Benedetti, 1502)*
   Synonym for macrodissected adult human *lacuna cerebri (Mondino, 1316)*, according to Soemmerring (1778) as quoted by Burdach (1822, p. 328), though Soemmerring actually listed *conchularem concavitatem*.
11. *third ventricle (Bell, 1802)*
   Bell wrote that he followed Vieussens (1684) in restricting it to *rima* or gutter-like cavity ventral to ***interthalamic adhesion (>1840)***; that is, to macrodissected adult human ***hypothalamic part of third ventricle (Swanson, 2004)***; Plates V-*M*, X-*P*.
12. *inferior wall of middle ventricle (Gerdy, 1838)*
   For macrodissected adult human, essentially ***hypothalamic part of third ventricle (Swanson, 2004)***; in the original French, *paroi inférieur*, p. 263.

PARTLY CORRESPONDS:

1. *rima ad infundibulum (Ridley, 1695)*
   Ridley explained that ***third ventricle (Galen, c173)*** consists of a rostral and a caudal channel [the *vulva (Vieussens, 1684)* and *anus (Ridley, 1695)*, respectively], and the *rima ad infundibulum*, or simply *rima*, between the two channels; pp. 83, 122, 124–125. This is a very precise reformulation of *infundibulum (Galen, c173)*. Thus, *rima ad infundibulum* probably corresponds roughly to intermediate rostrocaudal regions of ***hypothalamic part of third ventricle (Swanson, 2004)***.
2. *rima (Ridley, 1695)*
   Synonym for *rima ad infundibulum (Ridley, 1695)*; p. 124.
3. *ductus ad infundibulum (Ridley, 1695)*
   Synonym for *rima ad infundibulum (Ridley, 1695)*; p. 126.
4. *vulva (Salmon, 1714)*
   Clearly corresponds to caudal "canal" of *infundibulum (Galen, c173)*; that is, caudal end of ***hypothalamic part of third ventricle (Swanson, 2004)***; ventral to *foramen ani (Salmon, 1714)* or ***opening of cerebral aqueduct (>1840)***; p. 410. Also see *vulva (Colombo, 1559)*.

5. *striae medullares of third ventricle (Arnold, 1838b)*
   In macrodissected adult human, Arnold described set of dorsoventral (vertical) striations in wall of ***hypothalamic part of third ventricle (Swanson, 2004)***, just rostral to ***mammillary body (Ludwig, 1779)***; in the original Latin, *striae medullares ventriculi tertii*, Table VII, Figure 1-*θ*,*ϑ*. Their identity is unclear.
6. *blind hole of middle ventricle (Gerdy, 1838)*
   For macrodissected adult human, dorsal tip of ***hypothalamic part of third ventricle (Swanson, 2004)***, just dorsal to ***anterior commissure (Lieutaud, 1742)***; in the original French, *trou borgne du ventricule médian*, p. 261.

hypothalamic postcommissural fornix (>1840)

As described in macrodissected adult human, and mammal generally with histological methods for ***axons (Kölliker, 1896)***, the caudal and ventral segment of the ***postcommissural fornix (Loo, 1931)*** in the ***hypothalamus (Kuhlenbeck, 1927)***, between ***septal postcommissural fornix (>1840)*** segment dorsally and rostrally and ***mammillary body (Ludwig, 1779)*** ventrally and caudally. It has two major branches, ***subiculothalamic tract (Swanson et al. 1987)*** dorsally and ***medial corticohypothalamic tract (Gurdjian, 1927)*** ventrally. The rostral and dorsal part of the ***hypothalamic postcommissural fornix (>1840)*** was probably first recognized by Vieussens—see *columnas anteriores veri fornicis (Vieussens, 1684)*—and its extension to the ***mammillary body (Ludwig, 1779)*** was discovered by Pourfour du Petit, see *pillar of fornix (Pourfour du Petit, 1710)*.

EARLIER REFERENCES:

Earlier synonyms:

1. *exortus crurum fornicis (Santorini, 1724)*
   According to Burdach (1822, p. 356), synonym for macrodissected adult human ***hypothalamic postcommissural fornix (>1840)***; p. 60.
2. *root of anterior pillar of fornix (Winslow, 1733)*
   Synonym for macrodissected adult human ***hypothalamic postcommissural fornix (>1840)***, apparently based on *root of fornix (Willis, 1664)*; Section X, p. 43.
3. *fornicis crurum anteriorum ad tubercula mammillaria descensus (Haase, 1781)*
   Synonym for macrodissected adult human ***hypothalamic postcommissural fornix (>1840)***; p. 31.
4. *anterior crus of fornix (Monro, 1783)*
   Synonym for macrodissected adult human *root of anterior pillar of fornix (Winslow, 1733)*; Table II-Q.
5. *column of white matter (Vicq d'Azyr, 1786)*
   Synonym for macrodissected adult human ***hypothalamic postcommissural fornix (>1840)***. Vicq d'Azyr suggested it arises from junction of *anterior column of medullary triangle (Vicq d'Azyr, 1786)* and ***medullary stria (Wenzel & Wenzel, 1812)***; Plate XXV-*d*,*e*.
6. *ascending root of fornix (Burdach, 1822)*
   Essentially synonymous with macrodissected adult human *anterior crus of fornix (Monro, 1783)*; in the original Latin (plural), *radix adscendens*, p. 138.
7. *crura of corpora candicantia (Knox, 1832)*
   Synonym for macrodissected adult human right and left ***hypothalamic postcommissural fornix (>1840)***; Supplemental Plate IV-*b*.
8. *covered part of fornix column (His, 1895)*
   Essentially synonymous with macrodissected adult human ***hypothalamic postcommissural fornix (>1840)***; in the original Latin, *pars tecta columnae fornicis*, p. 86. For English form, see Ranson (1920, p. 272).
9. *sagittal part of fornix (Cajal, 1904)*
   Synonym for macrodissected adult human ***hypothalamic postcommissural fornix (>1840)***; in the original Spanish, *porción sagital del fornix*, p. 1044. Also called *sagittal segment of fornix* (*segmento sagital del fornix* in the original Spanish) on p. 1045.
10. *hypothalamic part of fornix (Cajal, 1904)*
    Synonym for macrodissected adult human ***hypothalamic postcommissural fornix (>1840)***; in the original Spanish, *porción hipothalámica*, pp. 1044–1045.
11. *inferior segment of fornix (Cajal, 1904)*
    Synonym for macrodissected adult human ***hypothalamic postcommissural fornix (>1840)***; in the original Spanish, *segmento inferior del fornix*, p. 1045.

PARTLY CORRESPONDS:

1. *root of fornix (Willis, 1664)****Postcommissural fornix (Loo, 1931)*** in general region caudal and ventral to ***anterior commissure (Lieutaud, 1742)*** where right and left bundles are clearly separated, probably corresponding roughly to initial dorsal part of ***hypothalamic postcommissural fornix (>1840)*** in macrodissected adult sheep; see Pordage translation (1681, p. 61, Fig. VII-*F*). Ridley (1695) noted that it extends farther caudally in macrodissected adult human than described by Vieussens; see *anterior column of true fornix (Vieussens, 1684)*.
2. *twofold root of fornix (Willis, 1664)*
   Right and left *root of fornix (Willis, 1664)*; see Pordage translation (1681, p. 61).
3. *straight roots of fornix (Willis, 1664)*
   Synonym for *twofold root of fornix (Willis, 1664)* in macrodissected adult sheep; see Pordage translation (1681, p. 102, Tab. 7-*F*).

hypothalamic sulcus (>1840)

The embryonic and adult longitudinal groove in the wall of the vertebrate ***third ventricle (Galen, c173)*** indicating the border between ***thalamus (His, 1893a)*** dorsally and ***hypothalamus (Kuhlenbeck, 1927)*** ventrally. In many species it is partly obliterated by the ***interthalamic adhesion (>1840)***; see Nieuwenhuys et al. (2008, pp. 47–48, Fig. 3.8). It was not clearly identified by 1840.

hypothalamohypophysial tract (>1840)

As described primarily with immunohistochemical methods in mammal, a somewhat diffusely organized ***central nervous system white matter tract (>1840)*** from neuroendocrine motor ***neurons (Waldeyer, 1891)*** in the

hypothalamus (Kuhlenbeck, 1927) to the ***neurohypophysis (Rioch et al., 1940)***, with ***axons (Kölliker, 1896)*** of parvicellular neuroendocrine ***neurons (Waldeyer, 1891)*** ending in the ***median eminence (Tilney, 1936)***, and ***axons (Kölliker, 1896)*** of magnocellular neuroendocrine ***neurons (Waldeyer, 1891)*** ending in the ***posterior lobe of pituitary gland (Haller, 1762)***; see Swanson (1986). For correct spelling see Rioch et al. (1940, p. 3 note *1*). It may first have been identified partly as the *spicarum fascis cum plumula annexa (Bergmann, 1831)*.

PARTLY CORRESPONDS:

1. *spicarum fascis cum plumula annexa (Bergmann, 1831)*
   Enigmatic feature illustrated for macrodissected adult human has roughly shape and location of ***paraventricular hypothalamic nucleus (Malone, 1910)*** component of ***hypothalamohypophysial tract (>1840)***, as unlikely as Bergmann's ability to identify it might seem; see Table II-*x*, shown but not labeled in Table I; also see pp. 22, 75. A translation might be *sheaf of grain with small feathers attached*. Also see *pennatula (Bergmann, 1831)*. It is remotely possible that Willis glimpsed the ***hypothalamohypophysial tract (>1840)*** earlier; see ***[supraoptic decussations (>1840)] (Willis, 1672)***.
2. *plumula (Bergmann, 1831)*
   Synonym for *spicarum fascis cum plumula annexa (Bergmann, 1831)*, or at least the feathery attachments; also see p. 26 and Table VIII, Figure 3.
3. *pennatula (Bergmann, 1831)*
   In macrodissected adult horse, apparently end of *spicarum fascis cum plumula annexa (Bergmann, 1831)* ventral to (below) ***third ventricle (Galen, c173)***; that is, in ***median eminence (Tilney, 1936)***; pp. 27, 42, 77 and Table VIII, Figure 4-*a*.

hypothalamus (Kuhlenbeck, 1927)

The ventral topographic division of the vertebrate ***interbrain (Baer, 1837)*** including the ***hypothalamic part of third ventricle (Swanson, 2004)***, ***periventricular hypothalamic zone (Nauta & Haymaker, 1969)***, ***medial hypothalamic zone (Nauta & Haymaker, 1969)***, and ***lateral hypothalamic zone (Nauta & Haymaker, 1969)***; the dorsal topographic division is the ***thalamus (His, 1893a)***. See Swanson & Bota (2010) for these definitions. For Kuhlenbeck's description based on comparative embryology, see p. 67 and Chapter 9; it is quite distinct from *hypothalamus (His, 1893a)* and *hypothalamus (His, 1893b)*. Also see Christ (1969, p. 23) and Nauta & Haymaker (1969, Tab. 4-*1*). The general region of the ***hypothalamus (Kuhlenbeck, 1927)*** was identified long ago; see *pelvis (Rufus of Ephesus, fl. c90–120)*. Bauhin (1605, pp. 604–605) specifically included the *base of brain (Varoli, 1573)* within the *pelvis (Rufus of Ephesus, fl. c90–120)* or *infundibulum (Galen, c173)*; see Crooke translation (1615, p. 469). Wharton (1656) apparently first stated clearly that the walls of the macrodissected adult human *infundibulum (Galen, c173)* are formed by *gray substance (Vesalius, 1543a)*, covered with ***pia (Galen, c192)***, "...the *funnel* [*infundibulum (Galen, c173)*] is perfectly matched at its own upper end to the size of the excretory passage of the fourth ventricle [either the ***cerebral aqueduct (>1840)*** or part of the ***third ventricle (Galen, c173)***], to which it is connected all round its circumference by means of a certain medullary substance very like the cortex of the brain. Now, it is established that the funnel is of two substances, membranous without and medullary within..." (translation, p. 170). Shortly thereafter, Willis (1664; see Pordage translation, 1681, p. 66) and Malpighi (1665; see Meyer, 1967, p. 186) made similar observations without citing Wharton. Steno (1669) provided the first realistic illustrations of the macrodissected adult human ***hypothalamus (Kuhlenbeck, 1927)*** in the first printed midsagittal views of the ***brain (Smith Papyrus, c1700 BC)***—his Plates I & II—as well as in two transverse sections, his Plates III & IV. Illustrated (with no legends or commentary) are the ***postcommissural fornix (Loo, 1931)***, crossing of the ***anterior commissure (Lieutaud, 1742)***, ***terminal lamina (Burdach, 1822)***, ***median eminence (Tilney, 1936)***, two lobes of the *pituitary gland (Galen, c192)*, ***mammillary body (Ludwig, 1779)***, and ***interthalamic adhesion (>1840)***—as well as the ***hypothalamic part of third ventricle (Swanson, 2004)*** and ***thalamic part of third ventricle (Swanson, 2004)***. Tarin (1750) provided a very clear frontal (horizontal) section through the macrodissected adult human ***hypothalamus (Kuhlenbeck, 1927)*** showing the ***anterior commissure (Lieutaud, 1742)*** and ***posterior commissure (Winslow, 1733)***, ***mammillary body (Ludwig, 1779)***, and ***hypothalamic part of third ventricle (Swanson, 2004)***; Table I, Figure 3.

EARLIER REFERENCES:

Earlier synonyms:

1. *pelvis (Rufus of Ephesus, fl. c90–120)*
   Perhaps referred roughly to all or majority of ***hypothalamus (Kuhlenbeck, 1927)*** and containing *hollow (Rufus of Ephesus, fl. c90–120)*, *infundibulum (Rufus of Ephesus, fl. c90–120)*, or ***hypothalamic part of third ventricle (Swanson, 2004)***; see Wiberg translation (1914, pp. 19, 91), May translation (1968, p. 429), Meyer (1971, p. 7). Also see ***[median eminence (Tilney, 1936)] (Vesalius, 1543a)***.
2. *basin (Rufus of Ephesus, fl. c90–120)*
   English form of *pelvis (Rufus of Ephesus, fl. c90–120)*; see May translation (1968, p. 429).
3. *infundibulum (Galen, c173)*
   Apparently synonym for *pelvis (Rufus of Ephesus, fl. c90–120)*. Galen also referred to two canals or channels leading down (ventrally) to base of *infundibulum (Galen, c173)*, one starting dorsally and rostrally near ***interventricular foramen (>1840)***, and the other starting dorsally and caudally near ***opening of cerebral aqueduct (>1840)***. He believed *infundibulum (Galen, c173)* acts as "funnel" for residues or waste products in ***ventricles (Hippocrates)*** to reach *pituitary gland (Galen, c192)*, which filters them before

passing through perforations of palate into mouth as *pituita*, *mucus*, or *phlegm*; see Duckworth (1962, p. 4), May translation (1968, pp. 428–430), and Ridley (1695, pp. 124, 125). Basically, Galen apparently regarded *infundibulum (Galen, c173)* as a cavity extending to *pituitary gland (Galen, c192)* and surrounded by a wall formed by ***pia (Galen, c192)*** and blood vessels, at least as his work has been translated into English; see May (1968, p. 429). Galen's description was probably based on macrodissected adult beef, pig, and/or macaque but not human.

4. *funnel (Galen, c173)*
Synonym for *infundibulum (Galen, c173)*; see May translation (1968, pp. 428, 429), Richardson & Carman (2009, p. 212).
5. *choane (Galen, c177)*
Greek form of *infundibulum (Galen, c173)*; see Singer translation (1999, p. 227).
6. *chone (Galen, c177)*
Alternate form of *choane (Galen, c177)*; another form is *choana*.
7. *base of third ventricle (Galen, c177)*
Synonym for *infundibulum (Galen, c173)*; see Singer translation (1999, p. 235). Later in the same chapter, Galen referred similarly to "the bottom of the [third] ventricle" indicating he associated *infundibulum (Galen, c173)* with ***third ventricle (Galen, c173)*** as a whole.
8. *caput rosae (Avicenna or Ibn Sina, c1030)*
Synonym for *infundibulum (Galen, c173)* because it resembles a rose calyx; see Meyer (1971, p. 9).
9. *head of rose (Avicenna or Ibn Sina, c1030)*
English form of *caput rosae (Avicenna or Ibn Sina, c1030)*; see Lind (1959, p. 143).
10. *infusorium (Avicenna or Ibn Sina, c1030)*
Synonym for *infundibulum (Galen, c173)*; see Meyer (1971, p. 9).
11. *large round eminences (Mondino, 1316)*
A passage in Mondino's *Anathomia* seems to describe vaguely the macrodissected adult human ***hypothalamus (Kuhlenbeck, 1927)***: "The *lacuna* [***hypothalamic part of third ventricle (Swanson, 2004)***] hath around it large round eminences [right and left ***hypothalamus (Kuhlenbeck, 1927)***?]. These are made to sustain the veins or arteries which ascend from the ***rete mirabile (Herophilus, c335–c280 BC)*** to the ventricles. In the base thereof do appear little glands [***mammillary body (Ludwig, 1779)***?] which project near the *rete mirable*." (Singer translation, 1925, p. 92).
12. *eminentia rotunda magna (Mondino, 1316)*
Latin form of *large round eminences (Mondino, 1316)* used, for example, in Ketham editions of Mondino; see Singer translation (1925, p. 55), Meyer (1971, p. 9).
13. *large round eminences (Manfredi, 1490)*
In *Anathomia*, Manfredi described *large round eminences (Mondino, 1316)* as part of macrodissected adult human ***brain (Smith Papyrus, c1700 BC)*** associated with *anterior ventricles (Galen, c173)* or ***lateral ventricles (Vesalius, 1543a)***, although Mondino clearly associated them with *middle ventricle (Galen, c173)* or ***third ventricle (Galen, c173)***. Thus, Manfredi's vague reference seemingly places ***hypothalamus (Kuhlenbeck, 1927)*** in ***endbrain (Kuhlenbeck, 1927)*** rather than ***interbrain (Baer, 1837)***. Some contemporary anatomists still place rostral components of *hypothalamus (His, 1893a)* and *hypothalamus (His, 1893b)* in *telencephalon (His, 1893a)* and *telencephalon (His 1893b)*.
14. *labrum (Berengario da Carpi, 1521)*
Probably synonym for macrodissected adult human *infundibulum (Galen, c173)*; f. 438, see Soemmerring (1778, p. 47), Burdach (1822, p. 328).
15. *embotum (Berengario da Carpi, 1521)*
Probably synonym for macrodissected adult human *infundibulum (Galen, c173)*; see Burdach (1822, p. 328).
16. *concha (Berengario da Carpi, 1521)*
Probably synonym for macrodissected adult human *infundibulum (Galen, c173)*; see Burdach (1822, p. 328).
17. *colatorium (Günther, 1536)*
Synonym for macrodissected adult human *infundibulum (Galen, c173)*; see Meyer (1971, p. 9). Burdach (1822, p. 328) quoted Günther as using the term *pelvis colatoria*, as noted by Soemmerring (1778, p. 47), although the latter actually listed *pelvim colatoriam*. According to Berengario da Carpi (1521, f. 427), as quoted by Burdach (1822, p. 328), Mondino (316) used the term *colatorium* to indicate *pituitary gland (Galen, c192)* and *infundibulum (Galen, c173)* considered together.
18. *pyelos (Vesalius, 1543a)*
Vesalius was more specific in his description of macrodissected adult human *infundibulum (Galen, c173)* than was Galen for other large mammals; see Singer translation (1952, pp. xvi, 52). Vesalius wrote that for some unnamed anatomists *pyelos* meant a "membranous body" forming upper part of *infundibulum (Galen, c173)*, and he illustrated it several times; see Singer translation (1952, pp. 114–117, Figs. 15, 16, and 18), Richardson & Carman translation (2009, p. 212 & Fig. 15 on p. 157). For other unnamed anatomists, he wrote, the term *pyelos* meant upper part of funnel just mentioned, along with lower part of funnel together forming the *infundibulum (Galen, c173)*. Lower part of funnel, or *tube of infundibulum (Vesalius, 1543a)*, roughly corresponds to *pituitary stalk (Lieutaud, 1842)*.
19. *funyil (Geminus, 1553)*
English form of *infundibulum (Galen, c173)*; see *The tables of the brayne*, Figure 6-Q, and *funnel (Galen, c173)*.
20. *basyn (Geminus, 1553)*
Early English form of *basin (Vesalius, 1543a)*, see *The tables of the brayne*, Fig. 6-Q). Elsewhere it was spelled *basyne* (see *The tables of the brayne*, Figs. 14-C, 15-*E*, 19-*B*); or *basine* (see *The tables of the brayne*, Fig. 16-*B*).

21. *pituitary flask (Vesalius, 1555)*
Synonym for macrodissected adult human *infundibulum (Galen, c173)*, see Singer translation (1952, p. 36).
22. *dropping pan (Hall, 1565)*
Hall noted that Dr. Langton "englisheth" *infundibulum (Galen, c173)* as *droppnge pan*; p. 42.
23. *tunnel (Crooke, 1615)*
English form of *infundibulum (Galen, c173)*, although it actually refers to ***hypothalamus (Kuhlenbeck, 1927)***; p. 469.
24. *pipe (Wharton, 1656)*
Synonym for macrodissected adult human *infundibulum (Galen, c173)*; translation p. 170. Wharton referred to it as a certain *vessel* or *pipe*.
25. *aqueduct (Brunn, 1753)*
Synonym for macrodissected adult human *infundibulum (Galen, c173)*; see Burdach (1822, p. 328).
26. *scyphum (Soemmerring, 1778)*
Synonym for macrodissected adult human *infundibulum (Galen, c173)*; p. 47.
27. *supersphenoidal peduncle (Burdin, 1803)*
Apparently synonym for macrodissected adult human *infundibulum (Galen, c173)*; see translation (1803, Vol. 1, p. 162). Burdin referred to *pituitary gland (Galen, c192)* as appendix of *supersphenoidal peduncle (Burdin, 1803)*; p. 162.
28. *pituitary peduncle (Burdin, 1803)*
Synonym for *supersphenoidal peduncle (Burdin, 1803)*; see translation (1803, Vol. 1, p. 162).
29. *structures under thalamus (Burdach, 1822)*
Description of then-known macrodissected adult human regions corresponding roughly to ***hypothalamus (Kuhlenbeck, 1927)***; p. 108, also see Schiller (1992, p. 248).
30. *pedicle of pituitary gland (Cloquet, 1828)*
Synonym for macrodissected adult human *pituitary peduncle (Burdin, 1803)*; in the original French, *pédicule de la glande pituitaire*, Plate CXLV, Figure 6-3.

PARTLY CORRESPONDS:

1. *tub (Vesalius, 1543a)*
Richardson & Carman's (2009, p. 212) translation of *pyelos (Vesalius, 1543a)*; in the same passage Vesalius wrote of the *infundibulum (Galen, c173)*, "Its upper part also resembles a dinghy or the shell-like shape in which we wash ourselves at the baths, and is therefore known as 'the tub' (the Greek word is *pyelos*)." Thus, *tub (Vesalius, 1543a)* corresponds roughly to macrodissected adult human ***hypothalamus (Kuhlenbeck, 1927)*** without ***infundibulum (Rioch et al., 1940)***.
2. *cyathus (Vesalius, 1543a)*
Vesalius used this term (meaning ladle) synonymously with *tub (Vesalius, 1543a)* and illustrated it clearly; see Singer translation (1952, p. 116, Fig. 18-*B*).
3. *foremost portion of basis of brain (Riolan, 1657)*
Term in English translation of Riolan indicating roughly *tuber cinereum (Soemmerring, 1788)*; Table 17, Figure 1-*P*.
4. *corpus cinereum (Albinus, 1744)*
In Albinus's explanation of Eustachius's plates, synonym for *tuber cinereum (Soemmerring, 1778)* at base of macrodissected adult human ***hypothalamus (Kuhlenbeck, 1927)***, surrounding bottom of *infundibulum (Rufus of Ephesus, fl. c90–120)*; Plate 18, Figures I, III, IV, and V-χ, p. 103. Volkmann (1831, Tab. XVII, Fig. 1-*e*) used it for macrodissected adult dolphin.
5. *pars infundibuli anterior (Tarin, 1750)*
Refers roughly to macrodissected adult human *preoptic level of hypothalamus (>1840)*; Table I, Figure 5-*V*. Burdach (1822, p. 327) listed full term as *pars infundibuli anterior, peculiari substantia circumscripta*. See Swanson (1987, p. 2).
6. *inferior olfactory tubercle (Haller, 1768)*
Macrodissected fish swelling from which ***pituitary gland (>1840)*** extends, thus similar to *tuber cinereum (Soemmerring, 1778)*; in the original Latin, *tuberculis olfactoriis inferioribus*, p. 203; also see Arsaky (1813, p. 36).
7. *tuber cinereum (Soemmerring, 1778)*
Corresponds to base of macrodissected adult human ***hypothalamus (Kuhlenbeck, 1927)***; Table II-*PSR*, also see Meyer (1971, p. 26). Anderson (1837, p. 20) gave an interesting historical account of this general region in fish.
8. *fundus of third ventricle (Günther, 1786)*
Synonym for macrodissected adult human *tuber cinereum (Soemmerring, 1778)*; in the original Latin, *fundus ventriculi tertii*, p. 15.
9. *cloison pulpeuse du troisieme ventricule (Bell, 1803b)*
Apparently roughly corresponds to macrodissected adult human *preoptic level of hypothalamus (>1840)*, with "striae which pass obliquely backwards and downwards, and some of which, while they adhere to the optic nerves, pass into them" (p. 93). The term's origin in the French literature was not indicated. See Swanson (1987, p. 2).
10. *ganglion of pituitary (Carus, 1814)*
Very roughly, region of mammalian ***mammillary body (Ludwig, 1779)*** in macrodissected adult fish ***hypothalamus (Kuhlenbeck, 1927)***; in the original German, *Ganglion des Hirnanhangs*, p. 114. Later on, Carus referred to it as *zitzenförmigen Erhabenheiten*, p. 156.
11. *gray mass of infundibulum (Carus, 1814)*
Synonym for *ganglion of pituitary (Carus, 1814)* in macrodissected adult amphibian and bird; in the original German, *graue Masse des Trichters (Infundibulum)*, pp. 184, 203, respectively.
12. *gray plate (Meckel, 1817)*
Translation of *tuber cinereum (Soemmerring, 1778)*; see translation (1832, Vol. 2, p. 439), where Meckel explained the gray plate "is continuous forward with the anterior extremity of the corpus callosum, where it forms on the surface of the anterior commissure a thin expansion, across which we perceive this cord." Here *gray substance (Vesalius, 1543a)* associated with ***terminal lamina (Burdach, 1822)*** is described. Follows similar description for macrodissected human by Gordon (1815, p. 131).
13. *gray optic thalamus (Sommé, 1824)*

Synonym for macrodissected adult vertebrate *tuber cinereum (Soemmerring, 1778)*, named for its "presumed functions"; in the original French, *couche optique grise*, p. 41.

14. *cineritious tubercle (Spurzheim, 1826)*
English form of *tuber cinereum (Soemmerring, 1778)* for macrodissected adult human; p. 231-17.

15. *floor of third ventricle (Langenbeck, 1826–1830)*
Synonym for macrodissected adult human *tuber cinereum (Soemmerring, 1778)*; in the original Latin, *pavimentum ventriculi tertii*, Fascicle I, Table XII-*q*.

16. *grey tubercle (Solly, 1836)*
English form of *tuber cinereum (Soemmerring, 1778)* for macrodissected adult human; p. 77.

17. *pons Tarini (Solly, 1836)*
Eponym for macrodissected adult human *tuber cinereum (Soemmerring, 1778)*; p. 121.

18. *inferior ganglion (Leuret, 1839)*
Synonym for macrodissected adult fish *inferior olfactory tubercle (Haller, 1768)*; in the original French (plural), *ganglions inférieurs*, p. 143.

19. *pars subthalamica of forebrain (His, 1892)*
Synonym for *hypothalamus (His, 1893a)*; in the original form, *pars subthalamica des Vorderhirns*, p. 346 and Figure 9.

20. *hypothalamus (His, 1893a)*
His's use of the term was based on macrodissected embryos and adults, including human, and is essentially as defined today except that he included the preoptic region or level (see Swanson, 1976, pp. 229–235; Swanson, 1987, p. 2) of the ***hypothalamus (Kuhlenbeck, 1927)*** in the corpus striatum part of the *telencephalon (His, 1893a)*; p. 159 and Figure 2-*Hth*; this was the interpretation in the *Basel Nomina Anatomica* (His, 1895, p. 158).

21. *hypothalamus (His, 1893b)*
Based on his interpretation of neural tube development, His defined hypothalamus here as having two major parts ventral to ***hypothalamic sulcus (>1840)***: *pars mamillaris hypothalami*, which he assigned to *diencephalon (His, 1893b)*; and *pars optica hypothalami* (see p. 178), which he assigned to *telencephalon (His, 1893b)*, along with *preoptic level of hypothalamus (>1840)*, which he assigned to corpus striatum part of *telencephalon (His, 1893b)*. This interpretation was adopted by the *Basel Nomina Anatomica* (His, 1895). The *pars optica hypothalami* corresponds roughly to anterior and tuberal regions or levels (see Swanson, 1987, p. 2) of ***hypothalamus (Kuhlenbeck, 1927)***.

I

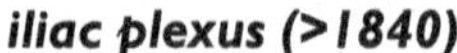

iliac plexus (>1840)

As described for macrodissected adult human, it surrounds the common iliac artery and is an extension mainly of the ***superior hypogastric plexus (Tiedemann, 1822)***, but also of the ***intermesenteric plexus (>1840)***; see Mitchell (1953, pp. 261–262), Williams & Warwick (1980, pp. 1134–1135 and Fig. 7.230). Meckel probably distinguished it first; see ***[iliac plexus (>1840)] (Meckel, 1817)***.

TRANSLATIONS:

1. *plexus iliacus (>1840)*
   Current Latin form of ***iliac plexus (>1840)***; see *Terminologia Anatomica* (1998, p. 143).

EARLIER REFERENCES:

Described, not named or illustrated:

1. ***[iliac plexus (>1840)] (Meckel, 1817)***
   Alluded to in macrodissected adult human; see translation (1832, Vol. 3, p. 88).

iliohypogastric nerve (Schmidt, 1794)

As described for macrodissected adult human, it arises from the first ***lumbar nerve (Diemerbroeck, 1672)*** and divides distally into a ***lateral cutaneous branch of iliohypogastric nerve (>1840)***, which distributes to skin of the dorsolateral (posterolateral) gluteal region, and an ***anterior cutaneous branch of iliohypogastric nerve (>1840)***, which distributes to the internal oblique and transversus muscles and abdominal skin rostral to (above) the pubis; see Hamilton (1976, Figs. 827, 828), Williams & Warwick (1980, p. 1106 and Fig. 7.209). For Schmidt's use in macrodissected adult human, see p. 31; he described external and internal branches (p. 33). It was first clearly delineated by Eustachi; see ***[iliohypogastric nerve (Schmidt, 1794)] (Eustachi, 1552)***.

TRANSLATIONS:

1. *nervus ilio-hypogastricus (Schmidt, 1794)*
   Original Latin form of ***iliohypogastric nerve (Schmidt, 1794)***; p. 31, including a history of earlier observations.
2. *nervi ileo-hypogastrici (Bock, 1827)*
   Latin form of ***iliohypogastric nerve (Schmidt, 1794)***; Table I, Figure 2-59.

EARLIER REFERENCES:

Illustrated, not named or described:

1. ***[iliohypogastric nerve (Schmidt, 1794)] (Eustachi, 1552)***
   Clearly illustrated initial part for macrodissected adult human; see Albinus edition (1761, Tab. 21-T). Vesalius (1543a) may have illustrated the initial part of it in a confused way for macrodissected adult human; see Richardson & Carman translation (2002, pp. 206, 207, 265).

Illustrated and described, not named:

1. ***[iliohypogastric nerve (Schmidt, 1794)] (Vieussens, 1684)***
   Described and illustrated, at least parts of it, for macrodissected adult human; Table 28.

Earlier synonyms:

1. *external anterior branch of first pair of lumbar nerves (Winslow, 1733)*
   Synonym for macrodissected adult human ***iliohypogastric nerve (Schmidt, 1794)***; Section VI, p. 86.
2. *third branch of first lumbar pair (Sabatier, 1775)*
   Synonym for macrodissected adult human ***iliohypogastric nerve (Schmidt, 1794)***; in the original French, *troisième branche de la premiere Paire lombaire*; p. 728. See Schmidt (1794, p. 31).
3. *third of four branches of first lumbar pair (Haase, 1781)*

Synonym for macrodissected adult human ***iliohypogastric nerve (Schmidt, 1794)***; in the original Latin, *ramorum quatuor primi paris tertius*; p. 104. See Schmidt (1794, p. 31).

4. *inguino-cutaneous nerve (Burdin, 1803)*
   Synonym for macrodissected adult human ***iliohypogastric nerve (Schmidt, 1794)***; see translation (1803, Vol. 1, p. 199).
5. *inferior musculocutaneous branch of lumbar plexus (Cloquet, 1816)*
   Synonym for macrodissected adult human ***iliohypogastric nerve (Schmidt, 1794)***; p. 662.
6. *internal cutaneous branch of lumbar plexus (Quain, 1828)*
   Synonym for macrodissected adult human ***iliohypogastric nerve (Schmidt, 1794)***; p. 285.
7. *abdominal branches of lumbar plexus (Cruveilhier, 1836)*
   Essentially synonym for macrodissected adult human ***iliohypogastric nerve (Schmidt, 1794)***; in the original French, *branches abdominale*, pp. 832–835.
8. *greater abdominal branch of lumbar plexus (Cruveilhier, 1836)*
   Synonym for macrodissected adult human ***iliohypogastric nerve (Schmidt, 1794)***; in the original French, *grande branche abdominale*, p. 833.
9. *superior musculocutaneous branch of lumbar plexus (Cruveilhier, 1836)*
   Synonym for *greater abdominal branch of lumbar plexus (Cruveilhier, 1836)*, attributed without citation to Bichat; in the original French, *branche musculo-cutanée supérieure*, p. 833.
10. *ilioscrotal branch of lumbar plexus (Cruveilhier, 1836)*
    Commonest synonym for *greater abdominal branch of lumbar plexus (Cruveilhier, 1836)* according to Cruveilhier; in the original French, *branche ilio-scrotale*, p. 833.
11. *internal musculo-cutaneous branch of lumbar plexus (Quain, 1837)*
    Synonym for macrodissected adult human ***iliohypogastric nerve (Schmidt, 1794)***; p. 786.
12. *internal musculo-cutaneous nerve (Quain & Wilson, 1839)*
    Synonym for *internal musculo-cutaneous branch of lumbar plexus (Quain, 1837)*; Plate XXI-*f*.
13. *inferior musculo-cutaneous nerve (Quain & Wilson, 1839)*
    Synonym for *internal musculo-cutaneous branch of lumbar plexus (Quain, 1837)*; Plate XXI-*f*.

PARTLY CORRESPONDS:

1. *internal branch of iliohypogastric nerve (Cloquet, 1828)*
   Macrodissected adult human medial branch of ***iliohypogastric nerve (Schmidt, 1794)***; in the original French, *rameau interne du nerf ilio-hypogastrique*, Plate CLXXII, Figure 1-*48*.
2. *external branch of iliohypogastric nerve (Cloquet, 1828)*
   Macrodissected adult human lateral branch of ***iliohypogastric nerve (Schmidt, 1794)***; in the original French, *rameau externe du nerf ilio-hypogastrique*, Plate CLXXII, Figure 1-*49*.
3. *lesser abdominal branch of lumbar plexus (Cruveilhier, 1836)*
   For macrodissected adult human, variable differentiation of *greater abdominal branch of lumbar plexus (Cruveilhier, 1836)* supplying skin in pubic region; in the original French, *petit branche abdominale*, p. 835.
4. *middle musculocutaneous branch of lumbar plexus (Cruveilhier, 1836)*
   Synonym for macrodissected adult human *lesser abdominal branch of lumbar plexus (Cruveilhier, 1836)*, attributed without citation to Bichat; in the original French, *branche musculo-cutanée moyenne*, p. 835.
5. *lesser ilioscrotal branch of lumbar plexus (Cruveilhier, 1836)*
   Synonym for macrodissected adult human *lesser abdominal branch of lumbar plexus (Cruveilhier, 1836)*; in the original French, *petite ilio-scrotale*, p. 835.

ilio-inguinal nerve (Schmidt, 1794)

As described for macrodissected adult human it arises from the first ***lumbar nerve (Diemerbroeck, 1672)*** and distributes small branches to the internal oblique muscle before innervating skin on proximal and medial areas of the thigh, skin on the root of the penis and upper part of the scrotum in male, and skin covering the mons pubis and adjoining part of the labium majus in female; see Williams & Warwick (1980, pp. 1106–1107), *Terminologia Anatomica* (1998, p. 139). It is sometimes considered a ***lumbar plexus ventral division (Peterson, 1887)***; see Durward (1951, Fig. 937), Carpenter (1976, Fig. 7.19). For Schmidt's use in macrodissected adult human, see p. 33; he described external and internal branches (p. 35). At least parts of it were probably first delineated in print by Vieussens; see ***[ilio-inguinal nerve (Schmidt, 1794)] (Vieussens, 1684)***, although Pietro da Cortona had drawn parts of it earlier (c1618).

TRANSLATIONS:

1. *nervus ilio-inguinalis (Schmidt, 1794)*
   Original Latin form of ***ilio-inguinal nerve (Schmidt, 1794)***; p. 33.
2. *nervus ileo-inguinalis (Bock, 1827)*
   Latin form of ***ilio-inguinal nerve (Schmidt, 1794)***; Table I, Figure 2-*64*.

EARLIER REFERENCES:

Illustrated and described, not named:

1. ***[ilio-inguinal nerve (Schmidt, 1794)] (Vieussens, 1684)***
   Vieussens described and illustrated at least parts of it for macrodissected adult human; Table 28. Distal part of ***nerve (Herophilus, c335–c280 BC)*** was illustrated by Pietro da Cortona (drawn c1618), and was labeled *nervi lumbalis, qui ad pudenda vergit* (Tab. I-*n.u.tt*) in the edition edited by Petrioli (1741).

Earlier synonyms:

1. *internal anterior branch of first pair of lumbar nerves (Winslow, 1733)*

Synonym for macrodissected adult human ***ilio-inguinal nerve (Schmidt, 1794)***; Section VI, p. 86.

2. *second branch of first lumbar pair (Sabatier, 1775)*
Synonym for macrodissected adult human ***ilio-inguinal nerve (Schmidt, 1794)***; in the original French, *seconde branche de la premiere Paire lombaire*, p. 718.
3. *second of four branches of first lumbar pair (Haase, 1781)*
Synonym for macrodissected adult human ***ilio-inguinal nerve (Schmidt, 1794)***; in the original Latin, *quatuor ramorum primi paris secundus*, p. 104.

LATER SYNONYMS:

1. *inguinal nerve (Burdin, 1803)*
Probably synonym for macrodissected adult human ***ilio-inguinal nerve (Schmidt, 1794)***; see translation (1803, Vol. 1, p. 201).
2. *ilioscrotal nerve (Chaussier, 1807)*
May correspond to ***ilio-inguinal nerve (Schmidt, 1794)***, although it was associated in adult human with second rather than first ***lumbar nerve (Diemerbroeck, 1672)***; also see Meckel (1832, Vol. 3, p. 14).
3. *superior musculocutaneous branch of lumbar plexus (Cloquet, 1816)*
Synonym for macrodissected adult human ***ilio-inguinal nerve (Schmidt, 1794)***; p. 661.
4. *abdominal branch of first lumbar nerve (Bock, 1827)*
Probably synonym for macrodissected adult human ***ilio-inguinal nerve (Schmidt, 1794)***; in the original Latin, *Ram. abdominalis nervi lumbaris primi*, Table I, Figure 2-*57*.
5. *external musculo-cutaneous branch of lumbar plexus (Quain, 1828)*
Synonym for macrodissected adult human ***ilio-inguinal nerve (Schmidt, 1794)***; p. 284.
6. *external inguinal branch of lumbar plexus (Cruveilhier, 1836)*
Synonym for macrodissected adult human ***ilio-inguinal nerve (Schmidt, 1794)***; in the original French, *branche inguinale externe*, p. 835.
7. *inguino-cutaneous branch of lumbar plexus (Cruveilhier, 1836)*
Synonym attributed without citation to Chaussier for *external inguinal branch of lumbar plexus (Cruveilhier, 1836)*; in the original French, *branche inguino-cutanée*, p. 835.
8. *inferior musculocutaneous branch of lumbar plexus (Cruveilhier, 1836)*
Synonym attributed without citation to Bichat for *external inguinal branch of lumbar plexus (Cruveilhier, 1836)*; in the original French, *branche musculo-cutanée inférieure*, p. 835.
9. *external musculo-cutaneous nerve (Quain & Wilson, 1839)*
Synonym for macrodissected adult human ***ilio-inguinal nerve (Schmidt, 1794)***; Plate XXI-*c*.
10. *superior musculo-cutaneous nerve (Quain & Wilson, 1839)*
Synonym for macrodissected adult human ***ilio-inguinal nerve (Schmidt, 1794)***; Plate XXI-*c*.

PARTLY CORRESPONDS:

1. *communicating branch of ilio-inguinal nerve with second lumbar nerve (Bock, 1827)*
Described for macrodissected adult human; in the original Latin, *ram. communicans nervi ileo-inguinalis*, Table II-*100*.
2. *internal branch of ilio-inguinal nerve (Cloquet, 1828)*
For macrodissected adult human, medial branch of ***ilio-inguinal nerve (Schmidt, 1794)***; in the original French, *rameau interne du nerf ilio-inguinal*, Plate CLXXII, Figure 1-*51*.
3. *external branch of ilio-inguinal nerve (Cloquet, 1828)*
For macrodissected adult human, lateral branch of ***ilio-inguinal nerve (Schmidt, 1794)***; in the original French, *rameau externe du nerf ilio-inguinal*, Plate CLXXII, Figure 1-*52*.
4. *external filament of internal branch of ilio-inguinal nerve (Cloquet, 1828)*
Small lateral branch of *internal branch of ilio-inguinal nerve (Cloquet, 1828)*; in the original French, *filet externe*, Plate CLXXII, Figure 2-*44*.
5. *internal filament of internal branch of ilio-inguinal nerve (Cloquet, 1828)*
Small medial branch of *internal branch of ilio-inguinal nerve (Cloquet, 1828)*; in the original French, *filet interne*, Plate CLXXII, Figure 2-*45*.
6. *internal musculo-cutaneous branch of lumbar plexus (Quain, 1828)*
For macrodissected adult human, mostly muscular branch of ***ilio-inguinal nerve (Schmidt, 1794)***; p. 284.
7. *posterior branch of external inguinal branch of lumbar plexus (Cruveilhier, 1836)*
For macrodissected adult human, dorsally directed branch of *external inguinal branch of lumbar plexus (Cruveilhier, 1836)*; in the original French, *rameau posterior*, p. 836.
8. *gluteal branch of external inguinal branch of lumbar plexus (Cruveilhier, 1836)*
Synonym for *posterior branch of external inguinal branch of lumbar plexus (Cruveilhier, 1836)*; in the original French, *rameau fessier*, p. 836.
9. *anterior branch of external inguinal branch of lumbar plexus (Cruveilhier, 1836)*
For macrodissected adult human, ventrally directed branch of *external inguinal branch of lumbar plexus (Cruveilhier, 1836)*; in the original French, *rameau antérieur*, p. 836. It in turn divides into external and internal ramifications; p. 836.
10. *cutaneous branch of external inguinal branch of lumbar plexus (Cruveilhier, 1836)*
Synonym for *anterior branch of external inguinal branch of lumbar plexus (Cruveilhier, 1836)*; in the original French, *rameau cutané*, p. 836.
11. *muscular branch of external musculo-cutaneous nerve (Quain & Wilson, 1839)*
For macrodissected adult human, branch of ***ilio-inguinal nerve (Schmidt, 1794)*** to internal oblique muscle; Plate XXI-c,*d*.

12. *muscular branch of superior musculo-cutaneous nerve (Quain & Wilson, 1839)*
    Synonym for *muscular branch of external musculo-cutaneous nerve (Quain & Wilson, 1839)*; Plate XXI-*c,d*.
13. *muscular branch of ilio-scrotal nerve (Quain & Wilson, 1839)*
    Synonym for *muscular branch of external musculo-cutaneous nerve (Quain & Wilson, 1839)*; Plate XXI-*c,d*.
14. *muscular branch of ilio-inguinal nerve (Quain & Wilson, 1839)*
    Synonym for *muscular branch of external musculo-cutaneous nerve (Quain & Wilson, 1839)*; Plate XXI-*c,d*.
15. *scrotal branch of external musculo-cutaneous nerve (Quain & Wilson, 1839)*
    Macrodissected adult human cutaneous branch of ***ilio-inguinal nerve (Schmidt, 1794)*** to internal oblique muscle; Plate XXI-*c,e*.
16. *scrotal branch of inferior musculo-cutaneous nerve (Quain & Wilson, 1839)*
    Synonym for *scrotal branch of external musculo-cutaneous nerve (Quain & Wilson, 1839)*; Plate XXI-*c,e*.
17. *scrotal branch of ilio-scrotal nerve (Quain & Wilson, 1839)*
    Synonym for *scrotal branch of external musculo-cutaneous nerve (Quain & Wilson, 1839)*; Plate XXI-*c,e*.
18. *scrotal branch of ilio-inguinal nerve (Quain & Wilson, 1839)*
    Synonym for *scrotal branch of external musculo-cutaneous nerve (Quain & Wilson, 1839)*; Plate XXI-*c,e*.

incisor nerve (>1840)

As described for macrodissected adult human, a common terminal branch of the ***inferior dental nerve (Meckel, 1817)*** forming an incisor ***plexus (Galen, c192)*** supplying the lower incisors and to some extent the canine tooth; see Starkie and Stewart (1931), Durward (1951, Fig. 899), Williams & Warwick (1980, p. 1067). Also see ***inferior dental plexus (>1840)***. It was perhaps first clearly described as the *incisor dental branch of inferior dental nerve (Cruveilhier, 1836)*.

EARLIER REFERENCES:

Earlier synonyms:

1. *incisor dental branch of inferior dental nerve (Cruveilhier, 1836)*
   Synonym for macrodissected adult human ***incisor nerve (>1840)***; in the original French, *rameau dentaire incisif du nerf dentaire inférieur*, p. 936; see Todd (1836–1839, p. 294).

indusium griseum (Valentin, 1841)

As described for macrodissected adult human, the tiny component of the ***hippocampal region (Swanson et al., 1987)*** extending between ***fasciola cinerea (Arnold, 1838b)*** caudally and ***tenia tecta (Swanson, 1992)*** rostrally, dorsal to the ***body of corpus callosum (Arnold, 1838a)*** and ventral to the ***sulcus of corpus callosum (>1840)***; see *Nomina Anatomica* (1983, p. A72), *Terminologia Anatomica* (1998, p. 127), Nieuwenhuys et al. (2008, Fig. 12.3). It is also known as the *supracallosal gyrus (>1840)* in human, and the ***indusium griseum (Valentin, 1841)*** in mammal generally. For Valentin's use in macrodissected adult human, see p. 244; also see Honegger (1890 p. 239). It was originally identified in print by Günz; see ***[indusium griseum (Valentin, 1841)] (Günz, 1750)***.

ALTERNATE SPELLINGS:

1. *induseum griseum (>1840)*
   Alternate (mis)spelling of ***indusium griseum (Valentin, 1841)***; see, for example, Brodmann (1909, Tab. 7, p. 247) and *Oxford Latin Dictionary* (1982, p. 889).

TRANSLATIONS:

1. *graue Schleier (Valentin, 1841)*
   Original German form of ***indusium griseum (Valentin, 1841)***; p. 244.

EARLIER REFERENCES:

Described, not named or illustrated:

1. ***[indusium griseum (Valentin, 1841)] (Günz, 1750)***
   Günz mentioned ***gray matter (Meckel, 1817)*** in what is now called ***indusium griseum (Valentin, 1841)*** of macrodissected adult human. Du Verney mentioned seeing it as early as 1729 in work not published until 1761; see Meyer (1971, p. 30), also see Vicq d'Azyr (1786, Pl. 4 legend).

Earlier synonyms:

1. *gray stria (Soemmerring, 1791)*
   Probably synonym for macrodissected adult human ***indusium griseum (Valentin, 1841)***; in the original German (plural), *grauliche Leisten*; p. 33.

LATER SYNONYMS:

1. *indusium griseum corporis callosi (Valentin, 1841)*
   Full term for ***indusium griseum (Valentin, 1841)***; in the original German, *graue Schleier des Balkens*, p. 244.
2. *gray stria of Lancisi (>1840)*
   Synonym for macrodissected adult human ***indusium griseum (Valentin, 1841)***; see Smith (1897), Crosby & Schnitzlein (1982, p. 493).
3. *supracallosal gyrus (>1840)*
   Synonym for macrodissected adult human ***indusium griseum (Valentin, 1841)***; see Williams & Warwick (1980, p. 998).

inferior branches of transverse nerve of neck (>1840)

As described for macrodissected adult human, they distribute to skin on the side and ventral part (front) of the neck, as caudal (low) as the sternum; see Williams & Warwick (1980, p. 1092), *Terminologia Anatomica* (1998, p. 137). They were perhaps first clearly described as the *inferior branch of subcutaneous nerve of neck (Meckel, 1753)*.

EARLIER REFERENCES:

Earlier synonyms:

1. *inferior branch of subcutaneous nerve of neck (Meckel, 1753)*
   Synonym for ***inferior branches of transverse nerve of neck (>1840)***; in the original French, *le rameau inférieur du nerf sous-cutané du cou*, p. 97.

2. *inferior cutaneous nerve of neck (Meckel, 1753)*
   Synonym for *inferior branch of subcutaneous nerve neck (Meckel, 1753)*; in the original French, *le cutané inférieur du cou*, Table 1-*286* and p. 97.
3. *inferior subcutaneous nerves of neck (Meckel, 1753)*
   Synonym for *inferior branch of subcutaneous nerve of neck (Meckel, 1753)*; in the original French, *les nerfs sous-cutané inférieurs du cou*, p. 94.
4. *interior branch of superficial nerve of neck (Bang, 1770)*
   Synonym for macrodissected adult human ***inferior branches of transverse nerve of neck (>1840)***; in the original Latin, *interior ramus*, Figure I-*45*. Probably typographical error for *inferior* ramus.
5. *lowest superficial branch of superficial nerve of neck (Bang, 1770)*
   Synonym for macrodissected adult human ***inferior branches of transverse nerve of neck (>1840)***; in the original Latin, *superficialis infimus ramus*, Figure I-*45*.
6. *middle and inferior cutaneous nerves of neck (Neubauer, 1772)*
   Synonym for macrodissected adult human ***inferior branches of transverse nerve of neck (>1840)***; in the original Latin, *nervum cutaneum medium colli* and *nervum cutaneum inferiorem colli*, Table 1-*171,187* and Table 1-*188*, Table 2-*31*, respectively.
7. *inferior branch of middle cutaneous nerve of neck (Peipers, 1793)*
   Roughly synonymous with ***inferior branches of transverse nerve of neck (>1840)***; in the original Latin, *ramus inferior subcutanei colli medii*, p. 34.
8. *descending branch of middle cutaneous nerve of neck (Peipers, 1793)*
   Synonym for ***inferior branches of transverse nerve of neck (>1840)***; in the original Latin, *ramus descendens subcutanei colli medii*, p. 34.
9. *middle and inferior subcutaneous cervical nerves (Meckel, 1817)*
   Synonym for ***inferior branches of transverse nerve of neck (>1840)***; in the original Latin, *nervi subcutanei colli medii et inferiores*, see translation (1832, Vol. 3, p. 32).
10. *descending branch of superficial cervical branch of cervical plexus (Cruveilhier, 1836)*
   Synonym for ***inferior branches of transverse nerve of neck (>1840)***; in the original French, *rameau descendant*, p. 782.

PARTLY CORRESPONDS:

1. *descending cutaneous nerve of neck (Peipers, 1793)*
   Macrodissected adult human ***inferior branch of transverse nerve of neck (>1840)*** near ventral (anterior) median plane; in the original Latin, *cutaneus colli descendens*, p. 34.
2. *inferior cutaneous nerves of neck (Peipers, 1793)*
   Several macrodissected adult human ***inferior branches of transverse nerve of neck (>1840)*** dorsal (posterior) to the ventral (anterior) median plane; in the original Latin, *cutaneus colli inferior*, p. 34.
3. *anterior superficial nerve of neck (Peipers, 1793)*
   Synonym for *descending cutaneous nerve of neck (Peipers, 1793)*; in the original Latin, *superficialis anterior*, p. 34.
4. *antilaryngeal cutaneous nerve of neck (Peipers, 1793)*
   Macrodissected adult human ***inferior branch of transverse nerve of neck (>1840)*** near ventral (anterior) median plane superficial to larynx; in the original Latin, *cutaneus antilaryngeus colli*, p. 34.
5. *cutaneous sublaryngeal nerve (Peipers, 1793)*
   Branch of *inferior branch of middle cutaneous nerve of neck (Peipers, 1793)* to skin caudal to (below) larynx; in the original Latin, *cutaneus sublaryngeus*, p. 34.

inferior cardiac nerve (Cloquet, 1816)

As described for macrodissected adult human, it usually consists of a variable number of small branches arising from the ***inferior cervical ganglion (Vieussens, 1684)*** or *cervicothoracic ganglion (>1840)*, and the ***ansa subclavia (>1840)***, extending caudally (descending) to the ***cardiac plexus (Keill, 1698)***; dorsal to (behind) the subclavian artery, it communicates with the ***recurrent laryngeal nerve (Albinus, 1744)*** and ***middle cardiac nerve (Cloquet, 1816)***; see Mitchell (1953, p. 250), Williams & Warwick (1980, p. 1129). For Cloquet's use in macrodissected adult human, see p. 696. It was illustrated first by Eustachi; see ***[inferior cardiac nerve (Cloquet, 1816)] (Eustachi, 1552)***.

TRANSLATIONS:

1. *nerf cardiaque inférieur (Cloquet, 1816)*
   Original French form of ***inferior cardiac nerve (Cloquet, 1816)***; p. 696.
2. *nervus cardiacus inferior (Meckel, 1817)*
   Original Latin form of ***inferior cardiac nerve (Cloquet, 1816)***; see translation (1832, Vol. 3, p. 95).

EARLIER REFERENCES:

Illustrated, not named or described:

1. ***[inferior cardiac nerve (Cloquet, 1816)] (Eustachi, 1552)***
   Illustrated for macrodissected adult human; see Albinus edition (1761, Tab. 18, Fig. 2-*x,y*), also see Haller (1762, p. 259 note *z*).

Described, not named or illustrated:

1. ***[inferior cardiac nerve (Cloquet, 1816)] (Winslow, 1733)***
   Described for macrodissected adult human; Section VI, no. 386, p. 96.

Earlier synonyms:

1. *major cardiac nerve (Neubauer, 1772)*
   Synonym for macrodissected adult human ***inferior cardiac nerve (Cloquet, 1816)***; in the original Latin, *nervum principem cardiacum*, Table 1-*68* and p. 169, where it is called a branch.
2. *nervos cervicales imos cardiacos (Haller, 1772)*
   Synonym for macrodissected adult human ***inferior cardiac nerve (Cloquet, 1816)***; p. 12.
3. *lowest cardiac nerve (Günther, 1786)*
   Synonym for macrodissected adult human ***inferior cardiac nerve (Cloquet, 1816)***; in the original Latin, *n. cordis infimi*, p. 93.

4. *smallest cardiac nerve (Chaussier, 1789)*
   Synonym for macrodissected adult human ***inferior cardiac nerve (Cloquet, 1816)***; in the original French, *le plus petit des nerfs cardiaques*, in *Table synoptique du nerf tri-splanchnic*.
5. *third cardiac nerve (Chaussier, 1789)*
   Synonym for macrodissected adult human ***inferior cardiac nerve (Cloquet, 1816)***; in the original French, *le troisième des nerfs cardiaques*, in *Table synoptique du nerf tri-splanchnic*.
6. *smaller cardiac nerve (Scarpa, 1794)*
   Synonym for macrodissected adult human ***inferior cardiac nerve (Cloquet, 1816)***; in the original Latin, *cardiacus nervus minor*, Table III-*112*; for English translation see Knox (1832, Pl. III-*152*). It is also translated *lesser cardiac nerve*.
7. *deep smaller cardiac nerves (Scarpa, 1794)*
   Synonym for macrodissected adult human ***inferior cardiac nerve (Cloquet, 1816)***; in the original Latin, *cardiaci nervi minores profundi*, Table III-*121*; for English translation see Knox (1832, Pl. III-*160*). It is also translated *deep lesser cardiac nerves*.
8. *superficial aortic cardiac nerve (Fyfe, 1800)*
   Synonym for macrodissected adult human right ***inferior cardiac nerve (Cloquet, 1816)***; in the original Latin, *cardiacus aortae superficialis*, Vol. 2. p. 317. Cloquet (1816, p. 699) attributed the term without citation to Scarpa.

inferior caroticotympanic nerve (>1840)

As described for macrodissected adult human, one of the two ***caroticotympanic nerves (>1840)*** extending from the ***internal carotid plexus (>1840)***; see Durward (1951, Figs. 901, 905), Williams & Warwick (1980, p. 1200, Fig. 7.184). Jacobson first described it; see ***[inferior caroticotympanic nerve (>1840)] (Jacobson, 1818)***.

EARLIER REFERENCES:

Described, not named or illustrated:

1. ***[inferior caroticotympanic nerve (>1840)] (Jacobson, 1818)***
   Clearly described for macrodissected adult human; see Lobstein translation (1831, p. 36).

inferior cerebellar peduncle (Günther, 1786)

As described for macrodissected adult human and other mammal, a caudal longitudinal extension of the ***arbor vitae (Winslow, 1733)*** along the dorsolateral surface of the ***medulla (Winslow, 1733)***. In macrodissected adult human, numerous ***central nervous system white matter tracts (>1840)*** merge with it; four of the more prominent include ***ventral external arcuate fibers (>1840)***, ***olivocerebellar tract (>1840)***, ***medullary striae (Scarpa, 1788)***, and ***dorsal spinocerebellar tract (1840)***; see Williams & Warwick (1980, pp. 916–917). For Günther's use in macrodissected adult human, see p. 23. It was first identified as the *lower tract of cerebellum (Vesalius, 1543a)*.

TRANSLATIONS:

1. *pedunculi cerebelli inferiores (Günther, 1786)*
   Original Latin form (plural) of ***inferior cerebellar peduncle (Günther, 1786)***; p. 23.

EARLIER REFERENCES:

Earlier synonyms:

1. *lower tract of cerebellum (Vesalius, 1543a)*
   Vesalius described vaguely, and illustrated, macrodissected adult human ***inferior cerebellar peduncle (Günther, 1786)***; see Singer translation (1952, p. 21 and Fig. 9-*F*,*G*).
2. *posterior cerebellar process (Willis, 1664)*
   Synonym for macrodissected adult human ***inferior cerebellar peduncle (Günther, 1786)***; see Pordage translation (1681, p. 113).
3. *processus medullares à cerebello ad medullam spinalem (Vieussens, 1684)*
   Latin synonym for macrodissected adult human ***inferior cerebellar peduncle (Günther, 1786)***; Table XIII-S. Soemmerring (1778, p. 178) gave *processus cerebelli ad medullam spinalem*.
4. *chordal process of cerebellum (Ridley, 1695)*
   Synonym for macrodissected adult human ***inferior cerebellar peduncle (Günther, 1786)***; p. 136. Derived from Willis's statement (1664; see Pordage translation, 1681, p. 68) that *posterior cerebellar process (Willis, 1664)* seems to add *cord* or *string* to ***medulla (Winslow, 1733)***; see Ridley (1695, Fig. VI-*f*).
5. *third process of cerebellum (Ridley, 1695)*
   Synonym for macrodissected adult human ***inferior cerebellar peduncle (Günther, 1786)***; Figure VI-*f*.
6. *processus ad medullam spinalem (Pourfour du Petit, 1710)*
   Abbreviated form of macrodissected adult human *processus medullares à cerebello ad medullam spinalem (Vieussens, 1684)*; p. 14.
7. *pedunculi cerebelli rami posteriores medullae oblongatae (Winslow, 1732)*
   Synonym for macrodissected adult human right and left ***inferior cerebellar peduncle (Günther, 1786)***; Section IV, pp. 170–172; see Burdach (1822, p. 288).
8. *crura posteriora medullae oblongatae (Winslow, 1733)*
   Synonym for macrodissected adult human right and left ***inferior cerebellar peduncle (Günther, 1786)***; Section X, p. 41.
9. *cerebellar peduncle (Winslow, 1733)*
   Synonym specifically for macrodissected adult human ***inferior cerebellar peduncle (Günther, 1786)***; Section X, pp. 41, 42. See *pedunculi cerebelli rami posteriores medullae oblongatae (Winslow, 1732)*.
10. *partes truncorum medullae cerebelli quae pertinent ad partem posteriorem medullae oblongatae (Albinus, 1744)*
    Synonym for macrodissected adult human ***inferior cerebellar peduncle (Günther, 1786)*** in Albinus's edition of the Eustachian plates; Table 17, Figure 2-*F*. Also see Burdach (1822, p. 288).

11. *restiform process (Tarin, 1750)*
Tarin's translation of *chordal process of cerebellum (Ridley, 1695)*, which was in English originally; in the original Latin, *restiformes processus*, p. 31. Also see Meckel (1753, p. 70).
12. *crurum medullae oblongatae cerebelli (Neubauer, 1772)*
Synonym for macrodissected adult human ***inferior cerebellar peduncle (Günther, 1786)***; p. 19.
13. *descending part of cerebellar brachia (Malacarne, 1776)*
Synonym for macrodissected adult human ***inferior cerebellar peduncle (Günther, 1786)***; in the original Italian, *le porzioni discendenti delle braccia del cervelletto*, p. 81. Burdach (1822, p. 324) gave the Latin, *portio adscendens brachiorum cerebelli.*
14. *posterior cerebellar crus (Mayer, 1779)*
Synonym for macrodissected adult human ***inferior cerebellar peduncle (Günther, 1786)***; in the original Latin, *crura cerebelli postica*, p. 19.
15. *crurum cerebelli ad medullam oblongatam (Haase, 1781)*
Variation on macrodissected adult human *processus medullares à cerebello ad medullam spinalem (Vieussens, 1684)*; p. 28. Arnold (1834, Tab. VI-*xx*) used *crus cerebelli ad medullam oblongatam.*
16. *peduncle of medulla oblongata (Vicq d'Azyr, 1784)*
Synonym for macrodissected adult human ***inferior cerebellar peduncle (Günther, 1786)***; p. 590 and Vicq d'Azyr (1786, Pls. XVII, Fig. I-*48/49*; XVIII:*55-x*).
17. *column of medulla oblongata (Vicq d'Azyr, 1784)*
Synonym for macrodissected adult human ***inferior cerebellar peduncle (Günther, 1786)***; p. 590, and Vicq d'Azyr (1786, Pl. XXX, Fig. I-*14*).

LATER SYNONYMS:

1. *processus á cerebello ad medullam oblongatum (Vicq d'Azyr, 1786)*
Variation on macrodissected adult human *processus medullares à cerebello ad medullam spinalem (Vieussens, 1684)*; p. 94, where Vicq d'Azyr attributed without citation the term to Haller, as did Gall & Spurzheim (1810, p. 180).
2. *inferior cerebellar process (Günther, 1786)*
Synonym for macrodissected adult human ***inferior cerebellar peduncle (Günther, 1786)***; in the original Latin, *processus cerebelli posteriores*, p. 19, see Burdach (1822, p. 288).
3. *restiform body (Günther, 1786)*
Synonym for macrodissected adult human ***inferior cerebellar peduncle (Günther, 1786)***; in the original Latin (plural), *corpora restiformia*, p. 23.
4. *anterior and lateral pyramid of Tarin (Günther, 1786)*
According to Günther, eponym for macrodissected adult human *restiform body (Günther, 1786)*, which is probably not entirely accurate; in the original Latin, *pyramidalia anteriora & lateralia Tarino*, p. 23. See *lateral pyramidal body (Tarin, 1750)* and *anterior pyramidal body (Tarin, 1750, Tab. I).*
5. *posterior cerebellar peduncle (Günther, 1786)*
Synonym for macrodissected adult human ***inferior cerebellar peduncle (Günther, 1786)***; in the original Latin (plural), *pedunculi cerebelli posteriores*; p. 23.
6. *pedunculus ad medullam spinalem (Soemmerring, 1791)*
Synonym for macrodissected adult human ***inferior cerebellar peduncle (Günther, 1786)***; p. 55.
7. *crus ad medullam spinalem (Soemmerring, 1791)*
Synonym for macrodissected adult human ***inferior cerebellar peduncle (Günther, 1786)***; p. 55.
8. *third cerebellar peduncle (Procháska, 1800)*
Synonym for macrodissected adult human ***inferior cerebellar peduncle (Günther, 1786)***; in the original Latin (plural), *pedunculi cerebelli tertii*; Vol. I, p. 387.
9. *posterior pyramidal body of medulla oblongata (Procháska, 1800)*
Synonym for macrodissected adult human ***inferior cerebellar peduncle (Günther, 1786)***; in the original Latin (plural), *corpora pyramidalia postica medullae oblongata*; Vol. I, p. 387.
10. *inferior prolongation of cerebellum (Burdin, 1803)*
Synonym for macrodissected adult human ***inferior cerebellar peduncle (Günther, 1786)***; see translation (1803, Vol. 3, p. 165).
11. *inferior column of cerebellum (Chaussier, 1807)*
Synonym for macrodissected adult human ***inferior cerebellar peduncle (Günther, 1786)***; in the original French (plural), *colonnes inférieures du cervelet*, p. 125.
12. *eminentiae posteriores bulbi rachidici (Chaussier, 1807)*
Synonym for macrodissected adult human right and left ***inferior cerebellar peduncle (Günther, 1786)***; p. 120.
13. *brachium of medulla oblongata (Reil, 1807–1808a)*
Synonym for macrodissected adult human ***inferior cerebellar peduncle (Günther, 1786)***, an obvious variation on *peduncle of medulla oblongata (Vicq d'Azyr, 1784)*; in the original German, *Arme zum Rückenmark*, see Mayo translation (1822, p. 24).
14. *faisceau primitif du cervelet (Gall & Spurzheim, 1810)*
Synonym for macrodissected adult human ***inferior cerebellar peduncle (Günther, 1786)***; pp. 184, 255, 262. See Burdach (1822, p. 288).
15. *pedunculi chordae spinalis (Gordon, 1815)*
Synonym for macrodissected adult human right and left ***inferior cerebellar peduncle (Günther, 1786)***; p. 178.
16. *restiform fasciculus (Tiedemann, 1816)*
Synonym for *restiform body (Reil, 1807–1808a)* in macrodissected, alcohol-hardened human fetus; see translation (1826, p. 143).
17. *cerebellar fasciculus (Tiedemann, 1816)*
Synonym for *restiform fasciculus (Tiedemann, 1816)*; spelled *cerebellic fasciculus* in translation (1826, p. 148).
18. *crus of cerebellum (Meckel, 1817)*
Synonym for macrodissected adult human ***inferior cerebellar peduncle (Günther, 1786)***; see translation (1832, Vol. 2, p. 422).
19. *eminentia pyramidalis lateralis Tarin (Meckel, 1817)*
Eponym listed for macrodissected adult human ***inferior cerebellar peduncle (Günther, 1786)***; see translation (1832, Vol. 2, p. 422).
20. *inferior descending prolongation of cerebellum (Meckel, 1817)*

Synonym listed for macrodissected adult human ***inferior cerebellar peduncle (Günther, 1786)***; see translation (1832, Vol. 2, p. 434).

21. *posterior prolongations of cerebellum (Meckel, 1817)*
Synonym for macrodissected adult human right and left ***inferior cerebellar peduncle (Günther, 1786)***; see translation (1832, Vol. 3, p. 45).
22. *spinal prolongation of cerebellum (Meckel, 1817)*
Synonym for macrodissected adult human ***inferior cerebellar peduncle (Günther, 1786)***; see translation (1832, Vol. 3, p. 52).
23. *rachidian prolongation of cerebellum (Meckel, 1817)*
Synonym for macrodissected adult human ***inferior cerebellar peduncle (Günther, 1786)***; see translation (1832, Vol. 3, p. 52).
24. *descending cerebellar crus (Meckel, 1817)*
Synonym for macrodissected adult human ***inferior cerebellar peduncle (Günther, 1786)***; in the original Latin (plural), *crura cerebelli descendentia*; see translation (1832, Vol. 3, p. 446).
25. *crus medullae posticum ad cerebellum ascendens (Tiedemann, 1821)*
Synonym for macrodissected adult monkey ***inferior cerebellar peduncle (Günther, 1786)***; Table I, Figure 6-*h*.
26. *posterior cord of spinal medulla (Rolando, 1825a)*
Synonym for macrodissected adult human ***inferior cerebellar peduncle (Günther, 1786)***; in the original French (plural), *cordons postérieurs de la moelle épinière*, Table I, Figure 1-*p.i*.
27. *inferior pedicle of cerebellum (Mayo, 1827)*
Synonym for macrodissected adult human ***inferior cerebellar peduncle (Günther, 1786)***; Plate IV-*a*.
28. *peduncle of spinal marrow (Meckel, 1832)*
English form (singular) of *pedunculi chordae spinalis (Gordon, 1815)*; Vol. 2, p. 422.
29. *posterior pyramidal bodies (Bell, 1834)*
Synonym for macrodissected adult human right and left ***inferior cerebellar peduncle (Günther, 1786)***; p. 476, note.
30. *processus cerebelli ad medullam (Cruveilhier, 1836)*
Synonym for macrodissected adult human ***inferior cerebellar peduncle (Günther, 1786)***; p. 633.
31. *restiform eminence (Arnold, 1838a)*
Synonym for macrodissected adult human ***inferior cerebellar peduncle (Günther, 1786)***; in the original Latin (plural), *eminentiae restiformia*, p. 17.

inferior cervical cardiac branches of vagus nerve (>1840)

As described for macrodissected adult human, 1–3 thin branches leaving the ***vagus nerve trunk (Wrisberg, 1786; Günther, 1786)*** in the caudal (lower) half of the neck and soon thereafter communicating with and/or joining the ***superior cardiac nerve (Neubauer, 1772)*** to reach eventually the ***cardiac plexus (Keill, 1698)***; see Durward (1951, Fig. 907-*Ca*[2]), Mitchell (1953, p. 181, called *middle group*), *Terminologia Anatomica* (1998, p. 136). They were perhaps first clearly delineated by Andersch (c1751–c1755); see Haller (1772).

EARLIER REFERENCES:

Illustrated and described, not named:

1. ***[inferior cervical cardiac branches of vagus nerve (>1840)] (Haller, 1772)***
Haller reproduced and provided explanatory text to accompany labeling of a plate prepared by Andersch for his thesis, conducted c1751–c1755 but not available publicly until Soemmerring & Andersch (1792), Andersch (1797). The ***inferior cervical cardiac branches of vagus nerve (>1840)*** were clearly illustrated for macrodissected adult human; see features labeled *9,10*. Also see Scarpa (1794; Tab. III-*3* and IV-*72*), where Andersch was cited.

inferior cervical ganglion (Vieussens, 1684)

As described for macrodissected adult human, the most caudal of the 3 ***cervical sympathetic ganglia (>1840)***, which is followed by the ***superior thoracic ganglion (Lieutaud, 1742)***. In about three-quarters of individuals the 2 ***ganglia (Galen, c173)*** are fused and called the *cervicothoracic ganglion (>1840)*; see Mitchell (1953, p. 227), Williams & Warwick (1980, p. 1129). For Vieussens's discovery and use in macrodissected adult human see Table XXIII-∇.

LATER SYNONYMS:

1. *plexus ganglioformis cervicalis inferior nervis intercostalis (Vieussens, 1684)*
Original long form of Latin term Vieussens used for ***inferior cervical ganglion (Vieussens, 1684)***; Table XXIII-∇ (in English, "inferior cervical ganglionic infolding of intercostal nerve"). Palfijn (1726, Part 2, p. 344) gave the French, *plexus ganglioforme cervical inférieur du nerf intercostal*.
2. *ganglion cervicale infimum (Winslow, 1733)*
Synonym for macrodissected adult human ***inferior cervical ganglion (Vieussens, 1684)***; Section VI, p. 96.
3. *lowest cervical ganglion (Winslow, 1733)*
English form of *ganglion cervicale infimum (Winslow, 1733)*; Section VI, p. 96.
4. *ganglion cervicale imum (Haller, 1762)*
Variation on *ganglion cervicale infimum (Winslow, 1733)*; p. 259, see Scarpa (1794, Tab. III-*100*).
5. *ganglion magnum cervicale imum (Haller, 1772)*
Apparently synonym for macrodissected adult human *ganglion cervicale imum (Haller, 1762)*; p. 9 note *84*.
6. *ganglion thoracicum supernum (Haller, 1772)*
Apparently synonym for macrodissected adult human *superior thoracic ganglion (Neubauer, 1772)*; p. 9 note *84*.
7. *ganglion ultimum cervicis (Neubauer, 1772)*
Synonym for macrodissected adult human ***inferior cervical ganglion (Vieussens, 1684)***; p. 117.
8. *superior thoracic ganglion (Neubauer, 1772)*
Unfortunate synonym for macrodissected adult human ***inferior cervical ganglion (Vieussens, 1684)***; in the original Latin, *ganglion thoracicum superius*, Table I-*60*, as pointed out by Scarpa (1794, Tab. III-*100*).

9. *great thoracic ganglion (Neubauer, 1772)*
Synonym for *superior thoracic ganglion (Neubauer, 1772)*; in the original Latin, *ganglion thoracicum magnum*, pp. 174–175.
10. *first dorsal ganglion (Neubauer, 1772)*
Synonym for *superior thoracic ganglion (Neubauer, 1772)*; in the original Latin, *ganglion dorsale primum*, Table I-60.
11. *great dorsal ganglion (Neubauer, 1772)*
Synonym for *superior thoracic ganglion (Neubauer, 1772)*; in the original Latin, *ganglion dorsale magnum*, Table I-60.
12. *thyroid ganglion (Haase, 1781)*
Synonym listed for macrodissected adult human ***inferior cervical ganglion (Vieussens, 1684)***; in the original Latin, *ganglion thyreoideum*, p. 120.
13. *third cervical ganglion (Günther, 1786)*
Günther's preferred term for macrodissected adult human ***inferior cervical ganglion (Vieussens, 1684)***; in the original Latin, *ganglion cervicale tertium*, p. 93.
14. *ganglion ultimum thyreoideum (Soemmerring, 1791)*
Synonym listed for macrodissected adult human ***inferior cervical ganglion (Vieussens, 1684)***; p. 321.
15. *cardiac ganglion (Soemmerring, 1791)*
Synonym for macrodissected adult human ***inferior cervical ganglion (Vieussens, 1684)***; in the original Latin, *ganglion cardiacum*, p. 321.
16. *lower cervical ganglion (Bell, 1803b)*
Variation on macrodissected adult human *lowest cervical ganglion (Winslow, 1733)*; p. 176.
17. *third cardiac ganglion (Bock, 1817)*
Synonym listed for macrodissected adult human ***inferior cervical ganglion (Vieussens, 1684)***; in the original Latin, *ganglion cardiacum tertium*, p. 71.
18. *stellate ganglion (Bock, 1817)*
Synonym listed for macrodissected adult human ***inferior cervical ganglion (Vieussens, 1684)***; in the original Latin, *ganglion stellatum*, p. 71.

inferior clunial nerves (>1840)

As described for macrodissected adult human, branches (usually 3 or 4) of the ***posterior cutaneous nerve of thigh (Günther, 1786)*** innervating skin over caudal (lower) and lateral parts of the gluteus maximus muscle; see Durward (1951, Figs. 941, 947), Williams & Warwick (1980, p. 1111, where they are referred to as *gluteal branches of posterior femoral cutaneous nerve*), *Terminologia Anatomica* (1998, p. 140). They were known to Vesalius; see ***[inferior clunial nerves (>1840)] (Vesalius, 1543a)***.

EARLIER REFERENCES:

Illustrated and described, not named:

1. ***[inferior clunial nerves (>1840)] (Vesalius, 1543a)***
Identified for macrodissected adult human; see Richardson & Carman translation (2002, p. 259).

Earlier synonyms:

1. *superior posterior cutaneous nerve (Fischer, 1791)*
Apparently synonym for macrodissected adult human ***inferior clunial nerves (>1840)***; in the original Latin, *nervum cutaneum posteriorem superiorem*, p. 28. In Table IV (Fig. 2-4,25,44,64) Fischer carefully documented four lateral branches.
2. *inferior gluteal cutaneous nerve (Fischer, 1791)*
Apparently synonym for macrodissected adult human ***inferior clunial nerves (>1840)***; in the original Latin, *nervum cutaneum gluteum inferiorem*, p. 28. Fischer there described in great detail five twigs from main ***nerve (Herophilus, c335–c280 BC)***.
3. *inferior gluteal branches of lesser sciatic nerve (Quain, 1828)*
Probably synonym for macrodissected adult human ***inferior clunial nerves (>1840)***; p. 291.
4. *posterior superior cutaneous nerve (Knox, 1832)*
Knox's translation of *superior posterior cutaneous nerve (Fischer, 1791)*; Plate XIV-73.
5. *external branch of recurrent branch of cutaneous branch of inferior gluteal nerve (Cruveilhier, 1836)*
Synonym for macrodissected adult human ***inferior clunial nerves (>1840)***; in the original French, *rameau externe*, p. 858.
6. *posterior and internal cutaneous nerve (Quain & Wilson, 1839)*
Basically synonym for macrodissected adult human ***inferior clunial nerves (>1840)***; Plate XXII-g.

inferior colliculus (Haller, 1762)

As described for adult mammal with gross dissection, and with cellular architecture and connections, a ***gray matter region (Swanson & Bota, 2010)*** in the caudal part of the right and left ***tectum (Baer, 1837)*** separated by the transverse arm of the ***cruciform sulcus (>1840)*** from the rostral part, the right and left ***superior colliculus (Haller, 1762)***; see Nieuwenhuys et al. (2008, p. 206 and Fig. 3.10). For Haller's original Latin term in macrodissected adult human, see p. 64 (*inferius par colliculorum*). It was first described (plural) as the *little buttocks (Galen, c173, definition 2)*.

EARLIER REFERENCES:

Earlier synonyms:

1. *little buttocks (Galen, c173, definition 2)*
Synonym in *On the Usefulness of the Parts* for ***inferior colliculi (Haller, 1762)*** of macrodissected adult beef, pig, and/or macaque but not human; see May translation (1968, p. 420). Also see *little buttocks (Galen, c173, definition 1)*.
2. *gloutia (Galen, c173, definition 2)*
Greek form of *little buttocks (Galen, c173, definition 2)*; see May translation (1968, p. 420). Singer (1999, p. 236) used *glouta* in his translation.
3. *buttocks (Galen, c173, definition 2)*
Alternate translation for *little buttocks (Galen, c173, definition 2)*; see Singer translation (1999, p. 236).
4. *nates (Galen, c173, definition 2)*
Alternate translation for *buttocks (Galen, c173, definition 2)*; see Singer translation (1999, p. 236).
5. *gloution (Vesalius, 1543a)*
Singular form of *gloutia (Galen, c173, definition 2)*, synonym for ***inferior colliculus (Haller, 1762)***; see Singer translation (1952, p. 47).

6. *natulae (Vesalius, 1543a)*
Singer's translation (1952, p. 47) of Vesalius's reference to *nates (Galen, c173, definition 2).*
7. *clunes (Vesalius, 1543a)*
Singer's translation (1952, p. 47) of Vesalius's reference to *nates (Galen, c173, definition 2).*
8. *eminentias inferiores (Guidi, 1611)*
Synonym for macrodissected adult human ***inferior colliculi (Haller, 1762)***; see Burdach (1822, p. 334).
9. *testicles (Crooke, 1615)*
Crooke referred to *buttocks (Galen, c173, definition 2)*, or ***inferior colliculi (Haller, 1762)***, as *testicles* (pp. 431–432), as well as *buttocks* (Tab. XII, Fig. 10-*F,G*), and discussed the nomenclature confusion (p. 468). Crooke's text was a rough translation of Bauhin (1605).
10. *testes (Willis, 1664)*
Synonym for macrodissected adult mammalian ***inferior colliculi (Haller, 1762)***; see Pordage translation (1681, p. 64, Figs. III, IV); simply alternate form of *testicles (Crooke, 1615).*
11. *stones of brain (Willis, 1664)*
Slang version of *testes (Willis, 1664)*; see Pordage translation (1681, p. 57).
12. *lesser protuberances (Willis, 1664)*
Synonym for macrodissected adult human ***inferior colliculi (Haller, 1762)***; see Pordage translation (1681, Fig. III-*H*).
13. *lesser orbicular protuberances (Willis, 1664)*
Synonym for macrodissected adult human ***inferior colliculi (Haller, 1762)***; see Pordage translation (1681, Figs. III-*H*, VII-*P*, VIII-*L*).
14. *head of anterior cerebellar process (Willis, 1664)*
Synonym for *testes (Willis, 1664)*; see Pordage translation (1681, p. 108). *Anterior cerebellar process (Willis, 1664)* is synonym for ***superior cerebellar peduncle (Procháska, 1800)***.
15. *corpora in turbinem acuminata (Vieussens, 1684)*
Latin synonym for macrodissected adult human ***inferior colliculi Haller, 1762)***; Table VIII-*H*.
16. *orbicular processes of cerebellum (Collins, 1685)*
Synonym for *lesser orbicular protuberances (Willis, 1664)*; p. 1010.
17. *testiforme process (Ridley, 1695)*
Synonym for macrodissected adult human ***inferior colliculus (Haller, 1762)***; p. 128, Figure VII-*d*.
18. *posterior tubercle (Winslow, 1733)*
Synonym for macrodissected adult human ***inferior colliculus (Haller, 1762)***; Section X, p. 37.
19. *corpora quadrigemina posteriora (Soemmerring, 1778)*
Synonym for macrodissected adult human ***inferior colliculi (Haller, 1762)***; Table III-*x*.
20. *inferior quadrigeminal tubercle (Vicq d'Azyr, 1786)*
Synonym for macrodissected adult human ***inferior colliculus (Haller, 1762)***; Plate VIII, Figure I-*21*, p. 23. Reil (1809c; see Mayo translation, 1823, p. 95) described it as "a gray and vascular prominence" where part of ***lateral lemniscus (Bechterew, 1885b)*** ends.
21. *inferior quadrigeminal eminences (Günther, 1786)*
Synonym for macrodissected adult human ***inferior colliculi (Haller, 1762)***; in the original Latin, *eminentia quadrigemina inferioribus*, p. 14.
22. *inferior midbrain tubercles (Chaussier, 1807)*
Synonym for macrodissected adult human ***inferior colliculi (Haller, 1762)***; in the original French, *les tubercules inférieurs du mésocéphale*, pp. 110–111.
23. *inferior quadrigeminal body (Wenzel & Wenzel, 1812)*
Synonym for macrodissected adult human ***inferior colliculi (Haller, 1762)***; in the original Latin (plural), *inferiora corpora quadrigemina*, Table I, Figure 4-*h*.
24. *gray nucleus of globular portions of cerebral nucleus (Reil, 1812c)*
Synonym for macrodissected adult human ***inferior colliculus (Haller, 1762)***; see Mayo translation (1823, p. 123, Tab. XI-*i,w*).
25. *gray nucleus (Reil, 1812c)*
Shortened form of *gray nucleus of globular portions of cerebral nucleus (Reil, 1812c)*. Arnold (1838, Tab. II, Fig. 9-*g*) gave the Latin (plural), *nuclei cinerei.*
26. *posterior eminence (Ramsay, 1813)*
Synonym listed for macrodissected adult human ***inferior colliculi (Haller, 1762)***; p. 46.
27. *lower corpora bigeminum (Gordon, 1815)*
Synonym for macrodissected adult human ***inferior colliculi (Haller, 1762)***; p. 91. Mayo (1827, Pl. IV, p. 10) supplied the Latin, *corpora bigeminum inferius.*
28. *posterior quadrigeminal bodies (Tiedemann, 1821)*
Synonym for macrodissected adult monkey ***inferior colliculi (Haller, 1762)***; in the original Latin, *corpora quadrigemina postica*, Table II, Figure 2-*h*.
29. *natiform eminences (Rolando, 1825a)*
Synonym for macrodissected adult beef ***inferior colliculi (Haller, 1762)***; in the original French, *éminences nates*; see Table VIII, Figure 5-*n*, where they are shown in transverse section.
30. *inferior bigeminal prominences (Rolando, 1831)*
Synonym for macrodissected adult human ***inferior colliculi (Haller, 1762)***; in the original Italian, *prominenze bigemine inferiori*; Figure 9-*1*.
31. *testiform eminences (Cruveilhier, 1836)*
Synonym for macrodissected adult human ***inferior colliculi (Haller, 1762)***; in the original French, *eminentiae testiformes*, p. 608.
32. *posterior bigeminal bodies (Owen, 1837)*
Synonym for macrodissected adult marsupial ***inferior colliculi (Haller, 1762)***; Plate VI-*6*.

inferior colliculus commissure (>1840)

As described for macrodissected adult human, and mammal generally with histological methods for ***axons (Kölliker, 1896)***, a short transverse ***central nervous system white matter tract (>1840)*** crossing the median plane between right and left ***inferior colliculus (Haller, 1762)***; see Mettler (1948, p. 316 and Fig. 248), Crosby et al. (1962, p. 226 and Figs. 172, 174), Swanson (2004,

Atlas Levels 46–48), Nieuwenhuys et al. (2008, Fig. 6.17). It was first described clearly as the *commissure of inferior quadrigeminal tubercles (Rolando, 1825a)*.

EARLIER REFERENCES:

Earlier synonyms:

1. *commissure of inferior quadrigeminal tubercles (Rolando, 1825a)*
   Synonym for ***inferior colliculus commissure (>1840)***, clearly illustrated in transverse section and described for macrodissected adult beef, and also described for human and various other mammals; Table VIII, Figure 6-*y*; also see Table VII, Figure 1-*n* (mislabeled *t* in drawing).

inferior dental branches of inferior dental plexus (>1840)

As described for macrodissected adult human, branches of the ***inferior dental plexus (>1840)*** to the inferior (lower or ventral) molar and premolar teeth; see Starkie and Stewart (1931), Durward (1951, p. 1028), Williams & Warwick (1980, p. 1067), *Terminologia Anatomica* (1998, p. 135). They were known to Galen; see ***[inferior dental branches of inferior dental plexus (>1840)] (Galen, c173)***.

EARLIER REFERENCES:

Described, not named or illustrated:

1. ***[inferior dental branches of inferior dental plexus (>1840)] (Galen, c173)***
   Alluded to for macrodissected adult beef, pig, and/or macaque but not human; see May translation (1968, p. 455).

Illustrated, not named or described:

1. ***[inferior dental branches of inferior dental plexus (>1840)] (Pietro da Cortona, c1618)***
   Clearly illustrated for macrodissected adult human; see first printing (1741) of the plates: Tables 7, Figure 1-*F*; 10, Figure 1-*B*; 13, Figure 1-*E*. Also see Meckel (1748, p. 89 note z).

Illustrated and described, not named:

1. ***[inferior dental branches of inferior dental plexus] (>1840)] (Vieussens, 1684)***
   Vieussens (p. 173, Tab. 22-7) referred to them in macrodissected adult human, as did Meckel (1817; see translation, 1832, Vol. 3, p. 74), attributing them to branch of ***inferior dental nerve (Meckel, 1817)***, the *dentar nerve (Meckel, 1817)*, an uncommon variant of the normal innervation pattern; see Starkie and Stewart (1931).

Earlier synonyms:

1. *dental branches of inferior maxillary branch (Loder, 1778)*
   Synonym for macrodissected adult human ***inferior dental branches of inferior dental plexus (>1840)***; in the original Latin, *dentales ramos*, p. 19.
2. *inferior dental branches of inferior maxillary nerve proper (Günther, 1786)*
   Synonym for macrodissected adult human ***inferior dental branches of inferior dental plexus (>1840)***; in the original Latin, *R. dentales inferiores*, p. 52.
3. *dental branches of maxillodental nerve (Chaussier, 1809)*
   Synonym for macrodissected adult human ***inferior dental branches of inferior dental plexus (>1840)***.
4. *dental branches of dental nerve (Arnold, 1834)*
   Synonym for macrodissected adult human ***inferior dental branches of inferior dental plexus (>1840)***; in the original Latin, *nervus dentalis, rami dentales*, p. 10.
5. *dental branches of dental nerve anastomosis (Arnold, 1834)*
   Synonym for macrodissected adult human ***inferior dental branches of inferior dental plexus (>1840)***; in the original Latin, *anastomosis nervorum dentalium rami dentales*, Table VIII-36,37.

PARTLY CORRESPONDS:

1. *posterior inferior dental branch of inferior maxillary nerve proper (Günther, 1786)*
   Macrodissected adult human caudal (posterior) branch of ***inferior dental branches of inferior dental plexus (>1840)***; in the original Latin, *R. dentales inferiores posteriores*, p. 52.
2. *anterior inferior dental branch of inferior maxillary nerve proper (Günther, 1786)*
   Macrodissected adult human rostral (anterior) branch of ***inferior dental branches of inferior dental plexus (>1840)***; in the original Latin, *R. dentales inferiores anteriorem*, p. 52.

inferior dental nerve (Meckel, 1817)

As described for macrodissected adult human, a branch of the ***posterior branch of mandibular nerve (>1840)*** most commonly giving off the ***mylohyoid nerve (Meckel, 1748)***, contributing to the ***inferior dental plexus (>1840)***, and generating two terminal differentiations, the ***incisor plexus (>1840)*** and ***mental nerve (Cheselden, 1726)***; see Starkie & Stewart (1931), Durward (1951, Fig. 899), Williams & Warwick (1980, p. 1067). For Meckel's use in macrodissected adult human, see translation (1832, Vol. 3, pp. 73–74). It was known to Galen; see ***[inferior dental nerve (Meckel, 1817)] (Galen, c173)***.

ALTERNATE SPELLINGS:

1. *inferior dentar nerve (Meckel, 1832)*
   Alternate form of ***inferior dental nerve (Meckel, 1817)***; Vol. 3, p. 73.

EARLIER REFERENCES:

Described, not named or illustrated:

1. ***[inferior dental nerve (Meckel, 1817)] (Galen, c173)***
   Described for macrodissected adult beef, pig, and/or macaque but not human; see May translation (1968, p. 454), Duckworth translation (1962, pp. 193, 195).

Earlier synonyms:

1. *fourth nerve of third pair of nerves arising from brain (Falloppio, 1561)*
   Roughly synonymous with macrodissected adult human ***inferior dental nerve (Meckel, 1817)*** according to Bauhin (1605); see Crooke translation (1615, p. 891).
2. *third branch of fourth conjugation of nerves of brain (Crooke, 1615)*
   Roughly synonymous with macrodissected adult human ***inferior dental nerve (Meckel, 1817)***; pp. 486– 487. Crooke's description is a translation of Bauhin (1605).
3. *secunda ac media propago rami majoris posterioris (Vieussens, 1684)*

Synonym for macrodissected adult human ***inferior dental nerve (Meckel, 1817)***; p. 173 and Table 22-5.

4. *inferior maxillary branch (Meckel, 1748)*
Synonym for macrodissected adult human ***inferior dental nerve (Meckel, 1817)***, branch of *inferior third branch of fifth pair (Meckel, 1748)*; in the original Latin, *ramus maxillaris inferior*, pp. 86–89, Figure 1-69.
5. *inferior maxillary nerve (Meckel, 1748)*
Synonym for macrodissected adult human ***inferior dental nerve (Meckel, 1817)***; in the original Latin, *nervo maxillari inferiori*, p. 92.
6. *inferior maxillary nerve proper (Schaarschmidt, 1750)*
Synonym for macrodissected adult human ***inferior dental nerve (Meckel, 1817)***; in the original Latin, *nervus maxillae inferiori proprius*, p. 28. Also see Monro (1783, Tab. 25-C).
7. *mandibulo-labial nerve (Soemmerring, 1798)*
Synonym for macrodissected adult human ***inferior dental nerve (Meckel, 1817)***; in the original Latin, *nervus mandibulo labialis*, p. 233. Bell (1803b, p. 145) spelled it, *mundibulo labrialis*.
8. *maxillo-dentary nerve (Burdin, 1803)*
Synonym for macrodissected adult human ***inferior dental nerve (Meckel, 1817)***; see translation (1803, Vol. 1, p. 177).
9. *inferior dental branch of inferior maxillary nerve (Cloquet, 1816)*
Synonym for macrodissected adult human ***inferior dental nerve (Meckel, 1817)***; in the original French, *rameau dentaire inférieur*, p. 607.
10. *proper lower maxillary nerve (Bell & Bell, 1816)*
Synonym for macrodissected adult mammalian ***inferior dental nerve (Meckel, 1817)***; Vol. 2, p. 497.
11. *nervus alveolaris maxillae inferioris (Meckel, 1817)*
Original Latin synonym for macrodissected adult human ***inferior dental nerve (Meckel, 1817)***; see translation (1832, Vol. 3, p. 73).

LATER SYNONYMS:

1. *maxillary branch of inferior maxillary branch of fifth pair of nerves (Bock, 1817)*
Synonym for macrodissected adult human ***inferior dental nerve (Meckel, 1817)***; in the original Latin, *ramus maxillaris*, p. 53.
2. *inferior alveolar branch of inferior maxillary branch of fifth pair of nerves (Bock, 1817)*
Synonym for macrodissected adult human ***inferior dental nerve (Meckel, 1817)***; in the original Latin, *ramus alveolaris inferior*, p. 53.
3. *mandibular branch of inferior maxillary branch of fifth pair of nerves (Bock, 1817)*
Synonym for macrodissected adult human ***inferior dental nerve (Meckel, 1817)***; in the original Latin, *ramus mandibularis*, p. 53.
4. *alveolar branch of inferior maxillary nerve (Jacobson, 1818)*
Synonym for macrodissected adult mammalian ***inferior dental nerve (Meckel, 1817)***; in the original Latin, *nervus maxillaris inferior ramus alveolaris*, p. 18.
5. *inferior alveolar surculus of inferior maxillary branch (Bellingeri, 1818)*
Synonym for macrodissected adult mammalian ***inferior dental nerve (Meckel, 1817)***; in the original Latin, *surculus alveolaris inferior*, see Table I.
6. *mandibulolabial branch of fifth nerve (Bell, 1829)*
Synonym for macrodissected adult human *mandibulolabial nerve (Soemmerring, 1798)*; in the original Latin, *[ramus] mandibulo-labralis*, p. 322, Plate VIII-*H*.
7. *inferior alveolar nerve (Arnold, 1834)*
Synonym for macrodissected adult human *mandibulolabial nerve (Soemmerring, 1798)*; in the original Latin, *nervus alveolaris inferior*, p. 10.
8. *dental nerve (Quain & Wilson, 1839)*
Synonym for macrodissected adult human *mandibulolabial nerve (Soemmerring, 1798)*; in the original Latin, *n. dentalis*, Plate XIII, Figure 2-*f**.

PARTLY CORRESPONDS:

1. *dentar nerve (Meckel, 1817)*
Described for macrodissected adult human as smaller, inferior branch of trunk of ***inferior dental nerve (Meckel, 1817)*** innervating molar teeth and gum associated with each; see translation (1832, Vol. 3, p. 74). It was later reported that in about a third of human dissections the ***inferior dental nerve (Meckel, 1817)*** divides into a *dentar nerve (Meckel, 1817)* and ***mental nerve (Cheselden, 1726)***, whereas about two-thirds of the time, branching is as described for the ***inferior dental nerve (Meckel, 1817)***; see Starkie & Stewart (1931).
2. *dental nerve (Meckel, 1817)*
Alternate form of *dentar nerve (Meckel, 1817)*; see translation (1832, Vol. 3, p. 74).
3. *dental branch of maxillary branch of inferior maxillary branch of fifth pair of nerves (Bock, 1817)*
Basically synonym for macrodissected adult human *dentar nerve (Meckel, 1817)*; in the original Latin, *ramus dentalis*, p. 54.

inferior dental plexus (>1840)

As described for macrodissected adult human, a series of ***communicating branches (Winslow, 1733)*** between branches of the ***inferior dental nerve (Meckel, 1817)***, distal to where the ***mylohyoid nerve (Meckel, 1748)*** branches off. The ***inferior dental plexus (>1840)*** in turn generates ***inferior dental branches of inferior dental plexus (>1840)*** and ***inferior gingival branches of inferior dental plexus (>1840)***; see Henle (1871, Fig. 248), Starkie and Stewart (1931) referring to *alveolar plexus (>1840)*, Williams & Warwick (1980, p. 1067), *Terminologia Anatomica* (1998, p. 135). Also see ***incisor plexus (>1840)***. It was known to Galen; see ***[inferior dental plexus (>1840)] (Galen, c173)***.

EARLIER REFERENCES:

Described, not named or illustrated:

1. ***[inferior dental plexus (>1840)] (Galen, c173)***
Existence suggested in macrodissected beef, pig, and/or macaque but not human; see May translation (1968, p. 455).

Earlier synonyms:

1. *dental nerve (Arnold, 1834)*
   Essentially synonym for macrodissected adult human ***inferior dental plexus (>1840)***; in the original Latin, *nervus dentalis*, p. 10.
2. *alveolar plexus (>1840)*
   Synonym for macrodissected adult human ***inferior dental plexus (>1840)***; see Starkie and Stewart (1931).

PARTLY CORRESPONDS:

1. *alveolar fascicles proper of inferior alveolar surculus of inferior maxillary branch (Bellingeri, 1818)*
   Caudal parts of macrodissected adult human ***inferior dental plexus (>1840)*** generating ***inferior dental branches of inferior dental plexus (1840)*** supplying two caudal molar teeth on each side; in the original Latin, *fasciculi alveolaris proprius*, see Table I.
2. *anterior dental fascicles of inferior alveolar surculus of inferior maxillary branch (Bellingeri, 1818)*
   Rostral parts of macrodissected adult human ***inferior dental plexus (>1840)*** generating ***inferior dental branches of inferior dental plexus (1840)*** to rostral molar, canine, and incisor teeth on right and left side; in the original Latin, *fasciculi dentalis anterior*, see Table I.

inferior fascicle of accessory optic system (Hayhow et al., 1960)

As described for adult mammal with degeneration and axonal transport pathway tracing methods, a caudally directed branch of the ***hypothalamic optic tract (>1840)*** ending in the ***medial terminal nucleus of accessory optic system (Hayhow et al., 1960)*** and distinguished from the ***superior fascicle of accessory optic system (Hayhow et al., 1960)***, a branch of the ***brachium of superior colliculus (>1840)***; see Nieuwenhuys et al. (2008, p. 781 and Fig. 19.13). For original use in rat by Hayhow et al., see p. 198 and Figure 2, where *fasciculus* not *fascicle* was used; the earlier literature was thoroughly reviewed. It was not identified by 1840.

EARLIER REFERENCES:

Earlier synonyms:

1. *anterior accessory optic tract (Bochenek, 1908)*
   Synonym for ***inferior fascicle of accessory optic system (Hayhow et al., 1960)***; see Hayhow et al. (1960, p. 195).

inferior frontal gyrus (>1840)

As described for macrodissected adult human, a topographic subdivision of the ***frontal region (Vicq d'Azyr, 1786)*** lying between ***middle frontal gyrus (>1840)*** dorsally and ***lateral orbital gyrus (>1840)*** ventrally; see Williams & Warwick (1980, p. 986, Figs. 7.111A, 7.116). Based on cellular architecture in adult human, it roughly consists, from rostral to caudal, of the *middle frontal area (Brodmann, 1909)*, *triangular area (Brodmann, 1909)*, and *opercular area (Brodmann, 1909)*. It was first clearly delineated by Vicq d'Azyr (1786); see ***[inferior frontal gyrus (>1840)] (Vicq d'Azyr, 1786)***.

EARLIER REFERENCES:

Illustrated, not named or described:

1. ***[inferior frontal gyrus (>1840)] (Vicq d'Azyr, 1786)***
   Clearly illustrated for macrodissected adult human; Plate XVI.

PARTLY CORRESPONDS:

1. *area frontalis media (Brodmann, 1909)*
   Original Latin form of *middle frontal area (Brodmann, 1909)*; p. 139.
2. *middle frontal area (Brodmann, 1909)*
   Based on cellular architecture in adult human, roughly rostral half of *inferior frontal gyrus (>1840)*, rostral to *triangular area (Brodmann, 1909)*; see Garey 1994 translaton p. 118 and Figure 85.
3. *area 46 (Brodmann, 1909)*
   Synonym for adult human *middle frontal area (Brodmann, 1909)*; in the original German, *Feld 46*, p. 139.

inferior frontal sulcus (>1840)

As described for macrodissected adult human, the groove between ***middle frontal gyrus (>1840)*** and ***inferior frontal gyrus (>1840)***; see Williams & Warwick (1980, Fig. 7.111A), *Terminologia Anatomica* (1998, p. 125). It was first clearly delineated by Vicq d'Azyr; see ***[inferior frontal sulcus (>1840)] (Vicq d'Azyr, 1786)***.

EARLIER REFERENCES:

Illustrated, not named or described:

1. ***[inferior frontal sulcus (>1840)] (Vicq d'Azyr, 1786)***
   Illustrated as clearly for macrodissected adult human as modern attempts; Plate III, where ***lateral cerebral fissure (>1840)*** is not quite exposed.

inferior gingival branches of inferior dental plexus (>1840)

As described for macrodissected adult human, branches of the ***inferior dental plexus (>1840)*** to gum associated with the inferior (lower or ventral) molar and premolar teeth; see Starkie and Stewart (1931), Durward (1951, p. 1028), Williams & Warwick (1980, p. 1067), *Terminologia Anatomica* (1998, p. 135). They were known to Galen; see ***[inferior gingival branches of inferior dental plexus (>1840)] (Galen, c173)***.

EARLIER REFERENCES:

Described, not named or illustrated:

1. ***[inferior gingival branches of inferior dental plexus (>1840)] (Galen, c173)***
   Described for macrodissected adult beef, pig, and/or macaque but not human; see May translation (1968, p. 455). Vieussens (1684, p. 173) apparently referred to them for macrodissected adult human, and Monro definitely observed them (1783, p. 65), as did Meckel (1817; see translation, 1832, Vol. 3, p. 74), attributing them to branch of ***inferior dental nerve (Meckel, 1817)***, *dentar nerve (Meckel, 1817)*, uncommon variant of normal innervation pattern; see Starkie and Stewart (1931).

Earlier synonyms:

1. *branches to gingiva of dental nerve anastomosis (Arnold, 1834)*
Synonym for macrodissected adult human ***inferior gingival branches of inferior dental plexus (>1840)***; in the original Latin, *anastomosis nervorum dentalium rami ad gingivam*, Table VIII-36,38.

inferior gluteal nerve (Martin, 1781)

As described for macrodissected adult human, it commonly arises from the fifth lumbar and first and second sacral ***sacral plexus dorsal divisions (Paterson, 1887)*** and supplies the gluteus maximus muscle; see Williams & Warwick (1980, p. 1111). For Martin's description in macrodissected adult human, see p. 237. It was known to Galen; see ***[inferior gluteal nerve (Martin, 1781)] (Galen, c177)***.

TRANSLATIONS:

1. *nervus gluteus inferior (Martin, 1781)*
Original Latin form of ***inferior gluteal nerve (Martin, 1781)***; p. 307.

EARLIER REFERENCES:

Described, not named or illustrated:

1. ***[inferior gluteal nerve (Martin, 1781)] (Galen, c177)***
Clearly described for macrodissected adult beef, pig, and/or macaque but not human; see Singer translation (1999, pp. 85–86); also see Duckworth translation (1962, p. 263). Vesalius (1543a) noted it in macrodissected adult human; see Richardson & Carman translation (2002, p. 255).

Earlier synonyms:

1. *nerve to gluteus maximus muscle (Jördens, 1788)*
Synonym for macrodissected adult human ***inferior gluteal nerve (Martin, 1781)***; in the original Latin, *nervus musculi glutei maximi*, p. 2, where Jördens described superior and inferior branches. Fischer (1791, p. 28) described at least five twigs arising from it.
2. *gluteal branches proper of inferior gluteal nerve (Cloquet, 1816)*
Synonym for macrodissected adult human ***inferior gluteal nerve (Martin, 1781)***; in the original French, *rameaux fessiers proprement dits*, p. 670. See *inferior gluteal nerve (Cloquet, 1816)*.
3. *inferior gluteal branches of small sciatic nerve (Quain, 1832)*
Synonym for macrodissected adult human ***inferior gluteal nerve (Martin, 1781)***; p. 702.
4. *muscular branches of inferior gluteal nerve (Cruveilhier, 1836)*
Synonym for macrodissected adult human ***inferior gluteal nerve (Martin, 1781)***; in the original French, *branches musculaires*, p. 857.

PARTLY CORRESPONDS:

1. *inferior part of gluteal plexus (Swan, 1830)*
For macrodissected adult human, roots from fifth lumbar and first and second sacral ***sacral plexus dorsal divisions (Paterson, 1887)*** joining distally to form ***inferior gluteal nerve (Martin, 1781)***; Plate XVIII-34,35.
2. *ascending and external branches of muscular branches of inferior gluteal nerve (Cruveilhier, 1836)*
Rostrolateral branches of macrodissected adult human ***inferior gluteal nerve (Martin, 1781)***; in the original French, *rameaux ascendants et externes*, p. 857.
3. *descending and internal branches of muscular branches of inferior gluteal nerve (Cruveilhier, 1836)*
Caudomedial branches of macrodissected adult human ***inferior gluteal nerve (Martin, 1781)***; in the original French, *rameaux descendants et internes*, p. 857.

inferior horn of lateral ventricle (Bell, 1802)

As described for macrodissected adult human, the part of the ***lateral ventricle (Vesalius, 1543a)*** extending ventrally from the ***atrium of lateral ventricle (>1840)*** into the ***temporal region (>1840)***; see Millen & Woollam (1962, pp. 33–39, Figs. 16–17), Carpenter & Sutin (1983, pp. 41–45, Fig. 2.20). For Bell's use in macrodissected adult human, see Plate III-O. It was known to Galen; see ***[inferior horn of lateral ventricle (Bell, 1802)] (Galen, c173)***.

EARLIER REFERENCES:

Described, not named or illustrated:

1. ***[inferior horn of lateral ventricle (Bell, 1802)] (Galen, c173)***
Galen alluded to it as *horn* in lower regions of *foremost ventricle (Galen, c177)*; see May translation (1968, p. 416), de Lacy translation (1980, pp. 449–450). More specifically, he referred to it as *thalamus (Galen, c173)* and *thalamic region (Galen, c192)*. And again, in *The Doctrines of Plato and Hippocrates*, he seemed to allude to ***inferior horn of lateral ventricle (Bell, 1802)*** as "inclining gradually downward toward the base" (May translation, 1968, p. 400 note 42). Galen macrodissected mostly adult beef, pig, and/or macaque, not human explicitly.

Earlier synonyms:

1. *thalamus (Galen, c173)*
In *On the Usefulness of the Parts*, Galen referred to *thalamus of the anterior [lateral] ventricle*, from whence the optic nerves grow. Galen's *thalamus* is quite likely ***inferior horn of lateral ventricle (Bell, 1802)***; see May translation (1968, p. 687), also see Polyak (1957, pp. 77–78), Savage-Smith (1971), de Lacy (1980, pp. 449–450), and Nieuwenhuys et al. (2008, Fig. 5.8). In a certain region it lies ventral to ***optic tract (Vicq d'Azyr, 1784)*** like an inner chamber or perhaps even a bed; see Nieuwenhuys et al. (2008, Figs. 6.36–6.38) and Jones (1985, pp. 5–8). However, some have (mis)interpreted it to mean ***interbrain (Baer, 1837)***; Schiller (1967, pp. 518–519), also see *optic thalamus (Riolan, 1618)*. Recall that Galen occasionally referred to ***ventricles (Hippocrates)*** in general as *chambers (Galen, c173)*. Most of Galen's neuroanatomical descriptions were based on macrodissected adult beef, pig, and/or macaque, never explicitly human.
2. *optic thalamus (Galen, c173)*

Variation on *thalamus (Galen, c173)*, although Galen did not use this precise term, as far as has been determined.

3. *thalamic region (Galen, c192)*
Synonym for *thalamus (Galen, c173)*; see Duckworth translation (1962, p. 187).
4. *horn of right and left ventricle (Vesalius, 1543a)*
Synonym for macrodissected adult human ***inferior horn of lateral ventricle (Bell, 1802)***, "...the right ventricle of the brain, like the left, narrows down like a horn as it advances from the back downwards and forwards through the substance of the brain" (Richardson & Carman translation, 2009, p. 139; also see p. 194).
5. *lower recess of ventricle (Vesalius, 1543a)*
Synonym for macrodissected adult human ***inferior horn of lateral ventricle (Bell, 1802)***; see Singer translation (1952, p. 98); Vesalius provided very nice diagram showing it along with *anterior horn of lateral ventricle (Vicq d'Azyr, 1786)*; see Richardson & Carman translation (2002, p. 180). It is not clear that his reference to posterior part of right and left ventricles indicates ***inferior horn of lateral ventricle (Bell, 1802)***, as suggested by Burdach (1822, p. 381).
6. *descending part of lateral ventricle (Valverde de Amusco, 1556)*
Synonym for macrodissected adult human ***inferior horn of lateral ventricle (Bell, 1802)***; f. 80, also see Burdach (1822, p. 382). Piccolomini (1586, p. 252) referred to *descending process of lateral ventricle* according to Burdach (1822, p. 382).
7. *hippocampal ventricle (Aranzi, 1587)*
Roughly synonymous with macrodissected adult human ***inferior horn of lateral ventricle (Bell, 1802)***; p. 43, also see Harvey (1961, p. 230 note 822), Clarke & O'Malley (1996, p. 720). According to du Laurens (1599, p. 408), Aranzi regarded hippocampal ventricle as separate from ***lateral ventricle (Vesalius, 1543a)***, and so counted a total of six ***ventricles (Hippocrates)***; see Crooke translation (1615, p. 528), also see *lower recess of lateral ventricle (Vesalius, 1543a)* and *fifth ventricle (Aranzi, 1587)*.
8. *sinus inferiores hippocampi (Aranzi, 1587)*
Synonym for *hippocampal ventricle (Aranzi, 1587)*; p. 46.
9. *silkworm ventricle (Aranzi, 1587)*
Synonym for ***inferior horn of lateral ventricle (Bell, 1802)*** in macrodissected adult human; see Clarke & O'Malley (1996, p. 720). According to Burdach (1822, p. 382), Duvernoy (1735, p. 134) named ***inferior horn of lateral ventricle (Bell, 1802)*** the *ventriculus bombycinus*.
10. *inferior cavity of foremost ventricle (Vesling, 1647)*
Synonym for macrodissected adult human ***inferior horn of lateral ventricle (Bell, 1802)***; see Culpeper translation (1653, p. 60).
11. *ram's horn (Winslow, 1733, p. 34)*
Winslow used it specifically in describing course in macrodissected adult human of ***inferior horn of lateral ventricle (Bell, 1802)***; Section X, p. 34. Later on, he also used it for *posterior pillar of fornix (Paré, 1564)*. The term was apparently used in the former sense by Morand (1748, p. 316), according to Burdach (1822, p. 376), who did not cite Winslow.
12. *minor crura of ventricle (Bergen, 1734)*
Synonym for macrodissected adult human right and left ***inferior horn of lateral ventricle (Bell, 1802)***; in the original Latin, *crura minora ventriculorum*; see Tarin (1750, Tab. XIII, Fig. 3-*b*).
13. *anterior horn of lateral ventricle (Haller, 1747)*
Synonym for macrodissected adult human ***inferior horn of lateral ventricle (Bell, 1802)***; see Mihles translation (1754b, pp. 292–293).
14. *descending horn of lateral ventricle (Haller, 1762)*
Synonym for macrodissected adult human ***inferior horn of lateral ventricle (Bell, 1802)***; in Latin, *cornu descendens*, p. 42.
15. *cornu ammonis (Malacarne, 1780)*
Synonym for macrodissected adult human ***inferior horn of lateral ventricle (Bell, 1802)***; p. 35, according to Burdach (1822, p. 382).
16. *long crus of lateral ventricle (Günther, 1786)*
Synonym for macrodissected adult human ***inferior horn of lateral ventricle (Bell, 1802)***; in the original Latin (plural), *crure longiori*, p. 10.
17. *inferior horn of tricornate ventricle (Soemmerring, 1791)*
Synonym for macrodissected adult human ***inferior horn of lateral ventricle (Bell, 1802)***; p. 47.
18. *inferior cornu of lateral ventricle (Fyfe, 1800)*
Synonym for macrodissected adult human ***inferior horn of lateral ventricle (Bell, 1802)***; p. 17.

LATER SYNONYMS:

1. *anterior lateral part of central fissure (Gordon, 1815)*
Synonym for macrodissected adult human ***inferior horn of lateral ventricle (Bell, 1802)***; p. 104 ff.
2. *middle horn of lateral ventricle (Tiedemann, 1816)*
Synonym for ***inferior horn of lateral ventricle (Bell, 1802)***, in Tiedemann's macroscopic dissection description of human fetus because of its association with *middle lobe of cerebrum (Winslow, 1733)*; see translation (1826, p. 262).
3. *lateral horn of lateral ventricle (Meckel, 1817)*
Synonym for macrodissected adult human ***inferior horn of lateral ventricle (Bell, 1802)***; see translation (1832, Vol. 2, p. 464).
4. *inferior sphenoidal horn of lateral ventricle (Cruveilhier, 1836)*
Synonym for macrodissected adult human ***inferior horn of lateral ventricle (Bell, 1802)***; in the original French, *corne inférieure sphénoïdale*, p. 691.
5. *inferior portion of lateral ventricle (Cruveilhier, 1836)*
Synonym for macrodissected adult human ***inferior horn of lateral ventricle (Bell, 1802)***; in the original French, *portion inférieure*, p. 691.

inferior hypogastric plexus (Tiedemann, 1822)

As described for macrodissected adult human, it is at the caudal or lower end of the ***prevertebral plexuses***

(Quain, 1832), caudal to the ***hypogastric nerve (Walter, 1783)***, and is unusual functionally because it is the only site in the ***peripheral nervous system (Meckel, 1817)*** containing a mixture of postganglionic sympathetic and parasympathetic ***neurons (Waldeyer, 1891)***—and thus, in a sense, is affiliated as well with the ***terminal plexuses (Swanson & Bota, 2010)***. Most preganglionic sympathetic ***axons (Kölliker, 1896)*** arrive via the ***hypogastric nerve (Walter, 1783)***, and most preganglionic parasympathetic ***axons (Kölliker, 1896)*** arrive via the ***pelvic splanchnic nerves (Gaskell, 1886)***; see Mitchell (1953, pp. 301–303 and Figs. 120, 131), Williams & Warwick (1980, p. 1135), Dail (1996). For Tiedemann's use in macrodissected adult human female, see Table II-*28,37*. It was probably known to Willis; see *two infoldings in pelvis (Willis, 1664)*.

TRANSLATIONS:

1. *plexum hypogastricum inferiorem (Tiedemann, 1822)*
   Original Latin form of ***inferior hypogastric plexus (Tiedemann, 1822)***; Table II-*28,37*.

EARLIER REFERENCES:

Earlier synonyms:

1. *plexus gemini intra pelvim (Willis, 1664)*
   Original Latin form of *double infolding within bason (Willis, 1664)*, that is, right and left ***inferior hypogastric plexus (Tiedemann, 1822)***; Table XI-*K*.
2. *two infoldings in pelvis (Willis, 1664)*
   Appears to indicate right and left ***inferior hypogastric plexus (Tiedemann, 1822)*** in macrodissected adult human and common quadrupeds; see Pordage translation (1681, p. 159).
3. *double infolding within bason (Willis, 1664)*
   English form of *plexus gemini intra pelvim (Willis, 1664)*; see Portage translation (1681, Tab. XI-*K*). Spelled today, *double infolding within basin*.
4. *plexus mesentericos infimus (Vieussens, 1684)*
   Apparently corresponds to macrodissected adult human *two infoldings in pelvis (Willis, 1664)*, or ***inferior hypogastric plexus (Tiedemann, 1822)***, although it is poorly described and illustrated as a single structure in median plane; p. 203, Table 23-*79*.
5. *inframesenteric plexus (Winslow, 1733)*
   Synonym for macrodissected adult human ***inferior hypogastric plexus (Tiedemann, 1822)***; in the original Latin, *plexus inframesentericus*, Section VI, p. 99.
6. *hypogastric plexus (Winslow, 1733)*
   Synonym for macrodissected adult human ***inferior hypogastric plexus (Tiedemann, 1822)***; in the original Latin, *plexus hypogastricus*, Section VI, p. 99. Langley & Anderson (1895, p. 71) noted that "there is a certain absurdity in applying the term 'hypogastric' to a plexus in the pelvic basin", and proposed using *pelvic plexus (Chaussier, 1789)* instead.
7. *submesenteric plexus (Winslow, 1733)*
   Synonym for macrodissected adult human ***inferior hypogastric plexus (Tiedemann, 1822)***; in the original Latin, *plexus submesentericus*, Section VI, p. 99.
8. *plexus mesentericus infimum (Haller, 1762)*
   Synonym for macrodissected adult human ***inferior hypogastric plexus (Tiedemann, 1822)***; p. 266, in English, *lowest mesenteric plexus*.
9. *pelvic plexus (Chaussier, 1789)*
   Synonym for macrodissected adult human ***inferior hypogastric plexus (Tiedemann, 1822)***; see *Table synoptique du nerf tri-splanchnique*. Also see Langley & Anderson (1895, p. 71), Mitchell (1953, p. 301).

LATER SYNONYMS:

1. *inferior uterine plexus (Tiedemann, 1822)*
   Apparently synonym for ***inferior hypogastric plexus (Tiedemann, 1822)*** in macrodissected adult human female; in the original Latin, *plexum uterinum inferiorem*, Table I-*76*, Table II-*28,37*.
2. *inferior ganglionic plexus (Tiedemann, 1822)*
   Synonym for ***inferior hypogastric plexus (Tiedemann, 1822)*** in macrodissected adult human female; in the original Latin, *plexus gangliosus inferior*, Table II-*29,37*.

PARTLY CORRESPONDS:

1. *pelvian nerves (Burdin, 1803)*
   Vaguely described ***nerves (Herophilus, c335–c280 BC)*** in macrodissected adult human associated with ***inferior hypogastric plexus (Tiedemann, 1822)***; in the original French, *nerfs pelviens*, see translation (1803, Vol. 1, p. 201).
2. *hypogastric nerves (Chaussier, 1809)*
   Synonym for *pelvian nerves (Burdin, 1803)*; in the original French, *nerfs hypogastriques*.

inferior labial branches of mental nerve (Meckel, 1753)

As described for macrodissected adult human, branches of the ***mental nerve (Cheselden, 1726)*** innervating skin of the lower lip and other related structures; see Williams & Warwick (1980, p. 1067), *Nomina Anatomica* (1983, p. A74). For Meckel's use in macrodissected adult human, see Table 1-*89,97*. They were known to Galen; see ***[inferior labial branches of mental nerve (>1840)] (Galen, c192)***.

EARLIER REFERENCES:

Described, not named or illustrated:

1. ***[inferior labial branches of mental nerve (>1840)] (Galen, c192)***
   Described for macrodissected adult beef, pig, and/or macaque but not human; see Duckworth translation (1962, p. 194). Vesalius (1543a) described them for macrodissected adult human; see Richardson & Carman translation (2002, p. 189).

Earlier synonyms:

1. *inferior labial nerves (Schaarschmidt, 1750)*
   Synonym for macrodissected adult human ***inferior labial branches of mental nerve (Meckel, 1753)***; in the original Latin, *nervi labiales inferiores*, p. 29. Schaarschmidt described two: exterior (larger) and interior (smaller).

LATER SYNONYMS:

1. *inferior labial branches of inferior maxillary nerve proper (Günther, 1786)*
   Synonym for macrodissected adult human ***inferior labial branches of mental nerve (Meckel, 1753)***; in the original Latin, *R. Labiales inferiores*, p. 52.
2. *inferior labial branches of inferior maxillary nerve (Todd, 1836–1839)*
   Synonym for macrodissected adult human ***inferior labial branches of mental nerve (Meckel, 1753)***; p. 295.

PARTLY CORRESPONDS:

1. *external inferior labial branch (Meckel, 1748)*
   Lateral component of macrodissected adult human ***inferior labial branches of mental nerve (Meckel, 1753)***; in the original Latin, *ramus labiales inferiores exterior (ramus maxillaris inferior)*, p. 90.
2. *internal inferior labial branch (Meckel, 1753)*
   Medial component of ***inferior labial branches of mental nerve (Meckel, 1753)*** with anterior, middle, and posterior branches to region of macrodissected adult human lower lip; in the original French, *le rameau labial inférieur du nerf mental (le rameau antérieur, le rameau moyen, le rameau postérieur)*, Table 1:89–94.
3. *external inferior labial nerve (Mayer, 1794)*
   Synonym for macrodissected adult human *external inferior labial branch (Meckel, 1748)*; in the original Latin, *nervus externus labii inferioris*; Part 5, Table VII-66 (p. 46).
4. *internal inferior labial nerve (Mayer, 1794)*
   Synonym for macrodissected adult human *internal inferior labial branch (Meckel, 1753)*; in the original Latin, *nervus internus labii inferioris*; Part 5, Table VII-59 (p. 46).
5. *internal labial thread of mental fascicle of inferior alveolar surculus of inferior maxillary branch (Bellingeri, 1818)*
   Medial branch of *mental fascicle of inferior alveolar surculus of inferior maxillary branch (Bellingeri, 1818)* sharing ***communicating branches (Winslow, 1733)*** with ***marginal mandibular branch of facial nerve (>1840)***; in the original Latin, *stamen labialis internus*, see Table I.
6. *external labial thread of mental fascicle of inferior alveolar surculus of inferior maxillary branch (Bellingeri, 1818)*
   Lateral branch of *mental fascicle of inferior alveolar surculus of inferior maxillary branch (Bellingeri, 1818)* sharing ***communicating branches (Winslow, 1733)*** with ***marginal mandibular branch of facial nerve (>1840)***; in the original Latin, *stamen labialis externus*, see Table I.

inferior laryngeal nerve (>1840)

As described for macrodissected adult human, terminal part of ***recurrent laryngeal nerve (Albinus, 1744)*** innervating the laryngeal muscles and continuous with the ***communicating branch of superior laryngeal nerve with inferior laryngeal nerve (>1840)***; see *Basel Nomina Anatomica* (His, 1895, p. 90), *Nomina Anatomica* (1983, p. A75).

EARLIER REFERENCES:

Described, not named or illustrated:

1. ***[inferior laryngeal nerve (>1840)] (Galen, c173)***
   Galen described, without naming, terminal part of *recurrent nerve (Galen, c173)* and its connection with ***[superior laryngeal nerve (Loder, 1778)] (Galen, c173)*** for macrodissected beef, pig, and macaque but not human; see May translation (1968, p. 371).

Illustrated and described, not named:

1. ***[inferior laryngeal nerve (>1840)] (Vesalius, 1543a)***
   Vesalius provided two illustrations of macrodissected adult human ***recurrent laryngeal nerve (Albinus, 1744)***, including its terminal branch(es) in larynx, ***inferior laryngeal nerve (>1840)***; see Richardson & Carman translation (2002, pp. 169, 196).

Earlier synonyms:

1. *ascending branches of recurrent nerve (Haase, 1781)*
   Synonym for macrodissected adult human ***inferior laryngeal nerve >1840)***; in the original Latin, *nervi recurrentis rami ascendentes*, p. 87.
2. *ascending branches of inferior laryngeal nerve (Günther, 1786)*
   Synonym for macrodissected adult human ***inferior laryngeal nerve (>1840)***; in the original Latin, *r. ascendentes*, p. 64.
3. *laryngeal branches of inferior laryngeal nerve (Arnold, 1834)*
   Synonym for macrodissected adult human ***inferior laryngeal nerve (>1840)***; in the original Latin, *rami laryngei nervus laryngeus inferior*, p. 14.
4. *laryngeal branches of recurrent laryngeal nerve (Arnold, 1834)*
   Synonym for macrodissected adult human ***inferior laryngeal nerve (>1840)***; in the original Latin, *rami laryngei nervus recurrens laryngeus*, p. 14.
5. *terminal branches of recurrent nerve (Cruveilhier, 1836)*
   Synonym for macrodissected adult human ***inferior laryngeal nerve (>1840)***; in the original French, *rameaux termineaux*, p. 963.

PARTLY CORRESPONDS:

1. *branches of inferior laryngeal nerve to posterior and lateral cricoarytenoid muscles (Langenbeck, 1826–1830)*
   Macrodissected adult human branches of ***inferior laryngeal nerve (>1840)*** to posterior and lateral cricoarytenoid muscles; in the original Latin, *rami nervi laryngei inferioris ad musculum cricoarytaenoideum posticum et lateralem*, Fascicle III, Table XVIII-35.
2. *nerve of posterior cricoarytenoid muscle (Cruveilhier, 1836)*
   Macrodissected adult human branch of ***inferior laryngeal nerve (>1840)*** to posterior cricoarytenoid muscle; in the original French, *nerf du muscle crico-arythénoïdien postérieur*, p. 963.
3. *nerve of arytenoid (Cruveilhier, 1836)*
   Macrodissected adult human branch of ***inferior laryngeal nerve (>1840)*** to arytenoid muscle; in the original French, *nerf de l'arythénoïdien*, p. 963.
4. *nerve of cricoarytenoid and thyroarytenoid together (Cruveilhier, 1836)*
   Macrodissected adult human branch of ***inferior laryngeal nerve (>1840)*** to lateral cricoarytenoid and thyroarytenoid

muscles together; in the original French, *nerf du crico-arythénoïdien et du thyro-arythénoïdien réunis*, p. 963.

inferior lateral cutaneous nerve of arm (>1840)

As described for macrodissected adult human, a small branch of the ***radial nerve (Du Verney, 1697)*** supplying skin on the lateral part of the distal half of the arm; see Williams & Warwick (1980, p. 1101 and Fig. 7.201), *Terminologia Anatomica* (1998, p. 138). It was initially identified as the *first branch of second nerve entering upper arm from spine (Galen, c177)*.

EARLIER REFERENCES:

Earlier synonyms:

1. *first branch of second nerve entering upper arm from spine (Galen, c177)*
   Synonym for ***inferior lateral cutaneous nerve of arm (>1840)*** in macrodissected adult beef, pig, and/or macaque but not human; see Singer translation (1999, p. 66) and *second nerve entering upper arm from spine (Galen, c177)*. Vesalius (1543a) mentioned without naming it for macrodissected adult human; see Richardson & Carman translation (2002, pp. 238, 242).
2. *external cutaneous nerve of arm (Mayer, 1794)*
   Synonym for macrodissected adult human ***inferior lateral cutaneous nerve of arm (>1840)***; in the original Latin, *nervus cutaneus brachii externus*; Part V, Table III, Figure 1-*31* (p. 25).
3. *external subcutaneous branch of radial nerve (Loder, 1803)*
   Probably synonym for macrodissected adult human ***inferior lateral cutaneous nerve of arm (>1840)***; in the original Latin, *ramulus nervi subcutanei externi ex radiali*, Table CLXXVIII-*90*.
4. *external subcutaneous nerve of radial nerve (Loder, 1803)*
   Synonym for *external subcutaneous branch of radial nerve (Loder, 1803); in* the original Latin, *nervi subcutanei externi ex nervo radiali*, Table CLXXVIII, Figure 2-*34,35*.

inferior longitudinal fascicle (Burdach, 1822)

As described for macrodissected adult human, a prominent longitudinally oriented system of long ***association fibers of cerebral cortex (>1840)*** interconnecting many parts of the ***occipital region (Vesalius, 1543a)*** and ***temporal region (>1840)***; see Crosby et al. (1962, Figs. 282, 283, 285), Williams & Warwick (1980, p. 1039, Fig. 7.148). For Burdach's use in macrodissected adult human, see p. 152. It was perhaps first clearly delineated by Reil; see ***[inferior longitudinal fascicle (Burdach, 1822] (Reil, 1809b)***.

TRANSLATIONS:

1. *fasciculus longitudinalis inferior (Burdach, 1822)*
   Original Latin form of ***inferior longitudinal fascicle (Burdach, 1822)***; p. 152.

EARLIER REFERENCES:

Illustrated and described, not named:

1. ***[inferior longitudinal fascicle (Burdach, 1822] (Reil, 1809b)***
   Clearly described for macrodissected adult human; see Mayo translation (1823, p. 62).

LATER SYNONYMS:

1. *longitudinal fascicle arising from inferior part of corona radiata (Arnold, 1838b)*
   Synonym for macrodissected adult human ***inferior longitudinal fascicle (Burdach, 1822)***; in the original Latin, *fasciculus longitudinalis, qui e parte inferioire coronae radiatae oritur*, Table X, Figure 4-*f* (also Tab. X, Fig. 1-*l*).

inferior mesenteric ganglion (>1840)

As described for macrodissected adult human, an obvious ***prevertebral ganglion (Quain, 1832)*** sometimes found in the ***inferior mesenteric plexus (Rau, 1720)***, although typically, small, discrete ***ganglia (Galen, c173)*** are scattered around the proximal part of the ***plexus (Galen, c192)*** near the origin of the inferior mesenteric artery; see Williams & Warwick (1980, p. 1134), *Terminologia Anatomica* (1998, p. 143). It was probably first described as the *least infolding of mesentery (Willis, 1664)*.

EARLIER REFERENCES:

Earlier synonyms:

1. *least infolding of mesentery (Willis, 1664)*
   Probably synonym for macrodissected adult human and quadruped ***inferior mesenteric ganglion (>1840)***; in the original Latin, *plexus mesenterii minimo*; see Pordage translation (1681, Tab. IX-*a*, and ☿).
2. *very little infolding of mesentery (Willis, 1664)*
   Synonym for *least infolding of mesentery (Willis, 1664)*; see Pordage translation (Tab. XI-*ω*).
3. *least infolding of abdomen (Willis, 1664)*
   Synonym for *least infolding of mesentery (Willis, 1664)*; see Pordage translation (1681, p. 159).

inferior mesenteric plexus (Rau, 1720)

As described for macrodissected adult human, a ***prevertebral plexus (Quain, 1832)*** derived mainly from the ***intermesenteric plexus (>1840)*** rostral to it, but also receiving branches from the second and third ***lumbar splanchnic nerves (Cruveilhier, 1836)***. It surrounds and distributes with the inferior mesenteric artery and its branches, and it contains tiny scattered ***ganglia (Galen, c173)*** as well, occasionally, as a clear ***inferior mesenteric ganglion (>1849)***; see Williams & Warwick (1980, p. 1134), Durward (1951, Fig. 968). For Rau's discovery and use in macrodissected adult human, see p. 110.

TRANSLATIONS:

1. *plexum mesaraicum inferiorem (Ludwig, 1772)*
   Latin form presumably of ***inferior mesenteric plexus (Rau, 1720)***; p. 10.
2. *plexum mesenterico inferiore (Haase, 1781)*
   Latin form of ***inferior mesenteric plexus (Rau, 1720)***; p. 125.

LATER SYNONYMS:

1. *plexus mesaraicus inferior (Schaarschmidt, 1750)*
   Synonym for macrodissected adult human ***inferior mesenteric plexus (Rau, 1720)***; p. 55.

2. *left colic plexus (Chaussier, 1789)*
   Synonym for macrodissected adult human ***inferior mesenteric plexus (Rau, 1720)***; in the original French, *colique gauche*, see *Table synoptique du nerf tri-splanchnique.*
3. *mesocolic plexus (Soemmerring, 1791)*
   Synonym for macrodissected adult human ***inferior mesenteric plexus (Rau, 1720)***; in the original Latin, *plexus mesocolicus*, p. 341.
4. *middle mesenteric plexus (Soemmerring, 1791)*
   Synonym for ***inferior mesenteric plexus (Rau, 1720)***; in the original Latin, *plexus mesentericus medius*; p. 341.
5. *lower mesenteric plexus (Bell & Bell, 1816)*
   Synonym for macrodissected adult human ***inferior mesenteric plexus (Rau, 1720)***; Vol. 2, p. 527.
6. *mesenteric plexus (Meckel, 1817)*
   Synonym listed for macrodissected adult human ***inferior mesenteric plexus (Rau, 1720)***; see translation (1832, Vol. 3, p. 87).
7. *plexus medius (Meckel, 1817)*
   According to Meckel, who provided no citation, term Vieussens used for macrodissected adult human ***inferior mesenteric plexus (Rau, 1720)***; see translation (1832, Vol. 3, p. 87).
8. *inferior mesenteric plexus proper (Meckel, 1817)*
   Synonym for ***inferior mesenteric plexus (Rau, 1720)***, to distinguish it from use of term *inferior mesenteric plexus (Haller, 1762)* for *hypogastric plexus (Haller, 1762)*; see translation (1832, Vol. 3, p. 88).
9. *inferior aortic plexus (Bock, 1827)*
   Apparently synonym for macrodissected adult human ***inferior mesenteric plexus (Rau, 1720)***; in the original Latin, *plex. aorticus inferior*; Table VI, Figure 1-8.

inferior occipital gyri (>1840)

As described for macrodissected adult human, a topographic subdivision on the ventrolateral face of the ***occipital region (Vesalius, 1543a)*** lying ventral to the ***lateral occipital sulcus (>1840)***; see Williams & Warwick (1980, p. 986, Fig. 7.111A). They were perhaps first clearly delineated by Gall & Spurzheim; see ***[inferior occipital gyri (>1840)] (Gall & Spurzheim, 1810)***.

EARLIER REFERENCES:

Illustrated, not named or described:

1. ***[inferior occipital gyri (>1840)] (Gall & Spurzheim, 1810)***
   Clearly illustrated for macrodissected adult human; Table VIII.

inferior olivary complex (>1840)

As described for macrodissected adult human, and for adult mammal in general based on cellular architecture and connections, a highly differentiated ***gray matter region (Swanson & Bota, 2010)*** in the ventromedial ***medulla (Winslow, 1733)***, caudal to the ***superior olivary complex (>1840)***, which is the only known source of climbing fibers that cross the median plane in the ***olivocerebellar tract (>1840)***, course through the contralateral ***inferior cerebellar peduncle (Günther, 1786)***, and enter the ***cerebellum (Aristotle)***; see Crosby et al. (1962, pp. 135–138), *Terminologia Anatomica* (1998, p. 110), Nieuwenhuys et al. (2008, p. 196, Fig. 6.14). It was first clearly delineated as the *olivary body gray matter (Santorini, 1775)*, although Pourfour de Petit (1710, Letter 1, p. 14) glimpsed it earlier. The first view with a simple microscope, in adult human, was provided by Rolando (1825a, Tab. V, Fig. 6).

EARLIER REFERENCES:

Earlier synonyms:

1. *olivary body gray substance (Santorini, 1775)*
   Santorini described *gray substance (Vesalius, 1543a)* or *cortical substance (Willis, 1664)* intermixed with *white substance (Vesalius, 1543a)* or *medullary substance (Colombo, 1559)* in and around the macrodissected adult human ***inferior olivary complex (>1840)***; p. 26, Table II-*v*. Earlier, a brown line—that is, *brown substance of brain (Vesalius, 1543a)* like that seen in *corpus rhomboïdeum (Vieussens, 1684)* or ***dentate nucleus (>1840)***, only smaller—was mentioned for macrodissected adult human by Pourfour du Petit (1710, Letter 1, p. 14).
2. *olivary body yellow substance (Malacarne, 1776)*
   Synonym for macrodissected adult human *olivary body gray substance (Santorini, 1775)*; in the original Italian, *di color giallo*, p. 88.
3. *serrated body of olivary eminence (Vicq d'Azyr, 1786)*
   Gray substance (Vesalius, 1543a) and associated *white substance (Vesalius, 1543a)* composition of macrodissected adult human ***inferior olivary complex (>1840)***; in the original French, *le corps festonné, dentelé ou rhomboïdal des éminences olivaires*, Plate XXXI, Figure V:*6–8*.
4. *dentate body of olivary eminence (Vicq d'Azyr, 1786)*
   Gray substance (Vesalius, 1543a) and associated *white substance (Vesalius, 1543a)* composition of macrodissected adult human ***inferior olivary complex (>1840)***; in the original French, *le corps festonné, dentelé ou rhomboïdal des éminences olivaires*, Plate XXXI, Figure V:*6–8*. Bell (1803b, p. 111) referred to *corpus dentatum emminentiae olivaris*, and Burdach (1822, p. 34) referred to *corpus dentatum olivae* in this regard.
5. *rhomboid body of olivary eminence (Vicq d'Azyr, 1786)*
   Gray substance (Vesalius, 1543a) and associated *white substance (Vesalius, 1543a)* composition of macrodissected adult human ***inferior olivary complex (>1840)***; in the original French, *le corps festonné, dentelé ou rhomboïdal des éminences olivaires*, Plate XXXI, Figure V:*6–8*.
6. *olivary body (Günther, 1786)*
   Gray substance (Vesalius, 1543a) and associated *white substance (Vesalius, 1543a)* composition of macrodissected adult human ***inferior olivary complex (>1840)***; in the original Latin (plural), *corpora olivaria*, p. 23.
7. *olivary tubercle (Günther, 1786)*
   Gray substance (Vesalius, 1543a) and associated *white substance (Vesalius, 1543a)* composition of

macrodissected adult human ***inferior olivary complex (>1840)***; in the original Latin (plural), *tubercula olivaria*, p. 23.

8. *ganglia ovalia intumescentiae magnae (Gall & Spurzheim, 1810)*
   Right and left macrodissected adult human ***inferior olivary complex (>1840)***; p. 346, according to Burdach (1822, p. 284).
9. *corpus olivae fimbriatum (Meckel, 1817)*
   Synonym for macrodissected adult human ***inferior olivary complex (>1840)***; see translation (1832, Vol. 2, p. 421), also referred to simply as *corpus fimbriatum*.
10. *corpus dentatum olivae (Burdach, 1822)*
   Synonym for macrodissected adult human ***inferior olivary complex (>1840)***; p. 34.
11. *olivary nucleus (Burdach, 1822)*
   Synonym for macrodissected adult human ***inferior olivary complex (>1840)***; p. 34, derived from *funiculus nuclei olivae (Burdach, 1822)*.
12. *olivary ganglion (Knox, 1832)*
   Knox's version of *ganglia ovalia intumescentiae magnae (Gall & Spurzheim, 1810)*; Supplemental Plate IV-*10*.
13. *pneumogastric ganglia (Solly, 1836)*
   Right and left macrodissected adult mammalian *olivary body (Günther, 1786)*; p. 92.
14. *nucleus of olivary fasciculus (Arnold, 1838b)*
   Synonym for macrodissected adult human ***inferior olivary complex (>1840)***, referring to *olivary fasciculus (Tiedemann, 1816)*; in the original Latin, *nucleus fasciculus olivaris*, Table IX, Figure 5-*d*.
15. *inferior corpora olivaria (Schroeder van der Kolk, 1854)*
   Synonym for macrodissected adult human ***inferior olivary complex (>1840)***, named as companion to *superior corpora olivaria (>1840)*, which he discovered; see translation (1859, p. 174). Also see Schiller (1967, p. 533).

inferior ovarian nerves (>1840)

As described for macrodissected adult human female, they arise from the ***inferior hypogastric plexus (Tiedemann, 1822)*** and sometimes the adjacent, caudal (lower) end of the ***hypogastric nerve (Walter, 1783)***. Near their origin they are associated with the *uterine nerves (Galen, c173)*—the ***uterovaginal plexus (>1840)***—to form the ***tubo-uterine plexus (>1840)***, from which they eventually diverge; see Mitchell (1953, pp. 295–296). Perhaps the first clear reference to them was *ovarian nerves (Cruveilhier, 1836)*.

EARLIER REFERENCES:

Earlier synonyms:

1. *ovarian nerves (Cruveilhier, 1836)*
   Probably synonym for ***inferior ovarian nerves (>1840)*** because mentioned in description of macrodissected adult human female ***inferior hypogastric plexus (Tiedemann, 1822)***; in the original French, *nerfs ovariques*, p. 1027.

inferior palpebral branches of infraorbital nerve (Meckel, 1748)

As described for macrodissected adult human they supply skin over the lower eyelid and communicate with ***zygomatic branches of facial nerve (>1840)*** and ***zygomaticofacial nerve (>1840)***; see Williams & Warwick (1980, p. 1064), *Terminologia Anatomica* (1998, p. 134). For Meckel's use in macrodissected adult human see Figure 1-*e*. They were first clearly alluded to by Winslow; see ***[inferior palpebral branches of infraorbital nerve (>1840)] (Winslow, 1733)***.

TRANSLATIONS:

1. *rami nervus infraorbitalis palpebrales inferiores (Meckel, 1748)*
   Original Latin form of ***inferior palpebral branches of infraorbital nerve (Meckel, 1748)***; Figure 1-*e*.

EARLIER REFERENCES:

Described, not named or illustrated:

1. ***[inferior palpebral branches of infraorbital nerve (>1840)] (Winslow, 1733)***
   Alluded to for macrodissected adult human; Section VI, p. 65.

LATER SYNONYMS:

1. *inferior palpebral nerves (Schaarschmidt, 1750)*
   Synonym and better term for macrodissected adult human ***inferior palpebral branches of infraorbital nerve (>1840)***; in the original Latin, *nervi palpebrales inferiores*, p. 25.
2. *internal inferior palpebral fascicle of infraorbital surculus (Bellingeri, 1818)*
   Synonym for macrodissected adult human ***inferior palpebral branches of infraorbital nerve (>1840)*** communicating with ***zygomatic branches of facial nerve (>1840)*** and ***infratrochlear nerve (Schaarschmidt, 1750)***, and supplying lower eyelid, orbicularis oculi muscle, "incisiv.", caruncle, and lacrimal sac; in the original Latin, *fasciculus palpebralis inf. inter.*, see Table 1.
3. *ascending filaments of superior maxillary nerve (Cruveilhier, 1836)*
   Synonym for macrodissected adult human ***inferior palpebral branches of infraorbital nerve (>1840)***; in the original French, *filets ascendans*, p. 928.
4. *palpebral filaments of superior maxillary nerve (Cruveilhier, 1836)*
   Synonym for macrodissected adult human ***inferior palpebral branches of infraorbital nerve (>1840)***; in the original French, *filets palpébraux*, p. 928.

PARTLY CORRESPONDS:

1. *interior palpebral branch of infraorbital nerve (Loder, 1778)*
   Medial branch of macrodissected adult human ***inferior palpebral branches of infraorbital nerve (Meckel, 1748)***; in the original Latin, *palpebralis interior*, p. 16.
2. *exterior palpebral branch of infraorbital nerve (Loder, 1778)*
   Lateral branch of macrodissected adult human ***inferior palpebral branches of infraorbital nerve (Meckel, 1748)***; in the original Latin, *palpebralis exterior*, p. 16.
3. *exterior palpebral nerve (Haase, 1781)*

Lateral branch of macrodissected adult human ***inferior palpebral branches of infraorbital nerve (Meckel, 1748)***; in the original Latin, *palpebralis nervus exterior*, p. 68.

4. *interior inferior palpebral nerve (Günther, 1786)*
Medial branch of macrodissected adult human ***inferior palpebral branches of infraorbital nerve (Meckel, 1748)***; in the original Latin, *palpebralis inferior interior*, p. 49.
5. *inferior internal palpebral nerve (Mayer, 1794)*
Medial branch of macrodissected adult human ***inferior palpebral branches of infraorbital nerve (Meckel, 1748)***; in the original Latin, *nervus palpebralis internus inferior*; Part 5, Table VII-*24* (p. 44).
6. *inferior external palpebral nerve (Mayer, 1794)*
Lateral branch of macrodissected adult human ***inferior palpebral branches of infraorbital nerve (Meckel, 1748)***; in the original Latin, *nervus palpebralis externus inferior*; Part 5, Table VII-*43* (p. 45).
7. *internal inferior palpebral nerve (Arnold, 1834)*
Medial branch of macrodissected adult human ***inferior palpebral branches of infraorbital nerve (Meckel, 1748)***; in the original Latin, *nervus palpebralis inferior, internus*, p. 9.
8. *external inferior palpebral nerve (Arnold, 1834)*
Lateral branch of macrodissected adult human ***inferior palpebral branches of infraorbital nerve (Meckel, 1748)***; in the original Latin, *nervus palpebralis inferior, externus*, p. 9.

inferior parietal lobule (>1840)

As described for macrodissected adult human, a topographic subdivision of the ***parietal region (>1840)*** lying ventral to the ***intraparietal sulcus (>1840)*** and caudal to the ***postcentral gyrus (>1840)***, and in turn subdivided into a rostral half, the ***supramarginal gyrus (>1840)***, and a caudal half, the ***angular gyrus (>1840)***; see Williams & Warwick (1980, p. 986, Fig. 7.111A). It was first delineated, at least partly, by Vicq d'Azyr; see ***[inferior parietal lobule (>1840)] (Vicq d'Azyr, 1786)***.

EARLIER REFERENCES:

Illustrated and described, not named:

1. ***[inferior parietal lobule (>1840)] (Vicq d'Azyr, 1786)***
Illustrated at least partly for macrodissected adult human; Plate III, ventral to part *l*.

inferior rectal nerves (>1840)

As described for adult human, branches of the ***pudendal nerve (Camper, 1762)*** distributing motor ***axons (Kölliker, 1896)*** to the external anal sphincter and sensory ***dendrites (His, 1889)*** to the distal (lower or ectodermal) part of the anal canal; see Durward (1951, Figs. 943, 944), Williams & Warwick (1980, pp. 1116, 1135), *Terminologia Anatomica* (1998, p. 140). They were known to Galen; see *nerve to rectum (Galen, c192)*.

EARLIER REFERENCES:

Earlier synonyms:

1. *nerve to rectum (Galen, c192)*
Galen mentioned without naming the ***inferior rectal nerves (>1840)*** for macrodissected adult beef, pig, and/or macaque but not human; see Duckworth translation (1962, p. 263). Eustachi indicated them in illustration of ***pudendal nerve (Camper, 1762)***; see Albinus edition (1761, Tab. 20/2-upper medial branch of ϕ). Willis illustrated them for macrodissected adult human and other common large mammals; see Pordage translation (pp. 159–160 and Tab. 11-*h,k*).
2. *hemorrhoidal nerves (Martin, 1781)*
Synonym for macrodissected adult human ***inferior rectal nerves (>1840)***, combining *external hemorrhoidal nerves (Walter, 1783)* and *internal hemorrhoidal nerves (Walter, 1783)*; in the original Latin, *nervi haemorrhoidales*, p. 234.
3. *inferior hemorrhoidal nerve (Meckel, 1817)*
Synonym for macrodissected adult human ***inferior rectal nerves (>1840)***; in the original Latin, *nervus haemorrhoideus inferior*, see translation (1832, Vol. 3, p. 15).
4. *inferior pudic nerve (Meckel, 1817)*
Synonym for *inferior hemorrhoidal nerve (Meckel, 1817)*; in the original Latin, *nervus pudendus inferior*, see translation (1832, Vol. 3, p. 15).
5. *external hemorrhoidal nerves (Bock, 1827)*
Probably synonym for *inferior hemorrhoidal nerve (Meckel, 1817)*; in the original Latin, *nervi haemorrhoidalis externi*, Table I, Figure 2-*76*.
6. *anal nerve (Cruveilhier, 1836)*
Synonym for macrodissected adult human ***inferior rectal nerves (>1840)***; in the original French, *nerf anal*, p. 852.
7. *external hemorrhoidal branch of internal pudic nerve (Quain & Wilson, 1839)*
Synonym for macrodissected adult human ***inferior rectal nerves (>1840)***; Plate XXII-C,*d*.
8. *external hemorrhoidal branch of pudendal nerve (Quain & Wilson, 1839)*
Synonym for macrodissected adult human ***inferior rectal nerves (>1840)***; Plate XXII-C,*d*.

PARTLY CORRESPONDS:

1. *perforating nerves (Walter, 1783)*
Synonym for macrodissected adult human *external hemorroidal nerves (Walter, 1783)*; in the original Latin, *nervi perforantes*, Table I-*484*.
2. *external hemorrhoidal nerves (Walter, 1783)*
One of two major components of ***inferior rectal nerves (>1840)***; in the original Latin, *nervi haemorrhoidales externi*, Table I-*486*. They arise from macrodissected adult human fourth ***sacral nerve (Camper, 1760)***; Table I-*484*.
3. *internal hemorrhoidal nerve (Walter, 1783)*
One of two major components of ***inferior rectal nerves (>1840)***; in the original Latin, *nervorum haemorrhoidalium interiorum*, Table I-*531*. It arises from macrodissected adult human third ***sacral nerve (Camper, 1760)***; Table I-*531*. Walter described a trunk (Tab. I-*531*) and three main branches (Tab. I:*532–534*).
4. *perineal cutaneous nerve (Walter, 1783)*
Branch of *internal hemorroidal nerve (Walter, 1783)*; in the original Latin, *nervum cutaneum perinaei*, Table 1-*542*.

5. *anal cutaneous nerve (Walter, 1783)*
   Branch of *internal hemorroidal nerve (Walter, 1783)*; in the original Latin, *nervum cutaneum ani*, Table 1-543,585.
6. *anterior branches of anal nerve (Cruveilhier, 1836)*
   Ventral (anterior) branches of *anal nerve (Cruveilhier, 1836)*; in the original French, *rameaux antérieurs*, p. 852.
7. *middle branches of anal nerve (Cruveilhier, 1836)*
   Between *anterior branches of anal nerve (Cruveilhier, 1836)* and *posterior branches of anal nerve (Cruveilhier, 1836)*; in the original French, *rameaux moyens*, p. 852.
8. *posterior branches of anal nerve (Cruveilhier, 1836)*
   Dorsal (posterior) branches of *anal nerve (Cruveilhier, 1836)*; in the original French, *rameaux postérieurs*, p. 852.

inferior root of ansa cervicalis (>1840)

As described for macrodissected adult human, it most commonly forms by the union of branches from the second and third cervical ***spinal nerve ventral branches (>1840)*** and then extends caudally (descends) lateral to the internal jugular vein to form a loop, the ansa cervicalis proper, in conjunction with the ***superior root of ansa cervicalis (>1840)***; see Williams & Warwick (1980, Figs. 7.193, 197), *Nomina Anatomica* (1983, p. A76), *Terminologia Anatomica* (1998, p. 137). It was probably first clearly delineated by Winslow; see ***[inferior root of ansa cervicalis (>1840)] (Winslow, 1733)***.

EARLIER REFERENCES:

Described, not named or illustrated:

1. ***[inferior root of ansa cervicalis (>1840)] (Winslow, 1733)***
   Described for macrodissected adult human; Section VI, p. 77.

Illustrated and described, not named:

1. ***[inferior root of ansa cervicalis (>1840)] (Asch, 1750)***
   Described and illustrated for macrodissected infant and adult human; see Figure 3-19.

Earlier synonyms:

1. *descending cervical branch (Neubauer, 1772)*
   Synonym for macrodissected infant human ***inferior root of ansa cervicalis (>1840)***; Table 3, Figure 3-ψ,1.
2. *external descending nerve of neck (Andersch & Soemmerring, 1792)*
   Synonym for macrodissected adult human ***inferior root of ansa cervicalis (>1840)***; in the original Latin, *nervus descendens colli externus*, p. 158. See Scarpa (1794, Tab. I-15).
3. *nervo musculos colli movente externo (Andersch, 1797)*
   Synonym for *external descending nerve of neck (Andersch & Soemmerring, 1792)*; p. 91.
4. *internal descending branch of cervical plexus (Cloquet, 1816)*
   Synonym for macrodissected adult human ***inferior root of ansa cervicalis (>1840)***; in the original French, *branche descendante interne*, p. 637.
5. *descending cervical nerve (Meckel, 1817)*
   Synonym for macrodissected adult human ***inferior root of ansa cervicalis (>1840)***; see translation (1832, Vol. 3, p. 40).

PARTLY CORRESPONDS:

1. *external descending nerve of neck of third nerves of neck (Andersch & Soemmerring, 1792)*
   Macrodissected adult human branch from third cervical ***spinal nerve ventral branch (>1840)*** contributing to formation of ***inferior root of ansa cervicalis (>1840)***; in the original Latin, *tertii nervi colli descendente nervo colli externo*, p. 146.
2. *internal descending nerve of neck of third nerves of neck (Andersch, 1797)*
   Apparently synonym for *external descending nerve of neck of third nerves of neck (Andersch & Soemmerring, 1792)*; in the original Latin, *nervus descendens colli internus tertii nervi colli*, p. 95. Apparently an error and should read *external* rather than *internal*; see Andersch & Soemmerring (1792, § XLV) and Andersch (1797, § 46).
3. *branch of anterior branch of second cervical nerve to descending nerve of hypoglossal nerve (Arnold, 1834)*
   The second cervical ***spinal nerve ventral branch (>1840)*** contribution to macrodissected adult human ***inferior root of ansa cervicalis (>1840)***; in the original Latin, *nervus cervicalis secundus ramus anterior ramus ad nervum descendentem nervi hypoglossi*, p. 16.

inferior salivatory nucleus (>1840)

As described for adult mammal based on cellular architecture and connections, a relatively indistinct ***gray matter region (Swanson & Bota, 2010)*** in ventral parts of the ***medulla (Winslow, 1733)*** lying roughly between the ***superior salivatory nucleus (>1840)*** rostrally and the ***ambiguus nucleus (>1840)*** and ***dorsal motor nucleus of vagus nerve (>1840)*** caudally, and generating a motor component of the ***glossopharyngeal nerve central root (>1840)*** continuing in the peripheral ***glossopharyngeal nerve root (>1840)***. Functionally, the ***inferior salivatory nucleus (>1840)*** contains preganglionic parasympathetic ***neurons (Waldeyer, 1891)*** preferentially influencing secretions of the parotid salivary gland; see Williams & Warwick (1980, pp. 1074, 1123), Nieuwenhuys et al. (2008, p. 191). It was not delineated by 1840.

inferior temporal gyrus (>1840)

As described for macrodissected adult human, a topographic subdivision of the ***temporal region (>1840)*** lying between ***middle temporal gyrus (>1840)*** dorsally and ***lateral occipitotemporal gyrus (>1840)*** ventrally and medially, with the border between ***inferior temporal gyrus (>1840)*** and ***lateral occipitotemporal gyrus (>1840)*** defined arbitrarily as running along the ventrolateral margin of the ***temporal region (>1840)***; see Williams & Warwick (1980, Figs. 7.111A, 7.114A), *Terminologia Anatomica* (1998, pp. 125–126), *Dorland's* (2003, p. 806). It was perhaps first clearly delineated by Vicq d'Azyr; see ***[inferior temporal gyrus (>1840)] (Vicq d'Azyr, 1786)***.

EARLIER REFERENCES:

Illustrated and described, not named:

1. ***[inferior temporal gyrus (>1840)] (Vicq d'Azyr, 1786)***

Pointed out and clearly illustrated for macrodissected adult human; Plates XVI-*24*, XVII-*17*.

Earlier synonyms:

1. *third process of middle lobe (Rolando, 1831)*
Synonym for macrodissected adult human ***inferior temporal gyrus (>1840)***; in the original Italian, *processo terzo del lobo di mezzo*, Figure 1-*b*. Also see *second process of middle lobe (Rolando, 1831)*.

PARTLY CORRESPONDS:

1. *sphenoidal lobe (Serres, 1824–1826)*
Rostral parts of ***inferior temporal gyrus (>1840)*** in macrodissected adult mandrill; in the original French, *lobe sphénoïdal*; Plate VIII, Figure 194-*G,D*; Plate XII, Figure 234-*H*.

inferior temporal sulcus (>1840)

As described for macrodissected adult human, a groove (often interrupted) between ***inferior temporal gyrus (>1840)*** ventrally and ***middle temporal gyrus (>1840)*** dorsally; see Mettler (1948, Fig. 76-*Inf. temp. s.*), Williams & Warwick (1980, Fig. 711A, mislabeled *mid. temp. sulc.*), *Terminologia Anatomica* (1998, pp. 125–126), Nieuwenhuys et al. (2008, Fig. 3.5-5). It was first delineated by Vicq d'Azyr; see ***[inferior temporal sulcus (>1840)] (Vicq d'Azyr, 1786)***.

EARLIER REFERENCES:

Illustrated, not named or described:

1. *[inferior temporal sulcus (>1840)] (Vicq d'Azyr, 1786)*
Illustrated for macrodissected adult human as clearly as various modern sources; Plate XVI.

inferior testicular nerves (>1840)

As described for macrodissected adult human male, they arise from ***nerve (Herophilus, c335–c280 BC)*** loops around the caudal (lower) end of the ureter and adjacent parts of the ***inferior hypogastric plexus (Tiedemann, 1822)*** and course to the nearby vas deferens and epididymis; see Mitchell (1953, pp. 295). Vesalius described ***nerves (Herophilus, c335–c280 BC)*** to the testicles as a group for macrodissected adult human; see *branch of sixth pair stretching along roots of ribs offshoots to testes (Vesalius, 1543a)*. The ***inferior testicular nerves (>1840)*** were perhaps first clearly described as *testicular nerves (Horne, 1707)*.

EARLIER REFERENCES:

Earlier synonyms:

1. *testicular nerves (Horne, 1707)*
Probably refers primarily to macrodissected adult human male ***inferior testicular nerves (>1840)***; in the original Latin, *nervi testiculorum*, see Index rerum.

inferior thalamic radiation peduncular loop (>1840)

As described in macrodissected adult human, and mammal generally with histological methods for ***axons (Kölliker, 1896)***, a dorsal branch of the ***peduncular loop (Gratiolet, 1857)*** to the ***dorsal part of thalamus (Herrick, 1910)***. It is the part of the ***inferior thalamic radiation (>1840)*** just medial to, rather than within, the ***internal capsule (Burdach, 1822)***; see Mettler (1948, Fig. 289, called *inferior thalamic peduncle*), Nauta & Haymaker (1969, Figs. 4.19-*ITP*, 4.22-*IP*). It was not known before 1840.

inferior ureteric nerves (>1840)

As described for macrodissected adult human, they arise from the ***hypogastric nerve (Walter, 1783)*** and rostral (upper) part of the ***inferior hypogastric plexus (Tiedemann, 1822)*** and end on the caudal (lower) part of the ureter; see Mitchell (1953, p. 293). They were probably first clearly delineated by Walter; see ***[inferior ureteric nerves (>1840)] (Walter, 1783)***.

EARLIER REFERENCES:

Illustrated and described, not named:

1. *[inferior ureteric nerves (>1840)] (Walter, 1783)*
Walter described but did not name one or two in macrodissected adult human; Table I-*462*.

infralimbic area (Rose & Woolsey, 1948)

As described with cellular architecture and connections in mammal, the most rostral and ventral subdivision of the ***cingulate region (>1840)***. Corresponds roughly to the adult human ***parolfactory gyrus (>1840)*** based on topographic macroarchitecture, and to *area 25 (Brodmann, 1909)* based on cellular architecture; see Rose & Woolsey (1948, p. 290). It was not identified by 1840.

EARLIER REFERENCES:

Earlier synonyms:

1. *area subgenualis (Brodmann, 1909)*
Original Latin form of *subgenual area (Brodmann, 1909)*; p. 148.
2. *subgenual area (Brodmann, 1909)*
Synonym for mammalian ***infralimbic area (Rose & Woolsey, 1948)***; see p. 148 for human.
3. *area 25 (Brodmann, 1909)*
Synonym for *subgenual area (Brodmann, 1909)* or *preterminal area (Brodmann, 1909)*; in the original German, *Feld 25*, see p. 148.
4. *area praeterminalis (Brodmann, 1909)*
Original Latin form of *preterminal area (Brodmann, 1909)*; Table 7 on p. 247.
5. *preterminal area (Brodmann, 1909)*
Synonym for mammalian ***infralimbic area (Rose & Woolsey, 1948)***; in the original Latin, *area praeterminalis*, see Table 7, p. 247.
6. *parolfactory area (Economo & Koskinas, 1925)*
Synonym for human *area 25 (Brodmann, 1909)*; p. 406. Also see Economo (1929, p. 48, Fig. 19).

infraorbital nerve (Schaarschmidt, 1750)

As described for macrodissected adult human, ***maxillary nerve (Meckel, 1753)*** assumes the name ***infraorbital nerve (Schaarschmidt, 1750)*** after giving off the ***posterior superior dental nerve (Haller, 1762)***, when it traverses the infraorbital fissure and then supplies the ala of the nose, lower eyelid, and skin and mucous membrane of the cheek and upper lip; see Durward (1951, p. 1025 and Figs. 895, 898), Williams & Warwick (1980, p. 1062). For Schaarschmidt's use in macrodissected adult human, see p. 24; also see *infraorbital nerve (Meckel, 1748)*. It was known to Galen; see ***[infraorbital nerve (Schaarschmidt, 1750)] (Galen, c192)***.

TRANSLATIONS:

1. *nervus infraorbitalis (Schaarschmidt, 1750)*
   Original Latin form of ***infraorbital nerve (Schaarschmidt, 1750)***; p. 24.

EARLIER REFERENCES:

Described, not named or illustrated:

1. ***[infraorbital nerve (Schaarschmidt, 1750)] (Galen, c192)***
   Vaguely described for macrodissected adult beef, pig, and/or macaque but not human; see Duckworth translation (1962, p. 194).

Illustrated, not named or described:

1. ***[infraorbital nerve (Schaarschmidt, 1750)] (Eustachi, 1552)***
   Clearly illustrated certain distal parts for macrodissected adult human; see Albinus edition (1761, Tab. 19/2-*b*, p. 111).

LATER SYNONYMS:

1. *infra orbitar nerve (Monro, 1783)*
   Synonym for macrodissected adult human ***infraorbital nerve (Schaarschmidt, 1750)***. Monro wrote that when it and, presumably, ***communicating branches of auriculotemporal nerve with facial nerve (>1840)***, communicate with branch of *hard part of seventh pair of nerves arising within skull (Willis, 1664)*, "both in man and in the ox, I have certainly found, that the small branches which come off beyond the union of two larger nerves, consist of fibres from both." (see p. 43 and Tab. 19).
2. *orbital nerve (Soemmerring, 1809)*
   Synonym for macrodissected adult human ***infraorbital nerve (Schaarschmidt, 1750)***; in the original German, *Augenhöhlnerve*, Table 3, Figure 1-*k*. Burdin (1803 translation, Vol. 1, p. 172) spelled it *orbitar* nerve.
3. *infraorbital branch of superior maxillary nerve (Jacobson, 1818)*
   Synonym for macrodissected adult mammalian ***infraorbital nerve (Schaarschmidt, 1750)***; in the original Latin, *nervus maxillaris superior ramus infraorbitalis*, p. 18.
4. *suborbital nerve (Bell, 1829)*
   Synonym for macrodissected adult mammalian ***infraorbital nerve (Schaarschmidt, 1750)***; p. 327.

PARTLY CORRESPONDS:

1. *superior external cutaneous nerve of infraorbital nerve (Meckel, 1753)*
   Branch of ***infraorbital nerve (Schaarschmidt, 1750)*** described and illustrated for macrodissected adult human; in the original French, *le nerf cutané externe supérieur de le nerf sous-orbitaire*, Table 1:32–35. It contributes ***inferior palpebral branches of infraorbital nerve (Meckel, 1748)*** and ***external nasal branches of infraorbital nerve (>1840)***.
2. *anterior alveolar nerve (Günther, 1786)*
   Macrodissected adult human ***middle superior dental nerve (Henle, 1871)*** and ***anterior superior dental nerve (Haller, 1762)*** considered together, with exterior and interior branches; p. 48.
3. *anterior dental nerve (Günther, 1786)*
   Synonym for *anterior alveolar nerve (Günther, 1786)*; p. 48.
4. *connection of infraorbital nerve with facial nerve (Arnold, 1834)****Communicating branch (Winslow, 1733)*** between macrodissected adult human ***infraorbital nerve (Schaarschmidt, 1750)*** and intermediate components of ***facial nerve trunk (>1840)***; in the original Latin, *conjunctio cum nervo faciali*, p. 9.
5. *facial branches of second division of fifth pair of nerves (Todd, 1836–1839)*
   Macrodissected adult human ***infraorbital nerve (Schaarschmidt, 1750)*** without ***middle superior dental nerve (Henle, 1871)*** and ***posterior superior dental nerve (Haller, 1762)***; p. 289.
6. *terminal branches of superior maxillary nerve (Cruveilhier, 1836)*
   Considered together, *ascending filaments of superior maxillary nerve (Cruveilhier, 1836)*, *internal filaments of superior maxillary nerve (Cruveilhier, 1836)*, and *descending filaments of superior maxillary nerve (Cruveilhier, 1836)*; in the original French, *branches terminales du nerf maxillaire supérieur*, p. 928.

infrapatellar branch of saphenous nerve (>1840)

As described for macrodissected adult human, it supplies skin in front of the patella and contributes to the ***patellar plexus (>1840)***; see Williams & Warwick (1980, p. 1109), *Nomina Anatomica* (1998, p. 140). It was known to Vesalius; see ***[infrapatellar branch of saphenous nerve (>1840)] (Vesalius, 1543a)***.

EARLIER REFERENCES:

Illustrated and described, not named:

1. ***[infrapatellar branch of saphenous nerve (>1840)] (Vesalius, 1543a)***
   Described and illustrated for macrodissected adult human; see Richardson & Carman translation (2002, p. 258).

Earlier synonyms:

1. *minor saphenous nerve (Fischer, 1791)*
   Synonym for macrodissected adult human ***infrapatellar branch of saphenous nerve (>1840)***; in the original Latin, *nervus saphenus minor*, p. 15. See Fyfe (1800, p. 328).
2. *anterior terminal branch of internal saphenous nerve (Cruveilhier, 1836)*
   Synonym for macrodissected adult human ***infrapatellar branch of saphenous nerve (>1840)***; in the original French, *branche antérieure*, p. 846.
3. *reflected terminal branch of internal saphenous nerve (Cruveilhier, 1836)*
   Synonym for *anterior terminal branch of internal saphenous nerve (Cruveilhier, 1836)*; in the original French, *branche réfléchie*, p. 846.

4. *patellar terminal branch of internal saphenous nerve (Cruveilhier, 1836)*
   Synonym for *anterior terminal branch of internal saphenous nerve (Cruveilhier, 1836)*; in the original French, *branche rotulienne*, p. 846.

PARTLY CORRESPONDS:

1. *ascending filaments of anterior terminal branch of internal saphenous nerve (Cruveilhier, 1836)*
   As described, for *anterior terminal branch of internal saphenous nerve (Cruveilhier, 1836)*; in the original French, *filets ascendans*, p. 847.
2. *descending filaments of anterior terminal branch of internal saphenous nerve (Cruveilhier, 1836)*
   As described, for *anterior terminal branch of internal saphenous nerve (Cruveilhier, 1836)*; in the original French, *filets descendans*, p. 847.
3. *middle filaments of anterior terminal branch of internal saphenous nerve (Cruveilhier, 1836)*
   As described, for *anterior terminal branch of internal saphenous nerve (Cruveilhier, 1836)*; in the original French, *filets moyens*, p. 847.

infratrochlear nerve (Schaarschmidt, 1750)

As described for macrodissected adult human, a branch of the ***nasociliary nerve (Meckel, 1817; Wutzer, 1817)*** arising at the same point as the ***anterior ethmoidal nerve (>1840)***, which is regarded as the continuation of the ***nasociliary nerve (Meckel, 1817; Wutzer, 1817)***. It supplies branches to skin of the eyelids and side of the nose above the medial angle of the eye, conjunctiva, lacrimal sac, and lacrimal caruncle; see Williams & Warwick (1980, pp. 1061–1062, Fig. 7.176), Hamilton (1976, Fig. 793). For Schaarschmidt's use in macrodissected adult human, see p. 15. Meckel (1753, see Tab. 1-*13 ff.*) provided a detailed description of its branches for macrodissected adult human. It was probably first recognized as the *surculus quartus crassioris ac interioris propaginis K (Vieussens, 1684)*.

TRANSLATIONS:

1. *nervus infratrochlearis (Schaarschmidt, 1750)*
   Original Latin form of ***infratrochlear nerve (Schaarschmidt, 1750)***; p. 15.
2. *nerf infra-trochléaire (Meckel, 1753)*
   Original French form of ***infratrochlear nerve (Schaarschmidt, 1750)***; p. 40.
3. *nerf sus-trochleaire (Meckel, 1753)*
   Original French form of ***infratrochlear nerve (Schaarschmidt, 1750)***; Table 1-*13,24*.

EARLIER REFERENCES:

Earlier synonyms:

1. *surculus quartus crassioris ac interioris propaginis K (Vieussens, 1684)*
   May correspond roughly to macrodissected adult human ***infratrochlear nerve (Schaarschmidt, 1750)***; p. 171 and Table 22-*o*.
2. *infratrochlear branch of nasal branch of first branch of fifth pair (Meckel, 1748)*
   Synonym for macrodissected adult human ***infratrochlear nerve (Schaarschmidt, 1750)***; pp. 31, 44.

LATER SYNONYMS:

1. *inner lesser frontal nerve (Meckel, 1753)*
   Synonym for macrodissected adult human ***infratrochlear nerve (Schaarschmidt, 1750)***; in the original French, *le petit nerf frontal intérieur*, Table 1-*17*.
2. *inferior frontal nerve (Martin, 1781)*
   Synonym for macrodissected adult human ***infratrochlear nerve (Schaarschmidt, 1750)***; in the original Latin, *frontalis inferior*, Table II.
3. *external nasal nerve (Meckel, 1817)*
   Synonym for macrodissected adult human ***infratrochlear nerve (Schaarschmidt, 1750)***; see translation (1832, Vol. 3, p. 64).
4. *superior nerve (Jacobson, 1818)*
   Synonym for macrodissected adult mammalian ***infratrochlear nerve (Schaarschmidt, 1750)***; in the original Latin, *nervus superior*, p. 17.
5. *infratrochlear branch of nasociliary nerve (Arnold, 1834)*
   Synonym for macrodissected adult mammalian ***infratrochlear nerve (Schaarschmidt, 1750)***; in the original Latin, *nervus nasociliaris, ramus infratrochlearis*, p. 8.
6. *infratrochlear branch of nasal nerve (Arnold, 1834)*
   Synonym for macrodissected adult mammalian ***infratrochlear nerve (Schaarschmidt, 1750)***; in the original Latin, *nervus nasalis, ramus infratrochlearis*, p. 8.
7. *external nasal branch of nasal nerve (Cruveilhier, 1836)*
   Synonym for macrodissected adult human ***infratrochlear nerve (Schaarschmidt, 1750)***; in the original French, *rameau nasal externe*, p. 915.
8. *palpebral nerve (Cruveilhier, 1836)*
   Synonym for macrodissected adult human ***infratrochlear nerve (Schaarschmidt, 1750)*** attributed without citation to Chaussier; in the original French, *palpébral*, p. 915.

PARTLY CORRESPONDS:

1. *anterior frontal branch of infratrochlear nerve (Meckel, 1753)*
   Branch of macrodissected adult human ***infratrochlear nerve (Schaarschmidt, 1750)***; in the original French, *le rameau frontal antérieur du nerf intra-trochleaire*, Table 1-*18*.
2. *frontal cutaneous branch of infratrochlear nerve (Meckel, 1753)*
   Branch of macrodissected adult human ***infratrochlear nerve (Schaarschmidt, 1750)***; in the original French, *le rameau cutané du front du nerf intra-trochleaire*, Table 1-*18*.
3. *superior interior palpebral nerve (Mayer, 1794)*
   Branch of macrodissected adult human ***infratrochlear nerve (Schaarschmidt, 1750)*** to medial regions of upper eyelid; in the original Latin, *nervus palpebralis internus superior*; Part 5, Table VII-*20* (p. 43).
4. *palpebro-frontal threads of infratrochlear fascicle (Bellingeri, 1818)*
   Branches of macrodissected adult human ***infratrochlear nerve (Schaarschmidt, 1750)*** to upper eyelid, frontalis and orbicularis oculi muscles, and skin of forehead; in the original Latin, *stamina palpebro-frontalis*, see Table I.

5. *oculo-nasal threads of infratrochlear fascicle (Bellingeri, 1818)*
   Branches of macrodissected adult human ***infratrochlear nerve (Schaarschmidt, 1750)*** to caruncle of eye, lacrimal sac, "m. pyramid." (probably corrugator supercilii muscle), and skin of nose; in the original Latin, *stamina oculo-nasalis*, see Table I.
6. *nasal filaments of external nasal branch of nasal nerve (Cruveilhier, 1836)*
   Branchlets of macrodissected adult human ***infratrochlear nerve (Schaarschmidt, 1750)*** to ridge (dorsum) of nose; in the original French, *filets nasaux*, p. 915.
7. *frontal filaments of external nasal branch of nasal nerve (Cruveilhier, 1836)*
   Small ***communicating branches (Winslow, 1733)*** of macrodissected adult human ***infratrochlear nerve (Schaarschmidt, 1750)*** with ***supratrochlear nerve (Schaarschmidt, 1750)***; in the original French, *filets frontaux*, p. 915.

infundibular recess (>1840)

As described for macrodissected adult mammal, the ventral extension of the ***hypothalamic part of third ventricle (Swanson, 2004)*** within the ***infundibulum (Rioch et al., 1940)***; see Williams & Warwick (1980, p. 981), *Terminologia Anatomica* (1998, p. 121). It was observed long ago by Galen; see ***[infundibular recess (>1840)] (Galen, c173)***.

EARLIER REFERENCES:

Described, not named or illustrated:

1. ***[infundibular recess (>1840)] (Galen, c173)***
   Clearly described in macrodissected adult large mammals like beef, pig, and/or macaque, but not human, as component of overall *infundibulum (Galen, c173)*; see May translation (1968, p. 429).

infundibular stem (Hanström, 1966)

As described histologically for adult human (and all other vertebrates), the part of the ***infundibulum (Rioch et al., 1940)*** distal to the ***median eminence (Tilney, 1936)***, characterized by ***axons (Kölliker, 1896)*** of magnocellular neuroendocrine ***neurons (Waldeyer, 1891)*** and components of the hypophysial portal system and often accompanied by the ***tuberal part of anterior lobe of pituitary (>1840)***; see Holmes & Ball (1974, pp. 5–6), Daniel & Pritchard (1975, Chs. 1, 3), *pituitary stalk (Lieutaud, 1742)*. It expands distally into the ***posterior lobe of pituitary gland (Haller, 1762)***. It was at least noted long ago by Rufus of Ephesus; see ***[infundibular stem (Hanström, 1996)] (Rufus of Ephesus, fl. c90–120)***.

EARLIER REFERENCES:

Described, not named or illustrated:

1. ***[infundibular stem (Hanström, 1996)] (Rufus of Ephesus, fl. c90–120)***
   Rufus of Ephesus described it vaguely, but could not have known about investment of ***tuberal part of anterior lobe (>1840)***; see *infundibulum (Rufus of Ephesus, fl. c90–120)*. Vesalius (1543a) described it more clearly for macrodissected adult human; see ***[median eminence (Tilney, 1936)] (Vesalius, 1543a)***.

PARTLY CORRESPONDS:

1. *infundibulum (Tilney, 1936)*
   Proximal part of mammalian ***infundibular stem (Hanström, 1966)***; p. 424.
2. *infundibular stem (Tilney, 1936)*
   Distal part of mammalian ***infundibular stem (Hanström, 1966)***; p. 425.

infundibulum (Rioch et al., 1940)

As described histologically in adult mammal, an unpaired ventral extension of the ***periventricular hypothalamic zone (Nauta & Haymaker, 1969)*** with two parts, ***median eminence (Tilney, 1936)*** and ***infundibular stem (Hanström, 1966)***. It is the proximal part of the ***neurohypophysis (Rioch et al., 1940)***, the distal part being the ***posterior lobe of pituitary gland (Haller, 1762)***; see Daniel & Pritchard (1975, Chs. 1, 3), Nauta & Haymaker (1969, pp. 136–141), Williams & Warwick (1980, p. 1439). For use by Rioch et al. in adult mammal, see p. 24. In early development ***infundibulum (>1840)*** has a different meaning, referring to what will become the entire ***neurohypophysis (Rioch et al., 1940)***. It was described at least partly by Vesalius; see ***[infundibulum (Rioch et al. (1940)] (Vesalius, 1543a)***.

EARLIER REFERENCES:

Described, not named or illustrated:

1. ***[infundibulum (Rioch et al. (1940)] (Vesalius, 1543a)***
   Described partly for macrodissected adult human; see ***[median eminence (Tilney, 1936)] (Vesalius, 1543a)***.

LATER SYNONYMS:

1. *neural stalk (Rioch et al., 1940)*
   Synonym for ***infundibulum (Rioch et al., 1940)***; Table 2.
2. *hypophysial stalk (Rioch et al., 1940)*
   Synonym for ***infundibulum (Rioch et al., 1940)***; p. 28.

infundibulum (>1840)

As described histologically in developing mammal, an unpaired ventral extension in the median plane of the ***primary forebrain vesicle (Baer, 1837)*** and then later the ***interbrain vesicle (Baer, 1837)*** going on to form the entire ***neurohypophysis (Rioch et al., 1940)*** in adult; see Hamilton & Mossman (1972, pp. 472–473, Fig. 445A), Alvarez-Bolado & Swanson (1996, Figs. 9, 13, 14). It was not identified by 1840.

inner part of transverse cerebral fissure (>1840)

As described for macrodissected adult human, the part of the ***transverse cerebral fissure (>1840)*** occupying the rostrocaudal (horizontal) space between the dorsal surfaces of the ***thalamus (His, 1893a)*** and ***tectum (Baer, 1837)*** on the ventral side, and the ventral surface of the ***fornix (Vesalius, 1543a)*** on the dorsal side. It contains the ***choroid membrane of third ventricle (>1840)***, and is filled with ***cerebrospinal fluid (Magendie, 1827)***; see

Carpenter (1976, pp. 65–66), illustrated beautifully by Rasmussen (1932, Fig. 1). It was first delineated clearly by Steno; see ***[inner part of transverse cerebral fissure (>1840)] (Steno, 1669)***.

EARLIER REFERENCES:

Illustrated, not named or described:

1. ***[inner part of transverse cerebral fissure (>1840)] (Steno, 1669)***
Clearly illustrated for macrodissected adult human in midsagittal view; Plate I.

Earlier synonyms:

1. *large transverse fissure (Bichat, 1802)*
Synonym for macrodissected adult human ***inner part of transverse cerebral fissure (>1840)***; in the original French, *un large fente transversale*, p. 24 and pp. 14–16. Also see Meckel (1817; and translation, 1832, Vol. 2, p. 459), who contrasted it with *small transverse fissure (Meckel, 1817)* or ***transverse cerebellar fissure (Burdach, 1822)***.
2. *middle fissure (Bichat, 1802)*
Synonym for *great transverse fissure (Bichat, 1802)*; in the original French, cette *fente moyenne*, p. 24.
3. *great cerebral fissure (Bichat, 1802)*
Synonym for *large transverse fissure (Bichat, 1802)*; in the original French, *grande fente cérébrale*, p, 73.
4. *fissura cerebralis magna (Bichat, 1802)*
Latin form of *great cerebral fissure (Bichat, 1802)*; see Burdach (1822, p. 386), Foster (1892, p. 1601).
5. *fissura posterior (Ramsay, 1813)*
Synonym for macrodissected adult human *fissura cerebralis magna (Bichat, 1802)*; p. 48, Plate XV, Figure 2-‡. Also see Burdach (1822, p. 387), who attributed to Ramsay the term *fissura magna posterior*.
6. *fissura cerebri transversa magna (Meckel, 1817)*
Synonym for macrodissected adult human *great cerebral fissure (Bichat, 1802)*; p. 522, see translation (1832, Vol. 2, p. 459).
7. *large transverse cerebral fissure (Meckel, 1817)*
English form of *fissura cerebri transversa magna (Meckel, 1817)*; see translation (1832, Vol. 2, p. 459).
8. *rima transversa cerebri (Burdach, 1822)*
Synonym for macrodissected adult human *great transverse fissure (Bichat, 1802)*; p. 165.
9. *fissure of Bichât (Quain, 1828)*
Eponym for macrodissected adult human *great transverse fissure (Bichat, 1802)*; p. 623.
10. *foramen of Bichat (Solly, 1836)*
Eponym for macrodissected adult human *great transverse fissure (Bichat, 1802)*; p. 177.
11. *cerebral fissure (Cruveilhier, 1836)*
Synonym for macrodissected adult human *great cerebral fissure (Bichat, 1802)*; in the original French, *fente cérébrale*, p. 695.
12. *mouth of ventricles (Gerdy, 1838)*
Synonym for macrodissected adult human *great cerebral fissure (Bichat, 1802)*; in the original French, *bouche des ventricules*, p. 259.
13. *great fissure of Bichat (Broca, 1878b)*
Eponym for *fissura cerebralis magna (Bichat, 1802)*; in the original French, *la grand fente de Bichat*, p. 404.
14. *transverse cerebral fissure (>1840)*
Essentially, synonym for macrodissected adult human ***inner part of transverse cerebral fissure (>1840)***; see Kuhlenbeck (1978, p. 150), *Dorland's* (2003, p. 704).

insular region (Brodmann, 1909)

As described for macrodissected adult human, a triangular topographic division of the ***cerebral cortex gray matter (>1840)*** lying deep in the floor of the ***lateral cerebral fossa (>1840)*** and separated from opercular parts of the ***frontal region (Vicq d'Azyr, 1786)***, ***parietal region (>1840)***, and ***temporal region (>1840)*** by the ***circular sulcus (Schwalbe, 1881)***. It usually consists of 3–4 ***short gyri of insula (Gall & Spurzheim, 1810)*** rostrally, separated by the ***central sulcus of insula (>1840)*** from the ***long gyrus of insula (Valentin, 1841)*** caudally. The triangle's apex is directed ventrally (inferiorly) toward the ***olfactory tubercle (Calleja, 1893)***, where the ***circular sulcus (Schwalbe, 1881)*** is lacking and the medial part of the apex is bounded by the ***ambient gyrus (>1840)***, corresponding to the histologically defined ***piriform area (Smith, 1919)***; see Nauta & Haymaker (1969, Fig. 4.10-*GA*). For modern overviews see Crosby et al. (1962, pp. 476–477, Figs. 316, 319), Williams & Warwick (1980, pp. 987, 988), Nieuwenhuys et al. (2008, p. 649 ff.). For Brodmann's use in cellular architecture studies of adult human, see p. 146 and Figure 89; for his use in all mammals, which included *areas 13–16 (Brodmann, 1909)*, see Table 7, p. 247. ***Insular region (>1840)*** is preferred to *insula (Reil, 1809b)* for the sake of uniformity with other *regions* of the ***cerebral cortex gray matter (>1840)***. It was first illustrated, at least partly, by Vesalius; see ***[insular region (Brodmann, 1909)] (Vesalius, 1543a)***.

TRANSLATIONS:

1. *regio insularis (Brodmann, 1909)*
Original Latin form of ***insular region (Brodmann, 1909)***; p. 146.

EARLIER REFERENCES:

Illustrated, not named or described:

1. ***[insular region (Brodmann, 1909)] (Vesalius, 1543a)***
Part of left ***insular region (Brodmann, 1909)*** illustrated in frontal (horizontal) slice through macrodissected adult human ***cerebrum (Obersteiner & Hill, 1900)***; see Singer translation (1952, Fig. 4, *E* and *F* on right side of figure, p. 95), Meyer (1971, p. 10). It was also illustrated by Eustachi (1552; see Albinus edition, 1761, Tab. 17, Fig. 2 near middle *D*), and very clearly illustrated by Bartholin (1641; see Clarke & Dewhurst, 1996, Fig. 90).

Described, not named or illustrated:

1. ***[insular region (Brodmann, 1909)] (Varoli, 1573)***
Varoli described it clearly for macrodissected adult human, pointing out that *middle cerebral prominence (Varoli, 1573)* and *anterior cerebral prominence (Varoli,*

1573), roughly ***temporal region (>1840)*** and ***frontal region (Vicq d'Azyr, 1786)*** respectively, are contiguous and can be separated; see Clarke & O'Malley (1996, p. 822).

Illustrated and described, not named:

1. ***[insular region (Brodmann, 1909)] (Bartholin, 1641)*** Footnote on p. 262 by Bartholin's teacher, Frans de Le Boë (Franciscus Sylvius), described accurately ***lateral cerebral sulcus (>1840)*** for first time, and it is illustrated, along with ***insular region (Brodmann, 1909)***, in Figure 5-*i,k*. According to Bartholin (1551), "The windings [*cerebral gyri (Vesalius, 1543a)*] of the brain [*cerebral cortex (Bauhin, 1605)*] (which I first learnt of *Fr. Sylvius* a great Anatomist) if you diligently examin the matter, you shall find to descend a good depth, & that the brain doth gape on each side, over & above that same middle division made by the Sickle, with a winding clift [***lateral cerebral sulcus (>1840)***] ["See *Tab. 3*." in accompanying margin note], which begins in the forepart, about the roots of the Eyes, whence according to the bones of the Temples, it goes back above the Root of the spinal Marrow [***cerebral nuclei (Swanson, 2000a)***], and divides the upper part of the brain [*cerebral cortex (Bauhin, 1605)*] from the lower part." (Culpeper translation, 1662, p. 134).

Earlier synonyms:

1. *convolutions of Sylvian sulcus (Vicq d'Azyr, 1786)*
   Refers to macrodissected adult human ***insular region (Brodmann, 1909)***; in the original French, *substance corticale des circonvolutions de la scissure de Sylvius*, Table 13 legend, see Meyer (1971, p. 127).
2. *insula (Reil, 1809b)*
   Macrodissected adult human ***insular region (Brodmann, 1909)*** described as "the oval floor of the fissura Sylvii, on which are placed small and low convolutions, surrounded by a furrow [***circular sulcus (Schwalbe, 1881)***]: the entrance [*limen insulae (>1840)*] of the fissura Sylvii is its lower and anterior extremity." (pp. 144, 196; see Mayo translation, 1823, p. 52). Also see Burdach (1822, p. 387). In the original German, *das Insel*.
3. *island (Reil, 1809b)*
   English form of *insula (Reil, 1809b)*.
4. *deep convolutions of great cerebral sulcus (Gall & Spurzheim, 1810)*
   Synonym for macrodissected adult human ***insular region (Brodmann, 1909)***; in the original French, *circonvolutions au fond de la grande scissure cérébrale*, Table 5-42 legend, see Meyer (1971, p. 127 note 8).
5. *island of Sylvian fissure (Meckel, 1817)*
   Synonym for macrodissected adult human *insula (Reil, 1809b)*; see translation (1832, Vol. 2, p. 442).
6. *lobus caudicis (Burdach, 1822)*
   Synonym for macrodissected adult human *insula (Reil, 1809b)*; in the original German, *Stammlappen*, p. 167, see Meyer (1971, p. 167).
7. *stem lobe (Burdach, 1822)*
   Translation of *lobus caudicis (Burdach, 1822)* provided by Meyer (1971, p. 167) from the fact that it lies close to what Burdach considered the rostral end of the stem of the brain, the *lenticular nucleus (Burdach, 1822)*.
8. *island of Reil (Cruveilhier, 1836)*
   Eponym for macrodissected adult human *insula (Reil, 1809b)*; in the original Latin, "*insula*, Reil", p. 657; and in the original French, *insula de Reil*, p. 660.
9. *lobule of Sylvian fissure (Cruveilhier, 1836)*
   Synonym for macrodissected adult human *insula (Reil, 1809b)*; in the original French, *lobule de la scissure de Sylvius*, p. 657.
10. *lobule of striate body (Cruveilhier, 1836)*
    Synonym for macrodissected adult human *insula (Reil, 1809b)*; in the original French, *lobule du corps strié*, pp. 657, 692.
11. *areas 13–16 (Brodmann, 1909)*
    Correspond to adult mammalian ***insular region (Brodmann, 1909)*** based on cellular architecture; in the original German, *Feld 13–16*, see p. 209 and Table 7 on p. 247.

interbrain (Baer, 1837)

The caudal unpaired topographic division of the vertebrate ***forebrain (Goette, 1873)***, the rostral division being the right and left ***endbrain (Kuhlenbeck, 1927)***. The ***midbrain (Baer, 1837)*** lies caudal to the ***interbrain (Baer, 1837)***, which contains the entire ***third ventricle (Galen, c173)*** and is divided into ***hypothalamus (Kuhlenbeck, 1927)*** ventrally and ***thalamus (His, 1893a)*** dorsally. For these precise definitions see Swanson & Bota (2010). Sharpey et al. (1867, p. 577) introduced the English translation *interbrain*, which was also used by Meynert (see 1872 translation, p. 653), Edinger (1890, p. 25), Barker (1899, p. 163), Emmel (1921, p. xxv) [using *interbrain (His, 1893b)*], Papez (1929, p. 129), Strong & Elwyn (1943, p. 11), Williams (1989, *Table of Contents*). Kuhlenbeck (1927, Chs. 3, 9) gave the currently accepted histological description of vertebrate ***interbrain (Baer, 1837)*** borders, especially with respect to the ***endbrain (Kuhlenbeck, 1927)***. The *interbrain (His, 1893b)* is quite different. The general region of the ***interbrain (Baer, 1837)*** was distinguished long ago as the *pars posterior medullae spinalis (Varoli, 1573)*.

TRANSLATIONS:

1. *Zwischenhirn (Baer, 1837)*
   Original German form of ***interbrain (Baer, 1837)***; p. 107. Sharpey et al. (1867, p. 577) introduced the English translation, *interbrain*.
2. *diencephalon (Sharpey et al., 1867)*
   Latin form of ***interbrain (Baer, 1837)***; p. 577.

EARLIER REFERENCES:

Earlier synonyms:

1. *pars posterior medullae spinalis (Varoli, 1591)*
   Rough synonym for macrodissected adult human ***interbrain (Baer, 1837)***; p. 13, see Burdach (1822, p. 340). Probably equivalent to *thalami nervorum opticorum (Riolan, 1618)*.

2. *thalami nervorum opticorum (Riolan, 1618)*
Riolan was apparently the first to use this Greek-Latin term for roughly the macrodissected adult human ***interbrain (Baer, 1837)***; p. 419, also see Polyak (1957, p. 105). Furthermore, he described how the *optic nerve (Galen, c173)*, that is, the ***optic tract (Vicq d'Azyr, 1784)***, wraps around the side of *thalami nervorum opticorum (Riolan, 1618)* to reach the ***inferior horn of lateral ventricle (Bell, 1802)***; see Bartholin (1662, pp. 324–325), also see *thalamus (Galen, c173)*. In early descriptions it was usually unclear how *infundibulum (Galen, c173)* was viewed in relation to *thalami nervorum opticorum (Riolan, 1618)*: was it a ventral part, a ventral extension, or a separate part ventral to it?
3. *thalamus nervi optici (Riolan, 1618)*
Singular Latin form of *thalami nervorum opticorum (Riolan, 1618)*; see Monro (1783, Tab. II-*T*).
4. *couchette des nerf optique (Riolan, 1628–1629)*
Riolan's own French form of *thalamus nervi optici (Riolan, 1618)*; p. 583.
5. *bed of optic nerve (Riolan, 1657)*
Culpeper's translation of *thalamus nervi optici (Riolan, 1618)*; p. 123.
6. *conjunction of round trunks (Bartholin, 1662)*
Bartholin's description of merged *round trunks (Bartholin, 1662)*, separated by ***third ventricle (Galen, c173)***, after they have proceeded out of *brain (Piccolomini, 1586, definition 2)* or ***cerebral cortex gray matter (>1840)***; corresponds roughly to macrodissected adult human ***interbrain (Baer, 1837)***; pp. 140–141.
7. *chambers of optic nerve (Willis, 1664)*
Synonym for macrodissected adult mammalian *thalami nervorum opticorum (Riolan, 1618)*; see Pordage translation (1681, pp. 63–64).
8. *second section of oblong marrow (Willis, 1664)*
Synonym for macrodissected adult mammalian *thalami nervorum opticorum (Riolan, 1618)*, roughly the ***interbrain (Baer, 1837)***; see Pordage translation (1681, p. 139).
9. *second pair of tubercles (Steno, 1669)*
Synonym for macrodissected adult human *thalami nervorum opticorum (Riolan, 1618)*, the ***interbrain (Baer, 1837)***; see translation (pp. 134, 137, 150) and Winslow 1733 (Sect. X, p. 61). Arnold (1838a, p. 62) gave the Latin, *secundum par gangliorum*, but this is not quite accurate.
10. *striatal protuberances (Diemerbroeck, 1672)*
Synonym for macrodissected adult human *thalami nervorum opticorum (Riolan, 1618)*, according to Burdach (1822, p. 340).
11. *thalamus (Malpighi, 1673)*
Simplified form of *thalami nervorum opticorum (Riolan, 1618)* Malpighi introduced for ***interbrain (Baer, 1837)***, based on his analysis of chick development; see Adelmann (1966, p. 967). Used thus as late as Papez (1929, p. 129). Bell noted (1802, p. 29) its precise identity is rather confused.
12. *couche optique (Saint Hilaire, 1680)*
French translation and shortening of *thalamus nervi optici (Riolan, 1618)* and *couchette des nerf optique (Riolan, 1628–1629)*; p. 30.
13. *striata corpora superna et posteriora (Vieussens, 1684)*
Synonym for macrodissected adult human ***interbrain (Baer, 1837)***; Table X-*E*, interpretation according to Haller (1762, p. 51), Chaussier (1807, p. 63), and Meyer (1971, p. 13).
14. *striata corpora posteriora interna (Vieussens, 1684)*
Haller (1762, p. 51) thought Vieussens used it synonymously with *striata corpora superna et posteriora (Vieussens, 1684)*, confirmed by Burdach (1822, p. 340).
15. *striata corpora posteriora et superna (Vieussens, 1684)*
Meckel's (1817) version of *striata corpora superna et posteriora (Vieussens, 1684)*; see translation (1832, Vol. 2, p. 452). Schreger (1803, p. 320) used the form *striata corp. posteriora superiora*.
16. *crura medullae oblongatae (Vieussens, 1684)*
Synonym for roughly right and left halves of ***interbrain (Baer, 1837)***; Table VIII-C, also see Haller (1762, p. 51), Meyer (1971, p. 13).
17. *nuptual chambers of optic nerves (Diemerbroeck, 1689)*
Translation of *thalami nervorum opticorum (Riolan, 1618)*; p. 400.
18. *juga crurum medullae oblongatae (Ridley, 1695)*
Synonym for macrodissected adult human ***interbrain (Baer, 1837)***; p. 120. Ridley wrote that the undermost side, roughly the ***hypothalamus (Kuhlenbeck, 1927)***, is quite different from roughly the ***thalamus (His, 1893a)***, which forms the uppermost segment of the *crura medulla oblongata (Vieussens, 1684)*; p. 121. *Juga* means *tops*; p. 121.
19. *capita medulla oblongata (Ridley, 1695)*
Synonym for macrodissected adult human *thalami nervorum opticorum (Riolan, 1618)*, roughly ***interbrain (Baer, 1837)***; pp. 120–121, also see Haller (1762, p. 51).
20. *thalamus opticus (Poupart, 1712)*
Latin form of *couche optique (Saint Hilaire, 1680)*; p. 644.
21. *optic bed (Poupart, 1712)*
English form of *thalamus opticus (Poupart, 1712)*; p. 644.
22. *optic eminence (Poupart, 1712)*
Apparently synonym for *thalamus opticus (Poupart, 1712)*; pp. 645, 647.
23. *stringy protuberance (Salmon, 1714)*
Apparently synonym for macrodissected adult human *thalami nervi optici (Riolan, 1618)*; p. 414.
24. *summitates medullae oblongatae (Steenbergen, 1731)*
Apparently synonym for macrodissected adult human *thalami nervi optici (Riolan, 1618)*; p. 30, according to Burdach (1822, p. 340).
25. *thalamos (Haller, 1747)*
Simplified form for macrodissected adult human of *thalami nervorum opticorum (Riolan, 1618)*, p. 181; Haller also used the plural, *thalami* (p. 181).

26. *thalamus ophthalmicis (Haase, 1781)*
Variation on macrodissected adult human *thalamus opticus (Poupart, 1712)*; Index, section 66.
27. *posterior striate body of Vieussens (Günther, 1786)*
Eponym for macrodissected adult human (plural) *striata corpora superna et posteriora (Vieussens, 1684)*; in the original Latin, *corpus striatum posterius Vieussenii*, p. 10.
28. *colliculi of optic nerve (Soemmerring, 1791)*
Synonym for macrodissected adult human *thalami nervi optici (Riolan, 1618)*; in the original Latin, *colliculi nervorum opticorum*, p. 39, according to Chaussier (1807, p. 63) and Burdach (1822, p. 340). Bock (1824) supplied singular form, *colliculus of optic nerve*; in the original Latin, *colliculus nervi optici*, p. 154.
29. *optic thalamus (Bell, 1802)*
English form of *couche optique (Saint Hilaire, 1680)*, p. 44; plural form, *optic thalami*.
30. *layers of ocular nerves (Burdin, 1803)*
Synonym for macrodissected adult human ***interbrain (Baer, 1837)***; see translation (1803, Vol. 1, p. 159).
31. *layers of optic nerves (Burdin, 1803)*
Synonym for macrodissected adult human ***interbrain (Baer, 1837)***; see translation (1803, Vol. 1, p. 159).
32. *bed of ocular nerve (Chaussier, 1807)*
Synonym for macrodissected adult human ***interbrain (Baer, 1837)***; in the original French, *couche du nerf oculaire*, pp. 56, 63.
33. *optic colliculus (Soemmerring, 1809)*
Synonym for *colliculi nervorum opticorum (Soemmerring, 1791)*; in the original Latin, *colliculorum opticorum*, p. 58.
34. *thalamus (Reil, 1809b)*
Reil used it to indicate roughly macrodissected adult human ***interbrain (Baer, 1837)***, and wrote that it consists of three layers, each with outer white part and inner gray part. These divisions were vaguely described and not clearly illustrated. In this vein he wrote, "Yet, must it not be expected, that in the tubercula [***tectum (Baer, 1837)***], and still less in the thalami, the different layers lie distinct: they are rather fused, and blended in one mass" (Reil, 1809c; see Mayo translation, 1823, p. 101). Nevertheless, in modern terms, superficial part of first layer is continuous caudally (posteriorly) with ***optic tract (Vicq d'Azyr, 1784)***; second layer is separated from first by ***mammillothalamic tract (>1840)***, and its gray part consists of ***medial geniculate complex (>1840)*** and ***anterior thalamic nuclei (>1840)*** and ***gray matter regions (Swanson & Bota, 2010)*** in between; and third layer is formed superficially by ***medial lemniscus (>1840)***; Reil (1809b), see Mayo translation (1823, pp. 57–58, 76). This interpretation is supported by Meckel's (1817) description; see translation (1832, Vol. 2, pp. 452–453).
35. *posterior cerebral ganglion (Gall & Spurzheim, 1810)*
One way Gall & Spurzheim referred to macrodissected adult human *thalamus nervi optici (Riolan, 1618)*; pp. 198–199.
36. *posterior and interior cerebral ganglion (Gall & Spurzheim, 1810)*
One way Gall & Spurzheim referred to macrodissected adult human *thalamus nervi optici (Riolan, 1618)*; pp. 198–199.
37. *great inferior cerebral ganglion (Gall & Spurzheim, 1810)*
Synonym for macrodissected adult human *thalamus nervi optici (Riolan, 1618)*; in the original French, *le grande ganglion inférieur*, pp. 204, 208. Also see Burdach (1822, p. 340) and Spurzheim (1826, p. 226), who also used *great inferior ganglion of brain*.
38. *colliculus opticus (Wenzel & Wenzel, 1812)*
Singular derivative of *colliculi nervorum opticorum (Soemmerring, 1800)*, thus referring to right or left half in macrodissected adult human; Table IV, Figure 1-*e*.
39. *posterior inner ganglia of optic tubercles (Carus, 1814)*
Synonym for ***interbrain (Baer, 1837)*** of macrodissected adult fish; in the original German, *hintern innern Ganglien des Sehhügels*, pp. 139, 155.
40. *optic tubercle (Carus, 1814, p. 176)*
Synonym for macrodissected adult amphibian and bird ***interbrain (Baer, 1837)***; in the original German, *Sehhügel*; pp. 176, 201.
41. *hemispheric ganglion (Carus, 1814)*
Synonym for macrodissected adult amphibian through human ***interbrain (Baer, 1837)***; in the original German, *Ganglien der Hemisphären*; e.g., pp. 176, 198, 223, Table VI-ç. Also see Carus (1818, Tab. XII, Fig. 4-*b* and Tab. XV, Fig. 3-*a**), Burdach (1822, p. 340).
42. *brain ganglia (Meckel, 1815)*
Synonym for macrodissected embryonic and adult mammalian ***interbrain (Baer, 1837)***; in the original German, *Hirnganglien*, pp. 380–383 and Tables I, II, part *d*.
43. *posterior medullary nucleus of Reil (Tiedemann, 1821)*
Eponym for macrodissected adult monkey ***interbrain (Baer, 1837)***; in the original Latin, *nuclei medullares posteriores Reili*, Table II, Figure 2-*d*. Citation to Reil not provided.
44. *ocular nerve colliculus (Burdach, 1822)*
Synonym for macrodissected adult human *bed of ocular nerve (Chaussier, 1807)*; in the original Latin (plural), *colliculi nervorum ocularium*, p. 340.
45. *great ganglions of affective powers (Spurzheim, 1826)*
Synonym for macrodissected adult mammalian ***interbrain (Baer, 1837)***; p. 208.
46. *inferior cerebral ganglion (Quain, 1828)*
Synonym for macrodissected adult mammalian ***interbrain (Baer, 1837)***; p. 625.
47. *posterior ganglion of spinal cord (Solly, 1836)*
Synonym for macrodissected adult human ***interbrain (Baer, 1837)***; p. 179.
48. *sensory ganglion of spinal cord (Solly, 1836)*
Synonym for macrodissected adult human ***interbrain (Baer, 1837)***; p. 179.

49. *posterior striated body (Solly, 1836)*
Synonym for macrodissected adult human ***interbrain (Baer, 1837)***; Figure 1-*E*, p. 180.

LATER SYNONYMS:

1. *opticos (Gerdy, 1838)*
Synonym for macrodissected adult human ***interbrain (Baer, 1837)***; p. 259.
2. *great ganglion of middle and posterior lobes (Combe et al., 1838)*
Synonym for macrodissected adult human ***interbrain (Baer, 1837)***; p. xxvi.
3. *great inferior ganglion (Arnold, 1838a)*
Synonym for macrodissected adult human *great inferior cerebral ganglion (Gall & Spurzheim, 1810)*; in the original Latin (plural), *ganglia magna inferiora*, p. 62.
4. *great posterior ganglion (Arnold, 1838a)*
Synonym for macrodissected adult human *great inferior cerebral ganglion (Gall & Spurzheim, 1810)*; in the original Latin (plural), *ganglia magna posteriora*, p. 62.
5. *optic nerve colliculus (Arnold, 1838b)*
Synonym for macrodissected adult human ***interbrain (Baer, 1837)***; in the original Latin (plural), *colliculi nervorum opticorum*, Table IV, Figure 3-*β*.

PARTLY CORRESPONDS:

1. *buttocks (Berengario da Carpi, 1522)*
In *A Short Introduction to Anatomy*, Berengario seemed to indicate that the walls of the ***third ventricle (Galen, c173)***, and thus the medial walls of the ***interbrain (Baer, 1837)***, look like human buttocks. He wrote, "In the [lateral] ventricle on both sides near the base is a pellicular red substance called a worm [***choroid plexus (Galen, c177)***], composed of veins and arteries, which reaches from one end to the other of each ventricle...*Below* [emphasis added] the worms at their sides is a certain eminent part of the brain which many compare to the human buttocks in its form. This part both in elongation and closing of the ventricles touches its two portions together and separates them in the shortening and dilation of the ventricles." (Lind translation, 1959, p. 143). And then, "Near this embotum [***hypothalamic part of third ventricle (Swanson, 2004)***] toward the rear also under the ventricles mentioned before is a certain somewhat oblong vacuity whose walls are like the aforesaid buttocks...Authors commonly regard this vacuity as the middle [third] ventricle..." (Lind translation, 1959, p. 144). This is a rather clear use of *buttocks (Mondino, 1316)*, although Mondino's description itself is ambiguous, as is a slightly later reference to Berengario da Carpi's work (Dryander, 1536; see Lind, 1975, p. 301).
2. *bed of gray substance (Reil, 1812c)*
Referred vaguely to posteromedial region of ***interbrain (Baer, 1837)*** associated with ***cerebral peduncle (Tarin, 1753)*** and is analogous to more dorsally placed *gray nucleus (Reil, 1811c)*, now called ***inferior colliculus (Haller, 1762)***. Rostrally *bed of gray substance (Reil, 1812c)* is connected to *medulla incognita (Reil, 1809b)* or ***substantia innominata (Meynert, 1872)*** by ***peduncular loop (Gratiolet, 1857)***; see Mayo translation (1823, p. 124).
3. *optic ganglion (Leuret, 1839)*
Macrodissected adult fish ***interbrain (Baer, 1837)*** without *inferior olfactory tubercle (Haller, 1768)*; in the original French (plural), *ganglions optiques*, p. 140.

interbrain corticospinal tract (>1840)

As described for macrodissected adult human, the longitudinal topographic segment of the ***corticospinal tract (>1840)*** in the ***posterior limb of internal capsule (>1840)***, between ***cerebral nuclei corticospinal tract (>1840)*** segment rostrally and ***cerebral peduncle (Tarin, 1753)*** caudally. It tends to be centered in more lateral parts of the ***posterior limb of internal capsule (>1840)*** and to avoid the ***sublentiform part of internal capsule (>1840)***; see Crosby et al. (1962, p. 394, Fig. 272), Williams & Warwick (1980, Fig. 7.154). Its existence was traced by Malpighi; see ***[interbrain corticospinal tract (>1840)] (Malpighi, 1666)***.

EARLIER REFERENCES:

Described, not named or illustrated:

1. ***[interbrain corticospinal tract (>1840)] (Malpighi, 1666)***
Clearly described the origin of "nerve fibers" in the ***cerebral cortex (>1840)*** coursing through the ***cerebral nuclei (Swanson, 2000a)*** and eventually reaching the ***spinal cord (Galen, c162–c166)***; see Meyer (1967, p. 189). Malpighi dissected a variety of mammals, including human, but the source of this observation is unclear. Willis (1664) thought these fibers arise in the *striated body (Willis, 1664)*, or ***cerebral nuclei (Swanson, 2000a)***, not the ***cerebral cortex (>1840)***; see Pordage translation (1681, pp. 62, 102).

Illustrated and described, not named:

1. ***[interbrain corticospinal tract (>1840)] (Vieussens, 1684)***
Clearly illustrated and described for macrodissected adult human with a scraping method; see Table XVI.

interbrain vesicle (Baer, 1837)

For macrodissected vertebrate embryo, the caudal division of the ***primary forebrain vesicle (Baer, 1837)*** developing into the adult ***interbrain (Baer, 1837)***—the ***hypothalamus (Kuhlenbeck, 1927)*** ventrally and ***thalamus (His, 1893a)*** dorsally; the rostral division is the ***endbrain vesicle (Baer, 1837)***. For Baer's use see p. 107. It was clearly recognized much earlier by Malpighi; see ***[interbrain vesicle (Baer, 1837)] (Malpighi, 1673)***.

EARLIER REFERENCES:

Illustrated and described, not named:

1. ***[interbrain vesicle (Baer, 1837)] (Malpighi, 1673)***
Clearly identified in 3-day macrodissected chick embryo; see Figure XVIII.

Earlier synonyms:

1. *optic thalamus vesicles (Serres, 1824–1826)*
Synonym for macrodissected vertebrate ***interbrain vesicle (Baer, 1837)***; in the original French, *vésicules de la couche optique*, Plate I, Figure 4-8.

LATER SYNONYMS:

1. *cell for optic thalamus and cerebral peduncle (Wagner, 1839)*
   Synonym for macrodissected embryonic chick ***inter-brain vesicle (Baer, 1837)***; in the original Latin, *cellula pro thalamis opticis et pedunculis cerebri*, Table IV, Figure 5-*c*.
2. *cerebrum medium (Wagner, 1839)*
   Synonym for macrodissected embryonic chick *cell for optic thalamus and cerebral peduncle (Wagner, 1839)*; Table IV, Figure 7-*f*; or just *optic thalamus*, Table IV, Figure 9-*c*.
3. *cell for third ventricle (Wagner, 1839)*
   Synonym for macrodissected embryonic chick *cell for optic thalamus and cerebral peduncle (Wagner, 1839)*; in the original Latin, *cellula pro ventriculo tertio*, Table XXII, Figure 2-*c*.
4. *cell for optic thalamus and third ventricle (Wagner, 1839)*
   Synonym for macrodissected embryonic human *cell for optic thalamus and cerebral peduncle (Wagner, 1839)*; in the original Latin, *cellula pro thalamis opticis et ventriculo tertio*, Table XXII, Figure 5-*c*.
5. *second cerebral cell (Wagner, 1839)*
   Synonym for macrodissected embryonic human *cell for optic thalamus and cerebral peduncle (Wagner, 1839)*; in the original Latin, *cellula cerebri secunda*, Table XXII, Figure 8-*c*[2].

intercostal nerves (Vesalius, 1543a)

As described for macrodissected adult human the first ***intercostal nerve (Vesalius, 1543a)*** is a small branch of the ***brachial plexus (Camper, 1760)***, whereas the second through last ***intercostal nerves (Vesalius, 1543a)*** constitute the ***spinal nerve ventral branches (>1840)*** for the 2nd–11th ***thoracic nerves (Diemerbroeck, 1672)***; see Durward (1951, p. 1084 and Figs. 924, 936). The ***spinal nerve ventral branch (>1840)*** for the last or twelfth ***thoracic nerve (Diemerbroeck, 1672)*** is the ***subcostal nerve (>1840)***. For Vesalius's use in macrodissected adult human, see Richardson & Carman translation (2002, pp. 171-*i*, 232-234). They were known to Galen; see *nerves in intercostal muscles (Galen, c173)*.

EARLIER REFERENCES:

Earlier synonyms:

1. *nerves in intercostal muscles (Galen, c173)*
   Synonym for *nerves of intercostal spaces (Galen, c177)* in macrodissected adult beef, pig, and/or macaque but not human; see May translation (1968, p. 703).
2. *nerves of intercostal spaces (Galen, c177)*
   Synonym for *nerves in intercostal muscles (Galen, c173)*; see Singer translation (1999, pp. 208–212, 217), Duckworth translation (1962, pp. 107, 218, 219, 222, 258, 260, 262).

LATER SYNONYMS:

1. *sinews between ribs (Geminus, 1553)*
   Synonym for macrodissected adult human ***intercostal nerves (Vesalius, 1543a)***; originally spelled *sinowes betwene ribbes*, see *The table of the figures of sinewes*.
2. *intercostal sinewes (Crooke, 1615)*
   Synonym for macrodissected adult human ***intercostal nerves (Vesalius, 1543a)***; p. 491.
3. *costal nerves (Camper, 1760)*
   Synonym for macrodissected adult human ***intercostal nerves (Vesalius, 1543a)***; in the original Latin, *nervi costales*, p. 13.
4. *anterior branch of proper intercostal nerve (Monro, 1783)*
   Synonym for macrodissected adult ox ***intercostal nerve (Vesalius, 1543a)***; Table 23-*NOP*.
5. *trunk of proper intercostal nerve (Monro, 1783)*
   Synonym for macrodissected adult ox ***intercostal nerve (Vesalius, 1543a)***; Table 23-*NOP*.
6. *intercostal branches proper (Günther, 1786)*
   Synonym for macrodissected adult human ***intercostal nerves (Vesalius, 1543a)***; in the original Latin, *r. intercostalis proprius*, p. 80.
7. *costal branch (Frotscher, 1788)*
   Synonym for macrodissected adult human ***intercostal nerve (Vesalius, 1543a)***; in the original Latin, *ramus costalis*, p. 90 of 1795 reprint.
8. *sub-costal branch of dorsal pairs (Burdin, 1803)*
   Synonym for macrodissected adult human ***intercostal nerves (Vesalius, 1543a)***; see translation (1803, Vol. 1, p. 197).
9. *subcostal nerves (Chaussier, 1809)*
   Synonym for macrodissected adult human ***intercostal nerves (Vesalius, 1543a)***; in the original French, *nerfs sous-costale*.
10. *proper intercostal nerve (Bell & Bell, 1816)*
   Synonym for macrodissected adult human ***intercostal nerve (Vesalius, 1543a)***; Vol. 2, p. 517.
11. *intercostal nerve properly so called (Bell & Bell, 1826)*
   Synonym for macrodissected adult human ***intercostal nerve (Vesalius, 1543a)***; Vol. 2, p. 594.
12. *anterior branches of thoracic nerves (Bock, 1827)*
   Synonym for macrodissected adult human ***intercostal nerves (Vesalius, 1543a)***; in the original Latin, *Ram. anterior nervi thoracici*, Table I, Figure 2-44,45.
13. *intercostal branch of costal nerve (Bock, 1827)*
   Synonym for macrodissected adult human ***intercostal nerve (Vesalius, 1543a)***; in the original Latin, *Ram. intercostalis nervi costalis*, Table I, Figure 2-49.
14. *anterior branches of dorsal nerves (Cruveilhier, 1836)*
   Synonym for macrodissected adult human ***intercostal nerves (Vesalius, 1543a)***; in the original French, *branches antérieures des nerfs dorsaux*, p. 823.
15 *intercostal branches of dorsal nerves (Cruveilhier, 1836)*
   Synonym for *anterior branches of dorsal nerves (Cruveilhier, 1836)*; in the original French, *branches intercostaux des nerfs dorsaux*, p. 823.
16. *intercostal branches of intercostal nerves (Quain & Wilson, 1839)*
   Synonym for macrodissected adult ox ***intercostal nerves (Vesalius, 1543a)***; Plate XX, Figure 1-*b*.

PARTLY CORRESPONDS:

1. *cutaneous nerve of armpit (Chaussier, 1809)*
   In macrodissected adult human,equals third ***intercostal nerve (Vesalius, 1543a)***; in the original French, *nerf cutané de l'aisselle*.

2. *intercostal branch of intercostal branches of dorsal nerves (Cruveilhier, 1836)*
   Macrodissected adult human segment of ***intercostal nerve (Vesalius, 1543a)*** distal to point where ***lateral cutaneous branch of intercostal nerve (>1840)*** arises; in the original French, *rameau intercostal*, p. 824.
3. *abdominal branch of intercostal branches of dorsal nerves (Cruveilhier, 1836)*
   In Cruveilhier's description, proper term for *intercostal branch of intercostal branches of dorsal nerves (Cruveilhier, 1836)* arising from 8th–12th ***thoracic nerves (Diemerbroeck, 1672)***; in the original Latin, *rameaux abdominaux*, p. 828.
4. *muscular filaments of abdominal branch of intercostal branches of dorsal nerves (Cruveilhier, 1836)*
   Branchlets to muscle from each *abdominal branch of intercostal branches of dorsal nerves (Cruveilhier, 1836)*; in the original French, *filets musculaires*, p. 828.
5. *cutaneous filaments of abdominal branch of intercostal branches of dorsal nerves (Cruveilhier, 1836)*
   Branchlets to skin from each *abdominal branch of intercostal branches of dorsal nerves (Cruveilhier, 1836)*; in the original French, *filets cutanés*, p. 828.

intercostobrachial nerves (>1840)

As described for macrodissected adult human, there is a large and constant ***lateral cutaneous branch of intercostal nerve (>1840)*** of the second ***intercostal nerve (Vesalius, 1543a)*** often joined by communications with ***medial cutaneous nerve of arm (>1840)*** and third ***intercostal nerve (Vesalius, 1543a)***. This ***intercostobrachial nerve (>1840)*** innervates skin and fascia stretching across the axilla and dorsal surface of the arm on the medial side as far as the elbow; see Durward (pp. 1085–1086 and Figs. 922, 924). In addition, a smaller and independent second ***intercostobrachial nerve (>1840)*** is often generated from the ***lateral cutaneous branch of intercostal nerve (>1840)*** of the third ***intercostal nerve (Vesalius, 1543a)*** and supplies small branches to the axilla and medial side of the arm; see Williams & Warwick (1980, p. 1104), *Terminologia Anatomica* (1998, p. 139). They were known to Galen; see ***[intercostobrachial nerves (>1840)] (Galen, c177)***.

EARLIER REFERENCES:

Described, not named or illustrated:

1. ***[intercostobrachial nerves (>1840)] (Galen, c177)***
   Galen clearly described for macrodissected adult beef, pig, and/or macaque but not human, even pointing out contribution from third ***intercostal nerve (Vesalius, 1543a)***; see Singer translation (1999, pp. 66, 67, 70) and Duckworth translation (1962, pp. 240, 243).

Illustrated, not named or described:

1. ***[intercostobrachial nerves (>1840)] (Eustachi, 1552)***
   Clearly illustrated for macrodissected adult human; see Albinus edition (1761, Tab. 21-8).

Earlier synonyms:

1. *intercosto-humeral nerves (Fyfe, 1800)*
   Synonym for macrodissected adult human ***intercostobrachial nerves (>1840)***; Vol. 2, p. 314. Fyfe described both of them, referred to as first and second.
2. *cutaneous nerve of axilla (Burdin, 1803)*
   Synonym for macrodissected adult human ***intercostobrachial nerve (>1840)***, described as arising from second and from third ***intercostal nerves (Vesalius, 1543a)***; see translation (1803, Vol. 1, p. 197).
3. *superior internal cutaneous nerve (Bell, 1803a)*
   Basically synonym for macrodissected adult human ***intercostobrachial nerve (>1840)***; Plate V-8. Meckel (1817) gave the Latin, *nervus cutaneus internus superior*, see translation (1832, Vol. 3, p. 29), where *internus* was left out, but compare with *inferior internal cutaneous nerve (Meckel, 1817)* in English and Latin on same page.
4. *upper and internal cutaneous nerve (Bell, 1803b)*
   Clearly macrodissected adult human ***intercostobrachial nerve (>1840)***; p. 195.
5. *cutaneous nerve of cubital side of arm (Chaussier, 1809)*
   Synonym for macrodissected adult human ***intercostobrachial nerve (>1840)***; in the original French, *nerf cutané du bord cubital du bras*.
6. *brachial nerve (Meckel, 1817)*
   Synonym for macrodissected adult human ***intercostobrachial nerve (>1840)***; see translation (1832, Vol. 3, p. 10).
7. *intercostal axillary nerves (Bell & Bell, 1826)*
   Synonym for macrodissected adult human *intercosto-humeral nerves (Fyfe, 1800)*; in the original Latin, *nervi axillares intercostales*, Vol. 2, p. 610.
8. *superior intercosto-humeral nerve (Knox, 1832)*
   Synonym for macrodissected adult human ***intercostobrachial nerve (>1840)***; Plate XIX-26.
9. *nerve of Wrisberg (Quain & Wilson, 1839)*
   Eponym for macrodissected adult human ***intercostobrachial nerve (>1840)***; Plate XVII-*x*.

PARTLY CORRESPONDS:

1. *brachial branch of anterior branch of second dorsal pair (Cloquet, 1815)*
   Major component of macrodissected adult human ***intercostobrachial nerve (>1840)***; in the original French, *rameau brachial du branche antérieure de la seconde paire dorsale*, p. 656.
2. *brachial branch of anterior branch of third dorsal pair (Cloquet, 1815)*
   Major component of macrodissected adult human ***intercostobrachial nerve (>1840)***; in the original French, *rameau brachial du branche antérieure de la troisième paire dorsale*, p. 656.
3. *external branch of perforating or cutaneous branch of second dorsal nerve (Cruveilhier, 1836)*
   Macrodissected adult human lateral branch of ***intercostobrachial nerve (>1840)***; in the original French, *rameau externe*, p. 826.
4. *internal branch of perforating or cutaneous branch of second dorsal nerve (Cruveilhier, 1836)*

Macrodissected adult human medial branch of ***intercostobrachial nerve (>1840)***; in the original French, *rameau interne*, p. 826.

5. *intercosto-humeral nerve from third dorsal nerve (Quain & Wilson, 1839)*
   Macrodissected adult human ***intercostobrachial nerve (>1840)*** from ***lateral cutaneous branch of intercostal nerve (>1840)*** of third ***intercostal nerve (Vesalius, 1543a)*** supplying small branches to axilla and medial side of arm; Plate XVII-*y*.

intermediate dorsal cutaneous nerve (>1840)

As described for macrodissected adult human, a branch of the ***superficial fibular nerve (Fyfe, 1800)*** supplying branches to the distal part of the leg and dorsum of the foot and then commonly dividing into two parts, in turn dividing into two smaller parts to help form ***dorsal digital nerves of intermediate dorsal cutaneous nerve (>1840)*** for the last three toes; see Durward (1951, p. 1108 and Figs. 948, 949; referred to as *musculo-cutaneous nerve*), *Terminologia Anatomica* (1998, p. 140). It was known to Galen; see ***[intermediate dorsal cutaneous nerve (>1840)] (Galen, c173)***.

EARLIER REFERENCES:

Described, not named or illustrated:

1. ***[intermediate dorsal cutaneous nerve (>1840)] (Galen, c173)***
   Alluded to for macrodissected adult beef, pig, and/or macaque but not human; see May translation (1968, p. 706), Singer translation (1999, pp. 86–87). Vieussens described and illustrated it for macrodissected adult human (1684, Tab. 29:92–95).

Earlier synonyms:

1. *external dorsal twig of foot of superficial branch of peroneal nerve (Jördens, 1788)*
   Synonym for macrodissected adult human ***intermediate dorsal cutaneous nerve (>1840)***; in the original Latin, *ramulus dorsalis pedis externus rami superficialis nervi peronei*, p. 7 and Table I-*102*.
2. *external branch of superficial peroneal nerve (Fischer, 1791)*
   Synonym for macrodissected adult human ***intermediate dorsal cutaneous nerve (>1840)***; in the original Latin, *ramus externum nervi peronei superficialis*, p. 32.
3. *external dorsal branch of superficial peroneal nerve (Fischer, 1791)*
   Synonym for *external branch of superficial peroneal nerve (Fischer, 1791)*; Table IV, Figure 1-*289*.
4. *external branches of metatarsal nerves (Bell, 1803b)*
   Synonym for macrodissected adult human ***intermediate dorsal cutaneous nerve (>1840)***; p. 210.
5. *external branches of dorsal branches of foot (Bell, 1803b)*
   Synonym for macrodissected adult human ***intermediate dorsal cutaneous nerve (>1840)***; p. 210.
6. *exterior branch of praetibio-digital nerve (Burdin, 1803)*
   Synonym for macrodissected adult human ***intermediate dorsal cutaneous nerve (>1840)***; see translation (1803, Vol. 1, p. 205).
7. *external and superficial branch to back of foot of musculocutaneous branch of external popliteal nerve (Cloquet, 1816)*
   Synonym for macrodissected adult human ***intermediate dorsal cutaneous nerve (>1840)***; in the original French, *rameau externe et superficiel du dos du pied*, p. 675. Cloquet further described internal and external branches of this branch.
8. *cutaneous peroneal nerve (Meckel, 1817)*
   Synonym for macrodissected adult human ***intermediate dorsal cutaneous nerve (>1840)***; in the original Latin, *nervus cutaneus peroneus*, see translation (1832, Vol. 3, p. 18).
9. *middle cutaneous nerve of back of foot (Meckel, 1817)*
   Synonym for macrodissected adult human ***intermediate dorsal cutaneous nerve (>1840)***; in the original Latin, *nervus cutaneus medius dorsi pedis*, see translation (1832, Vol. 3, p. 18).
10. *external cutaneous branch of peroneal nerve (Meckel, 1817)*
    Synonym for macrodissected adult human ***intermediate dorsal cutaneous nerve (>1840)***; in the original Latin, *nervus cutaneus peroneus externus*, see translation (1832, Vol. 3, p. 18).
11. *middle dorsal nerve of foot (Bock, 1827)*
    Synonym for *middle cutaneous nerve of back of foot (Bock, 1827)*; in the original Latin, *nerv. dorsalis pedis medius*; Table VI, Figure 3-3.
12. *external branch of fibular nerve (Quain, 1828)*
    Synonym for macrodissected adult human ***intermediate dorsal cutaneous nerve (>1840)***; p. 297.
13. *external branch of peroneal nerve (Quain, 1828)*
    Synonym for macrodissected adult human ***intermediate dorsal cutaneous nerve (>1840)***; p. 297.
14. *external branch of musculo-cutaneous nerve (Quain & Wilson, 1839)*
    Synonym for macrodissected adult human ***intermediate dorsal cutaneous nerve (>1840)***; Plate XXIV, Figure 1-*f*.

PARTLY CORRESPONDS:

1. *internal metatarsal twig of external dorsal twig of foot of superficial branch of peroneal nerve (Jördens, 1788)*
   Medial primary branch of ***intermediate dorsal cutaneous nerve (>1840)*** for macrodissected adult human; in the original Latin, *ramulus metatarsicus internus ramulus dorsalis pedis externus rami superficialis nervi peronei*, p. 7 and Table I-*103*.
2. *external metatarsal twig of external dorsal twig of foot of superficial branch of peroneal nerve (Jördens, 1788)*
   Lateral primary branch of ***intermediate dorsal cutaneous nerve (>1840)*** for macrodissected adult human; in the original Latin, *ramulus metatarsicus externus ramulus dorsalis pedis externus rami superficialis nervi peronei*, p. 8 and Table I-*103*.
3. *digital branch of superficial peroneal nerve (Mayer, 1794)*
   Essentially, major medial branch of macrodissected adult human ***intermediate dorsal cutaneous nerve (>1840)***;

in the original Latin, *ramus digitalis nervi peronei superficialis*; Part 5, Table V, Figure 1-31 (p. 26).

4. *digital branch of peroneal nerve (Mayer, 1794)*
Synonym for *digital branch of superficial peroneal nerve (Mayer, 1794)*; in the original Latin, *ramus digitalis nervi peronei*; Part 5, Table V, Figure 1-30 (p. 28).
5. *external cutaneous nerve of foot (Mayer, 1794)*
Essentially, major lateral branch of macrodissected adult human ***intermediate dorsal cutaneous nerve (>1840)***; in the original Latin, *nervus cutaneus externus pedis*; Part 5, Table V, Figure 1-G (p. 28).
6. *cutaneous peroneal nerve (Mayer, 1794)*
Synonym for *external cutaneous nerve of foot (Mayer, 1794)*; in the original Latin, *nervus peroneus cutaneus*; Part 5, Table V, Figure 1-G (p. 28).

intermediate ganglia (>1840)

As described for macrodissected adult human, small ***paravertebral ganglia (Durward, 1951)*** associated with ***spinal nerve trunks (Frotscher, 1788)***, ***communicating branches of sympathetic trunk (>1840)***, or nearby ***paravertebral nerves (Swanson & Bota, 2010)***; see Mitchell (1953, p. 31), Crosby et al. (1962, Fig. 338). They were first delineated as *accessory ganglia (Walter, 1783)*.

EARLIER REFERENCES:

Earlier synonyms:

1. *accessory ganglia (Walter, 1783)*
Synonym for macrodissected adult human ***intermediate ganglia (>1840)***. Walter used it in association with first three ***lumbar sympathetic ganglia (>1840)***; in the original Latin, *ganglii accessorii*, Table 1-322,328. Bell & Bell (1816, Vol. 2, p. 529) also used term for macrodissected adult human, using the original Latin form, *ganglia accessoria*.

PARTLY CORRESPONDS:

1. *first accessory lumbar ganglion (Walter, 1783)*
Small ***intermediate ganglion (>1840)*** just lateral to second and third ***lumbar sympathetic ganglia (>1840)*** and connected to them by ***communicating branches (Winslow, 1733)***, as observed in a macrodissected adult human; in the original Latin, *ganglion lumbare accessorium primum*, Table I-316.
2. *second accessory lumbar ganglion (Walter, 1783)*
Small ***intermediate ganglion (>1840)*** just lateral to third ***lumbar sympathetic ganglion (>1840)*** and connected to it by ***communicating branch (Winslow, 1733)***, as observed in a macrodissected adult human; in the original Latin, *ganglion lumbare accessorium secundum*, Table I-317.
3. *lateral ganglia (Soemmerring, 1791)*
Small ***intermediate ganglia (>1840)*** associated with ***inferior cervical ganglion (Vieussens, 1684)***, as observed in macrodissected adult human; in the original Latin, *ganglia lateralia*, p. 323, see Foster (1892, p. 1674).
4. *posterior ganglia (Soemmerring, 1791)*
Synonym for *lateral ganglia (Soemmerring, 1791)*; in the original Latin, *ganglia posteriora*, p. 323, see Foster (1892, p. 1674).
5. *first lateral ganglion (Soemmerring, 1798)*
Probably most rostral of *lateral ganglia (Soemmerring, 1791)*, if present, in macrodissected adult human; in the original Latin, *prius ganglion laterale*, p. 345.

intermediate hippocampal commissure (>1840)

As described in macrodissected adult human, and mammal generally with histological methods for ***axons (Kölliker, 1896)***, the middle and thinnest differentiation of the ***hippocampal commissures (Johnston, 1913)***, between ***ventral hippocampal commissure (>1840)*** rostrally and ***dorsal hippocampal commissure (Craigie, 1925)*** caudally and containing intermixed commissural ***axons (Kölliker, 1896)*** from both the ***hippocampal region (Swanson et al., 1987)*** and ***retrohippocampal region (Swanson et al., 1987)***; see Swanson and Cowan (1977), Swanson et al. (1978). It was not delineated by 1840.

EARLIER REFERENCES:

Earlier synonyms:

1. *thin part of dorsal hippocampal commissure (Craigie, 1925)*
Synonym for ***intermediate hippocampal commissure (>1840)*** as described in adult rat with normal histological stains; p. 103, Plate XXVI.
2. *hippocampal decussation (Demeter et al., 1985)*
Synonym for ***intermediate hippocampal commissure (>1840)*** as described in adult macaque monkey with normal myelin stains; see Figure 2-C. This account was confirmed in all essential details for adult human by Gloor et al. (1993).

intermediate nerve (>1840)

As described for macrodissected adult human, one of two ***intermediofacial nerve roots (>1840)***, the other being the ***facial nerve root*** (>1840). Proximally, the ***intermediate nerve (>1840)*** is attached to the surface of the ***medulla (Winslow, 1733)*** just caudal to the ***pons (Haller, 1747)*** as 1–4 ***intermediate nerve rootlets (>1840)***, together constituting the ***intermediate nerve root (>1840)*** that leads into the short distal part of the ***intermediate nerve (>1840)***, the ***intermediate nerve trunk (>1840)***. Its distal end converges with the distal end of the ***facial nerve root (>1840)*** to form the ***intermediofacial nerve trunk (>1840)***; for details see Meckel (1832, Vol. 3, p. 53), Henle (1871, pp. 400–401), Sapolini (1883), Hovelacque (1927, p. 153), Pearson (1947), Rhoton et al. (1968), Nieuwenhuys et al. (2008, p. 203). When there is only one ***intermediate nerve rootlet (>1840)***, it is equivalent to the ***intermediate nerve root (>1840)*** and ***intermediate nerve trunk (>1840)*** considered together. An excellent analysis of its development was provided by Streeter (1907). Although often described as the *sensory root of facial nerve (>1840)*, see Williams & Warwick (1980, Fig. 7.184), its central origin, course, and functional components are very different from the *facial nerve (Vicq d'Azyr, 1784)* and its ***facial nerve root (>1840)***; it carries sensory taste ***axons (Kölliker, 1896)*** from the tongue and preganglionic parasympathetic ***axons (Kölliker, 1896)*** to the lacrimal glands, submandibular and sublingual salivary glands, and glands of the nasal and palatine mucosae; see Williams & Warwick (1980, p. 1070, Fig. 7.184). Wrisberg is often credited with discovering this ***nerve (Herophilus, c335–c280 BC)*** in macrodissected adult human in 1777; for example, Garrison & McHenry (1969, p. 92). However, no description of it is given in the 1777 publication. According to Vicq d'Azyr (1784, p. 592), Wrisberg spoke of it before 1778 and the full names he gave, in Latin, were *portio media inter communicantem faciei et auditivum nervum* (see Vicq d'Azyr, 1784, p. 592) and *fibrillae nerveae ad par communicans faciei accessoriae* (see Vicq d'Azyr, 1786, Pl. 28–32). A footnote in Wrisberg's edition of Haller's *First Lines of Physiology* (Haller & Wrisberg, 1780; see Haller, Cullen, & Wrisberg translation, 1786, p. 208) states that "There are three portions of nerves, which are commonly taken under the seventh pair: *a*, the communicans faciei, or the portio dura, which we may also call the small sympathetic; *b*, a new intermediate portio; *c*, the auditory or acoustic properly so called. They are clearly represented by my ingenious pupil Sommering, Tab. 2 [1778]." Soemmerring (1778) referred to *fibrillae nerveae ad par communicans faciei accessoriae* Wrisbergii (Tab. 2-*Y*) or *portione inter par communicans faciei et auditorium media Wrisbergii* (Sect. 73, p. 151), and stated that Wrisberg had demonstrated it publicly (p. 152).

EARLIER REFERENCES:

Earlier synonyms:

1. *minor part of facial nerve (Soemmerring, 1778)*
   Synonym for macrodissected adult human ***intermediate nerve (>1840)***; in the original Latin, *portio minor facialis*, p. 93. In his translation of the *Fabrica*'s Book VII, Singer (1952, Fig. 14-*L*, pp. 112–113) suggested that Vesalius (1543a) may have identified the ***intermediate nerve (>1840)*** itself, whereas Richardson & Carman (2002, pp. 177, 193–195, and part *d* in the two figures on pp. 168–169) suggested it was instead the ***abducens nerve (Heister, 1717)***. However, Vesalius's own description makes it clear that he was describing part of the ***trigeminal nerve motor root (>1840)*** or *thinner root of fifth pair of cerebral nerves (Vesalius, 1543a)*; Richardson & Carman (2002, p. 193).
2. *portione inter par communicans faciei et auditorium media Wrisbergii (Soemmerring, 1778)*
   Eponym for macrodissected adult human ***intermediate nerve (>1840)***; p. 151.
3. *fibrillae nerveae ad par communicans faciei accessoriae Wrisbergii (Soemmerring, 1778)*
   Eponym for macrodissected adult human ***intermediate nerve (>1840)***; Table 2-*Y*.
4. *intermediate portio of seventh pair of nerves (Haller & Wrisberg, 1780)*
   Synonym for macrodissected adult human ***intermediate nerve (>1840)*** provided in footnote of his translation of Haller, later translated into English; see Haller, Cullen, & Wrisberg (1786, p. 208).
5. *nervus portio inter communicantem faciei et auditorium media (Haase, 1781)*
   Synonym for macrodissected adult human ***intermediate nerve (>1840)***; p. 39.
6. *portio media inter communicantem faciei et auditivum nervum (Vicq d'Azyr, 1784)*
   Term Vicq d'Azyr ascribed to Wrisberg for macrodissected adult human ***intermediate nerve (>1840)***; p. 592, also see Vicq d'Azyr (1786, p. 53).
7. *intermediate nervous filaments (Vicq d'Azyr, 1786)*
   Synonym for macrodissected adult human ***intermediate nerve (>1840)***; in the original French, *filets nerveux intermédiaires*, Table XXX, Figure 2:*8–10*.
8. *nerve of Wrisberg (Scarpa, 1788)*
   Eponym for macrodissected adult human ***intermediate nerve (>1840)***; in the original Latin, *nervae Wrisbergii*, Table X, Figure 1-*p*.
9. *external and posterior root of facial nerve (Meckel, 1817)*
   Synonym for macrodissected adult human ***intermediate nerve (>1840)***; see translation (1832, Vol. 3, p. 53).
10. *intermediate part of facial nerve (Arnold, 1834)*
    Synonym for macrodissected adult human ***intermediate nerve (>1840)***; in the original Latin, *nervus facialis portio intermedia*, Table I, Figure VII-*9*.
11. *nervus communicans faciei portio intermedia (Arnold, 1834)*
    Synonym for macrodissected adult human ***intermediate nerve (>1840)***; in the original Latin, *nervus communicans faciei portio intermedia*, Table I, Figure VII-*9*.
12. *sensory root of facial nerve (>1840)*
    Common synonym for macrodissected adult human ***intermediate nerve (>1840)***; see Cajal (1899–1904, Vol. 2, pt. 1, p. 171). Also see *motor root of facial nerve (>1840)*.
13. *glossopalatine nerve (>1840)*
    Synonym for macrodissected adult human ***intermediate nerve (>1840)***; see discussion in Durward (1951, p. 1033).

intermediate nerve root (>1840)

As described for macrodissected adult human, the set of ***intermediate nerve rootlets (>1840)*** between the ventral surface of the ***medulla (Winslow, 1733)*** and the region where they converge to form the single ***intermediate nerve trunk (>1840)***; see Williams & Warwick (1980, p. 1071 and Fig. 7.184.), also see ***intermediate nerve (>1840)***. It was first distinguished by Soemmerring; see ***[intermediate nerve root (>1840)] (Soemmerring, 1778)***.

EARLIER REFERENCES:

Illustrated, not named or described:

1. ***[intermediate nerve root (>1840)] (Soemmerring, 1778)***
   Clearly illustrated for macrodissected adult human; Table II. Also see Vicq d'Azyr (1784, pp. 592–593).

intermediate nerve rootlets (>1840)

As described for macrodissected adult human, the ***intermediate nerve trunk (>1840)*** forms distally from 1–4

intermediate nerve rootlets (>1840) emerging from the lateral side of the ***medulla (Winslow, 1733)***, just caudal to the ***pons (Haller, 1747)***. For anatomical descriptions see Meckel (1832, Vol. 3, p. 53), Hovelacque (1927, p. 153), and Pearson (1947, p. 143)—who specifically referred to a rootlet, as well as the synonymous bundle and fascicle. The rootlets together form the ***intermediate nerve root (>1840)***. They were probably first referred to as *fibrae ad facialem accessoriae (Soemmerring, 1778)*.

EARLIER REFERENCES:

Earlier synonyms:

1. *fibrae ad facialem accessoriae (Soemmerring, 1778)*
   Apparently synonym for macrodissected adult human ***intermediate nerve rootlets (>1840)***; p. 93.
2. *fibrillae nervaeae ad par communicans faciei accessoriae (Vicq d'Azyr, 1786)*
   Synonym for macrodissected adult human ***intermediate nerve rootlets (>1840)*** attributed without citation to Wrisberg; Plate XVIII-32.
3. *fibrils of nerve of Wrisberg (Scarpa, 1789)*
   Synonym for macrodissected adult human ***intermediate nerve rootlets (>1840)***; in the original Latin, *fibrillae nervae Wrisbergh*, Table VIII, Figure 5-*d,e*.
4. *filaments forming external and posterior root of facial nerve (Meckel, 1817)*
   Synonym for macrodissected adult human ***intermediate nerve rootlets (>1840)***; see translation (1832, Vol. 3, p. 53).

intermediate nerve trunk (>1840)

As described for macrodissected adult human, short segment of the ***intermediate nerve (>1840)*** extending distally from the ***intermediate nerve root (>1840)*** to the ***intermediofacial nerve trunk (>1840)***; see Rhoton et al. (1968). Probably first identified as *fasciculus of external root of facial nerve (Meckel, 1817)*.

EARLIER REFERENCES:

Earlier synonyms:

1. *fasciculus of external root of facial nerve (Meckel, 1817)*
   Synonym for macrodissected adult human ***intermediate nerve trunk (>1840)***; see translation (1832, Vol. 3, p. 53).

intermediate spinal zone (>1840)

As described for macrodissected adult human, and for mammal in general with cellular architecture and connections, the ***gray matter region (Swanson & Bota, 2010)*** of the ***spinal cord (Galen, c162–166)*** lying between ***ventral horn (>1840)*** ventrally and base of ***dorsal horn (>1840)*** dorsally. Some major differentiations include ***spinal central gray (>1840), central cervical nucleus (>1840), dorsal thoracic nucleus (>1840)***, and ***intermediolateral nucleus (>1840)***; see Carpenter (1976, p. 227), *Terminologia Anatomica* (1998, p. 106). For a good comparison of classical ***spinal cord (Galen, c162–166)*** parceling with the laminar scheme proposed by Rexed (1952) see Carpenter (1976, pp. 222–229); also see Cajal (1899–1904, Vol. 1, pp. 225–228), Swanson (1998–1999, pp. 212–213). The general outline of the ***intermediate spinal zone (>1840)***, except for the ***spinal central gray (>1840)***, was first delineated as the *body of lateral part of spinal ash-colored substance (Vicq d'Azyr, 1784)*.

EARLIER REFERENCES:

Earlier synonyms:

1. *lateral column of spinal medulla (>1840)*
   Synonym for macrodissected adult human ***intermediate spinal zone (>1840)***; see *Basel Nomina Anatomica* (His, 1895, p. 80).

PARTLY CORRESPONDS:

1. *body of lateral part of spinal ash-colored substance (Vicq d'Azyr, 1784)*
   Vicq d'Azyr wrote that *ash-colored substance (Winslow, 1733)* or *cortical substance (Willis, 1664)* of ***spinal cord (Galen, c162–c166)*** may be divided into middle and two lateral parts, with middle part being transverse and thus comparable to middle of letter ***H***. Then he divided lateral part of spinal *ash-colored substance (Winslow, 1733)* into anterior end, body or central part, and posterior end. Although his description was not entirely clear, body may thus correspond to ***intermediate spinal zone (>1840)***, without ***spinal central gray (>1840)***; pp. 600–601, see Clarke & O'Malley translation (1996, p. 269). Also see *posterior cineritious substance (Monro, 1783)*.
2. *central part of lateral part of spinal ash-colored substance (Vicq d'Azyr, 1784)*
   Synonym for *body of lateral part of spinal ash-colored substance (Vicq d'Azyr, 1784)*; pp. 600–601, see Clarke & O'Malley translation (1996, p. 269).

intermediate supraclavicular nerves (>1840)

As described for macrodissected adult human, they are derived from the ***cervical plexus (Molinetti, 1675)*** and innervate skin and fascia over the pectoralis major and deltoid muscles as caudal (low down) as the level of the second rib; see Durward (1951, p. 1064 and Fig. 921), Williams & Warwick (1980, p. 1092). They were first distinguished by Eustachi; see ***[intermediate supraclavicular nerves (>1840)] (Eustachi, 1552)***.

TRANSLATIONS:

1. *nervi supraclaviculares intermedii (>1840)*
   Current Latin form of ***intermediate supraclavicular nerves (>1840)***; see *Terminologia Anatomica* (1998, p. 137).

EARLIER REFERENCES:

Illustrated, not named or described:

1. ***[intermediate supraclavicular nerves (>1840)] (Eustachi, 1552)***
   Illustrated for macrodissected adult human; see Albinus edition (1761, Tab. 21-*i*).

Earlier synonyms:

1. *middle branch of anterior branch of fourth pair of cervical nerves (Bang, 1770)*
   Synonym for macrodissected adult human ***intermediate supraclavicular nerves (>1840)***; in the original Latin, *medius ramus*, Figure I-54.

2. *middle supraclavicular branches (Soemmerring, 1791)*
   Synonym for macrodissected adult human ***intermediate supraclavicular nerves (>1840)***; in the original Latin, *supraclaviculares medii*, p. 270.
3. *third supraclavicular branch (Peipers, 1793)*
   Synonym for macrodissected adult human ***intermediate supraclavicular nerves (>1840)***; in the original Latin, *ramus supraclavicularis tertius*, p. 35.
4. *external pectoral subcutaneous supraclavicular branch (Peipers, 1793)*
   Synonym for *third supraclavicular branch (Peipers, 1793)*; in the original Latin, *ramus supraclavicularis subcutaneus pectoris externus*, p. 35.
5. *middle superclavicular branches (Bell, 1803b)*
   Bell attributed term to Soemmerring; in the original Latin, *superclaviculares medii*, p. 166, see *middle supraclavicular branches (Soemmerring, 1791)*.
6. *acromian branch of thoracic part of trachelo-cutanean plexus (Burdin, 1803)*
   Synonym for macrodissected adult human *acromial branch of thoracic part of tracheosubcutaneous nerves (Chaussier, 1809)*; see translation (1803, Vol. 1, p. 188).
7. *acromial branch of thoracic part of tracheosubcutaneous nerves (Chaussier, 1809)*
   Probably synonym for macrodissected adult human ***intermediate supraclavicular nerves (>1840)***.
8. *middle superclavicular nerves (Bell & Bell, 1816)*
   Synonym for macrodissected adult human ***intermediate supraclavicular nerves (>1840)***; in the original Latin, *superclaviculares medii*, Vol. 2, p. 514.
9. *middle supraclavicular nerves (Bock, 1827)*
   Synonym for macrodissected adult human ***intermediate supraclavicular nerves (>1840)***; in the original Latin, *nervi supraclaviculares medii*, Table III-*11*.
10. *intermediate branches of supraclavicular branches (Cruveilhier, 1836)*
    Synonym for macrodissected adult human ***intermediate supraclavicular nerves (>1840)***; in the original French, *rameaux intermédiares*, p. 786.
11. *clavicular branches of supraclavicular branches (Cruveilhier, 1836)*
    Synonym for macrodissected adult human ***intermediate supraclavicular nerves (>1840)***; in the original French, *rameaux claviculaires*, p. 786.

PARTLY CORRESPONDS:

1. *acromial nerves (Bang, 1770)*
   Formed by terminal branches of one of the macrodissected adult human ***intermediate supraclavicular nerves (>1840)***; in the original Latin, *nervos acromiales*, Figure I-56.

intermediofacial nerve (Strong & Elwyn, 1943)

As described for macrodissected adult mammal, a ***cranial nerve (Soemmerring, 1791)*** consisting of the *facial nerve (Vicq d'Azyr, 1784)* and ***intermediate nerve (>1840)*** considered together, *facial nerve (Meckel, 1817)* being the most common synonym. At the surface of the ***medulla (Winslow, 1733)*** there are two ***intermediofacial nerve roots (>1840)—facial nerve root (>1840)*** and ***intermediate nerve (>1840)***—joining in the internal acoustic meatus, just proximal to the ***geniculate ganglion (Bischoff, 1832)***, to form the ***intermediofacial nerve trunk (>1840)*** that becomes the ***facial nerve trunk (>1840)*** distal to the point where the ***communicating branch of intermediofacial nerve trunk with vagus nerve (>1840)*** joins the ***intermediofacial nerve (Strong & Elwyn, 1943)***; see Durward (1951, Fig. 901), Hamilton (1976, pp. 628–629), Williams & Warwick (1980, p. 1071 and Fig. 7.184). For Strong & Elwyn's use in macrodissected adult human, see p. 208. Brodal (1948, p. 226) also pointed out that this term is preferable to *facial nerve (Meckel, 1817)*, defined as including the ***intermediate nerve (>1840)***. The term ***intermediofacial nerve (Strong & Elwyn, 1943)*** is preferable for the same basic reasons that the term ***vestibulocochlear nerve (>1840)*** is preferable (*Nomina Anatomica*, 1983, pp. A74-A75), and the same approach to topographic architecture (gross anatomy or macrodissection) is used here for both. Vicq d'Azyr (1784, p. 592) pointed out that since the work of Falloppio (1561), two distinct components of the *fifth pair of nerves from brain (Galen, c192)* were clearly distinguished—the *facial nerve (Vicq d'Azyr, 1784)* and ***vestibulocochlear nerve (>1840)***—and that it remained for Wrisberg to discover a third distinct ***nerve (Herophilus, c335–c280 BC)*** or component, the ***intermediate nerve (>1840)***. However, it is obvious that Galen himself distinguished the *facial nerve (Vicq d'Azyr, 1784)* and ***vestibulocochlear nerve (>1840)***; see *fifth pair of nerves from brain (Galen, c192)*. Gehuchten (1897, pp. 518, 531) may have been the first to insist that the *facial nerve (Meckel, 1817)* is actually two distinct ***nerves (Herophilus, c335–c280 BC)***; also see Gehuchten (1906, Fig. 499). The embryological condition of two clearly distinct ***nerves (Herophilus, c335–c280 BC)*** was documented by Streeter (1907, Fig. 7), who also outlined carefully the earlier literature. The ***intermediofacial nerve (Strong & Elwyn, 1943)*** was vaguely distinguished by Galen, see ***[intermediofacial nerve (Strong & Elwyn, 1943)] (Galen, c192)***, but was clearly distinguished as the *facial nerve (Meckel, 1817)*.

EARLIER REFERENCES:

Described, not named or illustrated:

1. ***[intermediofacial nerve (Strong & Elwyn, 1943)] (Galen, c192)***
   In macrodissected adult beef, pig, and/or macaque but not human, Galen clearly distinguished between *third and fourth pairs of nerves from brain (Galen, c192)*, corresponding approximately to the ***trigeminal nerve (Winslow, 1733)***, and ***intermediofacial nerve (Strong & Elwyn, 1943)***, roughly one component of *fifth pair of nerves from brain (Galen, c192)*, the other component being *acoustic nerve (Galen, c173)* or ***vestibulocochlear nerve (>1840)***; see Duckworth (1962, p. 195).

Earlier synonyms:

1. *facial nerve (Meckel, 1817)*
   Commonest synonym for macrodissected adult human ***intermediofacial nerve (Strong & Elwyn, 1943)***, with two distinct ***intermediofacial nerve roots (>1840)***—one large and often referred to now as *motor root of facial nerve (>1840)* or ***facial nerve root (>1840)***, and the other much smaller and often referred to as *sensory root of facial nerve (>1840)* or ***intermediate nerve (>1840)***; see translation (1832, Vol. 3, p. 53).

PARTLY CORRESPONDS:

1. *[facial nerve (Vicq d'Azyr, 1784)] (Herophilus, c335–c280 BC)*
   Herophilus, the founder of human anatomy, is credited with discovering most ***cranial nerves (Soemmerring, 1791)***, including *facial nerve (Vicq d'Azyr, 1784)*, which he apparently did not name or illustrate and may not have separated from ***vestibulocochlear nerve (>1840)***; see Solmsen (1961), von Staden (1969), Longrigg (1993), Clarke & O'Malley (1996, p. 261). He macrodissected large adult mammals and human cadavers. Also see *fifth pair of nerves from brain (Galen, c192)*.
2. *nerve issuing from blind perforation (Galen, c173)*
   Roughly synonymous with *facial nerve (Vicq d'Azyr, 1784)* in macrodissected adult beef, pig, and/or macaque but not human; see May translation (1968, pp. 700–701), Duckworth translation (1962, pp. 195–196).
3. *one-eyed nerve (Albertus Magnus, 13th century)*
   Apparently synonymous with *facial nerve (Vicq d'Azyr, 1784)*; that is, one of two parts of *fifth pair of nerves from brain (Galen, c192)*; in the original Latin, *monoculus*, see Kitchell & Resnick translation (1999, p. 182). Also see Duckworth (1962, p. 196).
4. *blind nerve (Albertus Magnus, 13th century)*
   According to Albertus Magnus, a name (*caecus* in Latin) for *facial nerve (Vicq d'Azyr, 1784)*, one of two parts of *fifth pair of nerves from brain (Galen, c192)*; see Kitchell & Resnick translation (1999, p. 182).
5. *[facial nerve (Vicq d'Azyr, 1784)] (Eustachi, 1552)*
   First adequate illustration of its distribution pattern for macrodissected adult human; see Albinus edition (1761, Tab. 21/2-*d*). Eustachi also illustrated clearly its separate origin from ***vestibulocochlear nerve (>1840)***; see Albinus edition (1761, Tab. 18, Figs. 1, 3, 4-*W* and Fig. 2-*a*).
6. *portio dura paris quinti (Falloppio, 1561)*
   Synonym for macrodissected adult human *facial nerve (Vicq d'Azyr, 1784)*; p. 148. Also see Meckel (1753, p. 32 and p. 71, where Falloppio's observations are documented). In English, *hard part of fifth pair.*
7. *hard part of seventh pair of nerves arising within skull (Willis, 1664)*
   Synonym for macrodissected adult mammalian *facial nerve (Vicq d'Azyr, 1784)*; see Pordage translation (1681, p. 144), where Willis suggested "hard part" arises from ***medullary striae (Scarpa, 1788)***. For Latinized form, *portio dura of seventh pair of nerves arising within skull (Willis, 1664)*, see *portio dura paris quinti (Falloppio, 1561)*. It was also referred to as *processus... durior* (1664, p. 295) or *hard process* (Pordage translation, 1681, p. 143).
8. *hard nerve (Willis, 1664)*
   Synonym for macrodissected adult human *hard part of seventh pair of nerves arising within skull (Willis, 1664)*—the *facial nerve (Vicq d'Azyr, 1784)*; in the original Latin, *durior nervus*, p. 296. For English form see Pordage translation (1681, p. 144). Haase (1781, p. 39) provided the Latin form, *nervus durus*.
9. *trunk of hard part of seventh pair of nerves arising within skull (Willis, 1664)*
   Roughly synonymous with macrodissected adult, presumably human and probably other large mammalian, ***intermediofacial nerve trunk (1840)*** and ***facial nerve trunk (>1840)*** considered together; see Pordage translation (1681, p. 144).
10. *portio dura nervi auditorii (Winslow, 1733)*
    Synonym for macrodissected adult human *hard part of seventh pair of nerves arising within skull (Willis, 1664)*; Section VI, p. 59.
11. *small sympathetic nerve (Winslow, 1733)*
    Synonym for macrodissected adult human *facial nerve (Vicq d'Azyr, 1784)*; in the original Latin, *nervus sympatheticus minor*, Section VI, p. 59. Also see Clarke & Jacyna (1987, p. 314).
12. *nervus communicans faciei (Soemmerring, 1778)*
    Synonym for macrodissected adult human *facial nerve (Vicq d'Azyr, 1784)*; see Vicq d'Azyr (1786, p. 49). Soemmerring attributed the term to Wrisberg, his mentor, who did not publish it prior to 1778; p. 145.
13. *seventh nerve (Soemmerring, 1778)*
    Synonym for macrodissected adult human *facial nerve (Vicq d'Azyr, 1784)*; in the original Latin, *nervus septimus*, p. 180.
14. *nervus dura portio nervi acustici (Haase, 1781)*
    Synonym for macrodissected adult human *hard part of seventh pair of nerves arising within skull (Willis, 1664)*—the *facial nerve (Vicq d'Azyr, 1784)*; p. 39.
15. *nervus sympathicus parvus (Haase, 1781)*
    Latin version of macrodissected adult human *small sympathetic nerve (Winslow, 1733)*; p. 40.
16. *facial nerve (Vicq d'Azyr, 1784)*
    Macrodissected adult human ***intermediofacial nerve (Strong & Elwyn, 1943)*** without ***intermediate nerve (>1840)***; that is, ***facial nerve root (>1840)*** and ***intermediofacial nerve trunk (>1840)*** with all its branches and extensions. For accounts of its origin, course, and distribution in macrodissected adult human see Durward (1951, pp. 1030–1034 and Figs. 901–903), Hamilton (1976, pp. 628–630 and Figs. 798, 800). Vicq d'Azyr noted without citations that others had used this term as well; p. 590. He also pointed out that Wrisberg had recently discovered a separate ***intermediate nerve (>1840)***; p. 592. Also see Vicq d'Azyr (1786, p. 49).
17. *first nerve of seventh pair (Vicq d'Azyr, 1784)*
    Synonym for macrodissected adult human *facial nerve (Vicq d'Azyr, 1784)*; p. 591 and Vicq d'Azyr (1786, Pl. XVII, Fig. I-48).

18. *hard nerve trunk (Günther, 1786)*
Probably synonym for macrodissected adult human *trunk of hard part of seventh pair of nerves arising within skull (Willis, 1664)*; p. 57.
19. *twelfth pair of nerves (Malacarne, 1791)*
Macrodissected adult human *facial nerve (Vicq d'Azyr, 1784)* listed as 12th of 17 *cerebral nerves (Malacarne, 1791)*.
20. *sympathicus minor par decimum tertium (Malacarne, 1791)*
Synonym for macrodissected adult human *facial nerve (Vicq d'Azyr, 1784)*, as provided in Latin by Burdach (1822, p. 312); based on *small sympathetic nerve (Winslow, 1733)*, or *lesser or minor sympathetic nerve*.
21. *seventh pair of cranial nerves (Soemmerring, 1791)*
Synonym for macrodissected adult human *facial nerve (Vicq d'Azyr, 1784)*; see ***cranial nerves (Soemmerring, 1791)***.
22. *seventh pair of cerebral nerves (Soemmerring, 1791)*
Synonym for *seventh pair of cranial nerves (Soemmerring, 1791)*; see p. 103 and *cerebral nerves (Soemmerring, 1791)*. In the original Latin, *par septimum nervorum cerebri*, Soemmerring (1798, p. 125).
23. *nervus consensorius parvus capitis (Andersch, 1797)*
Synonym for macrodissected adult human *facial nerve (Vicq d'Azyr, 1784)*; p. 1. Also see Burdach (1822, p. 312).
24. *nervus communis facili (Meckel, 1817)*
Synonym listed for macrodissected adult human *facial nerve (Vicq d'Azyr, 1784)*; see translation (1832, Vol. 3, p. 53).
25. *facial nerve trunk (Meckel, 1817)*
Synonym for macrodissected adult human *trunk of hard part of seventh pair of nerves arising within skull (Willis, 1664)*; see translation (1832, Vol. 3, pp. 54–55). Rhoton et al. (1968, p. 610) wrote that for adult human "the [***intermediate nerve (>1840)***] forms a common trunk with the facial motor root."
26. *respiratory nerve of face (Bell, 1821)*
Synonym for macrodissected adult mammalian *facial nerve (Vicq d'Azyr, 1784)*; p. 406.
27. *petrous part of seventh pair (Arnold, 1834)*
Macrodissected adult human segment of ***intermediofacial nerve (Strong & Elwyn, 1943)*** within petrous part of temporal bone, thus including distal parts of ***intermediofacial nerve roots (>1840)*** and proximal part of ***intermediofacial nerve trunk (>1840)***; in the original Latin, *par septimum, pars petrosa*, p. 11.
28. *petrous part of facial nerve (Arnold, 1834)*
Synonym for *petrous part of seventh nerve (Arnold, 1834)*; in the original Latin, *nervus facialis, pars petrosa*, p. 11.
29. *nervus communicans faciei pars petrosa (Arnold, 1834)*
Synonym for *petrous part of seventh nerve (Arnold, 1834)*; p. 11.
30. petrous part of middle sympathetic nerve (Arnold, 1834)
Synonym for *petrous part of seventh nerve (Arnold, 1834)*; in the original Latin, *nervus sympathicus medius, pars petrosa*, p. 11.
31. *petrous part of hard part of acoustic nerve (Arnold, 1834)*
Synonym for *petrous part of seventh nerve (Arnold, 1834)*; in the original Latin, *portio dura nervi acustici, pars petrosa*, p. 11.
32. *major part of facial nerve (Arnold, 1834)*
Synonym for macrodissected adult human *facial nerve (Vicq d'Azyr, 1784)*; in the original Latin, *nervus facialis portio major*, Table I:*VII-8*.
33. *nervus communicans faciei portio major (Arnold, 1834)*
Synonym for macrodissected adult human *facial nerve (Vicq d'Azyr, 1784)*; Table I-*VII*.
34. *collateral branches of facial nerve (Cruveilhier, 1836)*
Branches of macrodissected adult human ***intermediofacial nerve trunk (1840)*** and ***facial nerve trunk (>1840)*** proximal to **parotid plexus (Meckel, 1817)**; in the original French, *rameaux collatéraux du nerf facial*, p. 940.
35. *facial nerve proper (Kölliker, 1896)*
Synonym for *facial nerve (Vicq d'Azyr, 1784)*; in the original Latin, *facialis sensu stricto*; Vol. 2, p. 272.

intermediofacial nerve roots (>1840)

As described for macrodissected adult human there are two, the ***facial nerve root (>1840)*** and ***intermediate nerve (>1840)***, which join distally in the internal acoustic meatus to form the ***intermediofacial nerve trunk (>1840)***, which almost immediately forms the *genu of facial nerve (Langenbeck, 1826–1830)* in the facial canal of the temporal bone; see Williams & Warwick (1980, Figs. 7.184, 185). They were perhaps first clearly distinguished by Soemmerring; see ***[intermediofacial nerve roots (>1840)] (Soemmerring, 1778)***.

EARLIER REFERENCES:

Described, not named or illustrated:

1. ***[intermediofacial nerve roots (>1840)] (Soemmerring, 1778)***
Clearly distinguished in macrodissected adult human; see Table II.

PARTLY CORRESPONDS:

1. *cerebral part of seventh pair (Arnold, 1834)*
Proximal parts of macrodissected adult human ***intermediofacial nerve roots (>1840)***, proximal to reaching internal acoustic meatus; in the original Latin, *par septimum, pars cerebralis*, p. 11.
2. *cerebral part of facial nerve (Arnold, 1834)*
Synonym for *cerebral part of seventh nerve (Arnold, 1834)*; in the original Latin, *nervus facialis, pars cerebralis*, p. 11.
3. *nervus communicans faciei pars cerebralis (Arnold, 1834)*
Synonym for *cerebral part of seventh nerve (Arnold, 1834)*; p. 11.
4. *cerebral part of middle sympathetic nerve (Arnold, 1834)*
Synonym for *cerebral part of seventh nerve (Arnold, 1834)*; in the original Latin, *nervus sympathicus medius, pars cerebralis*, p. 11.
5. *cerebral part of hard part of acoustic nerve (Arnold, 1834)*
Synonym for *cerebral part of seventh nerve (Arnold, 1834)*; in the original Latin, *portio dura nervi acustici, pars cerebralis*, p. 11.

intermediofacial nerve trunk (>1840)

As described for macrodissected adult human, segment of the ***intermediofacial nerve (Strong & Elwyn, 1943)*** between ***intermediofacial nerve roots (>1840)*** proximally and ***facial nerve trunk (>1840)*** distally. Near its proximal end, the ***intermediofacial nerve trunk (>1840)*** makes a sharp bend in the facial canal of the temporal bone, and within this *genu of facial nerve (Langenbeck, 1826–1830)* lies the ***geniculate ganglion (Bischoff, 1832)***. The distal end of the ***intermediofacial nerve trunk (>1840)*** is defined as the point where the ***communicating branch of intermediofacial nerve trunk with vagus nerve (>1840)*** joins the ***intermediofacial nerve (Strong & Elwyn, 1943)*** and the ***facial nerve trunk (>1840)*** begins; see Durward (1951, pp. 1030–1034 and Figs. 901–903), Rhoton et al. (1968, pp. 610–612), Hamilton (1976, pp. 628–630 and Figs. 798, 800), Williams & Warwick (1980, p. 1071 and Figs. 7.184, 185). It was not recognized as such by 1840.

PARTLY CORRESPONDS:

1. *malleal filament of portio major and minor of facial nerve (Bellingeri, 1818)*
   Branch of ***intermediofacial nerve trunk (>1840)*** to part of tensor tympani muscle, the internal malleal muscle (*musculum internum mallei*; see Verheyen, 1693, p. 202); in the original Latin, *filamentum mallei*, see Table II.
2. *labyrinthine filament of portio major and minor of facial nerve (Bellingeri, 1818)*
   Questionable branch of macrodissected adult human ***intermediofacial nerve trunk (>1840)*** communicating with ***lingual nerve (Vesalius, 1543a)*** and going to vestibule of osseous labyrinth; in the original Latin, *filamentum labyrinthicum?*, see Table II.
3. *various filaments of portio major and minor of facial nerve (Bellingeri, 1818)*
   Basically macrodissected adult human ***communicating branch of intermediofacial nerve with tympanic plexus (>1840)*** and ***tympanic plexus (Müller, 1834)*** and its branches to mastoid air cells, tympanic membrane, and nearby structures; in the original Latin, *filamenta varia*, see Table II.
4. *anastomotic filament of portio major and minor of facial nerve with accessory nerve of Willis (Bellingeri, 1818)*
   Macrodissected adult human ***communicating branch (Winslow, 1733)*** of ***intermediofacial nerve trunk (>1840)*** with ***accessory nerve (Vieussens, 1684)***; in the original Latin, *filamentum anastomoticum*, see Table II.
5. *genu of facial nerve (Langenbeck, 1826–1830)*
   Approximately right turn of macrodissected adult human ***intermediofacial nerve trunk (1840)*** at site of ***geniculate ganglion (Bischoff, 1832)***; in the original Latin, *genu nervi facialis*, Fasc. III, Table XVIII-13. See Williams & Warwick (1980, Figs. 7.184, 185).

intermediolateral nucleus (>1840)

As described for macrodissected adult human, and for adult mammal in general with cellular architecture and connections, the thin longitudinal ***gray matter region (Swanson & Bota, 2010)*** forming a swelling on the lateral edge of the ***intermediate spinal zone (>1840)***. A rostral segment extends from the caudal end of the ***cervical part of spinal cord (>1840)*** rostrally, to about the middle of the ***lumbar part of spinal cord (>1840)*** caudaly, and a caudal segment is centered in the middle three levels of the ***sacral part of spinal cord (>1840)***. Functionally, the former contains preganglionic sympathetic motor ***neurons (Waldeyer, 1891)*** and the latter contains preganglionic parasympathetic motor ***neurons (Waldeyer, 1891)***; see Carpenter (1976, p. 230), *Terminologia Anatomica* (1998, p. 106), Nieuwenhuys et al. (2008, p. 180). It was not identified by 1840.

EARLIER REFERENCES:

Earlier synonyms:

1. *intermediolateral column (>1840)*
   Synonym for adult mammalian ***intermediolateral nucleus (>1840)***; see *Nomina Anatomica* (1983, p. A64).

intermesenteric plexus (>1840)

As described for macrodissected adult human, a ***prevertebral plexus (Quain, 1832)*** lying along the sides and ventral part (front) of the aorta, stretching between the ***superior mesenteric plexus (Rau, 1720)*** rostrally and ***inferior mesenteric plexus (Rau, 1720)*** caudally, and also receiving inputs from the first and second ***lumbar splanchnic nerves (Cruveilhier, 1836)***; see Williams & Warwick (1980, p. 1134), Durward (1951, Fig. 968 called *aortic plexus*). It was clearly differentiated by Willis; see ***[intermesenteric plexus (>1840)] (Willis, 1664)***.

EARLIER REFERENCES:

Illustrated and described, not named:

1. ***[intermesenteric plexus (>1840)] (Willis, 1664)***
   Illustrated and described for macrodissected adult human and other common large mammals, though not very accurately; see Pordage translation (1681, p. 159 and Tab. 11-*between* ⊙, ☽), Mitchell (1953, p. 4).

Earlier synonyms:

1. *fasciculi mesenterici posterioris (Winslow, 1733)*
   Synonym for macrodissected adult human ***intermesenteric plexus (>1840)***; Sect. VI, p. 99.
2. *nervos mesaraicos posteriores (Schaarschmidt, 1750)*
   Synonym for macrodissected adult human ***intermesenteric plexus (>1840)***; p. 55.
3. *aortic plexus (Cloquet, 1816)*
   Synonym for macrodissected adult human ***intermesenteric plexus (>1840)***; in the original French, *plexus aortique*, p. 711; also see Meckel (1832, Vol. 3, p. 90).
4. *lumboaortic plexus (Cruveilhier, 1836)*
   Synonym for macrodissected adult human ***intermesenteric plexus (>1840)***; in the original French, *plexus lumbo-aortique*, pp. 1020, 1025.

LATER SYNONYMS:

1. *abdominal aortic plexus (>1840)*
   Synonym for macrodissected adult human ***intermesenteric plexus (>1840)***; see Durward (1951, p. 1142), Williams & Warwick (1980, p. 1134).

internal arcuate fibers (>1840)

As described in macrodissected adult human, and mammal generally with histological methods for ***axons (Kölliker, 1896)***, a diffuse, obliquely dorsoventrally oriented ***central nervous system white matter tract (>1840)*** in the ***medulla (Winslow, 1733)***, between ***dorsal column nuclei (>1840)*** dorsolaterally and ***medial lemniscus decussation (>1840)*** ventromedially; see Williams & Warwick (1980, p. 901), Nieuwenhuys et al. (2008, p. 194 and Figs. 6.14, 6.22). They were not recognized by 1840.

internal branch of accessory nerve trunk (Meckel, 1817)

As described for macrodissected adult human, one of two major terminal branches of the ***accessory nerve trunk (Wrisberg, 1786)***, arising from the ***cranial root of accessory nerve (>1840)*** and distributing mainly to ***pharyngeal branches of vagus nerve (Wrisberg, 1786)*** and ***recurrent laryngeal nerve (Albinus, 1744)***; see Williams & Warwick (1980, p. 1082). For Meckel's use in macrodissected adult human, see translation (1832, Vol. 3, p. 44). It was first clearly delineated as the *internal branch of accessory nerve (Scarpa, 1788)*.

EARLIER REFERENCES:

Earlier synonyms:

1. *internal branch of accessory nerve (Scarpa, 1788)*
   Synonym for macrodissected adult human ***internal branch of accessory nerve trunk (Meckel, 1817)***; in the original Latin, *accessorii ramus internus*, Table X, Figure 1-5.
2. *internal branch of accessory vagal pair (Soemmerring, 1791)*
   Synonym for macrodissected adult human ***internal branch of accessory nerve trunk (Meckel, 1817)***; p. 255, also see Soemmerring (1798, p. 275).
3. *lesser internal branch of accessory eighth cranial nerve (Scarpa, 1794)*
   Basically synonym for macrodissected adult human *internal branch of accessory vagal pair (Soemmerring, 1791)*; in the original Latin, *accessorium nervus ad octavum cerebri ramus minor internus*, see Table II-27.
4. *smaller internal branch of spinal accessory (Knox, 1832)*
   Synonym for *lesser internal branch of accessory eighth cranial nerve (Scarpa, 1794)*; Plate II-61.
5. *internal branch of spinal nerve (Cruveilhier, 1836)*
   Synonym for macrodissected adult human ***internal branch of accessory nerve trunk (Meckel, 1817)***; in the original French, *branche interne du nerf spinal*, p. 956.
6. *anastomotic branch of spinal nerve (Cruveilhier, 1836)*
   Synonym for *internal branch of spinal nerve (Cruveilhier, 1836)*; in the original French, *branche anastomotique du nerf spinal*, p. 956.

PARTLY CORRESPONDS:

1. *anastomosis of internal branch of accessory nerve with eighth nerve fibers (Scarpa, 1788)*
   Scarpa described two ***communicating branches (Winslow, 1733)*** between macrodissected adult human ***internal branch of accessory nerve trunk (Meckel, 1817)*** and ***vagus nerve (Galen, c192)***; in the original Latin, *anastomosis rami interni nervi accessorii cum fibrilla octavi*, Table X, Figure 1-7,9.
2. *posterior filament of internal branch of accessory nerve (Bischoff, 1832)*
   Macrodissected adult human dorsal (posterior) branch of ***internal branch of accessory nerve trunk (Meckel, 1817)***; in the original Latin, *filum posterius rami interni Accessorii*, Table I, Figure 1-32.
3. *anterior filament of internal branch of accessory nerve (Bischoff, 1832)*
   Macrodissected adult human ventral (anterior) branch of ***internal branch of accessory nerve trunk (Meckel, 1817)***; in the original Latin, *filum anterius rami interni Accessorii*, Table I, Figure 1-33.

internal branch of superior laryngeal nerve (Fyfe, 1800)

As described for adult human, it mainly supplies sensory ***dendrites (His, 1889)*** to mucous membrane of the larynx caudally (down) to the level of the vocal folds, as well as to stretch receptors in various laryngeal muscles; see Williams & Warwick (1980, p. 1080), *Terminologia Anatomica* (1998, p. 136). For Fyfe's description in macrodissected adult human see Vol. 2, p. 295. It was known to Galen; see ***[internal branch of superior laryngeal nerve (Fyfe, 1800)] (Galen, c173)***.

EARLIER REFERENCES:

Described, not named or illustrated:

1. ***[internal branch of superior laryngeal nerve (Fyfe, 1800)] (Galen, c173)***
   Described for macrodissected adult beef, pig, and/or macaque, but not human; see May translation (1968, p. 689), Duckworth translation (1962, pp. 203–204). Willis (1664) probably mentioned it for macrodissected adult human; see Pordage translation (1681, p. 147 and Tab. IX-*h*).

Earlier synonyms:

1. *deep branchlets of superior laryngeal nerve (Loder, 1778)*
   Synonym for macrodissected adult human ***internal branch of superior laryngeal nerve (Fyfe, 1800)***; in the original Latin, *ramulum profundum*, p. 30.
2. *internal branch of laryngeal nerve (Haase, 1781)*
   Synonym for macrodissected adult human ***internal branch of superior laryngeal nerve (Fyfe, 1800)***; in the original Latin, *nervus laryngeus ramus internus*, p. 85.
3. *inner laryngeal nerve (Günther, 1786)*
   Synonym for macrodissected adult human ***internal branch of superior laryngeal nerve (Fyfe, 1800)***; in the original Latin, *nervus laryngeus interiorem*, p. 63.
4. *internal laryngeal nerve (Soemmerring, 1791)*
   Synonym for macrodissected adult human ***internal branch of superior laryngeal nerve (Fyfe, 1800)***; in the original Latin, *nervus laryngeus internus*, p. 246.

LATER SYNONYMS:

1. *internal laryngeal branch of vocal nerve (Bock, 1817)*
   Synonym for macrodissected adult human ***internal branch of superior laryngeal nerve (Fyfe, 1800)***; in the original Latin, *ramus laryngeus internus*, p. 69.
2. *internal branch of descending laryngeal nerve (Swan, 1830)*
   Synonym for macrodissected adult human ***internal branch of superior laryngeal nerve (Fyfe, 1800)***; p. 756.
3. *internal laryngeal nerve of pneumogastric (Knox, 1832)*
   Synonym for macrodissected adult human ***internal branch of superior laryngeal nerve (Fyfe, 1800)***; Plate III-176, in Knox's translation of Scarpa (1794).

PARTLY CORRESPONDS:

1. *posterior epiglottal nerve (Andersch & Soemmerring, 1792)*
   Described as fourth branch of macrodissected adult human *internal laryngeal nerve (Soemmerring, 1791)*; in the original Latin, *nervus epiglottideus posterior*, p. 130.
2. *anterior epiglottal nerve (Andersch & Soemmerring, 1792)*
   Branch of macrodissected adult human *internal laryngeal nerve (Soemmerring, 1791)*; in the original Latin, *nervus epiglottideus anterior*, p. 131.
3. *first epiglottal branch of posterior epiglottal nerve (Andersch & Soemmerring, 1792)*
   Rostral (superior or upper) branch of *posterior epiglottal nerve (Andersch & Soemmerring, 1792)* dividing into two primary branches; in the original Latin, *primum ramum epiglottideum*, p. 131.
4. *second epiglottal branch of posterior epiglottal nerve (Andersch & Soemmerring, 1792)*
   Middle branch of *posterior epiglottal nerve (Andersch & Soemmerring, 1792)*, in turn dividing into three major branches; in the original Latin, *secundum ramum epiglottideum*, p. 131.
5. *branches of superior laryngeal nerve to epiglottis (Langenbeck, 1826–1830)*
   Macrodissected adult human branches of ***internal branch of superior laryngeal nerve (Fyfe, 1800)*** to epiglottis; in the original Latin, *rami nervi laryngei superioris ad epiglottideum*, Fascicle III, Table XVI-8.
6. *branches of superior laryngeal nerve to mucosal tunic of larynx (Langenbeck, 1826–1830)*
   Macrodissected adult human branches of ***internal branch of superior laryngeal nerve (Fyfe, 1800)*** to laryngeal mucosa; in the original Latin, *rami nervi laryngei superioris ad tunicam mucosam laryngis*, Fascicle III, Table XVIII-29.
7. *branches of superior laryngeal nerve to tunica intima of trachea (Langenbeck, 1826–1830)*
   Macrodissected adult human branches of ***internal branch of superior laryngeal nerve (Fyfe, 1800)*** to inner layer of trachea; in the original Latin, *rami nervi laryngei superioris ad tunicam intimam tracheae*, Fascicle III, Table XVIII-38.
8. *anterior branches of superior laryngeal branches of pneumogastric nerve (Cruveilhier, 1836)*
   Macrodissected adult human branches of ***internal branch of superior laryngeal nerve (Fyfe, 1800)***, associated mostly with epiglottis; in the original French, *rameaux antérieurs*, p. 959.
9. *epiglottal branches of superior laryngeal branches of pneumogastric nerve (Cruveilhier, 1836)*
   Synonym for *anterior branches of superior laryngeal branches of pneumogastric nerve (Cruveilhier, 1836)*; in the original French, *rameaux épiglottiques*, p. 959.
10. *superior laryngeal filaments to tongue (Cruveilhier, 1836)*
    Macrodissected adult human *anterior branch of superior laryngeal branches of pneumogastric nerve (Cruveilhier, 1836)* to regions of base of tongue near median plane; in the original French, *filets linguaux du laryngé supérieur*, p. 960.
11. *posterior filaments of superior laryngeal branches of pneumogastric nerve (Cruveilhier, 1836)*
    Macrodissected adult human branches of ***internal branch of superior laryngeal nerve (Fyfe, 1800)***, associated mostly with larynx; in the original French, *filets postérieurs*, p. 960.
12. *laryngeal filaments of superior laryngeal branches of pneumogastric nerve (Cruveilhier, 1836)*
    Synonym for *posterior branches of superior laryngeal branches of pneumogastric nerve (Cruveilhier, 1836)*; in the original French, *filets laryngiens*, p. 960.
13. *mucous filaments of superior laryngeal branches of pneumogastric nerve (Cruveilhier, 1836)*
    Macrodissected adult human small branches of *posterior filaments of superior laryngeal branches of pneumogastric nerve (Cruveilhier, 1836)* associated with aryepiglottic fold; in the original French, *filets muqueux*, p. 960.
14. *arytenoid filament of superior laryngeal branches of pneumogastric nerve (Cruveilhier, 1836)*
    Macrodissected adult human small branch of *posterior filaments of superior laryngeal branches of pneumogastric nerve (Cruveilhier, 1836)* supplying arytenoid muscle; in the original French, *filet arythénoïdien*, p. 960.
15. *filament of arytenoid muscle (Cruveilhier, 1836)*
    Synonym for *arytenoid filament of superior laryngeal branches of pneumogastric nerve (Cruveilhier, 1836)*; in the original French, *filet du muscle arythénoïdien*, p. 960.

internal capsule (Burdach, 1822)

As described for macrodissected adult human, the main longitudinal, fanlike ***central nervous system white matter tract (>1840)*** of the ***forebrain (Goette, 1873)***, interposed between the transverse ***cerebral cortex white matter (>1840)*** rostrally and dorsally, and the longitudinal extension of the ***internal capsule (Burdach, 1822)***, the ***cerebral peduncle (Tarin, 1753)***, caudally and ventrally. Because the ***internal capsule (Burdach, 1822)*** has long been described most clearly in frontal (horizontal) sections, it is conventionally divided into an ***anterior limb of internal capsule (>1840)***, ***genu of internal capsule (>1840)***, and ***posterior limb of internal capsule (>1840)***, the latter having two ventral and caudal differentiations, the ***retrolentiform limb of internal capsule (>1840)*** and ***sublentiform limb of internal capsule***

(>1840). In addition, the ***thalamic radiations (>1840)*** and ***corticospinal tract (>1840)*** are incorporated into the ***internal capsule (Burdach, 1822)***; see Crosby et al. (1962, p. 394, Fig. 272), Carpenter (1976, pp. 462–465 and Fig. 15.18), *Terminologia Anatomica* (1998, p. 130). For Burdach's use in macrodissected adult human, see p. 127. Burdach (1822, p. 350) credited Reil with inspiring the term, based on his *inner wall of capsule (Reil, 1809b)*; p. 203. For the English form see Mayo translation (1823, p. 81). Also see Meyer (1971, p. 29). It was clearly illustrated by Vesalius; see ***[internal capsule (Burdach, 1822)] (Vesalius, 1543a)***.

EARLIER REFERENCES:

Illustrated, not named or described:

1. ***[internal capsule (Burdach, 1822)] (Vesalius, 1543a)***
   Very clearly illustrated for macrodissected adult human in frontal (horizontal) section, along with ***anterior limb of internal capsule (>1840)***, ***genu of internal capsule (>1840)***, and ***posterior limb of internal capsule (>1840)***; see Singer translation (1952, Fig. 7).

Earlier synonyms:

1. *corporis striati limbus posterior (Willis, 1672)*
   Synonym for macrodissected adult sheep and human right and left ***internal capsule (Burdach, 1822)***; Table VIII-*H*. Also see Ridley (1695, p. 122), Schiller (1967, pp. 526, 529).
2. *posterior limbus of corpus striatum (Willis, 1672)*
   English form (singular) of *corporis striati limbus posterior (Willis, 1672)*.
3. *latter border of streaked body (Willis, 1672)*
   English form of *corporis striati limbus posterior (Willis, 1672)* for macrodissected adult sheep; see Pordage translation (1683, Tab. V-*K*).
4. *hinder border of streaked body (Willis, 1672)*
   English form of *corporis striati limbus posterior (Willis, 1672)* for macrodissected adult sheep (Tab. VII-*E*) and human (Tab. VIII-*E*); see Pordage translation (1683).
5. *centrum semicirculare geminum (Vieussens, 1684)*
   Synonym for macrodissected adult human ***internal capsule (Burdach, 1822)***; Tables X-*D*, XIII-*G*, XIV-*E*. Also see Ridley (1695, p. 122), Schiller (1967, p. 526), and Meyer (1971, p. 14) who pointed out that the term refers to the fact that it surrounds the *thalamus (Malpighi, 1673)* in a semicircle. It is unclear whether *corpora striata media* (Tab. XIV-*D*; pp. 116, 122) refers to ***internal capsule (Burdach, 1822)***, a part of it, or a ***central nervous system white matter tract (>1840)*** including ***internal capsule (Burdach, 1822)***; see Burdach (1822, p. 350). Vieussens also used the form, *centrum geminum semicirculare*; p. 67, see Meyer (1971, p. 14).
6. *semicirculare centrum (Vieussens, 1684)*
   Synonym for *centrum semicirculare geminum (Vieussens, 1684)*.
7. *middle fluted body (Pourfour du Petit, 1710)*
   Roughly synonymous with macrodissected adult human ***internal capsule (Burdach, 1822)***; see Clarke & O'Malley translation (1996, p. 283).
8. *middle striated body (Pourfour du Petit, 1710)*
   Alternate form of *middle fluted body (Pourfour du Petit, 1710)*; in the original French, *les corps cannelez moi[y]ens*, pp. 7, 8, 10, 11, 14 (L. Kruger & L.W. Swanson, unpublished translation).
9. *inner wall of capsule (Reil, 1809b)*
   Synonym for macrodissected adult human ***internal capsule (Burdach, 1822)***; see Mayo translation (1823, pp. 69, 81).
10. *fascicle of great superior cerebral ganglion (Gall & Spurzheim, 1810)*
   Synonym for macrodissected adult human ***internal capsule (Burdach, 1822)***; in the original French (plural), *faisceaux du grand ganglion cérébral supérieur*, Tables V, VI-S.
11. *base of corona radiata (Burdach, 1822)*
   Synonym for macrodissected adult human ***internal capsule (Burdach, 1822)***; in the original Latin, *basis coronae radiatae*, p. 132. According to Schiller (1969, p. 529), foundation of term "*basal*" *ganglia*.

LATER SYNONYMS:

1. *layer of peduncle of hemisphere (Rolando, 1831)*
   Synonym for macrodissected adult human ***internal capsule (Burdach, 1822)***; in the original Italian, *strato de' pedoncoli degli emisferi*, p. 118.
2. *process of greater and superior ganglion of brain (Knox, 1832)*
   Synonym for macrodissected adult human ***internal capsule (Burdach, 1822)***; Supplemental Plate IV-24.
3. *meditullium album (Arnold, 1838b)*
   Synonym for macrodissected adult human ***internal capsule (Burdach, 1822)***; Table VIII, Figure 1-*n*. Arnold recognized anterior, middle, and posterior parts; see Table X, Figure 1-*f,g,h* and Figure 2-*b,c,d*.
4. *lateral forebrain bundle (Edinger, 1893)*
   Synonym for macrodissected adult human ***internal capsule (Burdach, 1822)***; see Nauta & Haymaker (1969, pp. 164–165).

PARTLY CORRESPONDS:

1. *flabellum (Bergmann, 1831)*
   Apparently component of macrodissected adult human *corona radiata (Reil, 1809b)* associated with *head of striated body (Willis, 1664)*, roughly ***head of caudate nucleus (>1840)***, and thus part of ***internal capsule (Burdach, 1822)***; p. 5 and Table II-*u*. It means fan-shaped.
2. *appendix flabelli (Bergmann, 1831)*
   Apparently component of macrodissected adult human *corona radiata (Reil, 1809b)* associated with ***body of caudate nucleus (>1840)*** and thus part of ***internal capsule (Burdach, 1822)***; Table II-*v*.

internal carotid nerve (>1840)

As described for macrodissected adult human, the extension of the ***sympathetic trunk (Winslow, 1733)*** rostral to (above) the ***superior cervical ganglion (Vieussens, 1684)***. It is usually single and courses rostrally, dorsal to (behind) the internal carotid artery before entering the carotid canal, where it usually breaks up into the ***internal carotid***

plexus (>1840) around the internal carotid artery and where medial and lateral branches of the ***internal carotid nerve (>1840)*** can sometimes be distinguished before disappearing in the ***internal carotid plexus (>1840)***; see Mitchell (1953, pp. 207, 215–221), Williams & Warwick (1980, pp. 1127). Earlier research is thoroughly reviewed by Neubauer (1772). Its existence was known to Galen; see ***[internal carotid nerve (>1840)] (Galen, c192)***.

EARLIER REFERENCES:

Described, not named or illustrated:

1. *[internal carotid nerve (>1840)] (Galen, c192)*
   Described without naming for macrodissected adult beef, pig, and/or macaque but not human; see Duckworth translation (1962, p. 217).

Illustrated and described, not named:

1. *[internal carotid nerve (>1840)] (Lancisi, 1728)*
   Beautifully described and illustrated for macrodissected adult human; Table VI-*A*.

Earlier synonyms:

1. *root of intercostal nerve (Willis, 1664)*
   Corresponds roughly to ***internal carotid nerve (>1840)*** of macrodissected adult human and other common large quadrupeds; see Figure 1-*b,b* on p. 302. Term reflects Willis's mistaken view that ***sympathetic trunk (Winslow, 1733)*** arises from ***trigeminal nerve (Winslow, 1733)*** and ***abducens nerve (Heister, 1717)***; see Pourfour du Petit (1729).
2. *ascending branch of intercostal nerve (Winslow, 1733)*
   Synonym for macrodissected adult human ***internal carotid nerve (>1840)***; Section VI, no. 359, p. 94. Winslow also referred to it as an ascending trunk; Section VI, no. 370, p. 95.
3. *superior root of intercostal nerve (Mayer, 1794)*
   Synonym for macrodissected adult human ***internal carotid nerve (>1840)***, although Mayer did not clearly distinguish an ***internal carotid plexus (>1840)***; in the original Latin, *radix superior nervi intercostalis*; Part V, Table VIII, Figure 6-*u*.
4. *superior branches of superior cervical ganglion (Cloquet, 1816)*
   Synonym for macrodissected adult human ***internal carotid nerve (>1840)***; in the original French, *filets supérieurs du ganglion cervical supérieur*, p. 688. For macrodissected adult human, Cruveilhier (1836, p. 985) referred to it as a superior branch (*rameau supérieur*).
5. *ascending branches of superior cervical ganglion (Cloquet, 1816)*
   Synonym for macrodissected adult human ***internal carotid nerve (>1840)***; in the original French, *filets ascendans du ganglion cervical supérieur*, p. 688.
6. *filament of communication with superior cervical ganglion (Meckel, 1817)*
   Synonym for *superior branch of superior cervical ganglion (Cloquet, 1816)*; see translation (1832, Vol. 3, p. 91).
7. *carotid nerve (Lobstein, 1823)*
   Apparently synonym for macrodissected adult human ***internal carotid nerve (>1840)***; see translation (1831, p. 58).
8. *superior nervi molles (Knox, 1832)*
   Synonym for macrodissected adult human ***internal carotid nerve (>1840)***; Plate III-*171*, in Knox's translation of Scarpa (1794).
9. *carotid branch of superior cervical ganglion (Cruveilhier, 1836)*
   Synonym for macrodissected adult human ***internal carotid nerve (>1840)***; in the original French, *rameau carotidien*, p. 985.

internal carotid plexus (>1840)

As described for macrodissected adult human, the rostral (upper) continuation of the ***internal carotid nerve (>1840)***, which begins breaking up into the ***internal carotid plexus (>1840)*** in the carotid canal and has wide and varied extensions accompanying all branches of the internal carotid artery arising in the ***cavernous sinus (Winslow, 1733)***; see Durward (1951, pp. 1133–1134), Mitchell (1953, pp. 215–221), Williams & Warwick (1980, p. 1127). Bell (1803b, p. 173) noted that "It has been often observed, that the branches of the carotid artery have a peculiar provision of nerves, and that these nerves are more numerous and minutely distributed than in any other part of the body." It was perhaps first clearly described and illustrated by Pourfour du Petit; see ***[internal carotid plexus (>1840)] (Pourfour du Petit, 1729)***.

EARLIER REFERENCES:

Illustrated and described, not named:

1. *[internal carotid plexus (>1840)] (Pourfour du Petit, 1729)*
   Very clearly described and illustrated for macrodissected adult dog and wolf, although it was briefly mentioned earlier (Rau, 1720, p. 110); p. 3 and Plate 1, Figure 3-*F,I*. Bergen (1731, Tab. parts *a* and *C*) schematically illustrated the ***internal carotid plexus (>1840)*** for macrodissected adult human very nicely for the first time, including part in ***cavernous sinus (Winslow, 1733)***. Meckel (1748; Fig. 1-*γ,ο,π,ξ* and Figs. 2–6) illustrated its variable relationship to ***deep petrosal nerve (Meckel, 1817)*** in macrodissected adult human.

Earlier synonyms:

1. *plexiform filaments surround carotid artery (Winslow, 1733)*
   Essence of Winslow's description of macrodissected adult human ***internal carotid plexus (>1840)***; Section VI, no. 368, p. 95.
2. *superficial plexus of posterior carotid arteries (Andersch & Soemmerring, 1792)*
   Synonym for macrodissected adult human ***internal carotid plexus (>1840)***; in the original Latin, *plexum superficialem arteriae carotidis posterioris*, p. 166.
3. *carotid plexus (Bock, 1817)*
   Synonym for macrodissected adult human ***internal carotid plexus (>1840)***; in the original Latin, *plexus caroticus*, p. 63.
4. *carotic plexus (Lobstein, 1831)*
   Alternate form of *carotid plexus (Burdach, 1819)*; p. 35.

5. *retiform plexus (Arnold, 1834)*
   Synonym for macrodissected adult human ***internal carotid plexus (>1840)***; in the original Latin, *plexus retiformis*, Table VI-53.
6. *cavernous plexus (Quain, 1837)*
   Synonym for macrodissected adult human *carotid plexus (Bock, 1817)*; p. 807.

PARTLY CORRESPONDS:

1. *communicating branch from submaxillary branch of inferior submaxillary nerve to great sympathetic nerve (Andersch & Soemmerring, 1792)****Communicating branch (Winslow, 1733)*** in macrodissected adult human between ***internal carotid plexus (>1840)*** and ***mylohyoid nerve (Meckel, 1748)***; in the original Latin, *ramus communicatorius a ramo submaxillari nervi submaxillaris inferioris*, p. 170.
2. *communicating branch from submaxillary branches of inferior maxillary nerves to great harmonic nerve of body (Andersch, 1797)*
   Synonym for *communicating branch from submaxillary branch of inferior submaxillary nerve to great sympathetic nerve (Andersch & Soemmerring, 1792)*; in the original Latin, *ramum communicatorium rami submaxillaris nervi maxillaris inferioris*, Vol. 1, p. 115.
3. *pterygoid filament (Cloquet, 1816)*
   Extension of macrodissected adult human ***internal carotid plexus (>1840)*** communicating with ***deep petrosal nerve (Meckel, 1817)*** and sending filaments to pharynx; in the original French, *filet ptérygoïdien*, p. 689. Cloquet attributed without citation the term to Chaussier.
4. *anterior branch of sympathetic nerve (Langenbeck, 1826–1830)*
   For macrodissected adult human, probably corresponds to *internal branch of carotid nerve (Arnold, 1834)*; in the original Latin, *ramus nervi sympathici anterior*, Fascicle III, Table XVI-*13*.
5. *posterior branch of sympathetic nerve (Langenbeck, 1826–1830)*
   For macrodissected adult human, probably corresponds to *external branch of carotid nerve (Arnold, 1834)*; in the original Latin, *ramus nervi sympathici posterior*, Fascicle III, Table XVI-*14*.
6. *anastomosis of sympathetic nerve with second branch of trigeminal (Langenbeck, 1826–1830)*
   For macrodissected adult human, ***communicating branch (Winslow, 1733)*** of ***internal carotid plexus (>1840)*** with ***maxillary nerve (Meckel, 1753)***; in the original Latin, *anastomosis nervi sympathici cum ramo secundo Trigemini*, Fascicle III, Table XVIII-*R*.
7. *external carotid nerve (Arnold, 1834)*
   Synonym for *external branch of carotid nerve (Arnold, 1834)*; in the original Latin, *nervo carotico externo*, p. 13.
8. *external branch of carotid nerve (Arnold, 1834)*
   In macrodissected adult human, rostral (superior) of two clear branches of ***internal carotid nerve (>1840)*** lying within broader ***internal carotid plexus (>1840)***, proximal to *cavernous plexus (Arnold, 1834)* and generating *connection of carotid nerve with tympanic nerve (Arnold, 1834)*, *connection of carotid nerve with nasal ganglion (Arnold, 1834)*, and *connection of carotid nerve with abducens nerve (Arnold, 1834)*; in the original Latin, *nervo carotico ramus externus*, p. 18. See Williams & Warwick (1980, Fig. 7.184).
9. *internal branch of carotid nerve (Arnold, 1834)*
   In macrodissected adult human, caudal (inferior) of two clear branches of ***internal carotid nerve (>1840)*** lying within the broader ***internal carotid plexus (>1840)***, and corresponding at least partly to *cavernous plexus (Arnold, 1834)*; in the original Latin, *nervo carotico ramus internus*, p. 18.
10. *external superior carotid nerve (Arnold, 1834)*
    Synonym for *external branch of carotid nerve (Arnold, 1834)*; in the original Latin, *nervus caroticus externus superior*, Table VI-*129*.
11. *internal inferior carotid nerve (Arnold, 1834)*
    Synonym for *internal branch of carotid nerve (Arnold, 1834)*; in the original Latin, *nervus caroticus internus inferior*, Table VI-*132*.
12. *cavernous plexus (Arnold, 1834)*
    In macrodissected adult human, segment of ***internal carotid plexus (>1840)*** associated with ***cavernous sinus (Winslow, 1733)***; in the original Latin, *plexus cavernosus*, p. 18.
13. *connections of internal branch of carotid nerve with external carotid nerve (Arnold, 1834)*
    In macrodissected adult human, ***communicating branch (Winslow, 1733)*** between *internal branch of carotid nerve (Arnold, 1834)* and *external branch of carotid nerve (Arnold, 1834)*; in the original Latin, *conjunctiones nervus caroticus ramus internus cum nervo carotico externo*, p. 18.
14. *plexus nervoso-arteriosus of Walter (Cruveilhier, 1836)*
    Eponym for macrodissected adult human *cavernous plexus (Arnold, 1834)*, attributed without citation to Walter; pp. 987–988.
15. *filament from sympathetic to third division of fifth pair of nerves (Todd, 1836–1839)*
    For macrodissected adult human, ***communicating branch (Winslow, 1733)*** from ***internal carotid plexus (>1840)*** to ***mandibular nerve (>1840)***; p. 289, where Todd noted that Munniks, Laumonier, and Bock had already mentioned it.

internal medullary lamina (>1840)

As described in macrodissected adult human, and mammal generally with histological methods for ***axons (Kölliker, 1896)***, a somewhat diffusely organized, wing-shaped ***central nervous system white matter tract (>1840)*** centered in the ***intralaminar thalamic nuclei (>1840)***; see Crosby et al. (1962, p. 273), Jones (1985, p. 607). It was delineated vaguely by Vesalius; see ***[internal medullary lamina (>1840)] (Vesalius, 1543a)***.

EARLIER REFERENCES:

Illustrated, not named or described:

1. ***[internal medullary lamina (>1840)] (Vesalius, 1543a)***
   Apparently indicated as streak of *white substance (Vesalius, 1543a)* through roughly middle of macrodissected adult

human ***thalamus (His, 1893a)*** as viewed in frontal (horizontal) section; see Singer translation (1952, Fig. 8, 'C' in ***thalamus (His, 1893a)*** on left side of figure).

2. ***[internal medullary lamina (>1840)] (Reil, 1809b)***
   Reil noted that by following ***mammillothalamic tract (Kölliker, 1896)*** from its origin, interval between two inner gray masses of *thalamus (Malpighi, 1672)* is found at once; see Mayo translation (1823, p. 57).

Earlier synonyms:

1. *thalamic medullary lamina (Burdach, 1822)*
   Synonym for macrodissected adult human ***internal medullary lamina (>1840)***; in the original Latin, *lamina medullaris thalami*, p. 122. Burdach noted (1822, p. 345) it is one of two *entrelacemens transversau* described and illustrated by Gall & Spurzheim (1810).

internal nasal branches of anterior ethmoidal nerve (>1840)

As described for macrodissected adult human, it usually has two branches, ***lateral nasal branches of internal nasal branches of anterior ethmoidal nerve (>1840)*** and ***medial nasal branches of internal nasal branches of anterior ethmoidal nerve (>1840)***; see Williams & Warwick (1980, p. 1061), *Terminologia Anatomica* (1998, p. 134). They were probably first identified by Willis; see ***[internal nasal branches of anterior ethmoidal nerve (>1840)] (Willis, 1664)***.

EARLIER REFERENCES:

Illustrated and described, not named:

1. ***[internal nasal branches of anterior ethmoidal nerve (>1840)] (Willis, 1664)***
   Probably illustrated and alluded to for macrodissected adult human and other common large mammals; p. 302, Figure 1-*c*.

Earlier synonyms:

1. *interior branch of nasal nerve (Scarpa, 1785)*
   Synonym for macrodissected adult human ***internal nasal branches of anterior ethmoidal nerve (>1840)***; in the original Latin, *nervi nasalis ramus interior*, Table I, Figure 1-*.
2. *internal branch of nasal nerve (Scarpa, 1785)*
   Synonym for macrodissected adult human ***internal nasal branches of anterior ethmoidal nerve (>1840)***; in the original Latin, *nervi nasalis ramus internus*, Table II, Figure 2-o.
3. *internal superior nasal nerves (Günther, 1786)*
   Synonym for macrodissected adult human ***internal branches of anterior ethmoidal nerve (>1840)***; in the original Latin, *N. nasales superiores interni*, p. 44.
4. *internal filament of internal nasal branch of nasal nerve (Cruveilhier, 1836)*
   Synonym for macrodissected adult human ***internal nasal branches of anterior ethmoidal nerve (>1840)***; in the original French, *filet interne*, p. 915.
5. *internal filament of ethmoidal branch of nasal nerve (Cruveilhier, 1836)*
   Synonym for macrodissected adult human ***internal nasal branches of anterior ethmoidal nerve (>1840)***; in the original French, *filet interne*, p. 915.
6. *nerve of nasal septum (Cruveilhier, 1836, p. 916)*
   Synonym for macrodissected adult human ***internal nasal branches of anterior ethmoidal nerve (>1840)***; in the original French, *nerf de la cloison*, p. 916.

PARTLY CORRESPONDS:

1. *minor branch of interior nasal nerve (Scarpa, 1785)*
   Smaller of two branches described for *interior branch of nasal nerve (Scarpa, 1785)*; in the original Latin, *nervi nasalis interioris ramus minor*, Table I, Figure 1-*k*.
2. *major branch of interior nasal nerve (Scarpa, 1785)*
   Larger of two branches described for *interior branch of nasal nerve (Scarpa, 1785)*; in the original Latin, *nervi nasalis interioris ramus major*, Table I, Figure 1-*l*.

internal nasal branches of infraorbital nerve (>1840)

As described for macrodissected adult human, they innervate skin on the moveable part of the nasal septum and communicate with the ***external nasal branch of anterior ethmoidal nerve (>1840)***; see Williams & Warwick (1980, p. 1064), *Terminologia Anatomica* (1998, p. 134). They were first clearly described by Meckel; see ***[internal nasal branches of infraorbital nerve (>1840)] (Meckel, 1748)***.

EARLIER REFERENCES:

Described, not named or illustrated:

1. ***[internal nasal branches of infraorbital nerve (>1840)] (Meckel, 1748)***
   Described for macrodissected adult human; p. 75.

Earlier synonyms:

1. *internal superior superficial nasal nerve (Meckel, 1817)*
   Synonym for macrodissected adult human ***internal nasal branches of infraorbital nerve (>1840)***; see translation (1832, Vol. 3, p. 70).
2. *internal superior cutaneous nasal nerve (Meckel, 1817)*
   Synonym for macrodissected adult human ***internal nasal branches of infraorbital nerve (>1840)***; see translation (1832, Vol. 3, p. 70).
3. *superior nasal subcutaneous branch of infraorbital nerve (Bock, 1817)*
   Synonym for macrodissected adult human ***internal nasal branches of infraorbital nerve (>1840)***; in the original Latin, *ramus subcutaneus nasi superior*, p. 36.
4. *interior and superior nasal nerve (Arnold, 1834)*
   Synonym for macrodissected adult human ***internal nasal branches of infraorbital nerve (>1840)***; in the original Latin, *nervus nasalis superior et inferior*, p. 9.

PARTLY CORRESPONDS:

1. *nerve of subseptum (Cruveilhier, 1836)*
   Meaning for macrodissected adult human unclear, but apparently related to ***internal nasal branches of infraorbital nerve (>1840)***; in the original French, *nerf de la sous-cloison*, p. 946.

interosseal nerve of leg (>1840)

As described for macrodissected adult human, a branch of the ***nerve to popliteus (>1840)*** coursing along the interosseous membrane of leg as far distally as the inferior tibiofibular joint; see Durward (1951, p. 1109), *Terminologia Anatomica* (1998, p. 141). It was perhaps first clearly identified by Murray; see ***[interosseal nerve of leg (>1840)] (Murray, 1780)***.

EARLIER REFERENCES:

Described, not named or illustrated:

1. ***[interosseal nerve of leg (>1840)] (Murray, 1780)***
 Murray identified it in macrodissected adult human, according to Fischer (1791, p. 35).

Illustrated and described, not named:

1. ***[interosseal nerve of leg (>1840)] (Jördens, 1788)***
 Described and illustrated for macrodissected adult human; p. 10 and Table III-*161*.

interpeduncular fossa (>1840)

As described for macrodissected adult human, a depression between the right and left ***cerebral peduncle (Tarin, 1753)***, with the other two walls formed by the caudal end of the ***mammillary body (Ludwig, 1779)*** rostrally and the rostoventral end of the ***pons (Haller, 1747)*** caudally, and the floor formed by the ventral surface of the ***interpeduncular nucleus (>1840)*** or *posterior perforated substance (>1840)*; see Mettler (1948, p. 76), Crosby et al. (1962, Fig. 98), *Dorland's* (2003, p. 731), Nieuwenhuys et al. (2008, Fig. 3.8-*16*). With accompanying ***cerebrospinal fluid (Magendie, 1827)***, it is called the *interpeduncular cistern (>1840)*; see Williams & Warwick (1980, p. 1049), *Dorland's* (2003, p. 370). By another definition its rostral end is formed instead by the ***optic chiasm (Galen, c173)*** and its extensions, the proximal ends of the ***optic tracts (Vicq d'Azyr, 1784)***; see Williams & Warwick (1980, pp. 996, 981 and Fig. 7.104). The ***interpeduncular fossa (>1840)*** was first clearly distinguished by Casserio; see ***[interpeduncular fossa (>1840)] (Casserio, 1609)***.

EARLIER REFERENCES:

Illustrated, not named or described:

1. ***[interpeduncular fossa (>1840)] (Casserio, 1609)***
 Clearly illustrated for macrodissected adult human; p. 123, Figure 2.

Earlier synonyms:

1. *parietum foveae inter corpora orbicularia & protuberantiam annularem (Tarin, 1750)*
 Synonym for ***interpeduncular fossa (>1840)***, being walls of *spatium triangulare inter crura (Tarin, 1750)* or *interpeduncular cistern (>1840)*; Table II, Figure 1-*v*.
2. *foveae inter corpora orbicularia & protuberantiam annularem (Tarin, 1750)*
 Synonym for macrodissected adult human ***interpeduncular fossa (>1840)***; Table II, Figure 1-*v*.
3. *antrum nervorum motoriorum communium oculorum (Malacarne, 1776)*
 Synonym for macrodissected adult human ***interpeduncular fossa (>1840)***; p. 89, see Burdach (1822, p. 322).
4. *fossa of oculo-muscular nerves (Vicq d'Azyr, 1786)*
 Synonym for macrodissected adult human ***interpeduncular fossa (>1840)***; Plate XVII-*38*. Also see *nervi oculo-musculares (Winslow, 1733)*.
5. *fovea of Tarin (Günther, 1786)*
 Eponym for macrodissected adult human *parietum foveae inter corpora orbicularia & protuberantiam annularem (Tarin, 1750)*; in the original Latin, *fovea Tarini*, p. 16.
6. *anterior foramen coecum of pons (Mayer, 1794)*
 Synonym for macrodissected adult human ***interpeduncular fossa (>1840)***; in the original Latin, *foramina coeca anteriora pontis*; Part 5, Table III, Figure 2-*ε*.
7. *triangular furrow (Gordon, 1815)*
 Synonym for macrodissected adult human ***interpeduncular fossa (>1840)***; pp. 84, 90.
8. *triangular space (Tiedemann, 1816)*
 Synonym for macrodissected ***interpeduncular fossa (>1840)*** observed in 4-month human fetus; see translation (1826, p. 45).
9. *interpeduncular space (Cruveilhier, 1836)*
 Synonym for macrodissected adult human ***interpeduncular fossa (>1840)***; in the original French, *espace interpédonculaire*, p. 606.

PARTLY CORRESPONDS:

1. *foramen caecum anterius (Soemmerring, 1778)*
 Large pit in caudal tip of macrodissected adult human ***interpeduncular fossa (>1840)***, near ventral median plane at junction of ***midbrain (Baer, 1837)*** and ***pons (Haller, 1747)***; Table II, legend on p. 177. See Nieuwenhuys et al. (2008, Fig. 3.8).
2. *foramen pontis coecum anterius (Günther, 1786)*
 Synonym for macrodissected adult human *foramen caecum anterius (Soemmerring, 1778)*; p. 20. It could be translated *anterior foramen cecum of pons*, and is contrasted with *foramen coecum posterius (Soemmerring, 1778)*.
3. *triangular surface (Laurencet, 1825)*
 Surface of macrodissected adult human ***interpeduncular nucleus (>1840)***; in the original French, *surface triangulaire*, Figure 14-*9*.

interpeduncular nucleus (>1840)

As described for macrodissected adult human, and for adult mammal in general with cellular architecture and connections, an unpaired ***gray matter region (Swanson & Bota, 2010)*** in the ventral median plane of the ***tegmentum (Swanson, 2000b)*** lying between the medial borders of the right and left ***cerebral peduncle (Tarin, 1753)***; see Williams & Warwick (1980, p. 966), Nieuwenhuys et al. (2008, p. 209 and Fig. 312-*30* for surface view). Also see ***interpeduncular fossa (>1840)***. Its first description as a ***gray matter region (Swanson & Bota, 2010)*** was as the *middle perforated substance (Vicq d'Azyr, 1784)*.

EARLIER REFERENCES:

Earlier synonyms:

1. *middle perforated substance (Vicq d'Azyr, 1784)*

Roughly the macrodissected adult human ***interpeduncular nucleus (>1840)***, or at least its ventral part near ***interpeduncular fossa (>1840)***; in the original Latin, *substantia perforata media*, p. 545. Also see Burdach (1822, p. 322) and *parietum foveae inter corpora orbicularia & protuberantiam annularem (Tarin, 1750)*. Meckel (1817) pointed out it is formed by ***gray matter (Meckel, 1817)*** and numerous blood vessels pass through it; see translation (1832, Vol. 2, p. 436).

2. *pons Tarini (Vicq d'Azyr, 1786)*
   Eponym for *middle perforated substance (Vicq d'Azyr, 1784)*; roughly, macrodissected adult human ***interpeduncular nucleus (>1840)***; Plate XVIII-52. Also see *spatium triangulare inter crura (Tarin, 1750)*.
3. *perforated substance of Vicq d'Azyr (Bell, 1803b)*
   Eponym for macrodissected adult human *middle perforated substance (Vicq d'Azyr, 1784)*; Bell used the French, *substance perforée* of Vicq d'Azyr, p. 107.
4. *gray perforated space (Cloquet, 1816)*
   Synonym for macrodissected adult human *middle perforated substance (Vicq d'Azyr, 1784)*; in the original French, *espace cendré perforé*, p. 592.
5. *gray cribriform plate (Meckel, 1817)*
   Synonym for macrodissected adult human *middle perforated substance (Vicq d'Azyr, 1784)*; see translation (1832, Vol. 3, p. 76).
6. *medial fascicles (Rolando, 1825a)*
   Roughly synonymous with macrodissected adult beef ***interpeduncular nucleus (>1840)*** as observed in transverse section; in the original French, *faisceaux moyens*, Table VIII, Figures 4, 7-*f.m*. Their relation to Rolando's median fascicle between peduncles of hemispheres (*faisceaux moyens situés entre les pédoncules des hémisphères*; Tab. VI, Fig. 1-*f.m*) is unclear.
7. *locus perforatus (Quain, 1828)*
   Synonym for macrodissected adult human *middle perforated substance (Vicq d'Azyr, 1784)*; p. 614.
8. *substantia perforata (Solly, 1836)*
   Synonym for macrodissected adult human *middle perforated substance (Vicq d'Azyr, 1784)*; p. 122.
9. *posterior perforated substance (>1840)*
   Synonym for macrodissected adult human *middle perforated substance (Vicq d'Azyr, 1784)*, roughly ***interpeduncular nucleus (>1840)***; see Williams & Warwick (1980, p. 966), *Dorland's* (2003, pp. 1781, 1782).

interposed nucleus (>1840)

As described with cellular architecture and connections in mammal, the middle component of the ***cerebellar nuclei (>1840)***, lying between ***fastigial nucleus (>1840)*** medially and ***dentate nucleus (>1840)*** laterally. In some species like human it can be differentiated into a more medial ***emboliform nucleus (>1840)*** and a more lateral ***globose nucleus (>1840)***; see Nieuwenhuys et al. (2008, pp. 200, 820 and Fig. 5.12-20,22). Not clearly described by 1840.

interthalamic adhesion (>1840)

The macrodissected topographic site where the right and left ***thalamus (His, 1893a)*** merge in the median plane to exclude the ***third ventricle (Galen, c173)***. It includes the ***middle commissure (>1840)*** and at least part of the ***midline thalamic nuclei (>1840)*** and ***intralaminar thalamic nuclei (>1840)***, and is thus a mixture of ***central nervous system gray matter regions (>1840)*** and a ***central nervous system white matter tract (>1840)***. In adult human it is occasionally absent, or even more occasionally double; see Meckel (1832, Vol. 2, p. 453); Crosby et al. (1962, p. 304). Its extent is quite variable in other mammals. The most common synonym is *massa intermedia (>1840)*; also see *soft commissure of optic thalamus (Vicq d'Azyr, 1784)*. It was probably known to Galen; see ***[interthalamic adhesion (>1840)] (Galen, c177)***.

TRANSLATIONS:

1. *adhesio interthalamica (>1840)*
   Current Latin form of ***interthalamic adhesion (>1840)***; see *Terminologia Anatomica* (1998, p. 120).

EARLIER REFERENCES:

Described, not named or illustrated:

1. ***[interthalamic adhesion (>1840)] (Galen, c177)***
   Almost certainly described, without naming, for macrodissected adult ox ***thalamus (His, 1893a)***; see Woollam (1958, pp. 15–16), Meyer (1971, p. 16), Rocca (2003, pp. 139, 140 note *126*, 142 note *135*). Willis (1664) vaguely but definitely described it for macrodissected adult mammal, though it is not clear whether he included human; see Pordage translation (1681, p. 64).

Illustrated, not named or described:

1. ***[interthalamic adhesion (>1840)] (Eustachi, 1552)***
   According to Burdach (1822, p. 341) and Meyer (1971, p. 10), Eustachi first illustrated it for macrodissected adult human, but this is not entirely obvious; see Albinus edition (1744, Plate XVIII).

Illustrated and described, not named:

1. ***[interthalamic adhesion (>1840)] (Steno, 1669)***
   Described, including the presence of a ***central nervous system white matter tract (>1840)***, and very clearly illustrated for macrodissected adult human in the first accurate midsagittal renderings of the ***brain (Smith Papyrus, c1700 BC)***; see translation pp. 134, 137, 149–150, Plates I–IV.

Earlier synonyms:

1. *commissura communi posterior (Bonhomme, 1748)*
   Synonym for macrodissected adult human ***interthalamic adhesion (>1840)***; pp. 55, 62; according to Burdach (1822, p. 341).
2. *inferior thalamic commissure (Günz, 1753)*
   Synonym for macrodissected adult human ***interthalamic adhesion (>1840)***; according to Schreger (1803, p. 320), Burdach (1822, p. 341).
3. *nexus thalamorum nervorum opticorum (Santorini, 1775)*
   Synonym for macrodissected adult human ***interthalamic adhesion (>1840)***, pointing out that it

contains both *gray substance (Vesalius, 1543a)* and *white substance (Vesalius, 1543a)*; p. 39, according to Burdach (1822, p. 341).

4. *thalamic commissure (Chaussier, 1807)*
   Synonym for macrodissected adult human ***interthalamic adhesion (>1840)***; p. 69, according to Burdach (1822, p. 342).
5. *commissura mediana (Gall & Spurzheim, 1810)*
   Synonym for macrodissected adult human ***interthalamic adhesion (>1840)***; p. 289, according to Burdach (1822, p. 342); Gordon (1815, p. 98) gave the French as *commissure médiane.*
6. *optic colliculus commissure (Wenzel & Wenzel, 1812)*
   Probably synonym for macrodissected adult human ***interthalamic adhesion (>1840)***; in the original Latin, *commissura colliculus opticis*, p. 309.
7. *commissure of thalami optici (Gordon, 1815)*
   Synonym for macrodissected adult human ***interthalamic adhesion (>1840)***; p. 98.
8. *middle commissure of optic chambers (Tiedemann, 1816)*
   Synonym for macrodissected fetal human ***interthalamic adhesion (>1840)***; see translation (1826, pp. 81, 114).
9. *middle cerebral commissure (Tiedemann, 1821)*
   Synonym for macrodissected adult lemur ***interthalamic adhesion (>1840)***; in the original Latin, *commissura cerebri media*, Table IV, Figure 3-*o*.
10. *transverse commissure uniting optic thalami (Cloquet, 1828)*
   Synonym for macrodissected adult human ***interthalamic adhesion (>1840)***; in the original French, *commissure transversale qui réuiit les couches optiques*, Plate CXXXVII-*17*.
11. *intermediate commissure (Bergmann, 1831)*
   Synonym for macrodissected adult human ***interthalamic adhesion (>1840)***; in the original Italian, *commissura intermedia*, p. 18.
12. *vascular commissure of optic thalamus (Cruveilhier, 1836)*
   Synonym for macrodissected adult human ***interthalamic adhesion (>1840)***; in the original French, *commissure vasculaire des couches optiques*, p. 683.
13. *middle commissure of third ventricle (Quain, 1838)*
   Synonym for macrodissected adult human ***interthalamic adhesion (>1840)***; Figure 152-*i*.
14. *commissure of posterior cerebral ganglia (Combe et al., 1838)*
   Synonym for macrodissected adult human *soft commissure of optic thalamus (Vicq d'Azyr, 1784)*; p. xxix.
15. *massa intermedia (>1840)*
   Synonym for mammalian ***interthalamic adhesion (>1840)***; see *Dorland's* (2003, p. 1103).

interventricular foramen (>1840)

A short canal between the medial wall of the ***lateral ventricle (Vesalius, 1543a)*** and the lateral wall of the ***third ventricle (Galen, c173)***; in macrodissected adult human there are separate right and left foramina that do not join to form a transverse canal, they are distinct; see Last & Tompsett (1953, p. 535), Millen & Woollam (1962, p 44). It has long been known; see ***[interventricular foramen (>1840)] (Erasistratus, c310–c250 BC)***.

EARLIER REFERENCES:

Described, not named or illustrated:

1. ***[interventricular foramen (>1840)] (Erasistratus, c310–c250 BC)***
   In *The Doctrines of Hippocrates and Plato* (c162–c166), Galen quoted from a now lost book of Erasistratus where the human ***brain (Smith Papyrus, c1700 BC)*** "...had a ventricle placed longitudinally on each side, and these were pierced through into one at the junction of the parts [***interventricular foramen (>1840)***]." (see Clarke & O'Malley, 1996, p. 12). This is the first clear description of the *foramen of Monro (Ramsay, 1813)*.

Earlier synonyms:

1. *inferior opening (Galen, c173)*
   In *On the Usefulness of the Parts*, Galen alluded to ***interventricular foramen (>1840)*** in a phrase translated *inferior opening* by Clarke & O'Malley (1996, p. 711) or *channel opening downward* by May (1968, p. 413). Galen dissected a variety of common large mammals but not explicitly human.
2. *hole (Galen, c177)*
   In *On Anatomical Procedures*, Galen described holes between ***anterior ventricles (Galen, c173)*** and ***third ventricle (Galen, c192)***, a clear description of right and left ***interventricular foramen (>1840)***; see Singer translation (1999, p. 234).
3. *aperture (Galen, c177)*
   Alternate translation of *hole (Galen, c177)*; see Wiberg (1914, p. 26).
4. *commissure of two ventricles (Haly Abbas or Ali ibn' ul-Abbas, d. 994)*
   In *The Complete Book of Medical Art, Called the Royal Book*, Haly Abbas referred to right and left ***interventricular foramen (>1840)*** as forming a commissure between the two *anterior ventricles (Galen, c173)* or ***lateral ventricles (Vesalius, 1543a)***; his book seems entirely derived from Galen's *On Anatomical Procedures*; see Wiberg translation (1914, p. 32).
5. *meatus (Vicary, 1548)*
   Synonym for macrodissected adult human ***interventricular foramen (>1840)*** in his English text; p. 31.
6. *oriface of third ventricle (Bartholin, 1662)*
   Synonym for macrodissected adult human ***interventricular foramen (>1840)***; p. 140.
7. *foramen commune anterius (Winslow, 1733)*
   Synonym for macrodissected adult human ***interventricular foramen (>1840)***; Section X, p. 38. Burdach (1822, p. 380) gave the Latin form, *orificium commune anticum.*
8. *foramen profundum (Lieutaud, 1742)*
   Roughly synonymous with macrodissected adult human ***interventricular foramen (>1840)***; see Burdach (1822, p. 380).

9. *ostium anterius ventriculi tertii (Haller, 1762)*
Synonym for macrodissected adult human ***interventricular foramen (>1840)***; p. 57, see Burdach (1822, p. 380).
10. *apertura anterior ventriculi tertii (Malacarne, 1780)*
Synonym for macrodissected adult human ***interventricular foramen (>1840)***; p. 60, see Burdach (1822, p. 380).
11. *aditus ad ventriculum tertium (Haase, 1781)*
Synonym for macrodissected adult human ***interventricular foramen (>1840)***; p. 22, see Burdach (1822, p. 380).
12. *apertura ad ventriculum tertium (Haase, 1781)*
Synonym for macrodissected adult human ***interventricular foramen (>1840)***; p. 22, see Burdach (1822, p. 380).
13. *orificium anticum ventriculi tertii (Haase, 1781)*
Synonym for macrodissected adult human ***interventricular foramen (>1840)***; p. 22, see Burdach (1822, p. 380).
14. *anterior aperture of third ventricle (Haase, 1781)*
Synonym for macrodissected adult human ***interventricular foramen (>1840)***; in the original Latin, *apertura ventriculus tertius anterior*, p. 22.
15. *anterior oriface of third ventricle (Haase, 1781)*
Synonym for macrodissected adult human ***interventricular foramen (>1840)***; in the original Latin, *orificium ventriculi tertii anterius*, p. 22.
16. *aditus ad infundibulum (Haase, 1781)*
Synonym for macrodissected adult human ***interventricular foramen (>1840)***; p. 22.
17. *passage by which lateral ventricles communicate with each other and with third ventricle (Monro, 1783)*
Monro provided good description of macrodissected adult human ***interventricular foramen (>1840)***; Tables III-*F*, IV-*F*.
18. *anterior ventricular oriface (Günther, 1786)*
Synonym for macrodissected adult human ***interventricular foramen (>1840)***; in the original Latin, *orificia ventriculi anterius*, p. 13.
19. *anterior ventricular aperture (Günther, 1786)*
Synonym for macrodissected adult human ***interventricular foramen (>1840)***; in the original Latin, *aperturae ventriculi anterius*, p. 13.
20. *vulva (Günther, 1786)*
Synonym for *anterior ventricular oriface (Günther, 1786)*; p. 13.
21. *iter ad infundibulum (Fyfe, 1800)*
Synonym for macrodissected adult human ***interventricular foramen (>1840)***; Vol. 2, p. 20.
22. *iter ad tertium ventriculum (Fyfe, 1800)*
Synonym for macrodissected adult human ***interventricular foramen (>1840)***; Vol. 2, p. 20. This was Fyfe's preferred term, and his English translation was *passage to third ventricle*.
23. *foramen of Monro (Ramsay, 1813)*
Eponym for macrodissected adult human ***interventricular foramen (>1840)***, "This was first described as present in the human species, by the justly celebrated anatomist Dr. Monro, under whom I had the honour and advantage of studying." (p. 41).
23. *fissure of Monro (Quain, 1828)*
Eponym for macrodissected adult human ***interventricular foramen (>1840)***; p. 637.

intralaminar thalamic nuclei (>1840)

As described for macrodissected adult human, and based on cellular architecture and connections in mammal, a component of the ***dorsal part of thalamus (Herrick, 1910)*** embedded within the rather diffuse, narrow, wing-shaped ***internal medullary lamina (>1840)***. Its main ***gray matter regions (Swanson & Bota, 2010)*** are the ***central medial thalamic nucleus (>1840)*** and ***rhomboid nucleus (>1840)*** in the medial plane separating the ventral and dorsal components of the ***midline thalamic nuclei (>1840)***, and progressively more laterally on the right and left sides the ***paracentral thalamic nucleus (>1840), central lateral thalamic nucleus (>1840)***, and ***parafascicular nucleus (>1840)*** and/or ***centromedian nucleus (>1840)***; see Carpenter (1976, Figs. 15.10, 15.11), Jones (1985, p. 607), Swanson (2004, Table B, p. 172), Nieuwenhuys et al. (2008, pp. 266–268 and Figs. 5.30-6, 6.36-9,*10*, 6.37-5). Parts near the median plane were vaguely identified early on as a component of the *lacunar (Vieussens, 1684)*.

intraparietal sulcus (>1840)

As described for macrodissected adult human, the groove between ***superior parietal lobule (>1840)*** and ***inferior parietal lobule (>1840)***; see Williams & Warwick (1980, Fig. 7.111A), *Terminologia Anatomica* (1998, p. 125). It was first clearly delineated by Vicq d'Azyr; see ***[intraparietal sulcus (>1840)] (Vicq d'Azyr, 1786)***.

EARLIER REFERENCES:

Illustrated and described, not named:

1. ***[intraparietal sulcus (>1840)] (Vicq d'Azyr, 1786)***
Clearly illustrated for macrodissected adult human; Plate III-*l*, which extends to the left into *m*.

intrinsic cardiac plexus (>1840)

A ***terminal plexus (Swanson & Bota, 2010)*** associated with cardiac muscle fibers and associated capillaries, sometimes accompanied by tiny ***ganglia (Galen, c173)*** in the subepicardial connective tissue; see Mitchell (1953, pp. 253–254). It was unequivocally described by Scarpa; see ***[intrinsic cardiac plexus (>1840)] (Scarpa, 1794)***.

EARLIER REFERENCES:

Described, not named or illustrated:

1. ***[intrinsic cardiac plexus (>1840)] (Scarpa, 1794)***
Scarpa first demonstrated unequivocally that cardiac muscle is innervated, based on macrodissected adult human; see Gillispie (1970–1980, Vol. 12, p. 138). Lobstein (1823) clearly discussed innervation of macrodissected adult human heart muscle tissue; see translation (1831, pp. 19–22).

intrinsic renal nerves (>1840)

As described for macrodissected adult human they arise from the ***renal plexus (Drake, 1707)*** and accompany branches of the renal artery into the kidney; see Mitchell (1953, pp. 291–292). They were first delineated by Willis; see ***[intrinsic renal nerves (>1840)] (Willis, 1664)***.

EARLIER REFERENCES:

Described, not named or illustrated:

1. ***[intrinsic renal nerves (>1840)] (Willis, 1664)***
   Willis illustrated for macrodissected adult human and other common large mammals a distinction between ***renal nerves (Haase, 1781)***, ***renal plexus (Drake, 1707)***, and ***intrinsic renal nerves (>1840)***; see Table XI-*v,y*.

Earlier synonyms:

1. *anterior renal nerves (Walter, 1783)*
   Synonym for macrodissected adult human ***intrinsic renal nerves (>1840)***; Walter described and illustrated at least five of them; in the original Latin, *nervi renalis anteriori*, Tables I-*268*, III:*353-362*.

PARTLY CORRESPONDS:

1. *trunk of anterior renal nerves (Walter, 1783)*
   Origin or trunk of *anterior renal nerves (Walter, 1783)* in macrodissected adult human; in the original Latin, *truncus nervi renalis anterioris*, Table I-*268*.
2. *anterior renal nerves (Mayer, 1794)*
   Macrodissected adult human ***intrinsic renal nerves (>1840)*** lying ventrally (anteriorly) and supplying the length of the kidney; in the original Latin, *nervi renales anteriores*; Part 6, Table VI-*241* (p. 43).
3. *posterior renal nerves (Mayer, 1794)*
   Macrodissected adult human ***intrinsic renal nerves (>1840)*** lying dorsally (posteriorly) and supplying the length of the kidney; in the original Latin, *nervi renales posteriores*; Part 6, Table VII-*3* (p. 50).

intrinsic vesical plexus (>1840)

As described for macrodissected adult human, the extension of the ***extrinsic vesical plexus (>1840)*** into the muscular wall of the urinary bladder; see Mitchell (1953, p. 305). It was perhaps first clearly identified by Walter; see ***[intrinsic vesical plexus (>1840)] (Walter, 1783)***. See *Terminologia Anatomica* (1998, p. 143) and *Oxford English Dictionary* (Online) for spelling of vesical.

EARLIER REFERENCES:

Described, not named or illustrated:

1. ***[intrinsic vesical plexus (>1840)] (Walter, 1783)***
   Walter mentioned branches from lower part of *hypogastric plexus (Haller, 1762)* implanting in urinary vesical; Table I-*444,445*.

invertebrate brain (>1840)

Brain (Smith Papyrus, c1700 BC) is a general term for the rostral topographic division of the ***central nervous system (Carus, 1814)***. ***Invertebrate brain (>1840)*** and ***vertebrate brain (Cuvier, 1800)*** are distinguished and treated separately because the evolutionary relationship between the two is not established and because whereas there is a common basic plan for the ***vertebrate brain (Cuvier, 1800)*** based on development, there are multiple basic plans for the ***invertebrate brain (>1840)*** and many invertebrates have nothing resembling a ***brain (Smith Papyrus, c1700 BC)***. The ***invertebrate brain (>1840)*** is typically the most rostral, largest, most differentiated ***central ganglion (>1840)***—or ganglia if multiple cords are involved—of a ***central nerve cord (Serres, 1824–1826)***; see Bullock & Horridge (1965, pp. 542–550). The ***invertebrate brain (>1840)*** was discovered long ago, see *brain (Aristotle)*. Swammerdam (see 1758, Tab. XX, Fig. V-*s*) noted it consists of *cortical substance (Willis, 1664)*, and Cuvier (1800, lecture 11) discussed both invertebrates and their brains without using the term explicitly—in contrast, he coined the term ***vertebrate brain (Cuvier, 1800)***.

EARLIER REFERENCES:

Earlier synonyms:

1. *brain (Aristotle)*
   Synonym for ***invertebrate brain (>1840)*** Aristotle used for molluscs, where he noted it is bilateral; see Clarke & O'Malley (1996, p. 8). He was responsible for the first broad comparative examination of the ***brain (Smith Papyrus, c1700 BC)*** in a range of animals; in antiquity the only Greco-Roman scientific dissection of the human body, including the ***nervous system (Monro, 1783)***, took place in Alexandria and was carried out by Herophilus and Erasistratus about 300 BC; see von Staden (1989), Rocca (2003). It is unclear in exactly which animals Aristotle observed particular ***nervous system (Monro, 1783)*** features, although he did write in *The Account of Animals* that all animals with blood he examined, including molluscs, have a ***brain (Smith Papyrus, c1700 BC)***. Thus he observed both the ***vertebrate brain (Cuvier, 1800)*** and the ***invertebrate brain (>1840)***.
2. *head ganglion (Lyonnet, 1762)*
   Synonym for ***invertebrate brain (>1840)*** Lyonnet used for goat moth larva; in the original French, *ganglion de la tête*, pp. 576, 589.
3. *central ganglion (Mangili, 1804)*
   Synonym for ***invertebrate brain (>1840)*** Mangili used for bivalves; in the original Italian, *ganglion centrale*, Figure 2-*T*, p. 31. He described it as bilobed (*bilobo*); see *brain (Aristotle)*. Carus (1814, pp. 66. 87, 103, 254) used the German, *Centralknoten*.
4. *so-called brain of invertebrate animals (Carus, 1814)*
   Synonym for ***invertebrate brain (>1840)***; in the original German, *sogenannten Gehirn der wirbellowen Thiere*, p. 121.
5. *brain ganglion (Carus, 1814)*
   Synonym for ***invertebrate brain (>1840)*** Carus used for snails; in the original German, *Hirnknoten*, Table III, Figure III-*1*.
6. *anterior ganglion (Bell, 1821)*
   Synonym for ***invertebrate brain (>1840)*** Bell used for leeches; p. 409.

PARTLY CORRESPONDS:

1. *head of oblong marrow (Willis, 1672)*
   Region of lobster ***invertebrate brain (>1840)*** in median plane Willis described as associated with *mammillary processes (Willis, 1672)* [presumably corresponding to olfactory nerves] and *optic nerves (Malpighi, 1669)*, in a farfetched analogy with vertebrate ***cerebral nuclei (Swanson, 2000)*** and ***interbrain (Baer, 1837)***; in the original Latin, *medulla oblongata caput*, Table III, Figure 1-*B*.
2. *cerebellum (Willis, 1672)*
   Caudal swelling of lobster ***invertebrate brain (>1840)*** Willis compared on strictly topographic grounds to vertebrate ***cerebellum (Aristotle)***; Table III, Figure 1-C.
3. *hemispheres (Swammerdam, c1675)*
   Swammerdam described the ***invertebrate brain (>1840)*** of Cossus (Rhinoceros beetle larva) as having two hemispheres together forming one body; see translation (1758; Tab. XXVIII, Fig. 1).
4. *ganglia of brain (Carus, 1814)*
   Clear subdivisions of macrodissected ***invertebrate brain (>1840)*** viewed under the microscope; in the original German, *Ganglien des Gehirns*, p. 63.
5. *pulpous nucleus (Dutrochet, 1824)*
   In molluscs, the center of each *hemisphere (Swammerdam, c1675)* of the ***invertebrate brain (>1840)*** was described using a simple microscope as formed by this feature, which in turn consisted of numerous globular cells (*cellules globuleuses*); in the original French, *noyau pulpeux*, pp. 165–166.

invertebrate nerves (>1840)

Nerves (Herophilus, c335–c280 BC) in the invertebrate ***peripheral nervous system (Carus, 1814)***; see Bullock & Horridge (1965). Perhaps first described as *nerves (Malpighi, 1669)*.

EARLIER REFERENCES:

Earlier synonyms:

1. *nerves (Malpighi, 1669)*
   Synonym for ***invertebrate nerves (>1840)*** viewed with a microscope in silkworm; in the original Latin, *nervorum*, p. 46, Table VI.

PARTLY CORRESPONDS:

1. *optic nerve (Malpighi, 1669)****Invertebrate nerve (>1840)*** between eye and *brain (Aristotle)* of adult silk moths viewed with a microscope; in the original Latin, *opticus nervus*, p. 90.
2. *mammillary process (Willis, 1672, Tab. III)*
   Extension of lobster ***invertebrate brain (>1840)*** Willis regarded as similar to mammalian *mammillary process (Willis, 1664)* or more broadly *olfactory sense instrument (Galen, c173)*; Table III, Figure 1-*B*.
3. *recurrent nerves (Swammerdam, c1675)*
   Paired ***invertebrate nerves (>1840)*** extending rostrally from ***invertebrate brain (>1840)*** and then curving caudally to join and descend to stomach; in the original Latin, *nervi recurrentes*, see translation (1758, pp. 138–139 and Tab. XXVIII, Fig. 2). Here it is described and illustrated for rhinoceros beetle larva and compared to larger animals and humans. Müller (1828a) provided a thorough review and analysis of this feature in insects.
4. *spinal nerves (Swammerdam, c1675)*
   Regular nerves extending from *spinal medulla (Malpighi, 1669)* in, for example, the snail viewed under a microscope; see translation (1758; Part I, p. 61, Ch. X).
5. *nerve ring (Lyonnet, 1762)*
   In macrodissected caterpillars viewed with magnification, ***invertebrate nerve (>1840)*** from *ganglion of head (Lyonnet, 1762)* encircling esophagus; in the original French, *anneau nerveux*, p. 534, Plate XVI, Figure 9 near *u*.
6. *cerebral nerves (Straus Durckheim, 1828)*
   In macrodissected beetle, *Melolontha*, ***invertebrate nerves (>1840)*** extending from ***supraesophageal ganglion (Grant, 1834a)***; in the original French, *nerfs cérébraux*, pp. 392–394. Straus Durckheim described five pairs, the first being *antennal nerve (Straus Durckheim, 1828)* and the second the *optic nerve (Malpighi, 1669)*. He suggested the last three may be analogous to vertebrate ***trigeminal nerve (Winslow, 1733)***.
7. *antennal nerve (Straus Durckheim, 1828)*
   In macrodissected beetle, *Melolontha*, large *cerebral nerve (Straus Durckheim, 1828)* extending to antenna; in the original French, *nerf antennal*, pp. 392–393.
8. *acoustic nerve (Straus Durckheim, 1828)*
   Synonym for *antennal nerve (Straus Durckheim, 1828)*; in the original French, *nerf acoustique*, p. 392.
9. *mandibular nerve (Straus Durckheim, 1828)*
   In macrodissected beetle, *Melolontha*, first of three pairs of ***invertebrate nerves (>1840)*** arising from *suboesophageal ganglia (Straus Durckheim, 1828)*; in the original French, *nerf mandibulaire*, p. 396.
10. *maxillary nerve (Straus Durckheim, 1828)*
    In macrodissected beetle, *Melolontha*, second of three pairs of ***invertebrate nerves (>1840)*** arising from *suboesophageal ganglia (Straus Durckheim, 1828)*; in the original French, *nerf maxillaire*, p. 396.
11. *crural nerve of forelegs (Straus Durckheim, 1828)*
    In macrodissected beetle, *Melolontha*, first of two pairs of ***invertebrate nerves (>1840)*** arising from "des Ganglions du corselet"; in the original French, *nerf crural des pattes antérieures*, p. 397.
12. *nerve of carapace (Straus Durckheim, 1828)*
    In macrodissected beetle, *Melolontha*, first of six pairs of thoracic *invertebrate nerves (>1840)*; in the original French, *nerf de l'Élytre*, p. 400.
13. *middle crural nerve (Straus Durckheim, 1828)*
    In macrodissected beetle, *Melolontha*, second of six pairs of thoracic *invertebrate nerves (>1840)*; in the original French, *nerf Crural moyen*, p. 401.
14. *nerve of wing (Straus Durckheim, 1828)*
    In macrodissected beetle, *Melolontha*, third of six pairs of thoracic ***invertebrate nerves (>1840)***; in the original French, *nerf de l'Aile*, p. 401.
15. *posterior crural nerve (Straus Durckheim, 1828)*

In macrodissected beetle, *Melolontha*, fourth of six pairs of thoracic ***invertebrate nerves (>1840)***; in the original French, *nerf Crural postérieur*, p. 402.

16. *vagus or pneumogastric nerve (Newport, 1834)*
As discussed for macrodissected hawkmoth, synonym for *recurrent nerve (Swammerdam, c1675)*; p. 399 and Plate 13, Figure 3-*g,e*.

invertebrate peripheral ganglia (Swanson & Bota, 2010)

Ganglia (Galen, c173) of the invertebrate ***peripheral nervous system (Meckel, 1817)***; see Bullock & Horridge (1965). For this usage see Swanson & Bota, 2010, Thesaurus); Swammerdam first described several instances of it; see ***[invertebrate peripheral ganglia (Swanson & Bota, 2010)] (Swammerdam, c1675)***.

EARLIER REFERENCES:

Illustrated and described, not named:

1. ***[invertebrate peripheral ganglia (Swanson & Bota, 2010)] (Swammerdam, c1675)***
Swammerdam described and illustrated several instances of them for rhinoceros beetle larva; see Table XXVIII, Figures 2-*d,f* and 3-*i*.

Earlier synonyms:

1. *collateral ganglia (Straus Durckheim, 1828)*
Essentially synonym for ***invertebrate peripheral ganglia (Swanson & Bota, 2010)***; in the original French, *ganglions collatéraux*, p. 374.

PARTLY CORRESPONDS:

1. *small ganglia of head (Lyonnet, 1762)*
In macrodissected adult caterpillar viewed with magnification, ***invertebrate peripheral ganglion (Swanson & Bota, 2010)*** on either side of esophagus, just caudal to *ganglion of head (Lyonnet, 1762)*; in the original French, *petits ganglions de la téte*, pp. 537, 541.

isthmus of cingulate region (>1840)

As described for macrodissected adult human, the caudal topographic subdivision of the ***cingulate region (>1840)*** extending to the dorsal (posterior, septal) end of the ***parahippocampal gyrus (>1840)***. Based on cellular architecture and connections in mammal, it corresponds to the ***retrosplenial region (>1840)***; see Williams & Warwick (1980, Fig. 7.114A), Nieuwenhuys et al. (2008, Fig. 12.13). It was first clearly illustrated by Soemmerring; see ***[isthmus of cingulate region (>1840)] (Soemmerring, 1778)***.

EARLIER REFERENCES:

Illustrated, not named or described:

1. ***[isthmus of cingulate region (>1840)] (Soemmerring, 1778)***
Clearly illustrated for macrodissected adult human; Table III.

Earlier synonyms:

1. *cingulate gyrus behind splenium of corpus callosum (Burdach, 1822)*
Roughly synonymous with macrodissected adult human ***isthmus of cingulate region (>1840)***; in the original German, described as *Randwülste der Zwinge, hinter der Balkenwulst*, p. 151 and Table VIII-*w*.
2. *lip of mouth of ventricles (Gerdy, 1838)*
Roughly synonymous with macrodissected adult human ***isthmus of cingulate region (>1840)***; in the original French, *lévre de la bouche ventriculaire*, p. 259.
3. *rim of mouth of ventricles (Gerdy, 1838)*
Synonym for *lip of mouth of ventricles (Gerdy, 1838)*; in the original French, *le bord de la bouche ventriculaire*, p. 259.
4. *isthmus gyri cinguli (>1840)*
Current Latin form of *isthmus of cingulate gyrus (>1840)*; see *Terminologia Anatomica* (1998, p. 126).
5. *isthmus of cingulate gyrus (>1840)*
Synonym for macrodissected adult human ***isthmus of cingulate region (>1840)***; see *Nomina Anatomica* (1983, p. A71), *Terminologia Anatomica* (1998, p. 126).

isthmus of fauces branches of lingual nerve (>1840)

As described for macrodissected adult human, 2–4 branches of the ***lingual nerve (Vesalius, 1543a)*** arising between the junction of the ***chorda tympani (Falloppio, 1559)*** with the ***lingual nerve (Haase, 1781)*** proximally and the origin of the ***sublingual nerve (Henle, 1871)*** distally; see Henle (1871, p. 390 and Fig. 247), *Terminologia Anatomica* (1998, p. 135), *Dorland's* (2003, p. 1574). They were perhaps first mentioned by Soemmerring; see ***[isthmus of fauces branches of lingual nerve (>1840)] (Soemmerring, 1791)***. Henle (1871, p. 390) attributed the term without citation to Arnold.

TRANSLATIONS:

1. *nervus lingualis rami isthmi faucium (>1840)*
Current Latin form of ***isthmus of fauces branches of lingual nerve (>1840)***; see *Terminologia Anatomica* (1998, p. 135). Also see Henle (1871, p. 390).

EARLIER REFERENCES:

Described, not named or illustrated:

1. ***[isthmus of fauces branches of lingual nerve (>1840)] (Soemmerring, 1791)***
Mentioned for macrodissected adult human; p. 214, also see Soemmerring (1798, p. 235).

jejunal and ileal plexuses (>1840)

As described for macrodissected adult human, they extend along the jejunal and ileal arteries from the ***superior mesenteric plexus (Rau, 1720)*** to supply the arteries and all but the proximal half of the small intestine; see Mitchell (1953, p. 283). They were perhaps first indicated as *filaments from superior mesenteric plexus to small intestine (Meckel, 1817)*.

EARLIER REFERENCES:

Earlier synonyms:

1. *filaments from superior mesenteric plexus to small intestine (Meckel, 1817)*
   Refers vaguely to ***jejunal and ileal plexuses (>1840)*** in macrodissected adult human; see translation (1832, Vol. 3, p. 87).

jugular nerves (>1840)

As described for macrodissected adult human, one or more branches of ***superior cervical ganglion (Vieussens, 1684)*** and/or adjacent ***internal carotid nerve (>1840)*** coursing to ***distal glossopharyngeal ganglion (>1840)***, ***distal vagal ganglion (>1840)***, ***proximal vagal ganglion (>1840)***, superior jugular bulb, and meninges of posterior cranial fossa. They or associated branches also go to the ***hypoglossal nerve (Winslow, 1733)***; see Mitchell (1953, p. 221), Williams & Warwick (1980, p. 1127). They were probably known to Galen; see ***[jugular nerves (>1840)] (Galen, c192)***. Hovelacque (1927, p. 687) assigned them eponymously to Arnold without citation.

EARLIER REFERENCES:

Described, not named or illustrated:

1. ***[jugular nerves (>1840)] (Galen, c192)***
   Probably identified by Galen but mistakenly thought to arise from ***vagus nerve (Galen, c192)*** in macrodissected adult beef, pig, and/or macaque but not human; see Duckworth translation (1962, p. 203).

Illustrated and described, not named:

1. ***[jugular nerves (>1840)] (Vieussens, 1684)***
   Vieussens described and illustrated for macrodissected adult human branch of ***sympathetic trunk (Winslow, 1733)*** to jugular vein, but had it arising near ***inferior cervical ganglion (Vieussens, 1684)***; Table 23-33.
2. ***[jugular nerves (>1840)] (Morgagni, 1719)***
   Morgagni described for macrodissected adult human branches of *intercostal nerve (Willis, 1664)* to ***glossopharyngeal nerve (Huber, 1744)*** and ***vagus nerve (Galen, c192)***; p. 105, according to Neubauer (1772, pp. 38-39).
3. ***[jugular nerves (>1840)] (Lancisi, 1728)***
   Lancisi described and illustrated for macrodissected adult human branch of ***superior cervical ganglion (Vieussens, 1684)*** to jugular vein; Table 6, Figure 1-*m*.
4. ***[jugular nerves (>1840)] (Huber, 1744)***
   Huber described in macrodissected adult human branch of ***internal carotid nerve (>1840)*** arising just rostral to (above) ***superior cervical ganglion (Vieussens, 1684)*** and extending as far as ***distal glossopharyngeal ganglion (>1740)***; pp. 12, 18, see Neubauer (1772, p. 46).

Earlier synonyms:

1. *ganglioform branches (Neubauer, 1772)*
   Neubauer described and illustrated in detail a number of such ventral (anterior) and dorsal (posterior) branches in macrodissected adult human, corresponding roughly to ***jugular nerves (>1840)***; in the original Latin, *anterior, posterior ramus gangliformis*, see Table 2, Figure 2.

PARTLY CORRESPONDS:

1. *highest soft nerve (Andersch & Soemmerring, 1792)*
   In macrodissected adult human, most rostral (uppermost), medially directed branch emerging from ***superior cervical ganglion (Vieussens, 1684)***, probably a ***jugular nerve (>1840)***; in the original Latin, *nervus mollis supremus, supremo nervus mollis*, p. 171.
2. *second soft nerve (Andersch & Soemmerring, 1792)*
   In macrodissected adult human, second branch emerging from ***superior cervical ganglion (Vieussens, 1684)***, with rostral (ascending) branch associated with *labial soft nerves (Andersch & Soemmerring, 1792)*, so probably a ***jugular nerve (>1840)***; in the original Latin, *nervus mollis secundus, secundo nervo molli*; p. 171.
3. *temporal soft nerve (Andersch & Soemmerring, 1792)*
   In macrodissected adult human, third branch emerging from ***superior cervical ganglion (Vieussens, 1684)***, forming association with *reverse nerve of superior thyroid artery (Andersch & Soemmerring, 1792)*, so probably a ***jugular nerve (>1840)***; in the original Latin, *nervus mollis temporalis, nervi mollis temporalis*; pp. 171–172.
4. *lowest soft nerve (Andersch & Soemmerring, 1792)*
   In macrodissected adult human, fourth branch emerging laterally from ***superior cervical ganglion (Vieussens, 1684)***, so probably a ***jugular nerve (>1840)***; in the original Latin, *infimus nervus mollis, infimo nervo molli, infimi nervi mollis*; pp. 176–177.
5. *second to sixth soft nerves from lowest (Andersch & Soemmerring, 1792)*
   Branches of ***sympathetic trunk (Winslow, 1733)*** or first two ***sympathetic trunk ganglia (Winslow, 1733)*** arising caudal to (below) the *lowest soft nerve (Andersch & Soemmerring, 1792)*, so probably ***jugular nerves (>1840)***; in the original Latin, *secundus nervus mollis ab infimo, tertius nervus mollis, quartus, quintus nervus mollis, sexto nervo molli*; pp. 177–179.
6. *lowest soft branch (Andersch, 1797)*
   Synonym for *lowest soft nerve (Andersch & Soemmerring, 1792)*; in the original Latin, *infimo ramo molli, infimi rami mollis*, pp. 127–128.
7. *anastomosis between supreme cervical ganglion and vagus nerve (Langenbeck, 1826-1830)*
   Macrodissected adult human ***communicating branch (Winslow, 1733)*** between ***superior cervical ganglion (Vieussens, 1684)*** and ***vagus nerve trunk (Wrisberg, 1786; Günther, 1786)*** at or just distal to ***distal vagal ganglion (>1840)***. As such, associated with ***jugular nerves (>1840)***; in the original Latin, *anastomosis inter ganglion cervicale supremum et nervum vagum*, Fascicle III, Table XVI-27.
8. *communicating branch between supreme cervical ganglion and second vagal ganglion (Bischoff, 1832)*
   Macrodissected adult fox ***communicating branch (Winslow, 1733)*** between ***superior cervical ganglion (Vieussens, 1684)*** and ***distal vagal ganglion (>1840)***. As such, associated with ***jugular nerves (>1840)***; in the original Latin, *ramus communicans inter ganglion cervicale supremum Sympathici et ganglion secundum Vagi*; Table II, Figure 3-20.
9. *connection of petrous part of ninth pair with supreme cervical ganglion (Arnold, 1834)*
   Macrodissected adult human ***jugular nerve (>1840)*** between ***superior cervical ganglion (Vieussens, 1684)*** and ***glossopharyngeal nerve (Huber, 1744)***; in the original Latin, *par nonum pars petrosa conjunctio cum ganglio cervicali supremo*, pp. 12–13.
10. *connection of petrous part of glossopharyngeal nerve with supreme cervical ganglion (Arnold, 1834)*
    Synonym for *connection of petrous part of ninth pair with supreme cervical ganglion (Arnold, 1834)*; in the original Latin, *nervus glossopharyngeus pars petrosa conjunctio cum ganglio cervicali supremo*, pp. 12–13.
11. *connection of petrous part of tenth pair with supreme cervical ganglion (Arnold, 1834)*
    Macrodissected adult human ***jugular nerve (>1840)*** between ***superior cervical ganglion (Vieussens, 1684)*** and ***vagus nerve (Galen, c192)***; in the original Latin, *par decimum pars petrosa conjunctio cum ganglio cervicale supremo*, p. 13.
12. *connection of petrous part of pneumogastric nerve with supreme cervical ganglion (Arnold, 1834)*
    Synonym for *connection of petrous part of tenth pair with supreme cervical ganglion (Arnold, 1834)*; in the original Latin, *nervus pneumogastricus pars petrosa conjunctio cum ganglio cervicale supremo*, p. 13.
13. *connection of petrous part of vagus nerve with supreme cervical ganglion (Arnold, 1834)*
    Synonym for *connection of petrous part of tenth pair with supreme cervical ganglion (Arnold, 1834)*; in the original Latin, *nervus vagus pars petrosa conjunctio cum ganglio cervicale supremo*, p. 13.
14. *connection of supreme cervical ganglion with ganglioform plexus of vagus nerve (Arnold, 1834)*
    Macrodissected adult human ***jugular nerve (>1840)*** between ***superior cervical ganglion (Vieussens, 1684)*** and *ganglioform plexus of vagus nerve (Arnold, 1834)*, a *pseudoganglion (>1840)* near origin of **superior laryngeal nerve (Loder, 1778)**; in the original Latin, *conjunctio ganglii cervicalis supremi cum plexu ganglioformi nervi vagi*, Table IV-34.
15. *connection of external branch of superior laryngeal nerve with filaments of superior cervical ganglion (Arnold, 1834)*
    Macrodissected adult human ***jugular nerve (>1840)*** between ***superior cervical ganglion (Vieussens, 1684)*** and ***external branch of superior laryngeal nerve (Fyfe, 1800)***; in the original Latin, *nervus laryngeus superior, ramus externus, conjungens cum filamento e ganglio cervicale superiore*, p. 14.
16. *connection of hypoglossal nerve with supreme cervical ganglion (Arnold, 1834)*
    Macrodissected adult human ***jugular nerve (>1840)*** between ***superior cervical ganglion (Vieussens, 1684)*** and ***hypoglossal nerve trunk (Günther, 1786)***; in the original Latin, *conjunctio nervus hypoglossus cum ganglio cervicali supremo*, p. 15. See Williams & Warwick (1980, Fig. 7.189).

lacrimal nerve (Meckel, 1748; Bonhomme, 1748)

As described for macrodissected adult human, branch of the ***ophthalmic nerve (Winslow, 1733)*** entering the lacrimal gland and giving off several small branches to it and the conjunctiva before continuing on to end in skin of the upper eyelid and then join with small ***zygomatic branches of facial nerve (>1840)***; see Williams & Warwick (1980, p. 1061 and Fig. 7.187). Meckel (p. 47) and Bonhomme (Pl. 10-9) used the term for macrodissected adult human. It was probably first clearly delineated as the *second branch of second division of fifth pair of nerves arising within skull (Willis, 1664)*.

ALTERNATE SPELLINGS:

1. *lachrymal nerve (Swan, 1830)*
   English form of macrodissected adult human ***lacrimal nerve (Meckel, 1748; Bonhomme, 1748)***; Plate XII, Figure 6-*11*.

TRANSLATIONS:

1. *lacrymalis nervus (Meckel, 1748)*
   Original Latin form (singular; plural, *nervo lacrymali*) for ***lacrimal nerve (Meckel, 1748; Bonhomme, 1748)***; p. 47.
2. *nerf lachrymal (Bonhomme, 1748)*
   Original French form of ***lacrimal nerve (Meckel, 1748; Bonhomme, 1748)***; Plate 10-9.
3. *lacrumalis nervus (Haller, 1762)*
   Latin form of ***lacrimal nerve (Meckel, 1748; Bonhomme, 1748)***; p. 211.

EARLIER REFERENCES:

Earlier synonyms:

1. *second branch of second division of fifth pair of nerves arising within skull (Willis, 1664)*
   Roughly synonymous with macrodissected adult, presumably human, ***lacrimal nerve (Meckel, 1748; Bonhomme, 1748)***; see Pordage translation (1681, p. 144, Fig. 1-*D*).
2. *ramulus tertius rami minoris superioris nervus quintae conjugationis (Vieussens, 1684)*
   Roughly synonymous with macrodissected adult human ***lacrimal nerve (Meckel, 1748; Bonhomme, 1748)***; p. 171 and Table 22-*p*.
3. *external ramus of ophthalmic nerve (Winslow, 1733)*
   Synonym for macrodissected adult human ***lacrimal nerve (Meckel, 1748; Bonhomme, 1748)***; Section VI, p. 64.
4. *lacrymal ramus of ophthalmic nerve (Winslow, 1733)*
   Synonym for macrodissected adult human ***lacrimal nerve (Meckel, 1748; Bonhomme, 1748)***; Section VI, p. 64.
5. *exterior branch of first branch of fifth pair (Haller, 1743)*
   Synonym for macrodissected adult human ***lacrimal nerve (Meckel, 1748; Bonhomme, 1748)***; in the original Latin, *primi rami quinti paris ramus exterior*, Fascicle 1, p. 46-23.

LATER SYNONYMS:

1. *lacrimal gland nerve (Meckel, 1748)*
   Synonym for macrodissected adult human ***lacrimal nerve (Meckel, 1748; Bonhomme, 1748)***; in the original Latin, *nervos glandulae lacrymalis*, p. 121.
2. *internal superior palpebral nerve (Meckel, 1753)*
   Synonym for macrodissected adult human ***lacrimal nerve (Meckel, 1748; Bonhomme, 1748)***; in the original French, *le nerf supérieur intérieur de la paupiere*, p. 47.
3. *internal palpebral branch (Meckel, 1753)*
   Synonym for macrodissected adult human ***lacrimal nerve (Meckel, 1748; Bonhomme, 1748)***; in the original French, *le rameau palpébral interne*, Table 1-25 (see p. 47).
4. *external lacrimal nerve (Le Cat, 1768)*
   Synonym for macrodissected adult human ***lacrimal nerve (Meckel, 1748; Bonhomme, 1748)***; Plate VIII, Figure 1-*S*.

5. *lacrimal branch of first branch of fifth pair (Bock, 1817)*
   Synonym for macrodissected adult human ***lacrimal nerve (Meckel, 1748; Bonhomme, 1748)***; in the original Latin, *ramus lacrymalis*, p. 18.
6. *lachrimopalpebral nerve (Cruveilhier, 1836)*
   Synonym for macrodissected adult human ***lacrimal nerve (Meckel, 1748; Bonhomme, 1748)***; in the original French, *nerf lacrymo-palpébral*, p. 910.
7. *external branch of first division of fifth pair of nerves (Todd, 1836–1839)*
   Synonym for macrodissected adult human ***lacrimal nerve (Meckel, 1748; Bonhomme, 1748)***; p. 279.

PARTLY CORRESPONDS:

1. *malo-temporal fascicle of lacrimal surculus (Bellingeri, 1818)*
   Macrodissected adult human ***communicating branch (Winslow, 1733)*** of ***lacrimal nerve (Meckel, 1748; Bonhomme, 1748)*** with ***mandibular nerve (>1840)***; in the original Latin, *fasciculus malo-temporalis*, see Table I.
2. *lacrimal threads of lacrimal fascicle proper (Bellingeri, 1818)*
   Three branches of macrodissected adult human ***lacrimal nerve (Meckel, 1748; Bonhomme, 1748)*** to lacrimal gland; in the original Latin, *tres stamina lacrymales*, see Table I.
3. *conjunctival filaments of lacrimal fascicle proper (Bellingeri, 1818)*
   Macrodissected adult human branches of ***lacrimal nerve (Meckel, 1748; Bonhomme, 1748)*** to conjunctiva; in the original Latin, *filamenta conjunctivae*, see Table I.
4. *palpebral filaments of lacrimal fascicle proper (Bellingeri, 1818)*
   Macrodissected adult human branches of ***lacrimal nerve (Meckel, 1748; Bonhomme, 1748)*** to upper eyelid; in the original Latin, *filamenta palpebralia*, see Table I.
5. *internal branch of lacrimal nerve (Arnold, 1834)*
   Macrodissected adult human medial branch of ***lacrimal nerve (Meckel, 174); Bonhomme, 1748)*** to conjunctiva and skin around lateral angle of eye; in the original Latin, *nervus lacrymalis, ramus internus*, p. 7.
6. *palpebral branch of lacrimal nerve (Cruveilhier, 1836)*
   Macrodissected adult human cutaneous branch of ***lacrimal nerve (Meckel, 1748; Bonhomme, 1748)*** running along lower border of tarsal cartilage; in the original French, *rameau palpébral*, p. 911.
7. *temporal branch of lacrimal nerve (Cruveilhier, 1836)*
   Macrodissected adult human ascending cutaneous branch of ***lacrimal nerve (Meckel, 1748; Bonhomme, 1748)*** to anterior temporal region; in the original French, *rameau temporal*, p. 911.
8. *malar branch of lacrimal nerve (Cruveilhier, 1836)*
   Macrodissected adult human branch of ***lacrimal nerve (Meckel, 1748; Bonhomme, 1748)*** communicating with *zygomatic branches of facial nerve (>1840)*; in the original French, *rameau malaire*, p. 911.

lamina affixa (>1840)

As described for macrodissected adult human, the thickened ***ependyma (>1840)*** of the ***lateral ventricle (Vesalius, 1543a)*** overlying the ***terminal stria (Wenzel & Wenzel, 1812)*** and adjacent ***dorsal part of thalamus (Herrick, 1910)***, including the thalamostriate vein—basically associated with the length of the ***body of lateral ventricle (Bell, 1803b)***; see His (1895, p. 86) and Eycleshymer translation (1917, p. 163 and Fig. 21-*L*), Mettler (1948, p. 147), *Terminologia Anatomica* (1998, p. 127), *Dorland's* (2003, p. 993). It was probably first described as *membrana cornea (Tarin, 1750)*.

EARLIER REFERENCES:

Earlier synonyms:

1. *membrana cornea (Tarin, 1750)*
   Probably first reference to macrodissected adult human *lamina cornea (Meckel, 1817)*; Table I, Figure 1-*U*.
2. *substantia cornea (Wenzel & Wenzel, 1812)*
   Synonym for macrodissected adult human *lamina cornea (Meckel, 1817)*; p. 82.
3. *lamina cornea (Meckel, 1817)*
   Refers to hard and solid brownish layer over macrodissected adult human ***terminal stria (Wenzel & Wenzel, 1812)*** as subjects get older or cerebral afflictions occur, now known as ***lamina affixa (>1840)***; see translation (1832, Vol. 2, p. 457).

laryngopharyngeal branches of superior cervical ganglion (>1840)

As described for macrodissected adult human, medial branches of the ***superior cervical ganglion (Vieussens, 1684)*** supplying the carotid body and passing to the side of the pharynx, where they join with branches of the ***glossopharyngeal nerve (Huber, 1744)*** and ***vagus nerve (Galen, c192)*** to form the ***pharyngeal plexus (Neubauer, 1772)***; see Mitchell (1953, p. 215), Williams & Warwick (1980, p. 1128). They were known to Willis; see ***[laryngopharyngeal branches of superior cervical ganglion (>1840)] (Willis, 1664)***.

EARLIER REFERENCES:

Described, not named or illustrated:

1. ***[laryngopharyngeal branches of superior cervical ganglion (>1840)] (Willis, 1664)***
   Willis mentioned and illustrated "A shoot sent down to the Sphincter of the throat" for macrodissected adult human; see Pordage translation (1681, Fig. 9-*y* and p. 157). Beautifully illustrated for macrodissected adult human by Lancisi (1728, Tab. 6, Fig. 2-*F*).

Earlier synonyms:

1. *laryngeal branch of cervical intercostal trunk (Neubauer, 1772)*
   Refers basically to at least one ***laryngopharyngeal branch of superior cervical ganglion (>1840)*** in macrodissected adult human; in the original Latin, *ramo laryngeo ex trunco intercostali cervicali*, Table 1-*14,16*. Also see Haller (1772, p. 8 note *f*).
2. *superior soft nerve (Neubauer, 1772)*
   Essentially ***communicating branch (Winslow, 1733)*** between ***superior cervical ganglion (Vieussens, 1684)*** and ***superior laryngeal nerve (Loder, 1778)*** in

macrodissected adult human; that is, an early synonym for ***laryngopharyngeal branches of superior cervical ganglion (>1840)***; in the original Latin, *superiorem nervum mollem*, p. 77, Table 3, Figure 2-*r*.

3. *soft branch of superior cervical ganglion (Lobstein, 1823)*
Basically synonym for macrodissected (with the aid of a microscope) adult human ***laryngopharyngeal branches of superior cervical ganglion (>1840)*** and *superior soft nerve (Neubauer, 1772)*; the Latin *mollis* was used for "soft," see translation (1831, pp. 13–14).

PARTLY CORRESPONDS:

1. *intercostal pharyngeal nerves (Wrisberg, 1786)*
As described for macrodissected adult human, at least pharyngeal branches of ***laryngopharyngeal branches of superior cervical ganglion (>1840)*** with superior and inferior secondary branches; in the original Latin, *nervei, pharyngaei intercostalis*, see Wrisberg (1800, pp. 433–434).
2. *pharyngeal branches of superior ganglion (Chaussier, 1789)*
As described for macrodissected adult human, pharyngeal branches of ***laryngopharyngeal branches of superior cervical ganglion (>1840)***; *Table synoptique du nerf tri-splanchnique*.
3. *laryngeal branches of superior ganglion (Chaussier, 1789)*
As described for macrodissected adult human, pharyngeal branches of ***laryngopharyngeal branches of superior cervical ganglion (>1840)***; *Table synoptique du nerf tri-splanchnique*.
4. *pharyngeal soft nerve (Andersch, 1797)*
In macrodissected adult human, ***communicating branch (Winslow, 1733)*** of ***superior cervical ganglion (Vieussens, 1684)*** to *second pharyngeal nerve (Andersch & Soemmerring, 1792)*; in the original Latin, *nervus mollis pharyngeus*, p. 28. Thus, a ***laryngopharyngeal branch of superior cervical ganglion (>1840)***.
5. *branch from first cervical ganglion to pharyngeal plexus (Swan, 1830)*
For macrodissected adult human, thick branch of ***superior cervical ganglion (Vieussens, 1684)*** to ***pharyngeal plexus (Neubauer, 1772)***; Plate I-*f*. Thus, a ***laryngopharyngeal branch of superior cervical ganglion (>1840)***.
6. *nerve from supreme cervical ganglion joining with external branch of superior laryngeal nerve (Arnold, 1834)*
In macrodissected adult human, ***communicating branch (Winslow, 1733)*** of ***superior cervical ganglion (Vieussens, 1684)*** to ***external branch of superior laryngeal nerve (Fyfe, 1800)***; in the original Latin, *nervus ganglion cervicale supremum cohaerens cum ramo externo nervi laryngei superioris*, p. 18. Thus, a ***laryngopharyngeal branch of superior cervical ganglion (>1840)***.
7. *branch of supreme cervical ganglion to intercarotid ganglion (Arnold, 1834)*
In macrodissected adult human, branch of ***superior cervical ganglion (Vieussens, 1684)*** to carotid body; in the original Latin, *ramus ganglion cervicale supremum ad ganglion intercaroticum*, Table VI:*XXI-123*. Thus, a ***laryngopharyngeal branch of superior cervical ganglion (>1840)***.
8. *pharyngeal branches of superior cervical ganglion (Cruveilhier, 1836)*
As described for macrodissected adult human, pharyngeal branches of ***laryngopharyngeal branches of superior cervical ganglion (>1840)*** to ***pharyngeal plexus (Neubauer, 1772)***; in the original French, *rameaux pharyngiens*, p. 994.
9. *laryngeal branches of superior cervical ganglion (Cruveilhier, 1836)*
As described for macrodissected adult human, laryngeal branches of ***laryngopharyngeal branches of superior cervical ganglion (>1840)*** joining ***superior laryngeal nerve (Loder, 1778)*** and extending through its branches; in the original French, *rameaux laryngiens*, p. 994.

lateral ampullary nerve (>1840)

As described for macrodissected adult human, commonly a branch of the ***utriculoampullary nerve (>1840)*** to the ampulla of the lateral (horizontal) semicircular canal; see Durward (1951, Fig. 904), *Terminologia Anatomica* (1998, p. 136). It was probably first accurately described as the *branch of anterior branch of vestibular nerve to ampulla of external semicircular canal (Langenbeck, 1826–1830)*.

EARLIER REFERENCES:

Earlier synonyms:

1. *branch of anterior branch of vestibular nerve to ampulla of external semicircular canal (Langenbeck, 1826–1830)*
Synonym for macrodissected adult human ***lateral ampullary nerve (>1840)***; in the original Latin, *ramus rami anterioris nervi vestibuli ad ampullam canalis semicircularis externi*; Fascicle III, Table XXIX, Figure I-8.
2. *branch of anterior vestibular nerve to ampulla of external membranous semicircular canal (Langenbeck, 1826–1830)*
Synonym for macrodissected adult human ***lateral ampullary nerve (>1840)***; in the original Latin, *ramus nervi vestibuli anterior ad ampullam canalis semicircularis membranacei externi*; Fascicle III, Table XXIX, Figure IX-5.

lateral aperture of fourth ventricle (>1840)

As described for macrodissected adult human, the opening between ***lateral recess of fourth ventricle (>1840)*** and ***subarachnoid space (Magendie, 1827)***, one on the right and one on the left side; see Millen & Woollam (1962, Fig. 36), Williams & Warwick (1980, p. 932). It was first clearly described by Haller; see ***[lateral aperture of fourth ventricle (>1840)] (Haller, 1747)***.

TRANSLATIONS:

1. *apertura lateralis ventriculi quarti (>1840)*
Current Latin form of ***lateral aperture of fourth ventricle (>1840)***; see *Dorland's* (2003, p. 112).

EARLIER REFERENCES:

Described, not named or illustrated:

1. ***[lateral aperture of fourth ventricle (>1840)] (Haller, 1747)***

First clear published description, in macrodissected adult human; see Millen & Woollam (1962, p. 18).

lateral branch of spinal nerve dorsal branch (>1840)

As described for macrodissected adult human, a lateral and a medial branch are found on all but the first cervical, fourth and fifth sacral, and coccygeal ***spinal nerve dorsal branches (Meckel, 1817)***. The lateral branch supplies dorsal skin and muscle lateral to that supplied by a corresponding ***medial branch of spinal nerve dorsal branch (>1840)***; see Durward (1951, Fig. 913), Williams & Warwick (1980, pp. 1089–1091), *Terminologia Anatomica* (1998, pp. 137–139). It was delineated first by Eustachi; see ***[lateral branch of spinal nerve dorsal branch (>1840)] (Eustachi, 1552)***.

EARLIER REFERENCES:

Illustrated, not named or described:

1. ***[lateral branch of spinal nerve dorsal branch (>1840)] (Eustachi, 1552)***
   Systematically illustrated for macrodissected adult human; see Albinus edition (1761, Tab. 23).

Earlier synonyms:

1. *external branch of spinal nerve dorsal branch (Meckel, 1817)*
   Synonym for ***lateral branch of spinal nerve dorsal branch (>1840)***, described for macrodissected adult human ***thoracic nerves (Diemerbroeck, 1672)***; see translation (1832, Vol. 3, p. 9).

PARTLY CORRESPONDS:

1. *subcutaneous branch of dorsal branch of thoracic nerve (Bock, 1827)*
   As indicated for macrodissected adult human, ***lateral branch of spinal nerve dorsal branch (>1840)*** for 2nd– 11th ***thoracic nerves (Diemerbroeck, 1672)***; in the original Latin, *ram. subcutaneus rami dorsalis nervi thoracici*; Table IV-47.
2. *common gluteal cutaneous nerve (Bock, 1827)*
   Macrodissected adult human ***lateral branch of spinal nerve dorsal branch (>1840)*** for first 4 ***sacral nerves (Camper, 1769)*** joining with one another and with ***lateral branch of spinal nerve dorsal branch (>1840)*** of last ***lumbar nerve (Diemerbroeck, 1672)*** to form loops on dorsal surface of sacrum; see (Williams & Warwick, 1980, p. 1091). Apparently Bock named and illustrated it; in the original Latin, *nerv. cutaneus glutaeus communis*, Table IV-66.
3. *posterior gluteal cutaneous branches (Bock, 1827)*
   Macrodissected adult human terminal branches of *common gluteal cutaneous nerve (Bock, 1827)*; in the original Latin, *rami cutanei glutaei posteriores*, Table IV-67. Also see Williams & Warwick (1980, p. 1091), referred to as *gluteal branches*.
4. *posterior gluteal cutaneous nerves (Bock, 1827)*
   Synonym for *posterior gluteal cutaneous branches (Bock, 1827)*; in the original Latin, *nervi cutanei glutaei posteriores*, Table IV-67.
5. *external branch of posterior branch of lumbar nerve (Bock, 1827)*
   Synonym for macrodissected adult human *external branch of spinal nerve dorsal branch (Meckel, 1817)* for ***lumbar nerves (Diemerbroeck, 1672)***; in the original Latin, *ram. externus posterior*; Table VII, Figure 1-5. Cruveilhier (1836, p. 771 ff.) used term systematically for all ***spinal nerve dorsal branches (Meckel, 1817)***.
6. *external branch of dorsal branch of thoracic nerve (Bock, 1827)*
   Synonym for macrodissected adult human *external branch of spinal nerve dorsal branch (Meckel, 1817)* for 11th and 12th ***thoracic nerves (Diemerbroeck, 1672)***; in the original Latin, *ram. externus dorsalis nervi thoracis*; Table VII, Figure 2-2,4.
7. *external branch of posterior branch of abdominal nerve (Bock, 1827)*
   Synonym for *external branch of posterior branch of lumbar nerve (Bock, 1827)*; in the original Latin, *ram. externus posterior nervi abdominalis*; Table VII, Figure 2-6.

lateral branch of supraorbital nerve (>1840)

As described for macrodissected adult human it and the smaller ***medial branch of supraorbital nerve (>1840)*** together supply skin of the scalp almost as far caudally (back) as the lambdoid suture, along with some branches to the frontal sinus mucus membrane and pericranium; see Williams & Warwick (1980, p. 1061 and Fig. 7.186), *Terminologia Anatomica* (1998, p. 133), and Henle (1871, Fig. 234, distal and lateral to part *f*). It was first clearly distinguished by Winslow; see ***[lateral branch of supraorbital nerve (>1840)] (Winslow, 1733)***.

EARLIER REFERENCES:

Described, not named or illustrated:

1. ***[lateral branch of supraorbital nerve (>1840)] (Winslow, 1733)***
   Winslow noted for macrodissected adult human that after passing through foramen superciliare [supraorbital foramen], end of *frontal ramus of ophthalmic nerve (Winslow, 1733)* is divided toward each side [presumably medial and lateral branches] to be spent in part on neighboring skin; Section VI, p. 63.

Earlier synonyms:

1. *external supraorbital branch of greater frontal nerve (Meckel, 1753)*
   Synonym for macrodissected adult human ***lateral branch of supraorbital nerve (>1840)***; in the original French, *le rameau sus-orbitaire externe du grand nerf frontal*, p. 40.
2. *external branch of greater frontal nerve (Meckel, 1753)*
   Synonym for macrodissected adult human ***lateral branch of supraorbital nerve (>1840)***; in the original French, *le rameau externe du grand nerf frontal*, Table 1-*1*.
3. *exterior branch of supraorbital nerve (Günther, 1786)*
   Synonym for macrodissected adult human ***lateral branch of supraorbital nerve (>1840)***; in the original Latin, *nervis supraorbitalis ramus exteriorem*, p. 42.

4. *deep branch of supraorbital nerve (Günther, 1786)*
Synonym for macrodissected adult human ***lateral branch of supraorbital nerve (>1840)***; in the original Latin, *nervis supraorbitalis ramus profundum*, p. 42.
5. *external branch of palpebro-frontal nerve (Burdin, 1803)*
Synonym for macrodissected adult human ***lateral branch of supraorbital nerve (>1840)***; see translation (1803, Vol. 1, p. 170).
6. *superficial branches of frontal branches of external frontal nerve (Todd, 1836–1839)*
Apparently synonym for macrodissected adult human *external branch of greater frontal nerve (Meckel, 1753)*; p. 280.
7. *long branches of frontal branches of external frontal nerve (Todd, 1836–1839)*
Apparently synonym for macrodissected adult human *external branch of greater frontal nerve (Meckel, 1753)*; pp. 280–281.
8. *external branch of ascending branch of external frontal nerve (Cruveilhier, 1836)*
Synonym for macrodissected adult human ***lateral branch of supraorbital nerve (>1840)***; in the original French, *rameau externe*, pp. 912–913.
9. *external branch of ascending branch of supraorbital nerve (Cruveilhier, 1836)*
Synonym for *external branch of ascending branch of external frontal nerve (Cruveilhier, 1836)*; pp. 912–913.
10. *external branch of frontal branch of external frontal nerve (Cruveilhier, 1836)*
Synonym for *external branch of ascending branch of external frontal nerve (Cruveilhier, 1836)*; pp. 912–913.
11. *external branch of frontal branch of supraorbital nerve (Cruveilhier, 1836)*
Synonym for *external branch of ascending branch of external frontal nerve (Cruveilhier, 1836)*; pp. 912–913.

lateral calcaneal branches of sural nerve (>1840)

As described for macrodissected adult human, cutaneous branches of the ***sural nerve (Pietro da Cortona, 1741)*** to the lateral and dorsal (back) sides of the ankle and heel, and the dorsolateral sole; see Durward (1951, p. 1110 and Fig. 950), *Terminologia Anatomica* (1998, p. 141). First clearly delineated by Eustachi; see ***[lateral calcaneal branches of sural nerve (>1840)] (Eustachi, 1552)***.

ALTERNATE SPELLINGS:

1. *lateral calcanean branches of sural nerve (>1840)*
Alternate form of ***lateral calcaneal branches of sural nerve (>1840)***; see Durward (1951, p. 1110).

EARLIER REFERENCES:

Illustrated, not named or described:

1. ***[lateral calcaneal branches of sural nerve (>1840)] (Eustachi, 1552)***
Clearly illustrated for macrodissected adult human; Table 23.

Illustrated and described, not named:

1. ***[lateral calcaneal branches of sural nerve (>1840)] (Vieussens, 1684)***
Described and illustrated for macrodissected adult human; see Table 29:*112–114*.

Earlier synonyms:

1. *exterior dorsal twig of foot of tibial communicating branch (Jördens, 1788)*
Probably synonym for macrodissected adult human ***lateral calcaneal branches of sural nerve (>1840)***; in the original Latin, *ramulus dorsalis pedis exterior rami communicantis tibiei*, p. 9 and Table I-*139*. Jördens there described, illustrated, and named 10 branches of it, p. 9 and Table I:*140–149*.
2. *external calcanean nerves (Cruveilhier, 1836)*
Synonym for macrodissected adult human ***lateral calcaneal branches of sural nerve (>1840)***; in the original French, *nerfs calcaniens externes*, p. 869.

PARTLY CORRESPONDS:

1. *supramalleolar twig of tibial communicating branch (Jördens, 1788)*
A macrodissected adult human ***lateral calcaneal branch of sural nerve (>1840)*** innervating skin in region just proximal (above) to lateral malleolus; in the original Latin, *ramulus supramalleolaris rami communicantis tibiei*, p. 8 and Table 1-*111*. Jördens there described, illustrated, and named eight branches of it, Table 1:*113–120*.
2. *supramalleolar nerve (Fischer, 1791)*
Synonym for macrodissected adult human *supramalleolar twig of tibial communicating branch (Jördens, 1788)*; in the original Latin, *nervus supramalleolaris*, p. 34.
3. *calcaneal cutaneous branch of tibial nerve (Bock, 1827)*
Synonym for a macrodissected adult human ***lateral calcaneal branch of sural nerve (>1840)*** to the heel; in the original Latin, *ram. cutaneus calcis nerv. tibialis*, Table VI, Figure 4-2.
4. *posterior plantar cutaneous branch of tibial nerve (Bock, 1827)*
Synonym for a macrodissected adult human ***lateral calcaneal branch of sural nerve (>1840)*** to back end of sole; in the original Latin, *ram. cutaneus plantaris posterior nerv. tibialis*, Table VI, Figure 4-3.

lateral cerebral fossa (>1840)

As described for macrodissected adult human, the dorsoventral (vertical) part or floor of the ***lateral cerebral sulcus(>1840)*** at the surface of the ***insular region (Brodmann, 1909)***; see Mettler (1948, p. 123), Nieuwenhuys et al. (2008, Fig. 5.6, unlabeled but space to left of *1-4*). It was first partly indicated by Vesalius; see ***[lateral cerebral fossa (>1840)] (Vesalius, 1543a)***.

EARLIER REFERENCES:

Illustrated, not named or described:

1. ***[lateral cerebral fossa (>1840)] (Vesalius, 1543a)***
Partly illustrated for macrodissected adult human in frontal (horizontal) section; see Singer translation (Fig. 4 near *E*). More fully illustrated in surface view by Bartholin (1641, Fig. 5-*k*) and in transverse section by Steno (1669, Pl. III).

Earlier synonyms:

1. *Sylvian fossa (Vicq d'Azyr, 1784)*
   Eponym for macrodissected adult human ***lateral cerebral fossa (>1840)***; p. 505.

lateral cerebral sulcus (>1840)

As described for macrodissected adult human, a deep longitudinal cleft starting on the lateral surface of the ***cerebral cortex gray matter (>1840)*** and extending medially with ventral and dorsal walls eventually extending dorsally and ventrally (vertically) at right angles to form the ***lateral cerebral fossa (>1840)*** covering the ***insular region (Brodmann, 1909)***. Viewed from the lateral surface, it has a short ***stem of lateral cerebral sulcus (>1840)*** that ends by dividing rostrally into the ***anterior branch of lateral cerebral sulcus (>1840)*** and ***ascending branch of lateral cerebral sulcus (>1840)***, and by extending caudally and dorsally as the ***posterior branch of lateral cerebral sulcus (>1840)***. The surface of its dorsal wall is formed by the ***frontal operculum (>1840)*** and ***parietal operculum (>1840)***, the surface of its ventral wall is formed by the ***temporal operculum (>1840)***, and all three are separated from the ***insular region (Brodmann, 1909)*** by the ***circular sulcus (Schwalbe, 1881)***; see Williams & Warwick (1980, pp. 984–986, Figs. 7.111–114), *Nomina Anatomica* (1983, p. A70), *Terminologia Anatomica* (1998, pp. 124–125). It was first indicated by Vesalius; see ***[lateral cerebral sulcus (>1840)] (Vesalius, 1543a)***.

EARLIER REFERENCES:

Described, not named or illustrated:

1. ***[lateral cerebral sulcus (>1840)] (Vesalius, 1543a)***
   Alluded to for macrodissected adult human; see Singer translation (1952, p. 70).

Earlier synonyms:

1. *great cerebral fissure (Bartholin, 1641)*
   A footnote by Bartholin's teacher, Frans de Le Boë (Franciscus Sylvius), in the 1641 book (p. 262) described the ***lateral cerebral sulcus (>1840)*** for the first time, and it was illustrated and labeled in the original Latin, *magna cerebri fissura* in Figure 5-*i*.
2. *winding cleft (Bartholin, 1662)*
   Synonym for macrodissected adult human ***lateral cerebral sulcus (>1840)***; p. 134.
3. *great cleft of brain (Bartholin, 1662)*
   Synonym for macrodissected adult human ***lateral cerebral sulcus (>1840)***; Tables 2-*V*, 3-*i*.
4. *great chink of brain (Bartholin, 1662)*
   Synonym for macrodissected adult human ***lateral cerebral sulcus (>1840)***; Table VI-*h*.
5. *fissure (Le Böe, 1663)*
   Le Boë (Franciscus Sylvius) also published an earlier footnote describing macrodissected adult human ***lateral cerebral sulcus (>1840)***, in Bartholin (1641, p. 262); see *great cerebral fissure (Bartholin, 1641)* and Baker (1909, p. 224).
6. *fissura cerebri (Winslow, 1733)*
   Synonym for macrodissected adult human ***lateral cerebral sulcus (>1840)***; Section X, p. 33.
7. *fissura magna Silvii (Winslow, 1733)*
   Eponym for macrodissected adult human ***lateral cerebral sulcus (>1840)***; Section X, p. 33.Winslow named it for Frans de Le Boë (Franciscus Sylvius); see *great cerebral fissure (Bartholin, 1641)*, *fissure (Le Böe, 1663)* and Meyer (1971, p. 130).
8. *great Sylvian fissure (Winslow, 1733)*
   English form of *fissura magna Silvii (Winslow, 1733)*.
9. *anfractuosa cerebri fissura (Tarin, 1753)*
   Synonym listed for macrodissected adult human ***lateral cerebral sulcus (>1840)***; pp. 22–23.
10. *Sylvian fossa (Tarin, 1753)*
    Eponym listed for macrodissected adult human ***lateral cerebral sulcus (>1840)***; in the original Latin, *fossa Sylvii*, p. 23.
11. *fissura major Sylvii (Tarin, 1753)*
    Eponym listed for macrodissected adult human ***lateral cerebral sulcus (>1840)***; p. 23.
12. *Sylvian fissure (Vicq d'Azyr, 1784)*
    Eponym for macrodissected adult human ***lateral cerebral sulcus (>1840)***; p. 506.
13. *inter-lobar scissure (Burdin, 1803)*
    Synonym for macrodissected adult human ***lateral cerebral sulcus (>1840)***; see translation (1803, Vol. 1, p. 217).
14. *great interlobar fissure (Chaussier, 1807)*
    Synonym for macrodissected adult human ***lateral cerebral sulcus (>1840)***; p. 38, see Dejerine & Dejerine-Klumpke (1895, p. 246).
15. *valley (Reil, 1809b)*
    Synonym for macrodissected adult human ***lateral cerebral sulcus (>1840)***; in the original German, *das Thal* or *das Tal*, p. 195 ff. See Burdach (1822, p. 387).
16. *fissura magna anterior (Ramsay, 1813)*
    Synonym for macrodissected adult human ***lateral cerebral sulcus (>1840)***; p. 48; Plate XV, Figure 2-*y*. See Burdach (1822, p. 387).
17. *inferior fissure (Burdach, 1822)*
    Synonym for macrodissected adult human ***lateral cerebral sulcus (>1840)***; p. 166.See Burdach (1822, p. 166).
18. *temporal fissure (Gerdy, 1838)*
    Synonym for macrodissected adult human ***lateral cerebral sulcus (>1840)***; in the original French, *scissure temporale*, p. 259.
19. *lateral fissure (>1840)*
    Synonym for macrodissected adult human ***lateral cerebral sulcus (>1840)***; see Crosby et al. (1962, p. 344 and Fig. 233).

PARTLY CORRESPONDS:

1. *cruciform sulcus (Rolando, 1831)*
   Apparently included macrodissected adult human ***anterior branch of lateral cerebral sulcus (>1840)***, ***ascending branch of lateral cerebral sulcus (>1840)***, and ventral (descending) extension of ***ascending branch of***

lateral cerebral sulcus (>1840); in the original Italian, *solco crociforme*, Figure 1-8.

lateral cutaneous branch of iliohypogastric nerve (>1840)

As described for macrodissected adult human, it corresponds to a ***lateral cutaneous branch of intercostal nerves (>1840)***, is small or sometimes absent, and supplies skin and fascia over the rostral (upper) part of the lateral side of the gluteal region; see Durward (1951, p. 1091 and Fig. 937), Hamilton (1976, Figs. 811, 812, 827) *Terminologia Anatomica* (1998, p. 139). It was first clearly delineated by Eustachi; see ***[lateral cutaneous branch of iliohypogastric nerve (>1840)] (Eustachi, 1552)***.

EARLIER REFERENCES:

Illustrated, not named or described:

1. ***[lateral cutaneous branch of iliohypogastric nerve (>1840)] (Eustachi, 1552)***
Clearly illustrated for macrodissected adult human; see Albinus edition (1761, Tabs. 19-υ and 20-ζ).

Earlier synonyms:

1. *external branch of iliohypogastric nerve (Bock, 1827)*
Synonym for macrodissected adult human ***lateral cutaneous nerve of iliohypogastric nerve (>1840)***; in the original Latin, *Ram. externus nervi ileo-hypogastrici*, Table I, Figure 2-59.
2. *pubic branch of greater abdominal branch of lumbar plexus (Cruveilhier, 1836)*
Synonym for macrodissected adult human ***lateral cutaneous nerve of iliohypogastric nerve (>1840)***; in the original French, *rameau pubien*, p. 834. Cruveilhier also described there its internal or pubic and its external branchlets.
3. *gluteal cutaneous branch of greater abdominal branch of lumbar plexus (Cruveilhier, 1836)*
In macrodissected adult human, not infrequent branching pattern of ***iliohypogastric nerve (Schmidt, 1794)*** generating ***lateral cutaneous nerve of iliohypogastric nerve (>1840)***; in the original French, *branche cutanée fessière*, p. 835. Other branching pattern generates *pubic branch of greater abdominal branch of lumbar plexus (Cruveilhier, 1836)*.

lateral cutaneous branch of intercostal nerves (>1840)

As described for macrodissected adult human, they supply skin on the lateral and dorsal body wall, with pectoral and abdominal components from the rostral (through 7th) and caudal ***intercostal nerves (Vesalius, 1543a)*** respectively; see Williams & Warwick (1980, pp. 1103–1105), *Nomina Anatomica* (1983, p. A77), *Terminologia Anatomica* (1998, p. 139). They were known to Galen; see ***[lateral cutaneous branch of intercostal nerves (>1840)] (Galen, c192)***.

TRANSLATIONS:

1. *ramus cutaneus lateralis nervi intercostalis (>1840)*
Current Latin form of ***lateral cutaneous branch of intercostal nerves (>1840)***; see *Nomina Anatomica* (1983, p. A77).

EARLIER REFERENCES:

Described, not named or illustrated:

1. ***[lateral cutaneous branch of intercostal nerves (>1840)] (Galen, c192)***
Mentioned for macrodissected adult beef, pig, and/or macaque but not human; see Duckworth translation (1962, pp. 242–243, 258–259).

Illustrated and described, not named:

1. ***[lateral cutaneous branch of intercostal nerves (>1840)] (Vesalius, 1543a)***
Alluded to in macrodissected adult human; see Richardson & Carman translation (2002, p. 234). Beautifully illustrated by Eustachi (1552); see Albinus edition (1761, Tabs. 21, 23).

Earlier synonyms:

1. *external thoracic nerves (Meckel, 1817)*
Synonym for macrodissected adult human ***lateral cutaneous branches of intercostal nerves (>1840)***; see translation (1832, Vol. 3, p. 9).
2. *rami pectorales externi (Meckel, 1817)*
Latin form given for *external thoracic nerves (Meckel, 1817)*; see translation (1832, Vol. 3, p. 9).
3. *lateral subcutaneous branch of intercostal branch of thoracic nerve (Bock, 1827)*
Synonym for macrodissected adult human ***lateral cutaneous branch of intercostal nerves (>1840)***; in the original Latin, *ram. subcutaneus lateralis*, Table I, Figure 2-47.
4. *posterior subcutaneous branch of intercostal branch of thoracic nerve (Bock, 1827)*
Synonym for *lateral subcutaneous branch of intercostal branch of thoracic nerve (Bock, 1827)*; in the original Latin, *ram. subcutaneus posterior*, Table I, Figure 2-47.
5. *lateral cutaneous nerve (Bock, 1827)*
Synonym for macrodissected adult human ***lateral cutaneous branch of intercostal nerves (>1840)***; in the original Latin, *nerv. cutaneus lateralis*, Table II-75.
6. *lateral cutaneous nerve of intercostal nerve (Bock, 1827)*
Synonym for *lateral cutaneous nerve (Bock, 1827)*; in the original Latin, *nervi cutanei lateralis intercostalis*, Table III-27.
7. *external branch of dorsal nerve (Swan, 1830)*
Synonym for macrodissected adult human ***lateral cutaneous branch of intercostal nerves (>1840)***; Plate XVII.
8. *perforating branch of intercostal branches of dorsal nerves (Cruveilhier, 1836)*
Synonym for macrodissected adult human ***lateral cutaneous branch of intercostal nerves (>1840)***; in the original French, *rameau perforant*, p. 824.
9. *cutaneous branch of intercostal branches of dorsal nerves (Cruveilhier, 1836)*
Synonym for macrodissected adult human ***lateral cutaneous branch of intercostal nerves (>1840)***; in the original French, *rameau cutané*, p. 824.

10. *perforating branches of dorsal nerves (Cruveilhier, 1836)*
Synonym for macrodissected adult human ***lateral cutaneous branches of intercostal nerves (>1840)***; in the original French, *rameaux perforans*, p. 830.
11. *cutaneous branches of dorsal nerves (Cruveilhier, 1836)*
Synonym for *perforating branches of dorsal nerves (Cruveilhier, 1836)*; in the original French, *rameaux cutanés*, p. 830.
12. *middle branches of dorsal nerves (Cruveilhier, 1836)*
Synonym for *perforating branches of dorsal nerves (Cruveilhier, 1836)*; in the original French, *rameaux moyens*, p. 830.
13. *short cutaneous nerves (Quain & Wilson, 1839)*
Synonym for macrodissected adult human ***lateral cutaneous branches of intercostal nerves (>1840)***; Plate XVII-*i*.

PARTLY CORRESPONDS:

1. *lateral pectoral nerves (Bock, 1827)*
Synonym for macrodissected adult human ***lateral cutaneous branches of intercostal nerves (>1840)*** for 3rd– 7th ***intercostal nerves (Vesalius, 1543a)***; in the original Latin, *nervi lateralis pectoris*, see Table II:*80-90*.
2. *lateral pectoral cutaneous nerve (Bock, 1827)*
Synonym for *lateral pectoral nerve (Bock, 1827)*; in the original Latin, *nerv. cutaneus lateralis pectoris*, Table II:*82-90*.
3. *lateral abdominal cutaneous nerves (Bock, 1827)*
Synonym for macrodissected adult human ***lateral cutaneous branch of intercostal nerves (>1840)*** for eighth and more caudal ***intercostal nerves (Vesalius, 1543a)***; in the original Latin, *nervi cutanei abdominis lateralis*, see Table II-*92*.

lateral cutaneous nerve of calf (>1840)

As described for macrodissected adult human, its origin and distribution are inconsistent; usually it arises from the ***common fibular nerve (>1840)***, either from its ***sciatic nerve (Keill, 1698)*** segment or from the proximal part of its free segment, and distributes small branches to ventral (anterior), dorsal (posterior), and lateral parts of the proximal leg; see Williams & Warwick (1980, p. 1115). Rarely its terminal end continues on as the ***sural nerve (Pietro da Cortona, 1741)***; see *Dorland's* (2003, p. 1234). It was known to Galen; see ***[lateral cutaneous nerve of calf (>1840)] (Galen, c177)***.

TRANSLATIONS:

1. *nervus cutaneus surae lateralis (>1840)*
Current Latin form of ***lateral cutaneous nerve of calf (>1840)***; see *Dorland's* (2003, p. 1238).

EARLIER REFERENCES:

Described, not named or illustrated:

1. ***[lateral cutaneous nerve of calf (>1840)] (Galen, c177)***
Described for macrodissected adult beef, pig, and/or macaque but not human; see Singer translation (1999, pp. 83–84). Vesalius (1543a) described and illustrated it for macrodissected adult human; see Richardson & Carman translation (2002, p. 260).

Earlier synonyms:

1. *posterior ramus of small sciatic branch (Winslow, 1733)*
Synonym for macrodissected adult human ***lateral cutaneous nerve of calf (>1840)***; Section VI, no. 344, p. 92.
2. *cutaneous peroneal nerve (Martin, 1781)*
Apparently synonym for macrodissected adult human ***lateral cutaneous nerve of calf (>1840)***; in the original Latin, *nervus peroneus cutaneus*, p. 245.
3. *external cutaneous branch of peroneal nerve (Martin, 1781)*
Apparently synonym for macrodissected adult human ***lateral cutaneous nerve of calf (>1840)***; in the original Latin, *nervus peroneus ramus cutaneus exterior*, Table XI.
4. *inferior posterior cutaneous branch of exterior branch of sciatic nerve (Günther, 1786)*
May correspond roughly to macrodissected adult human ***lateral cutaneous nerve of calf (>1840)***; in the original Latin, *ramus cutaneum posteriorem inferiorem*, p. 86.
5. *external cutaneous nerve (Jördens, 1788)*
Probably synonym for macrodissected adult human ***lateral cutaneous nerve of calf (>1840)***; in the original Latin, *nervo cutaneo externo*, p. 2. Cloquet (1828; Pl. CLXXI, Fig. 2-*30*) used the French, *nerf cutané externe*.
6. *external and superior posterior femoral cutaneous nerve (Mayer, 1794)*
Probably synonym for macrodissected adult human ***lateral cutaneous nerve of calf (>1840)***; in the original Latin, *nervus cutaneus posterior superior et externus femoris*; Part 5, Table VI-ε (p. 36). Later given as *nervus cutaneus posterior, superior et externus femoris*; Part 5, Table VI, Figure 3-ζ (p. 39).
7. *peroneo-cutaneous nerve (Burdin, 1803)*
Synonym for macrodissected adult human ***lateral cutaneous nerve of calf (>1840)***; see translation (1803, Vol. 1, p. 205).
8. *middle posterior cutaneous nerve (Meckel, 1817)*
Probably corresponds, at least partly, to macrodissected adult human ***lateral cutaneous nerve of calf (>1840)***; see translation (1832, Vol. 3, pp. 17–18).
9. *external cutaneous nerve of leg (Bock, 1827)*
Synonym for macrodissected adult human ***lateral cutaneous nerve of calf (>1840)***; in the original Latin, *nerv. cutaneus externus cruris*, Table III-*53*.
10. *long cutaneous branch of peroneal nerve (Swan, 1830)*
Probably synonym for macrodissected adult human ***lateral cutaneous nerve of calf (>1840)***; Plate XXV, Figure 1-*30*.
11. *peroneal cutaneous branch of external popliteal sciatic nerve (Cruveilhier, 1836)*
Synonym for macrodissected adult human ***lateral cutaneous nerve of calf (>1840)***; in the original French, *branche cutanée péronière*, p. 862.

lateral cutaneous nerve of forearm (>1840)

As described for macrodissected adult human, the continuation of the ***musculocutaneous nerve (Du Verney, 1697)***. It supplies skin over the lateral half of the ventral (anterior) surface of the forearm and distributes branches turning around the radial border of the forearm to communicate with the ***posterior cutaneous nerve of forearm (>1840)*** and terminal branch of the ***radial nerve (Du Verney, 1697)***, and then ends over the base of the thenar eminence; see Williams & Warwick (1980, p. 1097 and Fig. 7.201), *Terminologia Anatomica* (1998, p. 138). It was known to Galen; see ***[lateral cutaneous nerve of forearm (>1840)] (Galen, c177)***.

TRANSLATIONS:

1. *nervus cutaneus antebrachii lateralis (>1840)*
   Current Latin form of ***lateral cutaneous nerve of forearm (>1840)***; see *Terminologia Anatomica* (1998, p. 138).

EARLIER REFERENCES:

Described, not named or illustrated:

1. ***[lateral cutaneous nerve of forearm (>1840)] (Galen, c177)***
   Mentioned for macrodissected adult beef, pig, and/or macaque but not human; see Singer translation (1999, p. 70). Vesalius (1543a) provided very detailed description for macrodissected adult human; see Richardson & Carman translation (2002, pp. 240–241). Winslow called it "a true Nervus Cutaneus" because of its distribution; Section VI, p. 82.

Earlier synonyms:

1. *cutaneous branch of musculocutaneous nerve (Camper, 1760)*
   Synonym for macrodissected adult human ***lateral cutaneous nerve of forearm (>1840)***; Table 1, Figure 1-63,64. Also see Meckel (1832, Vol. 3, p. 26).
2. *superficial branch of musculocutaneous nerve (Soemmerring, 1791)*
   Synonym for macrodissected adult human ***lateral cutaneous nerve of forearm (>1840)***; pp. 280–281.
3. *cutaneous branch of external cutaneous nerve (Soemmerring, 1791)*
   Synonym for macrodissected adult human ***lateral cutaneous nerve of forearm (>1840)***; pp. 280–281.
4. *superficial branch of external cutaneous nerve (Soemmerring, 1791)*
   Synonym for macrodissected adult human ***lateral cutaneous nerve of forearm (>1840)***; pp. 280–281.
5. *inferior external cutaneous nerve of arm (Mayer, 1794)*
   Synonym for macrodissected adult human ***lateral cutaneous nerve of forearm (>1840)***; in the original Latin, *nervus cutaneus externus brachii inferior*; Part 5, p. 23.
6. *external branch of external cutaneous nerve of arm (Cloquet, 1816)*
   Synonym for macrodissected adult human ***lateral cutaneous nerve of forearm (>1840)***; p. 646.
7. *external branch of musculocutaneous nerve (Bock, 1827)*
   Synonym for macrodissected adult human ***lateral cutaneous nerve of forearm (>1840)***; in the original Latin, *ram. externus nervi musculo-cutanei*, Table III-*21*.
8. *anterior branch of musculocutaneous nerve (Bock, 1827)*
   Synonym for macrodissected adult human ***lateral cutaneous nerve of forearm (>1840)***; in the original Latin, *ram. anterior nervi musculo-cutanei*, Table V, Figure 4-*1*.

PARTLY CORRESPONDS:

1. *greater cutaneous branch of musculocutaneous nerve (Loder, 1803)*
   Larger of two branches described as forming macrodissected adult human ***lateral cutaneous nerve of forearm (>1840)***; in the original Latin, *ramus cutaneus major nervi musculocutanei*; Table CLXXIX, Figure 2-*96*.
2. *lesser cutaneous branch of musculocutaneous nerve (Loder, 1803)*
   Smaller of two branches described as forming macrodissected adult human ***lateral cutaneous nerve of forearm (>1840)***; in the original Latin, *ramus cutaneus minor nervi musculocutanei*; Table CLXXIX, Figure 2-*104*.
3. *communications between musculocutaneous nerve and middle cutaneous nerve (Caldani, 1813, 1814)*
   For macrodissected adult human, two ***communicating branches (Winslow, 1733)*** between ***lateral cutaneous nerve of forearm (>1840)*** and ***anterior branch of medial cutaneous nerve of forearm (>1840)***; in the original Latin, *communicationes inter nervum musculo-cutaneum et nervum cutaneum medium*, Table CCLVIII, Figure 1-*30*.
4. *branches of musculocutaneous nerve inserted into volar branch of median nerve (Caldani, 1813, 1814)*
   For macrodissected adult human, three branches of ***lateral cutaneous nerve of forearm (>1840)*** to ***palmar branch of median nerve (Bock, 1827)***; in the original Latin, *rami a nervo musculo-cutaneo prodeuntes et in ramum volarem nervi mediani inserti*, Table CCLVIII, Figure 1-*36*.
5. *external branch of musculocutaneous nerve (Cruveilhier, 1836)*
   Synonym for macrodissected adult human *lesser cutaneous branch of musculocutaneous nerve (Loder, 1803)*; in the original French, *rameau externe*, p. 801.
6. *internal branch of musculocutaneous nerve (Cruveilhier, 1836)*
   Synonym for macrodissected adult human *greater cutaneous branch of musculocutaneous nerve (Loder, 1803)*; in the original French, *rameau interne*, p. 801.
7. *articular branch of internal branch of musculocutaneous nerve (Cruveilhier, 1836)*
   Branch of macrodissected adult human ***lateral cutaneous nerve of forearm (>1840)*** to radiocarpal joint; in the original French, *rameau articulaire*, p. 801.
8. *posterior branch of external cutaneous nerve (Quain & Wilson, 1839)*
   Synonym for macrodissected adult human *greater cutaneous branch of musculocutaneous nerve (Loder, 1803)*; Plate XVIII-*e*.

9. *anterior branch of external cutaneous nerve (Quain & Wilson, 1839)*
   Synonym for macrodissected adult human *lesser cutaneous branch of musculocutaneous nerve (Loder, 1803)*; Plate XVIII-*f*.
10. *branch of communication from radial nerve to external cutaneous nerve (Quain & Wilson, 1839)*
   Probably macrodissected adult human ***communicating branch (Winslow, 1733)*** between ***lateral cutaneous nerve of forearm (>1840)*** and ***superficial branch of radial nerve (Martin, 1781)***; Plate XVIII-*g*.
11. *filaments of communication of internal cutaneous nerve with external cutaneous nerve (Quain & Wilson, 1839)*
   Synonym for macrodissected adult human *communications between musculocutaneous nerve and middle cutaneous nerve (Caldani, 1813, 1814)*; Plate XVIII-*c*.

lateral cutaneous nerve of thigh (>1840)

As described for macrodissected adult human, it arises from the ***lumbar plexus dorsal divisions (Paterson, 1887)*** of the second and third ***lumbar nerves (Diemerbroeck, 1672)*** and supplies branches to the parietal peritoneum of the iliac fossa, then continues eventually to form an *anterior branch* supplying skin of the ventral (anterior) and lateral parts of the thigh as far distally as the knee and a *posterior branch* supplying skin on the lateral surface of the limb from the level of the greater trochanter to about the middle of the thigh; see Durward (1951, p. 1092), Williams & Warwick (1980, pp. 1107–1108), *Terminologia Anatomica* (1998, p. 140). It was initially described and known as the *first cutaneous nerve of thigh (Galen, c177)*.

TRANSLATIONS:

1. *nervus cutaneus femoris lateralis (>1840)*
   Current Latin form of ***lateral cutaneous nerve of thigh (>1840)*** and *lateral femoral cutaneous nerve (>1840)*; see *Terminologia Anatomica* (1998, p. 140).

EARLIER REFERENCES:

Earlier synonyms:

1. *first cutaneous nerve of thigh (Galen, c177)*
   Synonym for ***lateral cutaneous nerve of thigh (>1840)*** in macrodissected adult beef, pig, and/or macaque but not human; see Singer translation (1999, p. 83). Vesalius (1543a) described but did not name it for macrodissected adult human; see Richardson & Carman translation (2002, p. 257). Part of *first nerve entering leg (Vesalius, 1543a)*.
2. *outer cutaneous nerve (Martin, 1781)*
   Synonym for macrodissected adult human ***lateral cutaneous nerve of thigh (>1840)***; in the original Latin, *cutaneum exteriorem nervum*, p. 231.
3. *external cutaneous nerve (Styx, 1782)*
   Synonym for macrodissected adult human ***lateral cutaneous nerve of thigh (>1840)***; in the original Latin, *nervum cutaneum externum*, p. 26.Cloquet (1828, Pl. CLXXII, Figs. 1:67–70, 2:67–73) described for macrodissected adult human external, internal, superior, and inferior branches of it.
4. *posterior femoral cutaneous branch of second lumbar nerve (Günther, 1786)*
   Apparently poor choice for describing badly macrodissected adult human ***lateral cutaneous nerve of thigh (>1840)***; in the original Latin, *r. cutaneus femoris posterior*, p. 81.
5. *outer and anterior crural cutaneous nerve (Fischer, 1791)*
   Synonym Fischer attributed without citation to Antoine Petit for macrodissected adult human ***lateral cutaneous nerve of thigh (>1840)***; in the original Latin, *cutaneum cruralem anteriorem et exteriorem nervum*, p. 3.
6. *superior and external inferior femoral cutaneous nerve (Mayer, 1794)*
   Probably synonym for macrodissected adult human ***lateral cutaneous nerve of thigh (>1840)***; in the original Latin, *nervus cutaneus femoris inferior externus et superior*; Part 5, Table V, Figure 1-***.
7. *superior and anterior external femoral cutaneous nerve (Mayer, 1794)*
   Probably synonym for macrodissected adult human ***lateral cutaneous nerve of thigh (>1840)***; in the original Latin, *nervus cutaneus externus anterior et superior femoris*; Part 6, Table VI-*88* (p. 38).
8. *external cutaneous nerve of thigh (Bell, 1803a)*
   Synonym for macrodissected adult human ***lateral cutaneous nerve of thigh (>1840)***; Plate VII-*1*. For French, see Chaussier (1809), *nerf cutané externe de la cuisse*.
9. *anterior external femoral cutaneous nerve (Bock, 1827)*
   Probably synonym for macrodissected adult human ***lateral cutaneous nerve of thigh (>1840)***; in the original Latin, *nerv. cutaneus femoris externus anterior*; Table 1, Figure 2-*65*.
10. *external anterior femoral cutaneous nerve (Bock, 1827)*
   Synonym for *anterior external femoral cutaneous nerve (Bock, 1827)*; in the original Latin, *nerv. cutaneus femoris anterior externus*, Table II-*102*. Listed elsewhere as *nerv. cutaneus anterior externus femoris*, Table III-*45*.
11. *superficial branches of crural nerve (Quain, 1828)*
   Apparently roughly synonymous with ***lateral cutaneous nerve of thigh (>1840)***; p. 287.
12. *external cutaneous branch of lumbar plexus (Quain, 1832)*
   Probably synonym for macrodissected adult human ***lateral cutaneous nerve of thigh (>1840)***; p. 695.
13. *inguino-cutaneous nerve (Quain & Wilson, 1839)*
   Synonym for macrodissected adult human ***lateral cutaneous nerve of thigh (>1840)***; Plate XXI-*k*.

PARTLY CORRESPONDS:

1. *posterior branch of external cutaneous nerve (Fischer, 1791)*
   Macrodissected adult human branch of ***lateral cutaneous nerve of thigh (>1840)*** supplying skin on lateral surface of limb from level of greater trochanter to about middle of thigh; Table II, Figure 1-*47*.
2. *anterior branch of external cutaneous nerve (Fischer, 1791)*
   Macrodissected adult human branch of ***lateral cutaneous nerve of thigh (>1840)*** supplying skin on ventral

(anterior) and lateral parts of thigh as far distally as knee; Table II, Figure 1-69.

3. *inferior branch of crural plexus (Meckel, 1817)*
Corresponds to terminal branches of ***lateral cutaneous nerve of thigh (>1840)*** according to Meckel, who attributed term to Bichat without citation; see translation (1832, Vol. 3, p. 15).

4. *posterior branches of external anterior femoral cutaneous nerve (Bock, 1827)*
Dorsal branches of macrodissected adult human ***lateral cutaneous nerve of thigh (>1840)***; in the original Latin, *rami posteriores nervi cutanei anterioris externi femoris*, Table IV-*80*.

lateral dorsal cutaneous nerve (>1840)

As described for macrodissected adult human, terminal branch of the ***sural nerve (Pietro da Cortona, 1741)*** supplying the lateral border of the foot and communicating with the ***superficial fibular nerve (Fyfe, 1800)***, reinforcing the latter's branches to the intervals between the 4th and 5th and the 3rd and 4th toes; see Durward (1951, p. 1110 and Fig. 949), *Terminologia Anatomica* (1998, p. 141). It was known to Galen; see ***[lateral dorsal cutaneous nerve (>1840)] (Galen, c177)***.

EARLIER REFERENCES:

Described, not named or illustrated:

1. ***[lateral dorsal cutaneous nerve (>1840)] (Galen, c177)***
Mentioned for macrodissected adult macaque but not human; see Singer translation (1999, p. 87).

Illustrated, not named or described:

1. ***[lateral dorsal cutaneous nerve (>1840)] (Eustachi, 1552)***
Clearly illustrated for macrodissected adult human; see Albinus edition (1761, Tab. 23).

Illustrated and described, not named:

1. ***[lateral dorsal cutaneous nerve (>1840)] (Vieussens, 1684)***
Described and illustrated for macrodissected adult human; see Table 29-*117*.

Earlier synonyms:

1. *inframalleolar nerve (Fischer, 1791)*
Essentially synonym for macrodissected adult human ***lateral dorsal cutaneous nerve (>1840)***; in the original Latin, *nervus inframalleolaris*, p. 34.

2. *dorsal peroneal nerve of fifth toe (Meckel, 1817)*
Roughly synonymous with macrodissected adult human ***lateral dorsal cutaneous nerve (>1840)***; see translation (1832, Vol. 3, p. 20).

3. *external cutaneous nerve of back of foot (Bock, 1827)*
Synonym for macrodissected adult human ***lateral dorsal cutaneous nerve (>1840)***; in the original Latin, *nerv. cutaneus externus dorsi pedis*, Tables I, Figure 2-*93* & II-*120*.

4. *external nerve of back of foot (Bock, 1827)*
Synonym for *external cutaneous nerve of back of foot (Bock, 1827)*; in the original Latin, *nerv. externus dorsi pedis*, Table III-*54*.

5. *external dorsal nerve of foot (Bock, 1827)*
Synonym for *external cutaneous nerve of back of foot (Bock, 1827)*; in the original Latin, *nerv. dorsalis externus pedis*, Table VI, Figure 3-*13*.

PARTLY CORRESPONDS:

1. *internal dorsal branch of inframalleolar nerve (Fischer, 1791)*
Synonym for *internal metatarsal branch of inframalleolar nerve (Fischer, 1791)*; in the original Latin, *ramus dorsalis internus*, p. 34.

2. *internal metatarsal branch of inframalleolar nerve (Fischer, 1791)*
Medial branch of macrodissected adult human ***lateral dorsal cutaneous nerve (>1840)*** contributing to dorsal digital nerves of lateral side of third, both sides of fourth, and medial side of little (5th) toe; in the original Latin, *ramus metatarsicus internus*, p. 34.Its presence is inconsistent compared to *external metatarsal branch of inframalleolar nerve (Fischer, 1791)*.

3. *external dorsal branch of inframalleolar nerve (Fischer, 1791)*
Synonym for *external metatarsal branch of inframalleolar nerve (Fischer, 1791)*; in the original Latin, *ramus dorsalis externus*, p. 34.

4. *external metatarsal branch of inframalleolar nerve (Fischer, 1791)*
Lateral branch of macrodissected adult human ***lateral dorsal cutaneous nerve (>1840)***, in turn contributing to dorsal digital nerve on lateral side of little toe; in the original Latin, *ramus metatarsicus externus*, p. 34.

5. *internal branch of external dorsal nerve of foot (Bock, 1827)*
Macrodissected adult human medial branch of ***lateral dorsal cutaneous nerve (>1840)*** generating ***dorsal digital nerves of lateral dorsal cutaneous nerve (>1840)*** to third and fourth toes, and medial side of little (5th) toe; in the original Latin, *ram. internus nervi dorsalis externi*; Table VI, Figure 3-*17*.

lateral funiculus (Burdach, 1822)

As described for macrodissected adult human and other mammal, the lateral topographic division of the ***funiculi of spinal cord (Burdach, 1822)***, between ***ventral root central parts (>1840)*** and ***ventral funiculus (>1840)*** ventrally and ***dorsal root central parts (>1840)*** and ***dorsal funiculus (>1840)*** dorsally; see Carpenter (1976, pp. 214–216 and Fig. 9.2), Williams & Warwick (1980, p. 868 and Fig. 7.36), *Terminologia Anatomica* (1998, p. 107). For Burdach's use in macrodissected adult human, see p. 35. It was first identified in illustration by Blasius; see ***[lateral funiculus (>1840)] (Blasius, 1666)***. Blasius (1674, p. 59) may have mentioned the lateral funiculus.

TRANSLATIONS:

1. *Seitenstrang (Burdach, 1822)*
Original German form of ***lateral funiculus (Burdach, 1822)***; p. 35.

EARLIER REFERENCES:

Illustrated, not named or described:

1. ***[lateral funiculus (Burdach, 1822)] (Blasius, 1666)***
   First clear illustration, in macrodissected adult human; Figures 10, 11, 18.

   Earlier synonyms:

   1. *posterior bundle of anterior funiculus (Rosenthal, 1815)*
      Synonym for macrodissected adult human ***lateral funiculus (Burdach, 1822)***; in the original German *hintres Bündel des vordern Strangs*, p. 27, see Burdach (1822, p. 284).

LATER SYNONYMS:

1. *lateral fascicle of spinal medulla (Bellingeri, 1823)*
   Synonym for macrodissected adult human and other mammalian ***lateral funiculus (Burdach, 1822)***; in the original Latin (plural), *fasciculi laterales medullae spinalis*, Table 1, Figure 1-*f*.
2. *restiform fascicle (Bellingeri, 1823)*
   Synonym for *lateral fascicle of spinal cord (Bellingeri, 1823)*; p. 9. Named because it appears to extend from *restiform body (Reil, 1807–1808a)*.
3. *lateral column (Bell, 1835)*
   Synonym for macrodissected adult human ***lateral funiculus (Burdach, 1822)***; p. 256. Also see *posterior column descending from hemisphere (Bell, 1834)*.
4. *sensitive column (Bell, 1835)*
   Synonym for *lateral column (Bell, 1835)*; Plate III, Figure 4-C. Alternately (plural), *columns of sensation*; Plate III, Figure 5-C.
5. *lateral column of spinal marrow (Bell, 1835)*
   Synonym for *lateral column (Bell, 1835)*; Plate III, Figure 5-C.
6. *lateral part of white substance of spinal medulla (Arnold, 1838b)*
   Synonym for macrodissected adult human ***lateral funiculus (Burdach, 1822)***; in the original Latin (plural), *substantiae albae pars lateralis*, Plate II, Figure 16-*d*.
7. *anterolateral column (>1840)*
   Synonym for macrodissected adult human ***lateral funiculus (Burdach, 1822)***; see *Dorland's* (2003, p. 744 under *funiculus lateralis medullae spinalis*).

lateral globus pallidus (>1840)

As described for macrodissected adult human, and with cellular architecture and connections for all mammals, the lateral component of the ***globus pallidus (Burdach, 1822)***, separated from the ***medial globus pallidus (>1840)*** by the ***medial medullary lamina (>1840)***; see Nieuwenhuys et al. (2008, Fig. 5.32-23, called *external part*), *Nomina Anatomica* (1983, p. A72), *Terminologia Anatomica* (1998, p. 130). It was probably first clearly delineated as the *third arcade of striate body (Vicq d'Azyr, 1786)*.

EARLIER REFERENCES:

Earlier synonyms:

1. *third arcade of striate body (Vicq d'Azyr, 1786)*
   Clearly illustrated synonym for macrodissected adult human ***lateral globus pallidus (>1830)***, although description somewhat confused; in the original French, *troisième arcade de [corps] stries*, Plate XIII-17,25; also see Plate XII. Arnold (1838b, Tab. VIII, Fig. 2) illustrated it even more accurately.

lateral hypothalamic zone (Nauta & Haymaker, 1969)

As described in macrodissected adult human, and with cellular architecture in mammal as well as vertebrate generally, the most lateral of three longitudinal divisions of the ***hypothalamus (Kuhlenbeck, 1927)***, lying lateral to the ***medial hypothalamic zone (Nauta & Haymaker, 1969)***. For a current parcellation in rat, see Swanson et al. (2005). The concept derived from the submammalian comparative histological work of Crosby & Woodbourne (1940), but the term was Nauta and Haymaker's, see p. 141. It was not clearly described before 1840.

lateral intersegmental tract (>1840)

As described in macrodissected adult human, and mammal generally with histological methods for ***axons (Kölliker, 1896)***, a narrow ***central nervous system white matter tract (>1840)*** in the deepest part of the ***lateral funiculus (Burdach, 1822)***, predominantly but not exclusively formed by ***axons (Kölliker, 1896)*** connecting different ***gray matter regions (Swanson & Bota, 2010)*** within the ***spinal cord (Galen, c162–c166)***; see Mettler (1948, pp. 236–237), Crosby et al. (1962, p. 108), Williams & Warwick (1980, p. 881 and Figs. 7.43, 44), and *Dorland's* (2003, p. 678 under *fasciculus proprius lateralis medullae spinalis*). It was not identified by 1840.

EARLIER REFERENCES:

Earlier synonyms:

1. *lateral fasciculus proprius (>1840)*
   Synonym for macrodissected adult human ***lateral intersegmental tract (>1840)***; see *Terminologia Anatomica* (1998, p. 107).

lateral lemniscus (Bechterew, 1885b)

As described for macrodissected adult human, and mammal generally with histological methods for ***axons (Kölliker, 1896)***, the ***central nervous system white matter tract (>1840)*** extending diagonally through the ***pons (Haller, 1747)*** between ***trapezoid body (Treviranus, 1820)*** caudally and ventrally, and ***inferior colliculus (Haller, 1762)*** rostrally and dorsally; see Nieuwenhuys et al. (2008, pp. 737–741 and Figs. 6.15–17). For Bechterew's use in human, see Meyer (1971, p. 51). It was perhaps first clearly alluded to as the *internal part of lemniscus (Reil, 1809c)*.

EARLIER REFERENCES:

Earlier synonyms:

1. *internal part of lemniscus (Reil, 1809c)*
   Initial, rough description of ***lateral lemniscus (Bechterew, 1885b)*** in macrodissected adult human: "following this process of the fillet, a gray and vascular prominence is found, corresponding with each inferior tubercle [***inferior colliculus (Haller,***

1762)]" (Mayo translation,1823, p. 95). Also see *lemniscus (Reil, 1809b)* and *fillet (Reil, 1809b)*.

2. *laqueus (Burdach, 1822)*
   Synonym for macrodissected adult human ***lateral lemniscus (Bechterew, 1885b)***; in the original German, *Schleife*, pp. 101, 323. Beautifully illustrated by Arnold (1838b; Tab. IX, Fig. 5-*s*).
3. *triangular fascicle (Cruveilhier, 1836)*
   Synonym for *lateral triangular fascicle of isthmus (Cruveilhier, 1836)*; in the original French, *faisceau triangulaire*, p. 602.
4. *lateral triangular fascicle of isthmus (Cruveilhier, 1836)*
   Synonym for macrodissected adult human ***lateral lemniscus (Bechterew, 1885b)*** according to Henle (1871, p. 124); in the original French, *faisceau triangulaire latéral de l'isthme*, p. 609. The term *trigonum lemnisci* has been attributed without citation to Haller.
5. *ribbon of Reil (Cruveilhier, 1836)*
   Eponym for macrodissected adult human ***lateral lemniscus (Bechterew, 1885b)***, or at least the part entering the ***inferior colliculus (>1840)***; in the original French, *ruban de Reil*, p. 613. Cruveilhier also referred to it here as *ganse de Reil*.
6. *posterior part of olivary fasciculus (Arnold, 1838b)*
   Synonym for macrodissected adult human *laqueus (Burdach, 1822)*; in the original Latin, *fasciculi olivaris pars posterior*; Table IX, Figure 5-*s*.

lateral longitudinal stria (Arnold, 1838a)

As described for macrodissected adult human, the lateral component of the ***longitudinal striae (>1840)*** extending rostrocaudally along the dorsal surface and both ends of the ***corpus callosum (Galen, c177)*** just lateral to ***medial longitudinal stria (>1840)***, from which it is separated by a narrow gap; see Williams & Warwick (1980, p. 998, Fig. 7.138), Nieuwenhuys et al. (2008, Fig. 3.18). For Arnold's use in macrodissected adult human, see p. 76. It was first identified as the *lateral longitudinal cord (Lancisi, 1713)*.

TRANSLATIONS:

1. *stria lateralis longitudinalis (Arnold, 1838a)*
   Original Latin form of ***lateral longitudinal stria (Arnold, 1838a)***; plural, *striae laterales longitudinales*, p. 76.

EARLIER REFERENCES:

Earlier synonyms:

1. *lateral longitudinal cord (Lancisi, 1713)*
   Synonym for macrodissected adult human ***lateral longitudinal stria (Arnold, 1838a)***; p. 153.
2. *limbi medullares (Lancisi, 1718)*
   Synonym for right and left macrodissected adult human *lateral longitudinal cord (Lancisi, 1713)*; the entire Latin description, used in figure legend for *limbi medullares (Lancisi, 1718)*, was *Limbi medullares, nervos referentes, corporis callosi*, p. 316.
3. *two lateral longitudinal nerves of corpus callosum (Tarin, 1753)*
   Synonym for macrodissected adult human *lateral longitudinal cords (Lancisi, 1713)*; in the original Latin, *nervi duo longitudinales laterales corporis callosi*, p. 23.

LATER SYNONYMS:

1. *lateral stria (Arnold, 1838b)*
   Synonym for macrodissected adult human ***lateral longitudinal stria (Arnold, 1838a)***; in the original Latin, *stria lateralis*, Table V, Figure 3-*i*.
2. *tectal stria (Arnold, 1838b)*
   Synonym for *lateral stria (Arnold, 1838b)*; in the original Latin, *stria tecta*, Table V, Figure 3-*i*.

lateral mammary branches of intercostal nerves (>1840)

As described for macrodissected adult human, ***anterior branches of lateral cutaneous branches of intercostal nerves (>1840)*** commonly arising from the fourth and fifth ***thoracic nerves (Diemerbroeck, 1672)*** and innervating the breast and nipple; see Durward (1951, Fig. 918), Williams & Warwick (1980, Fig. 7.206). They were known to Vesalius; see ***[lateral mammary branches of intercostal nerves (>1840)] (Vesalius, 1543a)***.

EARLIER REFERENCES:

Illustrated and described, not named:

1. ***[lateral mammary branches of intercostal nerves (>1840)] (Vesalius, 1543a)***
   Clearly described and illustrated for macrodissected adult human, ascribed to fourth ***intercostal nerve (Vesalius, 1543a)***; see Richardson & Carman translation (2002, p. 234). Vesalius noted their critical survival value for individuals and the species.

PARTLY CORRESPONDS:

1. *branch to mammary papilla from anterior branch of lateral pectoral cutaneous nerve of intercostal nerve (Bock, 1827)*
   Macrodissected adult human male branches of ***lateral mammary branches of intercostal nerve (>1840)*** to nipple; in the original Latin, *ram. papillae mammae*, Table III-33.

lateral medullary lamina (>1840)

As described for macrodissected adult human, the thin ***central nervous system white matter tract (>1840)*** between ***putamen (Burdach, 1822)*** laterally and ***lateral globus pallidus (>1840)*** medially; see Nieuwenhuys et al. (2008, Fig. 5.32-7), *Nomina Anatomica* (1983, p. A72), *Terminologia Anatomica* (1998, p. 130). It was perhaps first clearly delineated by Arnold; see ***[lateral medullary lamina (>1840)] (Arnold, 1838b)***.

EARLIER REFERENCES:

Illustrated and described, not named:

1. ***[lateral medullary lamina (>1840)] (Arnold, 1838b)***
   Clearly illustrated for macrodissected adult human; Table VIII, Figure 2.

lateral midbrain sulcus (>1840)

As described for macrodissected adult human, a longitudinal groove on the ventrolateral surface of the ***tegmentum (Swanson, 2000b)*** of the ***midbrain (Baer, 1837)*** running along the dorsal border of the ***cerebral peduncle (Tarin, 1753)***, whereas the ***medial midbrain sulcus (>1840)*** runs longitudinally along the ventromedial border of the ***cerebral peduncle (Tarin, 1753)*** and is the site of exit of the ***oculomotor nerve central rootlets (>1840)***; see Crosby et al. (1962, Fig. 170 unlabeled), Williams & Warwick (1980, p. 935). It was perhaps first clearly delineated by Vicq d'Azyr; see ***[lateral midbrain sulcus (>1840)] (Vicq d'Azyr, 1786)***.

EARLIER REFERENCES:

Illustrated, not named or described:

1. ***[lateral midbrain sulcus (>1840)] (Vicq d'Azyr, 1786)***
   Illustrated for macrodissected adult human in transverse section; Plates XV and XXI, Figure 1.

Earlier synonyms:

1. *ventrolateral fissure (>1840)*
   Synonym for macrodissected adult human ***lateral midbrain sulcus (>1840)***; see Crosby et al. (1962, p. 221).

lateral nasal branches of internal nasal branches of anterior ethmoidal nerve (>1840)

As described for macrodissected adult human, they supply mainly the rostral (anterior) part of the lateral wall of the nasal cavity; see Williams & Warwick (1980, p. 1061), *Terminologia Anatomica* (1998, p. 134). They were probably first clearly delineated as the *external nasal threads of ethmoidal fascicle (Bellingeri, 1818)*.

EARLIER REFERENCES:

Earlier synonyms:

1. *external nasal threads of ethmoidal fascicle (Bellingeri, 1818)*
   Synonym for macrodissected adult human ***lateral nasal branches of internal nasal branches of anterior ethmoidal nerve (>1840)***; in the original Latin, *stamina nasalis externus*, see Table I.
2. *lateral nasal branch of ethmoidal branch of nasociliary nerve (Arnold, 1834)*
   Synonym for macrodissected adult human ***lateral nasal branches of internal nasal branches of anterior ethmoidal nerve (>1840)***; in the original Latin, *nervus nasociliaris, ramus ethmoidalis, ramus lateralis narium*, p. 8.
3. *lateral nasal branch of ethmoidal branch of nasal nerve (Arnold, 1834)*
   Synonym for macrodissected adult human ***lateral nasal branches of internal nasal branches of anterior ethmoidal nerve (>1840)***; in the original Latin, *nervus nasalis, ramus ethmoidalis, ramus lateralis narium*, p. 8.

lateral occipital sulcus (>1840)

As described for macrodissected adult human, a longitudinal groove on the lateral surface of the ***occipital region (Vesalius, 1543a)*** dividing it generally into ***superior occipital gyri (>1840)*** and ***inferior occipital gyri (>1840)***; see Carpenter (1976, p. 24, Fig. 2.2), Williams & Warwick (1980, p. 986, Fig. 7.111A). It was first clearly delineated by Gall & Spurzheim; see ***[lateral occipital sulcus (>1840)] (Gall & Spurzheim, 1810)***.

EARLIER REFERENCES:

Illustrated, not named or described:

1. ***[lateral occipital sulcus (>1840)] (Gall & Spurzheim, 1810)***
   Clearly illustrated for macrodissected adult human; Table VIII.

lateral occipitotemporal gyrus (>1840)

As described for macrodissected adult human, a topographic subdivision of the ***temporal region (>1840)*** lying between ***inferior temporal gyrus (>1840)*** dorsally and ***medial occipitotemporal gyrus (>1840)*** medially, with the border between ***inferior temporal gyrus (>1840)*** and ***lateral occipitotemporal gyrus (>1840)*** defined arbitrarily as running along the ventrolateral margin of the ***temporal region (>1840)***; see Clark (1951, Fig. 872), Williams & Warwick (1980, Fig. 7.114A), *Terminologia Anatomica* (1998, pp. 125–126), *Dorland's* (2003, p. 806). It was perhaps first clearly delineated by Vicq d'Azyr; see ***[lateral occipitotemporal gyrus (>1840)] (Vicq d'Azyr, 1786)***.

EARLIER REFERENCES:

Illustrated, not named or described:

1. ***[lateral occipitotemporal gyrus (>1840)] (Vicq d'Azyr, 1786)***
   Illustrated for macrodissected adult human as clearly as many modern attempts; Plate XVI-*23,25*.

lateral olfactory tract (>1840)

As described for macrodissected adult human and other mammal, the thin ***central nervous system white matter tract (>1840)*** extending caudally from the ***olfactory bulb (Weitbrecht, 1751)*** along the medial surface of the ***piriform area (Smith, 1919)***; see Swanson (2004, Atlas Levels 3–25), Nieuwenhuys et al. (2008, Fig. 11.3). It was known to Eustachi; see ***[lateral olfactory tract (>1840)] (Eustachi, 1552)***.

EARLIER REFERENCES:

Illustrated, not named or described:

1. ***[lateral olfactory tract (>1840)] (Eustachi, 1552)***
   In plates not published until 1714, Eustachi clearly illustrated it for macrodissected adult human, although it is not distinguished from more rostral, classical *outgrowth of encephalon to nose (Galen, c173)*, the ***olfactory bulb (Weitbrecht, 1751)*** and ***olfactory peduncle (Solly, 1836)*** considered together. Illustrated near its caudal end to fan out in a way that could be interpreted to show medial and intermediate roots in addition to ***lateral olfactory tract (>1840)*** itself. See Albinus edition (1744, Pl. XVIII, Figs. I and II) and Meyer (1971, p. 77). Varoli (1573) may have provided a written description of it (Meyer 1971, p. 77 note 6). In human anatomy the ***olfactory peduncle (Solly, 1836)*** is often called the *olfactory nerve (Bartholin, 1611)* or *olfactory tract (Burdach, 1822)*, which caudally splits into lateral, medial, and sometimes intermediate roots or stria in the region of the *anterior perforated substance (Vicq d'Azyr, 1784)*; see Meyer (1971, p. 77, Fig. 4-*H*) and

lateral olfactory tract (>1840), *intermediate olfactory stria (>1840)*, *medial olfactory stria (>1840)*. Also see *double origination of olfactory nerve (Collins, 1685)*.

2. ***[lateral olfactory tract (>1840)] (Casseri, 1609)*** First published illustration, including several tiny medial roots; see Meyer (1971, p. 77, Fig. 4-*H*) and ***[lateral olfactory tract (>1840)] (Eustachi, 1552)***.
3. ***[lateral olfactory tract (>1840)] (Rolfinck, 1656)*** In macrodissected adult human ***olfactory peduncle (Solly, 1836)***, Rolfinck described gray and white stripes (Meyer 1971, p. 76), ***anterior olfactory nucleus (Herrick, 1910)***, and associated segment of ***lateral olfactory tract (>1840)***, respectively; see *nervos odoratorios (Rolfinck, 1656)*.

Earlier synonyms:

1. *long external root of olfactory nerve (Soemmerring, 1778)* Synonym for macrodissected adult human ***lateral olfactory tract (>1840)***; in the original Latin, *radix externa*, or *exterior, longior*, see p. 173, Table II-*a*.
2. *external medullary root of olfactory nerve (Haase, 1781)* Synonym for macrodissected adult human ***lateral olfactory tract (>1840)***; in the original Latin, *radix medullaris externa*, p. 35.
3. *external root of olfactory nerve (Swan, 1830)* Synonym for macrodissected adult human ***lateral olfactory tract (>1840)***; p. 14 and Plate X, Figure 3-*a*.
4. *medullary root of olfactory nerve (Owen, 1837)* Synonym for macrodissected adult mammalian ***lateral olfactory tract (>1840)***; p. 95.
5. *lateral olfactory stria (>1840)* Synonym for macrodissected adult human ***lateral olfactory tract (>1840)***; see His (1895, p. 177), *Terminologia Anatomica* (1998, p. 129), Nieuwenhuys et al. (2008, Fig. 11.3).

PARTLY CORRESPONDS:

1. *short internal root of olfactory nerve (Soemmerring, 1778)* Synonym for macrodissected adult human *intermediate olfactory stria (>1840)*, although Soemmerring illustrated *medial olfactory stria (>1840)* as well; pp. 173, 179 and Table I-*b*.
2. *internal medullary root of olfactory nerve (Haase, 1781)* Apparently synonym for macrodissected adult human *short internal root of olfactory nerve (Soemmerring, 1778)*; in the original Latin, *radix medullaris interna*, p. 35. Also see *external medullary root of olfactory nerve (Haase, 1781)*.
3. *stria alba accedens radici brevi (Scarpa, 1785)* Synonym for macrodissected adult human *intermediate olfactory stria (>1840)*; Table II, Figure 3-*c*.
4. *long internal root of olfactory nerve (Vicq d'Azyr, 1786)* Synonym for macrodissected adult human *intermediate olfactory stria (>1840)*; Plate XVII, Figure I-23.
5. *middle root of olfactory nerve (Swan, 1830)* Synonym for macrodissected adult human *intermediate olfactory stria (>1840)*; Plate X, Figure 3-*b*. Arnold (1834, Tab. 1-2) gave the Latin, *nervous olfactorius radix media*.
6. *internal root of olfactory nerve (Knox, 1832)* Knox's form of *short internal root of olfactory nerve (Soemmerring, 1778)*; Supplemental Plate I-15*b*.
7. *intermediate olfactory stria (>1840)* As described for macrodissected adult human, sometimes visible branch of ***lateral olfactory tract (>1840)*** ending in ***olfactory tubercle (Calleja, 1893)***. Horne (1662) first emphasized three *roots* associated with macrodissected adult human ***olfactory peduncle (Solly, 1836)***; see Meyer (1971, p. 77) and ***[lateral olfactory tract (>1840)] (Eustachi, 1552)***.

lateral orbital gyrus (>1840)

As described for macrodissected adult human, the lateral topographic subdivision of the ***orbital gyri (>1940)***, separated from the others by the ***orbital sulci (>1840)***; see Williams & Warwick (1980, Fig. 7.116). It was first clearly

delineated by Soemmerring; see ***[lateral orbital gyrus (>1840)] (Soemmerring, 1778)***.

EARLIER REFERENCES:

Illustrated, not named or described:

1. ***[lateral orbital gyrus (>1840)] (Soemmerring, 1778)*** Illustrated clearly for macrodissected adult human; Table II.

Earlier synonyms:

1. *area orbitalis (Brodmann, 1909)* Original Latin form of *orbital area (Brodmann, 1909)*; p. 139.
2. *orbital area (Brodmann, 1909)* Roughly corresponds to macrodissected adult human ***lateral orbital gyrus (>1840)***; p. 139.
3. *area 47 (Brodmann, 1909)* Synonym for adult human *orbital area (Brodmann, 1909)*; in the original German, *Feld 47*, p. 139.

lateral palatine nerve (Henle, 1871)

As described for macrodissected adult human, usually the smaller of the ***lesser palatine nerves (Meckel, 1817)*** supplying the soft palate and adjacent part of the tonsil; see Durward (1951, p. 1023). For Henle's use in macrodissected adult human, see p. 378. It was probably first described as the *least external branch of palatine nerve (Meckel, 1748)*.

EARLIER REFERENCES:

Earlier synonyms:

1. *least external branch of palatine nerve (Meckel, 1748)* Synonym for macrodissected adult human ***lateral palatine nerve (Henle, 1871)***; in the original Latin, *ramus nervi palatini exterior minimus*, Figure 1-*φ*.
2. *external branch of palatine nerve (Bang, 1770)* Synonym for macrodissected adult human ***lateral palatine nerve (Henle, 1871)***; in the original Latin, *nervus palatinus ramus exterior*, Figure II-*g*.
3. *external palatine nerve (Scarpa, 1785)* Synonym for macrodissected adult human ***lateral palatine nerve (Henle, 1871)***; in the original Latin, *palatinus nervus externus*, Table II, Figure II-32.

4. *exterior palatine nerve (Günther, 1786)*
Synonym for macrodissected adult human ***lateral palatine nerve (Henle, 1871)***; in the original Latin, *nervus palatinus exteriorem*, p. 48.
5. *lesser external palatine nerve (Mayer, 1794)*
Synonym for macrodissected adult human ***lateral palatine nerve (Henle, 1871)***; in the original Latin, *nervus palatinus externus minor*; Part 5, Table VIII-*φ* (p. 59).
6. *smallest exterior palatine nerve (Mayer, 1794)*
Presumably synonym for *lesser external palatine nerve (Mayer, 1794)*; in the original Latin, *nervus palatinus exterior minimus*; Part 5, Table VIII, Figure 3-*x*. Bell & Bell (1829, p. 496) called it *nervus palatinus minimus exterior*.
7. *small palatine nerve (Cloquet, 1816)*
Synonym for macrodissected adult human ***lateral palatine nerve (Henle, 1871)***; in the original French, *petit nerf palatin*, p. 685.
8. *least palatine nerve (Bock, 1817)*
Synonym for macrodissected adult human ***lateral palatine nerve (Henle, 1871)***; in the original Latin, *nervus palatinus minimus*, p. 31.
9. *external palatine fascicle of sphenopalatine ganglion (Bellingeri, 1818)*
Synonym for macrodissected adult human ***lateral palatine nerve (Henle, 1871)***; in the original Latin, *fasciculus palatinus externus*, see Table I.
10. *middle palatine nerve (Todd, 1836–1839)*
Synonym for macrodissected adult human ***lateral palatine nerve (Henle, 1871)***; p. 286.

PARTLY CORRESPONDS:

1. *uvular thread of external palatine fascicle (Bellingeri, 1818)*
Macrodissected adult human branch of ***lateral palatine nerve (Henle, 1871)*** to uvula; in the original Latin, *stamen uvularis*, see Table I.
2. *palato-tonsillar threads of external palatine fascicle (Bellingeri, 1818)*
Macrodissected adult human branches of ***lateral palatine nerve (Henle, 1871)*** to tonsil and palatine glands; in the original Latin, *stamina palato-tonsillaris*, see Table I.
3. *palato-pharyngeal threads of external palatine fascicle (Bellingeri, 1818)*
Macrodissected adult human branches of ***lateral palatine nerve (Henle, 1871)*** to junctional region of palate and pharynx; in the original Latin, *stamina palato-pharyngei*, see Table I.

lateral pectoral nerve (>1840)

As described for macrodissected adult human, it usually arises either as two roots from the ***brachial plexus ventral divisions (Paterson, 1887)*** of the ***brachial plexus upper trunk (>1840)*** and ***brachial plexus middle trunk (>1840)***, or by a single root from the point where these divisions merge to form the ***brachial plexus lateral cord (Schwalbe, 1881)***, and supplies mainly the pectoralis major muscle; see Durward (1951, pp. 1071–1072 and Fig. 925), Williams & Warwick (1980, p. 1096). It was known to Galen; see ***[lateral pectoral nerve (>1840)] (Galen, c173)***.

EARLIER REFERENCES:

Described, not named or illustrated:

1. ***[lateral pectoral nerve (>1840)] (Galen, c173)***
Clearly described for macrodissected adult pig, beef, and/or macaque but not human; see May translation (1968, p. 703), Singer translation (1999, p. 221), Duckworth translation (1962, pp. 248, 250, 255). Vesalius (1543a) alluded to it in macrodissected adult human; see Richardson & Carman translation (2002, pp. 228, 234).

Illustrated, not named or described:

1. ***[lateral pectoral nerve (>1840)] Eustachi (1552)***
Illustrated for macrodissected adult human; see Albinus edition (1761, Tab. 19-23).

Earlier synonyms:

1. *nerve to pectoral muscle (Camper, 1760)*
Synonym for macrodissected adult human ***lateral pectoral nerve (>1840)***; p. 13 and Table I, Figure 2:*51–56*.
2. *lesser thoracic nerve (Bang, 1770)*
Probably refers to macrodissected adult human ***lateral pectoral nerve (>1840)***; in the original Latin, *nervus thoracicus minor*, Figure I-*77*.
3. *greater anterior thoracic nerve (Günther, 1786)*
Probably refers to macrodissected adult human ***lateral pectoral nerve (>1840)***; in the original Latin, *nervus thoracicus anterior major*, p. 73.
4. *posterior pectoral nerve (Bock, 1827)*
Synonym for macrodissected adult human ***lateral pectoral nerve (>1840)***; in the original Latin, *nervi pectoralis posterior*, Table II-*22*.
5. *anterior thoracic branch of brachial plexus (Cruveilhier, 1836)*
Synonym for macrodissected adult human ***lateral pectoral nerve (>1840)***; in the original French, *branche thoraciques anterior du plexus brachial*, p. 794.
6. *pectoralis major branch of brachial plexus (Cruveilhier, 1836)*
Synonym for macrodissected adult human ***lateral pectoral nerve (>1840)***; in the original French, *branche du grand pectoral du plexus brachial*, p. 794.

PARTLY CORRESPONDS:

1. *pectoral nerves (Camper, 1760)*
Branches of *nerve to pectoral muscle (Camper, 1760)*; p. 13.
2. *long anterior thoracic nerve (Loder, 1803)*
Macrodissected adult human branch of seventh ***cervical nerve (Galen, c173)*** supplying pectoralis major muscle, and thus a ***lateral pectoral nerve (>1840)***; in the original Latin, *nervus thoracicus anterior longus*, Table CLXXVII-*123*.
3. *greater root of posterior pectoral nerve (Bock, 1827)*
Presumably larger or largest root of macrodissected adult human ***lateral pectoral nerve (>1840)***; in the original Latin, *radix major nervi pectoralis posterior*; Table V, Figure 2-*54*.

4. *anterior thoracic nerve (Cloquet, 1828)*
   Macrodissected adult human shorter root than *long anterior thoracic nerve (Loder, 1803)*, thus component of ***lateral pectoral nerve (>1840)***; in the original French, *nerf thoracique antérieur*, Plate CLXVII, Figure 1-24,26.
5. *anastomosis between anterior thoracic nerve and long anterior thoracic nerve (Cloquet, 1828)*
   Macrodissected adult human ***communicating branch (Winslow, 1733)*** between *anterior thoracic nerve (Cloquet, 1828)* and *long anterior thoracic nerve (Loder, 1803)*; in the original French, *anastomose entre le nerf thoracique antérieur et le long nerf thoracique antérieur*, Plate CLXVII, Figure 1-25.

lateral plantar nerve (>1840)

As described for macrodissected adult human, the smaller of two deep terminal branches of the ***tibial nerve (Haase, 1781)*** supplying muscular, cutaneous, and vascular branches to lateral parts of the sole of the foot, including the ***common plantar digital nerves of lateral plantar nerve (>1840)*** and ***proper plantar digital nerves of lateral plantar nerve (>1840)***; see Durward (1951, Figs. 951, 952), Williams & Warwick (1980, p. 1114), *Terminologia Anatomica* (1998, p. 141). It corresponds to the ***ulnar nerve (Cheselden, 1726)*** for the hand; see Durward (1951, p. 1110). It was known to Galen; see ***[lateral plantar nerve (>1840)] (Galen, c173)***.

EARLIER REFERENCES:

Described, not named or illustrated:

1. ***[lateral plantar nerve (>1840)] (Galen, c173)***
   Vaguely identified in macrodissected adult beef, pig, and/or macaque but not human; see May translation (1968, p. 192 with note 74, p. 706) and Singer translation (1999, p. 87).

Illustrated, not named or described:

1. ***[lateral plantar nerve (>1840)] (Eustachi, 1552)***
   Clearly illustrated course, but not origin, in macrodissected adult human; see Albinus edition (1761, Tab. 20-20).

Illustrated and described, not named:

1. ***[lateral plantar nerve (>1840)] (Vieussens, 1684)***
   Beautifully described and illustrated for macrodissected adult human; see Table 30-Q.

Earlier synonyms:

1. *external plantar nerve (Winslow, 1733)*
   Synonym for macrodissected adult human ***lateral plantar nerve (>1840)***; in the original Latin, *nervus plantaris externus*, Section VI, p. 92.
2. *external plantar branch of tibial nerve (Martin, 1781)*
   Synonym for macrodissected adult human ***lateral plantar nerve (>1840)***; in the original Latin, *nervus tibialis ramus plantaris exterior*, p. 242 and Table XI.
3. *exterior branch of tibial nerve (Burdin, 1803)*
   Synonym for macrodissected adult human ***lateral plantar nerve (>1840)***; see translation (1803, Vol. 1, p. 207).
4. *outer plantar nerve (Swan, 1830)*
   Synonym for macrodissected adult human ***lateral plantar nerve (>1840)***; Plate XXV, Figure 3-2.

PARTLY CORRESPONDS:

1. *nerve to calcaneal periosteum (Jördens, 1788)*
   Jördens's first branch of trunk of ***lateral plantar nerve (>1840)*** in macrodissected adult human; in the original Latin, *nervus ad periostium calcanei*, p. 12 and Table III-210.
2. *nerve to abductor digiti minimi and flexor digiti minimi brevis muscles (Jördens, 1788)*
   Macrodissected adult human ***nerve (Herophilus, c335–c280 BC)*** to these muscles of foot, arising according to Jördens's account from two roots—one from ***deep branch of lateral plantar nerve (>1840)***, see Table III-214, and one from ***superficial branch of lateral plantar nerve (>1840)***, see Table III-219. In the original Latin, *nervus ad musculum abductorem digiti minimi et flexorem brevem eiusdem digiti*, p. 12 and Table III-220.
3. *subcutaneous twig of external plantar nerve (Fischer, 1791)*
   Branch of macrodissected adult human ***lateral plantar nerve (>1840)*** to skin on lateral side of sole of foot; in the original Latin, *ramulus subcutaneus nervus plantaris externus*, p. 37.
4. *terminal branches of external plantar nerve (Cruveilhier, 1836)*
   Macrodissected adult human ***superficial branch of lateral plantar nerve (>1840)*** and ***deep branch of lateral plantar nerve (>1840)*** considered together; in the original French, *branches terminales*, p. 875.

lateral posterior superior nasal nerves (>1840)

As described for macrodissected adult human, around six branches of the ***posterior superior nasal nerves (>1840)*** supplying mucous membrane covering caudal (posterior) parts of the superior and middle nasal conchae and lining the posterior ethmoidal sinus. Histologically they contain predominantly sensory ***dendrites (His, 1889)*** simply passing through the ***pterygopalatine ganglion (>1840)*** from the ***lateral posterior superior nasal nerves (>1840)*** to the ***pterygopalatine nerves (Wrisberg, 1786)*** and then the ***maxillary nerve (Meckel, 1753)*** and the ***trigeminal ganglion (>1840)***; see Williams & Warwick (1980, pp. 1064–1065). They were first clearly identified as the *anterior superior nasal branches of Vidian nerve (Meckel, 1748)*.

EARLIER REFERENCES:

Earlier synonyms:

1. *anterior superior nasal branches of Vidian nerve (Meckel, 1748)*
   Synonym for macrodissected adult human ***lateral posterior superior nasal nerves (>1840)***; p. 51 for description and Figure 1-θ for origins. Also see Meckel (1751, p. 87).
2. *external sphenopalatine nerves (Cruveilhier, 1836)*
   Synonym for macrodissected adult human ***lateral posterior superior nasal nerves (>1840)***; in the original French, *nerfs sphéno-palatins externes*, p. 924.

3. *superior nasal nerves (Cruveilhier, 1836)*
   Synonym for *external sphenopalatine nerves (Cruveilhier, 1836)*; in the original French, *nerfs nasaux supérieure*, p. 924.
4. *posterior superior lateral nasal branches of pterygopalatine ganglion* (>1840)
   Synonym for macrodissected adult human ***lateral posterior superior nasal nerves (>1840)***; see *Terminologia Anatomica* (1998, p. 134).

lateral pterygoid nerve (>1840)

As described for macrodissected adult human, a branch of the ***anterior branch of mandibular nerve (>1840)*** that together with the ***buccal nerve (Meckel, 1748)*** enters the deep surface of the lateral pterygoid to supply the muscle; see Williams & Warwick (1980, p. 1066), *Terminologia Anatomica* (1998, p. 134). It was perhaps first delineated by Eustachi; see ***[lateral pterygoid nerve (>1840)] (Eustachi, 1552)***.

EARLIER REFERENCES:

Illustrated, not named or described:

1. ***[lateral pterygoid nerve (>1840)] (Eustachi, 1552)***
   Illustrated for macrodissected adult human; see Albinus edition (1761, Tab. 18, Figs. 1, 4, 5-O).

Illustrated and described, not named:

1. ***[lateral pterygoid nerve (>1840)] (Willis, 1664)***
   Possibly illustrated and vaguely described for macrodissected adult, presumably human; see Pordage translation (1681, p. 145, Fig. 1-*n*). Vieussens specifically referred to it for macrodissected adult human; Table 22-2. Meckel (1748, pp. 83, 85, 86) and the grandson Meckel (1817; see translation, 1832, Vol. 3, p. 72) described it as branch of ***buccal nerve (Meckel, 1748)***.

Earlier synonyms:

1. *pterygoid nerve (Schaarschmidt, 1750)*
   Synonym for macrodissected adult human ***lateral pterygoid nerve (>1840)***; *nervus pterygoideus*, p. 28.
2. *pterygoid branch of third branch of fifth pair (Loder, 1778)*
   Synonym for macrodissected adult human ***lateral pterygoid nerve (>1840)***; in the original Latin, *ramus pterygoideus*, p. 18.
3. *pterygo-muscular nerve (Burdin, 1803)*
   Synonym for macrodissected adult human ***lateral pterygoid nerve (>1840)***; see translation (1803, Vol. 1, p. 176).
4. *minor superior branch of inferior maxillary branch of fifth pair of nerves (Bock, 1817)*
   Apparently synonym for macrodissected adult human ***lateral pterygoid nerve (>1840)***; in the original Latin, *ramus superior minor*, p. 46.
5. *external pterygoid branch of buccal nerve (Arnold, 1834)*
   Synonym for macrodissected adult human ***lateral pterygoid nerve (>1840)***; in the original Latin, *nervus buccinatorius, ramus pterygoideus externus*, p. 9.
6. *external pterygoid branch of inferior maxillary nerve (Quain & Wilson, 1839)*
   Synonym for macrodissected adult human ***lateral pterygoid nerve (>1840)***; Plate XIII, Figure 2-*a**.
7. *external pterygoid nerve (Quain & Wilson, 1839)*
   Synonym for macrodissected adult human ***lateral pterygoid nerve (>1840)***; in the original Latin, *nervus pterygoideus externus*, Plate XIII, Figure 2-*a**.

lateral recess of fourth ventricle (>1840)

As described for macrodissected adult human, a narrow lateral extension of the ***fourth ventricle (Galen, c192)*** ending in the ***lateral aperture of fourth ventricle (>1840)***; see *Dorland's* (2003, p. 1596), Nieuwenhuys et al. (2008, Fig. 3.10-40). Its presence was indicated by Haller; see ***[lateral recess of fourth ventricle (>1840)] (Haller, 1747)***.

EARLIER REFERENCES:

Described, not named or illustrated:

1. ***[lateral recess of fourth ventricle (>1840)] (Haller, 1747)***
   In clearly describing macrodissected adult human ***[lateral aperture of fourth ventricle (>1840)] (Haller, 1747)***, Haller provided first published indication of lateral recess leading up to it; see Millen & Woollam (1962, p. 18).

lateral reticulospinal tract (>1840)

As described for adult mammal with normal and experimental pathway tracing methods, a caudally directed, diffusely organized, heterogeneous and poorly characterized longitudinal ***central nervous system white matter tract (>1840)*** arising primarily from the ***medulla (Winslow, 1733)*** but perhaps with minor contributions from the ***pons (Haller, 1747)*** and ***tegmentum (Swanson, 2000b)***. It has both crossed and uncrossed components and extends caudally through the ***spinal cord (Galen, c162–c166)***, centered in ventral deeper regions of the ***lateral funiculus (Burdach, 1822)***; see Mettler (1948, p. 238), Crosby et al. (1962, p. 105 and Figs. 85, 120, 133, 140, 145), Williams & Warwick (1980, pp. 875–876 and Fig. 7.44), *Terminologia Anatomica* (1998, p. 107, also gave synonym, *bulboreticulospinal tract*). For topographic description there are major ***medullary lateral reticulospinal tract (>1840)*** and ***spinal lateral reticulospinal tract (>1840)*** segments. It was not described by 1840.

EARLIER REFERENCES:

Earlier synonyms:

1. *medullary reticulospinal tract (>1840)*
   Synonym for macrodissected adult human ***lateral reticulospinal tract (>1840)***; see Carpenter (1976, pp. 267–269), *Terminologia Anatomica* (1998, p. 107).
2. *dorsal spinoreticular tract (>1840)*
   Synonym for macrodissected adult human ***lateral reticulospinal tract (>1840)***; see Mettler (1948, p. 238).
3. *crossed reticulospinal tract (>1840)*
   Synonym for macrodissected adult human ***medial reticulospinal tract (>1840)***; see Mettler (1948, p. 238).

lateral retinohypothalamic tract (>1840)

As described in mammal generally with histological methods for ***axons (Kölliker, 1896)***, a branch of the proximal ***hypothalamic optic tract (Vicq d'Azyr, 1786)*** near the ***optic chiasm (Galen, c173)*** to certain ***central nervous system gray matter regions (>1840)*** in the ***lateral hypothalamic zone (Nauta & Haymaker, 1969)***; see Canteras et al. (2011). It was not identified by 1840.

lateral root of median nerve (>1840)

As described for macrodissected adult human, a branch of the ***brachial plexus lateral cord (Schwalbe, 1881)*** joining the ***medial root of median nerve (>1840)*** to form the ***median nerve (Du Verney, 1697)***; see Durward (1951, p. 1073), *Terminologia Anatomica* (1998, p. 138). It was probably known to Vesalius; see ***[lateral root of median nerve (>1840)] (Vesalius, 1543a)***.

EARLIER REFERENCES:

Illustrated and described, not named:

1. ***[lateral root of median nerve (>1840)] (Vesalius, 1543a)***
   Apparently discussed and illustrated for macrodissected adult human; see Richardson & Carman translation (2002, p. 240).

Earlier synonyms:

1. *external head of median nerve (Quain & Wilson, 1839)*
   Synonym for macrodissected adult human ***lateral root of median nerve (>1840)***; Plate XVII-*r*.

lateral septal arcuate fibers (>1840)

As described in mammal with normal and experimental histological methods for ***axons (Kölliker, 1896)***, diffusely organized, arching ***axons (Kölliker, 1896)*** between the ***lateral septal complex (Risold & Swanson, 1997)*** rostrodorsally and the rostral end of the ***lateral hypothalamic zone (Nauta & Haymaker, 1969)*** caudoventrally; essentially a rostral branch of the ***medial forebrain bundle (Edinger, 1893)***. At the border between ***cerebral nuclei (Swanson, 2000a)*** and ***hypothalamus (Kuhlenbeck, 1927)***, they mostly join the ***medial forebrain bundle (Edinger, 1893)*** in the ***lateral preoptic area (>1840)*** before fanning out into many parts of the ***hypothalamus (Kuhlenbeck, 1927)*** and to limited parts of the ***thalamus (His, 1893a)*** as well. In addition, connections associated with more rostral parts of the ***cerebral cortex (>1840)***, especially in and around the ***infralimbic area (Rose & Woolsey, 1948)***, participate in this ***central nervous system white matter tract (>1840)***. For clear early description see *external arcuate fibers of septum (Cajal, 1901–1902)*; also see Brittain (1988), Risold & Swanson (1997). They were not known before 1840.

EARLIER REFERENCES:

Described, not named or illustrated:

1. *external arcuate fibers of septum (Cajal, 1901–1902)*
   Synonym for ***lateral septal arcuate fibers (>1840)*** described in Golgi material from young mouse and rat; in the original Spanish, *fibras arciformes externas*, see Figure 11-*B*, p. 187. Also see *internal arcuate fibers of septum (Cajal, 1901–1902)*.

lateral septal complex (Risold & Swanson, 1997)

As described for macrodissected adult human, the medial component of the ***striatum (Swanson, 2000a)***, separated from the ***caudoputamen (Heimer & Wilson, 1975)*** by the ***lateral ventricle (Vesalius, 1543a)***. Based on cellular architecture and connections in mammal, it includes the ***lateral septal nucleus (>1840)***, ***septohippocampal nucleus (>1840)***, and ***septofimbrial nucleus (>1840)***, and it receives its major ***cerebral cortex (>1840)*** input from the ***hippocampal formation (Swanson & Cowan, 1977)***. Not clearly described by 1840. For Risold & Swanson's use in rat with cellular architecture and connections, see p. 183 (and p. 121).

lateral spinothalamic tract (>1840)

As described for adult human most clearly with experimental pathway tracing methods, two adjacent components of the ***spinothalamic tract (>1840)*** in the ***spinal cord (Galen, c162–c166)*** are distinguished for clinical and descriptive purposes: ***ventral spinothalamic tract (>1840)*** centered in deeper regions of the ***ventral funiculus (>1840)***, and ***lateral spinothalamic tract (>1840)*** centered in adjacent ventral deeper regions of the ***lateral funiculus (Burdach, 1840)***; see Williams & Warwick (1980, pp. 876–877, 879–880, and Fig. 743), *Terminologia Anatomica* (1998, p. 107), Nieuwenhuys et al. (2008, pp. 697–701). Rostrally, in the ***medulla (Winslow, 1733)*** they merge and become essentially indistinguishable in the ***ventrolateral fascicle (>1840)***, where they form the ***medullary spinothalamic tract (>1840)*** segment. It was not known by 1840.

lateral supraclavicular nerves (>1840)

As described for macrodissected adult human, they are derived from the ***cervical plexus (Molinetti, 1675)*** and innervate skin and fascia of rostral (upper) and dorsal (posterior) parts of the shoulder; see Durward (p. 1064 and Fig. 921), Williams & Warwick (1980, p. 1092). They were distinguished by Eustachi; see ***[lateral supraclavicular nerves (>1840)] (Eustachi, 1552)***.

TRANSLATIONS:

1. *nervi supraclaviculares laterales (>1840)*
   Current Latin form of ***lateral supraclavicular nerves (>1840)***; see *Terminologia Anatomica* (1998, p. 137).

EARLIER REFERENCES:

Illustrated, not named or described:

1. ***[lateral supraclavicular nerves (>1840)] (Eustachi, 1552)***
   Illustrated for macrodissected adult human; see Albinus edition (1761, Tab. 21-*i*).

Earlier synonyms:

1. *posterior branch of anterior branch of fourth pair of cervical nerves (Bang, 1770)*
   Synonym for macrodissected adult human ***lateral supraclavicular nerves (>1840)***; in the original Latin, *superficialis scapulae ramus*, Figure I-51.
2. *superficial scapular branch of anterior branch of fourth pair of cervical nerves (Bang, 1770)*

Synonym for macrodissected adult human ***lateral supraclavicular nerves (>1840)***; in the original Latin, *superficialis scapulae ramus*, Figure I-*51*.

3. *posterior subclavicular branches (Soemmerring, 1791)* Synonym for macrodissected adult human ***lateral supraclavicular nerves (>1840)***; in the original Latin, *subclaviculares posteriores*, p. 271.
4. *superficial scapular nerve (Mayer, 1794)* Synonym for macrodissected adult human ***lateral supraclavicular nerves (>1840)***; in the original Latin, *nervus superficialis scapulae*; Part 6, Table II, Figure 1-*130* (p. 14).
5. *posterior scapular nerve (Mayer, 1794)* Synonym for macrodissected adult human ***lateral supraclavicular nerves (>1840)***; in the original Latin, *nervus posterior scapulae*; Part 6, Table II, Figure 1-*130* (p. 14).
6. *posterior superclavicular branches (Bell, 1803b)* Synonym for macrodissected adult human ***lateral supraclavicular nerves (>1840)***; in the original Latin, *superclaviculares posteriores*, p. 166.
7. *scapulary branch of thoracic part of trachelo-cutanean plexus (Burdin, 1803)* Synonym for macrodissected adult human *scapular branch of thoracic part of tracheosubcutaneous nerves (Chaussier, 1809)*; see translation (1803, Vol. 1, p. 189).
8. *scapular branch of thoracic part of tracheosubcutaneous nerves (Chaussier, 1809)* Probably synonym for macrodissected adult human ***lateral supraclavicular nerves (>1840)***.
9. *supra-acromial branches of cervical plexus (Cloquet, 1816)* Probably synonym for macrodissected adult human ***lateral supraclavicular nerves (>1840)***; in the original French, *rameaux sus-acromiens*, p. 639.
10. *posterior superclavicular nerves (Bell & Bell, 1816)* Synonym for macrodissected adult human ***lateral supraclavicular nerves (>1840)***; in the original Latin, *superclaviculares posteriores*, Vol. 2, p. 514.
11. *posterior supraclavicular nerves (Meckel, 1817)* Synonym for macrodissected adult human ***lateral supraclavicular nerves (>1840)***; in the original Latin, *nervi supraclaviculares posteriores*, see translation (1832, Vol. 3, p. 31).
12. *acromial branch of descending superficial branches of cervical plexus (Quain, 1828)* Synonym for macrodissected adult human ***lateral supraclavicular nerves (>1840)***; in the original Latin, *acromiales*, p. 490.
13. *acromial nerve (Quain, 1832)* Synonym for macrodissected adult human ***lateral supraclavicular nerves (>1840)***; in the original Latin, *n. acromiales*, p. 681.
14. *supra-acromial nerves (Cruveilhier, 1836)* Synonym for macrodissected adult human *lateral supraclavicular nerves (>1840)*; in the original French, *nerfs sus-acromiens*, p. 780.
15. *supra-acromial branch of supraclavicular branches (Cruveilhier, 1836)* Synonym for macrodissected adult human ***lateral supraclavicular nerves (>1840)***; in the original French, *branche sus-acromiale*, p. 785.

PARTLY CORRESPONDS:

1. *first exterior supraclavicular branch (Peipers, 1793)* Lateral member of macrodissected adult human ***lateral supraclavicular nerves (>1840)***; in the original Latin, *ramus supraclavicularis exterior primus*, p. 35.
2. *humeral subcutaneous supraclavicular branch (Peipers, 1793)* Synonym for macrodissected adult human *first exterior branch of supraclavicular nerve (Peipers, 1793)*; in the original Latin, *ramus supraclavicularis subcutaneus humeri*, p. 35.
3. *acromial supraclavicular branch (Peipers, 1793)* Synonym for macrodissected adult human *first exterior branch of supraclavicular nerve (Peipers, 1793)*; in the original Latin, *ramus supraclavicularis acromialis*, p. 35.
4. *second supraclavicular branch (Peipers, 1793)* Medial member of macrodissected adult human ***lateral supraclavicular nerves (>1840)***; in the original Latin, *ramus supraclavicularis secundus*, p. 35.
5. *subcutaneous deltoid supraclavicular branch (Peipers, 1793)* Synonym for *second supraclavicular branch (Peipers, 1793)*; in the original Latin, *ramus supraclavicularis subcutaneus deltoidei*, p. 35.
6. *deep posterior supraclavicular nerves (Bock, 1827)* Deep branch of ***lateral supraclavicular nerves (>1840)***; in the original Latin, *nervi supraclaviculares posteriores profundi*, Table V, Figure 1-*37*.
7. *acromial branch of descending superficial branches of cervical plexus (Quain, 1834)* Synonym for macrodissected adult human *acromial supraclavicular branch (Peipers, 1793)*; in the original Latin, *r. acromiales*, p. 730.

lateral thalamic nuclei (>1840)

As described for macrodissected adult human, and based on cellular architecture and connections in mammal, a lateral and dorsal component of the ***dorsal part of thalamus (Herrick, 1910)***. Its major ***gray matter region (Swanson & Bota, 2010)*** is the ***pulvinar (Burdach, 1822)*** and/or the ***lateral posterior thalamic nucleus (>1840)***; see Jones (1985, Ch. 10), Nieuwenhuys et al. (2008, pp. 265–266 and Figs. 5.9, 5.23, 5.31). Different authors place the ***lateral dorsal thalamic nucleus (>1840)*** either here or in the ***anterior thalamic nuclei (>1840)***; based on connections it is more appropriate in the latter. They were not recognized as a group by 1840.

lateral ventricle (Vesalius, 1543a)

The ***ventricle (Hippocrates)*** associated with the ***endbrain vesicle (Kuhlenbeck, 1927)*** of the vertebrate ***neural tube (Baer, 1837)*** both during development and in adult. In macrodissected adult human it is divided somewhat arbitrarily into an ***anterior horn of lateral ventricle (Bell, 1803b)*** with a variable rostral extension called the **olfactory ventricle (>1840)**, a ***body of lateral ventricle (Bell, 1803b)*** with a variable extension called the ***posterior horn of lateral ventricle (Haller, 1747)***, an ***atrium of lateral ventricle (>1840)*** when a ***posterior horn of lateral ventricle (Haller, 1747)*** is present, and an ***inferior horn of lateral ventricle (Bell, 1802)***. The border between ***anterior horn of lateral ventricle (Bell, 1803b)*** and ***body of lateral ventricle (Bell, 1803b)*** is set arbitrarily at the level of the ***interventricular foramen (>1840)***; see Millen & Woollam (1962, pp. 33–44, Figs. 13, 16) and Carpenter & Sutin (1983, pp. 41–45, Fig. 2.20). It may have been known very early on; see ***[lateral ventricle (Vesalius, 1543a)] (Anaxagoras of Athens, c488– c428 BC)***. Wiberg's translation (1914, p. 23) of Galen's *On Anatomical Procedures* (c177) contains a reference to lateral ventricle, but this interpretation is doubtful because it is not in Singer's translation of the same passage (1999, p. 231) or in other English translations of Galen. According to Singer's translation (1952, pp. 41, 68), Vesalius used the specific term *lateral ventricle* in describing macrodissected adult human, and provided a very nice schematic diagram showing the ***anterior horn of lateral ventricle (Bell, 1803b)*** and ***inferior horn of lateral ventricle (Bell, 1802)***; see Richardson & Carman translation (2002, p. 180). Burdach (1822, p. 380) attributed the term to Le Böe (1695).

EARLIER REFERENCES:

Described, not named or illustrated:

1. ***[lateral ventricle (Vesalius, 1543a)] (Anaxagoras of Athens, c488–c428 BC)***
According to Mettler (1947, p. 10) Anaxagoras identified it, but the source of this attribution is unclear and it is not widely acknowledged.

Earlier synonyms:

1. *longitudinal ventricle (Erasistratus, c310–c250 BC)*
In *The Doctrines of Hippocrates and Plato*, c162–166), Galen quoted from a now lost book of Erasistratus where the human ***brain (Smith Papyrus, c1700 BC)***, "...had a ventricle placed longitudinally on each side, and these were pierced through into one at the junction of the parts [***interventricular foramen (>1840)***]." (Clarke & O'Malley, 1996, p. 12). This is the first clear reference to ***lateral ventricle (Vesalius, 1543a)***.
2. *anterior ventricle (Galen, c173)*
Synonym Galen commonly used for ***lateral ventricle (Vesalius, 1543a)***; see May translation (1968, pp. 414–415).
3. *foreward ventricle (Galen, c173)*
Crooke translation (1615, p. 462) of *anterior ventricle (Galen, c173)*.
4. *ventricles one and two (Galen, c173, c177)*
Galen explained that two (anterior) ***ventricles (Hippocrates)*** lead into ***third ventricle (Galen, c173)***, which then leads into ***fourth ventricle (Galen, c192)***; see May translation (1968, pp. 414–415), Clarke & O'Malley (1996, p. 712), and Singer translation (1999, p. 235).
5. *cellula fantastica (Anatomia Magistri Nicolai physici, early 12th century; Guillaume de Conches, c1100–1154)*
According to the most popular version of the cell theory of ***brain (Smith Papyrus, c1700 BC)*** function, the ***lateral ventricle (Vesalius, 1543a)*** is the "cell of the imagination"; see Corner translation (1927, p. 71), Manzoni (1998, p. 125).
6. *venter anterior (Berengario da Carpi, 1521)*
Alternate Latin form of macrodissected adult human *anterior ventricle (Galen, c173)*; f. 436. Also see Berengario da Carpi (1523, bottom figure on f. 56).
7. *superior ventricle (Berengario da Carpi, 1521)*
Synonym for macrodissected adult human ***lateral ventricle (Vesalius, 1543a)***; f. 436, also see Burdach (1822, p. 380).
8. *anterior sinus (de Laguna, 1535)*
Synonym for macrodissected adult ***lateral ventricle (Vesalius, 1543a)***; see Lind translation (1975, p. 287).
9. *right and left ventricles (Vesalius, 1543a)*
Synonym for macrodissected adult human ***lateral ventricles (Vesalius, 1543a)*** on right and left side; see Singer translation (1952, p. 2).

LATER SYNONYMS:

1. *former ventricle (Hall, 1565)*
Synonym for macrodissected adult human ***lateral ventricle (Vesalius, 1543a)***, probably in reference to another synonym, *anterior ventricle (Galen, c173)*; pp. 37–38.
2. *great ventricles (Varoli, 1573)*
Synonym for right and left macrodissected adult human ***lateral ventricles (Vesalius, 1543a)***; in the original Latin, *ventriculi magni*, f. 4v; also see Burdach (1822, p. 380). In Latin, Haase (1781, p. 16) provided *ventriculi majores*.
3. *former pans of braine (Nemesius, 1636)*
English synonym for right and left ***lateral ventricles (Vesalius, 1543a)*** in this translation of Nemesius's 4th-century work, *On the Nature of Man*; p. 306.
4. *foremore and uppermore ventricle (Bartholin, 1662)*
Synonym for macrodissected adult human ***lateral ventricle (Vesalius, 1543a)***, based on *foreward ventricle (Galen, c173)* and *upper ventricle (Avicenna, c1030)*; see p. 140.
5. *infolding of brain (Willis, 1664)*
Synonym for macrodissected adult mammalian ***lateral ventricle (Vesalius, 1543a)***, which Willis regarded simply as a vacuity resulting from folding up of *cerebrum (Willis, 1664)*; see Pordage translation (1681, pp. 65, 96, 138, Fig. IV-*D*).
6. *ventricle of brain (Willis, 1664)*
Synonym for macrodissected adult mammalian ***lateral ventricle (Vesalius, 1543a)*** (see Pordage translation, 1681, p. 100), with *brain* an English translation of *cerebrum (Willis, 1664)*, which includes **cerebral cortex (>1840)** and ***lateral ventricle (Vesalius, 1543a)***.
7. *foremost ventricle (Salmon, 1714)*
Variation on macrodissected adult human *foreward ventricle (Galen, c173)*; p. 408.
8. *anterior superior ventricle of cerebrum (Winslow, 1733)*
Winslow wrote that this is the name generally given to ***lateral ventricle (Vesalius, 1543a)***; Section X, p. 34; also see *foremore and uppermore ventricle (Bartholin, 1662)*.

9. *tricornate ventricle (Bergen, 1734)*
Synonym for macrodissected adult human ***lateral ventricle (Vesalius, 1543a)***, according to Haller (1762, p. 40); in Latin, *ventriculus tricornis*; literally in English, three-horned ventricle.
10. *triangular ventricle (Haller, 1747)*
Version of *tricornate ventricle (Bergen, 1734)*; see Mihles translation (1754b, p. 290).
11. *two semilunar ventricles (Günther, 1786)*
Synonym for macrodissected adult human right and left ***lateral ventricles (Vesalius, 1543a)***; in the original Latin, *semilunares ventriculi duo*, p. 9.
12. *space within hemisphere (Gall & Spurzheim, 1810)*
Translation of a way Gall & Spurzheim referred to macrodissected adult human ***lateral ventricle (Vesalius, 1543a)***, according to Burdach (1822, pp. 380–381), who gave the Latin equivalent (plural) as *intervalla in interioribus hemisphaeriis*.

PARTLY CORRESPONDS:

1. *upper ventricle (Avicenna, c1030)*
According to du Laurens (1599, p. 408), Avicenna referred to *ventricles one and two (Galen, c173, c177)*, and regarded them as a unit rather than two separate ***ventricles (Hippocrates)***; see Crooke translation (1615, p. 528). By extension, for him, the right and left ***lateral ventricles (Vesalius, 1543a)*** together constituted the *first ventricle*; see *cerebral ventricles (Galen, c192)* and *cells (Anatomia Magistri Nicolai physici, early 12th century)*.
2. *great fore ventricle (Mondino, 1316)*
Synonym for macrodissected adult human *upper ventricle (Avicenna, c1030)*; see Singer (1925, p. 91).
3. *lacuna (Manfredi, 1490)*
In *Anothomia*, Manfredi seemed to regard *pyelos (Galen, c177)* as part of ***lateral ventricle (Vesalius, 1543a)***, see Singer translation (1917, p. 109), although Galen and Mondino [see *lacuna cerebri (Mondino, 1316)*] clearly equated it roughly with ***hypothalamic part of third ventricle (Swanson, 2004)***. The source of Manfredi's confusion is unknown, but some anatomists still regard rostral half of ***hypothalamic part of third ventricle (Swanson, 2004)*** as component of ***endbrain (Kuhlenbeck, 1927)*** rather than ***interbrain (Baer, 1837)***, following His (1895, p. 84).
4. *lower hinder seat of ventricle (Geminus, 1553)*
Corresponds to combination of macrodissected adult human *hind recess of ventricle (Vesalius, 1543a)* and *lower recess of ventricle (Vesalius, 1543a)*; originally spelled *lower and hinder seate of the ventricle*, see *The tables of the brayne*, Figure 6-*F*.
5. *head of former ventricle (Willis, 1664)*
Synonym for macrodissected adult mammalian *anterior horn of lateral ventricle (Vicq d'Azyr, 1786)*; see Pordage translation (1681, p. 63), also see *former ventricle (Willis, 1664)*.
6. *major crura of ventricle (Bergen, 1734)*
Synonym for macrodissected adult human right and left *anterior horn of lateral ventricle (Vicq d'Azyr, 1786)*; in the original Latin, *crura majora ventriculorum*; see Tarin (1750, Tab. XIII, Fig. 3-*a*).
7. *anterior horn of lateral ventricle (Vicq d'Azyr, 1786)*
Macrodissected adult human ***anterior horn of lateral ventricle (Bell, 1803b)*** and ***body of lateral ventricle (Bell, 1803b)*** considered together; in the original French, *cornes antérieures* for right and left; Plate V.
8. *anterior sinus of superior ventricle (Vicq d'Azyr, 1786)*
Synonym for *anterior horn of lateral ventricle (Vicq d'Azyr, 1786)*, or at least its rostral end, ***anterior horn of lateral ventricle (Bell, 1803b)***; p. 8, also see Burdach (1822, p. 381).
9. *anterior crus of lateral ventricle (Günther, 1786)*
Synonym for macrodissected adult human *anterior horn of lateral ventricle (Vicq d'Azyr, 1786)*; in the original Latin (plural), *crure anteriori*, p. 9.
10. *anterior horn of tricornate ventricle (Soemmerring, 1791)*
Synonym for macrodissected adult human *anterior horn of lateral ventricle (Vicq d'Azyr, 1786)*; p. 46.
11. *anterior sinus of lateral ventricle (Bell, 1802)*
Synonym for macrodissected adult human *anterior horn of lateral ventricle (Vicq d'Azyr, 1786)*; Plate III-*E*.
12. *superior portion of lateral ventricle (Chaussier, 1807)*
Basically synonym for macrodissected adult human *anterior horn of lateral ventricle (Vicq d'Azyr, 1786)*; p. 51.
13. *inferior portion of lateral ventricle (Chaussier, 1807)*
Basically synonym for macrodissected adult human ***posterior horn of lateral ventricle (Haller, 1747)***, ***collateral triangle (>1840)***, and ***inferior horn of lateral ventricle (Bell, 1802)*** considered together; p. 51.
14. *middle part of central fissure (Gordon, 1815)*
Basically synonym for macrodissected adult human *anterior horn of lateral ventricle (Vicq d'Azyr, 1786)*; p. 96 ff.
15. *anterior frontal horn of lateral ventricle (Cruveilhier, 1836)*
Synonym for macrodissected adult human *anterior horn of lateral ventricle (Vicq d'Azyr, 1786)*; in the original French, *corne antérieure frontale*, p. 691.
16. *superior ventricles (Gerdy, 1838)*
Basically part of macrodissected adult human ***lateral ventricles (Vesalius, 1543a)*** separated by *septum lucidum (Galen, c177)*; in the original Latin, *ventricules supérieurs*, p. 261.
17. *inferior ventricle (Gerdy, 1838)*
Basically part of macrodissected adult human ***lateral ventricles (Vesalius, 1543)*** caudal to *superior ventricles (Gerdy, 1838)*, and excluding *posterior prolongation of lateral ventricles (Vicq d'Azyr, 1786)*; in the original Latin, *ventricule inférieur*, p. 263.
18. *roof of lateral ventricle (Arnold, 1838b)*
Ventral (inner) face of lateral part of ***corpus callosum (Galen, c177)*** forming dorsal (upper) wall of ***anterior horn of lateral ventricle (Bell, 1803b)*** and ***body of lateral ventricle (Bell, 1803b)***; in the original Latin, *tectum ventriculi lateralis*, Table IV, Figure 2-*m*.

lateral vestibulospinal tract (>1840)

As described for macrodissected adult human, an uncrossed longitudinal ***central nervous system white matter tract (>1840)*** extending from the ***lateral vestibular***

nucleus (>1840) caudally along the length of the ***spinal cord (Galen, c162–c166)***, centered in ventral regions of the ***lateral funiculus (Burdach, 1822)***. See Carpenter (1976, p. 342 and Figs. 10.18–19), called simply *vestibulospinal tract (>1840)*; *Terminologia Anatomica* (1998, p. 110); Nieuwenhuys et al. (2008, p. 725 and Fig. 17.6). For topographic description it has ***medullary lateral vestibulospinal tract (>1840)*** and ***spinal lateral vestibulospinal tract (>1840)*** segments. It was not clearly delineated by 1840.

EARLIER REFERENCES:

Earlier synonyms:

1. *vestibulospinal tract (>1840)*
   Often synonymous with ***lateral vestibulospinal tract (>1840)***; see Carpenter (1976, p. 342 and Figs. 10.18– 19). The "medial vestibulospinal tract" descends in the ***medial longitudinal fascicle (>1840)***; see Williams & Warwick (1980, p. 875).

least splanchnic nerve (>1840)

As described for macrodissected adult human, it arises from the last (most caudal) ***thoracic sympathetic ganglion (>1840)***, is usually smaller than the ***greater splanchnic nerve (Walter, 1783)*** and ***lesser splanchnic nerve Haller, 1762)***, and typically ends in the ***renal ganglia (Walther, 1735)*** and adjacent part of the ***renal plexus (Drake, 1707)***; see Mitchell (1953, p. 245, Fig. 104). It was probably first distinguished by Willis; see ***[least splanchnic nerve (>1840)] (Willis, 1664)***.

TRANSLATIONS:

1. *nervus splanchnicus imus (>1840)*
   Current Latin form of ***least splanchnic nerve (>1840)***; see *Terminologia Anatomica* (1998, p. 142).

EARLIER REFERENCES:

Illustrated and described, not named:

1. ***[least splanchnic nerve (>1840)] (Willis, 1664)***
   Probably described and illustrated for macrodissected adult human; Table XI-*β,K*; see Pordage translation for English form, also see Mitchell (1953, p. 4). It was very clearly described and illustrated (but not named) by Vieussens (1684, Tab. 23-*67*) and Mayer (1794, Part 6, Tab. VII-*52*, p. 57).

Earlier synonyms:

1. *posterior renal nerve (Walter, 1783)*
   Synonym for macrodissected adult human ***least splanchnic nerve (>1840)***; in the original Latin, *nervus renalis posterior*, see Table I:*236–245*. Walter divided it into *superior posterior renal nerve (Walter, 1783)* and *inferior posterior renal nerve (Walter, 1783)* and described a common trunk for them; Table I-*245*.
2. *small suprarenal nerve (Chaussier, 1789, definition 2)*
   Synonym for macrodissected adult human ***least splanchnic nerve (>1840)***; in the original French, *petit nerf surrenal*, see *Table synoptique du nerf tri-splanchnique*. Also see *small suprarenal nerve (Chaussier, 1789, definition 1)*.
3. *small splanchnic nerve (Portal, 1803a; Burdin, 1803)*
   Synonym for macrodissected adult human ***least splanchnic nerve (>1840)***; Portal: in the original French, *petit nerf splanchnique*, p. 198; Burdin: see translation, 1803, Vol. 1, p. 211. Also see Meckel (1832, Vol. 3, p. 97).
4. *inferior splanchnic nerves (Tiedemann, 1822)*
   Synonym for macrodissected adult human right and left ***least splanchnic nerve (>1840)***; in the original Latin, *nervi splanchnici inferioris*, see Table I-*1*.
5. *renal nerve (Lobstein, 1823)*
   Synonym for ***least splanchnic nerve (>1840)***; see translation (1831, p. 24), also see Williams & Warwick (1980, p. 1131).

PARTLY CORRESPONDS:

1. *superior posterior renal nerve (Walter, 1783)*
   Corresponds to major rostral (upper) part of macrodissected adult human ***least splanchnic nerve (>1840)***; in the original Latin, *nervi renalis posterioris superioris*, Table I-*236*.
2. *superior posterior renal nerve roots (Walter, 1783)*
   Two segments of macrodissected adult human ***least splanchnic nerve (>1840)*** arising from 10th and 11th ***thoracic sympathetic ganglia (>1840)***—Walter's superior and inferior roots, respectively—to form *superior posterior renal nerve trunk (Walter, 1783)*; in the original Latin, *radix superior nervi posterioris superioris renalis*, Table I-*233* and *radix inferior nervi posterioris renalis superioris*, Table I-*234*.
3. *superior posterior renal nerve trunk (Walter, 1783)*
   Segment of macrodissected adult human ***least splanchnic nerve (>1840)*** distal to region where *superior posterior renal nerve roots (Walter, 1783)* join; in the original Latin, *truncus nervi posterioris superioris renalis*, Table I-*239*. Knox (1832, Pl. VII-*45*) called it *posterior and superior renal nerve* in English.
4. *inferior posterior renal nerve (Walter, 1783)*
   Term for minor caudal (lower) part of macrodissected adult human ***least splanchnic nerve (>1840)*** described as arising from ***sympathetic trunk (Winslow, 1733)***, just rostral to (above) first ***lumbar sympathetic ganglion (>1840)***; in the original Latin, *nervo renali posteriori inferiori*, Table I-*241*. Knox (1832, Pl. VII-*46*) called it the *posterior and inferior renal nerve* in English.

left colic plexus (Meckel, 1817)

As described for macrodissected adult human, it extends from the ***inferior mesenteric plexus (Rau, 1720)*** along the left colic artery to supply it and the left part of the transverse colon, descending colon, and sigmoid colon; see Williams & Warwick (1980, p. 1134). For Meckel's vague use of the term, see translation (1832, Vol. 3, p. 87). Long before, it was distinguished by Willis; see ***[left colic plexus (Meckel, 1817)] (Willis, 1664)***.

EARLIER REFERENCES:

Illustrated and described, not named:

1. ***[left colic plexus (Meckel, 1817)] (Willis, 1664)***
   Mentioned and illustrated for macrodissected adult human and other common large mammals; see Pordage translation (1681, p. 159, Tab. 11-*a*).

left coronary plexus (Scarpa, 1794)

As described for macrodissected adult human, the larger of the two ***coronary plexuses (Meckel, 1817)***, accompanying the left coronary artery and supplying the left atrium and ventricle; see Williams & Warwick (1980, p. 1132). For Scarpa's use in macrodissected adult human, see Table III-*129*; also see Mitchell (1953, p. 253). It was distinguished by Neubauer; see ***[left coronary plexus (Scarpa, 1794)] (Neubauer, 1772)***.

TRANSLATIONS:

1. *plexus coronarii sinistri (Scarpa, 1794)*
   Original Latin form of ***left coronary plexus (Scarpa, 1794)***; Table III-*129*.

EARLIER REFERENCES:

Illustrated and described, not named:

1. ***[left coronary plexus (Scarpa, 1794)] (Neubauer, 1772)***
   Alluded to in macrodissected adult human; p. 185-*86,87*.

Earlier synonyms:

1. *left coronary artery nerve (Behrends, 1792)*
   Synonym for macrodissected adult human ***left coronary plexus (Scarpa, 1794)***; in the original Latin, *nervorum arteriae coronariae sinistrae*, see 1793 reprint, pp. 7, 23. Behrends also referred to *nerve net (Behrends, 1792)* surrounding artery; in the original Latin, *reti nervorum circumdata*, p. 7.
2. *superficial nerve of left artery of septum of heart (Andersch, 1797)*
   Essentially macrodissected adult human ***left coronary plexus (Scarpa, 1794)*** arising from *lowest trunk of superficial nerve of nerve layers of septum of heart (Andersch, 1797)*; in the original Latin, *nervum superficialem dextrum arteriae septi cordis*, Volume 2, p. 60. Recall this was first printed c1751–c1755.

LATER SYNONYMS:

1. *posterior coronary plexus (Scarpa, 1794)*
   Synonym for macrodissected adult human ***left coronary plexus (Scarpa, 1794)***; in the original Latin, *plexum coronarium posteriorem*, Table IV:*45–48*, also see Mitchell (1953, p. 253).

left gastric plexus (>1840)

As described for macrodissected adult human, an extension of the ***celiac plexus (Winslow, 1733)*** accompanying the left gastric artery along the lesser curvature of the stomach. It is joined by ***gastric branches of anterior vagal trunk (>1840)*** and ***gastric branches of posterior vagal trunk (>1840)***, and distally joins the end of the ***right gastric plexus (>1840)***; see Durward (1951, p. 1142), Mitchell (1953, pp. 277–278), Williams & Warwick (1980, p. 1134). It was known to Willis; see ***[left gastric plexus (>1840)] (Willis, 1664)***.

EARLIER REFERENCES:

Illustrated and described, not named:

1. ***[left gastric plexus (>1840)] (Willis, 1664)***
   Clearly described and illustrated for macrodissected adult human and other common large mammals; see Pordage translation (1681, p. 158 and Tab. 11-*η*).

Earlier synonyms:

1. *nerveum plexum stomachium (Vieussens, 1684)*
   Roughly synonymous with macrodissected adult human ***left gastric plexus (>1840)***; Table 23-*25*.
2. *nerveus plexus stomachius (Vieussens, 1684)*
   Alternate form of *nerveum plexum stomachium (Vieussens, 1684)*; Table 23-*63*.
3. *nerveo plexu stomachico (Vieussens, 1684)*
   Alternate form of *nerveum plexum stomachium (Vieussens, 1684)*; Table 23-*65*.
4. *plexus stomachicus posterior (Haase, 1781)*
   Probably synonym for macrodissected adult human ***left gastric plexus (>1840)***; p. 89.
5. *plexum coronariostomachicum posteriorem (Haase, 1781)*
   Apparently synonym for macrodissected adult human *plexus stomachicus posterior (Haase, 1781)*; p. 124.
6. *plexum coronariostomachicum posteriorem (Haase, 1781)*
   Apparently synonym for macrodissected adult human *plexus stomachicus posterior (Haase, 1781)*; p. 124.
7. *gastric plexus (Walter, 1783)*
   Probably used to describe macrodissected adult human ***left gastric plexus (>1840)***; original Latin forms included *plexus gastricus* (Tab. III-after *285*), *plexum gastricum* (Tab. III-*508,509*), *plexu gastrico* (Tab. IV-after *32*), and *plexus stomachicus* (Tab. IV-*106*).
8. *nervos ventriculi sinisteriores (Soemmerring, 1798)*
   Probably synonym for macrodissected adult human ***left gastric plexus (>1840)***; p. 358.
9. *superior anterior gastric plexus (Langenbeck, 1826–1830)*
   Roughly synonymous with macrodissected adult human ***left gastric plexus (>1840)***; in the original Latin, *plexus gastricus anterior superior*, Fascicle III, Table III-*18*.
10. *coronary plexus of stomach (Cruveilhier, 1836)*
    Synonym for macrodissected adult human ***left gastric plexus (>1840)***; in the original French, *plexus coronaire-stomachique*, p. 1016.

PARTLY CORRESPONDS:

1. *trunk of gastro-hepatic nerve (Walter, 1783)*
   Small ***nerve (Herophilus, c335–c280 BC)*** from macrodissected adult human ***celiac ganglion (Walter, 1783)***; essentially component of ***left gastric plexus (>1840)*** dividing to supply on the order of five branches to cardia of stomach and nearby parts of ***hepatic plexus (Rau, 1720)***; in the original Latin, *truncus nervi hepatico-gastrici*; Table IV:*274,279–283*.

left gastroepiploic plexus (Wrisberg, 1800)

As described for macrodissected adult human, an extension of the ***splenic plexus (Palfijn, 1726)*** accompanying the left gastroepiploic artery along the upper left part of the greater curvature of the stomach, extending branches onto the greater omentum, and meeting distally the ***right gastroepiploic plexus (Wrisberg, 1800)***; see Mitchell (1953, pp. 280–282, Fig. 122). For Wrisberg's use in macrodissected adult human, see p. 569. It was known earlier as the *left gastroepiploic nerve (Mayer, 1794)* generating the *left omental nerves (Mayer, 1794)*.

TRANSLATIONS:

1. *plexus gastro-epiploicus sinister (Wrisberg, 1800)*
Original Latin form of ***left gastroepiploic plexus (Wrisberg, 1800)***; p. 569.

PARTLY CORRESPONDS:

1. *left gastroepiploic nerve (Mayer, 1794)*
As described for macrodissected adult human, single ***nerve (Herophilus, c335–c280 BC)*** stretching along proximal half of lesser curvature of stomach and generating *left omental nerves (Mayer, 1794)*; in the original Latin, *nervus gastro-epiploicus sinister*; Part 6, Table IV-*V* (p. 27). It is a component of the ***left gastroepiploic plexus (Wrisberg, 1800)***.
2. *left omental nerves (Mayer, 1794)*
As described for macrodissected adult human, branches of *left gastroepiploic nerve (Mayer, 1794)* extending transversely across stomach to greater omentum; in the original Latin, *nervi omentales sinistri*; Part 6, Table IV-*31* (p. 27). They are components of the ***left gastroepiploic plexus (Wrisberg, 1800)***.

lesser occipital nerve (Mayer, 1794)

As described for macrodissected adult human, it commonly arises from the second and, to a more variable extent, third cervical ***spinal nerve ventral branches (>1840)*** as an ***ascending superficial branch of cervical plexus (Quain, 1828)*** supplying skin and fascia of the rostral (upper) part of the neck, cranial surface of the auricle, and adjoining scalp; see Durward (1951, p. 1062 and Fig. 919). For Mayer's use in macrodissected adult human, see Part 5, Table VI-*γ* (p. 33); in the original Latin (plural), *nervi occipitales minores*. It was probably known to Galen; see ***[lesser occipital nerve (Mayer, 1794)] (Galen, c173)***.

EARLIER REFERENCES:

Described, not named or illustrated:

1. *[lesser occipital nerve (Mayer, 1794)] (Galen, c173)*
Apparently alluded to for macrodissected adult beef, pig, and/or macaque but not human; see May translation (1968, p. 597), Duckworth translation (1962, p. 226).

Illustrated, not named or described:

1. *[lesser occipital nerve (Mayer, 1794)] (Eustachi, 1552)*
Illustrated for macrodissected adult human; see Albinus edition (1761, Tab. 21/2-*c*).

Illustrated and described, not named:

1. *[lesser occipital nerve (Mayer, 1794)] (Vieussens, 1684)*
Illustrated and described for macrodissected adult human; Table 24-*h*.

Earlier synonyms:

1. *occipital nerve (Winslow, 1733)*
Probably synonym for macrodissected adult human ***lesser occipital nerve (Mayer, 1794)***; Section VI, p. 76.
2. *small posterior auricular nerve (Meckel, 1753)*
Synonym for macrodissected adult human ***lesser occipital nerve (Mayer, 1794)***; in the original French, *le petit nerf auriculaire postérieur*, Table 1-*II* (also see p. 101).
3. *small occipital nerve (Bang, 1770)*
Synonym for macrodissected adult human ***lesser occipital nerve (Mayer, 1794)***; in the original Latin, *nervus occipitalis parvus*, Figure I-*26*, see 1791 reprint.
4. *small occipital branch of third cervical nerve (Haase, 1781)*
Synonym for macrodissected adult human ***lesser occipital nerve (Mayer, 1794)***; in the original Latin, *nervus cervicalis tertii ramus occipitalis parvus*, p. 94 and *Index*.
5. *recurrent occipitoauricular nerve (Peipers, 1793)*
Synonym for macrodissected adult human ***lesser occipital nerve (Mayer, 1794)***; in the original Latin, *occipito-auricularis recurrens*, p. 33.

LATER SYNONYMS:

1. *superior and lesser posterior auricular nerve (Mayer, 1794)*
Synonym for macrodissected adult human ***lesser occipital nerve (Mayer, 1794)***; in the original Latin, *nervus auricularis posterior minor et superior*; Part 5, Table VII-*VIII* (p. 53).
2. *occipito-auricular branch of cephalic part of trachelo-cutanean plexus (Burdin, 1803)*
Synonym for *occipitoauricular branch of cephalic part of tracheosubcutaneous nerves (Chaussier, 1809)*; see translation (1803, Vol. 1, p. 188).
3. *occipitoauricular branch of cephalic part of tracheosubcutaneous nerves (Chaussier, 1809)*
Synonym for macrodissected adult human ***lesser occipital nerve (Mayer, 1794)***; in the original French, *branche occipito-oriculaire*.
4. *mastoid branch of cervical plexus (Cloquet, 1816)*
Synonym for macrodissected adult human ***lesser occipital nerve (Mayer, 1794)***; in the original French, *branche mastoïdienne*, p. 639.
5. *anterior occipital nerve (Meckel, 1817)*
Synonym for macrodissected adult human ***lesser occipital nerve (Mayer, 1794)***; see translation (1832, Vol. 3, p. 33).
6. *posterior ascending superficial branch of cervical plexus (Quain, 1828)*
Synonym for macrodissected adult human ***lesser occipital nerve (Mayer, 1794)***; p. 489.
7. *posterior branch of superficial branches of cervical plexus (Quain, 1832)*
Synonym for macrodissected adult human ***lesser occipital nerve (Mayer, 1794)***; p. 680.
8. *lesser occipital branch of cervical plexus (Quain, 1832)*
Synonym for macrodissected adult human ***lesser occipital nerve (Mayer, 1794)***; in the original Latin, *r. occipitalis minor*, p. 680.
9. *external occipital branch of cervical plexus (Cruveilhier, 1836)*
Synonym for macrodissected adult human ***lesser occipital nerve (Mayer, 1794)***; in the original French, *branche*

occipitale externe, p. 784. Cruveilhier described external and internal secondary branches.

10. *posterior branch of cervical plexus (Quain & Wilson, 1839)*
Synonym for macrodissected adult human ***lesser occipital nerve (Mayer, 1794)***; Plate XIV-*o*.

PARTLY CORRESPONDS:

1. *occipital branch of lesser posterior auricular nerve (Meckel, 1753)*
Dorsal (posterior) branch of *small posterior auricular nerve (Meckel, 1753)*; in the original French, *le rameau occipital du petit nerf auriculaire postérieur*, Table 1-278.
2. *lesser occipital nerve (Meckel, 1753)*
Indicates terminal end of ***lesser occipital nerve (Mayer, 1794)*** in regions dorsal (posterior) to ear, synonymous with *occipital branch of lesser posterior auricular nerve (Meckel, 1753)*; p. 101.
3. *occipital branch of occipitoauricular nerve (Peipers, 1793)*
Dorsal (posterior) branch of macrodissected adult human ***lesser occipital nerve (Mayer, 1794)***; in the original Latin, *ramus occipitalis nervi occipito-auricularis*, p. 33.
4. *occipital branch of lesser occipital nerve (Peipers, 1793)*
Dorsal (posterior) branch of macrodissected adult human ***lesser occipital nerve (Mayer, 1794)***; in the original Latin, *ramus occipitalis nervi occipitalis minor*, p. 33.
5. *superior auricular branch of occipitoauricular nerve (Peipers, 1793)*
Ventral (anterior) branch of macrodissected adult human ***lesser occipital nerve (Mayer, 1794)***; in the original Latin, *ramus auricularis superior nervi occipito-auricularis*, p. 33.
6. *superior auricular branch of lesser occipital nerve (Peipers, 1793)*
Ventral (anterior) branch of macrodissected adult human ***lesser occipital nerve (Mayer, 1794)***; in the original Latin, *ramus auricularis superior nervi occipitalis minor*, p. 33.
7. *auricular branch of lesser occipital nerve (Bock, 1827)*
Ventral (anterior) branch of macrodissected adult human ***lesser occipital nerve (Mayer, 1794)***; in the original Latin, *ram. auricularis nerv. occipitalis minor*, Table III-3.

lesser palatine nerves (Meckel, 1817)

As described for macrodissected adult human, two branches of the ***pterygopalatine nerves (Wrisberg, 1786)*** extending ventrally (descending) from the ***pterygopalatine ganglion (>1840)*** are usually delineated: ***lateral palatine nerve (Henle, 1871)*** and ***posterior palatine nerve (Günther, 1786)***. They supply the uvula, tonsil, and soft palate; see Henle (1871, pp. 377–378), Durward (1951, p. 1023), Williams & Warwick (1980, p. 1065), *Terminologia Anatomica* (1998, p. 134). For Meckel's use in macrodissected adult human, where 2–3 were described, see translation (1832, Vol. 3, p. 69). They were first accurately described by Meckel's grandfather; see ***[lesser palatine nerves (Meckel, 1817)] (Meckel, 1748)***.

EARLIER REFERENCES:

Illustrated and described, not named:

1. ***[lesser palatine nerves (Meckel, 1817)] (Meckel, 1748)***
Described for first time with modern precision, in macrodissected adult human; pp. 60–64.

Earlier synonyms:

1. *posterior lesser branch of palatine nerve (Loder, 1778)*
Synonym for macrodissected adult human ***lesser palatine nerves (Meckel, 1817)***; in the original Latin, *minorem posteriorem*, p. 15.
2. *gutturo-palatine nerve (Burdin, 1803)*
Synonym for macrodissected adult human ***lesser palatine nerves (Meckel, 1817)***; see translation (1803, Vol. 1, p. 174).
3. *palatine nerve (Burdin, 1803)*
Synonym for *gutturo-palatine nerve (Burdin, 1803)*; see translation (1803, Vol. 1, p. 3). Quain & Wilson (1839; Pl. XIII, Fig. 2-*r*) used *palatine nerves* for macrodissected adult human.
4. *posterior palatine nerve (Soemmerring, 1809)*
Synonym for macrodissected adult human ***lesser palatine nerves (Meckel, 1817)***; in the original German, *hinterer Gaumennerve*, Table 3, Figure 1-*u*.
5. *descending branches of spheno-palatine ganglion (Quain, 1828)*
Synonym for macrodissected adult human ***lesser palatine nerves (Meckel, 1817)***; p. 666.

PARTLY CORRESPONDS:

1. *superior palatine nerves (Burdin, 1803)*
Macrodissected adult human terminal branches of ***lesser palatine nerves (Meckel, 1817)*** to palatine arch; see translation (1803, Vol. 1, p. 174).
2. *outer palatine nerve (Soemmerring, 1809)*
Possibly a macrodissected adult human ***lesser palatine nerve (Meckel, 1817)*** with branches to uvula and orifice of auditory (Eustachian) tube; in the original Latin, *aeusserer Gaumennerve*, Table 3, Figure 1-*v,w,x,z*.

lesser petrosal nerve (>1840)

As described for macrodissected adult human, it extends between ***tympanic plexus (Müller, 1834)*** and ***otic ganglion (Arnold, 1828)***, and its main functional component is secretomotor (preganglionic parasympathetic) ***axons (Kölliker, 1896)***; see Durward (1951, Fig. 901), Williams & Warwick (1980, p. 175 and Figs. 7.79, 184), *Terminologia Anatomica* (1998, p. 136), ***tympanic nerve (Arnold, 1834)***. It was probably first identified by Winslow (1733); see ***[lesser petrosal nerve (>1840)] (Winslow, 1733)***.

EARLIER REFERENCES:

Described, not named or illustrated:

1. ***[lesser petrosal nerve (>1840)] (Winslow, 1733)***
Existence in macrodissected adult human apparently at least implied; Section VI, no. 81, p. 68. Also see ***[communicating branch of intermediofacial nerve with tympanic plexus (>1840)] (Drake, 1727)***. It was described more clearly for macrodissected adult human by Jacobson (1818); see Lobstein translation (1831, p. 37).

Earlier synonyms:

1. *lesser superficial petrosal nerve (Arnold, 1828)*
Long used synonym for macrodissected adult human ***lesser petrosal nerve (>1840)***; in the original Latin, *nervus petrosus superficialis minor*, p. 14. See Durward (1951, p. 1036 and Fig. 901). It has also been translated as *small superficial petrosal nerve*; see Cruveilhier (1844, p. 838).
2. *small petrosal nerve from tympanic branch of glosso-pharyngeal nerve (Quain, 1837)*
Synonym for macrodissected adult human ***lesser petrosal nerve (>1840)***; p. 813.
3. *communicating filament between otic ganglion and nervus tympanicus (Quain & Wilson, 1839)*
Synonym for macrodissected adult human ***lesser petrosal nerve (>1840)***; Plate XIII, Figure 1-*q*.

lesser splanchnic nerve (Haller, 1762)

As described for macrodissected adult human, it arises as 1–3 roots from the 9th and 10th, or less often the 10th and 11th, ***thoracic sympathetic ganglia (>1840)***, or from the ***communicating branches of sympathetic trunk (>1840)*** associated with them, pierces the diaphragmatic crus, and divides into several small branches entering the ***aorticorenal ganglion (>1840)*** and/or adjacent parts of the ***celiac plexus (Winslow, 1733)*** and more often than not the dorsal (posterior) part of the ***renal plexus (Drake, 1707)***; see Mitchell (pp. 243–245 and Fig. 104), Williams & Warwick (1980, p. 1131). For Haller's use in macrodissected adult human, see p. 261. Haller (1762, p. 261) and Wrisberg (1780, pp. 30–31) may not have clearly distinguished the ***least splanchnic nerve (>1840)***. It was first illustrated by Eustachi; see ***[lesser splanchnic nerve (Haller, 1762)] (Eustachi, 1552)***.

TRANSLATIONS:

1. *nervus splanchnicum minorem (Haller, 1762)*
Original Latin form of ***lesser splanchnic nerve (Haller, 1762)***; p. 261; *nervus splanchnicus minor* was provided by Soemmerring (1798, p. 355).

EARLIER REFERENCES:

Illustrated, not named or described:

1. ***[lesser splanchnic nerve (Haller, 1762)] (Eustachi, 1552)***
Illustrated for macrodissected adult human; see Albinus edition (1761, Tab. 18, Fig. 2-Θ). Willis (1664) illustrated it more clearly for macrodissected adult human; see Pordage translation (1681, Tab. XI-*β*,*K*).

Described, not named or illustrated:

1. ***[lesser splanchnic nerve (Haller, 1762] (Winslow, 1733)***
Described for macrodissected adult human (Sect. VI, p. 97) as fifth, last, and thickest branch arising from thoracic levels of ***sympathetic trunk (Winslow, 1733)***; also see Haller (1762, p. 261 note *r*).

Earlier synonyms:

1. *secondary trunk (Schmidel, 1754)*
Synonym for macrodissected adult human ***lesser splanchnic nerve (Haller, 1762)***; in the original Latin, *secondarius truncus*, p. 21, see Haller (1762, p. 261 note *r*).
2. *secondary splanchnic nerve (Haller, 1762)*
Apparently synonym for ***lesser splanchnic nerve (Haller, 1762)***; in the original Latin, *secundo splanchnico*, p. 261 note *a*. Also used thus by Günther (1786, p. 94).

LATER SYNONYMS:

1. *accessory splanchnic nerve (Walter, 1783)*
Synonym for macrodissected adult human ***lesser splanchnic nerve (Haller, 1762)***; in the original Latin, *nervum splanchnicum accessorium*, Tables I-*212*, III-*229*.
2. *accessory sympathetic nerve (Walter, 1783)*
Synonym for macrodissected adult human ***lesser splanchnic nerve (Haller, 1762)***; in the original Latin (plural), *nervi sympathici accessorii*, Table III-*227,228*.
3. *secondary sympathetic nerve (Walter, 1783)*
Synonym for macrodissected adult human ***lesser splanchnic nerve (Haller, 1762)***; in the original Latin (plural), *nervi sympathici accessorii seu secundarii*, Table III-*227,228*.
4. *small suprarenal nerve (Chaussier, 1789, definition 1)*
Synonym listed for macrodissected adult human ***lesser splanchnic nerve (Haller, 1762)***; in the original French, *le petit nerf surrénal*; see *Table synoptique du nerf tri-splanchnique*. Also see *small suprarenal nerve (Chaussier, 1789, definition 2)*.
5. *middle suprarenal nerve (Chaussier, 1789)*
Synonym listed for macrodissected adult human ***lesser splanchnic nerve (Haller, 1762)***; in the original French, *un moyen nerf surrénal*; see *Table synoptique du nerf tri-splanchnique*.
6. *inferior splanchnic nerve (Mayer, 1794)*
Synonym listed for macrodissected adult human ***lesser splanchnic nerve (Haller, 1762)***; in the original Latin, *nervus splanchnicus inferior*; Part 6, Table VI-*204* (p. 41).
7. *minor splanchnic nerve (Bell, 1803b)*
Synonym for macrodissected adult human ***lesser splanchnic nerve (Haller, 1762)***; in the original Latin, *splanchnicus minor*, p. 178.
8. *small splanchnic nerve (Meckel, 1817)*
Synonym for macrodissected adult human ***lesser splanchnic nerve (Haller, 1762)***; see translation (1832, Vol. 3, p. 97).
9. *smaller splanchnic nerve (Knox, 1832)*
Synonym for macrodissected adult human ***lesser splanchnic nerve (Haller, 1762)***; Plate VII-*42*.

PARTLY CORRESPONDS:

1. *accessory splanchnic nerve roots (Walter, 1783)*
Segments of macrodissected adult human ***lesser splanchnic nerve (Haller, 1762)*** arising from 9th and 10th ***thoracic sympathetic ganglia (>1840)*** to form *accessory splanchnic nerve trunk (Walter, 1783)* distally; in the original Latin, *radices nervus splanchnicus accessorius*, Table 1-*212*.
2. *accessory splanchnic nerve trunk (Walter, 1783)*
Segment of macrodissected adult human ***lesser splanchnic nerve (Haller, 1762)*** distal to (after) region where *accessory splanchnic nerve roots (Walter, 1783)* join; in the original Latin, *nervus splanchnicus accessorius truncus*, Table I-*214*.
3. *accessory sympathetic nerve trunk (Walter, 1783)*
Synonym for *accessory splanchnic nerve trunk (Walter, 1783)*; in the original Latin, *truncus nervi sympathici accessorii*, Table III-*227,228*.

4. *secondary sympathetic nerve trunk (Walter, 1783)*
Synonym for *accessory splanchnic nerve trunk (Walter, 1783)*; in the original Latin, *truncus nervi sympathici secondarii*, Tables II-*215*, III-*227,228*; described as dividing into superior and inferior branches, Table II-*216,217*.

limbic region (>1840)

As described for macrodissected adult human, a topographic division forming a ring just inside the topologically and developmentally medial border (limbus) of the ***cerebral cortex gray matter (>1840)***. It has three divisions: ***olfactory region (>1840)*** centered rostroventrally, ***hippocampal formation (Swanson & Cowan, 1977)*** centered caudally, and ***cingulate region (>1840)*** centered dorsally. For general modern overviews see Williams & Warwick (1980, p. 990 ff.), Nieuwenhuys et al. (2008, p. 617 ff.). ***Limbic region (>1840)*** is preferred to, for example, *limbic lobe (Broca, 1878b)* because an actual lobe cannot be distinguished and because the term *region* applies equally to gyrencephalic and lissencephalic species. Its vague outlines were glimpsed by Bartholin; see *limbus of brain (Bartholin, 1651)* and it was described rather accurately as the *limbic lobe (Broca, 1878b)*.

EARLIER REFERENCES:

Earlier synonyms:

1. *great limbic lobe (Broca, 1878b)*
Broadly synonymous with macrodissected adult mammalian ***limbic region (>1840)***; in the original French, *le grand lobe limbique*, p. 385. Also see Schwalbe (1881, p. 536), His (1895, pp. 169–170).
2. *limbic lobe (Broca, 1878b)*
Synonym for *great limbic lobe (Broca, 1878b)*, p. 386.

PARTLY CORRESPONDS:

1. *limbus of brain (Bartholin, 1651)*
Burdach (1822, p. 369) noted it is difficult to know what early anatomists meant by the term, although it was a vague forerunner of ***limbic region (>1840)***. Bartholin used it in explaining Le Boë's (unpublished) human ***brain (Smith Papyrus, c1700 BC)*** macrodissection method, and it apparently refers to the medial edge of ***cerebral cortex gray matter (>1840)*** bordering ***corpus callosum (Galen, c177)*** and ***brainstem (Schwalbe, 1881)***; see translation, 1662, pp. 140, 142. Bartholin used *limbus* in the original 1651 Latin edition, and *lace* was used in the 1662 translation (see Fig. 6-*m,n*). Molinetti (1675) suggested that to early anatomists it perhaps referred to ***fimbria (Honegger, 1890)***; see Burdach (1822, p. 374) and *limbus Sylvii (Haller, 1762)*.
2. *limbus cerebri (Willis, 1664)*
Term describing medial (and caudal) regions of macrodissected adult human ***cerebral cortex gray matter (>1840)***; Figure III-*A*. Willis did not illustrate or describe its full extent. As Burdach pointed out (1822, pp. 369, 372), it is difficult to know exactly what Willis meant by the term, although it is a vague precursor of ***limbic region (>1840)***, as was *limbus of brain (Bartholin, 1651)*, which may have been the source of Willis's term.
3. *border of brain (Willis, 1664)*
English form of *limbus cerebri (Willis, 1664)*; see Pordage translation (1681, Fig. III-*A*, p. 61).
4. *limbus of brain (Gibson, 1682)*
Gibson's translation of *limbus cerebri (Willis, 1664)*; see Table XI, Figure 1-*A*; also see *border of brain (Willis, 1664)*.
5. *limbus posterior (Vieussens, 1684)*
Synonym for macrodissected adult human *limbus cerebri (Willis, 1664)*; Tables III-*C* and XII-*F*, also see Burdach (1822, p. 372).
6. *natiform protuberance (Malacarne, 1780)*
Synonym for macrodissected adult human *piriform eminence (Laurencet, 1825)*; in the original Italian, *protuberanze natiforme*, Vol. 2, p. 9; see Meyer (1971, p. 85). Owen (1837, p. 95 and Pl. V, Figs. 8, 9-*1a*) used it for macrodissected adult opossum and wombat.
7. *piriform protuberance (Treviranus, 1820)*
Synonym for macrodissected adult mammalian *piriform eminence (Laurencet, 1825)*; in the original German, *Birnförmige*, p. 6. Tiedemann (1821, Tab. 3, Fig. 4-*o*) provided the Latin, *protuberantias pyriformes*, for macrodissected adult lion.
8. *piriform eminence (Laurencet, 1825)*
Apparently corresponds roughly to continuous part of macrodissected adult mammalian ***limbic region (>1840)*** including histologically defined ***piriform area (Smith, 1919)***, ***cortical amygdalar complex (>1840)***, and ***entorhinal area (Brodmann, 1909)***; in the original French, *eminence pyriforme*, Figure 13-*17*.
9. *processo cristato (Rolando, 1831)*
Major part of *great limbic lobe (Broca, 1878b)* in macrodissected adult human, consisting of ***cingulate region (>1840)***, ***parahippocampal gyrus (>1840)***, ***Ammon's horn (Vicq d'Azyr, 1784)***, and ***dentate gyrus (>1840)***; for original Italian term, see p. 125, Figure 2-*a*; also see Schiller (1992, pp. 256–257). Meyer stated (1971, p. 126) without citation that term was used by Rolando (1809).
10. *crested process (Rolando, 1831)*
English form of *processo cristato (Rolando, 1831)*.
11. *processo enteriodeo cristato (Rolando, 1831)*
Synonym for *processo cristato (Rolando, 1831)*; Figure 2-*a*. English form is *crested enteroid process*.
12. *convolution of corpus callosum (Cruveilhier, 1836)*
Synonym for macrodissected adult human *processo enteriodeo cristato (Rolando, 1831)*; in the original French, *circonvolution du corps calleux*, p. 662.
13. *annular convolution (Gerdy, 1838)*
In macrodissected adult human, an apparently closed oval ring of medial ***cerebral cortex gray matter (>1840)*** similar to, though somewhat less expansive than, *great limbic lobe (Broca, 1878b)* and consisting of ***cingulate region (>1840)***, ***parahippocampal gyrus (>1840)***, and ***straight gyrus (Valentin, 1841)***; in the original French, *circonvolution annulaire*, p. 259; see Broca (1878b, p. 387).
14. *lobar ring (Gerdy, 1838)*
Synonym for *annular convolution (Gerdy, 1838)*; in the original French, *anneau lobaire*, p. 260.

15. *fornicate gyrus (Arnold, 1838a)*
Macrodissected adult human ***cingulate region (>1840)*** and ***parahippocampal gyrus (>1840)*** considered together; in the original Latin, *gyrus fornicatus*, p. 52, and Arnold (1838b, Tab. IV, Fig. 4-χ).
16. *unciform gyri (Arnold, 1838a)*
Synonym for *fornicate gyrus (Arnold, 1838a)*; in the original Latin, *gyri unciformes*, p. 52.
17. *covered gyri (Arnold, 1838a)*
Synonym for *fornicate gyrus (Arnold, 1838a)*; in the original Latin, *gyri operti*, p. 52.
18. *internal convolution (Leuret, 1839)*
Synonym for macrodissected adult mammalian *annular convolution (Gerdy, 1838)*; in the original French, *circonvolution interne*, p. 379 ff.
19. *limbic convolution (Foville, 1844)*
Similar to macrodissected adult human *fornicate gyrus (Arnold, 1838a)*, consisting of ***cingulate region (>1840)*** and ***hippocampal formation (Swanson & Cowan, 1997)***; in the original French, *circonvolution de l'ourlet*; p. 381 and Plate 8, Figure 1. Also see Dejerine & Dejerine-Klumpke (1895, p. 297). Schiller (1992, pp. 256–257) gave the form *great aperture of hemisphere*.
20. *retrosplenial region (Brodmann, 1909)*
As described with cellular architecture in adult mammal, the most caudal subdivision of the ***cingulate region (>1840)***, further subdivided into dorsal or outer ***agranular retrosplenial area (>1840)***, or *area 30 (Brodmann, 1909)*; middle ***granular retrosplenial area (>1840)***, or *area 29 (Brodmann, 1909)*, together forming ***retrosplenial region (>1840)***; and tiny ventral or inner *ectosplenial area (Brodmann, 1909)*, or *area 26 (Brodmann, 1909)*, probably corresponding to ***fasciola cinerea (Arnold, 1838b)***; see Brodmann (1909, pp. 129, 148–149, 209, Fig. 86, Tab. 7 on p. 247), Nieuwenhuys et al. (2008, Fig. 12.13).
21. *precingulate subregion (Brodmann, 1909)*
Similar to adult human ***anterior cingulate region (>1840)*** except also includes *pregenual area (Brodmann, 1909)*; in the original Latin, *subregio praecingularis*, see pp. 147–148, Table 7 on p. 247.
22. *pyriform lobe (>1840)*
Modern definitions vary somewhat but generally include macrodissected adult human ***ambient gyrus (>1840)***, ***semilunar gyrus (>1840)***, and ***parahippocampal gyrus (>1840)***; see Carpenter (1976, p. 525), Williams & Warwick (1980, pp. 990–991). It was first described as *piriform protuberance (Treviranus, 1820)*.

limiting sulcus (>1840)

As described for the developing vertebrate ***neural tube (Baer, 1837)***, a continuous longitudinal groove in the luminal surface of the ***hindbrain vesicle (Baer, 1837)***, ***afterbrain vesicle (Baer, 1837)***, and ***spinal cord part of neural tube (>1840)*** separating the ***basal plate (>1840)*** ventrally and ***alar plate (>1840)*** dorsally. Its rostral extension into the ***midbrain vesicle (Baer, 1840)*** and beyond is controversial; see Alvarez-Bolado & Swanson (1996, p. 13 ff.). It is clear in the adult as the ***limiting sulcus of fourth ventricle (>1840)***, which was observed long ago by Ridley; see ***[limiting sulcus of fourth ventricle (>1840)] (Ridley, 1695)***.

TRANSLATIONS:

1. *sulcus limitans (>1840)*
Latin form of ***limiting sulcus (>1840)***.

limiting sulcus of fourth ventricle (>1840)

As described for macrodissected adult human, the groove in the ***floor of fourth ventricle (Reil, 1807–1808a)*** just lateral to the ***medial eminence (>1840)*** rostrally, just lateral to the ***facial colliculus (>1840)*** at intermediate levels, and just lateral to the ***hypoglossal triangle (>1840)*** caudally; see Crosby et al. (1962, Fig. 97), Williams & Warwick (1980, p. 933). It is the adult remnant of the segment of the embryonic ***limiting sulcus (>1840)*** in the ***medulla (Winslow, 1733)***; see Hamilton & Mossman (1972, Fig. 437). It was first noted by Ridley; see ***[limiting sulcus of fourth ventricle (>1840)] (Ridley, 1695)***.

EARLIER REFERENCES:

Illustrated, not named or described:

1. ***[limiting sulcus of fourth ventricle (>1840)] (Ridley, 1695)***
Vaguely illustrated in macrodissected adult human, separating ***medial eminence (>1840)*** from ***vestibular area of fourth ventricle (>1840)***; Figure VII between *k* and *l*. Soemmerring (1796, Tab. II) also vaguely illustrated it, whereas Rolando (1825a) illustrated it very clearly for macrodissected calf (Tab. VII, Fig. 1) in dorsal view, and for adult cattle (Tab. IX, Figs. 2–6) in transverse sections.

lingual branches of glossopharyngeal nerve (Haller, 1762)

As described for macrodissected adult human, the major terminal branch of the ***glossopharyngeal nerve trunk (Wrisberg, 1786, Günther, 1786)*** commonly generating two further branches, one supplying the vallate papillae and mucus membrane near the tongue's terminal sulcus and the other supplying mucous membrane of the caudal (posterior) region of the tongue; see Mettler (1948, Fig. 57), Hamilton (1976, Figs. 802, 803), Williams & Warwick (1980, p. 1976). Haller used the singular form in macrodissected adult human; p. 232. Scarpa (1794, Tab. II:*18–24*) named them individually for macrodissected adult human. They were known to Galen; see ***[lingual branches of glossopharyngeal nerve (Haller, 1762)] (Galen, c192)***.

EARLIER REFERENCES:

Described, not named or illustrated:

1. ***[lingual branches of glossopharyngeal nerve (Haller, 1762)] (Galen, c192)***
Described vaguely for macrodissected adult beef, pig, and/or macaque but not human; see Duckworth translation (1962, p. 201).

Illustrated, not named or described:

1 ***[lingual branches of glossopharyngeal nerve (Haller, 1762)] (Casseri, 1601)***
Clearly illustrated for macrodissected adult human; see *tractus primo* in Table I, Figure 1-*g* and Table XV, Figures 1-*I*, 2-*F*.

LATER SYNONYMS:

1. *lingual nerves of eighth pair (Loder, 1778)*
Synonym for macrodissected adult human ***lingual branches of glossopharyngeal nerve (Haller, 1762)***; in the original Latin, *nervi lingualis ex octavo pare*, p. 29.
2. *lingual branch of eighth pair (Monro, 1783)*
Synonym for macrodissected adult human ***lingual branches of glossopharyngeal nerve (Haller, 1762)***; Table 26*-*M*.
3. *fifth branch of glossopharyngeal nerve (Wrisberg, 1786)*
Synonym for macrodissected adult human ***lingual branches of glossopharyngeal nerve (Haller, 1762)***; see Wrisberg reprint (1800, p. 420).
4. *deep lingual branches of glossopharyngeal nerve (Bell, 1803b)*
Synonym listed for macrodissected adult human ***lingual branches of glossopharyngeal nerve (Haller, 1762)***; in the original Latin, *rami linguales profundi*, p. 153.
5. *lateral lingual branches of glossopharyngeal nerve (Bell, 1803b)*
Synonym listed for macrodissected adult human ***lingual branches of glossopharyngeal nerve (Haller, 1762)***; in the original Latin, *rami linguales laterales*, p. 153.

PARTLY CORRESPONDS:

1. *lateral lingual branches of eighth nerves of head (Andersch & Soemmerring, 1792)*
Topographically named ***lingual branches of glossopharyngeal nerve (Haller, 1762)*** for macrodissected adult human; in the original Latin, *linguales ramos laterales octavi nervi capitis*, p. 120.
2. *posterior lateral lingual branch of eighth pair of nerves of head (Andersch & Soemmerring, 1792)*
Topographically named *lateral lingual branch of eighth nerves of head (Andersch & Soemmerring, 1792)* for macrodissected adult human; in the original Latin, *posteriorem lateralem lingualem ramum*, p. 119.
3. *external lateral lingual branch of eighth pair of nerves of head (Andersch & Soemmerring, 1792)*
Topographically named *lateral lingual branch of eighth nerves of head (Andersch & Soemmerring, 1792)* for macrodissected adult human; in the original Latin, *externum lateralem lingualem ramum*, p. 120.
4. *internal lateral lingual branch of eighth pair of nerves of head (Andersch & Soemmerring, 1792)*
Topographically named *lateral lingual branch of eighth nerves of head (Andersch & Soemmerring, 1792)* for macrodissected adult human; in the original Latin, *lingualis lateralis internus ramus* or *ramus lingualis lateralis internus*, p. 120.
5. *lateral lingual branches of ninth nerves of head (Andersch, 1797)*
Topographically named ***lingual branches of glossopharyngeal nerve (Haller, 1762)*** for macrodissected adult human; in the original Latin, *ramos linguales laterales noni nervi capitis*, p. 14.
6. *posterior lateral lingual branch of ninth nerves of head (Andersch, 1797)*
Topographically named *lateral lingual branch of ninth nerves of head (Andersch & Soemmerring, 1792)* for macrodissected adult human; in the original Latin, *ramum lingualem lateralem posteriorem noni nervi capitis*, p. 14.
7. *external lateral lingual branch of ninth nerves of head (Andersch, 1797)*
Topographically named *lateral lingual branch of ninth nerves of head (Andersch & Soemmerring, 1792)* for macrodissected adult human; in the original Latin, *ramum lingualem lateralem externum noni nervi capitis*, p. 14.
8. *internal lateral lingual branch of ninth nerves of head (Andersch, 1797)*
Topographically named *lateral lingual branch of ninth nerves of head (Andersch & Soemmerring, 1792)* for macrodissected adult human; in the original Latin, *ramus lingualis lateralis internus noni nervi capitis*, p. 15.
9. *exterior minor lingual branch of glossopharyngeal nerve (Cloquet, 1828)*
Small branch named and illustrated for macrodissected adult human; in the original Latin, *ramus lingualis minor exterior*, Plate CLIX-53.
10. *lateral lingual branches of glossopharyngeal (Knox, 1832)*
Synonym for macrodissected adult human *lateral lingual branches of ninth nerves of head (Andersch, 1797)*; Plate II-56.

lingual branches of hypoglossal nerve (Cloquet, 1816)

As described for macrodissected adult human, muscular branches of the ***hypoglossal nerve (Winslow, 1733)*** supplying the styloglossus, hyoglossus, and genioglossus muscles, and the intrinsic muscles of the tongue. Another branch to the geniohyoid muscle arises from the first ***cervical nerve (Galen, c173)***; see Durward (1953, Fig. 909), Williams & Warwick (1980, p. 1083). For Cloquet's use in macrodissected adult human, see p. 630. It was known to Galen; see ***[lingual branches of hypoglossal nerve (Cloquet, 1816)] (Galen, c173)***.

TRANSLATIONS:

1. *branche linguale du nerf hypoglosse (Cloquet, 1816)*
Original French form (singular) of ***lingual branches of hypoglossal nerve (Cloquet, 1816)***; p. 630.

EARLIER REFERENCES:

Described, not named or illustrated:

1. ***[lingual branches of hypoglossal nerve (Cloquet, 1816)] (Galen, c173)***
Described for macrodissected adult beef, pig, and/or macaque but not human, "these motor nerves of the seventh pair are resolved into many fibers and are interwoven to fill all the muscles [of the tongue]" (May translation, 1968, p. 451).

Illustrated and described, not named:

1. ***[lingual branches of hypoglossal nerve (Cloquet, 1816)] (Vesalius, 1543a)***
Described and crudely illustrated for macrodissected adult human; see Richardson & Carman translation (2002, p. 204). Eustachi illustrated them more clearly for macrodissected adult human; see *trunci noni paris nervorum cerebri finis (Albinus, 1744)*.

Earlier synonyms:

1. *trunci noni paris nervorum cerebri finis (Albinus, 1744)*
Synonym for macrodissected adult human ***lingual branches of hypoglossal nerve (Cloquet, 1816)***; Table 18, Figure 2-*11*.
2. *lingual branches of ninth pair (Haller, 1762)*
Synonym for macrodissected adult human ***lingual branches of hypoglossal nerve (Cloquet, 1816)***; pp. 582 (and 239).
3. *muscular branches of ninth pair (Günther, 1786)*
Synonym for macrodissected adult human ***lingual branches of hypoglossal nerve (Cloquet, 1816)***; in the original Latin, *rami musculares*, p. 68; *par nonum*, p. 66.
4. *muscular branches of hypoglossal nerve (Günther, 1786)*
Synonym for macrodissected adult human ***lingual branches of hypoglossal nerve (Cloquet, 1816)***; in the original Latin, *rami musculares*, p. 68; *n. hypoglossum*, p. 66.

LATER SYNONYMS:

1. *lingual part of twelfth pair (Arnold, 1834)*
Synonym for macrodissected adult human ***lingual branches of hypoglossal nerve (Cloquet, 1816)***; in the original Latin, *par duodecimum, pars lingualis*, p. 15.
2. *lingual part of hypoglossal nerve (Arnold, 1834)*
Synonym for macrodissected adult human ***lingual branches of hypoglossal nerve (Cloquet, 1816)***; in the original Latin, *nervus hypoglossus, pars lingualis*, p. 15.
3. *lingual part of speaking nerve (Arnold, 1834)*
Synonym for macrodissected adult human ***lingual branches of hypoglossal nerve (Cloquet, 1816)***; in the original Latin, *nervus loquens, pars lingualis*, p. 15.

PARTLY CORRESPONDS:

1. *branch to ceratoglossus muscle (Andersch & Soemmerring, 1792)*
Macrodissected adult human ***lingual branch of hypoglossal nerve (Cloquet, 1816)*** to hyoglossus muscle; in the original Latin, *ramus musculi ceratoglossi*, p. 149.
2. *ceratobasiostyloglossus plexus (Andersch & Soemmerring, 1792)*
Communicating branches (Winslow, 1733) between certain ***lingual branches of hypoglossal nerve (Cloquet, 1816)*** for macrodissected adult human; in the original Latin, *plexum ceratobasiostyloglossum*, pp. 151–153. See Scarpa (1794, Tab. I-35).
3. *ceratobasioglossus nerve (Andersch & Soemmerring, 1792)*
Macrodissected adult human ***lingual branch of hypoglossal nerve (Cloquet, 1816)*** to hyoglossus muscle; in the original Latin, *nervus ceratobasioglossius*, p. 152. Basioglossus muscle is part of hyoglossus muscle arising from body of hyoid bone. Winslow (1733, Sect. VI, p. 75) mentioned filaments from ***hypoglossal nerve (Winslow, 1733)*** to "musculus cerato-basio-glossus."
4. *right nerve to geniohyoid muscle (Andersch & Soemmerring, 1792)*
Macrodissected adult human right ***lingual branch of hypoglossal nerve (Cloquet, 1816)*** to geniohyoid muscle; in the original Latin, *nervus geniohyoidei dextri*, p. 156.
5. *nerve to geniohyoid muscle (Andersch & Soemmerring, 1792)*
Macrodissected adult human ***lingual branch of hypoglossal nerve (Cloquet, 1816)*** to geniohyoid muscle; in the original Latin, *nervus geniohyoidei dextri*, p. 156.
6. *nerve to genioglossus muscle (Andersch & Soemmerring, 1792)*
Synonym for one of the *genioglossus nerves (Andersch & Soemmerring, 1792)*; in the original Latin, *nervus musculi genioglossi*, p. 150.
7. *genioglossus nerves (Andersch & Soemmerring, 1792)*
Macrodissected adult human ***lingual branch of hypoglossal nerve (Cloquet, 1816)*** to genioglossus muscle; in the original Latin, *nervum genioglossicum*, p. 156.
8. *right genioglossus nerves of tenth pair of nerves of head (Andersch & Soemmerring, 1792)*
Synonym for right *genioglossus nerves (Andersch & Soemmerring, 1792)*; in the original Latin, *nervi genioglossi decimus nervus capitis dexter*, p. 157.
9. *intermuscular branch to genioglossus muscle (Andersch & Soemmerring, 1792)*
Macrodissected adult human ***lingual branch of hypoglossal nerve (Cloquet, 1816)*** associated with genioglossus muscle; in the original Latin, *ramus intermuscularis musculi genioglossi*, p. 157.
10. *right genioglossus nerves (Andersch, 1797)*
Synonym for right *genioglossus nerves (Andersch & Soemmerring, 1792)*; in the original Latin, *nervum genioglossicum dextrum*, p. 87.
11. *ceratoglossal plexus of hypoglossal (Knox, 1832)*
Macrodissected adult human ***plexus (Galen, c192)*** formed on hyoglossus muscle by ***lingual branches of hypoglossal nerve (Cloquet, 1816)***; Plate I-69e, Knox's translation of Scarpa (1794).
12. *branchlet to geniohyoid muscle from hypoglossal nerve (Arnold, 1834)*
Synonym for *nerve to geniohyoid muscle (Andersch & Soemmerring, 1792)*; in the original Latin, *nervus hypoglossus ramulus ad musculum geniohyiodeum*, p. 15.
13. *branchlet to styloglossus muscle from hypoglossal nerve (Arnold, 1834)*
Macrodissected adult human ***lingual branch of hypoglossal nerve (Cloquet, 1816)*** to styloglossus muscle; in the original Latin, *nervus hypoglossus ramulus ad musculum styloglossum*, p. 15.
14. *branches to hyoglossus muscle from hypoglossal nerve (Arnold, 1834)*

Macrodissected adult human ***lingual branch of hypoglossal nerve (Cloquet, 1816)*** to hyoglossus muscle; in the original Latin, *nervus hypoglossus rami ad musculum hyoglossum*, p. 15.

15. *branch to genioglossus muscle from hypoglossal nerve (Arnold, 1834)*
 Macrodissected adult human ***lingual branch of hypoglossal nerve (Cloquet, 1816)*** to genioglossus muscle; in the original Latin, *nervus hypoglossus ramus ad musculum genioglossum*, p. 15.
16. *branches of great hypoglossal for hyoglossal and styloglossal (Cruveilhier, 1836)*
 Macrodissected adult human ***lingual branch of hypoglossal nerve (Cloquet, 1816)*** to hyoglossus and styloglossus muscles; in the original French, *branches de l'hyoglosse et du styloglosse*, p. 977.

lingual branches of lingual nerve (Arnold, 1834)

As described for macrodissected adult human, terminal branches of the ***lingual nerve (Vesalius, 1543a)*** supplying predominantly mucous membrane of the pre-sulcal part of the tongue; see Henle (1871, pp. 388–390 and Fig. 247), Mettler (1948, Fig. 57), Williams & Warwick (1980, p. 1067), *Terminologia Anatomica* (1998, p. 135). For Arnold's use in macrodissected adult human see p. 11. They were known to Vesalius; see ***[lingual branches of lingual nerve (>1840)] (Vesalius, 1543a)***.

TRANSLATIONS:

1. *nervus lingualis rami linguales (Arnold, 1834)*
 Original Latin form of ***lingual branches of lingual nerve (Arnold, 1834)***; p. 11.

EARLIER REFERENCES:

Described, not named or illustrated:

1. ***[lingual branches of lingual nerve (>1840)] (Vesalius, 1543a)***
 Vesalius wrote that the ***lingual nerve (Vesalius, 1543a)*** "joins up with the lingual nerve on the other side to form a tunic that functions as the proper organ of recognizing flavors." (Richardson & Carman translation, 2002, p. 189). They were described relatively thoroughly for macrodissected adult human by Meckel (1748, pp. 96–97).

LATER SYNONYMS:

1. *lingual branches of gustatory nerve (Arnold, 1834)*
 Synonym for ***lingual branches of lingual nerve (Arnold, 1834)***; in the original Latin, *nervus gustatorius, rami linguales*, p. 11.

lingual gyrus (>1840)

As described for macrodissected adult human, a topographic subdivision on the medial face of the ***occipital region (Vesalius, 1543a)*** lying ventral to the ***calcarine sulcus (>1840)*** and dorsal to the ***collateral sulcus (>1840)***, with the rostral (anterior) end merging with the caudal end of the ***parahippocampal gyrus (>1840)***; see Crosby et al. (1962, p. 349); Williams & Warwick (1980, Fig. 7.114A). It was perhaps first clearly delineated by Soemmerring; see ***[lingual gyrus (>1840)] (Soemmerring, 1778)***.

EARLIER REFERENCES:

Illustrated and described, not named:

1. ***[lingual gyrus (>1840)] (Soemmerring, 1778)***
 Clearly illustrated for macrodissected adult human; Table III. Vicq d'Azyr (1786) also clearly illustrated and drew attention to it for macrodissected adult human; Plate XVI-*18*.

Earlier synonyms:

1. *Randwülste des innern Grundbündls (Burdach, 1822)*
 Apparently general region of macrodissected adult human ***lingual gyrus (>1840)***; Table VIII-*4*, also see Table VII-*ç*.

lingual nerve (Vesalius, 1543a)

As described for adult human, a sensory component of the ***posterior branch of mandibular nerve (>1840)*** supplying mucous membrane of the presulcal part of the tongue, floor of the mouth, and mandibular gums. Three ***nerves (Herophilus, c335–c280 BC)*** communicate with it on the way to the tongue: ***chorda tympani (Falloppio, 1561)***, ***inferior dental nerve (Meckel, 1817)***, and ***hypoglossal nerve (Winslow, 1733)***; see Durward (1951, p. 1028), Williams & Warwick (1980, p. 1067). For Vesalius's use in macrodissected adult human, see Richardson & Carman translation (2002, p. 189). In 1559, Colombo reported the congenital absence of taste in a patient where the ***lingual nerve (Vesalius, 1543a)*** went to the occiput rather than to the tongue; see Meckel (1832, Vol. 3, p. 41). Henle (1871, Fig. 247) illustrated it especially well. It was first described as the *sensory nerve for tongue (Galen, c173)*.

TRANSLATIONS:

1. *nervus lingualis (Vesalius, 1543a)*
 Latin form of ***lingual nerve (Vesalius, 1543a)***; see Richardson & Carman (2002, p. 189).
2. *nervo linguae (Haase, 1781)*
 Latin form of ***lingual nerve (Vesalius, 1543a)***; p. 74 note *e*.

EARLIER REFERENCES:

Earlier synonyms:

1. *sensory nerve for tongue (Galen, c173)*
 Galen often wrote about ***nerve (Herophilus, c335–c280 BC)*** to tongue mediating taste, as observed primarily in macrodissected adult beef, pig, and/or macaque but not explicitly human; it corresponds to ***lingual nerve (Vesalius, 1543a)***; see May translation (1968, pp. 439–440, and pp. 391, 397, 401, 404, 451, 454, 552, 686). Also see Duckworth translation (1962, pp. 54, 193), *nerve of taste (Galen, c173)*, and *motor nerve for tongue (Galen, c173)*.
2. *nerve of taste (Galen, c173)*
 Synonym for *sensory nerve for tongue (Galen, c173)*; see May translation (1968, p. 439).
3. *gustatory nerve (Galen, c180)*
 Synonym for *sensory nerve for tongue (Galen, c173)*; see Goss (1966, p. 329) translation of *On Anatomy*

of Nerves. Galen noted that *third pair of nerves from brain (Galen, c192)* was first called thus by Marinus of Pergamum and was sometimes referred to as *gustatory nerve (Galen, c180)*; see Burdach (1822, p. 314), Goss (1966, p. 329), and *third and fourth pairs of nerves from brain (Galen, c192)*.

LATER SYNONYMS:

1. *fifth nerve of third pair of nerves arising from brain (Falloppio, 1561)*
   Roughly synonymous with macrodissected adult human ***lingual nerve (Vesalius, 1543a)*** according to Bauhin (1605); see Crooke translation (1615, p. 891).
2. *trunk itself of fourth conjugation of nerves of brain (Crooke, 1615)*
   Synonym for macrodissected adult human ***lingual nerve (Vesalius, 1543a)***; p. 487. Crooke's description is a translation of Bauhin (1605).
3. *trunk of first division of fifth pair of nerves arising within skull (Willis, 1664)*
   Roughly synonymous with macrodissected adult, presumably human, ***lingual nerve (Vesalius, 1543a)***; see Pordage translation (1681, p. 145, Fig. 1-*H*).
4. *prima ac interior propago rami majoris posterioris (Vieussens, 1684)*
   Synonym for macrodissected adult human ***lingual nerve (Vesalius, 1543a)***; Table 22-3.
5. *nervus hypoglossus minor (Winslow, 1733)*
   Synonym for macrodissected adult human ***lingual nerve (Vesalius, 1543a)***; Section VI, p. 66.
6. *internal lingual nerve (Schaarschmidt, 1750)*
   Synonym for macrodissected adult human ***lingual nerve (Vesalius, 1543a)***; in the original Latin, *nervus lingualis internus*, p. 28.
7. *lingual maxillary nerve (Le Cat, 1768)*
   Synonym for macrodissected adult human ***lingual nerve (Vesalius, 1543a)***; Plate VII, Figure 1-4.
8. *lingual branch of third branch of fifth pair (Loder, 1778)*
   Synonym for macrodissected adult human ***lingual nerve (Vesalius, 1543a)***; in the original Latin, *ramus lingualis*, p. 20.
9. *medial and internal branch of third branch of fifth pair (Comparetti, 1789)*
   Synonym for macrodissected adult human ***lingual nerve (Vesalius, 1543a)***; in the original Latin, *ramum internum & medium*, p. 53.
10. *superior lingual nerve (Andersch & Soemmerring, 1792)*
    Synonym for macrodissected adult human ***lingual nerve (Vesalius, 1543a)***; in the original Latin, *nervus lingualis superior (quinti nervi capitis)*, p. 154.
11. *lingual branch of inferior maxillary branch of fifth pair of nerves (Bock, 1817)*
    Synonym for macrodissected adult human ***lingual nerve (Vesalius, 1543a)***; in the original Latin, *ramus lingualis*, p. 50.
12. *lingual surculus with chorda tympani (Bellingeri, 1818)*
    Synonym for macrodissected adult human ***lingual nerve (Vesalius, 1543a)***; in the original Latin, *surculus lingualis cum chorda tympani*, see Table I.
13. *lingual branch of third division of fifth pair of nerves (Todd, 1836–1839)*
    Synonym for macrodissected adult human ***lingual nerve (Vesalius, 1543a)***; p. 291.

PARTLY CORRESPONDS:

1. *submaxillary nerves (Chaussier, 1809)*
   Apparently macrodissected adult human ***communicating branches of lingual nerve with submandibular ganglion (>1840)***, ***sublingual nerve (Henle, 1871)***, and branches of latter to sublingual artery; in the original French, *nerfs sous-maxillaires*.
2. *muscular fascicles of lingual surculus with chorda tympani (Bellingeri, 1818)*
   Macrodissected adult human branches of ***lingual nerve (Vesalius, 1543a)*** to tonsils, mylopharyngeal part of superior pharyngeal constrictor muscle, and medial pterygoid muscle; in the original Latin, *fasciculi musculares*, see Table I.
3. *gingival fascicles of lingual surculus with chorda tympani (Bellingeri, 1818)*
   Macrodissected adult human branches of ***lingual nerve (Vesalius, 1543a)*** to lingual gingiva and associated oral mucosa; in the original Latin, *fasciculi gingivales*, see Table I.
4. *lingual fascicles proper of lingual surculus with chorda tympani (Bellingeri, 1818)*
   Macrodissected adult human ***lingual branches of lingual nerve (Arnold, 1834)*** and ***communicating branches of lingual nerve with hypoglossal nerve (>1840)***, except for *lingual muscular fascicle of lingual surculus with chorda tympani (Bellingeri, 1818)*, considered together; in the original Latin, *fasciculi linguales proprii*, see Table I.
5. *conjunction of lingual nerve with chorda tympani (Arnold, 1834)*
   Macrodissected adult human point of union between ***lingual nerve (Vesalius, 1543a)*** and ***chorda tympani (Falloppio, 1561)***; in the original Latin, *conjunctio cum chorda tympani*, p. 10.
6. *connection of gustatory nerve with chorda tympani (Arnold, 1834)*
   Synonym for *conjunction of lingual nerve with chorda tympani (Arnold, 1834)*; p. 10.

lingula (Malacarne, 1776)

As described for macrodissected adult human, rostral and ventral end of the ***cerebellar vermis (Meckel, 1817)***, lying just ventral and caudal to the ***central lobule (Burdach, 1822)*** on the dorsal surface of the ***rostral medullary velum (>1840)***; see Angevine et al. (1961, Fig. 24), Larsell & Jansen (1972, Fig. 118), Carpenter (1976, Figs. 2.25, 2.26, 14.1), *Terminologia Anatomica* (1998, p. 118), Nieuwenhuys et al. (2008, Fig. 3.8-24). For Malacarne's original use in macrodissected adult human, see p. 40 and Clarke & O'Malley (1996, pp. 644, 646). It was first pointed out by Vesalius; see ***[lingula (Malacarne, 1776)] (Vesalius, 1543a)***.

TRANSLATIONS:

1. *Züngelchen (Burdach, 1822)*
   German form of ***lingula (Malacarne, 1776)***; p. 56.

EARLIER REFERENCES:

Described, not named or illustrated:

1. ***[lingula (Malacarne, 1776)] (Vesalius, 1543a)***
   Briefly described for macrodissected adult human; see Singer translation (1952, p. 23).

Earlier synonyms:

1. *laminated lingula (Malacarne, 1776)*
   Full expression used for ***lingula (Malacarne, 1776)***; in the original Italian, *linguetta laminosa*, p. 40.

locus ceruleus (Wenzel & Wenzel, 1812)

As described for adult human with gross dissection, and for adult mammal in general with cellular architecture and connections, a small ***gray matter region (Swanson & Bota, 2010)*** lying laterally and caudally in the ***pontine central gray (>1840)*** just medial to the ***pontine segment of midbrain tract of trigeminal nerve (>1840)***. In macrodissected adult human it is a *blue place (Meckel, 1832)* lying just ventral to the rostral end of the ***floor of fourth ventricle (Reil, 1807–1808a)***; see Carpenter (1996, A-9 on p. 684, labeled *pigmented nucleus*), Nieuwenhuys et al. (2008, pp. 204, 898 and Fig. 6.28). For the Wenzel brother's use in macrodissected adult human, see pp. 168, 194, and Meyer (1971, p. 30). It was discovered by Vicq d'Azyr; see ***[locus ceruleus (Wenzel & Wenzel, 1812)] (Vicq d'Azyr, 1784)***.

ALTERNATE SPELLINGS:

1. *loculos caeruleos (Wenzel & Wenzel, 1812)*
   Original spelling of ***locus ceruleus (Wenzel & Wenzel, 1812)***; p. 194. Other plural forms were *loculi caerulei* (p. 168) and *loci caerulei* (Tab. X, Fig. 4-*f*).
2. *locus caeruleus (Burdach, 1822)*
   Alternate form of *loculos caeruleos (Wenzel & Wenzel, 1812)*; p. 79.
3. *locus coeruleus (Arnold, 1838a)*
   Alternate form of *loculos caeruleos (Wenzel & Wenzel, 1812)*; p. 26.

TRANSLATIONS:

1. *blue place (Meckel, 1832)*
   English form of ***locus ceruleus (Wenzel & Wenzel, 1812)***; Vol. 2, p. 460. Meckel commented it is probably only present in human.

EARLIER REFERENCES:

Described, not named or illustrated:

1. ***[locus ceruleus (Wenzel & Wenzel, 1812)] (Vicq d'Azyr, 1784)***
   Discovered in macrodissected adult human and referred to as blackish substance; p. 585. See Meckel (1817; and 1832 translation, Vol. 2, p. 460), Meyer (1971, p. 30).

Earlier synonyms:

1. *black matter (Reil, 1809c)*
   Reil described vaguely dark substance in region of ***locus ceruleus (Wenzel & Wenzel, 1812)*** lying along ***superior cerebellar peduncle (Procháska, 1800)***; see Mayo translation (1823, p. 98). Burdach (1822, p. 306) provided Reil's term in German as *schwarzer Substanz*.

LATER SYNONYMS:

1. *substantia ferruginea (Arnold, 1838a)*
   Synonym for macrodissected adult human ***locus ceruleus (Wenzel & Wenzel, 1812)***; p. 26.

long ciliary nerves (Soemmerring, 1801)

As described for macrodissected adult human, usually 2–3 branches of the ***nasociliary nerve (Meckel, 1817; Wutzer, 1817)*** accompanying the ***short ciliary nerves (>1840)*** and distributing to the ciliary body, iris, and cornea; see Williams & Warwick (1980, p. 1061 and Figs. 7.173, 176). They also contain ***axons (Kölliker, 1896)*** from the ***superior cervical ganglion (Vieussens, 1684)***, and from the ***Edinger-Westphal nucleus (>1840)***, some of whose ***axons (Kölliker, 1896)*** may be carried by the ***oculomotor nerve (Estienne, 1545)***, ***trochlear nerve (Molinetti, 1669)***, ***trigeminal nerve (Winslow, 1733)***, and ***abducens nerve (Heister, 1717)***; see Mitchell (1952, pp. 155–157, 203–204), Durward (1951, Fig. 890). The first illustration to distinguish clearly between ***long ciliary nerves (Soemmerring, 1801)*** and ***short ciliary nerves (>1840)***, and even show a ***communicating branch (Winslow, 1733)*** between them, was provided by Zinn (1755, Tab. 6, Figs. 1 and 2). For Soemmerring's use in macrodissected adult human, see Table III, Figure VIII-*x*. Estienne may have provided the first delineation of at least part of them; see ***[long ciliary nerves (Soemmerring, 1801)] (Estienne, 1545)***.

TRANSLATIONS:

1. *lang Ciliarnerven (Soemmerring, 1801)*
   Original German for ***long ciliary nerves (Soemmerring, 1801)***; Table III, Figure VIII-*x*.

EARLIER REFERENCES:

Illustrated and described, not named:

1. ***[long ciliary nerves (Soemmerring, 1801)] (Estienne, 1545)***
   Estienne provided first brief description and illustration of their terminal parts for macrodissected adult human; Book 3, Chapter 10, Figure 1-C; see Zinn (1755, p. 202 note *d*). According to Albinus (1744), Eustachi (1552) may have indicated their origin and course for macrodissected adult human in his Table 18, Figure 5-*t*. They were described somewhat more fully by Falloppio (1561); see Zinn (1755, pp. 202, 209 note *p*).

Described, not named or illustrated:

1. ***[long ciliary nerves (Soemmerring, 1801)] (Willis, 1664)***
   Apparently two described for macrodissected adult, presumably human; see Pordage translation (1681, p. 142) and *lesser nerves out of infolding of third pair (Willis, 1664)*.

Earlier synonyms:

1. *minor ac exterior propago ramuli secundi rami minoris superioris nervorum quintae conjugationis (Vieussens, 1684)*

Corresponds roughly to macrodissected adult human ***long ciliary nerves (Soemmerring, 1801)***; p. 171 and Table 22-*g*. Also included may well be the curious *surculus primus crassioris ac interioris propago K...*; p. 171 and Table 22-*l*.

2. *internal ciliary nerve (Günther, 1786)*
   Apparently synonym for macrodissected adult human ***long ciliary nerves (Soemmerring, 1801)***; in the original Latin, *ciliaris internus*, p. 44.
3. *ciliary fascicle of nasal surculus (Bellingeri, 1818)*
   Synonym for macrodissected adult human ***long ciliary nerves (Soemmerring, 1801)***; in the original Latin, *fasciculus ciliaris*, see Table I.
4. *ciliary branches of nasal nerve (Todd, 1836–1839)*
   Synonym for macrodissected adult human ***long ciliary nerves (Soemmerring, 1801)***; p. 282.

long gyrus of insula (Valentin, 1841)

As described for macrodissected adult human, the caudal one or sometimes two *cerebral gyri (Vesalius, 1543a)* of the ***insular region (Brodmann, 1909)***, separated from the more rostral ***short gyri of insula (Gall & Spurzheim, 1810)*** by the ***central sulcus of insula (>1840)***; see Crosby et al. (1962, pp. 476–477, Fig. 319), Williams & Warwick (1980, pp. 987–988, Fig. 7.113A), *Terminologia Anatomica* (1998, p. 125), Nieuwenhuys et al. (2008, p. 649 ff.). For Valentin's use in macrodissected adult human see p. 169. It was perhaps first clearly identified as the *longer circumvolutions of island of Sylvian fissure (Meckel, 1817)*.

EARLIER REFERENCES:

Earlier synonyms:

1. *longer circumvolutions of island of Sylvian fissure (Meckel, 1817)*
   Synonym for macrodissected adult human ***long gyrus of insula (Valentin, 1841)***; see translation (1832, Vol. 2, p. 442).

long thoracic nerve (Quain & Wilson, 1839)

As described for macrodissected adult human it is usually formed by the rostral three ***brachial plexus roots (Schwalbe, 1881)***—that is, the 5th–7th ***cervical nerves (Galen, c173)***—and innervates each digitation of the serratus anterior muscle; see Williams & Warwick (1980, p. 1096). For Quain & Wilson's use in macrodissected adult human, see Plate XVII-*g*. It was known to Galen; see ***[long thoracic nerve (>1840)] (Galen, c192)***.

EARLIER REFERENCES:

Described, not named or illustrated:

1. ***[long thoracic nerve (>1840)] (Galen, c192)***
   Described for macrodissected adult beef, pig, and/or macaque but not human; see Duckworth translation (1962, p. 255). Vesalius (1543a) mentioned it for macrodissected adult human; see Richardson & Carman translation (2002, p. 234).

Earlier synonyms:

1. *nervus abscissus (Vieussens, 1684)*
   Term used in describing clear illustrations of macrodissected adult human ***long thoracic nerve (Quain & Wilson, 1839)*** shown arising from sixth and seventh ***cervical nerves (Galen, c173)***; Tables 23-*100* and 24-*n*.
2. *great thoracic nerve (Bang, 1770)*
   Synonym for macrodissected adult human ***long thoracic nerve (Quain & Wilson, 1839)***; in the original Latin, *[nervus] thoracicus major*, Figure I-*67*.
3. *lesser posterior thoracic nerve (Günther, 1786)*
   Synonym for macrodissected adult human ***long thoracic nerve (Quain & Wilson, 1839)***; in the original Latin, *nervus thor. post. minor*, p. 73.
4. *sterno-thoracic nerve (Burdin, 1803)*
   Apparently synonym for macrodissected adult human ***long thoracic nerve (Quain & Wilson, 1839)***; see translation (1803, Vol. 1, p. 191). Also see Meckel (1832, Vol. 3, p. 24).
5. *thoracic nerve (Burdin, 1803)*
   Synonym for *sterno-thoracic nerve (Burdin, 1803)*; see translation (1803, Vol. 1, p. 191).
6. *posterior thoracic branch of brachial plexus (Cloquet, 1816)*
   Synonym for macrodissected adult human ***long thoracic nerve (Quain & Wilson, 1839)***; in the original French, *branche thoracique postérieure*, p. 643.
7. *posterior thoracic nerve (Meckel, 1817)*
   Synonym for macrodissected adult human ***long thoracic nerve (Quain & Wilson, 1839)***; see translation (1832, Vol. 3, p. 24).
8. *external respiratory nerve (Bell, 1821)*
   Synonym for macrodissected adult mammalian ***long thoracic nerve (Quain & Wilson, 1839)***; p. 407, see Foster (1894, p. 2395).
9. *external thoracic nerve (Bell, 1821)*
   Synonym for *external respiratory nerve (Bell, 1821)*; p. 290.
10. *inferior external respiratory nerve (Bell & Bell, 1826)*
    Synonym for *external respiratory nerve (Bell, 1821)*; Vol. 2, p. 400.
11. *great dentate branch of brachial plexus (Cruveilhier, 1836)*
    Synonym for macrodissected adult human ***long thoracic nerve (Quain & Wilson, 1839)***; in the original French, *branche du grand dentelé du plexus brachial*, p. 793.

LATER SYNONYMS:

1. *Bell's nerve (>1840)*
   Eponym for ***long thoracic nerve (Quain & Wilson, 1839)*** or *external respiratory nerve (Bell, 1821)*; see *Terminologia Anatomica* (1998, p. 163).

PARTLY CORRESPONDS:

1. *greater thoracic nerve (Haase, 1781)*
   Apparently part of ***long thoracic nerve (Quain & Wilson, 1839)*** arising from fifth ***cervical nerve (Galen,***

c173) in macrodissected adult human; in the original Latin, *nervus thoracicus major*, p. 96.

2. *lesser thoracic nerve (Haase, 1781)*
Apparently part of ***long thoracic nerve (Quain & Wilson, 1839)*** arising from sixth ***long thoracic nerve (Quain & Wilson, 1839)*** in macrodissected adult human; in the original Latin, *nervus thoracicus minorem*, p. 96.
3. *superior root of posterior thoracic nerve (Bock, 1827)*
Macrodissected adult human root of ***long thoracic nerve (Quain & Wilson, 1839)*** arising from fifth ***cervical nerve (Galen, c173)***; in the original Latin, *radix superior nerv. thoracicus posterior*; Table V, Figure 1-42.
4. *inferior root of posterior thoracic nerve (Bock, 1827)*
Macrodissected adult human root of ***long thoracic nerve (Quain & Wilson, 1839)*** arising from sixth ***cervical nerve (Galen, c173)***; in the original Latin, *radix inferior nerv. thoracicus posterior*; Table V, Figure 1-43.

longitudinal cerebral fissure (Gordon, 1815)

As described for macrodissected adult human, the dorsoventral (vertical) space between right and left ***cerebral cortex gray matter (>1840)*** lying rostral, dorsal, and caudal to the ***corpus callosum (Galen, c177)*** in the median plane; see Nieuwenhuys et al. (2008, Figs. 3.1-*1*, 5.3-*1*, 5.8-*12*, 5.28). For Gordon's use in macrodissected adult human, see p. 80, also see Burdach (1822, p. 386). It was first clearly described by Vesalius; see ***[longitudinal cerebral fissure (Gordon, 1815)] (Vesalius, 1543a)***.

EARLIER REFERENCES:

Described, not named or illustrated:

1. ***[longitudinal cerebral fissure (Gordon, 1815)] (Vesalius, 1543a)***
Although a longitudinal membrane separating the ***brain (Smith Papyrus, c1700 BC)*** into right and left halves was known since Hippocrates [see ***anterior part of brain (Aristotle)***], Vesalius first wrote clearly about a *groove* separating the two *lobes of brain (Vesalius, 1543a)*, and accompanying ***cerebral falx (Vesalius, 1543a)*** and two layers of ***pia (Galen, c192)***; see Singer translation (1952, p. 24 and Fig. 3 on p. 93).

Earlier synonyms:

1. *interstitium between hemispheres (Willis, 1664)*
Synonym for macrodissected adult human ***longitudinal cerebral fissure (Gordon, 1815)***; see Pordage translation (1681, p. 75) and *cerebral hemisphere (Willis, 1664)*.

LATER SYNONYMS:

1. *interlobar fissure (Cloquet, 1816)*
Synonym for macrodissected adult human ***longitudinal cerebral fissure (Gordon, 1815)***; in the original French, *scissure inter-lobar*, p. 528; Cloquet attributed the term without citation to Chaussier.
2. *incisura pallii (Burdach, 1822)*
Synonym for macrodissected adult human ***longitudinal cerebral fissure (Gordon, 1815)***; p. 165.
3. *great median fissure of cerebrum (Cruveilhier, 1836)*
Synonym for macrodissected adult human ***longitudinal cerebral fissure (Gordon, 1815)***; in the original French, *grande scissure médiane du cerveau*, p. 648.
4. *longitudinal fissure (Arnold, 1838a)*
Synonym for macrodissected adult human ***longitudinal cerebral fissure (Gordon, 1815)***; in the original Latin, *fissura longitudinalis*, p. 49.

longitudinal pontine fibers (Arnold, 1838b)

As described for macrodissected adult human, and mammal generally with histological methods for ***axons (Kölliker, 1896)***, the longitudinal ***white matter (Meckel, 1817)*** bundles between ***cerebral peduncle (Tarin, 1573)*** rostrally and ***pyramid (Willis, 1664)*** caudally, and contrasted with ***transverse pontine fibers (>1840)***; see Clark (1951, p. 898), *Terminologia Anatomica* (1998, p. 112), *Dorland's* (2003, p. 694). For Arnold's use in macrodissected adult human see Table IX, Figure 4-*h*. They were perhaps first clearly delineated by Malpighi; see ***[longitudinal pontine fibers (>1840)] (Malpighi, 1666)***.

TRANSLATIONS:

1. *fibrae longitudinales pontis (Arnold, 1838b)*
Original Latin form of ***longitudinal pontine fibers (Arnold, 1838b)***; Table IX, Figure 4-*h*.

EARLIER REFERENCES:

Described, not named or illustrated:

1. ***[longitudinal pontine fibers (>1840)] (Malpighi, 1666)***
Clearly included in description of "nerve fibers" from ***cerebral cortex gray matter (>1840)*** coursing through ***cerebral nuclei (Swanson, 2000a)*** and eventually ending in ***spinal cord (Galen, c162–c166)***; see Meyer (1967, p. 189). Malpighi dissected a variety of mammals including human, but the species used for this observation is unclear.

Illustrated and described, not named:

1. ***[longitudinal pontine fibers (>1840)] (Vieussens, 1684)***
Clearly illustrated and described for macrodissected adult human; see Table XVI between *D,G,F*. Also see Bell (1834, Pl. XIX).

Earlier synonyms:

1. *longitudinal tract (Vicq d'Azyr, 1786)*
Synonym for macrodissected adult human ***longitudinal pontine fibers (>1840)***; Plate XXII-*16/17*. Bell (1834, p. 474) wrote of "the longitudinal striated matter which passes from the crus cerebri and is prolonged to the corpus pyramidale" in macrodissected adult human, echoing an earlier statement by Mayo (1827; Pl. II, Fig. 5-*l*).
2. *pyramidal fibers in pons Varolii (Langenbeck, 1826–1830)*
Synonym for macrodissected adult human ***longitudinal pontine fibers (>1840)***; in the original Latin, *fibrae pyramidis in ponte Varolii*, Fascicle I, Table XXX, Figure 3-*b*.
3. *pyramidal bundles (>1840)*
Synonym for macrodissected adult human ***longitudinal pontine fibers (>1840)***; see Clark (1951, Fig. 784).

4. *pyramidal tracts (>1840)*
   Synonym for ***longitudinal pontine fibers (>1840)***, contrasted with ***pyramid (Willis, 1964)***; see Crosby et al. (1962, Fig. 134; and Fig. 127 for *pyramid*).

longitudinal striae (>1840)

As described for macrodissected adult human, tiny differentiations of the ***fimbria (Honegger, 1890)*** coursing along the dorsal surface of the ***corpus callosum (Galen, c177)*** near the median plane. There is a ***medial longitudinal stria (>1840)*** and a ***lateral longitudinal stria (Arnold, 1838a)*** on the right and on the left sides, and they are associated with the still obscure rostral ***gray matter (Meckel, 1817)*** remnants of the ***hippocampal region (Swanson et al., 1987)*** that are currently divided, from caudal to rostral, into ***fasciola cinerea (Arnold, 1838b)***, ***indusium griseum (Valentin, 1841)***, and ***tenia tecta (Swanson, 1992)***. For a very clear account of the earlier literature see Zuckerkandl (1887, p. 47 ff.); also see Dejerine & Dejerine-Klumpke (1895, Fig. 199 and p. 699 ff.) and Smith (1897). For more recent views see Wyss & Sripanidkulchai (1983), Künzle (2004), Nieuwenhuys et al. (2008, Fig. 3.18). For early human development see Hines (1922). They were first clearly delineated as the *longitudinal funiculi (Lancisi, 1713)*.

EARLIER REFERENCES:

Earlier synonyms:

1. *longitudinal funiculi (Lancisi, 1713)*
   Synonym for macrodissected adult human ***longitudinal striae (>1840)***; in the original Latin, *funiculi longitudinales*, p. 153; see Burdach (1822, p. 365). Lancisi distinguished a medial and a lateral funiculus or cord—the ***medial longitudinal stria (>1840)*** and ***lateral longitudinal stria (Arnold, 1838a)***, respectively; see Zuckerkandl (1887, p. 47 and Schema 7).
2. *longitudinal cords (Lancisi, 1713)*
   English form of *funiculi longitudinales*, or *longitudinal funiculi (Lancisi, 1713)*.
3. *small medullary cords (Winslow, 1733)*
   Synonym for macrodissected adult human *longitudinal cords (Lancisi, 1713)*; Section X, p. 34. Also see *raphe of corpus callosum (Winslow, 1733)*.
4. *tractes medullares (Haller, 1762)*
   Synonym for macrodissected adult human *longitudinal cords (Lancisi, 1713)*; p. 34 ff.; see Burdach (1822, p. 366).
5. *longitudinal cords of Lancisi (Mayer, 1779)*
   Eponym for macrodissected adult human *longitudinal cords (Lancisi, 1713)*; p. 6. Mayer used the German, *laenglichte Saite des Lanzisius*, and gave the Latin, *chordae longitudinales Lancisii*.
6. *raphe (Mayer, 1779)*
   Synonym for *longitudinal cords of Lancisi (Mayer, 1779)*; p. 6.
7. *longitudinal medullary tracts of corpus callosum (Vicq d'Azyr, 1786)*
   Synonym for macrodissected adult human *longitudinal cords (Lancisi, 1713)*; in the original French, *tractus médullaires longitudinaux du corps calleux*, Plate IV, Figure II-*x*.
8. *pyramidal process of corpus callosum (Günther, 1786)*
   Synonym for macrodissected adult human *longitudinal cords of Lancisi (Mayer, 1779)*; in the original Latin, *processus corporis callosi pyramidales*, p. 9.
9. *suture of corpus callosum (Günther, 1786)*
   Synonym for macrodissected adult human *longitudinal cords of Lancisi (Mayer, 1779)*; in the original Latin, *suturam corporis callosi*, p. 9.
10. *linea media mesolobii (Chaussier, 1807)*
    Synonym for macrodissected adult human *longitudinal cords (Lancisi, 1713)*; p. 47, see Burdach (1822, p. 365).
11. *striae of Lancisi (Reil, 1812c)*
    Eponym for macrodissected adult human ***longitudinal striae (>1840)***; in the original Latin, *linea Lancisii*, see translation (1823, p. 120). *Striae of Lancisi* is an English form of *linea Lancissi*. The most accurate description to date of these ***central nervous system white matter tracts (>1840)*** was given in Reil (1809b); see Burdach (1822, p. 365).
12. *linea Lancisii (Reil, 1812c)*
    Original Latin form of *striae of Lancisi (Reil, 1812c)*.
13. *longitudinal stria of Lancisi (Tiedemann, 1821)*
    Eponym for macrodissected adult human (singular) ***longitudinal striae (>1840)***; in the original Latin, *stria longitudinalis Lancisii*, Table II, Figure 1-*d*.
14. *external suture of corpus callosum (Bock, 1824)*
    Synonym for macrodissected adult human *suture of corpus callosum (Günther, 1786)*; in the original Latin, *sutura externa corporis callosi*, pp. 147–148.
15. *longitudinal tract of corpus callosum (Cruveilhier, 1836)*
    Synonym for macrodissected adult human ***longitudinal striae (>1840)***; in the original French, *tractus longitudinaux du corps calleux*, p. 673.
16. *longitudinal nerve of Lancisi (Cruveilhier, 1836)*
    Eponym for macrodissected adult human ***longitudinal striae (>1840)***; in the original French, *nerf longitudinal de Lancisi*, p. 673.

longitudinal tectal sulcus (>1840)

As described for macrodissected adult human, the arm of the ***cruciform sulcus (>1840)*** in the median plane, separating right ***superior colliculus (Haller, 1762)*** and ***inferior colliculus (Haller, 1762)*** from left ***superior colliculus (Haller, 1762)*** and ***inferior colliculus (Haller, 1762)***; see Williams & Warwick (1980, p. 935). It was known to Galen; see ***[longitudinal tectal sulcus (>1840)] (Galen, c173)***.

EARLIER REFERENCES:

Described, not named or illustrated:

1. ***[longitudinal tectal sulcus (>1840)] (Galen, c173)***
   In describing ***superior colliculi (Haller, 1762)*** and ***inferior colliculi (Haller, 1762)*** of macrodissected adult beef, pig, and/or macaque but not human, Galen must have observed it; see *little buttocks (Galen, c173, definition 1)*.

Illustrated and described, not named:

1. ***[longitudinal tectal sulcus (>1840)] (Vesalius, 1543a)***
   Clearly described and illustrated for macrodissected adult human; see Singer translation (1952, p. 106, Fig. 10).

Earlier synonyms:

1. *longitudinal furrow of corpora bigemina (Gordon, 1815)*
   Synonym for macrodissected adult human ***longitudinal tectal sulcus (>1840)***; p. 91.
2. *longitudinal groove of quadrigeminal tubercles (Tiedemann, 1816)*
   Synonym for macrodissected embryonic human ***longitudinal tectal sulcus (>1840)***; in the original German, *die Vierhügelmassen mit ihrer Längsfurche*, Table II, Figure 6-*f*. See translation (1826, Plate 4, Fig. 3-*f*).

lower subscapular nerve (>1840)

As described for macrodissected adult human, a branch of the ***brachial plexus dorsal cord (Paterson, 1887)*** innervating the caudal (lower) part of the subscapular muscle and ending by innervating the teres major muscle; see Williams & Warwick (1980, p. 1096). It was known to Galen; see ***[lower subscapular nerve (>1840)] (Galen, c173)***.

EARLIER REFERENCES:

Described, not named or illustrated:

1. ***[lower subscapular nerve (>1840)] (Galen, c173)***
   Galen clearly described innervation of subscapular muscle in macrodissected adult beef, pig, and/or macaque but not human; see May translation (1968, pp. 598–599), Duckworth translation (1962, pp. 243, 253, 257). Vesalius (1543a) also mentioned this supply for macrodissected adult human; see Richardson & Carman translation (2002, pp. 228–229, 233).

Earlier synonyms:

1. *subscapular nerve (Günther, 1786)*
   Synonym for macrodissected adult human ***lower subscapular nerve (>1840)***; in the original Latin, *nervus subscapularis*, p. 73.
2. *internal scapular nerve (Günther, 1786)*
   Synonym for macrodissected adult human ***lower subscapular nerve (>1840)***; in the original Latin, *nervus internus scapularis*, p. 73.
3. *third subscapular branch of brachial plexus (Cloquet, 1816)*
   Synonym for macrodissected adult human ***lower subscapular nerve (>1840)***; p. 644.

PARTLY CORRESPONDS:

1. *nerve to teres major muscle (Langenbeck, 1826–1830)*
   For macrodissected adult human, variable feature associated often with ***lower subscapular nerve (>1840)*** and innervating teres major muscle; in the original Latin, *nerv. ad musculum teretem majorem*, Fascicle III, Table XIII-3.
2. *nerve of teres major (Cruveilhier, 1836)*
   For macrodissected adult human, variable feature associated often with ***lower subscapular nerve (>1840)*** and innervating teres major muscle; in the original French, *nerf du grand rond*, p. 797.
3. *inferior subscapular nerve (Cruveilhier, 1836)*
   For macrodissected adult human, variable feature associated with ***lower subscapular nerve (>1840)*** innervating, together with *nerve of teres major (Cruveilhier, 1836)*, teres major muscle and lower part of subscapular muscle; in the original French, *nerf sous-scapulaire inférieur*, p. 797.

lumbar nerves (Diemerbroeck, 1672)

As described for macrodissected adult human, the five pairs of ***spinal nerves (Camper, 1760–1762)*** associated with the ***lumbar part of spinal cord (>1840)***; see Carpenter (1976, pp. 213–216). For Diemerbroeck's use in macrodissected adult human see p. 874. They were first clearly described by Galen; see ***[lumbar nerves (Diemerbroeck, 1672)] (Galen, c173)***.

EARLIER REFERENCES:

Described, not named or illustrated:

1. ***[lumbar nerves (Diemerbroeck, 1672) (Galen, c173)***
   In *On the Usefulness of the Parts*, Galen wrote about five ***nerves (Herophilus, c335–c280 BC)*** associated with five lumbar vertebrae in adult human; see May translation (1968, pp. 602–603). He used the specific terms ***cervical nerves (Galen, c173)*** and *sacral nerves (Galen, c173)*, but apparently not *lumbar nerves*. He dissected many mammalian species including monkey, but not explicitly human.

Earlier synonyms:

1. *nerves from medulla of kidney (Achillini, 1520)*
   Synonym for macrodissected adult human ***lumbar nerves (Diemerbroeck, 1672)***; see Lind translation (1975, p. 63).
2. *nerves of nape of kidney (Berengario da Carpi, 1523)*
   Synonym for macrodissected adult human ***lumbar nerves (Diemerbroeck, 1672)***; see Lind translation (1959, p. 160).

LATER SYNONYMS:

1. *nerves of loins (Diemerbroeck, 1689)*
   Synonym for macrodissected adult human ***lumbar nerves (Diemerbroeck, 1672)***; p. 560.
2. *lumbar intervertebral nerves (Schaarschmidt, 1750)*
   Synonym for macrodissected adult human ***lumbar nerves (Diemerbroeck, 1672)***; in the original Latin, *nervi intervertebrales lumborum*, p. 60.
3. *abdominal nerves (Bock, 1827)*
   Synonym for macrodissected adult human ***lumbar nerves (Diemerbroeck, 1672)***; in the original Latin, *nervi abdominalis*, Table VII, Figure 2-5.

lumbar part of spinal cord (>1840)

As described for macrodissected adult vertebrate, the longitudinal ***spinal cord part (>1840)*** generating the *lumbar nerves*; see Carpenter (1976, pp. 213–216). As described for macrodissected adult human, the longitudinal ***spinal cord part (>1840)*** generating the five

lumbar nerves (Diemerbroeck, 1672); see *Nomina Anatomica* (1983, p. A64), *Terminologia Anatomica* (1998, p. 105). It was first described as the *lumbar spinal medulla (Galen, c173)*.

EARLIER REFERENCES:

Earlier synonyms:

1. *lumbar spinal medulla (Galen, c173)*
   In *On the Usefulness of the Parts*, Galen specifically referred to macrodissected adult common large mammal (but not human) ***lumbar part of spinal cord (>1840)***; see May translation (1968, p. 651).
2. *medulla of kidney (Achillini, 1520)*
   Synonym for macrodissected adult human ***lumbar part of spinal cord (>1840)***; see Lind translation (1975, p. 63).
3. *nape of kidney (Berengario da Carpi, 1523)*
   Synonym for macrodissected adult human ***lumbar part of spinal cord (>1840)***; see Lind translation (1975, p. 160).
4. *lumbar part of spinal medulla (Tiedemann, 1821)*
   Synonym for macrodissected adult monkey ***lumbar part of spinal cord (>1840)*** with five ***lumbar nerves (Diemerbroeck, 1672)***; in the original Latin, *pars lumbaris medullae spinalis*, Table I, Figure 5-*f*.

lumbar plexus (Vesalius, 1543a)

As described for macrodissected adult human, it is commonly formed by the ***spinal nerve ventral branches (>1840)*** of the first three and the greater part of the fourth ***lumbar nerves (Diemerbroeck, 1672)***, although its arrangement is variable; see Durward (1951, p. 1089), Williams & Warwick (1980, p. 1106). The term has its origins in the passage quoted under ***lumbosacral plexus (Vesalius, 1543a)***; also see Richardson & Carman translation (2002, pp. 252, 257).

EARLIER REFERENCES:

Earlier synonyms:

1. *lumbo-abdominal plexus (Schmidt, 1794)*
   Synonym for macrodissected adult human ***lumbar plexus (Vesalius, 1543a)*** according to Meckel (1832, Vol. 3, p. 12).
2. *crural plexus (Reil, 1796)*
   Synonym for macrodissected adult human ***lumbar plexus (Vesalius, 1543a)***; in the original Latin, *plexum cruralem*, p. 31.
3. *lumbar part of crural plexus (Chaussier, 1809)*
   Synonym for macrodissected adult human ***lumbar plexus (Vesalius, 1543a)***.

PARTLY CORRESPONDS:

1. *second ansa lumbalis (Bock, 1827)*
   Macrodissected adult human part of ***lumbar plexus (Vesalius, 1543a)*** formed by roots of ***femoral nerve (Haller, 1762)*** from ***spinal nerve ventral branches (>1840)*** of second and third ***lumbar nerves (Diemerbroeck, 1672)***; in the original Latin, *ansa lumbalis secunda*, Table VI, Figure 1-*14*.
2. *third ansa lumbalis (Bock, 1827)*
   Macrodissected adult human part of ***lumbar plexus (Vesalius, 1543a)*** formed by roots of ***femoral nerve (Haller, 1762)*** from ***spinal nerve ventral branches (>1840)*** of third and fourth ***lumbar nerves (Diemerbroeck, 1672)***; in the original Latin, *ansa tertia lumbalis*, Table VI, Figure 1-*16*.
3. *fourth ansa lumbalis (Bock, 1827)*
   Macrodissected adult human part of ***lumbar plexus (Vesalius, 1543a)*** that is a ***communicating branch (Winslow, 1733)*** between fourth and fifth ***lumbar nerves (Diemerbroeck, 1672)***; in the original Latin, *ansa tertia lumbalis*, Table VI, Figure 1-*18*.
4. *communicating branch of first lumbar nerve with second lumbar nerve (Bock, 1827)*
   Apparently inconsistent feature of macrodissected adult human as described in term itself, shown on right but not left side; in the original Latin, *ram. communicans*, Table VII, Figure 1-*12*.
5. *communicating branch of second lumbar nerve with third lumbar nerve (Bock, 1827)*
   Rostral (upper) half of *second ansa lumbalis (Bock, 1827)*; in the original Latin, *ram. communicans*, Table VII, Figure 1-*15*. See Williams & Warwick (1980, Fig. 7.209).
6. *lumbo-dorsal communicating branch (Quain, 1828)*
   Macrodissected adult human delicate ***communicating branch (Winslow, 1733)*** at rostral end of ***lumbar plexus (Vesalius, 1543a)***, between 12th ***thoracic nerve (Diemerbroeck, 1672)*** and first ***lumbar nerve (Diemerbroeck, 1672)***; p. 284.
7. *dorsi-lumbar communicating branch (Quain, 1832)*
   Synonym for macrodissected adult human *lumbo-dorsal communicating branch (Quain, 1828)*; p. 694.
8. *dorsi-lumbar nerve (Quain & Wilson, 1839)*
   Synonym for macrodissected adult human *lumbo-dorsal communicating branch (Quain, 1828)*; Plate XXI-*a*.

lumbar plexus dorsal divisions (Paterson, 1887)

As described for macrodissected adult mammal, the ***lumbar plexus ventral branches (>1840)*** divide into ***lumbar plexus dorsal divisions (Paterson, 1887)*** and ***lumbar plexus ventral divisions (Paterson, 1887)*** related evolutionarily and developmentally (rather loosely in adult) to the dorsal (extensor) and ventral (flexor) musculature of the leg; see Durward (1951, p. 1115 and Fig. 937). It is not certain whether the first ***lumbar nerve (Diemerbroeck, 1672)*** typically participates in this arrangement; see Williams & Warwick (1980, p. 1119 and Fig. 7.209). For Paterson's use in mammal, see p. 621. They were known to Galen; see ***[lumbar plexus dorsal divisions (Paterson, 1887)] (Galen, c192)***.

EARLIER REFERENCES:

Described, not named or illustrated:

1. ***[lumbar plexus dorsal divisions (Paterson, 1887)] (Galen, c192)***
   Galen mentioned or alluded to, without naming, all of them in macrodissected adult beef, pig, and/or macaque but not human; see Duckworth translation (1962, pp. 262–263).

Illustrated and described, not named:

1. ***[lumbar plexus dorsal divisions (Paterson, 1887)] (Vesalius, 1543a)***
   Compared to Galen, Vesalius provided a poor description, clearly mentioning only those from second and third ***lumbar nerves (Diemerbroeck, 1672)*** in macrodissected adult human; see Richardson & Carman translation (2002, pp. 257–258). Vieussens probably illustrated all of them for macrodissected adult human (1684, Tab. 28).

PARTLY CORRESPONDS:

1. *first nerve entering thigh (Vesalius, 1543a)*
   Synonym for *first nerve entering leg (Vesalius, 1543a)*; see Richardson & Carman translation (2002, pp. 214, 215, items 57.1 and 58.1).
2. *first nerve entering leg (Vesalius, 1543a)*
   Consists of ***lateral cutaneous nerve of thigh (>1840)*** and lateral ***muscular branches of femoral nerve (Quain & Wilson, 1839)*** to sartorius, vastus lateralis, and rectus femoris muscles, for macrodissected adult human; see Richardson & Carman translation (2002, pp. 257 and 268-&).
3. *first sinew going under thigh (Geminus, 1553)*
   Synonym for macrodissected adult human *first nerve entering thigh (Vesalius, 1543a)*; originally spelled *firste synowe goynge under thigh*, see *The table of the figures of synowes*.
4. *first sinew of leg (Geminus, 1553)*
   Synonym for macrodissected adult human *first nerve entering leg (Vesalius, 1543a)*; originally spelled *firste synowe of legge*, see *The table of the figures of synwes*.
5. *nervus accessorius to cruralis (Winslow, 1733)*
   Macrodissected adult human branch of ***spinal nerve ventral branch (>1840)*** of third ***lumbar nerve (Diemerbroeck, 1672)***, or its continuation as ***lumbar plexus dorsal division (Paterson, 1887)***, joining ***femoral nerve (Haller, 1762)*** near distal end of psoas major muscle; Section VI, no. 287, p. 87.
6. *accessory crural nerve (Styx, 1782)*
   Synonym for macrodissected adult human *nervus accessorius to cruralis (Winslow, 1733)*; in the original Latin, *nervus cruralis accessorius*, pp. 7, 30. Also see Frotscher (1788; p. 95 of 1795 reproduction), Schmidt (1794, pp. 74–75), Meissner (1830, Vol. 3, p. 286).

lumbar plexus ventral branches (>1840)

As described for macrodissected adult human, the ***spinal nerve ventral branches (>1840)*** of the first four ***lumbar nerves (Diemerbroeck, 1672)*** involved in forming the ***lumbar plexus (Vesalius, 1543a)***; see Durward (1951, Fig. 937), Williams & Warwick (1980, p. 1106). They were first known as *anterior branches of nerves coming forth from lumbar vertebrae (Vesalius, 1543a)*.

EARLIER REFERENCES:

Earlier synonyms:

1. *anterior branches of nerves coming forth from lumbar vertebrae (Vesalius, 1543a)*
   Synonym for ***lumbar plexus ventral branches (>1840)*** mentioned in a not very straightforward way for macrodissected adult human; see Richardson & Carman translation (2002, pp. 252, 257 ff.).
2. *lumbar plexus anterior branches (Meckel, 1817)*
   Synonym for macrodissected adult human ***lumbar plexus ventral branches (>1840)***; see translation (1832, Vol. 3, p. 13).
3. *lumbar plexus abdominal branches (Meckel, 1817)*
   Synonym for macrodissected adult human ***lumbar plexus ventral branches (>1840)***; see translation (1832, Vol. 3, p. 13).

PARTLY CORRESPONDS:

1. *abdominal branches of first lumbar pair (Cruveilhier, 1836)*
   Apparently macrodissected adult human ***iliohypogastric nerve (Schmidt, 1794)*** and ***ilio-inguinal nerve (Schmidt, 1794)*** considered together; in the original French, *branches abdominales*, p. 831.
2. *ilio-scrotal branches of first lumbar pair (Cruveilhier, 1836)*
   Synonym for *abdominal branches of first lumbar pair (Cruveilhier, 1836)*; in the original French, *branches ilio-scrotal*, p. 831.

lumbar plexus ventral divisions (Paterson, 1887)

As described for macrodissected adult mammal, the ***lumbar plexus ventral branches (>1840)*** divide distally into ***lumbar plexus dorsal divisions (Paterson, 1887)*** and ***lumbar plexus ventral divisions (Patterson, 1887)*** related primitively and rather loosely in adult to the dorsal (extensor) and ventral (flexor) musculature of the leg; see Durward (1951, p. 1115 and Fig. 937). It is not certain whether the first ***lumbar nerve (Diemerbroeck, 1672)*** typically participates in this division; see Williams & Warwick (1980, p. 1119 and Fig. 7.209). For Patterson's use in macrodissected adult mammal, see p. 621. They were first described by Galen; see ***[lumbar plexus ventral divisions (Paterson, 1887)] (Galen, c192)***.

EARLIER REFERENCES:

Described, not named or illustrated:

1. ***[lumbar plexus ventral divisions (Paterson, 1887)] (Galen, c192)***
   All of them mentioned or alluded to, without naming, in macrodissected adult beef, pig, and/or macaque but not human; see Duckworth translation (1962, pp. 262–263). Compared to Galen, Vesalius (1543a) provided a poor description of them in macrodissected adult human; see Richardson & Carman translation (2002, pp. 257–258). In contrast, Vieussens probably illustrated all of them for macrodissected adult human (1684, Tab. 28).

Earlier synonyms:

1. *most anterior fasciculi of second–fourth lumbar nerves (Meckel, 1817)*
   Synonym for macrodissected adult human ***lumbar plexus ventral divisions (Paterson, 1887)*** used in describing origin of ***obturator nerve (Cheselden, 1726)***; see translation (1832, Vol. 3, p. 15) and Williams & Warwick (1980, Fig. 7.209).

PARTLY CORRESPONDS:

1. *middle musculocutaneous branch of lumbar plexus (Cloquet, 1816)*
   Probably macrodissected adult human branch of ***lumbar plexus ventral divisions (Paterson, 1887)*** associated with ***ilio-inguinal nerve (Schmidt, 1794)*** and/or ***iliohypogastric nerve (Schmidt, 1794)***; p. 662.
2. *musculo-cutaneous branches of lumbar plexus (Quain, 1828)*
   Macrodissected adult human ***ilio-inguinal nerve (Schmidt, 1794)*** and ***iliohypogastric nerve (Schmidt, 1794)*** considered together; p. 284.
3. *collateral branches of lumbar plexus (Cruveilhier, 1836)*
   Macrodissected adult human *abdominal branches of lumbar plexus (Cruveilhier, 1836)* and *inguinal branches of lumbar plexus (Cruveilhier, 1836)* considered together; in the original French, *branches collatérales*, p. 832.
4. *inguinal branches of lumbar plexus (Cruveilhier, 1836)*
   Macrodissected adult human ***ilio-inguinal nerve (Schmidt, 1794)*** and ***genitofemoral nerve (>1840)*** considered together; in the original French, *branches inguinales*, p. 833.

lumbar spinal ganglia (>1840)

As described for macrodissected adult human, there is one ***spinal nerve ganglion (Burdach, 1819)*** for each ***dorsal root (Spurzheim, 1826)*** of the five pairs of ***lumbar nerves (Diemerbroeck, 1672)***. They are numbered sequentially from rostral to caudal; see Williams & Warwick (1980, p. 1086). They were discovered by Coiter; see ***[lumbar spinal ganglia (>1840)] (Coiter, 1572)***.

EARLIER REFERENCES:

Described, not named or illustrated:

1. ***[lumbar spinal ganglia (>1840)] (Coiter, 1572)***
   Coiter stated there is a *knot (Coiter, 1572)*, or ***spinal nerve ganglion (Burdach, 1819)***, for each *spinal nerve (Vesalius, 1543a)* in macrodissected adult human; see translation (1955, p. 115).

lumbar splanchnic nerves (Cruveilhier, 1836)

As described for macrodissected adult human, there are commonly four of these medial, visceral branches arising from ***lumbar sympathetic ganglia (>1840)***, with the first ***lumbar splanchnic nerve (Cruveilhier, 1836)*** issuing from the first (rostralmost or upper) ***lumbar sympathetic ganglion (>1840)*** and joining the ***celiac plexus (Winslow, 1733)***, ***renal plexus (Drake, 1707)***, and ***intermesenteric plexus (>1840)***; the second ***lumbar splanchnic nerve (Cruveilhier, 1836)*** leaving the second and sometimes third ***lumbar sympathetic ganglion (>1840)*** and passing to the caudal (lower) part of the ***intermesenteric plexus (>1840)***; the third ***lumbar splanchnic nerve (Cruveilhier, 1836)*** leaving the third or fourth ***lumbar sympathetic ganglion (>1840)*** to join the ***superior hypogastric plexus (Tiedemann, 1822)***; and the fourth ***lumbar splanchnic nerve (Cruveilhier, 1836)*** arising from the last ***lumbar sympathetic ganglion (>1840)*** and ending in the caudal (lower) part of the ***superior hypogastric plexus (Tiedemann, 1822)*** or the ***hypogastric nerve (Walter, 1783)***; see Durward (1951, p. 1137 and Fig. 967), Mitchell (1953, pp. 259–261 and Figs. 110, 111), Williams & Warwick (1980, p. 1131). For Cruveilhier's use in macrodissected adult human, see p. 1024. They were vaguely distinguished by Vesalius; see ***[lumbar splanchnic nerves (Cruveilhier, 1836)] (Vesalius, 1543a)***.

TRANSLATIONS:

1. *nerfs splanchniques lombaires (Cruveilhier, 1836)*
   Original French form of ***lumbar splanchnic nerves (Cruveilhier, 1836)***; p. 1024.

EARLIER REFERENCES:

Illustrated and described, not named:

1. ***[lumbar splanchnic nerves (Cruveilhier, 1836)] (Vesalius, 1543a)***
   Referred to and illustrated in very general and confused way for macrodissected adult human: "As soon as this branch [***sympathetic trunk (Winslow, 1733)***], along with the great artery, has passed beyond the transverse septum [diaphragm], it begins to send out offshoots" (Richardson & Carman translation, 2002, p. 199). Willis (1664) described and illustrated three major ***lumbar splanchnic nerves (Cruveilhier, 1836)*** from ***sympathetic trunk (Winslow, 1733)*** to ***inferior mesenteric ganglion (Rau, 1720)*** of macrodissected adult human and quadruped; see Pordage translation (pp. 159, 170 and Tab. 11- ϕ). Vieussens illustrated them clearly for macrodissected adult human; Table 23-83.

Earlier synonyms:

1. *anterior branches of lumbar ganglia of intercostal nerve (Günther, 1786)*
   Synonym for macrodissected adult human ***lumbar splanchnic nerves (Cruveilhier, 1836)***; in the original Latin, *r. anteriores*, p. 96.
2. *internal branches of lumbar ganglia (Cruveilhier, 1836)*
   Synonym for macrodissected adult human ***lumbar splanchnic nerves (Cruveilhier, 1836)***; in the original French, *rameaux internes des ganglions lombaires*, p. 1025.
3. *lumbar aortic and splanchnic branches (Cruveilhier, 1836)*
   Synonym for macrodissected adult human ***lumbar splanchnic nerves (Cruveilhier, 1836)***; in the original French, *rameaux aortiques et splanchniques lombaires*, p. 1025.
4. *pelvic aortic and splanchnic branches (Cruveilhier, 1836)*
   Synonym for macrodissected adult human ***lumbar splanchnic nerves (Cruveilhier, 1836)***; in the original French, *rameaux aortiques et splanchniques pelviens*, p. 1025.

PARTLY CORRESPONDS:

1. *hypogastric branch of first accessory lumbar ganglion (Walter, 1783)*
   First macrodissected adult human ***lumbar splanchnic nerve (Cruveilhier, 1836)***; in the original Latin, *ramus hypogastricus ganglii accessorii lumbaris primi*, Table I-322.

2. *hypogastric branch of second accessory lumbar ganglion (Walter, 1783)*
Second macrodissected adult human ***lumbar splanchnic nerve (Cruveilhier, 1836)***; in the original Latin, *ramus hypogastricus ganglii accessorii lumbaris secundi*, Table I-*328*.
3. *internal branch of hypogastric nerve of second accessory lumbar ganglion (Walter, 1783)*
Internal branch of *hypogastric branch of second accessory lumbar ganglion (Walter, 1783)*; in the original Latin, *ramus internus nervi hypogastrici ganglii lumbaris accessorii secundi*, Table I-*330*.
4. *external branch of hypogastric nerve of second accessory lumbar ganglion (Walter, 1783)*
External branch of *hypogastric branch of second accessory lumbar ganglion (Walter, 1783)*; in the original Latin, *ramus externus nervi hypogastrici ganglii lumbaris accessorii secundi*, Table I-*333*.
5. *hypogastric branch of third lumbar ganglion (Walter, 1783)*
Third macrodissected adult human ***lumbar splanchnic nerve (Cruveilhier, 1836)***; in the original Latin, *ramus hypogastricus ganglii lumbaris tertii*, Table I-*338*. Distally called arterial or anterior branch of *hypogastric branch of third lumbar ganglion (Walter, 1783)*; in the original Latin, *nervi hypogastrici 338 ramus arteriosus seu anterior*, Table I-*341*.
6. *hypogastric branches of great sympathetic (Cloquet, 1828)*
As described for macrodissected adult human, ***lumbar splanchnic nerves (Cruveilhier, 1836)*** associated specifically with third and fourth ***lumbar sympathetic ganglia (>1840)***; in the original French, *rameaux hypogastriques du grand sympathique*, Plate CLXX, Figure 2-*67,70,71*.
7. *hypogastric branches of great sympathetic forming hypogastric plexus (Cloquet, 1828)*
Synonym for macrodissected adult human *hypogastric branches of great sympathetic (Cloquet, 1828)*; in the original French, *rameaux hypogastriques du grand sympathique qui forment le plexus du même nom*, Plate CLXXVI-*86*.
8. *splanchnic nerves of lumbar ganglia (Cruveilhier, 1836)*
For macrodissected adult human, ***lumbar splanchnic nerves (Cruveilhier, 1836)*** contributing to ***intermesenteric plexus (>1840)***; in the original French, *nerfs splanchniques des ganglions lombaires*, p. 1024.

lumbar sympathetic ganglia (>1840)

As described for macrodissected adult human, ***sympathetic trunk ganglia (Winslow, 1733)*** having ***gray communicating branches (>1840)*** with all ***lumbar nerves (Diemerbroeck, 1672)***, and ***white communicating branches (>1840)*** only with the first two, or occasionally three. There are typically four ***lumbar sympathetic ganglia (>1840)***, numbered sequentially from rostral (superior) to caudal (inferior); see Mitchell (1953, Ch. 17), Williams & Warwick (1980, p. 1131). The first accurate full account was probably given for each *lumbar ganglion of great sympathetic nerve (Walter, 1783)*.

EARLIER REFERENCES:

Earlier synonyms:

1. *lumbar ganglion of great sympathetic nerve (Walter, 1783)*
Five ***lumbar sympathetic ganglia (>1840)*** described for macrodissected adult human; in the original Latin, *ganglion lumbare nervi sympathici magni*, Table I:*61–148*.
2. *lumbar ganglion (Walter, 1783)*
Synonym for *lumbar ganglion of great sympathetic nerve (Walter, 1783)*; in the original Latin, *ganglion lumbare*, Table I:*78–148*.
3. *lumbar ganglia of intercostal nerve (Günther, 1786)*
Five macrodissected adult human ***lumbar sympathetic ganglia (>1840)*** identified; in the original Latin, *ganglia lumbaria nervus intercostalis*, p. 96 (and p. 92).
4. *ganglia lumbalia (Soemmerring, 1791)*
Alternate spelling (in Latin) of *lumbar ganglia (Walter, 1783)*; p. 329.
5. *lumbo-intercostal ganglia (Schmidt, 1794)*
Five macrodissected adult human ***lumbar sympathetic ganglia (>1840)*** identified; in the original French (singular), *ganglion lumbo-intercostale*, Table II:*1-5*.
6. *prelumbar ganglia (Cloquet, 1816)*
Synonym for macrodissected adult human ***lumbar sympathetic ganglia (>1840)*** attributed to Chaussier without citation; in the original French, *ganglions prélombaires*, p. 710.
7. *lumbar ganglions of limiting cord (Meckel, 1817)*
Synonym for macrodissected adult human ***lumbar sympathetic ganglia (>1840)***; see translation (1832, Vol. 3, p. 98).

PARTLY CORRESPONDS:

1. *ganglion hordeiforme (Günther, 1786)*
Fused ***lumbar sympathetic ganglia (>1840)*** with longitudinal orientation as described for macrodissected adult human; p. 96.

lumbosacral enlargement (>1840)

As described for macrodissected adult human, the ***spinal cord differentiation (>1840)*** associated with attachment of the ***spinal nerves (Camper, 1760–1762)*** to the legs, most commonly from the first ***lumbar nerve (Diemerbroeck, 1672)*** to the third ***sacral nerve (Camper, 1760)***; see Carpenter (1976, Fig. 9.1), *Terminologia Anatomica* (1998, p. 105), *Dorland's* (2003, p. 947). It was first clearly distinguished by Estienne; see ***[lumbosacral enlargement (>1840)] (Estienne, 1545)***.

TRANSLATIONS:

1. *intumescentia lumbosacralis (>1840)*
Latin form of ***lumbosacral enlargement (>1840)***; see *Terminologia Anatomica* (1998, p. 105).

EARLIER REFERENCES:

Illustrated, not named or described:

1. ***[lumbosacral enlargement (>1840)] (Estienne, 1545)***
Very clearly illustrated for macrodissected adult human; p. 338. According to Diemerbroeck (1689,

p. 406), Falloppio (1561) described it clearly, and Willis (1664) certainly described it; see Pordage translation (1681, pp. 124–125).

Earlier synonyms:

1. *lumbar prominence (Meckel, 1817)*
   Synonym for macrodissected adult human ***lumbosacral enlargement (>1840)***; see translation (1832, Vol. 2, p. 411). Arnold (1838b; Tab. I, Fig. 2-*q*) gave the Latin, *intumescentia lumbalis*.
2. *inferior enlargement (Serres, 1824–1826)*
   Synonym for macrodissected vertebrate ***lumbosacral enlargement (>1840)***; in the original French, *renflement inférieur*, Plate I, Figure 21-2 and later. Also see Quain & Wilson (1839, Pl. I, Fig. 2-*11*).
3. *lumbar swelling of spinal cord (Quain & Wilson, 1839)*
   Synonym for macrodissected adult human ***lumbosacral enlargement (>1840)***; Plate I, Figure 2-*11*.

lumbosacral plexus (Vesalius, 1543a)

As described for macrodissected adult human, it innervates the lower limb as well as generating the ***pudendal nerve (Camper, 1762)*** and ***perineal nerve (Camper, 1762)***, and commonly arises predominantly from the ***spinal nerve ventral branches (>1840)*** of the first ***lumbar nerve (Diemerbroeck, 1672)*** through the greater part of the third ***sacral nerve (Camper, 1760)***. When the ***plexus (Galen, c192)*** is supplied predominantly by the 12th ***thoracic nerve (Diemerbroeck, 1672)*** through the second ***sacral nerve (Camper, 1760)***, it is called *prefixed*; when it is supplied predominantly by the second ***lumbar nerve (Diemerbroeck, 1672)*** through the fourth ***sacral nerve (Camper, 1760)***, it is called *postfixed*; see Durward (1951, p. 1089), Williams & Warwick (1980, p. 1106). It is conventionally divided into ***lumbar plexus (Vesalius, 1543a)*** and ***sacral plexus (Vesalius, 1543a)*** connected by the ***lumbosacral trunk (Cruveilhier, 1836)***. The same basic plan underlies the organization of limb ***plexuses (Galen, c192)*** in mammals generally (Paterson, 1887). Vesalius (1543a) described it for macrodissected adult human: "Four nerves travel to the leg. They originate at the top of the femur from the pairs of nerves that arise from the spinal marrow within the lumbar vertebrae and sacrum, and emerge from a sort of netlike plexus, in the same way as described above with reference to the principal nerves traveling to the arm, though the plexus in the neck shows more variation than the one at the loins and sacrum." (Richardson & Carman translation, 2002, p. 257). Thus, in the passage he referred to a ***plexus (Galen, c192)*** associated with the loins (or lumbar vertebrae) and sacrum, a "lumbosacral plexus." It was known to Galen; see ***[lumbosacral plexus (Vesalius, 1543a)] (Galen, c173)***.

EARLIER REFERENCES:

Described, not named or illustrated:

1. ***[lumbosacral plexus (Vesalius, 1543a)] (Galen, c173)***
   In *On the Usefulness of the Parts*, Galen described but did not name this communication of ***nerves (Herophilus, c335–c280 BC)*** to the lower limb in macrodissected beef, pig, and/or macaque but not human; see May translation (1968, pp. 602–603), Duckworth translation (1962, pp. 260–264). He wrote that "It is from these nerves that, in part, sensation, and in part, sensation accompanied by voluntary movement, is imparted to the urinary bladder, to the genital organs, that is to say, in the woman the uteri and in the man the penis, to the rectum, to all the various fasciae found there, to the muscles of these organs which we have mentioned, and to the skin which envelops them." (Duckworth translation, 1962, p. 263).

LATER SYNONYMS:

1. *plexus of nerves traveling to leg (Vesalius, 1543a)*
   Synonym for ***lumbosacral plexus (Vesalius, 1543a)*** and illustrated for macrodissected adult human; see Richardson & Carman translation (2002, pp. 238, 257 ff., and figure following p. 263).
2. *sacral or lumbar plexus (Molinetti, 1675)*
   Apparently synonym for macrodissected adult human ***lumbosacral plexus (Vesalius, 1543a)***; p. 203.
3. *net-resembling fold for thighs and feet (Diemerbroeck, 1689)*
   Synonym for macrodissected adult human ***lumbosacral plexus (Vesalius, 1543a)***; p. 563.
4. *crural plexus (Chaussier, 1809)*
   Synonym for macrodissected adult human ***lumbosacral plexus (Vesalius, 1543a)***; in the original French, *plexus crural*.
5. *femoral plexus (Meckel, 1817)*
   Synonym for macrodissected adult human ***lumbosacral plexus (Vesalius, 1543a)***; in the original Latin, *plexus femoralis*, see translation (1832, Vol. 3, p. 12).

PARTLY CORRESPONDS:

1. *nerves to leg (Galen, c177)*
   Galen described four major cutaneous ***nerves (Herophilus, c335–c280 BC)*** and four major ***nerves (Herophilus, c335–c280 BC)*** to muscles of lower limb in macrodissected adult beef, pig, and/or macaque but not human arising from ***lumbosacral plexus (Vesalius, 1543a)***; see Singer translation (1999, pp. 83–87), Duckworth translation (1962, pp. 262–264). Vesalius (1543a) referred to them in macrodissected adult human; in the original Latin, *nervos crus petere*, see Richardson & Carman translation (2002, p. 257).
2. *nerves to foot (Bauhin, 1605)*
   Synonym for macrodissected adult human *nerves to leg (Galen, c177)*; see Crooke translation (1615, p. 904), where it is spelled *foote*.
3. *crural nerve (Crooke, 1615)*
   Refers to a macrodissected adult human *nerve to leg (Galen, c177)*; originally spelled *crurall nerve*, p. 492. Cooke's passage was translation of Bauhin (1605).
4. *nerves of thigh (Bartholin, 1651)*
   Synonym for macrodissected adult human *nerves to leg (Galen, c177)*; see Culpeper translation (1662, p. 333).
5. *terminal branches of lumbar plexus (Cruveilhier, 1836)*

Macrodissected adult human ***obturator nerve (Cheselden, 1726)***, ***femoral nerve (Haller, 1762)***, and ***lumbosacral trunk (Cruveilhier, 1836)***, considered together; in the original French, *branches terminales du plexus lombaire*, p. 838.

lumbosacral trunk (Cruveilhier, 1836)

As described for macrodissected adult human, the caudally directed (descending) ***communicating branch (Winslow, 1733)*** of the fourth ***lumbar plexus ventral branch (>1840)*** divides after emerging from the border of the psoas major muscle into a ***sacral plexus dorsal division (Paterson, 1887)*** and ***sacral plexus ventral division (Paterson, 1887)***, each joining a corresponding part of the first ***sacral plexus ventral branch (>1840)*** arising from the fifth ***lumbar spinal nerve (Diemerbroeck, 1762)***. The two resulting trunks are together called ***lumbosacral trunk (Cruveilhier, 1836)***; see Durward (1951, p. 1099), Williams & Warwick (1980, p. 1110 and Figs. 7.209, 213). For Cruveilhier's use in macrodissected adult human, see p. 839. It was first mentioned by Winslow; see ***[lumbosacral trunk (Cruveilhier, 1836)] (Winslow, 1733)***.

TRANSLATIONS:

1. *tronc lombo-sacré (Cruveilhier, 1836)*
   Original French form of ***lumbosacral trunk (Cruveilhier, 1836)***; p. 839.

EARLIER REFERENCES:

Described, not named or illustrated:

1. ***[lumbosacral trunk (Cruveilhier, 1836)] (Winslow, 1733)***
   Mentioned but not named for macrodissected adult human; Section VI, nos. 292 & 296, p. 88.

Earlier synonyms:

1. *lumbosacral cord (Bichat et al., 1801–1803)*
   Synonym for macrodissected adult human ***lumbosacral trunk (Cruveilhier, 1836)***; in the original French, *cordon lombo-sacré*, Vol. 3, p. 298.
2. *lumbo-sacral communicating branch (Quain, 1828)*
   Synonym for macrodissected adult human ***lumbosacral trunk (Cruveilhier, 1836)***; p. 284.
3. *communicating nerve (Quain, 1828)*
   Synonym for *lumbo-sacral communicating branch (Quain, 1828)*; p. 289.
4. *iliosacral nerve (Cloquet, 1828)*
   Synonym for macrodissected adult human ***lumbosacral trunk (Cruveilhier, 1836)***; in the original French, *nerf ilio-sacré*, Plate CLXX, Figure 1-*18*.
5. *lumbosacral nerve (Cruveilhier, 1836)*
   Synonym for macrodissected adult human ***lumbosacral trunk (Cruveilhier, 1836)***; in the original French, *nerf lombo-sacré*, pp. 832, 848.

lunate sulcus (>1840)

As described for macrodissected adult human, when present a short, dorsoventrally (vertically) oriented, slightly curved groove convex rostrally on the lateral surface of the ***occipital region (Vesalius, 1543)*** near the ***occipital pole (Broca, 1878a)***; see Williams & Warwick (1980, p. 986 and Fig. 7.111A), *Terminologia Anatomica* (1998, p. 125), *Dorland's* (2003, p. 1787). Kuhlenbeck (1928) found it in less than a third of the European ***brains (Smith Papyrus, c1700 BC)*** examined. It was perhaps first clearly delineated by Gall & Spurzheim; see ***[lunate sulcus (>1840)] (Gall & Spurzheim, 1810)***.

EARLIER REFERENCES:

Illustrated, not named or described:

1. ***[lunate sulcus (>1840)] (Gall & Spurzheim, 1810)***
   Clearly illustrated for macrodissected adult human; Plate VIII.

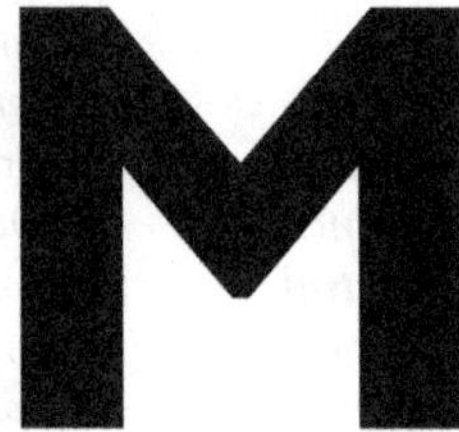

main olfactory bulb (>1840)

As described for adult human with macrodissection but primarily with histological methods, identical to the ***olfactory bulb (Weitbrecht, 1751)***, defined by an input from the ***olfactory nerve (Winslow, 1733)*** and classically divided into an ***olfactory nerve layer of main olfactory bulb (>1840)*** on the outside and five concentric and poorly differentiated ***gray matter (Meckel, 1817)*** layers on the inside. The ***cerebral cortex white matter (>1840)*** of the ***main olfactory bulb (>1840)*** is formed by the distal end of the ***olfactory limb of anterior commissure (>1840)*** surrounding a core ***subependymal zone (>1840)*** associated with the obliterated ***olfactory ventricle (>1840)***; see Crosby et al. (1962, pp. 414–416). In embryonic human the ***olfactory bulb (Weitbrecht, 1751)*** also contains a poorly differentiated ***accessory olfactory bulb (>1840)*** defined by input from the ***vomeronasal nerve (>1840)***, the ***gray matter (Meckel, 1817)*** layers are more clearly differentiated than in adult, and the ***olfactory ventricle (>1840)*** is open; see Crosby et al. (1962, pp. 414–416), Hamilton & Mossman (1972, Fig. 475). In macrosmatic adult mammal the ***main olfactory bulb (>1840)*** concentric layers are quite distinct histologically; in some species like ox, the ***olfactory ventricle (>1840)*** is open and a clear ***accessory olfactory bulb (>1840)*** is usually present; see Woollam (1958, p. 15), Shipley et al. (1996). ***Main olfactory bulb (>1840)*** and ***accessory olfactory bulb (>1840)*** were not distinguished by 1840.

mammillary body (Ludwig, 1779)

As described for macrodissected adult human, and based on cellular architecture and connections for mammals generally, the most caudal part of the ***medial hypothalamic zone (Nauta & Haymaker, 1969)*** lying caudal to the ***ventral premammillary nucleus (>1840)*** and ***dorsal premammillary nucleus (>1840)***. All recent accounts include at least two parts, ***medial mammillary nucleus (>1840)*** and ***lateral mammillary nucleus (>1840)***, which are the major contributors to the ***mammillothalamic tract (>1840)***, whereas the addition of other nearby ***gray matter regions (Swanson & Bota, 2010)*** varies greatly between authors; see Swanson (2004, Tab. B note *201*). For Ludwig's use in macrodissected adult human, see p. 73. Meyer (1971, p. 18) incorrectly credited Gall & Spurzheim (1810, pp. 222–223); in the original French (plural), *corps mammillaires*. Arnold (1838b, Pl. II, Fig. 34) showed its organization in transverse section of macrodissected adult human. It was probably first identified as the *little glands (Mondino, 1316)*.

TRANSLATIONS:

1. *corpora mammillaria (Ludwig, 1779)*
   Original Latin form (plural) of ***mammillary body (Ludwig, 1779)***; it was also used by Günther (1786, p. 16).

EARLIER REFERENCES:

Earlier synonyms:

1. *little glands (Mondino, 1316)*
   Two passages in Mondino's *Anathomia* apparently describe vaguely the ***mammillary body (Ludwig, 1779)***: **"The lacuna [*third ventricle (Galen, c173)*]** hath around it large round eminences [probably right and left ***hypothalamus (Kuhlenbeck, 1927)***]. These are made to sustain the veins or arteries which ascend from the *rete mirable* to the ventricles. In the base thereof do appear little glands [probably ***mammillary body (Ludwig, 1779)***] which project near the *rete mirable*." (Singer translation, 1925, p. 92). And, "The *rete* is supported by two glandular pieces of flesh made principally to support it..." (Singer translation, 1925, p. 94). Singer specifically identified these two structures as forming the ***mammillary body (Ludwig, 1779)***. Mondino dissected human cadavers. It was first illustrated for macrodissected adult human by Eustachi (1552), though not published until 1714 (see Pl. 18).

2. *two glandular pieces of flesh (Mondino, 1316)*
Synonym for *little glands (Mondino, 1316)*; see Singer translation (1925, p. 94).
3. *organa olfaciendi (Falloppio, 1561)*
Synonym for macrodissected adult human ***mammillary body (Ludwig, 1779)***; according to Schreger (1803, p. 324).
4. *cerebral testicles (Casseri, 1609)*
Synonym for macrodissected adult human ***mammillary body (Ludwig, 1779)*** in the first published illustration; p. 124, see Burdach (1822, p. 355), Meyer (1971, p. 18).
5. *testiculi cerebri (Casseri, 1609)*
Original Latin form of *cerebral testicles (Casseri, 1609)*; p. 124.
6. *glandulae duae candidae (Bartholin, 1651)*
Synonym for macrodissected adult human ***mammillary body (Ludwig, 1779)***; Table I-*ff*, p. 459.
7. *glandulae sub infundibulo (Marchetti, 1652)*
Synonym for macrodissected adult human ***mammillary body (Ludwig, 1779)***; p. 124.
8. *two white kernels (Bartholin, 1662)*
Culpeper's translation of *glandulae duae candidae (Bartholin, 1651)*; Table 1-*f*, p. 326. *Kernel* is synonym for *gland*; see *Oxford English Dictionary* (Online).
9. *glandulae candicantes (Willis, 1664)*
Synonym for macrodissected adult human ***mammillary body (Ludwig, 1779)***; p. 16, see Meyer (1971, p. 18). Willis pointed out that it lies behind (caudal to) thin membrane of *infundibulum (Galen, c173)*, whereas ***optic chiasm (Galen, c173)*** lies in front (rostral), and suggested that together they serve to protect the delicate *infundibulum (Galen, c173)*. He also observed that ***mammillary body (Ludwig, 1779)*** is double in human and single but larger in other mammals; see Pordage translation (1681, p. 66).
10. *glandula behind tunnel (Willis, 1664)*
Synonym for macrodissected adult human ***mammillary body (Ludwig, 1779)***; see Pordage translation (1681, Fig. I-*Y*) and *glandulae candicantes (Willis, 1664)*. Listed by Soemmerring as *glandulas pone infundibulum* (1778, p. 46), also see *glandulae sub infundibulo (Marchetti, 1652)*.
11. *kernel behind tunnel (Willis, 1664)*
Synonym for macrodissected adult human ***mammillary body (Ludwig, 1779)***; see Pordage (1681, translation Fig. I-*Y*) and *glandulae candicantes (Willis, 1664)*.
12. *two white glands behind tunnel (Willis, 1664)*
Synonym for macrodissected adult human ***mammillary body (Ludwig, 1779)***; see Pordage translation (1681, p. 66, Figs. I-*Y*, II-*X*), *glandulae candicantes (Willis, 1664)*, *glandulae duae albae ponè infundibulum (Willis, 1664)*. Based on comparative anatomy, Collins (1685, p. 1022) wrote, "About the middle region of the *Infundibulum* are seated *two whitish Glands* in Humane Brains, but in Brutes only one [***mammillary body (Ludwig, 1779)***], but far exceeding the other in magnitude, and seem to be constituted on this account instead of two soft Pillows made to secure the thin tender Membrane of the *Infundibulum* to rest upon, and to conserve it in its proper place on the one side, being supported on the other by the united Caudex of the Optic Nerves [***optic chiasm (Galen, c173)***]."
13. *glandulae duae albae ponè infundibulum (Willis, 1664)*
Latin form of *white glands behind tunnel (Willis, 1664)*; see Meyer (1971, p. 18).
14. *albicantes prominentiae duae pone infundibulum (Vieussens, 1684)*
Synonym for macrodissected adult human ***mammillary body (Ludwig, 1779)***; Table IV-*c*, see Meyer (1971, p. 20). Listed as *prominentias albicantes* by Soemmerring (1778, p. 47) and Burdach (1822, p. 355).
15. *two soft pillows (Collins, 1685)*
Synonym for *two white glands behind tunnel (Willis, 1664)*; p. 1022.
16. *two white protuberances behind infundibulum (Ridley, 1695)*
English form of *albicantes prominentiae duae pone infundibulum (Vieussens, 1684)*; Figure 1-*b*.
17. *two medullary protuberances behind infundibulum (Tyson, 1699)*
Synonym for *two white protuberances behind infundibulum (Ridley, 1695)*, from Tyson's description of macrodissected infant chimpanzee; Figure 13-*l*.
18. *small white bodies near infundibulum (Pourfour du Petit, 1710)*
Synonym for macrodissected adult human ***mammillary body (Ludwig, 1779)***; in the original French, *les petits corps blancs qui sont prés l'Antonnoir*, p. 13.
19. *orbicular protuberances (Heister, 1717)*
Synonym for macrodissected adult human ***mammillary body (Ludwig, 1779)***; p. 79. Burdach (1822, p. 355) attributed the term without citation to Munniks.
20. *bulbi fornicis (Santorini, 1724)*
Synonym for macrodissected adult human ***mammillary body (Ludwig, 1779)***; see Winslow (1733, Sect. X, p. 43), although simply an abbreviated form of *bulbi priorum crurum fornicis (Santorini, 1724)*. Santorini observed that ***mammillary body (Ludwig, 1779)*** has *white substance (Vesalius, 1543a)* on surface and *gray substance (Vesalius, 1543a)* within; see Burdach (1822, p. 356), Meyer (1971, p. 61). English form is *bulbs of fornix*; see Meckel (1832, Vol. 2, p. 451).
21. *bulbi priorum crurum fornicis (Santorini, 1724)*
Synonym for macrodissected adult human ***mammillary body (Ludwig, 1779)***; p. 60, see *bulbi fornicis (Santorini, 1724)*.
22. *protuberantiae crurum medullae oblongatae (Ruysch, 1728)*
Synonym for macrodissected adult human ***mammillary body (Ludwig, 1779)***; see Burdach (1822, p. 355).
23. *tubercula mammillaria (Winslow, 1733)*
Synonym for macrodissected adult human ***mammillary body (Ludwig, 1779)***; Section X, p. 43.

24. *mammillary tubercles (Winslow, 1733)*
English form of *tubercula mammillaria (Winslow, 1733)*; see Section X, p. 43.
25. *papillae medullares (Winslow, 1733)*
Winslow preferred *tubercula mammillaria (Winslow, 1733)* to this synonym; Section X, p. 43.
26. *mammillary protuberances (Lieutaud, 1742)*
Synonym for macrodissected adult human ***mammillary body (Ludwig, 1779)***; in the original French, *les protuberances mammillaires*, p. 399.
27. *eminentia candicans (Albinus, 1744)*
Synonym for macrodissected adult human ***mammillary body (Ludwig, 1779)*** in Albinus's description of Eustachian plates, referring back to *glandulae candicantes (Willis, 1664)*; Table 18, Figures 1, 3, 4, 5-*ϕ*. Listed by Soemmerring (1778) as *eminentiarum candicantium* (p. 47) and *eminentiae candicantes* (Tab. II-*R*). Burdach (1822, p. 355) attributed the term without citation to Lampers.
28. *orbicular eminence (Tarin, 1750)*
Synonym for macrodissected adult human ***mammillary body (Ludwig, 1779)***; Table I, Figure 4-*I*.
29. *orbicular body (Tarin, 1750)*
Synonym for macrodissected adult human ***mammillary body (Ludwig, 1779)***; Table II, Figure 1-*t*.
30. *protuberantia mammillares Santorini (Tarin, 1753)*
Eponym for macrodissected adult human ***mammillary body (Ludwig, 1779)***; p. 25.
31. *mamillary eminences (Haller, 1754a)*
Synonym for macrodissected adult human ***mammillary body (Ludwig, 1779)***; in the original Latin, *eminentiae mamillares*, Table I-*I*.
32. *globuli albicantia (Santorini, 1775)*
Synonym for macrodissected adult human ***mammillary body (Ludwig, 1779)***; p. 37.
33. *corpora albicantia (Santorini, 1775)*
Synonym for macrodissected adult human ***mammillary body (Ludwig, 1779)***; p. 37.
34. *glandulas albas (Soemmerring, 1778)*
Synonym for macrodissected adult human ***mammillary body (Ludwig, 1779)***; p. 46.
35. *protensiones glandulares (Soemmerring, 1778)*
Synonym listed for macrodissected adult human ***mammillary body (Ludwig, 1779)***, which Soemmerring attributed without citation to Ortlob; pp. 33, 46, see Burdach (1822, p. 355).
36. *protuberantias glandulosas (Soemmerring, 1778)*
Synonym listed for macrodissected adult human ***mammillary body (Ludwig, 1779)***, which Soemmerring attributed without citation to Petrioli; pp. 33, 45, see Burdach (1822, p. 355).
37. *eminentias glandulosas (Soemmerring, 1778)*
Synonym listed for macrodissected adult human ***mammillary body (Ludwig, 1779)***, which Soemmerring attributed without citation to Tarin; pp. 33, 45, see Burdach (1822, p. 355).
38. *corpora glandularia (Soemmerring, 1778)*
Synonym for macrodissected adult human ***mammillary body (Ludwig, 1779)***, which Soemmerring attributed without citation to Petrioli; pp. 33, 46–47, see Burdach (1822, p. 355).
39. *processus glandulosos (Soemmerring, 1778)*
Synonym listed for macrodissected adult human ***mammillary body (Ludwig, 1779)***, which Soemmerring attributed without citation to Petrioli; pp. 33, 47, see Burdach (1822, p. 355).
40. *processus mamillares (Soemmerring, 1778)*
Synonym listed for macrodissected adult human ***mammillary body (Ludwig, 1779)***, which Soemmerring attributed without citation to Andre; p. 47, see Burdach (1822, p. 355).
41. *mamillary process (Soemmerring, 1778)*
English form of *processus mamillares (Soemmerring, 1778)*.
42. *processus papillares (Soemmerring, 1778)*
Synonym for macrodissected adult human ***mammillary body (Ludwig, 1779)***, which Soemmerring attributed without citation to Andre; p. 47, see Burdach (1822, p. 355).
43. *cerebri portionem albam qua spinali medullae principium exporrigit (Soemmerring, 1778)*
Synonym for macrodissected adult human ***mammillary body (Ludwig, 1779)***, which Soemmerring attributed without citation to Cortesi; pp. 33, 47, see Burdach (1822, p. 355).
44. *eminentias papillares (Soemmerring, 1778)*
Synonym for macrodissected adult human ***mammillary body (Ludwig, 1779)***, which Soemmerring attributed without citation to Munniks; pp. 33, 47, see Burdach (1822, p. 355).
45. *hemisphaericorum tuberculorum (Soemmerring, 1778)*
Synonym Soemmerring suggested for macrodissected adult human ***mammillary body (Ludwig, 1779)***; plural, *tubercula hemisphaerica*, pp. 33, 47, see Burdach (1822, p. 355).

LATER SYNONYMS:

1. *bulbi Santorini (Haase, 1781)*
Eponym for macrodissected adult human ***mammillary body (Ludwig, 1779)***; p. 25.
2. *mammillary bodies of Willis (Günther, 1786)*
Eponym for macrodissected adult human ***mammillary body (Ludwig, 1779)***; evidently a careless mistake, "*Corpora mammillaria* WILLISII s. *eminentiae candicantes* [Willis's term], s. *bulbi* SANTORINI..." (p. 16).
3. *pyriform tubercles (Burdin, 1803)*
Synonym for macrodissected adult human ***mammillary body (Ludwig, 1779)***; see translation (1803, Vol. 1, p. 164).
4. *pisiform tubercles (Burdin, 1803)*
Synonym for macrodissected adult human ***mammillary body (Ludwig, 1779)***; see translation (1803, Vol. 1, p. 220).
5. *bulbs of vault with three pillars (Chaussier, 1807)*

Synonym listed for macrodissected adult human ***mammillary body (Ludwig, 1779)***; in the original French, *les bulbes de la voûte à trois piliers*, p. 42. Cruveilhier (1836, p. 679) simply used *bulbe de la voûte*, that is, *bulb of vault*.

6. *onions of vault with three pillars (Chaussier, 1807)*
   Synonym listed for macrodissected adult human ***mammillary body (Ludwig, 1779)***; in the original French, *les oignons de la voûte à trois piliers*, p. 42.
7. *eminentiae candicantes (Chaussier, 1807)*
   Synonym for macrodissected adult human ***mammillary body (Ludwig, 1779)***; p. 42.
8. *nodule of anterior root of crus of fornix (Reil, 1812c)*
   Synonym for macrodissected adult human ***mammillary body (Ludwig, 1779)***; see Mayo translation (1823, p. 52, Tab. XIII-*i*).
9. *medullary eminences (Meckel, 1817)*
   Synonym listed for macrodissected adult human ***mammillary body (Ludwig, 1779)***; in the original Latin, *eminentiae medullares*, see translation (1832, Vol. 2, p. 437).
10. *globuli (Burdach, 1822)*
    Synonym for macrodissected adult human ***mammillary body (Ludwig, 1779)***; p. 137.
11. *optic lobule (Serres, 1824–1826)*
    Synonym for macrodissected adult human ***mammillary body (Ludwig, 1779)***, and for a similarly placed eminence that may or may not be the same in all vertebrates; in the original French, *lobule optique*, pp. 498–513. Serres noted without citation that in bird Haller equated it with *mammillary eminences (Haller, 1754a)* and that Malacarne used *apophyses médullaires des nerfs optiques*.
12. *optic tubercle (Serres, 1824–1826)*
    Synonym for *optic lobule (Serres, 1824–1826)*; in the original French, *tubercule optique*, p. 504.
13. *maxillary eminences (Desmoulins, 1825)*
    Synonym for macrodissected adult human ***mammillary body (Ludwig, 1779)***; in the original French, *éminences maxillaires*, Plate XIII, Figure 1-*m*.
14. *mamillary body (His, 1895)*
    Alternate spelling of ***mammillary body (Ludwig, 1779)***; in the original Latin, *corpus mamillary*, p. 85. Also note singular rather than plural form in original usage.

mammillary peduncle (>1840)

As described in adult human and other mammals with histological methods for ***axons (Kölliker, 1896)***, a small longitudinal ***central nervous system white matter tract (>1840)*** extending between the caudal and lateral end of the ***mammillary body (Ludwig, 1779)*** rostrally and ventrally, and the ***tegmentum (Swanson, 2000b)*** of the ***midbrain (Baer, 1837)*** caudally and more dorsolaterally; see Nauta & Haymaker (1969, p. 172), Nieuwenhuys et al. (2008, p. 293). It was not known by 1840.

EARLIER REFERENCES:

Earlier synonyms:

1. *mamillary body peduncle (Honegger, 1890)*
   Synonym for adult mammalian ***mammillary peduncle (>1840)*** observed with histological methods for ***axons (Kölliker, 1896)***; in the original Latin, *pedunculus corporis mamillaris*, see p. 353 ff. Kölliker (1896, p. 491) spelled it *pedunculus corporis mammillaris*.

mammillary recess (>1840)

As described for macrodissected adult human and certain other mammals, a narrow caudoventral extension of the ***hypothalamic part of third ventricle (Swanson, 2004)*** into the ***mammillary body (Ludwig, 1779)***. For an early use of the term and illustration for macrodissected adult human, see Edinger (1893, Fig. 67, abbreviated *Recess. Mam.*). For rat see Swanson (2004, Atlas Levels 33–35). It was first delineated by Steno; see ***[mammillary recess (>1840)] (Steno, 1669)***.

EARLIER REFERENCES:

Illustrated, not named or described:

1. ***[mammillary recess (>1840)] (Steno, 1669)***
   Illustrated clearly in first accurate midsagittal view of macrodissected adult human ***brain (Smith Papyrus, c1700 BC)***; Plates I & II. Tiedemann (1816) described and illustrated it for 5-month human fetus; see translation (1826, p. 71 and Pl. VI, Fig. 1-*q*).

mammillary sulcus (>1840)

As described for macrodissected adult human, the longitudinal groove in the median plane dividing the ***mammillary body (Ludwig, 1779)*** into right and left superficial eminences; see Nauta & Haymaker (1969, Fig. 4.2). It was known to Mondino; see ***[mammillary sulcus (>1840)] (Mondino, 1316)***.

EARLIER REFERENCES:

Described, not named or illustrated:

1. ***[mammillary sulcus (>1840)] (Mondino, 1316)***
   In describing macrodissected adult human ***mammillary body (Ludwig, 1779)*** as *two glandular pieces of flesh (Mondino, 1316)*, Mondino must have observed the groove distinguishing them; see Singer translation (1925, p. 94).

Earlier synonyms:

1. *longitudinal groove separating mammillary bodies (Tiedemann, 1816)*
   Synonym for ***mammillary sulcus (>1840)***; in the original German, *eine schwache Längsvertiefung*, see translation (1826, p. 265).

mammillotegmental tract (Kölliker, 1896)

As described in macrodissected adult human, and mammal generally with histological methods for ***axons (Kölliker, 1896)***, a longitudinal ***central nervous system white matter tract (>1840)*** between the dorsal (distal) end of the ***principal mammillary tract (Kölliker, 1896)*** and certain more caudal ***central nervous system gray matter regions (>1840)***, including ***dorsal tegmental nucleus (>1840)*** and ***ventral tegmental nucleus (>1840)***; see Hayakawa & Zyo (1989, Fig. 12), Allen & Hopkins (1990). For topographic description, it has ***hypothalamic mammillothalamic tract (>1840)*** and ***tegmental mammillotegmental tract (>1840)*** segments. For Kölliker's use in adult rabbit with histological methods for ***axons (Kölliker, 1896)***, see p. 517 and Figure 643-*Ftm*. Cajal (1895, p. 99 and Fig. 26-C) discovered its axonal relationship with the ***principal mammillary tract (Kölliker, 1896)***. It was first clearly delineated by Vicq d'Azyr; see ***[mammillotegmental tract (>1840)] (Vicq d'Azyr, 1786)***.

TRANSLATIONS:

1. *fasciculus tegmento-mammillaris (Kölliker, 1896)*
   Original Latin form of ***mammillotegmental tract (Kölliker, 1896)***; p. 517 and Figure 643.

EARLIER REFERENCES:

Illustrated and described, not named:

1. ***[mammillotegmental tract (>1840)] (Vicq d'Azyr, 1786)***
   Described and illustrated clearly in macrodissected adult human, although ***principal mammillary tract (Kölliker, 1896)*** not distinguished; Plate XXV, Figure II-*41*.

Earlier synonyms:

1. *Hauben-Bündel (Gudden, 1889)*
   German synonym for ***mammillotegmental tract (>1840)*** in histological sections of adult rabbit; see Table XXX, Figure 5-*HB*, where *Gudden'sches Ganglion* or ***ventral tegmental nucleus (>1840)*** and *dorsales Ganglion* or ***dorsal tegmental nucleus (>1840)*** are also shown. An English form is *tegmental bundle*.

mammillothalamic tract (Kölliker, 1896)

As described in macrodissected adult human, and mammal generally with histological methods for ***axons (Kölliker, 1896)***, a transverse ***central nervous system white matter tract (>1840)*** between the dorsal (distal) end of the ***principal mammillary tract (Kölliker, 1896)*** ventrally and the ***anterior thalamic nuclei (>1840)*** dorsally. For topographic description it has a ***hypothalamic mammillothalamic tract (>1840)*** segment ventrally and a ***thalamic mammillothalamic tract (>1840)*** segment dorsally, ending in the right and left ***anterior thalamic nuclei (>1840)*** with a commissural part of the ***thalamic mammillothalamic tract (>1840)*** crossing the median plane in the ***middle commissure (>1840)***. For Kölliker's use in adult rabbit with histological methods for ***axons (Kölliker, 1896)***, see p. 517 and Figure 643-*Fthm*. Cajal (1895, p. 99 and Fig. 26-*V*) discovered its axonal relationship with the ***principal mammillary tract (Kölliker, 1896)***; also see Hayakawa & Zyo (1989, Fig. 12), Szabó et al. (2011). It was first clearly described by Pourfour du Petit; see ***[mammillothalamic tract (>1840)] (Pourfour du Petit, 1710)***. Willis may have dissected but misinterpreted it; see ***[mammillothalamic tract (>1840)] (Willis, 1672)***.

TRANSLATIONS:

1. *fasciculus thalamo-mammillaris (Kölliker, 1896)*
   Original Latin form of ***mammillothalamic tract (Kölliker, 1896)***; p. 517 and Figure 643.

EARLIER REFERENCES:

Illustrated, not named or described:

1. ***[mammillothalamic tract (>1840)] (Willis, 1672)***
   Possibly macrodissected but misinterpreted in adult human; see Pordage translation (1683, Tab. VIII-S).

Described, not named or illustrated:

1. ***[mammillothalamic tract (>1840)] (Pourfour du Petit, 1710)***
   Pourfour du Petit described for macrodissected adult human a ***central nervous system white matter tract (>1840)*** between ***mammillary body (Ludwig, 1779)*** and ***anterior thalamic nuclei (>1840)***; p. 13, see Meyer (1971, p. 20). He did not distinguish the ***principal mammillary tract (Kölliker, 1896)***. Also see *subrotunda corpora alba (Vieussens, 1684)* and ***[postcommissural fornix (Loo, 1931)] (Pourfour du Petit, 1710)***.

Illustrated and described, not named:

1. ***[mammillothalamic tract (>1840)] (Vicq d'Azyr, 1786)***
   Clearly described and illustrated for macrodissected adult human; Plate XII-*12*; Plate XXV, Figure II-*a*. Also see Vicq d'Azyr (1784, pp. 527, 561).

Earlier synonyms:

1. *root of fornix (Reil, 1809b)*
   Synonym for macrodissected adult human ***mammillothalamic tract (>1840)***; p. 144, see Mayo translation (1823, p. 52). In the original German, *umgekehrte Wurzel der Zwillingsbinde*; see Burdach (1822, p. 355).
2. *root of anterior pillar of fornix (Tiedemann, 1816)*
   Synonym for *root of fornix (Reil, 1809b)* in macrodissected fetal human; see translation (1826, p. 108), where it is misspelled *roof of anterior pillar of fornix* on p. 102.
3. *descending root of fornix (Burdach, 1822)*
   Synonym for macrodissected adult human ***mammillothalamic tract (>1840)***; in the original Latin (plural), *radix descendens*, p. 137.
4. *medullary cord (Rolando, 1825a)*
   Synonym for macrodissected adult beef ***mammillothalamic tract (>1840)*** seen in transverse section; in the original French (plural), *cordons médullaires*, Table VIII, Figures 1–4 part *x*. However, later in the Table the same term is applied to other structures; in Figure 6 it might possibly indicate ***mammillotegmental tract (>1840)***, whereas in Figure 7 it clearly indicates ***medial longitudinal fascicle (>1840)***. It is unknown whether Rolando regarded these features as part of one tract, although it is not indicated in Figure 5, possibly suggesting a discontinuity.
5. *internal posterior cord of mammillary bodies (Spurzheim, 1826)*
   Synonym for macrodissected adult human ***mammillothalamic tract (>1840)***; p. 227.
6. *descending root of mammillary body (Arnold, 1838a)*
   Synonym for macrodissected adult human ***mammillothalamic tract (>1840)***; in the original Latin (and German), *radix descendens* des *corporus mammillare*, p. 62.
7. *radix descendens corporum candicantium (Arnold, 1838a)*
   Synonym for *descending root of mammillary body (Arnold, 1838a)*; p. 81.
8. *ascending branch of crus fornicis (Meynert, 1872)*
   Synonym for macrodissected adult human ***mammillothalamic tract (>1840)***; Figure 269-*Fa*.

9. *Vicq d'Azyr's fascicle (Forel, 1877)*
   Eponym for macrodissected adult human ***mammillothalamic tract (>1840)***; in the original German, *Vicq d'Azyr'sches Bündle*, abbreviated *F. Vc.* on p. 491.
10. *ascending root of trigone (Dejerine & Dejerine-Klumpke, 1895)*
   Synonym for macrodissected adult human ***mammillothalamic tract (>1840)***; p. 347.

mandibular nerve (>1840)

As described for macrodissected adult human, the ventral (lower) and largest of the three primary ***trigeminal nerve branches (Winslow, 1733)***, both sensory and motor in function, with the ***trigeminal nerve motor root (Bell, 1829)*** joining the ***mandibular nerve sensory root (>1840)*** to form the ***mandibular nerve trunk (>1840)***. It supplies the teeth and gums of the mandible; skin of the temporal region, part of the auricle, lower lip, and lower part of the face; muscles of mastication; and mucous membrane of the rostral (anterior) part of the tongue and floor of the mouth; see Williams & Warwick (1980, p. 1066 and Fig. 7.177), *Terminologia Anatomica* (1998, p. 134). It was known to Galen; see ***[mandibular nerve (>1840)] (Galen, c173)***.

EARLIER REFERENCES:

Described, not named or illustrated:

1. ***[mandibular nerve (>1840)] (Galen, c173)***
   Described for macrodissected adult beef, pig, and/or macaque but not human; see May translation (1968, pp. 440, 686), Duckworth translation (1992, p. 193).

Illustrated, not named or described:

1. ***[mandibular nerve (>1840)] (Eustachi, 1552)***
   Clearly illustrated for macrodissected adult human; see Albinus edition (1761; Tab. 18, Figs. 1, 3, 4-*I* and 2-*Y*).

Earlier synonyms:

1. *fifth pair of nerves from brain (Benedetti, 1502)*
   Corresponds roughly to macrodissected adult human ***mandibular nerve (>1840)***; see Lind translation (1975, pp. 117, 118).
2. *third trunk of third pair (Falloppio, 1561)*
   Synonym for macrodissected adult human ***mandibular nerve (>1840)***; Falloppio also referred to it as one of three *shoots of third pair*; see Harvey (1961, notes 830 and 844) and *third pair of nerves from brain (Falloppio, 1561)*.
3. *third branch of third pair (Marchetti, 1652)*
   Synonym for macrodissected adult human *third trunk of third pair (Falloppio, 1561)*; p. 122.
4. *lower branch of fifth pair of nerves arising within skull (Willis, 1664)*
   Roughly synonymous with macrodissected adult, presumably human, ***mandibular nerve (>1840)***; see Pordage translation (1681, p. 141).
5. *first division of fifth pair of nerves arising within skull (Willis, 1664)*
   Roughly synonymous with macrodissected adult, presumably human, ***mandibular nerve (>1840)***; see Pordage translation (1681, p. 145, Fig. 1-*G*).
6. *ramus major posterior nervus quintae conjugationis (Vieussens, 1684)*
   Synonym for macrodissected adult human ***mandibular nerve (>1840)***; p. 172 and Table 22-*H*.
7. *third trunk of fifth pair (Rau, 1694)*
   Synonym for *third trunk of third pair (Falloppio, 1561)*; in the original Latin, *truncus tertius, quinti paris*, p. 193.
8. *posterior branch of fifth pair (Rau, 1694)*
   Synonym for ***mandibular nerve (>1840)***; in the original Latin, *posterior ramus, quinti paris*, p. 193.
9. *posterior largest branch of fifth pair (Ridley, 1695)*
   Translation of macrodissected adult human *ramus major posterior nervus quintae conjugationis (Vieussens, 1684)*; p. 147.
10. *inferior maxillary branch of fifth nerve (La Charrère, 1703)*
   Synonym for macrodissected adult human ***mandibular nerve (>1840)***; in the original French, *la branche maxillarre inferieure*, p. 221.
11. *inferior maxillary nerve (Heister, 1717)*
   Synonym for macrodissected adult human ***mandibular nerve (>1840)***; in the original Latin, *nervus maxillaris inferior*, see translation (1721, p. 245).
12. *inferior branch of trigeminal nerve (Winslow, 1733)*
   Synonym for macrodissected adult human ***mandibular nerve (>1840)***; Section VI, pp. 61–63.
13. *inferior branch of fifth pair (Winslow, 1733)*
   Synonym for macrodissected adult human ***mandibular nerve (>1840)***; Section VI, p. 63.
14. *third branch of fifth pair of nerves (Meckel, 1753)*
   Synonym for macrodissected adult human ***mandibular nerve (>1840)***; in the original French, *le troisième rameau de la cinquième paire des nerfs*, p. 26.
15. *third nerve of fifth pair (Meckel, 1753)*
   Synonym for *third branch of fifth pair of nerves (Meckel, 1753)*; in the original French, *le troisième nerf de la cinquième paire*, p. 88.
16. *inferior masticatory nerve (Malacarne, 1791)*
   Synonym for macrodissected adult human ***mandibular nerve (>1840)***; p. 233.
17. *ninth pair of nerves (Malacarne, 1791)*
   Inferior masticatory nerve (Malacarne, 1791) listed as 9th of 17 pairs of *cerebral nerves (Malacarne, 1791)*; p. 233.
18. *gustatory nerve (Soemmerring, 1791)*
   Synonym for macrodissected adult human ***mandibular nerve (>1840)***; in the original Latin, *nervus gustatorius*, p. 210.
19. *third division of fifth nerve (Bell, 1803a)*
   Synonym for macrodissected adult human ***mandibular nerve (>1840)***; Plate 1-*N*.
20. *lower maxillary nerve (Bell, 1803b)*
   Synonym for macrodissected adult human ***mandibular nerve (>1840)***; p. 144.
21. *maxillary nerve (Burdin, 1803)*
   Synonym for macrodissected adult human ***mandibular nerve (>1840)***; see translation (1803, Vol. 1, p. 170).

22. *third principal branch of fifth pair (Meckel, 1817)*
    Minor variation on *posterior largest branch of fifth pair (Ridley, 1695)*; see translation (1832, Vol. 3, p. 71).
23. *inframaxillary branch of trigeminal nerve (Bojanus, 1819–1821)*
    Synonym for macrodissected adult turtle ***mandibular nerve (>1840)***; in the original Latin, *ramus inframaxillaris nervus trigeminus*, Figure 87:V-*y*.
24. *third trunk of three-fold nerve (Swan, 1830)*
    Synonym for macrodissected adult human ***mandibular nerve (>1840)***; p. 17.
25. *third trunk of fifth nerve (Swan, 1830)*
    Synonym for macrodissected adult human ***mandibular nerve (>1840)***; Plate XII, Figure 1-3.
26. *inframaxillary nerve (Quain & Wilson, 1839)*
    Synonym for macrodissected adult human ***mandibular nerve (>1840)***; in the original Latin, *n. infra-maxillaris*, Plate XIII, Figure 2-*D*.

PARTLY CORRESPONDS:

1. *thicker root of third pair of cerebral nerves (Vesalius, 1543a)*
   Probably sensory component of macrodissected adult human ***mandibular nerve (>1840)***; see Richardson & Carman translation (2002, pp. 188–189).
2. *roots of inferior masticatory nerve (Malacarne, 1791)*
   Unclear feature of macrodissected adult human ***mandibular nerve (>1840)***; pp. 233–234.
3. *collateral branches of inferior maxillary nerve (Cruveilhier, 1836)*
   Macrodissected adult human ***deep temporal nerves (Haase, 1781)***, ***masseteric nerve (Meckel, 1748)***, ***buccal nerve (Meckel, 1748)***, ***medial pterygoid nerve (>1840)***, and ***auriculotemporal nerve (Haller, 1762)***, considered together; in the original French, *branches collatérales*, p. 930.
4. *inferior branches of inferior maxillary nerve (Cruveilhier, 1836)*
   Macrodissected adult human ***lingual nerve (Vesalius, 1543a)*** and ***inferior dental nerve (Meckel, 1817)*** considered together; in the original French, *rameaux inférieurs*, p. 929.
5. *terminal branches of inferior maxillary nerve (Cruveilhier, 1836)*
   Synonym for *inferior branches of inferior maxillary nerve (Cruveilhier, 1836)*; in the original French, *branches terminales*, p. 933.

mandibular nerve sensory root (>1840)

As described for macrodissected adult human, short distal extension of the ***trigeminal ganglion (>1840)*** passing with the ***trigeminal nerve motor root (Bell, 1829)*** in ***dura (Galen, c177)*** of the middle cranial fossa to the foramen ovale, through which they both emerge into the infratemporal fossa; as they leave the skull they combine to form a single, short ***mandibular nerve trunk (>1840)***; see Durward (1951, p. 1026), Williams & Warwick (1980, p. 1066 and Fig. 7.181), *Dorland's* (2003, p. 1641). It was probably known to Vesalius; see *greater or thicker root of third pair of nerves (Vesalius, 1543a)*.

EARLIER REFERENCES:

Earlier synonyms:

1. *greater or thicker root of third pair of nerves (Vesalius, 1543a)*
   From description and illustration probably corresponds to macrodissected adult human ***mandibular nerve sensory root (>1840)*** that passes through foramen ovale; see Richardson & Carman translation (2008, pp. 170, 189). Also see Geminus (1553, *The table of the figure of synowes*).
2. *thicker and greater root of third pair of sinews of brain (Geminus, 1553)*
   Synonym for macrodissected adult human *greater or thicker root of third pair of nerves (Vesalius, 1543a)*; originally spelled *thycker and greater roote of thyrde payre of synowes of brayne*, see *The tables of the brayne*, Figure 14-*I*. Also see *The table of the figures of sinowes*, Figure 7-*L*.
3. *greater and grosser root of third pair of sinews of brain (Geminus, 1553)*
   Synonym for macrodissected adult human *greater or thicker root of third pair of nerves (Vesalius, 1543a)*; originally spelled *greater and grosser roote of thirde payre of synowes of brayne*, see *The tables of the brayne*, Figure 14-*K*. Also see *The table of the figures of sinowes*, Figure 7-*L*.

mandibular nerve trunk (>1840)

As described for macrodissected adult human, short segment of the ***mandibular nerve (>1840)*** starting where the ***trigeminal nerve motor root (Bell, 1829)*** and ***mandibular nerve sensory root (>1840)*** merge, giving off the ***nervus spinosus (>1840)*** and ***medial pterygoid nerve (>1840)*** before splitting distally into ***anterior branch of mandibular nerve (>1840)*** and ***posterior branch of mandibular nerve (>1840)***; see Durward (1951, p. 1026), Williams & Warwick (1980, p. 1066). It was probably first identified by Falloppio; see ***[mandibular nerve trunk (>1840)] (Falloppio, 1561)***.

EARLIER REFERENCES:

Described, not named or illustrated:

1. ***[mandibular nerve trunk (>1840)] (Falloppio, 1561)***
   Described for macrodissected adult human; p. 453, according to Meckel (1748, p. 78 note *p*).

Illustrated and described, not named:

1. ***[mandibular nerve trunk (>1840)] (Vieussens, 1684)***
   Fairly clearly described and illustrated for macrodissected adult human; p. 172 and Table 22 (at label *H*).

Earlier synonyms:

1. *ramus tertius quinti paris fortissimus (Meckel, 1748)*
   Synonym for macrodissected adult human ***mandibular nerve trunk (>1840)***; Figure 1-54.
2. *inferior maxillary nerve trunk (Meckel, 1817)*
   Synonym for macrodissected adult human ***mandibular nerve trunk (>1840)***, although Meckel's

description was vague; see translation (1832, Vol. 3, pp. 72–73).

PARTLY CORRESPONDS:

1. *lesser superior branch of third branch of fifth pair (Meckel, 1748)*
   Corresponds to macrodissected adult human ***anterior branch of mandibular nerve (>1840)***, except Meckel also included ***medial pterygoid nerve (>1840)***; in the original Latin, *tertio ramo nervi quinti paris ramus superiorem minorem*, p. 79 and Figure 1:62–67.
2. *superior branches of third branch of fifth pair (Meckel, 1748)*
   Synonym for *lesser superior branch of third branch of fifth pair (Meckel, 1748)*; in the original Latin, *tertio ramo nervi quinti rami superiores*; Figure 1:62–67.
3. *pterygoid surculus of ganglioform plexus with inferior maxillary branch (Bellingeri, 1818)*
   Macrodissected adult human branches of ***mandibular nerve trunk (>1840)*** to pterygoid muscles; in the original Latin, *surculus pterygoideus*, see Table I.
4. *anterior branch of inferior maxillary nerve (Todd, 1836–1839)*
   Macrodissected adult human ***anterior branch of mandibular nerve (>1840)*** and ***medial pterygoid nerve (>1840)*** considered together; p. 291.
5. *masticatory nerve (>1840)*
   Synonym for macrodissected adult human ***anterior branch of mandibular nerve (>1840)*** and ***medial pterygoid nerve (>1840)*** considered together; see His (1895, p. 89).

marginal ganglia (>1840)

A ***marginal ganglion (>1840)*** is a small condensation of ***neurons (Waldeyer, 1891)***, outside a ***nerve ring (Tiedemann, 1815)***, in a ***nerve net (>1840)*** of at least some active Coelenterate medusae, Ctenophora, and Echinoderms; see Bullock & Horridge (1965, Ch. 8), Cobb (1995), and Swanson & Bota (2010) for this precise definition. Not clearly described before 1840.

marginal mandibular branch of facial nerve (>1840)

As described for macrodissected adult human, a ventral or descending terminal branch of the ***facial nerve trunk (>1840)*** supplying the risorius muscle and muscles of the lower lip and chin; see Williams & Warwick (1980, p. 1072 and Fig. 7.186), *Terminologia Anatomica* (1998, p. 135). It was known to Galen; see ***[marginal mandibular branch of facial nerve (>1840)] (Galen, c173)***.

EARLIER REFERENCES:

Described, not named or illustrated:

1. ***[marginal mandibular branch of facial nerve (>1840)] (Galen, c173)***
   Alluded to for macrodissected adult beef, pig, and/or macaque but not human; see May translation (1968, p. 537). Winslow (1733, Sect. VI, no. 102, p. 70) vaguely described it for macrodissected adult human.

Illustrated, not named or described:

1. ***[marginal mandibular branch of facial nerve (>1840)] (Eustachi, 1552)***
   Illustrated for macrodissected adult human; see Albinus edition (1761, Table 21, first branch below *f*).

Earlier synonyms:

1. *marginal branch of lower jaw of inferior facial branch of hard nerve (Meckel, 1753)*
   Synonym for macrodissected adult human ***marginal mandibular branch of facial nerve (>1840)***; in the original French, *le rameau marginal de la machoire inférieure du rameau facial inférieur du nerf dur*, p. 94. Meckel further described some six extensions of it, Table 1:246–259.
2. *angular branch of lower jaw of inferior facial branch of hard nerve (Meckel, 1753)*
   Synonym for macrodissected adult human ***marginal mandibular branch of facial nerve (>1840)***; in the original French, *le rameau angulaire de la machoire inférieure du rameau facial inférieur du nerf dur*, p. 94.
3. *inferior maxillary branch of hard nerve (Meckel, 1753)*
   Synonym for *marginal branch of lower jaw of inferior facial branch of hard nerve (Meckel, 1753)*; in the original French, *le rameau maxillaire inférieur du dur*, Table 1-244.
4. *inferior maxillary nerve (Meckel, 1753)*
   Synonym for *marginal branch of lower jaw of inferior facial branch of hard nerve (Meckel, 1753)*; in the original French, *le nerf maxillaire inférieur*, Table 1-253. Meckel further described some six extensions of it, Table 1:246–259.
5. *inferior facial branch of inferior branch of anterior branch of hard nerve (Loder, 1778)*
   Synonym for macrodissected adult human ***marginal mandibular branch of facial nerve (>1840)***; in the original Latin, *ramus facialis inferior*, p. 27.
6. *superficial maxillary branch of inferior branch of anterior branch of hard nerve (Loder, 1778)*
   Synonym for macrodissected adult human ***marginal mandibular branch of facial nerve (>1840)***; in the original Latin, *ramus maxillaris superficialis*, p. 27.
7. *marginal branch of lower facial branches of descending branch of superficial branch of hard nerve (Günther, 1786)*
   Synonym for macrodissected adult human ***marginal mandibular branch of facial nerve (>1840)***; in the original Latin, *ramus marginalem*, p. 60. Günther described superior and inferior divisions of marginal branch.
8. *inferior maxillary angular branch of lower facial branches of descending branch of superficial branch of hard nerve (Günther, 1786)*
   Synonym for macrodissected adult human ***marginal mandibular branch of facial nerve (>1840)***; in the original Latin, *ramus angularem maxillae inferioris*,

p. 60. Günther described superior and inferior divisions of inferior maxillary angular branch.

9. *inferior maxillary marginal branch (Soemmerring, 1791)* Synonym for macrodissected adult human ***marginal mandibular branch of facial nerve (>1840)***; in the original Latin, *ramus marginalis maxillae inferioris*, p. 238.
10. *inferior maxillary angular branch (Soemmerring, 1791)* Synonym for macrodissected adult human ***marginal mandibular branch of facial nerve (>1840)***; in the original Latin, *ramus angularis maxillae inferioris*, p. 238.
11. *marginal branch of hard nerve (Peipers, 1793)* Synonym for macrodissected adult human ***marginal mandibular branch of facial nerve (>1840)***; in the original Latin, *ramus marginalis duri*, p. 35.
12. *marginal nerve (Mayer, 1794)* Synonym for macrodissected adult human ***marginal mandibular branch of facial nerve (>1840)***; in the original Latin, *nervus marginalis*; Part 5, Table VII-169 (p. 51).
13. *marginal inferior maxillary nerve (Soemmerring, 1798)* Synonym for macrodissected adult human ***marginal mandibular branch of facial nerve (>1840)***; in the original Latin, *nervus marginalis maxillae inferioris*, p. 253.
14. *mentonniar branches of facial nerve (Burdin, 1803)* Synonym for macrodissected adult human ***marginal mandibular branch of facial nerve (>1840)***; see translation (1803, Vol. 1, p. 180).
15. *mental branches of facial nerve (Chaussier, 1809)* Form of *mentonniar branches of facial nerve (Burdin, 1803)*.
16. *marginal surculus of inferior branch of portio major and minor of facial nerve (Bellingeri, 1818)* Synonym for macrodissected adult human ***marginal mandibular branch of facial nerve (>1840)***; in the original Latin, *surculus marginalis*, see Table II.
17. *marginal surculus of cervico-facial branch of portio major and minor of facial nerve (Bellingeri, 1818)* Synonym for macrodissected adult human ***marginal mandibular branch of facial nerve (>1840)***; in the original Latin, *surculus marginalis*, see Table II.
18. *subcutaneous branch of lower jaw of facial nerve (Cloquet, 1828)* Synonym for macrodissected adult human ***marginal mandibular branch of facial nerve (>1840)***; in the original French, *rameau sous-cutané de la màchoire inférieure*, Plate CLVII-73.
19. *mental branches of cervicofacial branch of facial nerve (Cruveilhier, 1836)* Synonym for macrodissected adult human ***marginal mandibular branch of facial nerve (>1840)***; in the original French, *rameaux mentonniers*, p. 947.

PARTLY CORRESPONDS:

1. *communicating branch of inferior maxillary branch of hard nerve with superior cutaneous nerves of neck (Meckel, 1753)* ***Communicating branch (Winslow, 1733)*** between *inferior maxillary branch of hard nerve (Meckel, 1753)* and *superior cutaneous nerves of neck (Meckel, 1753)*; in the original French, *le rameau [du le rameau maxillaire inférieur du dur] qui communique avec les cutanés supérieurs du col*, Table 1-246,[244].
2. *superior cutaneous branches of neck of inferior branch of hard nerve (Meckel, 1753)* Three such branches of *inferior branch of hard nerve (Meckel, 1753)* described for macrodissected adult human; in the original French, *le premier rameau cutané du col, le second rameau cutané supérieur du col, le troisième cutané supérieur du col de l'inférieur du dur*, Table 1:250–252.
3. *inferior branch of external branch of inferior maxillary nerve (Meckel, 1753)* Ventral (inferior) branch of lateral branch of *inferior maxillary nerve (Meckel, 1753)*; in the original French, *le rameau inférieur du nerf maxillaire inférieur externe*, Table 1-253.
4. *communicating branch of inferior maxillary branch of hard nerve with medial cutaneous nerve of neck (Meckel, 1753)* ***Communicating branch (Winslow, 1733)*** between *inferior maxillary branch of hard nerve (Meckel, 1753)* and *middle cutaneous nerve of neck (Meckel, 1753)*; in the original French, *le rameau [du le rameau] maxillaire inférieur [du dur] qui communique avec le cutané moyen du col*, Table 1-259.
5. *superior branch of inferior facial branch of inferior branch of anterior branch of hard nerve (Loder, 1778)* Dorsally directed (ascending) branch of *inferior facial branch of inferior branch of anterior branch of hard nerve (Loder, 1778)*; p. 27.
6. *marginal branch of inferior facial branch of inferior branch of anterior branch of hard nerve (Loder, 1778)* Branch of *inferior facial branch of inferior branch of anterior branch of hard nerve (Loder, 1778)*; p. 27.
7. *inferior maxillary angle branch of inferior facial branch of inferior branch of anterior branch of hard nerve (Loder, 1778)* Synonym for *marginal branch of inferior facial branch of inferior branch of anterior branch of hard nerve (Loder, 1778)*; p. 27.
8. *major inferior branch of inferior maxillary branch of fifth pair of nerves (Bock, 1817)* Apparently synonym for macrodissected adult human *inferior branch of external branch of inferior maxillary nerve (Meckel, 1753)*, although Bock mistook *inferior maxillary nerve (Meckel, 1753)* of ***facial nerve trunk (>1840)*** for *inferior maxillary nerve (Heister, 1717)* of ***trigeminal nerve (Winslow, 1733)***; in the original Latin, *ramus inferior major*, p. 45.
9. *descending branch of inferior maxillary branch of fifth pair of nerves (Bock, 1817)* Synonym for *major inferior branch of inferior maxillary branch of fifth pair of nerves (Bock, 1817)*; in the original Latin, *ramus descendens*, p. 47.

10. *branch of inferior maxillary marginal nerve to buccinator muscle (Arnold, 1834)*
Macrodissected adult human branch of ***marginal mandibular branch of facial nerve (>1840)*** to buccinator muscle; in the original Latin, *nervus marginalis maxillae inferioris ramus ad musculum buccinatorium*, Table IX:*VII-30,31*.
11. *branch of inferior maxillary marginal nerve to depressor muscle (Arnold, 1834)*
Macrodissected adult human branch of ***marginal mandibular branch of facial nerve (>1840)*** to depressor labii inferioris muscle; in the original Latin, *nervus marginalis maxillae inferioris ramus ad musculum depressoris*, Table IX:*VII-32*.
12. *branch of inferior maxillary marginal nerve to quadrati muscle (Arnold, 1834)*
Macrodissected adult human branch of ***marginal mandibular branch of facial nerve (>1840)***, apparently to depressor anguli oris muscle; in the original Latin, *nervus marginalis maxillae inferioris ramus ad musculum quadrati*, Table IX:*VII-32*.
13. *branch of inferior maxillary marginal nerve to levator menti muscle (Arnold, 1834)*
Macrodissected adult human branch of ***marginal mandibular branch of facial nerve (>1840)*** to mentalis muscle; in the original Latin, *nervus marginalis maxillae inferioris ramus ad musculum levator menti*, Table IX:*VII-32*.

marginal sulcus (>1840)

As described for macrodissected adult human, the terminal, dorsally directed end of the ***cingulate sulcus (>1840)*** between ***posterior paracentral gyrus (>1840)*** rostrally and ***precuneus (Burdach, 1822)*** caudally; see Williams & Warwick (1980, Fig. 7.114A, unlabeled), *Terminologia Anatomica* (1998, p. 126). It was perhaps first clearly distinguished by Soemmerring; see ***[marginal sulcus (>1840)] (Soemmerring, 1778)***.

EARLIER REFERENCES:

Illustrated, not named or described:

1. ***[marginal sulcus (>1840)] (Soemmerring, 1778)***
Clearly illustrated for macrodissected adult human; Table III, just to the right of *Δ*.

masseteric nerve (Meckel, 1748)

As described for macrodissected adult human, branch of the ***anterior branch of mandibular nerve (>1840)*** eventually ramifying in the deep surface of the masseter muscle and sending a small branch to the temporomandibular joint; see Williams & Warwick (1980, p. 1066). For Meckel's use in macrodissected adult human, see p. 80. It was known to Galen; see ***[masseteric nerve (Meckel, 1748)] (Galen, c192)***.

TRANSLATIONS:

1. *nervus massetericus (Meckel, 1748)*
Original Latin form of ***masseteric nerve (Meckel, 1748)***; p. 80.

EARLIER REFERENCES:

Described, not named or illustrated:

1. ***[masseteric nerve (Meckel, 1748)] (Galen, c192)***
Alluded to in macrodissected adult beef, pig, and/or macaque but not human; see Duckworth translation (1962, p. 194). Vesalius (1543a) mentioned it for macrodissected adult human; see Richardson & Carman translation (2002, p. 189). Falloppio (1561, p. 453) also mentioned it for macrodissected adult human; see Meckel (1748, p. 80 note *v*).

Illustrated and described, not named:

1. ***[masseteric nerve (Meckel, 1748)] (Willis, 1664)***
Possibly illustrated for macrodissected adult, presumably human, although probably mistakenly shown as branch of ***maxillary nerve (Meckel, 1753)***; see Pordage translation (1681, pp. 144–145, Fig. 1-*E,e*). Du Verney (1683, Pl. 13-2) clearly and accurately illustrated its origin in macrodissected adult human.

LATER SYNONYMS:

1. *masseteric branch of inferior maxillary nerve (Loder, 1778)*
Synonym for macrodissected adult human ***masseteric nerve (Meckel, 1748)***; in the original Latin, *ramus massetericus*, p. 17.
2. *sub-zygomatic nerve (Burdin, 1803)*
Synonym for macrodissected adult human ***masseteric nerve (Meckel, 1748)***; see translation (1803, Vol. 1, p. 175).
3. *masseteric surculus of ganglioform plexus with inferior maxillary branch (Bellingeri, 1818)*
Synonym for macrodissected adult human ***masseteric nerve (Meckel, 1748)***; in the original Latin, *surculus massetericus*, see Table I.
4. *masseteric branch of superior primary branch of inferior maxillary nerve (Quain, 1832)*
Synonym for macrodissected adult human ***masseteric nerve (Meckel, 1748)***; p. 676.

PARTLY CORRESPONDS:

1. *external deep temporal branch of masseteric branch (Loder, 1778)*
Branch of *masseteric branch of inferior maxillary nerve (Loder, 1778)* described as distributing to temporal muscle; in the original Latin, *ramum temporalem profundum externum*, p. 17.

maxillary nerve (Meckel, 1753)

As described for macrodissected adult human, in size and position the intermediate of the three primary ***trigeminal nerve branches (Winslow, 1733)***, wholly sensory in function. It was superbly illustrated by Henle (1871, Fig. 238); also see Durward (1951, Fig. 898), Williams & Warwick (1980, pp. 1062–1066), *Terminologia Anatomica* (1998, p. 134). For Meckel's use in macrodissected adult human, see p. 34. It was discovered by Galen; see ***[maxillary nerve (Meckel, 1753)] (Galen, c173)***.

TRANSLATIONS:

1. *nerf maxillaire (Meckel, 1753)*
Original French form of ***maxillary nerve (Meckel, 1753)***; p. 35.

EARLIER REFERENCES:

Described, not named or illustrated:

1. ***[maxillary nerve (Meckel, 1753)] (Galen, c173)***
Described for macrodissected adult beef, pig, and/or macaque but not human; see May translation (1968, pp. 440, 454, 455, 686), Duckworth translation (1962, p. 194).

Illustrated, not named or described:

1. ***[maxillary nerve (Meckel, 1753)] (Eustachi, 1552)***
Clearly illustrated for macrodissected adult human; see Albinus edition (1761, Tab. 18, Figs. 1, 3, 4-*C* and Fig. 2-*X*).

Earlier synonyms:

1. *fourth pair of nerves from brain (Benedetti, 1502)*
Corresponds roughly to macrodissected adult human ***maxillary nerve (Meckel, 1753)***; see Lind translation (1975, p. 117).
2. *second trunk of third pair (Falloppio, 1561)*
Synonym for macrodissected adult human ***maxillary nerve (Meckel, 1753)***. Falloppio also referred to it as one of three *shoots of third pair*; see Harvey (1961, notes 830 and 844). Also see *third pair of nerves from brain (Falloppio, 1561)* and Meckel (1748, p. 46 note *q*).
3. *second branch of third pair (Marchetti 1652)*
Synonym for macrodissected adult human *second trunk of third pair (Falloppio, 1561)*; p. 122.
4. *third and fourth branches of second division of fifth pair of nerves arising within skull (Willis, 1664)*
Roughly synonymous with macrodissected adult, presumably human, ***maxillary nerve (Meckel, 1753)***; see Pordage translation (1681, pp. 144–145, Fig. 1-*E,F*).
5. *ramus minor inferior nervus quintae conjugationis (Vieussens, 1684)*
Synonym for macrodissected adult human ***maxillary nerve (Meckel, 1753)***; pp. 171–172 and Table 22-*F*.
6. *middle branch of fifth pair (Rau, 1694)*
Synonym for ***maxillary nerve (Meckel, 1753)***; in the original Latin, *quinti paris medius ramus*, p. 191.
7. *superior maxillary branch of fifth pair (Rau, 1694)*
Synonym for ***maxillary nerve (Meckel, 1753)***; in the original Latin, *quinti paris maxillaris superior ramus*, p. 191.
8. *major branch of fifth pair (Rau, 1694)*
Synonym for ***maxillary nerve (Meckel, 1753)***; in the original Latin, *quinti paris majori ramo*, p. 191.
9. *inferior smaller branch of fifth pair (Ridley, 1695)*
English form of macrodissected adult human *ramus minor inferior nervus quintae conjugationis (Vieussens, 1684)*; p. 147.
10. *superior maxillary nerve (Heister, 1717)*
Synonym for macrodissected adult human ***maxillary nerve (Meckel, 1753)***; in the original Latin, *nervus maxillaris superior*, see translation (1721, p. 245).
11. *middle branch of trigeminal nerve (Winslow, 1733)*
Synonym for macrodissected adult human ***maxillary nerve (Meckel, 1753)***; Section VI, pp. 61–63. Meckel (1748, Figs. 2–6) illustrated fascicles in cross-sections from macrodissected adult human.

LATER SYNONYMS:

1. *second branch of fifth pair of nerves (Meckel, 1753)*
Synonym for macrodissected adult human ***maxillary nerve (Meckel, 1753)***; in the original French, *le second rameau de la cinquième paire des nerfs*, p. 26.
2. *superior masticatory nerve (Malacarne, 1791)*
Synonym for macrodissected adult human ***maxillary nerve (Meckel, 1753)***; p. 232.
3. *eighth pair of nerves (Malacarne, 1791)*
Synonym for *superior masticatory nerve (Malacarne, 1791)*, listed as eighth of 17 pairs of *cerebral nerves (Malacarne, 1791)*; p. 232.
4. *second division of fifth pair (Bell, 1803a)*
Synonym for macrodissected adult human ***maxillary nerve (Meckel, 1753)***; Table 1-*E*.
5. *sub-maxillary nerve (Burdin, 1803)*
Synonym for macrodissected adult human ***maxillary nerve (Meckel, 1753)***; see translation (1803, Vol. 1, p. 170).
6. *second principal branch of fifth pair (Meckel, 1817)*
Synonym listed for macrodissected adult human ***maxillary nerve (Meckel, 1753)***; see translation (1832, Vol. 3, p. 65) and Meckel (1748, p. 45 note *n*).
7. *second trunk of three-fold nerve (Swan, 1830)*
Synonym for macrodissected adult human ***maxillary nerve (Meckel, 1753)***; p. 17.
8. *second trunk of fifth pair (Swan, 1830)*
Synonym for macrodissected adult human ***maxillary nerve (Meckel, 1753)***; p. 17.
9. *second trunk of fifth nerve (Swan, 1830)*
Synonym for macrodissected adult human ***maxillary nerve (Meckel, 1753)***; Plate XII, Figure 1-3,*11*.

PARTLY CORRESPONDS:

1. *second offshoot of thinner root of third pair (Vesalius, 1543a)*
Probably corresponds roughly to *infraorbital nerve (Meckel, 1748)*, partly described and illustrated for macrodissected adult human; see Richardson & Carman translation (2002, p. 188 and Figure on p. 169, part *O*).
2. *second branch of third conjugation of nerves of brain (Crooke, 1615)*
Synonym for macrodissected adult human *infraorbital nerve (Meckel, 1748)*, following terminology of *second offshoot of thinner root of third pair (Vesalius, 1543a)*; p. 486. Crooke's description is a translation of Bauhin (1605).
3. *second branch of fourth conjugation of nerves of brain (Crooke, 1615)*
Roughly combination in macrodissected adult human of ***posterior superior dental nerve (Haller, 1762)*** and ***superior gingival branches of superior dental plexus (>1840)***; p. 486. Crooke's description is a translation of Bauhin (1605).
4. *lower branch of second division of fifth pair of nerves arising within skull (Willis, 1664)*
Apparently combination of ***superior gingival branches of superior dental plexus (>1840)*** and ***palatine nerves (Schaarschmidt, 1750)***, which, however, do not usually arise from the same ***nerve (Herophilus, c335–c280 BC)*** trunk; see Pordage translation (1681, p. 145, Fig. 1-*F,h,i*).

5. *fourth branch of second division of fifth pair of nerves arising within skull (Willis, 1664)*
   Synonym for *lower branch of second division of fifth pair of nerves arising within skull (Willis, 1664)*; see Pordage translation (1681, p. 145, Fig. 1-*F,h,i*).
6. *ramulus primus rami minoris inferioris F (Vieussens, 1684)*
   Probably corresponds roughly to macrodissected adult human *infraorbital nerve (Meckel, 1748)*; p. 172 and Table 22-*r*.
7. *sub-orbitary ramus of superior maxillary nerve (Winslow, 1733)*
   Description apparently corresponds most closely to macrodissected adult human *infraorbital nerve (Meckel, 1748)*; in the original Latin, *ramus suborbitarius*, Section VI, p. 64.
8. *soft medullary branches of second branch of fifth pair (Meckel, 1748)*
   Macrodissected adult human proximal branches of ***maxillary nerve (Meckel, 1753)*** of uncertain identity; in the original Latin, *rami molles medullares secundi rami Quinti paris*, p. 46, Section LVIII. See Bell & Bell (1826, p. 514).
9. *infraorbital nerve (Meckel, 1748)*
   Macrodissected adult human terminal part of ***maxillary nerve (Meckel, 1753)*** distal to origin of ***posterior superior dental nerve (Haller, 1762)*** but including origin of ***anterior superior dental nerve (Haller, 1762)***; in the original Latin, *nervus infraorbitalis*, p. 67 and Figure 1-62. Modern usage for ***infraorbital nerve (Schaarschmidt, 1750)*** is slightly different, referring to terminal part of ***maxillary nerve (Meckel, 1753)*** distal to origin of ***anterior superior dental nerve (Haller, 1762)***.
10. *superior branch of superior maxillary branch of nerve of fifth pair (Bonhomme, 1748)*
    Corresponds to all branches of macrodissected adult human ***maxillary nerve (Meckel, 1753)*** distal to ***pterygopalatine nerves (Wrisberg, 1786)***; in the original French, *le nerf supérieur de la branche maxillaire supérieur de l'nerf de la cinquième paire*, pp. 73–74, Plate 10-*10*. Also see Williams & Warwick (1980, Fig. 7.177).
11. *inferior branch of superior maxillary branch of nerve of fifth pair (Bonhomme, 1748)*
    Corresponds to macrodissected adult human ***pterygopalatine nerves (Wrisberg, 1786)*** and ***palatine nerves (Schaarschmidt, 1750)*** considered together; in the original French, *le nerf inférieur de la branche maxillaire supérieur de l'nerf de la cinquième paire*, pp. 73–74, Plate 10-*11*.
12. *palatine nerve (Bonhomme, 1748)*
    Synonym for *inferior branch of superior maxillary branch of nerve of fifth pair (Bonhomme, 1748)*; in the original French, *le nerf palatin*, p. 74, Plate 10-*11*.
13. *superior dental nerves (Haller, 1762)*
    Macrodissected adult human ***posterior superior dental nerve (Haller, 1762)*** and ***anterior superior dental nerve (Haller, 1762)*** considered together; in the original Latin, *nervi dentales superiores*, p. 214.
14. *roots of superior masticatory nerve (Malacarne, 1791)*
    Uncertain feature of macrodissected adult human ***maxillary nerve (Meckel, 1753)***; p. 227.
15. *nervus infraorbitalis (Meckel, 1817)*
    Defined for macrodissected adult human as starting immediately caudal to ***pterygopalatine nerves (Wrisberg, 1786)***; see translation (1832, Vol. 3, p. 66) and *infraorbital nerve (Meckel, 1748)*. Also see Henle (1871, Fig. 238 and pp. 367–373). In English, *infraorbital nerve*.
16. *infraorbitar nerve (Meckel, 1832)*
    English form of *nervus infraorbitalis (Meckel, 1817)*; Vol. 3, p. 66.
17. *posterior dental branches of superior maxillary nerve (Quain, 1832)*
    Macrodissected adult human ***posterior superior dental nerve (Haller, 1762)*** and ***middle superior dental nerve (Henle, 1871)*** considered together; p. 674.
18. *collateral branches of superior maxillary nerve (Cruveilhier, 1836)*
    All branches of macrodissected adult human ***maxillary nerve (Meckel, 1753)*** except *terminal branches of superior maxillary nerve (Cruveilhier, 1836)*; in the original French, *branches collatérales du nerf maxillaire supérieur*, p. 919.
19. *posterior superior dental branches of superior maxillary nerve (Todd, 1836–1839)*
    Synonym for macrodissected adult human *superior dental nerves (Haller, 1762)*; p. 289.

medial amygdalar nucleus (Johnston, 1923)

As described for macrodissected adult human, and with cellular architecture and connections for all mammals, the most caudal and ventral differentiation of the ***striatum (Swanson, 2000a)***, ventral and medial to the ***central amygdalar nucleus (Johnston, 1923)***; see Price et al. (1987). For Johnston's use in mammal, based on phylogeny and histology, see pp. 340, 410, 456, where it was spelled *medial amygdaloid nucleus*; current spelling was introduced by Swanson & Petrovich (1998, p. 324). Not clearly described by 1840.

medial branch of spinal nerve dorsal branch (>1840)

As described for macrodissected adult human, a medial and lateral branch are found on all but the first cervical, fourth and fifth sacral, and coccygeal ***spinal nerve dorsal branches (Meckel, 1817)***. The medial branch supplies skin and muscle closest to the dorsal median plane (middle of the back); see Durward (1951, Fig. 913), Williams & Warwick (1980, pp. 1089–1091), *Terminologia Anatomica* (1998, pp. 137–139). It was perhaps first clearly delineated as *internal branch of spinal nerve dorsal branch (Meckel, 1817)*.

EARLIER REFERENCES:

Earlier synonyms:

1. *internal branch of spinal nerve dorsal branch (Meckel, 1817)*
   Synonym for ***medial branch of spinal nerve dorsal branch (>1840)***, described for macrodissected adult

human ***thoracic nerves (Diemerbroeck, 1672)***; see translation (1832, Vol. 3, p. 9).

PARTLY CORRESPONDS:

1. *internal branch of posterior branch of lumbar nerve (Bock, 1827)*
   Synonym for macrodissected adult human *internal branch of spinal nerve dorsal branch (Meckel, 1817)* for ***lumbar nerves (Diemerbroeck, 1672)***; in the original Latin, *ram. internus posterior*; Table VII, Figure 1-4. Cruveilhier (1836, p. 771 ff.) used the term systematically for all ***spinal nerve dorsal branches (Meckel, 1817)***.
2. *internal branch of dorsal branch of thoracic nerve (Bock, 1827)*
   Synonym for macrodissected adult human *internal branch of spinal nerve dorsal branch (Meckel, 1817)* for 11th and 12th ***thoracic nerves (Diemerbroeck, 1672)***; in the original Latin, *ram. internus dorsalis nervi thoracis*; Table VII, Figure 2-2,3.

medial branch of supraorbital nerve (>1840)

As described for macrodissected adult human, it and the larger ***lateral branch of supraorbital nerve (>1840)*** together supply skin of the scalp almost as far dorsally (back) as the lambdoid suture, along with some branches to the frontal sinus mucus membrane and pericranium; see Williams & Warwick (1980, p. 1061 and Fig. 7.186), *Terminologia Anatomica* (1998, p. 133), and Henle (1871, Fig. 234-*f*, where it is called *frontal nerve*). It was perhaps first clearly distinguished by Winslow; see ***[medial branch of supraorbital nerve (>1840)] (Winslow, 1733)***.

EARLIER REFERENCES:

Described, not named or illustrated:

1. ***[medial branch of supraorbital nerve (>1840)] (Winslow, 1733)***
   Winslow noted for macrodissected adult human that after passing through the foramen superciliare [supraorbital foramen], the end of the *frontal ramus of ophthalmic nerve (Winslow, 1733)* is divided toward each side [presumably medial and lateral branches] to be spent in part on neighboring skin; Section VI, p. 63.

Earlier synonyms:

1. *internal branch of greater frontal nerve (Meckel, 1753)*
   Synonym for macrodissected adult human ***medial branch of supraorbital nerve (>1840)***; in the original French, *le rameau interne du grand nerf frontal*, Table 1-2.
2. *interior branch of supraorbital nerve (Günther, 1786)*
   Synonym for macrodissected adult human ***medial branch of supraorbital nerve (>1840)***; in the original Latin, *nervis supraorbitalis ramus interiorem*, p. 42.
3. *superficial branch of supraorbital nerve (Günther, 1786)*
   Synonym for macrodissected adult human ***medial branch of supraorbital nerve (>1840)***; in the original Latin, *nervis supraorbitalis ramus superficialem*, p. 42. Bellingeri (1818) described for macrodissected adult human three fine branches of it; see Table I.
4. *internal branch of palpebro-frontal nerve (Burdin, 1803)*
   Synonym for macrodissected adult human ***medial branch of supraorbital nerve (>1840)***; see translation (1803, Vol. 1, p. 170).
5. *deep branches of frontal branches of external frontal nerve (Todd, 1836–1839)*
   Apparently synonym for macrodissected adult human *internal branch of greater frontal nerve (Meckel, 1753)*; p. 280.
6. *short branches of frontal branches of external frontal nerve (Todd, 1836–1839)*
   Apparently synonym for macrodissected adult human *internal branch of greater frontal nerve (Meckel, 1753)*; pp. 280–281.
7. *internal branch of ascending branch of external frontal nerve (Cruveilhier, 1836)*
   Synonym for macrodissected adult human ***medial branch of supraorbital nerve (>1840)***; in the original French, *rameau interne*, pp. 912–913.
8. *internal branch of ascending branch of supraorbital nerve (Cruveilhier, 1836)*
   Synonym for *internal branch of ascending branch of external frontal nerve (Cruveilhier, 1836)*; pp. 912–913.
9. *internal branch of frontal branch of external frontal nerve (Cruveilhier, 1836)*
   Synonym for *internal branch of ascending branch of external frontal nerve (Cruveilhier, 1836)*; pp. 912–913.
10. *internal branch of frontal branch of supraorbital nerve (Cruveilhier, 1836)*
    Synonym for *internal branch of ascending branch of external frontal nerve (Cruveilhier, 1836)*; pp. 912–913.
11. *frontal nerve (>1840)*
    Synonym for macrodissected adult human ***medial branch of supraorbital nerve (>1840)***; see Henle (1871, Fig. 234-*f*), where the Latin was *nervus frontalis*.
12. *frontal branch of supraorbital nerve (>1840)*
    Synonym for macrodissected adult human ***medial branch of supraorbital nerve (>1840)***; see *Basel Nomina Anatomica* (His, 1895, p. 88), where the Latin was *ramus frontalis n. supraorbitalis*.

medial calcaneal nerve (>1840)

As described for macrodissected adult human, a terminal cutaneous branch of the ***tibial nerve (Haase, 1781)*** supplying medial parts of the heel and dorsomedial parts of the sole of the foot; see Durward (1951, p. 1110 and Fig. 950), Hamilton (1976, Fig. 833), Williams & Warwick (1980, Fig. 7.216). It was perhaps first clearly delineated by Vieussens; see ***[medial calcaneal nerve (>1840)] (Vieussens, 1684)***.

ALTERNATE SPELLINGS:

1. *medial calcanean nerve (>1840)*
   Alternate form of ***medial calcaneal nerve (>1840)***; see Durward (1951, Fig. 950), Williams & Warwick (1980, Fig. 7.216).

EARLIER REFERENCES:

Illustrated and described, not named:

1. ***[medial calcaneal nerve (>1840)] (Vieussens, 1684)***

Described and illustrated branches of ***tibial nerve (Haase, 1781)*** to region of distribution of ***medial calcaneal nerve (>1840)*** in macrodissected adult human; Table 30-*1,2*.

Earlier synonyms:

1. *interior dorsal twig of foot from tibial communicating branch (Jördens, 1788)*
   Probably synonym for macrodissected adult human ***medial calcaneal nerve (>1840)***; in the original Latin, *ramulus dorsalis pedis interior a ramo communicante tibiei*, p. 9 and Table I-*121*. Jördens there described, illustrated, and named about 17 branches of this twig, p. 9 and Table I:*122–138*.
2. *calcaneus bone cutaneous nervelet (Fischer, 1791)*
   Probably synonym for macrodissected adult human ***medial calcaneal nerve (>1840)***; in the original Latin, *nervulus subcutaneus ossis calcis*, p. 36.
3. *external tibial nerve (Meckel, 1817)*
   Synonym for macrodissected adult human ***medial calcaneal nerve (>1840)***; see translation (1832, Vol. 3, p. 20).
4. *proper cutaneous plantar nerve (Meckel, 1817)*
   Synonym for macrodissected adult human ***medial calcaneal nerve (>1840)***; in the original Latin, *nervus cutaneus plantaris proprius*, see translation (1832, Vol. 3, p. 20).
5. *internal calcanean nerve (Cruveilhier, 1836)*
   Synonym for macrodissected adult human ***medial calcaneal nerve (>1840)***; in the original French, *nerf calcanien interne*, p. 871.
6. *medial calcaneal branches of tibial nerve (>1840)*
   Synonym for macrodissected adult human ***medial calcaneal nerve (>1840)***; see *Terminologia Anatomica* (1998, p. 141).

medial clunial nerves (>1840)

As described for macrodissected adult human, branches of the ***lateral branches of spinal nerve dorsal branches (>1840)*** arising from the 1st–3rd ***sacral nerves (Camper, 1760)*** and innervating skin caudally (inferiorly) and medially in the gluteal region; see Williams & Warwick (1980, Fig. 7.196), *Terminologia Anatomica* (1998, p. 139). They were known to Vesalius; see ***[medial clunial nerves (>1840)] (Vesalius, 1543a)***.

EARLIER REFERENCES:

Described, not named or illustrated:

1. ***[medial clunial nerves (>1840)] (Vesalius, 1543a)***
   Mentioned for macrodissected adult human; see Richardson & Carman translation (2002, pp. 254–255).

medial corticohypothalamic tract (Gurdjian, 1927)

As described in mammal with histological methods for demonstrating ***axons (Kölliker, 1896)***, a thin ***central nervous system white matter tract (>1840)*** splitting off from the proximal (rostrodorsal) end of the ***hypothalamic postcommissural fornix (>1840)*** and coursing ventrally in the ***periventricular hypothalamic zone (>1840)*** to the region of the ***suprachiasmatic nucleus (>1840)*** before turning and extending caudally. For Gurdjian's use in adult rat based on histological methods for ***axons (Kölliker, 1896)***, see pp. 102–103. It was discovered by Cajal and called *Ammonic bundle of tuber cinereum (Cajal, 1901–1902)*.

EARLIER REFERENCES:

Earlier synonyms:

1. *Ammonic bundle of tuber cinereum (Cajal, 1901–1902)*
   Synonym for ***medial corticohypothalamic tract (Gurdjian, 1927)*** observed in newborn mouse with Golgi method; in the original Spanish, *cordón amónico del tuber cinereum*, pp. 175–177. See Cajal (1909–1911, and translation, 1995, Vol. 2, pp. 654–656).

medial cutaneous nerve of arm (>1840)

As described for macrodissected adult human, it arises from the ***brachial plexus medial cord (Schwalbe, 1881)*** and supplies skin on the medial side of the arm; see Hamilton (1976, Fig. 819), Williams & Warwick (1980, p. 1097 and Figs. 7.200, 204), *Terminologia Anatomica* (1998, p. 138). It was known to Galen; see ***[medial cutaneous nerve of arm (>1840)] (Galen, c177)***.

TRANSLATIONS:

1. *nervus cutaneus brachii medialis (>1840)*
   Current Latin form of ***medial cutaneous nerve of arm (>1840)***; see *Terminologia Anatomica* (1998, p. 138).

EARLIER REFERENCES:

Described, not named or illustrated:

1. ***[medial cutaneous nerve of arm (>1840)] (Galen, c177)***
   Clearly described for macrodissected adult beef, pig, and/or macaque but not human; see Singer translation (1999, pp. 67, 69–70).

Illustrated and described, not named:

1. ***[medial cutaneous nerve of arm (>1840)] (Vesalius, 1543a)***
   Mentioned for macrodissected adult human; see Richardson & Carman translation (2002, p. 246). Eustachi (1552) illustrated clearly its distribution in macrodissected adult human; see Albinus edition (1761, Tab. 21-6).

Earlier synonyms:

1. *nervus cutaneus minor internus vel ulnaris Wrisbergii (Klint, 1784)*
   Eponym for macrodissected adult human ***medial cutaneous nerve of arm (>1840)***; pp. 36, 63. Klint did not provide citation for Wrisberg's use of term.
2. *internal minor cutaneous nerve (Klint, 1784)*
   Synonym for macrodissected adult human ***medial cutaneous nerve of arm (>1840)***; in the original Latin, *nervus cutaneus minor internus*, pp. 36, 63.
3. *ulnar nerve of Wrisberg (Klint, 1784)*
   Eponym for macrodissected adult human ***medial cutaneous nerve of arm (>1840)***; in the original Latin, *nervus ulnaris Wrisbergii*, pp. 36, 63. Also see

Günther (1786, p. 77). They attributed it to Wrisberg without citation (presumably from his lectures).

4. *minor cutaneous nerve (Günther, 1786, p. 77)*
Synonym for macrodissected adult human ***medial cutaneous nerve of arm (>1840)***; in the original Latin, *nervus cutaneus minor*, p. 77. Günther described a posterior, minor branch and an anterior major and interior branch of this ***nerve (Herophilus, c335–c280 BC)***; p. 77.

5. *minor internal musculo-cutaneous nerve (Frotscher, 1788)*
Synonym for macrodissected adult human ***medial cutaneous nerve of arm (>1840)***; in the original Latin, *nervus musculo-cutaneus internus minor*, p. 92.

6. *internal cutaneous nerve of arm (Mayer, 1794)*
Synonym for macrodissected adult human ***medial cutaneous nerve of arm (>1840)***. In the original Latin, *nervus cutaneus internus brachii*; Part 5, Table III, Figure 1-*B* (p. 21). Under this term, Cloquet (1828, Pl. CLXVII, Fig. 1:*67–71*) described and illustrated five major branches for macrodissected adult human.

7. *cutaneous nerve of Wrisberg (Bell, 1803b)*
As vaguely described for macrodissected adult human, appears to be eponym for ***medial cutaneous nerve of arm (>1840)*** and may be branch of *great internal cutaneous nerve (Bell, 1803b)*, or may arise from *axillary plexus (Salmon, 1714)* itself or even from *intercostal nerves (Bell, 1803b)*; p. 195. Attributed to Wrisberg without citation.

8. *superior humeral cutaneous nerve (Loder, 1803)*
Probably synonym for macrodissected adult human ***medial cutaneous nerve of arm (>1840)***; in the original Latin, *nervus cutaneus humeri superior*, Table CLXXVIII-*161*.

9. *external branch of internal cutaneous nerve of arm (Cloquet, 1816)*
Synonym for macrodissected adult human ***medial cutaneous nerve of arm (>1840)***; p. 645.

10. *nerve of Wrisberg (Bell & Bell, 1816)*
Eponym for *cutaneous nerve of Wrisberg (Bell, 1803b)*; Vol. 2, p. 534.

11. *small internal cutaneous nerve (Swan, 1830)*
Synonym for macrodissected adult human ***medial cutaneous nerve of arm (>1840)***; p. 26.

PARTLY CORRESPONDS:

1. *minor thoracic nerve (Frotscher, 1788)*
Meaning for macrodissected adult human is very obscure but may be synonym for *minor cutaneous nerve (Günther, 1786, p. 77)*, or some more restricted component of ***medial cutaneous nerve of arm (>1840)***; in the original Latin, *nervus thoracicus minor*, p. 89 of 1795 reprint, where Frotscher referred to Günther (1786, p. 77).

2. *anterior external branch of internal cutaneous nerve of arm (Cruveilhier, 1836)*
For macrodissected adult human, one of two terminal branches of ***medial cutaneous nerve of arm (>1840)***; in the original French, *branche externe antérieure*, p. 798.

3. *cubital branch of internal cutaneous nerve of arm (Cruveilhier, 1836)*
Synonym for *anterior external branch of internal cutaneous nerve of arm (Cruveilhier, 1836)*; in the original French, *branchè cubitale*, p. 798.

4. *posterior internal branch of internal cutaneous nerve of arm (Cruveilhier, 1836)*
For macrodissected adult human, one of two terminal branches of ***medial cutaneous nerve of arm (>1840)***; in the original French, *branche interne postérieure*, p. 798.

5. *epitrochlear branch of internal cutaneous nerve of arm (Cruveilhier, 1836)*
Synonym for *posterior internal branch of internal cutaneous nerve of arm (Cruveilhier, 1836)*; in the original French, *branchè épitrochléenne (or épitrokléenne)*, p. 798.

6. *accessory internal cutaneous nerve of arm (Cruveilhier, 1836)*
As described for macrodissected adult human, difficult to identify branch associated with ***medial cutaneous nerve of arm (>1840)*** generating secondary external and internal branches ending near elbow; in the original French, *accessoire du branchial cutané interne*, p. 799.

medial cutaneous nerve of calf (>1840)

As described for macrodissected adult human, a branch of the ***tibial nerve (Haase, 1781)*** usually joining the ***sural communicating branch of common fibular nerve (>1840)*** to form the ***sural nerve (Pietro da Cortona, 1741)***—that is, its proximal segment often forms the ***tibial root of sural nerve (>1840)***; see *Dorland's* (2003, p. 1238 under *nervus cutaneus surae medialis*) and Williams & Warwick (1980, Fig. 7.215), where the ***medial cutaneous nerve of calf (>1840)*** and its ***tibial root of sural nerve (>1840)*** are unlabeled above the junction, and the ***sural nerve ((Pietro da Cortona, 1741)*** is labeled distally. It is often called the *medial sural cutaneous nerve (>1840)* or is subsumed under the ***sural nerve (Pietro da Cortona, 1741)***. It was probably known to Galen; see ***[medial cutaneous nerve of calf (>1840)] (Galen, c177)***.

TRANSLATIONS:

1. *nervus cutaneus surae medialis (>1840)*
Current Latin form of ***medial cutaneous nerve of calf (>1840)***; see *Dorland's* (2003, p. 1238).

EARLIER REFERENCES:

Described, not named or illustrated:

1. ***[medial cutaneous nerve of calf (>1840)] (Galen, c177)***
Probably mentioned for macrodissected beef, pig, and/or macaque but not human; see Singer translation (1999, p. 87). Vesalius (1543a) mentioned it for macrodissected adult human; see Richardson & Carman translation (2002, p. 260).

Earlier synonyms:

1. *peroneo-digital nerve (Burdin, 1803)*
Synonym for macrodissected adult human ***medial cutaneous nerve of calf (>1840)***; see translation (1803, Vol. 1, p. 206).

2. *medial cutaneous nerve of leg (Bock, 1827)*

Synonym for macrodissected adult human ***medial cutaneous nerve of calf (>1840)***; in the original Latin, *nerv. cutaneus medius cruris*, Table IV-92.

3. *inferior and internal cutaneous nerve (Cloquet, 1828)*
   Synonym for macrodissected adult human ***medial cutaneous nerve of calf (>1840)***; in the original French, *nerf cutané interne et inférieur*, Plate CLXXI, Figure 2-28.
4. *internal inferior cutaneous nerve (Cloquet, 1828)*
   Synonym for *inferior and internal cutaneous nerve (Cloquet, 1828)*; in the original French, *N. cutané inférieur interne*, Plate CLXXIII, Figure 2-34. Cloquet described three branches; Plate CLXXIII, Figure 2-35,36.
5. *inferior internal cutaneous nerve (Cloquet, 1828)*
   Synonym for *inferior and internal cutaneous nerve (Cloquet, 1828)*; in the original French, *N. cutané interne inférieur*, Plate CLXXIV, Figure 2-38.
6. *medial sural cutaneous nerve (>1840)*
   Synonym for macrodissected adult human ***medial cutaneous nerve of calf (>1840)***; see *Dorland's* (2003, p. 1238).

medial cutaneous nerve of forearm (>1840)

As described for macrodissected adult human, it arises from the ***brachial plexus medial cord (Schwalbe, 1881)*** and supplies skin covering part of the biceps, then eventually divides into ***anterior branch of medial cutaneous nerve of forearm (>1840)*** and ***posterior branch of medial cutaneous nerve of forearm (>1840)***; see Williams & Warwick (1980, p. 1097), *Terminologia Anatomica* (1998, p. 138). It was known to Galen; see ***[medial cutaneous nerve of forearm (>1840)] (Galen, c177)***.

TRANSLATIONS:

1. *nervus cutaneus antebrachii medialis (>1840)*
   Current Latin form of ***medial cutaneous nerve of forearm (>1840)***; see *Terminologia Anatomica* (1998, p. 138).

EARLIER REFERENCES:

Described, not named or illustrated:

1. ***[medial cutaneous nerve of forearm (>1840)] (Galen, c177)***
   Clearly described in macrodissected adult beef, pig, and/or macaque but not human; see Singer translation (1999, pp. 69–70, 82). Vesalius (1543a) mentioned it for macrodissected adult human; see Richardson & Carman translation (2002, p. 246).

Earlier synonyms:

1. *internal cutaneous nerve (Du Verney, 1697)*
   Synonym for macrodissected adult human ***medial cutaneous nerve of forearm (>1840)***; in Latin, *nervus cutaneus internus*. According to Winslow (1733, Sect. VI, p. 79), his mentor Du Verney gave this name to the macrodissected adult human ***nerve (Herophilus, c335–c280 BC)*** in 1697.
2. *cutaneous nerve (Cheselden, 1726)*
   Apparently corresponds more or less to macrodissected adult human ***medial cutaneous nerve of forearm (>1840)***; in the original Latin, *nervus cutaneus*. See p. 265, essentially written by Monro *primus* as stated in Preface.
3. *subcutaneous basilic nerves (Monro, 1783)*
   Synonym for macrodissected adult human ***medial cutaneous nerve of forearm (>1840)***; Table 15-20.
4. *major internal cutaneous nerve (Klint, 1784)*
   Synonym for macrodissected adult human ***medial cutaneous nerve of forearm (>1840)***; in the original Latin, *nervus cutaneus internus major*, p. 49.
5. *middle cutaneous nerve of Wrisberg (Klint, 1784)*
   Eponym for macrodissected adult human ***medial cutaneous nerve of forearm (>1840)***, without a citation for Wrisberg; in the original Latin, *nervus cutaneus medius Wrisbergii*, p. 51.
6. *middle cutaneous nerve (Klint, 1784)*
   Synonym for macrodissected adult human ***medial cutaneous nerve of forearm (>1840)***; in the original Latin, *nervus cutaneus medius*, pp. 63, 64.
7. *major internal musculo-cutaneous nerve (Frotscher, 1788)*
   Synonym for macrodissected adult human ***medial cutaneous nerve of forearm (>1840)***; in the original Latin, *nervus musculo-cutaneus internus major*, p. 92. Frotscher described here two subcutaneous branches proximal to the bifurcation.
8. *middle musculo-cutaneous nerve (Frotscher, 1788)*
   Synonym for macrodissected adult human ***medial cutaneous nerve of forearm (>1840)***; in the original Latin, *nervus musculo-cutaneus medius*, p. 92.
9. *middle cutaneous nerve of arm (Soemmerring, 1791)*
   Synonym for macrodissected adult human ***medial cutaneous nerve of forearm (>1840)***; in the original German, *Mittlerer Hautnerve des Arms*, p. 289.
10. *great internal cutaneous nerve (Bell, 1803b)*
    Synonym for macrodissected adult human *major internal cutaneous nerve (Klint, 1784)*; p. 194.
11. *internal branch of internal cutaneous nerve of arm (Cloquet, 1816)*
    Synonym for macrodissected adult human ***medial cutaneous nerve of forearm (>1840)***; p. 645.
12. *inferior internal cutaneous nerve (Meckel, 1817)*
    Basically synonym for macrodissected adult human ***medial cutaneous nerve of forearm (>1840)***; in the original Latin, *nervus cutaneus internus inferior*, see translation (1832, Vol. 3, p. 29).

PARTLY CORRESPONDS:

1. *palmar cutaneous branch of medial cutaneous nerve trunk (Loder, 1803)*
   Short distal segment of trunk of macrodissected adult human ***medial cutaneous nerve of forearm (>1840)*** before dividing into ***anterior branch of medial cutaneous nerve of forearm (>1840)*** and ***posterior branch of medial cutaneous nerve of forearm (>1840)***; in the original Latin, *ramus cutaneus palmaris*, Table CLXXVIII-121.
2. *internal cutaneous nerve branches to biceps muscle (Caldani, 1813, 1814)*

Macrodissected adult human branches of ***medial cutaneous nerve of forearm (>1840)*** to biceps brachii muscle; in the original Latin, *nervus cutaneus internus rami ad musculum bicipitem*, Table CCLVIII, Figure 1-24.

3. *internal cutaneous nerve branch to triceps (Caldani, 1813, 1814)*
   Macrodissected adult human branch of ***medial cutaneous nerve of forearm (>1840)*** to triceps brachii muscle; in the original Latin, *nervus cutaneus internus ramus ad tricipitem*, Table CCLVIII, Figure 1-25.

medial cutaneous nerve of thigh (>1840)

As described for macrodissected adult human, a branch of the ***femoral nerve (Haller, 1762)*** supplying skin and fascia on the distal two-thirds of the medial side of the thigh; see Durward (1951, p. 1097 and Fig. 940), Williams & Warwick (1980, p. 1109 and Figs. 7.211, 212). It was delineated by Eustachi; see ***[medial cutaneous nerve of thigh (>1840)] (Eustachi, 1552)***.

EARLIER REFERENCES:

Illustrated, not named or described:

1. ***[medial cutaneous nerve of thigh (>1840)] (Eustachi, 1552)***
   Clearly illustrated for macrodissected adult human; see Albinus edition (1761, Tab. 21-*L*).

Illustrated and described, not named:

1. ***[medial cutaneous nerve of thigh (>1840)] (Vieussens, 1684)***
   Described and illustrated for macrodissected adult human; Table 28-94.

Earlier synonyms:

1. *internal branch of crural nerve (Winslow, 1733)*
   Synonym for macrodissected adult human ***medial cutaneous nerve of thigh (>1840)***; Section VI, p. 90.
2. *superior cutaneous branch of crural nerve (Martin, 1781)*
   Apparently synonym for ***medial cutaneous nerve of thigh (>1840)***; in the original Latin, *nervus cruralis ramus cutaneus superior*, p. 233 and Table X. Also see Fischer (1791, p. 7).
3. *internal cutaneous nerve of crural nerve (Styx, 1782)*
   Synonym for macrodissected adult human ***medial cutaneous nerve of thigh (>1840)***; in the original Latin, *nervus cutaneus internus*, p. 8.
4. *short cutaneous nerve (Günther, 1786)*
   Apparently synonym for macrodissected adult human ***medial cutaneous nerve of thigh (>1840)***; in the original Latin, *nervus cutaneus brevis*, p. 83.
5. *superior cutaneous nerve (Günther, 1786)*
   Apparently synonym for macrodissected adult human ***medial cutaneous nerve of thigh (>1840)***; in the original Latin, *nervus cutaneus superior*, p. 83.
6. *minor cutaneous nerve (Günther, 1786, p. 83)*
   Apparently synonym for macrodissected adult human ***medial cutaneous nerve of thigh (>1840)***; in the original Latin, *nervus cutaneus minor*, p. 83.
7. *internal lateral cutaneous nerve (Fischer, 1791)*
   Name Fischer gave to Vieussens's (1684) tenth branch of ***femoral nerve (Haller, 1762)***, synonym for macrodissected adult human ***medial cutaneous nerve of thigh (>1840)***; in the original Latin, *nervus cutaneus lateris interni*, p. 7.
8. *internal cutaneous nerve (Fischer, 1791)*
   Synonym for macrodissected adult human ***medial cutaneous nerve of thigh (>1840)***; in the original Latin, *nervus cutaneus internus*, pp. 7, 15. Also see Schmidt (1794, p. 61). Cloquet (1828, Pl. CLXXI, Fig. 1-*41*) used the French, *nerf cutané moyen*, and described (Pl. CLXXII, Fig. 1-*76,78*) internal and external branches of it.
9. *inner cutaneous branch of anterior femoral nerve (Soemmerring, 1791)*
   Synonym for macrodissected adult human ***medial cutaneous nerve of thigh (>1840)***; in the original German, *Innere Hautaeste*, p. 300, also see Soemmerring (1798, p. 318).
10. *superior internal femoral cutaneous nerve (Mayer, 1794)*
    Synonym for macrodissected adult human ***medial cutaneous nerve of thigh (>1840)***; in the original Latin, *nervus cutaneus internus superior femoris*; Part 5, Table V, Figure 1-*12* (p. 25).
11. *internal and superior posterior femoral cutaneous nerve (Mayer, 1794)*
    Synonym for macrodissected adult human ***medial cutaneous nerve of thigh (>1840)***; in the original Latin, *nervus cutaneus posterior superior et internus femoris*; Part 5, Table VI-*ζ* (p. 36).
12. *internal cutaneous branch of crural nerve (Fyfe, 1800)*
    Synonym for macrodissected adult human ***medial cutaneous nerve of thigh (>1840)***; Vol. 2, p. 328.
13. *internal cutaneous nerve of thigh (Bell, 1803a)*
    Synonym for macrodissected adult human ***medial cutaneous nerve of thigh (>1840)***; Plate VII-4.
14. *inferior and internal cutaneous nerve (Bell, 1803b)*
    Apparently synonym for macrodissected adult human ***medial cutaneous nerve of thigh (>1840)***; pp. 204–205.
15. *internal anterior femoral cutaneous nerve (Bock, 1827)*
    Apparently synonym for macrodissected adult human ***medial cutaneous nerve of thigh (>1840)***; in the original Latin, *nerv. cutaneus femoris internus anterior*, Table I, Figure 2-*77*. Also gave as *nerv. cutaneus anterior internus femoris*, Table II-*112*.
16. *superior internal cutaneous nerve (Cloquet, 1828)*
    Synonym for macrodissected adult human ***medial cutaneous nerve of thigh (>1840)***; in the original French, *nerf cutané interne supérieur*, Plate CLXXI, Figure 2-*27*.
17. *internal cutaneous nerve from second lumbar (Swan, 1830)*
    Synonym for macrodissected adult human ***medial cutaneous nerve of thigh (>1840)***; Plate XVIII-*29*.
18. *inferior cutaneous perforant branch of crural musculo-cutaneous nerve (Cruveilhier, 1836)*
    Probably synonym for macrodissected adult human ***medial cutaneous branches of femoral nerve***

(>1840); in the original French, *perforante cutanée inférieure*, p. 842.

PARTLY CORRESPONDS:

1. *accessory branch of saphenous nerve (Cruveilhier, 1836)*
   Probably a particular macrodissected adult human ***medial cutaneous branch of femoral nerve (>1840)***; in the original French, *branche accessoire du nerf saphène*, p. 842.
2. *accessory cutaneous branch of internal saphenous nerve (Cruveilhier, 1836)*
   Synonym for *accessory branch of saphenous nerve (Cruveilhier, 1836)*; in the original French, *branche cutanée accessoire du nerf saphène interne*, p. 843.
3. *superficial branch of accessory cutaneous branch of internal saphenous nerve (Cruveilhier, 1836)*
   For macrodissected adult human, Cruveilhier referred to this first branch of *accessory cutaneous branch of internal saphenous nerve (Cruveilhier, 1836)* as accompanying the saphenous vein; in the original French, *rameau superficiel*, p. 843.
4. *satellite branch of saphenous vein of accessory cutaneous branch of internal saphenous nerve (Cruveilhier, 1836)*
   Synonym for *superficial branch of accessory cutaneous branch of internal saphenous nerve (Cruveilhier, 1836)*; in the original French, *rameau satellite de la veine saphène*, p. 843.
5. *satellite branch of femoral artery of accessory cutaneous branch of internal saphenous nerve (Cruveilhier, 1836)*
   For macrodissected human, Cruveilhier referred to this second branch of *accessory cutaneous branch of internal saphenous nerve (Cruveilhier, 1836)* as accompanying the femoral artery; in the original French, *rameau satellite de l'artère fémorale*, p. 843.

medial dorsal cutaneous nerve (>1840)

As described for macrodissected adult human, a branch of the ***superficial fibular nerve (Fyfe, 1800)*** supplying smaller branches to skin and fascia of the distal third of the leg and dorsum of the foot. It commonly divides into three smaller branches, the medial supplying the dorsum of the foot and medial side of the big toe and communicating with the ***saphenous nerve (Haase, 1781)***, the intermediate branch passing to the interval between the big toe and second toe and dividing into two branches communicating with the ***medial plantar nerve (>1840)***, and the lateral branch passing to the interval between the second and third toes, where it divides into ***dorsal digital nerves of medial dorsal cutaneous nerve (>1840)***; see Durward (1951, p. 1108 and Figures 948, 949, where it is called *medial branch of musculo-cutaneous nerve*), *Terminologia Anatomica* (1998, p. 140). It was known to Galen; see ***[medial dorsal cutaneous nerve (>1840)] (Galen, c173)***.

EARLIER REFERENCES:

Described, not named or illustrated:

1. ***[medial dorsal cutaneous nerve (>1840)] (Galen, c173)***
   Alluded to for macrodissected adult beef, pig, and/or macaque but not human; see May translation (1968, p. 706), Singer translation (1999, pp. 86–87).

Illustrated, not named or described:

1. ***[medial dorsal cutaneous nerve (>1840)] (Eustachi, 1552)***
   Eustachi illustrated it for macrodissected adult human, but did not distinguish ***dorsal digital nerves of medial dorsal cutaneous nerve (>1840)*** and associated lateral branch more closely with ***intermediate dorsal cutaneous nerve (>1840)***; see Albinus edition (1761, Tab. 21-4).

Illustrated and described, not named:

1. ***[medial dorsal cutaneous nerve (>1840)] (Vieussens, 1684)***
   Described and illustrated for macrodissected adult human; Table 29-*u*.

Earlier synonyms:

1. *internal dorsal twig of foot of superficial branch of peroneal nerve (Jördens, 1788)*
   Synonym for macrodissected adult human ***medial dorsal cutaneous nerve (>1840)***; in the original Latin, *ramulus dorsalis pedis internum rami superficialis nervi peronei*, pp. 5, 14. Jördens described and illustrated a comprehensive fourth order branching pattern, and named all 19 segments; see pp. 5–7 and Table 1:*82–101*.
2. *internal branch of superficial peroneal nerve (Fischer, 1791)*
   Synonym for macrodissected adult human *internal dorsal twig of foot of superficial branch of peroneal nerve (Jördens, 1788)*; in the original Latin, *ramus internus nervi peronei superficialis*, p. 31.
3. *internal dorsal branch of superficial peroneal nerve (Fischer, 1791)*
   Synonym for macrodissected adult human *internal dorsal twig of foot of superficial branch of peroneal nerve (Jördens, 1788)*; in the original Latin, *ramus dorsalem internum nervi peronei superficialis*, p. 31.
4. *superficial cutaneous branch of peroneal nerve (Mayer, 1794)*
   Synonym for macrodissected adult human ***medial dorsal cutaneous nerve (>1840)***; in the original Latin, *ramus cutaneous nervi peronei superficialis*; Part 5, Table V, Figure 1-*30* (p. 26).
5. *internal branch of metatarsal nerves (Bell, 1803b)*
   Synonym for macrodissected adult human ***medial dorsal cutaneous nerve (>1840)***; p. 210.
6. *internal branch of dorsal branches of foot (Bell, 1803b)*
   Synonym for macrodissected adult human ***medial dorsal cutaneous nerve (>1840)***; p. 210.
7. *interior branch of praetibio-digital nerve (Burdin, 1803)*
   Synonym for macrodissected adult human ***medial dorsal cutaneous nerve (>1840)***; see translation (1803, Vol. 1, p. 205).
8. *internal and superficial branch to back of foot of musculocutaneous branch of external popliteal nerve (Cloquet, 1816)*
   Synonym for macrodissected adult human ***medial dorsal cutaneous nerve (>1840)***; in the original

French, *rameau interne et superficiel du dos du pied*, p. 674. Cloquet further described internal and external branches of this branch.

9. *anterior nerve of back of foot (Meckel, 1817)*
   Synonym for macrodissected adult human ***medial dorsal cutaneous nerve (>1840)***; in the original Latin, *nervus dorsi pedis anticus communis*, see translation (1832, Vol. 3, p. 18).
10. *anterior peroneal nerve (Meckel, 1817)*
    Synonym for macrodissected adult human ***medial dorsal cutaneous nerve (>1840)***; in the original Latin, *nervus peroneus anticus*, see translation (1832, Vol. 3, p. 18).
11. *anterior nerve of foot (Meckel, 1817)*
    Synonym for macrodissected adult human ***medial dorsal cutaneous nerve (>1840)***; in the original Latin, *nervus pedis anticus*, see translation (1832, Vol. 3, p. 18).
12. *internal cutaneous nerve of back of foot (Bock, 1827)*
    Synonym for macrodissected adult human ***medial dorsal cutaneous nerve (>1840)***; in the original Latin, *Nerv. cutaneus internus dorsi pedis*, Table I, Figure 2-*89*.
13. *internal dorsal nerve of foot (Bock, 1827)*
    Synonym for *internal cutaneous nerve of back of foot (Bock, 1827)*; in the original Latin, *nerv. dorsalis pedis internus*, Table VI, Figure 3-*4*.
14. *internal branch of fibular nerve (Quain, 1828)*
    Synonym for macrodissected adult human ***medial dorsal cutaneous nerve (>1840)***; p. 297.
15. *internal branch of peroneal nerve (Quain, 1828)*
    Synonym for macrodissected adult human ***medial dorsal cutaneous nerve (>1840)***; p. 297.
16. *internal branch of musculo-cutaneous nerve (Quain & Wilson, 1839)*
    Synonym for macrodissected adult human ***medial dorsal cutaneous nerve (>1840)***; Plate XXIV, Figure 1-*e*.
17. *medial branch of musculocutaneous nerve (>1840)*
    Synonym for macrodissected adult human ***medial dorsal cutaneous nerve (>1840)***; see Durward (1951, p. 1108), Williams & Warwick (1980, p. 1115).

PARTLY CORRESPONDS:

1. *trunk of internal dorsal twig of foot of superficial peroneal nerve (Jördens, 1788)*
   Proximal undivided segment of macrodissected adult human ***medial dorsal cutaneous nerve (>1840)***; in the original Latin, *ramulus dorsalis pedis internum rami superficialis nervi peronei, trunculum*, pp. 5, 14.
2. *internal metatarsal twig of internal branch of superficial peroneal nerve (Fischer, 1791)*
   Branch of ***medial dorsal cutaneous nerve (>1840)*** supplying dorsal digital nerve to medial side of big toe; in the original Latin, *ramulus metatarsicus internus*, p. 31.
3. *external metatarsal twig of internal branch of superficial peroneal nerve (Fischer, 1791)*
   Branch of ***medial dorsal cutaneous nerve (>1840)*** supplying dorsal digital nerves to lateral side of big toe and medial side of second toe; in the original Latin, *ramulus metatarsicus externus*, p. 32.

medial eminence (>1840)

As described for macrodissected adult human, the longitudinal raised surface of the ***floor of fourth ventricle (Reil, 1807–1808b)*** just lateral to the ***median sulcus of fourth ventricle (>1840)*** and rostral to the ***hypoglossal triangle (>1840)***. The ***facial colliculus (>1840)*** lies just lateral to the region where the ***medial eminence (>1840)*** abuts the ***hypoglossal triangle (>1840)***; see Millen & Woollam (1962, p. 54), Crosby et al. (1962, p. 113), Carpenter (1976, Fig. 11.2). It was identified long ago; see ***[medial eminence (>1840)] (Ridley, 1695)***.

EARLIER REFERENCES:

Illustrated and described, not named:

1. ***[medial eminence (>1840)] (Ridley, 1695)***
   Described and illustrated for macrodissected adult human; p. 198, Figure VII-*k*; it was very clearly illustrated for macrodissected adult human by Santorini (1775, Tab. III, Fig. II).

Earlier synonyms:

1. *crura medullae oblongatae ad corpora quadrigemina (Langenbeck, 1826–1830)*
   Synonym for macrodissected adult human right and left ***medial eminence (>1840)***; Fascicle I, Table XXIX, Figure 1-*m*.
2. *scala rhythmica (Bergmann, 1831)*
   Apparently synonym for macrodissected adult human ***medial eminence (>1840)***; Table V-*i,k*.

medial forebrain bundle (Edinger, 1893)

As described in macrodissected adult human, and vertebrate generally with histological methods for ***axons (Kölliker, 1896)***, the most complex of the longitudinal ***central nervous system white matter tracts (>1840)***, with rostrally and caudally directed components. For ease of topographic description, it extends from the ***lateral hypothalamic zone (Nauta & Haymaker, 1969)*** rostrally, where it is largest, to the ***lateral funiculus (Burdach, 1822)*** of the ***spinal cord (Galen, c162– c166)*** caudally, where it is smallest, and it has five segments: ***hypothalamic medial forebrain bundle (>1840)***, ***tegmental medial forebrain bundle (>1840)***, ***pontine medial forebrain bundle (>1840)***, ***medullary medial forebrain bundle (>1840)***, and ***spinal medial forebrain bundle (>1840)***. Osborn (1888, p. 78) probably first described the ***medial forebrain bundle (>1840)*** as extending all the way to the ***spinal cord (Galen, c162–c166)*** in amphibian; also see Saper et al. (1976). Along with many branches, it has been called the "medial forebrain bundle system"; see Swanson (2004, Tab. C, p. 178). For Edinger's use in histological sections of adult human and other mammal see Figure 67, where he referred to "medial fascicles of forebrain bundle." It was probably first identified, at least in part, by Meckel; see ***[medial forebrain bundle (Edinger, 1893)] (Meckel, 1817)***.

EARLIER REFERENCES:

Described, not named or illustrated:

1. ***[medial forebrain bundle (Edinger, 1893)] (Meckel, 1817)***
Meckel probably described for macrodissected adult human a major branched component of it, with the caudal end near the ***mammillary body (Ludwig, 1779)*** and the rostral end entering the ***terminal stria (Wenzel & Wenzel, 1812)*** and ***medullary stria (Wenzel & Wenzel, 1812)***—basically the ***hypothalamic medial forebrain bundle (>1840)***; see translation (1832, Vol. 2, pp. 451–452).

PARTLY CORRESPONDS:

1. *ventral reticulospinal tract (>1840b)*
Appears to form part of the ***pontine medial forebrain bundle (>1840)*** and ***medullary medial forebrain bundle (>1840)***; see Crosby et al. (1962, p. 105), who also refer to a ventrolateral reticulospinal tract in the same vicinity but more lateral.

medial frontal gyrus (>1840)

As described for macrodissected adult human, a topographic subdivision of the ***frontal region (Vicq d'Azyr, 1786)*** on the medial face of the *cerebral hemisphere (Tiedemann, 1816)*, medial and ventral to the ***superior frontal gyrus (>1840)*** and rostral to the ***paracentral sulcus (>1840)***; see Williams & Warwick (1980, Fig. 7.114A), *Terminologia Anatomica* (1998, p. 126), *Dorland's* (2003, p. 806). It was first clearly delineated by Soemmerring; see ***[medial frontal gyrus (>1840)] (Soemmerring, 1778)***.

EARLIER REFERENCES:

Illustrated, not named or described:

1. ***[medial frontal gyrus (>1840)] (Soemmerring, 1778)***
Clearly illustrated for macrodissected adult human; Table III.

PARTLY CORRESPONDS:

1. *peripheral cingulate gyrus (Burdach, 1822)*
Apparently indicates at least part of macrodissected adult human ***medial frontal gyrus (1840)***; in the original German, *peripherischen Randwulst der Zwinge*, p. 150, Table VIII-*ψ*.

medial geniculate complex (>1840)

As described for macrodissected adult human, and based on cellular architecture and connections in mammal generally, a ***gray matter region (Swanson & Bota, 2010)*** in the caudal and medial end of the ***dorsal part of thalamus (Herrick, 1910)*** receiving a massive auditory input from the ***inferior colliculus (Haller, 1762)*** and projecting to the *primary auditory area (>1840)* and surrounding auditory areas of ***cerebral cortex gray matter (>1840)***; see Jones (1985, p. 425 ff.), Nieuwenhuys et al. (2008, p. 742, Fig. 18.3). It was probably first roughly delineated by Willis; see ***[medial geniculate complex (>1840)] (Willis, 1664)***.

EARLIER REFERENCES:

Described, not named or illustrated:

1. ***[medial geniculate complex (>1840)] (Willis, 1664)***
According to Burdach (1822, p. 342), Willis described without naming specifically its general location; Chapter 3, p. 21.

Earlier synonyms:

1. *geniculate body (Santorini, 1724)*
Synonym for macrodissected adult human ***medial geniculate complex (>1840)***; p. 63, see Polyak (1957, p. 115).
2. *corpus geniculatum (Santorini, 1724)*
Latin form of *geniculate body (Santorini, 1724)*; p. 63.
3. *tuberculum thalami inferius (Soemmerring, 1778)*
Synonym for macrodissected adult human ***medial geniculate complex (>1840)***; Table II-*O,i*. See Polyak (1957, p. 115) and *tuberculo thalamorum inferiore* in Table II-*i*.
4. *internal geniculate body (Reil, 1809b)*
Synonym for macrodissected adult human ***medial geniculate complex (>1840)***; see Mayo translation (1823, p. 58). Burdach (1822, p. 118) provided Latin form, *corpus geniculatum internum*. Gordon (1815, p. 90) used English form, *inner corpus geniculatum*.
5. *tuberculum thalami posticum medium (Meckel, 1817)*
Synonym for macrodissected adult human ***medial geniculate complex (>1840)***; p. 511.
6. *nodose tubercle (Rolando, 1831)*
Apparently synonym for macrodissected adult human ***medial geniculate complex (>1840)***; in the original Italian, *tuberculo nodoso*, pp. 121–122, Figure 9-*1,2,11*.
7. *posterior geniculate (Gerdy, 1838)*
Synonym for macrodissected adult human ***medial geniculate complex (>1840)***; in the original French, *genouillé postérieur*, p. 262.
8. *internal geniculate tubercle (Arnold, 1838b)*
Synonym for macrodissected adult human ***medial geniculate complex (>1840)***; in the original Latin, *tuberculum geniculatum internum*, Table IV, Figure 3-*ε*.

medial globus pallidus (>1840)

As described for macrodissected adult human, and with cellular architecture and connections for all mammals, the medial component of the ***globus pallidus (Burdach, 1822)***, separated from the ***lateral globus pallidus (>1840)*** by the ***medial medullary lamina (>1840)***; see Nieuwenhuys et al. (2008, Fig. 5.32-24, where it is called *internal part*), *Nomina Anatomica* (1983, p. A72), *Terminologia Anatomica* (1998, p. 130). It was probably first clearly delineated as the *innermost arcade of striate body (Vicq d'Azyr, 1786)*.

EARLIER REFERENCES:

Earlier synonyms:

1. *innermost arcade of striate body (Vicq d'Azyr, 1786)*
Clearly illustrated synonym for macrodissected adult human ***medial globus pallidus (>1840)***; in the original French, *arcade la plus intérieure des [corps] stries*, Plate XIII-29; also see Plate XII. Arnold (1838b, Tab. VIII, Fig. 2) illustrated it even more accurately.

medial hypothalamic zone (Nauta & Haymaker, 1969)

As described in macrodissected adult human, and with cellular architecture in mammal as well as vertebrate generally, the middle of three longitudinal divisions of the ***hypothalamus (Kuhlenbeck, 1927)***, between ***periventricular hypothalamic zone (Nauta & Haymaker, 1969)*** medially and ***lateral hypothalamic zone (Nauta & Haymaker, 1969)*** laterally. Based most clearly on cellular architecture, it is characterized by a longitudinal series of well-defined nuclei, from rostral to caudal the ***medial preoptic nucleus (>1840)***, ***anterior hypothalamic nucleus (>1840)***, ***descending division of paraventricular hypothalamic nucleus (Swanson, 1991)***, ***ventromedial hypothalamic nucleus (>1840)***, ***ventral premammillary nucleus (>1840)*** and ***dorsal premammillary nucleus (>1840)***, and ***mammillary body (Ludwig, 1779)***; see Swanson (1998, Table B, p. 206). The concept was derived from the submammalian comparative histological work of Crosby & Woodbourne (1940), but the term was Nauta and Haymaker's, see p. 141. It was not clearly described before 1840.

medial lemniscus (>1840)

As described in macrodissected adult human, and mammal generally with histological methods for ***axons (Kölliker, 1896)***, the rostral extension of the ***medial lemniscus decussation (>1840)*** ending in the ***ventral posterolateral nucleus (>1840)*** of the ***ventral thalamic nuclei (>1840)***; see Carpenter (1996, Fig. 10.1). For topographic description, it has ***thalamic medial lemniscus (>1840)***, ***tegmental medial lemniscus (>1840)***, ***pontine medial lemniscus (>1840)***, and ***medullary medial lemniscus (>1840)*** segments. It was first delineated as the *external part of lemniscus (Reil, 1809c)*.

EARLIER REFERENCES:

Earlier synonyms:

1. *external part of lemniscus (Reil, 1809c)*
   Initial, rough description of macrodissected adult human ***medial lemniscus (>1840)***; see Mayo translation (1823, p. 95); also see *internal part of lemniscus (Reil, 1809c)*.
2. *outer portion of fillet (Reil, 1809c)*
   Synonym for *external part of lemniscus (Reil, 1809c)*; see Mayo translation (1823, p. 96).
3. *anterior part of olivary fasciculus (Arnold, 1838b)*
   Synonym for macrodissected adult human ***medial lemniscus (>1840)***; in the original Latin, *fasciculi olivaris pars anterior*, Table IX, Figure 5-*t*.

medial lemniscus decussation (>1840)

As described for macrodissected adult human, and mammal generally with histological methods for ***axons (Kölliker, 1896)***, a transverse ***central nervous system white matter tract (>1840)*** in the median plane of the ventral ***medulla (Winslow, 1733)***, between ***internal arcuate fibers (>1840)*** dorsally and ***medial lemniscus (>1840)*** rostrally; see Carpenter (1976, pp. 291–293), *Terminologia Anatomica* (1998, p. 109). It was perhaps first clearly delineated as the *decussation of posterior column (Bell, 1834)*.

EARLIER REFERENCES:

Earlier synonyms:

1. *decussation of posterior part (Bell, 1834)*
   Synonym for macrodissected adult human *decussation of posterior column (Bell, 1834)*; p. 477.
2. *decussation of sensitive part (Bell, 1834)*
   Synonym for macrodissected adult human *decussation of posterior column (Bell, 1834)*; p. 477.
3. *decussation of posterior column (Bell, 1834)*
   Synonym for macrodissected adult human ***medial lemniscus decussation (>1840)***; p. 478.
4. *decussation of posterior tract (Bell, 1834)*
   Synonym for macrodissected adult human *decussation of posterior column (Bell, 1834)*; Table XX, Figure 2-C.

medial longitudinal fascicle (>1840)

As described in macrodissected adult human, and mammal generally with histological methods for ***axons (Kölliker, 1896)***, a thin, heterogeneous, longitudinal ***central nervous system white matter tract (>1840)*** extending from the ***midbrain (Baer, 1837)*** level of the ***interstitial nucleus (>1840)*** rostrally to join the ***ventral funiculus (>1840)*** of the ***spinal cord (>Galen, c162–c166)*** caudally. Main components of the ***medial longitudinal fascicle (>1840)*** include vestibulospinal ***axons (Kölliker, 1896)*** of the ***medial vestibular nucleus (>1840)***, the *interstitiospinal tract (>1840)* from the ***interstitial nucleus (>1840)***, and the *tectobulbar tract (>1840)*, sometimes considered together with the ***tectospinal tract (>1840)*** as the *pretectal bundle (>1840)*; see Carpenter (1976, pp. 269–270, 342–344), Nieuwenhuys et al. (2008, p. 182). For topographic description, it has ***tegmental medial longitudinal fascicle (>1840)***, ***pontine medial longitudinal fascicle (>1840)***, ***medullary medial longitudinal fascicle (>1840)***, and ***spinal medial longitudinal fascicle (>1840)*** segments. It was probably first noted by Soemmerring; see ***[medial longitudinal fascicle (>1840)] (Soemmerring, 1778)***.

EARLIER REFERENCES:

Illustrated and described, not named:

1. ***[medial longitudinal fascicle (>1840)] (Soemmerring, 1778)***
   Soemmerring apparently indicated its approximate location ventral to the ***cerebral aqueduct (>1840)*** and rostral ***fourth ventricle (Galen, c192)*** in macrodissected adult human; Table III-*.
2. ***[medial longitudinal fascicle (>1840)] (Vicq d'Azyr, 1786)***
   Probably illustrated as ***central nervous system white matter tract (>1840)*** extending caudally from approximate region where ***oculomotor nerve***

(Estienne, 1545) originates in ***tegmentum (Swanson, 2000b)*** to rostral part of ***pons (Haller, 1747)***, roughly same extent as ***[medial longitudinal fascicle (>1840)] (Soemmerring, 1778)***; Plate XXXI, Figure II-2 toward *6*.

Earlier synonyms:

1. *cylindrical fascicle (Reil, 1809c)*
   May correspond to macrodissected adult human ***medial longitudinal fascicle (>1840)***. Although not illustrated, described as stretching from level of ***pyramidal decussation (Reil, 1809c)***, through *gray substance (Vesalius, 1543a)* ventral to ***fourth ventricle (Galen, c192)*** and ***cerebral aqueduct (>1840)*** to level of ***superior cerebellar peduncle decussation (>1840)***; see Mayo translation (1823, pp. 87, 102).
2. *longitudinal fascicle (Gall & Spurzheim, 1810)*
   Central nervous system white matter tract (>1840) described as forming part of ***fourth ventricle (Galen, c192)***, probably corresponding to at least part of macrodissected adult human ***medial longitudinal fascicle (>1840)***; p. 192 and Plate VI-*m*.
3. *round bundle (Burdach, 1822)*
   Term attributed to Reil (1809c), apparently synonym for macrodissected adult human *cylindrical fascicle (Reil, 1809c)*; in the original German, *runde Bündel*, p. 493, also see p. 285.
4. *funiculus terete (Burdach, 1822)*
   Latin form of *round bundle (Burdach, 1822)*; pp. 37, 285; Table IV-*v*.

medial longitudinal stria (>1840)

As described for macrodissected adult human, the medial component of the ***longitudinal striae (>1840)*** extending rostrocaudally along the dorsal surface and both ends of the ***corpus callosum (Galen, c177)*** just lateral to the median plane and separated by a narrow gap from the ***lateral longitudinal stria (Arnold, 1838a)***; see Williams & Warwick (1980, p. 998 and Fig. 7.139), Nieuwenhuys et al. (2008, Fig. 3.18). It was first identified as the *medial longitudinal cord (Lancisi, 1713)*.

EARLIER REFERENCES:

Earlier synonyms:

1. *medial longitudinal cord (Lancisi, 1713)*
   Synonym for macrodissected adult human ***medial longitudinal stria (>1840)***; p. 153.
2. *longitudinal nerve (Lancisi, 1718)*
   Synonym for macrodissected adult human *medial longitudinal cord (Lancisi, 1713)*; the entire Latin description, used in figure legend for right and left *longitudinal nerve (Lancisi, 1718)*, was *Nervuli longitudinales ab anterioribus ad posteriora excurrentes*, p. 316.
3. *raphe of corpus callosum (Arnold, 1838b)*
   Synonym for macrodissected adult human ***medial longitudinal stria (>1840)***; in the original Latin, *raphe corporis callosi*, Table V, Figure 3-*h*.

medial mammary branches of intercostal nerves (>1840)

As described for macrodissected adult human, branches of the ***anterior cutaneous branches of intercostal nerves (>1840)*** commonly arising from the fourth and fifth ***thoracic nerves (Diemerbroeck, 1672)*** and innervating the breast and nipple; see Durward (1951, Fig. 918), Williams & Warwick (1980, Fig. 7.206), *Nomina Anatomica* (1998, p. 139). They were known to Vesalius; see ***[medial mammary branches of intercostal nerves (>1840)] (Vesalius, 1543a)***.

EARLIER REFERENCES:

Described, not named or illustrated:

1. ***[medial mammary branches of intercostal nerves (>1840)] (Vesalius, 1543a)***
   Clearly illustrated for macrodissected adult human and ascribed to fourth ***intercostal nerve (Vesalius, 1543a)***; see Richardson & Carman translation (2002, p. 206-v) and ***lateral mammary branches of intercostal nerves (>1840)***.

Earlier synonyms:

1. *mammary nerves (Horne, 1707)*
   Probably refers to macrodissected adult human ***medial mammary branches of intercostal nerves (>1840)***; in the original Latin, *nervi mammarum*, see *Index rerum*.

medial medullary lamina (>1840)

As described for macrodissected adult human, the thin ***central nervous system white matter tract (>1840)*** between ***lateral globus pallidus (>1840)*** laterally and ***medial globus pallidus (>1840)*** medially; see Nieuwenhuys et al. (2008, Fig. 5.32-8), *Nomina Anatomica* (1983, p. A72), *Terminologia Anatomica* (1998, p. 130). It was perhaps first clearly delineated by Arnold; see ***[medial medullary lamina (>1840)] (Arnold, 1838b)***.

EARLIER REFERENCES:

Illustrated and described, not named:

1. ***[medial medullary lamina (>1840)] (Arnold, 1838b)***
   Clearly illustrated for macrodissected adult human; Table VIII, Figure 2.

medial midbrain sulcus (>1840)

As described for macrodissected adult human, a shallow longitudinal groove on the surface of the ***tegmentum (Swanson, 2000b)*** of the ***midbrain (Baer, 1837)***, running along the ventromedial border of the ***cerebral peduncle (Tarin, 1753)*** and indicating the site of exit of the ***oculomotor nerve central rootlets (>1840)*** continuing as peripheral ***oculomotor nerve rootlets (>1840)***; see Williams & Warwick (1980, p. 935), Nieuwenhuys et al. (2008, Fig. 3.12). The ***lateral midbrain sulcus (>1840)*** runs along the dorsal border of the ***cerebral peduncle (Tarin, 1753)***. The ***medial midbrain sulcus (>1840)*** was perhaps first delineated by Vicq d'Azyr; see ***[medial midbrain sulcus (>1840)] (Vicq d'Azyr, 1786)***.

EARLIER REFERENCES:

Illustrated, not named or described:

1. ***[medial midbrain sulcus (>1840)] (Vicq d'Azyr, 1786)***
   Illustrated for macrodissected adult human; Plate XXXI, Figure 2, between *2* and *4*, on either side of *3*. Very clearly illustrated by Gall & Spurzheim (1810, Pl. V, medial side of *9*).

medial nasal branches of internal nasal branches of anterior ethmoidal nerve (>1840)

As described for macrodissected adult human, they supply primarily mucus membrane of the rostral (front) part of the nasal septum; see Williams & Warwick (1980, p. 1061), *Terminologia Anatomica* (1998, p. 134).They were probably first clearly delineated as the *internal nasal threads of ethmoidal fascicle (Bellingeri, 1818).*

EARLIER REFERENCES:

Earlier synonyms:

1. *internal nasal threads of ethmoidal fascicle (Bellingeri, 1818)*
   Synonym for macrodissected adult human ***medial nasal branches of internal nasal branches of anterior ethmoidal nerve (>1840)***; in the original Latin, *stamina nasalis internus*, see Table I.
2. *branch to nasal septum of ethmoidal branch of nasociliary nerve (Arnold, 1834)*
   Synonym for macrodissected adult human ***medial nasal branches of internal nasal branches of anterior ethmoidal nerve (>1840)***; in the original Latin, *nervus nasociliaris, ramus ethmoidalis, ramus septi narium*, p. 8.
3. *branch to nasal septum of ethmoidal branch of nasal nerve (Arnold, 1834)*
   Synonym for macrodissected adult human ***medial nasal branches of internal nasal branches of anterior ethmoidal nerve (>1840)***; in the original Latin, *nervus nasalis, ramus ethmoidalis, ramus septi narium*, p. 8.
4. *septal branch of nasal branch of ophthalmic nerve (Quain, 1837)*
   Synonym for macrodissected adult human ***medial nasal branches of internal nasal branches of anterior ethmoidal nerve (>1840)***; pp. 761–763.

medial occipitotemporal gyrus (>1840)

As described for macrodissected adult human, a topographic subdivision of the ***temporal region (>1840)*** lying between ***lateral occipitotemporal gyrus (>1840)*** laterally and ***parahippocampal gyrus (>1840)*** medially; see Clark (1951, Fig. 872), Williams & Warwick (1980, Fig. 7.114A). It was perhaps first clearly delineated by Vicq d'Azyr; see ***[medial occipitotemporal gyrus (>1840)] (Vicq d'Azyr, 1786).***

EARLIER REFERENCES:

Illustrated and described, not named:

1. ***[medial occipitotemporal gyrus (>1840)] (Vicq d'Azyr, 1786)***
   Vicq d'Azyr illustrated and drew attention to this "longitudinal convolution" of macrodissected adult human; Plate XVI-*18*.

PARTLY CORRESPONDS:

1. *area perirhinalis (Brodmann, 1909)*
   Original Latin form of *perirhinal area (Brodmann, 1909)*; p. 149.
2. *perirhinal area (Brodmann, 1909)*
   Based on cellular architecture in adult human, a narrow medial zone of ***medial occipitotemporal gyrus (>1840)*** between ***entorhinal area (Brodmann, 1909)*** medially and *ectorhinal area (Brodmann, 1909)* laterally; see Garey translation (1994, p. 129 and Fig. 86). Brodmann considered it an extended part of ***hippocampal formation (Swanson & Cowan, 1977)***.
3. *area 35 (Brodmann, 1909)*
   Synonym for adult human *perirhinal area (Brodmann, 1909)*; in the original German, *Feld 35*, p. 149.
4. *area ectorhinalis (Brodmann, 1909)*
   Original Latin form of *ectorhinal area (Brodmann, 1909)*; p. 143.
5. *ectorhinal area (Brodmann, 1909)*
   Based on cellular architecture in adult human, a narrow lateral zone of the ***medial occipitotemporal gyrus (>1840)*** surrounded by *perirhinal area (Brodmann, 1909)* medially, *inferior temporal area (Brodmann, 1909)* laterally, and *temporopolar area (Brodmann, 1909)* rostrally (anteriorly); see Garey translation (1994, p. 122 and Fig. 86).
6. *area 36 (Brodmann, 1909)*
   Synonym for adult human *ectorhinal area (Brodmann, 1909)*; in the original German, *Feld 36*, p. 143.

medial orbital gyrus (>1840)

As described for macrodissected adult human, the medial topographic subdivision of the ***orbital gyri (>1940)***, separated from the others by the ***orbital sulci (>1840)***; see Williams & Warwick (1980, Fig. 7.116). It was first clearly delineated by Soemmerring; see ***[medial orbital gyrus (>1840)] (Soemmerring, 1778).***

EARLIER REFERENCES:

Illustrated, not named or described:

1. ***[medial orbital gyrus (>1840)] (Soemmerring, 1778)***
   Illustrated clearly for macrodissected adult human; Table II.

Earlier synonyms:

1. *external olfactory convolution (Gerdy, 1838)*
   Synonym for macrodissected adult human ***medial orbital gyrus (>1840)***; in the original French, *circonvolution olfactive externe*, p. 259.

medial pectoral nerve (>1840)

As described for macrodissected adult human, it arises from the ***brachial plexus medial cord (Schwalbe, 1881)*** and primarily supplies the pectoralis minor muscle; see Durward (1951, p. 1071 and Fig. 925), Williams & Warwick (1980, p. 1096), *Terminologia Anatomica* (1998,

p. 138). It was known to Galen; see ***[medial pectoral nerve (>1840)] (Galen, c173)***.

EARLIER REFERENCES:

Described, not named or illustrated:

1. ***[medial pectoral nerve (>1840)] (Galen, c173)***
   Clearly described in macrodissected adult beef, pig, and/or macaque but not human; see May translation (1968, p. 703), Duckworth translation (1962, pp. 250, 253, 255); also see Singer translation (1999, p. 221).

Illustrated and described, not named:

1. ***[medial pectoral nerve (>1840)] (Vesalius, 1543a)***
   Alluded to in macrodissected adult human; see Richardson & Carman translation (2002, p. 234).

Earlier synonyms:

1. *internal cutaneous nerve (Neubauer, 1772)*
   Probably refers to macrodissected adult human ***medial pectoral nerve (>1840)***; in the original Latin, *nervus cutaneus internus*, Table 1-*228*; compare with Williams & Warwick (1980, Fig. 7.200).
2. *lesser anterior thoracic nerve (Günther, 1786)*
   Probably refers to macrodissected adult human ***medial pectoral nerve (>1840)***; in the original Latin, *nervus thoracicus anterior minor*, p. 73. Cloquet (1828, Pl. CLXVII, Fig. 1-*28*) used the French, *nerf petit thoracique antérieur*.
3. *anterior thoracic branch of brachial plexus (Cloquet, 1816)*
   Synonym for macrodissected adult human ***medial pectoral nerve (>1840)***; in the original French, *branche thoracique antérieure*, p. 643.
4. *anterior pectoral nerves (Bock, 1827)*
   Synonym for macrodissected adult human ***medial pectoral nerve (>1840)***; in the original Latin, *nervi pectoralis anteriores*, Table II-*21*.
5. *posterior thoracic branch of brachial plexus (Cruveilhier, 1836)*
   Synonym for macrodissected adult human ***medial pectoral nerve (>1840)***; in the original French, *branche thoraciques postérieure du plexus brachial*, p. 795.
6. *pectoralis minor branch of brachial plexus (Cruveilhier, 1836)*
   Synonym for macrodissected adult human ***medial pectoral nerve (>1840)***; in the original French, *branche du petit pectoral du plexus brachial*, p. 795.

medial plantar nerve (>1840)

As described for macrodissected adult human, the larger of two deep terminal branches of the ***tibial nerve (Haase, 1781)*** supplying muscular, cutaneous, articular, and vascular branches to medial parts of the sole of the foot, including the ***common plantar digital nerves of medial plantar nerve (>1840)*** and ***proper plantar digital nerves of medial plantar nerve (>1840)***; see Durward (1951, Figs. 951, 952), Williams & Warwick (1980, p. 1114), *Terminologia Anatomica* (1998, p. 141). It corresponds to the ***median nerve (Du Verney, 1697)*** for the hand; see Durward (1951, p. 1110). It was known to Galen; see ***[medial plantar nerve (>1840)] (Galen, c173)***.

EARLIER REFERENCES:

Described, not named or illustrated:

1. ***[medial plantar nerve (>1840)] (Galen, c173)***
   Vaguely identified in macrodissected adult beef, pig, and/or macaque but not human; see May translation (1968, pp. 192 with note *74*, 706), Singer translation (1999, p. 87).

Illustrated, not named or described:

1. ***[medial plantar nerve (>1840)] (Eustachi, 1552)***
   Clearly illustrated distribution, though not origin, for macrodissected adult human; see Albinus edition (1761, Tab. 20-*26*).

Illustrated and described, not named:

1. ***[medial plantar nerve (>1840)] (Vieussens, 1684)***
   Beautifully described and illustrated for macrodissected adult human; see Table 30-C.

Earlier synonyms:

1. *internal plantar nerve (Winslow, 1733)*
   Synonym for macrodissected adult human ***medial plantar nerve (>1840)***; in the original Latin, *nervus plantaris internus*, Section VI, p. 92.
2. *internal plantar branch of tibial nerve (Martin, 1781)*
   Synonym for macrodissected adult human ***medial plantar nerve (>1840)***; in the original Latin, *nervus tibialis ramus plantaris interior*, p. 242 and Table XI.
3. *interior branch of tibial nerve (Burdin, 1803)*
   Synonym for macrodissected adult human ***medial plantar nerve (>1840)***; see translation (1803, Vol. 1, p. 207).
4. *internal plantar branch of posterior tibial nerve (Quain, 1828)*
   Synonym for macrodissected adult human ***medial plantar nerve (>1840)***; p. 295.
5. *inner plantar nerve (Swan, 1830)*
   Synonym for macrodissected adult human ***medial plantar nerve (>1840)***; Plate XXV, Figure 2-*12*.

PARTLY CORRESPONDS:

1. *cutaneous nervelet of internal plantar nerve (Fischer, 1791)*
   Small branch of macrodissected adult human ***medial plantar nerve (>1840)*** to skin on medial side of heel; in the original Latin, *nervulus cutaneus nervi plantaris interni*, p. 36 and Table IV, Figure 3-*5* (where it is also referred to as a twig; *ramulus*).
2. *internal branch of internal plantar nerve (Fischer, 1791)*
   Medial branch of macrodissected adult human ***medial plantar nerve (>1840)*** ending as *internal plantar digital twig of big toe (Fischer, 1791)*; in the original Latin, *ramus internus nervi plantaris interni*, p. 36.
3. *ligamentous twig of internal branch of internal plantar nerve (Fischer, 1791)*
   Small branch of *internal branch of internal plantar nerve (Fischer, 1791)* to ligamentous fibers associated with calcaneus bone; in the original Latin, *ramulus ligamentosus ramus internus nervi plantaris interni*, p. 36.

4. *cutaneous twig of internal branch of internal plantar nerve (Fischer, 1791)*
   Small branch of *internal branch of internal plantar nerve (Fischer, 1791)* to medial side of foot; in the original Latin, *ramulus cutaneus ramus internus nervi plantaris interni*, p. 36.
5. *external branch of internal plantar nerve (Fischer, 1791)*
   Lateral branch of macrodissected adult human ***medial plantar nerve (>1840)*** in turn generating two *tarsal nerves (Fischer, 1791)*; in the original Latin, *ramum externum nervi plantaris interni*, p. 36.
6. *tarsal nerves (Fischer, 1791)*
   In macrodissected adult human, two branches (internal and external) of *external branch of internal plantar nerve (Fischer, 1791)* in turn generating lateral four *metatarsal nerves (Fischer, 1791)*; in the original Latin, *nervos tarsicos*, pp. 36–37.
7. *collateral branches of internal plantar nerve (Cruveilhier, 1836)*
   Considered together, *cutaneous nerves of collateral branches of internal plantar nerve (Cruveilhier, 1836)*, *muscular nerves of collateral branches of internal plantar nerve (Cruveilhier, 1836)*, and *plantar internal collateral nerve of big toe (Cruveilhier, 1836)*; in the original French, *rameaux collatéraux*, p. 872.
8. *cutaneous nerves of collateral branches of internal plantar nerve (Cruveilhier, 1836)*
   Cutaneous calcanean nerve (Cruveilhier, 1836) and *plantar cutaneous nerve (Cruveilhier, 1836)* considered together; in the original French, *nerfs cutanés*, p. 872.
9. *cutaneous calcanean nerve (Cruveilhier, 1836)*
   Synonym for macrodissected adult human *cutaneous nervelet of internal plantar nerve (Fischer, 1791)*; in the original French, *nerf calcanien cutané*, p. 872.
10. *plantar cutaneous nerve (Cruveilhier, 1836)*
   Macrodissected adult human branch of ***medial plantar nerve (>1840)*** to skin on plantar surface of foot that itself produces branch proceeding forward and branch proceeding backward; in the original French, *nerf cutané plantaire*, p. 872.

medial posterior superior nasal nerves (>1840)

As described for macrodissected adult human, 2–3 of the ***posterior superior nasal nerves (>1840)*** supplying mucous membrane covering the caudal (posterior) part of the roof of the nasal cavity and of the nasal septum. Histologically they contain predominantly sensory ***dendrites (His, 1889)*** simply passing through the ***pterygopalatine ganglion (>1840)*** from the ***medial posterior superior nasal nerves (>1840)*** to the ***pterygopalatine nerves (Wrisberg, 1786)*** and then the ***maxillary nerve (Meckel, 1753)*** and ***trigeminal ganglion (>1840)***; see Williams & Warwick (1980, pp. 1064–1065 and Fig. 7.171). The largest and longest component is the ***nasopalatine nerve (Scarpa, 1785)***. They were probably first clearly delineated as the *internal sphenopalatine nerve (Cruveilhier, 1836)*.

EARLIER REFERENCES:

Earlier synonyms:

1. *internal sphenopalatine nerve (Cruveilhier, 1836)*
   Synonym for macrodissected adult human ***medial posterior superior nasal nerves (>1840)***; in the original French, *nerf sphéno-palatin interne*, p. 923.
2. *nerve of nasal septum (Cruveilhier, 1836, p. 923)*
   Synonym for *internal sphenopalatine nerve (Cruveilhier, 1836)*; in the original French, *nerf de la cloison*, p. 923. Also see Cruveilhier (1844, p. 832).
3. *posterior superior medial nasal branches of pterygopalatine ganglion (>1840)*
   Synonym for macrodissected adult human ***medial posterior superior nasal nerves (>1840)***; see *Terminologia Anatomica* (1998, p. 134).

medial preoptic nucleus (>1840)

Based primarily on cellular architecture and connections in mammal, the most rostral component of the ***medial hypothalamic zone (Nauta & Haymaker, 1969)***, rostral to the ***anterior hypothalamic nucleus (>1840)***; see Swanson (1998, Table B, p. 206). It was not described by 1840.

medial pterygoid nerve (>1840)

As described for macrodissected adult human, a tiny branch of the ***mandibular nerve trunk (>1840)*** entering the deep surface of the medial pterygoid muscle after giving off the ***nerve to tensor veli palatini (>1840)*** and ***nerve to tensor tympani (Arnold, 1834)***, both of which pass uninterrupted through the ***otic ganglion (Arnold, 1828)***; see Williams & Warwick (1980, p. 1066 and Fig. 7.181), *Nomina Anatomica* (1983, p. A74). It may have been identified first by Willis; see ***[medial pterygoid nerve (>1840)] (Willis, 1664)***.

EARLIER REFERENCES:

Illustrated and described, not named:

1. ***[medial pterygoid nerve (>1840)] (Willis, 1664)***
   Possibly illustrated for macrodissected adult, presumably human, although description is quite vague; see Pordage translation (1681, p. 145, Fig. 1-*l*). Its origin in macrodissected adult human was clearly illustrated by Du Verney (1683, Pl. 13-4) and Vieussens (1684, Tab. 22-2).

Earlier synonyms:

1. *pterygoid branch of superior branch of inferior maxillary nerve (Meckel, 1748)*
   Synonym for macrodissected adult human ***medial pterygoid nerve (>1840)***; p. 86.
2. *pterygoid nerve (Haase, 1781)*
   Synonym for macrodissected adult human ***medial pterygoid nerve (>1840)***; in the original Latin, *nervus pterygoideus*; see Index, section 136. Also see Bock (1817, pp. 46–47), Meckel (1832, Vol. 3, p. 73).

3. *pterygoid muscle nerve (Soemmerring, 1798)*
   Synonym for macrodissected adult human ***medial pterygoid nerve (>1840)***; in the original Latin, *nervus musculi pterygoidei*, p. 233.
4. *internal pterygoid nerve (Arnold, 1834)*
   Synonym for macrodissected adult human ***medial pterygoid nerve (>1840)***; in the original Latin, *nervus pterygoideus internus*, p. 10.
5. *internal branch of inferior maxillary nerve (Cruveilhier, 1836)*
   Synonym for macrodissected adult human ***medial pterygoid nerve (>1840)***; in the original French, *branche interne*, p. 932.
6. *nerve of internal pterygoid muscle (Cruveilhier, 1836)*
   Synonym for macrodissected adult human ***medial pterygoid nerve (>1840)***; in the original French, *nerf du muscle ptérigoïdien*, p. 932.

PARTLY CORRESPONDS:

1. *pharyngeal surculus of inferior maxillary branch (Bellingeri, 1818)*
   Apparently branch of macrodissected adult human ***medial pterygoid nerve (>1840)*** ending deep within pharynx; in the original Latin, *surculus pharyngeus*, see Table 1.
2. *short root of otic ganglion (Arnold, 1834)*
   Probably synonym for macrodissected adult human *communicating branch from medial pterygoid nerve to otic ganglion (>1840)*; in the original Latin, *ganglion oticum, radix brevis*, p. 10. See Williams & Warwick (1980, Figs. 7.181, 184).
3. *short root of auricular ganglion (Arnold, 1834)*
   Synonym for *short root of otic ganglion (Arnold, 1834)*; in the original Latin, *ganglion auriculare, radix brevis*, p. 10.
4. *communicating branch from medial pterygoid nerve to otic ganglion (>1840)*
   Macrodissected adult human short proximal segments of ***nerve to tensor veli palatini (>1840)*** and ***nerve to tensor tympani (Arnold, 1834)***, or the common trunk for them, between origin from ***mandibular nerve (>1840)*** and ***otic ganglion (Arnold, 1828)***, through which, based on histology, both of them pass uninterrupted on their way to their corresponding muscles; see Williams & Warwick (1980, p. 1066 and Fig. 7.181), *Nomina Anatomica* (1983, p. A74).
5. *sensory root of otic ganglion (>1840)*
   Synonym for macrodissected adult human *communicating branch from medial pterygoid nerve to otic ganglion (>1840)*; see *Terminologia Anatomica* (1998, p. 134), where term *branches to otic ganglion from mandibular nerve* was also used. The origin of this term has not been traced; possibly an error that should read *motor root of otic ganglion*.

medial reticulospinal tract (>1840)

As described for adult mammal with normal and experimental pathway tracing methods, a caudally directed, diffusely organized, heterogeneous and poorly characterized longitudinal ***central nervous system white matter tract (>1840)*** arising predominantly from the ***pons (Haller, 1747)***, but also to some extent from the ***tegmentum (Swanson, 2000b)*** and ***medulla (Winslow, 1733)***. It is mostly ipsilateral and extends caudally through the ***spinal cord (Galen, c162–c166)*** in the ***ventral funiculus (>1840)***; see Mettler (1948, p. 238), Crosby et al. (1962, p. 105 and Figs. 85, 120, 133, 140, 145, 148), Williams & Warwick (1980, p. 875–876 and Fig. 7.44), *Terminologia Anatomica* (1998, p. 107, also gave synonym, *pontoreticulospinal tract*). For topographic description, there are major ***pontine medial reticulospinal tract (>1840)***, ***medullary medial reticulospinal tract (>1840)***, and ***spinal medial reticulospinal tract (>1840)*** segments. It was not described by 1840.

EARLIER REFERENCES:

Earlier synonyms:

1. *pontine reticulospinal tract (>1840)*
   Synonym for macrodissected adult human ***medial reticulospinal tract (>1840)***; see Carpenter (1976, p. 267 and Figs. 10.11, 10.21).
2. *ventral reticulospinal tract (>1840a)*
   Synonym for macrodissected adult human ***medial reticulospinal tract (>1840)***; see Mettler (1948, p. 238).
3. *direct spinoreticular tract (>1840)*
   Synonym for macrodissected adult human ***medial reticulospinal tract (>1840)***, "direct" meaning uncrossed; see Mettler (1948, p. 238).

medial retinohypothalamic tract (>1840)

As described in macrodissected adult human, and mammal generally with histological methods for ***axons (Kölliker, 1896)***, a branch of the ***optic chiasm (Galen, c173)*** to certain ***central nervous system gray matter regions (>1840)*** in the ***periventricular hypothalamic zone (Nauta & Haymaker, 1969)*** and ***medial hypothalamic zone (Nauta & Haymaker, 1969)***; see Canteras et al. (2011). It was first identified in macrodissected adult human by Solly and by Cruveilhier; see ***[medial retinohypothalamic tract (>1840)] (Solly, 1836; Cruveilhier, 1836)***.

EARLIER REFERENCES:

Described, not named or illustrated:

1. ***[medial retinohypothalamic tract (>1840)] (Solly, 1836; Cruveilhier, 1836)***
   "Tracing the fibres of the optic nerve in man from its commissure [***optic chiasm (Galen, c173)***], we find it sending a few fibres into the tuber cinereum." (Solly, p. 245). Cruveilhier (p. 889) made essentially the same statement, referring to white fibers passing between *tuber cinereum (Soemmerring, 1778)* and ***optic chiasm (Galen, c173)***.

medial root of median nerve (>1840)

As described for macrodissected adult human, the ***median nerve (Du Verney, 1697)*** commonly arises by two roots: one from the ***brachial plexus medial cord***

(Schwalbe, 1881), the ***medial root of median nerve (>1840)***, and one from the ***brachial plexus lateral cord (Schwalbe, 1881)***, the ***lateral root of median nerve (>1840)***; see Williams & Warwick (1980, p. 1098 and Fig. 7.200), *Terminologia Anatomica* (1998, p. 138). It was probably first delineated by Eustachi; see ***[medial root of median nerve (>1840)] (Eustachi, 1552)***.

EARLIER REFERENCES:

Illustrated, not named or described:

1. ***[medial root of median nerve (>1840)] (Eustachi, 1552)***
   Possibly illustrated for macrodissected adult human; see Albinus edition (1761, Tab. 18) where it may be indicated near the left ***brachial plexus (Camper, 1760)*** on the right side of Figure 2. Camper clearly illustrated it for macrodissected adult human (1760, Tab. 1, Fig. 1-near *m*).

Earlier synonyms:

1. *internal head of median nerve (Quain & Wilson, 1839)*
   Synonym for macrodissected adult human ***medial root of median nerve (>1840)***; Plate XVII-*s*.

medial septal complex (Swanson et al., 1987)

As described for macrodissected adult human, and with cellular architecture and connections for all mammals, a ventromedial component of the mammalian ***pallidum (Swanson, 2000a)*** closely associated connectionally with the ***lateral septal complex (Risold & Swanson, 1997)*** and ***hippocampal formation (Swanson & Cowan, 1977)*** and having two arbitrarily separated parts, the more dorsal ***medial septal nucleus (>1840)*** and the more ventrolateral ***diagonal band nucleus (>1840)***. For use in rat by Swanson et al., see p. 650; also see Swanson & Cowan (1979).

PARTLY CORRESPONDS:

1. *basis septi (Burdach, 1822)*
   Indicates at least part of external surface of adult human ***medial septal complex (Swanson et al., 1987)***; p. 146. Also see *paraterminal gyrus >1840)*.
2. *paraterminal gyrus (>1840)*
   As described for macrodissected adult human, external medial surface of ***medial septal complex (Swanson et al., 1987)***, but may also include smaller, ill-defined adjacent parts of ***lateral septal complex (Risold & Swanson, 1997)*** on the surface; see Nauta & Haymaker (1969, p. 158), Williams & Warwick (1980, p. 997, Fig. 7.117A). Common synonym in macrodissected adult human is *precommissural septum* as used by Crosby & Humphrey (1941); see Nauta & Haymaker (1969, p. 158). "Paraterminal gyrus" is a misnomer because it is not a component of the ***cerebral cortex (>1840)***. It is the main component of the *subcallosal area (>1840)*.

medial supraclavicular nerves (>1840)

As described for macrodissected adult human, they are derived from the ***cervical plexus (Molinetti, 1675)*** and innervate skin and fascia of the neck and chest as far caudally (down) as the angle of the sternum; see Durward (1951, p. 1064). They were first distinguished by Eustachi; see ***[medial supraclavicular nerves (>1840)] (Eustachi, 1552)***.

TRANSLATIONS:

1. *nervi supraclaviculares mediales (>1840)*
   Current Latin form of ***medial supraclavicular nerves (>1840)***; see *Terminologia Anatomica* (1998, p. 137).

EARLIER REFERENCES:

Illustrated, not named or described:

1. ***[medial supraclavicular nerves (>1840)] (Eustachi, 1552)***
   Illustrated for macrodissected adult human; see Albinus edition (1761, Tab. 21-*i*).

Earlier synonyms:

1. *anterior branch of anterior branch of fourth pair of cervical nerves (Bang, 1770)*
   Synonym for macrodissected adult human ***medial supraclavicular nerves (>1840)***; in the original Latin, *anterior ramus*, Figure I-57.
2. *internal supraclavicular branches (Soemmerring, 1791)*
   Synonym for macrodissected adult human ***medial supraclavicular nerves (>1840)***; in the original Latin, *supraclaviculares interni*, p. 270.
3. *interior superclavicular branches (Soemmerring, 1798)*
   Alternate form of *internal supraclavicular nerves (Soemmerring, 1791)*; in the original Latin, *superclaviculares interiores*, p. 289.
4. *sternal branch of thoracic part of trachelo-cutanean plexus (Burdin, 1803)*
   Synonym for macrodissected adult human *sternal branch of thoracic part of tracheosubcutaneous nerves (Chaussier, 1809)*; see translation (1803, Vol. 1, p. 188).
5. *sternal branch of thoracic part of tracheosubcutaneous nerves (Chaussier, 1809)*
   Probably synonym for macrodissected adult human ***medial supraclavicular nerves (>1840)***.
6. *anterior superclavicular nerves (Bell & Bell, 1816)*
   Synonym for macrodissected adult human ***medial supraclavicular nerves (>1840)***; in the original Latin, *superclaviculares anteriores*, Vol. 2, p. 514.
7. *anterior supraclavicular nerves (Meckel, 1817)*
   Synonym for macrodissected adult human ***medial supraclavicular nerves (>1840)***; see translation (1832, Vol. 3, p. 31).
8. *sternal branch of supraclavicular branches (Cruveilhier, 1836)*
   Synonym for macrodissected adult human ***medial supraclavicular nerves (>1840)***; in the original French, *rameaux sternaux*, p. 785.

PARTLY CORRESPONDS:

1. *fourth supraclavicular branch (Peipers, 1793)*
   Lateral member of macrodissected adult human ***medial supraclavicular nerves (>1840)***; in the original Latin, *ramus supraclavicularis quartus*, p. 35.

2. *internal pectoral subcutaneous supraclavicular branch (Peipers, 1793)*
   Synonym for *fourth supraclavicular branch (Peipers, 1793)*; in the original Latin, *ramus supraclavicularis subcutaneus pectoris externus*, p. 35.
3. *minor internal fifth supraclavicular branch (Peipers, 1793)*
   Medial member of macrodissected adult human ***medial supraclavicular nerves (>1840)***; in the original Latin, *ramus supraclavicularis quintus internus minor*, p. 35.
4. *innermost supraclavicular branch (Peipers, 1793)*
   Synonym for *minor internal fifth supraclavicular branch (Peipers, 1793)*; in the original Latin, *ramus supraclavicularis intimus*, p. 35.

medial thalamic nuclei (>1840)

As described for macrodissected adult human, and based on cellular architecture and connections in mammal, a medial and dorsal component of the ***dorsal part of thalamus (Herrick, 1910)***. Its major ***gray matter region (Swanson & Bota, 2010)*** is the ***mediodorsal thalamic nucleus (>1840)***, with much smaller ones including the ***submedial thalamic nucleus (>1840)*** and ***perireuniens nucleus (>1840)***; see Swanson (2004, Table B, pp. 171–172), Nieuwenhuys et al. (2008, p. 264 and Fig. 5.31-25). Their main projections to ***cerebral cortex (>1840)*** involve the rostral half of the ***cingulate region (>1840)***. They were first identified, at least generally, as the *internal gray nucleus (Burdach, 1822)*.

EARLIER REFERENCES:

Earlier synonyms:

1. *internal gray nucleus (Burdach, 1822)*
   Roughly synonymous with ***medial thalamic nuclei (>1840)*** as observed in slabs of alcohol-hardened macrodissected adult human; in the original Latin, *nucleus cinereus internus*, p. 121. See Jones (1985, p. 11); also see Meyer (1971, p. 31).
2. *internal nucleus of thalamus of optic nerve (Arnold, 1838b)*
   Synonym for macrodissected adult human *internal gray nucleus (Burdach, 1822)*; in the original Latin, *nucleus internus thalami nervi optici*, Table IV, Figure 5-*k*.
3. *internal nucleus of colliculus of optic nerve (Arnold, 1838b)*
   Synonym for macrodissected adult human *internal gray nucleus (Burdach, 1822)*; in the original Latin, *nucleus internus colliculi nervi optici*, Table VIII, Figure 2-*h*.

median aperture of fourth ventricle (>1840)

As described for macrodissected adult human, the single opening in the median plane between the caudal end of the ***roof of fourth ventricle (Vesalius, 1543a)*** and ***subarachnoid space (Magendie, 1827)***; see Millen & Woollam (1962, pp. 18–19, 55–58), Williams & Warwick (1980, p. 932). Credit for discovery usually goes to Magendie; see ***[median aperture of fourth ventricle (>1840)] (Magendie, 1828)***.

TRANSLATIONS:

1. *apertura mediana ventriculi quarti (>1840)*
   Current Latin form of ***median aperture of fourth ventricle (>1840)***; see *Dorland's* (2003, p. 112).

EARLIER REFERENCES:

Described, not named or illustrated:

1. ***[median aperture of fourth ventricle (>1840)] (Magendie, 1828)***
   First clear published description, for macrodissected adult human; p. 222, see Millen & Woollam (1962, p. 18).

Earlier synonyms:

1. *inferior orifice of fourth ventricle (Cruveilhier, 1836)*
   Synonym for macrodissected adult human ***median aperture of fourth ventricle (>1840)***; in the original French, *oriface inférieur du quatrième ventricule*, p. 628. Cruveilhier credited its description to Magendie without citation.

median eminence (Tilney, 1936)

As described histologically for adult vertebrate, the unpaired proximal part of the ***infundibulum (Rioch et al., 1940)*** lying ventral to the ***hypothalamic part of third ventricle (Swanson, 2004)*** and characterized by the proximal capillary bed associated with the long portal vessels of the hypophysial portal system and by the ***axons (Kölliker, 1896)*** of magnocellular neuroendocrine ***neurons (Waldeyer, 1891)*** passing to the ***posterior lobe of pituitary gland (Haller, 1762)***. It extends as the ***infundibular stem (Hanström, 1966)***, the distal part of the ***infundibulum (Rioch et al., 1940)***; see Hanström (1966), Holmes & Ball (1974, pp. 5–6), Daniel & Pritchard (1975). For Tilney's use in adult mammal, see p. 388. It was at least partly identified by Vesalius; see ***[median eminence (Tilney, 1936)] (Vesalius, 1543a)***.

EARLIER REFERENCES:

Illustrated and described, not named:

1. ***[median eminence (Tilney, 1936)] (Vesalius, 1543a)***
   Illustrated and described for macrodissected adult human, "The first part of this process is exactly like the top of the funnel that we use to pour wine into containers with narrow orifices; it is a wide circle [part of the ***hypothalamus (Kuhlenbeck, 1927)*** and ***hypothalamic part of third ventricle (Swanson, 2004)***]. From this point, still like a funnel, it gradually becomes narrower [***median eminence (Tilney, 1936)***] until eventually, again like a funnel, it ends in a long, narrow pipe [***infundibular stem (Hanström, 1966)***], which extends downwards through a foramen in the hard cerebral membrane that exists specifically for its benefit, so that its tip ends at the gland that receives cerebral pituita." (Richardson & Carman translation, 2009, p. 212, and Fig. 15 on p. 157). Steno (1669, Pl. IV) first clearly illustrated it in a transverse section of macrodissected adult human.

LATER SYNONYMS:

1. *median eminence of tuber cinereum (Tilney, 1936)*
   Synonym for ***median eminence (Tilney, 1936)***; p. 388.

median nerve (Du Verney, 1697)

As described for macrodissected adult human, the largest ***nerve (Herophilus, c335–c280 BC)*** of the upper limb, typically arising from the junction of two main roots, a ***lateral root of median nerve (>1840)*** from the ***brachial plexus lateral cord (Schwalbe, 1881)*** and a ***medial root of median nerve (>1840)*** from the ***brachial plexus medial cord (Schwalbe, 1881)***. The resulting *trunk* of the ***median nerve (Du Verney, 1697)***—for this strictly correct terminology, see Meckel (1832, Vol. 3, p. 27)—commonly generates ***muscular branches of median nerve (Martin, 1781)***, the ***anterior interosseous nerve (Quain, 1832)***, the ***palmar branch of median nerve (Bock, 1827)***, a ***communicating branch of median nerve with ulnar nerve (Bock, 1827)***, ***common palmar digital nerves of median nerve (>1840)***, and ***proper palmar digital nerves of median nerve (>1840)***; see Durward (1951, Fig. 923), Williams & Warwick (1980, pp. 1098–1099). According to Winslow (1733, Sect. VI, p. 79), his mentor Du Verney gave this name in 1697 to the ***nerve (Herophilus, c335–c280 BC)*** in macrodissected adult human. It was first described as the *fifth nerve from spine to upper arm (Galen, c177)*.

TRANSLATIONS:

1. *nervus medianus (Du Verney, 1697)*
   Original Latin form of ***median nerve (Du Verney, 1697)***; see Winslow (1733, Sect. VI, p. 79).

EARLIER REFERENCES:

Earlier synonyms:

1. *fifth nerve from spine to upper arm (Galen, c177)*
   Synonym for ***median nerve (Du Verney, 1697)*** in macrodissected adult beef, pig, and/or macaque but not human; see Singer translation (1999, pp. 69–71, 73–74, 82). Also see May translation (1968, pp. 599 note 24, 704–705).
2. *third nerve entering arm (Vesalius, 1543a)*
   Synonym for macrodissected adult human ***median nerve (Du Verney, 1697)***; see Richardson & Carman translation (2002, p. 239).
3. *largest nerve of arm (Paré, 1550)*
   Synonym for macrodissected adult human ***median nerve (Du Verney, 1697)***; in the original French, *le plus grand nerf du bras*, see Salomon & Trouilloud (2003, pp. 254, 255).
4. *third sinew coming to arm (Geminus, 1553)*
   Synonym for macrodissected adult human *third nerve entering arm (Vesalius, 1543a)*; originally spelled, *thyrde synowe comynge to arme*, see *The table of the figures of sinowes*.
5. *third nerve of hand (Bauhin, 1605)*
   Synonym for macrodissected adult human *third nerve entering arm (Vesalius, 1543a)*; see Crooke translation (1615, p. 903).

LATER SYNONYMS:

1. *muscularis nerve (Cheselden, 1713)*
   According to Klint (1784, p. 11), synonym for macrodissected adult human ***median nerve (Du Verney, 1697)***; in the original Latin, *nervus muscularis*, p. 243.
2. *superior cubital nerve (Cheselden, 1713)*
   In obscure description of ***nerves (Herophilus, c335–c280 BC)***, ***median nerve (Du Verney, 1697)*** may be referred to thus; in the original Latin, *nervus cubitalis superior*, p. 143.
3. *radial nerve (Cheselden, 1726)*
   Apparently corresponds roughly to macrodissected adult human ***median nerve (Du Verney, 1697)***; in the original Latin, *nervus radialis*, p. 266, which was essentially written by Monro *primus* as stated in Preface.
4. *nervum brachialem medium (Pietro da Cortona, 1741)*
   Synonym for macrodissected adult human ***median nerve (Du Verney, 1697)***; p. 3-ε, also see Klint (1784, p. 11).
5. *nervum axillarem (Pietro da Cortona, 1741)*
   Synonym for macrodissected adult human ***median nerve (Du Verney, 1697)***; p. 6-χ, also see Klint (1784, p. 11).
6. *second great brachial nerve (Albinus, 1744)*
   Synonym for macrodissected adult human ***median nerve (Du Verney, 1697)***; in the original Latin, *nervorum brachium magni secundi*, Table 19-29. Also see Camper (1760, p. 11).
7. *digital median nerve (Burdin, 1803)*
   Synonym for macrodissected adult human ***median nerve (Du Verney, 1697)***; see translation (1803, Vol. 1, p. 194).

PARTLY CORRESPONDS:

1. *superficial branch of median nerve (Langenbeck, 1826–1830)*
   Macrodissected adult human continuation of ***median nerve (Du Verney, 1697)*** distal to point ***anterior interosseous nerve (Quain, 1832)*** branches off; in the original Latin, *ramus superficialis nervi mediani*, Fascicle III, Table XIV-6.
2. *branch of median nerve to muscles of deep layer (Cruveilhier, 1836)*
   Macrodissected adult human branch of ***median nerve (Du Verney, 1697)*** with external branch to flexor pollicis longus muscle (*long fléchisseur propre du pounce*), two internal branches to flexor digitorum profundus muscle (*fléchisseur profond*), and middle branch, the *interosseous nerve (Quain, 1828)*; in the original French, *branche des muscles de la couche profonde*, p. 805. Also see Todd (1839, Vol. 2, p. 368).
3. *terminal branches of median nerve (Cruveilhier, 1836)*
   Macrodissected adult human *median nerve terminal branch to thenar muscles (Cruveilhier, 1836)* and ***common palmar digital nerves of median nerve (>1840)***, considered together; in the original French, *branches terminales du médian*, p. 807.
4. *first terminal branch of median nerve (Cruveilhier, 1836)*
   Macrodissected adult human branch of ***median nerve (Du Verney, 1697)*** to muscles of thenar eminence; in the original French, *1re branche terminale du médian*, p. 807.
5. *median nerve terminal branch to thenar muscles (Cruveilhier, 1836)*
   Synonym for *first terminal branch of median nerve (Cruveilhier, 1836)*; in the original French, *branche terminale du médian des muscles du thénar*, p. 807.
6. *collateral nerves of fingers (Cruveilhier, 1836)*

Macrodissected adult human branches of ***median nerve (Du Verney, 1697)*** following collateral blood vessels in palm and fingers; in the original French, *nerfs collatéraux des doigts*, p. 809.

median sulcus of fourth ventricle (>1840)

As described for macrodissected adult human, the longitudinal groove in the median plane running the length of the ***floor of fourth ventricle (Reil, 1807–1808a)***; see Nieuwenhuys et al. (2008, Fig. 3.10), *Nomina Anatomica* (1983, p. A66). It was mentioned by Galen long ago; see ***[median sulcus of fourth ventricle (>1840)] (Galen, c177)***.

EARLIER REFERENCES:

Described, not named or illustrated:

1. ***[median sulcus of fourth ventricle (>1840)] (Galen, c177)***
   In *On Anatomical Procedures*, Galen described it briefly for macrodissected adult large mammal, but not human specifically, as a "hollow like an incision"; see Singer translation (1999, p. 237).

Illustrated, not named or described:

1. ***[median sulcus of fourth ventricle (>1840)] (Vesalius, 1543a)***
   Illustrated beautifully for macrodissected adult human; see Singer translation (1952, p. 104 and Figs. 9,10).

Earlier synonyms:

1. *longitudinal sulcus of fourth ventricle (Huber, 1741)*
   Synonym for macrodissected adult human ***median sulcus of fourth ventricle (>1840)***; in the original Latin, *ventriculus quartus sulcus longitudinalis*, Figure 2-*c*.
2. *calamus scriptorius (Haller, 1762)*
   Synonym for macrodissected adult human ***median sulcus of fourth ventricle (>1840)***: p. 76, as noted by Burdach (1822, p. 303).
3. *calamus (Mayer, 1779)*
   Synonym for macrodissected adult human ***median sulcus of fourth ventricle (>1840)***; p. 21, as noted by Burdach (1822, p. 303); Vicq d'Azyr also used it thus (1786, p. 93).
4. *anterior rima of medulla oblongata (Monro, 1783)*
   Synonym for macrodissected adult human ***median sulcus of fourth ventricle (>1840)***; p. 28.
5. *sulcus of cerebellar ventricle (Vicq d'Azyr, 1786)*
   Synonym for macrodissected adult human ***median sulcus of fourth ventricle (>1840)***; p. 93, as noted by Burdach (1822, p. 303), who gave the Latin, *sulcus ventriculi cerebelli*.
6. *longitudinal sulcus of medulla oblongata (Günther, 1786)*
   Synonym for macrodissected adult human ***median sulcus of fourth ventricle (>1840)***; in the original Latin, *sulcus longitudinalis medulla oblongata*, p. 22.
7. *median furrow of lozenge (Reil, 1809c)*
   Synonym for macrodissected adult human ***median sulcus of fourth ventricle (>1840)***; see Mayo translation (1823, p. 98). Also see *lozenge-shaped field (Reil, 1809c)*.
8. *longitudinal sulcus of cerebellar ventricle (Gordon, 1815)*
   Synonym for macrodissected adult human ***median sulcus of fourth ventricle (>1840)***; p. 119, as noted by Burdach (1822, p. 303), who gave the Latin, *sulcus longitudinalis ventriculi cerebelli*.

medulla (Winslow, 1733)

The most caudal topographic division of the ***vertebrate brain (Cuvier, 1800)***, caudal to the ***pons (Haller, 1747)*** and rostral to the ***spinal cord (Galen, c162–c166)***; see Swanson & Bota (2010). Winslow used this contraction of *medulla oblongata (Collins, 1685)* twice in his description of the *cauda of medulla oblongata (Winslow, 1733)*, that is, the region of the human ***brainstem (Schwalbe, 1881)*** between the ***pons (Haller, 1747)*** and ***spinal cord (Galen, c162–c166)***; Section X, p. 42. Haller (1747) also used the contraction; see Mihles translation (1753, pp. 287, 296). In recent times it was used by, for example, Mettler (1948, p. 76), Carpenter (1976, p. 60). It was clearly identified (illustrated) early on by Vesalius; see ***[medulla (Winslow, 1733)] (Vesalius, 1543a)***.

EARLIER REFERENCES:

Illustrated, not named or described:

1. ***[medulla (Winslow, 1733)] (Vesalius, 1543a)***
   In his illustration of ventral surface of macrodissected adult human ***brain (Smith Papyrus, c1700 BC)***, Vesalius clearly though crudely depicted *pons (Varoli, 1573)*; see Richardson & Carman translation (2002, p. 168). He also wrote that *spinal marrow proper (Vesalius, 1543a)* is cut at the point where it slips into first cervical vertebra. The region shown between the two is ***medulla (Winslow, 1733)***, along with ***abducens nerve (Heister, 1717)*** through ***hypoglossal nerve (Winslow, 1733)*** emerging.

Earlier synonyms:

1. *intracranial medulla oblongata (Piccolomini, 1586)*
   Synonym for macrodissected adult human ***medulla (Winslow, 1733)***. As Bauhin explained (1605, p. 625), it is the part of the *medulla oblongata (Piccolomini, 1586)* within the skull [*medulla oblongata intracranium*], as opposed to the *spinal medulla oblongata (Piccolomini, 1586)*; see translation of Bauhin in Crooke (1615, p. 479). Piccolomini illustrated the *intracranial medulla oblongata* in his schematic midsagittal drawing of the ***brain (Smith Papyrus, c1700 BC)*** (p. 265; also see Clarke and Dewhurst, 1996, Fig. 88-*E*) and described his views on p. 259. Burdach (1822, p. 279) noted that Piccolomini's actual references were to *medulla, quae oblongari incipit* (p. 252) or *medulla cerebri, quae oblongata est* (p. 254).
2. *pons (Casseri, 1609)*
   Synonym for macrodissected adult human ***medulla (Winslow, 1733)***; p. 124, according to Burdach (1822, p. 279).
3. *principium medullae spinalis (Spiegel, 1627)*

Synonym for macrodissected adult human ***medulla (Winslow, 1733)***; p. 290, according to Burdach (1822, p. 279). This term was used by Tyson (1699, Fig. 13-*D*) for infant chimpanzee brain, "…that part of the *Caudex Medullaris*, where the *Corpora Pyramidalia* and *Olivaria* are placed, as in an Humane Brain."

4. *medulla oblongata intra calvariam (Bartholin, 1651)* Synonym for macrodissected adult human ***medulla (Winslow, 1733)***; p. 317, according to Burdach (1822, p. 279).
5. *lowest foot of oblong marrow (Willis, 1664)* Probably synonym for ***medulla (Winslow, 1733)*** in macrodissected adult human and other mammals; p. 58.
6. *inferior portion of oblong marrow (Willis, 1664)* Term clearly refers to ***medulla (Winslow, 1733)*** in macrodissected adult human and other mammals; p. 124.
7. *medulla oblongata (Collins, 1685)* Synonym for macrodissected adult human ***medulla (Winslow, 1733)***; Table 48-*M*. As acknowledged in figure legend, drawing is based on a dissection by Tyson. Cowper (1698, f. C2) also used the term in this way, as did Bell (1802, Pl. VII-*10*), who regarded it as upper part of *medulla spinalis (Bauhin, 1605)* and formed by union of *cerebrum (Vesalius, 1543a)* and ***cerebellum (Aristotle)***. Rasmussen (1947, p. 14) mistakenly attributed the term to Haller.
8. *caudex medullaris (Cowper, 1698)* Synonym for macrodissected adult human *medulla oblongata (Collins, 1685)*; Appendix Figure 28-*n*.
9. *anterior part of tail of medulla oblongata (Pourfour du Petit, 1710)* Synonym for macrodissected adult human ***medulla (Winslow, 1733)***; in the original French, *la queuë de la moelle allongée, partie anterieure*, p. 14.
10. *extremity of medulla oblongata (Winslow, 1733)* Synonym for macrodissected adult human ***medulla (Winslow, 1733)***; Section X, pp. 41, 42.
11. *cauda of medulla oblongata (Winslow, 1733)* Synonym for macrodissected adult human ***medulla (Winslow, 1733)***; Section X, pp. 41, 42.A complete translation is *tail of medulla oblongata*; Rolando (1825a) gave in French, *queue de la moelle allongée*.

LATER SYNONYMS:

1. *medulla oblongata properly so-called (Soemmerring, 1778)* A specific way of referring to the macrodissected adult human ***medulla (Winslow, 1733)***; in Latin, *medulla oblongata proprie sic dicta*, p. 178.
2. *pars suprema medullae spinalis (Soemmerring, 1778)* Synonym for macrodissected adult human ***medulla (Winslow, 1733)***; p. 16, according to Burdach (1822, p. 279).
3. *cephalic part of spinal marrow (Haase, 1781)* Synonym for macrodissected adult human ***medulla (Winslow, 1733)***; in the original Latin, *pars cephalica medullae spinalis*, pp. 2, 29–31; see Chaussier (1807, p. 120 note *1*). Günther (1786, p. 21) gave *pars medullae spinalis cephalica*.
4. *cerebral prolongation (Burdin, 1803)* Synonym for macrodissected adult vertebrate ***medulla (Winslow, 1733)***; see translation (1803, Vol. 1, pp. 143, 167).
5. *rachidian prolongation (Burdin, 1803)* Synonym for macrodissected adult vertebrate ***medulla (Winslow, 1733)***; see translation (1803, Vol. 1, pp. 143, 167).
6. *superior extremity of spinal prolongation (Chaussier, 1807)* Synonym for macrodissected adult human ***medulla (Winslow, 1733)***; in the original French, *l'extrémité supérieure du prolongement rachidien*, p. 120.
7. *cephalic part of spinal prolongation (Chaussier, 1807)* Synonym for *superior extremity of spinal prolongation (Chaussier, 1807)*; in the original French, *la portion céphalique du prolongement rachidien*, p. 120.
8. *superior bulb of spinal prolongation (Chaussier, 1807)* Synonym for *superior extremity of spinal prolongation (Chaussier, 1807)*; in the original French, *le bulb supérieur du prolongement rachiedien*, p. 120
9. *spinal bulb (Chaussier, 1807)* Chaussier's shortened form of *superior bulb of spinal prolongation (Chaussier, 1807)*, macrodissected adult human ***medulla (Winslow, 1733)***; in the original French, *le bulb rachidien*, p. 120.
10. *bulb (Chaussier, 1807)* Shortened form of *spinal bulb (Chaussier, 1807)*.
11. *grand renflement au dessus des nerfs cervicaux (Gall & Spurzheim, 1810)* Synonym for macrodissected adult human ***medulla (Winslow, 1733)***; p. 250, according to Burdach (1822, p. 279).
12. *cranial portion of spinal cord (Gordon, 1815)* Synonym for macrodissected adult human ***medulla (Winslow, 1733)***; p. 175.
13. *top of spinal cord (Gordon, 1815)* Synonym for *cranial portion of spinal cord (Gordon, 1815)*, following *pars suprema medullae spinalis (Soemmerring, 1778)*; p. 175.
14. *superior extremity of vertebral marrow (Cloquet, 1816)* Synonym for macrodissected adult human *rachidian bulb (Chaussier, 1807)*; in the original French, *extrémité supérieure*, p. 539.
15. *superior rachidian bulb (Meckel, 1817)* Synonym for macrodissected adult human *rachidian bulb (Chaussier, 1807)*; see translation (1832, Vol. 2, p. 419).
16. *cephalic part of medulla oblongata (Meckel, 1817)* Synonym for macrodissected adult human *rachidian bulb (Chaussier, 1807)*; see translation (1832, Vol. 2, p. 419); for the Latin form, Meckel gave *medulla oblongata, pars cephalica*.
17. *medulla oblongata brainstem (Burdach, 1822)* Synonym for macrodissected adult human ***medulla (Winslow, 1733)*** part of *brainstem (Burdach, 1822)*; in the original German, *Das verlängerte Mark ist der Hirnstamm*, p. 28.
18. *bulb of medulla oblongata (Serres, 1824–1826)* Synonym for macrodissected embryonic mammalian ***medulla (Winslow, 1733)***; in the original French, *bulbe de la moelle allongée*, Plate I.

19. *rachidian bulb (Meckel, 1832)*
Translation of macrodissected adult human *spinal bulb (Chaussier, 1807)*; Vol. 2, p. 419.
20. *chorda oblongata (Quain, 1832)*
Synonym for macrodissected adult human ***medulla (Winslow, 1733)***; p. 636. In English, *oblong cord*.
21. *cranial bulb (Cruveilhier, 1836)*
Synonym for macrodissected adult human ***medulla (Winslow, 1733)***; in the original French, *bulbe crânien*, p. 583.
22. *superior portion of spinal cord (Anderson, 1837)*
Synonym for macrodissected vertebrate ***medulla (Winslow, 1733)***; p. 17.

PARTLY CORRESPONDS:

1. *oblong inferior eminences (Winslow, 1733)*
Synonym for macrodissected adult human ***inferior olivary complex (>1840)*** and ***pyramid (Willis, 1664)*** considered together; Section X, p. 48.
2. *pyramidal eminences (Burdin, 1803)*
As described for macrodissected adult human ***medulla (Winslow, 1733)***, apparently combination of ***gracile fascicle (Müller, 1834)***, ***cuneate fascicle (Müller, 1834)***, and ***inferior cerebellar peduncle (Günther, 1786)*** on right and left side; see translation (1803, Vol. 1, p. 166).
3. *peduncle of spinal cord (Gordon, 1815)*
Surface of macrodissected adult human ***medulla (Winslow, 1733)*** extending from just dorsal to ***olive (Tiedemann, 1821)*** all the way to ***dorsal median sulcus of medulla (>1840)***; p. 178.
4. *gray substance of restiform body (Arnold, 1838b)*
Basically, macrodissected adult human ***central nervous system gray matter region (>1840)*** in ***medulla (Winslow, 1733)*** dorsal and rostral to ***inferior olivary complex (>1840)***; in the original Latin (plural), *substantia cinerea corpora restiformia*; Table II, Figures 10-*e*, 11,12-*f*.
5. *anterior gray bodies (Arnold, 1838b)*
Basically, macrodissected adult human ***central nervous system gray matter region (Swanson & Bota, 2010)*** in ***medulla (Winslow, 1733)*** caudal to ***inferior olivary complex (>1840)*** and ventral to ***dorsal column nuclei (>1840)*** and ***spinal nucleus of trigeminal nerve (>1840)***; in the original Latin, *corpora cinerea anteriora*; Table II, Figures 13, 14-*i*. Considered an extension of right and left ***inferior olivary complex (>1840)*** and ***ventral horn (>1840)***.
6. *posterior gray bodies (Arnold, 1838b)*
For macrodissected adult human, roughly the ***dorsal column nuclei (>1840)*** and ***spinal nucleus of trigeminal nerve (>1840)*** considered together as rostral continuation of ***dorsal horns (>1840)***; in the original Latin, *corpora cinerea posteriora*, Table II, Figure 13-*k*.
7. *central gray of medulla oblongata (Arnold, 1838b)*
For macrodissected adult human, relatively narrow and elongated ***central nervous system gray matter region (>1840)*** surrounding ***central canal of medulla (>1840)***; in the original Latin, *centrum cinereum medullae oblongatae*, Table IX, Figure 4-*c*.

medullary branch of nerve to popliteus (>1840)

As described for macrodissected adult human, it courses to the shaft of the tibia from the ***nerve to popliteus (>1840)***; see Durward (1951, p. 1110). It was postulated by Massa; see ***[medullary branch of nerve to popliteus (>1840)] (Massa, 1536)***.

EARLIER REFERENCES:

Described, not named or illustrated:

1. ***[medullary branch of nerve to popliteus (>1840)] (Massa, 1536)***
In a remarkable passage Massa wrote, "I swear to God that I have seen a man who had an ulcer in his leg where the bone was visible. In this bone there was painful sensation to such a degree that he did not permit it to be touched by a rough instrument; the bone was denuded of its panniculus. Nevertheless I perforated the bone; inside there was the same feeling of pain. I wished to make this explanation so that anatomists might discover whether or not some scattering of nerves penetrates to the substance of the bone." (Lind translation, 1975, p. 222).

medullary central tegmental tract (>1840)

As described in macrodissected adult human, and mammal generally with histological methods for ***axons (Kölliker, 1896)***, the topographic segment of the ***central tegmental tract (Bechterew, 1889)*** in the ***medulla (Winslow, 1733)***, between ***pontine central tegmental tract (>1840)*** segment rostrally and ***amiculum of olive (>1840)*** caudally; see Riley (1943, pp. 693–694), Crosby et al. (1962, pp. 256–257), Nieuwenhuys et al. (2008, Figs. 6.22–24). It was not clearly described by 1840.

medullary cone (Bock, 1827)

As described for macrodissected adult human, the cone-shaped ***spinal cord differentiation (>1840)*** between ***lumbosacral enlargement (>1840)*** rostrally and ***terminal filament (Tiedemann, 1821)*** caudally. The ***medullary cone (Bock, 1827)*** most commonly extends from the fourth ***sacral nerve (Camper, 1760)*** to the last ***coccygeal nerve (Camper, 1762)***; see Mettler (1948, p. 31), *Terminologia Anatomica* (1998, p. 105). For Bock's use in macrodissected adult human see Table I, Figure 1-*v*. It was first clearly distinguished by Estienne; see ***[medullary cone (Bock, 1827)] (Estienne, 1545)***.

TRANSLATIONS:

1. *conus medullaris (Bock, 1827)*
Original Latin form of ***medullary cone (Bock, 1827)***; Table I, Figure 2-*v*.

EARLIER REFERENCES:

Illustrated, not named or described:

1. ***[medullary cone (Bock, 1827)] (Estienne, 1545)***
Very clearly illustrated for macrodissected adult human; p. 338.

Earlier synonyms:

1. *inferior extremity of spinal prolongation (Chaussier, 1807)*

Synonym for macrodissected adult human ***medullary cone (Bock, 1827)***; in the original French, *extrémité inférieure du prolongement rachidien*, see p. 120 and Plate V, Figure 1-*B,C*.

2. *lumbar extremity of spinal prolongation (Chaussier, 1807)*
   Synonym for *inferior extremity of spinal prolongation (Chaussier, 1807)*; in the original French, *extrémité lombaire du prolongement rachidien*, p. 120.
3. *apex of spinal medulla (Tiedemann, 1821)*
   Synonym for macrodissected adult monkey ***medullary cone (>1840)***; in the original Latin, *apex medullae spinalis*, Table I, Figure 5-*h*.
4. *cone of spinal medulla (Bock, 1824)*
   Synonym for macrodissected adult human ***medullary cone (>1840)***; Table 3, Figure 1-*a*. Arnold (1838b; Tab. I, Figure 2-*o*) gave the Latin, *conus medullae spinalis*.

medullary cuneate fascicle (>1840)

As described in macrodissected adult human, and mammal generally with histological methods for ***axons (Kölliker, 1896)***, the rostral topographic segment of the ***cuneate fascicle (Müller, 1834)*** in the ***medulla (Winslow, 1733)***, rostral to the ***spinal cuneate fascicle (>1840)*** segment; see Williams & Warwick (1980, p. 881), Nieuwenhuys et al. (2008, Figs. 3.10, 6.21–22). It was clearly delineated by Santorini; see ***[medullary cuneate fascicle (>1840)] (Santorini, 1775)***.

EARLIER REFERENCES:

Illustrated, not named or described:

1. ***[medullary cuneate fascicle (>1840)] (Santorini, 1775)***
   Clearly illustrated for macrodissected adult human; Table III, Figure 2.

medullary dorsal spinocerebellar tract (>1840)

As described in macrodissected adult human, and mammal generally with histological methods for ***axons (Kölliker, 1896)***, the rostral topographic segment of the ***dorsal spinocerebellar tract (>1840)*** extending rostrally in the ***medulla (Winslow, 1733)*** between ***inferior cerebellar peduncle (Günther, 1786)*** rostrally and ***spinal dorsal spinocerebellar tract (>1840)*** segment caudally; see Mettler (1948, Figs. 182, 185, 187, 189, 195, 198, 200), Nieuwenhuys et al. (2008, Fig. 6.21). It was not delineated clearly by 1840.

medullary gracile fascicle (>1840)

As described in macrodissected adult human, and mammal generally with histological methods for ***axons (Kölliker, 1896)***, the rostral topographic segment of the ***gracile fascicle (Müller, 1834)*** in the ***medulla (Winslow, 1733)***, rostral to the ***spinal gracile fascicle (>1840)*** segment; see Nieuwenhuys et al. (2008, Fig. 3.10-*18*). Its surface is called the ***gracile tubercle (>1840)***. It was delineated clearly by Santorini; see ***[medullary gracile fascicle (>1840)] (Santorini, 1775)***.

EARLIER REFERENCES:

Illustrated, not named or described:

1. ***[medullary gracile fascicle (>1840)] (Santorini, 1775)***
   Clearly illustrated for macrodissected adult human; Table III, Figure 2.

medullary lateral reticulospinal tract (>1840)

As described for adult human and other mammal most clearly with experimental pathway tracing methods, the major rostral topographic segment of the ***lateral reticulospinal tract (>1840)*** extending caudally in the ***medullary ventrolateral fascicle (>1840)***, rostral to the ***spinal lateral reticulospinal tract (>1840)*** segment. It may have minor contributions from ***pons (Haller, 1747)*** and ***tegmentum (Swanson, 2000b)*** more rostrally; see Mettler (1948, p. 238), Crosby et al. (1962, p. 105 and Figs. 120, 133, 140, 145), Williams & Warwick (1980, pp. 875–876). It was not described by 1840.

medullary lateral vestibulospinal tract (>1840)

As described in macrodissected adult human, and mammal generally with histological methods for ***axons (Kölliker, 1896)***, the rostral topographic segment of the ***lateral vestibulospinal tract (>1840)*** in the ***medulla (Winslow, 1733)***, rostral to the ***spinal lateral vestibulospinal tract (>1840)*** segment; see Carpenter (1976, p. 342 and Figs. 10.18–19), called simply *vestibulospinal tract (>1840)*, and Nieuwenhuys et al. (2008, p. 725 and Fig. 17.6). It was not clearly delineated by 1840.

medullary medial forebrain bundle (>1840)

As described in mammal generally with experimental histological methods for ***axons (Kölliker, 1896)***, the topographic segment of the ***medial forebrain bundle (Edinger, 1893)*** in the ***medulla (Winslow, 1733)***, between ***pontine medial forebrain bundle (>1840)*** segment rostrally and ***spinal medial forebrain bundle (>1840)*** segment caudally. It is diffusely distributed near the ventral surface of the ***medulla (Winslow, 1733)*** and has a major dorsal branch to the ***dorsal motor nucleus of vagus nerve (>1840)*** and adjacent ***nucleus of solitary tract (>1840)***; see Saper et al. (1976). It was not known by 1840.

medullary medial lemniscus (>1840)

As described in macrodissected adult human, and mammal generally with histological methods for ***axons (Kölliker, 1896)***, the caudal topographic segment of the ***medial lemniscus (>1840)*** in the ***medulla (Winslow, 1733)***, between ***pontine medial lemniscus (>1840)*** segment rostrally and ***medial lemniscus decussation (>1840)*** caudally; see Nieuwenhuys et al. (2008, Figs. 6.14, 6.22–24). It was known to Reil; see ***[medullary medial lemniscus (>1840)] (Reil, 1809c)***.

EARLIER REFERENCES:

Described, not named or illustrated:

1. ***[medullary medial lemniscus (>1840)] (Reil, 1809c)***
   Segment of *external part of lemniscus (Reil, 1809c)* in ***medulla (Winslow, 1733)***, vaguely described; see Mayo translation (1823, p. 95).

medullary medial longitudinal fascicle (>1840)

As described in macrodissected adult human, and mammal generally with histological methods for ***axons (Kölliker, 1896)***, the topographic segment of the ***medial longitudinal fascicle (>1840)*** in the ***medulla (Winslow, 1733)***, between ***pontine medial longitudinal fascicle (>1840)*** segment rostrally and ***spinal medial longitudinal fascicle (>1840)*** segment caudally; see Nieuwenhuys et al. (2008, Figs. 6.14–15). It was not known by 1840.

medullary medial reticulospinal tract (>1840)

As described in macrodissected adult human, and mammal generally with histological methods for ***axons (Kölliker, 1896)***, the topographic segment of the ***medial reticulospinal tract (>1840)*** in the ***medulla (Winslow, 1733)***, between ***pontine medial reticulospinal tract (>1840)*** segment rostrally and ***spinal medial reticulospinal tract (>1840)*** segment caudally; see Crosby et al. (1962, p. 105 and Figs. 85, 120, 133), Williams & Warwick (1980, pp. 875–876). It was not described by 1840.

medullary rubrospinal tract (>1840)

As described in adult human and other mammals most clearly with experimental pathway tracing methods, the topographic segment of the ***rubrospinal tract (>1840)*** extending caudally in the ***medullary ventrolateral fascicle (>1840)***, between ***pontine rubrospinal tract (>1840)*** segment rostrally and ***spinal rubrospinal tract (>10840)*** segment caudally. See Mettler (1948, Figs. 185, 189, 191, 195, 200, 202, 205, 210, 212, 214), Swanson (2004, Atlas Levels 53–73). It was not identified by 1840.

medullary segment of spinal tract of trigeminal nerve (>1840)

As described in macrodissected adult human, and mammal generally with histological methods for ***axons (Kölliker, 1896)***, the topographic segment of the ***spinal tract of trigeminal nerve (>1840)*** in the ***medulla (Winslow, 1733)***, between ***pontine segment of spinal tract of trigeminal nerve (>1840)*** rostrally and ***spinal segment of spinal tract of trigeminal nerve (>1840)*** caudally; see Carpenter (1976, Fig. 12.20), Nieuwenhuys et al. (2008, Figs. 6.14–15). It was known to Rolando; see *root of fifth pair of nerves (Rolando, 1825a)*.

medullary spinothalamic tract (>1840)

As described for adult human and other mammal most clearly with experimental pathway tracing methods, a topographic segment of the ***spinothalamic tract (>1840)*** extending rostrally in the ***medullary ventrolateral fascicle (>1840)***, between the ***pontine spinothalamic tract (>1740)*** segment rostrally and ***lateral spinothalamic tract (>1840)*** and ***ventral spinothalamic tract (>1840)*** components in the ***spinal cord (Galen, c162–c166)*** caudally; see Carpenter (1976, Figs. 10.7–8), Nieuwenhuys et al. (2008, p. 698 and Figs. 6.13, 14-*FAL red*). It was not identified as a differentiable part of the ***ventrolateral fascicle (>1840)*** before 1840.

medullary stria (Wenzel & Wenzel, 1812)

As described in macrodissected adult human, and mammal generally with histological methods for ***axons (Kölliker, 1896)***, a ***central nervous system white matter tract (>1840)*** of the ***interbrain (Baer, 1837)***. For topographic description, it has two segments: the ***hypothalamic medullary stria (>1840)*** is a dorsal branch of the ***hypothalamic medial forebrain bundle (>1840)*** and it joins the rostral end of the ***epithalamic medullary stria (>1840)***, which extends longitudinally in the ***epithalamus (His, 1893b)***, medial and dorsal to the ***habenular nuclei (>1840)***. The caudal ends of the right and left ***epithalamic medullary stria (>1840)*** are connected across the median plane by the ***habenular commissure (>1840)*** associated with the dorsal lamina of the ***pineal stalk (Burdach, 1822)***. For Wenzel & Wenzel's use in macrodissected adult human and other mammals, see pp. 86, 320; also see Meyer (1971, p. 107). For English form see *Dorland's* (2003, p. 1773, under *stria medullaris*), Nieuwenhuys et al. (2008, p. 209). It was known to Vesalius; see ***[medullary stria (Wenzel & Wenzel, 1812)] (Vesalius, 1543a)***.

TRANSLATIONS:

1. *stria medullaris (Wenzel & Wenzel, 1812)*
   Original Latin form of ***medullary stria (Wenzel & Wenzel, 1812)***; pp. 86, 320.

EARLIER REFERENCES:

Illustrated, not named or described:

1. ***[medullary stria (Wenzel & Wenzel, 1812)] (Vesalius, 1543a)***
   Very clearly illustrated for macrodissected adult human; see Singer translation (1952, p. 107, Fig. 10).

Earlier synonyms:

1. *tractus medullaris nervorum opticorum thalamus intermedius (Vieussens, 1684)*
   Synonym for macrodissected adult human ***medullary stria (Wenzel & Wenzel, 1812)***; Table VII-G, see Meyer (1971, p. 107).
2. *tractus medullaris nervorum opticorum thalamus interjectus (Vieussens, 1684)*
   Alternate form of *tractus medullaris nervorum opticorum thalamus intermedius (Vieussens, 1684)*; p. 64. See Ridley (1695, p. 84) who suggested it arises from *anterior column of true fornix (Vieussens, 1684)*.
3. *medullary tract (Ridley, 1695)*
   Synonym for macrodissected adult human *tractus medullaris nervorum opticorum thalamus interjectus (Vieussens, 1684)*; p. 84.
4. *processus medullares (Lancisi, 1718)*
   Probably synonym for macrodissected adult human *tractus medullaris nervorum opticorum thalamus intermedius (Vieussens, 1684)*; p. 318, Figure 4-*f*, see Burdach (1822, p. 333).
5. *columna medullaris (Tarin, 1750)*

Synonym for macrodissected adult human ***medullary stria (Wenzel & Wenzel, 1812)***; Table I, Figure 2-*K*; Table II, Figure 1-*r*. Soemmerring (1778, Tab. III-*p*) gave the full eponym, *columna medullaris glandulam pinealem alligans thalamo, Tarini*.

6. *linea alba (Haller, 1754a)*
   Synonym for macrodissected adult human ***medullary stria (Wenzel & Wenzel, 1812)***; Vol. VII, p. 19; see Burdach (1822, p. 333).
7. *pedicelli glandulae pinealis (Haller, 1762)*
   Synonym for macrodissected adult human right and left ***medullary stria (Wenzel & Wenzel, 1812)***; p. 66, see Burdach (1822, p. 333). According to Meyer (1971, p. 107) it may have included ***habenular commissure (>1840)*** and ***pineal stalk (Burdach, 1822)***; also see Vicq d'Azyr (1786, Pl. VIII, p. 8).
8. *petioli glandulae pinealis (Haller, 1762)*
   Synonym for *pedicelli glandulae pinealis (Haller, 1762)*; p. 66, see Burdach (1822, p. 333).
9. *pedunculi glandulae pinealis (Soemmerring, 1778)*
   Alternate form of macrodissected adult human *petioli glandulae pinealis (Haller, 1762)*; Table III-*p,q*.
10. *crura medullaria glandulae pinealis (Mayer, 1779)*
   Variation on macrodissected adult human *petioli glandulae pinealis (Haller, 1762)*; p. 14, see Burdach (1822, p. 338).
11. *processus glandulae pinealis (Mayer, 1779)*
   Variation on macrodissected adult human *petioli glandulae pinealis (Haller, 1762)*; p. 14, see Burdach (1822, p. 338).
12. *markiger Streisen (Soemmerring, 1791)*
   German synonym for macrodissected adult human ***medullary stria (Wenzel & Wenzel, 1812)***, similar to *lineae albae (Haller, 1762)*; p. 39.
13. *markigen Leistchen der Zirbel (Soemmerring, 1791)*
   German synonym for macrodissected adult human ***medullary stria (Wenzel & Wenzel, 1812)***, similar to *lineae albae (Haller, 1762)*; p. 40.
14. *peduncles of conarium (Burdin, 1803)*
   Synonym for right and left macrodissected adult human ***medullary stria (Wenzel & Wenzel, 1812)***; see translation (1803, Vol. 1, p. 162). Burdach (1822, p. 334) gave the Latin, *pedunculi conarii*.

LATER SYNONYMS:

1. *anterior peduncles of pineal gland (Serres, 1824–1826)*
   Synonym for macrodissected embryonic human right and left ***medullary stria (Wenzel & Wenzel, 1812)***; in the original French, *pédoncules antérieurs de la glande pinéale*, Plate II, Figure 74-3.
2. *superior peduncles of conarium (Cruveilhier, 1836)*
   Synonym for right and left macrodissected adult human ***medullary stria (Wenzel & Wenzel, 1812)***; in the original French, *pédoncules supérieurs*, p. 687.
3. *superior peduncles of pineal body (Cruveilhier, 1836)*
   Synonym for right and left macrodissected adult human ***medullary stria (Wenzel & Wenzel, 1812)***; in the original French, *pédoncules supérieurs*, p. 687.
4. *reins (Cruveilhier, 1836)*
   Synonym for right and left macrodissected adult human ***medullary stria (Wenzel & Wenzel, 1812)***; in the original French, *rénes*, p. 687.
5. *brakes of pineal gland (Cruveilhier, 1836)*
   Synonym for right and left macrodissected adult human ***medullary stria (Wenzel & Wenzel, 1812)***; in the original French, *freins de la glande pinéale*, p. 687.
6. *habenae (Cruveilhier, 1836)*
   Original Latin form of *reins (Cruveilhier, 1836)*; p. 687.
7. *medullary stria of colliculus of optic nerve (Arnold, 1838a)*
   Synonym for macrodissected adult human ***medullary stria (Wenzel & Wenzel, 1812)***; in the original Latin, *stria medullaris colliculi nervi optici*, p. 71.

medullary striae (Scarpa, 1788)

As described for macrodissected adult human, variable numbers of narrow bands stretching diagonally across the caudal half of the ***floor of fourth ventricle (Reil, 1807–1808a)***; the associated ***axons (Kölliker, 1896)*** enter the ***inferior cerebellar peduncle (Günther, 1786)***; see Mettler (1948, Figs. 210, 212, 214; called *arcuocerebellar tract* or *medullary stria*), Crosby et al. (1962, p. 131 and Figs. 97, 115), Williams & Warwick (1980, p. 910), *Terminologia Anatomica* (1998, p. 113). For Scarpa's use in macrodissected adult human, see Table X, Figure 1-*c*; also see Burdach (1822, p. 305), Meckel (1832, Vol. 2, p. 423). They were first described by Piccolomini; see ***[medullary striae (Scarpa, 1788)] (Piccolomini, 1586)***.

TRANSLATIONS:

1. *medullares striae (Scarpa, 1788)*
   Original Latin form of ***medullary striae (Scarpa, 1788)***; Table X, Figure 1-*c*.
2. *strias medullares (Procháska, 1800)*
   Latin form of ***medullary striae (Scarpa, 1788)*** for macrodissected adult human; Vol. 1, p. 387 ff. See Burdach (1822, p. 305).
3. *striae medullosae (Wenzel & Wenzel, 1812)*
   Latin form of ***medullary striae (Scarpa, 1788)*** for macrodissected adult human; p. 169.
4. *striae medullares (>1840)*
   Current Latin form of ***medullary striae (Scarpa, 1788)***; see *Terminologia Anatomica* (1998, p. 113).

EARLIER REFERENCES:

Described, not named or illustrated:

1. ***[medullary striae (Scarpa, 1788)] (Piccolomini, 1586)***
   Piccolomini is usually credited with first describing them in macrodissected adult human; p. 300, see Wenzel & Wenzel (1812, p. 169). He related them to origin of ***vestibulocochlear nerve (>1840)*** according to Mettler (1947, p. 49) and Clarke & O'Malley (1996, p. 387).

Earlier synonyms:

1. *root of auditory nerve (Willis, 1664)*
   Synonym for macrodissected adult human ***medullary striae (Scarpa, 1788)***; see Pordage translation (1681, p. 68).

2. *white medullary line covering fourth ventricle (Willis, 1664)*
Synonym for one of the macrodissected adult human ***medullary striae (Scarpa, 1788)***; in the original Latin, *linea alba medullari ventriculi quarti*, p. 45, see Haller (1762, p. 225 note *p*). Willis suggested that *facial nerve (Vicq d'Azyr, 1784)*, or *hard part of seventh pair of nerves arising within skull (Willis, 1664)*, arises from ***medullary striae (Scarpa, 1788)***, referred to as "the medullar whitish line leading about the bottom of the fourth Ventricle" (Pordage translation, 1681, p. 144).
3. *transverse medullary process of fourth ventricle (Ridley, 1695)*
Synonym for macrodissected adult human ***medullary striae (Scarpa, 1788)***; Figure VII-*i*.
4. *medullary tract of fourth ventricle (Drake, 1707)*
Synonym for macrodissected adult human ***medullary striae (Scarpa, 1788)***; p. 513.

LATER SYNONYMS:

1. *oblique medullary striae from calamus scriptorius (Bell, 1802)*
Synonym for macrodissected adult human ***medullary striae (Scarpa, 1788)***; Plate IX-*T*.
2. *transverse medullary fibers of calamus scriptorius (Reil, 1809c)*
Synonym for macrodissected adult human ***medullary striae (Scarpa, 1788)***; see Mayo translation (1823, p. 89).
3. *white ridges of triangular fossa (Gordon, 1815)*
Synonym for macrodissected adult human ***medullary striae (Scarpa, 1788)***; p. 179.
4. *transverse medullary striae (Meckel, 1817)*
Synonym for macrodissected adult human ***medullary striae (Scarpa, 1788)***; see translation (1832, Vol. 3, p. 53).
5. *taeniae foveae rhomboidalis (Burdach, 1822)*
Synonym for macrodissected adult human ***medullary striae (Scarpa, 1788)***; p. 77.
6. *roots of acoustic nerve (Rolando, 1831)*
Synonym for macrodissected adult human ***medullary striae (Scarpa, 1788)***; in the original Italian, *radici del nervo acustico*, Figure 10-32.
7. *anterior division of auditory nerve (Bergmann, 1831)*
Synonym for macrodissected adult human ***medullary striae (Scarpa, 1788)***; in the original German, *vordere Abtheilung des Hörnerven*, Taf. V-*g*, where Bergmann referred to them as *Chorden*. There are a number of fascinating drawings illustrating variations on bundles associated with ***medullary striae (Scarpa, 1788)*** in Table VII.
8. *lineae transversae of calamus scriptorius (Quain, 1837)*
Synonym for macrodissected adult human ***medullary striae (Scarpa, 1788)***; Figure 154-*l*.
9. *taeniae medullares (Arnold, 1838a)*
Synonym for macrodissected adult human ***medullary striae (Scarpa, 1788)***; p. 24.
10. *striae medullares ventriculi quarti (>1840)*
Synonym for macrodissected adult human ***medullary striae (Scarpa, 1788)***; see *Terminologia Anatomica* (1998, p. 113).

medullary tectospinal tract (>1840)

As described in macrodissected adult human, and mammal generally with histological methods for ***axons (Kölliker, 1896)***, a topographic segment of the ***tectospinal tract (>1840)*** in the ***medulla (Winslow, 1733)***, between ***pontine tectospinal tract (>1840)*** segment rostrally and ***spinal tectospinal tract (>1840)*** segment caudally; see Mettler (1948, Figs. 193, 195, 200, 202, 210, 212, 214), Crosby et al. (1962, Figs. 120, 133, called *medial tectospinal tract*), Swanson (2004, Atlas Levels 48–73). It was not recognized by 1840.

medullary ventral spinocerebellar tract (>1840)

As described in macrodissected adult human, and mammal generally with histological methods for ***axons (Kölliker, 1896)***, the topographic segment of the ***ventral spinocerebellar tract (>1840)*** extending rostrally in the ***medullary ventrolateral fascicle (>1840***, between ***pontine ventral spinocerebellar tract (>1840)*** segment rostrally and ***spinal ventral spinocerebellar tract (>1840)*** segment caudally; see Mettler (1948, Figs. 182, 185, 187, 189, 195, 198, 202, 210, 212, 214, 216). It was known to Reil; see ***[medullary ventral spinocerebellar tract (>1840)] (Reil, 1809c)***.

EARLIER REFERENCES:

Described, not named or illustrated:

1. ***[medullary ventral spinocerebellar tract (>1840)] (Reil, 1809c)***
Described vaguely in macrodissected adult sheep; see Mayo translation (1823, p. 99).

medullary ventrolateral fascicle (>1840)

As described in macrodissected adult human, and mammal generally with histological methods for ***axons (Kölliker, 1896)***, the caudal topographic segment of the ***ventrolateral fascicle (>1840)*** in the ***medulla (Winslow, 1733)*** between the ***pontine ventrolateral fascicle (>1840)*** segment rostrally and a continuous zone of the ***ventral funiculus (>1840)*** and ***lateral funiculus (Burdach, 1822)*** caudally; see Nieuwenhuys et al. (2008, Figs. 6.1, 6.3, 6.14). Its five most obvious partly overlapping components are the ***medullary spinothalamic tract (>1840)***, ***medullary ventral spinocerebellar tract (>1840)***, ***medullary rubrospinal tract (>1840)***, ***medullary lateral reticulospinal tract (>1840)***, and ***medullary dorsal spinocerebellar tract (>1840)***; see Crosby et al. (1962, Figs. 120, 133), where terminology and interpretation varies somewhat. It was observed but not separately named by Rolando; see ***[medullary ventrolateral tract (>1840)] (Rolando, 1825a)***.

EARLIER REFERENCES:

Illustrated and described, not named:

1. ***[medullary ventrolateral tract (>1840)] (Rolando, 1825a)***
Rolando observed segment of *anterolateral cord of oblong medulla (Rolando, 1825a)* or ***ventrolateral fascicle (>1840)*** in the ***medulla (Winslow, 1733)*** without separately naming it; see Table VIII, Figure 1-*z*.

medullopontine sulcus (>1840)

As described for macrodissected adult human, the transverse groove between the caudal end of the ***pons (Haller, 1747)*** and rostral end of the ***medulla (Winslow, 1733)***, and occupied by the ***abducens nerve (Heister, 1717)***, ***intermediofacial nerve (Strong & Elwyn, 1943)***, and ***vestibulocochlear nerve (>1840)***; see Riley (1943, p. 535), Williams & Warwick (1980, Fig. 7.55), *Terminologia Anatomica* (1998, p. 112). It lies just ventral to the ***cerebellopontine angle (>1840)*** and was first clearly delineated by Eustachi; see ***[medullopontine sulcus (>1840)] (Eustachi, 1552)***.

EARLIER REFERENCES:

Illustrated, not named or described:

1. ***[medullopontine sulcus (>1840)] (Eustachi, 1552)***
   Beautifully illustrated for macrodissected adult human by Eustachi in 1552 but not published until 1714; see Albinus edition (1761, Pl. 18, Fig. II, between *I* and *G,H*). Varoli indicated it for macrodissected adult human in Figure 1, published in 1573.

Earlier synonyms:

1. *posterior pontine sulcus (Günther, 1786)*
   Synonym for macrodissected adult human ***medullopontine sulcus (>1840)***; in the original Latin, *sulcus posterior*, p. 20. See Nieuwenhuys et al. (2008, Figs. 3.8, 3.9, 3.12).
2. *transverse sulcus separating annular protuberance from superior end of medulla oblongata (Cloquet, 1828)*
   Synonym for macrodissected adult human ***medullopontine sulcus (>1840)***; in the original French, *sillon transversal qui sépar la protubérance annulaire de l'extrémité supérieure de la moëlle alongée*, p. 384 and Table CXXXV-14.
3. *inferior pontine sulcus (>1840)*
   Synonym for macrodissected adult human ***medullopontine sulcus (>1840)***; see Mettler (1948, p. 186).

PARTLY CORRESPONDS:

1. *fossa of olivary body (Vicq d'Azyr, 1786)*
   Small triangular region on surface of macrodissected adult human ***medulla (Winslow, 1733)***, basically limited by ***medullopontine sulcus (>1840)*** rostrally and ***olive (Tiedemann, 1821)*** caudally; in the original French, *fosse des corps olivaires*; Plates XVII, Figure I-*48,49*; XXX, Figure II, between *5–7*.
2. *quadrilateral fovea (Malacarne, 1791)*
   Feature recognized on ventral surface of ***medulla (Winslow, 1733)*** between rostral end of ***olive (Tiedemann, 1821)*** and exit point of ***intermediofacial nerve (Strong & Elwyn, 1943)***; in the original Italian, *cavità quadrilatere*, p. 235. Also see Rolando (1825, p. 18 and Tab. I, Fig. 1-7), where he gave the Latin, *fovea quadrilatera*. It is similar if not identical to *fossa of olivary body (Vicq d'Azyr, 1786)*.
3. *triangular pit (Gordon, 1815)*
   Synonym for macrodissected adult human *fossa of olivary body (Vicq d'Azyr, 1786)*; p. 180.
4. *fossa eminentiae olivaris (Burdach, 1822)*
   Latin form of macrodissected adult human *fossa of olivary body (Vicq, d'Azyr, 1786)*; p. 284.

meningeal branch of maxillary nerve (>1840)

As described for macrodissected adult human, it leaves the ***maxillary nerve (Meckel, 1753)*** near the foramen rotundum, receives a ***communicating branch (Winslow, 1733)*** from the ***internal carotid plexus (>1840)***, and accompanies the frontal branch of the middle meningeal artery to supply ***dura (Galen, c177)*** of the middle cranial fossa, with rostral (anterior) branchlets reaching the anterior cranial fossa; see Williams & Warwick (1980, pp. 1062–1063), *Terminologia Anatomica* (1998, p. 134). It was discovered by Winslow; see ***[meningeal branch of maxillary nerve (>1840)] (Winslow, 1733)***.

EARLIER REFERENCES:

Described, not named or illustrated:

1. ***[meningeal branch of maxillary nerve (>1840)] (Winslow, 1733)***
   Mentioned without naming for macrodissected adult human; Section VI, p. 64.

Earlier synonyms:

1. *meningeal nerve (>1840)*
   Synonym for macrodissected adult human ***meningeal branch of maxillary nerve (>1840)***; see His (1895, p. 88), Williams & Warwick (1980, p. 1062).
2. *middle meningeal nerve (>1840)*
   Synonym for macrodissected adult human ***meningeal branch of maxillary nerve (>1840)***; see Williams & Warwick (1980, p. 1062) where Latin form, *nervus meningeus medius*, was given.

meningeal branch of spinal nerve trunk (>1840)

As described for macrodissected adult human, there is usually one for every ***spinal nerve (Camper, 1760–1762)*** and it arises as several small branches from the ***spinal nerve trunk (Frotscher, 1788)*** and ***communicating branches of spinal nerves (Wutzer, 1817)*** before reentering the corresponding intervertebral foramen to supply the ***meninges (Smith Papyrus, c1700 BC)***, blood vessels, and vertebral column; see Carpenter (1975, p. 162), Williams & Warwick (1980, p. 1089), *Terminologia Anatomica* (1988, p. 133). They were not described clearly by 1840.

meningeal branch of vagus nerve (>1840)

As described for macrodissected adult human, proximal branch or branches of the ***vagus nerve trunk (Wrisberg, 1786; Günther, 1786)*** appearing to arise from the ***distal vagal ganglion (>1840)***, joined by the ***communicating branch of glossopharyngeal nerve with meningeal branch of vagus nerve (>1840)***, and distributing to ***dura (Galen, c177)*** of the posterior cranial fossa; see Durward (1951, Fig. 907-*F*), Mitchell (1953, p. 178), Williams & Warwick (1980, p. 1079), *Terminologia Anatomica* (1998, p. 136). Functionally, the branch may actually contain sensory ***dendrites (His, 1889)*** from rostral (upper) ***cervical spinal ganglia (>1840)*** and sympathetic ***axons (Kölliker, 1896)*** from ***superior cervical ganglion (Vieussens, 1684)***; see Kimmel (1961). It was not identified by 1840.

meninges (Smith Papyrus, c1700 BC)

The three concentric membranes covering the tetrapod ***central nervous system (Carus, 1814)***: the inner ***pia (Galen, c192)***, middle ***arachnoid (Blasius, 1666)***, and outer ***dura (Galen, c177)***, with a ***subarachnoid space (Magendie, 1827)*** between ***arachnoid (Blasius, 1666)*** and ***pia (Galen, c192)***, and a vascular ***epipial layer (Key & Retzius, 1875–1876)*** just outside the largely avascular ***pia (Galen, c192)*** that is a differentiation of ***arachnoid trabeculae (>1840)*** in the ***subarachnoid space (Magendie, 1827)***; see Millen & Woollam (1962). The ***pia (Galen, c192)*** and ***arachnoid (Blasius, 1666)*** are now considered differentiations of a histologically homogeneous layer, the ***pia-arachnoid (>1840)*** or *leptomeninges (>1840)*, whereas the ***dura (Galen, c177)*** is referred to as the *pachymeninges (>1840)*. Thus, the ***meninges (Smith Papyrus, c1700 BC)*** are now considered as two primary membranes—***pia-arachnoid (>1840)*** and ***dura (Galen, c177)***—with three main parts. A term equivalent to the Greek *meninx (Hippocrates)*—a membrane, in the present context a fibrous membrane around the ***central nervous system (Carus, 1814)***—was used to describe a human head wound in the Edwin Smith Surgical Papyrus, a c1700 BC copy of a manuscript composed c3200 BC; see Breasted (1930, pp. 65, 167, 171–172), Clarke & O'Malley (1996, p. 384), Allen (2005, p. 75). In *Places in Man*, Hippocrates referred to two membranes (the plural in Greek is *meninges*) around the ***brain (Smith Papyrus, c1700 BC)***, "Of the brain, there are two membranes; the fine one cannot be healed, when once it is injured." (Potter, 1995, p. 23). In *The Account of Animals*, Aristotle clearly described two membranes (*meninges*): a strong one near the skull, the ***dura (Galen, c177)***, and a finer one around the ***brain (Smith Papyrus, c1700 BC)*** itself, the ***pia (Galen, c192)***; see Thompson translation (1962, p. 494). In *On the Names of the Parts of the Human Body*, Rufus of Ephesus (fl. c90–120) used the term "meninges" in text that has survived (see Clarke & O'Malley, 1996, p. 13). He used it specifically for the membranes surrounding the ***nervous system (Monro, 1783)***; see Galen's comment in *On Anatomical Procedures* (Singer translation, 1999, p. 230). Galen pointed out that "the name meninx [is] being somehow now reserved for the membranes round the brain. For our predecessors used to call all membranes MÊNINGES, not only these brain membranes..." (Singer translation, 1999, p. 230).

TRANSLATIONS:

1. *netnet (Smith Papyrus, c1700 BC)*
   English form of Egyptian hieroglyph for ***meninges (Smith Papyrus, c1700 BC)***; see Nunn (2002, pp. 51, 223).
2. *membranes (Smith Papyrus, c1700 BC)*
   English translation of *meninges*; see ***meninges (Smith Papyrus, c1700 BC)***.
3. *meninx (Hippocrates)*
   In *On the Sacred Disease* (see Adams translation, 1972, p. 351) and *On Injuries of the Head* (Adams translation, 1972, p. 152), the Hippocratic Corpus refers to a membrane (in Greek, *meninx*) surrounding the ***brain (Smith Papyrus, c1700 BC)***. In one vague passage from *Places in Man*, the Corpus refers to two membranes—***meninges (Smith Papyrus, c1700 BC)***, the plural of *meninx*—around the ***brain (Smith Papyrus, c1700 BC)***, which may refer to the ***dura (Galen, c177)*** and ***pia (Galen, c192)***; see Lloyd (1975, p. 135).
4. *membrane (Hippocrates)*
   English form of *meninx (Hippocrates)*.

LATER SYNONYMS:

1. *tunic (Hippocrates)*
   Synonym Hippocratic Corpus used in *Fleshes* for ***meninges (Smith Papyrus, c1700 BC)***, "Thus the brain, having the least fat but the most gluey material, cannot be burnt up by heat, but after a time engenders a tunic, the thick membrane [***dura (Galen, c177)***], and around the membrane, bones..." (Potter translation, 1995, p. 139). In *Places in Man*, the Corups referred to two membranes (the plural in Greek is *meninges*) around the ***brain (Smith Papyrus, c1700 BC)***: "Of the brain, there are two membranes; the fine one cannot be healed, when once it is injured." (Potter translation, 1995, p. 23).
2. *sheaths (Hippocrates)*
   In *On the Articulations*, "sheaths" probably refers to two ***meninges (Smith Papyrus, c1700 BC)***; see Adams translation (1972, p. 234), also see ***dura (Galen, c177)***.
3. *sheaths (Galen, c192)*
   Clearly synonym for ***meninges (Smith Papyrus, c1700 BC)***; see Duckworth translation (1962, p. 157).
4. *omenta (Macrobius, 5th century)*
   Synonym for ***meninges (Smith Papyrus, c1700 BC)***, according to Bauhin (1605, p. 547).
5. *umm (Haly Abbas or Ali ibn' ul-Abbas, d. 994)*
   Haly Abbas applied the Arabic word for "mothers" to the ***meninges (Smith Papyrus, c1700 BC)***; see Wiberg translation (1914, pp. 86–99). The Latin word *matres* (singular, *mater*) was introduced for *umm* by Stephen of Antioch in his translation of Haly Abbas; see Singer (1957, p. 81). *Matres* was used in the sense of mother-of-pearl (Millen and Woollam, 1962, p. 21), and Haly Abbas—following Galen (see May translation, 1968, pp. 409–412)—compared them with two other major membrane systems, the mesentery and chorion, and noted that one part, *dura mater (Haly Abbas or Ali ibn' ul-Abbas, d. 994)*, protects the other part, *pia mater (Haly Abbas or Ali ibn' ul-Abbas, d. 994)*, from hard bones of cranium, whereas *pia mater (Haly Abbas or Ali ibn' ul-Abbas, d. 994)* protects ***brain (Smith Papyrus, c1700 BC)*** from *dura mater (Haly Abbas or Ali ibn' ul-Abbas, d. 994)*; see Wiberg translation (1914, pp. 88–89). In the Second Salernitan Demonstration (c1070–1100), which was based on Constantine the African's *Pantegni* (late 11th century), *pia mater (Haly Abbas or Ali ibn' ul-Abbas, d. 994)* was said to protect ***brain (Smith Papyrus, c1700 BC)*** from harshness of *dura mater (Haly Abbas or Ali ibn' ul-Abbas, d. 994)* "like a devoted mother", whereas the latter protects ***brain (Smith Papyrus, c1700 BC)*** and *pia mater (Haly Abbas*

or Ali ibn' ul-Abbas, d. 994) from harshness of cranium; see Corner (1927, p. 66). It was also common in medieval and early modern times to ascribe nourishing as well as protective qualities to the "devoted mother" (Millen and Woollam, 1962, p. 21), and the idea was even mooted that "These Skins are called Maters, i.e., Mothers, by the Arabians, as if all the other Membranes of the Body took their rise from or were propagated by them" (see Riolan, 1657, p. 121; Phillips & Kersey, 1706; Millen and Woollam, 1962, p. 21).

6. *matres (Stephen of Antioch, 1127)*
The Latin word *matres* (singular, *mater*), a synonym for ***meninges (Smith Papyrus, c1700 BC)***, was introduced for the Arabic *umm (Haly Abbas or Ali ibn' ul-Abbas, d. 994)* by Stephen of Antioch in his translation of Haly Abbas; see Singer (1957, p. 81). Also see Berengario da Carpi (1521, f. 421), Burdach (1822 p. 273).
7. *heterocrania (Benedetti, 1502)*
Synonym for macrodissected adult human ***meninges (Smith Papyrus, c1700 BC)***; see Lind translation (1975, p. 115).
8. *double panniculus (Benedetti, 1502)*
Synonym for macrodissected adult human ***meninges (Smith Papyrus, c1700 BC)***; see Lind translation (1975, p. 113). In Latin, *panniculus* refers to a small piece of cloth.
9. *pannicles (Geminus, 1553)*
Synonym for macrodissected adult human *double panniculus (Benedetti, 1502)*; see *The tables of the brayne*, Figures 1–4.
10. *veils (Hall, 1565)*
English synonym for macrodissected adult human ***meninges (Smith Papyrus, c1700 BC)***; p. 41.
11. *kelles (Crooke, 1615)*
English form of *omenta (Macrobius, 5th century)*; p. 444.
12. *films (Willis, 1664)*
Synonym for ***meninges (Smith Papyrus, c1700 BC)***, usually in the singular when referring to one of them, such as the ***dura (Galen, c177)***; see Pordage translation (1681, p. 57).
13. *tunicles (Diemerbroeck, 1689)*
Early English spelling (plural) of *tunic (Hippocrates)*, a synonym for ***meninges (Smith Papyrus, c1700 BC)***; p. 387.

PARTLY CORRESPONDS:

1. *meninx vasculosa (Ruysch, 1737)*
Pia (Galen, c192) and ***epipial layer (Key & Retzius, 1875)*** considered together; see Epistola VII, Responsio (pp. 6–8). The two parts of the thesis were written in 1696, with the first part by Albrecht Graetz and the response by Ruysch.
2. *vasculosae membranae (Haller & Wrisberg, 1780)*
Synonym for macrodissected adult human *meninx vasculosa (Ruysch, 1737)*, provided by Wrisberg in a footnote; p. 176 note 92.
3. *vasculosa cerebri membrana (Haase, 1781)*
Synonym for macrodissected adult human *meninx vasculosa (Ruysch, 1737)*; p. 12.
4. *membrana vasculosa (Soemmerring, 1791)*
Synonym for macrodissected adult human *meninx vasculosa (Ruysch, 1737)*; p. 11, see Burdach (1822, p. 274).
5. *meninx interior (Soemmerring, 1798)*
Synonym for macrodissected adult human *meninx vasculosa (Ruysch, 1737)*; p. 32.
6. *tunica vasculosa (Bell, 1803b)*
Synonym for macrodissected adult human *meninx vasculosa (Ruysch, 1737)*; p. 21.
7. *proper pia mater (Bell, 1803b)*
Synonym for *tunica vasculosa (Bell, 1803b)*; p. 22.

mental branches of mental nerve (Arnold, 1834)

As described for macrodissected adult human, branches of the ***mental nerve (Cheselden, 1726)*** supplying skin of the chin and other related structures; see Williams & Warwick (1980, p. 1067), *Terminologia Anatomica* (1998, p. 135). For Arnold's use in macrodissected adult human, see p. 10. They were known to Eustachi; see ***[mental branches of mental nerve (>1840)] (Eustachi, 1552)***.

TRANSLATIONS:

1. *nervus mentalis rami mentales (Arnold, 1834)*
Original Latin form of ***mental branches of mental nerve (Arnold, 1834)***; p. 10.

EARLIER REFERENCES:

Illustrated, not named or described:

1. ***[mental branches of mental nerve (>1840)] (Eustachi, 1552)***
Clearly illustrated for macrodissected adult human; see Albinus edition (1761, Tab. 19/2-c, p. 111).

Illustrated and described, not named:

1. ***[mental branches of mental nerve (>1840)] (Willis, 1664)***
Illustrated and vaguely described for macrodissected adult, presumably human; see Pordage translation (1681, p. 145, Fig. 1-*t*).

Earlier synonyms:

1. *mental subcutaneous branch of mental branch of maxillary branch of third branch of fifth pair of nerves (Bock, 1817)*
Synonym for macrodissected adult human ***mental branches of mental nerve (>1840)***; in the original Latin, *ramus subcutaneus menti*, p. 55.
2. *sympathetic labial threads of mental fascicle of inferior alveolar surculus of inferior maxillary branch (Bellingeri, 1818)*
Synonym for macrodissected adult human ***mental branches of mental nerve (>1840)*** and sharing ***communicating branches (Winslow, 1733)*** with ***marginal mandibular branch of facial nerve (>1840)***; in the original Latin, *stamina labialis sympathicus*, see Table I.

PARTLY CORRESPONDS:

1. *inferior filaments of sympathetic labial threads of mental fascicle of inferior alveolar surculus of inferior maxillary branch (Bellingeri, 1818)*
Ventral branches of *sympathetic labial threads of mental fascicle of inferior alveolar surculus of inferior maxillary*

branch (Bellingeri, 1818); in the original Latin, *filamentum inferius*, see Table I.

2. *superior filaments of sympathetic labial threads of mental fascicle of inferior alveolar surculus of inferior maxillary branch (Bellingeri, 1818)*
   Dorsal branches of *sympathetic labial threads of mental fascicle of inferior alveolar surculus of inferior maxillary branch (Bellingeri, 1818)*; in the original Latin, *filamentum superius*, see Table I.

mental nerve (Cheselden, 1726)

As described for macrodissected adult human, most commonly a terminal branch of the ***inferior dental nerve (Meckel, 1817)*** emerging through the mental foramen and dividing into three branches, as well as communicating with the ***marginal mandibular branch of facial nerve (>1840)***; see Williams & Warwick (1980, p. 1067), Hamilton (1976, Fig. 792). For Cheselden's use in macrodissected adult human, see p. 262 (and p. 255); Alexander Monro *primus* wrote the chapter on the ***nerves (Herophilus, c335- c280 BC)*** in Cheselden. It was known to Galen; see ***[mental nerve (Cheselden, 1726)] (Galen, c173)***.

TRANSLATIONS:

1. *nervus mentalis (Cheselden, 1726)*
   Original Latin form of ***mental nerve (Cheselden, 1726)***; p. 262.

EARLIER REFERENCES:

Described, not named or illustrated:

1. ***[mental nerve (Cheselden, 1726)] (Galen, c173)***
   Alluded to in macrodissected beef, pig, and/or macaque but not human; see May translation (1968, p 539). Vesalius (1543a) described it for macrodissected adult human; see Richardson & Carman translation (2002, p. 189).

LATER SYNONYMS:

1. *mental branch of maxillary branch of inferior maxillary branch of fifth pair of nerves (Bock, 1817)*
   Synonym for macrodissected adult human ***mental nerve (Cheselden, 1726)***; in the original Latin, *ramus mentalis*, p. 55.
2. *mental fascicle of inferior alveolar surculus of inferior maxillary branch (Bellingeri, 1818)*
   Synonym for macrodissected adult human ***mental nerve (Cheselden, 1726)***; in the original Latin, *fasciculus mentalis*, see Table I.
3. *mental branch of inferior dental nerve (Cruveilhier, 1836)*
   Synonym for macrodissected adult human ***mental nerve (Cheselden, 1726)***; in the original French, *rameau mentonnier*, p. 936.

PARTLY CORRESPONDS:

1. *muscular branch of mental nerve (Meckel, 1753)*
   Branch of macrodissected adult human ***mental nerve (Cheselden, 1726)***; in the original French, *le rameau musculaire de le nerf mental*, Table 1-85.
2. *sympathetic branch of mental nerve (Meckel, 1753)*
   Synonym for *muscular branch of mental nerve (Meckel, 1753)*; Table 1-85.
3. *connection of mental nerve with facial nerve (Arnold, 1834)*
   Macrodissected adult human ***communicating branch (Winslow, 1733)*** between ***mental nerve (Cheselden, 1726)*** and ***marginal mandibular branch of facial nerve (>1840)***; in the original Latin, *conjunctio cum nervo faciali*, p. 10.

midbrain (Baer, 1837)

The topographic division of the ***vertebrate brain (Cuvier, 1800)*** between ***forebrain (Goette, 1873)*** rostrally and ***rhombicbrain (His, 1893b)*** caudally; see Swanson & Bota (2010). Malpighi first identified the *cristate vesicle of brain (Malpighi, 1675)* in the chick ***neural tube (Baer, 1837)***, and Baer named it the ***primary midbrain vesicle (Baer, 1837)*** for vertebrates in general. He also named the corresponding adult structure ***midbrain (Baer, 1837)***, see *Mittelhirn (Baer, 1837)*, and Sharpey et al. (1867, p. 577) gave the first English translation, *midbrain*.

TRANSLATIONS:

1. *Mittelhirn (Baer, 1837)*
   Original German form of ***midbrain (Baer, 1837)***; p. 107.
2. *mesencephalon (Sharpey et al., 1867)*
   Latin form of *Mittelhirn (Baer, 1837)* was introduced here for macrodissected adult human; p. 577.

PARTLY CORRESPONDS:

1. *tegmentum (Reil, 1809c)*
   Here Reil seemed to use the term for *gray substance (Vesalius, 1543a)* limited to macrodissected adult human ***midbrain (Baer, 1837)***, apparently including ***tectum (Baer, 1837)***; see Mayo translation (1823, p. 96). Earlier, he used *tegmentum (Reil, 1809b)*. in a broader sense to also include ***interbrain (Baer, 1837)*** and ***cerebral nuclei (Swanson, 2000)***.
2. *cylinder of crus cerebri (Reil, 1809c)*
   Synonym for *tegmentum (Reil, 1809c)*; see Mayo translation (1823, p. 96). Also see *cylinder of crus cerebri (Reil, 1809b)*.

midbrain reticular nucleus (>1840)

As described for macrodissected adult human, and for adult mammal in general with cellular architecture and connections, the largest ***gray matter region (Swanson & Bota, 2010)*** of the ***tegmentum (Swanson, 2000b)***, regarded as relatively undifferentiated and separated from the median plane by (from rostral to caudal) the unpaired ***rostral linear nucleus (>1840)***, ***central linear nucleus (>1840)***, and ***superior central nucleus (>1840)*** or ***median raphe nucleus (>1840)***; see Brodal (1957b, p. 10), Swanson (2004, Atlas Levels 34–46 and Table B, notes *206* and *291*). It was first roughly delineated as the *gray equally rounded spaces (Vicq d'Azyr, 1786)*.

EARLIER REFERENCES:

Earlier synonyms:

1. *gray equally rounded spaces (Vicq d'Azyr, 1786)*
   Vicq d'Azyr described and illustrated roughly the right and left ***midbrain reticular nucleus (>1840)*** as seen in macrodissected adult human transverse section;

in the original French, *espaces également arrondis et de la même [grise] couleur*, Plate XV-53. Also see *gray rounded spaces (Vicq d'Azyr, 1786)*, which refer to ***tectum (Baer, 1837)***. Rolando (1825a, Tab. VIII, Figs. 4–7, indicated by *) illustrated the same feature in transverse sections of macrodissected adult beef.

midbrain tract of trigeminal nerve (>1840)

As described in macrodissected adult human, and mammal generally with histological methods for ***axons (Kölliker, 1896)***, the thin longitudinal ***central nervous system white matter tract (>1840)*** associated with the ***midbrain nucleus of trigeminal nerve (>1840)*** and appearing as a branch of the ***trigeminal nerve central motor root (>1840)***; see Carpenter (1976, p. 359), Williams & Warwick (1980, p. 1060 and Fig. 7.175), Nieuwenhuys et al. (2008, p. 203 and Fig. 16.8). For topographic description it has a ***tegmental segment of midbrain tract of trigeminal nerve (>1840)*** and ***pontine segment of midbrain tract of trigeminal nerve (>1840)***. It was not discovered by 1840.

EARLIER REFERENCES:

Earlier synonyms:

1. *mesencephalic tract of trigeminal nerve (>1840)*
   Synonym for macrodissected adult human ***midbrain tract of trigeminal nerve (>1840)***; see *Terminologia Anatomica* (1998, p. 116).

midbrain vesicle (Baer, 1837)

For macrodissected vertebrate embryo, the ***primary midbrain vesicle (Baer, 1837)*** matures into the ***midbrain vesicle (Baer, 1837)*** during Baer's (1837) second stage of ***vertebrate brain (Cuvier, 1800)*** development with five ***secondary brain vesicles (>1840)***, and then goes on to become the adult ***midbrain (Baer, 1837)***; see description on p. 107. It was clearly differentiated early on by Malpighi; see ***[midbrain vesicle (Baer, 1837)] (Malpighi, 1673)***.

EARLIER REFERENCES:

Illustrated and described, not named:

1. ***[midbrain vesicle (Baer, 1837)] (Malpighi, 1673)***
   Clearly illustrated for 3-day-old chick embryo; see Figure XVIII.

middle cerebellar peduncle (Rolando, 1819)

As described for macrodissected adult mammal, the transverse crossed pontocerebellar ***central nervous system white matter tract (>1840)*** extending on the lateral surface of the ***pons (Haller, 1747)*** from the region of the ***pontine nuclei (Jacobsohn, 1909)*** ventrally to the ***arbor vitae (Winslow, 1733)*** dorsally; see Crosby et al. (1962, p. 206), Carpenter (1976, Fig. 14.22), Williams & Warwick (1980, p. 917). Within the ***pontine nuclei (Jacobsohn, 1909)***, its dispersed fascicles are called ***transverse pontine fibers (>1840)***. Earlier, it often referred to the segment of the ***middle cerebellar peduncle (Rolando, 1819)*** between ***arbor vitae (Winslow, 1733)*** dorsally and about the level where the ***trigeminal nerve motor root (Bell, 1829)*** and ***trigeminal nerve sensory root (>1840)*** emerge ventrolaterally: the *crus cerebelli (Vicq d'Azyr, 1786)* or *middle cerebellar peduncle (Reil, 1809b)*. For Rolando's use in macrodissected adult human, see Part 2, pp. 15–16. It was observed by Varoli; see ***[middle cerebellar peduncle (Rolando, 1819)] (Varoli, 1573)***.

EARLIER REFERENCES:

Illustrated and described, not named:

1. ***[middle cerebellar peduncle (Rolando, 1819)] (Varoli, 1573)***
   Its surface was illustrated and described crudely for macrodissected adult human; see *pons of cerebellum (Varoli, 1573)*.

Earlier synonyms:

1. *middle cerebellar process (Willis, 1664)*
   Synonym for macrodissected adult mammalian ***middle cerebellar peduncle (Rolando, 1819)***; see Pordage translation (1681, pp. 68, 113).
2. *posterior appendix of cerebellum (Willis, 1664)*
   Synonym for macrodissected adult mammalian ***middle cerebellar peduncle (Rolando, 1819)***; see Pordage translation (1681, p. 121).
3. *processus medullares a cerebello recta descendentes (Willis, 1664)*
   Synonym for macrodissected adult mammalian ***middle cerebellar peduncle (Rolando, 1819)***, as noted by Burdach (1822, p. 298).
4. *processus medullares à cerebello ad medullam oblongatam (Vieussens, 1684)*
   Synonym for macrodissected adult human ***middle cerebellar peduncle (Rolando, 1819)***; Table XIV-*L*.
5. *second process of cerebellum (Ridley, 1695)*
   Synonym for macrodissected adult human ***middle cerebellar peduncle (Rolando, 1819)***; Figure VI-*k*.
6. *first medullary process of cerebellum (Cowper, 1698)*
   Roughly synonymous with macrodissected adult human ***middle cerebellar peduncle (Rolando, 1819)***; Table 10, Figure 1-*S* and Appendix Figures 28-*s* and 29-*a*, where also referred to as *second process of cerebellum*.
7. *processus ad medullam oblongatam (Pourfour du Petit, 1710)*
   Abbreviated form of *processus medullares à cerebello ad medullam oblongatam (Vieussens, 1684)*; p. 14.
8. *crura cerebri posteriora (Tarin, 1750)*
   Although somewhat ambiguous, probably corresponds to macrodissected adult human ***middle cerebellar peduncles (Rolando, 1819)***, though it might indicate set of ***cerebellar peduncles (Ridley, 1695)*** emerging from ***arbor vitae (Winslow, 1733)***; Table I, Figure 4-*A*.
9. *inferior cerebellar peduncle (Santorini, 1775)*
   Synonym for macrodissected adult human ***middle cerebellar peduncle (Rolando, 1819)***; p. 42. In Latin (plural), *pedunculi cerebelli inferiores*, see Burdach (1822, p. 299).

10. *crura cerebelli ad pontem (Soemmerring, 1778)*
Synonym for macrodissected adult human right and left ***middle cerebellar peduncle (Rolando, 1819)***; p. 63. Arnold (1834, Tab. VI-*yy*) had *crus cerebelli ad pontem*.
11. *middle cerebellar medullary process (Soemmerring, 1778)*
Synonym for macrodissected adult human ***middle cerebellar peduncle (Rolando, 1819)***; in the original Latin, *processus cerebelli medullaris medius*, Table II-*V*.
12. *anterior cerebellar crus (Mayer, 1779)*
Synonym for macrodissected adult human ***middle cerebellar peduncle (Rolando, 1819)***; p. 20. In Latin (plural), *crura cerebelli anteriora*, see Burdach (1822, p. 299).
13. *anterior cerebellar process (Haase, 1781)*
Synonym for macrodissected adult human ***middle cerebellar peduncle (Rolando, 1819)***; p. 27.
14. *processus ad pontem Varolii (Haase, 1781)*
Variation (singular) on macrodissected adult human *crura cerebelli ad pontem (Soemmerring, 1778)*; p. 28.
15. *crus cerebelli (Bell, 1803b)*
Synonym for macrodissected adult human ***middle cerebellar peduncle (Rolando, 1819)***; p. 107. Plural is *crura cerebelli*, p. 107.
16. *middle prolongation of cerebellum (Burdin, 1803)*
Synonym for macrodissected adult human ***middle cerebellar peduncle (Rolando, 1819)***; see translation (1803, Vol. 3, p. 165).
17. *anterior cerebellar peduncle (Chaussier, 1807)*
Synonym for macrodissected adult human ***middle cerebellar peduncle (Rolando, 1819)***; in the original French (plural), *pédoncules antérieurs du cervelet*, p. 113. Tiedemann (1816) used it for macrodissected 6-month human fetus; see translation (1826, p. 79).
18. *great cerebellar commissure (Gall & Spurzheim, 1810)*
Synonym for macrodissected adult human ***middle cerebellar peduncle (Rolando, 1819)***; p. 258. In Latin, *commissura magna cerebelli*, see Burdach (1822, p. 298).
19. *pars anterior corporis cerebralis adscendentis (Gall & Spurzheim, 1810)*
Synonym for macrodissected adult human ***middle cerebellar peduncle (Rolando, 1819)***; p. 350.
20. *pons cerebri (Wenzel & Wenzel, 1812)*
Synonym for macrodissected adult human ***middle cerebellar peduncle (Rolando, 1819)***; p. 203; Table XV, Figure 5-*o*.
21. *lower commissure of cerebellum (Carus, 1814)*
Synonym for macrodissected adult mammalian ***middle cerebellar peduncle (Rolando, 1819)***; in the original German, *untere Commissur des kleinen Hirns*, p. 249.
22. *middle cord (Tiedemann, 1816)*
Synonym for *anterior cerebellar peduncle (Chaussier, 1807)*; see translation (1826, p. 173).

LATER SYNONYMS:

1. *greater pons (Serres, 1824–1826)*
Synonym for macrodissected adult brown bear ***middle cerebellar peduncle (Rolando, 1819)***; in the original French, *grand pont*; Plate XI, Figure 231-*P*.
2. *cerebellar commissure (Spurzheim, 1826)*
Synonym for macrodissected adult human *great cerebellar commissure (Gall & Spurzheim, 1810)*; p. 138. Bell & Bell (1829, p. 383) used *commissure of cerebellum*.
3. *middle pedicle of cerebellum (Mayo, 1827)*
Synonym for macrodissected adult human ***middle cerebellar peduncle (Rolando, 1819)***; Plate IV, p. 8.
4. *crura of cerebellum (Swan, 1830)*
English form of *crura cerebelli (Bell, 1803b)*; Plate X, Figure 1-*K*. Swan also gave the singular, *crus of cerebellum*; Plate X, Figure 4.
5. *greater cerebellar commissure (Knox, 1832)*
Knox's version of macrodissected adult human *great cerebellar commissure (Gall & Spurzheim, 1810)*; Supplemental Plate IV-*17*.
6. *great cerebellic commissure (Grant, 1834c)*
Grant's version of macrodissected adult vertebrate *great cerebellar commissure (Gall & Spurzheim, 1810)*; p. 546.
7. *posterior peduncle (Cruveilhier, 1836)*
Synonym for macrodissected adult human *posterior appendix of cerebellum (Willis, 1664)*; in the original French (plural), *pédoncules postérieurs*, p. 603.
8. *corpus callosum of cerebellum (Cruveilhier, 1836)*
Synonym for macrodissected adult human ***middle cerebellar peduncle (Rolando, 1819)***; in the original French, *corps calleux du cervelet*, p. 605.
9. *cerebellar peduncle (Cruveilhier, 1836)*
Synonym for macrodissected adult human ***middle cerebellar peduncle (Rolando, 1819)***; in the original French (plural), *pédoncules cérébelleux*, p. 633.
10. *crura of medulla oblongata (Cruveilhier, 1836)*
Synonym for macrodissected adult human ***middle cerebellar peduncle (Rolando, 1819)***; in the original French, *cuisses de la moelle allongée*, p. 633.

PARTLY CORRESPONDS:

1. *lingula quaedam pontis intercedens inter has portiones (Wrisberg, 1777)*
Corresponds to medial region on ventral surface of macrodissected adult human right and left ***middle cerebellar peduncles (Rolando, 1819)*** between right and left ***trigeminal nerves (Winslow, 1733)***; see Vicq d'Azyr (1786, Pl. XVIII-63), Nieuwenhuys et al. (2008, Fig. 3.12).
2. *crus cerebelli (Vicq d'Azyr, 1786)*
Latin form of term corresponding to segment of ***middle cerebellar peduncle (Rolando, 1819)*** between ***arbor vitae (Winslow, 1733)*** dorsally and about the level of the ***trigeminal nerve (Winslow, 1733)*** ventrally; in the original French, *jambe du cervelet*; p. 54; Plate XXX, Figure II-23. Also see Quain (1837, p. 760), Crosby et al. (1962, Fig. 170).
3. *middle cerebellar crus (Günther, 1786)*

Synonym for macrodissected adult human *crus cerebelli (Vicq d'Azyr, 1786)*; in the original Latin, *crus cerebelli medii*, p. 19. Also see Burdach (1822, p. 299).

4. *middle cerebellar process (Günther, 1786)*
   Synonym for macrodissected adult human *crus cerebelli (Vicq d'Azyr, 1786)*; in the original Latin, *processus cerebelli medii*, p. 19. Also see Burdach (1822, p. 299).
5. *second cerebellar crus (Günther, 1789)*
   Synonym for macrodissected adult human *crus cerebelli (Vicq d'Azyr, 1786)*; in the original Latin, *crus cerebelli secundi*, p. 19. Also see Burdach (1822, p. 299).
6. *second cerebellar process (Günther, 1789)*
   Synonym for macrodissected adult human *crus cerebelli (Vicq d'Azyr, 1786)*; in the original Latin, *processus cerebelli secundi*, p. 19. Also see Burdach (1822, p. 299).
7. *anterior cerebellar peduncle (Procháska, 1800, p. 372)*
   Synonym for macrodissected adult human *crus cerebelli (Vicq d'Azyr, 1786)*; pp. 372, 387. In Latin (plural), *pedunculi cerebelli anteriores*, see Burdach (1822, p. 299).
8. *second cerebellar peduncle (Procháska, 1800)*
   Synonym for macrodissected adult human *crus cerebelli (Vicq d'Azyr, 1786)*; pp. 372, 387. In Latin (plural), *pedunculi cerebelli secundi*, see Burdach (1822, p. 299).
9. *middle cerebellar peduncle (Procháska, 1800)*
   Synonym for macrodissected adult human *crus cerebelli (Vicq d'Azyr, 1786)*; pp. 372, 387. In Latin (plural), *pedunculi cerebelli medii*, see Burdach (1822, p. 299). Reil (1809b) used it the same way; see Mayo translation (1823, p. 55).
10. *processus posteriores (Bichat et al., 1801–1803)*
    Synonym for macrodissected adult human *crus cerebelli (Vicq d'Azyr, 1786)*; Vol. 3, p. 114. See Burdach (1822, p. 299).
11. *processus cerebellares protuberantiae cerebralis (Bichat et al., 1801–1803)*
    Synonym for macrodissected adult human *crus cerebelli (Vicq d'Azyr, 1786)*; Vol. 3, p. 114. See Burdach (1822, p. 299).
12. *brachium of pons (Reil, 1807–1808a)*
    Apparently synonym for *middle cerebellar peduncle (Procháska, 1800)*; in the original German, *Arme dur Brucke*, see Mayo translation (1822, p. 24).
13. *lateral cerebellar peduncle (Reil, 1809b)*
    Synonym for *middle cerebellar peduncle (Procháska, 1800)*; see Mayo translation (1823, pp. 56–57).
14. *peduncle of annular protuberance (Reil, 1809b)*
    Synonym for *middle cerebellar peduncle (Procháska, 1800)*; see Mayo translation (1823, pp. 68, 89; Tab. VI, Fig. 2-*h*).
15. *peduncle of cerebellum (Gordon, 1815)*
    Synonym for macrodissected adult human *peduncle of annular protuberance (Reil, 1809b)*; p. 116. Quain (1837, p. 737) gave the Latin (plural), *crura cerebelli*.
16. *middle lateral cord (Tiedemann, 1816)*
    Essentially synonym for *crus cerebelli (Vicq d'Azyr, 1786)* in macrodissected 4-month and older fetal human. Tiedemann claimed it arises from ***dentate nucleus (>1840)*** and ***arbor vitae (Winslow, 1733)***; see translation (1826, p. 164).
17. *brachium pontis (Burdach, 1822)*
    Latin form of macrodissected adult human *brachium of pons (Reil, 1807–1808a)*; p. 67.
18. *posterior prolongation of cerebral protuberance (Cloquet, 1828)*
    Synonym for macrodissected adult human *crus cerebelli (Vicq d'Azyr, 1786)*; in the original French, *prolongemens postérieurs de la protubérance cérébrale*, p. 384 and Plate CXXXV-15.
19. *cerebellar prolongation of cerebral protuberance (Cloquet, 1828)*
    Synonym for *posterior prolongation of cerebral protuberance (Cloquet, 1828)*; in the original French (plural), *prolongemens cérébelleux de la protubérance cérébrale*, p. 384.
20. *chordae verticillatae (Bergmann, 1831)*
    Probably superficial aspect of macrodissected adult human ***middle cerebellar peduncle (Rolando, 1819)*** along wall of ***fourth ventricle (Galen, c192)***; Table V-*f*.
21. *verticillum (Bergmann, 1831)*
    Synonym for *chordae verticillatae (Bergmann, 1831)*; Table V-*f*.
22. *brachia cerebelli ad pontem (Arnold, 1838a)*
    Essentially synonym (plural) for macrodissected adult human *crus cerebelli (Vicq d'Azyr, 1786)*; p. 35.

middle cerebral artery plexus (>1840)

As described for macrodissected adult human, an extension of the ***internal carotid plexus (>1840)*** along the middle cerebral artery and its branches; see Mitchell (1953, pp. 219–220). It was pointed out at least as early as ***[middle cerebral artery plexus (>1840)] (Cloquet, 1816)***.

EARLIER REFERENCES:

Described, not named or illustrated:

1. ***[middle cerebral artery plexus (>1840)] (Cloquet, 1816)***
   Existence mentioned in macrodissected adult human; p. 690.

middle cervical ganglion (Haller, 1762)

As described for macrodissected adult human, the smallest of the three ***cervical sympathetic ganglia (>1840)*** associated with the ***sympathetic trunk (Winslow, 1733)***, not always observed macroscopically; see Henle (1871, Fig. 307), Mitchell (1953, pp. 223–224), Williams & Warwick (1980, pp. 1128–1129). For Haller's use in macrodissected adult human, see p. 257. It was probably first described as the *middle infolding in trunk of intercostal nerve (Willis, 1664)*.

TRANSLATIONS:

1. *ganglion cervicale medium (Haller, 1762)*
   Original Latin form of ***middle cervical ganglion (Haller, 1762)***; p. 257.

EARLIER REFERENCES:

Earlier synonyms:

1. *middle infolding in trunk of intercostal nerve (Willis, 1664)*

Synonym for macrodissected adult human ***middle cervical ganglion (Haller, 1762)***; in the original Latin, *plexus medius in trunco nervi intercostalis*; see Pordage translation (1681, Tab. IX-*Γ*). A modern rough translation is *middle ganglion of sympathetic trunk*.

2. *cervical infolding in trunk of intercostal nerve (Willis, 1664)*
   Synonym for macrodissected adult human ***middle cervical ganglion (Haller, 1762)***; in the original Latin, *plexus cervicalis in trunco nervi intercostalis*; see Pordage translation (1681, Tab. IX-*Γ*). A modern rough translation is *cervical ganglion of sympathetic trunk*.

LATER SYNONYMS:

1. *inferior cervical ganglion (Neubauer, 1772)*
   Unfortunate synonym for macrodissected adult human ***middle cervical ganglion (Haller, 1762)***; Table I-33 (but see p. 11 note *4*) as pointed out by Scarpa (1794, Tab. III-*91*).
2. *last cervical ganglion (Neubauer, 1772)*
   Synonym for macrodissected adult human *inferior cervical ganglion (Neubauer, 1772)*; in the original Latin, *ganglion ultimum cervicis*, p. 117.
3. *middle thyroid ganglion (Neubauer, 1772)*
   Synonym for macrodissected adult human ***middle cervical ganglion (Haller, 1762)***; in the original Latin, *ganglion thyroideum medium*, p. 111.
4. *thyroid ganglion (Neubauer, 1772; Haller, 1772)*
   Synonym listed for macrodissected adult human ***middle cervical ganglion (Haller, 1762)***, named because it lies near origin of inferior thyroid artery; in the original Latin, *ganglion thyroideum*; see Neubauer p. 111 and Haller p. 9 note *v*. The term was attributed without citation to Haller by Scarpa (1794, Tab. III-*91*).
5. *thyroid cervical ganglion (Haller, 1772)*
   Synonym for macrodissected adult human *inferior cervical ganglion (Neubauer, 1772)*; in the original Latin, *ganglio cervicali thyreoideo*, p. 8 note *p*.
6. *middle cervical plexus (Burdin, 1803)*
   Synonym for macrodissected adult human *inferior cervical ganglion (Neubauer, 1772)*; see translation (1803, Vol. 1, p. 209).
7. *central cervical ganglion (Meckel, 1817)*
   Synonym for macrodissected adult human ***middle cervical ganglion (Haller, 1762)***; see translation (1832, Vol. 3, p. 95).
8. *second cervical ganglion of sympathetic nerve (Swan, 1830)*
   Synonym for macrodissected adult human ***middle cervical ganglion (Haller, 1762)***; Plate I-*II*.

middle colic plexus (>1840)

As described for macrodissected adult human, it extends from the ***superior mesenteric plexus (Rau, 1720)*** along the middle colic artery to supply it and the transverse colon; see Mitchell (1953, p. 283). It was known to Vesalius; see ***[middle colic plexus (>1840)] (Vesalius, 1543a)***.

EARLIER REFERENCES:

Described, not named or illustrated:

1. ***[middle colic plexus (>1840)] (Vesalius, 1543a)***
   Mentioned and vaguely illustrated for macrodissected adult human, combined with ***right colic plexus (>1840)***; see Richardson & Carman translation (2002, p. 200 and Fig. on p. 169, part *κ*).

middle commissure (>1840)

As described in macrodissected adult human, and mammal generally with histological methods for ***axons (Kölliker, 1896)***, the part of the ***internal medullary lamina (>1840)*** crossing the median plane through regions of the ***intralaminar thalamic nuclei (>1840)*** associated with the ***interthalamic adhesion (>1840)***. It is sometimes absent or even double in adult human; see Meckel (1832, Vol. 2, p. 453) and *middle cerebral commissure (Tiedemann, 1821)*. It was first identified by Steno; see ***[middle commissure (>1840)] (Steno, 1669)***.

EARLIER REFERENCES:

Illustrated and described, not named:

1. ***[middle commissure (>1840)] (Steno, 1669)***
   Indicated for macrodissected adult human, in particular the presence of *white substance (Vesalius, 1543a)* in the ***interthalamic adhesion (>1840)***; see translation pp. 134, 137, 149–150, Plates I–IV.

Earlier synonyms:

1. *transverse tract of third ventricle (Santorini, 1724)*
   Synonym for macrodissected adult human ***middle commissure (>1840)***; in the original Latin, *tractus transversus tertii ventriculi*, p. 59, according to Burdach (1822, p. 341).

middle deep temporal nerve (>1840)

As described for macrodissected adult human, a very small and not always present component of the ***deep temporal nerves (Haase, 1781)***. When present as a separate entity it supplies intermediate regions of the temporalis muscle; see Williams & Warwick (1980, p. 1066). It was discovered by Meckel; see ***[middle deep temporal nerve (>1840)] (Meckel, 1748)***.

EARLIER REFERENCES:

Described, not named or illustrated:

1. ***[middle deep temporal nerve (>1840)] (Meckel, 1748)***
   Meckel indicated that a third (middle) ***deep temporal nerve (Haase, 1781)*** is sometimes present in macrodissected adult human; p. 220.

middle frontal gyrus (>1840)

As described for macrodissected adult human, a topographic subdivision of the ***frontal region (Vicq d'Azyr, 1786)*** lying between ***superior frontal gyrus (>1840)*** dorsally and ***inferior frontal gyrus (>1840)*** ventrally; see Williams & Warwick (1980, Fig. 7.111A), *Terminologia Anatomica* (1998, p. 125). It was clearly delineated by Vicq d'Azyr; see ***[middle frontal gyrus (>1840)] (Vicq d'Azyr, 1786)***.

EARLIER REFERENCES:

Illustrated, not named or described:

1. ***[middle frontal gyrus (>1840)] (Vicq d'Azyr, 1786)***

Illustrated as clearly for macrodissected adult human as modern attempts; Plate III, where ***lateral cerebral sulcus (>1840)*** is not quite exposed.

middle ovarian nerves (>1840)

As described for macrodissected adult human female, they arise by a series of rootlets from the side of the ***superior hypogastric plexus (Tiedemann, 1822)*** or rostral (upper) end of the homolateral ***hypogastric nerve (Walter, 1783)*** and are often partly blended with the ***middle ureteric nerves (>1840)*** and ***genitofemoral nerve (>1840)***. They follow the ovarian artery to the ovary, uterine tube, and uterus, where they communicate with the ***tubo-uterine nerve (>1840)***; see Mitchell (1953, p. 295). They were apparently known to Haller; see ***[middle ovarian nerves (>1840)] (Haller, 1762)***.

EARLIER REFERENCES:

Described, not named or illustrated:

1. ***[middle ovarian nerves (>1840)] (Haller, 1762)***
   Apparently mentioned for macrodissected adult human female; p. 266 note *a*.

middle rectal plexus (>1840)

As described for macrodissected adult human, an extension, perhaps arbitrary (Mitchell, 1953, p. 304), of the rostral (upper) part of the ***inferior hypogastric plexus (Tiedemann, 1822)*** accompanying the middle rectal artery and communicating rostrally (above) with the ***superior rectal plexus (>1840)*** and extending caudally (below) as far as the internal anal sphincter; see Williams & Warwick (1980, p. 1135). It was known to Willis; see ***[middle rectal plexus (>1840)] (Willis, 1664)***.

EARLIER REFERENCES:

Illustrated and described, not named:

1. ***[middle rectal plexus (>1840)] (Willis, 1664)***
   Alluded to for macrodissected adult human and other common large mammals; see Pordage translation (1681, p. 159 and Table 11-*d*).

Earlier synonyms:

1. *hemorrhoidal plexus (Mayer, 1794)*
   Essentially synonym for macrodissected adult human ***middle rectal plexus (>1840)***; in the original Latin, *plexus haemorhoidalis*; Part 6, Table VI-*189* (p. 41).
2. *internal hemorrhoidal plexus (Mayer, 1794)*
   Based on Mayer's illustrations of macrodissected adult human, apparently synonym for *hemorrhoidal plexus (Mayer, 1794)*, although the latter was described for male and *internal hemorrhoidal plexus (Mayer, 1794)* was described for female; in the original Latin, *plexus haemorrhoidalis internus*, Part 6, Table VIII, p. 57.
3. *hemorrhoidal nerves (Bock, 1827)*
   Synonym for macrodissected adult human *hemorrhoidal plexus (Mayer, 1794)*; in the original Latin, *nervi haemorrhoidales*, Table VI, Figure 1-*28*.
4. *inferior hemorrhoidal plexus (Cruveilhier, 1836)*
   Synonym for macrodissected adult human ***middle rectal plexus (>1840)***; in the original French (plural), *plexus hémorroïdaux inférieurs*, p. 1026.
5. *superior hemorrhoidal nerves (Quain, 1837)*
   Synonym for macrodissected adult human *hemorrhoidal nerves (Bock, 1827)*; in the original Latin, *nervi haemorrhoidales superiores*, p. 793.

middle superior dental nerve (Henle, 1871)

As described for macrodissected adult human, a variably present branch of the ***maxillary nerve (Meckel, 1753)*** supplying upper premolar teeth and contributing to the ***superior dental plexus (>1840)***; see Durward (1951, p. 1025), Williams & Warwick (1980, p. 1064 and Fig. 7.177, unlabeled *middle superior dental nerve*). For Henle's use in macrodissected adult human, see p. 370, including note *1*. Perhaps first delineated as the *middle dental nerve (Le Cat, 1768)*.

TRANSLATIONS:

1. *nervus dentalis superiores medialis (Henle, 1871)*
   Original Latin form of ***middle superior dental nerve (Henle, 1871)***; p. 370, including note *1*.

EARLIER REFERENCES:

Earlier synonyms:

1. *middle dental nerve (Le Cat, 1768)*
   Probably synonym for macrodissected adult human ***middle superior dental nerve (Henle, 1871)***; in the original French, *nerf dentale moyen*, Plate VIII, Figure 1-*21*.
2. *second dental nerve of second trunk of fifth nerve (Swan, 1830)*
   Synonym for macrodissected adult human ***middle superior dental nerve (Henle, 1871)***; Plate XII, Figure 5-*3*.
3. *lesser anterior dental nerve (Arnold, 1834)*
   Synonym for macrodissected adult human ***middle superior dental nerve (Henle, 1871)***; in the original Latin, *nervus dentalis anterior minor*, p. 9.

middle temporal gyrus (>1840)

As described for macrodissected adult human, a topographic subdivision of the ***temporal region (>1840)*** lying between ***superior temporal gyrus (>1840)*** dorsally and ***inferior temporal gyrus (>1840)*** ventrally; see Williams & Warwick (1980, Fig. 7.111A), Nieuwenhuys et al. (2008, Fig. 3.2). It was clearly delineated by Vicq d'Azyr; see ***[middle temporal gyrus (>1840)] (Vicq d'Azyr, 1786)***.

EARLIER REFERENCES:

Illustrated, not named or described:

1. ***[middle temporal gyrus (>1840)] (Vicq d'Azyr, 1786)***
   Clearly illustrated for macrodissected adult human; Plate XVII, between *17* and *14*.

Earlier synonyms:

1. *second process of middle lobe (Rolando, 1831)*
   Synonym for macrodissected adult human ***middle temporal gyrus (>1840)***; in the original Italian, *processo secondo del lobo di mezzo*, Figure 1-*a*.

Also see *superior enteroid processes of middle lobe (Rolando, 1831)*.

PARTLY CORRESPONDS:

1. *area temporalis media (Brodmann, 1909)*
   Original Latin form of *middle temporal area (Brodmann, 1909)*; p. 144.
2. *middle temporal area (Brodmann, 1909)*
   Based on cellular architecture in adult human, roughly corresponds to ***middle temporal gyrus (>1840)*** except for rostral (anterior) end occupied by *temporopolar area (Brodmann, 1909)*; see Garey translation (1994, p. 124 and Fig. 85).
3. *area 21 (Brodmann, 1909)*
   Synonym for adult human *middle temporal area (Brodmann, 1909)*; in the original German, *Feld 21*, p. 114.

middle testicular nerves (>1840)

As described for macrodissected adult human male, they arise by a series of rootlets from the side of the ***superior hypogastric plexus (Tiedemann, 1822)*** or rostral (upper) end of the homolateral ***hypogastric nerve (Walter, 1873)*** and are often partly blended with the ***middle ureteric nerves (>1840)*** and ***genitofemoral nerve (>1840)***. They follow the testicular artery to the testicle, where they distribute mainly or completely to the epididymis and beginning of the vas deferens; see Mitchell (1953, p. 295). Vesalius described the ***nerves (Herophilus, c335–c280 BC)*** to the testicles as a group for macrodissected adult human; see *branch of sixth pair stretching along roots of ribs offshoots to testes (Vesalius, 1543a)*. The ***middle testicular nerves (>1840)*** specifically were known to Haller; see ***[middle testicular nerves (>1840)] (Haller, 1762)***.

EARLIER REFERENCES:

Described, not named or illustrated:

1. ***[middle testicular nerves (>1840)] (Haller, 1762)***
   Mentioned for macrodissected adult human (presumably male and female); p. 266 note *a*.

middle ureteric nerves (>1840)

As described for macrodissected adult human, they arise by two or more rootlets from the side of the ***superior hypogastric plexus (Tiedemann, 1822)*** and rostral (upper) end of the homolateral ***hypogastric nerve (Walter, 1783)***, alongside or in conjunction with the ***middle testicular nerves (>1840)*** or ***middle ovarian nerves (>1840)***, and they are often united or interconnected with branches passing to the vas deferens in male; they supply the intermediate part of the ureter; see Mitchell (1953, p. 293). At least one was identified by Walter; see ***[middle ureteric nerves (>1840)] (Walter, 1783)***.

EARLIER REFERENCES:

Illustrated and described, not named:

1. ***[middle ureteric nerves (>1840)] (Walter, 1783)***
   At least one described but not named in macrodissected adult human; Table I-*464*.

midline thalamic nuclei (>1840)

Based on cellular architecture and connections, a component of the mammalian ***dorsal part of thalamus (Herrick, 1910)*** formed by small ***gray matter regions (Swanson & Bota, 2010)*** between the ***thalamic part of third ventricle (Swanson, 2004)*** and ***hypothalamic part of third ventricle (Swanson, 2004)***. Parts of the ***intralaminar thalamic nuclei (>1840)*** near the median plane divide the ***midline thalamic nuclei (>1840)*** into ventral parts dominated by the ***nucleus reuniens (>1840)*** and dorsal parts including mainly the ***paraventricular thalamic nucleus (>1840)*** and laterally adjacent ***paratenial nucleus (>1840)***; see Carpenter (Figs. 15.10, A15, A16), Swanson (2004, Table B, p. 172), Nieuwenhuys et al. (2008, p. 267), and ***interthalamic adhesion (>1840)***. Their main projections to the ***cerebral cortex (>1840)*** involve the ***cingulate region (>1840)*** and ***hippocampal formation (>1840)***. They were at least partly identified early on as a component of the *lacunar (Vieussens, 1684)*.

motor nucleus of trigeminal nerve (>1840)

As described for adult mammal based on cellular architecture and connections, the ***gray matter region (Swanson & Bota, 2010)*** in lateral parts of the ***pons (Haller, 1747)***, lying just medial to the ***principal sensory nucleus of trigeminal nerve (>1840)*** and generating the ***trigeminal nerve central motor root (>1840)*** continuing as the peripheral ***trigeminal nerve motor root (Bell, 1829)***; see Nieuwenhuys et al. (2008, pp. 203, 863–864 and Fig. 6.27-9). It was not identified by 1840.

muscular branches of anterior branch of obturator nerve (>1840)

As described for macrodissected adult human, they supply the adductor longus, gracilis, usually the adductor brevis, and often the pectineus muscles; see Williams & Warwick (1980, p. 1108), *Terminologia Anatomica* (1998, p. 140). At least one, to the gracilis muscle, was known to Galen; see ***[muscular branches of anterior branch of obturator nerve (>1840)] (Galen, c177)***.

EARLIER REFERENCES:

Described, not named or illustrated:

1. ***[muscular branches of anterior branch of obturator nerve (>1840)] (Galen, c177)***
   Galen described branch to gracilis muscle in macrodissected adult beef, pig, and/or macaque but not human; see Singer translation (1999, p. 85). Vesalius (1543a) did the same for macrodissected adult human; see Richardson & Carman translation (2002, p. 258).

Earlier synonyms:

1. *internal branch of anterior branch of obturator nerve (Cloquet, 1816)*
   Synonym for macrodissected adult human ***muscular branches of anterior branch of obturator nerve (>1840)***; p. 665.

PARTLY CORRESPONDS:

1. *branch of anterior branches of obturator nerve to adductor brevis muscle (Styx, 1782)*
   Macrodissected adult human branch of ***muscular branches of anterior branch of obturator nerve (>1840)***; in the original Latin, *ramus rami anterioris nervi obturatorii ad musculum adductorem brevem*, p. 24.
2. *branch of anterior branches of obturator nerve to gracilis muscle (Styx, 1782)*
   Macrodissected adult human branch of ***muscular branches of anterior branch of obturator nerve (>1840)***; in the original Latin, *ramus rami anterioris nervi obturatorii ad musculum gracilem*, p. 24. Also see ***[muscular branches of anterior branch of obturator nerve (>1840)] (Galen, c177)***.
3. *branch of obturator nerve to adductor longus muscle (Styx, 1782)*
   Macrodissected adult human branch of ***muscular branches of anterior branch of obturator nerve (>1840)***; in the original Latin, *ramus nervi obturatorii ad musculum adductorem longum*, p. 25.
4. *nerve to gracilis muscle (Fischer, 1791)*
   Macrodissected adult human branch of ***muscular branches of anterior branch of obturator nerve (>1840)*** named by Fischer, who noted that Berrettini (see Pietro da Cortona, 1741) illustrated it; in the original Latin, *nervus musculi gracilis*, p. 7.
5. *branch of obturator nerve to short head of triceps muscle (Swan, 1830)*
   Macrodissected adult human ***muscular branch of anterior branch of obturator nerve (>1840)*** probably to adductor brevis muscle; Plate XXIV, Figure 1-26.
6. *branch of obturator nerve to long head of triceps muscle (Swan, 1830)*
   Macrodissected adult human ***muscular branch of anterior branch of obturator nerve (>1840)*** probably to adductor longus muscle (or adductor magnus muscle); Plate XXIV, Figure 1-27.
7. *branch of obturator nerve to gracile muscle (Swan, 1830)*
   Macrodissected adult human ***muscular branch of anterior branch of obturator nerve (>1840)*** to gracilis muscle; Plate XXIV, Figure 1-28.
8. *terminal branches of obturator nerve (Cruveilhier, 1836)*
   For macrodissected adult human, four ***muscular branches of anterior branch of obturator nerve (>1840)*** considered together: *internal terminal branch of obturator nerve (Cruveilhier, 1836)*, *external terminal branch of obturator nerve (Cruveilhier, 1836)*, *middle terminal branch of obturator nerve (Cruveilhier, 1836)*, and *fourth terminal branch of obturator nerve (Cruveilhier, 1836)*; in the original French, *branches terminales*, p. 839.
9. *internal terminal branch of obturator nerve (Cruveilhier, 1836)*
   Macrodissected adult human ***muscular branch of anterior branch of obturator nerve (>1840)*** to gracilis muscle (*droit interne*); p. 839.
10. *external terminal branch of obturator nerve (Cruveilhier, 1836)*
   Macrodissected adult human ***muscular branch of anterior branch of obturator nerve (>1840)*** to pectineus muscle (*premier adducteur ou adducteur superficiel*); p. 839.
11. *middle terminal branch of obturator nerve (Cruveilhier, 1836)*
   Macrodissected adult human ***muscular branch of anterior branch of obturator nerve (>1840)*** to adductor brevis muscle (*petit adducteur*); p. 839.
12. *fourth terminal branch of obturator nerve (Cruveilhier, 1836)*
   Macrodissected adult human ***muscular branch of anterior branch of obturator nerve (>1840)*** to adductor longus muscle (*grand adducteur*); p. 839.

muscular branches of axillary nerve (>1840)

As described for macrodissected adult human, they supply mainly the deltoid and teres minor muscles; see Williams & Warwick (1980, p. 1097), *Terminologia Anatomica* (1998, p. 139). They were known to Galen; see ***[muscular branches of axillary nerve (>1840)] (Galen, c173)***.

EARLIER REFERENCES:

Described, not named or illustrated:

1. ***[muscular branches of axillary nerve (>1840)] (Galen, c173)***
   Alluded to for macrodissected adult beef, pig, and/or macaque but not human; see May translation (1968, pp. 703–704), Duckworth translation (1962, pp. 243, 247). Meckel described them carefully for macrodissected adult human; see translation (1832, Vol. 3, p. 24).

Illustrated, not named or described:

1. ***[muscular branches of axillary nerve (>1840)] (Eustachi, 1552)***
   Clearly illustrated innervation of macrodissected adult human deltoid muscle; see Albinus edition (1761, Tab. 20-39).

Illustrated and described, not named:

1. ***[muscular branches of axillary nerve (>1840)] (Vieussens, 1684)***
   Clearly illustrated and described innervation of macrodissected adult human deltoid muscle; Table 25-*11*.

PARTLY CORRESPONDS:

1. *branch of axillary nerve partly to deltoid and partly to teres minor muscle (Caldani, 1813, 1814)*
   Macrodissected adult human ***muscular branch of axillary nerve (>1840)*** splitting and going partly to deltoid muscle and partly to teres minor muscle; in the original Latin, *ramus partim deltoidem pererrans partim musculum teretam minorem*; Table CCLX, Figure 1-22.
2. *branch of axillary nerve to long belly of triceps (Caldani, 1813, 1814)*
   Macrodissected adult human ***muscular branch of axillary nerve (>1840)*** to long head of triceps muscle; in the

original Latin, *ramus pro ventre longiore tricipitis*; Table CCLX, Figure 1-23.

3. *branch of axillary nerve to infraspinatus muscle (Caldani, 1813, 1814)*
   Macrodissected adult human ***muscular branch of axillary nerve (>1840)*** to infraspinatus muscle; in the original Latin, *ramus musculo infraspinato tributus*, Table CCLX, Figure 1-24.
4. *branch of humeral circumflex nerve to teres minor muscle (Langenbeck, 1826–1830)*
   Macrodissected adult human ***muscular branch of axillary nerve (>1840)*** to teres minor muscle; in the original Latin, *ramus nervi circumflexi humeri ad musculum teretem minorem*, Fascicle III, Table XIII-*8*.
5. *branches of humeral circumflex nerve to deltoid muscle (Langenbeck, 1826–1830)*
   Macrodissected adult human ***muscular branches of axillary nerve (>1840)*** to deltoid muscle; in the original Latin, *rami nervi circumflexi humeri ad musculum deltoidem*, Fascicle III, Table XIII-*8*.
6. *branch to teres minor muscle (Bock, 1827)*
   Macrodissected adult human ***muscular branch of axillary nerve (>1840)***; in the original Latin, *ram. musculi teretis minoris*, Table V, Figure 2-*70*.
7. *nerve of teres minor (Cruveilhier, 1836)*
   Synonym for macrodissected adult human *branch to teres minor muscle (Bock, 1827)*; in the original French, *nerf du petit rond*, p. 796.
8. *terminal branch of axillary nerve (Cruveilhier, 1836)*
   Synonym for *deltoid branch of axillary nerve (Cruveilhier, 1836)*; in the original French, *rameaux de terminaison de l'axillaire*, p. 796.
9. *deltoid branch of axillary nerve (Cruveilhier, 1836)*
   Macrodissected adult human ***muscular branch of axillary nerve (>1840)*** to deltoid muscle; in the original French, *rameaux deltoïdiens de l'axillaire*, p. 796. Cruveilhier further described ascending and descending branches of this branch.

muscular branches of brachial plexus roots (>1840)

As described for macrodissected adult human, they innervate primarily the scaleni and longus colli muscles; see Williams & Warwick (1980, p. 1095). They were probably at least mentioned by Vieussens; see ***[muscular branches of brachial plexus roots (>1840)] (Vieussens, 1684)***.

EARLIER REFERENCES:

Described, not named or illustrated:

1. ***[muscular branches of brachial plexus roots (>1840)] (Vieussens, 1684)***
   Probably mentioned for macrodissected adult human; Table 24-*c*. Haase (1781, pp. 94–97) mentioned a number of them for macrodissected adult human.

muscular branches of cervical plexus (Cruveilhier, 1836)

As described for macrodissected adult human, they include branches to the rectus capitis lateralis and rectus capitis anterior, longus capitis and longus colli, sternocleidomastoid, trapezius, levator scapulae, and scalenus medius muscles; the ***inferior root of ansa cervicalis (>1840)*** and ***phrenic nerve (Galen c173)*** are described separately; see Durward (1951, Fig. 919) and Williams & Warwick (1980, pp. 1092–1094), who divide the muscular branches into medial and lateral groups, as is common. For Cruveilhier's use in macrodissected adult human, see p. 781. Essentially all of them were known to Galen; see ***[muscular branches of cervical plexus (Cruveilhier, 1836)] (Galen, c173)***.

EARLIER REFERENCES:

Described, not named or illustrated:

1. ***[muscular branches of cervical plexus (Cruveilhier, 1836)] (Galen, c173)***
   Galen mentioned essentially all major currently recognized branches for adult human based on macrodissected adult beef, pig, and/or macaque but not human; see May translation (1968, pp. 696–704) and Duckworth translation (1962, p. 230 ff.).

Illustrated and described, not named:

1. ***[muscular branches of cervical plexus (Cruveilhier, 1836)] (Vesalius, 1543a)***
   Vesalius accounted for most of them in macrodissected adult human; see Richardson & Carman translation (2002, pp. 224–227).

Earlier synonyms:

1. *deep branches of cervical plexus (Quain, 1828)*
   Synonym for macrodissected adult human ***muscular branches of cervical plexus (Cruveilhier, 1836)***; p. 490.

PARTLY CORRESPONDS:

1. *posterior branches of third cervical pair (Winslow, 1733)*
   Refers to some ***muscular branches of cervical plexus (Cruveilhier, 1836)*** arising from fourth cervical ***spinal nerve ventral branch (>1840)*** in macrodissected adult human; Section VI, p. 79.
2. *muscular branch of third cervical nerve (Haller, 1772)*
   Clear precursor synonym for macrodissected adult human ***muscular branches of cervical plexus (Cruveilhier, 1836)***; p. 9-*β,β*.
3. *deep branch of fourth pair of cervical nerves (Neubauer, 1772)*
   Synonym for macrodissected adult human *posterior branches of third cervical pair (Winslow, 1733)*; in the original Latin, *ramus profundus paris quarti nervorum*, Table 1-*200*, where Neubauer also referred to it as posterior branch.
4. *subclavicular branches of cervical plexus (Cloquet, 1816)*
   Macrodissected adult human ***muscular branches of cervical plexus (Cruveilhier, 1836)*** to omohyoid muscle and superior part of subscapular and anterior serratus muscles; in the original French, *rameaux sous-claviculaires*, p. 639.
5. *deep cervical branches of cervical plexus (Cloquet, 1816)*
   Macrodissected adult human ***muscular branches of cervical plexus (Cruveilhier, 1836)*** to trapezius, longus

capitis, and rhomboid muscles; in the original French, *rameaux cervicaux profonds*, p. 639.

muscular branches of deep fibular nerve (>1840)
As described for macrodissected adult human they supply the tibialis anterior, extensor hallucis, extensor digitorum longus, and peroneus tertius muscles; see Williams & Warwick (1980, p. 1115) and Durward (1951, Fig. 948; referred to there as *anterior tibial nerve*), *Terminologia Anatomica* (1998, p. 140). They were known to Galen; see ***[muscular branches of deep fibular nerve (>1840)] (Galen, c173)***.

EARLIER REFERENCES:

Described, not named or illustrated:

1. ***[muscular branches of deep fibular nerve (>1840)] (Galen, c173)***
Alluded to as group for macrodissected adult beef, pig, and/or macaque but not human; see May translation (1968, p. 706), Singer translation (1999, p. 86). Meckel (1817) described all of them for macrodissected adult human without naming group; see translation (1832, Vol. 3, p. 19).

Illustrated, not named or described:

1. ***[muscular branches of deep fibular nerve (>1840)] (Eustachi, 1552)***
Eustachi illustrated at least the beginnings of some for macrodissected adult human; see Albinus edition (1761, Tab. 19/2-*17,18*).

Illustrated and described, not named:

1. ***[muscular branches of deep fibular nerve (>1840)] (Vieussens, 1684)***
Described and illustrated at least two for macrodissected adult human (1684, Tab. 29-*81,82*).

Earlier synonyms:

1. *superior anterior branches of muscular branch of peroneal nerve (Martin, 1781)*
Synonym for macrodissected adult human ***muscular branches of deep fibular nerve (>1840)***; in the original Latin, *nervus peroneus ramus muscularis ramus anterior superior*, p. 248 and Table XI.
2. *muscular branches of anterior tibial nerve (Quain & Wilson, 1839)*
Synonym for macrodissected adult human ***muscular branches of deep fibular nerve (>1840)***; Plate XXIV, Figure 2-*C,b*.
3. *muscular branches of interosseous nerve (Quain & Wilson, 1839)*
Synonym for macrodissected adult human ***muscular branches of deep fibular nerve (>1840)***; Plate XXIV, Figure 2-*C,b*.

PARTLY CORRESPONDS:

1. *posterior twig of deep branch of peroneal nerve (Jördens, 1788)*
Macrodissected adult human ***muscular branch of deep fibular nerve (>1840)*** to tibialis anterior muscle; in the original Latin, *ramulus huius rami profundi [ramus nervi peronei profundus], posterior*, pp. 4, 14.
2. *anterior twig of deep branch of peroneal nerve (Jördens, 1788)*
Macrodissected adult human ***muscular branch of deep fibular nerve (>1840)*** to tibialis anterior muscle; in the original Latin, *ramulus anterior rami profundi*, pp. 4, 14.
3. *first internal lateral twig of deep branch of peroneal nerve (Jördens, 1788)*
Macrodissected adult human ***muscular branch of deep fibular nerve (>1840)*** to tibialis anterior muscle; in the original Latin, *ramulus lateralis internus primus rami profundi nervi peronei*, pp. 4, 14.
4. *first external lateral twig of deep branch of peroneal nerve (Jördens, 1788)*
Macrodissected adult human ***muscular branch of deep fibular nerve (>1840)*** to extensor digitorum longus muscle; in the original Latin, *ramulus lateralis internus primus rami profundi nervi peronei*, pp. 4, 14.
5. *second internal lateral twig of deep branch of peroneal nerve (Jördens, 1788)*
Macrodissected adult human ***muscular branch of deep fibular nerve (>1840)*** to tibialis anterior muscle; in the original Latin, *ramulus lateralis internus secundus rami profundi nervi peronei*, pp. 4, 14.
6. *second external lateral twig of deep branch of peroneal nerve (Jördens, 1788)*
Macrodissected adult human ***muscular branch of deep fibular nerve (>1840)*** to tibialis anterior muscle; in the original Latin, *ramulus lateralis internus secundus rami profundi nervi peronei*, pp. 4, 14.
7. *third internal lateral twig of deep branch of peroneal nerve (Jördens, 1788)*
Macrodissected adult human ***muscular branch of deep fibular nerve (>1840)*** to tibialis anterior muscle; in the original Latin, *ramulus lateralis internus tertius rami profundi nervi peronei*, pp. 4, 14.
8. *fourth internal lateral twig of deep branch of peroneal nerve (Jördens, 1788)*
Macrodissected adult human ***muscular branch of deep fibular nerve (>1840)*** to tibialis anterior muscle; in the original Latin, *ramulus lateralis internus quartus rami profundi nervi peronei*, pp. 4, 14.
9. *fifth internal lateral twig of deep branch of peroneal nerve (Jördens, 1788)*
Macrodissected adult human ***muscular branch of deep fibular nerve (>1840)*** to tibialis anterior muscle; in the original Latin, *ramulus lateralis internus quintus rami profundi nervi peronei*, pp. 4, 14.
10. *first nerve to tibialis anterior muscle (Fischer, 1791)*
Macrodissected adult human ***muscular branch of deep fibular nerve (>1840)*** to tibialis anterior muscle; in the original Latin, *nervum musculi tibialis antici primum*, p. 32.
11. *second nerve to peroneus longus muscle (Fischer, 1791)*
Macrodissected adult human ***muscular branch of deep fibular nerve (>1840)*** to peroneus longus muscle; in the original Latin, *nervus musculi peronei longi secundum*, p. 32.

12. *common nerve to extensor digitorum longus and extensor pollicis longus muscles (Fischer, 1791)*
Macrodissected adult human ***muscular branch of deep fibular nerve (>1840)*** to extensor digitorum longus and extensor hallucis longus muscles; in the original Latin, *nervus communis musculi extensoris digitorum longi et extensoris pollicis longi*, p. 32.
13. *first nerve to extensor digitorum longus muscle (Fischer, 1791)*
Branch of *common nerve to extensor digitorum longus and extensor pollicis longus muscles (Fischer, 1791)*; in the original Latin, *nervus musculum extensorem digitorum longum primus*, p. 32.
14. *second nerve to extensor pollicis longus muscle (Fischer, 1791)*
Branch of *common nerve to extensor digitorum longus and extensor pollicis longus muscles (Fischer, 1791)* to extensor hallucis longus muscle; in the original Latin, *nervus musculi extensori pollicis longo secundus*, p. 32.
15. *common nerve to tibialis anterior, extensor digitorum longus, and extensor pollicis longus muscles (Fischer, 1791)*
Macrodissected adult human ***muscular branch of deep fibular nerve (>1840)*** to tibialis anterior, extensor digitorum longus, and extensor hallucis longus muscles; in the original Latin, *nervus communis musculi tibialis antici, extensoris digitorum longi et extensoris pollicis longi*, p. 33.
16. *second nerve to tibialis anterior muscle (Fischer, 1791)*
Branch of *common nerve to tibialis anterior, extensor digitorum longus, and extensor pollicis longus muscles (Fischer, 1791)*; in the original Latin, *nervum musculi tibialis antici secundum*, p. 33.
17. *second nerve to extensor digitorum longus muscle (Fischer, 1791)*
Branch of *common nerve to tibialis anterior, extensor digitorum longus, and extensor pollicis longus muscles (Fischer, 1791)*; in the original Latin, *nervum musculi extensori digitorum longo secundus*, p. 33.
18. *third nerve to extensor pollicis longus muscle (Fischer, 1791)*
Branch of *common nerve to tibialis anterior, extensor digitorum longus, and extensor pollicis longus muscles (Fischer, 1791)* to extensor hallucis longus muscle; in the original Latin, *nervum musculi extensorem pollicis longus tertius*, p. 33.
19. *third nerve to tibialis anterior muscle (Fischer, 1791)*
A macrodissected adult human ***muscular branch of deep fibular nerve (>1840)***; in the original Latin, *nervus musculi tibialis antici tertius*, p. 33.
20. *first nerve to posterior tibial muscle (Fischer, 1791)*
A macrodissected adult human ***muscular branch of deep fibular nerve (>1840)***; in the original Latin, *nervus musculi tibialis postici primus*, p. 33.
21. *common twig to extensor digitorum brevis muscle and superior interossei muscles (Fischer, 1791)*
Branch of *internal branch of deep peroneal nerve (Fischer, 1791)* that may be considered ***muscular branch of deep fibular nerve (>1840)*** to extensor digitorum brevis muscle and dorsal interossei muscles of foot; in the original Latin, *ramulum communem musculi extensoris brevis digitorum et musculorum interosseorum superiorum*, p. 33. It generates *third nerve to tibialis anterior muscle (Fischer, 1791)*; p. 33.
22. *external branch of deep peroneal nerve (Fischer, 1791)*
Fischer described for macrodissected adult human two terminal branches of ***deep fibular nerve (Fyfe, 1800)***, external and internal. External branch was said to generate common branch to extensor digitorum brevis muscle and dorsal interossei muscles, distinct from *common twig to extensor digitorum brevis muscle and superior interossei muscles (Fischer, 1791)*. Thus, *external branch of deep peroneal nerve (Fischer, 1791)* may be considered ***muscular branch of deep fibular nerve (>1840)***. In the original Latin, *ramum externum nervi peronei profundi*, p. 33.
23. *external dorsal branch of deep peroneal nerve (Fischer, 1791)*
Synonym for *external branch of deep peroneal nerve (Fischer, 1791)*; Table IV, Figure 1-*361*.
24. *deep branch of deep peroneal nerve (Fischer, 1791)*
Synonym for *external branch of deep peroneal nerve (Fischer, 1791)*; Table IV, Figure 1-*361*.
25. *deep dorsal branch of foot of deeper seated branch of fibular nerve (Bell & Bell, 1816)*
Term emerging from Bell & Bell's description of a macrodissected adult human ***muscular branch of deep fibular nerve (>1840)*** to extensor digitorum brevis and "interossei" muscles; in the original Latin, *ramus dorsalis pedis profundus*, Vol. 2, p. 551.
26. *branches of peroneal nerve to anterior tibial muscle (Swan, 1830)*
Macrodissected adult human ***muscular branches of deep fibular nerve (>1840)*** to tibialis anterior muscle; Plate XXIII, Figure 4-5.
27. *tibialis anterior branches of external popliteal sciatic nerve (Cruveilhier, 1836)*
For macrodissected adult human, two ***muscular branches of deep fibular nerve (>1840)*** to tibialis anterior muscle; in the original French, *branches du jambier antérieur*, p. 864.
28. *superior branches of external popliteal sciatic nerve (Cruveilhier, 1836)*
Synonym for *tibialis anterior branches of external popliteal sciatic nerve (Cruveilhier, 1836)*; in the original French, *branches supérieures*, p. 864.
29. *recurrent branches of external popliteal sciatic nerve (Cruveilhier, 1836)*
Synonym for *tibialis anterior branches of external popliteal sciatic nerve (Cruveilhier, 1836)*; in the original French, *branches récurrentes*, p. 864.
30. *branches of anterior tibial nerve to extensor brevis digitorum muscle (Quain & Wilson, 1839)*
Macrodissected adult human ***muscular branches of deep fibular nerve (>1840)*** to extensor brevis digitorum muscle; Plate XXIV, Figure 2-C,*d*.
31. *branches of interosseous nerve to extensor brevis digitorum muscle (Quain & Wilson, 1839)*
Macrodissected adult human ***muscular branches of deep fibular nerve (>1840)*** to extensor brevis digitorum muscle; Plate XXIV, Figure 2-C,*d*.

32. *interosseous branches of anterior tibial nerve (Quain & Wilson, 1839)*
    Macrodissected adult human ***muscular branches of deep fibular nerve (>1840)*** to interossei muscles of foot; Plate XXIV, Figure 2-C,*e*.
33. *interosseous branches of interosseous nerve (Quain & Wilson, 1839)*
    Macrodissected adult human ***muscular branches of deep fibular nerve (>1840)*** to interossei muscles of foot; Plate XXIV, Figure 2-C,*e*.

muscular branches of external branch of accessory nerve trunk (>1840)

As described for macrodissected adult human, small terminal branches of the ***external branch of accessory nerve trunk (Meckel, 1817)*** supplying primarily the sternocleidomastoid muscle and trapezius muscle; see Williams & Warwick (1980, p. 1082), *Terminologia Anatomica* (1998, p. 137). They were first described by Galen; see ***[muscular branches of external branch of accessory nerve trunk (>1840)] (Galen, c192)***.

EARLIER REFERENCES:

Described, not named or illustrated:

1. ***[muscular branches of external branch of accessory nerve trunk (>1840)] (Galen, c192)***
   Distribution to trapezius and sternocleidomastoid muscles clearly described for macrodissected adult beef, pig, and/or macaque but not human; see Duckworth translation (1962, p. 202).

Illustrated and described, not named:

1. ***[muscular branches of external branch of accessory nerve trunk (>1840)] Willis (1664)***
   Described and illustrated for macrodissected adult human; see Pordage translation (1681, p. 173, Tab. 9-☽).

PARTLY CORRESPONDS:

1. *branches to sternocleidomastoid muscle from external ramus of accessory nerve of Willis (Arnold, 1834)*
   Macrodissected adult human ***muscular branches of external branch of accessory nerve trunk (>1840)*** to sternocleidomastoid muscle; in the original Latin, *nervi accessorii Willisii ramus externus rami ad musculum sternocleidomastoideum*; Table VIII:*XI-62*.
2. *branches to cucullaris muscle from external ramus of accessory nerve of Willis (Arnold, 1834)*
   Macrodissected adult human ***muscular branches of external branch of accessory nerve trunk (>1840)*** to trapezius muscle; in the original Latin, *nervi accessorii Willisii ramus externus rami ad musculum cucullarem*; Table VIII:*XI-64*. Sometimes translated, *cowl muscle*.

muscular branches of femoral nerve (Quain & Wilson, 1839)

As described for macrodissected adult human, main branches supply the pectineus, sartorius, iliopsoas, and quadriceps (the rectus femoris, vastus lateralis, vastus medialis, and vastus intermedius) muscles; see Durward (1951, p. 1094), Williams & Warwick (1980, p. 1109). For Quain & Wilson's use in macrodissected adult human see Plate XI-*F,w,y* and Plate XXIII-*c*. They were known generally to Galen, see ***[muscular branches of femoral nerve (Quain & Wilson, 1839)] (Galen, c177)***, and they were carefully described and named for macrodissected adult human by Styx (1782, p. 8).

EARLIER REFERENCES:

Described, not named or illustrated:

1. ***[muscular branches of femoral nerve (Quain & Wilson, 1839)] (Galen, c177)***
   Referred to generally for macrodissected adult beef, pig, and/or macaque but not human; see Singer translation (1999, pp. 84–85). Vesalius (1543a) described most of them in macrodissected adult human, although he ascribed a lateral group to *first nerve entering leg (Vesalius, 1543a)* and a medial group to larger part of *second nerve entering leg (1543a)*; see Richardson & Carman translation (2002, pp. 257–258). Fischer (1791, pp. 6–7) reviewed in detail earlier references to them in macrodissected adult human.

Earlier synonyms:

1. *muscular branches of crural nerve (Günther, 1786)*
   Synonym for macrodissected adult human ***muscular branches of femoral nerve (Quain & Wilson, 1839)***; in the original Latin, *r. musculares*, p. 83.
2. *muscular nerves of crural nerve (Bock, 1827)*
   Synonym for macrodissected adult human ***muscular branches of femoral nerve (Quain & Wilson, 1839)***; in the original Latin, *nervi musculares nervi cruralis*, Table I, Figure 2-*82*.
3. *external and internal deep-seated branches of crural nerve (Quain, 1828)*
   Basically synonym for macrodissected adult human ***muscular branches of femoral nerve (Quain & Wilson, 1839)***, as Quain divided them into two major parts; p. 288.

PARTLY CORRESPONDS:

1. *second deep nerve of thigh (Galen, c177)*
   Femoral flexor ***nerve (Herophilus, c335–c280 BC)***, a ***muscular branch of femoral nerve (Quain & Wilson, 1839)*** found in macrodissected adult monkey but not human, according to Singer (1999, p. 84).
2. *short nerve to sartorius muscle (Styx, 1782)*
   Macrodissected adult human ***muscular branch of femoral nerve (Quain & Wilson, 1839)*** to proximal end of sartorius muscle; in the original Latin, *nervus musculi sartorii brevis*, p. 8. Styx summarized earlier observations on p. 10.
3. *long nerve to sartorius muscle (Styx, 1782)*
   Macrodissected adult human ***muscular branch of femoral nerve (Quain & Wilson, 1839)*** to distal part of sartorius muscle; in the original Latin, *nervus musculi sartorii longus*, p. 8. Styx summarized earlier observations on p. 10.
4. *nerve to pectineus muscle (Styx, 1782)*
   Macrodissected adult human ***muscular branch of femoral nerve (Quain & Wilson, 1839)***; in the original Latin,

nervus musculi pectinei sive liuidi, p. 8. Styx noted it was illustrated by Eustachi (1552) in his Plate XIII; see Albinus edition (1744).

5. *nerve to livid muscle (Styx, 1782)*
Synonym for *nerve to pectineus muscle (Styx, 1782)*; in the original Latin, *nervus musculi lividi*, p. 8. For translation see Knox (1832, Pl. XV-*109*).
6. *short nerve to crural muscle (Styx, 1782)*
Macrodissected adult human ***muscular branch of femoral nerve (Quain & Wilson, 1839)*** to proximal part of rectus femoris muscle; in the original Latin, *nervus brevis musculi crurei*, p. 8.
7. *short nerve to vastus externus muscle (Styx, 1782)*
Macrodissected adult human ***muscular branch of femoral nerve (Quain & Wilson, 1839)*** to proximal part of vastus lateralis muscle; in the original Latin, *nervus brevis musculi vasti externi*, p. 8.
8. *long nerve to vastus externus muscle (Styx, 1782)*
Macrodissected adult human ***muscular branch of femoral nerve (Quain & Wilson, 1839)*** to distal part of vastus lateralis muscle; in the original Latin, *nervus longus musculi vasti externi*, p. 8. Styx also summarized earlier observations on p. 16.
9. *long nerve to crural muscle (Styx, 1782)*
Macrodissected adult human ***muscular branch of femoral nerve (Quain & Wilson, 1839)*** to distal part of rectus femoris muscle; in the original Latin, *nervus longus musculi crurei*, p. 9. Styx also summarized earlier observations on p. 17.
10. *short nerve to vastus internus muscle (Styx, 1782)*
Macrodissected adult human ***muscular branch of femoral nerve (Quain & Wilson, 1839)*** to proximal part of vastus medialis muscle; in the original Latin, *nervus brevis musculi vasti interni*, p. 9.
11. *long nerve to vastus internus muscle (Styx, 1782)*
Macrodissected adult human ***muscular branch of femoral nerve (Quain & Wilson, 1839)*** to distal part of vastus medialis muscle; in the original Latin, *nervus longus musculi vasti interni*, p. 9. Styx also summarized earlier observations on pp. 18–19.
12. *nerve to recti cruris muscle (Styx, 1782)*
Macrodissected adult human ***muscular branch of femoral nerve (Quain & Wilson, 1839)*** to rectus femoris muscle; in the original Latin, *nervus musculi recti cruris*, p. 15. Styx also summarized earlier observations on p. 15.
13. *nerve to rectus muscle (Styx, 1782)*
Synonym for *nerve to recti cruris muscle (Styx, 1782)*; in the original Latin, *nervus musculi recti*, p. 34.
14. *nerve to rectus femoris muscle (Frotscher, 1788)*
Synonym for macrodissected adult human *nerve to recti cruris muscle (Styx, 1782)*; in the original Latin, *nervum recti femoris*, p. 95 of 1795 reprint.
15. *superior nerve to sartorius muscle (Fischer, 1791)*
Synonym for macrodissected adult human *short nerve to sartorius muscle (Styx, 1782)*; in the original Latin, *nervus musculi sartorii superior*, p. 6.
16. *middle nerve to sartorius muscle (Fischer, 1791)*
Macrodissected adult human ***muscular branch of femoral nerve (Quain & Wilson, 1839)*** between *short nerve to sartorius muscle (Styx, 1782)* and *long nerve to sartorius muscle (Styx, 1782)*; in the original Latin, *nervus musculi sartorii medius*, p. 6.
17. *superior nerve for vastus externus muscle (Fischer, 1791)*
Synonym for macrodissected adult human *short nerve to vastus externus muscle (Styx, 1782)*; in the original Latin, *nervus superior pro musculo vasto externo*, p. 6.
18. *first nerve for vastus externus muscle (Fischer, 1791)*
Synonym for *superior nerve for vastus externus muscle (Fischer, 1791)*; in the original Latin, *nervus primus pro musculo vasto externo*, p. 6.
19. *middle nerve for vastus externus muscle (Fischer, 1791)*
Fischer described for macrodissected adult human four ***nerves (Herophilus, c335–c280 BC)*** to vastus externus muscle, this being the second; in the original Latin, *nervus musculi vasto externo medius*, p. 6. A ***muscular branch of femoral nerve (Quain & Wilson, 1839)***.
20. *second nerve for vastus externus muscle (Fischer, 1791)*
Synonym for *middle nerve to vastus externus muscle (Fischer, 1791)*; in the original Latin, *nervus secundus pro musculo vasto externo*, p. 6.
21. *third nerve for vastus externus muscle (Fischer, 1791)*
Fischer described for macrodissected adult human four ***nerves (Herophilus, c335–c280 BC)*** to vastus externus muscle, this being the third; in the original Latin, *nervus tertius pro musculo vasto externo*, p. 6. A ***muscular branch of femoral nerve (Quain & Wilson, 1839)***.
22. *inferior nerve for vastus externus muscle (Fischer, 1791)*
Synonym for *third nerve of vastus externus muscle (Fischer, 1791)*; in the original Latin, *nervus inferior pro musculo vasto externo*, p. 6.
23. *fourth nerve for vastus externus muscle (Fischer, 1791)*
Synonym for macrodissected adult human *long nerve to vastus externus muscle (Styx, 1782)*; in the original Latin, *nervus quartus pro musculo vasto externo*, p. 6.
24. *superior nerve to crural muscle (Fischer, 1791)*
Synonym for macrodissected adult human *short nerve to crural muscle (Styx, 1782)*; in the original Latin, *nervus musculi cruralis superior*, p. 6.
25. *inferior nerve for sartorius muscle (Fischer, 1791)*
Synonym for macrodissected adult human *long nerve to sartorius muscle (Styx, 1782)*; in the original Latin, *nervus pro musculo sartorio inferior*, p. 6.
26. *nerve to abductor brevis muscle of Albinus (Fischer, 1791)*
Macrodissected adult human ***muscular branch of femoral nerve (Quain & Wilson, 1839)***; in the original Latin, *nervus musuculi abductoris brevis Albini*, p. 6.
27. *inferior nerve for crural muscle (Fischer, 1791)*
Synonym for macrodissected adult human *long nerve to crural muscle (Styx, 1782)*; in the original Latin, *nervus pro musculo crurali inferior*, p. 6.
28. *superior nerve to vastus internus muscle (Fischer, 1791)*
Synonym for macrodissected adult human *short nerve to vastus internus muscle (Styx, 1782)*; in the original Latin, *nervus musculi vasti interni superior*, p. 6.

29. *inferior nerve to vastus internus muscle (Fischer, 1791)* Synonym for macrodissected adult human *long nerve to vastus internus muscle (Styx, 1782)*; in the original Latin, *nervus musculi vasti interni inferior*, p. 6.
30. *nerve to longissimi tibiae muscle (Fischer, 1791)* Macrodissected adult human ***muscular branch of femoral nerve (Quain & Wilson, 1839)*** to rectus femoris muscle, identified by Vieussens (1684) and named by Fischer; in the original Latin, *nervus musculi longissimi tibiae*, p. 6.
31. *nerve to gracilis antici muscle (Fischer, 1791)* Macrodissected adult human ***muscular branch of femoral nerve (Quain & Wilson, 1839)*** to rectus femoris muscle, identified by Vieussens (1684) and named by Fischer; in the original Latin, *nervus musculi gracilis antici*, p. 6.
32. *iliac plexus (Fischer, 1791)* In macrodissected adult human, ***plexus (Galen, c192)*** formed on surface of iliacus muscle by a ***muscular branch of femoral nerve (Quain & Wilson, 1839)***; in the original Latin, *plexum iliacum*, Table II, Figure 1-*105*.
33. *long nerve (Bell, 1803b)* Synonym for macrodissected adult human *long nerve to vastus internus muscle (Styx, 1782)*; Bell noted it is possible to regard ***saphenous nerve (Haase, 1781)*** as one of its branches, p. 199. See Hamilton (1976, Fig. 830B).
34. *first branch of anterior crural nerve to straight muscle of thigh (Swan, 1830)* Macrodissected adult human ***muscular branch of femoral nerve (Quain & Wilson, 1839)*** to rectus femoris muscle; Plate XXIV, Figure 1-*10*.
35. *second branch of anterior crural nerve to external vast and crural muscles (Swan, 1830)* Macrodissected adult human ***muscular branch of femoral nerve (Quain & Wilson, 1839)*** to vastus lateralis and vastus intermedius muscles; Plate XXIV, Figure 1-*11*.
36. *third branch of anterior crural nerve to crural and internal vast muscles (Swan, 1830)* Macrodissected adult human ***muscular branch of femoral nerve (Quain & Wilson, 1839)*** to vastus intermedius and vastus medialis muscles; Plate XXIV, Figure 1-*12*.
37. *fourth branch of anterior crural nerve to sartorius muscle (Swan, 1830)* Macrodissected adult human ***muscular branch of femoral nerve (Quain & Wilson, 1839)*** to sartorius muscle; Plate XXIV, Figure 1-*13*.
38. *eighth branch of anterior crural nerve to saphena vein (Swan, 1830)* Macrodissected adult human ***muscular branch of femoral nerve (Haller, 1762)*** to great saphenous vein; Plate XXIV, Figure 1-*21*.
39. *ninth branch of anterior crural nerve to pectineal muscle (Swan, 1830)* Macrodissected adult human ***muscular branch of femoral nerve (Quain & Wilson, 1839)*** to pectineus muscles; Plate XXIV, Figure 1-*22*.
40. *collateral branches of crural nerve (Cruveilhier, 1836)* Macrodissected adult human ***muscular branches of femoral nerve (Quain & Wilson, 1839)*** to iliopsoas muscles; in the original French, *rameaux collatéraux du nerf crural*, p. 841.
41. *iliacus branches of crural nerve (Cruveilhier, 1836)* Synonym for *collateral branches of crural nerve (Cruveilhier, 1836)*; in the original French, *rameaux iliaques*, p. 841.
42. *muscular branches of crural musculocutaneous nerve (Cruveilhier, 1836)* Macrodissected adult human ***muscular branches of femoral nerve (Quain & Wilson, 1839)*** to sartorius muscle (*muscle couturier*); in the original French, *branches musculaires*, p. 842.
43. *nerve of vastus externus (Cruveilhier, 1836)* Macrodissected adult human ***muscular branch of femoral nerve (Quain & Wilson, 1839)*** to vastus lateralis muscle; in the original French, *nerf du vaste externe*, p. 844.
44. *nerves of vastus internus (Cruveilhier, 1836)* Cruveilhier described two, *external nerve of vastus internus (Cruveilhier, 1836)* and *internal nerve of vastus internus (Cruveilhier, 1836)*; in the original French, *nerfs du vaste interne*, p. 845.
45. *external nerve of vastus internus (Cruveilhier, 1836)* Macrodissected adult human lateral ***muscular branch of femoral nerve (Quain & Wilson, 1839)*** to vastus medialis muscle; in the original French, *nerf externe du vaste interne*, p. 845.
46. *periosteal and articular filaments of external nerve of vastus internus (Cruveilhier, 1836)* In macrodissected adult human, various small branches of *external nerve of vastus internus (Cruveilhier, 1836)* to nearby bones and joints; in the original French, *filets périostiques et articulaires*, p. 845.
47. *internal nerve of vastus internus (Cruveilhier, 1836)* Macrodissected adult human medial ***muscular branch of femoral nerve (Quain & Wilson, 1839)*** to vastus medialis muscle; in the original French, *nerf interne du vaste interne*, p. 845.
48. *articular and periosteal filaments of internal nerve of vastus internus (Cruveilhier, 1836)* In macrodissected adult human, various small branches of *internal nerve of vastus internus (Cruveilhier, 1836)* to nearby joints and bones; in the original French, *filets articulaires et périostiques*, p. 845.

muscular branches of intercostal nerves (Quain & Wilson, 1839)

As described for macrodissected adult human, they supply primarily the intercostal and abdominal muscles; see Durward (1951, pp. 1084–1087). For Quain & Wilson's use in macrodissected adult human, see Plate XX, Figure 1-*e*. They were known to Galen; see ***[muscular branches of intercostal nerves (Quain & Wilson, 1839)] (Galen, c192)***.

EARLIER REFERENCES:

Described, not named or illustrated:

1. ***[muscular branches of intercostal nerves (Quain & Wilson, 1839)] (Galen, c192)***

Mentioned for macrodissected adult beef, pig, and/or macaque but not human; see Duckworth translation (1962, p. 258–259). Vesalius (1543a) described them for macrodissected adult human without naming the group; see Richardson & Carman translation (2002, p. 234).

Earlier synonyms:

1. *muscular branches of dorsal nerves (Cruveilhier, 1836)*
   Synonym for macrodissected adult human ***muscular branches of intercostal nerves (Quain & Wilson, 1839)***; in the original French, *rameaux musculaires*, p. 830.

muscular branches of lateral plantar nerve (>1840)

As described for macrodissected adult human, they arise from the trunk of the ***lateral plantar nerve (>1840)*** before it splits into ***superficial branch of lateral plantar nerve (>1840)*** and ***deep branch of lateral plantar nerve (>1840)***; they innervate the flexor digitorum accessorius (quadratus plantae) and abductor digiti minimi of foot muscles; see Durward (1951, p. 1112 and Fig. 951), Williams & Warwick (1980, p. 1114). They were probably first clearly delineated, at least partly, by Jördens; see *flexor digitorum brevis nerve from external plantar nerve (Jördens, 1788)*, *quadrate flesh nerve from external plantar nerve (Jördens, 1788)*.

EARLIER REFERENCES:

Earlier synonyms:

1. *collateral branches of external plantar nerve (Cruveilhier, 1836)*
   Synonym for macrodissected adult human ***muscular branches of lateral plantar nerve (>1840)***; in the original French, *branches collatérales*, p. 875.
2. *muscular branches of external plantar nerve (Quain & Wilson, 1839)*
   Synonym for macrodissected adult human ***muscular branches of lateral plantar nerve (>1840)***; Plate XXVI, Figure 1-*c*.

PARTLY CORRESPONDS:

1. *flexor digitorum brevis nerve from external plantar nerve (Jördens, 1788)*
   First of Jördens's macrodissected adult human ***muscular branches of lateral plantar nerve (>1840)***; in the original Latin, *nervus flexoris digitorum brevis ex nervus plantaris externus*, p. 12 and Table III-*211*.
2. *quadrate flesh nerve from external plantar nerve (Jördens, 1788)*
   Second of Jördens's macrodissected adult human ***muscular branches of medial plantar nerve (>1840)***, presumably to abductor digiti minimi of foot muscle and perhaps its environs; in the original Latin, *nervus carnis quadratae ex nervus plantaris externus*, p. 12 and Table III-*212*.
3. *third branch of external plantar nerve (Fischer, 1791)*
   Macrodissected adult human ***muscular branch of lateral plantar nerve (>1840)*** with branches supplying abductor digiti minimi of foot, flexor digiti minimi brevis, dorsal interosseus digiti quinti, and flexor digitorum accessorius (quadratus plantae) muscles; in the original Latin, *ramulus tertius*, p. 38.
4. *twig to abductor digiti minimi muscle from third branch of external plantar nerve (Fischer, 1791)*
   Macrodissected adult human ***muscular branch of lateral plantar nerve (>1840)*** from *third branch of external plantar nerve (Fischer, 1791)* to abductor digiti minimi of foot muscle; in the original Latin, *ramulus musculi abductoris digiti minimi*, p. 38.
5. *twig to flexor brevis and interosseus digiti quinti (Fischer, 1791)*
   Macrodissected adult human ***muscular branch of lateral plantar nerve (>1840)*** from *third branch of external plantar nerve (Fischer, 1791)* to flexor digiti minimi brevis of foot and dorsal interosseus digiti quinti muscles; in the original Latin, *ramulus flexoris brevis et interossei digiti quinti*, p. 38.
6. *twig to carne quadrata Sylvii (Fischer, 1791)*
   Macrodissected adult human ***muscular branch of lateral plantar nerve (>1840)*** from *third branch of external plantar nerve (Fischer, 1791)* to flexor digitorum accessorius (quadratus plantae) muscle; in the original Latin, *ramulus carnis quadratae Sylvii*, p. 38.
7. *transverse branch of abductor digiti minimi muscle of external plantar nerve (Cruveilhier, 1836)*
   Macrodissected adult human ***muscular branch of lateral plantar nerve (>1840)*** to abductor digiti minimi of foot muscle; in the original French, *rameau transverse du muscle abducteur du petit orteil*, p. 875.
8. *nerves of accessory muscle of common long flexor (Cruveilhier, 1836)*
   Macrodissected adult human ***muscular branches of lateral plantar nerve (>1840)*** to flexor digitorum accessorius (quadratus plantae) muscle; in the original French, *nerfs du muscle accessoire du long fléchisseur commun*, p. 875.

muscular branches of lumbar plexus ventral branches (>1840)

As described for macrodissected adult human, they supply the quadratus lumborum muscle from the 12th ***thoracic nerve (Diemerbroeck, 1672)***, and first 3–4 ***lumbar nerves (Diemerbroeck, 1672)***; the psoas minor muscle from the first ***lumbar nerve (Diemerbroeck, 1672)***; the psoas major muscle from the second, third, and sometimes fourth ***lumbar nerves (Diemerbroeck, 1672)***; and the iliacus muscle from the second and third ***lumbar nerves (Diemerbroeck, 1672)***; see Williams & Warwick (1980, p. 1106). They were perhaps first clearly described by Meckel; see ***[muscular branches of lumbar plexus ventral branches (>1840)] (Meckel, 1817)***.

EARLIER REFERENCES:

Described, not named or illustrated:

1. ***[muscular branches of lumbar plexus ventral branches (>1840)] (Meckel, 1817)***
   All major branches recognized today described, without naming as group, for macrodissected adult human; see translation (1832, Vol. 3, pp. 13–14).

PARTLY CORRESPONDS:

1. *recurrent nerve of psoas magnus muscle (Fischer, 1791)*
   Macrodissected adult human ***muscular branch of lumbar plexus ventral branches (>1840)*** to psoas major muscle; in the original Latin, *nervus musculi psoae recurrens*, Table II, Figure 1-*106*. Cloquet (1828, Tab. CLXXIII, Fig. 1-42) referred simply to *recurrent nerve of psoas muscle (N. récurrent du M. psoas)*.

muscular branches of medial plantar nerve (>1840)

As described for macrodissected adult human, they arise from proximal regions of the trunk of the ***medial plantar nerve (>1840)*** and supply the abductor hallucis, flexor hallucis brevis, and flexor digitorum brevis muscles; see Durward (1951, Fig. 951), Williams & Warwick (1980, p. 1114). They were first identified as the *muscular nerves of collateral branches of internal plantar nerve (Cruveilhier, 1836)*.

EARLIER REFERENCES:

Earlier synonyms:

1. *muscular nerves of collateral branches of internal plantar nerve (Cruveilhier, 1836)*
   Synonym for macrodissected adult human ***muscular branches of medial plantar nerve (>1840)***; in the original French, *nerfs musculaires*, p. 872.
2. *muscular branches of internal plantar nerve (Quain & Wilson, 1839)*
   Synonym for macrodissected adult human ***muscular branches of medial plantar nerve (>1840)***; Plate XXVI, Figure 1-*a*.

PARTLY CORRESPONDS:

1. *nerve to abductor pollicis muscle (Jördens, 1788)*
   Macrodissected adult human ***muscular branch of medial plantar nerve (>1840)*** to abductor hallucis muscle; in the original Latin, *nervus musculi abductoris pollicis*, p. 10 and Table III-*182*. Jördens had it arising just proximal to, or near, origin of ***medial plantar nerve (>1840)***.
2. *twig to flexor digitorum brevis muscle (Jördens, 1788)*
   Macrodissected adult human ***muscular branch of medial plantar nerve (>1840)***; in the original Latin, *surculus ad musculum flexorem digitorum brevem*, p. 11 and Table III-*184*.
3. *nerve of flexor hallucis brevis muscle (Cruveilhier, 1836)*
   Macrodissected adult human ***muscular branch of medial plantar nerve (>1840)***; in the original French, *nerf du muscle court fléchisseur du gros orteil*, p. 872.
4. *nerve of common flexor digitorum brevis muscle (Cruveilhier, 1836)*
   Macrodissected adult human ***muscular branch of medial plantar nerve (>1840)*** to flexor digitorum brevis muscle; in the original French, *nerf du muscle court fléchisseur commun des orteils*, p. 872.

muscular branches of median nerve (Martin, 1781)

As described for macrodissected adult human, branches of the ***median nerve (Du Verney, 1697)*** supplying superficial flexor forearm muscles: pronator teres, flexor carpi radialis, palmaris longus, and flexor digitorum superficialis. For Martin's use in macrodissected human see p. 213. They were known to Galen; see ***[muscular branches of median nerve (Martin, 1781)] (Galen, c177)***.

EARLIER REFERENCES:

Described, not named or illustrated:

1. ***[muscular branches of median nerve (Martin, 1781)] (Galen, c177)***
   Branches described to flexor carpi radialis, flexor digitorum superficialis, pronator teres, palmaris longus, and pronator quadratus muscles in macrodissected adult beef, pig, and/or macaque but not human; see Singer translation (1999, pp. 71, 73). Vesalius (1543a) described branches to abductor pollicis brevis, first dorsal interosseous, flexor pollicis brevis, opponens pollicis, abductor pollicis, lumbrical, interossei, flexor digitorum superficialis, and flexor carpi radialis muscles in macrodissected adult human; see Richardson & Carman translation (2002, pp. 243–244).

PARTLY CORRESPONDS:

1. *internal interosseous plexus (Caldani, 1813, 1814)*
   Basically, macrodissected adult human differentiation in forearm of ***muscular branches of median nerve (Martin, 1781)***; in the original Latin, *plexus interosseus internus*, Table CCLIX, Figure 1-*20*.
2. *branch of median nerve to origin of round pronator muscle of radius and radial flexor of wrist (Swan, 1830)*
   Macrodissected adult human ***muscular branch of median nerve (Martin, 1781)*** to pronator teres and flexor carpi radialis muscles; Plate XXII, Figure 2-2.
3. *branch of median nerve to round pronator muscle of radius (Swan, 1830)*
   Macrodissected adult human ***muscular branch of median nerve (Martin, 1781)*** to pronator teres muscle; Plate XXII, Figure 2-3.
4. *branches of median nerve to radial flexor muscle of wrist (Swan, 1830)*
   Macrodissected adult human ***muscular branches of median nerve (Martin, 1781)*** to flexor carpi radialis muscle; Plate XXII, Figure 2-4,5.
5. *branches of median nerve to sublime flexor muscle of fingers (Swan, 1830)*
   Macrodissected adult human ***muscular branches of median nerve (Martin, 1781)*** to flexor digitorum superficialis muscle; Plate XXII, Figure 2-6,9.
6. *branch of median nerve to abductor and opponent muscles of thumb (Swan, 1830)*
   Macrodissected adult human ***muscular branch of median nerve (Martin, 1781)*** to abductor pollicis brevis and opponens pollicis muscles; Plate XXII, Figure 2-*11*. Sometimes known today as *recurrent branch of median nerve*.
7. *branch of median nerve to short flexor muscle of thumb (Swan, 1830)*
   Macrodissected adult human ***muscular branch of median nerve (Martin, 1781)*** to flexor pollicis brevis muscle; Plate XXIII, Figure 3-3.
8. *branches of median nerve to lumbrical muscles (Swan, 1830)*

Macrodissected adult human ***muscular branches of median nerve (Martin, 1781)*** to first three lumbrical muscles of hand; Plate XXIII, Figure 3-5.

9. *pronator teres branch of median nerve (Cruveilhier, 1836)*
   Macrodissected adult human ***muscular branch of median nerve (Martin, 1781)*** to pronator teres muscle; in the original French, *rameau du rond pronateur*, p. 804.
10. *articular filaments of elbow from pronator teres branch of median nerve (Cruveilhier, 1836)*
   Macrodissected adult human small branches of *pronator teres branch of median nerve (Cruveilhier, 1836)* to elbow-joint; in the original French, *filets articulaires du coude*, p. 805.
11. *branch of median nerve to muscles of superficial layer (Cruveilhier, 1836)*
   Macrodissected adult human ***muscular branch of median nerve (Martin, 1781)*** to pronator teres (*rond pronateur*), flexor carpi radialis (*radial antérieur*), palmaris longus (*palmaire grêle*), and flexor digitorum superficialis (*flechisseur sublime*) muscles; in the original French, *branche des muscles de la couche superficielle*, p. 805. Also see Todd (1839, Vol. 2, p. 366).

muscular branches of musculocutaneous nerve (Günther, 1786)

As described for macrodissected adult human, they typically innervate the coracobrachialis, both heads of the biceps, and most of the brachialis muscles; see Williams & Warwick (1980, p. 1097). For Günther's listing of macrodissected adult human branches, see p. 73. They were known to Galen; see ***[muscular branches of musculocutaneous nerve (Günther, 1786)] (Galen, c177)***.

TRANSLATIONS:

1. *nervus musculo-cutaneus ramus musculoris (Soemmerring, 1798)*
   Original Latin form (singular) of ***muscular branches of musculocutaneous nerve (Günther, 1786)***; p. 73.

EARLIER REFERENCES:

Described, not named or illustrated:

1. ***[muscular branches of musculocutaneous nerve (Günther, 1786)] (Galen, c177)***
   Relationships with both heads of biceps and brachialis muscles described for macrodissected adult beef, pig, and/or macaque but not human; see Singer translation (1999, p. 68). Vesalius (1543a) described branches to both heads of biceps and brachialis muscles in macrodissected adult human; see Richardson & Carman translation (2002, p. 239).

Earlier synonyms:

1. *nervus perforans (Cheselden, 1713)*
   Probably refers to macrodissected adult human ***muscular branches of musculocutaneous nerve (Günther, 1786)***; p. 143, also see Cheselden (1722, p. 209), Quain & Wilson (1839, Pl. XVII-*m*).

LATER SYNONYMS:

1. *deep branch of musculocutaneous nerve (Soemmerring, 1791)*
   Synonym for macrodissected adult human ***muscular branches of musculocutaneous nerve (Günther, 1786)***; pp. 280–281.
2. *deep branch of external cutaneous nerve (Soemmerring, 1791)*
   Synonym for macrodissected adult human ***muscular branches of musculocutaneous nerve (Günther, 1786)***; pp. 280–281.
3. *muscular branch of external cutaneous nerve (Soemmerring, 1791)*
   Synonym for macrodissected adult human ***muscular branches of musculocutaneous nerve (Günther, 1786)***; pp. 280–281.
4. *internal branch of external cutaneous nerve of arm (Cloquet, 1816)*
   Synonym for macrodissected adult human ***muscular branches of musculocutaneous nerve (Günther, 1786)***; p. 647.

PARTLY CORRESPONDS:

1. *perforans nerve (Cheselden, 1722)*
   In vaguely worded and unillustrated account of macrodissected adult human ***nerves (Herophilus, c335–c280 BC)***, *perforans nerve (Cheselden, 1722)* to coracobrachialis muscle mentioned as branch of *axillary nerve (Cheselden, 1722)*; p. 209. Perhaps synonym for *coracobrachialis muscle branch of musculocutaneous nerve (Scarpa, 1794)*. Monro (1732) claimed in his Note to the Reader that he provided account of ***nerves (Herophilus, c335–c280 BC)*** in Cheselden (1722).
2. *coracobrachialis muscle branch of musculocutaneous nerve (Scarpa, 1794)*
   Macrodissected adult human ***muscular branch of musculocutaneous nerve (Günther, 1786)***; in the original Latin, *nervi musculo-cutanei ramus coraco-brachiali musculo traditus*, Table III-*176*. Cruveilhier (1836, p. 800) described for macrodissected adult human two such branches, superior and inferior.
3. *musculocutaneous nerve twigs for subscapularis muscle (Caldani, 1813, 1814)*
   Macrodissected adult human ***muscular branches of musculocutaneous nerve (Günther, 1786)*** to subscapularis muscle; in the original Latin, *nervus musculo-cutaneus surculi pro musculo subscapulari*, Table CCLVIII, Figure 1-*21*.
4. *musculocutaneous nerve branches for pectoral muscle (Caldani, 1813, 1814)*
   Macrodissected adult human ***muscular branches of musculocutaneous nerve (Günther, 1786)*** to rostral (upper) intercostal muscles and serratus anterior muscle; in the original Latin, *nervus musculo-cutaneus rami per musculum pectoralem*, Table CCLVIII, Figure 1-*22*.
5. *branch of musculocutaneous nerve to biceps muscle (Langenbeck, 1826–1830)*
   Macrodissected adult human ***muscular branch of musculocutaneous nerve (Günther, 1786)*** to biceps brachii muscle; in the original Latin, *ramus nervi musculocutanei ad musculum bicipitem*, Fascicle III, Table XIII-*10*.

6. *branch of musculocutaneous nerve to internal brachial muscle (Langenbeck, 1826–1830)*
   Macrodissected adult human ***muscular branch of musculocutaneous nerve (Günther, 1786)*** to brachialis muscle; in the original Latin, *ramus nervi musculocutanei ad musculum brachialem internum*, Fascicle III, Table XIII-*11*.
7. *biceps branches of musculocutaneous nerve (Cruveilhier, 1836)*
   Multiple macrodissected adult human ***muscular branches of musculocutaneous nerve (Günther, 1786)*** to biceps brachii muscle; in the original French, *rameaux du biceps*, p. 800.
8. *articular branch of biceps branches of musculocutaneous nerve (Cruveilhier, 1836)*
   Macrodissected adult human branch of *biceps branches of musculocutaneous nerve (Cruveilhier, 1836)* to elbow joint; in the original French, *rameau articulaire*, p. 800.
9. *anterior brachial branches of musculocutaneous nerve (Cruveilhier, 1836)*
   Macrodissected adult human ***muscular branches of musculocutaneous nerve (Günther, 1786)*** to biceps brachii and brachialis muscles; in the original French, *rameaux du brachial antérieur*, p. 800.
10. *branch of musculocutaneous nerve to short head of biceps muscle (Quain & Wilson, 1839)*
   Macrodissected adult human ***muscular branch of musculocutaneous nerve (Günther, 1786)*** to short head of biceps brachii muscle; Plate XVII-*m*.
11. *branch of musculocutaneous nerve to brachialis anticus muscle (Quain & Wilson, 1839)*
   Macrodissected adult human ***muscular branch of musculocutaneous nerve (Günther, 1786)*** to brachialis muscle; Plate XVII-*p*.

muscular branches of perineal nerve (>1840)

As described for macrodissected adult human, they supply the transversus perinei superficialis, bulbospongiosus, ischiocavernosus, transversus perinei profundus, sphincter urethrae and ventral (anterior) parts of the external sphincter and levator ani muscles; see Durward (1951, Figs. 943, 944), Williams & Warwick (1980, p. 1116), *Terminologia Anatomica* (1998, p. 140). They were known to Galen; see ***[muscular branches of perineal nerve (>1840)] (Galen, c192)***.

EARLIER REFERENCES:

Described, not named or illustrated:

1. ***[muscular branches of perineal nerve (>1840)] (Galen, c192)***
   Galen mentioned ***nerve (Herophilus, c335–c280 BC)*** to muscles of genital organs and related viscera; see Duckworth translation (1962, p. 263). Vesalius (1543a) described ***nerve (Herophilus, c335–c280 BC)*** branch to ischiocavernosus muscle in macrodissected adult human but ascribed it to *third nerve entering leg (Vesalius, 1543a)*; see Richardson & Carman translation (2002, p. 258). Meckel (1817) described for macrodissected adult human just branch to bulbospongiosus, which he called bulbocavernosus muscle; see translation (1832, Vol. 3, p. 15).

PARTLY CORRESPONDS:

1. *superior branch of perineal branch of internal pudendal nerve (Cruveilhier, 1836)*
   Macrodissected adult human ***muscular branch of perineal nerve (>1840)*** to bulbospongiosus muscle; in the original French, *rameau supérieur*, p. 853.
2. *bulbo-urethral branch of perineal branch of internal pudendal nerve (Cruveilhier, 1836)*
   Synonym for *superior branch of perineal branch of internal pudendal nerve (Cruveilhier, 1836)*; in the original French, *rameau bulbo-urétral*, pp. 853, 854.

muscular branches of posterior branch of obturator nerve (>1840)

As described for macrodissected adult human, they supply the obturator externus and adductor magnus muscles, and the adductor brevis muscle when it does not receive a branch from the ***anterior branch of obturator nerve (Haase, 1781; Martin, 1781)***; see Durward (1951, Fig. 939), Williams & Warwick (1980, p. 1108), *Terminologia Anatomica* (1998, p. 140). They were known to Galen; see ***[muscular branches of posterior branch of obturator nerve (>1840)] (Galen, c177)***.

EARLIER REFERENCES:

Described, not named or illustrated:

1. ***[muscular branches of posterior branch of obturator nerve (>1840)] (Galen, c177)***
   Galen described major branches to adductor magnus and adductor brevis muscles in macrodissected adult beef, pig, and/or macaque but not human; see Singer translation (1999, p. 85). Vesalius (1543a) described in macrodissected adult human branches to adductor magnus and obturator externus muscles without clearly describing posterior branch itself; see Richardson & Carman translation (2002, p. 258). Eustachi (1552) clearly illustrated them for macrodissected adult human; see Albinus edition (1761, Tab. 19-3,4).

PARTLY CORRESPONDS:

1. *nerve of obturator externus (Cruveilhier, 1836)*
   Macrodissected adult human ***muscular branch of posterior branch of obturator nerve (>1840)*** to obturator externus muscle; in the original French, *nerf de l'obturateur externe*, p. 839.

muscular branches of radial nerve (>1840)

As described for macrodissected adult human, they mainly supply the triceps, anconeus, brachioradialis, extensor carpi radialis longus, and brachialis muscles; see Williams & Warwick (1980, p. 1101), *Terminologia Anatomica* (1998, p. 138). At least one was known to Galen; see ***[muscular branches of radial nerve (>1840)] (Galen, c177)***.

EARLIER REFERENCES:

Described, not named or illustrated:

1. ***[muscular branches of radial nerve (>1840)] (Galen, c177)***
Galen described branch to triceps muscle in macrodissected adult beef, pig, and/or macaque but not human; see Singer translation (1999, p. 68). Vesalius (1543a) described without naming as a group branches to triceps, brachioradialis, and extensor carpi radialis muscles in macrodissected adult human; see Richardson & Carman translation (2002, pp. 241–242).

Earlier synonyms:

1. *muscular branches of spiral nerve (Quain & Wilson, 1839)*
Synonym for macrodissected adult human ***muscular branches of radial nerve (>1840)***; p. 43.

PARTLY CORRESPONDS:

1. *supinator longus muscle branch of radial nerve (Bock, 1827)*
Macrodissected adult human ***muscular branch of radial nerve (>1840)*** to brachioradialis muscle; in the original Latin, *ramus musculi supinatoris longi*, Table II-56.
2. *branches of radial nerve to anterior brachial muscle (Cloquet, 1828)*
Macrodissected adult human ***muscular branch of radial nerve (>1840)*** to brachialis muscle; in the original French, *rameaux du nerf radial allant au M. brachial antérieur*, Plate CLXVIII, Fig 2-81.
3. *branch of spiral nerve to internal brachial muscle (Swan, 1830)*
Macrodissected adult human ***muscular branch of radial nerve (>1840)*** to brachialis muscle; Plate XXII, Figure 2-34.
4. *branch of spiral nerve to long supinator muscle of radius and longer radial extensor of wrist (Swan, 1830)*
Macrodissected adult human ***muscular branch of radial nerve (>1840)*** to brachioradialis and extensor carpi radialis longus muscles; Plate XXII, Figure 2-35.
5. *branch of spiral nerve to long supinator muscle of radius (Swan, 1830)*
Macrodissected adult human ***muscular branch of radial nerve (>1840)*** to brachioradialis muscle; Plate XXII, Figure 2-36.
6. *branches to long portion of triceps of radial nerve (Cruveilhier, 1836)*
Macrodissected adult human ***muscular branches of radial nerve (>1840)*** to long head of triceps brachii muscle; in the original French, *rameaux à la longue portion du triceps*, p. 816.
7. *branch to vastus internus of radial nerve (Cruveilhier, 1836)*
Macrodissected adult human ***muscular branch of radial nerve (>1840)*** to medial head of triceps brachii muscle; in the original French, *rameau au vaste interne*, p. 816.
8. *branch of vastus externus and anconeus muscles of radial nerve (Cruveilhier, 1836)*
Macrodissected adult human ***muscular branch of radial nerve (>1840)*** to lateral head of triceps brachii and anconeus muscles; in the original French, *rameau du vaste externe et de l'anconé*, p. 816.
9. *branch of long supinator of radial nerve (Cruveilhier, 1836)*
Macrodissected adult human ***muscular branch of radial nerve (>1840)*** to brachioradialis muscle; in the original French, *rameau du long supinateur*, p. 816.
10. *branch of first external radial muscle of radial nerve (Cruveilhier, 1836)*
Macrodissected adult human ***muscular branch of radial nerve (>1840)*** to extensor carpi radialis longus muscle; in the original French, *rameau du premier radial externe*, p. 816.

muscular branches of superficial fibular nerve (>1840)

As described for macrodissected adult human, they supply the fibularis longus and fibularis brevis muscles, and skin of the distal (lower) part of the leg; see Williams & Warwick (1980, p. 1115), *Terminologia Anatomica* (1998, p. 140). They were known to Vesalius; see ***[muscular branches of superficial fibular nerve (>1840)] (Vesalius, 1543a)***.

EARLIER REFERENCES:

Described, not named or illustrated:

1. ***[muscular branches of superficial fibular nerve (>1840)] (Vesalius, 1543a)***
Alluded to for macrodissected adult human; see Richardson & Carman translation (2002, p. 260). Jördens (1788, pp. 5, 14) described and illustrated them clearly for macrodissected adult human.

Earlier synonyms:

1. *collateral branches of musculocutaneous branch of external popliteal sciatic nerve (Cruveilhier, 1836)*
Synonym for macrodissected adult human ***muscular branches of superficial fibular nerve (>1840)***; in the original French, *rameaux collatéraux*, p. 865.
2. *muscular branches of musculo-cutaneous nerve (Quain & Wilson, 1839)*
Synonym for macrodissected adult human ***muscular branches of superficial fibular nerve (>1840)***; Plate XXIV, Figure 2-*B,a*.

PARTLY CORRESPONDS:

1. *common trunk for nerves to extensor pollicis longus and anterior peroneal muscles (Fischer, 1791)*
Trunk for several macrodissected adult human ***muscular branches of superficial fibular nerve (>1840)***; in the original Latin, *trunculum communem nervi musculi extensoris pollicis longi et peronei antici*, p. 31.
2. *nerve to extensor pollicis longus muscle (Fischer, 1791)*
Branch of *common trunk for nerves to extensor pollicis longus and anterior peroneal muscles (Fischer, 1791)* to extensor hallucis longus muscle; p. 31.
3. *nerve to anterior peroneal muscle (Fischer, 1791)*
Branch of *common trunk for nerves to extensor pollicis longus and anterior peroneal muscles (Fischer, 1791)* to fibularis tertius muscle; p. 31.
4. *branches of peroneal nerve to long peroneal muscle (Swan, 1830)*

Macrodissected adult human ***muscular branches of superficial fibular nerve (>1840)*** to fibularis longus muscle; Plate XXIII, Figure 4-*9*.

5. *branch of dorsal branch of peroneal nerve to middle peroneal muscle (Swan, 1830)*
   Macrodissected adult human ***muscular branch of superficial fibular nerve (>1840)*** to fibularis brevis muscle; Plate XXIII, Figure 4-*10*.
6. *branches of lateral peroneus longus of musculocutaneous branch of external popliteal sciatic nerve (Cruveilhier, 1836)*
   For macrodissected adult human, two ***muscular branches of superficial fibular nerve (>1840)*** to fibularis longus muscle; in the original French, *rameaux du long péronier latéral*, p. 865.
7. *branch of lateral peroneus brevis of musculocutaneous branch of external popliteal sciatic nerve (Cruveilhier, 1836)*
   Macrodissected adult human ***muscular branch of superficial fibular nerve (>1840)*** to fibularis brevis muscle; in the original French, *rameaux du court péronier latéral*, p. 865.
8. *external maleolar filament of musculocutaneous branch of external popliteal sciatic nerve (Cruveilhier, 1836)*
   Macrodissected adult human cutaneous branch of ***muscular branches of superficial fibular nerve (>1840)*** to skin associated with lateral maleolus; in the original French, *filet mallèolaire externe*, p. 865.

muscular branches of tibial nerve (>1840)

As described for macrodissected adult human, they include the ***nerve to plantaris (>1840)***, ***nerves to gastrocnemius (>1840)***, ***nerve to popliteus (>1840)***, ***nerve to soleus (>1840)***, ***nerve to flexor digitorum longus (>1840)***, and ***nerve to flexor hallucis longus (>1840)***; see Durward (1951, pp. 1109–1110). The gastrocnemius and soleus muscles are sometimes considered together as the triceps surae muscle. The ***nerve to hamstring muscles (>1840)*** is described under ***sciatic nerve (Keill, 1698)***. They were known to Galen; see ***[muscular branches of tibial nerve (>1840)] (Galen, c177)***.

EARLIER REFERENCES:

Described, not named or illustrated:

1. ***[muscular branches of tibial nerve (>1840)] (Galen, c177)***
   Alluded to in macrodissected adult beef, pig, and/or macaque but not human; see Singer translation (1999, p. 86). Vesalius (1543a) described and illustrated most of them (without naming the group) for macrodissected adult human; see Richardson & Carman translation (2002, p. 259). Meckel (1817) described all of them without naming the group; see translation (1832, Vol. 3, pp. 17, 20).

PARTLY CORRESPONDS:

1. *common nerve to gastrocnemius and plantaris muscles (Fischer, 1791)*
   Macrodissected adult human ***muscular branch of tibial nerve (>1840)*** generating branches to the two named muscles; in the original Latin, *nervus communis musculi gastrocnemii et plantaris*, p. 33.
2. *common nerve to left head of gastrocnemius muscle, soleus muscle, and tibial communicating nerve (Fischer, 1791)*
   Macrodissected adult human ***muscular branch of tibial nerve (>1840)*** generating branches to the two named muscles, and to the *tibial communicating nerve (Jördens, 1788)*; in the original Latin, *[nervus] communis capiti sinistro musculi gastrocnemii, musculo soleo, et nervo communicanti tibieo*, p. 34.
3. *nerve trunk to soleus and popliteus muscles and right head of gastrocnemius muscle (Fischer, 1791)*
   Macrodissected adult human ***muscular branch of tibial nerve (>1840)*** generating branches to the three named muscles; in the original Latin, *truncus nervi musculi solei, poplitei et dextri capitis musculi gastrocnemii*, p. 34.
4. *common nerve to popliteus muscle and interosseous ligament (Fischer, 1791)*
   Macrodissected adult human ***muscular branch of tibial nerve (>1840)*** generating two branches, to popliteus muscle and to interosseous membrane of leg—the ***interosseal nerve of leg (>1840)***; in the original Latin, *nervum communem musculi poplitei et ligamenti interossei*, p. 34.
5. *common nerve to soleus and flexor longus of big toe muscles (Fischer, 1791)*
   Macrodissected adult human ***muscular branch of tibial nerve (>1840)*** generating two branches, to soleus and flexor hallucis longus muscles; in the original Latin, *nervus communis musculi solei et flexoris pollicis pedis longi*, p. 35 and Table III, Figure 2-*446*. Fischer also called it a common branch (Tab. IV-*446*).
6. *common nerve to tibialis posterior, flexor digitorum longus, and flexor longus of big toe muscles and first internal inferior posterior cutaneous nerve (Fischer, 1791)*
   Macrodissected adult human ***muscular branch of tibial nerve (>1840)*** generating branches to tibialis posterior, flexor digitorum longus, and flexor hallucis longus muscles, and to *tibial communicating nerve (Jördens, 1788)*; in the original Latin, *nervum communem musculi tibialis postici, flexoris longi digitorum, flexoris longi pollicis et nervi cutanei posterioris inferioris interni primi*, p. 35.
7. *trunk for nerves to soleus muscle, popliteal muscle and gastrocnemius muscle (Fischer, 1791)*
   Synonym for *nerve trunk to soleus and popliteus muscles and right head of gastocnemius muscle (Fischer, 1791)*; Table III, Figure 2-*425*.
8. *common nerve for soleus, popliteus, and gastrocnemius muscles (Fischer, 1791)*
   Macrodissected adult human ***muscular branch of tibial nerve (>1840)*** generating branches to three muscles named; in the original Latin, *nervus communis pro musculo soleo, popliteo et gastrocnemio*, Table IV, Figure 2-*425*.
9. *nerve for soleus muscle and flexor pollicis pedis longus (Fischer, 1791)*
   Synonym for *common nerve to soleus and flexor longus of big toe muscles (Fischer, 1791)*; in the original Latin, *nervus pro musculo soleo et flexore pollicis pedis longo*, Table III, Figure 2-*446*.

10. *proper branch for soleus and flexor longus of big toe muscles (Fischer, 1791)*
    Synonym for *common nerve to soleus and flexor longus of big toe muscles (Fischer, 1791)*; in the original Latin, *ramus proprio pro musculo soleo et flexore pollicis pedis longo*, Table IV, Figure 2-*446*.
11. *trunk of nerve for soleus, popliteal and gastrocnemii muscles (Knox, 1832)*
    Synonym for macrodissected adult human *trunk for nerves to soleus muscle, popliteal muscle and gastrocnemius muscle (Fischer, 1791)*; Plate XVI-*425*.
12. *nerve of soleus muscle and flexor longus pollicis pedis (Knox, 1832)*
    Synonym for macrodissected adult human *nerve for soleus muscle and flexor pollicis pedis longus (Fischer, 1791)*; Plate XVI-*446*.
13. *muscular branches of popliteal nerve (Quain & Wilson, 1839)*
    Macrodissected adult human muscular branches of *popliteal nerve (Quain & Wilson, 1839)*; Plate XXV, Figure 2-*a*.
14. *muscular branches of posterior tibial nerve (Quain & Wilson, 1839)*
    Macrodissected adult human muscular branches of *posterior tibial nerve (Quain, 1828)*; Plate XXV, Figure 2-*c*.

muscular branches of ulnar nerve (Quain & Wilson, 1839)

As described for macrodissected adult human, they supply the flexor carpi ulnaris and medial half of the flexor digitorum profundus muscles; see Williams & Warwick (1980, p. 1100), *Terminologia Anatomica* (1998, p. 138). For Quain & Wilson's use in macrodissected adult human see Plate XVIII, Figure 2-*m*. They were known to Galen; see ***[muscular branches of ulnar nerve (Quain & Wilson, 1839)] (Galen, c177)***.

EARLIER REFERENCES:

Described, not named or illustrated:

1. ***[muscular branches of ulnar nerve (Quain & Wilson, 1839)] (Galen, c177)***
   Branches described to flexor carpi ulnaris and flexor digitorum profundus muscles for macrodissected adult beef, pig, and/or macaque but not human; see Singer translation (1999, p. 73). Vesalius (1543a) described branches to flexor carpi radialis, palmaris longus, flexor carpi ulnaris, and pronator teres muscles in macrodissected adult human; see Richardson & Carman translation (2002, pp. 243–244).

Earlier synonyms:

1. *muscular branches of cubital nerve (Cruveilhier, 1836)*
   Synonym for macrodissected adult human ***muscular branches of ulnar nerve (Quain & Wilson, 1839)***; in the original French, *branches musculaires*, p. 814.

PARTLY CORRESPONDS:

1. *branches of ulnar nerve to ulnar flexor muscle of wrist (Swan, 1830)*
   Macrodissected adult human ***muscular branches of ulnar nerve (Quain & Wilson, 1839)*** to flexor carpi ulnaris muscle; Plate XXII, Figure 2-*19,20*.
2. *branch of ulnar nerve to deep flexor muscle of fingers (Swan, 1830)*
   Macrodissected adult human ***muscular branch of ulnar nerve (Quain & Wilson, 1839)*** to flexor digitorum profundus muscle; Plate XXII-*21*.
3. *cubital nerve branches of anterior cubital muscle (Cruveilhier, 1836)*
   Macrodissected adult human ***muscular branches of ulnar nerve (Quain & Wilson, 1839)*** to flexor carpi ulnaris muscle; in the original French, *rameaux du cubital antérieur*, p. 811.
4. *cubital nerve branch of deep flexor muscle (Cruveilhier, 1836)*
   Macrodissected adult human ***muscular branch of ulnar nerve (Quain & Wilson, 1839)*** to flexor digitorum profundus muscle; in the original French, *rameau du fléchisseur profond*, p. 811.
5. *muscular branches of ulnar nerve to triceps muscle (Quain & Wilson, 1839)*
   Macrodissected adult human ***muscular branches of ulnar nerve (Quain & Wilson, 1839)*** to triceps muscle; Plate XVII-*v*.

musculocutaneous nerve (Du Verney, 1697)

As described in macrodissected adult human, a branch of the ***brachial plexus lateral cord (Schwalbe, 1881)*** generating distally ***muscular branches of musculocutaneous nerve (Günther, 1786)*** and the ***lateral cutaneous nerve of forearm (>1840)***; see Durward (1951, Fig. 923), Williams & Warwick (1980, p. 1097). According to Winslow (1733, Sect. VI, p. 79), his mentor Du Verney gave it this name in 1697 for macrodissected adult human. It was described originally as the *first nerve from spine to upper arm (Galen, c177)*.

TRANSLATIONS:

1. *nervus musculo-cutaneus (Du Verney, 1697)*
   Original Latin form of ***musculocutaneous nerve (Du Verney, 1697)***; see Winslow (1733, Sect. VI, p. 79).

EARLIER REFERENCES:

Earlier synonyms:

1. *first nerve from spine to upper arm (Galen, c177)*
   Synonym for ***musculocutaneous nerve (Du Verney, 1697)*** in macrodissected adult beef, pig, and/or macaque but not human; see Singer translation (1999, p. 68).
2. *second nerve entering arm (Vesalius, 1543a)*
   Synonym for macrodissected adult human ***musculocutaneous nerve (Du Verney, 1697)***; see Richardson & Carman translation (2002, p. 239). In a figure legend, Vesalius wrote, "In my excessive devotion to Galen I have depicted it thinner than it should be, but it is correct in the figure sewn in at the end of this book." (Richardson & Carman translation, 2002, p. 212).
3. *second sinew going to arm (Geminus, 1553)*
   Synonym for macrodissected adult human *second nerve entering arm (Vesalius, 1543a)*; originally spelled *seconde synnowe goynge to arme*, see *The table of the figures of sinowes*.
4. *second nerve of hand (Bauhin, 1605)*

Synonym for macrodissected adult human *second nerve entering arm (Vesalius, 1543a)*; see Crooke translation (1615, p. 901).

LATER SYNONYMS:

1. *external cutaneous nerve (Du Verney, 1697)*
According to Winslow (1733, Sect. VI, p. 79), his mentor Du Verney used this synonym for ***musculocutaneous nerve (Du Verney, 1697)***; in Latin, *nervus cutaneus externus*.
2. *axillary nerve (Cheselden, 1722)*
Brief, rather obscure account (p. 209) of ***nerves (Herophilus, c335–c280 BC)*** stated that *axillary nerve (Cheselden, 1722)* has large perforans branch to coracobrachialis muscle—apparently making *axillary nerve (Cheselden, 1722)* synonym for ***musculocutaneous nerve (Du Verney, 1697)***, which has ***muscular branch of musculocutaneous nerve (Günther, 1786)*** to coracobrachialis muscle. Monro *primus* (1732) claimed in his Note to the Reader that he provided the account of the ***nerves (Herophilus, c335–c280 BC)*** in Cheselden (1722).
3. *nervus perforans Casserii (Cheselden, 1726)*
Listed as eponym for ***musculocutaneous nerve (Du Verney, 1697)*** in chapter essentially written by Monro *primus* as stated in Preface; p. 265, also see Monro (1732, p. 27). Translation, *perforating nerve of Casseri*, in Meckel (1832, Vol. 3, p. 26).
4. *first great brachial nerve (Albinus, 1744)*
Probably synonym for macrodissected adult human ***musculocutaneous nerve (Du Verney, 1697)*** in annotated Eustachian plates; in the original Latin, *nervorum brachium magni primus*, Table 19-28.
5. *cutaneus externus et radialis (Klint, 1784)*
Synonym for macrodissected adult human ***musculocutaneous nerve (Du Verney, 1697)***. Ascribed to Wrisberg without citation by Klint (1784, p. 3). Günther (1786, p. 73) also listed it as synonym.
6. *musculocutaneous nerve of arm (Mayer, 1794)*
Synonym for macrodissected adult human ***musculocutaneous nerve (Du Verney, 1697)***; in the original Latin, *nervus musculo-cutaneus brachii;* Part 5, Table V, Figure 1-*F* (p. 25).
6. *radio-cutaneous nerve (Burdin, 1803)*
Synonym for macrodissected adult human ***musculocutaneous nerve (Du Verney, 1697)***; see translation (1803, Vol. 1, p. 191).
7. *external cutaneous nerve of arm (Cloquet, 1816)*
Synonym for macrodissected adult human ***musculocutaneous nerve (Du Verney, 1697)***; in the original French, *nerf brachial cutané externe*, p. 646.
8. *perforans of Casser (Knox, 1832)*
Eponym for macrodissected adult human *nervus perforans Casserii (Cheselden, 1726)*; Plate III-210*i*.

mylohyoid nerve (Meckel, 1748)

As described for macrodissected adult human, branch of the ***inferior dental nerve (Meckel, 1817)*** supplying the inferior surface of the mylohyoid muscle and anterior belly of the digastric muscle; see Williams & Warwick (1980, p. 1067, Fig. 7.177). For Meckel's clear description in macrodissected adult human, see p. 88. It was known to Vieussens; see ***[mylohyoid nerve (Meckel, 1748)] (Vieussens, 1684)***.

EARLIER REFERENCES:

Illustrated and described, not named:

1. ***[mylohyoid nerve (Meckel, 1748)] (Vieussens, 1684)***
Described rather vaguely for macrodissected adult human; p. 173 and Table 22-6,7.

LATER SYNONYMS:

1. *mylohyoid branch of inferior maxillary branch (Loder, 1778)*
Synonym for macrodissected adult human ***mylohyoid nerve (Meckel, 1748)***; in the original Latin, *ramum mylohyoideum*, p. 19.
2. *mylohyoid branch of inferior maxillary nerve proper (Haase, 1781)*
Synonym for macrodissected adult human ***mylohyoid nerve (Meckel, 1748)***; in the original Latin, *nervus maxillae inferiori proprius ramus mylohyoideus*, p. 72 and Index, section 138.
3. *submaxillary branch of inferior maxillary nerve (Andersch, 1797)*
Synonym for macrodissected adult human ***mylohyoid nerve (Meckel, 1748)***; in the original Latin, *nervus maxillaris inferior ramum submaxillarem*, Vol. 2, p. 121.
4. *mylohyoid fascicle of inferior alveolar surculus of inferior maxillary branch (Bellingeri, 1818)*
Synonym for macrodissected adult human ***mylohyoid nerve (Meckel, 1748)***; in the original Latin, *fasciculus mylo-hyoideus*, see Table I.
5. *mylohyoid branch of inferior dental nerve (Quain, 1828)*
Synonym for macrodissected adult human ***mylohyoid nerve (Meckel, 1748)***; p. 651.

PARTLY CORRESPONDS:

1. *communicating branch of submaxillary branches of inferior maxillary nerves and lingual nerves of fifth pair of nerves of head (Andersch, 1797)*
Macrodissected adult human ***communicating branch (Winslow, 1733)*** between ***mylohyoid nerve (Meckel, 1748)*** and ***lingual nerve (Vesalius, 1543a)***; in the original Latin, *ramus communicatorius rami submaxillaris nervi maxillaris inferioris et nervi lingualis quinti nervi capitis*, Vol. 2, p. 122.
2. *digastric branch of submaxillary branch of inferior maxillary nerve (Andersch, 1797)*
Macrodissected adult human branch of ***mylohyoid nerve (Meckel, 1748)*** to anterior belly of digastric muscle; in the original Latin, *ramus digasticus*, Vol. 2, p. 125.
3. *mental branch of submaxillary branch of inferior maxillary nerve (Andersch, 1797)*
Macrodissected adult human branch of ***mylohyoid nerve (Meckel, 1748)*** to mylohyoid and mental muscles; in the original Latin, *ramus mentalis*, Vol. 2, p. 125.

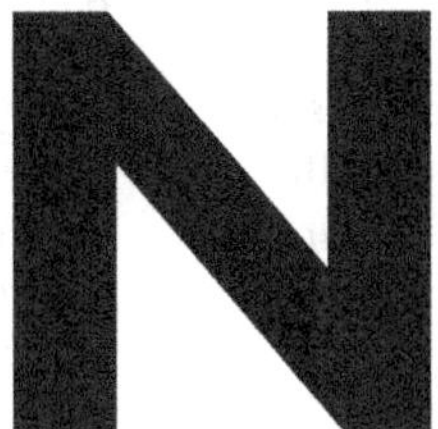

nasal branch of anterior superior dental nerve (>1840)

As described for macrodissected adult human, it supplies mucous membrane of the rostral (anterior) part of the lateral wall and floor of the nasal cavity, communicates with the ***posterior superior nasal nerves (Soemmerring, 1791)***, and ends in the part of the nasal septum near the root of the anterior nasal spine; see Durward (1951, Fig. 898), Williams & Warwick (1980, p. 1064). It was probably discovered by Falloppio; see ***[nasal branch of anterior superior dental nerve (>1840)] (Falloppio, 1561)***.

EARLIER REFERENCES:

Described, not named or illustrated:

1. ***[nasal branch of anterior superior dental nerve (>1840)] (Falloppio, 1561)***
   According to Haller (1762, p. 216 note *m*), Falloppio described it for macrodissected adult human (p. 144), as did Winslow (1733, Sect. VI, pp. 64–65). Meckel (1748, p. 69) clearly described innervation of macrodissected adult human nasal cavity from *anterior dental branch of infraorbital nerve (Meckel, 1748)*.

Earlier synonyms:

1. *filaments into nose from anterior dentar nerves (Meckel, 1817)*
   Vaguely described synonym for macrodissected adult human ***nasal branch of anterior superior dental nerve (>1840)***; see translation (1832, Vol. 3, p. 69).
2. *nasal branch of greater anterior alveolar nerve (Arnold, 1834)*
   Synonym for macrodissected adult human ***nasal branch of anterior superior dental nerve (>1840)***; in the original Latin, *nervus alveolaris anterior major, ramus nasalis*, p. 9.
3. *nasal branch of greater anterior dental nerve (Arnold, 1834)*
   Synonym for macrodissected adult human ***nasal branch of anterior superior dental nerve (>1840)***; in the original Latin, *nervus dentalis anterior major, ramus nasalis*, p. 9.
4. *ascending filaments of anterior alveolo-dental nerve (Cruveilhier, 1836)*
   Synonym for macrodissected adult human ***nasal branch of anterior superior dental nerve (>1840)***; in the original French, *filets ascendans*, p. 928.

nasal branches of anterior ethmoidal nerve (>1840)

As described for macrodissected adult human, the ***anterior ethmoidal nerve (>1840)*** enters the nasal cavity through the nasal slit and ends by dividing into ***internal nasal branches of anterior ethmoidal nerve (>1840)*** and an ***external nasal branch of anterior ethmoidal nerve (>1840)***; see Durward (1951, pp. 1019–1022), *Nomina Anatomica* (1983, p. A74). They were first clearly delineated by Willis; see ***[nasal branches of anterior ethmoidal nerve (>1840)] (Willis, 1664)***.

EARLIER REFERENCES:

Illustrated and described, not named:

1. ***[nasal branches of anterior ethmoidal nerve (>1840)] (Willis, 1664)***
   Illustrated for macrodissected adult human and presumably other common large mammals; p. 302, Figure 1-*c*.

Earlier synonyms:

1. *surculus tertius crassioris ac interioris propaginis K (Vieussens, 1684)*
   Probably corresponds roughly to macrodissected adult human ***nasal branches of anterior ethmoidal nerve (>1840)***; p. 171 and Table 22-*n*. They were described clearly for macrodissected adult human by Meckel (1753, Tab. 1:*28–31*).

2. *nasal branch of first branch of fifth pair (Monro, 1783)*
   Presumably ***nasal branches of anterior ethmoidal nerve (>1840)*** in macrodissected adult ox and human; p. 63.
3. *nasal nerve from ophthalmic nerve of fifth pair (Scarpa, 1785)*
   Presumably macrodissected adult human ***nasal branches of anterior ethmoidal nerve (>1840)***; in the original Latin, *nervus nasalis ab ophthalmico paris quinti*, Table I, Figure 1-*h*.

nasociliary nerve (Meckel, 1817; Wutzer, 1817)

As described for macrodissected adult human, lateral branch of the ***ophthalmic nerve (Winslow, 1733)*** changing name to ***anterior ethmoidal nerve (>1840)*** distal to where the ***infratrochlear nerve (Schaarschmidt, 1750)*** branches off; see Durward (1951, Fig. 892), Williams & Warwick (1980, p. 1061 and Fig. 7.174). For Meckel's use in macrodissected adult human, see translation (1832, Vol. 3, p. 63); for Wutzer (1817, Fig. 3-*a*). It was first clearly identified by Falloppio; see ***[nasociliary nerve (Meckel, 1817; Wutzer, 1817)] (Falloppio, 1561)***.

TRANSLATIONS:

1. *nervus nasociliaris (Meckel, 1817)*
   Original Latin form of ***nasociliary nerve (Meckel, 1817; Wutzer, 1817)***; see translation (1832, Vol. 3, p. 63).

EARLIER REFERENCES:

Described, not named or illustrated:

1. ***[nasociliary nerve (Meckel, 1817; Wutzer, 1817)] (Falloppio, 1561)***
   Described as branch of *third pair of nerves from brain (Falloppio, 1561)*; p. 452, see Meckel (1748, p. 37 note *l*).

Earlier synonyms:

1. *inferior branch of first and superior branch of third pair (Marchetti, 1652)*
   Roughly synonymous with macrodissected adult human ***nasociliary nerve (Meckel, 1817; Wutzer, 1817)***; p. 122.
2. *first shoot of uppermost branch of second division of fifth pair of nerves arising within skull (Willis, 1664)*
   Corresponds roughly to macrodissected adult, presumably human, ***nasociliary nerve (Meckel, 1817; Wutzer, 1817)***; see Pordage translation (1681, p. 144, Fig. 1-C,*c*).
3. *ramulus secundus rami minoris superioris nervorum quintae conjugationis (Vieussens, 1684)*
   Corresponds roughly to macrodissected adult human ***nasociliary nerve (Meckel, 1817; Wutzer, 1817)***; p. 170 and Table 22-*f*.
4. *internal ramus of orbitary nerve (Winslow, 1733)*
   Synonym for macrodissected adult human ***nasociliary nerve (Meckel, 1817; Wutzer, 1817)***; Section VI, p. 63.
5. *nasal ramus of orbitary nerve (Winslow, 1733)*
   Synonym for macrodissected adult human ***nasociliary nerve (Meckel, 1817; Wutzer, 1817)***; Section VI, p. 63.
6. *inner ramus of ophthalmic nerve (Winslow, 1733)*
   Synonym for macrodissected adult human ***nasociliary nerve (Meckel, 1817; Wutzer, 1817)***; Section X, p.102.
7. *inferior branch of first branch of fifth pair (Haller, 1743)*
   Synonym for macrodissected adult human ***nasociliary nerve (Meckel, 1817; Wutzer, 1817)***; in the original Latin, *primi rami quinti paris ramus inferior*, Fascicle 1, p. 46-26.
8. *nasal branch of first branch of fifth pair (Meckel, 1748)*
   Synonym for macrodissected adult human ***nasociliary nerve (Meckel, 1817; Wutzer, 1817)***; in the original Latin, *rami nasalis primi Quinti paris*, pp. 31, 42.
9. *nasal branch of ophthalmic branch of nerve of fifth pair (Bonhomme, 1748)*
   Synonym for macrodissected adult human ***nasociliary nerve (Meckel, 1817; Wutzer, 1817)***; in the original French, *la branche* (or *le filet) nasal de la branche ophthalmique de l'nerf de la cinquième paire*, p. 72, Plate 10-5.
10. *nasal nerve (Meckel, 1753)*
    Synonym for macrodissected adult human ***nasociliary nerve (Meckel, 1817; Wutzer, 1817)***; in the original French, *nerf nasal (du premier rameau de la cinquième paire)*, Table 1-28.
11. *nasolacrymal nerve (Le Cat, 1768)*
    Synonym for macrodissected adult human ***nasociliary nerve (Meckel, 1817; Wutzer, 1817)***; Plate VIII, Figure 1-S.
12. *naso-ocular nerve (Soemmerring, 1791)*
    Synonym for macrodissected adult human ***nasociliary nerve (Meckel, 1817; Wutzer, 1817)***; in the original Latin, *nervus naso-ocularis*, p. 193. Quain & Wilson (1839, Pl. XIII, Fig. 2-*e*) gave it as *n. oculo-nasalis*.
13. *naso-palpebral nerve (Burdin, 1803)*
    Synonym for macrodissected adult human ***nasociliary nerve (Meckel, 1817; Wutzer, 1817)***; see translation (1803, Vol. 1, p. 171).

LATER SYNONYMS:

1. *nasociliary branch of supraorbital branch of first branch of fifth pair of nerves (Bock, 1817)*
   Synonym for macrodissected adult human ***nasociliary nerve (Meckel, 1817; Wutzer, 1817)***; in the original Latin, *ramus nasociliaris*, p. 11.
2. *nasal branch of supraorbital branch of first branch of fifth pair of nerves (Bock, 1817)*
   Synonym for *nasociliary branch of supraorbital branch of first branch of fifth pair of nerves (Bock, 1817)*; in the original Latin, *ramus nasalis*, p. 11.
3. *nasal branch of first trunk of fifth nerve (Swan, 1830)*
   Synonym for macrodissected adult human ***nasociliary nerve (Meckel, 1817; Wutzer, 1817)***; Plate XII, Figure 6-8.
4. *ramus oculo-nasalis of ophthalmic nerve (Quain, 1832)*
   Synonym for macrodissected adult human ***nasociliary nerve (Meckel, 1817; Wutzer, 1817)***; p. 673.
5. *internal branch of first division of fifth pair of nerves (Todd, 1836–1839)*

Synonym for macrodissected adult human ***nasociliary nerve (Meckel, 1817; Wutzer, 1817)***; p. 279.
6. *inferior branch of first division of fifth pair of nerves (Todd, 1836–1839)*
Synonym for macrodissected adult human ***nasociliary nerve (Meckel, 1817; Wutzer, 1817)***; p. 279.

PARTLY CORRESPONDS:
1. *nasal infratrochlear nerve (Günther, 1786)*
Branch of macrodissected adult human *ethmoidal nerve (Günther, 1786)* with branches to upper and lower eyelids, also generating *external superior nasal nerves (Günther, 1786)*; in the original Latin, *infratrochlearis nasalis*, p. 44.

nasopalatine nerve (Scarpa, 1785)

As described for macrodissected adult human, the largest of the ***medial posterior superior nasal nerves (>1840)*** supplying a few small branches to the nasal septum before ending in mucus membrane of the rostral (anterior) part of the hard palate and communicating with the ***greater palatine nerve (Cloquet, 1816)***; see Williams & Warwick (1980, pp. 1065–1066), and Durward (1951, Figs. 893–894, labeled *long spheno-palatine nerve*). For Scarpa's use in macrodissected adult human, see Table I, Figure 1-*s,u* and Table II, Figure 2-*t,7*. According to Castiglioni (1947, p. 601), Scarpa first described it in his 1772 study on the *Round Window of the Ear*, but this is erroneous. It was discovered by Galen; see ***[nasopalatine nerve (Scarpa, 1785)] (Galen, c173)***.

TRANSLATIONS:
1. *nervus naso-palatinus (Scarpa, 1785)*
Original Latin form of ***nasopalatine nerve (Scarpa, 1785)***; Table I, Figure 1-*s*.

EARLIER REFERENCES:

Described, not named or illustrated:
1. ***[nasopalatine nerve (Scarpa, 1785)] (Galen, c173)***
Described in macrodissected adult beef, pig, and/or macaque but not human; see May translation (1968, pp. 456, 540 note 53).

LATER SYNONYMS:
1. *nasopalatine branch of Scarpa (Wrisberg, 1786)*
Eponym for macrodissected adult human ***nasopalatine nerve (Scarpa, 1785)***; in the original Latin, *ramus naso-palatinus Scarpae*, see Wrisberg translation (1800, p. 374).
2. *nasopalatine branch of sphenopalatine nerves (Cloquet, 1816)*
Synonym for macrodissected adult human ***nasopalatine nerve (Scarpa, 1785)***; in the original French, *rameau naso-palatin*, p. 683.
3. *nerve of septum of nose (Meckel, 1817)*
Synonym for macrodissected adult human ***nasopalatine nerve (Scarpa, 1785)***; in the original Latin, *nervus septi narium*, see translation (1832, Vol. 3, pp. 66, 68).
4. *nasopalatine nerve of Scarpa (Bock, 1817)*
Eponym for macrodissected adult human ***nasopalatine nerve (Scarpa, 1785)***; in the original Latin, *nervus naso-palatinus Scarpae*, p. 27.
5. *nasopalatine fascicle of sphenopalatine ganglion (Bellingeri, 1818)*
Synonym for macrodissected adult human ***nasopalatine nerve (Scarpa, 1785)***; in the original Latin, *fasciculus naso-palatinus*, see Table I.
6. *nerve of Cotunnius (Todd, 1836–1839, p. 287)*
Todd noted that while this eponym is sometimes used for macrodissected adult human ***nasopalatine nerve (Scarpa, 1785)***, it is incorrect because Scarpa (and John Hunter) described it earlier; p. 287.
7. *long spheno-palatine nerve (Quain & Wilson, 1839)*
Synonym for macrodissected adult human ***nasopalatine nerve (Scarpa, 1785)***; Plate XI, Figure 2-*F*. See Durward (1951, Figs. 893–894), Williams & Warwick (1980, p. 1065).
8. *Scarpa's nerve (>1840)*
Eponym for macrodissected adult human ***nasopalatine nerve (Scarpa, 1785)***; see *Dorland's* (2003, p. 1236).

PARTLY CORRESPONDS:
1. *nasopalatine ganglion (Cloquet, 1815)*
As described for macrodissected adult human, this small feature lies in common anterior palatine foramen (incisive foramen) and receives right and left ***nasopalatine nerves (Scarpa, 1785)*** before giving off filaments to palate; in the original French, *ganglion naso-palatin*, see Cloquet (1816, p. 687), Clark (1836, p. 333), Wilson (1838, Fig. 49-*), Dunglison (1874, p. 687). Foster (1892) listed it but referred to the "nasopalatine plexus". It is not recognized today and if anything is probably a *pseudoganglion (>1840)*.
2. *nasopalatine nerve (Meckel, 1817)*
Meckel indicated it is more appropriate to use the term in adult human for peripheral (distal) segment of ***nasopalatine nerve (Scarpa, 1785)*** associated just with membrane of palate; see translation (1832, Vol. 3, p. 68), where he wrote that "In passing through the palatine canal the nerves of the two sides unite, sometimes form a small prominence termed the *naso-palatine ganglion* (*G. naso-palatinum*) [*nasopalatine ganglion (Cloquet, 1815)*], and expand on a prominence situated below the anterior palatine foramen."
3. *nasal ganglion (Blainville, 1821)*
Synonym for macrodissected adult human *nasopalatine ganglion (Cloquet, 1815)*; in the original French, *ganglion nasal*, p. 218.
4. *anterior palatine nerves (Quain & Wilson, 1839)*
Macrodissected adult human terminal branches of ***nasopalatine nerve (Scarpa, 1785)***; Plate XI, Figure 2-*H*.
5. *Cloquet's ganglion (Quain & Wilson, 1839)*
Eponym for macrodissected adult human *nasopalatine ganglion (Cloquet, 1815)*; Plate XXVII-*F*.
6. *anterior palatine branches of naso-palatine ganglion (Quain & Wilson, 1839)*
Anterior palatine nerves (Quain & Wilson, 1839) distal to *nasopalatine ganglion (Cloquet, 1815)*; Plate XXVII-*j*.
7. *naso-palatine ganglion filament of communication with Meckel's ganglion (Quain & Wilson, 1839)*
Macrodissected adult human segment of ***nasopalatine nerve (Scarpa, 1785)*** between **pterygopalatine ganglion**

(>1840) and *nasopalatine ganglion (Cloquet, 1815)*; Plate XXVII-*k*.

nerve cord (Serres, 1824–1826)

A topographic division of the ***nervous system (Monro, 1783)*** including scattered ***ganglia (Galen, c173)*** separated by ***communicating branches (Winslow, 1733)***, commonly called connectives, of more or less predictable lengths; see Swanson & Bota (2010). Gross anatomically it has the appearance of a beaded string. Examples include ***radial nerve cord (>1840)***, ***central nerve cord (Serres, 1824–1826)***, ***ventral cord (Anderson, 1837)***, and ***peripheral nerve cord (Swanson & Bota, 2010)***. At the systems architecture level, it is a series of ***gray matter regions (Swanson & Bota, 2010)***, or ***ganglia (Galen, c173)***, attached to a ***white matter tract (Bell & Bell, 1826)*** called a ***nerve cord trunk (>1840)***. For Serres's use in the molluscan ***central nerve cord (Serres, 1824–1826)***, see Vol. 2, p. 13. It was first described as the *spinal medulla (Malpighi, 1669)*, the ***ventral cord (>1840)***, of the silkworm.

nerve cord trunk (>1840)

A ***white matter tract (Bell & Bell, 1826)*** for a ***nerve cord (Serres, 1824–1826)***; see Swanson & Bota (2010). For examples, see ***central nerve cord trunk (>1840)*** and ***peripheral nerve cord trunk (Swanson & Bota, 2010)***. Not clearly described before 1840.

nerve net (>1840)

A longitudinally arranged ***nervous system (Monro, 1783)*** with radial symmetry and relatively evenly and diffusely distributed ***neurons (Waldeyer, 1891)***, characteristic of Coelenterates, Ctenophores, Hemichordates, Pogonophores, and adult Echinoderms. While small condensations called ***marginal ganglia (>1840)*** and circular zones called ***nerve rings (Tiedemann, 1815)***, both with a higher concentration of ***neurons (Waldeyer, 1891)*** and ***neuron extensions (Swanson & Bota, 2010)***, can be present, ***nerves (Herophilus, c335–c280 BC)*** are not clearly differentiated, and nothing like a ***central nervous system (Carus, 1814)*** is present; see Bullock & Horridge (1965, p. 12 and Ch. 8), Cobb (1995), and Swanson & Bota (2010) for this precise definition. It is thus a ***nervous system (Monro, 1783)*** with no clear topographic divisions—a slightly differentiated but divisionless ***nervous system (Monro, 1783)***. The ***nervous system (Monro, 1783)*** of hydra (a Coelenterate) is an example of a relatively simple diffuse ***nerve net (>1840)***, whereas the ***terminal plexuses (Swanson & Bota, 2010)*** in the wall of the mammalian digestive system, the ***enteric plexuses (Hill, 1927)***, can be viewed as analogous to a well differentiated ***nerve net (>1840)***. The ***nerve net (>1840)*** was not clearly described by 1840.

nerve of pterygoid canal (>1840)

As described for macrodissected adult human, rostral continuation of the ***greater petrosal nerve (>1840)***, after the ***deep petrosal nerve (Meckel, 1817)*** joins the latter, to the caudal (posterior) end of the ***pterygopalatine ganglion (>1840)***; see Williams & Warwick (1980, Fig. 7.179). It was probably first mentioned by Guido; see ***[nerve of pterygoid canal (>1840)] (Guido, 1611)***.

EARLIER REFERENCES:

Described, not named or illustrated:

1. ***[nerve of pterygoid canal (>1840)] (Guido, 1611)***
   Guido is credited with first mentioning it for macrodissected adult human; pp. 88–91, known eponymously as *Vidian nerve (Meckel, 1748)*.

Earlier synonyms:

1. *Vidian branch of second branch of fifth pair (Meckel, 1748)*
   Eponym for macrodissected adult human ***nerve of pterygoid canal (>1840)***; in the original Latin, *ramus vidianus secundi rami Quinti pairs*, Figure 1-57,*η*.
2. *Vidian nerve (Meckel, 1748)*
   Eponym for macrodissected adult human ***nerve of pterygoid canal (>1840)***; in the original Latin, *nervi Vidiani*, Figure 1-57,*κ*. It is referred to as recurrent; in the original Latin, *recurrentem*, p. 50. Also see *retrograde Vidian nerve (Meckel, 1751)*.
3. *recurrent Vidian nerve (Meckel, 1748)*
   Synonym for *Vidian nerve (Meckel, 1748)*; in the original Latin, *nervi Vidiani recurrentem*, p. 50. Haase (1781, p. 62 and Index section 116) gave the Latin form, *nervi vidiani recurrentis*.
4. *recurrent pterygoid nerve (Schaarschmidt, 1750)*
   Synonym for macrodissected adult human ***nerve of pterygoid canal (>1840)***; in the original Latin, *nervus pterygoideus recurrens*, p. 19.
5. *retrograde Vidian nerve (Meckel, 1751)*
   Synonym for macrodissected adult human *Vidian nerve (Meckel, 1748)*; in the original French, *le nerf vidien rétrograde*, p. 85.
6. *pterygoid branch of superior maxillary branch of fifth pair (Haller, 1762)*
   Roughly synonymous with macrodissected adult human *Vidian nerve (Meckel, 1748)*. Haller described its various "branches" as well—***greater petrosal nerve (>1840)***, ***deep petrosal nerve (Meckel, 1817)***, and ***posterior superior nasal nerves (Soemmerring, 1791)***; in the original Latin, *ramus pterygoideus, paris quinti ramus maxillaris superior*, pp. 213–214.
7. *cordon pterigoïdien (Le Cat, 1768)*
   French synonym for macrodissected adult human ***nerve of pterygoid canal (>1840)***; Plate VIII, Figure 1-*u*.
8. *sphenopalatine nerve (Haase, 1781)*
   Synonym for macrodissected adult human ***nerve of pterygoid canal (>1840)***; in the original Latin, *nervus sphenopalatinus*; Index section 116.
9. *pterygoid nerve (Soemmerring, 1791)*
   Synonym for macrodissected adult human ***nerve of pterygoid canal (>1840)***; in the original Latin, *nervus pterygoideus*, which Soemmerring ascribed to Haller,

p. 201. Spelled *pterygoidian nerve* in Burdin translation (1803, Vol. 1, p. 174).

10. *recurrent fifth nerve (Meckel, 1817)*
Synonym for macrodissected adult human ***nerve of pterygoid canal (>1840)***; in the original Latin, *nervus quinti recurrens*, see translation (1832, Vol. 3, pp. 67, 90).
11. *anastomotic fifth nerve (Meckel, 1817)*
Synonym for macrodissected adult human ***nerve of pterygoid canal (>1840)***; in the original Latin, *nervus quinti anastomoticus*, see translation (1832, Vol. 3, p. 67).
12. *Vidian fascicle of sphenopalatine ganglion (Bellingeri, 1818)*
Synonym for macrodissected adult human ***nerve of pterygoid canal (>1840)***; in the original Latin, *fasciculus Vidianus*, see Table I.
13. *posterior branch of Meckel's ganglion (Quain, 1828)*
Synonym for macrodissected adult human ***nerve of pterygoid canal (>1840)***; p. 666.
14. *posterior branch of spheno-palatine ganglion (Quain & Wilson, 1839)*
Synonym for macrodissected adult human ***nerve of pterygoid canal (>1840)***; Plate XXVII-*G,o*.

PARTLY CORRESPONDS:

1. *posterior superior nasal branches of Vidian nerve (Meckel, 1748)*
Probably synonym for macrodissected adult human *posterior superior nasal nerves (Günther, 1786)*; p. 52 for description of distribution and Figure 1-*ι* for illustration of origins. Also see Todd (1836–1839, p. 288). They also supply mucous membrane of the vomer; see Meckel (1751, p. 87).
2. *nasal branch to septum from Vidian nerve (Scarpa, 1785)*
Synonym for macrodissected adult human *pharyngeal nerves from Vidian nerve (Wrisberg, 1786)*; in the original Latin, *ramus nasalis ad septum e nervo Vidiano*, Table I, Figure I-*u* and Table II, Figure II-*10*.
3. *twigs from Vidian nerve to sphenoid sinus membrane (Scarpa, 1785)*
Scarpa described two thin branches from ***nerve of pterygoid canal (>1840)*** to sphenoid sinus membrane in macrodissected adult human; in the original Latin, *surculi e nervo Vidiano ad membranam sinus sphoenoidei*, Table II, Figure II-9.
4. *pharyngeal nerves from Vidian nerve (Wrisberg, 1786)*
Wrisberg described several branches of ***nerve of pterygoid canal (>1840)*** to pharynx in macrodissected adult human and noted two were well illustrated by Scarpa (1785, Tab. II, Fig. II-*10*); in the original Latin, *nervi pharyngis ex Vidiano*, see Wrisberg reprint (1800, pp. 410–411).
5. *posterior superior nasal nerves (Günther, 1786)*
Macrodissected adult human branches from ***nerve of pterygoid canal (>1840)*** complementing ***posterior superior nasal nerves (Soemmerring, 1791)***; in the original Latin, *nasales superiores posteriores*, p. 46. Todd (1836–1839, p. 287) discussed how most authors follow this description, whereas a minority (including Bock, J.F. Meckel, and Hirzel) stated that sometimes the ***nerve of pterygoid canal (>1840)*** and ***posterior superior nasal nerves (Soemmerring, 1791)*** connect separately to ***pterygopalatine ganglion (>1840)***.
6. *salpingo-pharyngeal threads of Vidian fascicle* (Bellingeri, 1818)
Two branches from macrodissected adult human ***nerve of pterygoid canal (>1840)*** to pharyngeal palate; in the original Latin, *stamina salpingo-pharyngei*, see Table I.
7. *anastomotic petrosal thread of Vidian fascicle with trunk of facial nerve (Bellingeri, 1818)*
Macrodissected adult human ***communicating branch (Winslow, 1733)*** between ***nerve of pterygoid canal (>1840)*** and *facial nerve (Vicq d'Azyr, 1784)*; in the original Latin, *stamina petrosus anastomoticus cum trunco nervi facialis*, see Table I.

nerve ring (Tiedemann, 1815)

The relatively vague differentiation of a circular zone in a ***nerve net (>1840)***, with a higher concentration of ***neurons (Waldeyer, 1891)*** and ***neuron extensions (Swanson & Bota, 2010)***; see Bullock & Horridge (1965, p. 475), Cobb (1995, p. 411). For Tiedemann's use in starfish, see p. 170.

TRANSLATIONS:

1. *Nervenring (Tiedemann, 1815)*
Original German form of ***nerve ring (Tiedemann, 1815)***; p. 170. Tiedemann referred to Cuvier (1800, Vol. 2, p. 360) who described a similar feature in starfish, but described it as more tendonous than nervous, raising doubt about its identity.

nerve to flexor digitorum longus (>1840)

As described for macrodissected adult human, it innervates the flexor digitorum longus muscle and is a ***muscular branch of tibial nerve (>1840)***; see Williams & Warwick (1980, p. 1113 and Fig. 7.216). It was known to Eustachi; see ***[nerve to flexor digitorum longus (>1840)] (Eustachi, 1552)***.

EARLIER REFERENCES:

Illustrated, not named or described:

1. ***[nerve to flexor digitorum longus (>1840)] (Eustachi, 1552)***
Illustrated for macrodissected adult human; see Albinus edition (1761, Tab. 20-χ, p. 121).

Earlier synonyms:

1. *branch of posterior tibial nerve to long flexor muscle of toes (Swan, 1830)*
Synonym for macrodissected adult human ***nerve to flexor digitorum longus (>1840)***; Plate XXV, Figure 2-5.
2. *nerve of common flexor (Cruveilhier, 1836)*
Synonym for macrodissected adult human ***nerve to flexor digitorum longus (>1840)***; in the original French, *nerf du flechisseur commun*, p. 871.

PARTLY CORRESPONDS:

1. *first branch of tibial nerve to flexor digitorum longus muscle (Jördens, 1788)*
   One of two components of ***nerve to flexor digitorum longus (>1840)*** identified in macrodissected adult human; in the original Latin, *ramus primus [nervus tibieus] ad musculum flexorem digitorum longum*, p. 10 and Table III-*173*.
2. *second branch to flexor digitorum longus muscle (Jördens, 1788)*
   Second of two components of ***nerve to flexor digitorum longus (>1840)*** identified in macrodissected adult human; in the original Latin, *ramo secundo ad musculum flexorem digitorum longum*, p. 10 and Table III-*175*. Jördens identified two small branches of this branch; Table III-*176,177*.
3. *first nerve to flexor digitorum longus muscle (Fischer, 1791)*
   Macrodissected adult human ***nerve to flexor digitorum longus (>1840)*** from one of two branches of *common nerve to tibialis posterior, flexor digitorum longus, and flexor longus of big toe muscles and first internal inferior posterior cutaneous nerve (Fischer, 1791)*; in the original Latin, *nervum musculi flexoris longi digitorum primum*, p. 35.
4. *second nerve to flexor digitorum longus muscle (Fischer, 1791)*
   Macrodissected adult human ***nerve to flexor digitorum longus (>1840)*** from one of two branches of *common nerve to tibialis posterior, flexor digitorum longus, and flexor longus of big toe muscles and first internal inferior posterior cutaneous nerve (Fischer, 1791)*; in the original Latin, *nervum musculi flexoris longi digitorum secundum*, p. 35.
5. *third nerve to flexor digitorum longus of foot muscle (Fischer, 1791)*
   Macrodissected adult human ***nerve to flexor digitorum longus (>1840)*** from trunk of ***tibial nerve (Haase, 1781)***; in the original Latin, *nervus musculi flexoris longi digitorum pedis tertius*, p. 35.

nerve to flexor hallucis longus (>1840)

As described for macrodissected adult human, it innervates the flexor hallucis longus muscle and is a ***muscular branch of tibial nerve (>1840)***; see Williams & Warwick (1980, p. 1113 and Fig. 7.216). It was known to Eustachi; see ***[nerve to flexor hallucis longus (>1840)] (Eustachi, 1552)***.

EARLIER REFERENCES:

Illustrated, not named or described:

1. ***[nerve to flexor hallucis longus (>1840)] (Eustachi, 1552)***
   Illustrated for macrodissected adult human; see Albinus edition (1761, Tab. 20-*17,18* and p. 121).

Illustrated and described, not named:

1. ***[nerve to flexor hallucis longus (>1840)] (Vieussens, 1684)***
   Described and illustrated for macrodissected adult human; see Table 29-*125*.

Earlier synonyms:

1. *nerve to flexor pollicis proper (Jördens, 1788)*
   Synonym for macrodissected adult human ***nerve to flexor hallucis longus (>1840)***; in the original Latin, *nervus flexoris pollicis proprii*, p. 10 and Table III-*166*. Jördens identified six smaller branches from it; Table III:*167–172*.
2. *branch of posterior tibial nerve to long flexor muscle of great toe (Swan, 1830)*
   Synonym for macrodissected adult human ***nerve to flexor hallucis longus (>1840)***; Plate XXV, Figure 2-*6*.
3. *nerve of flexor hallucis longus proper (Cruveilhier, 1836)*
   Synonym for macrodissected adult human ***nerve to flexor hallucis longus (>1840)***; in the original French, *nerf du long fléchisseur propre du gros orteil*, p. 871.

PARTLY CORRESPONDS:

1. *first nerve to flexor longus of big toe muscle (Fischer, 1791)*
   A ***nerve to flexor hallucis longus (>1840)*** described for macrodissected adult human as branch of *common nerve to soleus and flexor longus of big toe muscles (Fischer, 1791)*; p. 35.
2. *second nerve to flexor longus of big toe muscle (Fischer, 1791)*
   A ***nerve to flexor hallucis longus (>1840)*** described for macrodissected adult human as branch of *common nerve to tibialis posterior, flexor digitorum longus, and flexor longus of big toe muscles and first internal inferior posterior cutaneous nerve (Fischer, 1791)*; in the original Latin, *nervum musculi flexoris longi pollicis secundum*, p. 35.
3. *inferior nerve to flexor longus of big toe muscle (Fischer, 1791)*
   Synonym for *second nerve to flexor longus of big toe muscle (Fischer, 1791)*; in the original Latin, *nervum musculi flexoris longi pollicis inferiorem*, p. 35.

nerve to hamstring muscles (>1840)

As described for macrodissected adult human, it commonly arises from all the ***sacral plexus ventral divisions (Paterson, 1887)*** contributing to the ***tibial nerve (Haase, 1781)*** and forms a trunk in the caudal (lower) part of the buttock before branching to supply the semitendinosus, long head of biceps femoris, ischial head of adductor magnus, and semimembranosus muscles. Occasionally, however, a series of branches to the various muscles may be given off instead by the ***sciatic nerve (Keill, 1698)***; see Durward (1951, pp. 1105–1106 and Figs. 937, 947). It was known to Galen; see ***[nerve to hamstring muscles (>1840)] (Galen, c177)***.

EARLIER REFERENCES:

Described, not named or illustrated:

1. ***[nerve to hamstring muscles (>1840)] (Galen, c177)***
   Mentioned for macrodissected adult beef, pig, and/or macaque but not human; see Singer translation (1999, p. 84).

Illustrated and described, not named:

1. ***[nerve to hamstring muscles (>1840)] (Vesalius, 1543a)***

Described and illustrated for macrodissected adult human; see Richardson & Carman translation (2002, p. 259).

Earlier synonyms:

1. *branches of sciatic nerve trunk to flexor muscles of thigh (Meckel, 1817)*
   Synonym for macrodissected adult human ***nerve to hamstring muscles (>1840)***; see translation (1832, Vol. 3, p. 17).

PARTLY CORRESPONDS:

1. *common trunk to major belly of biceps and superior internal cutaneous nerve (Jördens, 1788)*
   Component of macrodissected adult human ***nerve to hamstring muscles (>1840)***; in the original Latin, *truncus communis ventris majoris bicipitis et nervi cutanei interni superioris*, p. 2.
2. *superior internal cutaneous nerve (Jördens, 1788)*
   Branch of *common trunk to major belly of biceps and superior internal cutaneous nerve (Jördens, 1788)* in turn a branch of ***nerve to hamstring muscles (>1840)***; in the original Latin, *nervi cutanei interni superioris*, p. 2.
3. *inferior and internal cutaneous nerve (Jördens, 1788)*
   Apparently component of ***nerve to hamstring muscles (>1840)*** part of which innervates semitendinosus muscle; in the original Latin, *nervo cutaneo interno et inferiore*, p. 2.
4. *nerve to seminervosi muscle (Fischer, 1791)*
   Branch of macrodissected adult human ***nerve to hamstring muscles (>1840)*** misidentified as usually arising from ***femoral nerve (Haller, 1762)*** by Winslow (1733) and ending in semitendinosus muscle, and named as here by Fischer; in the original Latin, *nervus musculi seminervosi*, p. 7.
5. *nerve to semitendinosus muscle (Fischer, 1791)*
   Synonym for *nerve to seminervosi muscle (Fischer, 1791)*, identified by Coopmans (1789) and named as here by Fischer; in the original Latin, *nervus musculi semitendinosi*, pp. 8, 29.
6. *trunk of superior internal cutaneous nerve and nerve to long head of crural biceps muscle (Fischer, 1791)*
   Synonym for macrodissected adult human *common trunk to major belly of biceps and superior internal cutaneous nerve (Jördens, 1788)*; in the original Latin, *trunculus nervi cutanei interni superioris et nervi capitis longi musculi bicipitis cruris*, p. 29.
7. *first nerve to long head of crural biceps muscle (Fischer, 1791)*
   Branch of macrodissected adult human ***nerve to hamstring muscles (>1840)*** to long head of biceps femoris muscle, in the original Latin, *nervi primi capitis longi musculi bicipitis cruris*, p. 29.
8. *common trunk for nerves to adductor femoris magnus, semimembranosus, biceps, and semitendinosus muscles (Fischer, 1791)*
   Branch of macrodissected adult human ***nerve to hamstring muscles (>1840)***; in the original Latin, *trunculum communem pro nervis musculi adductoris femoris magni, semimembranosi, bicipitis et semitendinosi*, p. 29. It supplies *second branch to long head of biceps femoris muscle* and *first nerve to short head of biceps muscle (Fischer, 1791)*.
9. *nerve to adductor femoris magnus muscle (Fischer, 1791)*
   Branch of *common trunk for nerves to adductor femoris magnus, semimembranosus, biceps, and semitendinosus muscles (Fischer, 1791)* to adductor magnus muscle; p. 29.
10. *nerve to semimembranosus muscle (Fischer, 1791)*
    Branch of *common trunk for nerves to adductor femoris magnus, semimembranosus, biceps, and semitendinosus muscles (Fischer, 1791)*; p. 29.
11. *first nerve to short head of biceps muscle (Fischer, 1791)*
    Branch of *common trunk for nerves to adductor femoris magnus, semimembranosus, biceps, and semitendinosus muscles (Fischer, 1791)* to short head of biceps femoris muscle; in the original Latin, *nervum primum capitis brevis musculi bicipitis*, p. 30.
12. *second nerve to short head of biceps muscle (Fischer, 1791)*
    Branch of macrodissected adult human ***nerve to hamstring muscles (>1840)*** to short head of biceps femoris muscle; in the original Latin, *nervus secundus capitis brevis musculi bicipitis*, p. 30.
13. *third nerve to long head of biceps muscle (Fischer, 1791)*
    Branch of macrodissected adult human ***nerve to hamstring muscles (>1840)*** to long head of biceps femoris muscle; in the original Latin, *nervus tertius capitis longi musculi bicipitis*, p. 30. Also see *common trunk for nerves to adductor femoris magnus, semimembranosus, biceps, and semitendinosus muscles (Fischer, 1791)*.
14. *fourth nerve to short head of biceps muscle (Fischer, 1791)*
    Branch of macrodissected adult human ***nerve to hamstring muscles (>1840)*** from ***tibial nerve (Haase, 1781)*** to short head of biceps femoris muscle; in the original Latin, *nervus capitis brevis musculi bicipitis quartus*, p. 33.
15. *common branch to semitendinosus, semimembranosus, and abductor femoris magnus muscles (Bock, 1827)*
    Synonym for macrodissected adult human *common trunk for nerves to adductor femoris magnus, semimembranosus, biceps, and semitendinosus muscles (Fischer, 1791)*; in the original Latin, *ram. communis musculi semitendinosi, semimembranosi et abductoris [sic] magni femoris*; Table VII, Figure 2-43.
16. *branch to semitendinosus muscle (Bock, 1827)*
    Branch of macrodissected adult human ***nerve to hamstring muscles (>1840)*** to semitendinosus muscle; in the original Latin, *ram. musculi semitendinosi*, Table VII, Figure 2-44.
17. *branch of sciatic nerve to semi-membranous muscle (Swan, 1830)*
    Macrodissected adult human branch of ***nerve to hamstring muscles (>1840)*** to semimembranosus muscle; Plate XXV, Figure 1-14.
18. *branch of sciatic nerve to long head of biceps muscle (Swan, 1830)*
    Macrodissected adult human branch of ***nerve to hamstring muscles (>1840)*** to long head of biceps femoris muscle; Plate XXV, Figure 1-15.

19. *branch of sciatic nerve to semi-tendinous muscle (Swan, 1830)*
Macrodissected adult human branch of ***nerve to hamstring muscles (>1840)*** to semitendinosus muscle; Plate XXV, Figure 1-*15*.
20. *internal superior cutaneous nerve (Knox, 1832)*
Knox's form of *superior internal cutaneous nerve (Jördens, 1788)*; see Table XVIII-*124*.
21. *nerve of long portion of biceps (Cruveilhier, 1836)*
Macrodissected adult human branch of ***nerve to hamstring muscles (>1840)*** to long head of biceps femoris muscle; in the original French, *nerf de la longue portion du biceps*, p. 861, where Cruveilhier described two ascending branches and one descending branch of it.
22. *nerve of semitendinosus (Cruveilhier, 1836)*
Macrodissected adult human branch of ***nerve to hamstring muscles (>1840)*** to semitendinosus muscle; in the original French, *nerf du demi-tendineux*, p. 861.
23. *nerves of semimembranosus (Cruveilhier, 1836)*
For macrodissected adult human,two branches of ***nerve to hamstring muscles (>1840)*** to semimembranosus muscle; in the original French, *nerf du demi-membraneux*, p. 861.
24. *nerve of adductor magnus (Cruveilhier, 1836)*
Macrodissected adult human branch of ***nerve to hamstring muscles (>1840)*** to adductor magnus muscle; in the original French, *nerf du grand adducteur*, p. 861.

nerve to inferior oblique (>1840)

As described for macrodissected adult human, branch of the ***oculomotor nerve inferior branch (Haase, 1781)*** to the inferior oblique muscle of the eye, also generating the ***branch of oculomotor nerve to ciliary ganglion (>1840)***; see Williams & Warwick (1980, p. 1057). It was first delineated by Eustachi; see ***[nerve to inferior oblique (>1840)] (Eustachi, 1552)***.

EARLIER REFERENCES:

Illustrated, not named or described:

1. ***[nerve to inferior oblique (>1840)] (Eustachi, 1552)***
Clearly illustrated for macrodissected adult human; see Albinus edition (1761, Tab. XVII, Figs. 1, 3, 4-*h*).

Described, not named or illustrated:

1. ***[nerve to inferior oblique (>1840)] (Vieussens, 1684)***
Described for macrodissected adult human; pp. 167–168.

Earlier synonyms:

1. *long inferior branch of third pair of nerves (Winslow, 1733)*
Synonym for macrodissected adult human ***nerve to inferior oblique (>1840)***; Section VI, pp. 61–62.
2. *long inferior branch of nervi motores oculorum communes (Winslow, 1733)*
Synonym for macrodissected adult human ***nerve to inferior oblique (>1840)***; Section VI, pp. 61–62.
3. *branch to inferior oblique from third pair (Haller, 1743)*
Synonym for macrodissected adult human ***nerve to inferior oblique (>1840)***; in the original Latin, *ramus ad obliquum inferiorem*, p. 45.
4. *external branch of third pair (Haller, 1743)*
Synonym for macrodissected adult human ***nerve to inferior oblique (>1840)***; in the original Latin, *ramus externus*, p. 45.
5. *external inferior twig of common motor nerve (Meckel, 1817)*
Synonym for macrodissected adult human ***nerve to inferior oblique (>1840)***; see translation (1832, Vol. 3, p. 77).
6. *external branch of common motor nerve inferior terminal branch (Cruveilhier, 1836)*
Synonym for macrodissected adult human ***nerve to inferior oblique (>1840)***; in the original French, *rameau externe*, p. 906.

nerve to inferior rectus (>1840)

As described for macrodissected adult human, branch of the ***oculomotor nerve inferior branch (Haase, 1781)*** to the inferior rectus muscle of the eye; see Williams & Warwick (1980, p. 1057). It was first delineated by Eustachi; see ***[nerve to inferior rectus (>1840)] (Eustachi, 1552)***.

EARLIER REFERENCES:

Illustrated, not named or described:

1. ***[nerve to inferior rectus (>1840)] (Eustachi, 1552)***
Clearly illustrated for macrodissected adult human; see Albinus edition (1761, Tab. XVII, Figs. 1, 3, 4-*i*).

Described, not named or illustrated:

1. ***[nerve to inferior rectus (>1840)] (Vieussens, 1684)***
Described for macrodissected adult human; pp. 167–168.

Earlier synonyms:

1. *short inferior branch of third pair of nerves (Winslow, 1733)*
Synonym for macrodissected adult human ***nerve to inferior rectus (>1840)***; Section VI, pp. 61–62.
2. *short inferior branch of nervi motores oculorum communes (Winslow, 1733)*
Synonym for macrodissected adult human ***nerve to inferior rectus (>1840)***; Section VI, pp. 61–62.
3. *branch to inferior rectus from third pair (Haller, 1743)*
Synonym for macrodissected adult human ***nerve to inferior rectus (>1840)***; in the original Latin, *ramus ad rectum inferiorem*, p. 45.
4. *middle branch of third pair (Haller, 1743)*
Synonym for macrodissected adult human ***nerve to inferior rectus (>1840)***; in the original Latin, *ramus medius*, p. 45.
5. *middle twig of common motor nerve (Meckel, 1817)*
Synonym for macrodissected adult human ***nerve to inferior rectus (>1840)***; see translation (1832, Vol. 3, p. 77).
6. *middle branch of common motor nerve inferior terminal branch (Cruveilhier, 1836)*
Synonym for macrodissected adult human ***nerve to inferior rectus (>1840)***; in the original French, *rameau moyen*, p. 906.

nerve to medial rectus (>1840)

As described for macrodissected adult human, branch of the ***oculomotor nerve inferior branch (Haase, 1781)*** to the medial rectus muscle of the eye; see Williams & Warwick (1980, p. 1057). It was first delineated by Eustachi; see ***[nerve to medial rectus (>1840)] (Eustachi, 1552)***.

EARLIER REFERENCES:

Illustrated, not named or described:

1. ***[nerve to medial rectus (>1840)] (Eustachi, 1552)***
Clearly illustrated for macrodissected adult human; see Albinus edition (1761, Tab. XVII, Figs. 1, 3, 4-*g*).

Described, not named or illustrated:

1. ***[nerve to medial rectus (>1840)] (Vieussens, 1684)***
Described for macrodissected adult human; pp. 167–168.

Earlier synonyms:

1. *internal branch of third pair of nerves (Winslow, 1733)*
Synonym for macrodissected adult human ***nerve to medial rectus (>1840)***; Section VI, pp. 61–62.
2. *internal branch of nervi motores oculorum communes (Winslow, 1733)*
Synonym for macrodissected adult human ***nerve to medial rectus (>1840)***; Section VI, pp. 61–62.
3. *branch to internal rectus from third pair (Haller, 1743)*
Synonym for macrodissected adult human ***nerve to medial rectus (>1840)***; in the original Latin, *ramus ad rectum internum*, p. 45.
4. *internal branch of third pair (Haller, 1743)*
Synonym for macrodissected adult human ***nerve to medial rectus (>1840)***; in the original Latin, *ramus internus*, p. 45.
5. *internal twig of common motor nerve (Meckel, 1817)*
Synonym for macrodissected adult human ***nerve to medial rectus (>1840)***; see translation (1832, Vol. 3, p. 77).
6. *internal branch of common motor nerve inferior terminal branch (Cruveilhier, 1836)*
Synonym for macrodissected adult human ***nerve to medial rectus (>1840)***; in the original French, *rameau interne*, p. 906.

nerve to obturator internus (>1840)

As described for macrodissected adult human, it arises from the fifth lumbar and first two sacral ***sacral plexus ventral divisions (Paterson, 1887)*** and supplies the obturator internus and gemellus superior muscles; see Williams & Warwick (1980, p. 1111), *Terminologia Anatomica* (1998, p. 140). It was known to Galen; see ***[nerve to obturator internus (>1840)] (Galen, c177)***.

EARLIER REFERENCES:

Described, not named or illustrated:

1. ***[nerve to obturator internus (>1840)] (Galen, c177)***
Alluded to in macrodissected adult beef, pig, and/or macaque but not human; see Singer translation (1999, p. 85).

Illustrated, not named or described:

1. ***[nerve to obturator internus (>1840)] (Eustachi, 1552)***
Illustrated for macrodissected adult human; see Albinus edition (1761, Tab. 20-χ).

Earlier synonyms:

1. *nerve to gemellus and internal obturator muscles (Jördens, 1788)*
Synonym for macrodissected adult human ***nerve to obturator internus (>1840)***; in the original Latin, *nervus musculorum geminum et obturatoris interni*, p. 2.
2. *common trunk for nerves to gemellus superior, obturator internus, gemellus inferior, and quadratus femoris muscles (Fischer, 1791)*
Synonym for macrodissected adult human ***nerve to obturator internus (>1840)***; in the original Latin, *trunculus communis nervi musculi gemini superioris, obturatorii internis, gemini inferioris et quadratus femoris*, p. 28.
3. *branch of sciatic nerve to obturator internus (Meckel, 1817)*
Synonym for macrodissected adult human ***nerve to obturator internus (>1840)***; see translation (1832, Vol. 3, p. 17).
4. *branch to obturator internus muscle (Bock, 1827)*
Synonym for macrodissected adult human ***nerve to obturator internus (>1840)***; in the original Latin, *ram. musculi obturatorii interni*; Table VII, Figure 2-39.

PARTLY CORRESPONDS:

1. *nerve of obturator internus muscle (Cruveilhier, 1836)*
Arises from macrodissected adult human ***sacral plexus (Vesalius, 1543a)*** and supplies just obturator internus muscle, although the muscle is more commonly described now as supplied by one of two branches of ***nerve to obturator internus (>1840)***; in the original French, *nerf du muscle obturateur interne*, p. 852.
2. *nerve of gemellus superior (Cruveilhier, 1836)*
Arises from macrodissected adult human ***sacral plexus (Vesalius, 1543a)*** and supplies gemellus superior muscle, although it is more commonly described now as component of ***nerve to obturator internus (>1840)***; in the original French, *nerf du jumeau supérieur*, p. 858.

nerve to plantaris (>1840)

As described for macrodissected adult human, it innervates the plantaris muscle and is a ***muscular branch of tibial nerve (>1840)***; see Durward (1951, p. 1109), Hamilton (1976, Fig. 833). It was known to Vesalius; see ***[nerve to plantaris (>1840)] (Vesalius, 1543a)***.

EARLIER REFERENCES:

Illustrated and described, not named:

1. ***[nerve to plantaris (>1840)] (Vesalius, 1543a)***
Identified for macrodissected adult human; see Richardson & Carman translation (2002, p. 259).

Earlier synonyms:

1. *branch to plantaris muscle from internal popliteal nerve (Bock, 1827)*
Synonym for macrodissected adult human ***nerve to plantaris (>1840)***; in the original Latin, *ram. musculi plantaris*, Table IV-99.
2. *branch of sciatic nerve to plantar muscle (Swan, 1830)*
Synonym for macrodissected adult human ***nerve to plantaris (>1840)***; Plate XXV, Figure 1-24.

3. *nerve of plantaris longus (Cruveilhier, 1836)*
   Synonym for macrodissected adult human ***nerve to plantaris (>1840)***; in the original French, *nerf du plantaire gréle*, p. 870.

PARTLY CORRESPONDS:

1. *first nerve to plantaris muscle (Fischer, 1791)*
   Dorsal (posterior) branch of *common nerve to gastrocnemius and plantaris muscles (Fischer, 1791)*; p. 34.

nerve to popliteus (>1840)

As described for macrodissected adult human, it innervates the popliteus muscle and is a ***muscular branch of tibial nerve (>1840)***. As it winds around the ventral border of the muscle before ending, it gives off the ***nerve to tibialis posterior (Cruveilhier, 1836)***, ***interosseal nerve of leg (>1840)***, ***articular branch of nerve to popliteus (>1840)***, and ***medullary branch of nerve to popliteus (>1840)***; see Durward (1951, p. 1109), Hamilton (1976, Fig. 833). Eustachi may have delineated it first; see ***[nerve to popliteus (>1840)] (Eustachi, 1552)***.

EARLIER REFERENCES:

Illustrated, not named or described:

1. ***[nerve to popliteus (>1840)] (Eustachi, 1552)***
   Possibly illustrated for macrodissected adult human; see Albinus edition (1761, Tab. 20-*14*, p. 120).

Illustrated and described, not named:

1. ***[nerve to popliteus (>1840)] (Vieussens, 1684)***
   Clearly identified for macrodissected adult human; Table 29-*103,119*.

Earlier synonyms:

1. *inferior popliteal nerve (Günther, 1786)*
   Synonym for macrodissected adult human ***nerve to popliteus (>1840)***; in the original Latin, *nervus popliteus inferior*, p. 87.
2. *nerve for popliteus muscle (Fischer, 1791)*
   Synonym for macrodissected adult human ***nerve to popliteus (>1840)***; in the original Latin, *nervus pro musculo popliteo*, Table III, Figure 2-*439*. Swan (1830, Pl. XXV, Fig. 1-*25*) specifically used *nerve of popliteal muscle*.

PARTLY CORRESPONDS:

1. *first nerve to popliteus muscle from tibial nerve trunk (Jördens, 1788)*
   First of two components described for macrodissected adult human ***nerve to popliteus (>1840)***; in the original Latin, *nervus musculi poplitei primus ex trunco nervi tibiei*, p. 9 and Table II-*157*.
2. *second nerve to popliteus muscle (Jördens, 1788)*
   Second of two components described for macrodissected adult human ***nerve to popliteus (>1840)***; in the original Latin, *nervus musculi poplitei secundus*; p. 10 and Table III-*160*.
3. *first nerve to popliteus muscle (Fischer, 1791)*
   First component described for macrodissected adult human ***nerve to popliteus (>1840)***, from *nerve trunk to soleus and popliteus muscles and right head of gastrocnemius muscle (Fischer, 1791)*; p. 34.

nerve to quadratus femoris (>1840)

As described for macrodissected adult human, it arises from the fourth and fifth lumbar and first sacral ***sacral plexus ventral divisions (Paterson, 1887)*** and supplies the gemellus inferior and quadratus femoris muscles, and the hip joint via an ***articular branch of nerve to quadratus femoris (>1840)***; see Williams & Warwick (1980, p. 1111), *Terminologia Anatomica* (1998, p. 140). It was known to Galen; see ***[nerve to quadratus femoris (>1840)] (Galen, c177)***.

EARLIER REFERENCES:

Described, not named or illustrated:

1. ***[nerve to quadratus femoris (>1840)] (Galen, c177)***
   Alluded to for macrodissected adult beef, pig, and/or macaque but not human; see Singer translation (1999, p. 85).

Illustrated, not named or described:

1. ***[nerve to quadratus femoris (>1840)] (Eustachi, 1552)***
   Illustrated for macrodissected adult human; see Albinus edition (1761, Tab. 20-*ψ*).

Illustrated and described, not named:

1. ***[nerve to quadratus femoris (>1840)] (Vieussens, 1684)***
   Described and illustrated for macrodissected adult human; Table 29-*27*.

Earlier synonyms:

1. *nerve to quadratus femoris muscle (Fischer, 1791)*
   Synonym for macrodissected adult human ***nerve to quadratus femoris (>1840)***. Fischer's second branch to muscle, for first branch see *common trunk for nerves to gemellus superior, obturator internus, gemellus inferior, and quadratus femoris muscle (Fischer, 1791)*. In the original Latin, *nervum musculi quadrati femoris*, p. 29.
2. *branch of sciatic nerve distributing to quadratus femoris (Meckel, 1817)*
   Synonym for ***nerve to quadratus femoris (>1840)***, described accurately for macrodissected adult human, except for ***articular branch of nerve to quadratus femoris (>1840)***; see translation (1832, Vol. 3, p. 17).
3. *branch to muscles of femoral trochlea (Bock, 1827)*
   Apparently synonym for macrodissected adult human ***nerve to quadratus femoris (>1840)***; in the original Latin, *ram. musculorum trochlearium femoris*, Table IV-*79*.
4. *branch to gemellus and quadratus femoris muscles (Bock, 1827)*
   Synonym for macrodissected adult human ***nerve to quadratus femoris (>1840)***; in the original Latin, *ram. musculorum gemellorum et quadrati femoris*, Table VII, Figure 2-*40*.
5. *nerve of quadratus femoris and gemellus inferior (Cruveilhier, 1836)*
   Synonym for macrodissected adult human ***nerve to quadratus femoris (>1840)***; in the original French, *nerf du carré crural et du jumeau inférieur*, p. 859.

PARTLY CORRESPONDS:

1. *periosteal and osseous external branches of nerve of quadratus femoris and gemellus inferior (Cruveilhier, 1836)*
   Macrodissected adult human branches of ***nerve to quadratus femoris (>1840)*** to region of ischial tuberosity; in the original French, *rameaux externes périostiques et osseux*, p. 859.
2. *gemellus inferior branch of nerve of quadratus femoris and gemellus inferior (Cruveilhier, 1836)*
   Macrodissected adult human branch of ***nerve to quadratus femoris (>1840)*** to gemellus inferior muscle; in the original French, *rameau jumeau inférieur*, p. 859.

nerve to short head of biceps femoris (>1840)

As described for macrodissected adult human, it usually arises from the ***common fibular nerve (>1840)*** segment associated with the ***sciatic nerve (Keill, 1698)***; see Durward (1951, p. 1106 and Fig. 947), Williams & Warwick (1980, p. 1112). It was known to Vesalius; see ***[nerve to short head of biceps femoris (>1840)] (Vesalius, 1543a)***.

EARLIER REFERENCES:

Illustrated and described, not named:

1. ***[nerve to short head of biceps femoris (>1840)] (Vesalius, 1543a)***
   Identified for macrodissected adult human; see Richardson & Carman translation (2002, p. 259).

Earlier synonyms:

1. *branch of exterior branch of sciatic nerve to short head of biceps (Günther, 1786)*
   Synonym for macrodissected adult human ***nerve to short head of biceps femoris (>1840)***; p. 86.
2. *third nerve to short head of biceps muscle (Fischer, 1791)*
   Synonym for macrodissected adult human ***nerve to short head of biceps femoris (>1840)***; in the original Latin, *nervus tertium capitis brevis musculi bicipitis*, p. 30.
3. *branch of sciatic nerve trunk to short head of biceps (Meckel, 1817)*
   Synonym for macrodissected adult human ***nerve to short head of biceps femoris (>1840)***; see translation (1832, Vol. 3, p. 17).
4. *branch of sciatic nerve to short head of biceps muscle (Swan, 1830)*
   Synonym for macrodissected adult human ***nerve to short head of biceps femoris (>1840)***; Plate XXV, Figure 1-*18*.
5. *nerve of short portion of biceps (Cruveilhier, 1836)*
   Synonym for macrodissected adult human ***nerve to short head of biceps femoris (>1840)***; in the original French, *nerf de la courte portion du biceps*, p. 861.

nerve to soleus (>1840)

As described for macrodissected adult human, one or more innervate the soleus muscle as ***muscular branches of tibial nerve (>1840)***; see Durward (1951, p. 1109 and Fig. 950), Williams & Warwick (1980, p. 1113). It was known to Eustachi; see ***[nerve to soleus (>1840)] (Eustachi, 1552)***.

EARLIER REFERENCES:

Illustrated, not named or described:

1. ***[nerve to soleus (>1840)] (Eustachi, 1552)***
   Illustrated for macrodissected adult human; see Albinus edition (1761, Tab. 20/2-*11* combined with 20/1-*D* and 21/1-*G*) and specific reference to *ischiadicorum rami... ad capita exteriora gemellorum*.

Illustrated and described, not named:

1. ***[nerve to soleus (>1840)] (Vieussens, 1684)***
   Described and illustrated for macrodissected adult human; see Table 29-*108,122*.

Earlier synonyms:

1. *nerve to soleus muscle (Fischer, 1791)*
   Synonym for macrodissected adult human ***nerve to soleus (>1840)***; in the original Latin, *nervus ad musculum soleum*, Table IV, Figure 2-*375*.
2. *soleus branch of internal popliteal nerve (Bock, 1827)*
   Synonym for macrodissected adult human ***nerve to soleus (>1840)***; in the original Latin, *ram. solei*, Table IV-*101*.
3. *nerve of soleus (Cruveilhier, 1836)*
   Synonym for macrodissected adult human ***nerve to soleus (>1840)***; in the original French, *nerf du soléaire*, p. 870.

PARTLY CORRESPONDS:

1. *superior nerve to soleus muscle from tibial nerve trunk (Jördens, 1788)*
   Proximal of two components described for macrodissected adult human ***nerve to soleus (>1840)***; in the original Latin, *nervus superior musculi solei ex trunco nervi tibiei*, Table II-*150*.
2. *inferior nerve to soleus muscle (Jördens, 1788)*
   Distal of two components described for macrodissected adult human ***nerve to soleus (>1840)***; in the original Latin, *nervus inferior musculi solei*, Table III-*162*. Jördens identifiedtwo branches of it; Table III-*163,164*.
3. *first nerve to soleus muscle (Fischer, 1791)*
   The first of five components of ***nerve to soleus (>1840)*** described in macrodissected adult human, from trunk of ***tibial nerve (Haase, 1781)***; in the original Latin, *nervum musculi solei primum*, p. 33.
4. *second nerve to soleus muscle (Fischer, 1791)*
   The second of five components of ***nerve to soleus (>1840)*** described in macrodissected adult human, from *common nerve to left head of gastrocnemius muscle, soleus muscle, and tibial communicating nerve (Fischer, 1791)*; p. 34.
5. *third nerve to soleus muscle (Fischer, 1791)*
   The third of five components of ***nerve to soleus (>1840)*** described in macrodissected adult human, from *nerve trunk to soleus and popliteus muscles and right head of gastrocnemius muscle (Fischer, 1791)*; p. 34.
6. *fourth nerve to soleus muscle (Fischer, 1791)*
   The fourth of five components of ***nerve to soleus (>1840)*** described in macrodissected adult human, from *common nerve to soleus and flexor longus of big toe muscles (Fischer, 1791)*; p. 35.

7. *fifth nerve to soleus muscle (Fischer, 1791)*
The last of five components of ***nerve to soleus (>1840)*** described in macrodissected adult human, from trunk of ***tibial nerve (Haase, 1781)***; in the original Latin, *nervum musculi solei quintum*, p. 35.

nerve to tensor tympani (Arnold, 1834)

As described for macrodissected adult human, commonly a branch of the ***medial pterygoid nerve (>1840)*** of the ***mandibular nerve (>1840)***, or less commonly a branch of a common trunk for it and the ***nerve to tensor veli palatini (>1840)***; see Williams & Warwick (1980, p. 1066 and Fig. 7.181). For Arnold's use in macrodissected adult human, see p. 10. It was perhaps first delineated by Le Cat; see ***[nerve to tensor tympani (>1840)] (Le Cat, 1768)***.

TRANSLATIONS:

1. *nervus ad tensorem tympani (Arnold, 1834)*
Original Latin form of ***nerve to tensor tympani (Arnold, 1834)***; p. 10.

EARLIER REFERENCES:

Described, not named or illustrated:

1. ***[nerve to tensor tympani (>1840)] (Le Cat, 1768)***
Beautifully illustrated for macrodissected adult human but misidentified as branch of ***intermediofacial nerve (Strong & Elwyn, 1943)***; Volume 3, Plate VIII, Figure IV-*g,5*. Soemmerring (1806, Tab. II, Fig. XX-*k*) made the same mistake.

Earlier synonyms:

1. *nervus communicans faciei ramus ad musculus tensorem tympani (Günther, 1786)*
Synonym for macrodissected adult human *branch of hard nerve to tensor tympani muscle (Günther, 1786)*; p. 56.
2. *branch of hard nerve to tensor tympani muscle (Günther, 1786)*
Synonym for macrodissected adult human ***nerve to tensor tympani (>1840)***; in the original Latin, *nervus durus r. ad musc. tensorem tympani*, p. 56.
3. *nervus communicans faciei ramus ad musculo Eustachii (Günther, 1786)*
Synonym for *branch of hard nerve to tensor tympani muscle (Günther, 1786)*; p. 56.
4. *branch of hard nerve to Eustachian muscle (Günther, 1786)*
Synonym for macrodissected adult human ***nerve to tensor tympani (>1840)***; in the original Latin, *nervus durus r. ad musc. Eustachii*, p. 56.
5. *branch of facial nerve to internal malleus muscle (Langenbeck, 1826–1830)*
Synonym for macrodissected adult human ***nerve to tensor tympani (>1840)***; in the original Latin, *ramus nervi facialis ad musculum mallei internum*, Fascicle III, Table XXV-*r*. Also see Fascicle III, Table XXVI-*a*.

LATER SYNONYMS:

1. *filament to tensor tympani muscle (Quain & Wilson, 1839)*
Synonym for macrodissected adult human ***nerve to tensor tympani (>1840)***; Plate XIII, Figure 1-*p*.

nerve to tensor veli palatini (>1840)

As described for macrodissected adult human, commonly a branch of the ***medial pterygoid nerve (>1840)*** of the ***mandibular nerve (>1840)***, or less commonly a branch of a common trunk for it and the ***nerve to tensor tympani (Arnold, 1834)***; see Williams & Warwick (1980, p. 1066 and Fig. 7.181). It was probably first clearly described by Wrisberg; see ***[nerve to tensor veli palatini (>1840)] (Wrisberg, 1786)***.

EARLIER REFERENCES:

Described, not named or illustrated:

1. ***[nerve to tensor veli palatini (>1840)] (Wrisberg, 1786)***
Wrisberg described it for macrodissected adult human and mentioned relevant earlier observations; see Wrisberg reprint (1800, pp. 412–413).

Earlier synonyms:

1. *palato-pharyngeal surculus of inferior maxillary branch (Bellingeri, 1818)*
Synonym for macrodissected adult human ***nerve to tensor veli palatini (>1840)***; in the original Latin, *surculus palato-pharyngeus*, see Table I.
2. *nerve of tensoris palati mollis (Arnold, 1834)*
Synonym for macrodissected adult human ***nerve to tensor veli palatini (>1840)***; in the original Latin, *nervus tensoris palati mollis*, Table V:*V-24*.

nerve to tibialis posterior (Cruveilhier, 1836)

As described for macrodissected adult human, it innervates the tibialis posterior muscle and is a branch of the ***nerve to popliteus (>1840)***, in turn a ***muscular branch of tibial nerve (>1840)***; see Durward (1951, p. 1109 and Fig. 950). For Cruveilhier's use in macrodissected adult human, see p. 871. It was perhaps first clearly delineated by Eustachi; see ***[nerve to tibialis posterior (>1840)] (Eustachi, 1552)***.

TRANSLATIONS:

1. *nerf du jambier postérieur (Cruveilhier, 1836)*
Original French version of ***nerve to tibialis posterior (Cruveilhier, 1836)***; p. 871.

EARLIER REFERENCES:

Illustrated, not named or described:

1. ***[nerve to tibialis posterior (>1840)] (Eustachi, 1552)***
Clearly illustrated for macrodissected adult human; see Albinus edition (1761, Tab. 20-*15*).

Illustrated and described, not named:

1. ***[nerve to tibialis posterior (>1840)] (Vieussens, 1684)***
Described and illustrated for macrodissected adult human; see Table 29-*121*.

Earlier synonyms:

1. *branch of tibial nerve to tibialis posterior muscle (Günther, 1786)*
Synonym for macrodissected adult human ***nerve to tibialis posterior (>1840)***; in the original Latin, *r. ad m. tibialem posticum*, p. 87.

PARTLY CORRESPONDS:

1. *first nerve to tibialis posterior muscle (Fischer, 1791)*
A ***nerve to tibialis posterior (>1840)*** from *common nerve to tibialis posterior, flexor digitorum longus, and*

flexor longus of big toe muscles and first internal inferior posterior cutaneous nerve (Fischer, 1791); in the original Latin, *nervum musculi tibialis postici primum*, p. 35.

2. *second nerve to tibialis posterior muscle (Fischer, 1791)* A ***nerve to tibialis posterior (>1840)*** from trunk of macrodissected adult human ***tibial nerve (Haase, 1781)***; in the original Latin, *nervum musculi tibialis postici secundum*, p. 35.

nerves (Herophilus, c335–c280 BC)

Macrodissected bundles of ***neuron extensions (Swanson & Bota, 2010)*** in the ***peripheral nervous system (Meckel, 1817)***. Histologically they include associated glial cells, connective tissue, and vascular cells, especially related to capillaries, in addition to ***neuron extensions (Swanson & Bota, 2010)***. Most ***neuron extensions (Swanson & Bota, 2010)*** in ***nerves (Herophilus, c335–c280 BC)*** are *nerve fibers (Ehrenberg, 1833)*, which are myelinated and unmyelinated ***axons (Kölliker, 1896)***, although many ***nerves (Herophilus, c335–c280 BC)*** contain sensory ***neuron (Waldeyer, 1891)*** peripheral ***neuron extensions (Swanson & Bota, 2010)***, which are ***dendrites (His, 1889)*** based on phylogenetic and developmental analysis. From systems architecture and connectivity perspectives ***nerves (Herophilus, c335–c280 BC)*** are ***peripheral nervous system white matter tracts (>1840)***. In general, the major vertebrate ***nerves (Herophilus, c335–c280 BC)*** are currently named after nearby bones and blood vessels; early on they were referred to by numbers; for example, see Diemerbroeck (1689). In addition, vertebrate ***nerves (Herophilus, c335–c280 BC)*** generally have one or more *central roots* and *peripheral roots*, which do not imply direction of impulse conduction in the component ***neuron extensions (Swanson & Bota, 2010)***. *Central roots* are within the ***central nervous system (Carus, 1814)***, whereas *peripheral roots* are between the external surface of the ***central nervous system (Carus, 1814)*** and either the cranium—for ***cranial nerves (Soemmerring, 1791)***—or a ***spinal nerve trunk (>1840)***—for ***spinal nerves (Camper, 1760–1762)***. For macroscopic descriptive purposes, two topographic divisions, ***cerebrospinal nerves (Herrick, 1915)*** and ***autonomic nerves (Langley, 1898)***, are distinguished.

Herophilus, the founder of human anatomy, is credited with discovering ***nerves (Herophilus, c335–c280 BC)***, including most of the ***cranial nerves (Soemmerring, 1791)*** and ***spinal nerves (Camper, 1760–1762)***; see Solmsen (1961, p. 185), von Staden (1969, pp. 250–252), Longrigg (1993, pp. 192, 211). He was the first person to distinguish both anatomically and functionally between ***nerves (Herophilus, c335–c280 BC)***, tendons, ligaments, and blood vessels; his teacher, Praxagoras of Cos (fl. c.320 BC), thought that arteries transmit pneuma from ***brain (Smith Papyrus, c1700 BC)*** and ***spinal cord (Galen, c162–c166)*** to muscle; see Longrigg (1993, p. 192). In the Hippocratic Corpus (c460–c370 BC), nerves, tendons, ligaments, arteries, and veins were often confused, and the Greek word *neuron* was used for all of them; see Clarke & O'Malley (1996, p. 141). According to Rufus of Ephesus (fl. c90–120), Herophilus also distinguished between sensory and motor ***nerves (Herophilus, c335–c280 BC)***, see von Staden (1989, pp. 250–252), and suggested that ***nerves (Herophilus, c335–c280 BC)*** are hollow for transmitting pneuma—see Clarke (1968), Clarke & O'Malley (1996, pp. 139–144)—a notion Alcmaeon possibly introduced for the ***optic nerve (Vicq d'Azyr, 1786)***. Herophilus dissected animals and human cadavers. Galen mentioned in *The Doctrines of Hippocrates and Plato* (c162–c166) that Erasistratus (c310–c250 BC) first showed that ***nerves (Herophilus, c335–c280 BC)*** arise from the substance of the ***brain (Smith Papyrus, c1700 BC)***, rather than from the ***meninges (Smith Papyrus, c1700 BC)***, see Longrigg (1993, p. 212), and Galen referred specifically to sensory and motor ***nerves (Herophilus, c335–c280 BC)***; see May translation (1968, pp. 453–454). As he explained, "Hippocrates named the nerves collectively from the Greek *tenōn*, which means 'to stretch'. And this name for the nerves is derived from the fact that some individuals believe that the nerve stretches. In Greek, too, the nerves were also called *neura*, which comes from *neuein* and means 'to bend'. The term is used because the limbs of the animal extend and flex themselves in this or that direction primarily by means of the nerves, since it is the nerves alone, when they have joined the muscles and grown into them, which bestow upon them voluntary movement" (Duckworth translation, 1962, p. 185). In one passage, Galen also mentioned in passing that "each of these [ligaments, membranes, and nerves] consists of numerous fibers" (Clarke translation, 1968, p. 124). Based on macrodissection, Vesalius (1543a, p. 633) observed that ***nerves (Herophilus, c335–c280 BC)*** consist of "a thick cord, twisted from many threads" (Clarke & Jacyna translation, 1987, p. 388 note *10*). Coiter first generalized that all ***nerves (Herophilus, c335–c280 BC)*** consist of multiple smaller fibers, stated they consist of *medullary substance (Coiter, 1572)*, and wrote that "the substance of the [spinal] cord must necessarily contribute to the formation of the nerves", noting that the outer substance of the cord is white; Coiter (1572, see translation pp. 113–117). Vicq d'Azyr (1784, p. 508) noted that ***central nervous system gray matter regions (>1840)*** are usually accumulated near the origins of ***nerves (Herophilus, c335–c280 BC)***, and this was amplified by Reil, who wrote that "To me it seems that the origins of nerves are uniformly in the grey matter; that the optic nerve rises from the corpus geniculatum, the third from the black matter [***substantia nigra (Soemmerring, 1791)***], the fifth, seventh, and eighth, from the chamber just described [***pons (Haller, 1747)*** and ***medulla (Winslow, 1733)***], and the spinal nerves from the grey matter in the axis of the spinal chord." (Reil, 1809c; see Mayo translation, 1823, p. 87; also see Meckel, 1832, Vol. 2, p. 167). Meckel (1817) noted that ***nerves (Herophilus, c335–c280 BC)*** are formed by variable numbers of *fasciculi* visible to the naked eye, which in turn are composed of smaller *chords*, which finally are made up of *filaments*; see translation, 1832, Vol. 1, p. 156).

TRANSLATIONS:

1. *neura (Herophilus, c335–c280* **BC***)*
   According to Galen (c177, c192), the Greek term for ***nerves (Herophilus, c335–c280 BC)***—springing from ***brain (Smith Papyrus, c1700 BC)*** and ***spinal cord (Galen, c162–c166)*** and thus clearly distinguished from tendons, ligaments, and blood vessels; see Singer translation (1999, p. 8), Duckworth translation (1962, pp. 185, 186); also see *nerve (Hippocrates)*.
2. *neuris (Herophilus, c335–c280* **BC***)*
   In Greek, ***nerve (Herophilus, c335–c280 BC)*** is *neuris* or *neuron (Hippocrates)*, as noted by Berengario da Carpi (1522); see Lind translation (1959, p. 145).
3. *neuron (Herophilus, c335–c280* **BC***)*
   Singular form of *neura (Herophilus, c335–c280 BC)*, that is, ***nerve (Herophilus, c335–c280 BC)***.

EARLIER REFERENCES:

Earlier synonyms:

1. *channels (Alcmaeon, c490–c430 BC)*
   In *De Sensu*, Aristotle's successor Theophrastus (c327–c287 BC) wrote that Alcmaeon postulated the existence of channels (alternate translations: *passages, ducts*) between most of major sense organs (eyes, ears, nostrils, and probably tongue) and ***brain (Smith Papyrus, c1700 BC)***. It has been claimed that Alcmaeon discovered the first ***nerve (Herophilus, c335–c280 BC)***—*optic nerve (Galen, c173)*—by dissection, but this is far from certain; see Solmsen (1961, pp. 151–152), Lloyd (1975), and *ducts (Aristotle)*.

LATER SYNONYMS:

1. *passages (Herophilus, c335–c280 BC)*
   Galen wrote in *On the Usefulness of the Parts* (c173) that Herophilus called ***nerves (Herophilus, c335–c280 BC)*** "passages" (in Greek, *poroi*; alternate translations: *channels, ducts*) because they alone have a visible passage for pneuma to pass through; see von Staden (1989, p. 318). Herophilus based his statements on macrodissected large mammals and human cadavers.
2. *cords (Rufus of Ephesus (fl. c90–120)*
   Synonym for ***nerves (Herophilus, c335–c280 BC)***; the term itself derives from Hippocrates, who did not distinguish clearly between ***nerves (Herophilus, c335–c280 BC)***, tendons, ligaments, and blood vessels; see May translation (1968, p. 30).
3. *nerves properly so-called (Galen, c173)*
   In *On the Usefulness of the Parts*, used for extensions from ***brain (Smith Papyrus, 1700 BC)*** and ***spinal cord (Galen, c162–c166)*** to distinguish them clearly from tendons, ligaments, and blood vessels; see May translation (1968, pp. 656, 681–683). Also see ***nerves (Herophilus, c335–c280 BC)*** and *neura (Herophilus, c335–c280 BC)*. The term is equally well translated simply *nerves proper*.
4. *sinews (Brunschwig, 1525)*
   Synonym in English for macrodissected adult human ***nerves (Herophilus, c335–c280 BC)***, in the original text spelled either *senewes* (p. [5]) or *senowes* (p. [8]). In Geminus (1553, *The table of the figure of synowes*) spelled *synowes, synnowes*, or *sinowes*; in Hall (1565, p. 6) spelled *synewes* and *synews*.
5. *nervous ropes (Winslow, 1733)*
   Synonym for macrodissected adult human ***nerves (Herophilus, c335–c280 BC)***; Section X, p. 55.
6. *nervous cords (Spurzheim, 1826)*
   Synonym for macrodissected *nervous ropes (Winslow, 1733)* in "the more perfect animals" (p. 1).

PARTLY CORRESPONDS:

1. *nerves (Hippocrates)*
   In this and other contemporary writing, the word "nerve" (*neuron* in Greek) was used indiscriminately for what were later recognized as ***nerve (Herophilus, c335–c280 BC)***, tendon, ligament, artery, and vein; see Clarke & O'Malley (1996, p. 141). In the 4th edition of his *Dictionary*, Blancard (1702, p. 215) wrote under *Nervus*, "A Nerve, a Tendon, and a Ligament are impertinently taken for one and the same thing by Chyrurgeons."
2. *neuron (Hippocrates)*
   Greek translation of *nerve (Hippocrates)*; Singer (1999, p. xix); singular of *neura*. Vesalius (1543a) wrote that *neuron* is derived from the verb *neuein*, "to nod", because it is to nerves that muscles owe their capability of nodding, although this may not be entirely correct; see Richardson & Carman translation (2002, pp. 160, 166).
3. *tenōn (Hippocrates)*
   According to Galen, a term Hippocrates used for ***nerves (Herophilus, c335–c280 BC)***, although they were not clearly distinguished from tendons, ligaments, arteries, and veins; see Duckworth translation (1962, p. 185).
4. *tonos (Hippocrates)*
   See *tenōn (Hippocrates)*. According to Vesalius (1543a) *tonos* is derived from the verb *teinein*, "to stretch" because it is to ***nerves (Herophilus, c335–c280 BC)*** that muscles owe their capability of stretching; see Richardson & Carman translation (2002, p. 160).
5. *roots (Galen, c192)*
   Galen referred to the roots of ***spinal nerves (Camper, 1760–1762)***, and more generally the root of a ***nerve (Herophilus, c335–c280 BC)***, in the following passage, "...the nerves spring out on both sides of [the vertebrae], and the nerve-roots pass out through perfectly rounded foramina, the width of each single foramen corresponding to the thickness of the nerve which passes out through it." (Duckworth translation, 1962, p. 21).
6. *tactile nerves (Anatomia Magistri Nicolai physici, early 12th century)*
   Functional term used in very general way for certain ***nerves (Herophilus, c335–c280 BC)***; see Corner translation (1927, p. 73).
7. *involuntary nerves (Willis, 1664)*
   Willis divided ***nerves (Herophilus, c335–c280 BC)*** into those subserving involuntary functions (including instinctive and emotional) and ultimately deriving from ***cerebellar cortex (Willis, 1664)***, and those

subserving voluntary or spontaneous functions and ultimately deriving from ***cerebral cortex gray matter (>1840)***. In his scheme the ***trigeminal nerve (Winslow, 1733)***, ***abducens nerve (Heister, 1717)***, *facial nerve (Vicq d'Azyr, 1784)*, ***vestibulocochlear nerve (>1840)***, ***glossopharyngeal nerve (Huber, 1744)***, ***vagus nerve (Galen, c192)***, and ***accessory nerve (Vieussens, 1684)***, and ***sympathetic trunk (Winslow, 1733)*** and all ***nerves (Herophilus, c335–c280 BC)*** derived from it, constituted the *involuntary nerves (Willis, 1664)*; see Pordage translation (1681, Chapters 15–18, p. 137) and *voluntary nerves (Willis, 1664)*. One passage is particularly clear, "…some nerves, as it were Clients and Servants of the Brain, perform only spontaneous Acts, and others, Ministers and Servants of the Cerebel, are imployed only about the exercises of the involuntary function." (Pordage translation, 1681, p. 127). The origins of the term *sympathetic system (Langley, 1900)* are found in passages such as, "We have already shewn, that the Nerve of the wandring pair, and others belonging to its family, do serve almost only to the involuntary Function. Wherefore it may be thought, that as there are many shoots and fibres, which going out distinctly from the same origine, are carried to divers parts, that indeed those Bowels and Members, into which these nerves are inserted, do perform their particular actions, stirred up either by the instinct of Nature, or by the force of the Passions, the Animal in the mean time scarce knowing it: yea also, that when certain other nerves, arising afar off, are joyned to this Trunk of the wandring pair, and communicate with it near the very origine of it; this seems to be therefore done, that those nerves, an affinity with the wandring pair being begun, may be drawn into Sympathy with it, and into an unity of action of the involuntary Function." (Pordage translation, 1681, p. 149). Further on he wrote, "For as the nerve of the wandring pair distributes shoots chiefly to the *Praecordia*, and the Stomach, and the intercostal Nerve to the rest of the *Viscera* of the lower Belly; we may observe, that between all these there are not only some commerces, but Sympathies, and a consent of Actions and Passions; wherefore there is a necessity, that the nerves designed to either parts, should communicate among themselves." (Pordage translation, 1681, p. 150). And then he wrote, "…the nerves which are the Executors of the spontaneous, and those of the involuntary Function, might have both a more certain commerce together, and might be sometimes excited into mutual succors. Hence Respiration and some other Acts, especially what concerns the Act of *Venus*, participate of either Regiment, so that sometimes they follow the will, and sometimes draw it even by force or unwilling." (Pordage translation, 1681, p. 161).

8. *voluntary nerves (Willis, 1664)*
Willis divided ***nerves (Herophilus, c335–c280 BC)*** into those subserving involuntary functions and ultimately deriving from ***cerebellar cortex (Willis, 1664)***, and those subserving voluntary or spontaneous functions and ultimately deriving from ***cerebral cortex gray matter (>1840)***. In his scheme the *organ of smell (Willis, 1664)*, *optic nerve (Galen, 173)*, ***oculomotor nerve (Estienne, 1545)***, ***trochlear nerve (Molinetti, 1669)***, and ***hypoglossal nerve (Winslow, 1733)***, and the ***spinal nerves (Camper, 1760–1762)***, constituted voluntary nerves; see Pordage translation (1681, Chapters 15–18, p. 137), also see *involuntary nerves (Willis, 1664)*.
9. *cardiac nerves (Willis, 1664)*
As applied to macrodissected adult human, they included a combination of ***[middle cardiac nerve (Cloquet, 1816] (Willis, 1664)***, *cardiac branch of wandring pair (Willis, 1664)* or ***thoracic cardiac branches of vagus nerve (>1840)***, and ***[inferior cervical cardiac branches of recurrent laryngeal nerve (>1840)] (Willis, 1664)***; see Pordage translation (1681, pp. 147–148, 150–154, 163, 176; and Tab. IX). Willis (1664) claimed that the human heart receives many more fibers from ***sympathetic trunk (Winslow, 1733)*** than from ***vagus nerve (Galen, c192)***, whereas the opposite is true for large mammals he dissected; see Pordage translation (1681, p. 148).
10. *pulmonary nerves (Horne, 1707)*
Combination of macrodissected adult human ***pulmonary branches of vagus nerve (Cloquet, 1828)*** and ***thoracic pulmonary nerves (>1840)***; in the original Latin, *nervi pulmonum*, see *Index rerum*.
11. *ciliary plexus (Meckel, 1748)*
Set of ***communicating branches (Winslow, 1733)*** between macrodissected adult human ***short ciliary nerves (>1840)*** and ***long ciliary nerves (Soemmerring, 1801)***; in the original Latin, *plexum ciliarem*, p. 40. Called *retro-orbital plexus* by Ruskell (1971), who added branches from ***internal carotid nerve (>1840)***.
12. *insulas (Meckel, 1753)*
Latin term for spaces or islands between ***communicating branches (Winslow, 1733)*** of a ***plexus (Galen, c192)***, in this particular instance the ***plexus (Galen, c192)*** in macrodissected adult human formed between ***zygomaticotemporal nerve (>1840)*** and ***infraorbital nerve (Schaarschmidt, 1750)***, which is quite striking in Table 1-*146,147*.
13. *laryngeal plexus (Neubauer, 1772)*
Interaction in macrodissected adult human larynx of branches from ***sympathetic trunk (Winslow, 1773)***, ***superior laryngeal nerve (Loder, 1778)***, and ***recurrent laryngeal nerve (Albinus, 1761)***; in the original Latin, *laryngeus plexus*, p. 65.
14. *mixed nerves (Haase, 1781)****Nerves (Herophilus, c335–c280 BC)*** with clearly distinct multiple origins in macrodissected adult human. The three Haase included in this category were ***accessory nerve (Vieussens, 1684)***, ***phrenic nerve (Galen, c173)***, and ***sympathetic trunk (Winslow, 1733)*** with all its branches; see pp. 35, 49, 114 ff. For the French, Chaussier (1809) gave *nerfs composés*.
15. *highest lateral plexus of neck (Andersch & Soemmerring, 1792)*
As described for macrodissected adult human, possibly laterally directed branches of ***superior cervical ganglion***

(Vieussens, 1684) associated with nearby segments of ***vagus nerve (Galen, c192)*** and ***cervical nerves (Galen, c173)***; in the original Latin, *supremum lateralem plexum colli*, p. 125. The term did not catch on, but see Mitchell (1953, p. 214).

16. *superior lateral plexus of neck (Andersch & Soemmerring, 1792)*
   Synonym for *highest lateral plexus of neck (Andersch & Soemmerring, 1792)*; in the original Latin, *plexus lateralis colli superioris*, p. 180.
17. *posterior layer of superior lateral plexus of neck (Andersch & Soemmerring, 1792)*
   Dorsal layer of *superior lateral plexus of neck (Andersch & Soemmerring, 1792)*; in the original Latin, *stratum posterius plexus lateralis colli superioris*, p. 180.
18. *rete nervorum mollium (Mayer, 1794)*
   A ***plexus (Galen, c192)*** described in macrodissected adult human lying medial to ***superior cervical ganglion (Vieussens, 1684)*** and formed by *soft nerves (Haller, 1762)* and associated branches of ***vagus nerve (Galen, c192)***; Part 6, Table III-8 (p. 18).
19. *network of soft nerves (Mayer, 1794)*
   English form of *rete nervorum mollium (Mayer, 1794)*.
20. *visceral nerves (Johnstone, 1795)*
   Johnstone seemed to use it broadly to include perhaps ***vagus nerve (Galen, c192)***, ***sympathetic trunk (Winslow, 1733)***, and ***paravertebral nerves (Swanson & Bota, 2010)*** in general; p. 97 ff. It was foreshadowed by *involuntary nerves (Willis, 1664)*, which were basically defined as supplying the viscera, and was a forerunner of *nervous system of organic life (Bichat, 1801)*. Its use was revived in modern times by Gaskell around 1886–1889; see Langley (1921, pp. 4–5).
21. *tracheoesophageal plexus (Andersch, 1797)*
   In macrodissected adult human, basically extension of ***esophageal plexus (Haller, 1762)*** rostrally (superiorly) and ventrally (in front) to include trachea; in the original Latin, *plexum tracheooesophageum*, Vol. 2, p. 136.
22. *pharyngeal nerves (Chaussier, 1809)*
   Essentially all ***nerves (Herophilus, c335–c280 BC)*** into ***pharyngeal plexus (Neubauer, 1772)***, from ***glossopharyngeal nerve (Huber, 1744)***, ***vagus nerve (Galen, c192)***, ***cervical plexus (Molinetti, 1675)***, and ***sympathetic trunk (Winslow, 1733)***; in the original French, *nerfs pharyngiens*.
23. *iridic nerves (Chaussier, 1809)*
   Synonym for *ciliary nerves (Chaussier, 1809)*; in the original French, *nerfs iriens*.
24. *ciliary nerves (Chaussier, 1809)*
   For macrodissected adult human, combination of ***short ciliary nerves (>1840)***, ***long ciliary nerves (Soemmerring, 1801)***, and ***sympathetic root of ciliary ganglion (>1840)***; in the original French, *nerfs ciliares*.
25. *gutturo-palatine nerves (Chaussier, 1809)*
   Basically various ***nerves (Herophilus, c335–c280 BC)*** associated with macrodissected adult human ***pterygopalatine ganglion (>1840)***, including ***nerve of pterygoid canal (>1840)***, ***deep petrosal nerve (Meckel, 1817)***, ***pterygopalatine nerves (Wrisberg, 1786)***, ***posterior superior nasal nerves (Soemmerring, 1791)***, and ***palatine nerves (Schaarschmidt, 1750)***; in the original French, *nerfs gutturo-palatins*.
26. *primary nerves (Gordon, 1815)*
   All ***nerves (Herophilus, c335–c280 BC)*** arising directly from ***central nervous system (Monro, 1783)***, as described for macrodissected adult human; p. 195.
27. *secondary nerves (Gordon, 1815)*
   All ***nerves (Herophilus, c335–c280 BC)*** arising directly from a ***plexus (Galen, c192)***, ***ganglion (Galen, c173)***, or larger ***nerve (Herophilus, c335–c280 BC)***, as described for macrodissected adult human; p. 195.
28. *inferior pharyngeal plexus (Bock, 1817)*
   Probably roughly synonymous with macrodissected adult human *laryngeal plexus (Neubauer, 1772)*; in the original Latin, *plexus pharyngeus inferior, sive plexus laryngeus*, p. 69.
29. *simple nerve (Bell, 1826)*
   A ***nerve (Herophilus, c335–c280 BC)*** that is either sensory or motor in function but not both; "a pure or simple nerve has the influence propagated along it in one direction only, and not backwards and forwards; it has no reflected operation or power retrograde; it does not both act from and to the sensorium" (p. 168). This is Cajal's functional (dynamic) polarity hypothesis for whole ***nerves (Herophilus, c335–c280 BC)*** rather than individual ***neurons (Waldeyer, 1891)***. See *compound nerve (Bell, 1826)*.
30. *compound nerve (Bell, 1826)*
   A ***nerve (Herophilus, c335–c280 BC)*** that has both sensory and motor functions; pp. 165–166. Also see *mixed nerves (Haase, 1781)*.
31. *ganglion annulare (Cruveilhier, 1836)*
   Synonym for macrodissected adult human *ciliary plexus (Günther, 1786)*, term attributed without citation to Soemmerring; p. 918.
32. *annulus gangliformis (Cruveilhier, 1836)*
   Synonym for *ganglion annulare (Cruveilhier, 1836)*; p. 918.
33. *laryngeal plexus (Cruveilhier, 1836)*
   For macrodissected adult human, described as meshwork formed by branches of ***external branch of superior laryngeal nerve (Fyfe, 1800)*** and ***superior cardiac nerve (Neubauer, 1772)***, a definition ascribed without citation to Haller; in the original French, *plexus larynge*, p. 959.
34. *pseudoganglion (>1840)*
   Connective tissue thickening of a ***nerve (Herophilus, c335–c280 BC)*** simulating a ***ganglion (Galen, c173)***; see Williams & Warwick (1980, p. 1115), *Dorland's* (2003, p. 1533).

nerves to gastrocnemius (>1840)

As described for macrodissected adult human, they innervate both the medial and lateral heads of the gastrocnemius muscle and are ***muscular branches of***

tibial nerve (>1840); see Durward (1951, p. 1109). They were known to Vesalius; see ***[nerves to gastrocnemius (>1840)] (Vesalius, 1543a)***.

EARLIER REFERENCES:

Illustrated and described, not named:

1. ***[nerves to gastrocnemius (>1840)] (Vesalius, 1543a)***
   Identified for macrodissected adult human; see Richardson & Carman translation (2002, p. 259).

Earlier synonyms:

1. *nerve to gastrocnemius muscle from tibial nerve trunk (Jördens, 1788)*
   Synonym for macrodissected adult human ***nerves to gastrocnemius (>1840)***; in the original Latin, *nervus musculorum gastrocnemiorum ex trunco nervi tibiei*, Table II-151. Jördens described, illustrated, and named five of them; Table II:152–156.

PARTLY CORRESPONDS:

1. *first nerve to right head of gastrocnemius muscle (Fischer, 1791)*
   One of the ***nerves to gastrocnemius (>1840)***, a ventral (anterior) branch of *common nerve to gastrocnemius and plantaris muscles (Fischer, 1791)* to right (presumably lateral) head of gastrocnemius muscle; p. 34.
2. *first nerve to left head of gastrocnemius muscle (Fischer, 1791)*
   One of the ***nerves to gastrocnemius (>1840)***, a branch of *common nerve to left head of gastrocnemius muscle, soleus muscle, and tibial communicating nerve (Fischer, 1791)* to left (presumably medial) head of gastrocnemius muscle, p. 34.
3. *second nerve to right head of gastrocnemius muscle (Fischer, 1791)*
   One of the ***nerves to gastrocnemius (>1840)***, a branch of *nerve trunk to soleus and popliteus muscles and right head of gastrocnemius muscle (Fischer, 1791)* to right (presumably lateral) head of gastrocnemius muscle; p. 34.
4. *internal gastrocnemius branch of internal popliteal nerve (Bock, 1827)*
   Macrodissected adult human ***nerve to gastrocnemius (>1840)*** to medial head; in the original Latin, *ram. gastrocnemii interni*, Table IV-98.
5. *external gastrocnemius branch of internal popliteal nerve (Bock, 1827)*
   Macrodissected adult human ***nerve to gastrocnemius (>1840)*** to lateral head; in the original Latin, *ram. gastrocnemii externi*, Table IV-100.
6. *nerve of internal gastrocnemius (Cruveilhier, 1836)*
   Macrodissected adult human ***nerve to gastrocnemius (>1840)*** to medial head; in the original French, *nerf du jumeau interne*, p. 870.
7. *nerve of external gastrocnemius (Cruveilhier, 1836)*
   Macrodissected adult human ***nerve to gastrocnemius (>1840)*** to lateral head; in the original French, *nerf du jumeau externe*, p. 870.

nervous system (Monro, 1783)

One of the set of body structure-functional systems, like the circulatory system, respiratory system, and digestive system. According to Bullock & Horridge, "A nervous system may be defined as an organized constellation of cells (neurons) specialized for the repeated conduction of an excited state from receptor sites or from other neurons to effectors or to other neurons." (1965, p. 6; also see Brusca & Brusca, 1990, p. 81). The structural organization of connections between these ***neurons (Waldeyer, 1891)***, or more generally nodes, forms a neural network that is described by the wiring diagram of the ***nervous system (Monro, 1783)***. In many animals the ***nervous system (Monro, 1783)*** also contains ***glia (Virchow, 1846)***, and is invaded by the *circulatory system*. It is the chief system integrating adjustments and reactions of the organism to internal and environmental conditions; see *Dorland's* (2003, p. 1843). In all animals with a ***nervous system (Monro, 1783)*** it probably differentiates from the embryonic ectodermal layer; see Brusca & Brusca (1990, p. 103). There are two ways of parceling ***nervous system (Monro, 1783)*** parts (Swanson & Bota, 2010). The first is topographic architecture dealing with topographic divisions created in principle by cutting the organ system with a knife at the gross anatomical level (naked eye resolution) and with supporting structures—***meninges (Smith Papyrus, c1700 BC)*** and ***ventricular-subarachnoid space (Swanson & Bota, 2010)***. The second way of parceling is systems architecture dealing with distinctions between ***gray matter regions (Swanson & Bota, 2010)*** and ***white matter tracts (Bell & Bell, 1826)***, and with connections formed by them at both the gross anatomical and cellular levels. There are no known isolated parts of the adult ***nervous system (Monro, 1783)*** in a particular species; every part is connected to at least one other part. The ***nervous system (Monro, 1783)*** as such was probably first recognized (in writings that survive) by Rufus of Ephesus (fl. c90–120; see Clarke & O'Malley (1996, p. 13). Monro (1783, p. 1) introduced the term as now used; he wrote for macrodissected adult human, "The brain [***cerebrum (Obersteiner & Hill, 1900)***], cerebellum, medulla oblongata, medulla spinalis, and the nerves, with their ganglia, form this [nervous] system." Meckel then divided it into ***central nervous system (Carus, 1814)*** and ***peripheral nervous system (Meckel, 1817)*** for macrodissected adult human, as done now.

EARLIER REFERENCES:

Described, not named or illustrated:

1. ***[nervous system (Monro, 1783)] (Rufus of Ephesus, fl. c90–120)***
   In *On the Names of the Parts of the Human Body*, Rufus clearly viewed for the first time the ***brain (Smith Papyrus, c1700 BC)***, ***spinal cord (Galen, c162–c166)***, and ***craniospinal nerves (Herrick, 1915)*** as an anatomical unit, although he wrote little about its function; see Clarke & O'Malley (1996, p. 13). His work was based on macrodissected adult monkey. For Galen, who macrodissected adult large mammals but not human, the ***[nervous system (Monro, 1783)] (Rufus of Ephesus, fl. c90–120)*** is organized such

that the ***brain (Smith Papyrus, c1700 BC)*** generates the ***spinal cord (Galen, c162–c166)***, which generates the ***nerves (Herophilus, c335–c280 BC)***, as in *The Construction of the Embryo*; Singer (1997, p. 193).

LATER SYNONYMS:

1. *innervation organs (Cloquet, 1828)*
Synonym for macrodissected adult human ***nervous system (Monro, 1783)***; in the original French, *organes de l'innervation*, p. 325.
2. *innervation apparatus (Cruveilhier, 1836)*
Synonym for macrodissected adult human ***nervous system (Monro, 1783)***; in the original French, *appareil de l'innervation*, p. 527.

PARTLY CORRESPONDS:

1. *pairs of nerves from brain (Theophilos Protospatharios, fl. 610–641)*
Compared to *pairs of nerves from brain (Galen, c192)*, Theophilos Protospatharios counted eight rather than seven because he referred to *olfactory sense instrument (Galen, c173)* as first pair; 1540 edition, f. 40v; see Meyer (1971, p. 75). This was the first real break on the topic with Galen, who considered *optic nerves (Galen, c173)* the first pair because they exit the cranial cavity. However, Galen pointed out clearly that other contemporaries counted eight pairs, starting with the olfactory as the first; see *pairs of nerves from skull (Galen, c192)*. Early in the 16th century, Massa (1536; see Lind translation, 1975, p. 240) followed Theophilos Protospatharios's enumeration and wrote, "...although Galen, *On the Use of the Parts IX* was unwilling to call these substances nerves, for if anyone correctly recognizes the instruments of sense-perception I do not know by what other name he may call these substances than nerves. Our question here, however, does not concern names. Let us see whether these substances are similar to the substance of other nerves of sense. Indeed they are in shape, color, and other features since their substance is similar to that of the brain in color and softness, as the optic nerves are also similar as well as those nerves which ascend to the ears...As to their operations these nerves are instruments of the sense of smell as the other nerves are of vision, taste, and hearing...Add further that these nerves pass through two foramina in the basilar bone to the nostrils. They form the first pair of nerves which descend to the nostrils, as you have seen..." Thus, he also apparently observed ***olfactory nerve (Winslow, 1733)***, along with ***olfactory bulb (Weitbrecht, 1751)*** and ***olfactory peduncle (Solly, 1836)***—including all three in *first pair of nerves from brain (Massa, 1536)*.
2. *pairs of nerves from brain (Benedetti, 1502)*
Benedetti had a very idiosyncratic account compared to the seven *pairs of nerves from brain (Galen, c192)*; see Lind translation (1975, pp. 117–118). It was: first pair, *optic nerves (Galen, c173)* and ***oculomotor nerves (Estienne, 1545)*** considered together; second pair, ***vestibulocochlear nerves (>1840)***; third pair, roughly *olfactory peduncles (Solly, 1836)*; fourth pair, roughly ***maxillary nerves (Meckel, 1753)***; fifth pair, roughly ***mandibular nerves (>1840)***; sixth pair, ***spinal cord (Galen, c162–c166)***; and seventh pair, ***glossopharyngeal nerves (Huber, 1744)***, ***vagus nerves (Galen, c192)***, and ***accessory nerves (Vieussens, 1684)*** considered together.
3. *first pair of nerves from brain (Massa, 1536)*
For macrodissected adult human, appears to include right and left ***olfactory nerves (Winslow, 1733)***, along with ***olfactory bulbs (Weitbrecht, 1751)*** and ***olfactory peduncles (Solly, 1836)***; see Lind translation (1975, p. 240), and *pairs of nerves from brain (Theophilos Protospatharios, fl. 610–641)*.
4. *pairs of nerves from brain (Piccolomini, 1586)*
Piccolomini counted eight pairs in macrodissected adult human because, unlike Galen, he included *nerves of smelling (Piccolomini, 1586)* as a *pair of nerves from brain (Piccolomini, 1586)*; see *pairs of nerves from skull (Galen, c192)* and Bartholin (1662, p. 323). He counted *nerves of smelling (Piccolomini, 1586)* as second pair, the *optic nerves (Galen, c173)* as the first pair; p. 262. Also see Soemmerring (1778, p. 73).
5. *pairs of nerves from brain (Bartholin, 1611)*
An account in English of Bartholin's ten pairs for macrodissected adult human is in Bartholin (1662, pp. 138, 323–326): first pair was *olfactory sense instruments (Galen, c173)*; second pair was *optic nerves (Galen, c173)*; third pair was ***oculomotor nerves (Estienne, 1545)***; fourth pair included ***trochlear nerves (Molinetti, 1669)*** and parts of ***trigeminal nerves (Winslow, 1733)*** and *facial nerves (Vicq d'Azyr, 1784)*; fifth pair was mixture of ***trigeminal nerve sensory roots (>1840)*** and ***trigeminal nerve motor roots (Bell, 1829)***, and parts of *facial nerves (Vicq d'Azyr, 1784)*; sixth pair included ***palatine nerves (Schaarschmidt, 1750)***; seventh pair was ***abducens nerves (Heister, 1717)***; eighth pair was mostly ***vestibulocochlear nerves (>1840)***; ninth pair was ***glossopharyngeal nerves (Huber, 1744)***, ***vagus nerves (Galen, c192)***, and ***accessory nerves (Vieussens, 1684)*** considered together; and tenth pair was ***hypoglossal nerves (Winslow, 1733)***. All of them arise from *part within skull of medulla oblongata (Bartholin, 1662)*. For the original description, see Bartholin (1611, p. 399 ff.).
6. *pairs of nerves from brain (Spiegel, 1627)*
Like *pairs of nerves from brain (Piccolomini, 1586)*, Spiegel counted eight pairs for macrodissected adult human, but put the *olfactory sense instruments (Galen, c173)* at the end instead of second; see *pairs of nerves from brain (Piccolomini, 1586)* and *eighth pair of nerves from brain (Spiegel, 1627)*.
7. *sinews proceeding from brain (Read, 1650)*
Read's account had eight pairs for macrodissected adult human; the first seven are basically the same as *pairs of nerves from skull (Galen, c192)*, but his eighth was simply the paired *olfactory sense instrument (Galen, c173)* added on to the end of the list, rather than placed at the beginning; p. 229 ff. This followed *eighth pair of nerves from*

brain (Spiegel, 1627). Also see *pairs of nerves from brain (Piccolomini, 1586)*.

8. *pairs of nerves arising within skull (Willis, 1664)*
Willis's ten pairs for macrodissected adult large mammals including human were as follows: first pair included ***olfactory nerves (Winslow, 1733)***, ***olfactory bulbs (Weitbrecht, 1751)***, and ***olfactory peduncles (Solly, 1836)*** considered together; second pair was *optic nerves (Galen, c173)*; third pair was ***oculomotor nerves (Estienne, 1545)***; fourth pair he named *pathetic nerves (Willis, 1664)*, the ***trochlear nerves (Molinetti, 1669)***; fifth pair, ***trigeminal nerves (Winslow, 1733)***; sixth pair, ***abducens nerves (Heister, 1717)***; seventh pair with two separate pairs, ***vestibulocochlear nerves (>1840)*** and *facial nerves (Vicq d'Azyr, 1784)*; eighth pair, ***glossopharyngeal nerves (Huber, 1744)***, ***vagus nerves (Galen, c192)***, and ***accessory nerves (Vieussens, 1684)*** considered together; ninth pair, ***hypoglossal nerves (Winslow, 1733)***; tenth pair, from first and second ***cervical nerves (Galen, c173)***; see Pordage translation (1681, p. 137 ff., Tabs. 1, 2, and 9-*H*), also see Ridley (1695, p. 142 ff.). Willis wrote that the same basic set of ten *pairs of nerves arising within skull (Willis, 1664)* is found in human and other mammals, birds, and fish, except that fish lack his seventh pair; see Pordage translation (1681, pp. 76, 77). Vesalius used a similar way of referring generally to ***cranial nerves (Soemmerring, 1791)***: "...nerve outgrowths that come forth from the skull" (Richardson & Carman translation, 2001, p. 177).

9. *first pair of nerves arising within skull (Willis, 1664)*
Willis's macrodissected adult human *organ of smell (Willis, 1664)* included *nerve fibers (Ehrenberg, 1833)* passing through right and left parts of the cribriform plate, ***[olfactory nerves (Winslow, 1733)] (Willis, 1664)***, as well as ***olfactory bulb (Weitbrecht, 1751)*** and ***olfactory peduncles (Solly, 1836)***, all three paired parts considered together; see Pordage translation (1681, pp. 137–139).

10. *organ of smell (Willis, 1664)*
Synonym for *first pair of nerves arising within skull (Willis, 1664)*; see Pordage translation (1681, p. 139).

11. *combinationibus nervorum (Molinetti, 1675)*
Molinetti's Latin synonym for macrodissected adult human eight *pairs of nerves arising from brain (Spiegel, 1627)*; p. 188, also see Burdach (1822, pp. 265–266).

12. *pairs of nerves arising within skull (Gibson, 1682)*
Gibson generally followed for macrodissected adult human the ten *pairs of nerves arising within skull (Willis, 1664)*, except for ninth pair he replaced Willis's designation of ***hypoglossal nerve (Winslow, 1733)*** with ***sympathetic trunk (Winslow, 1733)***, and he left off Willis's tenth; he thus had here (p. 330 ff.) a total of nine pairs.

13. *pairs of nerves arising within skull (Gibson, 1684)*
Gibson generally followed for macrodissected adult human the ten *pairs of nerves arising within skull (Willis, 1664)*, except for the ninth pair he replaced Willis's designation of ***hypoglossal nerve (Winslow, 1733)*** with ***sympathetic trunk (Winslow, 1733)***; pp. 374–389.

14. *olfactory nerve (Cowper, 1698)*
It included very clear description of macrodissected adult human ***olfactory peduncle (Solly, 1836)***, ***olfactory bulb (Weitbrecht, 1751)***, and ***olfactory nerve (Winslow, 1733)*** considered together, "The First Pair of Nerves of the Brain, call'd *Par Olfactorium*, they are much Larger in Brutes, and are Hollow; which Hollownesses Communicate with the Ventricles of their Brains, but do not Appear so in Humane Bodies. They are call'd *Processus Mammillares*, from their Appearance in Quadrupedes. By the utmost Scrutiny that Exact Anatomizer of these Parts, Dr. *Ridley* and my Self could make, we never Discover'd but One Original to each of these Nerves; which is from the Under and Foremost Part of the *Crura Medulla Oblongata* [base of the *corpus striatum (Willis, 1664)*], whence they pass in an Oblique Manner for some Space between the Fore and Hindmost Lobes of the Brain, and March from thence as Appears in the Figure: As they pass thro' the *Os Ethmoides* these Medullary Bodies are Converted into as many Nervous *Fasciculi*, as there are Perforations in that Bone, which are afterwards Expanded on the Glandulous Membrane that Invests the *Foramina Narium*." (Appendix Fig. 28-*1*). Around the same time, Jean Mery (1698, p. 25) used the term *olfactory nerve* in the same way, and claimed that postmortem examination of three or four adult humans with an intact sense of smell had the filaments associated with the cribriform plate either hardened or disconnected from the nasal mucosa, whereas a branch of the fifth nerve, the ***trigeminal nerve (Winslow, 1733)***, was intact. From this he concluded that "olfactory nerve" was a misnomer and that the sense of smell is conveyed by the ***trigeminal nerve (Winslow, 1733)***.

15. *pairs of nerves of medulla oblongata (Winslow, 1733)*
Winslow's ten pairs are basically synonymous with macrodissected adult human *pairs of nerves arising within skull (Willis, 1664)*; Section VI, p. 59 ff.; Vicq d'Azyr (1784) also followed this scheme.

16. *nerves of medulla oblongata (Le Cat, 1768)*
Le Cat provided a unique listing of ten pairs for macrodissected adult human; pp. 300–301, illustrated in Plate X. The first six pairs generally correspond to first seven *pairs of nerves arising within skull (Willis, 1664)*. But then his eighth corresponds to ***glossopharyngeal nerve (Huber, 1744)*** and ***vagus nerve (Galen, c192)***, considered together, his ninth was ***hypoglossal nerve (Winslow, 1733)***, and his tenth was ***cranial root of accessory nerve (>1840)***.

17. *nervorum per ossa capitis egredientium (Soemmerring, 1778)*
Soemmerring's account of what was adapted as the ***cranial nerves (Soemmerring, 1791)*** in macrodissected adult human was exceptionally accurate and scholarly. First was *olfactory nerve (Soemmerring, 1778)*, including ***olfactory peduncle (Solly, 1836)*** and ***olfactory bulb (Weitbrecht, 1751)***; second was *optic nerve (Galen, c173)*; third was ***oculomotor nerve (Estienne, 1545)***; fourth was

trochlear nerve (Molinetti, 1669); fifth was ***trigeminal nerve (Winslow, 1733)*** with major [sensory] and minor [motor] parts; sixth was ***abducens nerve (Heister, 1717)***; seventh was *facial nerve (Vicq d'Azyr, 1784)*; eighth was ***vestibulocochlear nerve (>1840)***, ninth was ***glossopharyngeal nerve (Huber, 1744)***; tenth was ***vagus nerve (Galen, c192)***; and 11th was ***hypoglossal nerve (Winslow, 1733)***; he mentioned ***accessory nerve (Vieussens, 1684)*** and illustrated it, but did not fully incorporate it into his enumeration. In addition, he stated that the first eight ***nerves (Herophilus, c335–c280 BC)*** arise from the *encephalon (Soemmerring, 1778)*, and the last four from the *medulla spinalis (Bauhin, 1605)*, which included the ***medulla (Winslow, 1733)*** and ***spinal cord (Galen, c162–c166)***. Nevertheless, Burdach (1822, p. 266) stated that Soemmerring brought the number of cerebral nerves to 12 (which he did in 1791), and noted that Bichat (1801) regarded the first two pairs as arising from *cerebrum (Vesalius, 1543a)*, the next six from ***pons (Haller, 1747)***, and the final four from *medulla spinalis (Bauhin, 1605)*; and that Gordon (1815) thought the first three pairs arise from *cerebrum (Vesalius, 1543a)*, the next five from *cerebellum (Gordon, 1815)*, and the last four from *medulla spinalis (Bauhin, 1605)*.

18. *cranial nerves (Haller & Wrisberg, 1780)*
In a footnote by the distinguished editor, H.A. Wrisberg (p. 195 note 99), the term "cranial nerves" was used explicitly in referring to the work of Soemmerring, Camper, and Mayer in macrodissected adult human, but he did not adopt Soemmerring's scheme and it was not used in the main text. In the same footnote "spinal nerves" were also mentioned, without a numbering system.

19. *cerebral nerves (Haase, 1781)*
For macrodissected adult human, Haase considered nine pairs: first included *olfactory nerves (Soemmerring, 1778)*, second included *optic nerves (Galen, c173)*, third included ***oculomotor nerves (Estienne, 1545)***, fourth included ***trochlear nerves (Molinetti, 1669)***, fifth included ***trigeminal nerves (Winslow, 1733)***, sixth included ***abducens nerves (Heister, 1717)***, seventh included ***vestibulocochlear nerves (>1840)*** and *facial nerves (Vicq d'Azyr, 1784)* considered together, eighth included ***glossopharyngeal nerves (Huber, 1744)*** and ***vagus nerves (Galen, c192)*** considered together, and ninth included ***hypoglossal nerves (Winslow, 1733)***. He considered the ***accessory nerve (Vieussens, 1684)*** a *mixed nerve (Haase, 1781)*, with a *cerebral nerve (Vesalius, 1543a)* component and a ***spinal nerve (Camper, 1760–1762)*** component; in the original Latin, *nervi cerebri*, see pp. 35–43.

20. *cerebral nerves (Malacarne, 1791)*
Malacarne listed 17 pairs for macrodissected adult human; in the original Italian, *N. dell' Encefalo*, p. xix. First included *olfactory nerves (Soemmerring, 1778)*, p. 227; second included *optic nerves (Galen, c173)*, p. 228; third included ***oculomotor nerves (Estienne, 1545)***, pp. 171, 230 and Burdach (1822, p. 391); fourth included right and left *nervus accessorius motorum communium (Palletta, 1784)*, whose identity is unclear, p. 230; fifth included ***trochlear nerves (Molinetti, 1669)***, pp. 172, 230, and Burdach (1822, p. 389); sixth included right and left *nervus accessorius ad patheticum (Palletta, 1784)*, an "accessory trochlear nerve" that has not been confirmed, pp. 174, 231, and Burdach (1822, p. 390); seventh through ninth included three divisions of right and left ***trigeminal nerve (Winslow, 1733)***, pp. 174–186, 232–233; tenth included ***abducens nerves (Heister, 1717)***, p. 234 and Burdach (1822 p. 313); 11th included ***sympathetic trunks (Winslow, 1733)***, p. 234; 12th included ***intermediofacial nerves (Strong & Elwyn, 1943)***, p. 235; 13th included ***vestibulocochlear nerves (>1840)***, pp. 193, 236; 14th included *intermediate sympathetic nerves (Malacarne, 1791)*, corresponding to ***glossopharyngeal nerves (Huber, 1744)*** and ***vagus nerves (Galen, c192)*** considered together, pp. 193, 237; 15th included ***accessory nerve (Vieussens, 1684)***, p. 238 and Burdach (1822, p. 309); 16th included ***hypoglossal nerves (Winslow, 1733)***, pp. 193, 239; and 17th included ***suboccipital nerves (Winslow, 1733)***, pp. 211, 240.

21. *olfactory pair of cranial nerves (Soemmerring, 1791)*
Synonym for macrodissected adult human *first pair of cerebral nerves (Arnold, 1834)*; see Sections 128, 203–272.

22. *olfactory pair of cerebral nerves (Soemmerring, 1791)*
Synonym for *olfactory pair of cranial nerves (Soemmerring, 1791)*; see p. 103 and Sections 203–272. In the original Latin, *par olfactorium nervorum cerebri*, Soemmerring (1798, p. 125).

23. *nervous system of animal life (Bichat, 1801)*
Refers in general to part of ***nervous system (Monro, 1783)*** associated with ***brain (Smith Papyrus, c1700 BC)*** and ***spinal cord (Galen, c162–c166)***, along with ***cranial nerves (Soemmerring, 1791)*** and ***spinal nerves (Camper, 1760–1762)***, mediating voluntary actions; in the original French, *système nerveux de la vie animale*, pp. 115, 168 ff. Compare with *nervous system of organic life (Bichat, 1801)*.

24. *cerebral nerves (Bichat, 1801)*
Only two in Bichat's scheme: ***olfactory nerve (Winslow, 1733)*** and ***optic nerve (Vicq d'Azyr, 1786)***; he listed nine other ***cranial nerves (Soemmerring, 1791)*** as *nerves from tuber annulare and its elongations (Bichat, 1801)*, excluding ***accessory nerve (Vieussens, 1684)***, assigned to *nerves from spinal marrow (Bichat, 1801)*; see translation (1822, Vol. 1, pp. 172–173).

25. *cerebral nervous system (Bichat et al., 1801–1803)*
Synonym for *nervous system of animal life (Bichat, 1801)*, in a volume of the work finished by Buisson after Bichat's death; in the original French, *système nerveux cérébral*, p. 367.

26. *ethmoidal pair of nerves (Burdin, 1803)*
Synonym for macrodissected adult human *olfactory pair of cranial nerves (Soemmerring, 1791)*; see translation (1803, Vol. 1, pp. 143, 167–168).

27. *nerves of head (Gall & Spurzheim, 1810)*
For macrodissected adult human, Gall & Spurzheim listed and discussed 12 in this order: ***accessory nerve***

(Vieussens, 1684), ***hypoglossal nerve (Winslow, 1733)***, *vocal nerve (Gall & Spurzheim, 1810)*, ***glossopharyngeal nerve (Huber, 1744)***, *abductor nerve of eye (Gall & Spurzheim, 1810)*, *facial nerve (Vic d'Azyr, 1784)*, *auditory nerve (Galen, c192)*, ***trigeminal nerve (Winslow, 1733)***, *nerve of superior oblique muscle of eye (Gall & Spurzheim, 1810)*, *common oculomotor nerve (Malacarne, 1791)*, *optic nerve (Galen, c173)*, and *olfactory nerve (Soemmerring, 1778)*. In the original French, *des nerfs de la tête*, p. 66.

28. *nervous matter (Gordon, 1815)*
Gordon described it for macrodissected adult human ***nervous system (Monro, 1783)*** as consisting of *white nervous matter (Gordon, 1815)* and *brown nervous matter (Gordon, 1815)*; p. 120.
29. *cerebral nerves (Gordon, 1815)*
Gordon listed eight pairs for macrodissected adult human and purposefully did not number them: *olfactory nerves (Cowper, 1698)*, ***optic nerves (Vicq d'Azyr, 1786)***, *common oculo-muscular nerves (Chaussier, 1807)*, *internal oculo-muscular nerves (Chaussier, 1807)*, *external oculo-muscular nerves (Winslow, 1733)*, ***trigeminal nerves (Winslow, 1733)***, *facial nerves (Vicq d'Azyr, 1786)*, and *auditory nerves (Galen, c192)*; p. 202 ff.
30. *cerebral proper nerves (Gordon, 1815)*
Three pairs of *cerebral nerves (Gordon, 1815)* arising from *brain proper (Gordon, 1815)*: *olfactory nerves (Cowper, 1698)*, ***optic nerves (Vicq d'Azyr, 1786)***, and *common oculo-muscular nerves (Chaussier, 1807)*; p. 202.
31. *nerves of head (Bell, 1823)*
Synonym for *pairs of nerves arising within skull (Willis, 1664)*, but considered functionally rather than topographically; p. 299. "In our books of Anatomy, the nerves are numbered according to the method of Willis, an arrangement which was made in ignorance of the distinct functions of the nerves, and merely in correspondence with the order of succession in which they appear in dissection." (p. 300). Bell went on to list the functions; pp. 300–301.
32. *nerves of encephalon (Bell, 1834)*
Synonym for *nerves of head (Bell, 1823)*; p. 479, illustrated cleverly in Plate XIX.
33. *nervous masses of phrenic life (Spurzheim, 1826)*
Essentially synonym for vertebrate *nervous system of animal life (Bichat, 1801)*, which Spurzheim claimed is responsible for handling external senses, and affective and intellectual functions; p. 25.
34. *first pair of cerebral nerves (Arnold, 1834)*
Synonym for macrodissected adult human *first pair of nerves arising within skull (Willis, 1664)*, *external root of olfactory nerve (Knox, 1832)*, *middle root of olfactory nerve (Arnold, 1834)*, and *internal root of olfactory nerve (Arnold, 1834)*, considered together; in the original Latin, *par primum nervi cerebralis*, p. 6.
35. *supraoesophageal ganglia (Newport, 1834)*
For the hawkmoth, Newport's *cerebral ganglia (Newport, 1834)*, *anterior lateral ganglia*, and *ganglion of vagus*, considered together; p. 389 and Plate 13, Figure 3.
36. *rachidian nerves (Cruveilhier, 1836)*
Synonym for *cranial nerves (Cruveilhier, 1836)*; in the original French, *nerfs rachidiens*, p. 759.
37. *cranial nerves (Cruveilhier, 1836)*
For macrodissected adult humans, the nine *cerebral nerves (Haase, 1781)*; in the original French, *nerfs crâniens*, pp. 759, 882 ff.
38. *internal portion of fifth pair of nerves (Todd, 1836–1839)*
In macrodissected adult human, ***trigeminal nerve trunk (Winslow, 1733)***, ***trigeminal nerve central sensory root (>1840)***, and ***trigeminal nerve central motor root (>1840)***, considered together; p. 269 ff.
39. *encephalic portion of fifth pair of nerves* (Todd, 1836–1839)
Synonym for *internal portion of fifth pair of nerves (Todd, 1835–1859)*; p. 269.

nervus spinosus (>1840)

As described for macrodissected adult human, the most proximal branch of the ***mandibular nerve trunk (>1840)*** entering the cranium through the foramen spinosum with the middle meningeal artery before dividing into anterior and posterior branches accompanying corresponding branches of the artery. The branches supply mainly ***dura (Galen, c177)*** of the middle cranial fossa, and to a lesser extent of the anterior cranial fossa and calvarium. The posterior branch also sends a twig to mucous lining of the mastoid air cells, and the anterior branch communicates with the ***meningeal branch of maxillary nerve (>1840)***; see Durward (1952, p. 1026), Williams & Warwick (1980, p. 1066 and Fig. 7.181), *Dorland's* (2003, p. 1576 under *r. meningeus nerve mandibularis*). It was probably first identified as the *surculi rami majoris posterioris crassam meningem penetrantes (Vieussens, 1684)*.

EARLIER REFERENCES:

Earlier synonyms:

1. *surculi rami majoris posterioris crassam meningem penetrantes (Vieussens, 1684)*
Probably synonym for macrodissected adult human ***nervus spinosus (>1840)***; p. 172, Table 22-*z*.
2. *meningeal branch of mandibular nerve (>1840)*
Synonym for ***nervus spinosus (>1840)***; see Williams & Warwick (1980, p. 1066), *Terminologia Anatomica* (1998, p. 134) where the Latin form, *ramus meningeus nervus mandibularis*, is given.

neural crest (>1840)

During early vertebrate development, the narrow differentiation of ectoderm lying between ***neural plate (Stricker, 1860)*** medially and somatic ectoderm laterally; among many other things, it eventually generates most of the ***neurons (Waldeyer, 1891)*** in ***peripheral ganglia (>1840)***, although some sensory ***neurons (Waldeyer, 1891)*** of the ***peripheral nervous system (Meckel, 1817)*** are generated by ***neural placodes (>1840)***. It was identified in the embryonic chick as the *dorsal crest of plate (Wagner, 1839)*.

EARLIER REFERENCES:

Earlier synonyms:

1. *dorsal crest of plate (Wagner, 1839)*
Synonym for macrodissected embryonic chick ***neural crest (>1840)***; in the original Latin (plural), *laminarum dorsalium cristas*, Table III, Figures IX, XII-*b*.

Illustrated for macrodissected chick embryo; Table I from a chick embryo younger than 36 hours of incubation; also see Malpighi (1675, Tab. III, Fig. XVI-*B,D*) from a chick embryo of 24–36 hours.

neural folds (>1840)

The right and left halves of the vertebrate ***neural plate (Stricker, 1860)***, lateral to the ***neural groove (>1840)*** in the median plane. They eventually fuse dorsally to form the ***neural tube (Baer, 1837)*** by the process of neurulation; see Williams & Warwick (1980, p. 112). They were illustrated by Serres; see ***[neural folds (>1840)] (Serres, 1824–1826)***.

EARLIER REFERENCES:

Illustrated and described, not named:

1. ***[neural folds (>1840)] (Serres, 1824–1826)***
Illustrated for macrodissected amphibian, bird, mammalian, including human, embryos; Plate I.

Earlier synonyms:

1. *medullary plates (Baer, 1837)*
In macrodissected vertebrate embryo, right and left *medullary plates (Baer, 1837)* form ***neural plate (Stricker, 1860)***, thus synonym for ***neural folds (>1840)***; in the original German, *Markplatten*, p. 104. Also see Sharpey et al. (1867, Fig. 387C-2,3).

neural groove (>1840)

The longitudinal indentation in the dorsal surface of the vertebrate ***neural plate (Stricker, 1860)*** dividing it into symmetrical right and left ***neural folds (>1840)***; see Hamilton & Mossman (1972, pp. 437–441). It was clearly illustrated by Serres, see ***[neural groove (>1840)] (Serres, 1824–1826)***.

EARLIER REFERENCES:

Illustrated and described, not named:

1. ***[neural groove (>1840)] (Serres, 1824–1826)***
Illustrated for macrodissected amphibian, bird, mammalian, including human, embryos; Plate I.

neural placodes (>1840)

Small islands of specialized ectoderm outside the contiguous region of the ***neural plate (Stricker, 1860)*** and ***neural crest (>1840)*** generating ***neurons (Waldeyer, 1891)***; see Schlosser (2006). They were not clearly described by 1840.

neural plate (Stricker, 1860)

The medial differentiation of the embryonic vertebrate ectodermal layer, dorsal to the notochord, going on by the process of neurulation to form the ***neural tube (Baer, 1837)***. For Stricker's use in toad embryo with histology, see p. 474. For Malpighi's discovery see ***[neural plate (Stricker, 1860)] (Malpighi, 1673)***.

EARLIER REFERENCES:

Illustrated and described, not named:

1. ***[neural plate (Stricker, 1860)] (Malpighi, 1673)***

neural tube (Baer, 1837)

The embryonic primordium of the adult ***cerebrospinal axis (Meckel, 1817)*** or vertebrate ***central nervous system (Carus, 1814)*** formed from the ***neural plate (Stricker, 1860)*** by the process of neurulation; see Nieuwenhuys et al. (2008, pp. 7–9). Galen probably glimpsed the macrodissected mammalian ***[neural tube (Baer, 1837] (Galen, c170–c172)*** and Baer (1837, p. 59) introduced the term for macrodissected vertebrate embryos in general. Coiter observed three *transparent globules (Coiter, 1572)* in the 9-day macrodissected chick embryo and Baer called them the three ***primary brain vesicles (Baer, 1837)*** for vertebrates in general.

EARLIER REFERENCES:

Described, not named or illustrated:

1. ***[neural tube (Baer, 1837)] (Galen, c170–c172)***
Galen probably glimpsed and described it in *On Semen*; see De Lacy translation (1992, e.g., p. 93), Adelmann (1966, p. 747).

LATER SYNONYMS:

1. *medullary tube (Baer, 1837)*
Synonym for ***neural tube (Baer, 1837)***; in the original German, *Medullarröhre*, p. 106.

neurohypophysis (Rioch et al., 1940)

As described histologically for adult vertebrate, the ***infundibulum (Rioch et al., 1940)*** and ***posterior lobe of pituitary gland (Haller, 1762)*** considered together; see Holmes & Ball (1974, pp. 5–6), Daniel & Pritchard (1975, p. 4). Developmentally the ***neurohypophysis (Rioch et al., 1940)*** is a ventral and median, ventrally directed extension of the ***periventricular hypothalamic zone (Nauta & Haymaker, 1969)*** and is thus neural tissue, the ***infundibulum (>1840)***. The ***adenohypophysis (Rioch et al., 1940)***, by contrast, develops from Rathke's pouch, and has an ***anterior lobe of pituitary gland (Haller, 1762)*** derived from the rostral wall of the pouch, and an ***intermediate lobe of pituitary gland (>1840)*** derived from the caudal wall and is thus non-neural tissue; see Simmons et al. (1990). For use of ***neurohypophysis (Rioch et al., 1940)*** by Rioch et al. in mammal see Table 2. It was not recognized as such by 1840.

EARLIER REFERENCES:

Earlier synonyms:

1. *neural lobe of hypophysis (Tilney, 1936)*
Synonym for mammalian ***neurohypophysis (Rioch et al., 1940)***; pp. 424–425.
2. *pars nervosa (Tilney, 1936)*
Synonym for *neural lobe of hypophysis (Tilney, 1936)*; p. 425.

nidus (Reil, 1809c)

As described for macrodissected adult human, a depression on the ventral surface of the ***cerebellum (Aristotle)*** lying between the ***uvula (Malacarne, 1776)*** and ***caudal medullary velum (>1840)*** and indicating the location of the ***tonsil (Malacarne, 1776)***; see Clark (1951, Fig. 795 top, labeled *bed of tonsil*), Williams & Warwick (1980, Fig. 7.75, labeled *inferior medullary velum*), *Dorland's* (2003, p. 1264). For Reil's use in macrodissected adult human, see Mayo translation (1823, p. 89). It was perhaps first drawn attention to as the *swallow's nest (Reil, 1807–1808a)*.

EARLIER REFERENCES:

Earlier synonyms:

1. *swallow's nest (Reil, 1807–1808a)*
   Synonym for macrodissected adult human ***nidus (Reil, 1809c)***; see Mayo translation (1822, p. 49).
2. *nidus hirundinus (Reil, 1807–1808c)*
   Latin form of *swallow's nest (Reil, 1807–1808a)*.

LATER SYNONYMS:

1. *nidus avis (>1840)*
   Synonym for macrodisssected adult human ***nidus (Reil, 1809c)***; see *Dorland's* (2003, p. 1264). *Bird's nest* in English.

nodule (Reil, 1807–1808a)

As described for macrodissected adult human, caudal and ventral end of the ***cerebellar vermis (Meckel, 1817)***, lying just rostral to the ***uvula (Malacarne, 1776)***, between right and left ***flocculus (Meckel, 1817)***, and at least partly on the ***caudal medullary velum (>1840)***; see Angevine et al. (1961, Fig. 24), Larsell & Jansen (1972, Fig. 118), Carpenter (1976, Figs. 2.25, 2.26, 14.1), Nieuwenhuys et al. (2008, Fig. 3.8-40). For Reil's use in macrodissected adult human, see Mayo translation (1822, p. 24). It was first clearly delineated as the *laminated tubercle (Malacarne, 1776)*.

EARLIER REFERENCES:

Earlier synonyms:

1. *laminated tubercle (Malacarne, 1776)*
   Synonym for macrodissected adult human ***nodule (Reil, 1807–1808a)***; p. 61, see Clarke & O'Malley translation (1996, p. 645).
2. *tuberculum laminosum (Malacarne, 1776)*
   Latin form of *laminated tubercle (Malacarne, 1776)*; see Burdach (1822, p. 297).
3. *laminated tubercle of fourth ventricle (Chaussier, 1807)*
   Chaussier credited Malacarne, without citation, with this full term for macrodissected adult human *laminated tubercle (Malacarne, 1776)*; p. 103.

LATER SYNONYMS:

1. *head of inferior vermiform process (Gordon, 1815)*
   Synonym for macrodissected adult human ***nodule (Reil, 1807–1808a)***; p. 115. Burdach (1822, p. 297) gave Latin form, *caput processus vermiformis inferioris*.
2. *anterior part of inferior vermiform process (Gordon, 1815)*
   Synonym for macrodissected adult human ***nodule (Reil, 1807–1808a)***; pp. 114–115.

nucleus of solitary tract (>1840)

As described for macrodissected adult human, and for adult mammal in general with cellular architecture and connections, a ***gray matter region (Swanson & Bota, 2010)*** lying dorsomedially in the caudal ***medulla (Winslow, 1733)***, essentially between ***dorsal motor nucleus of vagus nerve (>1840)*** medially and ***dorsal column nuclei (>1840)*** laterally. It is the primary sensory nucleus for taste (rostrally) and visceral sensation (caudally); see Swanson (2004, Tab. B, p. 173), Nieuwenhuys et al. (2008, pp. 193, 705 and Figs. 6.22–24). It was probably first identified as the *tubercula striata (Haller, 1762)*.

EARLIER REFERENCES:

Earlier synonyms:

1. *tubercula striata (Haller, 1762)*
   Synonym for macrodissected adult fish *vagal ganglia (Carus, 1814)*; pp. 594, 596.
2. *vagal ganglia (Carus, 1814)*
   Right and left macrodissected adult fish ***nucleus of solitary tract (>1840)***; in the original German, *Ganglien des Vagus*, Table 2-χ.
3. *gray lanceolate leaves (Desmoulins, 1825)*
   Roughly region in and around macrodissected adult human ***nucleus of solitary tract (>1840)*** on right and left sides; in the original French, *feuilles lancéolées*, pp. 243–244 and Plate XIII, Figures 5-*p*, 12-*p*. Rolando (1825a; Tab. IV, Figs. 2–5; Tab. V, Fig. 2-*b*; Tab. VII, Fig. 1-*f*) indicated it (*feuilles de substance cendrée*) in transverse section and dorsal view of macrodissected adult and juvenile beef, or adult human.
4. *ganglia of pneumogastric nerve (Leuret, 1839)*
   Synonym for macrodissected adult fish *vagal ganglia (Carus, 1814)*; in the original French, *ganglions des nerfs pneumo-gastriques*, p. 142. Leuret also gave synonyms *lobus vagi* and *lobus striatus [tubercula striata]* of Haller, without citation.
5. *vagal lobes (Leuret, 1839)*
   Synonym for macrodissected adult fish *vagal ganglia (Carus, 1814)*; in the original Latin, *lobus vagi*, p. 142.
6. *lobus striatus (Leuret, 1839)*
   Synonym for macrodissected adult fish *tubercula striata (Haller, 1762)*; p. 142.

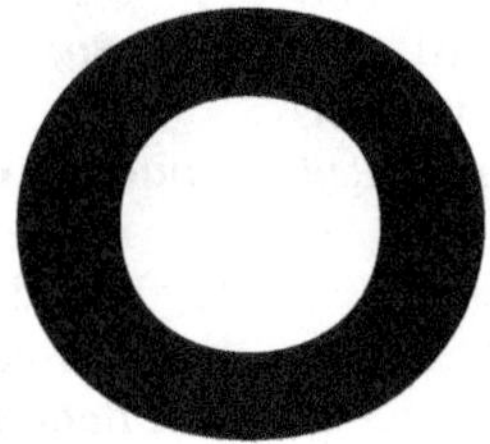

obex (Burdach, 1822)

As described for adult human, a small curved margin forming a landmark at the caudal tip of the ***floor of fourth ventricle (Reil, 1807–1808a)*** just dorsal to the ***area postrema (>1840)***, and covered by ***ependyma (>1840)*** on both sides; see Crosby et al. (1962, Fig. 97), Williams & Warwick (1980, p. 932, Fig. 7.89). For Burdach's use in macrodissected adult human, see p. 77. It was clearly illustrated by Vesalius; see ***[obex (Burdach, 1822)] (Vesalius, 1543a)***.

EARLIER REFERENCES:

Illustrated, not named or described:

1. *[obex (Burdach, 1822)] (Vesalius, 1543a)*
   Very clearly illustrated in macrodissected adult human; see Singer translation (1952, p. 107, Fig. 10-O).

Earlier synonyms:

1. *nib of calamus scriptorius (Vicq d'Azyr, 1786)*
   Basically synonym for macrodissected adult human ***obex (Burdach, 1822)***; in the original French, *le bec de la plume à écrire*; Plate XXX, Figures I-27, III-*a*; also see *calamus scriptorius (Vicq d'Azyr, 1786)*.

LATER SYNONYMS:

1. *commissure between gracile fascicles* (Arnold, 1839)
   Synonym for macrodissected adult human ***obex (Burdach, 1822)***; in the original Latin, *commissura inter fasciculos graciles*, Table XXVII, Figure 5-**.

obturator nerve (Cheselden, 1726)

As described for macrodissected adult human, it arises from the 2nd–4th ***lumbar plexus ventral divisions (Paterson, 1887)*** and divides distally into ***anterior branch of obturator nerve (Haase, 1781; Martin, 1781)*** and ***posterior branch of obturator nerve (Haase, 1781; Martin, 1781)***; see Durward (1951, Fig. 939), Williams & Warwick (1980, p. 1108 and Fig. 7.209). Cheselden indicated it is the common name given to the ***nerve (Herophilus, c335–c280 BC)*** in macrodissected adult human; p. 267, which was essentially written by Monro *primus* as stated in the Preface. It was first described as the *third deep nerve of thigh (Galen, c177)*.

TRANSLATIONS:

1. *nervus obturator (Cheselden, 1726)*
   Original Latin form of ***obturator nerve (Cheselden, 1726)***; p. 267.
2. *nervus obturatorius (Meckel, 1817)*
   Latin form of ***obturator nerve (Cheselden, 1726)***; see translation (1832, Vol. 3, p. 15).

EARLIER REFERENCES:

Earlier synonyms:

1. *third deep nerve of thigh (Galen, c177)*
   Synonym for ***obturator nerve (Cheselden, 1726)*** in macrodissected adult beef, pig, and/or macaque but not human; see Singer translation (1999, p. 84). Also see May translation (1968, p. 707), Duckworth translation (1962, pp. 262–263).
2. *third nerve traveling to thigh (Vesalius, 1543a)*
   Synonym for *third nerve entering leg (Vesalius, 1543a)*; see Richardson & Carman translation (2002, p. 215).
3. *third nerve entering leg (Vesalius, 1543a)*
   Synonym for macrodissected adult human *third deep nerve of thigh (Galen, c177)*; see Richardson & Carman translation (2002, p. 258).
4. *third sinew pertaining to thigh (Geminus, 1553)*
   Synonym for macrodissected adult human *third nerve traveling to thigh (Vesalius, 1543a)*; originally spelled *thyrde synowe parteynyng to thyghe*, see *The table of the figures of synowes*.
5. *third sinew going to leg (Geminus, 1553)*
   Synonym for macrodissected adult human *third nerve entering leg (Vesalius, 1543a)*; originally spelled *thyrde synowe goyng to legge*, see *The table of the figures of synowes*.

LATER SYNONYMS:

1. *posterior crural nerve (Monro, 1732)*
   Synonym for macrodissected adult human ***obturator nerve (Cheselden, 1726)***; p. 30, also see Haase (1781, p. 106). Camper (1762, p. 7) gave the Latin form, *nervus cruralis posterior*.
2. *internal crural nerve (Schmidt, 1794)*
   Synonym for macrodissected adult human ***obturator nerve (Cheselden, 1726)***; in the original Latin, *nervus cruralis internus*, p. 76.
3. *subpubial nerve (Cuvier, 1800)*
   Synonym for macrodissected adult human ***obturator nerve (Cheselden, 1726)***; in the original French, *nerf sous-pubien*, Vol. 2, p. 275.
4. *sub-pubio-femoral nerve (Burdin, 1803)*
   Synonym for macrodissected adult human ***obturator nerve (Cheselden, 1726)***; see translation (1803, Vol. 1, p. 203).

PARTLY CORRESPONDS:

1. *roots of obturator nerve (Walter, 1783)*
   Walter described three roots of ***obturator nerve (Cheselden, 1726)*** arising from 2nd–4th ***lumbar plexus ventral divisions (Paterson, 1887)*** in macrodissected adult human; in the original Latin, *prima, secunda, tertia radix nervi obturarorii*; Table III:*179–183*.
2. *nerve to triceps muscle (Fischer, 1791)*
   Branches of macrodissected adult human ***obturator nerve (Cheselden, 1726)*** apparently to adductor magnus, adductor brevis, and adductor longus muscles identified and inaccurately attributed to ***femoral nerve (Haller, 1762)*** by Winslow (1733, Sect. III, pp. 51, 56); given this name by Fischer, in the original Latin, *nervum musculi tricipitis*, p. 7.
3. *long descending branch of obturator nerve communicating with internal saphenous nerve (Quain & Wilson, 1839)*
   Macrodissected adult human long descending ***communicating branch (Winslow, 1733)*** from ***obturator nerve (Cheselden, 1726)*** to ***saphenous nerve (Haase, 1781)***; Plate XXIII-*k*.

occipital branch of posterior auricular nerve (Arnold, 1834)

As described for macrodissected adult human, a secondary branch of the ***facial nerve trunk (>1840)*** supplying the occipital belly of the occipitofrontalis muscle and extending caudal (posterior) to the ***auricular branch of posterior auricular nerve (Arnold, 1834)***; see Hamilton (1976, Fig. 798). For Arnold's use in macrodissected adult human, see p. 12. It was discovered by Du Verney; see ***[occipital branch of posterior auricular nerve (Arnold, 1834)] (Du Verney, 1683)***.

TRANSLATIONS:

1. *nervus auricularis posterior ramus occipitalis (Arnold, 1834)*
   Original Latin form of ***occipital branch of posterior auricular nerve (Arnold, 1834)***; p. 12.

EARLIER REFERENCES:

Illustrated, not named or described:

1. ***[occipital branch of posterior auricular nerve (Arnold, 1834)] (Du Verney, 1683)***
   Clearly illustrated for macrodissected adult human; Plate 12, Figure 3, extending toward *B*.

Earlier synonyms:

1. *occipital branch of external deep branch of hard nerve (Meckel, 1753)*
   Synonym for macrodissected adult human ***occipital branch of posterior auricular nerve (Arnold, 1834)***; in the original French, *le rameau occipital du rameau profond externe du nerf dur*, p. 75.
2. *occipital branch of hard nerve (Meckel, 1753)*
   Synonym for ***occipital branch of posterior auricular nerve (Arnold, 1834)***; in the original French, *le rameau occipital du dur*, Table 1-*275*.
3. *posterior auricular branch of hard nerve (Bang, 1770)*
   Synonym for macrodissected adult human ***occipital branch of posterior auricular nerve (Arnold, 1834)***; in the original Latin, *auriculari nervi duri posteriori*, Figure I-*38*.
4. *posterior branch of external deep branch of hard nerve (Haase, 1781)*
   Synonym for macrodissected adult human ***occipital branch of posterior auricular nerve (Arnold, 1834)***; p. 81.
5. *posterior branch of auricular portion of hard part of acoustic nerve (Frotscher, 1788)*
   Synonym for macrodissected adult human ***occipital branch of posterior auricular nerve (Arnold, 1834)***; in the original Latin, *auriculari portionis durae nervi acustici posteriori*, see p. 87 of 1795 reprint.
6. *posterior branch of posterior auricular nerve (Meckel, 1817)*
   Synonym for macrodissected adult human ***occipital branch of posterior auricular nerve (Arnold, 1834)***; see translation (1832, Vol. 3, p. 54).
7. *occipital surculus of external deep branch of portio major and minor of facial nerve (Bellingeri, 1818)*
   Synonym for macrodissected adult human ***occipital branch of posterior auricular nerve (Arnold, 1834)***; in the original Latin, *surculus occipitalis*, see Table II.
8. *horizontal filament of posterior auricular branch of facial nerve (Cruveilhier, 1836)*
   Synonym for macrodissected adult human ***occipital branch of posterior auricular nerve (Arnold, 1834)***; in the original French, *filet horizontal*, p. 943.
9. *occipital filament of posterior auricular branch of facial nerve (Cruveilhier, 1836)*
   Synonym for *horizontal filament of posterior auricular branch of facial nerve (Cruveilhier, 1836)*; in the original French, *filet occipital*, p. 943.

occipital forceps (>1840)

As described for macrodissected adult human, extension of the ***splenium of corpus callosum (Burdach, 1822)*** into the region of the ***occipital pole (Broca, 1878a)*** and thus a ***radiation of corpus callosum (Dejerine & Dejerine-Klumpke, 1895)*** in the ***cerebral cortex white matter (>1840)***; see Crosby et al. (1962, Fig. 277, called *posterior forceps*), *Nomina Anatomica* (1983, p. A72), *Terminologia Anatomica* (1998, p. 127), *Dorland's* (2003, p. 726). It was probably first clearly delineated as one of the two *forceps of corpus callosum (Reil, 1809b)*, and first separately named the *radiation of posterior fold of corpus callosum (Reil, 1812c)*.

TRANSLATIONS:

1. *forceps occipitalis (>1840)*
   Current Latin form of ***occipital forceps (>1840)***; see *Terminologia Anatomica* (1998, p. 127).

EARLIER REFERENCES:

Earlier synonyms:

1. *radiation of posterior fold of corpus callosum (Reil, 1812c)*
   Synonym for macrodissected adult human ***occipital forceps (>1840)***; see Mayo translation (1823, Tab. XIII-*y,z*). Also see *posterior fold of corpus callosum (Reil, 1809b)*.
2. *forceps (Arnold, 1838a)*
   Synonym for macrodissected adult human ***occipital forceps (>1840)***; in the original German, *Zange*, p. 77.
3. *forceps major (Arnold, 1838a)*
   Synonym for macrodissected adult human *forceps (Arnold, 1838a)*; in the original German, *grosse Zange*, p. 77.

LATER SYNONYMS:

1. *posterior forceps (>1840)*
   Synonym for macrodissected adult human ***occipital forceps (>1840)***; see Carpenter (1976, p. 26).

PARTLY CORRESPONDS:

1. *fasciculus baseosis interni (Burdach, 1822)*
   A sweep of ***axons (Kölliker, 1896)*** between macrodissected adult human ***corpus callosum (Galen, c177)*** and ***occipital region (Vesalius, 1543a)***, lying deep to ***cuneus (Burdach, 1822)***, so probably component of ***occipital forceps (>1840)***; in the original German, *das innre Grundbündle*, p. 151. See Henle (1871, Fig. 85-*Fep*), Foster (1892, p. 1548).

occipital pole (Broca, 1878a)

As described for macrodissected adult human, the caudal tip of the ***occipital region (Vesalius, 1543a)*** of the ***cerebral cortex gray matter (>1840)***; see Williams & Warwick (1980, p. 982), *Terminologia Anatomica* (1998, p. 125). For Broca's use in macrodissected adult human, see p. 209. Attention was first drawn to it by Vesalius; see ***[occipital pole (Broca, 1878a)] (Vesalius, 1543a)***.

EARLIER REFERENCES:

Illustrated, not named or described:

1. ***[occipital pole (Broca, 1878a)] (Vesalius, 1543a)***
   Indicated and illustrated for macrodissected adult human; see Richardson & Carman translation (2002, figure following p. 263, indicated by *C*).

Earlier synonyms:

1. *occipital horn (Cruveilhier, 1836)*
   Synonym for macrodissected adult human ***occipital pole (>1840)***; in the original French, *corne occipitale*, p. 658.

occipital region (Vesalius, 1543a)

As described for macrodissected adult human, a topographic division of the ***cerebral cortex gray matter (>1840)*** lying caudal to the ***parietal region (>1840)***. Its main parts are the ***lingual gyrus (>1840)*** and ***cuneus (Burdach, 1822)*** on the medial surface of the *cerebral hemisphere (Tiedemann, 1816)*, and the ***superior occipital gyri (>1840)*** and ***inferior occipital gyri (>1840)*** on the lateral surface; for general modern overview see Nieuwenhuys et al. (2008, p. 600 ff.). ***Occipital region (Vesalius, 1543a)*** is preferred to *occipital lobe (Arnold, 1838a)*, because an actual lobe cannot be distinguished and because the term *region* applies to all mammals, whether gyrencephalic or lissencephalic. Vesalius coined this term for macrodissected adult human ***cerebral cortex gray matter (>1840)***, which he first clearly drew attention to, lying under occipital bone; Book 7, Figure 1-*I* and Richardson & Carman translation (2002, part *C* in figure following p. 263). Also see Vicq d'Azyr (1786, Pl. III-*o*), Bell (1802, p. 4 and Pl. XI-*N*), Arnold (1838a, p. 52), and Brodmann (1909, p. 140).

TRANSLATIONS:

1. *occipitij regionis (Vesalius, 1543a)*
   Original Latin form of ***occipital region (Vesalius, 1543a)***; Book 7, Figure 1-*I*.
2. *regio occipitalis (Brodmann, 1909)*
   Latin form of ***occipital region (Vesalius, 1543a)***; p. 140.

EARLIER REFERENCES:

Earlier synonyms:

1. *posterior part of cerebrum (Galen, c177)*
   In *On Anatomical Procedures*, Galen may refer to general region of ***cerebral cortex gray matter (>1840)*** lying over ***cerebellum (Aristotle)***, roughly ***occipital region (Vesalius, 1543a)***; see Clarke & O'Malley (1996, p. 712). However, it is more likely Galen referred in this passage to ***cerebellum (Aristotle)*** itself; see Singer translation (1999, p. 236).

LATER SYNONYMS:

1. *keel of brain (Willis, 1664)*
   Roughly synonymous with ***occipital region (Vesalius, 1543a)*** in macrodissected adult human and other large mammal; see Pordage translation (1681, p. 60).
2. *occipital cerebral lobule (Chaussier, 1807)*
   Synonym for macrodissected adult human ***occipital region (Vesalius, 1543a)***; pp. 37–38; see Burdach (1822, p. 389), Meyer (1971, p. 122).
3. *posterior lobe (Burdach, 1822)*
   Synonym for macrodissected adult human ***occipital region (Vesalius, 1543a)***; p. 175; in the original Latin, *lobus posterior*, and in the original German, *der Hinterlappen*.

4. *occipital lobe (Arnold, 1838a)*
   Synonym for macrodissected adult human ***occipital region (Vesalius, 1543a)***; in the original Latin, *lobus occipitalis*, p. 52.

PARTLY CORRESPONDS:

1. *posterior lobe (Fyfe, 1800)*
   Ventral (inferior) surface or base of macrodissected adult human ***occipital region (Vesalius, 1543a)***; p. 15.
2. *posterior process (Fyfe, 1800)*
   Synonym for *posterior lobe (Fyfe, 1800)*; p. 15.
3. *area occipitalis (Brodmann, 1909)*
   Original Latin form of *occipital area (Brodmann, 1909)*; p. 142.
4. *occipital area (Brodmann, 1909)*
   Based on cellular architecture in adult human, a middle zone of ***occipital region (Vesalius, 1543a)*** between *striate area (Brodmann, 1909)* or *primary visual area (>1840)* caudally and *preoccipital area (Brodmann, 1909)* rostrally. In macrodissected adult human it includes parts of ***lingual gyrus (>1840)***, ***cuneus (Burdach, 1822)***, ***superior occipital gyri (>1840)***, and ***inferior occipital gyri (>1840)***; see Garey translation (1994, p. 120 and Figs. 85, 86).
5. *area 18 (Brodmann, 1909)*
   Synonym for adult human *occipital area (Brodmann, 1909)*; in the original German, *Feld 18*, p. 142. Talbott (1942) referred to it as *visual area 2* in cat based on electrophysiology.
6. *area praeoccipitalis (Brodmann, 1909)*
   Original Latin form of *preoccipital area (Brodmann, 1909)*; p. 142.
7. *preoccipital area (Brodmann, 1909)*
   Based on cellular architecture in adult human, the rostral and outer zone of the ***occipital region (Vesalius, 1543a)***, rostral to and outside the *occipital area (Brodmann, 1909)* or *area 18 (Brodmann, 1909)*. In macrodissected adult human, it includes parts of ***lingual gyrus (>1840)***, ***cuneus (Burdach, 1822)***, ***superior occipital gyri (>1840)***, and ***inferior occipital gyri (>1840)***; see Garey translation (1994, p. 120 and Figs. 85, 86).
8. *area 19 (Brodmann, 1909)*
   Synonym for adult human *preoccipital area (Brodmann, 1909)*; in the original German, *Feld 19*, p. 142.

occipitotemporal sulcus (>1840)

As described for macrodissected adult human, a groove between ***lateral occipitotemporal gyrus (>1840)*** and ***medial occipitotemporal gyrus (>1840)***; see Williams & Warwick (1980, p. 990 and Fig. 7.114A), *Nomina Anatomica* (1983, p. A71), *Terminologia Anatomica* (1998, p. 126). It was first clearly delineated by Vicq d'Azyr; see ***[occipitotemporal sulcus (>1840)] (Vicq d'Azyr, 1786)***.

EARLIER REFERENCES:

Illustrated, not named or described:

1. ***[occipitotemporal sulcus (>1840)] (Vicq d'Azyr, 1786)***
   Illustrated clearly for macrodissected adult human; Plate XVI.

oculomotor nerve (Estienne, 1545)

As described for macrodissected adult human, a ***cranial nerve (Soemmerring, 1791)*** attached to the ventral surface of the ***tegmentum (Swanson, 2000b)*** of the ***midbrain (Baer, 1837)*** and supplying all the extraocular muscles (except superior oblique and lateral rectus), the levator palpebrae superioris muscle, and through the ***branch of oculomotor nerve to ciliary ganglion (>1840)*** the pupillary sphincter and ciliary muscle; see Williams & Warwick (1980, p. 1056). For Estienne's use in macrodissected adult human, see part *C* in plate on p. 236; for an historical review of early research see Zinn (1755, pp. 194–198). It was probably known to Herophilus; see ***[oculomotor nerve (Estienne, 1545)] (Herophilus, c335–c280 BC)***.

TRANSLATIONS:

1. *nervi oculorum motorii (Estienne, 1545)*
   Original plural Latin form of ***oculomotor nerve (Estienne, 1545)***. In Read's account (1638, pp. 411–412), "The second paire is framed of those called *motorii oculorum*, this paire springeth from the innermost part of the beginning of the prolongation of the *spinalis medulla*."

EARLIER REFERENCES:

Described, not named or illustrated:

1. ***[oculomotor nerve (Estienne, 1545)] (Herophilus, c335–c280 BC)***
   Herophilus, the founder of human anatomy, is credited with discovering most of the ***cranial nerves (Soemmerring, 1791)***; see Solmsen (1961), von Staden (1969), Longrigg (1993), and Clarke & O'Malley (1996, p. 261). This included the ***oculomotor nerve (Estienne, 1545)***, which he apparently did not name, in macrodissected adult mammal and human cadavers.

Earlier synonyms:

1. *second pair of nerves from brain (Galen, c173)*
   Roughly synonymous with macrodissected adult pig, beef, and/or macaque but not human ***oculomotor nerves (Estienne, 1545)***. Opinions vary as to whether Galen included ***trochlear nerve (Molinetti, 1669)*** and/or ***abducens nerve (Heister, 1717)*** with his second pair, but on the whole it seems unlikely; see May translation (1968, p. 507), Savage-Smith (1971, p. 87 ff.). Varolio (1573, Fig. I-*c,d* on f. 17v) first showed correctly in print its origin from the ventral ***tegmentum (Swanson, 2000b)***, although Eustachi (1552) illustrated this in plates not published until 1714; see Albinus edition (1744, Pl. XVIII) and Roberts & Tomlinson (1992, Pl. 46).
2. *nerves that move muscles of eyes (Galen, c173)*
   Synonym for *second pair of nerves from brain (Galen, c173)*; see May translation (1968, p. 439), Burdach (1822, p. 390).
3. *third pair of nerves from brain (Theophilos Protospatharios, fl. 610–641)*
   Synonym for ***oculomotor nerves (Estienne, 1545)***; see *pairs of nerves from brain (Theophilos Protospatharios, fl. 610–641)*. Massa (1536) also regarded them as the third pair; see Lind translation (1975, p. 240).

LATER SYNONYMS:

1. *second pair of sinews of brain (Geminus, 1553)*
Synonym for macrodissected adult human *second pair of nerves from brain (Galen, c173)*; originally spelled, *seconde payre of the synowes of the brayne*, see *The table of the figure of synowes.*
2. *nervorum oculosmoventium (Casseri, 1627)*
Variation in Latin on ***oculomotor nerve (Estienne, 1545)*** for macrodissected adult human; see Book X, Table X-G.
3. *eye-mover pair of nerves from brain (Bartholin, 1662)*
Culpeper's form (from original Latin, *motorium oculorum*) of ***oculomotor nerves (Estienne, 1545)*** for macrodissected adult human; p. 325.
4. *combinatio tertia (Molinetti, 1675)*
Latin variation on *third pair of nerves from brain (Theophilos Protospatharios, fl. 610–641)* for macrodissected adult human; p. 188, see Soemmerring (1778, p. 115).
5. *nervi musculares communes (Winslow, 1733)*
Synonym for macrodissected adult human ***oculomotor nerves (Estienne, 1545)***; Section VI, p. 59.
6. *nervi motores oculi (Winslow, 1733)*
Synonym for macrodissected adult human ***oculomotor nerves (Estienne, 1545)***; Section X, p. 47. In Section X, p. 59 it was spelled *nervi motores oculorum*. The singular, *motor oculi*, was given in Section VI, p. 62.
7. *nervi oculares communes (Winslow, 1733)*
Synonym for macrodissected adult human ***oculomotor nerves (Estienne, 1545)***; Section X, p. 47.
8. *nervi oculo-musculares (Winslow, 1733)*
Synonym for macrodissected adult human ***oculomotor nerves (Estienne, 1545)***; Section X, p. 47.
9. *third pair of nerves from medulla oblongata (Winslow, 1733)*
Synonym for macrodissected adult human ***oculomotor nerves (Estienne, 1545)***; see Soemmerring (1778 p. 114).
10. *nervorum motorium opticum (Pietro da Cortona, 1741)*
Synonym Petrioli used for ***oculomotor nerve (Estienne, 1545)***, in explaining tables Pietro da Cortona drew around 1618 but never published; Table XVIII, Figure V-G. See Soemmerring (1778, p. 115).
11. *common motor nerve of eye (Malacarne, 1791)*
Synonym for macrodissected adult human ***oculomotor nerve (Estienne, 1545)***; in the original Italian, *N. motori comuni degli occhi*, p. xxx (Roman 30). Gall & Spurzheim (1810, p. 79) used the French, *nerf oculo-moteur commun*; in English, *common oculomotor nerve*.
12. *third pair of cranial nerves (Soemmerring, 1791)*
Synonym for macrodissected adult human ***oculomotor nerves (Estienne, 1545)***; see ***cranial nerves (Soemmerring, 1791)***.
13. *third pair of cerebral nerves (Soemmerring, 1791)*
Synonym for *third pair of cranial nerves (Soemmerring, 1791)*; see p. 103 and *cerebral nerves (Soemmerring, 1791)*. For original Latin form, *par tertium nervorum cerebri*, see Soemmerring (1798, p. 125).
14. *nervus motorius medius oculi (Andersch, 1797)*
Synonym for macrodissected adult human ***oculomotor nerve (Estienne, 1545)***; p. 1, see Burdach (1822, p. 390).
15. *common oculo-muscular pair of nerves (Burdin, 1803)*
Synonym for macrodissected adult human ***oculomotor nerves (Estienne, 1545)***; see translation (1803, Vol. 1, p. 143). Burdach (1822, p. 390) gave the Latin, *nervus oculomuscularis communis*.
16. *nervus oculomuscularis inferior (Meckel, 1817)*
Synonym for macrodissected adult human ***oculomotor nerve (Estienne, 1545)***; p. 740, see Burdach (1822, p. 390).
17. *nervus oculomuscularis medius (Meckel, 1817)*
Synonym for macrodissected adult human ***oculomotor nerve (Estienne, 1545)***; see translation (1832, Vol. 3, p. 76).
18. *common motor nerve (Meckel, 1817)*
Synonym for macrodissected adult human ***oculomotor nerve (Estienne, 1545)***; see translation (1832, Vol. 3, p. 76).
19. *nervus oculomuscularis communis (Burdach, 1822)*
Synonym for macrodissected adult human ***oculomotor nerve (Estienne, 1545)***; p. 390.
20. *motor nerve of eye (Spurzheim, 1826)*
Synonym for macrodissected adult human ***oculomotor nerve (Estienne, 1545)***; p. 75.

PARTLY CORRESPONDS:

1. *nervus accessorius motorum communium (Palletta, 1784)*
Palletta identified this "accessory oculomotor nerve" in macrodissected adult human (p. 124), as did Malacarne (1791, pp. 171, 230); see Burdach (1822, p. 391), and *nervus accessorius ad patheticum (Palletta, 1784)*. Its identity is unclear.
2. *fourth pair of nerves (Malacarne, 1791)*
Synonym for *nervus accessorius motorum communium (Palletta, 1784)*; see Burdach (1822, p. 391).
3. *cerebral part of third pair (Arnold, 1834)*
Proximal segment of macrodissected adult human ***oculomotor nerve (Estienne, 1545)*** before piercing ***dura (Galen, c177)*** to enter ***cavernous sinus (Winslow, 1733)***; in the original Latin, *par tertium, pars cerebralis*, p. 6. It includes the ***oculomotor nerve root (>1840)***.
4. *cerebral part of oculomotor nerve (Arnold, 1834)*
Synonym for *cerebral part of third pair (Arnold, 1834)*; in the original Latin, *nervus oculomotorius, pars cerebralis*, p. 6.
5. *orbital part of third pair (Arnold, 1834)*
Segment of macrodissected adult human ***oculomotor nerve (Estienne, 1545)*** distal to piercing ***dura (Galen, c177)*** to enter ***cavernous sinus (Winslow, 1733)*** and proximal to splitting into ***oculomotor nerve superior branch (Winslow, 1733)*** and ***oculomotor nerve inferior branch (Haase, 1781)***; in the original Latin, *par tertium, pars orbitalis*, p. 6.
6. *orbital part of oculomotor nerve (Arnold, 1834)*
Synonym for *orbital part of third pair (Arnold, 1834)*; in the original Latin, *nervus oculomotorius, pars orbitalis*, p. 6.

oculomotor nerve central root (>1840)

As described in macrodissected adult human, and mammal generally with histological methods for ***axons (Kölliker, 1896)***, the central root *nerve fibers (Ehrenberg,

1833) of the ***oculomotor nucleus (>1840)*** form bundles coursing ventrally through the ***tegmentum (Swanson, 2000b)*** to its surface; see Strong & Elwyn (1943, p. 247 and Fig. 220), Nieuwenhuys et al. (2008, Fig. 6.31-26, called *oculomotor nerve*). The bundles are ***oculomotor nerve central rootlets (>1840)*** together forming the ***oculomotor nerve central root (>1840)*** that on leaving the ventral surface of the ***tegmentum (Swanson, 2000b)*** at the ***medial midbrain sulcus (>1840)*** becomes the peripheral ***oculomotor nerve root (>1840)***. It was discovered by Vieussens; see ***[oculomotor nerve central root (>1840)] (Vieussens, 1684)***.

EARLIER REFERENCES:

Illustrated and described, not named:

1. ***[oculomotor nerve central root (>1840)] (Vieussens, 1684)***
   Clearly illustrated and described for macrodissected adult human; see Table XIV-*a2* and p. 167.

Earlier synonyms:

1. *roots of motor nerve of eye (Vicq d'Azyr, 1786)*
   Clearly illustrated and described synonym (plural) for macrodissected adult human ***oculomotor nerve central root (>1840)***; Plate XXXI, Figure II-*a* toward *7*. Meckel (1817) traced it to region just ventral to (below) macrodissected adult human ***cerebral aqueduct (>1840)***; see translation (1832, Vol. 3, p. 76). Rolando (1825a, Tab. VIII, Fig. 5-*r.3*) clearly illustrated it for macrodissected adult beef in transverse section.

oculomotor nerve central rootlets (>1840)

As described in macrodissected adult human, and mammal generally with histological methods for ***axons (Kölliker, 1896)***, the central root *nerve fibers (Ehrenberg, 1833)* of the ***oculomotor nucleus (>1840)*** form bundles coursing ventrally through the ***tegmentum (Swanson, 2000b)*** to its surface; see Strong & Elwyn (1943, p. 247 and Fig. 220). The bundles are ***oculomotor nerve central rootlets (>1840)*** together forming the ***oculomotor nerve central root (>1840)***. On leaving the ventral surface of the ***tegmentum (Swanson, 2000b)*** at the ***medial midbrain sulcus (>1840)***, the ***oculomotor nerve central rootlets (>1840)*** become peripheral ***oculomotor nerve rootlets (>1840)***. They were known to Meckel; see ***[oculomotor nerve central rootlets (>1840)] (Meckel, 1817)***.

EARLIER REFERENCES:

Described, not named or illustrated:

1. ***[oculomotor nerve central rootlets (>1840)] (Meckel, 1817)***
   Meckel clearly traced macrodissected adult human ***oculomotor nerve (Estienne, 1545)*** from its emergence on ventral surface of ***tegmentum (Swanson, 2000b)*** to region just ventral to ***cerebral aqueduct (>1840)*** and wrote that in places it forms fasciculi (*rootlets*); see translation (1832, Vol. 3, p. 76).

Earlier synonyms:

1. *real origin of common motor nerve of eye (Cruveilhier, 1836)*
   Synonym for macrodissected adult human ***oculomotor nerve central rootlets (>1840)***, referred to as filaments (*filamens*); in the original French, *origine réelle*, p. 891.

oculomotor nerve inferior branch (Haase, 1781)

As described for macrodissected adult human, the larger of the two main branches of the ***oculomotor nerve (Estienne, 1545)*** generating three smaller branches to three of the extraocular muscles—the ***nerve to medial rectus (>1840)***, ***nerve to inferior rectus (>1840)***, and ***nerve to inferior oblique (>1840)***—with the latter giving off the ***branch of oculomotor nerve to ciliary ganglion (>1840)***; see Williams & Warwick (1980, p. 1057). For Haase's use in macrodissected adult human, including its three branches, see p. 51. It was first delineated by Eustachi; see ***[oculomotor nerve inferior branch (>1840)] (Eustachi, 1552)***.

TRANSLATIONS:

1. *par oculorem motorium ramus inferior (Haase, 1781)*
   Original Latin form (plural referring to pair) of ***oculomotor nerve inferior branch (Haase, 1781)***; p. 51.

EARLIER REFERENCES:

Illustrated, not named or described:

1. ***[oculomotor nerve inferior branch (>1840)] (Eustachi, 1552)***
   Illustrated for macrodissected adult human; Table 18, Figures 1, 3; see Albinus edition (1761), Zinn (1755, p. 196 note *x*).

Described, not named or illustrated:

1. ***[oculomotor nerve inferior branch (>1840)] (Vieussens, 1684)***
   Described for macrodissected adult human; pp. 167– 168, see Zinn (1755, p. 196 note *x*).

Earlier synonyms:

1. *common motor nerve inferior branch (Meckel, 1817)*
   Synonym for macrodissected adult human ***oculomotor nerve inferior branch (>1840)***; see translation (1832, Vol. 3, p. 77).
2. *common motor nerve inferior terminal branch (Cruveilhier, 1836)*
   Synonym for macrodissected adult human ***oculomotor nerve inferior branch (>1840)***; in the original French, *branche terminale inférieure*, p. 906.

oculomotor nerve root (>1840)

As described for macrodissected adult human, the set of multiple ***oculomotor nerve rootlets (>1840)*** condensing distally to form the ***oculomotor nerve trunk (>1840)***; see Durward (1951, p. 1016), Hamilton (1976, p. 617). The ***oculomotor nerve root (>1840)*** lies distal to the ***oculomotor nerve central root (>1840)***. It was first delineated by Du Verney; see ***[oculomotor nerve root (>1840)] (Du Verney, 1683)***.

EARLIER REFERENCES:

Illustrated, not named or described:

1. ***[oculomotor nerve root (>1840)] (Du Verney, 1683)***
   Because Du Verney illustrated ***oculomotor nerve rootlets (>1840)*** he also illustrated this feature of macrodissected adult human; Plate 11, Figure 1-*K*.

Earlier synonyms:

1. *third nerve root (Soemmerring, 1778)*
   Synonym for macrodissected adult human ***oculomotor nerve root (>1840)***; Soemmerring noted that it often consists of a short, anterior root and a long posterior root; see p. 174, Table I-5; and p. 179, Table II-*q,r*.

oculomotor nerve rootlets (>1840)

As described for macrodissected adult human, on emerging from the ventral surface of the ***midbrain (Baer, 1837)*** just medial to the ***cerebral peduncle (Tarin, 1753)***, the ***oculomotor nerve (Estienne, 1545)*** has the form of multiple small fascicles condensing distally into the ***oculomotor nerve trunk (>1840)*** itself, which courses rostrally through the **interpeduncular fossa (>1840)** lateral to the posterior communicating artery; the ***oculomotor nerve rootlets (>1840)*** (multiple small fascicles) together form the ***oculomotor nerve root (>1840)***; see Durward (1951, p. 1016), Hamilton (1976, p. 617). They were first delineated by Du Verney; see ***[oculomotor nerve rootlets (>1840)] (Du Verney, 1683)***.

EARLIER REFERENCES

Illustrated, not named or described:

1. ***[oculomotor nerve rootlets (>1840)] (Du Verney, 1683)***
   Illustrated for macrodissected adult human; Plate 11, Figure 1-*K*.

Earlier synonyms:

1. *root fibers of third nerve (Soemmerring, 1778)*
   Synonym mentioned and illustrated for macrodissected adult human ***oculomotor nerve rootlets (>1840)***; in the original Latin, *nervus tertius...filamenta radicalia*, p. 174, Table I-4.
2. *roots of common motor nerve of eye (Malacarne, 1791)*
   Malacarne mentioned this synonym for ***oculomotor nerve rootlets (>1840)*** in macrodissected adult human and noted they are composed of fibrillae; pp. 227, 229.
3. *radical filaments of third pair (Knox, 1832)*
   Synonym for macrodissected adult human ***oculomotor nerve rootlets (>1840)***; Supplemental Plate I-19.
4. *apparent origin of common motor nerve of eye (Cruveilhier, 1836)*
   Synonym for macrodissected adult human ***oculomotor nerve rootlets (>1840)***; in the original French, *origine apparente*, p. 891.

oculomotor nerve superior branch (Winslow, 1733)

As described for macrodissected adult human, the smaller of the two main branches of the ***oculomotor nerve (Estienne, 1545)*** supplying the superior rectus and levator palpabrae superior muscles; see Williams & Warwick (1980, p. 1057), *Terminologia Anatomica* (1998, p. 133). Winslow described it accurately for macrodissected adult human, referring to a superior branch of motor oculi nerve; Section VI, p. 62. It was known to Eustachi; see ***[oculomotor nerve superior branch (Winslow, 1733)] (Eustachi, 1552)***.

EARLIER REFERENCES:

Illustrated, not named or described:

1. ***[oculomotor nerve superior branch (Winslow, 1733)] (Eustachi, 1552)***
   Illustrated for macrodissected adult human; Table 18, Figures 1, 3; see Albinus edition (1761). Also see Haller (1743, p. 44 note 34), Zinn (1755, p. 196 note *x*).

Described, not named or illustrated:

1. ***[oculomotor nerve superior branch (Winslow, 1733)] (Vieussens, 1684)***
   Described for macrodissected adult human; p. 167, see Zinn (1755, p. 196 note *x*).

Earlier synonyms:

1. *common motor nerve superior branch (Meckel, 1817)*
   Synonym for macrodissected adult human ***oculomotor nerve superior branch (>1840)***; see translation (1832, Vol. 3, p. 77).
2. *common motor nerve superior terminal branch (Cruveilhier, 1836)*
   Synonym for macrodissected adult human ***oculomotor nerve superior branch (>1840)***; in the original French, *branche terminale supérieure*, p. 906.

oculomotor nerve trunk (>1840)

As described for macrodissected adult human, segment of the ***oculomotor nerve (Estienne, 1545)*** between the ***oculomotor nerve root (>1840)*** proximally and the point where the trunk splits into ***oculomotor nerve superior branch (Winslow, 1733)*** and ***oculomotor nerve inferior branch (Haase, 1781)*** distally; see Williams & Warwick (1980, p. 1057). It was known to Galen; see ***[oculomotor nerve trunk (>1840)] (Galen, c192)***.

EARLIER REFERENCES:

Described, not named or illustrated:

1. ***[oculomotor nerve trunk (>1840)] (Galen, c192)***
   Galen alluded to it for macrodissected adult pig, beef, and/or macaque but not human, "Next you find, as the second pair, the two nerves which ramify in the eye-muscles", that is, each ***nerve (Herophilus, c335-c280 BC)*** has a trunk before it branches; see Duckworth translation (1962, p. 8; also see p. 188) and *second pair of nerves from brain (Galen, c173)*. It was illustrated for macrodissected adult (presumably human) by Willis (1664); see Pordage translation (1681, p. 302 Fig. 2-*A*).

Earlier synonyms:

1. *trunk of third pair of nerves (Haller, 1743)*
   Synonym for macrodissected adult human ***oculomotor nerve trunk (>1840)***; in the original Latin, *nervi tertii truncus*, p. 48 note *p*.

PARTLY CORRESPONDS:

1. *communicating twigs between oculomotor nerve and abducens nerve (Langenbeck, 1826-1830)*
   For macrodissected adult human Langenbeck described and illustrated small ***communicating branches (Winslow, 1733)*** between ***oculomotor nerve trunk (>1840)*** and ***abducens nerve trunk (>1840)***; in the original Latin,

surculi communicantes inter nervum oculomotorium et nervum abducentem; Fascicle III, Table XVI-*17*.

oculomotor nucleus (>1840)

As described for vertebrate with cellular architecture and connections, the ***gray matter region (Swanson & Bota, 2010)*** in the ***tegmentum (Swanson, 2000b)*** lying just ventral to the ventromedial corner of the ***periaqueductal gray (>1840)*** and generating the ***oculomotor nerve central rootlets (>1840)*** continuing as the peripheral ***oculomotor nerve rootlets (>1840)***; see Nieuwenhuys et al. (2008, p. 208 and Figs. 6.31, 6.32). It was first identified as the *ganglia of third nerves (Carus, 1814)* on the right and left side.

EARLIER REFERENCES:

Earlier synonyms:

1. *ganglia of third nerves (Carus, 1814)*
   Refers however vaguely to right and left macrodissected adult fish ***oculomotor nucleus (>1840)***; in the original German, *Ganglien des dritten nerven*, p. 140.
2. *ganglia of oculomuscular nerves (Carus, 1814)*
   Synonym for *ganglia of third nerves (Carus, 1814)*; in the original German, *Ganglien des Augenmuskelnerven*, p. 140.

olfactory bulb (Weitbrecht, 1751)

As described with cellular architecture in adult mammal, a part of the ***olfactory region (>1840)*** rostral (distal) to the ***anterior olfactory nucleus (Herrick, 1910)***, and having a ***main olfactory bulb (>1840)*** and usually, though not always, an ***accessory olfactory bulb (>1840)***; see Brodmann (1909, Tab. 7 on p. 247), Shipley et al. (1996). Like all regions or areas of the ***cerebral cortex gray matter (>1840)***, it has underlying ***cerebral cortex white matter (>1840)***—here the distal end of the ***olfactory limb of anterior commissure (>1840)***. Although a swelling on the distal end of the ***olfactory peduncle (Solly, 1836)***, the gross anatomical equivalent of the ***anterior olfactory nucleus (Herrick, 1910)***, had long been described—see *caruncle (Anatomia Magistri Nicolai physici, early 12th century)*]—Weitbrecht first called it a "bulb"; p. 283, see Meyer (1971, p. 75). Belon (1551) noted regression of what is now called the ***olfactory bulb (Weitbrecht, 1751)*** and ***olfactory peduncle (Solly, 1836)*** during development in the dolphin (Cole, 1944, p. 62), and Ray (1671, p. 2277) emphasized their absence in a young porpoise. According to Meyer (1971, p. 76), Santorini (1724) first noted *gray substance (Vesalius, 1543a)* within the ***olfactory bulb (Weitbrecht, 1751)*** specifically, although Collins (1685, p. 1040) identified both *gray substance (Vesalius, 1543a)* and *white substance (Vesalius, 1543a)* in the *mammillary process (Vesalius, 1543a)*—that is, the ***olfactory bulb (Weitbrecht, 1751)*** and ***olfactory peduncle (Solly, 1836)*** considered together—"These Mammillary Processes cannot be truly accounted Nerves, by reason they are not constituted as the Nerves are, of many filaments, mutually conjoyned by thin Membranes, but are only Processes of the Brain, made up of a *Cortex* and a Medullary substance, deriving themselves (not as Nerves) from the *Medulla oblongata* [of Willis] but from the anterior [lateral] Ventricle of the Brain..."

TRANSLATIONS:

1. *Riechkolben (Carus, 1814)*
   German form of macrodissected adult mammalian ***olfactory bulb (Weitbrecht, 1751)***; Table 5-*p*.

EARLIER REFERENCES:

Earlier synonyms:

1. *pap (Anatomia Magistri Nicolai physici, early 12th century)*
   The work refers to macrodissected adult human "nerves", presumably the ***olfactory peduncles (Solly, 1836)***, to the caruncles of the nose, which are spongy and formed like paps; that is, ***olfactory bulbs (Weitbrecht, 1751)***; see Corner translation (1927, p. 72). According to the *Oxford English Dictionary* (Online), *pap* formerly referred to either the breast as a whole, or to the nipple; see *nipple (Haly Abbas or Ali ibn' ul-Abbas, d. 994)* and *mammillary carunculae (Benedetti, 1502)*. Hall (1565, p. 45) wrote that "the organes of smellynge…have at their extreme endes wythin the forheade, at the upper end of the nose…certeine eminences lyke in forme to the tetes or neples of womens brestes," while Du Laurens (1600) explained that they are "processes which are like to the nipples of a woman's paps", or alternately "because they are somewhat like the nipples of a Dugge"; see Crooke translations (1615, pp. 528 and 619, respectively).
2. *caruncle (Anatomia Magistri Nicolai physici, early 12th century)*
   Synonym for *pap (Anatomia Magistri Nicolai physici, early 12th century)*; see Corner translation (1927, p. 72).
3. *heads of instruments of smell (Berengario da Carpi, 1522)*
   Clear reference to macrodissected adult human ***olfactory bulbs (Weitbrecht, 1751)***; see Lind translation (1959, p. 145).
4. *mammillary carunculae (Berengario da Carpi, 1522)*
   Synonym for *heads of instruments of smell (Berengario da Carpi, 1522)*; see Lind translation (1959, p. 145).
5. *extremitas vaccinis papillis similis (Casseri, 1609)*
   Synonym for macrodissected adult ***olfactory bulbs (Weitbrecht, 1751)***; p. 302, see Schreger (1803, p. 332). English form is *nipples like blueberries at end*.
6. *processus papillares (Bartholin, 1611)*
   Synonym for macrodissected adult human ***olfactory bulbs (Weitbrecht, 1751)***, harking back to *pap (Anatomia Magistri Nicolai physici, early 12th century)*; p. 399.
7. *processus mammillares (Bartholin, 1611)*
   Synonym for *processus papillares (Bartholin, 1611)*; p. 399.
8. *vaccarum mammis (Spiegel, 1627)*
   Apparently synonym for macrodissected adult human ***olfactory bulbs (Weitbrecht, 1751)***; p. 329; also see Soemmerring (1778, p. 89). English form is *cow tits*.

9. *teatlike processes (Read, 1638)*
 Synonym for macrodissected adult human ***olfactory bulbs (Weitbrecht, 1751)***; p. 420.
10. *partes papillares (Rolfinck, 1656)*
 Synonym for macrodissected adult human ***olfactory bulbs (Weitbrecht, 1751)***, clearly distinguished from ***olfactory peduncles (Solly, 1836)*** or *nervos odoratorios (Rolfinck, 1656)*; see Meyer (1971, p. 75) and *processus papillares (Bartholin, 1651)*.
11. *dug-like process (Riolan, 1657)*
 Synonym for macrodissected adult human ***olfactory bulb (Weitbrecht, 1751)***; Table 18, Figure 3-*aa*.
12. *knobs of brain (Bartholin, 1662)*
 English form of macrodissected adult human *processus mammillares (Read, 1638)*, the ***olfactory bulbs (Weitbrecht, 1751)***; p. 134.
13. *mammillares (Bartholin, 1662)*
 Synonym by contraction for *processus mammillares (Read, 1638)*; p. 324.
14. *mammillary process (Willis, 1664)*
 Synonym for macrodissected adult mammalian ***olfactory bulb (Weitbrecht, 1751)***; see Pordage translation (1681, pp. 57, 137–139, Figs. II-*D*, V-C, VI-*B*). Distinguished from ***olfactory peduncle (Solly, 1836)***, which Willis called *olfactory nerve (Willis, 1664)*; simply English form of *processus mammillares (Bartholin, 1611)*.
15. *papillary process (Diemerbroeck, 1689)*
 Simply English form of *processus papillares (Bartholin, 1611)* for macrodissected adult human; p. 408.
16. *protuberantia cinereae substantiae similis (Santorini, 1724)*
 Synonym for macrodissected adult human ***olfactory bulb (Weitbrecht, 1751)***; p. 62, see Schreger (1803, p. 332), Burdach (1822, p. 395). Santorini was apparently the first to note *gray substance (Vesalius, 1543a)* specifically in the ***olfactory bulb (Weitbrecht, 51)***; see Meyer (1971, p. 76).

LATER SYNONYMS:

1. *cortical tubercle (Weitbrecht, 1751)*
 Synonym for macrodissected adult human ***olfactory bulb (Weitbrecht, 1751)***; in the original Latin, *tuberculum corticale*, p. 280, see Schreger (1803, p. 332).
2. *bulbum cinereum (Soemmerring, 1778)*
 Synonym for macrodissected adult human ***olfactory bulb (Weitbrecht, 1751)***; p. 88, see Meyer (1971, p. 75) and alternate form on p. 90, *bulbo cinereo*. Wenzel & Wenzel (1812, Tab. XV, Fig. 5-*c*) referred to *bulbus cinereus*.
3. *bulbum cinereum oblongum (Soemmerring, 1778)*
 Synonym for macrodissected adult human ***olfactory bulb (Weitbrecht, 1751)***; p. 173.
4. *head of olfactory nerve (Vicq d'Azyr, 1786)*
 Synonym for macrodissected adult human ***olfactory bulb (Weitbrecht, 1751)***; Plate XX-*10*.
5. *bulb of olfactory nerves (Soemmerring, 1798)*
 Synonym for macrodissected adult human ***olfactory bulb (Weitbrecht, 1751)***, referring to *olfactory nerve (Soemmerring, 1778)*; in the original Latin, *bulbo nervi olfactorii*, p. 213.
6. *ganglion of olfactory nerve (Gall & Spurzheim, 1810)*
 Synonym for macrodissected adult human ***olfactory bulb (Weitbrecht, 1751)***; p. 245. According to Cruveilhier (1836, p. 887), who provided no citation, Malacarne first applied *ganglion* to it.
7. *orbicular eminence (Tiedemann, 1816)*
 Synonym for macrodissected fetal human ***olfactory bulb (Weitbrecht, 1751)***; see translation (1826, p. 45).
8. *olfactory ganglion (Meckel, 1817)*
 English form of Meckel's German term, *Riechganglion* (p. 754), for macrodissected adult human ***olfactory bulb (Weitbrecht, 1751)***. For use in fish see Leuret (1839, p. 139).
9. *olfactory lobe (Serres, 1824–1826)*
 Synonym for ***olfactory bulb (Weitbrecht, 1751)*** in macrodissected bony fish, amphibian, reptile, bird, and mammal—where Serres distinguished it from *cerebral lobe (Serres, 1824–1826)* or *cerebral hemisphere (Serres, 1824–1826)* and thus laid groundwork for concept of *rhinencephalon (Turner, 1891)*; in the original French, *lobe olfactif*, Vol. 2, p. 208 ff.
10. *olfactory lobule (Serres, 1824–1826)*
 Synonym for *olfactory lobe (Serres, 1824–1826)*; in the original French (plural), *lobules olfactifs*; p. 208 ff.; Plate II, Figure 44-*8*.
11. *gray bulb of olfactory nerve (Langenbeck, 1826–1830)*
 Synonym for macrodissected adult human ***olfactory bulb (Weitbrecht, 1751)***; in the original Latin, *nerv. olfactorii bulbus cinereus*, Fascicle I, Table XIII-*f*.
12. *bulbous extremity of olfactory nerve (Swan, 1830)*
 Synonym for macrodissected adult human ***olfactory bulb (Weitbrecht, 1751)***; Plate XI, Figure 1-*1*.
13. *olfactory tubercle (Grant, 1834c)*
 Synonym for ***olfactory bulb (Weitbrecht, 1751)*** in macrodissected adult vertebrate, applied first to fish; p. 547.
14. *ethmoidal bulb (Quain, 1837)*
 Synonym for macrodissected adult human ***olfactory bulb (Weitbrecht, 1751)***; in the original Latin, *bulbus ethmoidalis*, p. 742.
15. *caruncula mammilaris (Arnold, 1838a)*
 Synonym for macrodissected adult human ***olfactory bulb (Weitbrecht, 1751)***; p. 50.

olfactory limb of anterior commissure (>1840)

As described in macrodissected adult human, and mammal generally with histological methods for ***axons (Kölliker, 1896)***, the rostrally directed division of the ***anterior commissure (Lieutaud, 1742)*** interconnecting right and left ***olfactory bulb (Weitbrecht, 1751)*** and ***anterior olfactory nucleus (Herrick, 1910)*** considered together; see Nieuwenhuys et al. (2008, p. 596). It was first identified by Malpighi; see ***[olfactory limb of anterior commissure (>1840)] (Malpighi, 1665)***.

EARLIER REFERENCES:

Described, not named or illustrated:

1. ***[olfactory limb of anterior commissure (>1840)] (Malpighi, 1665)***

Malpighi briefly noted it, "A large fibre bundle has been observed—so far a puzzle to the mind—which courses transversally through the anterior part of the spinal medulla [*striate body (Willis, 1664)* or ***cerebral nuclei (Swanson, 2000a)***], to twine itself densely round like a girdle and finally to terminate in two roots, after it had been carried laterally." (Meyer translation, 1967, p. 187). The two roots are ***olfactory limb of anterior commissure (>1840)*** and ***temporal limb of anterior commissure (>1840)***; see Meyer (1971, p. 14). Malpighi dissected a variety of mammals, including human, but the species used for this observation is unclear.

2. ***[anterior commissure olfactory limb (>1840] (Malacarne, 1780)***
   Malacarne was the first to recognize an association of ***anterior commissure (Lieutaud, 1742)*** specifically with ***olfactory bulb (Weitbrecht, 1751)*** and ***anterior olfactory nucleus (Herrick, 1910)*** considered together; see Burdach (1822, p. 362), Meyer (1971, pp. 25, 109).

Earlier synonyms:

1. *anterior branch of anterior commissure (Reil, 1812a)*
   Reil clearly recognized ***olfactory limb of anterior commissure (>1840)*** in macrodissected adult sheep and rabbit, "In sheep, the anterior commissure, as if composed of two cylinders in apposition, divides at either end into an anterior and posterior branch: the anterior branch bends itself forward at the foremost fasciculus of the fibrous cone [*corona radiata (Reil, 1809b)*] towards the processus mammillaris [***olfactory bulb (Weitbrecht, 1751)***] and its outer wall, and is lost where the latter meets by a narrow opening the anterior horn, in radiated fibres which surround this opening... in the hare a similar organization is seen." (Mayo translation, 1823, p. 110).
2. *commissure of olfactory nerve (Spurzheim, 1826)*
   Synonym for ***olfactory limb of anterior commissure (>1840)*** in macrodissected "animals"; p. 232-31.
3. *real origin of olfactory nerve (Cruveilhier, 1836)*
   Synonym for macrodissected adult human ***olfactory limb of anterior commissure (>1840)***; in the original French, *origine réelle*, pp. 883, 885.
4. *anterior part of anterior commissure (>1840)*
   Synonym for macrodissected adult human ***olfactory limb of anterior commissure (>1840)***; in Latin, *commissura anterior pars anterior*, see *Terminologia Anatomica* (1998, p. 127).

olfactory nerve (Winslow, 1733)

As described for adult human, olfactory ***axons (Kölliker, 1896)*** originate from sensory ***neurons (Waldeyer, 1891)*** in the olfactory mucosa (olfactory Schneiderian membrane) of the nasal cavity, then form criss-crossing bundles before collecting into about 20 branches crossing the cribriform plate of the ethmoid bone in medial and lateral groups before entering the ***olfactory bulb (Weitbrecht, 1751)***, and more specifically the ***main olfactory bulb (>1840)***; see Durward (1951, pp. 1012–1013), Crosby et al. (1962, pp. 413–414), Williams & Warwick (1980, p. 1054). It is a ***cranial nerve (Soemmerring, 1791)***, usually considered along with the ***terminal nerve (>1840)*** and ***vomeronasal nerve (>1840)***. Winslow defined the macrodissected adult human ***olfactory nerve (Winslow, 1733)*** as filaments "which run down through the holes of the transverse lamina [cribriform plate] of the os ethmnoides, and are distributed to the common membrane of the internal nares" (Sect. X, p. 101; also see Sect. X, p. 46). Vicq d'Azyr (1784, p. 552) pointed out that there is some similarity between the olfactory mucosa and ***retina (Herophilus, c335–c280 BC)***. The ***olfactory nerve (Winslow, 1733)*** enters the **main olfactory bulb (>1840)** and the ends of the ***axons (Kölliker, 1896)*** course through the ***olfactory nerve layer of main olfactory bulb (>1840)*** terminating in glomeruli of the subjacent ***glomerular layer of main olfactory bulb (>1840)***; there is thus a very short *olfactory nerve central root (>1840)* in the outer part of the ***main olfactory bulb (>1840)***; for adult human, see Crosby et al. (1962, pp. 414–416). Also see *organ of smell (Willis, 1664)* and *olfactory nerve (Cowper, 1698)*. The ***olfactory nerve (Winslow, 1733)*** was postulated and perhaps observed long ago; see ***[olfactory nerve (Winslow, 1733)] (Alcmaeon, c490–c430 BC)***, ***[olfactory nerve (Winslow, 1733)] (Erasistratus, c310–c250 BC)***.

TRANSLATIONS:

1. *nervi olfactorii (Winslow, 1733)*
   Original Latin form of right and left ***olfactory nerve (Winslow, 1733)***; Section X, p. 101; also see Section X, p. 46.

EARLIER REFERENCES:

Described, not named or illustrated:

1. ***[olfactory nerve (Winslow, 1733)] (Alcmaeon, c490–c430 BC)***
   In *De Sensu*, Aristotle's successor, Theophrastus (c327–c287 BC), wrote that Alcmaeon postulated the existence of a channel, passage, or duct between nostrils and ***brain (Smith Papyrus, c1700 BC)***; see Solmsen (1961, pp. 151–152), Lloyd (1975, pp. 122–125).
2. ***[olfactory nerve (Winslow, 1733)] (Erasistratus, c310–c250 BC)***
   In *The Doctrines of Hippocrates and Plato* (c169–c176), Galen quoted from a now lost book of Erasistratus, "the sensory channels from the nostrils opened onto it [the ***brain (Smith Papyrus, c1700 BC)***]" (see Longrigg, 1998, p. 93). Erasistratus dissected animals and human cadavers.
3. ***[olfactory nerve (Winslow, 1733)] (Massa, 1536)***
   Apparently observed in macrodissected adult human; see Lind translation (1975, p. 240), and *pairs of nerves from brain (Theophilos Protospatharios, fl. 610–641)*.
4. ***[olfactory nerve (Winslow, 1733)] (Vesalius, 1543a)***
   Vesalius seemed clearly to refer to it in macrodissected adult human, "...have a view of the sinuses

of the olfactory organs [***olfactory bulb (Weitbrecht, 1751)***, along perhaps with the *olfactory peduncle (Solly, 1836)*], perforated by little foramina through which nerves everywhere emerge [foramina of cribriform plate of ethmoid bone]" (Singer translation, 1952, p. 71). Diemerbroeck (1689, p. 409) explicitly denied this observation.

5. ***[olfactory nerve (Winslow, 1733)] (Willis, 1664)***
Willis wrote "manifold nerve fibers pass through every one of its [cribriform plate of ethmoid bone] pores" (see Pordage translation, 1681, p. 100), and they go from the ***olfactory bulb (Weitbrecht, 1751)***, or *mammillary process (Willis, 1664)*, to the membrane of the nasal cavity for in effect the reception of odorants; see Pordage translation (1681, pp. 100, 137). Willis referred to the fascicles passing through the cribriform plate as *nervulets*, *filaments*, and *little strings*, and wrote that they are more numerous in hunting dogs than any other animal; see Pordage translation (1681, p. 139).

LATER SYNONYMS:

1. *nerve filaments of first pair (Scarpa, 1785)*
Synonym for macrodissected adult human ***olfactory nerves (Winslow, 1733)***; in the original Latin, *filamenta nervea paris primi*, Table I, Figure 1:*m-p*. Scarpa divided them into a number of groups, including anterior, middle, and posterior, and a long branch (Tab. I, Fig. I:*m-q*), as well as others (Tab. II, Fig. II, Fig. II:**,*g-m*).
2. *olfactory nerve fibers (Carus, 1814)*
Synonym for macrodissected adult mammalian ***olfactory nerve (Winslow, 1733)***; in the original German, *Riechnervenfäden*, p. 257. See Meyer (1971, p. 78).
3. *branches of olfactory nerve (Swan, 1830)*
Synonym for macrodissected adult human ***olfactory nerve (Winslow, 1733)***; Plate XI, Figure 2-*1*.
4. *olfactory nerves proper (Cruveilhier, 1836)*
Synonym for macrodissected adult mammalian ***olfactory nerves (Winslow, 1733)***; in the original French, *nerfs olfactifs proprement dits*, p. 887.

PARTLY CORRESPONDS:

1. *internal branches of olfactory nerves (Langenbeck, 1826–1830)*
Macrodissected adult human medial branches (fila) of ***olfactory nerve (Winslow, 1733)***; in the original Latin, *rami interni nervorum olfactoriorum*, Fascicle III, Table XXI-*1*.
2. *external branches of olfactory nerves (Langenbeck, 1826–1830)*
Macrodissected adult human lateral branches (fila) of ***olfactory nerve (Winslow, 1733)***; in the original Latin, *rami externi nervorum olfactoriorum*, Fascicle III, Table XXII-2.

olfactory nerve layer of main olfactory bulb (>1840)

As described for adult mammal, the outermost layer of the ***main olfactory bulb (>1840)*** containing the distal end of the ***olfactory nerve (Winslow, 1733)*** before it terminates in the subjacent ***glomerular layer of main olfactory bulb (>1840)***; see Williams & Warwick (1980, Fig. 7.118), Shipley et al. (1996, pp. 474–475), Nieuwenhuys et al. (2008, Fig. 11.4). It corresponds to most of the *olfactory nerve central root (>1840)* and was not clearly differentiated by 1840.

EARLIER REFERENCES:

Earlier synonyms:

1. *stratum of olfactory nerves of bulbus olfactorius (Meynert, 1872)*
Synonym for macrodissected adult human ***olfactory nerve layer of main olfactory bulb (>1840)***; see translation p. 672, Figure 262.

LATER SYNONYMS:

1. *olfactory nerve central root (>1840)*
Basically synonym for macrodissected adult mammalian ***olfactory nerve layer of main olfactory bulb (>1840)***, although ***axon terminals (Barker, 1899)*** of the ***olfactory nerve (Winslow, 1733)*** extend slightly deeper to end in the subjacent ***glomerular layer of main olfactory bulb (>1840)***; see Williams & Warwick (1980, Fig. 7.118), Shipley et al. (1996, pp. 474–475), Nieuwenhuys et al. (2008, Fig. 11.4).

olfactory peduncle (Solly, 1836)

As described for macrodissected adult human, a topographic subdivision of the ***cerebral cortex (>1840)*** forming a rostrally directed cylindrical stalk just proximal to the ***olfactory bulb (Weitbrecht, 1751)*** and just distal to the ***ambient gyrus (>1840)***; in the center is an obliterated ***olfactory ventricle (>1840)***. From a cellular architecture and connections perspective in mammal, it includes the ***anterior olfactory nucleus (Herrick, 1910)*** and adjacent segment of the ***lateral olfactory tract (>1840)***, and either an open or obliterated ***olfactory ventricle (>1840)*** with accompanying ***subependymal zone (>1840)***. Belon (1551) noted regression of the ***olfactory bulb (Weitbrecht, 1751)*** and ***olfactory peduncle (Solly, 1836)*** during development in the dolphin (see Cole, 1944, p. 62), and Ray (1671, p. 2277) emphasized their absence in a young porpoise. For Solly's use in macrodissected adult vertebrate, including human, see pp. 80, 86, 241. It was delineated separately as the *par olfactorium (Bartholin, 1611)*.

EARLIER REFERENCES:

Earlier synonyms:

1. *par olfactorium (Bartholin, 1611)*
The smelling pair, whose processes or ends are called *processes mammillares (Bartholin, 1611)*; p. 324. Synonym for macrodissected adult human *olfactory nerves (Bartholin, 1611)* or ***olfactory peduncles (Solly, 1836)***.
2. *olfactory nerve (Bartholin, 1611)*
Synonym for macrodissected adult human ***olfactory peduncle (Solly, 1836)***; p. 399. Labeled thus in later edition by his son (Bartholin, 1751, Book III, Tab. I-*A*) as opposed to ***olfactory bulb (Weitbrecht, 1751)***, which he called *processus papillares (Bartholin,*

1611)—p. 399; and Bartholin, 1651, Book III, Table I-*b*, p. 459—or *processus mammillares (Bartholin, 1611).*

3. *nervos odoratorios (Rolfinck, 1656)*
   Synonym for macrodissected adult human ***olfactory peduncles (Solly, 1836)***. Rolfinck noted it has gray and white stripes, vague reference to ***anterior olfactory nucleus (Herrick, 1910)*** and accompanying segment of ***lateral olfactory tract (>1840)***, respectively; see Meyer (1971, p. 76).
4. *smelling nerve (Bartholin, 1662)*
   Culpeper's English form of *olfactory nerve (Bartholin, 1611)*; p. 324.
5. *medullary rope (Winslow, 1733)*
   Synonym for macrodissected adult human ***olfactory peduncle (Solly, 1836)***; Section X, p. 46.
6. *trunk of olfactory nerve (Scarpa, 1785)*
   Synonym for macrodissected adult human ***olfactory peduncle (Solly, 1836)***; in the original Latin, *truncus olfactorii nervi*, Table II, Figure 3-*p*.
7. *olfactory tract (Burdach, 1822)*
   Synonym for macrodissected adult human ***olfactory peduncle (Solly, 1836)***; p. 179, still often used in this way; see Williams & Warwick (1980, p. 994); in the original Latin, *tractus olfactorius*, and the original German, *Riechstreifen*. Burdach also noted it was referred to in recent times as *der Stamm* [*stalk, stem, trunk*] *des Nerven*; p. 394.
8. *olfactory stalk (Burdach, 1822)*
   English synonym for *olfactory tract (Burdach, 1822)*; original German form, *Stamm*, p. 394. Derived from *trunk of olfactory nerve (Scarpa, 1785).*
9. *olfactory trunk (Burdach, 1822)*
   English synonym for *olfactory tract (Burdach, 1822)*; original German form, *Stamm*, p. 394. Derived from *trunk of olfactory nerve (Scarpa, 1785).*
10. *peduncle of olfactory lobule (Serres, 1824–1826)*
   Synonym for macrodissected adult reptilian and mammalian ***olfactory peduncle (Solly, 1836)***; in the original French, *pédoncule du lobule olfactif*, for example, Plate IV, Figure 109-*8*; Plate VIII, Figure 194-*I*.
11. *cerebral part of first pair (Arnold, 1834)*
   Synonym for macrodissected adult human ***olfactory peduncle (Solly, 1836)***; in the original Latin, *par primum, pars cerebralis*, p. 6.
12. *cerebral part of olfactory nerve (Arnold, 1834)*
   Synonym for macrodissected adult human ***olfactory peduncle (Solly, 1836)***; in the original Latin, *nervus olfactorius, pars cerebralis*, p. 6.

LATER SYNONYMS:

1. *olfactory commissure (Solly, 1836)*
   Synonym for macrodissected adult mammalian ***olfactory peduncle (Solly, 1836)***; p. 96.

olfactory region (>1840)

As described for macrodissected adult human, the rostroventral topographic subdivision of the ***limbic region (>1840)*** lying between ***hippocampal formation (Swanson & Cowan, 1977)*** caudally and ***cingulate region (>1840)*** dorsally. It has four macrotopographic parts, from rostral to caudal: ***olfactory bulb (Weitbrecht, 1751)***, ***olfactory peduncle (Solly, 1836)***, ***ambient gyrus (>1840)***, and ***semilunar gyrus (>1840)***. Based on cellular architecture and connections, they correspond to ***olfactory bulb (Weitbrecht, 1751)***, ***anterior olfactory nucleus (Herrick, 1910)***, ***piriform area (Smith, 1919)***, and ***cortical amygdalar complex (>1840)***, respectively. For general modern overviews see Shipley et al. (1996), Nieuwenhuys et al. (2008, p. 641 ff.). ***Olfactory region (>1840)*** is preferred to *olfactory lobe*, however defined, because a distinct lobe cannot be distinguished in human or other mammals. It was not delineated as here before 1840.

olfactory sulcus (Quain, 1834)

As described for macrodissected adult human, a groove between ***medial orbital gyrus (>1840)*** laterally and ***straight gyrus (Valentin, 1841)*** medially, cradling the underlying ***olfactory peduncle (Solly, 1836)*** and ***olfactory bulb (Weitbrecht, 1751)***; see Nieuwenhuys et al. (2008, Figs. 3.4, 3.5), *Terminologia Anatomica* (1998, p. 126). For Quain's use in macrodissected adult human, see p. 689. It was probably first described by Varoli; see ***[olfactory sulcus (Quain, 1834)] (Varoli, 1573)***.

TRANSLATIONS:

1. *sulcus olfactorius (Quain, 1834)*
   Original Latin form of ***olfactory sulcus (Quain, 1834)***; p. 689.

EARLIER REFERENCES:

Described, not named or illustrated:

1. ***[olfactory sulcus (Quain, 1834)] (Varoli, 1573)***
   Described for macrodissected adult human; f. 23, see Soemmerring (1778, p. 38).

Earlier synonyms:

1. *straight sulcus (Santorini, 1724)*
   Synonym for macrodissected adult human ***olfactory sulcus (Quain, 1834)***; in the original Latin, *rectum sulcum*, p. 62. See Soemmerring (1778, p. 39), Vicq d'Azyr (1786, Pl. XVII, Fig. II-3).
2. *first nerve sulcus (Soemmerring, 1778)*
   Synonym for macrodissected adult human ***olfactory sulcus (Quain, 1834)***; in the original Latin, *sulci nervo primo*, p. 40.
3. *sulcus insculptus basi lobi cerebri anterioris (Scarpa, 1785)*
   Synonym for macrodissected adult human ***olfactory sulcus (Quain, 1834)***; Table II, Figure 3-*n*.
4. *olfactory nerve sulcus (Vicq d'Azyr, 1786)*
   Synonym for macrodissected adult human ***olfactory sulcus (Quain, 1834)***; in the original French, *sillon du nerf olfactif*, Plate XVIII-9.
5. *sulcus longitudinalis (Günther, 1786)*
   Synonym for macrodissected adult human ***olfactory sulcus (Quain, 1834)***; p. 15, see Burdach (1822, p. 388).
6. *anfractuosity of olfactory nerves (Cruveilhier, 1836)*
   Synonym for macrodissected adult human ***olfactory sulcus (Quain, 1834)***; in the original French, *anfractuosité des nerfs olfactifs*, p. 883.

olfactory tubercle (Calleja, 1893)

As described for macrodissected adult human, and with cellular architecture and connections for all mammals, the most rostral and ventral differentiation of the ***striatum (Swanson, 2000a)***, ventral to the ***accumbens nucleus (Ziehen, 1897–1901)***; see Shipley et al. (1996). For Calleja's use based on adult mammalian histology, see p. 12. It was probably first indicated by Varoli; see ***[olfactory tubercle (Calleja, 1893)] (Varoli, 1573)***.

EARLIER REFERENCES:

Illustrated and described, not named:

1. ***[olfactory tubercle (Calleja, 1893)] (Varoli, 1573)*** Illustrated and described for macrodissected adult human as "locality where the olfactory apparatus originates" (Tab. II-*8*), also see Polyak (1957, p. 98).

PARTLY CORRESPONDS:

1. *olfactory trigone (Soemmerring, 1778)* Corresponds to rostral end of macrodissected adult human ***olfactory tubercle (Calleja, 1893)***, in region presenting origin of *short internal root of olfactory nerve (Soemmerring, 1778)* and *long external root of olfactory nerve (Soemmerring, 1778)*, and is derived from Soemmerring's work according to Meyer (1971, p. 194); also see Soemmerring (1798, p. 194), Beccari (1911, Fig. 2), Crosby and Humphrey (1941, p. 320), *olfactory tubercle (Meckel, 1817)*. Vicq d'Azyr (1784, p. 550) referred to a "flattened triangle" in this region of macrodissected adult human; in the original French, *un triangle aplati*.
2. *gray tubercle of first pair (Vicq d'Azyr, 1784)* Refers to small mound of *gray substance (Vesalius, 1543a)* in or near macrodissected adult human *olfactory trigone (Soemmerring, 1778)*; in the original French, *tubercule de la première paire*, pp. 549–550, and *tubercule d'où sort la première paire*, pp. 544, 546. Also see Vicq d'Azyr (1786, Pl. XVII, Fig. 1-*78*).
3. *tubercle generating first pair (Vicq d'Azyr, 1784)* Synonym for *gray tubercle of first pair (Vicq d'Azyr, 1784)*; pp. 544, 546.
4. *pyramidal eminence (Gordon, 1815)* Apparently synonym for macrodissected adult human *olfactory trigone (Soemmerring, 1778)*; p. 87.
5. *olfactory tubercle (Meckel, 1817)* Probably synonym for macrodissected adult human *olfactory trigone (Soemmerring, 1778)* and/or *gray tubercle of first pair (Vicq d'Azyr, 1784)*; see translation (1832, Vol. 2, p. 441), and Crosby and Humphrey (1941, pp. 320–321). Nicely defined by Foster (1894, p. 2968) as "A small projection of gray matter in front of the anterior perforated space from which arise the roots of the olfactory nerve [***olfactory peduncle (Solly, 1836)***]."
6. *gray pyramid (Cruveilhier, 1836)* Synonym for macrodissected adult human *gray tubercle of first pair (Vicq d'Azyr, 1784)*; in the original French, *pyramide grise*, p. 884.
7. *gray root of olfactory nerve (Cruveilhier, 1836)* Synonym for *gray pyramid (Cruveilhier, 1836)*; in the original French, *racine grise du nerf olfactif*, p. 884.

olfactory ventricle (>1840)

In early vertebrate development, an open rostral extension of the ***anterior horn of lateral ventricle (Bell, 1803b)*** into the olfactory evagination; in adult it may be open, as in ox, or it may be obliterated, as in human; see Woollam (1958, p. 15), Hamilton & Mossman (1972, Fig. 475). It was known to Galen; see ***[olfactory ventricle (>1840)] (Galen, c173)***.

EARLIER REFERENCES:

Earlier synonyms:

1. ***[olfactory ventricle (>1840)] (Galen, c173)*** Recognized in macrodissected adult ox; see Woollam (1958, p. 15); Duckworth translation (1962, pp. 3, 5, 186), May translation (1968, p. 401 note *44*). Vesalius (1543a) emphasized there is no such structure in macrodissected adult human; see Singer translation (1952, p. 34).
2. *organ of smelling (du Laurens, 1599)* Synonym for macrodissected adult human ***[olfactory ventricle (>1840)] (Galen, c173)***. Du Laurens wrote, "We answere for *Galen*, that the *anterior* ventricles are therefore called the Organs of smelling, because unto them are odours brought of which also they judge." (p. 408; see Crooke translation, 1615, p. 528).
3. *rhinocele (>1840)* Synonym for ***olfactory ventricle (>1840)***; see Craigie (1925, Pl. XXIV, XXV).

olive (Tiedemann, 1821)

As described for macrodissected adult human, the swelling on the ventrolateral surface of the ***medulla (Winslow, 1733)*** overlying the ***amiculum of olive (>1840)*** and then ***inferior olivary complex (>1840)***, just dorsal to the ***ventrolateral sulcus of medulla (>1840)***; see Clark (1951, p. 882), Williams & Warwick (1980, p. 898), *Nomina Anatomica* (1983, p. A65), *Terminologia Anatomica* (1998, p. 108, in Latin, *oliva*), Nieuwenhuys et al. (2008, Figs. 6.23–24). For Tiedemann's use in macrodissected adult monkey, see Table I, Figure 6-*i*. Burdach (1822, p. 34) used it for macrodissected adult human. It was first delineated by Eustachi; see ***[olive (Tiedemann, 1821)] (Eustachi, 1552)***.

TRANSLATIONS:

1. *oliva (Tiedemann, 1821)* Original Latin form of ***olive (Tiedemann, 1821)***; Table I, Figure 6-*i*.

EARLIER REFERENCES:

Illustrated, not named or described:

1. ***[olive (Tiedemann, 1821)] (Eustachi, 1552)*** First illustration, in macrodissected adult human, but not published until 1714; see Albinus edition (1761, Tab. XVIII), Haller (1762, p. 79).

Earlier synonyms:

1. *corpora teretia (Willis, 1664)* Synonym for and first published indication of macrodissected adult human ***olives (Tiedemann, 1821)***; see Pordage translation (1681, p. 123) and Meyer (1971, p. 12 note *4*).

2. *corpora olivaria (Vieussens, 1684)*
Synonym for macrodissected adult human ***olives (Tiedemann, 1821)***; Table IV-S. Vieussens wrote, "*Corpora olivaria sunt albae prominentiae duae olivae nucleum referentes, quae corporum pyramidalium lateribus adjacent.*" (p. 82). Also see Ridley (1695, p. 141).
3. *olivary body (Vieussens, 1684)*
Singular English form of *corpora olivaria (Vieussens, 1684)*.
4. *olivary eminences (Palfijn, 1726)*
Synonym for macrodissected adult human *corpora olivaria (Vieussens, 1684)*; in the original French, *éminences olivaires*, Part II, p. 23.
5. *corpora pyramidalia (Winslow, 1733)*
Synonym for macrodissected adult human ***olives (Tiedemann, 1821)***; Section X, p. 42. Based on Du Verney (1683), Winslow switched the ***pyramid (Willis, 1664)*** and ***olive (Tiedemann, 1821)***; see *corpora olivaria (Winslow, 1733)*.
6. *pyramidal body (Winslow, 1733)*
Singular English form of *corpora pyramidalia (Winslow, 1733)*.
7. *corpora pyramidalia posteriora (Tarin, 1750)*
Synonym for macrodissected adult human *corpora olivaria (Vieussens, 1684)*, according to Burdach (1822, p. 284).
8. *tubercula olivaria (Soemmerring, 1778)*
Synonym for macrodissected adult human *corpora olivaria (Vieussens, 1684)*; p. 178.
9. *prominentiae semiovales (Soemmerring, 1778)*
Synonym for macrodissected adult human *corpora olivaria (Vieussens, 1684)*; p. 103, according to Burdach (1822, p. 284).
10. *corpora ovalia (Soemmerring, 1791)*
Synonym for macrodissected adult human *corpora olivaria (Vieussens, 1684)*; p. 62.
11. *corpora ovata (Soemmerring, 1791)*
Synonym for *corpora ovalia (Soemmerring, 1791)*; p. 80.
12. *eminentiae medullae spinalis ovatae (Soemmerring, 1799)*
Synonym for macrodissected adult human *corpora ovalia (Soemmerring, 1791)*; p. 16, according to Burdach (1822, p. 284).
13. *tubercula ovalia (Soemmerring, 1799)*
Synonym for macrodissected adult human *corpora ovalia (Soemmerring, 1791)*; p. 16, according to Burdach (1822, p. 284).
14. *lateral eminences of spinal bulb (Chaussier, 1807)*
Synonym for macrodissected adult human *corpora olivaria (Vieussens, 1684)*; in the original French, *eminences latérales*, p. 123. Burdach (1822, p. 284) gave the Latin, *eminentiae laterales bulbi rachidici*.
15. *oval eminence (Gordon, 1815)*
Simplified English form of macrodissected adult human *eminentiae medullae spinalis ovatae (Soemmerring, 1799)*; p. 178.
16. *corpus pyramidale anticum laterale (Gordon, 1815)*
Synonym listed for macrodissected adult human ***olive (Tiedemann, 1821)***; p. 178.

LATER SYNONYMS:

1. *corpora pyramidalia lateralia (Burdach, 1822)*
Synonym for macrodissected adult human *corpora olivaria (Vieussens, 1684)*; p. 284. Burdach erroneously attributed the term to Tarin, see *lateral pyramidal body (Tarin, 1750)*.
2. *inferior olivary eminence (>1840)*
Synonym for macrodissected adult human ***olive (Tiedemann, 1821)***; see Crosby et al. (1962, p. 115).
3. *eminence of inferior olivary complex (>1840)*
Synonym for macrodissected adult human ***olive (Tiedemann, 1821)***; see Carpenter (1976, p. 39).

PARTLY CORRESPONDS:

1. *funiculus siliquae internus (Burdach, 1822)*
Rather vague term referring to ***white matter (Meckel, 1817)*** on ventral surface of macrodissected adult human ***inferior olivary complex (>1840)***, that is, the ***olive (Tiedemann, 1821)***, just lateral to the ***pyramid (Willis 1664)***; in the original German, *innere Hülsenstrangbahn*, Table III-*f*.

olivocerebellar tract (>1840)

As described for macrodissected adult human, and mammal generally with histological methods for ***axons (Kölliker, 1896)***, the ***central nervous system white matter tract (>1840)*** arising in the ***inferior olivary complex (>1840)***, immediately crossing the median plane, passing through the contralateral ***inferior olivary complex (>1840)***, and then coursing dorsolaterally to enter the ***inferior cerebellar peduncle (Günther, 1786)***; see Nieuwenhuys et al. (2008, Fig. 6.14), *Terminologia Anatomica* (1998, p. 109). At least its initial part was delineated as the *dull white nucleus inside olivary eminence (Vicq d'Azyr, 1784)* and *transverse fibers of medulla oblongata (Arnold, 1838a)*.

PARTLY CORRESPONDS:

1. *dull white nucleus inside olivary eminence (Vicq d'Azyr, 1784)*
Hilus and deeper *white substance (Vesalius, 1543a)* of macrodissected adult human ***inferior olivary complex (>1840)***, specifically of ***principal olivary nucleus (>1840)***, constituting initial segment of crossed ***olivocerebellar tract (>1840)***; p. 588. See Crosby et al. (1962, p. 137).
2. *funiculus nuclei olivae (Burdach, 1822)*
Synonym for macrodissected adult human *dull white nucleus inside olivary eminence (Vicq d'Azyr, 1784)*; p. 34, also see Foster (1892, p. 1656).
3. *funiculus olivae (Burdach, 1822)*
Synonym for *funiculus nuclei olivae (Burdach, 1822)*; p. 34.
4. *dentate body of olivary body (Langenbeck, 1826–1830)*
Synonym for macrodissected adult human *dull white nucleus inside olivary eminence (Vicq d'Azyr, 1784)*; in the original Latin, *corpus dentatum corporis olivaris*, Fascicle I, Table XV-*z*.

5. *transverse fibers of medulla oblongata (Arnold, 1838a)*
   Probably crossing segments of macrodissected adult human ***olivocerebellar tracts (>1840)*** between right and left ***inferior olivary complex (>1840)***; in the original Latin, *fibrae transversae*, p. 22, also see Arnold (1838b, Tab. IX, Fig. 5-*c*).

opening of cerebral aqueduct (>1840)

Aperture between caudal end of ***third ventricle (Galen, c173)*** and rostral end of ***cerebral aqueduct (>1840)***; see *Terminologia Anatomica* (1998, p. 118). The first name given to this region was probably *vulva (Colombo, 1559)*.

TRANSLATIONS:

1. *apertura aqueductus cerebri (>1840)*
   Current Latin form of ***opening of cerebral aqueduct (>1840)***; see *Terminologia Anatomica* (1998, p. 118).

EARLIER REFERENCES:

Earlier synonyms:

1. *vulva (Colombo, 1559)*
   Roughly macrodissected adult human ***opening of cerebral aqueduct (>1840)***; p. 192, also see Harvey (1961, p. 221). In contrast, Bell (1802, p. 30 note 2) and Chaussier (1807, p. 70) indicated that Colombo was referring to rostrodorsal end of ***third ventricle (Galen, c173)***, a general conclusion supported by Bauhin (1605, p. 594); in Crooke's translation, reference is made to "a certaine slitte or cleft, *Columbus* will needs liken the same unto the lap or priuity of a woman." (1615, p. 463). This alternate use of Bell, at least, is clearly that of *vulva (Casseri, 1627)*. Vieussens (1684, Tab. VII-*d*) used the term to indicate ***opening of cerebral aqueduct (>1840)***, although Burdach (1822, p. 379) stated that Vieussens used the term in referring to rostral end of ***third ventricle (Galen, c173)*** associated with ***interventricular foramen (>1840)***. Burdach (1822, p. 378) also stated that Colombo was referring to ***opening of fourth ventricle (>1840)***. Also see *vulva (Salmon, 1714)*.
2. *anus (Bauhin, 1605)*
   Synonym for macrodissected adult human ***opening of cerebral aqueduct (>1840)***; Book III, Chapter 14, p. 600; according to Chaussier (1807, p. 70) and Burdach (1822, p. 378). It is probably thus synonymous with *vulva (Colombo, 1559)*. It was clearly described by Ridley (1695, p. 124).
3. *aditus ad aquaeductum (Bartholin, 1654)*
   Synonym for macrodissected adult human ***opening of cerebral aqueduct (>1840)***; Book III, Chapter 3, p. 334; according to Burdach (1822, p. 378).
4. *anus (Willis, 1664)*
   For its ambiguous use by Willis on p. 65 of Pordage 1681 translation, see *rima (Willis, 1664)*.
5. *arse-hole (Willis, 1664)*
   For its ambiguous use by Willis on p. 65 of Pordage 1681 translation, see *rima (Willis, 1664)*.
6. *chink (Willis, 1664)*
   For its ambiguous use by Willis on p. 65 of Pordage 1681 translation, see *rima (Willis, 1664)*.
7. *apertura declivis (Willis, 1664)*
   Synonym for macrodissected adult human and sheep *vulva (Colombo, 1559)*; Figure VII-*M*; in English (Pordage 1881 translation, pp. 65, 123) the term was *declining aperture* (of tunnel or infundibulum). Also see Burdach (1822, p. 378).
8. *hiatus ad canalem natibus et testibus substratum ducens (Vieussens, 1684)*
   Synonym for macrodissected adult human *anus (Bauhin, 1605)*; p. 68, see Burdach (1822, p. 378).
9. *womb of Colombo (Diemerbroeck, 1689)*
   English eponym for *vulva (Colombo, 1559)*; p. 400.
10. *anterior foramen (Tyson, 1699)*
    Synonym for macrodissected infant chimpanzee ***opening of cerebral aqueduct (>1840)***; Figure 14-*k*.
11. *foramen ani (Salmon, 1714)*
    Synonym for macrodissected adult human ***opening of cerebral aqueduct (>1840)***; p. 402.
12. *foramen commune posterius (Winslow, 1733)*
    Synonym for macrodissected adult human ***opening of cerebral aqueduct (>1840)***; Section X, p. 37.
13. *posterior aperture of third ventricle (Haase, 1781)*
    Synonym for macrodissected adult human ***opening of cerebral aqueduct (>1840)***; in the original Latin, *apertura posterior ventriculi tertii*, p. 24.
14. *aditus ad aquaeductum Sylvii (Haase, 1781)*
    Synonym for *posterior aperture of third ventricle (Haase, 1781)*; p. 24.
15. *posterior ventricular oriface (Günther, 1786)*
    Synonym for macrodissected adult human *anus (Bauhin, 1605)*; in the original Latin, *orificia ventriculi posterius*, p. 13.
16. *posterior ventricular aperture (Günther, 1786)*
    Synonym for macrodissected adult human *anus (Bauhin, 1605)*; in the original Latin, *aperturae ventriculi posterius*, p. 13.
17. *anterior opening of aqueduct of Sylvius (Mayer, 1794)*
    Synonym for macrodissected adult human *anus (Bauhin, 1605)*; in the original Latin, *aditus anterior aquaeductus Sylvii*; Part 5, Table III, Figure 2-*v*.
18. *anterior aperture of aqueduct of Sylvius (Mayer, 1794)*
    Synonym for macrodissected adult human *anus (Bauhin, 1605)*; in the original Latin, *apertura anterior aquaeductus Sylvii*; Part 5, Table III, Figure 2-*v*.

opening of fourth ventricle (>1840)

Aperture between the caudal end of the ***cerebral aqueduct (>1840)*** and rostral end of the ***fourth ventricle (Galen, c192)***; named by analogy with ***opening of cerebral aqueduct (>1840)***. It was specifically pointed out by Vesalius; see *anus (Vesalius, 1543a)*.

EARLIER REFERENCES:

Earlier synonyms:

1. *anus (Vesalius, 1543a)*
   Synonym for macrodissected adult human ***opening of fourth ventricle (>1840)***. Vesalius noted that caudal opening of ***cerebral aqueduct (>1840)***, as it leads into

fourth ventricle (Galen, c192), bears some resemblance to the anus in so far as it lies between *buttocks (Galen, c177)*, or ***inferior colliculi (Haller, 1762)***; see Singer translation (1952, p. 47), Harvey (1961, p. 230, note *823*).

2. *fundament (Vesalius, 1543a)*
   Synonym for *anus (Vesalius, 1543)*; see Singer translation (1952, p. 106 and Fig. 10-C).
3. *arse-hole (Riolan, 1657)*
   Culpeper translation of *anus (Vesalius, 1543a)* for macrodissected adult human; p. 123.
4. *alveus (Le Böe, 1663)*
   Apparently roughly synonymous with *anus (Vesalius, 1543a)* for macrodissected adult human; p. 20, also see Burdach (1822, p. 302).
5. *posterior foramen (Tyson, 1699)*
   Synonym for *anus (Vesalius, 1543a)* in macrodissected infant chimpanzee; Figure 14-*r*.
6. *inferior foramen (Tyson, 1699)*
   Synonym for *posterior foramen (Tyson, 1699)*; Figure 14-*r*.

opercular part of inferior frontal gyrus (>1840)

As described for macrodissected adult human, a ventral topographic zone of the ***inferior frontal gyrus (>1840)*** caudal to the ***ascending branch of lateral cerebral sulcus (>1840)*** and associated with the ***frontal operculum (>1840)***; see Williams & Warwick (1980, Fig. 7.111A). According to Brodmann (1909, p. 138), it corresponds quite well to Broca's speech area. It was perhaps first clearly delineated by Rolando; see ***[opercular part of inferior frontal gyrus (>1840)] (Rolando, 1831)***.

EARLIER REFERENCES:

Illustrated, not named or described:

1. ***[opercular part of inferior frontal gyrus (>1840)] (Rolando, 1831)***
   Clearly illustrated for macrodissected adult human; Figure 1.

Earlier synonyms:

1. *area opercularis (Brodmann, 1909)*
   Original Latin form of *opercular area (Brodmann, 1909)*; p. 138.
2. *opercular area (Brodmann, 1909)*
   Based on cellular architecture in adult human, roughly synonymous with ***opercular part of inferior frontal gyrus (>1840)***; see Garey translation (1994, p. 117 and Fig. 85).
3. *area 44 (Brodmann, 1909)*
   Synonym for adult human *opercular area (Brodmann, 1909)*; in the original German, *Feld 44*, p. 138.

ophthalmic nerve (Winslow, 1733)

As described for macrodissected adult human, the most dorsal (upper) and smallest of the three primary ***trigeminal nerve branches (Winslow, 1733)***, wholly sensory in function. It was superbly illustrated by Henle (1871, Fig. 234), also see Durward (1951, Fig. 892), Williams & Warwick (1980, Figs. 7.176, 177). For Winslow's use in macrodissected adult human, see Sections VI, p. 63, and X, pp. 47, 102. It was first clearly delineated by Eustachi; see ***[ophthalmic nerve (Winslow, 1733)] (Eustachi, 1552)***.

EARLIER REFERENCES:

Illustrated, not named or described:

1. ***[ophthalmic nerve (Winslow, 1733)] (Eustachi, 1552)***
   Clearly illustrated for macrodissected adult human; see Albinus edition (1761, Tab. 18, Figs. 1, 3, 4-*r* and Fig. 2-*W*).

Earlier synonyms:

1. *first trunk of third pair (Falloppio, 1561)*
   Synonym for macrodissected adult human ***ophthalmic nerve (Winslow, 1733)***; see Meckel (1748, pp. 29 note *r*, 30 note *y*), who pointed out Falloppio omitted ***lacrimal nerve (Meckel, 1748)***. Falloppio also referred to it as one of three *shoots of third pair* according to Harvey (1961, notes *830*, *844*).
2. *first and superior branch of third pair (Marchetti, 1652)*
   Synonym for macrodissected adult human ***ophthalmic nerve (Winslow, 1733)***; p. 122.
3. *uppermost and second branches of second division of fifth pair of nerves arising within skull (Willis, 1664)*
   Synonym for macrodissected adult, presumably human, ***ophthalmic nerve (Winslow, 1733)***; see Pordage translation (1681, p. 144, Fig. 1-*C,D*).
4. *ophthalmic branches of second division of fifth pair of nerves arising within skull (Willis, 1664)*
   Synonym for *uppermost and second branches of second division of fifth pair of nerves arising within skull (Willis, 1664)* or ***ophthalmic nerve (Winslow, 1733)***; see Pordage translation (1681, p. 144, Fig. 1-*C,D*), where it is spelled *ophthalmick*.
5. *ramus minor superior nervus quintae conjugationis (Vieussens, 1684)*
   Synonym for macrodissected adult human ***ophthalmic nerve (Winslow, 1733)***; p. 170 and Table 22-*E*.
6. *superior branch of fifth pair (Rau, 1694)*
   Synonym for ***ophthalmic nerve (Winslow, 1733)***; p. 190.
7. *anterior branch of fifth pair (Rau, 1694)*
   Synonym for ***ophthalmic nerve (Winslow, 1733)***; p. 190.
8. *superior small branch of fifth pair (Ridley, 1695)*
   Synonym for macrodissected adult human *ramus minor superior nervus quintae conjugationis (Vieussens, 1684)*; p. 125.

LATER SYNONYMS:

1. *orbitary nerve (Winslow, 1733)*
   Synonym for macrodissected adult human ***ophthalmic nerve (Winslow, 1733)***; in the original Latin, *nervus orbitarius*, Section VI, pp. 59, 63.
2. *ophthalmic nerve of Willis (Winslow, 1733)*
   Eponym for macrodissected adult human ***ophthalmic nerve (Winslow, 1733)***; in the original Latin, *nervus ophthalmicus Willisii*, Section VI, p. 63.
3. *superior branch of trigeminal nerve (Winslow, 1733)*
   Synonym for macrodissected adult human ***ophthalmic nerve (Winslow, 1733)***; Section VI, pp. 61–63.

4. *first branch of fifth pair of nerves (Meckel, 1753)*
Synonym for macrodissected adult human ***ophthalmic nerve (Winslow, 1733)***; in the original French, *le premier rameau de la cinquième paire des nerfs*, p. 26.
5. *superior palpebral nerve (Meckel, 1753)*
Apparently synonym for macrodissected adult human ***ophthalmic nerve (Winslow, 1733)***; in the original French, *le nerf de la paupiere supérieure*, p. 40.
6. *ocular branch of fifth pair (Monro, 1783)*
Synonym for macrodissected adult human ***ophthalmic nerve (Winslow, 1733)***; Table 8, Figure 1-*N*.
7. *ophthalmicofrontal branch of trigeminal nerve (Günther, 1786)*
Synonym listed for macrodissected adult human ***ophthalmic nerve (Winslow, 1733)***; p. 42.
8. *first division of fifth pair (Bell, 1803a)*
Synonym for macrodissected adult human ***ophthalmic nerve (Winslow, 1733)***; Plate 1-*A*.
9. *ophthalmic branch of fifth pair (Bell, 1803a)*
Synonym for macrodissected adult human ***ophthalmic nerve (Winslow, 1733)***; Plate 1-*A*.
10. *orbito-frontal nerve (Burdin, 1803)*
Synonym for macrodissected adult human ***ophthalmic nerve (Winslow, 1733)***; see translation (1803, Vol. 3, p. 170).
11. *first trunk of three-fold nerve (Swan, 1830)*
Synonym for macrodissected adult human ***ophthalmic nerve (Winslow, 1733)***; p. 16.
12. *first trunk of fifth pair (Swan, 1830)*
Synonym for macrodissected adult human ***ophthalmic nerve (Winslow, 1733)***; p. 16.
13. *first trunk of fifth nerve (Swan, 1830)*
Synonym for macrodissected adult human ***ophthalmic nerve (Winslow, 1733)***; Plate XII, Figure 1-3,13.
14. *ophthalmic branch of Willis (Cruveilhier, 1836)*
Eponym for macrodissected adult human ***ophthalmic nerve (Winslow, 1733)***; in the original French, *branche ophthalmique de Willis*, p. 910.

PARTLY CORRESPONDS:

1. *uppermost branch of second division of fifth pair of nerves arising within skull (Willis, 1664)*
Corresponds roughly to macrodissected adult, presumably human, ***nasociliary nerve (Meckel, 1817; Wutzer, 1817)*** and ***frontal nerve (Cheselden, 1726)*** considered together; see Pordage translation (1681, p. 144, Fig. 1-C).
2. *roots of ophthalmic nerve (Malacarne, 1791)*
Unclear feature of macrodissected adult human ***ophthalmic nerve (Winslow, 1733)***; p. 232.
3. *middle branch of orbital nerve (Jacobson, 1818)*
Macrodissected adult mammal branch of ***ophthalmic nerve (Winslow, 1733)*** ending in region of levator palpebrae superioris muscle; in the original Latin, *nervus orbitarius ramus medius*, p. 17.
4. *external branch of orbital nerve (Jacobson, 1818)*
Essentially macrodissected adult human ***lacrimal nerve (Meckel, 1748; Bonhomme, 1748)*** and ***frontal nerve (Cheselden, 1726)*** considered together; in the original Latin, *nervus orbitarius ramus externus*, p. 17.
5. *ophthalmic branch of fifth pair communicates with third and fourth nerves (Bell & Bell, 1829)*
Macrodissected adult human ***communicating branches (Winslow, 1733)*** between proximal part of ***ophthalmic nerve (Winslow, 1733)***, and ***oculomotor nerve (Estienne, 1545)*** and ***trochlear nerve (Molinetti, 1669)***; p. 490, where earlier corroborative observations are quoted.

ophthalmic plexus (>1840)

As described for macrodissected adult human, an extension of the ***internal carotid plexus (>1840)*** along the ophthalmic artery (a branch of the internal carotid artery) and its many branches; see Mitchell (1953, p. 219), *Dorland's* (2003, p. 1455). It was described clearly perhaps for the first time by Ribes; see ***[ophthalmic plexus (>1840)] (Ribes, 1811)***.

EARLIER REFERENCES:

Described, not named or illustrated:

1. ***[ophthalmic plexus (>1840)] (Ribes, 1811)***
Described for macrodissected adult human, including an extension along the central retinal artery; p. 97, see Meckel (1832, Vol. 3, pp. 91–92).

optic chiasm (Galen, c173)

As described for macrodissected adult human, and vertebrate generally, the ***central nervous system white matter tract (>1840)*** on the ventral side or base of the ***hypothalamus (Kuhlenbeck, 1927)*** where the right and left ***optic nerves (Vicq d'Azyr, 1786)*** decussate to a greater or lesser extent in different species and continue on as the right and left ***optic tracts (Vicq d'Azyr, 1784)***; see Williams & Warwick (1980, pp. 974–975), Nieuwenhuys et al. (2008, p. 757). Aristotle probably knew of its existence; see ***[optic chiasm (Galen, c173)] (Aristotle)***. In *On the Usefulness of the Parts*, Galen described how the two *optic nerves (Galen, c173)* diverge toward the eyes from a region that resembles *X*); see May translation (1968, pp. 491–502). Rufus of Ephesus (fl. c90–120) believed that fibers in the *optic nerve (Galen, c173)* cross in the ***optic chiasm (Galen, c173)***, which he did not name, unlike Galen; see Singer (1917, p. 110), Duckworth translation (1962, p. 187), and May translation (1968, pp. 491–502). Much if not all of Galen's neuroanatomical work was done on beef, pig, and/or macaque but not human; Woollam (1958, p. 15). According to Singer (1957, p. 145), the term *optic chiasma* in its modern application was introduced by du Laurens (1595). Wenzel & Wenzel (1812, p. 109) demonstrated convincingly in macrodissected adult human a partial decussation of the ***optic nerves (Vicq d'Azyr, 1786)*** in the ***optic chiasm (Galen, c173)***.

EARLIER REFERENCES:

Described, not named or illustrated:

1. ***[optic chiasm (Galen, c173)] (Aristotle)***
In *The Account of Animals*, Aristotle may refer to it in terms of ducts from eyes meeting behind ***brain (Smith Papyrus, c1700 BC)***; see Thompson translation (1919, p. 494), Lloyd (1975, p. 120).

2. ***[optic chiasm (Galen, c173)] (Rufus of Ephesus, fl. c90–120)***
   Clearly referred to, though precise term for it is unknown; see May (1968, p. 30), Clarke & O'Malley (1996, p. 14).

LATER SYNONYMS:

1. *meeting of optic nerves (Galen, c173)*
   Synonym for ***optic chiasm (Galen, c173)***; see May translation (1968, p. 499).
2. *union of optic nerves (Galen, c173)*
   Synonym for ***optic chiasm (Galen, c173)***; see May translation (1968, p. 500).
3. *conjoining of optic nerves (Galen, c192)*
   Synonym for ***optic chiasm (Galen, c173)***; see Duckworth translation (1962, p. 6).
4. *common station for optic nerves (Mondino, 1316)*
   Synonym for macrodissected adult human ***optic chiasm (Galen, c173)***; see Singer translation (1925, p. 93).
5. *incruciatio (Berengario da Carpi, 1521)*
   Synonym for macrodissected adult human ***optic chiasm (Galen, c173)***, according to Burdach (1822, p. 392). Alternately, Berengario da Carpi used Latin form *incruciari*, according to Soemmerring (1778, p. 101).
6. *visoriorum nervorum coitus (Vesalius, 1543a)*
   Synonym for macrodissected adult human ***optic chiasm (Galen, c173)***; Book IV, Figure I-*H*.
7. *junction of optic nerves (Vesalius, 1543a)*
   English form of *visoriorum nervorum coitus (Vesalius, 1543a)*; see Richardson & Carman translation (2002, Fig. on p. 168, part *H*). Vesalius also described and illustrated the case of a macrodissected adult human where the two ***optic nerves (Vicq d'Azyr, 1786)*** did not cross or even touch; see Richardson & Carman translation (2002, p. 184).
8. *visoriorum nervorum congressus (Vesalius, 1543a)*
   Synonym for *visoriorum nervorum coitus (Vesalius, 1543a)*; see Book IV, Chapter IV and Book VII, Chapter XVIII.
9. *congress of optic nerves (Vesalius, 1543a)*
   English form of *visoriorum nervorum congressus (Vesalius, 1543a)*; see Richardson & Carman translation (2002, p. 183).
10. *conjunction of optic nerves (Vesalius, 1543a)*
    Singer translation (1952, p. 70) of *visoriorum nervorum congressus (Vesalius, 1543a)*.
11. *conjunction of nerves of vision (Vesalius, 1543a)*
    Singer translation (1952, p. 110) of *visoriorum nervorum congressus (Vesalius, 1543a)*.
12. *going together of sinews of sight (Geminus, 1553)*
    English form of *visoriorum nervorum congressus (Vesalius, 1543a)*; originally spelled *goyng together of the synowes of syght*, see *The table of the figures of sinowes*, Figure 7-*G*.
13. *joining together of sinews of sight (Geminus, 1553)*
    English form of *visoriorum nervorum congressus (Vesalius, 1543a)*; originally spelled *yoynge together of the synowes of sight*, see *The tables of the brayne*, Figure 13-*M*; or *joynynge together of the synowes of syght*, see *The tables of the brayne*, Figure 14.
14. *coition of optic nerves (Crooke, 1615)*
    English form of *visoriorum nervorum coitus (Vesalius, 1543a)*; p. 476, Table XIV, Figure 19-*O*.
15. *concourse of optic nerves (Crooke, 1615)*
    Synonym for *coition of optic nerves (Crooke, 1615)*; p. 495, Table XXV, Figure 1-*c*.
16. *coalitu nervorum opticorums (Bartholin, 1651)*
    Synonym for macrodissected adult human ***optic chiasm (Galen, c173)***; p. 456.
17. *coalition of optic nerves (Willis, 1664)*
    Synonym for macrodissected adult human ***optic chiasm (Galen, c173)***; see Pordage translation (1681, Fig. II-*E*).
18. *contactus lateralis (Blasius, 1674)*
    Synonym for macrodissected adult mammalian ***optic chiasm (Galen, c173)***, according to Burdach (1822, p. 392).
19. *copula (Blasius, 1674)*
    Synonym for macrodissected adult mammalian ***optic chiasm (Galen, c173)***, according to Burdach (1822, p. 392).
20. *decussation of optic nerves (Collins, 1685)*
    Synonym for macrodissected adult vertebrate ***optic chiasm (Galen, c173)***; p. 1045.
21. *united caudex of optic nerves (Collins, 1685)*
    Synonym for macrodissected adult vertebrate ***optic chiasm (Galen, c173)***; p. 1022. *Caudex* is an old form of *codex*, or *trunk*.
22. *reunion of optic nerves (Winslow, 1733)*
    Synonym for macrodissected adult human ***optic chiasm (Galen, c173)***; Section X, p. 46.
23. *commissure of optic nerves (Tarin, 1753)*
    Synonym for macrodissected adult human ***optic chiasm (Galen, c173)***; in the original French, *la Commissure des nerfs optiques*, p. 28.
24. *quadrangular space (Zinn, 1755)*
    Synonym for macrodissected adult human ***optic chiasm (Galen, c173)***; see Vicq d'Azyr (1786, Pl. XXI-*46*).
25. *continuitas (Albinus, 1768)*
    Synonym for macrodissected adult human ***optic chiasm (Galen, c173)*** in Chapter IV, according to Burdach (1822, p. 392).
26. *joining of optic nerves (Monro, 1783)*
    Synonym for macrodissected adult human ***optic chiasm (Galen, c173)***; Monro wrote, "unless I am much deceived, I have seen, in man, an intermixture and partial decussation of the cords which compose the optic nerves." (p. 43).
27. *optic commissure (Vicq d'Azyr, 1786)*
    Occasional synonym for macrodissected adult human ***optic chiasm (Galen, c173)***; Plate XXI-*46*.
28. *coitus nervorum opticorum (Schreger, 1803)*
    Synonym for macrodissected adult human ***optic chiasm (Galen, c173)***; p. 332.
29. *commissure of optic tracts (Reil, 1809b)*
    Synonym for macrodissected adult human ***optic chiasm (Galen, c173)***; see Mayo translation (1823, p. 74).

30. *intercrossing (Meckel, 1817)*
Synonym for macrodissected adult human ***optic chiasm (Galen, c173)***; see translation (1832, Vol. 3, p. 78).
31. *quadrate area (Rolando, 1825a)*
Synonym for macrodissected adult human ***optic chiasm (Galen, c173)***; in the original Latin, *area quadrata*, Table I, Figure 1-*a*.
32. *corpus quadrilaterum (Knox, 1832)*
Synonym for macrodissected adult human ***optic chiasm (Galen, c173)***; Supplemental Plate IV-27.

optic nerve (Vicq d'Azyr, 1786)

As described for macrodissected adult mammal, the ***cranial nerve (Soemmerring, 1791)*** segment between ***retina (Herophilus, c335–c280 BC)*** and ***optic chiasm (Galen, c173)***; see Williams & Warwick (1980, p. 1055). Early views on the origins and other ***white matter (Meckel, 1817)*** contributions to the ***optic nerve (Vicq d'Azyr, 1786)***, ***optic chiasm (Galen, c173)***, and ***optic tract (Vicq d'Azyr, 1784)*** were reviewed by Burdach (1822, pp. 392–394); also see *optic nerve (Galen, c173)*. For Vicq d'Azyr's use in macrodissected adult human, see Plate XVII, Figure I-31. Its discovery is usually credited to Alcmaeon; see ***[optic nerve (Vicq d'Azyr, 1786)] (Alcmaeon, c490–c430 BC)***.

EARLIER REFERENCES:

Described, not named or illustrated:

1. ***[optic nerve (Vicq d'Azyr, 1786)] (Alcmaeon, c490–c430 BC)***
Alcmaeon is often credited with discovering it by using scientific animal dissections for the first time in recorded history, but the supporting passage from Chalcidius (c300 BC) is quite ambiguous; see Polyak (1957, p. 77), May (1968, p. 13), von Staden (1989, p. 155 ff.), Rocca (2003, pp. 22–23). However, in *De Sensu*, Aristotle's successor Theophrastus (c327–c287 BC) clearly stated that Alcmaeon at least postulated the existence of a channel, passage, or duct between eye and ***brain (Smith Papyrus, c1700 BC)***; see Solmsen (1961, pp. 151–152), Lloyd (1975).

LATER SYNONYMS:

1. *orbital part of second pair (Arnold, 1834)*
Synonym for macrodissected adult human ***optic nerve (Vicq d'Azyr, 1786)***; in the original Latin, *par secundum, pars orbitalis*, p. 6.
2. *orbital part of optic nerve (Arnold, 1834)*
Synonym for *orbital part of second pair (Arnold, 1834)*; in the original Latin, *nervus opticus, pars orbitalis*, p. 6.
3. *orbital part of optic nerve chiasm (Arnold, 1838b)*
Synonym for macrodissected adult human ***optic nerve (Vicq d'Azyr 1786)***; in the original Latin, *chiasma nervorum opticorum partes orbitales*, Table IV, Figure 1-*o*.

optic radiation (>1840)

As described for macrodissected adult human, a topographic division of ***cerebral cortex white matter (>1840)*** between ***sublentiform part of internal capsule (>1840)***, specifically its ***posterior thalamic radiation (>1840)*** component, and ***primary visual area (>1840)*** or *area 17 (Brodmann, 1909)*. A major component is the projection from ***dorsal lateral geniculate nucleus (>1840)*** to ***primary visual area (>1840)***, often called the geniculocalcarine tract; see Mettler (1948, p. 141), Polyak (1957, pp. 196–197, 405–409 and Figs. 235, 236), Crosby et al. (1962, p. 279 and Fig. 262). It was perhaps first clearly delineated by Reil; see ***[optic radiation (>1840)] (Reil, 1809b)***.

EARLIER REFERENCES:

Illustrated and described, not named:

1. ***[optic radiation (>1840)] (Reil, 1809b)***
Clearly illustrated and described for macrodissected adult human; see Mayo translation (1823, pp. 58–59, 65 and Tab. IX-*t*).

optic tract (Vicq d'Azyr, 1784)

As described for macrodissected adult human and other vertebrates, the extension of the ***optic nerve (Vicq d'Azyr, 1786)***, between ***optic chiasm (Galen, c173)*** ventrally and ***brachium of superior colliculus (>1840)*** dorsally, a change in name occurring at the level of the ***dorsal lateral geniculate nucleus (>1840)***. For Vicq d'Azyr's use in macrodissected adult human, see p. 523; also see Vicq d'Azyr (1786, Pls. XIV, Fig. IV-*8*; XVII, Fig. I-*30*). He noted (1784, p. 529) that Santorini (1775, p. 32) identified its origin as the ***superior colliculus (Haller, 1762)***, whereas Meckel (1817) later identified it as the ***inferior colliculus (Haller, 1762)***, see translation (1832, Vol. 3, p. 77). It was first named separately from the *optic nerve (Galen, c173)* as the *cerebral part of optic nerve (Casseri, 1609)* although it was obviously known to Galen.

EARLIER REFERENCES

Earlier synonyms:

1. *cerebral part of optic nerve (Casseri, 1609)*
Synonym for macrodissected adult human ***optic tract (Vicq d'Azyr, 1784)***; see Tables on p. 123, Figure 2-*E* and p. 259, Figure 2-*E*. For dog, cat, and cow see Table on p. 123.
2. *first part of optic nerve (Perrault, 1688)*
Origin of *optic nerve (Galen, c173)*, the ***optic tract (Vicq d'Azyr, 1784)***, from eminence of ***brain (Smith Papyrus, c1700 BC)*** in chameleon, before joining ***optic chiasm (Galen, c173)***; p. 26. Tarin (1750, Tab. I, Fig. 5-*N*.) used it for macrodissected adult human.
3. *great cornu of optic nerve (Winslow, 1733)*
Apparently synonym for macrodissected adult human ***optic tract (Vicq d'Azyr, 1784)***; see Section X, p. 43.
4. *great curvature of optic nerve (Winslow, 1733)*
Apparently synonym for macrodissected adult human ***optic tract (Vicq d'Azyr, 1784)***; Section X, p. 46.

LATER SYNONYMS:

1. *optic band (Meckel, 1832)*
English form of macrodissected adult human ***optic tract (Vicq d'Azyr, 1784)***; Vol. 3, p. 80.
2. *band of optic nerves (Cruveilhier, 1836)*
Synonym for macrodissected adult human ***optic tract (Vicq d'Azyr, 1784)***; in the original French, *bandelette des nerfs optiques*, p. 649.

3. *central end of optic nerves (Cruveilhier, 1836)*
Synonym for macrodissected adult human ***optic tract (Vicq d'Azyr, 1784)***; in the original French, *extrémité centrale des nerfs optiques*, p. 887.
4. *origin of optic nerve (Cruveilhier, 1836)*
Synonym for *central end of optic nerve (Cruveilhier, 1836)*; p. 887.
5. *cerebral part of optic nerve chiasm (Arnold, 1838b)*
Synonym for macrodissected adult human ***optic tract (Vicq d'Azyr, 1784)***; in the original Latin, *chiasma nervorum opticorum partes cerebrales*, Table IV, Figure 1-*n*.

PARTLY CORRESPONDS:

1. *root of optic nerve (Galen, c192)*
In *On Anatomical Procedures*, Galen may refer to at least distal segment of ***optic tract (Vicq d'Azyr, 1784)***, near ***dorsal lateral geniculate nucleus (>1840)***, in this way for macrodissected adult beef, pig, and/or macaque but not human; see Duckworth translation (1962, pp. 3, 19).
2. *root of great arch of optic nerve (Winslow, 1733)*
Apparently synonym for macrodissected adult human *root of optic nerve (Galen, c192)*, see Section X, p. 47.
3. *root of great body of optic nerve (Winslow, 1733)*
Apparently synonym for macrodissected adult human *root of optic nerve (Galen, c192)*; see Section X, p. 47.

orbital branches of pterygopalatine ganglion (>1840)

As described for macrodissected adult human, 2–3 delicate branches between the periosteum and orbitalis muscle and sphenoidal and ethmoidal sinuses, and the ***pterygopalatine ganglion (>1840)***. Histologically they are formed mostly by sensory ***dendrites (His, 1889)*** simply extending proximally through the ***pterygopalatine ganglion (>1840)*** to the ***pterygopalatine nerves (Wrisberg, 1786)*** and then the ***maxillary nerve (Meckel, 1753)*** and ***trigeminal ganglion (>1840)***; see Williams & Warwick (1980, pp. 1064–1065), *Terminologia Anatomica* (1998, p. 134). The ***orbital branches of pterygopalatine ganglion (>1840)*** join with branches of the ***internal carotid nerve (>1840)*** in contributing to the *ciliary plexus (Meckel, 1748)*, more recently called the *retro-orbital plexus* by Ruskell (1970, p. 237; 1971). It was probably first noted, at least in part, by Meckel; see ***[orbital branches of pterygopalatine ganglion (>1840)] (Meckel, 1817)***.

EARLIER REFERENCES:

Described, not named or illustrated:

1. ***[orbital branches of pterygopalatine ganglion (>1840)] (Meckel, 1817)***
Meckel at least mentioned without naming a branch of ***pterygopalatine ganglion (>1840)*** to sphenoidal sinus; see translation (1832, Vol. 3, p. 66). They were considered more fully by Todd (1836–1839, p. 286).

Earlier synonyms:

1. *orbital branch of superior maxillary nerve (Cruveilhier, 1836)*
Synonym for macrodissected adult human ***orbital branches of pterygopalatine ganglion (>1840)***; in the original French, *rameau orbitaire*, p. 919.
2. *orbital nerve (Cruveilhier, 1836)*
Synonym for *orbital branch of superior maxillary nerve (Cruveilhier, 1836)*; in the original French, *nerf orbitaire*, p. 920.

PARTLY CORRESPONDS:

1. *lacrimal branch of orbital branch of superior maxillary nerve (Cruveilhier, 1836)*
Branch of macrodissected adult human *orbital branch of superior maxillary nerve (Cruveilhier, 1836)* passing through lacrimal gland and ending in external angle of upper eyelid; in the original French, *rameau lacrymal de l'orbitaire*, p. 919.
2. *temporo-malar branch of orbital branch of superior maxillary nerve (Cruveilhier, 1836)*
Branch of macrodissected adult human *orbital branch of superior maxillary nerve (Cruveilhier, 1836)* entering a canal in the zygomatic bone; in the original French, *rameau temporo-malaire*, p. 920.
3. *malar filament of temporo-malar branch of orbital branch of superior maxillary nerve (Cruveilhier, 1836)*
Branch of macrodissected adult human *temporo-malar branch of orbital branch of superior maxillary nerve (Cruveilhier, 1836)* supplying skin of cheek; in the original French, *filet malaire*, p. 920.
4. *temporal filament of temporo-malar branch of orbital branch of superior maxillary nerve (Cruveilhier, 1836)*
Branch of macrodissected adult human *temporo-malar branch of orbital branch of superior maxillary nerve (Cruveilhier, 1836)* entering rostral (anterior) part of temporalis muscle; in the original French, *filet temporal*, p. 920.

orbital gyri (>1840)

As described for macrodissected adult human, a topographic subdivision of the ***orbital region (Rolando, 1831)*** lying lateral to the other subdivision, the ***straight gyrus (Valentin, 1841)***, and often having four parts surrounding the roughly ***H***-shaped ***orbital sulci (>1840)***: ***medial orbital gyrus (>1840)***, **anterior orbital gyrus** (>1840), ***posterior orbital gyrus (>1840)***, and ***lateral orbital gyrus (>1840)***; see Williams & Warwick (1980, Fig. 7.116), *Terminologia Anatomica* (1998, p. 126). They were first clearly delineated by Soemmerring; see ***[orbital gyri (>1840)] (Soemmerring, 1778)***.

EARLIER REFERENCES:

Illustrated, not named or described:

1. ***[orbital gyri (>1840)] (Soemmerring, 1778)***
Clearly illustrated for macrodissected adult human; Table II.

PARTLY CORRESPONDS:

1. *supraorbital convolution (Gerdy, 1838)*
Roughly macrodissected adult human ***anterior orbital gyrus (>1840)***, ***posterior orbital gyrus (>1840)***, and ***lateral orbital gyrus (>1840)***, considered together; in the original French, *circonvolution sus-orbitaire*, p. 259.

orbital part of inferior frontal gyrus (>1840)

As described for macrodissected adult human, a rostral and ventral topographic zone of the ***inferior frontal gyrus (>1840)*** between ***anterior branch of lateral cerebral fissure (>1840)*** and ***lateral orbital gyrus (>1840)***; see Williams & Warwick (1980, Figs. 7.111A, 7.116), *Terminologia Anatomica* (1998, p. 125). It was clearly delineated by Rolando; see ***[orbital part of inferior frontal gyrus (>1840)] (Rolando, 1831)***.

EARLIER REFERENCES:

Illustrated, not named or described:

1. ***[orbital part of inferior frontal gyrus (>1840)] (Rolando, 1831)***
   Clearly illustrated for macrodissected adult human; Figure 1.

orbital region (Rolando, 1831)

As described for macrodissected adult human, the most ventral and rostral topographic subdivision of the ***frontal region (Vicq d'Azyr, 1786)***, lying ventral to the ***inferior frontal gyrus (>1840)*** and including ***straight gyrus (Valentin, 1841)*** and ***orbital gyri (>1840)***; see Williams & Warwick (1980, Fig. 7.116). Based on cellular architecture in human, it corresponds roughly with the *prefrontal area (Brodmann, 1909)* and *orbital area (Brodmann, 1909)* considered together. For Rolando's use in macrodissected adult human, see Figure 4:1–3 and Meyer (1971, p. 126). It was perhaps first clearly indicated by Soemmerring; see ***[orbital region (Rolando, 1831)] (Soemmerring, 1778)***.

TRANSLATIONS:

1. *regione orbitale (Rolando, 1831)*
   Original Italian form of ***orbital region (Rolando, 1831)***; Figure 4:1–3.

EARLIER REFERENCES:

Illustrated and described, not named:

1. ***[orbital region (Rolando, 1831)] (Soemmerring, 1778)***
   Soemmerring carefully illustrated each major component for macrodissected adult human; Table II.
2. ***[orbital region (Rolando, 1831)] (Vicq d'Azyr, 1786)***
   Vicq d'Azyr explicitly associated it with macrodissected adult human orbital convexity of frontal bone; Plates XVI, XVII-*80*.

Earlier synonyms:

1. *anterior lobe (Fyfe, 1800)*
   Ventral (under) surface of macrodissected adult human ***frontal region (Vicq d'Azyr, 1786)*** corresponding roughly to ***orbital region (Rolando, 1831)***; p. 15.
2. *anterior process (Fyfe, 1800)*
   Synonym for *anterior lobe (Fyfe, 1800)*; p. 15.

LATER SYNONYMS:

1. *inferior region of anterior lobe (Rolando, 1831)*
   Synonym for ***orbital region (Rolando, 1831)***; in the original Italian, *regione inferiore del lobo anteriore*, Figure 4:1–3.

PARTLY CORRESPONDS:

1. *area praefrontalis (Brodmann, 1909)*
   Original Latin form of *prefrontal area (Brodmann, 1909)*; p. 137.
2. *prefrontal area (Brodmann, 1909)*
   Based on cellular architecture in adult human, roughly corresponds to ***straight gyrus (Valentin, 1841)***, ***medial orbital gyrus (>1840)***, **anterior orbital gyrus (>1840)**, and ***posterior orbital gyrus (>1840)***, considered together; see p. 137 and Figures 85, 86. Also see Williams & Warwick (1980, Fig. 7.116).
3. *area 11 (Brodmann, 1909)*
   Synonym for *prefrontal area (Brodmann, 1909)*; in the original German, *Feld 11*, p. 137.

orbital sulci (>1840)

As described for macrodissected adult human, often roughly ***H***-shaped grooves distinguishing the various and variable ***orbital gyri (>1840)*** of the ***orbital region (Rolando, 1831)***, lying medial to the ***straight gyrus (Valentin, 1841)***; see Williams & Warwick (1980, Fig. 7.116), *Terminologia Anatomica* (1998, p. 126). They were first clearly delineated by Soemmerring; see ***[orbital sulci (>1840)] (Soemmerring, 1778)***.

EARLIER REFERENCES:

Illustrated, not named or described:

1. ***[orbital sulci (>1840)] (Soemmerring, 1778)***
   Clearly illustrated for macrodissected adult human; Table II.

otic ganglion (Arnold, 1828)

As described for macrodissected adult human, a ***terminal ganglion (Gaskell, 1886)*** lying just ventral to (below) the foramen ovale of the sphenoid bone and having complex neural relationships, although best known for controlling salivation from the parotid gland; see Durward (1951, Fig. 906), Hamilton (1976, Fig. 793), Williams & Warwick (1980, p. 1076 and Fig. 7.181). Its connecting branches were magnificently illustrated in Schwalbe (1881, Fig. 450). For Arnold's use in macrodissected adult mammal, see p. 11 ff.; for an historical analysis, see Arnold (1838a, p. 188 ff.). Arnold first described it accurately in 1826; see ***[otic ganglion (Arnold, 1828)] (Arnold, 1826)***. It may have been alluded to earlier by Winslow although Arnold is usually given credit for the discovery; see ***[otic ganglion (Arnold, 1828)] (Winslow, 1733)***.

TRANSLATIONS:

1. *Ohrknoten (Arnold, 1828)*
   Original German form of ***otic ganglion (Arnold, 1828)***; p. 11.
2. *auricular ganglion (Arnold, 1828)*
   Alternate translation of *Ohrknoten (Arnold, 1828)*; see Bendz (1833, p. 10), who gave the Latin, *ganglion auriculare*.

EARLIER REFERENCES:

Described, not named or illustrated:

1. ***[otic ganglion (Arnold, 1828)] (Winslow, 1733)***
   Possibly alluded to vaguely in macrodissected adult human as "short collateral Branch which is sometimes plexiform [ganglionated]" (Sect. VI, no. 67, p. 66).

Illustrated and described, not named:

1. ***[otic ganglion (Arnold, 1828)] (Arnold, 1826)***
   Carefully illustrated and described for macrodissected adult human but not named; pp. 15–17, Figure III-*12*.

LATER SYNONYMS:

1. *ganglion of Arnold (Bendz, 1833)*
   Eponym for macrodissected adult mammalian ***otic ganglion (Arnold, 1828)***; in the original Latin, *ganglion Arnoldi*; see Table I, Figure 2-*1*.

outer part of transverse cerebral fissure (>1840)

As described for macrodissected adult human, the extension of the ***inner part of transverse cerebral fissure (>1840)*** lying between the ventral surface of the ***occipital region (Vesalius, 1543a)*** and the nearby face of the ***cerebellum (Aristotle)***, and occupied partly by the ***cerebellar tentorium (Winslow, 1733)***; see Carpenter (1976, pp. 65–66), and illustrated beautifully by Rasmussen (1932, Fig. 1). It was first delineated clearly by Steno; see ***[outer part of transverse cerebral fissure (>1840)] (Steno, 1669)***.

EARLIER REFERENCES:

Illustrated, not named or described:

1. ***[outer part of transverse cerebral fissure (>1840)] (Steno, 1669)***
   Clearly illustrated for macrodissected adult human in midsagittal view; Plate I.

Earlier synonyms:

1. *transverse cerebral fissure (Todd, 1845)*
   Essentially synonym for macrodissected adult human ***outer part of transverse cerebral fissure (>1840)***; p. 26, also see Mettler (1948, p. 113), Crosby et al. (1962, p. 571).

ovarian plexus (Cruveilhier, 1836)

As described for macrodissected adult human female, it arises from the ***superior ovarian nerves (>1840), middle ovarian nerves (>1840)***, and perhaps ***inferior ovarian nerves (>1840)*** and supplies the ovary and uterine tube; see Mitchell (1953, pp. 293–295), Williams & Warwick (1980, p. 1134). For Cruveilhier's use in macrodissected adult human female, see p. 1021. It was known to Willis; see ***[ovarian plexus (Cruveilhier, 1836)] (Willis, 1664)***.

TRANSLATIONS:

1. *plexus ovarique (Cruveilhier, 1836)*
   Original French form of ***ovarian plexus (Cruveilhier, 1836)***; p. 1021.

EARLIER REFERENCES:

Illustrated and described, not named:

1. ***[ovarian plexus (Cruveilhier, 1836)] (Willis, 1664)***
   Described and illustrated for macrodissected adult human and other large female mammals; see Pordage translation (1681, p. 159 and Tab. 11-*τ,ν,χ*). Also see *spermatic plexus (Haller, 1762)*.

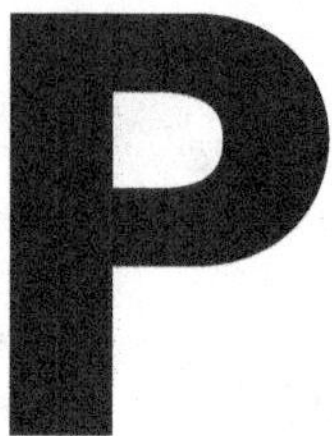

palatine nerves (Schaarschmidt, 1750)

As described for macrodissected adult human, they extend ventrally (descend) from the ***pterygopalatine ganglion (>1840)***, either as a short common trunk (palatine nerve) or as 2–3 separate ***nerves (Herophilus, c335–c280 BC)***, to supply the roof of the mouth, soft palate, tonsil, and lining membrane of the nasal cavity. Most commonly three parts are recognized: ***greater palatine nerve (Cloquet, 1816)*** and two ***lesser palatine nerves (Meckel, 1817)***; see Henle (1871, Fig. 241), Williams & Warwick (1980, Fig. 7.178). Histologically they are formed mostly by sensory ***dendrites (His, 1889)*** simply passing through the ***pterygopalatine ganglion (>1840)*** to the ***pterygopalatine nerves (Wrisberg, 1786)*** and then ***maxillary nerve (Meckel, 1753)*** and ***trigeminal ganglion (>1840)***; see Williams & Warwick (1980, p. 1065). For Schaarschmidt's use in macrodissected adult human, see p. 21. They were known to Galen; see ***[palatine nerves (Schaarschmidt, 1750)] (Galen, c173)***.

EARLIER REFERENCES:

Described, not named or illustrated:

1. ***[palatine nerves (Schaarschmidt, 1750)] (Galen, c173)***
   Alluded to in macrodissected adult beef, pig, and/or macaque but not human, and assigned to *fourth pair of nerves from brain (Galen, c192)*; see May translation (1968, pp. 444, 525, 686), Duckworth translation (1962, p. 194), Meckel (1748, p. 2 note *i*).

Earlier synonyms:

1. *second branch of lower branch of second division of fifth pair of nerves arising within skull (Willis, 1664)*
   Synonym for macrodissected adult, presumably human, ***palatine nerves (Schaarschmidt, 1750)***; see Pordage translation (1681, p. 145, Fig. 1-*F,i*).
2. *second branch of fourth branch of second division of fifth pair of nerves arising within skull (Willis, 1664)*
   Synonym for macrodissected adult, presumably human, ***palatine nerves (Schaarschmidt, 1750)***; see Pordage translation (1681, p. 145, Fig. 1-*F,i*).

LATER SYNONYMS:

1. *odonto-palatino-nasal nerve (Le Cat, 1768)*
   Synonym for macrodissected adult human ***palatine nerves (Schaarschmidt, 1750)***; in the original French, *nerf odonto-palatino-nasal*; Plate VIII, Figure 1-*22(5)* and Plate VIII, Figure 2-*7*. See Neubauer (1772, p. 27).
2. *descending branch of pterygopalatine nerve (Meckel, 1817)*
   Synonym for macrodissected adult human ***palatine nerves (Schaarschmidt, 1750)***; see translation (1832, Vol. 3, pp. 67–68).
3. *pterygopalatine nerve (Bock, 1817)*
   Synonym for macrodissected adult human ***palatine nerves (Schaarschmidt, 1750)***; in the original Latin, *nervus pterygopalatinus*, p. 29, Table II-*75*.
4. *posterior palatine nerves from Meckel's ganglion (Quain & Wilson, 1839)*
   Synonym for macrodissected adult human ***palatine nerves (Schaarschmidt, 1750)***; Plate XI, Figure 2-*I*. See *posterior palatine nerves (Quain & Wilson, 1839)*.
5. *descending branches of spheno-palatine ganglion (Quain & Wilson, 1839)*
   Synonym for macrodissected adult human ***palatine nerves (Schaarschmidt, 1750)***; Plate XXVII-*G,m*.
6. *posterior palatine nerves (Quain & Wilson, 1839)*
   Synonym for macrodissected adult human ***palatine nerves (Schaarschmidt, 1750)***; Plate XXVII-*G,m*.

pallidum (Swanson, 2000a)

Based on histology and development, a ***gray matter region (Swanson & Bota, 2010)*** forming the ventral of two major divisions of the mammalian ***cerebral nuclei (Swanson, 2000a)***, with the dorsal division being the ***striatum (Swanson, 2000a)***. The major components are ***globus pallidus (Burdach, 1822)***, ***substantia innominata (Meynert, 1872)***, ***medial septal complex (Swanson & Cowan, 1979)***, and ***bed nuclei of terminal stria (Gurdjian, 1925)***; see Swanson (2004, Table B) for detailed list in rat. For Swanson's original use in rat, generalized to all mammals, see pp. 127–130, Figure 19. It was not recognized as such by 1840.

palmar branch of median nerve (Bock, 1827)

As described for macrodissected adult human, this cutaneous branch supplies skin over the thenar eminence and central part of the palm; see Williams & Warwick (1980, p. 1098, Fig. 7.201). For Bock's use in macrodissected adult human, see description in Table II-*28*. It was first clearly delineated as the *nervus cutaneus longus volae (Günther, 1786)*.

EARLIER REFERENCES:

Earlier synonyms:

1. *nervus cutaneus longus volae (Günther, 1786)*
   Synonym for *long palmar nerve (Günther, 1786)*; p. 74.
2. *long palmar nerve (Günther, 1786)*
   Clear description of macrodissected adult human ***palmar branch of median nerve (Bock, 1827)***; in the original Latin, *nervus palmaris longus*, p. 74. Winslow probably mentioned it for macrodissected adult human, but his description was too vague to be certain; Section VI, no. 230, p. 82.
3. *volar long cutaneous nerve of median nerve (Loder, 1803)*
   Synonym for macrodissected adult human ***palmar branch of median nerve (Bock, 1827)***; in the original Latin, *nervo cutaneo longo volae ex mediano*, Table CLXXVIII-*87*.
4. *volar long cutaneous branch of median nerve (Loder, 1803)*
   Synonym for macrodissected adult human ***palmar branch of median nerve (Bock, 1827)***; in the original Latin, *ramus cutaneus longus volae*, Table CLXXX-*49*.
5. *long palmar cutaneous branch of median nerve (Loder, 1803)*
   Synonym for macrodissected adult human ***palmar branch of median nerve (Bock, 1827)***; in the original Latin, *ramus cutaneus palmaris longus*, Table CLXXX-*49*.
6. *volar cutaneous branch of median nerve (Caldani, 1813, 1814)*
   Synonym for macrodissected adult human ***palmar branch of median nerve (Bock, 1827)***; in the original Latin, *ramus cutaneus volaris nervi mediani*, Table CCLVIII, Figure 1-*34*.
7. *cutaneous palmar branch of median nerve (Cloquet, 1816)*
   Synonym for macrodissected adult human ***palmar branch of median nerve (Bock, 1827)***; in the original French, *rameau palmaire cutané*, p. 648. Used by Durward (1951, p. 1076). Quain (1828, p. 423) called it *cutaneous palmar branch of median nerve* in English.
8. *long palmar branch of median nerve (Bock, 1827)*
   Synonym for macrodissected adult human ***palmar branch of median nerve (Bock, 1827)***; in the original Latin, *ram. palmaris longus*, Table I, Figure 2-*27*. Bock also showed it sometimes is associated with *superficial branch of radial nerve (Martin, 1781)*; see Table V, Figure 4-*6*.
9. *great cutaneous palmar branch of median nerve (Cloquet, 1828)*
   Glorified synonym for *cutaneous palmar branch of median nerve (Cloquet, 1816)*; in the original French, *grand rameau palmaire cutané du N. médian*, Plate CLXVIII, Figure 2-*95*.
10. *median volar nerve (Knox, 1832)*
    Synonym for macrodissected adult human ***palmar branch of median nerve (Bock, 1827)***; Plate XX-*9*.
11. *volar branch of median nerve (Knox, 1832)*
    Synonym for *median volar nerve (Knox, 1832)*; Plate 20-*11*.
12. *long volar cutaneous branch of median nerve (Knox, 1832)*
    Synonym for macrodissected adult human *volar long cutaneous nerve of median nerve (Loder, 1803)*; Plate 21, Figure 1-*22*.
13. *long cutaneous branch of median nerve (Knox, 1832)*
    Synonym for macrodissected adult human *volar long cutaneous nerve of median nerve (Loder, 1803)*; Plate 21, Figure 2-*8*.
14. *palmar cutaneous nerve (Quain & Wilson, 1839)*
    Synonym for macrodissected adult human ***palmar branch of median nerve (Bock, 1827)***; Plate XVIII, Figure 1-*i*.
15. *superficial palmar nerve (Quain & Wilson, 1839)*
    Synonym for macrodissected adult human ***palmar branch of median nerve (Bock, 1827)***; Plate XVIII, Figure 2-*f*.

PARTLY CORRESPONDS:

1. *volar long cutaneous branch of median nerve communications with musculocutaneous nerve (Caldani, 1813, 1814)*
   Macrodissected adult human ***communicating branches (Winslow, 1733)*** between ***palmar branch of median nerve (Bock, 1827)*** and ***musculocutaneous nerve (Du Verney, 1697)***; in the original Latin, *ramus mediani cutaneus longus volaris communicationes cum ramis nervi musculo-cutanei*, Table CCLIX, Figure 1-*23*.
2. *external branch of palmar cutaneous nerve (Cruveilhier, 1836)*
   Smaller, lateral branch of macrodissected adult human ***palmar branch of median nerve (Bock, 1827)***; in the original French, *rameau externe*, p. 806.
3. *internal branch of palmar cutaneous nerve (Cruveilhier, 1836)*
   Larger, medial branch of macrodissected adult human ***palmar branch of median nerve (Bock, 1827)***; in the original French, *rameau interne*, p. 806.

palmar branch of ulnar nerve (Soemmerring, 1791)

As described for macrodissected adult human, it arises about the middle of the forearm and ends in skin of the palm after communicating with the ***palmar branch of median nerve (Bock, 1827)***; see Hamilton (1976, Fig. 821), Williams & Warwick (1980, p. 1100 and Figs. 7.201, 204). For Soemmerring's discovery and use in macrodissected adult human, see p. 288, in the original German, *Palmarast*.

LATER SYNONYMS:

1. *palmar branch of cubital nerve (Soemmerring, 1791)*
   Synonym for *palmar branch of ulnar nerve (Soemmerring, 1791)*; pp. 286–288.
2. *volar branch of ulnar nerve (Mayer, 1794)*
   Synonym for macrodissected adult human ***palmar branch of ulnar nerve (Soemmerring, 1791)***; in the original Latin, *ramus volaris nervi ulnaris*; Part 5, Table 5, Figure 1-4 (p. 22).
3. *long palmar nerve of ulnar nerve (Meckel, 1817)*
   Synonym for macrodissected adult human ***palmar branch of ulnar nerve (Soemmerring, 1791)***; in the original Latin, *nervus ulnaris longus palmaris*, see translation (1832, Vol. 3, p. 28).
4. *long palmar branch of ulnar nerve (Bock, 1827)*
   Synonym for macrodissected adult human ***palmar branch of ulnar nerve (Soemmerring, 1791)***; in the original Latin, *ram. palmaris longus ulnaris*, Table I, Figure 2-33.
5. *cutaneous long palmar branch of ulnar nerve (Bock, 1827)*
   Synonym for macrodissected adult human ***palmar branch of ulnar nerve (Soemmerring, 1791)***; in the original Latin, *ram. palmaris longus cutaneus*, Table II-64.

palpebral branches of infratrochlear nerve (>1840)

As described for macrodissected adult human, they end in skin of the upper and lower eyelids; see Durward (1951, p. 1020), *Terminologia Anatomica* (1998, p. 134). Winslow first clearly indicated them; see ***[palpebral branches of infratrochlear nerve (>1840)] (Winslow, 1733)***.

EARLIER REFERENCES:

Described, not named or illustrated:

1. ***[palpebral branches of infratrochlear nerve (>1840)] (Winslow, 1733)***
   Alluded to for macrodissected adult human; Section VI, p. 64. Meckel (1817) mentioned twigs of ***infratrochlear nerve (Schaarschmidt, 1750)*** supplying "orbicularis palpebrarum" in macrodissected adult human; see translation (1832, Vol. 3, p. 60).

Earlier synonyms:

1. *superior and inferior branches of infratrochlear nerve (Haase, 1781)*
   Synonym for macrodissected adult human ***palpebral branches of infratrochlear nerve (>1840)***, designations adopted by the *Basel Nomina Anatomica* (His, 1895, p. 88); in the original Latin, *nervus infratrochlearem ramulos superior et inferior*, pp. 59–60.
2. *palpebral branches of naso-palpebral nerve (Burdin, 1803)*
   Synonym for macrodissected adult human ***palpebral branches of infratrochlear nerve (>1840)***; see translation (1803, Vol. 1, p 172).
3. *palpebral filaments of external nasal branch of nasal nerve (Cruveilhier, 1836)*
   Synonym for macrodissected adult human ***palpebral branches of infratrochlear nerve (>1840)***; in the original French, *filets palpébraux*, p. 915.

pancreatic branches of superior mesenteric plexus (>1840)

As described for macrodissected adult human, they accompany the superior mesenteric artery from the ***superior mesenteric plexus (Rau, 1720)*** to the ***pancreatic plexus (Cruveilhier, 1736)***; see Williams & Warwick (1980, p. 1134). They were known to Haller; see ***[pancreatic branches of superior mesenteric plexus (>1840)] (Haller, 1762)***.

EARLIER REFERENCES:

Described, not named or illustrated:

1. ***[pancreatic branches of superior mesenteric plexus (>1840)] (Haller, 1762)***
   Mentioned for macrodissected adult human; p. 264.

pancreatic plexus (Cruveilhier, 1836)

As defined for macrodissected adult human, mainly an extension of the ***celiac plexus (Winslow, 1733)*** following the pancreatic arteries; see *Dorland's* (2003, p. 1455). More specifically, contributions arise from the ***hepatic plexus (Rau, 1720)*** to the head and neck of the pancreas, ***splenic plexus (Palfijn, 1726)***, ***superior mesenteric plexus (Rau, 1720)***, and ***intermesenteric plexus (>1840)***; see Durward (1951, p. 1142), Mitchell (1953, pp. 278–280), Williams & Warwick (1980, p. 1134), Tiscornia et al. (1987). For Cruveilhier's use in macrodissected adult human, see p. 1018. It was known at least in part to Willis; see ***[pancreatic plexus (>1840)] (Willis, 1664)***.

TRANSLATIONS:

1. *plexus pancréatique (Cruveilhier, 1836)*
   Original French form of ***pancreatic plexus (Cruveilhier, 1836)***; p. 1018.

EARLIER REFERENCES:

Described, not named or illustrated:

1. ***[pancreatic plexus (>1840)] (Willis, 1664)***
   Willis described contributions from ***hepatic plexus (Rau, 1720)*** in macrodissected adult human and other large mammals; see Pordage translation (1681, p. 158 and Tab. 11-*o*).

Earlier synonyms:

1. *pancreatic nerves (Walter, 1783)*
   Essentially synonym for macrodissected adult human ***pancreatic plexus (Cruveilhier, 1836)***; in the original Latin, *nervi pancreatici*, Table III:*294–299*; singular, *nervus pancreaticus*, Table III-*314*.

PARTLY CORRESPONDS:

1. *anterior pancreatic nerves from splenic plexus (Walter, 1783)*
   Specific component of macrodissected adult human ***pancreatic plexus (Cruveilhier, 1836)***; in the original Latin, *nervi pancreatici anteriores ex plexu lienali*, Table IV:*114–116*.
2. *pancreatic nerves from hepatic plexus (Walter, 1783)*
   Specific component of macrodissected adult human ***pancreatic plexus (Cruveilhier, 1836)***; in the original Latin, *nervi pancreatici ex plexu hepatico*, Table IV:*125–128*.

3. *middle pancreatic nerves (Mayer, 1794)*
As described for macrodissected adult human, arise from region of ***hepatic plexus (Rau, 1720)*** and contribute to ***pancreatic plexus (Cruveilhier, 1836)***; in the original Latin, *nervi pancreatis medii*; Part 6, Table IV-38 (p. 27).
4. *left pancreatic nerves (Mayer, 1794)*
As described for macrodissected adult human, arise from region of ***splenic plexus (Palfijn, 1726)*** and contribute to ***pancreatic plexus (Cruveilhier, 1836)***; in the original Latin, *nervi pancreatis sinistri*; Part 6, Table IV-39 (p. 27).

pancreaticoduodenal plexus (Wrisberg, 1800)

As described for macrodissected adult human, it accompanies the superior and inferior pancreaticoduodenal arteries and is thus an extension of the ***right gastroepiploic plexus (Wrisberg, 1800)*** at one end and the ***superior mesenteric plexus (Winslow, 1733)*** at the other end, which join in the middle; see Mitchell (1953, p. 280 and Figs. 79, 122). For Wrisberg's use in macrodissected adult human, see p. 563. He was also the first to clearly distinguish it.

TRANSLATIONS:

1. *plexu pancreatico-duodenali (Wrisberg, 1800)*
Original Latin form of ***pancreaticoduodenal plexus (Wrisberg, 1800)***; p. 563.

parabrachial nucleus (>1840)

As described for adult human with gross dissection, and for adult mammal in general with cellular architecture and connections, a ***gray matter region (Swanson & Bota, 2010)*** in the dorsolateral ***pons (Haller, 1747)*** surrounding the ***superior cerebellar peduncle (Procháska, 1800)*** and receiving a major connection from the ***nucleus of solitary tract (>1840)***; see Nieuwenhuys et al. (2008, pp. 203, 892 and Fig. 6.28). It was first identified by Reil; see ***[parabrachial nucleus (>1840)] (Reil, 1809c)***.

EARLIER REFERENCES:

Described, not named or illustrated:

1. ***[parabrachial nucleus (>1840)] (Reil, 1809c)***
Reil vaguely though definitely alluded to it in macrodissected adult human as thin layer of *gray substance (Vesalius, 1543a)* on ventromedial (under) surface of *body of superior cerebellar peduncle (Reil, 1809c)*; see Mayo translation (1823, p. 97).

paracentral sulcus (>1840)

As described for macrodissected adult human, a dorsal extension of the ***cingulate sulcus (>1840)*** between ***medial frontal gyrus (>1840)*** rostrally and ***anterior paracentral gyrus (>1040)*** caudally; see Crosby et al. (1962, p. 348), Williams & Warwick (1980, Fig. 7.114A, unlabeled), *Terminologia Anatomica* (1998, p. 126). It was first clearly delineated by Soemmerring; see ***[paracentral sulcus (>1840)] (Soemmerring, 1778)***.

EARLIER REFERENCES:

Illustrated, not named or described:

1. ***[paracentral sulcus (>1840)] (Soemmerring, 1778)***
Illustrated clearly for macrodissected adult human; Table III.

paracervical ganglia (>1840)

As described for macrodissected adult human female, a variable number of small ***terminal ganglia (Gaskell, 1886)*** in the ***uterovaginal plexus (>1840)***; see Mitchell (1953, p. 309), Williams & Warwick (1980, p. 1136). At least one was first clearly delineated by Tiedemann; see ***[paracervical ganglia (>1840)] (Tiedemann, 1822)***.

EARLIER REFERENCES:

Illustrated and described, not named:

1. ***[paracervical ganglia (>1840)] (Tiedemann, 1822)***
At least one identified in macrodissected adult human female; see *ganglion of uterine plexus (Tiedemann, 1822)*.

paraflocculus (Stroud, 1895)

As described for macrodissected adult human, a lateral extension of the ***tonsil (Malacarne, 1776)*** of the ***cerebellar hemisphere (Willis, 1664)***; see Angevine et al. (1961, p. 24 under *paraflocculus accessorius*, and Figs. 5, 11, 13, 19, 20, 22), Larsell & Jansen (1972, Fig. 118), Carpenter (1976, Fig. 14.1), *Dorland's* (2003, p. 1362). For Stroud's use in macrodissected embryonic and adult mammal, see pp. 95–96. It was not distinguished by 1840.

parahippocampal gyrus (>1840)

As described for macrodissected adult human, the lateral topographic subdivision of the ***hippocampal formation (Swanson & Cowan, 1977)*** as opposed to the medial subdivision, the ***hippocampal region (Swanson et al., 1987)***. Based on cellular architecture and connections in mammal, the ***parahippocampal gyrus (>1840)*** corresponds to the ***retrohippocampal region (Swanson, et al. 1987)*** further subdivided into ***entorhinal area (Brodmann, 1909)*** laterally and ***subicular complex (Swanson& Cowan, 1977)*** medially; see Carpenter (1976, p. 531, Fig. 530), Williams & Warwick (1980, p. 995, Figs. 7.114A, 117A, 119), *Nomina Anatomica* (1983, p. A71), Nauta & Feirtag (1986, pp. 126, 228), Swanson et al. (1987), *Terminologia Anatomica* (1998, p. 126), Nieuwenhuys et al. (2008, p. 68). It is frequently called *hippocampal gyrus (>1840)*, in distinction to *hippocampus (Vicq d'Azyr, 1784)* or ***Ammon's horn (Vicq d'Azyr, 1784)***. For recent review in primate, see Van Hoesen (1982). It was first clearly illustrated by Steno; see ***[parahippocampal gyrus (>1840)] (Steno, 1669)***.

EARLIER REFERENCES:

Illustrated, not named or described:

1. ***[parahippocampal gyrus (>1840)] (Steno, 1669)***
Very clearly illustrated in transverse section through macrodissected adult human ***forebrain (Goette, 1873)***; Plate III.

Earlier synonyms:

1. *convolution of hippocampus major (Vicq d'Azyr, 1786)*
Synonym for macrodissected adult human ***parahippocampal gyrus (>1840)***; in the original French, *la circonvolution du grand hypocampe*, Plate XVI, p. 46. It is further described as "*circonvolutions situées près du grand hypocampe ou corne d'Ammon, et qui servent à former son étui.*" (Pl. XXV, Fig. III-*n,p*).

2. *inferior and superior floor of hippocampus major (Vicq d'Azyr, 1786)*
   Apparently synonym for *convolution of hippocampus major (Vicq d'Azyr, 1786)*; in the original French, *le plancher inférieur et le plancher supérieur des grands hypocampes*, Plate XV-25,26.
3. *accessories of cylindroid protuberances (Burdin, 1803)*
   Probably roughly synonymous with right and left macrodissected adult human ***parahippocampal gyrus (>1840)***; see translation (1803, Vol. 1, p. 160).
4. *accessories of cornua Ammonis (Burdin, 1803)*
   Synonym for *accessories of cylindroid protuberances (Burdin, 1803)*; see translation (1803, Vol. 1, p. 160).
5. *long internal convolution (Reil, 1812b)*
   Roughly synonymous with macrodissected adult human ***parahippocampal gyrus (>1840)***; see Mayo translation (1823, p. 116).
6. *inner margin of middle lobe (Gordon, 1815)*
   Although vaguely described, probably corresponds more or less to *convolution of hippocampus major (Vicq d'Azyr, 1786)*; p. 85. Like Vicq d'Azyr, Gordon apparently divided it into anterior and posterior parts; pp. 85–86, also see *inferior and superior floor of hippocampus major (Vicq d'Azyr, 1786)*.
7. *subiculum of Ammon's horn (Burdach, 1822)*
   Exact boundaries for macrodissected adult human not illustrated or described. Clearly includes histologically defined ***subiculum (>1840)*** and extends for unknowable distance laterally into rest of ***subicular complex (Swanson & Cowan, 1977)*** and adjacent ***entorhinal area Brodmann, 1909)***. Later German authorities, including Henle (1871, p. 165), Meynert (1872, p. 668, Fig. 259), Schwalbe (1881, pp. 734–735), and Kölliker (1896, p. 735), all regarded it as synonymous with entire ***parahippocampal gyrus (>1840)***. In the original Latin, *subiculum cornu ammonis*; p. 156. In Latin, *subiculum* is diminutive of *subex*, a base or support, here for ***Ammon's horn (Vicq d'Azyr, 1784)***; see Foster (1894, p. 2866).
8. *border of inferior lobe (Burdach, 1822)*
   Refers roughly to macrodissected adult human ***parahippocampal gyrus (>1840)***; p. 174 and Tables VII-λ, VIII-6, and XI, Figure 2-*i,l*; compare with Nieuwenhuys et al. (2008, Fig. 3.6). In the original German, *die Kante*.
9. *ora lobi inferioris (Burdach, 1822)*
   Original Latin form of *border of inferior lobe (Burdach, 1822)*.
10. *hippocampal lobe (Serres, 1824–1826)*
    Probably roughly synonymous with ***parahippocampal gyrus (>1840)*** in macrodissected adult mammal; in the original French, *lobe de l'hippocampe*; Vol. 2, pp. 468–469. Leuret (1839, Pl. XII, Fig. 2-*l.h.*; Pl. XVI, Fig. 3-*l.h.*; and p. 404) used it the same way. Serres also labeled it in certain macrodissected adult reptiles (crocodile and cobra), where its identity is even less certain; Figures 117-5, 118-3, 127-4.
11. *hippocampal lobule (Serres, 1824–1826)*
    Synonym for *hippocampal lobe (Serres, 1824–1826)*; in the original French, *lobule de l'hippocampe*, p. 548 ff.
12. *internal tuberosity of temporal lobe (Gerdy, 1838)*
    Probably roughly synonymous with macrodissected adult human ***parahippocampal gyrus (>1840)***; in the original French, *tubérosité interne du lobe temporal*, p. 259.
13. *hippocampal gyrus (>1840)*
    Can be synonym for macrodissected adult human ***parahippocampal gyrus (>1840)***; see Henle (1871, p. 165), Schwalbe (1881, pp. 734–735), Kölliker (1896, p. 735), Nauta & Haymaker (1969, Fig. 4.10, p. 151), *Nomina Anatomica* (1983, p. A71), Nauta & Feirtag (1986, p. 126).

paramedian fissure (>1840)

As described for macrodissected adult mammalian ***cerebellum (Aristotle)***, the longitudinal depression between ***cerebellar vermis (Burdach, 1822)*** medially and ***cerebellar hemisphere (Willis, 1664)*** laterally; see Nieuwenhuys et al. (2008, p. 70 and Figs. 3.11, 3.13). It was known to Galen; see ***[paramedian fissure (>1840)] (Galen, c173)***.

EARLIER REFERENCES:

Described, not named or illustrated:

1. ***[paramedian fissure (>1840)] (Galen, c173)***
   In distinguishing *vermiform epiphysis (Galen, c173)* Galen necessarily observed it; see May translation (1968, p. 420).

Illustrated, not named or described:

1. ***[paramedian fissure (>1840)] (Vesalius, 1543a)***
   Illustrated for macrodissected adult human; see Singer translation (1952, Figs. 8, 9, 11).

Earlier synonyms:

1. *isthmus (Reil, 1807–1808a)*
   Synonym for macrodissected adult human ***paramedian fissure (>1840)***; see Mayo translation (1822, Tab. III, Fig. III-*b*).

parasubiculum (>1840)

As described with cellular architecture and connections in mammal, the topologically and developmentally lateral division of the ***subicular complex (Swanson & Cowan, 1977)*** lying lateral to ***presubiculum (>1840)*** and medial to ***entorhinal area (>1840)***; see Swanson et al. (1987), Nieuwenhuys et al. (2008, p. 372 and Fig. 12.5). It was not identified by 1840.

TRANSLATIONS:

1. *area parasubicularis (Brodmann, 1909)*
   Synonym for ***parasubiculum (>1840)***; see pp. 182, 188.
2. *parasubicular area (Brodmann, 1909)*
   English form of *area parasubicularis (Brodmann, 1909)*: see translation (1994, p. 160).
3. *area 49 (Brodmann, 1909)*
   Synonym for ***parasubiculum (>1840)***, which he only observed in flying fox, rabbit, hedgehog, and kinkajou; in the original German, *Feld 49*, see p. 182.

paravertebral ganglia (Durward, 1951)

As described for macrodissected adult human, ***autonomic ganglia (Langley, 1900)*** associated with the ***sympathetic trunk (Winslow, 1733)*** and branches associated directly with it, and including the ***carotid ganglion (>1840)***, ***sympathetic trunk ganglia (Winslow, 1733)***, and ***intermediate ganglia (>1840)***; p. 1126. They are now commonly described sequentially from rostral (superior) to caudal (inferior). Perhaps the first reference to them was by Falloppio; see ***[paravertebral ganglia (Durward, 1951)] (Falloppio, 1561)***.

EARLIER REFERENCES:

Described, not named or illustrated:

1. ***[paravertebral ganglia (Durward, 1951)] (Falloppio, 1561)***
   Falloppio is credited with discovering the first members in thoracic regions of ***sympathetic trunk (Winslow, 1733)***; see Johnstone (1765, p. 177).

Earlier synonyms:

1. *limiting ganglions of ganglionnary nerve (Meckel, 1817)*
   Synonym for macrodissected adult human ***paravertebral ganglia (Durward, 1951)***; see translation (1832, Vol. 3, pp. 9, 84).
2. *great sympathetic part of nervous system (Blainville, 1821)*
   Essentially synonym for macrodissected ***paravertebral ganglia (Durward, 1951)*** in vertebrates generally; in the original French, *grand sympathetique*, p. 206. It relates *visceral part of nervous system (Blainville, 1821)* with *central part of nervous system (Carus, 1818)* via *ganglionated part of nervous system (Blainville, 1821)*.
3. *sympathetic nervous system (Blainville, 1821)*
   Synonym for *great sympathetic part of nervous system (Blainville, 1821)*; in the original French, *système nerveux sympathetique*, p. 217.
4. *intermediate nervous system (Blainville, 1821)*
   Synonym for *great sympathetic part of nervous system (Blainville, 1821)*; in the original French, *système nerveux intermédiare*, p. 217.
5. *lateral ganglia of sympathetic (Grant, 1834c)*
   Essentially synonym for macrodissected ***paravertebral ganglia (Durward, 1951)*** in vertebrate, applied here to reptile; p. 551.
6. *vertebral ganglia (Gaskell, 1886)*
   Synonym for ***paravertebral ganglia (Durward, 1951)***; p. 2.

paravertebral nerves (Swanson & Bota, 2010)

Autonomic nerves (Langley, 1898) macroscopically appearing to arise from ***paravertebral ganglia (Durward, 1951)*** and/or associated ***sympathetic trunk (Winslow, 1733)***. They are now commonly described sequentially from rostral (superior) to caudal (inferior). The first example was described long ago by Galen; see ***[greater splanchnic nerve (Walter, 1783)] (Galen, c177)***.

EARLIER REFERENCES:

Earlier synonyms:

1. *interior branches of sympathetic nerve (Lobstein, 1823)*
   Synonym for macrodissected adult human ***paravertebral nerves (Swanson & Bota, 2010)***; see translation (1831, p. 44).
2. *visceral nerves (Lobstein, 1823)*
   Synonym for macrodissected adult human ***paravertebral nerves (Swanson & Bota, 2010)***; see translation (1831, p. 70).
3. *ganglionic nerves (Cruveilhier, 1836)*
   Synonym for macrodissected adult human ***paravertebral nerves (Swanson & Bota, 2010)***; in the original French, *nerfs ganglionnaires*, pp. 759, 998.
4. *great sympathetic nerves (Cruveilhier, 1836)*
   Generally synonymous with macrodissected adult human ***paravertebral nerves (Swanson & Bota, 2010)***; in the original French, *nerfs du grand sympathique*, p. 759.
5. *splanchnic nerves (Cruveilhier, 1836)*
   Synonym for *visceral nerves (Cruveilhier, 1836)*; in the original French, *nerfs splanchniques*, p. 1031.

PARTLY CORRESPONDS:

1. *interiorem ramum credo esse splanchnicum (Lancisi, 1719)*
   Probably synonym for macrodissected adult human *splanchnic nerve (Haller, 1762)*; see Haller (1762, p. 260 note *l*).
2. *collateral rope of great sympathetic nerve (Winslow, 1733)*
   Refers to macrodissected adult human ***greater splanchnic nerve (Walter, 1783)***, ***lesser splanchnic nerve (Haller, 1762)***, and ***least splanchnic nerve (>1840)***, considered together, and formed from five branches; Section VI, pp. 98, 100.
3. *great trunk of great sympathetic nerve (Winslow, 1733)*
   Synonym for *collateral rope of great sympathetic nerve (Winslow, 1733)*; Section VI, p. 98.
4. *collateral trunk of great sympathetic nerve (Winslow, 1733)*
   Synonym for *collateral rope of great sympathetic nerve (Winslow, 1733)*; Section VI, p. 100.
5. *external trunk (Schmidel, 1754)*
   Synonym for macrodissected adult human *splanchnic nerve (Haller, 1762)*; in the original Latin, *truncus exterior*, p. 19, according to Haller (1762, p. 260).
6. *splanchnic nerve (Haller, 1762)*
   Haller used this general term for macrodissected adult human ***nerves (Herophilus, c335–c280 BC)*** from thoracic levels 5–12 of ***sympathetic trunk (Winslow, 1733)*** to subdiaphragmatic viscera, thus including ***greater splanchnic nerve (Walter, 1783)***, ***lesser splanchnic nerve (Haller, 1762)***, and ***least splanchnic nerve (>1840)***; in the original Latin, *nervus splanchnicum*, p. 260, where earlier accounts of it are reviewed in note *m*.
7. *nervi molles (Haller, 1762)*
   Original Latin form of *soft nerves (Haller, 1762)*; pp. 256–257.
8. *soft nerves (Haller, 1762)*
   Correspond roughly to ***jugular nerves (>1840)***, ***laryngopharyngeal branches of superior cervical ganglion (>1840)***, and ***superior cardiac nerve (Neubauer, 1772)*** of

macrodissected adult human; in the original Latin, *nervi molles*, pp. 256–257. Neubauer (1772; pp. 62, 87 ff., 133–136 and Tab. 1-6), Haase (1781, pp. 119–120), and Scarpa (1794, Tab. III) gave even more thorough accounts of them in macrodissected adult human, and Scarpa also included the ***internal carotid nerve (>1840)*** and its rostral extensions. Thus its use varied with authors, but it often referred to all extensions of ***superior cervical ganglion (Vieussens, 1684)***; also see Meckel (1832, Vol. 3, p. 92). According to Portal (1803a, p. 167; no citation provided), Vieussens first wrote of them. Quain (1828, p. 664) succinctly defined them as anterior branches of ***superior cervical ganglion (Vieussens, 1684)***. From the modern perspective they are ***paravertebral nerves (Swanson & Bota, 2010)*** consisting of mostly unmyelinated postganglionic ***axons (Kölliker, 1896)*** from ***superior cervical ganglion (Vieussens, 1684)***; in describing extensions of ***external carotid plexus (>1840)***, Cruveilhier (1836, p. 993) wrote, "These plexuses appear to me to be particularly remarkable for containing a mixture of white fibres and nervi molles, which proves their double origin." (translation, 1844, p. 859). Also see Quain (1837, p. 808).

9. *inferior splanchnic nerve (Haller, 1762)*
Corresponds roughly to lesser ***splanchnic nerve (Haller, 1762)*** and ***least splanchnic nerve (>1840)*** considered together because it arises from last three ***thoracic sympathetic ganglia (>1840)*** in macrodissected adult human; in the original Latin, *nervo splanchnico inferiori*; p. 264.
10. *soft intercostal nerve (Neubauer, 1772)*
Roughly synonymous with *soft nerves (Haller, 1762)*; in the original Latin, *nervum mollem intercostalis*, Table 2-*78* and p. 64.
11. *rete nervorum mollium (Haller, 1772)*
Network or ***plexus (Galen, c192)*** of macrodissected adult human *soft nerves (Haller, 1762)*; p. 9-*42*.
12. *roots of splanchnic nerve (Haase, 1781)*
Origins of *splanchnic nerve (Haller, 1762)* from thoracic levels of ***sympathetic trunk (Winslow, 1733)*** in macrodissected adult human; in the original Latin, *radicibus nervi splanchnici*, p. 122.
13. *anterior intercostal nerve (Haase, 1781)*
Synonym for macrodissected adult human *splanchnic nerve (Haller, 1762)*; in the original Latin, *anteriorem intercostalem nervus*, p. 123.
14. *rami splanchnici (Monro, 1783)*
Synonym for *splanchnic nerve (Haller, 1762)* in macrodissected adult ox and human; p. 53.
15. *aortic branch of ninth thoracic ganglion (Walter, 1783)*
For macrodissected adult human, branch of tenth ***thoracic sympathetic ganglion (>1840)*** to descending aorta; in the original Latin, *ramus aorticus ex ganglio thoracico nono*, Table III-*103*. Walter described without specifically naming such branches from 7th–10th ***thoracic sympathetic ganglia (>1840)***.
16. *soft nerves of Haller (Günther, 1786)*
Eponym for 2–3 macrodissected adult human *soft nerves (Haller, 1762)*; in the original Latin, *n. molles Halleri*, p. 92. For them, Günther listed a ***communicating branch (Winslow, 1733)*** with ***vagus nerve (Galen, c192)***, and branches to pharynx, longus colli muscle, thyroid gland, and external carotid artery.
17. *superficial branch of first nerve of trunk (Andersch, 1797)*
Synonym for *superficial communicating branch of first nerves of trunk and second nerves of trunk (Andersch, 1797)*; in the original Latin, *ramus superficialis primi nervi trunci*, Vol. 2, p. 4.
18. *superficial communicating branch of first nerves of trunk and second nerves of trunk (Andersch, 1797)*
Macrodissected adult human ***communicating branch (Winslow, 1733)*** between ***sympathetic trunk (Winslow, 1733)*** and ***phrenic nerve (Galen, c173)***; in the original Latin, *primi nervi trunci ramum communicatorium superficialem secundi nervi trunci*, Vol. 2, p. 5, also see Williams & Warwick (1980, p. 1094).
19. *inferior lateral plexus of neck (Andersch, 1797)*
Apparently, network of ***communicating branches (Winslow, 1733)*** of macrodissected adult human ***paravertebral nerves (Swanson & Bota, 2010)*** associated with and lateral to ***middle cervical ganglion (Haller, 1762)***; in the original Latin, *plexum lateralem colli inferiorem*, Vol. 2, p. 146.
20. *nervi vasorum (Bell, 1803b)*
Synonym for macrodissected adult human *soft nerves (Haller, 1762)*; p. 172. A translation is *nerves of vessels*.
21. *great splanchnic nerve (Burdin, 1803)*
Synonym for macrodissected adult human ***greater splanchnic nerve (Walter, 1783)*** and ***lesser splanchnic nerve (Haller, 1762)***, considered together; see translation (1803, Vol. 1, p. 211).
22. *great suprarenal nerve (Chaussier, 1807)*
Synonym for *splanchnic nerve (Meckel, 1817)*; in the original French, *nerf grand surrenal*, see Meckel (1832, Vol. 3, p. 97).
23. *splanchnic nerve (Meckel, 1817)*
As described for macrodissected adult human, it included ***greater splanchnic nerve (Walter, 1783)*** and ***lesser splanchnic nerve (Haller, 1762)***; see translation (1832, Vol. 3, p. 97).
24. *plexus of soft nerves (Bock, 1817)*
Apparently roughly synonymous with macrodissected adult human *soft nerves (Haller, 1762)*; in the original Latin, *plexus nervorum mollium*, p. 63. For good illustration see *glossopharyngeal nerve branches of plexus of soft nerves (Langenbeck, 1826–1830)*.
25. *abdominal nerves (Lobstein, 1823)*
Apparently synonym for macrodissected adult human *splanchnic nerve (Haller, 1762)*; see translation (1831, p. 98).
26. *glossopharyngeal nerve branches of plexus of soft nerves (Langenbeck, 1826–1830)*
For macrodissected adult human, branches of ***pharyngeal branches of glossopharyngeal nerve (Neubauer, 1772)*** to *plexus of soft nerves (Bock, 1817)*; in the original Latin, *rami nervi glossopharyngei ad plexum nervorum mollium*, Fascicle III, Table XVI-*22*.

27. *aortic filaments from thoracic ganglia of great sympathetic (Cloquet, 1828)*
   For macrodissected adult human, small branches from 7th–10th ***thoracic sympathetic ganglia (>1840)*** to descending aorta; in the original French, *filets aortiques*, Plate CLXXVII:*112–117* and *63–66*.
28. *right thoracic plexus (Swan, 1830)*
   For macrodissected adult human, basically right ***thoracic cardiac nerves (>1840)*** and ***thoracic pulmonary nerves (>1840)*** considered together; p. 7.
29. *left thoracic plexus (Swan, 1830)*
   For macrodissected adult human, basically left ***thoracic cardiac nerves (>1840)*** and ***thoracic pulmonary nerves (>1840)*** considered together; p. 7.
30. *carotid nerve (Arnold, 1834)*
   In macrodissected adult human, ***internal carotid nerve (>1840)*** and ***internal carotid plexus (>1840)*** considered together; in the original Latin, *nervus caroticus*, p. 18.
31. *visceral branches of superior cervical ganglion (Cruveilhier, 1836)*
   For macrodissected adult human, *pharyngeal branches of superior cervical ganglion (Cruveilhier, 1836)*, *laryngeal branches of superior cervical ganglion (Cruveilhier, 1836)*, and *cardiac branches of superior cervical ganglion (Cruveilhier, 1836)*, considered together; in the original French, *branches viscérales*, p. 994.
32. *pelvic visceral nerves (Cruveilhier, 1836)*
   From description on pp. 1031–1032 for macrodissected adult human, clearly ***lumbar splanchnic nerves (Cruveilhier, 1836)*** and ***sacral splanchnic nerves (>1840)*** considered together; in the original French, *nerfs viscéraux pelviens*, p. 1024.
33. *pelvic splanchnic nerves (Cruveilhier, 1836)*
   Synonym for *pelvic visceral nerves (Cruveilhier, 1836)*; in the original French, *nerfs splanchniques pelviens*, p. 1031.

parietal operculum (>1840)

As described for macrodissected adult human, the surface of the ***parietal region (>1840)*** lining the dorsal wall of the **lateral cerebral sulcus** (>1840) up to the ***circular sulcus (Schwalbe, 1881)***, and including the ventral (lower) end of the ***postcentral gyrus (>1840)*** and rostroventral (anterior and inferior) part of ***supramarginal gyrus (>1840)***; see Carpenter (1976, Fig. 2.3), *Terminologia Anatomica* (1998, p. 125), *Dorland's* (2003, p. 1316). It was perhaps first clearly distinguished by Rolando; see ***[parietal operculum (>1840)] (Rolando, 1831)***.

EARLIER REFERENCES:

Illustrated, not named or described:

1. ***[parietal operculum (>1840)] (Rolando, 1831)***
   Clearly illustrated for macrodissected adult human; Figure 3, caudal part of ventral surface of 2.

Earlier synonyms:

1. *operculum of superior lobe (Arnold, 1838b)*
   Synonym for macrodissected adult human ***parietal operculum (>1840)***; in the original Latin, *operculum lobi superioris*, Table IV, Figure 5-*c*.

parietal region (>1840)

As described for macrodissected adult human, a dorsal topographic division of the ***cerebral cortex gray matter (>1840)*** lying between ***frontal region (Vicq d'Azyr, 1786)*** rostrally and ***occipital region (Vesalius, 1543a)*** caudally. Its main parts are the ***postcentral gyrus (>1840)*** and ***posterior paracentral gyrus (>1840)***, and the ***precuneus (Burdach, 1822)***, ***superior parietal lobule (>1840)***, and ***inferior parietal lobule (>1840)***; for general modern overview see Nieuwenhuys et al. (2008, p. 605 ff.). ***Parietal region (>1840)*** is preferred to, for example, *parietal lobe (Arnold, 1838a)* because an actual lobe cannot be distinguished and because the term *region* applies to all mammals, whether gyrencephalic or lissencephalic. It was not recognized as such by 1840.

PARTLY CORRESPONDS:

1. *parietal lobe (Arnold, 1838a)*
   For macrodissected adult human, the ***parietal region (>1840)*** but specifically without ***cerebral cortex gray matter (>1840)*** associated with ***parietal operculum (>1840)***, which Arnold included in *intermediate lobe (Arnold, 1838a)*; in the original Latin, *lobus parietalis*, p. 51.
2. *area postcentralis oralis (Brodmann, 1909)*
   Original Latin form of *rostral postcentral area (Burdach, 1909)*; p. 132.
3. *rostral postcentral area (Brodmann, 1909)*
   Based on cellular architecture in adult human, the most rostral zone of ***parietal region (>1840)*** in rostral end of ***postcentral gyrus (>1840)*** and rostral end of medially adjacent ***posterior paracentral gyrus (>1840)***, between *giant pyramidal area (Brodmann, 1909)* rostrally and *intermediate postcentral area (Brodmann, 1909)* caudally; see Garey translation (1994, p. 112 and Figs. 85, 86).
4. *area 3 (Brodmann, 1909)*
   Synonym for adult human *rostral postcentral area (Brodmann, 1909)*; in the original German, *Feld 3*, p. 132.
5. *area postcentralis intermedia (Brodmann, 1909)*
   Original Latin form of *intermediate postcentral area (Burdach, 1909)*; p. 132.
6. *intermediate postcentral area (Brodmann, 1909)*
   Based on cellular architecture in adult human, rostral zone of ***parietal region (>1840)*** in ***postcentral gyrus (>1840)*** and medially adjacent ***posterior paracentral gyrus (>1840)***, between *rostral postcentral area (Brodmann, 1909)* rostrally and *caudal postcentral area (Brodmann, 1909)* caudally; see Garey translation (1994, pp. 111–112 and Figs. 85, 86).
7. *area 1 (Brodmann, 1909)*
   Synonym for adult human *intermediate postcentral area (Brodmann, 1909)*; in the original German, *Feld 1*, p. 132.
8. *area postcentralis caudalis (Brodmann, 1909)*
   Original Latin form of *caudal postcentral area (Burdach, 1909)*; p. 132.
9. *caudal postcentral area (Brodmann, 1909)*
   Based on cellular architecture in adult human, rostral zone of ***parietal region (>1840)*** centered caudally

in ***postcentral gyrus (>1840)*** and caudally in medially adjacent ***posterior paracentral gyrus (>1840)***, between *intermediate postcentral area (Brodmann, 1909)* rostrally and *preparietal area (Brodmann, 1909)* caudally; see Garey translation (1994, pp. 111–112 and Figs. 85, 86).

10. *area 2 (Brodmann, 1909)*
Synonym for adult human *caudal postcentral area (Brodmann, 1909)*; in the original German, *Feld* 2, p. 132.
11. *area praeparietalis (Brodmann, 1909)*
Original Latin form of *preparietal area (Brodmann, 1909)*; p. 139.
12. *preparietal area (Brodmann, 1909)*
Based on cellular architecture in adult human, rostral zone of ***parietal region (>1840)*** centered in caudal end of ***posterior paracentral gyrus (>1840)*** and extending laterally into dorsal and caudal end of ***postcentral gyrus (>1840)*** and adjacent rostral parts of ***superior parietal lobule (>1840)***; see Garey translation (1994, p. 118 and Figs. 85, 86).
13. *area 5 (Brodmann, 1909)*
Synonym for adult human *preparietal area (Brodmann, 1909)*; in the original German, *Feld* 5, p. 139.
14. *area parietalis superior (Brodmann, 1909)*
Original Latin form of *superior parietal area (Brodmann, 1909)*; p. 140.
15. *superior parietal area (Brodmann, 1909)*
Based on cellular architecture in adult human, a large zone of ***parietal region (>1840)*** including ***precuneus (>1840)*** medially and ***superior parietal lobule (>1840)*** dorsally, except rostrally where ***superior parietal lobule (>1840)*** is occupied by caudal end of *preparietal area (Brodmann, 1909)*; see Garey translation (1994, pp. 118–119 and Figs. 85, 86).
16. *area 7 (Brodmann, 1909)*
Synonym for adult human *superior parietal area (Brodmann, 1909)*; in the original German, *Feld* 7, p. 140.
17. *area 50 Brodmann, 1909)*
Based on cellular architecture Brodmann illustrated it just dorsal to *area 13 (Brodmann, 1909)* of ***insular region (Brodmann, 1909)*** in marmoset (Fig. 96), flying fox (Fig. 102), kinkajou (Fig. 104), rabbit (Fig. 106 and p. 190), and ground squirrel (Fig. 108), but not human. He could not decide whether to include it in ***insular region (Brodmann, 1909)*** or ***parietal region (>1840)***; see Garey translation (1994, p. 167).

parieto-occipital sulcus (>1840)

As described for macrodissected adult human, the groove centered on the medial surface of the ***cerebral cortex gray matter (>1840)*** between ***precuneus (Burdach, 1822)*** rostrally and ***cuneus (Burdach, 1822)*** caudally, and often extending slightly over onto the lateral surface; see Williams & Warwick (1980, Figs. 7.111, 7.114), *Terminologia Anatomica* (1998, p. 126). It was first delineated by Vesalius; see ***[parieto-occipital sulcus (>1840)] (Vesalius, 1543a)***.

EARLIER REFERENCES:

Illustrated, not named or described:

1. ***[parieto-occipital sulcus (>1840)] (Vesalius, 1543a)***
Clearly illustrated without comment for macrodissected adult human; see Singer translation (1952, p. 95, Fig. 4, left cortex on right side of figure).

Earlier synonyms:

1. *posterior sulcus (Soemmerring, 1778)*
Synonym for macrodissected adult human ***parieto-occipital sulcus (>1840)***; Table III, see Meyer (1971, p. 124).

parolfactory gyrus (>1840)

As described for macrodissected adult human, the most rostral and ventral topographic subdivision of the ***cingulate region (>1840)***, bounded by ***anterior parolfactory sulcus (>1840)*** rostrally and ***posterior parolfactory sulcus (>1840)*** caudally. Based on cellular architecture and connections in mammal it corresponds to the ***infralimbic area (Rose & Woolsey, 1948)*** or *area 25 (Brodmann, 1909)*; see Nauta and Haymaker (1969, Fig. 4.11, p. 158). It was first clearly illustrated by Soemmerring; see ***[parolfactory gyrus (>1840)] (Soemmerring, 1778)***.

ALTERNATE SPELLINGS:

1. *paraolfactory gyrus (>1840)*
Alternate spelling of ***parolfactory gyrus (>1840)***; see *Terminologia Anatomica* (1998, p. 126).

EARLIER REFERENCES:

Illustrated, not named or described:

1. ***[parolfactory gyrus (>1840)] (Soemmerring, 1778)***
Illustrated clearly for macrodissected adult human; Table III, rostral to *4* and caudoventral to *c*. Also very clearly depicted for macrodissected adult human in a wonderful drawing by Rolando (1831, Fig. 10-*15*).

parotid branches of auriculotemporal nerve (>1840)

As described for macrodissected adult human, branches of ***auriculotemporal nerve (Haller, 1762)*** supplying the parotid gland; see Mitchell (1953, Fig. 69), *Terminologia Anatomica* (1998, p. 134). They were known to Galen, see ***[parotid branches of auriculotemporal nerve (>1840)] (Galen, c173)***.

EARLIER REFERENCES:

Described, not named or illustrated:

1. ***[parotid branches of auriculotemporal nerve (>1840)] (Galen, c173)***
Described for macrodissected adult beef, pig, and/or macaque but not human; see May translation (1968, p. 455).

Illustrated and described, not named:

1. ***[parotid branches of auriculotemporal nerve (>1840)] (Willis, 1664)***
Illustrated and very briefly described for macrodissected adult, presumably human; see Pordage translation (1681, p. 145, Fig. 1-*k*). Todd (1836–1839, p. 293) noted they "establish upon the [external carotid]

artery a manifest communication with branches of the sympathetic."

Earlier synonyms:

1. *tertia ac exterior propago rami majoris posterioris (Vieussens, 1684)*
   Synonym for macrodissected adult human ***parotid branches of auriculotemporal nerve (>1840)***; p. 173 and Table 22-9.
2. *inferior auricular fascicle of cutaneous temporal surculus of inferior maxillary branch (Bellingeri, 1818)*
   Synonym for macrodissected adult human ***parotid branches of auriculotemporal nerve (>1840)*** including branches to parotid gland and ventral part of pinna; in the original Latin, *fasciculus auricularis inferior*, see Table I.

parotid plexus (Meckel, 1817)

As described for macrodissected adult human, the network within the parotid gland of ***communicating branches (Winslow, 1733)*** of the ***facial nerve trunk (>1840)*** generating its five terminal branches, ***temporal branches of facial nerve (Swan, 1830)***, ***zygomatic branches of facial nerve (>1840)***, ***buccal branch of facial nerve (>1840)***, ***marginal mandibular branch of facial nerve (>1840)***, and ***cervical branch of facial nerve (>1840)***; see Durward (1951, Fig. 902), Hamilton (1976, Fig. 798), Williams & Warwick (1980, p. 1071). For Meckel's use in macrodissected adult human, see translation (1832, Vol. 3, p. 55). It was first clearly described as the *plexus which resembles a goose's foot (Winslow, 1733)*.

TRANSLATIONS:

1. *plexus parotideus (Meckel, 1817)*
   Original Latin form of ***parotid plexus (Meckel, 1817)***; see translation (1832, Vol. 3, p. 55).

EARLIER REFERENCES:

Earlier synonyms:

1. *plexus which resembles a goose's foot (Winslow, 1733)*
   Synonym for macrodissected adult human ***parotid plexus (Meckel, 1817)***; Section VI, p. 69.
2. *pedem anserinum (Haller, 1762)*
   Latin form (plural) of *plexus which resembles a goose's foot (Winslow, 1733)* for macrodissected adult human; p. 229.
3. *pes anserinus (Mayer, 1794)*
   Singular Latin of *pedem anserinum (Haller, 1762)*; Part 5, Table VII-96,97 (p. 48).

LATER SYNONYMS:

1. *parotid filaments of portio major and minor of facial nerve (Bellingeri, 1818)*
   Synonym for macrodissected adult human ***parotid plexus (Meckel, 1817)***; in the original Latin, *filamenta parotidea*, see Table II.
2. *plexus anserinus (Arnold, 1834)*
   Synonym for macrodissected adult human ***parotid plexus (Meckel, 1817)***; p. 12.
3. *plexus intraparotideus (>1840)*
   Synonym for macrodissected adult human ***parotid plexus (Meckel, 1817)***; see *Nomina Anatomica* (1983, p. A75). *Terminologia Anatomica* (1998, p. 135) gave the English use of Latin term as "parotid plexus."

patellar plexus (>1840)

As described for macrodissected adult human, a network of fine ***communicating branches (Winslow, 1733)*** beneath the skin in front of the knee, receiving contributions mainly from the ***infrapatellar branch of saphenous nerve (>1840)***, ***medial cutaneous nerve of thigh (>1840)***, and ***anterior cutaneous branches of femoral nerve (Quain & Wilson, 1839)***, and sometimes from the ***lateral cutaneous nerve of thigh (>1840)*** as well; see Durward (1951, p. 1098 and Fig. 940). It was first clearly delineated by Cruveilhier; see ***[patellar plexus (>1840)] (Cruveilhier, 1836)***.

EARLIER REFERENCES:

Described, not named or illustrated:

1. ***[patellar plexus (>1840)] (Cruveilhier, 1836)***
   Described for macrodissected adult human; see p. 847.

peduncular loop (Gratiolet, 1857)

As described in macrodissected adult human, and mammal generally with histological methods for ***axons (Kölliker, 1896)***, a heterogenous, longitudinal, bidirectional, diffusely organized ***central nervous system white matter tract (>1840)*** between *amyglar region (>1840)* and ***globus pallidus (Burdach, 1822)*** rostrally and laterally, and ***interbrain (Baer, 1837)*** caudally and medially, passing through and to ***substantia innominata (Meynert, 1872)*** along the way; see Mettler (1948, pp. 361–362), Nauta & Haymaker (1969, p. 168). For topographic description, at the border between ***interbrain (Baer, 1837)*** and ***hypothalamus (Kuhlenbeck, 1927)*** it joins the rostral end of the ***medial forebrain bundle (Edinger, 1893)*** ventrally and the ***inferior thalamic radiation peduncular loop (>1840)*** dorsally. For the term in English see *Dorland's* (2003, p. 96, under *ansa peduncularis*). For Gratiolet's use in macrodissected adult baboon see Atlas Plate 26, Figures 5-*k*, 6; Plate 27, Figure 1-*c*. It was first clearly described by Reil; see ***[peduncular loop (Gratiolet, 1857)] (Reil, 1812c)***.

TRANSLATIONS:

1. *anse du pédoncule (Gratiolet, 1857)*
   Original French form of ***peduncular loop (Gratiolet, 1857)***; see Atlas Plate 26, Figure 6.
2. *ansa peduncularis (>1840)*
   Latin form of ***peduncular loop (Gratiolet, 1857)***; see Meynert (1872 translation, pp. 683–684, 689, 691).

EARLIER REFERENCES:

Described, not named or illustrated:

1. ***[peduncular loop (Gratiolet, 1857)] (Reil, 1812c)***
   First described, for macrodissected adult human, "The bed of gray substance analogous to them [the right and left *gray nucleus (Reil, 1812c)* or ***inferior colliculus (>1840)***] in either thalamus [***interbrain (Baer, 1837)***] occupies its internal and posterior

part: from this are derived fasciculi, which partly join the radiation of the fibrous cone [*corona radiata (Reil, 1809b)*], occupying its fore part; but some fasciculi internal to the others, bend round the margin of the crus cerebri [***cerebral peduncle (Tarin, 1753)***], forming the medulla incognita [***substantia innominata (Meynert, 1872)***]." (Mayo translation, 1823, p. 124).

LATER SYNONYMS:

1. *ansa peduncularis of Gratiolet (Dejerine & Dejerine-Klumpke, 1895)*
Eponym for macrodissected adult human ***peduncular loop (Gratiolet, 1857)***; in the original French, *anse pédonculaire de Gratiolet*, see p. 374. Also see Meynert (1872 translation, p. 689).

pelvic ganglia (>1840)

As described for macrodissected adult human, small ***terminal ganglia (Gaskell, 1886)*** in the ***inferior hypogastric plexus (Tiedemann, 1822)***; see Williams & Warwick (1980, p. 1135), *Nomina Anatomica* (1983, p. A79), *Terminologia Anatomica* (1998, p. 142). They were probably first clearly delineated by Cruveilhier; see ***[pelvic ganglia (>1840)] (Cruveilhier, 1836)***.

EARLIER REFERENCES:

Described, not named or illustrated:

1. ***[pelvic ganglia (>1840)] (Cruveilhier, 1836)***
Clearly identified in macrodissected adult human, referring to *hypogastric plexus (Winslow, 1733)* as consisting of "des nerfs et des ganglions" (p. 1032).

pelvic splanchnic nerves (Gaskell, 1886)

As described for macrodissected adult human, they arise from the second, third, and often fourth ***sacral plexus ventral divisions (Paterson, 1887)*** as so-called *visceral branches of sacral plexus (Cruveilhier, 1836)* and pass directly to the ***inferior hypogastric plexus (Tiedemann, 1822)***—or *pelvic plexus (Chaussier, 1789)*—that contains small ***ganglia (Galen, c173)***, as do the walls of the individual pelvic viscera. Functionally, these ***ganglia (Galen, c173)*** act as relays for parasympathetic preganglionic ***axons (Kölliker, 1896)*** in the ***pelvic splanchnic nerves (Gaskell, 1886)*** supplying the rectum with motor ***axons (Kölliker, 1896)***, the bladder wall with motor and its sphincter with inhibitory ***axons (Kölliker, 1896)***, the erectile tissue of the penis or clitoris with vasodilator ***axons (Kölliker, 1896)***, the testes or ovaries probably with vasodilator ***axons (Kölliker, 1896)***, and the uterine tubes and uterus with vasodilator and possibly inhibitory ***axons (Kölliker, 1896)***. Small branches from the ***pelvic splanchnic nerves (Gaskell, 1886)*** also pass rostrally (upwards) through the ***inferior hypogastric plexus (Tiedemann, 1822)*** to supply the sigmoid colon, descending colon, left colic flexure, and terminal part of the transverse colon with visceromotor ***axons (Kölliker, 1896)***; see Durward (1951, Fig. 962), Mitchell (1953, Fig. 131), Williams & Warwick (1980, pp. 1116,1123 and Figs. 7.224, 231). For Gaskell's use in macrodissected adult dog, see p. 9; also see ***sacral splanchnic nerves (>1840)***. At least some were known to Galen and Vesalius; see *nerve for urinary bladder (Galen, c173)*.

EARLIER REFERENCES:

Earlier synonyms:

1. *nerve for urinary bladder (Galen, c173)*
Almost certainly refers vaguely to ***pelvic splanchnic nerves (Gaskell, 1886)*** in macrodissected adult beef, pig, and/or macaque but not human; see May translation (1968, pp. 261–262), Duckworth translation (1962, p. 263). Vesalius (1543a) probably referred to some of them in macrodissected adult human when he wrote, "the bladder and uterus also have their own special nerves coming from the spinal marrow in the sacrum" (Richardson & Carman translation, 2002, pp. 200, 255).
2. *internal pudendal nerve (Mayer, 1794)*
Apparently synonym for macrodissected adult human ***pelvic splanchnic nerves (Gaskell, 1886)***; in the original Latin, *nervus pudendalis internus*; Part 6, Table VI-*160* (p. 40).
3. *middle hemorrhoidal nerves (Meckel, 1817)*
Synonym for macrodissected adult human ***pelvic splanchnic nerves (Gaskell, 1886)***; in the original Latin, *nervi haemorrhoidales medii*, see translation (1832, Vol. 3, p. 15).
4. *hypogastric branches of sacral nerves (Cloquet, 1828)*
Synonym for macrodissected adult human ***pelvic splanchnic nerves (Gaskell, 1886)***; in the original French, *rameaux hypogastriques des N. sacrés*, Plate CLXX, Figure 2-97.
5. *visceral branches of sacral plexus (Cruveilhier, 1836)*
Synonym for macrodissected adult human ***pelvic splanchnic nerves (Gaskell, 1886)***; in the original French, *branches viscérales*, p. 851. See Williams & Warwick (1980, pp. 1110, 1111, 1123).
6. *branches from sacral nerves communicating with lateral portion of hypogastric plexus (Quain & Wilson, 1839)*
Synonym for macrodissected adult human ***pelvic splanchnic nerves (Gaskell, 1886)***; Plate XXVIII-*n*.

LATER SYNONYMS:

1. *nervi erigentes* (>1840)
Synonym for ***pelvic splanchnic nerves (Gaskell, 1886)***; see Mitchell (1953, p. 190).
2. *parasympathetic roots of pelvic ganglion (>1840)*
Synonym for ***pelvic splanchnic nerves (Gaskell, 1886)***; see *Terminologia Anatomica* (1998, p. 142).

PARTLY CORRESPONDS:

1. *hypogastric branches of third sacral nerve (Walter, 1783)*
Walter described for a macrodissected adult human ten ***pelvic splanchnic nerves (Gaskell, 1886)*** from third ***sacral nerve (Camper, 1760)***; in the original Latin, *rami hypogastricus tertii nervi sacralis*, Table I:*405–418*. He also noted, however, that the number is quite variable and may be only a few in some cadavers.
2. *hypogastric branch of fourth sacral pair (Walter, 1783)*
Walter described for a macrodissected adult human one ***pelvic splanchnic nerve (Gaskell, 1886)*** from fourth

sacral nerve (Camper, 1760); in the original Latin, *ramus paris quarti sacralis hypogastricus*, Table I-*423*.

3. *uterine nerve (Cloquet, 1828)*
Macrodissected adult human ***pelvic splanchnic nerve (Gaskell, 1886)*** to uterus from fourth ***sacral nerve (Camper, 1760)***; in the original French, *nerf utérin*, Plate CLXX, Figure 2-*96*.
4. *hemorrhoidal branch of fifth sacral nerve (Cloquet, 1828)*
Macrodissected adult human ***pelvic splanchnic nerve (Gaskell, 1886)*** to rectum and adjacent regions from fifth ***sacral nerve (Camper, 1760)***; in the original French, *rameau hémorrhoïdal du cinquième nerf sacré*, Plate CLXX, Figure 2-*98,99*.
5. *hemorrhoidal branches of third and fourth sacral nerves (Cloquet, 1828)*
Macrodissected adult human ***pelvic splanchnic nerves (Gaskell, 1886)*** to anal sphincter and overlying skin from third and fourth ***sacral nerves (Camper, 1760)***; in the original French, *rameaux hémorrhoïdaux des troisième et quatrième N. sacré*, Plate CLXXV-*235*.
6. *internal hemorrhoidal nerve of third sacral nerve (Cloquet, 1828)*
Macrodissected adult human ***pelvic splanchnic nerve (Gaskell, 1886)*** to anal sphincter from third ***sacral nerve (Camper, 1760)***; in the original French, *N. hémorrhoïdaux internes venant du troisième N. sacrés*, Plate CLXXV-*241*.

perforating cutaneous nerve (>1840)

As described for macrodissected adult human, it most commonly arises from the second and third ***sacral plexus dorsal divisions (Paterson, 1887)*** and supplies skin over caudal (lower) and medial parts of the gluteus maximus muscle. However, it may be absent, when its place may be taken by a branch from the ***posterior cutaneous nerve of thigh (Günther, 1786)*** or by branches from the third and fourth or fourth and fifth ***sacral nerves (Camper, 1760)***; see Williams & Warwick (1980, p. 1115 and Figure 7.196), *Terminologia Anatomica* (1998, p. 140). It was first clearly indicated by Eustachi; see ***[perforating cutaneous nerve (>1840)] (Eustachi, 1552)***.

EARLIER REFERENCES:

Illustrated, not named or described:

1. ***[perforating cutaneous nerve (>1840)] (Eustachi, 1552)***
Clearly, if somewhat inaccurately, illustrated peripheral distribution in unpublished plates of macrodissected adult human; see Albinus edition (1761, Tab. 23-Ω).

Described, not named or illustrated:

1. ***[perforating cutaneous nerve (>1840)] (Colombo, 1559)***
Colombo is credited with first describing it in print, for macrodissected adult human; see Crooke (1615, p. 906).

PARTLY CORRESPONDS:

1. *inferior gluteal cutaneous nerve (Walter, 1783)*
Probably component of, or equivalent to part of, ***perforating cutaneous nerve (>1840)*** in macrodissected adult human; in the original Latin, *nervus cutaneus gluteus inferior*, Table I-*380*.
2. *inferior cutaneous nerves of buttocks (Walter, 1783)*
Probably component of, or equivalent to part of, ***perforating cutaneous nerve (>1840)*** in macrodissected adult human; in the original Latin, *nervi cutanei natium inferior*, Table I:*385–387*. Walter described a trunk and two branches. Bell (1803b, p. 203) translated it *inferior cutaneous nerve of nates*.
3. *trunk of inferior cutaneous nerves of buttocks (Walter, 1783)*
Trunk of *inferior cutaneous nerves of buttocks (Walter, 1783)*, dividing in two branches, for macrodissected adult human; in the original Latin, *truncus nervi cutanei natium inferior (in duos ramos divisus)*, Table I-*385*.
4. *middle cutaneous nerves of buttocks (Walter, 1783)*
Probably component of, or equivalent to part of, ***perforating cutaneous nerve (>1840)*** in macrodissected adult human; in the original Latin, *nervi cutanei natium medius*, Table I-*400*. Bell (1803b, p. 203) translated it *middle cutaneous nerve of nates*.
5. *superior cutaneous nerves of buttocks (Walter, 1783)*
Probably component of, or equivalent to part of, ***perforating cutaneous nerve (>1840)*** in macrodissected adult human; in the original Latin, *nervi cutanei natium superiorem*, Table I:*385–387*; singular, *nervum cutaneum natium superiorem*, Table I-*404*. Bell (1803b, p. 203) translated it *superior cutaneous nerve of nates*.
6. *inferior cutaneous nerve of haunches (Knox, 1832)*
Form of *inferior cutaneous nerves of buttocks (Walter, 1783)*; Plate XI-*90*.
7. *middle cutaneous nerve of haunches (Knox, 1832)*
Form of *middle cutaneous nerves of buttocks (Walter, 1783)*; Plate XI-*100*.
8. *superior cutaneous nerve of hips (Knox, 1832)*
Form of *superior cutaneous nerves of buttocks (Walter, 1783)*; Plate XI-*103*.

periaqueductal gray (>1840)

As described for macrodissected adult human, and for adult mammal in general with cellular architecture and connections, a ***gray matter region (Swanson & Bota, 2010)*** of the ***tegmentum (Swanson, 2000b)*** forming a cylinder around the ***cerebral aqueduct (>1840)***, just ventral to the ***tectum (Baer, 1837)*** and dorsomedial to the ***midbrain reticular nucleus (>1840)***; see Nieuwenhuys et al. (2008, Figs. 6.29–6.32) for human, and Swanson (2004, Table B, p. 174) for a list of parts including ***nucleus of Darkschewitch (>1840)*** and ***dorsal raphe nucleus (>1840)***, which are best known in rat. It was perhaps first clearly delineated by Vicq d'Azyr; see ***[periaqueductal gray (>1840)] (Vicq d'Azyr, 1786)***.

EARLIER REFERENCES:

Illustrated, not named or described:

1. ***[periaqueductal gray (>1840)] (Vicq d'Azyr, 1786)***
Clearly illustrated in macrodissected adult human transverse section; Plate XV-*17*.

Earlier synonyms:

1. *ring of gray substance (Rolando, 1825)*
   Synonym for macrodissected adult beef ***periaqueductal gray (>1840)*** illustrated in transverse section; in the original French, *cercle de substance cendrée*, Table VIII, Figure 6-*a.s.*

pericardial branch of phrenic nerve (>1840)

As described for adult human, the ***phrenic nerve (Galen, c173)*** as it courses through the thorax receives sensory branches from the fibrous pericardium and parietal layer of the serous pericardium; see Williams & Warwick (1980, p. 1094), *Terminologia Anatomica* (1998, p. 137). It was perhaps first clearly delineated as *pericardial twigs of diaphragmatic nerve (Vieussens, 1684)*.

EARLIER REFERENCES:

Earlier synonyms:

1. *pericardial twigs of diaphragmatic nerve (Vieussens, 1684)*
   Synonym for macrodissected adult human ***pericardial branch of phrenic nerve (>1840)***, "*Nervus diaphragmatis, qui aliquando pericardio surculos quofdam impertitur...*" (see * on p. 216).
2. *communicating branch from phrenic nerve to pericardium (Krüger, 1758)*
   Synonym for macrodissected adult human ***pericardial branch of phrenic nerve (>1840)***; Sections 13,14 and Table 2-*38,39*.

perineal branch of fourth sacral nerve (>1840)

As described for macrodissected adult human, it supplies the levator ani, coccygeus, and sphincter ani externus muscles; see Durward (1951, p. 1102, Figs. 937, 943). It was probably first indicated by Eustachi; see ***[perineal branch of fourth sacral nerve (>1840)] (Eustachi, 1552)***.

EARLIER REFERENCES:

Illustrated, not named or described:

1. ***[perineal branch of fourth sacral nerve (>1840)] (Eustachi, 1552)***
   Origin probably indicated for macrodissected adult human; see Albinus edition (1761, Tab. 20/2-Σ on left side of body) compared with Durward (1951, Fig. 937).

Illustrated and described, not named:

1. ***[perineal branch of fourth sacral nerve (>1840)] (Vieussens, 1684)***
   Described and illustrated for macrodissected adult human; Table 29-*16,17*.

Earlier synonyms:

1. *external hemorrhoidal branches of fourth sacral pair (Fischer, 1791)*
   Three described for macrodissected adult human, probably corresponding to ***perineal branch of fourth sacral nerve (>1841)***; in the original Latin, *ramulos haemorrhoidales externos*, p. 21.

PARTLY CORRESPONDS:

1. *branch to levator ani muscle (Bock, 1827)*
   Branch of macrodissected adult human ***perineal branch of fourth sacral nerve (>1840)*** to levator ani muscle; in the original Latin, *ram. musculi levatoris ani*; Table VII, Figure 1-*39*.

perineal branches of posterior cutaneous nerve of thigh (>1840)

As described for macrodissected adult human, they arise at the caudal (lower) border of the gluteus maximus muscle and sweep medially supplying collateral branches to the proximal (upper) medial part of the thigh and terminal branches to skin and fascia of the scrotum and root of the penis (male), or labium majus and clitoris (female); they also communicate with the ***ilio-inguinal nerve (Schmidt, 1794)*** and with two components of the ***pudendal nerve (Camper, 1762)***, the ***inferior rectal nerves (>1840)*** and ***perineal nerve (Camper, 1762)***; see Durward (1951, pp. 1103–1104 and Figs. 943, 947), *Terminologia Anatomica* (1998, p. 140). They were probably first delineated by Eustachi; see ***[perineal branches of posterior cutaneous nerve of thigh (>1840)] (Eustachi, 1552)***.

EARLIER REFERENCES:

Illustrated, not named or described:

1. ***[perineal branches of posterior cutaneous nerve of thigh (>1840)] (Eustachi, 1552)***
   Illustrated for macrodissected adult human; see Albinus edition (1761, Tab. 23/2-Ω, lower branch).

Illustrated and described, not named:

1. ***[perineal branches of posterior cutaneous nerve of thigh (>1840)] (Vieussens, 1684)***
   Described and illustrated for macrodissected adult human; see Table 29-*31*.

Earlier synonyms:

1. *posterior cutaneous branch of sciatic nerve (Soemmerring, 1791)*
   Probably synonym for macrodissected adult human ***perineal branches of posterior cutaneous nerve of thigh (>1840)***; p. 308, also see Soemmerring (1798, p. 327).
2. *internal branch of recurrent branch of cutaneous branch of inferior gluteal nerve (Cruveilhier, 1836)*
   Synonym for macrodissected adult human ***perineal branches of posterior cutaneous nerve of thigh (>1840)***; in the original French, *rameau interne*, p. 858.
3. *scrotal branch of recurrent branch of cutaneous branch of inferior gluteal nerve (Cruveilhier, 1836)*
   Synonym for macrodissected adult human ***perineal branches of posterior cutaneous nerve of thigh (>1840)***; in the original French, *rameau scrotal*, p. 858. Cruveilhier attributed to Soemmerring without citation the Latin synonym *pudendalis longus inferior*.
4. *middle posterior cutaneous nerve (Quain & Wilson, 1839)*
   Basically synonym for macrodissected adult human ***perineal branches of posterior cutaneous nerve of thigh (>1840)***; Plate XXII-*h*.

PARTLY CORRESPONDS:

1. *posterior cutaneous branches of thigh (Bock, 1827)*
   Terminal branches of macrodissected adult human ***perineal branches of posterior cutaneous nerve of thigh (>1840)*** to proximal (upper) and dorsal (posterior)

regions of thigh; in the original Latin, *rami cutanei posteriores femoris*, Table VII, Figure 3-*37*.

perineal nerve (Camper, 1762)

As described for macrodissected adult human, the caudal (inferior) and larger terminal branch of the ***pudendal nerve (Camper, 1762)***, dividing distally into ***posterior scrotal nerves (Mayer, 1794)*** or ***posterior labial nerves (>1840)*** and ***muscular branches of perineal nerve (>1840)***; see Durward (1951, Figs. 943, 944), Williams & Warwick (1980, p. 1116). For Camper's use in macrodissected adult human, see Table 1, Figure 1-*14,17,18*. It was first described as the *nerve to genital organs (Galen, c192)*.

EARLIER REFERENCES:

Earlier synonyms:

1. *nerve to genital organs (Galen, c192)*
Galen mentioned a ***nerve (Herophilus, c335–c280 BC)*** to skin and muscles of genital organs in macrodissected adult beef, pig, and/or macaque but not human—essentially the ***perineal nerve (Camper, 1762)***; see Duckworth translation (1962, p. 263, and pp. 110–111), also see May translation (1968, p. 651). Eustachi illustrated it for macrodissected adult human, see Albinus edition (1761, Tab. 20/2-lower 2 of 3 branches of Φ), and it was clearly illustrated by Vieussens (1684, Tab. 29-*13,20*) for macrodissected adult human.

LATER SYNONYMS:

1. *inferior pudendal nerve (Camper, 1762)*
Corresponds more or less to macrodissected adult human ***perineal nerve (Camper, 1762)***; p. 7.
2. *hemorrhoidal nerve (Günther, 1786)*
Apparently synonym for macrodissected adult human ***perineal nerve (Camper, 1762)***; in the original Latin, *haemorrhoidales*, p. 84.
3. *long pudendal nerve (Fischer, 1791)*
Synonym for macrodissected adult human ***inferior pudendal nerve (Camper, 1762)***; in the original Latin, *nervus pudendus inferior*, p. 21.
4. *inferior external pudendal nerve (Mayer, 1794)*
Synonym for macrodissected adult human ***inferior pudendal nerve (Camper, 1762)***; in the original Latin, *nervus pudendus externus inferior*; Part 6, Table VI-*178* (p. 40).
5. *external pudic nerve (Bell, 1803a)*
Synonym for macrodissected adult human ***perineal nerve (Camper, 1762)***; Plate VII-5. Meckel (1817) gave the Latin, *nervus pudendus externus*, see translation (1832, Vol. 3, p. 14).
6. *superior pudic nerve (Meckel, 1817)*
Synonym for macrodissected adult human ***perineal nerve (Camper, 1762)***; in the original Latin, *nervus pudendus superior*, see translation (1832, Vol. 3, p. 14).
7. *inferior branches of pudendal nerve (Bock, 1827)*
Synonym for macrodissected adult human ***perineal nerve (Camper, 1762)***; in the original Latin, *rami nervi pudendi inferioris*, Table IV-*112*.
8. *superficial pudendal nerve (Bock, 1827)*
Synonym for macrodissected adult human ***perineal nerve (Camper, 1762)***; in the original Latin, *nerv. pudendus superficialis*, Table VI, Figure 1-*36*.
9. *inferior branch of internal pudendal nerve (Cruveilhier, 1836)*
Synonym for macrodissected adult human ***perineal nerve (Camper, 1762)***; in the original French, *branche inférieure*, p. 853.
10. *perineal branch of internal pudendal nerve (Cruveilhier, 1836)*
Synonym for macrodissected adult human ***perineal nerve (Camper, 1762)***; in the original French, *branche périnéale*, p. 853. Alternate form of Quain & Wilson (1839, Pl. XXII-*e*), *perineal branch of internal pudic nerve*.

PARTLY CORRESPONDS:

1. *inferior nerve of penis (Soemmerring, 1798)*
Corresponds partly to macrodissected adult human ***perineal nerve (Camper, 1762)***; in the original Latin, *nervusque penis inferior*, p. 322.
2. *inferior branch of perineal branch of internal pudendal nerve (Cruveilhier, 1836)*
Branch of *perineal branch of internal pudendal nerve (Cruveilhier, 1836)* following superficial perineal artery; in the original French, *rameau inférieur*, p. 853.
3. *collateral branches of perineal branch of internal pudendal nerve (Cruveilhier, 1836)*
Synonym for *external perineal branch of perineal branch of internal pudendal nerve (Cruveilhier, 1836)*; in the original French, *rameaux collatéraux de la branche périnéale*, p. 853.
4. *external perineal branch of perineal branch of internal pudendal nerve (Cruveilhier, 1836)*
Branch of *perineal branch of internal pudendal nerve (Cruveilhier, 1836)* supplying ***muscular branch of perineal nerve (>1840)*** to ischiocavernosus muscle and apparently forming ***posterior labial nerves (>1840)*** or ***posterior scrotal nerves (Mayer, 1794)***; in the original French, *rameau périnéal externe*, p. 853.
5. *terminal branches of perineal branch of internal pudendal nerve (Cruveilhier, 1836)*
Two were described: *superficial perineal branch of perineal branch of internal pudendal nerve (Cruveilhier, 1836)* and *bulbo-urethral branch of perineal branch of internal pudendal nerve (Cruveilhier, 1836)*; in the original French, *rameaux de terminaison de la branche périnée*, p. 854.
6. *superficial perineal branch of perineal branch of internal pudendal nerve (Cruveilhier, 1836)*
Probably synonym for macrodissected adult human *inferior nerve of penis (Soemmerring, 1798)*; in the original French, *rameau superficiel du périnée*, p. 854.

peripheral ganglia (>1840)

Localized, macroscopically visible collections of ***neurons (Waldeyer, 1891)*** in the ***peripheral nervous system (Meckel, 1817)*** divided topographically into ***craniospinal ganglia (>1840)*** and ***autonomic ganglia (Langley,***

1900) and distinguished from ***central ganglia (>1840)*** of invertebrates; see Swanson & Bota (2010, Thesaurus). Galen introduced the term "ganglia" in referring to certain differentiations on the ***sympathetic trunk (Winslow, 1733)***; see May translation (1968, p. 695) and ***[autonomic ganglia (Langley, 1900] (Galen c173, c177, c192)***. He wrote that a ***ganglion (Galen, c173)*** has the consistency of ***nerve (Herophilus, c335–c280 BC)*** and is found on small ***nerves (Herophilus, c335–c280 BC)*** conducting over a long path; previous usage referred to an encapsulated tumor on a tendon or aponeurosis; see May translation (1968, p. 695). Morgagni (1719) is credited with describing for the first time a mixture of ***gray matter (Meckel, 1817)*** and ***white matter (Meckel, 1817)*** in ***peripheral ganglia (>1840)***, along with small blood vessels; see Clarke & Jacyna (1987, p. 330). "The term 'ganglion' is also sometimes used for nuclei or centers within the brain... but this usage is objectionable, for the use of the word ganglion in vertebrate neurology should be restricted to collections of neurons outside the central nervous system, such as the ganglia of the cranial and spinal nerves and the sympathetic [autonomic] ganglia." (Herrick, 1915, p. 108). Gaskell (1886, p. 3) advanced an influential generalization reflected in ***peripheral nervous system (Meckel, 1817)*** organization adapted here, "We have therefore four sets of ganglia in possible connection with each *ramus visceralis* [***gray communicating branch (>1840)*** and ***white communicating branch (>1840)***], two of which, viz. the root ganglia [***spinal nerve ganglia (Burdach, 1819)***] and the lateral ganglia [***paravertebral ganglia (Durward, 1951)***], may be spoken of as proximal, and two, the collateral [***prevertebral ganglia (Quain, 1837)***] and terminal ganglia [***(Gaskell, 1886)***], as distal."

EARLIER REFERENCES:

Earlier synonyms:

1. *plexus (Falloppio, 1561)*
   According to Johnstone (1795, pp. 1–2), Falloppio used for macrodissected adult human the terms ***ganglia (Galen, c173)***, *corpora olivaria* [see *olive body (Falloppio, 1561)*], and *plexus* interchangeably; in this usage, *plexus* would mean ***ganglion (Galen, c173)*** or ***peripheral ganglion (>1840)***. Johnston wrote further that this usage was common until the beginning of the 18th century.
2. *knots (Crooke, 1615)*
   Synonym for macrodissected adult human ***peripheral ganglia (>1840)***; Table 16, Figure 1-*MM*, p. 482.
3. *ganglioform infoldings (Willis, 1664)*
   Synonym for ***peripheral ganglia (>1840)*** in macrodissected adult large mammals and human; see Pordage translation (1681, p. 146).
4. *infoldings (Willis, 1664)*
   This word (in Latin, *plexus*) was usually used to indicate ***peripheral ganglia (>1840)***, e.g., *cervical infolding (Willis, 1664)* for ***middle cervical ganglion (Haller, 1762)***; but sometimes to indicate *plexuses*, e.g., *two infoldings in pelvis (>1664)* for right and left ***inferior hypogastric plexus (Tiedemann, 1822)***.
5. *nervous folds (Diemerbroeck, 1689)*
   Synonym for macrodissected adult human *infoldings (Willis, 1664)*; pp. 417, 561.
6. *tumors (Diemerbroeck, 1689)*
   Synonym for macrodissected adult human ***peripheral ganglia (>1840)***; p. 417.
7. *ganglions (Winslow, 1733)*
   Alternate spelling of ***ganglia (Galen, c173)***, specifically for macrodissected adult human ***peripheral ganglia (>1840)***; Section VI, p. 94.
8. *gangliaform tubercles (Winslow, 1733)*
   Synonym for macrodissected adult human ***peripheral ganglia (>1840)***; Section VI, p. 94.
9. *little brains (Winslow, 1733)*
   Synonym for macrodissected adult human ***peripheral ganglia (>1840)***; Section VI, p. 94.
10. *corpora olivaria Fallopii (Tarin, 1753)*
    Eponym for macrodissected adult human ***peripheral ganglia (>1840)***; p. 40.
11. *olivi-formia nervorum (Tarin, 1753)*
    Synonym for macrodissected adult human ***peripheral ganglia (>1840)***; p. 72.
12. *nervorum nodum (Neubauer, 1772)*
    Synonym for macrodissected adult human ***peripheral ganglion (>1840)***; basically a *nervous knot* or *node of nerve*, p. 43.
13. *node of nerve (Neubauer, 1772)*
    English form of *nervorum nodum (Neubauer, 1772)*, a ***peripheral ganglion (>1840)***. *Nerve node* is another obvious form.
14. *nervous ganglia (Cloquet, 1828)*
    Synonym for macrodissected adult human ***peripheral ganglia (>1840)***; in the original French, *ganglions nerveux*, p. 328.

peripheral longitudinal communicating branch (Swanson & Bota, 2010)

The segment of a ***peripheral nerve cord (Swanson & Bota, 2010)*** between two ***peripheral ganglia (>1840)***; for Swanson & Bota's use in all animals see their Thesaurus; it was clearly distinguished early on as ***[communicating branches of sympathetic trunk (>1840)] (Willis, 1664)***.

EARLIER REFERENCES:

Illustrated and described, not named:

1. ***[communicating branches of sympathetic trunk (>1840)] (Willis, 1664)***
   Clearly distinguished in macrodissected adult human and other large mammals; see Tables IX, X, and Pordage translation (1681, pp. 157–158).

peripheral nerve cord (Swanson & Bota, 2010)

A ***nerve cord (Serres, 1824–1826)*** in the ***peripheral nervous system (Meckel, 1817)***. As a topographic division, a series of more or less regularly spaced ***peripheral ganglia (>1840)*** separated by ***peripheral longitudinal***

communicating branches (Swanson & Bota, 2010). From a systems architecture perspective, a longitudinal ***peripheral nerve cord trunk (Swanson & Bota, 2010)*** equivalent to a ***white matter tract (Bell & Bell, 1826)***, with a series of more or less regularly spaced ***peripheral ganglia (>1840)*** equivalent to ***gray matter regions (Swanson & Bota, 2010)*** along its course. The prototypical vertebrate example is the ***sympathetic trunk (Winslow, 1733)*** with its ***sympathetic trunk ganglia (Winslow, 1733)***—together the ***sympathetic cord (>1840)***. For Swanson & Bota's use, see (2010, Thesaurus). It was first described by Galen; see ***[peripheral nerve cord (>1840)] (Galen, c173)***.

EARLIER REFERENCES:

Described, not named or illustrated:

1. *[peripheral nerve cord (>1840)] (Galen, c173)*
   First description, in macrodissected adult beef, pig, and/or macaque but not human; see ***[sympathetic cord (>1840)] (Galen, c173)***.

peripheral nerve cord trunk (Swanson & Bota, 2010)

The equivalent of a ***peripheral nervous system white matter tract (>1840)*** for a ***peripheral nerve cord (Swanson & Bota, 2010)***, with ***peripheral ganglia (>1840)*** distributed along its length; that is, the ***peripheral nerve cord (Swanson & Bota, 2010)*** without the associated ***peripheral ganglia (>1840)***, the ***white matter tract (Bell & Bell, 1826)*** without the ***gray matter regions (Swanson & Bota, 2010)***. The vertebrate instance is the ***sympathetic trunk (Winslow, 1733)***. For Swanson & Bota's use, see (2010, Thesaurus). The existence of such a feature was known to Galen; see *nerve extending along roots of ribs (Galen, c173)*.

peripheral nervous system (Meckel, 1817)

In adult animals with bilateral symmetry, a topographic division of the ***nervous system (Monro, 1783)*** consisting of ***nerves (Herophilus, c335–c280 BC)*** and ***ganglia (Galen, c173)***. When a ***peripheral nervous system (Meckel, 1817)*** is present, its obligate companion topographic division is a ***central nervous system (Carus, 1814)***. There is no known isolated part of the adult ***peripheral nervous system (Meckel, 1817)*** without a *connection* to the ***central nervous system (Carus, 1814)***; see Bullock & Horridge (1965, pp. 9–14), Swanson & Bota (2010). At the systems architecture level the ***peripheral nervous system (Meckel, 1817)*** consists of ***peripheral nervous system gray matter regions (>1840)*** and ***peripheral nervous system white matter tracts (>1840)***. Meckel apparently was the first to use the terms ***central nervous system (Carus, 1814)*** and ***peripheral nervous system (Meckel, 1817)*** together to describe the entire ***nervous system (Monro, 1783)*** as universally done now; see translation (1832, Vol. 1, p. 153). It was recognized long ago as ***[peripheral nervous system (Meckel, 1817)] (Herophilus, c335–c280 BC)***.

EARLIER REFERENCES:

Described, not named or illustrated:

1. *[peripheral nervous system (Meckel, 1817)] (Herophilus, c335c–c280 BC)*
   The founder of human anatomy is credited with discovering ***nerves (Herophilus, c335–c280 BC)***, including most of the ***cranial nerves (Soemmerring, 1791)*** and ***spinal nerves (Camper, 1760–1762)*** in macrodissected adult mammals and human cadavers; see Solmsen (1961), von Staden (1969).

Earlier synonyms:

1. *nervous system (Willis, 1664)*
   Synonym for macrodissected adult mammalian ***peripheral nervous system (Meckel, 1817)***; see Pordage translation (1681, p. 125 ff.).
2. *radiosa concretio (Willis, 1664)*
   Synonym for *nervous system (Willis, 1664)*, the ***peripheral nervous system (Meckel, 1817)***: "…if the Head containing in it self the chief part and power of the sensitive Soul [the ***brain (Smith Papyrus, c1700 BC)***], be taken for the body of some Luminary, as of the Sun or a Star; the [peripheral] nervous System shall be that radiant or beamy concretion (*radiosa concretio*) compassing it about. Because the animal Spirits flowing from the Brain and Cerebel, with the medullar Appendix of either, as it were from a double Luminary, irradiate the [peripheral] nervous System, and so constitute its several parts, the Organs of Motion or Sense, or of both together, as hath been said. The parts of the nervous System, as a radiant or beamy texture (*texturae radiosae*), are either primary…" (see Pordage translation, 1681, p. 126).
3. *radiant concretion (Willis, 1664)*
   English form of *radiosa concretio (Willis, 1664)*; see Pordage translation (1681, p. 126).
4. *texturae radiosae (Willis, 1664)*
   Synonym for *radiosa concretio (Willis, 1664)*; see Pordage translation (1681, p. 126).
5. *radiant texture (Willis, 1664)*
   English form of *texturae radiosae (Willis, 1664)*; see Pordage translation (1681, p. 126).

LATER SYNONYMS:

1. *external nervous system (Meckel, 1817)*
   Synonym for macrodissected adult human ***peripheral nervous system (Meckel, 1817)***; see translation (1832, Vol. 1, p. 153).
2. *lateral nervous system (Desmoulins, 1825)*
   Variation on *external nervous system (Meckel, 1817)* for vertebrates generally; in the original French, *systèmes nerveux latéraux*, Atlas p. 4.

PARTLY CORRESPONDS:

1. *plexus of sixth pair (Falloppio, 1561)*
   According to Bauhin (1605), complex network in macrodissected adult human neck of ***vagus nerve (Galen, c192)***, ***sympathetic trunk (Winslow, 1733)***, branches of ***cervical nerves (Galen, c173)***, and associated ***ganglia (Galen, c173)*** at least partly innervating the heart; see Crooke translation (1615, p. 893).

2. *plexus retiformis (Read, 1638)*
Appears to indicate roughly macrodissected adult human *solar plexus (Willis, 1664)*; also referred to as *net-like texture* (p. 167).
3. *nervous plexure of mesenterium (Vesling, 1647)*
Probably equivalent to *solar plexus (Willis, 1664)*; see 1653 translation, p. 11 and Table for Chapter 3, Figure VIII-δ.
4. *nervous plexure (Vesling, 1647)*
Synonym for *nervous plexure of mesenterium (Vesling, 1647)*; see 1653 translation, p. 11.
5. *mesenterical plexure (Vesling, 1647)*
Synonym for *nervous plexure of mesenterium (Vesling, 1647)*; see 1653 translation, p. 13.
6. *plexure of costals (Vesling, 1647)*
Synonym for *nervous plexure of mesenterium (Vesling, 1647)*; see 1653 translation, p. 17.
7. *nerve plexus of abdomen (Wharton, 1656)*
Probably equivalent to *solar plexus (Willis, 1664)*; in the original Latin, *nerveum plexum abdominis* (p. 85; for English translation see Freer, 1996, p. 85).
8. *primary nervous system (Willis, 1664)*
Major ***nerve (Herophilus, c335–c280 BC)*** trunks of ***peripheral nervous system (Meckel, 1817)***; see Pordage translation (1681, p. 126). Also see *nervous system (Willis, 1664)* and *secondary nervous system (Willis, 1664)*.
9. *secondary nervous system (Willis, 1664)*
Part of ***peripheral nervous system (Meckel, 1817)*** consisting of small branches of ***nerves (Herophilus, c335–c280 BC)***—"nervous fibres"—in tissues, although not all appear to arise from ***nerve (Herophilus, c335–c280 BC)*** trunks themselves; see Pordage translation (1681, pp. 126, 128). Also see *nervous system (Willis, 1664)* and *primary nervous system (Willis, 1664)*.
10. *plexus mesenterici (Willis, 1664)*
General term to indicate seven *infoldings (Willis, 1664)*—five great and superior, and two less and inferior—corresponding to much of the ***prevertebral plexuses (Quain, 1837)*** and including region in and around right and left ***celiac ganglion (Walter, 1783)*** (2), right and left ***aorticorenal ganglion (>1840)*** (2), and ***superior mesenteric ganglion (>1840)*** (1); and ***inferior mesenteric plexus (Rau, 1720)*** (1) and ***superior hypogastric plexus (Tiedemann, 1822)*** (1) respectively (pp. 342–343).
11. *mesenteric infoldings (Willis, 1664)*
English form of *plexus mesenterici (Willis, 1664)*; see Pordage translation (1681, p. 158).
12. *solar plexus (Willis, 1664)*
From vague description and illustration, apparently corresponds roughly to ***superior mesenteric plexus (Rau, 1720)*** and ***superior mesenteric ganglion (>1840)*** considered together; see Pordage translation (1681, pp. 159, 169). "The greatest Infolding of the Mesentery [*(Willis, 1664)*] being placed in the midst of the rest [of the infoldings or ***plexuses (Galen, c192)*** and ***ganglia (Galen, c173)***], like the sun, disperses every where round about nervous Fibres like rays, *Figure 11*-[⊙] and casts them not only on every one of those infoldings, as if so many Planets with a peculiar Aspect, or *Actinobolism* or Irridiation, but also it distributes them into many Intestines, sanguiferous Vessels, and other parts lying round about..." (Pordage translation, 1681, p. 169). Also see Table XI-⊙.
13. *greatest infolding of mesentery (Willis, 1664)*
Synonym for *solar plexus (Willis, 1664)*; in the original Latin, *plexum mesenterii maximum*; see Pordage translation (1681, p.169 and Table XI-⊙).
14. *greatest mesenteric infolding (Willis, 1664)*
Synonym for *greatest infolding of mesentery (Willis, 1664)*; see Table XI-⊙.
15. *upper plexure of abdomen (Diemerbroeck, 1672)*
Apparently synonym (see translation, 1689, p. 51) for *solar plexus (Willis, 1664)*; in the original Latin, *plexu superiore abdominus*, p. 71. Gibson (1684, p. 94) used essentially the same term, *upper nervous plexus of abdomen*.
16. *plexure of nerves between two kidneys (Diemerbroeck, 1672)*
Synonym for *upper plexure of abdomen (Diemerbroeck, 1672)*; see translation (1689, p. 126). Earlier, Riolan (1649) referred to "a complication of the Costal and Stomachical Nerves, disposed between the two Kidneis. From whence are derived Nerves, that are dispersed to al Parts of the Belly" (see translation, 1657, p. 53).
17. *cervical plexus (Diemerbroeck, 1672)*
Term used in margin note vaguely referring to interconnections established by macrodissected adult human ***vagus nerve (Galen, c192)*** and ***sympathetic trunk (Winslow, 1733)*** in the neck; in the original Latin, *plexus cervicalis*, p. 618.
18. *plexus mesentericus magnus (Drake, 1707)*
Variation on Willis's Latin form of *greatest infolding of mesentery (Willis, 1664)* in macrodissected adult human; p. 519.
19. *pupillary nerves (Pourfour du Petit, 1729)*
Pourfour du Petit suggested it might be a better term than *ciliary nerves (Ruysch, 1702)*, and went on to review carefully the earlier literature and conclude they are formed by branches of ***optic nerve (Vicq d'Azyr, 1786)***, ***trigeminal nerve (Winslow, 1733)***, ***abducens nerve (Heister, 1717)***, and ***sympathetic trunk (Winslow, 1733)*** in macrodissected adult human and quadrupeds; p. 12. Contributions from ***ciliary ganglion (Loder, 1778)*** were not clearly described. Based on this analysis, including contribution from ***trigeminal nerve (Winslow, 1733)***, it seems likely that the term includes ***short ciliary nerves (>1840)*** and ***long ciliary nerves (Soemmerring, 1801)*** considered together.
20. *ganglioform plexuses (Tarin, 1750)*
Tarin's definition is clear and corresponds to ***prevertebral plexuses (Quain, 1837)*** with associated ***prevertebral ganglia (Quain, 1837)***, and ***terminal plexuses (Swanson & Bota, 2010)*** with associated ***terminal ganglia (Gaskell, 1886)***; in the original French, *les plexus ganglio-formes*, and in the original Latin, *plexus ganglio-formes*, p. 72.

21. *anterior gastric plexus (Loder, 1778)*
As described for macrodissected adult human, basically ***gastric branches of anterior vagal trunk (>1840)*** and their contributions to ***left gastric plexus (>1840)***; in the original Latin, *plexum gastricum anteriorem*, p. 31.
22. *ganglio plexuque semilunari (Wrisberg, 1780)*
Macrodissected adult human ***celiac plexus (Winslow, 1733)*** and ***celiac ganglion (Walter, 1783)*** considered together; see Wrisberg (1800, pp. 268–269).
23. *plexus semilunaris et ganglii (Wrisberg, 1780)*
Synonym for *ganglio plexuque semilunari (Wrisberg, 1780)*; see Wrisberg (1780, p. 269).
24. *abdominal brain (Wrisberg, 1780)*
Synonym for macrodissected adult human ***celiac plexus (Winslow, 1733)*** and ***celiac ganglion (Walter, 1783)*** considered together; in the original Latin, *cerebrum abdominale*, p. 69 and Wrisberg (1780, pp. 269, 275, 551). Cruveilhier (1836, p. 103) gave the French, *cerveau abdominal*. Lobstein (1831, p. 82) provided the English form.
25. *nervi stomachici (Walter, 1783)*
May correspond to macrodissected adult human *gastric branches of anterior trunk of eighth pair of nerves (Walter, 1783)* or to distinct ***nerves (Herophilus, c335–c280 BC)*** in ***left gastric plexus (>1840)***; Table IV-*after 32*, where *nervi stomachicos* and *nervos stomachicos* were used. Other forms included *nervo stomachio*, Table IV-*81*; *nervum stomachium*, Table IV-*84*; and *nervus stomachicum*, Table IV-*105*.
26. *nervi ventriculi (Walter, 1783)*
Synonym for *nervi stomachi (Walter, 1783)*; Table IV-after 32. Another form is *nervorum ventriculi*, Table III-*456*.
27. *nervi gastrici (Walter, 1783)*
Synonym for *nervi stomachi (Walter, 1783)*; Table IV:*94,102-108*.
28. *common pudendal plexus (Frotscher, 1788)*
As described for macrodissected adult human, network formed by branches of ***inferior hypogastric plexus (Tiedemann, 1822)*** and ***pudendal nerve (Camper, 1762)*** in turn supplying branches to penis or clitoris, and associated genitalia; in the original Latin, *plexum pudendum communem*, p. 97. Frotscher further described two parts, superior pudendal plexus (*plexum pudendum superiorem*) and inferior pudendal plexus (*plexum pudendum inferiorem*).
29. *superior gastric plexus (Wrisberg, 1800)*
Synonym for *anterior gastric plexus (Loder, 1778)*; in the original Latin, *plexum gastricum superiorem*; p. 560.
30. *epiploic plexus (Wrisberg, 1800)*
As described for macrodissected adult human, it has three main parts considered together, caudally (inferiorly) the ***right gastroepiploic plexus (Wrisberg, 1800)*** and ***left gastroepiploic plexus (Wrisberg, 1800)***, and rostrally (superiorly) the *gastrohepatic plexus (Wrisberg, 1800)*; in the original Latin the term, which never caught on, was *plexus epiploici*, p. 567.
31. *omental plexus (Wrisberg, 1800)*
Uncommon synonym for *epiploic plexus (Wrisberg, 1800)*; in the original Latin, *plexus omentales*, pp. 559, 567.
32. *gastrohepatic plexus (Wrisberg, 1800)*
Rostral (superior) component of *epiploic plexus (Wrisberg, 1800)* and associated with *superior gastric plexus (Wrisberg, 1800)*; in the original Latin, *plexus gastro-hepatici*, p. 569.
33. *nervous system of organic life (Bichat, 1801)*
In today's terms refers specifically to ***ciliary ganglion (Loder, 1778)***, ***sympathetic trunk (Winslow, 1733)*** and ***prevertebral ganglia (Quain, 1837)***, and ***autonomic nerves (Langley, 1898)*** associated with both of the latter, in macrodissected adult human; see translation (1822, Vol. 1, p. 249); also see Bichat et al. (1801–1803, Vol. 3, p. 319 ff.). Compare with *nervous system of animal life (Bichat, 1801)*.
34. *nervous system of ganglions (Bichat, 1801)*
Synonym for *nervous system of organic life (Bichat, 1801)*; see translation (1822, Vol. 1, p. 249).
35. *nerves of organic life (Bichat et al., 1801–1803)*
Synonym for *nervous system of organic life (Bichat, 1801)*; Vol. 3, p. 319 ff.
36. *ganglionic nervous system (Bichat et al., 1801–1803)*
Synonym for *nervous system of organic life (Bichat et al., 1801–1803)*, used by Buisson, the editor of the final part of Volume 3, after Bichat had died; in the original French, *système nerveux des Ganglions*, p. 367.
37. *transverse plexus (Portal, 1803a)*
Synonym for macrodissected adult human *solar plexus (Willis, 1664)*; in the original French, *plexus transversal*, p. 192.
38. *ganglion system (Reil, 1807)*
Probably corresponds at least roughly to macrodissected adult human *ganglionic nervous system (Bichat et al., 1801–1803)*; in the original German, *Ganglien-system*, p. 189.
39. *vegetative nervous system (Reil, 1807)*
Reil introduced it for macrodissected adult human and whereas its exact meaning is unclear today, it undoubtedly corresponds at least roughly to *nervous system of organic life (Bichat, 1801)*; in the original German, *vegetativen Nerven-Systems* and *vegetative System*, p. 204. Also see Mitchell (1953, p. 7).
40. *vegetative nerves (Reil, 1807)*
Reil introduced it for macrodissected adult human and whereas its exact meaning is unclear today, it undoubtedly corresponds at least roughly to *visceral nerves (Johnstone, 1795)* and even more specifically *nerves of organic life (Bichat et al., 1801–1803)*; in the original German, *vegetativen Nerven*, p. 229.
41. *organic nerves (Ackermann, 1813)*
Generally corresponds to *nervous system of organic life (Bichat, 1801)*; p. 91 ff. Later used, for example, by Müller (1834), see translation (1838, p. 788).
42. *sympathetic system of nerves (Bell & Bell, 1816)*
Not clearly defined but probably roughly synonymous with macrodissected adult human *nervous system of organic life (Bichat, 1801)*; pp. 499, 519.

43. sympathetic nervous system (Wutzer, 1817)
Probably synonym for *vegetative nervous system (Reil, 1807)*; in the original German, *systema nervi sympathici (vegetativum)*, pp. 96, 97.

44. *ganglionnary system (Meckel, 1817)*
Synonym for macrodissected adult human *ganglionnary nerve (Meckel, 1817)* and *ganglion system (Reil, 1807)*; see translation (1832, Vol. 3, pp. 8, 84).

45. *ganglionnary nerve (Meckel, 1817)*
Essentially synonym for macrodissected adult human *nervous system of ganglions (Bichat, 1801)*, which Meckel divided into *limiting portion of ganglionnary nerve (Meckel, 1817)*, essentially *sympathetic chain (Gaskell, 1886)*, and *central portion of ganglionnary nerve (Meckel, 1817)*, essentially ***prevertebral ganglia (Quain, 1837)***, and ***autonomic nerves (Langley, 1898)*** associated with both parts; in the original Latin, *nervus gangliosus*, see translation (1832, Vol. 3, p. 83 ff.). "The chain of the limiting ganglions and of the nervous cords which unite them have been generally and until lately considered as its trunk and its upper extremity as its origin, admitting that prolongations proceed outward from these two points to the nervous system of animal life, inward to the thoracic and abdominal viscera. But now it is admitted to be more proper to describe first its most internal part, and to conclude with the history of the ganglions which connect it with the nervous system of animal life, and the filaments which establish this communication." (p. 85). "Our mode of describing the ganglionnary nerve differs from that hitherto adopted even by those anatomists who consider it as directly opposed to the rest of the system... Our course will at first view be more surprising, because we have several times mentioned that there is no manifest contrariety between the two nervous systems. In fact the ganglionnary nerve is only the highest development of a form which has passed through several gradations..." (pp. 98–99). "The ganglions of this nervous system divide in respect to their situation and mode of distribution into two classes which comprise, the first the *internal* or *central ganglions*, the second the *limiting ganglions*." (p. 84).

46. *nerves of vegetative life (Meckel, 1817)*
Alternate form of *nerves of organic life (Bichat et al., 1801–1803)*; see translation (1832, Vol. 3, p. 83), where Meckel gave the Latin, *systema vitae anatomaticae vegitativae*. Also see *ganglionnary nerve (Meckel, 1817)*.

47. *ganglionnary plexuses (Meckel, 1817)*
Corresponds basically to macrodissected adult human ***prevertebral plexuses (Quain, 1837)*** and ***prevertebral ganglia (Quain, 1837)*** considered together; see translation (1832, Vol. 3, p. 85). By way of distinction, it is worth noting: "...**perivascular plexuses**. All blood-vessels are accompanied by nerve-fibres, both medullated and non-medullated, some of which are afferent and others motor. Ganglion cells are not encountered in these plexuses" (Durward, 1951, p. 1145). These perivascular plexuses are usually described as extensions of ***craniospinal nerves (Herrick, 1915)***, ***autonomic nerves (Langley, 1898)***, ***prevertebral plexuses (Quain, 1837)***, or ***terminal plexuses (Swanson & Bota, 2010)***.

48. *spermatic plexus (Meckel, 1817)*
As described for macrodissected adult human, referred to combination of ***superior ureteric nerves (Walter, 1783)*** with in males ***superior testicular nerves (>1840)*** and ***testicular plexus (Cruveilhier, 1836)***, and in females ***superior ovarian nerves (>1840)*** and ***ovarian plexus (Cruveilhier, 1836)***; see translation (1832, Vol. 3, p. 87).

49. *Rumpfnervensystem (Burdach, 1819)*
Roughly synonymous with macrodissected adult human *nervous system of organic life (Bichat, 1801)*; pp. 70, 212.

50. *trunk nervous system (Burdach, 1819)*
English form of *Rumpfnervensystem (Burdach, 1819)*.

51. *visceral part of nervous system (Blainville, 1821)*
Essentially synonym for macrodissected *prae-vertebral part of tri-splanchnic nervous system (Quain & Wilson, 1839)* in animals generally; in the original French, *viscérale*, p. 206. Blainville described it as very deep, associated with digestive system, and forming special relationship with vascular system; he contrasted it with *great sympathetic part of nervous system (Blainville, 1821)*.

52. *visceral nervous system (Blainville, 1821)*
Synonym for *visceral part of nervous system (Blainville, 1821)*; in the original French, *système nerveux viscéral*, p. 216.

53. *nervous masses of vegetative life (Spurzheim, 1826)*
Basically synonym for macrodissected vertebrate *nerves of vegetative life (Meckel, 1817)*; p. 25. Compared to *nervous masses of phrenic life (Spurzheim, 1826)*.

54. *sympathetic nerves (Quain, 1828)*
For macrodissected adult human, basically ***autonomic ganglia (Langley, 1900)*** and ***autonomic nerves (Langley, 1898)*** considered together; p. 662 ff.

55. *visceral nervous system (Müller, 1828a)*
For macrodissected insects apparently analogous to *nervous system of organic life (Bichat, 1801)*; in the original German, *Nervensystem der eingeweide*; p. 71.

56. *cephalic part of vegetative nervous system (Arnold, 1834)*
Rostrally directed components of macrodissected adult human *vegetative nervous system (Reil, 1807)* in the head; in the original Latin, *pars cephalica systematis nervorum vegitativi*, p. 17.

57. *cyclo-ganglionic system (Solly, 1836)*
Essentially synonym for macrodissected adult human *ganglionic nervous system (Bichat et al., 1801–1803)*, reflecting organization of "cyclo-ganglionated or molluscous division of the animal kingdom" as opposed to cerebro-spinal; p. 28.

58. *great sympathetic (Cruveilhier, 1836)*
For macrodissected adult human, basically *sympathetic system of nerves (Bell & Bell, 1816)* but explicitly excluding ***autonomic ganglia (Langley, 1900)*** of the head; in the original French, *grand sympathique*, p. 981.

59. *central part of great sympathetic (Cruveilhier, 1836)*
Part of *great sympathetic (Cruveilhier, 1836)* associated with ***sympathetic trunk (Winslow, 1733)***, ***paravertebral***

ganglia (Durward, 1951), and ***paravertebral nerves (Swanson & Bota, 2010)***; in the original French, *partie centrale*, p. 981.

60. *visceral part of great sympathetic (Cruveilhier, 1836)*
Peripheral part of *great sympathetic (Cruveilhier, 1836)*, distal to *central part of great sympathetic (Cruveilhier, 1836)*; in the original French, *partie viscérale*, p. 981.
61. *median part of great sympathetic (Cruveilhier, 1836)*
Synonym for *visceral part of great sympathetic (Cruveilhier, 1836)*; in the original French, *partie médiane*, p. 981.
62. *tri-splanchnic nervous system (Quain & Wilson, 1839)*
For macrodissected adult human, basically *nervous system of organic life (Bichat, 1801)*; p. 4.
63. *prae-vertebral part of tri-splanchnic nervous system (Quain & Wilson, 1839)*
For macrodissected adult human, basically ***prevertebral plexuses (Quain, 1837)***, ***prevertebral ganglia (Quain, 1837)***, and ***prevertebral nerves (Swanson & Bota, 2010)***, considered together; p. 4. Quain & Wilson contrasted it with *great sympathetic part of nervous system (Blainville, 1821)*.
64. *sympathetic system (Cruveilhier, 1844)*
English form of the French *grand sympathique*, see *great sympathetic (Cruveilhier, 1836)*; p. 854.

peripheral nervous system gray matter regions (>1840)

Gray matter regions (Swanson & Bota, 2010) are divided topographically into two parts, ***central nervous system gray matter regions (>1840)*** and ***peripheral nervous system gray matter regions (>1840)***. ***Peripheral nervous system gray matter regions (>1840)*** are differentiations of ***gray matter (Meckel, 1817)*** now based essentially on cellular architecture and connections. The synonym specifically for gross anatomy (topographic architecture) is ***peripheral ganglia (>1840)***. Morgagni (1719) is credited with describing for the first time a mixture of ***gray matter (Meckel, 1817)*** and ***white matter (Meckel, 1817)*** in ***peripheral ganglia (>1840)***; see Clarke & Jacyna (1987, p. 330). This led Winslow to refer to ***peripheral ganglia (>1840)*** as *little brains (Winslow, 1733)*.

EARLIER REFERENCES:

Earlier synonyms:

1. *grey matter of ganglions (Grainger, 1837)*
Synonym for macrodissected adult vertebrate ***peripheral nervous system gray matter regions (>1840)***; p. 158.

peripheral nervous system white matter tracts (>1840)

White matter tracts (Bell & Bell, 1826) are divided topographically into two parts, ***central nervous system white matter tracts (>1840)*** and ***peripheral nervous system white matter tracts (>1840)***. ***Peripheral nervous system white matter tracts (>1840)*** are differentiations of ***white matter (Meckel, 1817)***, now based essentially on histologically defined connections. The synonym specifically for gross anatomy (topographic architecture) is ***nerves (Herophilus, c335–c280 BC)***, and Herophilus is credited with discovering them.

EARLIER REFERENCES:

Earlier synonyms:

1. *peripheral nerve mass (Carus, 1814)*
Probably synonym for macrodissected adult human ***peripheral nervous system white matter tracts (>1840)***; in the original German, *peripherischer Nervenmasse*, p. 296.
2. *fibres of nerves (Grainger, 1837)*
Synonym for macrodissected adult vertebrate ***peripheral nervous system white matter tracts (>1840)***; p. 158.

PARTLY CORRESPONDS:

1. *plexus on third nerve (Swan, 1830)*
As described for macrodissected adult human, network around ***oculomotor nerve (Estienne, 1545)***, formed by small branches of ***abducens nerve (Heister, 1717)***, ***nasociliary nerve (Meckel, 1817; Wutzer, 1817)***, and an orbital branch of ***pterygopalatine ganglion (>1840)***; Plate XV, Figure 3-6,7.

periventricular bundle of hypothalamus (>1840)

As described in mammal most clearly with histological methods for ***axons (Kölliker, 1896)***, a diffusely organized ***central nervous system white matter tract (>1840)*** dispersed throughout much of the ***periventricular hypothalamic zone (Nauta & Haymaker, 1969)***. It is continuous rostrally with the rostral end of the ***periventricular bundle of thalamus (>1840)*** and it is continuous caudally with the caudal end of the ***periventricular bundle of thalamus (>1840)*** and rostral end of the ***dorsal longitudinal fascicle (Schütz, 1891)***, all three together often regarded as forming the periventricular system, with most ***axons (Kölliker, 1896)*** tending to orient longitudinally; see Gurdjian (1927, pp. 103–104), Crosby et al. (1962, pp. 318–320), Sutin (1966), Nauta & Haymaker (1969, pp. 172–173, 197–198 and Fig. 4.26), Swanson (2004, p. 178 notes *125*, *130*). It was not recognized by 1840.

periventricular bundle of thalamus (>1840)

As described in mammal most clearly with histological methods for ***axons (Kölliker, 1896)***, a diffusely organized ***central nervous system white matter tract (>1840)*** coursing through the ***paraventricular thalamic nucleus (>1840)*** just ventral to the ***thalamic part of third ventricle (Swanson, 2004)*** near the median plane. It is continuous rostrally with the rostral end of the ***periventricular bundle of hypothalamus (>1840)*** and it is continuous caudally with the caudal end of the ***periventricular bundle of hypothalamus (>1840)*** and rostral end of the ***dorsal longitudinal fascicle (Schütz, 1891)***, all three together often regarded as forming the periventricular system, with most ***axons (Kölliker, 1896)*** tending to orient longitudinally; see Gurdjian (1927, pp. 103–104), Crosby et al.

(1962, pp. 318–320), Sutin (1966), Nauta & Haymaker (1969, pp. 172–173, 197–198 and Fig. 4.26), Swanson (2004, p. 178 notes *125*, *130*). It was not recognized by 1840.

periventricular hypothalamic zone (Nauta & Haymaker, 1969)

As described in macrodissected adult human, and with cellular architecture in mammal as well as vertebrate generally, the most medial of three longitudinal divisions of the ***hypothalamus (Kuhlenbeck, 1927)***, lying between ***hypothalamic part of third ventricle (Swanson, 2004)*** medially and ***medial hypothalamic zone (Nauta & Haymaker, 1969)*** laterally. Some of its more prominent ***gray matter regions (Swanson & Bota, 2010)*** include the ***neuroendocrine division of paraventricular hypothalamic nucleus (>1840)*** and closely related ***supraoptic nucleus (>1840)***, ***suprachiasmatic nucleus (>1840)***, ***arcuate nucleus of hypothalamus (>1840)***, and ***dorsomedial hypothalamic nucleus (>1840)***. For a complete list of parts in rat, see Swanson (1998, Table B, pp. 205–206). The concept was derived from the submammalian comparative histological work of Crosby & Woodbourne (1940), but the term was Nauta and Haymaker's, see p. 141. It was not delineated by 1840.

pharyngeal branches of glossopharyngeal nerve (Neubauer, 1772)

As described for macrodissected adult human, 3–4 branches of the ***glossopharyngeal nerve trunk (Wrisberg, 1786; Günther, 1786)*** uniting opposite the middle constrictor muscle of the pharynx with ***pharyngeal branches of vagus nerve (Wrisberg, 1786)*** and ***laryngopharyngeal branches of superior cervical ganglion (>1840)*** to form the ***pharyngeal plexus (Neubauer, 1772)***; see Williams & Warwick (1980, p. 1075), *Terminologia Anatomica* (1998, p. 136). For Neubauer's use in macrodissected human, see Table 2-*81*. Kilian (1822, pp. 94, 97) provided a very detailed account, naming four branches in macrodissected adult human. They were perhaps first identified by Winslow; see ***[pharyngeal branches of glossopharyngeal nerve (>1840)] (Winslow, 1733)***.

TRANSLATIONS:

1. *ramus glossopharyngei inferior sive pharyngeus dictus (Neubauer, 1772)*
   Original Latin reference to ***pharyngeal branches of glossopharyngeal nerve (Neubauer, 1772)***; see Table 2-*81*.

EARLIER REFERENCES:

Described, not named or illustrated:

1. ***[pharyngeal branches of glossopharyngeal nerve (>1840)] (Winslow, 1733)***
   Described but not named for macrodissected adult human; Section VI, p. 71.

LATER SYNONYMS:

1. *pharyngeal nerves (Kilian, 1822)*
   Essentially synonym for macrodissected adult human ***pharyngeal branches of glossopharyngeal nerve (Neubauer, 1772)***; in the original Latin, *nervos pharyngeos*, p. 94.
2. *pharyngeal branches of ninth pair trunk (Arnold, 1834)*
   Synonym for macrodissected adult human ***pharyngeal branches of glossopharyngeal nerve (Neubauer, 1772)***; in the original Latin, *rami pharyngei e trunco noni paris*, p. 13.
3. *branches of glosso-pharyngeal nerve to pharyngeal plexus (Quain & Wilson, 1839)*
   Synonym for macrodissected adult human ***pharyngeal branches of glossopharyngeal nerve (Neubauer, 1772)***; Plate XV-*n*.

PARTLY CORRESPONDS:

1. *circumflex glossopharyngeal branch (Scarpa, 1794)*
   Macrodissected adult human ***communicating branch (Winslow, 1733)*** between ***pharyngeal branches of glossopharyngeal nerve (Neubauer, 1772)*** and ***stylopharyngeal branch of glossopharyngeal nerve (>1840)***; in the original Latin, *ramus glossopharyngaei circumflexis*, Table II-*15*.
2. *first pharyngeal branch of main communicating branch of glossopharyngeal nerve (Kilian, 1822)*
   First of two pharyngeal branches of macrodissected adult human *main communicating branch of glossopharyngeal nerve (Kilian, 1822)*; in the original Latin, *ramus pharyngeus primus*, p. 93.
3. *pharyngeal nerve from ninth pair (Kilian, 1822)*
   Synonym for *first pharyngeal branch of main communicating branch of glossopharyngeal nerve (Kilian, 1822)*; in the original Latin, *nervus pharyngeis e pare nono*, pp. 94, [106]. A branch of *main communicating branch of glossopharyngeal nerve (Kilian, 1822)*.
4. *second pharyngeal branch of main communicating branch of glossopharyngeal nerve (Kilian, 1822)*
   Second of two pharyngeal branches of macrodissected adult human *main communicating branch of glossopharyngeal nerve (Kilian, 1822)*; in the original Latin, *ramus pharyngeus secundus*, p. 94.
5. *pharyngolingual branch of glossopharyngeal nerve (Kilian, 1822)*
   Substantial branch of macrodissected adult human ***glossopharyngeal nerve (Haller, 1762)*** supplying four almost exclusively pharyngeal branches and arising between *main communicating branch of glossopharyngeal nerve (Kilian, 1822)* and *superior lingual branch of glossopharyngeal nerve (Kilian, 1822)*; in the original Latin, *ramus pharyngo-lingualis*, p. 96.
6. *superior pharyngeal branch of pharyngolingual branch of glossopharyngeal nerve (Kilian, 1822)*
   First of four main branches of macrodissected adult human *pharyngolingual branch of glossopharyngeal nerve (Kilian, 1822)*; in the original Latin, *ramus pharyngeus superior*, p. 97.
7. *major pharyngeal branch of pharyngolingual branch of glossopharyngeal nerve (Kilian, 1822)*
   Synonym for *superior pharyngeal branch of pharyngolingual branch of glossopharyngeal nerve (Kilian, 1822)*; in the original Latin, *ramus pharygeus major*, p. 97.
8. *middle pharyngeal branch of pharyngolingual branch of glossopharyngeal nerve (Kilian, 1822)*
   Second of four main branches of macrodissected adult human *pharyngolingual branch of glossopharyngeal nerve*

(Kilian, 1822); in the original Latin, *ramus pharyngeus medius*, p. 97.

9. *smallest pharyngeal branch of pharyngolingual branch of glossopharyngeal nerve (Kilian, 1822)*
   Synonym for *middle pharyngeal branch of pharyngolingual branch of glossopharyngeal nerve (Kilian, 1822)*; in the original Latin, *ramus pharygeus minimus*, p. 97.
10. *inferior pharyngeal branch of pharyngolingual branch of glossopharyngeal nerve (Kilian, 1822)*
   Third of four main branches of macrodissected adult human *pharyngolingual branch of glossopharyngeal nerve (Kilian, 1822)*; in the original Latin, *ramus pharyngeus inferior*, p. 97. It in turn has four smaller branches: *tonsillaris, musculares, magnus*, and *ad membranam mucosam pharyngis*; see p. [106].
11. *largest pharyngeal branch of pharyngolingual branch of glossopharyngeal nerve (Kilian, 1822)*
   Synonym for *inferior pharyngeal branch of pharyngolingual branch of glossopharyngeal nerve (Kilian, 1822)*; in the original Latin, *ramus pharygeus maximus*, p. 97.
12. *fourth pharyngeal branch of pharyngolingual branch of glossopharyngeal nerve (Kilian, 1822)*
   Last of four main branches of macrodissected adult human *pharyngolingual branch of glossopharyngeal nerve (Kilian, 1822)*; in the original Latin, *ramus pharyngeus quartus*, p. 97.
13. *small pharyngeal branch of pharyngolingual branch of glossopharyngeal nerve (Kilian, 1822)*
   Synonym for *fourth pharyngeal branch of pharyngolingual branch of glossopharyngeal nerve (Kilian, 1822)*; in the original Latin, *ramus pharygeus parvus*, p. 97.

pharyngeal branches of recurrent laryngeal nerve (>1840)

As described for macrodissected adult human and other mammal, they provide a minor input to the inferior constrictor muscle of the pharynx derived at least in part from the ***cranial root of accessory nerve (>1840)***; see Williams & Warwick (1980, p. 1082), Kobler et al. (1994, p. 139), *Terminologia Anatomica* (1998, p. 136), *Dorland's* (2003, p. 1579). They were first mentioned by Winslow; see ***[pharyngeal branches of recurrent laryngeal nerve (>1840)] (Winslow, 1733)***.

EARLIER REFERENCES:

Described, not named or illustrated:

1. ***[pharyngeal branches of recurrent laryngeal nerve (>1840)] (Winslow, 1733)***
   Mentioned for macrodissected adult human; Section VI, p. 72.

Earlier synonyms:

1. *pharyngeal branches of recurrent nerve (Meckel, 1817)*
   Synonym for macrodissected adult human ***pharyngeal branches of recurrent laryngeal nerve (>1840)***; see translation (1832, Vol. 3, p. 48).
2. *pharyngeal filaments of recurrent nerve (Cruveilhier, 1836)*
   Synonym for macrodissected adult human ***pharyngeal branches of recurrent laryngeal nerve (>1840)***; in the original French, *filets pharyngiens*, p. 963.

pharyngeal branches of vagus nerve (Wrisberg, 1786)

As described for macrodissected adult human, 2–5 appear to arise from the ***distal vagal ganglion (>1840)***, and others arise from the ***vagus nerve trunk (Wrisberg, 1786; Günther, 1786)*** distal to it. Functionally, they are the chief motor innervation of the pharynx and soft palate, are derived primarily from the ***cranial root of accessory nerve (>1840)***, and contribute to the ***pharyngeal plexus (Neubauer, 1772)***; see Mitchell (1953, pp. 178–179), Williams & Warwick (1980, p. 1082). For Wrisberg's description based on more than 500 macrodissected adult human cadavers, and including at least five named branches, see Wrisberg reprint (1800, pp. 417, 423–428). They were first delineated by Eustachi; see ***[pharyngeal branches of vagus nerve (Wrisberg, 1786)] (Eustachi, 1552)***.

TRANSLATIONS:

1. *ramo pharyngaeo ex vago (Wrisberg, 1786)*
   Original Latin form of ***pharyngeal branches of vagus nerve (Wrisberg, 1786)***; see Wrisberg (1800, p. 417).

EARLIER REFERENCES:

Illustrated, not named or described:

1. ***[pharyngeal branches of vagus nerve (Wrisberg, 1786)] (Eustachi, 1552)***
   Illustrated for macrodissected adult human; see Albinus edition (1761, Tab. 18, Fig. 2-*m*, p. 105).

Described, not named or illustrated:

1. *[pharyngeal branches of vagus nerve (Wrisberg, 1786)] (Falloppio, 1561)*
   Mentioned for macrodissected adult human, "*tenues ad faucium ortum*" (p. 152); see Haller (1762, p. 233), Scarpa (1794, Tab. II).

Earlier synonyms:

1. *pharyngeal nerves from eighth pair (Asch, 1750)*
   Synonym for macrodissected infant and adult human ***pharyngeal branches of vagus nerve (Wrisberg, 1786)***; in the original Latin, *nervi pharyngei ex octavo pare*, see Figure 3-*13,14*. Asch also described an anastomosis or ***communicating branch (Winslow, 1733)*** between them (Fig. 3-*15*).
2. *pharyngeal nerve of vagal pair (Haase, 1781)*
   Synonym for macrodissected adult human ***pharyngeal branches of vagus nerve (Wrisberg, 1786)***; in the original Latin, *par vagum nervum pharyngeum*, p. 85.
3. *pharyngeal nerve proper (Günther, 1786)*
   Synonym for macrodissected adult human ***pharyngeal branches of vagus nerve (Wrisberg, 1786)***; in the original Latin, *pharyngeum proprium*, p. 63.

LATER SYNONYMS:

1. *pharyngeal branch of vocal nerve (Bock, 1817)*
   Synonym for macrodissected adult human ***pharyngeal branches of vagus nerve (Wrisberg, 1786)***; in the original Latin, *ramus pharyngeus*, p. 67.
2. *pharyngeal nerve of pneumogastric (Knox, 1832)*
   Synonym for macrodissected adult human ***pharyngeal branches of vagus nerve (Wrisberg, 1786)***; Plate II-63.

3. *pharyngeal branch of pneumo-gastric nerve (Quain & Wilson, 1839)*
Synonym for macrodissected adult human ***pharyngeal branches of vagus nerve (Wrisberg, 1786)***; Plate XV-*k*.

PARTLY CORRESPONDS:

1. *major pharyngeal nerve (Soemmerring, 1791)*
Major rostral (upper) ***pharyngeal branch of vagus nerve (Wrisberg, 1786)*** to ***pharyngeal plexus (Neubauer, 1772)*** of macrodissected adult human; in the original Latin, *nervus pharyngaeus primus*, p. 246.
2. *small pharyngeal nerves (Soemmerring, 1791)*
Several smaller, caudal (lower) ***pharyngeal branches of vagus nerve (Wrisberg, 1786)*** for macrodissected adult human; in the original Latin, *nervo pharyngeo secundo* (or *Kleiner* in the original German), p. 246. Also see Soemmerring (1798, p. 266).
3. *first pharyngeal nerve (Andersch & Soemmerring, 1792)*
Probably synonym for macrodissected adult human *major pharyngeal nerve (Soemmerring, 1791)*; in the original Latin, *primus nervus pharyngeus*, p. 126.
4. *second pharyngeal nerve (Andersch & Soemmerring, 1792)*
Probably a macrodissected adult human *minor pharyngeal nerve (Soemmerring, 1791)*; in the original Latin, *secundus nervus pharyngeus*, pp. 125–126.
5. *third pharyngeal nerve (Andersch & Soemmerring, 1792)*
Probably a macrodissected adult human *minor pharyngeal nerve (Soemmerring, 1791)*; in the original Latin, *tertium nervum pharyngeum*, p. 125.
6. *recurrent nerves of neck (Andersch & Soemmerring, 1792)*
Probably synonym for macrodissected adult human *ascending branches of pharyngeal nerves (Scarpa, 1794)*; in the original Latin, *nervi recurrentis colli*, p. 135.
7. *esophageal ring (Andersch & Soemmerring, 1792)*
Branches of macrodissected adult human *recurrent nerves of neck (Andersch & Soemmerring, 1792)* ringing esophagus; in the original Latin, *circulus oesophageus*, p. 136.
8. *tracheal branches from recurrent nerves (Andersch & Soemmerring, 1792)*
Tracheal branches from macrodissected adult human *recurrent nerves of neck (Andersch & Soemmerring, 1792)*; in the original Latin, *ramos tracheales, a principio nervi recurrentis*, p. 136.
9. *ascending esophageal branch of fourth branch of recurrent nerves of neck (Andersch & Soemmerring, 1792)*
Ascending esophageal branch of macrodissected adult human *recurrent nerves of neck (Andersch & Soemmerring, 1792)*; in the original Latin, *ramus oesophageus ascendens*, p. 137.
10. *descending esophageal branches of fourth branch of recurrent nerves of neck (Andersch & Soemmerring, 1792)*
Descending esophageal branches of macrodissected adult human *recurrent nerves of neck (Andersch & Soemmerring, 1792)*; in the original Latin, *rami oesophagei descendentis*, p. 137.
11. *ascending branches of pharyngeal nerves (Scarpa, 1794)*
Synonym for macrodissected adult human *major pharyngeal nerve (Soemmerring, 1791)*; in the original Latin, *rami adscendentes*, Table II:31–33.
12. *descending branch of pharyngeal nerves (Scarpa, 1794)*
Synonym for macrodissected adult human *minor pharyngeal nerve (Soemmerring, 1791)*; in the original Latin, *ramus descendens*, Table II-36.
13. *pharyngeal nerve (Meckel, 1817)*
Synonym for macrodissected adult human *major pharyngeal nerve (Soemmerring, 1791)*; see translation (1832, Vol. 3, p. 46). It is now usually considered a ***pharyngeal branch of vagus nerve (Wrisberg, 1786)***.
14. *superior pharyngeal nerve (Meckel, 1817)*
Synonym for macrodissected adult human *major pharyngeal nerve (Soemmerring, 1791)*; see translation (1832, Vol. 3, p. 46).
15. *inferior pharyngeal nerve (Meckel, 1817)*
Synonym for macrodissected adult human *minor pharyngeal nerve (Soemmerring, 1791)*; see translation (1832, Vol. 3, p. 46).
16. *trunk of pharyngeal branches of vagus (Bischoff, 1832)*
Bischoff illustrated a common trunk for macrodissected adult human ***pharyngeal branches of vagus nerve (Wrisberg, 1786)***; in the original Latin, *truncus rami Pharyngei Vagi*, Table I, Figure 1-35.
17. *interior branch of trunk of pharyngeal branches of vagus (Bischoff, 1832)*
First of two main branches described for *trunk of pharyngeal branches of vagus (Bischoff, 1832)*; in the original Latin, *ramus interior truncus rami Pharyngei Vagi*, Table I, Figure 1-36.
18. *pharyngeal nerve itself (Bischoff, 1832)*
Synonym for *interior branch of trunk of pharyngeal branches of vagus (Bischoff, 1832)*; in the original Latin, *nervus Pharyngeus ipse*, Table I, Figure 1-36.
19. *external branch of trunk of pharyngeal branches of vagus (Bischoff, 1832)*
Second of two main branches described for *trunk of pharyngeal branches of vagus (Bischoff, 1832)*; in the original Latin, *ramus externus truncus rami Pharyngei Vagi*, Table I, Figure 1-37.

pharyngeal nerve (Bock, 1817)

As described for macrodissected adult human, it is variable and small and extends caudally (descends) from the caudal (posterior) part of the ***pterygopalatine ganglion (>1840)***, or from the ***posterior superior nasal nerves (Soemmerring, 1791)***, through the palatinovaginal (pharyngeal) canal to supply mucus membrane of the nasal part of the pharynx behind the auditory (Eustachian) tube; see Williams & Warwick (1980, p. 1066). For Bock's use in macrodissected adult human, see pp. 27–28 where he referred to "der Nerve" earlier called *pharyngeal branch of Vidian nerve (Bock, 1817)*; also see Meckel (1832, Vol. 3, p. 67). It was perhaps first clearly delineated as the *palatino-pharyngeal nerve (Wrisberg, 1786)*.

EARLIER REFERENCES:

Earlier synonyms:

1. *palatino-pharyngeal nerve (Wrisberg, 1786)*
Synonym for macrodissected adult human ***pharyngeal nerve (Bock, 1817)***; see Wrisberg reprint (1800, p. 412).

2. *pharyngeal branch of Vidian nerve (Bock, 1817)*
Synonym for macrodissected adult human ***pharyngeal nerve (Bock, 1817)***; in the original German, *ramus pharyngeus*, p. 27.

pharyngeal plexus (Neubauer, 1772)

In adult human, its branches supply motor ***axons (Kölliker, 1896)*** to muscles of the pharynx and soft palate, sensory endings to certain parts of the pharyngeal mucosa, and autonomic ***axons (Kölliker, 1896)*** to pharyngeal vessels and glands. Tiny ***ganglia (Galen, c173)*** are scattered among its branches, and it communicates primarily with ***pharyngeal branches of glossopharyngeal nerve (Neubauer, 1772), pharyngeal branches of vagus nerve (Wrisberg, 1786), pharyngeal branches of recurrent laryngeal nerve (>1840), hypoglossal nerve (Winslow, 1733), laryngopharyngeal branches of superior cervical ganglion (>1840)***, and ***superior cardiac nerve (Neubauer, 1772)***, and with the ***internal carotid plexus (>1840)*** and ***external carotid plexus (>1840)***; see Mitchell (1953, p. 179), Williams & Warwick (1980, p. 1079). Importantly, the ***enteric plexuses (Hill, 1927)*** are not present in this segment of the ***digestive system***, see Mitchell (1953, p. 179), so it is a ***terminal plexus (Swanson & Bota, 2010)***. Neubauer used it for macrodissected adult human in its current general sense; p. 63, where a detailed earlier history is provided. Wrisberg (1786) gave an exceptionally detailed account for macrodissected adult human based on examination of over 500 cadavers; see Wrisberg reprint (1800). Scarpa (1794, Tab. III) attributed without citation the term to Haller; it might emerge from a sentence in Haller (1762, p. 232). At least part of it was known to Willis; see ***[pharyngeal plexus (Neubauer, 1772)] (Willis, 1664)***.

TRANSLATIONS:

1. *plexus pharyngeus (Neubauer, 1772)*
Original Latin form of ***pharyngeal plexus (Neubauer, 1772)***; p. 63.

EARLIER REFERENCES:

Illustrated and described, not named:

1. ***[pharyngeal plexus (Neubauer, 1772)] (Willis, 1664)***
Willis illustrated for macrodissected adult human one contribution to it—ramifications of ***[laryngopharyngeal branches of superior cervical ganglion (>1840)] (Willis, 1664)*** in "the Sphincter of the throat" (Pordage translation, 1681, Tab. 9-γ). Haller (1762, p. 233) gave a more complete description for macrodissected adult human.

LATER SYNONYMS:

1. *superior pharyngeal plexus (Bock, 1817)*
Synonym for macrodissected adult human ***pharyngeal plexus (Neubauer, 1772)***; in the original Latin, *plexus pharyngeus superior*, p. 69. Also see *inferior pharyngeal plexus (Bock, 1817)*.
2. *pharyngocarotid plexus of vagus nerves (Kilian, 1822)*
Synonym for macrodissected adult human ***pharyngeal plexus (Neubauer, 1772)***; in the original Latin, *plexus pharyngo-carotideus*, pp. 93–94. Arnold (1834, p. 18, Tab. VI-*123*) identified a [sympathetic] contribution from macrodissected adult human ***external carotid plexus (>1840)***.
3. *pharyngeal plexus of nerves (Todd, 1836–1839)*
Synonym for macrodissected adult human ***pharyngeal plexus (Neubauer, 1772)***; p. 497.

PARTLY CORRESPONDS:

1. *ganglioform plexus of pharyngeal nerves (Scarpa, 1794)*
Differentiation of macrodissected adult human ***pharyngeal plexus (Neubauer, 1772)***; in the original Latin, *plexu ganglioformi nervi pharyngaei*, Table II:*30–33*.
2. *pharyngeal plexus (Cruveilhier, 1836)*
Extension of macrodissected adult human ***external carotid plexus (>1840)*** along ascending pharyngeal artery, thus component of ***pharyngeal plexus (Neubauer, 1772)***; in the original French, *plexus pharyngien*, p. 993.

phrenic ganglia (Walter, 1783)

As described for macrodissected adult human, from no to several ***prevertebral ganglia (Quain, 1832)*** distributed in the ***phrenic plexus (Loder, 1778)***; see Mitchell (1953, p. 280), *Terminologia Anatomica* (1998, p. 143). For Walter's discovery and use in macrodissected adult human, see Table II-*19*; he described three of them (Tab. II-*470*) and a *phrenico-hepatic ganglion (Walter, 1783)*.

LATER SYNONYMS:

1. *small ganglion of second nerve of body (Andersch, 1797)*
Synonym for macrodissected adult human ***phrenic ganglion (Walter, 1783)***; in the original Latin, *gangliolum secundi nervi corporis*, Vol. 2, p. 118. Andersch's thesis work was competed about 1751–1755, but not published intact until 1797.

PARTLY CORRESPONDS:

1. *phrenico-hepatic ganglion (Walter, 1783)*
Small ***prevertebral ganglion (Quain, 1832)*** observed in macrodissected adult human that could be included either with ***phrenic ganglia (Walter, 1783)*** or ***hepatic ganglia (Walter, 1783)***; in the original Latin, *ganglion phrenico-hepaticum*, Tables II-*24*, III-*27*, IV-*27*.

phrenic nerve (Galen, c173)

As described functionally for adult human, it is the sole motor supply to the diaphragm, it carries sensory ***dendrites (His, 1889)*** with a wide distribution, and it often though not always has variable ***communicating branches (Winslow, 1733)*** from the ***cervical sympathetic ganglia (>1840)*** and/or their branches. Its chief origin is the 3rd– 5th (predominantly from the 4th) cervical ***spinal nerve ventral branches (>1840)*** associated with the ***cervical plexus (Molinetti, 1675)***; see Williams & Warwick (1980, pp. 1093–1094, Fig. 7.197). Galen apparently used the term *phrenic nerve* (in Greek; see May translation, 1968, pp. 598–600) and provided a brilliant description and experimental functional analysis of it in a variety of common large mammals; see Duckworth translation (1962, pp. 239, 255–256) and Singer translation (1999, p. 219). Galen referred to the origins of the ***phrenic nerve***

(Galen, c173) from the ***cervical nerves (Galen, c173)*** as *roots* or *heads*; see Duckworth translation (1962, pp. 255–256). Vieussens (1684, Tab. 23-97) described and illustrated a ***communicating branch (Winslow, 1733)*** with the ***sympathetic trunk (Winslow, 1733)***. The first detailed history, description, and illustration of the macrodissected adult human ***phrenic nerve (Galen, c173)*** was by Krüger (1758). Bell (1803b, p. 186) described its function thus: "When the nerve is stimulated, the diaphragm is excited to contraction; when cut, pressed, or tied, it becomes relaxed and inactive, and there is difficulty of respiration."

LATER SYNONYMS:

1. *nerve entering phrenes (Galen, c177)*
   Synonym for ***phrenic nerve (Galen, c173)***; see Singer translation (1999, p. 222).
2. *nerve of transverse septum (Vesalius, 1543a)*
   Synonym for macrodissected adult human ***phrenic nerve (Galen, c173)***; see Richardson & Carman translation (2002, pp. 226–227). Vesalius beautifully illustrated its origin in a small figure; see Richardson & Carman translation (2002, p. 210).
3. *sinew of midriff (Geminus, 1553)*
   Synonym for macrodissected adult human ***phrenic nerve (Galen, c173)***; originally spelled *synowe of the mydryfe*, see *The table of the figures of synowes*, Figures 5–7. Crooke (1615, p. 492) spelled it *sinewe of midriffe.*
4. *nerve of midriffe (Crooke, 1615)*
   Synonym for macrodissected adult human ***phrenic nerve (Galen, c 173)***; p. 488. Crook's description was a translation of Bauhin (1605).
5. *nerve of diaphragma (Willis, 1664)*
   Synonym in English for macrodissected adult human and other quadruped ***phrenic nerve (Galen, c173)***; in the original Latin, *diaphragmatis nervus* (Tab. X-*f*), see Pordage translation (1681, p. 175).
6. *diaphragmatic nerve (Diemerbroeck, 1689)*
   Synonym for macrodissected adult human ***phrenic nerve (Galen, c173)***; p. 558.
7. *forty-third nerve of body (Andersch & Soemmerring, 1792)*
   Synonym for macrodissected adult human ***phrenic nerve (Galen, c173)***; in the original Latin, *quadragesimum tertium nervum corporis*, p. 189.
8. *second nerve of trunk (Andersch, 1797)*
   Synonym for macrodissected adult human ***phrenic nerve (Galen, c173)***; in the original Latin, *secundum nervum trunci*, Vol. 1, p. 151.
9. *small nerve of body (Andersch, 1797)*
   Synonym for macrodissected adult human ***phrenic nerve (Galen, c173)***; in the original Latin, *parvo nervo corporis*, Vol. 2, p. 110.
10. *small harmonic nerve of body (Andersch, 1797)*
    Synonym for macrodissected adult human ***phrenic nerve (Galen, c173)***; in the original Latin, *parvo nervo harmonico corporis*, Vol. 2, p. 110.
11. *second nerve of body (Andersch, 1797)*
    Synonym for macrodissected adult human ***phrenic nerve (Galen, c173)***; in the original Latin, *secundi nervum corporis*, Vol. 2, p. 110.
12. *phrenic branch of cervical plexus (Cloquet, 1816)*
    Synonym for macrodissected adult human ***phrenic nerve (Galen, c173)***; in the original French, *branche phrénique*, p. 637.
13. *diaphragmatic branch of cervical plexus (Cloquet, 1816)*
    Synonym for macrodissected adult human ***phrenic nerve (Galen, c173)***; in the original French, *branche diaphragmatique*, p. 637.
14. *great internal respiratory nerve (Bell, 1821)*
    Synonym for macrodissected adult mammalian ***phrenic nerve (Galen, c173)***; p. 407.

PARTLY CORRESPONDS:

1. *phrenic nerve trunk (Neubauer, 1772)*
   Actually refers to root of ***phrenic nerve (Galen, c173)***, arising from major fourth cervical ***spinal nerve ventral branch (>1840)*** before joining with minor roots from nearby cervical ***spinal nerve ventral branches (>1840)*** in macrodissected infant human; in the original Latin, *truncus nervi phrenici (ex quarto paris ortus)*, Table 3, Figure 3-θ.
2. *phrenic nerve spinal roots (Günther, 1786)*
   Major origin of macrodissected adult human *phrenic nerve trunk (Neubauer, 1772)* and minor root from fifth cervical ***spinal nerve ventral branch (>1840)***; in the original Latin, *radicibus spinalibus*, p. 90.
3. *phrenic nerve cerebral roots (Günther, 1786)*
   Minor origin of macrodissected adult human ***phrenic nerve (Galen, c173)*** from *descending branch of hypoglossal nerve (Günther, 1786)*, which Günther claimed arises from ***vagus nerve (Galen, c192)*** and ***hypoglossal nerve (Winslow, 1733)***, as well as from second and third cervical ***spinal nerve ventral branches (>1840)***, and occasionally from ***middle cervical ganglion (Haller, 1762)***; in the original Latin, *radicibus cerebralibus*, p. 90.
4. *pulmonary nerve (Andersch, 1797)*
   Branch of macrodissected adult human ***phrenic nerve (Galen, c173)*** to mediastinal pleura; in the original Latin, *nervum pulmonarium*, Vol. 2, p. 115. Also see Williams & Warwick (1980, p. 1094).

phrenic plexus (Loder, 1778)

As described for macrodissected adult human, the asymmetric right and left ***phrenic plexuses (Loder, 1778)*** are rostral (upper) extensions of the ***celiac plexus (Haller, 1762)*** coursing along the right and left inferior phrenic artery to innervate the adjacent peritoneum and diaphragm, after supplying small branches to the cardiac end of the stomach and receiving branches from the ***phrenic nerves (Galen c173)***; see Mitchell (1953, pp. 280–281), Williams & Warwick (1980, pp. 1133–1134). For Loder's use in macrodissected adult human, see p. 31. It was perhaps first distinguished by Vieussens; see ***[phrenic plexus (Loder, 1778)] (Vieussens, 1684)***.

TRANSLATIONS:

1. *plexum phrenicum (Loder, 1778)*
   Original Latin form of ***phrenic plexus (Loder, 1778)***; p. 94.

EARLIER REFERENCES:

Illustrated and described, not named:

1. *[phrenic plexus (Loder, 1778)] (Vieussens, 1684)*
   Briefly described and illustrated for macrodissected adult human, extending from right ***celiac ganglion (Walter, 1783)***; Table 23-58.

LATER SYNONYMS:

1. *diaphragmatic plexus (Loder, 1778)*
   Synonym for macrodissected adult human ***phrenic plexus (Loder, 1778)***; in the original Latin, *plexum diaphragmaticum*, p. 31.
2. *subdiaphragmatic plexus (Chaussier, 1789)*
   Synonym for macrodissected adult human ***phrenic plexus (Loder, 1778)***; in the original French, *sus-diaphragmatiques*, see *Table synoptique du nerf tri-splanchnique.*

phrenico-abdominal branches of phrenic nerve (Günther, 1786)

As described for macrodissected adult human, branches of the ***phrenic nerve (Galen, c173)*** primarily to the ***celiac plexus (Winslow, 1733)*** and ***phrenic plexus (Loder, 1778)***; see Durward (1952, pp. 1065–1066), Williams & Warwick (1980, p. 1094). For Günther's use in macrodissected adult human, see p. 91. They were perhaps first noted by Winslow; see ***[phrenico-abdominal branches of phrenic nerve (Günther, 1786)] (Winslow, 1733)***.

TRANSLATIONS:

1. *ramus phrenicus abdominalis nervus phrenicus (Günther, 1786)*
   Original Latin form (singular) of ***phrenico-abdominal branches of phrenic nerve (Günther, 1786)***, p. 91; also see *Dorland's* (2003, p. 1579).

EARLIER REFERENCES:

Described, not named or illustrated:

1. ***[phrenico-abdominal branches of phrenic nerve (Günther)] (Winslow, 1733)***
   Mentioned for macrodissected adult human; Section VI, p. 79. Segment rostral to (above) diaphragm illustrated for macrodissected adult human by Walter (1783, Tab. 1-17), who also illustrated segment caudal to (below) diaphragm (Tab. 2-50).

LATER SYNONYMS:

1. *abdominal branch of second nerve of body (Andersch, 1797)*
   Synonym for macrodissected adult human ***phrenico-abdominal branches of phrenic nerve (Günther, 1786)***; in the original Latin, *ramum abdominalem secundi nervi corporis*, Vol. 2, p. 118. Andersch's work on thesis finished in c1751–c1755 but was not issued publicly in its entirety until 1797.

pia (Galen, c192)

As now commonly described for human, the thin innermost layer of the ***meninges (Smith Papyrus, c1700 BC)***, and more specifically of the ***pia-arachnoid (>1840)***, that is essentially avascular; the immediately overlying ***epipial layer (Key & Retzius, 1875)*** of the ***arachnoid (Blasius, 1666)*** and its ***subarachnoid space (Magendie, 1827)*** contain abundant blood vessels; see Millen & Woollam (1962). In the later books of *On Anatomical Procedures*, Galen probably used the term *pia* for the inner, thin membrane; see ***meninges (Smith Papyrus (c1700 BC)***] of the ***nervous system (Monro, 1783)***, Duckworth translation (1962, p. 6). However, also see *pia mater (Haly Abbas or Ali ibn' ul-Abbas, d. 994)*. It is impossible to know to what extent, if any, Galen included blood vessels and ***arachnoid trabeculae (>1840)*** of the ***subarachnoid space (Magendie, 1827)*** in ***pia (Galen, c192)***; see Millen & Woollam (1962, p. 20). Nevertheless, it is generally acknowledged that Blasius first distinguished clearly the ***arachnoid (Blasius, 1666)***. The first written indication of ***pia (Galen, c192)*** was probably in the Hippocratic Corpus; see *fine membrane (Hippocrates)*.

EARLIER REFERENCES:

Earlier synonyms:

1. *fine membrane (Hippocrates)*
   Synonym for ***pia (Galen, c192)***. In *Places in Man*, the Hippocratic Corpus referred to two membranes (the plural in Greek is *meninges*) around the ***brain (Smith Papyrus, c1700 BC)***, "Of the brain, there are two membranes; the fine [thin] one cannot be healed, when once it is injured." (Potter translation, 1995, p. 23).
2. *thin membrane (Hippocrates)*
   Alternate translation of *fine membrane (Hippocrates)*; Vesalius (1543a, p. 539) used the Latin term, *membrana tenuis*; see Burdach (1822, p. 274).
3. *inner membrane (Aristotle)*
   In *The Account of Animals*, Aristotle described two membranes around the ***brain (Smith Papyrus, c1700 BC)***, a stronger one nearer the skull [***dura (Galen, c177)***] and a finer one around the ***brain (Smith Papyrus, c1700 BC)*** itself [***pia (Galen, c192)***]; see Thompson translation (1962, Sect. 494b) and Clarke & O'Malley (1996, p. 8). He dissected a variety of animals, but not human cadavers. Many years later, Soemmerring (1798, p. 32) still used the Latin form, *meninx interior*, for ***pia (Galen, c192)***.
4. *tenuis meninx (Aristotle)*
   Latin term meaning *thin membrane*, referring to *fine membrane (Hippocrates)*; for example, see Vesalius (1543a; Singer translation, 1952, p. 17) and Hall (1565, p. 40). Ramsay (1813) referred to the term *mininx tenuis*.
5. *brain-caul (Aristotle)*
   Another way Aristotle referred to *inner membrane (Aristotle)* of ***brain (Smith Papyrus, c1700 BC)*** in *The Account of Animals*; see Thompson translation (1962, Sect. 494b) and Clarke & O'Malley, 1996, p. 8).
6. *skin-like membrane (Aristotle)*
   Another way Aristotle referred to *inner membrane (Aristotle)* of ***brain (Smith Papyrus, c1700 BC)*** in *The Account of Animals*; see Thompson translation (1962, Sect. 494b) and Clarke & O'Malley 1996, p. 8).
7. *tunica altera (Rufus of Ephesus, c90–120)*
   Synonym for ***pia (Galen, c192)***; see Burdach (1822, p. 273).

8. *choroid membrane (Galen, c173)*
Galen often used it when referring to ***pia (Galen, c192)*** in general; see May translation (1968, p. 410). He apparently thought mistakenly that ***pia (Galen, c192)*** lines ***lateral ventricles (Vesalius, 1543a)*** and ***third ventricle (Galen, c173)*** but not ***fourth ventricle (Galen, c192)***; see May translation (1968, p. 417).
9. *chorioeides (Galen, c173)*
Greek term Galen often used for ***pia (Galen, c192)*** or *choroid membrane (Galen, c173)*; see Singer and Rabin (1945, p. 14).
10. *delicate membrane (Galen, c177)*
Synonym for ***pia (Galen, c192)***; see Singer translation (1999, p. 226).
11. *soft membrane (Galen, c177)*
Synonym for ***pia (Galen, c192)***; see Singer translation (1999, p. 226). Falloppio used the Latin, *membrana mollis*; see Burdach (1822, p. 274).
12. *membranous membrane (Galen, c177)*
Synonym for ***pia (Galen, c192)***; see Singer translation (1999, p. 226). According to Wiberg (1914, p. 18), Galen also referred to ***dura (Galen, c177)*** as *membranous membrane* in the same passage; see *cuticular membrane (Galen, c177)*.

LATER SYNONYMS:

1. *pia mater (Haly Abbas or Ali ibn' ul-Abbas, d. 994)*
Haly Abbas clearly used the Arabic term for ***pia (Galen, c192)***, and apparently was responsible for adding *mater* (mother) to it; see Wiberg (1914, pp. 86–89). In the Second Salernitan Demonstration (c1070–1100), *pia mater (Haly Abbas or Ali ibn' ul-Abbas, d. 994)* was described as protecting ***brain (Smith Papyrus, c1700 BC)*** "like a devoted mother" from harshness of *dura mater (Haly Abbas or Ali ibn' ul-Abbas, d. 994)*, whereas the latter protects ***brain (Smith Papyrus, c1700 BC)*** and *pia mater (Haly Abbas or Ali ibn' ul-Abbas, d. 994)* from harshness of cranium (Corner 1927, p. 66). In Latin, *pia* can mean soft, tender, or devoted. The actual Latin term *pia mater* came from Stephen of Antioch's 1127 Latin translation of *Liber Regius*; see Singer (1957, p. 81). Use of the term *pia mater* in translations of Galen's *On Anatomical Procedures* is probably not strictly correct (Duckworth, 1962, p. 6; Singer, 1999, p. 230), but this should be checked against original Greek texts.
2. *panniculus subtilis (Averroes, 12th century)*
Synonym for *soft membrane (Galen, c177)*, the ***pia (Galen, c192)***; see Burdach (1822, p. 274).
3. *veil-like membrane (William of Saliceto, 1275)*
Synonym for macrodissected adult human ***pia (Galen, c192)***; see Rosenman translation (1998, p. 182).
4. *ilamide (Benedetti, 1502)*
According to Benedetti, term Julius Pollux (c134–192) used in *Onomasticon* for ***pia (Galen, c192)***; see Lind translation (1975, p. 115), also spelled *eilamides*.
5. *tegimen secundinale (Zerbi, 1502)*
Synonym for macrodissected adult human ***pia (Galen, c192)***; p. 112, see Burdach (1822, p. 274).
6. *mininga subtilis (Zerbi, 1502)*
Synonym for macrodissected adult human ***pia (Galen, c192)***; p. 112, see Burdach (1822, p. 274) and *panniculus subtilis (Averroes, 12th century)*.
7. *pellicula subtilis (Zerbi, 1502)*
Synonym for macrodissected adult human ***pia (Galen, c192)***; p. 112, see Burdach (1822, p. 274); also see *panniculus subtilis (Averroes, 12th century)*.
8. *secundina (Berengario da Carpi, 1522)*
Berengario da Carpi wrote that ***pia (Galen, c192)*** is sometimes referred to as *secundina* [*chorion*] because it nourishes ***brain (Smith Papyrus, c1700 BC)*** as *secundina* nourishes fetus; see Lind translation (1959, p. 141) and *tegimen secundinale (Zerbi, 1502)*.
9. *thin cerebral membrane (Vesalius, 1543a)*
Fairly clearly refers specifically to macrodissected adult human ***pia (Galen, c192)*** as now defined, "Its outer surface is covered with a sort of aqueous liquid [***cerebrospinal fluid (Magendie, 1827)***] and swells out to accommodate swellings in the parts that it surrounds. It is of equal thickness all over and everywhere presents the appearance of a very thin membrane covered with innumerable vessel ducts [blood vessels]" (Richardson & Carman translation, 2009, p. 176).
10. *thin pannicle (Geminus, 1553)*
Alternate form of *thin membrane (Hippocrates)* for macrodissected adult human; originally spelled *thyn pannicle*, f. BII; or *thynne pannicle*, see *The tables of the brayne, seconde fygure*. Geminus gave the Latin as *tenuis membrana* (f. BII).
11. *meek mother (Geminus, 1553)*
English form of *pia mater (Haly Abbas or Ali ibn' ul-Abbas, d. 994)* for macrodissected adult human, "because it is softe and tender over the brayne, and that it doth nourysche and feede the same as doeth a lovynge mother to her tender chylde" (f. BII).
12. *soft pannicle (Hall, 1565)*
Alternate form of *soft membrane (Galen, c177)*; actually spelled *softe pannicle*, p. 40.
13. *tender pannicle (Hall, 1565)*
Alternate form of *soft membrane (Galen, c177)* and *panniculus subtilis (Averroes, 12th century)*, and influenced by *soft mother (Hall, 1565)*; p. 40.
14. *soft mother (Hall, 1565)*
English form of *pia mater (Haly Abbas or Ali ibn' ul-Abbas, d. 994)*; actually spelled *softe mother*, p. 40.
15. *soft veil (Hall, 1565)*
Alternate form of *soft membrane (Galen, c177)*; actually spelled *softe veyle*, p. 41.
16. *subtle veil (Hall, 1565)*
Alternate form of *soft membrane (Galen, c177)*; actually spelled *subtill veyle*, p. 41.
17. *secundina cerebri (Bauhin, 1605)*
Synonym for macrodissected adult human ***pia (Galen, c192)***; see Burdach (1822, p. 274).
18. *holy mother (Diemerbroeck, 1689)*
English form of *pia mater (Haly Abbas or Ali ibn' ul-Abbas, d. 994)*; p. 387.

19. *tenuis membrana cerebrum involvens (Chaussier, 1807)*"Ancient synonym" for macrodissected adult human ***pia (Galen, c192)***; p. 29.
20. *membrana interna cerebri (Wenzel & Wenzel, 1812)*
Synonym for macrodissected adult human ***pia (Galen, c192)***; p. 6, see (Burdach 1822, p. 274). Simple variation on *inner membrane (Aristotle)*.
21. *localis membrana (Ramsay, 1813)*
Synonym for macrodissected adult human ***pia (Galen, c192)***; p. 33.
22. *tunica cerebri propria (Meckel, 1817)*
Synonym for macrodissected adult human ***pia (Galen, c192)***; see translation (1832, Vol. 2, p. 470).

PARTLY CORRESPONDS:

1. *tomentum cerebri (Ramsay, 1813)*
Refers to ***pia (Galen, c192)*** accompanying *cerebral sulci (Vesalius, 1543a)*: "The pia mater being raised from the convolutions, it assumes the appearance of a villous web, transmitting its vascular branches into the substance of the brain, and has on this account received the name of tomentum cerebri" (p. 33).
2. *internal pia mater (Meckel, 1817)*
External pia mater (Meckel, 1817) was ***pia (Galen, c192)*** investing external surface of ***brain (Smith Papyrus, c1700 BC)***, whereas *internal pia mater (Meckel, 1817)* was ***pia (Galen, c192)*** forming ***choroid membrane of lateral ventricle (>1840)***, ***choroid membrane of third ventricle (>1840)***, and ***choroid membrane of fourth ventricle (>1840)***, as well as an imaginary layer of ***pia (Galen, c192)*** lining ***lateral ventricles (Vesalius, 1543a)*** and ***third ventricle (Galen, c173)***; see translation (1832, Vol. 2, pp. 470–475) and *choroid membrane (Galen, c173)*.
3. *external pia mater (Meckel, 1817)*
See definition under *internal pia mater (Meckel, 1817)*.
4. *ventricular membrane (Cruveilhier, 1836)*
For macrodissected adult human, ***choroid membrane of third ventricle (>1840)*** and ***choroid membrane of lateral ventricle (>1840)*** considered together; in the original French, *membrane ventriculaire*, p. 699.

pia-arachnoid (>1840)

As described for macrodissected adult human, the ***pia (Galen, c192)*** and ***arachnoid (Blasius, 1666)*** are now considered differentiations of a histologically homogeneous layer, the ***pia-arachnoid (>1840)*** or *leptomeninges (>1840)*, whereas the ***dura (Galen, c177)*** is referred to as the *pachymeninges (>1840)*. The ***subarachnoid space (Magendie, 1827)*** filled with ***cerebrospinal fluid (Magendie, 1827)*** lies between ***arachnoid (Blasius, 1666)*** and ***pia (Galen, c192)***, and a vascular ***epipial layer (Key & Retzius, 1875–1876)***, just outside the largely avascular ***pia (Galen, c192)***, is a differentiation of ***arachnoid trabeculae (>1840)*** in the ***subarachnoid space (Magendie, 1827)***; see Millen & Woollam (1962; p. 90 ff.). The ***pia-arachnoid (>1840)*** as a clear unit was perhaps first described as the *pia mater (Lieutaud, 1742)*.

EARLIER REFERENCES:

Earlier synonyms:

1. *pia mater (Lieutaud, 1742)*
Clearly described in macrodissected adult human as having inner layer, ***pia (Galen, c192)***, and outer layer, ***arachnoid (Blasius, 1666)***, the ***pia-arachnoid (>1840)***; in the original French, *pie-mere*, p. 388. Also see *meningine (Burdin, 1803)*.
2. *meningine (Burdin, 1803)*
Macrodissected adult human ***pia (Galen, c192)*** and ***arachnoid (Blasius, 1666)*** distinguished but considered together as a single layer, the ***pia-arachnoid (>1840)***; see translation (1803, Vol. 1, pp. 155–156).
3. *meningeal layer (Meckel, 1817)*
Synonym for macrodissected adult human *meningine (Burdin, 1803)*; see translation (1832, Vol. 2, p. 469).
4. *meningina (Meckel, 1817)*
Latin form of *meningeal layer (Meckel, 1817)*; see translation (1832, Vol. 2, p. 469).
5. *leptomeninges (>1840)*
Synonym for ***pia-arachnoid (>1840)***; see Millen & Woollam (1962, p. 90).

pineal gland (Galen, c192)

As described for mammal, an unpaired dorsal and caudal extension of the caudal end of the ***epithalamus (>1840)*** in the median plane; see Crosby et al. (1962, pp. 268-269), Williams & Warwick (1980, p. 1445). For Galen's use in macrodissected adult beef, pig, and/or macaque but not human, see Duckworth translation (1962, p. 2). It was first described as the *little pine cone (Galen, c173)*.

EARLIER REFERENCES:

Earlier synonyms:

1. *little pine cone (Galen, c173)*
Synonym for ***pineal gland (Galen, c192)***; see May translation (1968, p. 392).
2. *pineal body (Galen, c177)*
Synonym for ***pineal gland (Galen, c192)***; see Singer translation (1999, p. 233).
3. *cone-like body (Galen, c177)*
Synonym for ***pineal gland (Galen, c192)***; see Singer translation (1999, p. 233).
4. *conarium (Galen, c177)*
Latin synonym for ***pineal gland (Galen, c192)***; see Singer translation (1999, p. 233). It means pine nut; see Singer (1952, p. 81 note 63).
5. *kōnarion (Galen, c177)*
Greek form of *conarium (Galen, c177)*; see Singer (1952, p. 81 note 63).
6. *pine nut (Galen, c177)*
English form of *conarium (Galen, c177)*; see Singer (1952, p. 81 note 63) and Singer (1952, p. 44) for Vesalius's (1543a) use of it.
7. *pine cone-like body (Galen, c177)*
Synonym for ***pineal gland (Galen, c192)***; see Singer translation (1999, p. 233).

8. *kōnoeidēs (Galen, c177)*
   Greek form of *pine cone-like body (Galen, c177)*; see Singer translation (1999, p. 233).
9. *corpus turbinatum (Galen, c177)*
   Latin form of term Galen used for ***pineal gland (Galen, c192)*** according to Soemmerring (1800, p. 50), also see Burdach (1822, p. 330).
10. *glandula turbinata (Galen, c177)*
   Latin form of term Galen used for ***pineal gland (Galen, c192)*** according to Soemmerring (1800, p. 50), also see Burdach (1822, p. 330).
11. *turbo (Galen, c177)*
   Latin form of term Galen used for ***pineal gland (Galen, c192)*** according to Soemmerring (1800, p. 50), also see Burdach (1822, p. 330).

LATER SYNONYMS:

1. *pineapple (Berengario da Carpi, 1522)*
   Synonym for macrodissected adult human ***pineal gland (Galen, c192)***; see Lind translation (1959, p. 144). Geminus referred to it in English as *a karnell not muche unlyke a pyne aple* or *apple* (1553, see *The tables of the brayne*, Figs. 7-*K*, 10-*D*).
2. *glandulous flesh (Berengario da Carpi, 1522)*
   Synonym for macrodissected adult human ***pineal gland (Galen, c192)***; see Lind translation (1959, p. 144).
3. *caro glandulosa (Berengario da Carpi, 1522)*
   Latin form of *glandulous flesh (Berengario da Carpi, 1522)*; see Huart & Imbault-Huart (1980, p. 29). According to Burdach (1822, p. 331), Berengario may have been following Avicenna's usage.
4. *gland like a penis (Vesalius, 1543a)*
   Vesalius noted that the ancients referred to right and left ***superior colliculi (Haller, 1762)*** collectively as *testes (Galen, c177)* because of the gland that looks like a penis [***pineal gland (Galen, c192)***] lying on top of them; see Singer translation (1952, p. 47). Burdach (1822, p. 331) gave Latin form, *glans quae peni assimilatur, s. glans nuci pineae similis*, also see Schiller (1967, p. 518).
5. *gland resembling spinning top (Vesalius, 1543a)*
   Description of macrodissected adult human ***pineal gland (Galen, c192)*** attributed to ancient Greeks by Vesalius; see Richardson & Carman translation (2009, p. 204).
6. *cerebri penis (Bauhin, 1605)*
   Bauhin explained (p. 598), "some have resembled it [adult human ***pineal gland (Galen, c192)***] to the end of the Virile member, and therfore call it *penis Cerebri*, the yarde of the brain." (Crooke translation,1615, p. 467).
7. *penis of brain (Bauhin, 1605)*
   English form of *cerebri penis (Bauhin, 1605)*; also see *gland like a penis (Vesalius, 1543a)*.
8. *pine-glandule (Crooke, 1615)*
   Bauhin (1605, p. 597) referred in Latin to macrodissected adult human ***pineal gland (Galen, c192)*** as *glandula pineali*, which Crooke (1615; p. 465, Table XI, Fig. 7-*L*) translated as *pine-glandule*.
9. *yard of brain (Crooke, 1615)*
   Crooke's English form of *cerebri penis (Bauhin, 1605)*; p. 467. Originally spelled *yarde of brain*. Also see *little prick (Read, 1638)*.
10. *little prick (Read, 1638)*
   English term for *gland like a penis (Vesalius, 1543a)*, actually spelled *little pricke*; p. 408. As Read explained in a later edition (1650, p. 215), "About the hindermost hole of the third ventricle, which passeth to the fourth ventricle, certain round bodies appear, small portions of the brain, having their denomination from those things which they resemble. The first is *glandula pinealis*, or *penis*; because it representeth the Pine-Nut, or a Prick."
11. *pine-apple kernel (Riolan, 1657)*
   Culpeper's English translation of term for ***pineal gland (Galen, c192)***; p. 123.
12. *pine-kernel-shaped glandule (Bartholin, 1662)*
   Culpeper's English translation of term for ***pineal gland (Galen, c192)***; Table V-*K*.
13. *button (Willis, 1664)*
   Synonym for macrodissected adult human ***pineal gland (Galen, c192)***; see Pordage translation (1681, p. 66).
14. *pineal kernel (Willis, 1664)*
   Synonym for macrodissected adult human ***pineal gland (Galen, c192)***; see Pordage translation (1681, pp. 65, 66).
15. *superior gland (Steno, 1669)*
   Synonym for macrodissected adult human ***pineal gland (Galen, c192)***; see translation p. 135.
16. *virga (Salmon, 1714)*
   Synonym for macrodissected adult human ***pineal gland (Galen, c192)***; p. 410. It is a Latin word for *rod*, referring to *penis*; see *gland like a penis (Vesalius, 1543a)*.
17. *cerebral epiphysis (Serres, 1824–1826)*
   Synonym for macrodissected adult vertebrate ***pineal gland (Galen, c192)***; in the original French, *épiphyse cérébrale*, Vol. 2, p. 483. The common Latin form is *epiphysis cerebri*.

pineal recess (>1840)

As described for macrodissected adult human, a narrow caudal extension of the ***thalamic part of third ventricle (Swanson, 2004)*** into the ***pineal stalk (Burdach, 1822)***; see Mettler (1948, Figs. 68, 100), Williams & Warwick (1980, p. 981). It was first described as the *chimney (Galen, c177)*.

EARLIER REFERENCES:

Earlier synonyms:

1. *chimney (Galen, c177)*
   From Millen & Woollam's analysis (1962, pp. 8–9) it seems obvious Galen described ***pineal recess (>1840)*** of macrodissected adult ox as resembling a chimney, and as "the duct on which the pineal gland is mounted." Cruveilhier (1836, p. 688) privided an update on observations related to human.

pineal stalk (Burdach, 1822)

As described for macrodissected adult human, and histologically for mammal generally, a proximal part of the

pineal gland (Galen, c192) consisting of two thin laminae, dorsal (superior) and ventral (inferior), separated by the ***pineal recess (>1840)*** of the ***thalamic part of third ventricle (Swanson, 2004)***. The base or proximal end of the dorsal lamina surrounds the ***habenular commissure (>1840)***, and the base of the ventral lamina surrounds the ***posterior commissure (Winslow, 1733)***; see Williams & Warwick (1980, p. 1445, Fig. 8.199A). For Burdach's use in macrodissected adult human see pp. 114, 338, where he also provided a detailed history of earlier work on relationships between the ***pineal gland (Galen, c192)*** and region of the ***posterior commissure (Winslow, 1733)***; pp. 338–339. It was first clearly delineated by Vesalius; see ***[pineal stalk (Burdach, 1822)] (Vesalius, 1543a)***.

EARLIER REFERENCES:

Described, not named or illustrated:

1. ***[pineal stalk (Burdach, 1822)] (Vesalius, 1543a)***
Observed in macrodissected lamb but not macrodissected adult human; see Richardson & Carman translation (2009, p. 204).

Earlier synonyms:

1. *nervous little string (Bartholin, 1662)*
According to Bartholin, Frans de Le Boë (Franciscus Sylvius) described "nervous little string", apparently ***pineal stalk (Burdach, 1822)*** fastening ***pineal gland (Galen, c192)*** as it lies between ***superior colliculi (Haller, 1762)***; p. 142.
2. *funiculus medullaris transversus (Haller, 1762)*
Synonym for macrodissected adult human ***pineal stalk (Burdach, 1822)***; pp. 52, 67. According to Burdach (1822, p. 338), Vieussens (1684, pp. 64, 66) referred to it as *tractus medullaris transversus ano et glandulae pineali intermedius, s. natibus antepositus*.
3. *trabecula fibrosa medullaris thalamos uniens (Haller, 1762)*
Synonym for macrodissected adult human ***pineal stalk (Burdach, 1822)***; pp. 52, 67. See Burdach (1822, p. 338).
4. *membrana medullaris (Haase, 1781)*
Apparently synonym for macrodissected adult human ***pineal stalk (Burdach, 1822)***; p. 24, see Burdach (1822, p. 338).
5. *taeniola conarii (Wenzel & Wenzel, 1812)*
Synonym for macrodissected adult human ***pineal stalk (Burdach, 1822)***; pp. 86, 151. See Burdach (1822, p. 338).
6. *peduncle of pineal body (Tiedemann, 1821)*
Synonym for macrodissected adult monkey ***pineal stalk (Burdach, 1822)***; in the original Latin, *pedunculi corporis pinealis*, Table II, Figure 2-*e*.
7. *peduncle of conarium (Arnold, 1838b)*
Synonym for macrodissected adult human ***pineal stalk (Burdach, 1822)***; in the original Latin, *pedunculus conarii*, Table VII, Fig. 1-*w*.

piriform area (Smith, 1919)

As described with cellular architecture and connections in mammal, a component of the ***olfactory region (>1840)*** between ***anterior olfactory nucleus (Herrick, 1910)*** rostrally and ***cortical amygdalar complex (>1840)*** caudally. In macrodissected adult human and some other primates, it corresponds to the ***ambient gyrus (>1840)***; see Nauta & Haymaker (1969, pp. 151, 156). For Smith's use based on phylogeny and histology in turtle and "primitive mammals," see pp. 284, 286 and Figures 15, 20. In the original Latin, *area pyriformis*. Also see *pyriform cortex (Johnston, 1923)*, *prepiriform cortex (>1840)*. It was not identified as such by 1840.

LATER SYNONYMS:

1. *area praepyriformis (Brodmann, 1909)*
Original Latin form of *prepyriform area (Brodmann, 1909)*; p. 177.
2. *prepyriform area (Brodmann, 1909)*
Based on cellular architecture in mammal, basically ***piriform area (Smith, 1919)***; in the original Latin, *area praepyriformis*, see pp. 177, 188, Table 7 on p. 247.
3. *area 51 (Brodmann, 1909)*
Synonym for *prepyriform area (Brodmann, 1909)*; in the original German, *Feld 51*; see p. 177.
4. *pyriform lobe (Johnston, 1923)*
Based on histology and phylogeny, synonym for mammalian ***piriform area (Smith, 1919)***; see p. 340.
5. *pyriform cortex (Johnston, 1923)*
Based on histology and phylogeny, synonym for mammalian ***piriform area (Smith, 1919)***; see p. 340. For adult rat, see Craigie (1925; for example, Pl. XXI). *Piriform cortex (>1840)* was preferred spelling for adult human by Nauta & Haymaker (1969, p. 151).
6. *piriform cortex (>1840)*
Alternate form of *pyriform cortex (Johnston, 1923)*; see Nauta & Haymaker (1969, p. 151).
7. *lateral olfactory gyrus (Craigie, 1925)*
Synonym for ***piriform area (Smith, 1919)*** in rat based on histology; see Plate XXI.
8. *prepiriform cortex (>1840)*
Synonym for ***piriform area (Smith, 1919)***, along with *piriform cortex*; see Nauta & Haymaker (1969, p. 151).

piriformis nerve (>1840)

As described for macrodissected adult human, it commonly arises from the first and second sacral ***sacral plexus dorsal divisions (Paterson, 1887)*** and enters the dorsal surface of the piriformis muscle; see Durward (1951, Fig. 947), *Nomina Anatomica* (1983, p. A78). It was known to Galen; see ***[piriformis nerve (>1840)] (Galen, c177)***.

EARLIER REFERENCES:

Described, not named or illustrated:

1. ***[piriformis nerve (>1840)] (Galen, c177)***
Alluded to for macrodissected adult beef, pig, and/or macaque but not human; see Singer translation (1999, pp. 85–86). Vieussens described and illustrated it for macrodissected adult human; see Table 29-*10*. Meckel (1817) described the adult human situation as follows, "From the *second* and *third* sacral nerve,

come some fasciculi which unite, then give filaments to the pyramidalis muscle, and coming from the pelvis below it, go to form the inferior gluteal nerve." (translation, 1832, Vol. 3, p. 14).

pituitary gland (>1840)

A hybrid gland with one part, the ***neurohypophysis (Rioch et al., 1940)***, a component of the ***hypothalamus (Kuhlenbeck, 1927)*** and thus neural tissue, and the other part, the ***adenohypophysis (Rioch et al., 1940)***, formed by Rathke's pouch and thus non-neural (endocrine) tissue. From a systems perspective, then, the ***pituitary gland (>1840)*** is an unusual hybrid: part ***nervous system (Monro, 1783)*** and part ***endocrine system***. *Pituitary stalk (>1840)* typically has varying amounts of each component in different species and is thus a term of limited value, except as defined in a particular species; see Daniel & Pritchard (1975, Chs. 1, 3). It was discovered by Galen and named *pituitary gland (Galen, c192)*, although he did not include the *pituitary stalk (Lieutaud, 1742)*.

PARTLY CORRESPONDS:

1. *gland at infundibulum (Galen, c173)*
   Synonym for macrodissected adult large mammal but not human *pituitary gland (Galen, c192)*; see May translation (1968, pp. 429–430, 457).
2. *gland (Galen, c173)*
   Synonym for macrodissected adult large mammal but not human *pituitary gland (Galen, c192)*; see May translation (1968, pp. 429–430, 457). As Crooke (1615, p. 469), translating Bauhin (1605, p. 605), put it, Galen, in Chapter 3 of Book 9, simply called the pituitary glandule, *glandule*; Burdach (1822, p. 328) quoted Berengario da Carpi (1521, f. 440) as having used *glandula*.
3. *pituitary gland (Galen, c192)*
   In *On the Usefulness of the Parts*, Galen referred to the *gland at infundibulum (Galen, c173)* and in the later Books of *On Anatomical Procedures*, which were not available in translation to Western scholars until the 19th century, he referred to the *pituitary (Galen, c192)*, writing in the next sentence that it is a gland; see Duckworth translation (1962, p. 7); also see Bauhin (1605, p. 605) and its translation in Crooke (1615, p. 469). The term is derived from the Latin, *pituita*, meaning phlegm or thick mucous secretion. Galen wrote, "As for the usefulness of the gland that comes after the pelvis [*infundibulum (Galen, c173)*], very evidently it filters the residues, a great truth entirely unknown to anatomists, who pass over in silence the reason why the residues do not fall from the infundibulum directly into the perforations at the palate (though it is a subject worthy of investigation), just as they also neglect this question in connection with the colanderlike bones [*ethmoid bone*] at the nostrils. For they do not tell that for the sake of which these bones have been formed, but consider it sufficient to say only that they filter the residues, and they pass over in complete silence the fact that it is better for the residues to be filtered rather than to escape directly." (May translation, 1968, pp. 429–430). He mostly dissected adult beef, pig, and/or macaque but not human. The *pituitary gland (Galen, c192)* was first illustrated, schematically, by Peyligk in 1499, see Clarke & Dewhurst (1996, p. 36). Also see *infundibulum (Galen, c173)* and ***[median eminence (>1840)] (Vesalius, 1543a)***.
4. *pituitary (Galen, c192)*
   Synonym in the later Books of *On Anatomical Procedures* for *pituitary gland (Galen, c192)*; see Duckworth translation (1962, p. 7).
5. *lupine-bean-shaped spongy flesh (Galen, c192)*
   Synonym in the later Books of *On Anatomical Procedures* for *pituitary gland (Galen, c192)*; see Duckworth translation (1962, p. 7). "Spongy flesh" is a term Galen used for glandular tissue; see Duckworth translation (1962, p. 110).
6. *tube of infundibulum (Vesalius, 1543a)*
   Roughly synonymous with macrodissected adult human *pituitary stalk (Lieutaud, 1742)*; see Singer (1952, p. xvi).
7. *choane (Vesalius, 1543a)*
   Vesalius wrote that some unnamed (and implicitly uninformed) authorities refer to macrodissected adult human *pituitary gland (Galen, c192)* as *choane* (Greek); see Singer translation (1952, p. xvii).
8. *infundibulum (Vesalius, 1543a)*
   Latin form of the Greek, *choane (Vesalius, 1543a)*; translated by Richardson & Carman (2009, p. 212) as "funnel".
9. *pipe of infundibulum (Vesalius, 1543a)*
   Synonym for *tube of infundibulum (Vesalius, 1543a)*; see Richardson & Carman translation (2009, p. 212). Willis used it for mammal generally, see Pordage translation (1681, p. 66).
10. *gland below extreme end of funnel (Vesalius, 1543a)*
    Synonym for *choane (Vesalius, 1543a)*; see Singer translation (1952, p. 98).
11. *straining gland (Estienne, 1545)*
    Synonym for macrodissected adult human *pituitary gland (Galen, c192)*; see Singer (1952, p. 138, Fig. 45). Spelled *strainynge glandule* in Hall (1565, p. 42).
12. *kernel put under this region of brain (Geminus, 1553)*
    Synonym for macrodissected adult human *gland below extreme end of funnel (Vesalius, 1543a)*; originally spelled *kernel put under thys region of braine*; see *The table of the figures of synowes*, Figure 1:1–3.
13. *kernel set under nethermost end of funnel (Geminus, 1553)*
    Synonym for macrodissected adult human *gland below extreme end of funnel (Vesalius, 1543a)*; originally spelled *carnell set under the neathermoste ende of the funyll*, see *The tables of the brayne*, Figure 6-Q.
14. *glandula in sphenoïdis sella posita (Colombo, 1559)*
    Synonym for macrodissected adult human *pituitary gland (Galen, c192)*; p. 192, see Burdach (1822, p. 329).
15. *aden colatorius (Hall, 1565)*
    Greek term listed for macrodissected adult human *pituitary gland (Galen, c192)*; p. 42.
16. *glans pituitaria (du Laurens, 1600)*
    Synonym for macrodissected adult human *pituitary gland (Galen, c192)*; p. 528, see (Burdach 1822, p. 329).

17. *flegmaticke glandule (Crooke, 1615)*
Synonym for macrodissected adult human *pituitary gland (Galen, c192)*; p. 469.
18. *pituitary glandule (Crooke, 1615)*
Synonym for macrodissected adult human *pituitary gland (Galen, c192)*; p. 471.
19. *kernel of flegm (Crooke, 1615)*
Synonym for macrodissected adult human *pituitary gland (Galen, c192)*; p. 471. Rendered *flegm-kernel* in Riolan (1657, p. 124).
20. *glandula cunearis (Wharton, 1656)*
Synonym for macrodissected adult human *pituitary gland (Galen, c192)*; see Burdach (1822, p. 329), who also listed *glandula sphenoïdes* for Wharton, a simple derivative of *glandula in sphenoïdis sella posita (Colombo, 1559)*.
21. *rheum-kernel (Bartholin, 1662)*
Synonym for macrodissected adult human *pituitary gland (Galen, c192)*; p. 138.
22. *pituitary kernel (Willis, 1664)*
Synonym for *pituitary gland (Galen, c192)*, which Willis clearly described as having two distinct *lobes* in macrodissected adult human, corresponding to ***posterior lobe of pituitary gland (Haller, 1762)*** and ***anterior lobe of pituitary gland (Haller, 1762)***; see Pordage translations (1681, pp. 66, 104; 1683, Tab. VI-*F*).
23. *snotty kernel (Willis, 1664)*
Synonym for *pituitary kernel (Willis, 1664)*; see Pordage translation (1681, pp. 70, 104).
24. *inferior gland (Steno, 1669)*
Synonym for macrodissected adult human *pituitary gland (Galen, c192)*; see Burdach (1822, p. 331).
25. *spittle kernel (Diemerbroeck, 1689)*
Synonym for macrodissected adult human *pituitary gland (Galen, c192)*; p. 385.
26. *spity kernel (Diemerbroeck, 1689)*
Synonym for macrodissected adult human *pituitary gland (Galen, c192)*; p. 419.
27. *beak of infundibulum (Winslow, 1733)*
Synonym for macrodissected adult human *pituitary stalk (Lieutaud, 1742)*; Section X, pp. 43, 46.
28. *production of infundibulum (Winslow, 1733)*
Synonym for macrodissected adult human *pituitary stalk (Lieutaud, 1742)*; Section X, p. 46.
29. *pituitary stalk (Lieutaud, 1742)*
For macrodissected adult mammal, the ***infundibular stem (Hanström, 1966)***—distal part of ***infundibulum (Haymaker, 1969)***—and any surrounding ***tuberal part of anterior lobe (>1840)***; it is especially prominent in human and other primates, and quite variable in mammals generally, and is a combination of neural and non-neural tissue; see Rioch et al. (1940, Tab. 2; referred to as *hypophysial stalk*), Daniel & Pritchard (1975, Ch. 3), ***anterior lobe of pituitary gland (Haller, 1762)***. For Lieutaud's use in macrodissected adult human, see p. 395. Vesalius wrote that some unnamed anatomists refer to lower tube-like part of "funnel as a whole [*infundibulum (Galen, c173)*]" as *choane*; see Singer (1952, pp. xvi, 52, and Fig. 14-*D*). This corresponds roughly to *pituitary stalk (Lieutaud, 1742)*, which may include distal end of ***infundibular recess (>1840)***, in some species. Vieussens (1684) stated correctly that at least lower or distal end of *infundibulum (Rufus of Ephesus, fl. c90–120)* is closed in adult human (see Burdach, 1822, p. 328; Meyer, 1971, p. 26), first calling into question the ancient theory that *infundibulum (Rufus of Ephesus, fl. c90–120)* channels residues or waste products from ***ventricles (Hippocrates)*** into *pituitary gland (Galen, c192)*, which acts as a filter, before they pass through channels in palate, and on into mouth; see *infundibulum (Galen, c173)*. Earlier, Vesalius had denied the existence of holes in skull deep to *pituitary gland (Galen, c192)* that would allow drainage and filtration of *pituita* or *phlegm* eventually into mouth; see Singer translation (1952, p. 54), also see *pituitary gland (Galen, c192)*.
30. *tige pituitaire (Lieutaud, 1742)*
Original French form of *pituitary stalk (Lieutaud, 1742)*; p. 395.
31. *columnae pituitariae (Tarin, 1750)*
Synonym for macrodissected adult human *pituitary stalk (Lieutaud, 1742)*; Table II, Figure 1-*.
32. *appendix cerebri (Haller, 1762)*
Synonym for macrodissected adult human *pituitary gland (Galen, c192)*; p. 59.
33. *pituitary cerebral gland (Günther, 1786)*
Synonym for macrodissected adult human *pituitary gland (Galen, c192)*; in the original Latin, *glandulam cerebri pituitariam*, p. 16.
34. *appendicula cerebri (Ebel, 1789)*
Variation on *appendix cerebri (Haller, 1762)*; p 22, also see Chaussier (1807, p. 41).
35. *hypophysis (Soemmerring, 1791)*
Synonym for macrodissected adult human *pituitary gland (Galen, c192)*; p. 50, and Soemmerring (1798, p. 70). Strictly, Soemmerring did not use the more complete *hypophysis cerebri (Arnold, 1834)*.
36. *cerebral infundibulum (Mayer, 1794)*
Synonym for macrodissected adult human *pituitary stalk (Lieutaud, 1742)*; in the original Latin, *infundibulum cerebri*; Part 5, Table III, Figure 2-*E*.
37. *suprasphenoidal appendix of cerebrum (Chaussier, 1807)*
Synonym for macrodissected adult human *pituitary gland (Galen, c192)*; in the original French, *appendice sus-sphénoïdale du cerveau*, pp. 17, 40.
38. *suprasphenoidal stalk (Chaussier, 1807)*
Synonym for macrodissected adult human *pituitary stalk (Lieutaud, 1742)*; in the original French, *la tige sus-sphénoïdale*, p. 40.
39. *root of pituitary (Chaussier, 1807)*
Synonym for macrodissected adult human *pituitary stalk (Lieutaud, 1742)*; in the original Latin, *radix pituitaria*, p. 41.
40. *lacuna (Chaussier, 1807)*
According to Chaussier, synonym for macrodissected adult human *pituitary gland (Galen, c192)*; p. 41 note *1*.

41. *basilar gland (Chaussier, 1807)*
According to Chaussier, synonym for macrodissected adult human *pituitary gland (Galen, c192)*; in the original French, *glande basilaire*, p. 41 note *1*.
42. *peduncle of pituitary gland (Desmoulins, 1825)*
Synonym for macrodissected adult vertebrate *pituitary stalk (Lieutaud, 1742)*; in the original French, *péduncle de la glande pituitaire*, Plate XIII, Figure 1-*e*.
43. *hypophysis cerebri (Arnold, 1834)*
For macrodissected adult human, Arnold used this exact term, only implied by *hypophysis (Soemmerring, 1791)*; Table III-*A*.
44. *pituitary body (Quain, 1834)*
Synonym for macrodissected adult human *pituitary gland (Galen, c192)*; p. 690. It seems likely the term was used earlier.

plexus (Galen, c192)

As a topographic division of the ***nervous system (Monro, 1783)***, a general term referring to a meshwork of communicating ***nerve (Herophilus, c335–c280 BC)*** or ***neuron (Waldeyer, 1891)*** components without or with ***ganglia (Galen, c173)***; see Swanson & Bota (2010, Thesaurus). Also see *Oxford English Dictionary* (Online), Bullock & Horridge (1965, p. 1606). Examples include ***nerve nets (>1840)***, ***prevertebral plexuses (Quain, 1837)***, and ***plexuses (Galen, c192)*** of ***spinal nerves (Camper, 1760–1762)*** like the ***brachial plexus (Camper, 1760)***, with postplexus ***spinal nerves (Camper, 1760–1762)*** distal to them. Galen used the term in describing macrodissected adult mammalian, but not human, ***brachial plexus (Camper, 1760)***; see Duckworth translation (1962, p. 243). In the context of systems architecture at the cellular level, the term refers to a meshwork of ***neuron extensions (>1840)*** that may or may not include the ***cell bodies (Deiters, 1865)*** of ***neurons (Waldeyer, 1891)***; see Bullock & Horridge (1965, p. 1606).

PARTLY CORRESPONDS:

1. *nerve net (Behrends, 1792)*
Used to describe arrangement of *left coronary artery nerve (Behrends, 1792)*, the ***left coronary plexus (Scarpa, 1794)***, in macrodissected adult human; in the original Latin, *reti nervorum*, p. 7.

pons (Haller, 1747)

The ventral topographic division of the vertebrate ***hindbrain (Baer, 1837)***, the dorsal topographic division being the ***cerebellum (Aristotle)***; see Swanson & Bota (2010). The name is derived from *pons of cerebellum (Varoli, 1573)*, the ***middle cerebellar peduncle (Rolando, 1819)*** on each side of the macrodissected adult human ***pons (Haller, 1747)***. This feature was long ago illustrated crudely as the ***[pons (Haller, 1747)] (Vesalius, 1543a)***. Haller used the term in the modern sense of a ***brainstem (Schwalbe, 1881)*** component between ***midbrain (Baer, 1837)*** rostrally and ***medulla (Winslow, 1733)*** caudally; see Mihles translation (1753, pp. 287, 296). He also noted a depression ventrally in the median plane, the ***basilar sulcus of pons (Gordon, 1815)***. Santorini (1775, p. 17) referred to a mixture of *gray substance (Vesalius, 1543a)* and *white substance (Vesalius, 1543a)* in the ***pons (Haller, 1747)***; see Burdach (1822, p. 301). The simple term *pons* was used in more recent times by, e.g., Carpenter (1976, p. 61), Nauta & Feirtag (1986, p. 41).

EARLIER REFERENCES:

Illustrated, not named or described:

1. ***[pons (Haller, 1747)] (Vesalius, 1543a)***
Clearly though crudely illustrated as swelling on base of macrodissected adult human *origin of dorsal medulla (Vesalius, 1543a)*, without comment in text; see Richardson & Carman translation (2002, part *D* in the figure on p. 169). It was beautifully illustrated for macrodissected adult human by Eustachi in 1552; see Albinus edition (1761, Pl. 18, Fig. II-*I* and Figs. I, III, and IV-*σ*).

Earlier synonyms:

1. *hinder part of trunk of long marrow (Diemerbroeck, 1689)*
Refers basically to macrodissected adult human ***pons (Haller, 1747)***; p. 403.

LATER SYNONYMS:

1. *pons Varolii (Bell, 1802)*
Eponym for macrodissected adult human ***pons (Haller, 1747)***; Plates VII-*8*, IX-*N*, X-*b*. Earlier authors restricted it to original meaning, part of ***middle cerebellar peduncle (Rolando, 1819)*** associated directly with ***pons (Haller, 1747)***; see *pons of cerebellum (Varoli, 1573)*.
2. *tuber annulare (Bell, 1802)*
Synonym for *pons Varolii (Bell, 1802)*; Plates VII-*8*, IX-*N*, X-*b*.
3. *metencephalon (Nomina Anatomica, 1983)*
Synonym for macrodissected adult human ***pons (Haller, 1747)***; note *128* on pp. A65, A66.

PARTLY CORRESPONDS:

1. *pons of cerebellum (Varoli, 1573)*
Varoli clearly described and illustrated this large bulge on ventral and lateral surfaces of macrodissected adult human ***pons (Haller, 1747)***, which includes ***middle cerebellar peduncle (Rolando, 1819)*** and its commissural part referred to as ***transverse pontine fibers (>1840)***, ***longitudinal pontine fibers (>1840)***, and ***pontine nuclei (Jacobsohn, 1909)*** embedded within these *nerve fiber (Ehrenberg, 1833)* bundles. In essence, he described a transverse *U*-shaped structure reminiscent of a bridge (*pons*) spanning the main part of the ***brainstem (Schwalbe, 1881)*** when viewed from the base; Figure I, f. 17v. Also see Clarke & O'Malley (1996, pp. 634–635, 821) and *ventral part of pons (>1840)*.
2. *transverse process of cerebellum (Varoli, 1573)*
Synonym for *pons of cerebellum (Varoli, 1573)*; in the original Latin, *processus transversalis cerebelli*, Figure 1-*h*.
3. *pons (Varoli, 1573)*
Synonym for *pons of cerebellum (Varoli, 1573)*; see Figure 1-*h*.
4. *ponticulus (Riolan, 1649)*
Riolan's variation on *pons (Varoli, 1573)* for macrodissected adult human; see translation (1657, p. 126).

5. *little bridge (Riolan, 1657)*
English form of *ponticulus (Riolan, 1649)*; p. 126.
6. *band of roots of spinal marrow (Riolan, 1657)*
Synonym for macrodissected adult human *pons (Varoli, 1573)*; p. 126.
7. *sconce (Bartholin, 1662)*
Proposed as more appropriate name for macrodissected adult human *pons (Varoli, 1573)*; p. 138.
8. *fence (Bartholin, 1662)*
Proposed as more appropriate name for *pons (Varoli, 1573)*; p. 138. Burdach (1822, p. 297) gave Latin, *sepimentum*.
9. *annulary protuberance (Willis, 1664)*
Synonym for macrodissected adult human *pons of cerebellum (Varoli, 1573)*; see Pordage translation (1681, pp. 57, 65, 68). Knox (1832, Suppl. Pl. V) spelled it *anular protuberance*.
10. *greater protuberance (Willis, 1664)*
Synonym for *annulary protuberance (Willis, 1664)*; see Pordage translation (1681, p. 68).
11. *greater ring (Willis, 1664)*
Synonym for *annulary protuberance (Willis, 1664)*; see Pordage translation (1681, pp. 68, 116).
12. *pons Varolii (Steno, 1669)*
Eponym for macrodissected adult human *pons of cerebellum (Varoli, 1573)*; see translation, p. 135.
13. *annulary process (Vieussens, 1684)*
Synonym for macrodissected adult human *annulary protuberance (Willis, 1664)*; in Latin, *processus annularis*, p. 85.
14. *circular protuberance (Gibson, 1684)*
Synonym for macrodissected adult human *annulary protuberance (Willis, 1664)*; p. 361.
15. *bridge of cerebel (Diemerbroeck, 1689)*
Early English form of *pons of cerebellum (Varoli, 1573)* for macrodissected adult human; p. 415.
16. *eminentia annularis (Palfijn, 1726)*
Synonym for macrodissected adult human *annulary protuberance (Willis, 1664)*; in the original French, *éminence annulaire*, Part 2, p. 20.
17. *corpus globosum (Ruysch, 1728)*
Probably synonym for *annulary protuberance (Willis, 1664)*; p. 24.
18. *transverse protuberance (Winslow, 1733)*
Synonym for macrodissected adult human *pons of cerebellum (Varoli, 1573)*; Section X, pp. 41, 42. Burdach (1822, p. 298) gave the Latin, *protuberantia transversalis*.
19. *great transverse protuberance (Winslow, 1733)*
Synonym for macrodissected adult human *pons of cerebellum (Varoli, 1573)*; Section X, p. 52.
20. *semi-annular protuberance (Winslow, 1753)*
Synonym for macrodissected adult human *pons of cerebellum (Varoli, 1573)*; Section X, pp. 41, 42.
21. *protuberantia annularis Willissi (Tarin, 1753)*
Eponym for macrodissected adult human *annulary protuberance (Willis, 1664)*; p. 25.
22. *pars media et anterior trunci medullaris (Haller, 1762)*
Synonym for macrodissected adult human *pons of cerebellum (Varoli, 1573)*; p. 72, see Burdach (1822, p. 299).
23. *crura magna cerebelli (Haller, 1762)*
Synonym for macrodissected adult human *pons of cerebellum (Varoli, 1573)*; p. 72, see Burdach (1822, p. 299).
24. *nodus encephali (Soemmerring, 1778)*
Essentially synonym for macrodissected adult human *pons of cerebellum (Varoli, 1573)*; p. 65. Burdach (1822, p. 298) noted without citation that Johann Rau (1668–1719) referred to it as *nodus*. As illustrated by Tiedemann for macrodissected adult monkey (1821, Tab. I, Fig. 7-g), it must have included ***pontine nuclei (Jacobsohn, 1909)***. An English form is *node of brain*.
25. *tuber annulare (Monro, 1783)*
Synonym for macrodissected adult human *annulary protuberance (Willis, 1664)*; p. 23.
26. *[pontine brainstem (Burdach (1822)] (Vicq d'Azyr, 1786)*
Region between ***pontine nuclei (Jacobsohn, 1909)*** and ***fourth ventricle (Galen, c192)*** in transverse section through adult human ***pons (Haller, 1747)*** was illustrated and described as roundish *gray substance (Vesalius, 1543a)* space forming ***floor of fourth ventricle (Reil, 1807–1808a)***; Plate XVI-47.
27. *basal protuberance (Hildebrand, 1803)*
Synonym for macrodissected adult human *annulary protuberance (Willis, 1664)*; Vol. 4, p. 302. For Latin form, *protuberantia basilaris*, see Schreger (1803, p. 327), Burdach (1822, p. 298).
28. *annular prominence (Schreger, 1803)*
Synonym for macrodissected adult human *annulary protuberance (Willis, 1664)*; in the original Latin, *prominentia annularis*, p. 327.
29. *transverse medullary process (Wenzel & Wenzel, 1812)*
Apparently synonym for macrodissected adult human *annulary protuberance (Willis, 1664)*; p. 22. For Latin form, *processus medullaris transversus*, see Burdach (1822, p. 298).
30. *nodus cerebri (Wenzel & Wenzel, 1812)*
Apparently macrodissected adult human *nodus encephali (Soemmerring, 1778)*; see illustration in Table XIV, Figure 4-*e*.
31. *encephalic protuberance (Meckel, 1817)*
Apparently synonym for macrodissected adult human *annulary protuberance (Willis, 1664)*; p. 459, also see translation (1832, Vol. 2, p. 425). For Latin form, *protuberantia encephalica*, see Burdach (1822, p. 298).
32. *commissura cerebri (Meckel, 1817)*
Apparently synonym for macrodissected adult human *annulary protuberance (Willis, 1664)*; see translation (1832, Vol. 2, p. 425).
33. *central gray layer (Meckel, 1817)*
Essentially synonym for macrodissected adult human *caudex encephali pontilis (Burdach, 1822)*; see translation (1832, Vol. 2, p. 426).
34. *transverse prolongation of cerebellum (Meckel, 1817)*
Synonym for *commissura cerebri (Meckel, 1817)*; see translation (1832, Vol. 3, p. 52).
35. *caudex encephali pontilis (Burdach, 1822)*
Refers to macrodissected adult human ***pons (Haller, 17473)*** without *pons of cerebellum (Varoli, 1573)*; in the

original German, *Brückenhirnstamm*, pp. 67, 70, 300. It has been called *pontine tegmentum (>1840)*.

36. *pontine brainstem (Burdach, 1822)*
Translation of *Brückenhirnstamm*; see *caudex encephali pontilis (Burdach, 1822)*. It was first identified as *[pontine brainstem (Burdach (1822)] (Vicq d'Azyr, 1786)*. It has been called *pontine tegmentum (>1840)*.
37. *cerebral protuberance (Rolando, 1825a)*
Synonym for macrodissected adult human *encephalic protuberance (Meckel, 1817)*; in the original French, *protubérance cérébrale*, Table III, Figure 5.
38. *annular tubercle (Swan, 1830)*
For macrodissected adult human, variation on *tuber annulare (Monro, 1783)*; Plate X, Figure 1-*H*.
39. *cerebral protuberance (Quain, 1832)*
As redefined for macrodissected adult human, synonym for *nodus cerebri (Wenzel & Wenzel, 1812)*; p. 649.
40. *hemispheric commissure (Arnold, 1838a)*
Synonym for macrodissected adult human *commissure of cerebellar hemispheres (Arnold, 1838a)*; in the original Latin (plural), *commissurae cerebelli*, p. 35.
41. *commissure of cerebellar hemispheres (Arnold, 1838a)*
Synonym for macrodissected adult human *nodus encephali (Soemmerring, 1778)*; in the original German, *Commissur der Hemisphären des kleinen HIrns*, p. 39.
42. *cerebellar commissure (Arnold, 1838a)*
Synonym for macrodissected adult human *commissure of cerebellar hemispheres (Arnold, 1838a)*; in the original Latin, *commissura cerebelli*, p. 39.
43. *trunk of cerebellar commissure (Arnold, 1838b)*
Synonym for macrodissected adult human *pons Varolii (Steno, 1669)*; in the original Latin, *truncus commissurae cerebelli*, Plate III, Figure 1-*u*.
44. *ventral part of pons (>1840)*
Common term now for macrodissected adult human ***pontine nuclei (Jacobsohn, 1909)***, ***longitudinal pontine fibers (Arnold, 1838b)***, and ***transverse pontine fibers (>1840)***, considered together and corresponding to *pons of cerebellum (Varoli, 1573)*. See Williams & Warwick (1980, p. 907), *Nomina Anatomica* (1983, p. A66).
45. *basilar part of pons (>1840)*
Synonym for macrodissected adult human *ventral part of pons (>1840)*; see *Terminologia Anatomica* (1998, p. 112).

pontine central gray (>1840)

As described for adult human with gross dissection, and for adult mammal in general with cellular architecture and connections, the ***gray matter region (Swanson & Bota, 2010)*** caudal extension of the ***periaqueductal gray (>1840)*** lying in the dorsomedial part of the ***pons (Haller, 1747)***, between the rostral half of the ***floor of fourth ventricle (Reil, 1807–1808a)*** dorsally and the **pontine reticular nucleus** (>1840) ventrally. It has a number of tiny differentiations including, from medial to lateral, the ***nucleus incertus (>1840)***, ***dorsal tegmental nucleus (>1840)***, ***laterodorsal tegmental nucleus (>1840)***, ***Barrington's nucleus (>1840)***, ***locus ceruleus (Wenzel & Wenzel, 1812)***, and ***suprageniculate nucleus (>1840)***; see Swanson (2004, Atlas Levels 48–54 and Table B, including note *241*). It was not distinguished as such by 1840.

pontine central tegmental tract (>1840)

As described in macrodissected adult human, and mammal generally with histological methods for ***axons (Kölliker, 1896)***, the topographic segment of the ***central tegmental tract (Bechterew, 1889)*** in the ***pons (Haller, 1747)***, between ***tegmental central tegmental tract (>1840)*** segment rostrally and ***medullary central tegmental tract (>1840)*** segment caudally; see Riley (1943, pp. 693–694), Crosby et al. (1962, pp. 256–257), Nieuwenhuys et al. (2008, Figs. 6.25–28). It was not clearly described by 1840.

pontine dorsal longitudinal fascicle (>1840)

As described in adult human with histological methods for ***axons (Kölliker, 1896)***, the caudal topographic segment of the ***dorsal longitudinal fascicle (Schütz, 1891)***, caudal to the ***tegmental dorsal longitudinal fascicle (>1840)*** segment and centered in the ***pontine central gray (>1840)***; see Mettler (1948, Figs. 233, 238, 240), Crosby et al. (1962, Figs. 145, 148). It was not recognized by 1840.

pontine medial forebrain bundle (>1840)

As described in mammal generally with experimental histological methods for ***axons (Kölliker, 1896)***, the topographic segment of the ***medial forebrain bundle (Edinger, 1893)*** in the ***pons (Haller, 1747)***, between ***tegmental medial forebrain bundle (>1840)*** segment rostrally and ***medullary medial forebrain bundle (>1840)*** segment caudally. It is diffusely distributed in ventral parts of the ***pontine reticular nucleus (>1840)***, just dorsal to the ***pontine nuclei (Jacobsohn, 1909)***; see Saper et al. (1976). It was not known by 1840.

pontine medial lemniscus (>1840)

As described in macrodissected adult human, and mammal generally with histological methods for ***axons (Kölliker, 1896)***, the topographic segment of the ***medial lemniscus (>1840)*** in the ***pons (Haller, 1747)***, between ***tegmental medial lemniscus (>1840)*** segment rostrally and ***medullary medial lemniscus (>1840)*** segment caudally; see Nieuwenhuys et al. (2008, Figs. 6.26–28). It was known to Reil; see ***[pontine medial lemniscus (>1840)] (Reil, 1809c)***.

EARLIER REFERENCES:

Described, not named or illustrated:

1. *[pontine medial lemniscus (>1840)] (Reil, 1809c)*
Segment of *external part of lemniscus (Reil, 1809c)* in ***pons (Haller, 1747)***, vaguely described; see Mayo translation (1823, p. 95).

pontine medial longitudinal fascicle (>1840)

As described in macrodissected adult human, and mammal generally with histological methods for ***axons (Kölliker, 1896)***, the topographic segment of the ***medial longitudinal fascicle (>1840)*** in the ***pons (Haller, 1747)***, between ***tegmental medial longitudinal fascicle (>1840)*** segment rostrally and ***medullary medial longitudinal fascicle (>1840)*** segment caudally; see Nieuwenhuys et al. (2008, Figs. 6.16, 16.18-*16*). It was probably known to Vicq d'Azyr; see ***[pontine medial longitudinal fascicle (>1840)] (Vicq d'Azyr, 1786)***.

EARLIER REFERENCES:

Illustrated, not named or described:

1. ***[pontine medial longitudinal fascicle (>1840)] (Vicq d'Azyr, 1786)***
   Apparently illustrated at least rostral part for macrodissected adult human; Plate XXXI, Figure II-2 toward *6*.

pontine medial reticulospinal tract (>1840)

As described in macrodissected adult human, and mammal generally with experimental histological methods for ***axons (Kölliker, 1896)***, the rostral topographic segment of the ***medial reticulospinal tract (>1840)*** in the ***pons (Haller, 1747)***, rostral to ***medullary medial reticulospinal tract (>1840)*** segment; see Crosby et al. (1962, p. 105 and Figs. 140, 145, 148), Williams & Warwick (1980, pp. 875–876). It was not described by 1840.

pontine nuclei (Jacobsohn, 1909)

As described for macrodissected adult human, and for adult mammal in general with cellular architecture and connections, the ***gray matter region (Swanson & Bota, 2010)*** lying in the ventral part of the ***pons (Haller, 1747)***, ventral to the ***pontine reticular nucleus (>1840)*** and dispersed among the ***longitudinal pontine fibers (Arnold, 1838b)*** and ***transverse pontine fibers (>1840)***. Histologically, the ***pontine nuclei (Jacobsohn, 1909)*** generate the crossed ***middle cerebellar peduncle (Rolando, 1819)*** and include a dorsomedial differentiation, the ***tegmental reticular nucleus (>1840)***; see Williams & Warwick (1980, p. 908), Nieuwenhuys et al. (208, p. 202). For Jacobsohn's use in macrodissected adult human, see p. 41; also see Masuda (1914, p. 11). They were probably first recognized by Malpighi; see ***[pontine nuclei (Jacobsohn, 1909)] (Malpighi, 1666)***.

TRANSLATIONS:

1. *Brückenkerns (Jacobsohn, 1909)*
   Original German form of ***pontine nuclei (Jacobsohn, 1909)***; p. 43.

EARLIER REFERENCES:

Described, not named or illustrated:

1. ***[pontine nuclei (Jacobsohn, 1909)] (Malpighi, 1666)***
   Malpighi referred to equivalent of ***gray matter region (Swanson & Bota, 2010)*** "beneath the pons of Varolius", that is, dispersed within ***middle cerebellar peduncles (Rolando, 1819)***; see Meyer (1967, p. 189). This is first vague reference to ***pontine nuclei (Jacobsohn, 1909)*** and Malpighi dissected a variety of mammals including human, though species used for this particular observation is unclear. In macrodissected adult human, Cowper (1698, Appendix Fig. 29-*b*) clearly showed and pointed out alternating *gray substance (Vesalius, 1543a)* and *white substance (Vesalius, 1543a)* striae associated with ***middle cerebellar peduncles (Rolando, 1819)***; that is, ***pontine nuclei (Jacobsohn, 1909)***.

Earlier synonyms:

1. *pontine gray (Reil, 1809b)*
   Synonym for macrodissected adult human ***pontine nuclei (Jacobsohn, 1909)***; in the original German, *der grauen Substanz in der Brücke*, p. 152. Also see Burdach (1822, p. 301), Masuda (1914, p. 7), Crosby et al. (1962, p. 159).

pontine raphe nucleus (>1840)

As described for macrodissected adult human, and for adult mammal in general with cellular architecture and connections, a thin, unpaired ***gray matter region (Swanson & Bota, 2010)*** in the median plane of the ***pons (Haller, 1747)***, between ***pontine nuclei (Jacobsohn, 1909)*** ventrally and ***pontine central gray (>1840)*** dorsally; see Nieuwenhuys et al. (2008, p. 204 and Fig. 6.27-*13*), *Terminologia Anatomica* (1998, p. 115). It was first delineated as the *raphe of annular protuberance (Vicq d'Azyr, 1784)*.

TRANSLATIONS:

1. *nucleus raphes pontis (>1840)*
   Current Latin form of ***pontine raphe nucleus (>1840)***; see *Terminologia Anatomica* (1998, p. 115).

EARLIER REFERENCES:

Earlier synonyms:

1. *raphe of annular protuberance (Vicq d'Azyr, 1784)*
   Vicq d'Azyr described (pp. 560, 562) and illustrated (1786, Pls. XVII-*38*, XXII-*19*) a median plane strip through full dorsoventral extent of macrodissected adult human ***pons (Haller, 1747)***, as viewed with the naked eye in transverse section—roughly ***pontine raphe nucleus (>1840)***. Chaussier (1807, p. 109) simply referred to a *raphé* in this region of macrodissected adult human.
2. *median line of midbrain (Chaussier, 1807)*
   Synonym for macrodissected adult human *raphe of annular protuberance (Vicq d'Azyr, 1784)*; *midbrain (Chaussier, 1807)* included ***midbrain (Baer, 1837)*** and ***pons (Haller, 1747)***; in the original French, *ligne médiane du mésocéphale*, pp. 109, 196.
3. *raphe pontis (Gordon, 1815)*
   Synonym for macrodissected adult human *raphe of annular protuberance (Vicq d'Azyr, 1784)*; p. 140, also see Burdach (1822 p. 299).

pontine reticular nucleus (>1840)

As described for macrodissected adult human, and for adult mammal in general with cellular architecture and connections, the major ***gray matter region (Swanson & Bota, 2010)*** of the ***pons (Haller, 1747)*** lying dorsal to the ***pontine nuclei (Jacobsohn, 1909)*** and lateral to the ***pontine raphe nucleus (>1840)***, and regarded as relatively undifferentiated except for generally recognized rostral (oral) and caudal parts; see Meessen & Olszewski (1949), Brodal (1957b, p. 12), Carpenter (1966, p. 322), Swanson (2004, Table B, notes *206*, *291*). It was not recognized by 1840.

pontine rubrospinal tract (>1840)

As described in adult human and other mammals most clearly with experimental pathway tracing methods, the topographic segment of the ***rubrospinal tract (>1840)*** extending caudally in the ***pontine ventrolateral fascicle (>1840)***, between ***tegmental rubrospinal tract (>1840)*** segment rostrally and ***medullary rubrospinal tract (>10840)*** segment caudally. See Mettler (1948, Figs. 229, 231, 236, 240), Swanson (2004, Atlas Levels 44–52). It was not identified by 1840.

pontine segment of midbrain tract of trigeminal nerve (>1840)

As described in macrodissected adult human, and mammal generally with histological methods for ***axons (Kölliker, 1896)***, the caudal segment of the ***midbrain tract of trigeminal nerve (>1840)***, caudal to the ***tegmental segment of midbrain tract of trigeminal nerve (>1840)*** segment and lying on the lateral edge of the rostral half of the ***pontine central gray (>1840)*** just lateral to the ***midbrain nucleus of trigeminal nerve (>1840)***; see Nieuwenhuys et al. (2008, Fig. 6.28). It was not known by 1840.

pontine segment of spinal tract of trigeminal nerve (>1840)

As described in macrodissected adult human, and mammal generally with histological methods for ***axons (Kölliker, 1896)***, the short rostral topographic segment of the ***spinal tract of trigeminal nerve (>1840)*** in the ***pons (Haller, 1747)***, between the bifurcation of the ***trigeminal nerve central root (>1840)*** rostrally and the ***medullary segment of spinal tract of trigeminal nerve (>1840)*** caudally; see Carpenter (1976, Fig. 12.20). It was known to Rolando; see *root of fifth pair of nerves (Rolando, 1825a).*

pontine spinothalamic tract (>1840)

As described for adult human and other mammals most clearly with experimental pathway tracing methods, a topographic segment of the ***spinothalamic tract (>1840)*** extending rostrally in the ***pons (Haller, 1747)***, between ***tegmental spinothalamic tract (>1840)*** segment rostrally and ***medullary spinothalamic tract (>1840)*** segment caudally. It lies within the ***pontine ventrolateral fascicle (>1840)*** and its largest branches are to the ***parabrachial nucleus (>1840)*** and ***pontine reticular nucleus (>1840)***; see Carpenter (1976, Fig. 10.8), Nieuwenhuys et al. (2008, p. 698 and Fig. 6.16-*FAL red*). It was not identified as a differentiable part of the ***ventrolateral fascicle (>1840)*** before 1840.

pontine sulcus (Soemmerring, 1778)

As described for macrodissected adult human, the transverse groove between the rostral and ventral end of the ***pons (Haller, 1747)*** with its ***middle cerebellar peduncle (Rolando, 1819)*** and the caudal end of the ***midbrain (Baer, 1837)***, and more specifically, its ***cerebral peduncle (Tarin, 1753)***; see Nieuwenhuys et al. (2008, Fig. 3.9 unlabeled between *21* and *26*). For Soemmerring's use in macrodissected adult human, see Table II-*T*.

TRANSLATIONS:

1. *sulcum pontem (Soemmerring, 1778)*
   Original Latin form of ***pontine sulcus (Soemmerring, 1778)***; Table II-*T*.

LATER SYNONYMS:

1. *anterior pontine sulcus (Günther, 1786)*
   Synonym for macrodissected adult human ***pontine sulcus (Soemmerring, 1778)***; in the original Latin, *sulcus anterior*, p. 20.
2. *lateral sulcus of isthmus (Cruveilhier, 1836)*
   Synonym for macrodissected adult human ***pontine sulcus (Soemmerring, 1778)***; in the original French, *sillon latéral de l'isthme*, p. 607.

pontine superior cerebellar peduncle (>1840)

As described in macrodissected adult human, and mammal generally with histological methods for ***axons (Kölliker, 1896)***, the caudal topographic segment of the ***superior cerebellar peduncle (Procháska, 1800)*** in the ***pons (Haller, 1747)***, between ***arbor vitae (Winslow, 1733)*** caudally and ***tegmental superior cerebellar peduncle (>1840)*** segment rostrally. Sometimes three components are distinguished near the ***arbor vitae (Winslow, 1733)***: the ***pontine ventral spinothalamic tract (>1840)*** dorsally, the thin ***uncinate fascicle of cerebellum (>1840)*** in the middle, and the superior cerebellar peduncle proper ventrally; see Carpenter (1976, pp. 417, 420–422 and Fig. 14.18). It was almost certainly known to Galen; see ***[pontine superior cerebellar peduncle (>1840)] (Galen, c177).***

EARLIER REFERENCES:

Described, not named or illustrated:

1. ***[pontine superior cerebellar peduncle (>1840)] (Galen, c177)***
   Almost certainly known to Galen, though not named separately; see ***[superior cerebellar peduncle (Procháska, 1800)] (Galen, c177).***

pontine tectospinal tract (>1840)

As described in macrodissected adult human, and mammal generally with histological methods for ***axons (Kölliker, 1896)***, a topographic segment of the ***tectospinal tract (>1840)*** in the ***pons (Haller, 1747)*** between the short longitudinal ***tegmental tectospinal tract (>1840)*** segment rostrally and the ***medullary tectospinal tract (>1840)*** segment caudally; see Mettler (1948, Fig. 229), Crosby et al. (1962, Fig. 145, called *medial tectospinal tract*), Swanson (2004, Atlas Levels 44–47), Nieuwenhuys et al. (2008, Fig. 6.28-*19*). It was not recognized by 1840.

pontine ventral spinocerebellar tract (>1840)

As described in macrodissected adult human, and mammal generally with histological methods for ***axons***

(Kölliker, 1896), the rostral topographic segment of the ***ventral spinocerebellar tract (>1840)*** extending rostrally in the ***pontine ventrolateral fascicle (>1840)***, between ***medullary ventral spinocerebellar tract (>1840)*** segment caudally and ventrally, and ***superior cerebellar peduncle (Procháska, 1800)*** rostrally and dorsally; see Mettler (1948, Figs. 229, 231, 236, 238, 240), Swanson (2004, Atlas Levels 45–48). It was known to Reil; see ***[pontine ventral spinocerebellar tract (>1840)] (Reil, 1809c)***.

EARLIER REFERENCES:

Described, not named or illustrated:

1. ***[pontine ventral spinocerebellar tract (>1840)] (Reil, 1809c)***
   Described vaguely in macrodissected adult sheep; see Mayo translation (1823, p. 99).

pontine ventrolateral fascicle (>1840)

As described for macrodissected adult human, the topographic segment of the ***ventrolateral fascicle (>1840)*** in the ***pons (Haller, 1747)***, between ***tegmental spinothalamic tract (>1840)*** segment rostrally and ***medullary ventrolateral fascicle (>1840)*** segment caudally; with two main components, ***pontine spinothalamic tract (>1840)*** and ***pontine rubrospinal tract (>1840)***; see Nieuwenhuys et al. (2008, Fig. 6.16-*FAL*). It was observed but not separately named by Rolando; see ***[pontine ventrolateral tract (>1840)] (Rolando, 1825a)***.

EARLIER REFERENCES:

Illustrated and described, not named:

1. ***[pontine ventrolateral tract (>1840)] (Rolando, 1825a)***
   Rolando observed the *anterolateral cord of oblong medulla (Rolando, 1825a)*, or ***ventrolateral fascicle (>1840)***, in the ***pons (Haller, 1747)*** without separately naming it; see Table VIII, Figure 1-*z*.

postcentral gyrus (>1840)

As described for macrodissected adult human, the rostral topographic subdivision of the ***parietal region (>1840)*** lying between ***central sulcus (Huschke, 1854)*** rostrally and ***postcentral sulcus (>1840)*** caudally; see Williams & Warwick (1980, Fig. 7.111A). Also see ***posterior paracentral gyrus (>1840)***. It was perhaps first clearly delineated by Vicq d'Azyr; see ***[postcentral gyrus (>1840)] (Vicq d'Azyr, 1786)***.

EARLIER REFERENCES:

Illustrated, not named or described:

1. ***[postcentral gyrus (>1840)] (Vicq d'Azyr, 1786)***
   Clearly illustrated for macrodissected adult human; Plate III, see Meyer (1971, p. 124), Clarke & Dewhurst (1996, p. 90).

postcentral sulcus (>1840)

As described for macrodissected adult human, the groove forming the caudal border of the ***postcentral gyrus (>1840)***; see Williams & Warwick (1980, Fig. 7.111A). It was first clearly delineated by Vicq d'Azyr; see ***[postcentral sulcus (>1840)] (Vicq d'Azyr, 1786)***.

EARLIER REFERENCES:

Illustrated, not named or described:

1. ***[postcentral sulcus (>1840)] (Vicq d'Azyr, 1786)***
   Clearly illustrated for macrodissected adult human; Plate III, see Meyer (1971, p. 124), Clarke & Dewhurst (1996, p. 90).

postcommissural fornix (Loo, 1931)

As described in macrodissected adult human, and mammal generally with histological methods for ***axons (Kölliker, 1896)***, one of two major subdivisions of the ***fornix (Vesalius, 1543a)*** lying rostral to the level of the ***subfornical organ (>1840)*** and ***interventricular foramen (>1840)***, the other subdivision being the ***precommissural fornix (Loo, 1931)***. The ***postcommissural fornix (Loo, 1931)*** "is the columna fornicis of the literature" (Loo, 1931, p. 81), and for topographic description has two segments: the ***septal postcommissural fornix (>1840)*** between ***subfornical organ (>1840)*** and ***anterior commissure (Lieutaud, 1742)***, and its extension the ***hypothalamic postcommissural fornix (>1840)*** between ***anterior commissure (Lieutaud, 1742)*** and ***mammillary body (Ludwig, 1779)***. It was known vaguely to Galen; see ***[postcommissural fornix (Loo, 1931)] (Galen, c177)***.

EARLIER REFERENCES:

Described, not named or illustrated:

1. ***[postcommissural fornix (Loo, 1931)] (Galen, c177)***
   In *On Anatomical Procedures*, Galen referred to extension of *fornix (Galen, c177)* passing down close to right and left ***interventricular foramen (>1840)***—right and left ***septal postcommissural fornix (>1840)***, considered together—just to the level where they pass caudal to the ***anterior commissure (Lieutaud, 1742)***; see Singer translation (1999, p. 234). Galen macrodissected mostly adult beef, pig, and/or monkey but not human; see Woollam (1958, p. 15).

Illustrated and described, not named:

1. ***[postcommissural fornix (Loo, 1931)] (Vesalius, 1543a)***
   Clearly illustrated for macrodissected adult human; see Singer translation (1952, pp. 41-42, 66 and Fig. 5). Eustachi (1552) illustrated very clearly macrodissected adult human right and left ***postcommissural fornix (Loo, 1931)*** just caudal to ***anterior commissure (Lieutaud, 1742)***, but his plates were not published until 1714, and then without his text; see Albinus edition (1744, Plate XVII, Fig. VI-*H*), where he referred to them as *radices fornicis (Willis, 1664)*. According to Burdach (1822, p. 356), an extension of ***postcommissural fornix (Loo, 1931)*** ventral to macrodissected adult human ***anterior commissure (Lieutaud, 1742)***, the ***hypothalamic postcommissural fornix (>1840)***, was first clearly indicated by Vieussens (1684, p. 82), and its extension to ***mammillary body (Ludwig, 1779)*** was discovered by Pourfour du Petit; see *pillar of fornix (Pourfour du Petit, 1710)*.

Earlier synonyms:

1. *ascending crus of fornix (Volkmann, 1831)*
Roughly synonymous with ***postcommissural fornix (Loo, 1931)*** in macrodissected adult "Simiae nemestrinae, Simiae sabaeae, and Talpae"; in the original Latin, *crus adscendens fornicis*, Table IV, Figures 3, 4, 8-*k*.
2. *descending cornu of fornix (Volkmann, 1831)*
Roughly synonymous with ***postcommissural fornix (Loo, 1931)*** in macrodissected adult "*Cervi capreoli*"; in the original Latin, *cornu descendens fornicis*, Table XIII, Figure 3-*k*.
3. *ascending root of mammillary body (Arnold, 1838b)*
Roughly synonymous with macrodissected adult human ***postcommissural fornix (Loo, 1931)***; in the original Latin, *radix ascendens corporis mammillaris*, Table X, Figure 5-*h*.
4. *anterior column of vault (Longet, 1842)*
Roughly synonymous with macrodissected adult human ***postcommissural fornix (Loo, 1931)***; in the original French, *colonnes antérieurs de la voûte*, p. 541.
5. *pillar of vault (Luys, 1865)*
Roughly synonymous with macrodissected adult human ***postcommissural fornix (Loo, 1931)***; in the original French, *piliers de la voûte*, p. 191 and Plates XXI-*10*, XXXII-*15*, XXXIII-*20*.
6. *fornix (Meynert, 1867)*
Synonym for macrodissected adult human ***postcommissural fornix (Loo, 1931)***; in the original German, *das Gewolbe*, p. 89.
7. *descending branch of crus fornicis (Meynert, 1872)*
Synonym for adult human ***postcommissural fornix (Loo, 1931)*** viewed in histological sections; p. 689, Figure 269-*Fd*.
8. *descending branch of anterior pillar of fornix (Meynert, 1872)*
Probably synonym for macrodissected adult human ***postcommissural fornix (Loo, 1931)***; p. 689.
9. *fornix column (Honegger, 1890)*
Synonym for macrodissected adult human ***postcommissural fornix (Loo, 1931)***; in the original Latin (plural), *columnae fornicis*, see p. 331 ff. Also see His (1895, p. 86).
10. *anterior crus of fornix (Beevor, 1891)*
Synonym for macrodissected adult human ***postcommissural fornix (Loo, 1931)***; p. 191.
11. *anterior pillar of fornix column (Dejerine & Dejerine-Klumpke, 1901)*
Synonym for macrodissected adult human ***postcommissural fornix (Loo, 1931)***; the original phrase (plural): *piliers antérieurs du columnae fornicis*, p. 272 ff.
12. *anterior column of fornix column (Dejerine & Dejerine-Klumpke, 1901)*
Synonym for macrodissected adult human ***postcommissural fornix (Loo, 1931)***; the original phrase (plural): *colonnes antérieurs du columnae fornicis*, p. 272 ff.
13. *anterior pillar of trigone (Dejerine & Dejerine-Klumpke, 1901)*
Synonym for macrodissected adult human ***postcommissural fornix (Loo, 1931)***; in the original French (plural), *piliers antérieurs du trigone*, p. 272 ff.
14. *anterior column of trigone (Dejerine & Dejerine-Klumpke, 1901)*
Synonym for macrodissected adult human ***postcommissural fornix (Loo, 1931)***; in the original French (plural), *colonnes antérieurs du trigone*, p. 272 ff.
15. *anterior pillar of fornix (Dejerine & Dejerine-Klumpke, 1901)*
Synonym for macrodissected adult macrosmatic mammalian ***postcommissural fornix (Loo, 1931)***; pp. 294, 297.
16. *inferior fornix (Cajal, 1904)*
Synonym for mammalian ***postcommissural fornix (Loo, 1931)***; in the original Latin, *fornix inferior*, p. 1044.
17. *column of fornix (Craigie, 1925)*
Alternate form of *fornix column (His, 1895)*; pp. 102–103. Used by Craigie for adult rat; for adult human see Nieuwenhuys et al. (2008, p. 379).
18. *descending column of fornix (Sprague & Meyer, 1950)*
Synonym for ***postcommissural fornix (Loo, 1931)***, p. 354. Based on description of Glees anterograde terminal degeneration in adult rabbit.
19. *anterior column of fornix (>1840)*
Synonym for macrodissected adult human ***postcommissural fornix (Loo, 1931)***; see Strong & Elwin (1942, pp. 348–349).

PARTLY CORRESPONDS:

1. *columnas anteriores veri fornicis (Vieussens, 1684)*
According to Burdach (1822, pp. 356–357), synonym for macrodissected adult human right and left *root of fornix (Willis, 1664)*; pp. 60; 65, Table VIII-*a*. However, Vieussens showed them extending much more caudally and ventrally in ***hypothalamus (Kuhlenbeck, 1927)*** than Willis, though not quite to ***mammillary body (Ludwig, 1779)***; see Table IX-*a*, where he suggested they connect with ***anterior commissure (Lieutaud, 1742)***. Also see Table X-*D*, where he suggested they connect with ***internal capsule (Burdach, 1822)***. Also see *fimbriatae veri fornicis appendix (Vieussens, 1684)*.
2. *anterior column of true fornix (Vieussens, 1684)*
English form (singular) of *columnas anteriores veri fornicis (Vieussens, 1684)*.
3. *pillar of fornix (Pourfour du Petit, 1710)*
Corresponds to indeterminate length of ventral part of ***septal postcommissural fornix (>1840)*** and ***hypothalamic postcommissural fornix (>1840)***, considered together for macrodissected adult human. Pourfour du Petit's very brief account of ***fornix (Vesalius, 1543a)*** vaguely described right and left [*anterior*] *pillar of fornix (Pourfour du Petit, 1710)* extending as two separated entities from rostral end of adjacent right and left *posterior pillar of fornix (Pourfour du Petit, 1710)*, a separation

occurring somewhere now impossible to determine in ***septal postcommissural fornix (Loo, 1931)***. More importantly, extension of ***postcommissural fornix (Loo, 1931)*** all the way to ***mammillary body (Ludwig, 1779)*** was described here for the first time, "The posterior pillars of this vault [***fornix (Vesalius, 1543a)***] take origin in the inferior part of the ventricles. They rise up under the corpus callosum, attach to it, and although flat before, now become round and unite; after that they leave the corpus callosum, separate by submerging into the anterior part of the cavity which is above the funnel [rostral end of ***third ventricle (Galen, c173)***]—and by their situation there recalls to mind the infant's vulva [*vulva (Casseri, 1627)*]. These pillars project to the small white bodies near the funnel; from these small white bodies [***mammillary body (Ludwig, 1779)***] leave medullary fibers or projections [***mammillothalamic tracts (>1840)***] that seem to be a continuation of these pillars, and rise up again through the optic thalamus, dividing in their superior aspect into a great number of fibers—some of which end in the *centrum semiovale*, others in the little eminence at the superior and anterior part of the optic thalamus [***anterior thalamic nuclei (>1840)***]." (1710, p. 13; L. Kruger and L.W. Swanson, unpublished translation; also see Meyer, 1971, p. 20).

posterior ampullary nerve (>1840)

As described for macrodissected adult human, a terminal branch of the ***caudal part of vestibular nerve (>1840)*** to the ampulla of the posterior semicircular canal; see Durward (1951, Fig. 904), *Terminologia Anatomica* (1998, p. 136). It was perhaps first clearly delineated as the *minor branch of anterior fascicles of acoustic nerve (Scarpa, 1789)*.

EARLIER REFERENCES:

Earlier synonyms:

1. *minor branch of anterior fascicles of acoustic nerve (Scarpa, 1789)*
   Description and illustration of macrodissected adult human ***posterior ampullary nerve (>1840)***; Table 8, Figure 2-*k*.
2. *minor twig of posterior branch of auditory nerve (Soemmerring, 1791)*
   Synonym for *minor branch of anterior fascicles of acoustic nerve (Scarpa, 1789)*; p. 227 and Soemmerring (1798, p. 260).
3. *posterior branch of vestibular nerve to ampulla of posterior semicircular canal (Langenbeck, 1826–1830)*
   Synonym for macrodissected adult human ***posterior ampullary nerve (>1840)***; in the original Latin, *ramus posterior nervi vestibuli ad ampullam canalis semicircularis posterior*, Fascicle III, Table XXIX-*10*.
4. *minor branch of posterior branch of acoustic nerve (Cloquet, 1828)*
   Synonym for macrodissected adult human ***posterior ampullary nerve (>1840)***; in the original French, *petit rameau de la branche postérieure du nerf acoustique*, Table CXXX, Figure 9-22.
5. *inferior branch of vestibular nerve (Arnold, 1839)*
   Synonym for macrodissected adult human ***posterior ampullary nerve (>1840)***; in the original Latin, *ramus inferior nervi vestibuli*, Table VII, Figure 9.

posterior auricular nerve (Meckel, 1753)

As described for macrodissected adult human, a branch of the ***facial nerve trunk (>1840)*** leaving near the stylomastoid foramen and coursing dorsally (upward), rostral to (in front of) the mastoid process. In its course it communicates with the ***great auricular nerve (Haase, 1781)***, ***lesser occipital nerve (Mayer, 1794)***, and ***auricular branch of vagus nerve (Arnold, 1834)***; see Durward (1951, p. 1032 and Fig. 902), Williams & Warwick (1980, p. 1072 and Fig. 7.186). For Meckel's use in macrodissected adult human, see Table 1-*114*. Unfortunately, he sometimes abbreviated the *great posterior auricular nerve (Meckel, 1753)*, the ***great auricular nerve (Haase, 1781)***, as *posterior auricular [nerve]*, see Table 1-*265*. It may have been noticed first by Willis; see ***[posterior auricular nerve (Meckel, 1753)] (Willis, 1664)***.

TRANSLATIONS:

1. *nerf auriculaire postérieur (Meckel, 1753)*
   Original French form of ***posterior auricular nerve (Meckel, 1753)***; Table 1-*114*.

EARLIER REFERENCES:

Illustrated and described, not named:

1. ***[posterior auricular nerve (Meckel, 1753)] (Willis, 1664)***
   Possibly mentioned and illustrated for macrodissected adult human, but description is vague; see Pordage translation (1681, p. 144 and Tab. IX-5).

Earlier synonyms:

1. *first ramification of trunk of portio dura (Du Verney, 1683)*
   Synonym for ***posterior auricular nerve (Meckel, 1753)***, beautifully illustrated for macrodissected adult human; see translation (1737, Pl. 12, Fig. 3-*D*).
2. *superior ramus of trunk of nerve of portio dura (Winslow, 1733)*
   Synonym for macrodissected adult human ***posterior auricular nerve (Meckel, 1753)***; Section VI, p. 68.

LATER SYNONYMS:

1. *occipital nerve (Meckel, 1753)*
   Synonym listed for macrodissected adult human ***posterior auricular nerve (Meckel, 1753)***; in the original French, *le nerf occipital*, Table 1-*114*.
2. *external deep nerve of hard nerve (Meckel, 1753)*
   Synonym Meckel preferred for macrodissected adult human ***posterior auricular nerve (Meckel, 1753)***; in the original French, *le nerf profond extérieur du dur*, Table 1-*114*.
3. *deep posterior auricular nerve (Meckel, 1753)*
   Synonym for macrodissected adult human ***posterior auricular nerve (Meckel, 1753)***; in the original French, *le nerf auriculaire postérieur profond (du dur)*, Table 1-*274*.
4. *external deep branch of hard nerve (Meckel, 1753)*
   Synonym Meckel preferred for macrodissected adult human ***posterior auricular nerve (Meckel, 1753)***; in

the original French, *le rameau profond extérieur du dur*, p. 75.

5. *auricular nerve of hard nerve (Bang, 1770)*
Synonym for macrodissected adult human ***posterior auricular nerve (Meckel, 1753)***; in the original Latin, *nervi auriculari nervi duri*, Figure I-34,38. Also see Haase (1781, p. 81).
6. *transverse occipital branch of hard nerve (Peipers, 1793)*
Synonym for macrodissected adult human ***posterior auricular nerve (Meckel, 1753)***; in the original Latin, *nervi duri ramus occipitalis transversus*, p. 35.
7. *posterior auricular branch of hard nerve (Mayer, 1794)*
Synonym for macrodissected adult human ***posterior auricular nerve (Meckel, 1753)***; in the original Latin, *ramus auricularis posterior nervi duri*; Part 5, Table VII-79 (p. 47).
8. *occipital branch of hard nerve (Mayer, 1794)*
Synonym for macrodissected adult human ***posterior auricular nerve (Meckel, 1753)***; in the original Latin, *ramus occipitalis nervi duri*; Part 5, Table VII-79 (p. 47).
9. *posterior auricular branchlets of facial nerve (Chaussier, 1809)*
Synonym for macrodissected adult human ***posterior auricular nerve (Meckel, 1753)***; in the original French, *filets oriculaires postérieurs*.
10. *inferior auricular nerve (Meckel, 1817)*
Synonym for macrodissected adult human ***posterior auricular nerve (Meckel, 1753)***; in the original Latin, *nervus auricularis inferior*, see translation (1832, Vol. 3, p. 54).
11. *deep auricular nerve (Meckel, 1817)*
Synonym for macrodissected adult human ***posterior auricular nerve (Meckel, 1753)***; in the original Latin, *nervus auricularis profundus*, see translation (1832, Vol. 3, p. 54).
12. *external deep branch of portio major and minor of facial nerve (Bellingeri, 1818)*
Synonym for macrodissected adult human ***posterior auricular nerve (Meckel, 1753)***; in the original Latin, *ramus profundus externus*, see Table II.
13. *posterior auricular branch of facial nerve (Cruveilhier, 1836)*
Synonym for macrodissected adult human ***posterior auricular nerve (Meckel, 1753)***; in the original French, *rameau auriculaire postérieur*, p. 942.
14. *auriculo-occipital branch of facial nerve (Cruveilhier, 1836)*
Synonym for macrodissected adult human ***posterior auricular nerve (Meckel, 1753)***; in the original French, *rameau auriculo-occipital*, p. 942.

PARTLY CORRESPONDS:

1. *posterior deep branch of hard nerve (Mayer, 1794)*
Apparently, short proximal segment of macrodissected adult human ***posterior auricular nerve (Meckel, 1753)***; in the original Latin, *ramus profundus posterior nervi duri*; Part 5, Table VII-79 (p. 47).
2. *connection of posterior auricular nerve with auricular branch of vagus nerve (Arnold, 1834)*
Macrodissected adult human ***communicating branch (Winslow, 1733)*** between ***posterior auricular nerve (Meckel, 1753)*** and ***auricular branch of vagus nerve (Arnold, 1834)***; in the original Latin, *nervus auricularis posterior conjunctio cum ramo auriculare nervi vagi*, pp. 12, 14.

posterior branch of great auricular nerve (Bock, 1827)

As described for macrodissected adult human, it innervates skin of the face over the mastoid process and of the back of the auricle (except its upper part), lobule, and concha, and it communicates with the ***lesser occipital nerve (Mayer, 1794)***, ***auricular branch of vagus nerve (Arnold, 1834)***, and ***posterior auricular nerve (Meckel, 1753)***; see Williams & Warwick (1980, p. 1092) and Schwalbe (1881, Fig. 468-9). For Bock's use in macrodissected adult human, see Table III-5. It was known to Galen; see ***[posterior branch of great auricular nerve (Bock, 1827)] (Galen, c192)***.

TRANSLATIONS:

1. *ramus posterior nervi auricularis magni (Bock, 1827)*
Original Latin form of ***posterior branch of great auricular nerve (Bock, 1827)***; Table III-5.

EARLIER REFERENCES:

Described, not named or illustrated:

1. ***[posterior branch of great auricular nerve (Bock, 1827)] (Galen, c192)***
Mentioned for macrodissected adult beef, pig, and/or macaque but not human; see Duckworth translation (1962, p. 225).

Illustrated, not named or described:

1. ***[posterior branch of great auricular nerve (Bock, 1827)] (Eustachi, 1552)***
Clearly illustrated for macrodissected adult human; see Albinus edition (1761, Tab. 21/2-*h*). Du Verney (1683, Pl. 14-*D,E*) published clear illustration for macrodissected adult human.

Earlier synonyms:

1. *posterior branch of auricular nerve of third pair of cervical nerves (Meckel, 1753)*
Synonym for macrodissected adult human ***posterior branch of great auricular nerve (Bock, 1827)***; p. 99.
2. *auricular branch proper of auricular nerve of third cervical pair (Meckel, 1753)*
Synonym for macrodissected adult human ***posterior branch of great auricular nerve (Bock, 1827)***; p. 99.
3. *great auricular branch of auricular nerve of third cervical pair (Meckel, 1753)*
Synonym for macrodissected adult human ***posterior branch of great auricular nerve (Bock, 1827)***; p. 100.
4. *posterior branch of principal auricular nerve (Bang, 1770)*
Synonym for macrodissected adult human ***posterior branch of great auricular nerve (Bock, 1827)***; in the original Latin, *posterior ramus nervus auricularis principalis*, Figure I-30,39.
5. *posterior branch of greater posterior auricular nerve (Bang, 1770)*

Synonym for macrodissected adult human ***posterior branch of great auricular nerve (Bock, 1827)***; in the original Latin, *posterior ramus nervus auricularis magnus posterior*, Figure I-30,39.

6. *great posterior auricular nerve (Neubauer, 1772)*
   Large component of macrodissected adult human *posterior auricular nerve (Neubauer, 1772)*, presumably ***posterior branch of great auricular nerve (Bock, 1827)***; in the original Latin, *magnum nervum auricularem posteriorem*, Table 1-159,189. Also see Schwalbe (1881, Fig. 468-9).
7. *posterior twig of great cervical auricular nerve (Soemmerring, 1791)*
   Synonym for macrodissected adult human ***posterior branch of great auricular nerve (Bock, 1827)***; p. 269.
8. *posterior branches of auricular branch of cervical plexus (Cloquet, 1816)*
   Synonym for macrodissected adult human ***posterior branch of great auricular nerve (Bock, 1827)***; p. 640.

LATER SYNONYMS:

1. *auricular branches of great auricular nerve (Arnold, 1834)*
   Synonym for macrodissected adult human ***posterior branch of great auricular nerve (Bock, 1827)***; in the original Latin, *nervus auricularis magnus rami auriculares*, Table IX-43,45.

PARTLY CORRESPONDS:

1. *anterior branch of posterior branch of auricular nerve (Meckel, 1753)*
   First of three branches described from macrodissected adult human ***posterior branch of great auricular nerve (Bock, 1827)***; in the original French, *le rameau antérieur de l'auriculaire postérieur*, Table 1-265.
2. *middle branch of posterior branch of auricular nerve (Meckel, 1753)*
   Second of three branches described from macrodissected adult human ***posterior branch of great auricular nerve (Bock, 1827)***; in the original French, *le rameau moyen de l'auriculaire postérieur*, Table 1-270.
3. *posterior branch of posterior branch of auricular nerve (Meckel, 1753)*
   Third of three branches described from macrodissected adult human ***posterior branch of great auricular nerve (Bock, 1827)***; in the original French, *le rameau postérieur de l'auriculaire postérieur*, Table 1-272.
4. *superficial auricular branch of auricular nerve (Cruveilhier, 1836)*
   More superficial branch of macrodissected adult human ***posterior branch of great auricular nerve (Bock, 1827)***; in the original French, *rameau auriculaire superficiel*, p. 783.
5. *deep auricular branch of auricular nerve (Cruveilhier, 1836)*
   Deeper branch of macrodissected adult human ***posterior branch of great auricular nerve (Bock, 1827)***; in the original French, *rameau auriculaire profond*, pp. 783–784.
6. *anterior mastoid branch of auricular nerve (Cruveilhier, 1836)*
   Synonym for *deep auricular branch of auricular nerve (Cruveilhier, 1836)*; in the original French, *rameau mastoïdien antérieur*, p. 784, where two secondary branches, posterior and anterior, were described.

posterior branch of lateral cerebral sulcus (>1840)

As described for macrodissected adult human, the caudal and somewhat dorsal extension of the ***lateral cerebral sulcus (>1840)*** ending in the ***parietal region (>1840)*** surrounded by the ***supramarginal gyrus (>1840)***; see Williams & Warwick (1980, p. 984, Fig. 7.111A). It was first delineated as the *posterior ramus of Sylvian fissure (Vicq d'Azyr, 1784)*.

EARLIER REFERENCES:

Earlier synonyms:

1. *posterior ramus of Sylvian fissure (Vicq d'Azyr, 1784)*
   Synonym for macrodissected adult human ***posterior branch of lateral cerebral sulcus (>1840)***; p. 506. Rolando (1831, Fig. 1) clearly illustrated it for macrodissected adult human.

posterior branch of lateral cutaneous branch of intercostal nerves (>1840)

As described for macrodissected adult human, the dorsally (posteriorly) directed branch of the ***lateral cutaneous branch of intercostal nerves (>1840)***; see Durward (1951, Fig. 935), Williams & Warwick (1980, p. 1103). It was probably first clearly described as the *posterior branch of lateral cutaneous nerve of intercostal nerve (Bock, 1827)*.

EARLIER REFERENCES:

Earlier synonyms:

1. *posterior branch of lateral cutaneous nerve of intercostal nerve (Bock, 1827)*
   Synonym for macrodissected adult human ***posterior branch of lateral cutaneous branch of intercostal nerve (>1840)***; in the original Latin, *ram. posterior nervi cutanei lateralis intercostalis*, Table III-28.
2. *posterior filament of perforating branch of intercostal branches of dorsal nerves (Cruveilhier, 1836)*
   Synonym for macrodissected adult human ***posterior branch of lateral cutaneous branch of intercostal nerves (>1840)***; in the original French, *filet postérieur*, p. 825.
3. *reflected filament of perforating branch of intercostal branches of dorsal nerves (Cruveilhier, 1836)*
   Synonym for *posterior filament of perforating branch of intercostal branches of dorsal nerves (Cruveilhier, 1836)*; in the original French, *filet réfléchi*, p. 825.

PARTLY CORRESPONDS:

1. *posterior branch of lateral pectoral cutaneous nerve (Bock, 1827)*
   Synonym for macrodissected adult human ***posterior branch of lateral cutaneous branch of intercostal nerve (>1840)*** of 3rd–7th ***lateral cutaneous branches of intercostal nerves (>1840)***; in the original Latin, *ram. posterior nervi cutanei lateralis pectoris*, see Table II:82–90.

2. *posterior branch of lateral pectoral cutaneous nerve of intercostal nerve (Bock, 1827)*
   Synonym for macrodissected adult human ***posterior branch of lateral cutaneous branch of intercostal nerve (>1840)*** of 3rd–7th ***lateral cutaneous branches of intercostal nerves (>1840)***; in the original Latin, *ram. posterior nervi cutanei lateralis pectoris intercostalis*, see Table III-30.

posterior branch of mandibular nerve (>1840)

As described for adult human, the larger of the two major divisions of the ***mandibular nerve (>1840)*** that is predominantly sensory, although it does receive some contribution from the ***trigeminal nerve motor root (Bell, 1829)***, and divides into ***auriculotemporal nerve (Haller, 1762)***, ***lingual nerve (Vesalius, 1543a)***, and ***inferior dental nerve (Meckel, 1817)***; see Durward (1951, pp. 1026–1029), and Williams & Warwick (1980, p. 1066), who called it a trunk instead of branch—Hamilton (1976, p. 624) called it a division. It was first delineated by Eustachi; see ***[posterior branch of mandibular nerve (>1840)] (Eustachi, 1552)***.

EARLIER REFERENCES:

Illustrated, not named or described:

1. ***[posterior branch of mandibular nerve (>1840)] (Eustachi, 1552)***
   Illustrated for macrodissected adult human; see *posterior branch of third branch of fifth pair of cerebral nerves (Albinus, 1744)*.

Earlier synonyms:

1. *posterior branch of third branch of fifth pair of cerebral nerves (Albinus, 1744)*
   Synonym for macrodissected adult human ***posterior branch of mandibular nerve (>1840)***; in the original Latin, *ramus posterior tertii rami nervi quinti paris cerebri*, Table 18, Figures 1, 3, 4, 5-*L*.
2. *greater inferior branch of third branch of fifth pair (Meckel, 1748)*
   Roughly synonymous with ***posterior branch of mandibular nerve (>1840)***; in the original Latin, *tertio ramo nervi quinti paris ramis inferiorem majorem*, p. 79.
3. *inferior third branch of fifth pair (Meckel, 1748)*
   Synonym for *greater inferior branch of third branch of fifth pair (Meckel, 1748)*; in the original Latin, *inferior tertii quinti paris ramus*, p. 86.
4. *descending third branch of fifth pair (Meckel, 1748)*
   Synonym for *greater inferior branch of third branch of fifth pair (Meckel, 1748)*; in the original Latin, *descendens tertii quinti paris ramus*, p. 86 note *q*, and Figure 1-*68*.
5. *major branches of inferior maxillary nerve (Loder, 1778)*
   Synonym for macrodissected adult human *posterior branch of mandibular nerve (>1840)*; in the original Latin, *ramos majores*, p. 17.
6. *inferior fascicle of inferior maxillary nerve (Günther, 1786)*
   Synonym for macrodissected adult human ***posterior branch of mandibular nerve (>1840)***; in the original Latin, *fasciculum inferiorem*, p. 51.
7. *descending fascicle of inferior maxillary nerve (Günther, 1786)*
   Synonym for macrodissected adult human ***posterior branch of mandibular nerve (>1840)***; in the original Latin, *fasciculum descendentem*, p. 51.
8. *posterior and inferior branch of inferior maxillary nerve (Meckel, 1817)*
   Synonym for macrodissected adult human ***posterior branch of mandibular nerve (>1840)***; see translation (1832, Vol. 3, p. 73).

posterior branch of medial cutaneous nerve of forearm (>1840)

As described for macrodissected adult human, it is smaller than the ***anterior branch of medial cutaneous nerve of forearm (>1840)*** and descends on the dorsal part (back) of the medial side of the forearm, supplying skin as far as the wrist, and communicating with the ***medial cutaneous nerve of arm (1840)***, ***posterior cutaneous nerve of forearm (>1840)***, and ***dorsal branch of ulnar nerve (Günther, 1786)***; see Williams & Warwick (1980, p. 1097 and Fig. 7.202), *Terminologia Anatomica* (1998, p. 138). It was first clearly delineated by Eustachi; see ***[posterior branch of medial cutaneous nerve of forearm (>1840)] (Eustachi, 1552)***.

EARLIER REFERENCES:

Illustrated, not named or described:

1. ***[posterior branch of medial cutaneous nerve of forearm (>1840)] (Eustachi, 1552)***
   Illustrated for macrodissected adult human; see Albinus edition (1761, Tab. 21/2-*16* lower branch).

Described, not named or illustrated:

1. ***[posterior branch of medial cutaneous nerve of forearm (>1840)] (Winslow, 1733)***
   Described for macrodissected adult human; Section VI, no. 241, p. 83.

Earlier synonyms:

1. *ulnar cutaneous nerve of Wrisberg (Frotscher, 1788)*
   Eponym for macrodissected adult human ***posterior branch of medial cutaneous nerve of forearm (>1840)***; in the original Latin, *nervus cutaneo-ulnaris [Wrisbergii]*, p. 92 of 1795 reprint, where Frotscher described two branches. Wrisberg citation not given, but presumably from his lectures.
2. *ulnar cutaneous nerve (Soemmerring, 1791)*
   Synonym for macrodissected adult human ***posterior branch of medial cutaneous nerve of forearm (>1840)***; in the original Latin, *cutaneo-ulnaris*, p. 290.
3. *internal branch of cutaneous nerve (Fyfe, 1800)*
   Synonym for macrodissected adult human ***posterior branch of medial cutaneous nerve of forearm (>1840)***; Vol. 2, p. 308.
4. *ramus magis ulnaris nervi (Loder, 1803)*
   Synonym for macrodissected adult human ***posterior branch of medial cutaneous nerve of forearm (>1840)***; Table CLXXVIII-*122*.
5. *posterior branch of internal cutaneous nerve (Loder, 1803)*

Synonym for macrodissected adult human ***posterior branch of medial cutaneous nerve of forearm (>1840)***; in the original Latin, *nervi cutanei interni ramus posterior*, Table CLXXVIII, Figure 2-*10*.

6. *ulnar branch of medial cutaneous nerve (Bock, 1827)*
Synonym for macrodissected adult human ***posterior branch of medial cutaneous nerve of forearm (>1840)***; in the original Latin, *nervus cutaneus medius ramus ulnaris*, Table II-29,34.
7. *ulnar branch of major internal cutaneous nerve (Bock, 1827)*
Synonym for macrodissected adult human ***posterior branch of medial cutaneous nerve of forearm (>1840)***; in the original Latin, *nervus cutaneus internus major ramus ulnaris*, Table II-29,34.
8. *posterior branch of medial cutaneous nerve (Bock, 1827)*
Synonym for macrodissected adult human ***posterior branch of medial cutaneous nerve of forearm (>1840)***; in the original Latin, *ram. posterior nervi cutanei medii*, Table IV-37.
9. *dorsal nerve from internal cutaneous nerve (Knox, 1832)*
Synonym for macrodissected adult human ***posterior branch of medial cutaneous nerve of forearm (>1840)***; Plate 21, Figure 1-34.

PARTLY CORRESPONDS:

1. *lesser volar branch of dorsal nerve from internal cutaneous nerve (Knox, 1832)*
Macrodissected adult human smaller and more medial of two branches of *dorsal nerve from internal cutaneous nerve (Knox, 1832)*; Plate 21, Figure 1-35.
2. *greater volar branch of dorsal nerve from internal cutaneous nerve (Knox, 1832)*
Macrodissected adult human larger and more lateral of two branches of *dorsal nerve from internal cutaneous nerve (Knox, 1832)*; Plate 21, Figure 1-36.

posterior branch of obturator nerve (Haase, 1781; Martin, 1781)

As described for macrodissected adult human, it generates ***muscular branches of posterior branch of obturator nerve (>1840)*** and an ***articular branch of posterior branch of obturator nerve (>1840)***; see Williams & Warwick (1980, p. 1108), *Terminologia Anatomica* (1998, p. 140). For Haase's use in macrodissected adult human, see p. 106; for Martin's see p. 231. It was probably first described as the *lower part of third deep nerve of thigh (Galen, c177)*.

TRANSLATIONS:

1. *nervus obturatorius ramus posterior (Haase, 1781)*
Original Latin form of ***posterior branch of obturator nerve (Haase, 1781; Martin, 1781)***; p. 106.

EARLIER REFERENCES:

Earlier synonyms:

1. *lower part of third deep nerve of thigh (Galen, c177)*
Probably corresponds to ***posterior branch of obturator nerve (Haase, 1781; Martin, 1781)***, with major branches to adductor magnus and adductor brevis muscles described for macrodissected adult beef, pig, and/or macaque but not human; see Singer translation (1999, p. 85). Eustachi (1552) illustrated part of it for macrodissected adult human; see Albinus edition (1761, Tab. 19-3,4).

LATER SYNONYMS:

1. *inferior branch of obturator nerve (Soemmerring, 1798)*
Synonym for macrodissected adult human ***posterior branch of obturator nerve (Haase, 1781; Martin, 1781)***; p. 320.

PARTLY CORRESPONDS:

1. *collateral branch of obturator nerve (Cruveilhier, 1836)*
Generates *nerve of obturator externus (Cruveilhier, 1836)* and is thus associated with macrodissected adult human ***posterior branch of obturator nerve (Haase, 1781; Martin, 1781)***; in the original French, *branche collatérale*, p. 839.

posterior cerebellar notch (Chaussier, 1807)

As described for macrodissected adult human, the depression in the median plane on the surface of the ***cerebellum (Aristotle)*** occupied by the ***cerebellar falx (Günther, 1786)***; see Carpenter (1976, Fig. 2.23, labeled *posterior incisure*), *Dorland's* (2003, pp. 920, 1280). For Chaussier's use in macrodissected adult human, see pp. 78–79. It was probably first identified as the *posterior notch in body of cerebellum (Winslow, 1733)*.

TRANSLATIONS:

1. *échancrure postérieure (du cervelet) (Chaussier, 1807)*
Original French form of ***posterior cerebellar notch (Chaussier, 1807)***; pp. 78–79.
2. *incisura posterior cerebelli (Burdach, 1822)*
Latin form of macrodissected adult human ***posterior cerebellar notch (Chaussier, 1807)***; p. 49.
3. *incisura cerebelli posterior (Burdach, 1822)*
Latin form of *incisura posterior cerebelli (Burdach, 1822)*, preferred now; see *Dorland's* (2003, p. 920).

EARLIER REFERENCES:

Earlier synonyms:

1. *posterior notch in body of cerebellum (Winslow, 1733)*
Apparently synonym for macrodissected adult human ***posterior cerebellar notch (Chaussier, 1807)***; Section X, p. 39.
2. *common perpendicular cavity (Malacarne, 1776)*
Synonym for macrodissected adult human ***posterior cerebellar notch (Chaussier, 1807)***; see Dejerine & Dejerine-Klumpke (1901, p. 437), Clarke & O'Malley (1996, p. 643).
3. *purse-like fissure of cerebellum (Reil 1807–1808a)*
Synonym for macrodissected adult human ***posterior cerebellar notch (Chaussier, 1807)***; Tables I, Figure I-*i,l*; II, Figure II-*r*.
4. *posterior fissure of cerebellum (Reil 1807-1808a)*
Synonym for macrodissected adult human ***posterior cerebellar notch (Chaussier, 1807)***; Tables I, Figure I-*i,l*; II, Figure II-*r*.
5. *posterior semilunar notch (Tiedemann, 1816)*
Synonym for macrodissected fetal human *posterior fissure of cerebellum (Reil, 1807–1808a)*; see translation (1826, p. 63).

6. *posterior notch of Reil (Tiedemann, 1816)*
   Eponym for macrodissected fetal human *posterior fissure of cerebellum (Reil, 1807–1808a)*; see translation (1826, pp. 157, 162).

posterior cerebral artery plexus (Chaussier, 1789)

As described for macrodissected adult human, an extension of the ***internal carotid plexus (>1840)*** along the posterior cerebral artery and its branches; see Mitchell (1953, pp. 219–220). For Chaussier's observations and use of name in macrodissected human, see *Table synoptic du nerf tri-splanchnique.*

posterior cingulate region (>1840)

As described with cellular architecture in adult human, a subdivision of the ***cingulate region (>1840)*** between ***anterior cingulate region (>1840)*** rostrally and ***retrosplenial region (>1840)*** caudally, and further divided into ***dorsal posterior cingulate area (Brodmann, 1909)*** or *area 31 (Brodmann, 1909)*, and ***ventral posterior cingulate area (Brodmann, 1909)*** or *area 23 (Brodmann, 1909)*. See Nieuwenhuys et al. (2008, Fig. 12.13). It was not identified by 1840.

EARLIER REFERENCES:

Earlier synonyms:

1. *postcingulate subregion (Brodmann, 1909)*
   Synonym for adult human ***posterior cingulate region (>1840)***; in the original Latin, *subregio postcingularis*, see p. 147, Fig 86 on p. 131, Table 7 on p. 247.

posterior commissure (Winslow, 1733)

As described for macrodissected adult human and other mammals, a small transverse ***central nervous system white matter tract (>1840)*** at the dorsal junction of ***interbrain (Baer, 1837)*** and ***midbrain (Baer, 1837)***, playing a particularly important functional role in optic reflexes mediated by ***central nervous system gray matter regions (>1840)*** in the ***midbrain (Baer, 1837)*** with crossed connections; see Nieuwenhuys et al. (2008, pp. 781–784 and Fig. 19.13). Winslow referred specifically in macrodissected adult human to the *posterior commissure of hemispheres of cerebrum* as lying below the ***pineal gland (Galen, c192)***, and conspicuously avoided mentioning any connection with the latter (Sect. X, p. 38). It is impossible to know whether it included the ***habenular commissure (>1840)***, but this seems unlikely because he apparently alluded to the latter earlier (Sect. X, p. 37). The ***posterior commissure (Winslow, 1733)*** was perhaps first detected as at least part of the *tractus medullaris transversus natibus antipositus (Vieussens, 1684)*.

EARLIER REFERENCES:

Earlier synonyms:

1. *tractus medullaris transversus natibus antipositus (Vieussens, 1684)*
   Probably refers to macrodissected adult human ***posterior commissure (Winslow, 1733)*** because Ridley later wrote that its diameter is about the same as the ***anterior commissure (Lieutaud, 1742)***; Table VIII-*f*, see Ridley (1695, pp. 84, 125–126), also see Meyer (1971, p. 16). However, it might refer to ***habenular commissure (>1840)*** because Vieussens indicated it interconnects right and left ***medullary stria (Wenzel & Wenzel, 1812)***; see Ridley (1695, pp. 84, 125–126). Close inspection of Table VIII-*f* indicates the presence of two parts of this feature, so perhaps Vieussens observed both ***posterior commissure (Winslow, 1733)***, caudal and thicker, and ***habenular commissure (>1840)***, rostral and thinner.
2. *processus natibus antepositus (Ridley, 1695)*
   Synonym for macrodissected adult human *tractus medullaris transversus natibus antipositus (Vieussens, 1684)*; p. 125.

LATER SYNONYMS:

1. *posterior cerebral commissure (Haller, 1762)*
   Synonym for macrodissected adult human ***posterior commissure (Winslow, 1733)***; in the original Latin, *commissura cerebri posterior*, p. 67.
2. *upper commissure of optic tubercles (Carus, 1814)*
   Synonym for macrodissected adult amphibian ***posterior commissure (Winslow, 1733)***; in the original German, *obern Commissur der Sehhügel*, Table 3-*y*.
3. *lamina connectens (Gordon, 1815)*
   Latin term Burdach (1822, p. 337) gave to Gordon's (p. 97) description of macrodissected adult human ***posterior commissure (Winslow, 1733)***: "a much broader white *lamina*, also connected laterally with the *Thalami*."
4. *posterior commissure of brain proper (Gordon, 1815)*
   Synonym for macrodissected adult human ***posterior commissure (Winslow, 1733)***; p. 97.
5. *commissure of optic nerve ganglia (Schönlein, 1816)*
   Synonym for ***posterior commissure (Winslow, 1733)***; in the original German, *Commissur der Sehnervenganglien*, p. 44.
6. *posterior small cerebral commissure (Meckel, 1817)*
   Synonym for macrodissected adult human ***posterior commissure (Winslow, 1733)***; see translation (1832, Vol. 2, p. 446).
7. *nervus thalamos conjugens (Burdach, 1822)*
   Latin term Burdach coined (p. 337) to summarize Ridley's (1695, pp. 125–126) description of *processus natibus antepositus (Ridley, 1695)*.
8. *trabecula (Bergmann, 1831)*
   Probably synonym for macrodissected adult human ***posterior commissure (Winslow, 1733)***; p. 36, Table III, Figure 2-*d*.

posterior cutaneous nerve of arm (>1840)

As defined for macrodissected adult human, a small branch of the ***radial nerve (Du Verney, 1697)*** supplying skin on the dorsal surface of the arm almost as far distally as the olecranon; see Williams & Warwick (1980, p. 1101 and Fig. 7.202), *Terminologia Anatomica* (1998, p. 138). It was recognized by Galen; see ***[posterior cutaneous nerve of arm (>1840)] (Galen, c177)***.

EARLIER REFERENCES:

Described, not named or illustrated:

1. ***[posterior cutaneous nerve of arm (>1840)] (Galen, c177)***
Alluded to for macrodissected adult beef, pig, and/or macaque but not human; see Singer translation (1999, pp. 65–66).

Illustrated and described, not named:

1. ***[posterior cutaneous nerve of arm (>1840)] (Vesalius, 1543a)***
Described and illustrated in macrodissected adult human; see Richardson & Carman translation (2002, p. 242).

Earlier synonyms:

1. *internal subcutaneous nerve (Klint, 1784)*
Probably synonym for macrodissected adult human ***posterior cutaneous nerve of arm (>1840)***; in the original Latin, *nervus subcutaneus internus*, p. 29.
2. *internal subcutaneous branch of radial nerve (Loder, 1803)*
Probably synonym for macrodissected adult human ***posterior cutaneous nerve of arm (>1840)***; in the original Latin, *ramus subcutaneus internus nervi radialis*, Table CLXXVIII-*98*.
3. *posterior internal cutaneous nerve (Bock, 1827)*
Probably synonym for macrodissected adult human ***posterior cutaneous nerve of arm (>1840)***; in the original German, *hintere innere Hautnerv des Oberarmes*, in the original Latin, *cutaneus internus posterior*, Table II-*37*.
4. *brachial cutaneous branch (Bock, 1827)*
Synonym for *posterior internal cutaneous nerve (Bock, 1827)*; in the original Latin, *ramus cutaneus brachialis*; in the original German, *Armhautast*; Table II-*37*.
5. *internal posterior cutaneous nerve (Bock, 1827)*
Alternate form of *posterior internal cutaneous nerve (Bock, 1827)*; in the original Latin, *nervi cutanei posterioris interni*, Table IV-*53*.
6. *superior external cutaneous nerve (Quain, 1828)*
Probably synonym for macrodissected adult human ***posterior cutaneous nerve of arm (>1840)***; in the original Latin, *nervus cutaneous externus superior*, p. 424.
7. *internal cutaneous branch of radial nerve (Cloquet, 1828)*
Synonym for macrodissected adult human ***posterior cutaneous nerve of arm (>1840)***; in the original French, *rameau cutané interne du nerf radial*, Plate CLXVII, Figure 2-*13*.
8. *internal radial cutaneous branch of radial nerve (Cruveilhier, 1836)*
Probably synonym for macrodissected adult human ***posterior cutaneous nerve of arm (>1840)***; in the original French, *rameau cutané radial interne*, p. 816.

posterior cutaneous nerve of forearm (>1840)

As described for macrodissected adult human, a branch of the ***radial nerve (Du Verney, 1687)*** innervating fascia and skin of the forearm dorsal surface including the region of the elbow; see Williams & Warwick (1980, Fig. 7.202), *Terminologia Anatomica* (1998, p. 138). It was known to Galen; see ***[posterior cutaneous nerve of forearm (>1840)] (Galen, c177)***.

EARLIER REFERENCES:

Described, not named or illustrated:

1. ***[posterior cutaneous nerve of forearm (>1840)] (Galen, c177)***
Described for macrodissected adult beef, pig, and/or macaque but not human; see Singer translation (1999, pp. 66, 72). Vesalius (1543a) described it for macrodissected adult human; see Richardson & Carman translation (2002, p. 242).

Earlier synonyms:

1. *major subcutaneous branch of radial nerve (Haase, 1781)*
Synonym for macrodissected adult human ***posterior cutaneous nerve of forearm (>1840)***; in the original Latin, *major ramus sub cute*, p. 101.
2. *external subcutaneous branch of radial nerve (Klint, 1784)*
Apparently synonym for macrodissected adult human ***posterior cutaneous nerve of forearm (>1840)***; in the original Latin, *subcutaneum externum ex radiali*, p. 29.
3. *external cutaneous branch of radial nerve (Günther, 1786)*
Synonym for macrodissected adult human ***posterior cutaneous nerve of forearm (>1840)***; in the original Latin, *r. cutaneum externum ex radiali*, p. 78.
4. *cutaneous branches of muscular spiral nerve (Bell, 1803a)*
Synonym for macrodissected adult human ***posterior cutaneous nerve of forearm (>1840)***; Plate VI-*1*.
5. *superficial dorsal branch of radial nerve (Caldani, 1813, 1814)*
Synonym for macrodissected adult human ***posterior cutaneous nerve of forearm (>1840)***; in the original Latin, *ramus superficialis dorsalis*, Table CCLX, Figure 1-*3*. See Knox (1832, Pl. XXII, Fig. 1-*3*) for translation.
6. *superior external cutaneous nerve (Meckel, 1817)*
Probably roughly synonymous with macrodissected adult human ***posterior cutaneous nerve of forearm (>1840)***; in the original Latin, *nervus cutaneus externus superior*, see translation (1832, Vol. 3, p. 25).
7. *superior posterior cutaneous nerve (Bock, 1827)*
Apparently synonym for macrodissected adult human ***posterior cutaneous nerve of forearm (>1840)***; in the original Latin, *nerv. cutaneus posterior superior*; Table III-*19*.
8. *posterior cutaneous branch of spiral nerve (Swan, 1830)*
Synonym for macrodissected adult human ***posterior cutaneous nerve of forearm (>1840)***; Plate XXII-*1*.
9. *external radial cutaneous branch of radial nerve (Cruveilhier, 1836)*
Synonym for macrodissected adult human ***posterior cutaneous nerve of forearm (>1840)***; in the original French, *rameau cutané radial externe*, p. 816.
10. *radial cutaneous nerve (Quain & Wilson, 1839)*
Synonym for macrodissected adult human ***posterior cutaneous nerve of forearm (>1840)***; Plate XVIII-*h*.

posterior cutaneous nerve of thigh (Günther, 1786)

As described for macrodissected adult human, it emerges both from the first and second ***sacral plexus dorsal divisions (Paterson, 1887)*** and from the second and third ***sacral plexus ventral divisions (Paterson, 1887)*** and generates purely cutaneous branches to the gluteal region, perineum, and flexor region of the thigh and leg; see Williams & Warwick (1980, p. 1111 and Figs. 7.215, 216), *Terminologia Anatomica* (1998, p. 140). For Günther's description in macrodissected adult human, see p. 86. It was first described as the *third cutaneous nerve of thigh (Galen, c177)*.

TRANSLATIONS:

1. *nervus cutaneus femoris posterior (Günther, 1786)*
   Original Latin form of ***posterior cutaneous nerve of thigh (Günther, 1786)***; p. 86.

EARLIER REFERENCES:

Earlier synonyms:

1. *third cutaneous nerve of thigh (Galen, c177)*
   Synonym for ***posterior cutaneous nerve of thigh (Günther, 1786)*** in macrodissected adult beef, pig, and/or macaque but not human; see Singer translation (1999, pp. 83, 87), also see Duckworth translation (1962, p. 263). Vesalius (1543a) described and illustrated it for macrodissected adult human; see Richardson & Carman translation (2002, p. 259).

LATER SYNONYMS:

1. *posterior femoral cutaneous nerve (Günther, 1786)*
   Alternate form of *nervus cutaneus femoris posterior (Günther, 1786)*.
2. *posterior cutaneous nerve (Jördens, 1788)*
   Synonym for macrodissected adult human ***posterior cutaneous nerve of thigh (Günther, 1786)***; in the original Latin, *nervus cutaneus posterior*, p. 1. Quain & Wilson (1839; Tab. XXV, Fig. 1-*a*) used *posterior cutaneous nerves* for macrodissected adult human.
3. *superior and posterior cutaneous nerve (Jördens, 1788)*
   Synonym for *posterior cutaneous nerve (Jördens, 1788)*; in the original Latin, *nervus cutaneus posterior et superior*, Table I-*10*; also see Bell (1803b, p. 204).
4. *external and posterior cutaneous nerve (Bell, 1803b)*
   Apparently synonym for macrodissected adult human *posterior cutaneous nerve of thigh (Günther, 1786)*; p. 205.
5. *posterior common cutaneous nerve of thigh (Bock, 1827)*
   Synonym for macrodissected adult human ***posterior cutaneous nerve of thigh (Günther, 1786)***; in the original Latin, *nervus cutaneus communis posterior femoris*, Table IV-*73*.
6. *cutaneous branch of inferior gluteal nerve (Cruveilhier, 1836)*
   Synonym for macrodissected adult human ***posterior cutaneous nerve of thigh (Günther, 1786)***; in the original French, *branche cutanée*, p. 857.

PARTLY CORRESPONDS:

1. *inferior posterior cutaneous nerve (Martin, 1781)*
   Probably branch of macrodissected adult human ***posterior cutaneous nerve of thigh (Günther, 1786)***; in the original Latin, *nervus cutaneus posterior inferior*, p. 240 and Table XI. Also see Soemmerring (1791, p. 308).
2. *superior first lateral branch of posterior cutaneous nerve (Fischer, 1791)*
   Most proximal of four lateral branches of macrodissected adult human ***posterior cutaneous nerve of thigh (Günther, 1786)***; in the original Latin, *nervi cutanei posterioris superioris ramus lateralis primus*, Table II, Figure 2-*164(4)*.
3. *middle posterior cutaneous nerve (Soemmerring, 1791)*
   Probably branch of macrodissected adult human ***posterior cutaneous nerve of thigh (Günther, 1786)***; in the original Latin, *nervus cutaneus posterior medius*, p. 308.
4. *superior inferior cutaneous nerve (Soemmerring, 1798)*
   Synonym for *middle posterior cutaneous nerve (Soemmerring, 1791)*; in the original Latin, *nervum cutaneum inferiorem superiorem*, p. 328.
5. *superior internal cutaneous nerve (Fyfe, 1800)*
   Synonym for macrodissected adult human *cutaneous sub-pelvian nerve (Burdin, 1803)*; in the original Latin, *cutaneus internus superior*, Vol. 2, p. 330.
6. *inferior internal cutaneous nerve (Fyfe, 1800)*
   Synonym for macrodissected adult human *posterior cutaneous nerve of thigh (Chaussier, 1809)*; in the original Latin, *cutaneus internus inferior*, Vol. 2, p. 330.
7. *cutaneous sub-pelvian nerve (Burdin, 1803)*
   Proximal part of macrodissected adult human ***posterior cutaneous nerve of thigh (Günther, 1786)*** distributing to subpelvic region and medial part of thigh; see translation (1803, Vol. 1, p. 204).
8. *posterior cutaneous nerve of thigh (Chaussier, 1809)*
   Distal part of macrodissected adult human ***posterior cutaneous nerve of thigh (Günther, 1786)*** distributing to flexor aspect of thigh; in the original French, *nerf cutané postérieur de la cuisse*.
9. *sciatic branch of inferior gluteal nerve (Cloquet, 1816)*
   Synonym for macrodissected adult human *cutaneous sub-pelvian nerve (Burdin, 1803)*; in the original French, *rameau sciatique*, p. 671. See *inferior gluteal nerve (Cloquet, 1816)*.
10. *crural branch of inferior gluteal nerve (Cloquet, 1816)*
    Synonym for macrodissected adult human *posterior cutaneous nerve of thigh (Chaussier, 1809)*; in the original French, *rameau crural*, p. 671. See *inferior gluteal nerve (Cloquet, 1816)*.
11. *posterior and superior cutaneous nerve (Cloquet, 1828)*
    Most lateral major branch of macrodissected adult human ***posterior cutaneous nerve of thigh (Günther, 1786)***; in the original French, *N. cutané supérieur et postérieur*, Plate CLXXIII, Figure 2-*32*.
12. *posterior and internal cutaneous branch of small sciatic nerve (Quain, 1832)*
    Probably major branch of macrodissected adult human ***posterior cutaneous nerve of thigh (Günther, 1786)***; p. 703.
13. *middle cutaneous branch of small sciatic nerve (Quain, 1832)*
    Probably minor branch of macrodissected adult human ***posterior cutaneous nerve of thigh (Günther, 1786)***; p. 703.

14. *posterior and external cutaneous branches of great sciatic nerve (Quain, 1832)*
Probably lateral branches of macrodissected adult human ***posterior cutaneous nerve of thigh (Günther, 1786)***; p. 704.
15. *recurrent branch of cutaneous branch of inferior gluteal nerve (Cruveilhier, 1836)*
Macrodissected adult human branch of ***posterior cutaneous nerve of thigh (Günther, 1786)*** in turn generating ***inferior clunial nerves (>1840)*** and ***perineal branches of posterior cutaneous nerve of thigh (>1840)***; in the original French, *rameau récurrent*, p. 857.

posterior deep temporal nerve (Arnold, 1834)

As described for macrodissected adult human, a small component of the ***deep temporal nerves (Haase, 1781)*** lying in the caudal (posterior) part of the temporal fossa, and sometimes arising in common with the ***masseteric nerve (Meckel, 1748)***; see Williams & Warwick (1980, p. 1066). It supplies caudal (posterior) regions of the temporalis muscle (see Kwak et al., 2003, p. 395) and was beautifully illustrated by Henle (1871, Fig. 243-*tpr*[2]). For Arnold's use in macrodissected adult human, see p. 10. It was perhaps first clearly delineated as the *external deep temporal branch of third branch of fifth pair (Meckel, 1748)*.

TRANSLATIONS:

1. *nervus temporalis profundus posterior (Arnold, 1834)*
Original Latin form of ***posterior deep temporal nerve (Arnold, 1834)***; p. 10.

EARLIER REFERENCES:

Earlier synonyms:

1. *external deep temporal branch of third branch of fifth pair (Meckel, 1748)*
Synonym for macrodissected adult human ***posterior deep temporal nerve (Arnold, 1834)***; in the original Latin, *ramus temporalis profundus exterior tertii rami quinti paris*, p. 81.
2. *external fascicle of crotaphitic surculus of ganglioform plexus of inferior maxillary branch (Bellingeri, 1818)*
Synonym for macrodissected adult human ***posterior deep temporal nerve (Arnold, 1834)***; in the original Latin, *fasciculus externus*, see Table I.

LATER SYNONYMS:

1. *posterior deep temporal branch of inferior maxillary nerve (Todd, 1836–1839)*
Synonym for macrodissected adult human ***posterior deep temporal nerve (Arnold, 1834)***; p. 291. Also see Quain (1837, p. 764).
2. *external deep temporal branch of inferior maxillary nerve (Todd, 1836–1839)*
Synonym for macrodissected adult human ***posterior deep temporal nerve (Arnold, 1834)***; p. 291.

posterior esophageal plexus (Haller, 1762)

As described for macrodissected adult human, a caudal (descending) extension of the ***esophageal plexus (Haller, 1762)*** derived predominantly, though by no means exclusively, from the right ***vagus nerve trunk (Wrisberg, 1786; Günther, 1786)***. It is concentrated around caudal (lower) thoracic parts of the dorsal (posterior) esophagus, it receives sympathetic ***axons (Kölliker, 1896)***, and some parts of it condense into the ***posterior vagal trunk (Wrisberg, 1780)*** extending caudally (descending) into the abdomen whereas other parts penetrate directly into the esophageal part of the ***enteric plexuses (Hill, 1927)***; see Mitchell (1953, pp. 184–185), Williams & Warwick (1980, p. 1079). For Haller's use in macrodissected adult human, see p. 235. It was known to Galen; see ***[posterior esophageal plexus (Haller, 1762)] (Galen, c173)***.

TRANSLATIONS:

1. *plexus oesophageus posterior (Haller, 1762)*
Original Latin form of ***posterior esophageal plexus (Haller, 1762)***; p. 235.
2. *plexus nervorum gulae posterior (Soemmerring, 1798)*
Latin form of *plexus oesophagus posterior (Haller, 1762)*; p. 270.
3. *posterior plexus gulae (Bell, 1803b)*
Mixed English-Latin form of *plexus nervorum gulae posterior (Soemmerring, 1798)*; p. 158.

EARLIER REFERENCES:

Described, not named or illustrated:

1. ***[posterior esophageal plexus (Haller, 1762)] (Galen, c173)***
Described briefly as part of entwined ***vagus nerves (Galen, c192)*** around distal (lower) part of esophagus in macrodissected adult beef, pig, and/or macaque but not human; see May translation (1968, pp. 290, 449), Duckworth translation (1962, p. 220). Winslow (1733, Sect. VI, p. 73) described it rather clearly for macrodissected adult human.

LATER SYNONYMS:

1. *smaller posterior esophageal plexus (Scarpa, 1794)*
Synonym for macrodissected adult human ***posterior esophageal plexus (Haller, 1762)***; in the original Latin, *plexus oesophagaeus minor posterior*, Table V-4. From Knox's translation (1832, Pl. V-4).

posterior ethmoidal nerve (>1840)

As described for macrodissected adult human, a tiny and often inconspicuous branch of the ***nasociliary nerve (Meckel, 1817; Wutzer, 1817)***—between ***long ciliary nerves (Soemmerring, 1801)*** and ***anterior ethmoidal nerve (>1840)***—supplying the ethmoidal and sphenoidal sinuses; see Williams & Warwick (1980, p. 1062), *Terminologia Anatomica* (1998, p. 134). It was probably first clearly delineated as the *posterior trunk of ethmoidal nerve (Meckel, 1817)*.

EARLIER REFERENCES:

Earlier synonyms:

1. *posterior trunk of ethmoidal nerve (Meckel, 1817)*
Synonym for macrodissected adult human ***posterior ethmoidal nerve (>1840)***; see translation (1832, Vol. 3, p. 64).

posterior horn of lateral ventricle (Haller, 1747)

As described for macrodissected adult human, the part of the ***lateral ventricle (Vesalius, 1543a)*** extending caudally from the ***atrium of lateral ventricle (>1840)*** into the ***occipital region (Vesalius, 1543a)***; see Millen & Woollam (1962, pp. 38–44, Figs. 13, 16–18), Carpenter & Sutin (1983, p. 45, Fig. 2.20). For Haller's use in macrodissected adult human, see Mihles translation (1754b, p. 292). It was illustrated clearly long ago; see ***[posterior horn of lateral ventricle (Haller, 1747)] (Berengario da Carpi, 1523)***.

EARLIER REFERENCES:

Illustrated, not named or described:

1. *[posterior horn of lateral ventricle (Haller, 1747)] (Berengario da Carpi, 1523)*
   In the 2nd edition of *A Short Introduction to Anatomy*, Berengario presented the first realistic drawings of the dissected ***brain (Smith Papyrus, c1700 BC)*** showing the ***ventricles (Hippocrates)***, and the bottom drawing clearly shows right and left macrodissected adult human ***posterior horn of lateral ventricle (Haller, 1747)***; see Singer translation (1952, p. xxiii), Clarke & O'Malley (1996, p. 721).

Earlier synonyms:

1. *digital cavity (Bartholin, 1641)*
   Synonym for macrodissected adult human ***posterior horn of lateral ventricle (Haller, 1747)***; in the original Latin, *ventriculi cavitas digitali similis*; Figure 7-*k*, p. 277. In Culpeper's translation of Bartholin (1662), referred to as "A roundish cavity of the right Ventricle resembling the finger of a glove."
2. *digital process (Bergen, 1734)*
   Synonym for macrodissected adult human ***posterior horn of lateral ventricle (Haller, 1747)***; in the original Latin, *processus digitalis*; see Tarin (1750, Tab. XIII, Fig. 3-*f*).
3. *posterior process of ventricle (Bergen, 1734)*
   Synonym for macrodissected adult human ***posterior horn of lateral ventricle (Haller, 1747)***; in the original Latin, *processus ventriculorum posteriores*; see Tarin (1750, Tab. XIII, Fig. 3-*c*).

LATER SYNONYMS:

1. *ancyroid cavity (Morand, 1748)*
   Synonym meaning "like the fluke of an anchor" for macrodissected adult human ***posterior horn of lateral ventricle (Haller, 1747)***; see Vicq d'Azyr (1786, Pl. V-*x*), also see *calcar avis (Morand, 1748)*. Haller (1762, p. 41) spelled it *ancyroideae cavitatis* in Latin (plural), and Burdach (1822, p. 382) *cavitas ancyroïdea*.
2. *ancyroïde (Morand, 1748)*
   Synonym of *ancyroid cavity (Morand, 1748)*; see Vicq d'Azyr (1786, Pl. V-*x*).
3. *anchyroïde (Morand, 1748)*
   Form of *ancyroïde (Morand, 1748)*; see Vicq d'Azyr (1786, Pl. V-*x*).
4. *posterior sinus of lateral ventricle (Tarin, 1750)*
   Synonym for macrodissected adult human ***posterior horn of lateral ventricle (Haller, 1747)***; Table I, Figure I.
5. *diverticulum (Günz, 1753)*
   Synonym for macrodissected adult human ***posterior horn of lateral ventricle (Haller, 1747)***, according to Burdach (1822, p. 382).
6. *posterior cavity of lateral ventricle (Haller, 1754a)*
   Synonym for ***posterior horn of lateral ventricle (Haller, 1747)***. Haller used the term in conjunction with *calcar avis (Morand, 1748)*: *colliculus, vel unguis caveae posterioris ventriculorum lateralium*; see Vicq d'Azyr (1786, pp. 7, 15). Also see *unguis (Haller, 1762)*, *colliculus (Haller, 1762)*.
7. *posterior prolongation of lateral ventricle (Vicq d'Azyr, 1786)*
   Synonym for macrodissected adult human ***posterior horn of lateral ventricle (Haller, 1747)***; Plate V-*x*. Vicq d'Azyr also mentioned use of the term *posterior cavity of lateral ventricle* (in the Latin phrase *unguis caveae posterioris ventriculorum lateralium*), which probably derives from Haller (1762); see *unguis (Haller, 1762)*.
8. *short crus of lateral ventricle (Günther, 1786)*
   Synonym for macrodissected adult human ***posterior horn of lateral ventricle (Haller, 1747)***; in the original Latin (plural), *crure breviori*, p. 10.
9. *posterior crus of lateral ventricle (Günther, 1786)*
   Synonym for macrodissected adult human ***posterior horn of lateral ventricle (Haller, 1747)***; in the original Latin (plural), *crure posteriori*, p. 10.
10. *posterior horn of tricornate ventricle (Soemmerring, 1791)*
    Synonym for macrodissected adult human ***posterior horn of lateral ventricle (Haller, 1747)***; p. 47.
11. *appendices of ventricles (Burdin, 1803)*
    Synonym for right and left macrodissected adult human ***posterior horn of lateral ventricle (Haller, 1747)***; see translation (1803, Vol. 1, p. 160).
12. *digital sinus of lateral ventricle (Ramsay, 1813)*
    Synonym for macrodissected adult human ***posterior horn of lateral ventricle (Haller, 1747)***; p. 42.
13. *posterior lateral part of central fissure (Gordon, 1815)*
    Synonym for macrodissected adult human ***posterior horn of lateral ventricle (Haller, 1747)***; p. 106 ff.
14. *digital fovea (Meckel, 1817)*
    Synonym for macrodissected adult human ***posterior horn of lateral ventricle (Haller, 1747)***; in Latin, *fovea digitata*, see translation (1832, Vol. 2, p. 463).
15. *posterior occipital horn of lateral ventricle (Cruveilhier, 1836)*
    Synonym for macrodissected adult human ***posterior horn of lateral ventricle (Haller, 1747)***; in the original French, *corne postérieure occipitale*, p. 691.
16. *posterior portion of lateral ventricle (Cruveilhier, 1836)*
    Synonym for macrodissected adult human ***posterior horn of lateral ventricle (Haller, 1747)***; in the original French, *portion postérieure*, p. 691.

PARTLY CORRESPONDS:

1. *anfractuosity of digital cavity (Cruveilhier, 1836)*
   One of several possible grooves in floor of macrodissected adult human ***posterior horn of lateral ventricle (Haller, 1747)***; in the original French, *anfractuosité de la cavité digitale*, p. 663.

posterior inferior nasal nerves (Günther, 1786)

As described for macrodissected adult human, branches of the ***greater palatine nerve (Cloquet, 1816)*** ramifying over the inferior nasal concha and walls of the middle and inferior meatuses and finally supplying both surfaces of the soft palate; see Williams & Warwick (1980, p. 1065), *Terminologia Anatomica* (1998, p. 134). For Günther's use in macrodissected adult human, see p. 47. They were perhaps first recognized as the *inferior nasal branch of anterior palatine nerve (Meckel, 1748)*.

TRANSLATIONS:

1. *nervi nasales inferiores posteriores (Günther, 1786)*
   Original Latin form of ***posterior inferior nasal nerves (Günther, 1786)***; p. 47.

EARLIER REFERENCES:

Earlier synonyms:

1. *inferior nasal branch of anterior palatine nerve (Meckel, 1748)*
   Term emerging from description of macrodissected adult human ***posterior inferior nasal nerves (Günther, 1786)***; see p. 61 (in the original Latin, *ramus nasalibus inferioribus...palatinus anterior nervus*) and Figure 1-*τ*.
2. *inferior anterior nasal nerves (Scarpa, 1785)*
   Synonym for macrodissected adult human ***posterior inferior nasal nerves (Günther, 1786)***; in the original Latin, *nervi nasalis anterioris inferioris*, Table II, Figure II-*13*.

LATER SYNONYMS:

1. *inferior nasal nerves (Soemmerring, 1791)*
   Synonym for macrodissected adult human ***posterior inferior nasal nerves (Günther, 1786)***; in the original German, *Untere Nasennerven*, pp. 204–205.
2. *nervi nasales posteriores medii et inferiores (Meckel, 1817)*
   Synonym for macrodissected adult human ***posterior inferior nasal nerves (Günther, 1786)***; see translation (1832, Vol. 3, p. 68). Meckel credited a description to Cloquet (1816, p. 687).
3. *inferior nasal branch of greater palatine nerve (Cruveilhier, 1836)*
   Synonym for macrodissected adult human ***posterior inferior nasal nerves (Günther, 1786)***; in the original French, *rameau nasal inférieur*, p. 921.

PARTLY CORRESPONDS:

1. *ascending minor branch of inferior anterior nasal nerves (Scarpa, 1785)*
   Small ascending branch of macrodissected adult human ***posterior inferior nasal nerves (Günther, 1786)***; in the original Latin, *ramus minor ascendens*, Table II, Figure II-*14*.
2. *descending major branch of inferior anterior nasal nerves (Scarpa, 1785)*
   Major branch of macrodissected adult human ***posterior inferior nasal nerves (Günther, 1786)***; in the original Latin, *ramus major descendens*, Table II, Figure II-*15*. It in turn divides into two branches, Table II, Figure II-*16*.
3. *posterior middle nasal nerve (Meckel, 1817)*
   Along with *posterior inferior nasal nerve (Meckel, 1817)*, forms ***posterior inferior nasal nerves (Günther, 1786)***; see translation (1832, Vol. 3, p. 68).
4. *posterior inferior nasal nerve (Meckel, 1817)*
   Along with *posterior middle nasal nerve (Meckel, 1817)*, forms ***posterior inferior nasal nerves (Günther, 1786)***; see translation (1832, Vol. 3, p. 68).
5. *anterior superior internal nerves of palatine nerve (Bell & Bell, 1826)*
   More dorsal of macrodissected adult human ***posterior inferior nasal nerves (Günther, 1786)***; Vol. 2, p. 515.
6. *inferior internal nerves of nose (Bell & Bell, 1826)*
   Essentially more ventral of macrodissected adult human ***posterior inferior nasal nerves (Günther, 1786)***; Vol. 2, p. 516.

posterior intercavernous sinus (>1840)

As described for macrodissected adult human, a component of the ***circulatory system***; the caudal transverse segment of the ***circular sinus (Ridley, 1695)*** caudal to the ***infundibulum (Rioch et al., 1940)*** and continuous with rostral parts of the right and left ***cavernous sinus (Winslow, 1733)***; see Williams & Warwick (1980, p. 748 and Figs. 6.126, 127B), *Terminologia Anatomica* (1998, p. 94). It was perhaps first clearly delineated as *posterior clinoid sinus (Vicq d'Azyr, 1786)*.

EARLIER REFERENCES:

Earlier synonyms:

1. *sinus clinoïdeus posterior (Vicq d'Azyr, 1786)*
   Synonym for macrodissected adult human ***posterior intercavernous sinus (>1840)***; p. 72, see Burdach (1822, p. 400).
2. *posterior clinoid sinus (Vicq d'Azyr, 1786)*
   English form of *sinus clinoïdeus posterior (Vicq d'Azyr, 1786)*.

posterior interosseous nerve (Quain & Wilson, 1839)

As described for macrodissected adult human, the continuation of the ***deep branch of radial nerve (Meckel, 1817)*** distal to where it crosses the supinator muscle and then supplies the following muscles—extensor carpi radialis brevis, supinator, extensor digitorum, extensor digiti minimi, extensor carpi ulnaris, extensor pollicis longus, extensor indicis, abductor pollicis longus, and extensor pollicis brevis—as well as ligaments and joints of the carpus; see Hamilton (1976, p. 651), Williams & Warwick (1980, p. 1102). For Quain & Wilson's use in macrodissected adult human, see Plate XVIII, Figure 2-*b*. It was known to Vesalius; see ***[posterior interosseous nerve (Quain & Wilson, 1839)] (Vesalius, 1543a)***.

EARLIER REFERENCES:

Illustrated and described, not named:

1. ***[posterior interosseous nerve (Quain & Wilson, 1839)] (Vesalius, 1543a)***
   Mentioned and crudely illustrated for macrodissected adult human; see Richardson & Carman translation (2002, p. 243). Monro (1783, p. 66) described in macrodissected adult human fibers to "the back-part of the ligament of the carpus" from an unnamed small branch corresponding to this ***nerve (Herophilus,***

c335–c280 BC) described by Vesalius; also see illustration in Table 26. The macrodissected adult human ***posterior interosseous nerve (Quain & Wilson, 1839)*** has associated with it a *pseudoganglion (>1840)* that Monro also described and illustrated, Table 26-*L*; see Williams & Warwick (1980, p. 1102).

Earlier synonyms:

1. *external interosseous nerve (Günther, 1786)*
   Synonym for macrodissected adult human ***posterior interosseous nerve (Quain & Wilson, 1839)***; in the original Latin, *nervus interossei externi*, p. 78.
2. *interosseous nerve (Fyfe, 1800)*
   Synonym for macrodissected adult human ***posterior interosseous nerve (Quain & Wilson, 1839)***; Vol. 2, p. 311.

PARTLY CORRESPONDS:

1. *branch of spiral nerve to short supinator muscle of radius (Swan, 1830)*
   Macrodissected adult human branch of ***posterior interosseous nerve (Quain & Wilson, 1839)*** to supinator muscle; Plate XXII, Figure 2-37.
2. *branch of spiral nerve to shorter radial extensor muscle of wrist (Swan, 1830)*
   Macrodissected adult human branch of ***posterior interosseous nerve (Quain & Wilson, 1839)*** to extensor carpi radialis brevis muscle; Plate XXII, Figure 2-38.
3. *branch of second external radial muscle of radial nerve (Cruveilhier, 1836)*
   Macrodissected adult human branch of ***posterior interosseous nerve (Quain & Wilson, 1839)*** to external carpi radialis brevis muscle; in the original French, *rameau du deuxième radial externe*, p. 817.
4. *branch of short supinator of radial nerve (Cruveilhier, 1836)*
   Macrodissected adult human branch of ***posterior interosseous nerve (Quain & Wilson, 1839)*** to supinator muscle; in the original French, *rameau du court supinateur*, p. 817.
5. *branches of superficial layer of posterior region of forearm of antibrachial deep branch of radial nerve (Cruveilhier, 1836)*
   Considered together, macrodissected adult human *branches of common extensor of digits of radial nerve (Cruveilhier, 1836)*, *branch of extensor of little finger of radial nerve (Cruveilhier, 1836)*, and *branch of posterior cubital muscle of radial nerve (Cruveilhier, 1836)*; in the original French, *rameaux de la couche superficielle*, p. 817.
6. *branches of common extensor of digits of radial nerve (Cruveilhier, 1836)*
   Macrodissected adult human branches of ***posterior interosseous nerve (Quain & Wilson, 1839)*** to extensor digitorum muscle; in the original French, *rameaux de l'extenseur commun des doigts*, p. 817.
7. *branch of extensor of little finger of radial nerve (Cruveilhier, 1836)*
   Macrodissected adult human branches of ***posterior interosseous nerve (Quain & Wilson, 1839)*** to extensor digiti minimi muscle; in the original French, *rameau de l'extenseur du petit doigt*, p. 817.
8. *branch of posterior cubital muscle of radial nerve (Cruveilhier, 1836)*
   Macrodissected adult human branches of ***posterior interosseous nerve (Quain & Wilson, 1839)*** to extensor carpi ulnaris muscle; in the original French, *rameau du cubital postérieur*, p. 817.
9. *branches of deep layer of posterior region of forearm of antibrachial deep branch of radial nerve (Cruveilhier, 1836)*
   Considered together, macrodissected adult human *branch of long extensor proper of thumb of radial nerve (Cruveilhier, 1836)*, *branch of extensor proper of index finger of radial nerve (Cruveilhier, 1836)*, and *articular filaments of radial nerve (Cruveilhier, 1836)*; in the original French, *rameaux de la couche profonde*, p. 817.
10. *branch of long extensor proper of thumb of radial nerve (Cruveilhier, 1836)*
    Macrodissected adult human branch of ***posterior interosseous nerve (Quain & Wilson, 1839)*** to extensor pollicis longus muscle; in the original French, *rameau au long extenseur propre du pouce*, p. 818.
11. *branch of extensor proper of index finger of radial nerve (Cruveilhier, 1836)*
    Macrodissected adult human branch of ***posterior interosseous nerve (Quain & Wilson, 1839)*** to extensor indicis muscle; in the original French, *rameau à l'extenseur propre de l'index*, p. 818.
12. *articular filaments of radial nerve (Cruveilhier, 1836)*
    Numerous terminal branches of macrodissected adult human ***posterior interosseous nerve (Quain & Wilson, 1839)*** to various joints of wrist; in the original French, *filets articulaires du nerf radial*, p. 818.

posterior labial nerves (>1840)

As described for macrodissected adult human female, usually two branches (medial and lateral) of the ***perineal nerve (Camper, 1840)*** innervating skin of the labium majus, and communicating with the ***inferior rectal nerves (>1840)*** and ***perineal branches of posterior cutaneous nerve of thigh (>1840)***; see Williams & Warwick (1980, p. 1116), *Terminologia Anatomica* (1998, p. 140). They were known to Galen; see ***[posterior labial nerves (>1840)] (Galen, c192)***.

EARLIER REFERENCES:

Described, not named or illustrated:

1. ***[posterior labial nerves (>1840)] (Galen, c192)***
   Galen mentioned ***nerve (Herophilus, c335–c280 BC)*** to skin of genital organs in macrodissected adult beef, pig, and/or macaque but not human; see Duckworth translation (1962, p. 263).

PARTLY CORRESPONDS:

1. *pudendal nerves (Walter, 1783)*
   Roughly the rostral (upper) three ***posterior labial nerves (>1840)***, described for a macrodissected adult human female; in the original Latin, *pudendales nervi*, Table I:551–553.

2. *long inferior pudendal nerve (Walter, 1783)*
Apparently most caudal (lowest) of ***posterior labial nerves (>1840)***, described for a macrodissected adult human female; in the original Latin, *nervus pudendalis inferior longus*, Table I, Figures 1, 2 part *570*.
3. *long pudendal nerve (Walter, 1783)*
Synonym for *long inferior pudendal nerve (Walter, 1783)*; in the original Latin, *nervus pudendalis longus*, Table I-*574*.
4. *inferior pudendal nerve (Walter, 1783)*
Synonym for *long inferior pudendal nerve (Walter, 1783)*; in the original Latin, *nervus pudendalis inferior*, Table I-*598*.

posterior limb of internal capsule (>1840)

As described for macrodissected adult human, typically in frontal (horizontal) section, the caudal ***internal capsule (Burdach, 1822)*** segment lying between ***cerebral nuclei (Swanson, 2000a)*** laterally and rostrally, and ***interbrain (Baer, 1837)*** medially and caudally; see Crosby et al. (1962, p. 394, Fig. 272). It was clearly illustrated by Vesalius; see ***[posterior limb of internal capsule (>1840)] (Vesalius, 1543a)***.

EARLIER REFERENCES:

Illustrated, not named or described:

1. ***[posterior limb of internal capsule (>1840)] (Vesalius, 1543a)***
Clearly illustrated in frontal (horizontal) section of macrodissected adult human; see Singer translation (1952, Fig. 7).

Earlier synonyms:

1. *middle part of base of corona radiata (Arnold, 1838b)*
Roughly synonymous with macrodissected adult human ***posterior limb of internal capsule (>1840)***; in the original Latin, *pars media basis corona radiata*, Table X, Figures 1-*g*, 2-*c*.

PARTLY CORRESPONDS:

1. *transverse band of great superior ganglion (Spurzheim, 1826)*
Roughly corresponds to part of macrodissected adult human ***posterior limb of internal capsule (>1840)***, p. 232-37, along with Spurzheim's *transverse band of bundles which go to middle lobe*, p. 232-36.
2. *chordis contortis (Bergmann, 1831)*
Apparently component of macrodissected adult human ***posterior limb of internal capsule (>1840)***; p. 75 and Table II-*s*. Also illustrated in Table VIII, Figure 1-*d*, where the plural, *chordulae contortae*, is given; on p. 19, *cordulae supercilia* is given for it.

posterior lobe of pituitary gland (Haller, 1762)

As described histologically for adult vertebrate, the expanded part of the ***neurohypophysis (Rioch et al., 1940)*** lying distal to the ***infundibular stem (Hanström, 1966)*** and the site where most magnocellular neuroendocrine ***axons (Kölliker, 1896)*** from the ***hypothalamus (Kuhlenbeck, 1927)*** end and release oxytocin or vasopressin into the general circulation; see Holmes & Ball (1974, pp. 5–6), Daniel & Pritchard (1975, pp. 3–4). For Haller's use in macrodissected adult human, see p. 60, in the original Latin, *lobus posterior*. It was first clearly described by Willis; see ***[posterior lobe of pituitary gland (Haller, 1762)] (Willis, 1664)***.

EARLIER REFERENCES:

Described, not named or illustrated:

1. ***[posterior lobe of pituitary gland (Haller, 1762)] (Willis, 1664)***
Two distinct lobes described for *pituitary gland (Galen, c192)*, one of which, ***posterior lobe of pituitary gland (Haller, 1762)***, is whitish, centrally located, and attached to *infundibulum (Galen, c173)*; see Pordage translation (1681, p. 104), and Willis (1672, Tab. VI-*F*). Riolan (1618, p. 421) mentioned without elaboration two glands (*duabus glandulis*) in macrodissected adult human sella turcica of sphenoid bone; also see Burdach (1822, p. 330).

Earlier synonyms:

1. *appendix (Morgagni, 1719)*
Synonym for macrodissected adult human ***posterior lobe of pituitary gland (Haller, 1762)***; p. 32, also see Burdach (1822, p. 330).
2. *appendix glandulae pituitariae (Santorini, 1724)*
Synonym for macrodissected adult human ***posterior lobe of pituitary gland (Haller, 1762)***; p. 70.

LATER SYNONYMS:

1. *posterior lobule of pituitary gland (Arnold, 1834)*
Synonym for macrodissected adult human ***posterior lobe of pituitary gland (Haller, 1762)***; in the original Latin, *glandula pituitaria lobulus anterior*, Table III-*n*.
2. *hypophysis cerebri lobulus posterior (Arnold, 1834)*
Synonym for macrodissected adult human ***posterior lobe of pituitary gland (Haller, 1762)***; Table III-*n*.
3. *infundibular process (Tilney, 1936)*
Essentially ***posterior lobe of pituitary (Haller, 1762)***; intrasellar part of ***neurohypophysis (>1840)***, distal to ***infundibulum (Rioch et al., 1940)***; p. 424.
4. *neural lobe of pituitary gland (Rioch et al., 1940)*
Synonym for mammalian ***posterior lobe of pituitary gland (Haller, 1762)***; p. 24, also see Daniel & Pritchard (1975, p. 3).
5. *distal part of neurohypophysis (Daniel & Pritchard, 1975)*
Synonym for ***posterior lobe of pituitary gland (Haller, 1762)***; see Daniel & Pritchard (1975, p. 4).
6. *pars distalis (Daniel & Pritchard, 1975)*
Latin form of *distal part of neurohypophysis (Daniel & Pritchard, 1975)*.

posterior nerve of lesser curvature (>1840)

As described for macrodissected adult human, it frequently presents as the largest of the ***gastric branches of posterior vagal trunk (>1840)***, coursing along the dorsal (posterior) margin of the lesser curvature of the stomach between layers of the lesser omentum; see Mitchell (1953, p. 187), *Terminologia Anatomica* (1998, p. 137). It was clearly illustrated by Eustachi; see ***[posterior nerve of lesser curvature (>1840)] (Eustachi, 1552)***.

EARLIER REFERENCES:

Illustrated, not named or described:

1. ***[posterior nerve of lesser curvature (>1840)] (Eustachi, 1552)***
Clearly illustrated for macrodissected adult human; see Albinus edition (1761, Tab. 18, Fig. 2-Ξ).

Earlier synonyms:

1. *right gastro-epiploic nerve (Albinus, 1744)*
Synonym for macrodissected adult human **posterior nerve of lesser curvature (>1840)**; in the original Latin, *nervus gastro-epiploïcus dexter*; Table 18, Figure 2-Ξ.
2. *greater posterior gastric nerve (>1840)*
Synonym for macrodissected adult human **posterior nerve of lesser curvature (>1840)**; see Mitchell (1953, p. 187).
3. *principal nerve of posterior curvature (>1840)*
Synonym for macrodissected adult human **posterior nerve of lesser curvature (>1840)**; see Mitchell (1953, p. 187). It should probably be *principal posterior nerve of lesser curvature*; see *principal anterior nerve of lesser curve (>1840)*.

posterior orbital gyrus (>1840)

As described for macrodissected adult human, the caudal topographic subdivision of the **orbital gyri (>1940)**, separated from the others by the **orbital sulci (>1840)**; see Williams & Warwick (1980, Fig. 7.116). It was first clearly delineated by Soemmerring; see ***[posterior orbital gyrus (>1840)] (Soemmerring, 1778)***.

EARLIER REFERENCES:

Illustrated, not named or described:

1. ***[posterior orbital gyrus (>1840)] (Soemmerring, 1778)***
Clearly illustrated for macrodissected adult human; Table II.

posterior palatine nerve (Günther, 1786)

As described for macrodissected adult human, usually the larger of the **lesser palatine nerves (Meckel, 1817)** supplying branches to the soft palate; see Durward (1951, p. 1023). For Günther's use in macrodissected adult human, see p. 47. It was probably first clearly delineated as the *lesser posterior palatine nerve (Meckel, 1748)*.

TRANSLATIONS:

1. *nervus palatinus posteriorem (Günther, 1786)*
Original Latin form of ***posterior palatine nerve (Günther, 1786)***; p. 47.

EARLIER REFERENCES:

Earlier synonyms:

1. *lesser posterior palatine nerve (Meckel, 1748)*
Synonym for macrodissected adult human ***posterior palatine nerve (Günther, 1786)***; in the original Latin, *minor posterior nervi palatini*, p. 63; or *palatinus nervus posterior minor*, p. 129-*u*. Scarpa (1785, Tab. II, Fig. II:26–31) described its branches in detail for macrodissected adult human.
2. *posterior branch of palatine nerve (Bang, 1770)*
Synonym for macrodissected adult human ***posterior palatine nerve (Günther, 1786)***; in the original Latin, *nervus palatinus ramus posterior*; Figure II-*f*.

LATER SYNONYMS:

1. *middle palatine nerve (Cloquet, 1816)*
Synonym for macrodissected adult human ***posterior palatine nerve (Günther, 1786)***; in the original French, *nerf palatin moyen*, p. 685.
2. *lesser palatine nerve (Bock, 1817)*
Synonym for macrodissected adult human ***posterior palatine nerve (Günther, 1786)***; in the original Latin, *nervus palatinus minor*, p. 30.
3. *internal palatine nerve (Bock, 1817)*
Synonym for macrodissected adult human ***posterior palatine nerve (Günther, 1786)***; in the original Latin, *nervus palatinus internus*, p. 30.
4. *posterior palatine fascicle of sphenopalatine ganglion (Bellingeri, 1818)*
Synonym for macrodissected adult human ***posterior palatine nerve (Günther, 1786)***; in the original Latin, *fasciculus palatinus posterior*, see Table I.
5. *little palatine nerve (Todd, 1836–1839)*
Synonym for macrodissected adult human ***posterior palatine nerve (Günther, 1786)***; p. 287.

PARTLY CORRESPONDS:

1. *tonsillar thread of posterior palatine fascicle (Bellingeri, 1818)*
Macrodissected adult human branch of ***posterior palatine nerve (Günther, 1786)*** to glandular part of palatine tonsil; in the original Latin, *stamen tonsillaris*, see Table I.
2. *palatine muscle threads of posterior palatine fascicle (Bellingeri, 1818)*
Macrodissected adult human branches of ***posterior palatine nerve (Günther, 1786)*** to several palatine muscles; in the original Latin, *stamina muscularis*, see Table I.
3. *middle palatine threads of posterior palatine fascicle (Bellingeri, 1818)*
Macrodissected adult human branches of ***posterior palatine nerve (Günther, 1786)*** to palatine musculature; in the original Latin, *stamina palatinus medius*, see Table I.
4. *palato-pharyngeal thread of posterior palatine fascicle (Bellingeri, 1818)*
Macrodissected adult human branch of ***posterior palatine nerve (Günther, 1786)*** to transitional region between palate and pharynx; in the original Latin, *stamen palato-pharyngei*, see Table I.

posterior paracentral gyrus (>1840)

As described for macrodissected adult human, a rostral topographic subdivision of the **parietal region (>1840)** on the medial surface of the *cerebral hemisphere (Tiedemann, 1816)*, medial to the **postcentral gyrus (>1840)**, caudal to the **central sulcus (Huschke, 1854)**, and rostral to the **marginal sulcus (>1840)**. It forms the caudal half of the *paracentral lobule (>1840)*; see Williams & Warwick (1980, Fig. 7.114A), *Terminologia Anatomica* (1998, p. 126), *Dorland's* (2003, p. 806). It was first clearly delineated by Soemmerring; see ***[posterior paracentral gyrus (>1840)] (Soemmerring, 1778)***.

EARLIER REFERENCES:

Illustrated, not named or described:

1. ***[posterior paracentral gyrus (>1840)] (Soemmerring, 1778)***
   Clearly illustrated for macrodissected adult human; Table III.

posterior parolfactory sulcus (>1840)

As described for macrodissected adult human, a roughly dorsoventrally oriented (vertical) groove between the ***parolfactory gyrus (>1840)*** rostrally and the ***tenia tecta (Swanson, 1992)*** part of the *subcallosal gyrus (>1840)* caudally; see Nauta & Haymaker (1969, Fig. 4.11), *Terminologia Anatomica* (1998, p. 126). It was first clearly distinguished by Soemmerring; see ***[posterior parolfactory sulcus (>1840)] (Soemmerring, 1778)***.

EARLIER REFERENCES:

Illustrated, not named or described:

1. ***[posterior parolfactory sulcus (>1840)] (Soemmerring, 1778)***
   Clearly illustrated for macrodissected adult human; Table III.

posterior pulmonary plexus (Haller, 1762)

As described for macrodissected adult human, a relatively large region of the ***pulmonary plexus (Winslow, 1733)*** arising from branches of the ***superior cervical cardiac branches of vagus nerve (>1840)*** and ***thoracic cardiac branches of vagus nerve (>1840)***, from the ***cardiac plexus (Keill, 1698)***, and from the second to fifth or sixth ***thoracic sympathetic ganglia (>1840)***, and lying on the dorsal (posterior) aspect of bronchial and vascular structures in the hila of the lungs; see Mitchell (1953, Fig. 105), Williams & Warwick (1980, p. 1133). For Haller's use in macrodissected adult human, see p. 235. The first clear delineation of it was probably by Vieussens; see ***[posterior pulmonary plexus (Haller, 1762)] (Vieussens, 1684)***. It was brilliantly illustrated by Scarpa (1794, Tab. V).

ALTERNATE SPELLINGS:

1. *posterior pulmonic plexus (Bell & Bell, 1816)*
   Alternate form of macrodissected adult human ***posterior pulmonary plexus (Haller, 1762)***; p. 507.

TRANSLATIONS:

1. *posterioris plexus pulmonis (Haller, 1762)*
   Original Latin form of ***posterior pulmonary plexus (Haller, 1762)***; p. 235.
2. *plexum pulmonalem posteriorem (Haase, 1781)*
   Early Latin form of ***posterior pulmonary plexus (Haller, 1762)***; p. 88.

EARLIER REFERENCES:

Illustrated and described, not named:

1. ***[posterior pulmonary plexus (Haller, 1762)] (Vieussens, 1684)***
   Origins described and illustrated for macrodissected adult human; Table 23-44.

PARTLY CORRESPONDS:

1. *superficial pulmonary plexus (Scarpa, 1794)*
   All or part of macrodissected adult human ***posterior pulmonary plexus (Haller, 1762)***; in the original Latin, *plexum pulmonalem superficialem*, Table III:43–47.

posterior renal ganglion (>1840)

As described for macrodissected adult human, the largest and most consistent of the ***renal ganglia (Walther, 1735)***; see Mitchell (1953, p. 288). It was probably discovered by Willis; see ***[posterior renal ganglion (>1840)] (Willis, 1664)***.

EARLIER REFERENCES:

Illustrated and described, not named:

1. ***[posterior renal ganglion (>1840)] (Willis, 1664)***
   Willis probably deserves credit for first identifying it, whereas Haller (1762) clearly described it; see Mitchell (1953, p. 288).

Earlier synonyms:

1. *Hirschfeld's ganglion (>1840)*
   Eponym for macrodissected adult human ***posterior renal ganglion (>1840)***; see Mitchell (1953, p. 288), referring to Hirschfeld & Léveillé (1853).

posterior scrotal nerves (Mayer, 1794)

As described for macrodissected adult human male, they are usually two branches (medial and lateral) of the ***perineal nerve (Camper, 1762)*** innervating skin of the scrotum and communicating with the ***inferior rectal nerves (>1840)*** and ***perineal branches of posterior cutaneous nerve of thigh (>1840)***; see Williams & Warwick (1980, p. 1116), *Terminologia Anatomica* (1998, p. 140). For Mayer's use in macrodissected adult human, see Part 5, Table VI-3 (p. 36). They were known to Galen; see ***[posterior scrotal nerves (Mayer, 1794)] (Galen, c192)***.

TRANSLATIONS:

1. *nervi scrotales posteriores (Mayer, 1794)*
   Original Latin form of ***posterior scrotal nerves (Mayer, 1794)***; Part 5, Table VI-3 (p. 36).

EARLIER REFERENCES:

Described, not named or illustrated:

1. ***[posterior scrotal nerves (Mayer, 1794)] (Galen, c192)***
   Galen mentioned ***nerve (Herophilus, c335–c280 BC)*** to skin of genital organs in macrodissected adult beef, pig, and/or macaque but not human; see Duckworth translation (1962, p. 263). Vieussens described and illustrated them for macrodissected adult human male (1684, Tab. 29-15).

Earlier synonyms:

1. *pudendal scrotal nerve (Günther, 1786)*
   Probably synonym for macrodissected adult human ***posterior scrotal nerves (Mayer, 1794)***; in the original Latin, *nervus scrotalis pudendalis*, p. 84.

posterior superior dental nerve (Haller, 1762)

As described for macrodissected adult human, branch of the ***maxillary nerve (Meckel, 1753)*** supplying the maxillary sinus and then dividing into smaller branches linking up to form the molar part of the ***superior dental plexus (>1840)***, as well as supplying a branch to the upper gum and adjoining part of the cheek; see Williams & Warwick (1980, p. 1063 and Fig. 7.177). For Haller's use in macrodissected adult human, see p. 214. It was first identified by Vesalius; see ***[posterior superior dental nerve (Haller, 1762)] (Vesalius, 1543a)***.

TRANSLATIONS:

1. *nervus dentalis posterior superior (Haller, 1762)*
   Original Latin form of ***posterior superior dental nerve (Haller, 1762)***; p. 214.
2. *upper and posterior dentar nerve (Meckel, 1832)*
   Alternate English form of ***posterior superior dental nerve (Haller, 1762)***; Vol. 3, p. 69.

EARLIER REFERENCES:

Described, not named or illustrated:

1. ***[posterior superior dental nerve (Haller, 1762)] (Vesalius, 1543a)***
   Described for macrodissected adult human but erroneously ascribed to ***mandibular nerve (>1840)***; see Richardson & Carman translation (2002, p. 189).

Earlier synonyms:

1. *ramulus secundus rami minoris inferioris (Vieussens, 1684)*
   Probably roughly synonymous with macrodissected adult human ***posterior superior dental nerve (Haller, 1762)***; p. 172 and Table 22-*T*.
2. *posterior alveolar branch of superior maxillary branch (Meckel, 1748)*
   Synonym for macrodissected adult human ***posterior superior dental nerve (Haller, 1762)***, which Meckel described as dividing into anterior and posterior branches; in the original Latin, *ramum alveolarem posteriorem*, p. 65.
3. *posterior dental branch of superior maxillary branch (Meckel, 1748)*
   Synonym for macrodissected adult human *posterior dental branch of superior maxillary branch (Meckel, 1748)*; in the original Latin, *ramum dentalem posteriorem*, p. 65.
4. *posterior alveolar nerve (Schaarschmidt, 1750)*
   Synonym for macrodissected adult human ***posterior superior dental nerve (Haller, 1762)***; in the original Latin, *nervus alveolaris posterior*, p. 23.
5. *posterior dental nerve (Meckel, 1751)*
   Synonym for macrodissected adult human ***posterior superior dental nerve (Haller, 1762)***; in the original French, *le nerf dental postérior*, p. 85.

LATER SYNONYMS:

1. *alveolar branch of second branch of fifth pair (Haase, 1781)*
   Synonym for macrodissected adult human *posterior alveolar branch of superior maxillary branch (Meckel, 1748)*; in the original Latin, *ramus rami secundi paris quinti alveolaris*, p. 66.
2. *superior maxillary posterior alveolar nerve (Mayer, 1794)*
   Synonym for macrodissected adult human ***posterior superior dental nerve (Haller, 1762)***; in the original Latin, *nervus alveolaris posterior maxillae superioris*; Part 5, Table VIII-χ (p. 59).
3. *alveolar branch of superior maxillary nerve (Cuvier, 1800)*
   Synonym for macrodissected adult human ***posterior superior dental nerve (Haller, 1762)***; in the original French, *rameau alvéolaire du nerf maxillaire supérieur*, Vol. 2, p. 208.
4. *posterior superior alveolar nerve (Meckel, 1817)*
   Synonym for macrodissected adult human ***posterior superior dental nerve (Haller, 1762)***; see translation (1832, Vol. 3, p. 69).
5. *first dental nerve of second trunk of fifth nerve (Swan, 1830)*
   Synonym for macrodissected adult human ***posterior superior dental nerve (Haller, 1762)***; Plate XII, Figure 5-2.
6. *posterior dentar nerves (Meckel, 1832)*
   Synonym for *upper and posterior dentar nerve (Meckel, 1832)*, probably plural because of branches Meckel described for it; Vol. 3, p. 69.
7. *posterior alveolo-dental nerves (Cruveilhier, 1836)*
   Synonym for macrodissected adult human ***posterior superior dental nerve (Haller, 1762)***; in the original French, *nerfs alvéolo-dentaires postérieurs*, p. 926. Cruveilhier described 2–3, sometimes arising from common trunk.
8. *posterior dental branches of superior maxillary nerve (Quain & Wilson, 1839)*
   Synonym for macrodissected adult human ***posterior superior dental nerve (Haller, 1762)***; Plate XIII, Figure 2-*t*.

PARTLY CORRESPONDS:

1. *internal dental fascicle of posterior dental surculus of superior maxillary branch (Bellingeri, 1818)*
   Major branch of macrodissected adult human ***posterior superior dental nerve (Haller, 1762)*** to ***superior dental plexus (>1840)***; in the original Latin, *fasciculus dentalis internus*, see Table I.
2. *dento-muscular fascicle of posterior dental surculus of superior maxillary branch (Bellingeri, 1818)*
   Minor branch of macrodissected adult human ***posterior superior dental nerve (Haller, 1762)*** supplying lateral pterygoid and buccinator muscles; in the original Latin, *fasciculus dentato-muscularis*, see Table I.
3. *buccal branches of posterior alveolar nerve (Arnold, 1834)*
   Branches of macrodissected adult human ***posterior superior dental nerve (Haller, 1762)*** to cheek; in the original Latin, *nervus alveolaris posterior, rami buccales*, p. 9.
4. *buccal branches of posterior dental nerve (Arnold, 1834)*
   Branches of macrodissected adult human ***posterior superior dental nerve (Haller, 1762)*** to cheek; in the original Latin, *nervus dentalis posterior, rami buccales*, p. 9.
5. *dental branches of posterior alveolar nerve (Arnold, 1834)*
   Branches of macrodissected adult human ***posterior superior dental nerve (Haller, 1762)*** to teeth; in the original Latin, *nervus alveolaris posterior, rami dentales*, p. 9.
6. *dental branches of posterior dental nerve (Arnold, 1834)*
   Branches of macrodissected adult human ***posterior superior dental nerve (Haller, 1762)*** to teeth; in the original Latin, *nervus dentalis posterior, rami dentales*, p. 9.

7. *posterior and superior dental nerve (Cruveilhier, 1836)*
   Smaller of two major branches of *posterior alveo-dental nerves (Cruveilhier, 1836)*; in the original French, *nerf dentaire postérieur et supérieur*, p. 926.
8. *posterior and inferior dental nerve (Cruveilhier, 1836)*
   Larger of two major branches of *posterior alveo-dental nerves (Cruveilhier, 1836)*; in the original French, *nerf dentaire postérieur et inférieur*, p. 926.

posterior superior fissure (>1840)

As described for macrodissected adult human, the groove between ***simple lobule (Jansen & Brodal, 1954)*** and ***ansiform lobule crus 1 (Bolk, 1906)*** of the ***cerebellar cortex (Willis, 1664)***, continuing across the median plane between ***declive (>1840)*** and ***folium vermis (>1840)*** of the ***cerebellar vermis (Meckel, 1817)***; see Flatau & Jacobsohn (1899), Angevine et al. (1961, Figs. 6, 14, 17, 18, 24), *Terminologia Anatomica* (1998, p. 119). It was perhaps first clearly delineated as the *superior cerebellar fissure (Vicq d'Azyr, 1784)* and *inferior cerebellar fissure (Vicq d'Azyr, 1784)* considered together.

EARLIER REFERENCES:

Earlier synonyms:

1. *postclival fissure (>1840)*
   Synonym for macrodissected adult human ***posterior superior fissure (>1840)***; see Crosby et al. (1962, p. 189, Tab. I), *Terminologia Anatomica* (1998, p. 119).

PARTLY CORRESPONDS:

1. *superior cerebellar fissure (Vicq d'Azyr, 1784)*
   Dorsal (superior) part of macrodissected adult human ***posterior superior fissure (>1840)***; in the original French, *sillon supérieur du cervelet*, p. 568. Also see Vicq d'Azyr (1786, p. 89; Pl. XXVIII, Figs. I:*7–12*, II:*26,27*), Larsell & Jansen (1972, p. 44). Burdach (1822, p. 294) gave the Latin form, *sulcus superior cerebelli*.
2. *inferior cerebellar fissure (Vicq d'Azyr, 1784)*
   Ventral (inferior) extension of macrodissected adult human *superior cerebellar fissure (Vicq d'Azyr, 1786)*; in the original French, *sillon inférieur du cervelet*, p. 568 and Vicq d'Azyr (1786, Pl. XVIII, Fig. III:*9-14*). Together they form the ***posterior superior fissure (>1840)***. Dejerine & Dejerine-Klumpke (1901, p. 465, Fig. 344) confused matters by indicating that *inferior cerebellar fissure of Vicq d'Azyr* corresponded with *semilunar fissure (Dejerine & Dejerine-Klumpke, 1901)* or ***ansoparamedian fissure (>1840)***.

posterior superior nasal nerves (Soemmerring, 1791)

As described for macrodissected adult human, they extend ventrally (descend) from the ***pterygopalatine ganglion (>1840)*** and divide into two sets, ***lateral posterior superior nasal nerves (>1840)*** and ***medial posterior superior nasal nerves (>1840)***. Histologically they are formed mostly by sensory ***dendrites (His, 1889)*** simply passing through the ***pterygopalatine ganglion (>1840)*** from the ***posterior superior nasal nerves (Soemmerring, 1791)*** before continuing in the ***pterygopalatine nerves (Wrisberg, 1786)*** to the ***maxillary nerve (Meckel, 1753)*** and then ***trigeminal ganglion (>1840)***; see Williams & Warwick (1980, p. 1065 and Fig. 7.181). For Soemmerring's use in macrodissected adult human, see p. 202. They were discovered by Galen; see ***[posterior superior nasal nerves (Soemmerring, 1791)] (Galen, c192)***.

TRANSLATIONS:

1. *nervos nasales superiores posteriores (Soemmerring, 1791)*
   Original Latin form of ***posterior superior nasal nerves (Soemmerring, 1791)***; p. 202.
2. *upper posterior nasal nerves (Meckel, 1832)*
   English form of ***posterior superior nasal nerves (Soemmerring, 1791)***; Vol. 3, p. 67.

EARLIER REFERENCES:

Described, not named or illustrated:

1. ***[posterior superior nasal nerves (Soemmerring, 1791)] (Galen, c192)***
   Alluded to in macrodissected adult beef, pigs, and/or macaque but not human; see Duckworth translation (1962, p. 194). Winslow (1733, Sect. VI, p. 65) mentioned them for macrodissected adult human.

Earlier synonyms:

1. *nasal nerves (Meckel, 1748)*
   Probably synonym for macrodissected adult human ***posterior superior nasal nerves (Soemmerring, 1791)***; in the original Latin, *nervorum nasalium* (singular), pp. 108–109. In the original French, *les nerfs nasaux*; Meckel (1751, p. 85). Also see Quain & Wilson (1839, Pl. XXVII-G,*n*).
2. *posterior superior nasal branches (Loder, 1778)*
   Synonym for macrodissected adult human ***posterior superior nasal nerves (Soemmerring, 1791)***; p. 14.
3. *nasal branch of second branch of fifth pair (Monro, 1783)*
   Presumably synonym for ***posterior superior nasal nerves (Soemmerring, 1791)***, described for macrodissected ox, sheep, and human; p. 63.
4. *anterior superior branches of nasal branches from fifth pair (Scarpa, 1785)*
   Synonym for macrodissected adult human ***posterior superior nasal nerves (Soemmerring, 1791)***; in the original Latin, *rami nasales superiores anteriores e pari quinto*, Table II, Figure II:*2-4*.

LATER SYNONYMS:

1. *sphenopalatine nerves (Cloquet, 1816)*
   Essentially macrodissected adult human ***posterior superior nasal nerves (Soemmerring, 1791)*** including ***nasopalatine nerve (Scarpa, 1785)***; in the original French, *nerfs sphéno-palatins*, p. 683.
2. *anterior superior nasal fascicles of sphenopalatine ganglion (Bellingeri, 1818)*
   Synonym for macrodissected adult human ***posterior superior nasal nerves (Soemmerring, 1791)***; in the original Latin, *ganglion sphoeno-palatinum fasciculi nasales sup. ant.*, see Table I.

3. *posterior nasal nerves (Cruveilhier, 1836)*
   Synonym for macrodissected adult human ***posterior superior nasal nerves (Soemmerring, 1791)***; in the original French, *nerfs nasaux postérieurs*, p. 922.
4. *nasal branches of Meckel's ganglion (Quain & Wilson, 1839)*
   Synonym for macrodissected adult human ***posterior superior nasal nerves (Soemmerring, 1791)***; Plate II, Figure 1-*E*.
5. *anterior branches of spheno-palatine ganglion (Quain & Wilson, 1839)*
   Synonym for macrodissected adult human ***posterior superior nasal nerves (Soemmerring, 1791)***; Plate XXVII-*G,n*.

PARTLY CORRESPONDS:

1. *anterior and superior nasal nerves (Schaarschmidt, 1750)*
   Component of ***posterior superior nasal nerves (Soemmerring, 1791)*** supplying rostral (anterior) part of nasal septum; in the original Latin, *nervi nasales superiores & anteriores*, p. 20. Todd (1736–1839, p. 287) used simply *anterior superior nasal nerves*.
2. *posterior and superior nasal nerves (Schaarschmidt, 1750)*
   Component of ***posterior superior nasal nerves (Soemmerring, 1791)*** supplying caudal (posterior) part of nasal septum; in the original Latin, *nervi nasales superiores & posteriores*, p. 20.
3. *internal anterior superior nasal nerves (Günther, 1786)*
   Major component of macrodissected adult human ***posterior superior nasal nerves (Soemmerring, 1791)*** extending ventrally (descending) from ***pterygopalatine ganglion (>1840)***; in the original Latin, *nasales superiores anteriores interni*, p. 46.
4. *superior nasal nerves (Arnold, 1834)*
   Major component of macrodissected adult human ***posterior superior nasal nerves (Soemmerring, 1791)*** notably excluding ***nasopalatine nerve (Scarpa, 1785)***; in the original Latin, *nervi nasales superiores*, p. 9.

posterior thalamic nuclei (>1840)

As described for macrodissected adult human, and based on cellular architecture and connections in mammal, a relatively ill-defined caudal component of the ***dorsal part of thalamus (Herrick, 1910)*** lying basically between ***lateral thalamic nuclei (>1840)*** and ***ventral thalamic nuclei (>1840)***, just rostral to the ***medial geniculate complex (>1840)***. Its main ***gray matter regions (Swanson & Bota, 2010)*** are the ***posterior thalamic nucleus (>1840)***, ***suprageniculate nucleus (>1840)***, and ***limiting nucleus (>1840)***; see Jones (1985, Ch. 11), Nieuwenhuys et al. (2008, p. 266). It is sometimes lumped with the ***lateral thalamic nuclei (>1840)***; see Swanson (2004, Table B, p. 171). Not clearly described before 1840.

posterior vagal trunk (Wrisberg, 1780)

As described for macrodissected adult human, it has contributions from the right and left ***vagus nerve trunk (Wrisberg, 1786; Günther, 1876)***, though predominantly from the right, and extends caudally from the distal part of the ***posterior esophageal plexus (Haller, 1762)***; see Williams & Warwick (1980, p. 1079). For Wrisberg's formulation of the term for macrodissected adult human, see reprint in Wrisberg (1800, p. 258). It was perhaps first known as the *right stomach nerve (Crooke, 1615)*, from Crooke's rough translation of Bauhin (1605).

EARLIER REFERENCES:

Earlier synonyms:

1. *right stomach nerve (Crooke, 1615)*
   Roughly synonymous with macrodissected adult human ***posterior vagal trunk (Wrisberg, 1780)***; originally spelled *right stomacke (or stomack) nerve*, and in Latin *nervus stomachichus dexter*, p. 365. Crooke's text was basically a translation of Bauhin (1605).
2. *inferior stomachical branch of wandring pair (Willis, 1664)*
   Probably corresponds to macrodissected adult human, and other common large mammal, ***posterior vagal trunk (Wrisberg, 1780)*** because of accompanying large ***celiac branch of posterior vagal trunk (>1840)***, although it is illustrated very inaccurately; see Pordage translation (1681, p. 156 and Fig. 11-*A*,*η*).
3. *lower stomachical branch of wandring pair (Willis, 1664)*
   Synonymous with *inferior stomachical branch of wandring pair (Willis, 1664)*; see Pordage translation (1681, p. 156 and Fig. 11-*A*,η).
4. *internal trunk of vagus nerve (Drake, 1707)*
   Probably corresponds to *inferior stomachical branch of wandring pair (Willis, 1664)*, or alternately *superior stomachical branch of wandring pair (Willis, 1664)*; p. 517.
5. *posterior rope of eighth pair (Winslow, 1733)*
   Synonym for ***posterior vagal trunk (Wrisberg, 1780)*** from Winslow's very clear description of macrodissected adult human; Section VI, p. 73.
6. *posterior stomachic nerve (Winslow, 1733)*
   Synonym for macrodissected adult human ***posterior vagal trunk (Wrisberg, 1780)***; Section VI, p. 73.

LATER SYNONYMS:

1. *posterior trunk of eighth pair of nerves (Wrisberg, 1780)*
   Synonym for ***posterior vagal trunk (Wrisberg, 1780)***; see Wrisberg reprint (1800, p. 258).
2. *right vagus nerve (Haase, 1781)*
   Synonym for macrodissected adult human ***posterior vagal trunk (Wrisberg, 1780)***; in the original Latin (plural), *nervi vagi dextri*, p. 89.
3. *posterior trunk of gastric and hepatic plexus (Walter, 1783)*
   Synonym for macrodissected adult human ***posterior vagal trunk (Wrisberg, 1780)***; in the original Latin, *truncus posterior plexus ventriculi et hepatis*, Table III-486.
4. *esophageal cord of right side (Cloquet, 1816)*
   Synonym for macrodissected adult human ***posterior vagal trunk (Wrisberg, 1780)***; in the original French, *cordon oesophagien du côté droit*, p. 625.
5. *right cord of pneumogastric nerve (Meckel, 1817)*
   Synonym for macrodissected adult human ***posterior vagal trunk (Wrisberg, 1780)***; see translation (1832, Vol. 3, p. 50).

posterolateral fissure (Larsell, 1937)

As described for macrodissected adult human, the groove between ***paraflocculus (Stroud, 1895)*** and ***flocculus (Meckel, 1817)*** of the ***cerebellar cortex (Willis, 1664)*** continuing across the median plane between ***uvula (Malacarne, 1776)*** and ***nodule (Reil, 1807–1808a)*** of the ***cerebellar vermis (Meckel, 1817)***; see Angevine et al. (1961, pp. 17–18 and Figs. 20, 23, 24), *Terminologia Anatomica* (1998, p. 119). For Larsell's use in comparative vertebrate anatomy see p. 583. It was first delineated by Vesalius; see ***[posterolateral fissure (Larsell, 1937)] (Vesalius, 1543a)***.

EARLIER REFERENCES:

Described, not named or illustrated:

1. ***[posterolateral fissure (Larsell, 1937)] (Vesalius, 1543a)***
 Clearly illustrated for macrodissected adult human; see Singer translation (1952, p. 107, Fig. 11).

Earlier synonyms:

1. *fissure of cerebellar peduncles (Vicq d'Azyr, 1784)*
 Synonym for at least medial parts of macrodissected adult human ***posterolateral fissure (Larsell, 1937)***; in the original French, *sillon des jambes du cervelet*, p. 569 and Vicq d'Azyr (1786, Pls. XVII, Fig. I-75/76, XXII-44).

postsubiculum (Swanson & Cowan, 1977)

As described with cellular architecture and connections in mammal, it is distinguished topologically and developmentally as the dorsal (septal) part of the ***presubiculum (>1840)***; see Swanson et al. (1987). For Swanson & Cowan's use in rat see p. 71. It was not identified by 1840. Earlier

1. *retrosubicular area (Brodmann, 1909)*Synonym for ***postsubiculum (Swanson & Cowan, 1977)***; see Table 7, p. 247.
2. *area 48 (Brodmann, 1909)*Synonym for ***postsubiculum (Swanson & Cowan, 1977)***; in the original German, *Feld 48*, see Table 7, p. 247.
3. *postsubicular area (Rose & Woolsey, 1948)*Synonym for ***postsubiculum (Swanson & Cowan, 1977)***; see pp. 292, 296 and Figures 1, 5, 54, 58.

preaortic plexus (Arnulf, 1939)

As described for macrodissected adult human, the only real topographically distinct region of the ***cardiac plexus (Keill, 1698)***, lying predominantly on the ventral (anterior) side of the aortic arch and ascending aorta and apparently formed by essentially all components contributing to the ***cardiac plexus (Keill, 1698)*** as a whole; see Mitchell (1953, pp. 249, 251). For Arnulf's use in macrodissected adult human and cat see Figures 1, 2. It was perhaps first distinguished as the *anterior aortic plexus (Andersch & Soemmerring, 1792)*.

TRANSLATIONS:

1. *plexus préaortique (Arnulf, 1939)*
 Original French form of ***preaortic plexus (Arnulf, 1939)***; see Figures 1, 2.

EARLIER REFERENCES:

Earlier synonyms:

1. *anterior aortic plexus (Andersch & Soemmerring, 1792)*
 Terminal part of *superficial aortic nerve (Andersch & Soemmerring, 1792)* and probably roughly synonymous with macrodissected adult human ***preaortic plexus (Arnulf, 1939)***; in the original Latin, *plexus aortici anterioris*, p. 192.

PARTLY CORRESPONDS:

1. *posterior aortic plexus (Andersch & Soemmerring, 1792)*
 Terminal part of *deep aortic nerve (Andersch & Soemmerring, 1792)* related to *anterior aortic plexus (Andersch & Soemmerring, 1792)* and may thus be part or extension of ***preaortic plexus (Arnulf, 1939)***; in the original Latin, *plexum aorticum posteriorem*, p. 198.
2. *reverse nerve of aorta (Andersch, 1797)*
 Probably component of macrodissected adult ***preaortic plexus (Arnulf, 1939)***; in the original Latin, *nervum aorticum reversiuum*, p. 46.

precentral fissure (>1840)

As described for macrodissected adult human, the groove between ***lingula (Malacarne, 1776)*** and ***central lobule (Burdach, 1822)*** of the ***cerebellar cortex (Willis, 1664)***; see Angevine et al. (1961, p. 18 and Figs. 7, 11, 14, 19, 20, 24), *Terminologia Anatomica* (1998, p. 119). It was probably not clearly recognized by 1840.

precentral gyrus (>1840)

As described for macrodissected adult human, the caudal topographic subdivision of the ***frontal region (Vicq d'Azyr, 1786)*** lying between ***central sulcus (Huschke, 1854)*** caudally and ***precentral sulcus (>1840)*** rostrally; see Williams & Warwick (1980, Fig. 7.111A). Also see ***anterior paracentral gyrus (>1840)***. It was perhaps first clearly delineated by Vicq d'Azyr; see ***[precentral gyrus (>1840] (Vicq d'Azyr, 1786)***.

EARLIER REFERENCES:

Illustrated, not named or described:

1. ***[precentral gyrus (>1840] (Vicq d'Azyr, 1786)***
 Clearly illustrated for macrodissected adult human; Plate III, see Meyer (1971, p. 124), Clarke & Dewhurst (1996, p. 90).

precentral sulcus (>1840)

As described for macrodissected adult human, an irregular groove forming the rostral border of the ***precentral gyrus (>1840)***; see Williams & Warwick (1980, Fig. 7.111A). It was perhaps first clearly delineated by Vicq d'Azyr; see ***[precentral sulcus (>1840)] (Vicq d'Azyr, 1786)***.

EARLIER REFERENCES:

Illustrated, not named or described:

1. ***[precentral sulcus (>1840)] (Vicq d'Azyr, 1786)***
 Clearly illustrated for macrodissected adult human; Plate III, see Meyer (1971, p. 124), Clarke & Dewhurst (1996, p. 90).

precommissural fornix (Loo, 1931)

As described in adult mammal with normal and experimental histological methods for ***axons (Kölliker, 1896)***, one of two major subdivisions of the ***fornix (Vesalius, 1543a)*** lying rostral to the level of the ***subfornical organ (>1840)*** and ***interventricular foramen (>1840)***, the other subdivision being the ***postcommissural fornix (Loo, 1931)***. The ***precommissural fornix (Loo, 1931)*** lies mainly within the ***lateral septal complex (Risold & Swanson, 1997)***, with small branches extending to the ***orbital region (Rolando, 1831)***, ***frontal region (Vicq d'Azyr, 1786)***, and ***olfactory region (>1840)***, and it merges ventromedially with the ***diagonal band (Broca, 1879)***, which is continuous caudally with the ***medial forebrain bundle (Edinger, 1893)***. For Loo's original use in adult opossum, see p. 81. It was perhaps first delineated, at least partly, by Bichat; see ***[precommissural fornix (Loo, 1931)] (Bichat et al., 1801–1803)***.

EARLIER REFERENCES:

Described, not named or illustrated:

1. ***[precommissural fornix (Loo, 1931)] (Bichat et al., 1801–1803)***
   Bichat described at least part of it for macrodissected adult human; Vol. 3, p. 81. Earlier observations related to it were summarized by Burdach (1822, p. 354). Beautifully illustrated by Luys (1865, Pl. XXI-*12,13*).

PARTLY CORRESPONDS:

1. *fornix obliquus (Honegger, 1890)*
   Dubious component of ***precommissural fornix (Loo, 1931)***. "The term 'fornix obliquus,' which Honegger [p. 332] and Koelliker [p. 778, Fig. 800-*F.obl*] applied to certain fibres of the pre-commissural bundle springing from the hippocampal flexure, is of doubtful significance and no obvious value, and might well be discarded." (Smith, 1898, p. 243).

preculminate fissure (Smith, 1903)

As described for macrodissected adult human, the groove between ***central lobule (Burdach, 1822)*** and ***culmen (Stroud, 1895)*** of the ***cerebellar cortex (Willis, 1664)***; see Angevine et al. (1961, p. 18 and Figs. 8, 19, 20, 24), *Terminologia Anatomica* (1998, p. 119). For Smith's use in macrodissected embryonic and adult human, see p. 634. It was probably not clearly recognized by 1840.

precuneus (Burdach, 1822)

A described for macrodissected adult human, a medial and caudal topographic subdivision of the ***parietal region (>1840)*** lying between ***posterior paracentral gyrus (>1840)*** rostrally and ***parieto-occipital sulcus (>1840)*** caudally; see Williams & Warwick (1980, p. 989, Fig. 7.114A). For Burdach's use in macrodissected adult human, see Table VII-*y*; also see Dejerine & Dejerine-Klumpke (1895, p. 290) and Meyer (1971, p. 130). It was perhaps first clearly delineated by Soemmerring; see ***[precuneus (Burdach, 1822)] (Soemmerring, 1778)***.

TRANSLATIONS:

1. *Vorzwickel (Burdach, 1822)*
   Original German form of ***precuneus (Burdach, 1822)***; see Table VII-*y*.

EARLIER REFERENCES:

Illustrated, not named or described:

1. ***[precuneus (Burdach, 1822)] (Soemmerring, 1778)***
   Accurately illustrated for macrodissected adult human; Table III.

preoccipital notch (>1840)

As described for macrodissected adult human, an indentation between the caudal end of the ***inferior temporal gyrus (>1840)*** and the adjacent rostral ventrolateral edge of the ***occipital region (Vesalius, 1543a)***; see Nieuwenhuys et al. (2008, Figs. 3.2-*15*, 3.5-*10*), *Terminologia Anatomica* (1998, p. 125), *Dorland's* (2003, p. 920 under Latin form, *incisura preoccipitalis*). It was first clearly distinguished by Vicq d'Azyr; see ***[preoccipital notch (>1840)] (Vicq d'Azyr, 1786)***.

EARLIER REFERENCES:

Illustrated and described, not named:

1. ***[preoccipital notch (>1840)] (Vicq d'Azyr, 1786)***
   Described and illustrated for macrodissected adult human; Plate XVII-*6*.

preoptic recess (>1840)

As described for macrodissected adult human, a triangular rostroventral extension of the ***hypothalamic part of third ventricle (Swanson, 2004)*** into the region overlying the ***optic chiasm (Galen, c173)***; see Mettler (1948, Figs. 68, 100), Carpenter (1976, Fig. 2.15A), Nauta & Haymaker (1969, Fig. 4.1). It was clearly illustrated long ago; see ***[preoptic recess (>1840)] (Steno, 1669)***.

EARLIER REFERENCES:

Illustrated, not named or described:

1. ***[preoptic recess (>1840)] (Steno, 1669)***
   Illustrated clearly in first accurate midsagittal view of macrodissected adult human ***brain (Smith Papyrus, c1700 BC)***; Plates I & II.

Earlier synonyms:

1. *foveola ante nervorum opticorum confluxum (Soemmerring, 1778)*
   Synonym for macrodissected adult human ***preoptic recess (>1840)***. Soemmerring quoted Haller's (1762) very clear description, as well as references (uncited) to it by Tarin and Günz; Table III-*3,4*.
2. *sulcus ante nervorum opticorum confluxum (Günther, 1786)*
   Synonym for macrodissected adult human *foveola ante nervorum opticorum confluxum (Soemmerring, 1778)*; p. 16.

prepyramidal fissure (Hayashi, 1924)

As described for macrodissected adult human, the groove between ***gracile lobule (>1840)*** and ***biventral lobule (>1840)*** of the ***cerebellar cortex (Willis, 1664)*** that may or may not be continuous with a medial segment of the fissure between ***tuber vermis (>1840)*** and ***pyramis (Malacarne, 1776)*** of the ***cerebellar vermis (Meckel, 1817)***; see *Terminologia Anatomica* (1998, p. 119) and Angevine et al. (1961, p. 18 and Figs. 15, 24), who preferred to distinguish between a vermal *prepyramidal fissure* and a hemispheric *prebiventral fissure* because Larsell suggested that the two are not necessarily continuous during mammalian development. It was perhaps first clearly distinguished by Reil; see ***[prepyramidal fissure (Hayashi, 1924)] (Reil, 1809a).***

EARLIER REFERENCES:

Illustrated and described, not named:

1. ***[prepyramidal fissure (Hayashi, 1924)] (Reil, 1809a)*** Clearly described for macrodissected adult human, noting it is an inconsistent feature not found in every individual; see Mayo translation (1822, p. 103).

Earlier synonyms:

1. *external inferior sulcus (Meckel, 1817)* Synonym for macrodissected adult human ***prepyramidal fissure (Hayashi, 1924)***; see Burdach (1822, p. 295).

presubiculum (>1840)

As described with cellular architecture and connections in mammal, the topologically and developmentally middle division of the ***subicular complex (Swanson & Cowan, 1977)*** lying between ***subiculum (>1840)*** medially and ***parasubiculum (>1840)*** laterally; see Swanson et al. (1987), Nieuwenhuys et al. (2008, p. 372 and Fig. 12.5). Often the dorsal part is considered separately as ***postsubiculum (Swanson & Cowan, 1977)***; see Swanson et al. (1987). It was not identified by 1840.

TRANSLATIONS:

1. *area praesubicularis (Brodmann, 1909)* Synonym for ***presubiculum (>1840)***; see pp. 149, 209 and Table 7 on p. 247.
2. *presubicular area (Brodmann, 1909)* English form of *area praesubicularis (Brodmann, 1909).*
3. *area 27 (Brodmann, 1909)* Synonym for ***presubiculum (>1840)***; in the original German, *Feld 27*, see p. 149 and Table 7 on p. 247.

pretectal brachium of superior colliculus (>1840)

As described in macrodissected adult human, and mammal generally with histological methods for ***axons (Kölliker, 1896)***, the caudal segment of the ***brachium of superior colliculus (>1840)***, between ***thalamic brachium of superior colliculus (>1840)*** segment ventrally and rostrally, and ***superior colliculus (Haller, 1762)*** dorsally and caudally. It lies adjacent to the ***pretectal region (>1840)***; see Swanson (2004, Atlas Levels 34–39). It was known to Willis; see ***[pretectal brachium of superior colliculus (>1840)] (Willis, 1664).***

EARLIER REFERENCES:

Illustrated and described, not named:

1. ***[pretectal brachium of superior colliculus (>1840)] (Willis, 1664)*** Clearly described and illustrated for macrodissected adult human and sheep, although not explicitly distinguished from ***thalamic brachium of superior colliculus (>1840)***; see *appendix of nates (Willis, 1664).*

pretectal region (>1840)

As described for macrodissected adult human, and for adult mammal in general with cellular architecture and connections, a rostral dorsomedial part of the ***tegmentum (Swanson, 2000b)***, essentially rostral to the ***superior colliculus (Haller, 1762)***, dorsal to the ***midbrain reticular nucleus (>1840)***, and caudal to the ***thalamus (His, 1893a)***; see Nieuwenhuys (2008, Fig. 5.32-30) for human and Scalia (1972) for account of parts in mammal. It was not clearly identified as such by 1840.

PARTLY CORRESPONDS:

1. *trigonon durum (Bergmann, 1831)* Apparently caudal surface or part of macrodissected adult human ***pretectal region (>1840)***; p. 31 and Table IV-*l*. See Arnold (1838a, p. 60).
2. *trigonon molle (Bergmann, 1831)* Apparently rostral surface or part of macrodissected adult human ***pretectal region (>1840)***; p. 31 and Table IV-*m*. See Arnold (1838a, p. 60).
3. *trigonon pensile (Bergmann, 1831)* Synonym for *trigonon molle (Bergmann, 1831)*; p. 32 and Table IV-*m*.
4. *trigonon fluctuans (Bergmann, 1831)* Synonym for *trigonon molle (Bergmann, 1831)*; p. 32.

prevertebral ganglia (Quain, 1832)

Autonomic ganglia (Langley, 1900) associated with the ***prevertebral plexuses (Quain, 1837)***. They are now commonly described sequentially from rostral (superior) to caudal (inferior), with the ***celiac ganglion (Walter, 1783)*** being the largest. For Quain's use in macrodissected adult human, see p. 725, also see p. 722; he spelled it *praevertebral*. Galen provided the first indication of this feature; see ***[celiac ganglion (Walter, 1783)] (Galen, c173)***. Gaskell (1886, p. 3) popularized the term and also referred to a prevertebral *chain* of ganglia (p. 11), complementing the paravertebral *sympathetic chain (Gaskell, 1886)*. His description was based on dog macrodissections.

EARLIER REFERENCES:

Earlier synonyms:

1. *internal ganglions of ganglionnary nerve (Meckel, 1817)* Synonym for macrodissected adult human ***prevertebral ganglia (Quain, 1832)***; see translation (1832, Vol. 3, p. 84).
2. *central ganglions of ganglionnary nerve (Meckel, 1817)* Synonym for macrodissected adult human ***prevertebral ganglia (Quain, 1832)***; see translation (1832, Vol. 3, p. 84).
3. *splanchnic ganglia of sympathetic (Grant, 1834c)* Essentially synonym for ***prevertebral ganglia (Quain, 1832)*** in macrodissected adult vertebrate; p. 551, specifically for reptile. Cruveilhier (1836, p. 748) applied it specifically to macrodissected adult human; in the original French, *ganglions splanchniques*.

LATER SYNONYMS:

1. *collateral ganglia (Gaskell, 1886)* Synonym for ***prevertebral ganglia (Quain, 1832)***; p. 3.

prevertebral nerves (Swanson & Bota, 2010)

Autonomic nerves (Langley, 1898) macroscopically appearing to arise from ***prevertebral ganglia (Quain, 1837)*** and/or ***prevertebral plexuses (Quain, 1837)***, and typically ending in ***terminal plexuses (Swanson & Bota, 2010)*** and/or ***terminal ganglia (Gaskell, 1886)***. They are now commonly described sequentially from rostral (superior) to caudal (inferior). The first hint of them was probably the *branch of sixth pair stretching along roots of ribs offshoots to testes (Vesalius, 1543a)*.

PARTLY CORRESPONDS:

1. *branch of sixth pair stretching along roots of ribs offshoots to testes (Vesalius, 1543a)*
As described for macrodissected adult human, probably corresponds to some combination of ***superior testicular nerves (Walter, 1783)***, ***middle testicular nerves (>1840)***, and ***inferior testicular nerves (>1840)***; see Richardson & Carman translation (2002, p. 200).
2. *spermatic plexus (Günther, 1786)*
For macrodissected adult human, combination of ***superior testicular nerves (Walter, 1783)***, ***middle testicular nerves (>1840)***, and ***inferior testicular nerves (>1840)*** in male; and ***superior ovarian nerves (>1840)***, ***middle ovarian nerves (>1840)***, and ***inferior ovarian nerves (>1840)*** in female; in the original Latin, *pl. spermaticum*, p. 95.
3. *testicular plexuses (Chaussier, 1789)*
Synonym for *spermatic plexuses (Günther, 1786)*; in the original French, *spermatiques*, see *Table synoptique du nerf tri-splanchnique*.
4. *ovarian plexus (Tiedemann, 1822)*
For macrodissected adult human female, equivalent of *spermatic plexus (Günther, 1786)*; see Table I-5.

prevertebral plexuses (Quain, 1832)

An interconnected series or chain of more or less distinguishable perivascular thoracic, abdominal, and pelvic ***plexuses (Galen, c192)*** of small anastomotic *nerve fiber (Ehrenberg, 1833)* bundles. The functional composition of bundles is complex and consists of varying mixtures of postganglionic sympathetic ***axons (Kölliker, 1896)*** from the ***prevertebral ganglia (Quain, 1832)***, preganglionic sympathetic ***axons (Kölliker, 1896)*** from ***paravertebral nerves (Swanson & Bota, 2010)***, preganglionic parasympathetic ***axons (Kölliker, 1896)***, and visceral afferent or sensory ***dendrites (His, 1889)***; see Durward (1951, pp. 1120, 1128, and 1138), Williams & Warwick (1980, pp. 1132–1137). Embedded within the ***prevertebral plexuses (Quain, 1832)*** are ***prevertebral ganglia (Quain, 1832)*** that are mostly sympathetic. The combination of a ***prevertebral plexus (Quain, 1832)*** and macroscopically identifiable ***prevertebral ganglia (Quain, 1832)*** was called a *ganglionnary plexus (Meckel, 1817)*. They are now commonly described sequentially from rostral (superior) to caudal (inferior), and are *autonomic plexuses (Strong & Elwyn, 1943)*. For Quain's use in macrodissected adult human, see p. 724, also see p. 722; he spelled it *praevertebral*. They were alluded to long ago by Galen; see *nerves for all intestines (Galen, c173)*.

PARTLY CORRESPONDS:

1. *nerves for all intestines (Galen, c173)*
Mentioned for macrodissected adult beef, pig, and/or macaque but not human; refers to source of innervation for intestines ultimately emerging from ***prevertebral plexuses (Quain, 1832)***; see May translation (1968, pp. 685, 711) and Duckworth translation (1962, p. 221).
2. *mesenteric plexus (Vieussens, 1684)*
Apparently refers to macrodissected adult human *superior mesenteric plexus (Vieussens, 1684)*; in the original Latin, *plexus mesentericos*, p. 199 and Table 23-25,*61*.
3. *nerveos plexus mesentericos (Vieussens, 1684)*
Synonym for *mesenteric plexus (Vieussens, 1684)*; Table 23-*65*.
4. *superior mesenteric plexus (Vieussens, 1684)*
From the illustration, corresponds roughly in macrodissected adult human to regions of ***celiac plexus (Winslow, 1733)*** and ***superior mesenteric plexus (Rau, 1720)*** near median plane; in the original Latin, *plexus mesentericos superior*, pp. 199, 202 and Table 23-*77*.
5. *middle mesenteric plexus (Vieussens, 1684)*
Apparently corresponds roughly to macrodissected adult human ***inferior mesenteric plexus (Rau, 1720)*** and ***superior hypogastric plexus (Tiedemann, 1822)*** considered together; in the original Latin, *plexus mesentericos medius*, p. 202 and Table 23-*78*.
6. *mesenteric plexus (Keill, 1698)*
From Keill's brief description of macrodissected adult human, may refer to combination of *superior mesenteric plexus (Vieussens, 1684)* and *middle mesenteric plexus (Vieussens, 1684)*; p. 293.
7. *plexus coronarius stomachicus (Winslow, 1733)*
Corresponds to all the various ***nerves (Herophilus, c335–c280 BC)*** and ***plexuses (Galen, c192)*** associated with macrodissected adult human stomach, including ***right gastric plexus (>1840)*** and ***left gastric plexus (>1840)***, and ***gastric branches of posterior vagal trunk (>1840)*** and ***gastric branches of anterior vagal trunk (>1840)***; Section VI, pp. 73, 99. Haase (1781, p. 124 and Index, section for p. 124) spelled it *plexum coronariostomachicum*.
8. *coronary plexus (Winslow, 1733)*
Synonym for *plexus coronarius stomachicus (Winslow, 1733)*; Section VI, p. 73.
9. *plexus stomachus (Winslow, 1733)*
Synonym for *plexus coronarius stomachicus (Winslow, 1733)*; Section VI, p. 98. Quain, (1837, p. 818) used English form, *stomachic plexus*.
10. *great mesenteric plexus (Winslow, 1733)*
Winslow apparently included in it specifically ***celiac plexus (Winslow, 1733)***, ***renal plexus (Drake, 1707)***, ***hepatic plexus (Rau, 1720)***, and ***splenic plexus (Palfijn, 1726)*** on both sides of macrodissected adult human; Section VI, no. 411, p. 99.
11. *solar plexus (Winslow, 1733)*
Corresponds in macrodissected adult human to part of ***celiac plexus (Winslow, 1733)*** surrounding root of superior mesenteric artery and its ***superior mesenteric plexus (Rau, 1720)***, where some filaments of ***celiac plexus (Winslow, 1733)*** appear to radiate out from trunk

of artery; in the original Latin, *plexus solaris*, Section VI, p. 99. "The right and left semilunar Ganglions [***celiac ganglia (Walter, 1783)***] send Nervous Fasciculi to each other, which by a particular Intertexture form a kind of flat Ganglion or Plexus, immediately under the Diaphragm, before the Articulation of the last Vertebra of the Back with the first of the Loins... From this Plexiform Union, called commonly Plexus Solaris, several filaments are detached in a radiated manner to the Mesocolon and Mesentery; and some of them go likewise to the Diaphragm." (Sect. VI, p. 99). Very clear definition of, though not necessarily synonym for, rather vaguely defined *solar plexus (Willis, 1664)*.

12. *solar ganglioform plexus (Tarin, 1753)*
   Probably synonym for macrodissected adult human *solar plexus (Winslow, 1733)*; in the original French, *le plexus ganglio-forme solaire*, p. 72.
13. *plexus mesocolicus (Haller, 1762)*
   Probably includes roughly ***intermesenteric plexus (>1840)*** and ***inferior mesenteric plexus (Rau, 1720)*** for macrodissected adult human; pp. 265–266.
14. *plexus mesentericus medius (Haller, 1762)*
   Synonym for *plexus mesocolicus (Haller, 1762)*; pp. 265–266.
15. *hypogastric plexus (Haller, 1762)*
   Probably includes ***superior hypogastric plexus (Tiedemann, 1822)***, ***inferior hypogastric plexus (Tiedemann, 1822)***, and ***hypogastric nerves (Walter, 1783)*** for macrodissected adult human; in the original Latin, *plexus hypogastricus*, pp. 266–267; also see alternate form, *plexum hypogastricum* (p. 253). This usage was followed by Walter, who divided it into five differentiations in macrodissected adult human (1783, Tab. I).
16. *inferior mesenteric plexus (Haller, 1762)*
   Synonym for *hypogastric plexus (Haller, 1762)*; in the original Latin, *plexum mesentericum infimum*, p. 266.
17. *abdominal plexus (Ludwig, 1772)*
   Synonym for *hypogastric plexus (Haller, 1762)*; in the original Latin, *plexuum abdominalium*, p. XI.
18. *phrenico-hepatic plexus (Günther, 1786)*
   Not clearly described, but essentially region in macrodissected adult human where ***phrenic plexus (Loder, 1778)*** merges with ***celiac plexus (Winslow, 1733)***; in the original Latin, *plexus phrenico-hepaticus*, p. 94.
19. *gastric plexus (Günther, 1786)*
   Synonym for macrodissected adult human *plexus coronarius stomachicus (Winslow, 1733)*; in the original Latin, *plexus gastricus*, p. 95.
20. *abdominal aortic plexus (Chaussier, 1789)*
   Apparently macrodissected adult human ***prevertebral plexuses (Quain, 1832)*** between ***celiac plexus (Winslow, 1733)*** and ***inferior hypogastric plexus (Tiedemann, 1822)***; in the original French, *l'aortique de l'abdomen*, see *Table synoptique du nerf tri-splanchnique*.
21. *stomogastric plexus (Chaussier, 1789)*
   Synonym for macrodissected adult human *coronary plexus (Winslow, 1733)*; in the original French, *stomogastrique*, see *Table synoptique du nerf tri-splanchnique*.
22. *superior gastric plexus (Chaussier, 1789)*
   Synonym for macrodissected adult human *coronary plexus (Winslow, 1733)*; in the original French, *gastrique supérieur*, see *Table synoptique du nerf tri-splanchnique*.
23. *aortic plexus (Fyfe, 1800)*
   Probably synonymous with macrodissected adult human *abdominal aortic plexus (Chaussier, 1789)*; Vol. 2, p. 323.
24. *inferior mesenteric plexus (Cruveilhier, 1836)*
   Description for macrodissected adult human is ambiguous but probably includes ***inferior mesenteric plexus (Rau, 1720)*** and ***superior hypogastric plexus (Tiedemann, 1822)*** considered together; in the original French, *plexus mésentérique inferieur*, pp. 1020–1025.
25. *aortic plexus (Quain, 1837, p. 819)*
   For macrodissected adult human, ***superior mesenteric plexus (Rau, 1720)***, ***intermesenteric plexus (>1840)***, and ***inferior mesenteric plexus (Rau, 1720)***, considered together; p. 819.
26. *pelvic plexus (Beck, 1846)*
   Mitchell (1953, p. 301) noted that many writers follow Beck and include ***hypogastric nerves (Walter, 1783)*** under this designation, along with ***inferior hypogastric plexus (Tiedemann, 1822)***, in macrodissected adult human.

primary brain vesicles (Baer, 1837)

For macrodissected vertebrate embryo, three sequential ***brain vesicles (Malpighi, 1673)*** arranged from rostral to caudal: ***primary forebrain vesicle (Baer, 1837)***, ***primary midbrain vesicle (Baer, 1837)***, and ***primary hindbrain vesicle (Baer, 1837)***; they in turn generate five ***secondary brain vesicles (>1840)***. For Baer's use see pp. 107, 303. They were first clearly described as *three vesicles (Malpighi, 1673)*.

TRANSLATIONS:

1. *primären Hirnbläschen (Baer, 1837)*
   Original German form of ***primary brain vesicles (Baer, 1837)***; pp. 107, 303.

EARLIER REFERENCES:

Earlier synonyms:

1. *three vesicles (Malpighi, 1673)*
   Synonym for ***primary brain vesicles (Baer, 1837)*** in macrodissected chick embryo at 40 hours of incubation; in the original Latin, *tres vesiculae*, see p. 7 for Figure VIII.

primary fissure (Smith, 1902)

As described for macrodissected adult human, the groove between the ***culmen*** on one side, and the ***simple lobule (Jansen & Brodal, 1954)*** of the ***cerebellar hemisphere (Willis, 1664)*** and ***declive (>1840)*** of the ***cerebellar vermis (Meckel, 1817)*** on the other side; see Angevine et al. (1961, pp. 19–20 and Figs. 8, 10, 15, 16, 19, 20, 22–24), *Terminologia Anatomica* (1998, p. 119). For Smith's use in macrodissected adult mammal, see p. 381, *fissura prima* in the original Latin. It was probably not clearly distinguished by 1840.

primary forebrain vesicle (Baer, 1837)

For macrodissected vertebrate embryo, the most rostral of the three ***primary brain vesicles (Baer, 1837)***, rostral to the ***primary midbrain vesicle (Baer, 1837)***; see Carpenter (1976, p. 38), Nieuwenhuys et al. (2008, Fig 2.2). For derivation of Baer's term, see passages on pp. 106–107, 303; he equated it with the adult *grosse Hirn*. It was first clearly distinguished and illustrated by Malpighi; see ***brain vesicles (Malpighi, 1673)***.

TRANSLATIONS:

1. *vorderes primären Hirnbläschen (Baer, 1837)*
One possible translation is ***primary forebrain vesicle (Baer, 1837)***, another is *anterior primary brain vesicle (Baer, 1837)*; see description on pp. 106–107, 303.

EARLIER REFERENCES:

Earlier synonyms:

1. *anterior brain vesicle (Baer, 1837)*
Synonym for ***primary forebrain vesicle (Baer, 1837)***; in the original German, *vordere HIrnbläschen*; p. 106.
2. *anterior brain cell (Baer, 1837)*
Synonym for *anterior brain vesicle (Baer, 1837)*; p. 106.

LATER SYNONYMS:

1. *anterior primary brain vesicle (Baer, 1837)*
Synonym for ***primary forebrain vesicle (Baer, 1837)***; in the original German, *vorderes primären Hirnbläschen*, see passages on pp. 106–107 and English form in Sharpey et al. (1867, p. 577).
2. *cell for eye and optic thalamus (Wagner, 1839)*
Synonym for macrodissected embryonic chick ***primary forebrain vesicle (Baer, 1837)***; in the original Latin, *cellula pro oculis ac thalamis opticis*, Table III, Figure 12-*d*[1].

primary hindbrain vesicle (Baer, 1837)

For macrodissected vertebrate embryo the most caudal of the three ***primary brain vesicles (Baer, 1837)***, between ***primary midbrain vesicle (Baer, 1837)*** rostrally and ***spinal cord part of neural tube (>1840)*** caudally; see Strong & Elwyn (1943, p. 11, Fig. 6). It subsequently divides into ***hindbrain vesicle (Baer, 1837)*** and ***afterbrain vesicle (Baer, 1837)***, which together generate the adult ***rhombicbrain (His, 1893b)***. For Baer's use see description on pp. 106–107. It was first clearly distinguished and illustrated by Malpighi, see ***brain vesicles (Malpighi, 1673)***.

TRANSLATIONS:

1. *hinteres primären Hirnbläschen (Baer, 1837)*
One possible translation is ***primary hindbrain vesicle (Baer, 1837)***, another is *posterior primary brain vesicle (Baer, 1837)*; see description on pp. 106–107.

EARLIER REFERENCES:

Earlier synonyms:

1. *common vesicle for medulla oblongata and cerebellum (Serres, 1824–1826)*
Synonym for ***primary hindbrain vesicle (Baer, 1837)*** in macrodissected chick on fourth day of incubation; in the original French, *vésicule commune à la moelle allongée et au cervelet*; Plate I, Figure 4-5,6.
2. *posterior brain vesicle (Baer, 1837)*
Synonym for ***primary hindbrain vesicle (Baer, 1837)***; in the original German, *hinteres Hirnbläshen*, see description on p. 106.
3. *posterior brain cell (Baer, 1837)*
Synonym for ***primary hindbrain vesicle (Baer, 1837)***; p. 106.

LATER SYNONYMS:

1. *posterior primary brain vesicle (Baer, 1837)*
Synonym for ***primary hindbrain vesicle (Baer, 1837)***; in the original German, *hinteres primären Hirnbläschen*, see passages on pp. 106–107 and English form in Sharpey et al. (1867, p. 577).
2. *cell for medulla oblongata (Wagner, 1839)*
Synonym for macrodissected embryonic chick ***primary hindbrain vesicle (Baer, 1837)***; in the original Latin, *cellula pro medulla oblongata*, Table III, Figure 12-*d*[3].
3. *cell for cerebellum and medulla oblongata (Wagner, 1839)*
Synonym for macrodissected embryonic human ***primary hindbrain vesicle (Baer, 1837)***; in the original Latin, *cellula pro cerebello et medulla oblongata*, Table XXII, Figure 5-*d*.

primary midbrain vesicle (Baer, 1837)

For macrodissected vertebrate embryo, the middle of the three ***primary brain vesicles (Baer, 1837)*** between ***primary forebrain vesicle (Baer, 1837)*** rostrally and ***primary hindbrain vesicle (Baer, 1837)*** caudally; it develops into the mature ***midbrain (Baer, 1837)***. For Baer's use, see p. 106. It was first clearly distinguished and illustrated by Malpighi, see ***brain vesicles (Malpighi, 1673)***, and named shortly thereafter, see *cristate vesicle of brain (Malpighi, 1675)*.

EARLIER REFERENCES:

Earlier synonyms:

1. *cristate vesicle of brain (Malpighi, 1675)*
Synonym for ***primary midbrain vesicle (Baer, 1837)*** in macrodissected developing chick embryo; in the original Latin, *cerebri cristata vesicula*, Table V, Figure XXXVI-*B*; see Adelmann (1966, p. 1003).
2. *optic lobes vesicle (Serres, 1824–1826)*
Synonym for ***primary midbrain vesicle (Baer, 1837)*** in macrodissected chick embryo on third day of incubation; in the original French, *vésicule des lobes optiques*; Plate I, Figure 3-7. Used later in the book for all vertebrates.
3. *middle brain vesicle (Baer, 1837)*
Synonym for ***middle primary brain vesicle (Baer, 1837)***; in the original German, *mittleres Hirnbläshen*, p. 106.
4. *middle brain cell (Baer, 1837)*
Synonym for *middle brain vesicle (Baer, 1837)*; p. 106.

LATER SYNONYMS:

1. *middle primary brain vesicle (Baer, 1837)*
Synonym for ***primary midbrain vesicle (Baer, 1837)***; in the original German, *mittleres primären Hirnbläschen*, see description on pp. 106–107 and English form in Sharpey et al. (1867, p. 577).

2. *cell for quadrigeminal body (Wagner, 1839)*
   Synonym for macrodissected embryonic ***primary midbrain vesicle (Baer, 1837)***; in the original Latin, *cellula pro corporibus quadrigeminis*, Table III, Figure 12-d^2.

primary visual area (>1840)

As defined with cellular architecture, connections, and functional analysis for adult human, the part of the caudal end of the ***occipital region (Vesalius, 1543a)*** receiving the major projection of the ***dorsal lateral geniculate nucleus (>1840)*** and abbreviated V1. In macrodissected adult human, it includes parts of the ***lingual gyrus (>1840)***, ***cuneus (Burdach, 1822)***, ***superior occipital gyri (>1840)***, and ***inferior occipital gyri (>1840)***; see Williams & Warwick (1980, p. 1018), Nieuwenhuys et al (2008, p. 760), and *striate area (Brodmann, 1909)*. The same term is used for all mammals. It was first identified by the presence of the *lineola albidior (Gennari, 1782)*.

LATER SYNONYMS:

1. *area striata (Brodmann, 1909)*
   Original Latin form of *striate area (Brodmann, 1909)*; p. 140.
2. *striate area (Brodmann, 1909)*
   Synonym for macrodissected adult human ***primary visual area (>1840)***; see Garey translation (1994, pp. 119–120 and Figs. 85, 86). It is surrounded by *occipital area (Brodmann, 1909)* or *area 18 (Brodmann, 1909)*.
3. *area 17 (Brodmann, 1909)*
   Synonym for macrodissected adult human ***primary visual area (>1840)***; in the original German, *Feld 17*, p. 140.
4. *visual area 1 (Talbot, 1942)*
   Synonym for *striate area (Brodmann, 1909)* based on histology and electrophysiology in adult cat.
5. *first visual area (Talbot, 1942)*
   Synonym for adult cat *visual area 1 (Talbot, 1942)*.

PARTLY CORRESPONDS:

1. *lineola albidior (Gennari, 1782)*
   In frozen adult human ***cerebral cortex (>1840)*** sectioned by hand, as a medical student Gennari observed by eye on February 2, 1776, and described in print in 1782, a little white line (*lineola albidior* in Latin) in the ***occipital region (Vesalius, 1543a)*** corresponding to layer 4b of ***primary visual area (>1840)***, *area 17 (Brodmann, 1909)*, or *striate area (Brodmann, 1909)*. Vicq d'Azyr was probably unaware of Gennari's observations and reported the same white line (*blanc linéaire* in French) for macrodissected adult human at a meeting of the Royal Academy in 1781, the proceedings of which were published in 1784 (p. 511). See Garrison & McHenry (1969, p. 104), Crosby et al. (1962, p. 438 and Fig. 303), Clarke & O'Malley (1996, p. 423). It is now often called *stria of Gennari (Obersteiner, 1888)*. Twenty years earlier, Haller described a superficial layer of *white substance (Vesalius, 1543a)*, the *columna anonyma (Haller, 1762)*, distinguishing another region of ***cerebral cortex gray matter (>1840)***, the ***parahippocampal gyrus (>1840)***.
2. *yellow substance of posterior lobe (Arnold, 1838b)*
   Synonym for macrodissected adult human *lineola albidior (Gennari, 1782)*; in the original Latin, *substantia flava lobi posterioris*, Table IV, Figure 1-*λ*.
3. *stria of Gennari (Obersteiner, 1888)*
   Eponym for *lineola albidior (Gennari, 1782)*; in the original German, *Gennari'schen Streifen*, p. 348. It can also be translated *stripe of Gennnari* or *line of Gennari*.

principal mammillary tract (Kölliker, 1896)

As described in macrodissected adult human, and mammal generally with histological methods for ***axons (Kölliker, 1896)***, a short ***central nervous system white matter tract (>1840)*** between the ***mammillary body (Ludwig, 1779)*** ventrally, and a branch point dorsally for the ***mammillotegmental tract (>1840)*** and ***mammillothalamic tract (>1840)***. For interpretation of axonal branching patterns in this system, see Hayakawa & Zyo (1989, Fig. 12), Szabó et al. (2011). For Kölliker's use in adult rabbit with histological methods for ***axons (Kölliker, 1896)***, see p. 517 and Figure 643-*Fmpr*. Cajal (1895, p. 99 and Fig. 26-*B*) discovered it.

TRANSLATIONS:

1. *fasciculus mammillaris princeps (Kölliker, 1896)*
   Original Latin form of ***principal mammillary tract (Kölliker, 1896)***; see Figure 643-*Fmpr*.

principal sensory nucleus of trigeminal nerve (>1840)

As described for adult mammal based on cellular architecture and connections, the ***gray matter region (Swanson & Bota, 2010)*** in lateral parts of the ***pons (Haller, 1747)***, lying just lateral to the ***motor nucleus of trigeminal nerve (>1840)*** and just rostral to the ***spinal nucleus of trigeminal nerve (>1840)***, and associated with the ***trigeminal nerve central sensory root (>1840)*** that is the continuation of the peripheral ***trigeminal nerve sensory root (Bell, 1829)***; see Nieuwenhuys et al. (2008, pp. 191, 794 and Figs. 6.26-*10*, 6.27-*8*). It was not identified by 1840.

proper palmar digital nerves of median nerve (>1840)

As described for macrodissected adult human, terminal branches of the ***common palmar digital nerves of median nerve (>1840)*** extending along the fingers; see Williams & Warwick (1980, p. 1099), *Terminologia Anatomica* (1998, p. 138). They were known to Galen; see ***[proper palmar digital nerves of median nerve (>1840)] (Galen, c177)***.

TRANSLATIONS:

1. *nervus medianus nervi digitales palmares proprii (>1840)*
   Current Latin form of ***proper palmar digital nerves of median nerve (>1840)***; see *Terminologia Anatomica* (1998, p. 138).

EARLIER REFERENCES:

Described, not named or illustrated:

1. ***[proper palmar digital nerves of median nerve (>1840)] (Galen, c177)***

Mentioned for macrodissected adult macaque but not human; see Singer translation (1999, p. 74).

Illustrated and described, not named:

1. ***[proper palmar digital nerves of median nerve (>1840)] Vesalius (1543a)***
   Vesalius clearly described five of them (2 to thumb, 2 to index finger, and one to inner part of middle finger) for macrodissected adult human without naming the group; see Richardson & Carman translation (2002, p. 244). Mayer (1794) described and named for macrodissected adult human the individual ***nerves (Herophilus, c335–c280 BC)*** without naming the group; see p. 24.

Earlier synonyms:

1. *digital nerves of median nerve (Schaarschmidt, 1750)*
   Synonym for macrodissected adult human ***proper palmar digital nerves of median nerve (>1840)***; in the original Latin, *(nervus medianus) nervi digitali,* pp. 71–72.
2. *volar digital nerves of median nerve (Bock, 1827)*
   Synonym for macrodissected adult human ***proper palmar digital nerves of median nerve (>1840)***; in the original Latin, *nervi digitales volares nervi mediani*; Table II-53. Langenbeck (1826–1830; Fasc. III, Tab. XIV-7) also used this term for macrodissected adult human, but Fascicle III was printed in 1830.

PARTLY CORRESPONDS:

1. *[radio-palmar nerve of thumb (Meckel, 1817)] (Vesalius, 1543a)*
   Clearly described without naming as ***proper palmar digital nerve of median nerve (>1840)*** to lateral part of thumb for macrodissected adult human; see Richardson & Carman translation (2002, p. 244).
2. *[cubito-palmar nerve of thumb (Meckel, 1817)] (Vesalius, 1543a)*
   Clearly described without naming as ***proper palmar digital nerve of median nerve (>1840)*** to medial part of thumb for macrodissected adult human; see Richardson & Carman translation (2002, p. 244).
3. *[radio-palmar nerve of index finger (Meckel, 1817)] (Vesalius, 1543a)*
   Clearly described without naming as ***proper palmar digital nerve of median nerve (>1840)*** to lateral part of index finger for macrodissected adult human; see Richardson & Carman translation (2002, p. 244).
4. *[cubito-palmar nerve of index finger (Meckel, 1817)] (Vesalius, 1543a)*
   Clearly described without naming as ***proper palmar digital nerve of median nerve (>1840)*** to medial part of index finger for macrodissected adult human; see Richardson & Carman translation (2002, p. 244).
5. *[radio-palmar nerve of third finger (Meckel, 1817)] (Vesalius, 1543a)*
   Clearly described without naming as ***proper palmar digital nerve of median nerve (>1840)*** to lateral part of middle finger for macrodissected adult human; see Richardson & Carman translation (2002, p. 244).
6. *[cubito-palmar nerve of third finger (Meckel, 1817)] (Vesalius, 1543a)*
   Clearly described without naming as ***proper palmar digital nerve of ulnar nerve (>1840)*** to medial part of middle finger for macrodissected adult human, though it is usually a ***proper palmar digital nerve of median nerve (>1840)***; see Richardson & Carman translation (2002, p. 244).
7. *[radio-palmar nerve of fourth finger (Meckel, 1817)] (Vesalius, 1543a)*
   Clearly described without naming as ***proper palmar digital nerve of ulnar nerve (>1840)*** to lateral part of ring finger for macrodissected adult human, though it is usually a ***proper palmar digital nerve of median nerve (>1840)***; see Richardson & Carman translation (2002, p. 244).
8. *external thumb nerve (Mayer, 1794)*
   Synonym for macrodissected adult human *cubito-palmar nerve of thumb (Meckel, 1817)*; in the original Latin, *nervus pollicaris externus*; Part 5, Table V, Figure 1-*17* (p. 22).
9. *external volar nerve of thumb (Mayer, 1794)*
   Synonym for *external thumb nerve (Mayer, 1794)*; in the original Latin, *nervus volaris externus pollicis*; Part 5, Table V, Figure 1-*14* (p. 24).
10. *internal volar nerve of thumb (Mayer, 1794)*
    Synonym for *cubito-palmar nerve of thumb (Meckel, 1817)*; in the original Latin, *nervus volaris internus pollicis*; Part 5, Table V, Figure 1-*15* (p. 24).
11. *external volar nerve of index finger (Mayer, 1794)*
    Synonym for *radio-palmar nerve of index finger (Meckel, 1817)*; in the original Latin, *nervus volaris externus indicis*; Part 5, Table V, Figure 1-*17* (p. 24).
12. *internal volar nerve of index finger (Mayer, 1794)*
    Synonym for *cubito-palmar nerve of index finger (Meckel, 1817)*; in the original Latin, *nervus volaris internus indicis*; Part 5, Table V, Figure 1-*20* (p. 24).
13. *external volar nerve of middle finger (Mayer, 1794)*
    Synonym for *radio-palmar nerve of third finger (Meckel, 1817)*; in the original Latin, *nervus volaris externus digiti medii*; Part 5, Table V, Figure 1-*21* (p. 24).
14. *internal volar nerve of middle finger (Mayer, 1794)*
    Synonym for *cubito-palmar nerve of third finger (Meckel, 1817)*; in the original Latin, *nervus volaris internus medii*; Part 5, Table V, Figure 1-*24* (p. 24).
15. *external volar nerve of ring finger (Mayer, 1794)*
    Synonym for *radio-palmar nerve of fourth finger (Meckel, 1817)*; in the original Latin, *nervus volaris externus digiti annularis*; Part 5, Table V, Figure 1-*25* (p. 24).
16. *radial volar nerve of thumb (Loder, 1803)*
    Synonym for macrodissected adult human *external volar nerve of thumb (Mayer, 1794)*; in the original Latin, *nervus volaris radialis pollicis*, Table CLXXX, Figure 1-*54*.
17. *ulnar volar nerve of thumb (Loder, 1803)*
    Synonym for macrodissected adult human *internal volar nerve of thumb (Mayer, 1794)*; in the original Latin, *nervus volaris ulnaris pollicis*, Table CLXXX, Figure 1-*65*.

18. *radial volar nerve of index finger (Loder, 1803)*
Synonym for macrodissected adult human *external volar nerve of index finger (Mayer, 1794)*; in the original Latin, *nervus volaris radialis indicis*, Table CLXXX, Figure 1-68.
19. *ulnar volar nerve of index finger (Loder, 1803)*
Synonym for macrodissected adult human *internal volar nerve of index finger (Mayer, 1794)*; in the original Latin, *nervus volaris ulnaris indicis*, Table CLXXX, Figure 1-77.
20. *radial volar nerve of middle finger (Loder, 1803)*
Synonym for macrodissected adult human *external volar nerve of middle finger (Mayer, 1794)*; in the original Latin, *nervus volaris radialis digiti medii*, Table CLXXX, Figure 1-82.
21. *ulnar volar nerve of middle finger (Loder, 1803)*
Synonym for macrodissected adult human *internal volar nerve of middle finger (Mayer, 1794)*; in the original Latin, *nervus volaris ulnaris digiti medii*, Table CLXXX, Figure 1-89.
22. *radial volar nerve of ring finger (Loder, 1803)*
Synonym for macrodissected adult human *external volar nerve of ring finger (Mayer, 1794)*; in the original Latin, *nervus volaris radialis digiti annularis*, Table CLXXX, Figure 1-90.
23. *radial volar branch of thumb of median nerve (Caldani, 1813, 1814)*
Synonym for macrodissected adult human *radial volar nerve of thumb (Loder, 1803)*; in the original Latin, *ramus volaris radialis pollicis*, Table CCLIX, Figure 2-11.
24. *communications between radial and ulnar volar nerves of thumb (Caldani, 1813, 1814)*
Macrodissected adult human ***communicating branches (Winslow, 1733)*** between *radial volar nerve of thumb (Loder, 1803)* and *ulnar volar nerve of thumb (Loder, 1803)*; in the original Latin, *communicationes inter nervum volarem radialem atque ulnarem pollicis*, Table CCLIX, Figure 2-13.
25. *radial volar nerve of third finger (Caldani, 1813, 1814)*
Synonym for macrodissected adult human *radial volar nerve of middle finger (Loder, 1803)*; in the original Latin, *nervus radialis volaris tertii digiti*, Table CCLIX, Figure 2-24.
26. *radio-palmar nerve of thumb (Meckel, 1817)*
A ***proper palmar digital nerve of median nerve (>1840)*** to lateral side of thumb as described for macrodissected adult human; see translation (1832, Vol. 3, p. 27). See *[radio-palmar nerve of thumb (Meckel, 1817)] (Vesalius, 1543a)*.
27. *cubito-palmar nerve of thumb (Meckel, 1817)*
A ***proper palmar digital nerve of median nerve (>1840)*** to medial side of thumb as described for macrodissected adult human; see translation (1832, Vol. 3, p. 27). See *[cubito-palmar nerve of thumb (Meckel, 1817)] (Vesalius, 1543a)*.
28. *radio-palmar nerve of index finger (Meckel, 1817)*
A ***proper palmar digital nerve of median nerve (>1840)*** to lateral side of index finger as described for macrodissected adult human; see translation (1832, Vol. 3, p. 27). See *[radio-palmar nerve of index finger (Meckel, 1817)] (Vesalius, 1543a)*.
29. *cubito-palmar nerve of index finger (Meckel, 1817)*
A ***proper palmar digital nerve of median nerve (>1840)*** to medial side of index finger as described for macrodissected adult human; see translation (1832, Vol. 3, p. 27). See *[cubito-palmar nerve of index finger (Meckel, 1817)] (Vesalius, 1543a)*.
30. *radio-palmar nerve of third finger (Meckel, 1817)*
A ***proper palmar digital nerve of median nerve (>1840)*** to lateral side of middle finger as described for macrodissected adult human; see translation (1832, Vol. 3, p. 27). See *[radio-palmar nerve of third finger (Meckel, 1817)] (Vesalius, 1543a)*.
31. *cubito-palmar nerve of third finger (Meckel, 1817)*
A ***proper palmar digital nerve of median nerve (>1840)*** to medial side of middle finger as described for macrodissected adult human; see translation (1832, Vol. 3, p. 27). See *[cubito-palmar nerve of third finger (Meckel, 1817)] (Vesalius, 1543a)*.
32. *radio-palmar nerve of fourth finger (Meckel, 1817)*
A ***proper palmar digital nerve of median nerve (>1840)*** to lateral side of ring finger as described for macrodissected adult human; see translation (1832, Vol. 3, p. 27). See *[radio-palmar nerve of fourth finger (Meckel, 1817)] (Vesalius, 1543a)*.
33. *superior dorsal branch of external volar nerve of index finger (Bock, 1827)*
Branch of *external volar nerve of index finger (Mayer, 1794)* coursing along intermediate regions of lateral surface of index finger; in the original Latin, *ram. dorsalis superior*; Table V, Figure 3-15.
34. *internal collateral nerve of thumb of median nerve (Cloquet, 1828)*
A ***proper palmar digital nerve of median nerve (>1840)*** to medial side of macrodissected adult human thumb; in the original French, *nerf collatéral interne du pouce fourni par le médian*, Plate CLXVIII, Figure 1-23.
35. *internal palmar branch of thumb of first common digital branch of median nerve (Cloquet, 1828)*
Synonym for *internal collateral nerve of thumb of median nerve (Cloquet, 1828)*; in the original French, *rameau palmaire interne du pouce*, Plate CLXIX, Figure 1-48.
36. *external palmar branch of index finger of first common digital branch of median nerve (Cloquet, 1828)*
A ***proper palmar digital nerve of median nerve (>1840)*** to lateral side of macrodissected adult human index finger; in the original French, *rameau palmaire externe de l'indicateur*, Plate CLXIX, Figure 1-49.
37. *internal palmar branch of index finger of second common digital branch of median nerve (Cloquet, 1828)*
A ***proper palmar digital nerve of median nerve (>1840)*** to medial side of macrodissected adult human index finger; in the original French, *rameau palmaire interne de l'indicateur*, Plate CLXIX, Figure 1-53,58.

38. *anastomosis between internal palmar branch and external palmar branch of index finger (Cloquet, 1828)* ***Communicating branch (Winslow, 1733)*** between *internal palmar branch of index finger of second common digital branch of median nerve (Cloquet, 1828)* and *external palmar branch of index finger of first common digital branch of median nerve (Cloquet, 1828)*; in the original French, *anastomose entre le rameau palmaire interne et le rameau palmaire externe de l'indicateur*, Plate CLXIX, Figure 1-53.
39. *anastomotic arcade of palmar nerves of index finger (Cloquet, 1828)*
Multiple ***communicating branches (Winslow, 1733)*** at distal ends of *internal palmar branch of index finger of second common digital branch of median nerve (Cloquet, 1828)* and *external palmar branch of index finger of first common digital branch of median nerve (Cloquet, 1828)*; in the original French, *arcade anastomotique des N. palmaires de l'index*, Plate CLXIX, Figure 1-55.
40. *external palmar branch of middle finger of second common digital branch of median nerve (Cloquet, 1828)*
A ***proper palmar digital nerve of median nerve (>1840)*** to lateral side of macrodissected adult human middle finger; in the original French, *rameau palmaire externe du doigt médius*, Plate CLXIX, Figure 1-59.
41. *internal palmar branch of middle finger of third common digital branch of median nerve (Cloquet, 1828)*
A ***proper palmar digital nerve of median nerve (>1840)*** to medial side of macrodissected adult human middle finger; in the original French, *rameau palmaire interne du doigt médius*, Plate CLXIX, Figure 1-66.
42. *external palmar branch of ring finger of third common digital branch of median nerve (Cloquet, 1828)*
A ***proper palmar digital nerve of median nerve (>1840)*** to lateral side of macrodissected adult human ring finger; in the original French, *rameau palmaire externe du doigt annulaire*, Plate CLXIX, Figure 1-67.
43. *dorsal branch of median nerve external collateral branch of index finger (Cruveilhier, 1836)*
Tiny dorsal branch or component of macrodissected adult human *external volar nerve of index finger (Mayer, 1794)*; in the original French, *rameau dorsal*, p. 808.
44. *palmar branch of median nerve external collateral branch of index finger (Cruveilhier, 1836)*
Substantial ventral branch or component of macrodissected adult human *external volar nerve of index finger (Mayer, 1794)*; in the original French, *rameau palmaire*, p. 808.
45. *internal collateral branch of index finger of fifth terminal branch of median nerve (Cruveilhier, 1836)*
Macrodissected adult human ***proper palmar digital nerve of median nerve (>1840)*** to medial side of index finger; in the original French, *collatéral interne de l'index*, p. 808.
46. *external collateral branch of middle finger of fifth terminal branch of median nerve (Cruveilhier, 1836)*
Macrodissected adult human ***proper palmar digital nerve of median nerve (>1840)*** to lateral side of middle finger; in the original French, *collatéral externe du médius*, p. 808.
47. *collateral branches to thumb of median nerve (Quain & Wilson, 1839)*
Macrodissected adult human ***proper palmar digital nerve of median nerve (>1840)*** to medial side of thumb; Plate XVIII, Figure 2-*h*.
48. *digital branch of first finger of median nerve (Quain & Wilson, 1839)*
Macrodissected adult human ***proper palmar digital nerve of median nerve (>1840)*** to lateral side of index finger; Plate XVIII, Figure 2-*h*.
49. *posterior branches of digital nerves of median nerve (Quain & Wilson, 1839)*
Macrodissected adult human ***proper palmar digital nerves of median nerve (>1840)*** to medial side of index finger, middle finger, and lateral side of ring finger; Plate XVIII, Figure 2-*l*.

proper palmar digital nerves of ulnar nerve (>1840)

As described for macrodissected adult human, these distal branches of the ***common palmar digital nerves of ulnar nerve (>1840)*** extend along the fingers; see Williams & Warwick (1980, p. 1100), *Terminologia Anatomica* (1998, p. 138). They were known to Galen; see ***[proper palmar digital nerves of ulnar nerve (>1840)] (Galen, c177)***.

EARLIER REFERENCES:

Described, not named or illustrated:

1. ***[proper palmar digital nerves of ulnar nerve (>1840)] (Galen, c177)***
Mentioned for macrodissected adult macaque; see Singer translation (1999, p. 74). Vesalius (1543a) described five individual ***nerves (Herophilus, c335–c280 BC)*** for macrodissected adult human without naming them as a group; see Richardson & Carman translation (2002, p. 245) and *[cubito-palmar nerve of fourth finger (Meckel, 1817)] (Vesalius, 1543a)*. Meckel (1817) described and named for macrodissected adult human three individual ***nerves (Herophilus, c335–c280 BC)*** without naming the group; see translation (1832, Vol. 3, p. 27).

Earlier synonyms:

1. *volar digital nerves of superficial branch of volar branch of ulnar nerve (Langenbeck, 1826–1830)*
Synonym for macrodissected adult human ***proper palmar digital nerves of ulnar nerve (>1840)***; in the original Latin, *nervi digitales volares ex ramo sublimi rami volaris nervi ulnaris*, Fascicle III, Table XIV-13.
2. *volar digital nerves of ulnar nerve (Bock, 1827)*
Synonym for macrodissected adult human *proper palmar digital nerves of ulnar nerve (>1840)*; in the original Latin, *nervi digitales volares nervus ulnaris*, Table II-62,66.

PARTLY CORRESPONDS:

1. *[cubito-palmar nerve of fourth finger (Meckel, 1817)] (Vesalius, 1543a)*
Clearly described without naming as ***proper palmar digital nerve of ulnar nerve (>1840)*** to medial part of ring

finger for macrodissected adult human; see Richardson & Carman translation (2002, p. 244). Also see *[cubito-palmar nerve of third finger (Meckel, 1817)] (Vesalius, 1543a)* and *[radio-palmar nerve of fourth finger (Meckel, 1817)] (Vesalius, 1543a)*.

2. *[radio-palmar nerve of fifth finger (Meckel, 1817)] (Vesalius, 1543a)*
Clearly described without naming as ***proper palmar digital nerve of ulnar nerve (>1840)*** to lateral part of little finger for macrodissected adult human; see Richardson & Carman translation (2002, p. 244).
3. *[cubito-palmar nerve of fifth finger (Meckel, 1817)] (Vesalius, 1543a)*
Clearly described without naming as ***proper palmar digital nerve of ulnar nerve (>1840)*** to medial part of little finger for macrodissected adult human; see Richardson & Carman translation (2002, p. 244).
4. *internal volar nerve of little finger (Mayer, 1794)*
Synonym for macrodissected adult human *cubito-palmar nerve of fifth finger (Meckel, 1817)*; in the original Latin, *nervus volaris internus digiti minimi*; Part 5, Table V, Figure 1-7 (p. 24).
5. *external volar nerve of little finger (Mayer, 1794)*
Synonym for macrodissected adult human *radio-palmar nerve of fifth finger (Meckel, 1817)*; in the original Latin, *nervus volaris externus digiti minimi*; Part 5, Table V, Figure 1-7 (p. 24).
6. *internal volar nerve of ring finger (Mayer, 1794)*
Synonym for macrodissected adult human *cubito-palmar nerve of fourth finger (Meckel, 1817)*; in the original Latin, *nervus volaris internus digiti annularis*; Part 5, Table V, Figure 1-9 (p. 24).
7. *ulnar volar nerve of ring finger (Loder, 1803)*
Synonym for macrodissected adult human *internal volar nerve of ring finger (Mayer, 1794)*; in the original Latin, *nervus volaris ulnaris digiti annularis*, Table CLXXX, Figure 1-*100*.
8. *radial volar nerve of auricular finger (Loder, 1803)*
Synonym for macrodissected adult human *external volar nerve of little finger (Mayer, 1794)*; in the original Latin, *nervus volaris radialis digiti auricularis*, Table CLXXX, Figure 1-*101*.
9. *ulnar volar branch of auricular finger (Loder, 1803)*
Synonym for *ulnar volar nerve of auricular finger (Loder, 1803)*; in the original Latin, *ramus volaris ulnaris digiti auricularis*, Table CLXXX, Figure 1-*102*.
10. *ulnar volar nerve of auricular finger (Loder, 1803)*
Synonym for macrodissected adult human *internal volar nerve of little finger (Mayer, 1794)*; in the original Latin, *nervus volaris ulnaris digiti auricularis*, Table CLXXX, Figure 1-*106*.
11. *ulnar volar nerve of fourth finger (Caldani, 1813, 1814)*
Synonym for macrodissected adult human *ulnar volar nerve of ring finger (Loder, 1803)*; in the original Latin, *nervus ulnaris volaris quarti digiti*, Table CCLIX, Figure 2-*36*.
12. *radial volar nerve of little finger (Caldani, 1813, 1814)*
Synonym for macrodissected adult human *external volar nerve of little finger (Mayer, 1794)*; in the original Latin, *nervus volaris radialis digiti minimi*, Table CCLIX, Figure 2-*37*.
13. *ulnar volar nerve of little finger (Caldani, 1813, 1814)*
Synonym for macrodissected adult human *internal volar nerve of little finger (Mayer, 1794)*; in the original Latin, *nervus volaris ulnaris digiti minimi*, Table CCLIX, Figure 2-*38*.
14. *cubito-palmar nerve of fourth finger (Meckel, 1817)*
A ***proper palmar digital nerve of ulnar nerve (>1840)*** to medial side of ring finger for macrodissected adult human; see translation (1832, Vol. 3, p. 28). See *[cubito-palmar nerve of fourth finger (Meckel, 1817)] (Vesalius, 1543a)*.
15. *radio-palmar nerve of fifth finger (Meckel, 1817)*
A ***proper palmar digital nerve of ulnar nerve (>1840)*** to lateral side of little finger for macrodissected adult human; see translation (1832, Vol. 3, p. 28). See *[radio-palmar nerve of fifth finger (Meckel, 1817)] (Vesalius, 1543a)*.
16. *cubito-palmar nerve of fifth finger (Meckel, 1817)*
A ***proper palmar digital nerve of ulnar nerve (>1840)*** to medial side of little finger for macrodissected adult human; see translation (1832, Vol. 3, p. 28). See *[cubito-palmar nerve of fifth finger (Meckel, 1817)] (Vesalius, 1543a)*.
17. *volar nerves of little finger (Bock, 1827)*
Macrodissected adult human *radio-palmar nerve of fifth finger (Meckel, 1817)* and *cubito-palmar nerve of fifth finger (Meckel, 1817)*; in the original Latin, *nervi volares digiti minimi*, Table II-*72*.
18. *internal palmar nerve of ring finger (Cloquet, 1828)*
Macrodissected adult human ***proper palmar digital nerve of ulnar nerve (>1840)*** to medial side of ring finger; in the original French, *nerf palmaire interne du doigt annulaire*, Plate CLXIX, Figure 1-*74*. Called in error *doigt indicateur*; see Plate CLXIX, Figure 1-*67*.
19. *external palmar nerve of little finger (Cloquet, 1828)*
Macrodissected adult human ***proper palmar digital nerve of ulnar nerve (>1840)*** to lateral side of little finger; in the original French, *nerf palmaire externe du petit doigt*, Plate CLXIX, Figure 1-*75*.
20. *internal palmar nerve of little finger (Cloquet, 1828)*
Macrodissected adult human ***proper palmar digital nerve of ulnar nerve (>1840)*** to medial side of little finger; in the original French, *nerf palmaire interne du doigt*, Plate CLXIX, Figure 1-*77*.
21. *palmar internal collateral branch of internal branch of superficial terminal branch of cubital nerve (Cruveilhier, 1836)*
Macrodissected adult human ***proper palmar digital nerve of ulnar nerve (>1840)*** to medial side of little finger; in the original French, *collatéral interne palmaire*, p. 813.
22. *palmar external collateral branch of little finger of external branch of superficial terminal branch of cubital nerve (Cruveilhier, 1836)*
Macrodissected adult human ***proper palmar digital nerve of ulnar nerve (>1840)*** to lateral side of little

finger; in the original French, *collatéral externe palmaire du petit doigt*, p. 813.

23. *palmar internal collateral branch of ring finger of external branch of superficial terminal branch of cubital nerve (Cruveilhier, 1836)*
 Macrodissected adult human ***proper palmar digital nerve of ulnar nerve (>1840)*** to medial side of ring finger; in the original French, *collatéral interne palmaire de l'annulaire*, p. 813.

proper plantar digital nerves of lateral plantar nerve (>1840)

As described for macrodissected adult human, there are commonly three of these branches of the ***common plantar digital nerves of lateral plantar nerve (>1840)*** running along the lateral part of the fourth toe, and medial and lateral parts of the fifth (little) toe; see Durward (1951, Figs. 951, 952), Hamilton (1976, Fig. 837), Williams & Warwick (p. 1114), *Terminologia Anatomica* (1998, p. 141). They were known to Vesalius; see ***[proper plantar digital nerves of lateral plantar nerve (>1840)] (Vesalius, 1543a)***.

EARLIER REFERENCES:

Illustrated and described, not named:

1. ***[proper plantar digital nerves of lateral plantar nerve (>1840)] (Vesalius, 1543a)***
 Identified for macrodissected adult human; see Richardson & Carman translation (2002, p. 261).

Earlier synonyms:

1. *external and internal plantar nerves of external plantar nerve (Meckel, 1817)*
 Synonym for the three macrodissected adult human ***proper plantar digital nerves of lateral plantar nerve (>1840)***; see translation (1832, Vol. 3, p. 21).
2. *digital filaments of external plantar nerve to dorsal surface of toes (Quain & Wilson, 1839)*
 Synonym for macrodissected adult human ***proper plantar digital nerves of lateral plantar nerve (>1840)***; Plate XXVI, Figure 2-*k*.

PARTLY CORRESPONDS:

1. *external plantar twig of fifth digit (Jördens, 1788)*
 Macrodissected adult human ***proper plantar digital nerve of lateral plantar nerve (>1840)*** for lateral part of fifth (little) toe; in the original Latin, *ramulus plantaris digiti quinti externus*, p. 12 and Table III-222. In Jördens's account, it arises from *superficial branch of external plantar nerve (Günther, 1786)*.
2. *external plantar nerve of fourth small toe (Mayer, 1794)*
 Macrodissected adult human ***proper plantar digital nerve of lateral plantar nerve (>1840)*** for lateral part of fifth (little) toe; in the original Latin, *nervus plantaris externus digiti quarti minoris pedis*; Part 5, Table VI-45 (p. 38).
3. *internal plantar nerve of little toe (Mayer, 1794)*
 Macrodissected adult human ***proper plantar digital nerve of lateral plantar nerve (>1840)*** for medial part of fifth (little) toe; in the original Latin, *nervus plantaris externus digiti minimi pedis*; Part 5, Table VI-46 (p. 38).
4. *external plantar nerve of little toe (Mayer, 1794)*
 Macrodissected adult human ***proper plantar digital nerve of lateral plantar nerve (>1840)*** for lateral part of fifth (little) toe; in the original Latin, *nervus plantaris internus digiti minimi pedis*, Part 5, Table VI-47 (p. 38).
5. *external plantar nerve of fourth toe (Bock, 1827)*
 Macrodissected adult human ***proper plantar digital nerve of lateral plantar nerve (>1840)*** for lateral part of fourth toe; in the original Latin, *nervus plantaris externus digiti quarti*, Table VI, Figure 4-23.
6. *external collateral nerve of little toe (Cruveilhier, 1836)*
 Macrodissected adult human ***proper plantar digital nerve of lateral plantar nerve (>1840)*** for lateral part of fifth (little) toe; in the original French, *nerf collatéral externe du petit orteil*, p. 875.
7. *internal collateral nerve of little toe (Cruveilhier, 1836)*
 Macrodissected adult human ***proper plantar digital nerve of lateral plantar nerve (>1840)*** for medial part of fifth (little) toe; in the original French, *nerf collatéral interne du petit orteil*, p. 875.
8. *external collateral nerve of fourth toe (Cruveilhier, 1836)*
 Macrodissected adult human ***proper plantar digital nerve of lateral plantar nerve (>1840)*** for lateral part of fourth toe; in the original French, *nerf collatéral externe du quatrième*, p. 875.

proper plantar digital nerves of medial plantar nerve (>1840)

As described for macrodissected adult human, there are commonly seven of these branches of the ***common plantar digital nerves of medial plantar nerve (>1840)*** running along the medial and lateral parts of the first three toes, and the medial part of the fourth; see Durward (1951, Figs. 951, 952), Hamilton (1976, Fig. 837), Williams & Warwick (p. 1114), *Terminologia Anatomica* (1998, p. 141). They were first clearly delineated by Vesalius; see ***[proper plantar digital nerves of lateral plantar nerve (>1840)] (Vesalius, 1543a)***.

EARLIER REFERENCES:

Illustrated and described, not named:

1. ***[proper plantar digital nerves of medial plantar nerve (>1840)] (Vesalius, 1543a)***
 Identified for macrodissected adult human; see Richardson & Carman translation (2002, p. 261).

Earlier synonyms:

1. *external and internal plantar nerves of internal plantar nerve (Meckel, 1817)*
 Synonym describing accurately for macrodissected adult human all seven ***proper plantar digital nerves of medial plantar nerve (>1840)***; see translation (1832, Vol. 3, p. 20).
2. *digital branches of internal plantar nerve (Quain & Wilson, 1839)*
 Synonym for macrodissected adult human ***proper plantar digital nerves of medial plantar nerve (>1840)***; Plate XXVI, Figure 2:*a–d*. Four were described.

PARTLY CORRESPONDS:

1. *internal plantar twig of big toe (Jördens, 1788)*
Macrodissected adult human ***proper plantar digital nerve of medial plantar nerve (>1840)*** to medial part of big toe; in the original Latin, *ramulum plantarem pollicis internum*, Table III-*183**.
2. *external plantar twig of big toe (Jördens, 1788)*
Macrodissected adult human ***proper plantar digital nerve of medial plantar nerve (>1840)*** to lateral part of big toe; in the original Latin, *ramulus plantaris pollicis externus*, Table III-*190*.
3. *internal plantar twig of second digit (Jördens, 1788)*
Macrodissected adult human ***proper plantar digital nerve of medial plantar nerve (>1840)*** to medial part of second toe; in the original Latin, *ramulus plantaris digiti secundi internus*, Table III-*193*.
4. *external plantar twig of second digit (Jördens, 1788)*
Macrodissected adult human ***proper plantar digital nerve of medial plantar nerve (>1840)*** to lateral part of second toe; in the original Latin, *ramulus plantaris digiti secundi externus*, Table III-*198*.
5. *internal plantar twig of third digit (Jördens, 1788)*
Macrodissected adult human ***proper plantar digital nerve of medial plantar nerve (>1840)*** to medial part of third toe; in the original Latin, *ramulus plantaris digiti tertii internus*, Table III-*197*.
6. *external plantar twig of third digit (Jördens, 1788)*
Macrodissected adult human ***proper plantar digital nerve of medial plantar nerve (>1840)*** to lateral part of third toe; in the original Latin, *ramulus plantaris digiti tertii externus*, Table III-*205*.
7. *internal plantar twig of fourth digit (Jördens, 1788)*
Macrodissected adult human ***proper plantar digital nerve of medial plantar nerve (>1840)*** to medial part of fourth toe; in the original Latin, *ramulus plantaris digiti quarti internus*, Table III-*204*.
8. *external plantar twig of fourth digit (Jördens, 1788)*
Macrodissected adult human small and variable ***proper plantar digital nerve of medial plantar nerve (>1840)*** to lateral part of fourth toe; in the original Latin, *ramulus plantaris digiti quarti externus*, Table III-*207*.
9. *internal plantar twig of fifth digit (Jördens, 1788)*
Macrodissected adult human small and variable ***proper plantar digital nerve of medial plantar nerve (>1840)*** to medial part of fifth (little) toe; in the original Latin, *ramulus plantaris digiti quinti internus*, Table III-*208*.
10. *internal plantar digital twig of big toe (Fischer, 1791)*
Macrodissected adult human ***proper plantar digital nerve of medial plantar nerve (>1840)*** to medial part of big toe; in the original Latin, *ramulus plantaris digitalis pollicis internus*, p. 36.
11. *external plantar digital twig of big toe (Fischer, 1791)*
Macrodissected adult human ***proper plantar digital nerve of medial plantar nerve (>1840)*** to lateral part of big toe; in the original Latin, *ramulus plantaris digitalis pollicis externus*, p. 36.
12. *internal plantar digital twig of second toe (Fischer, 1791)*
Macrodissected adult human ***proper plantar digital nerve of medial plantar nerve (>1840)*** to medial part of second toe; in the original Latin, *ramulus plantaris digitalis digiti secundi internus*, p. 36.
13. *external plantar digital twig of second toe (Fischer, 1791)*
Macrodissected adult human ***proper plantar digital nerve of medial plantar nerve (>1840)*** to lateral part of second toe; in the original Latin, *ramulus plantaris digitalis digiti secundi externus*, p. 37.
14. *internal plantar digital twig of third toe (Fischer, 1791)*
Macrodissected adult human ***proper plantar digital nerve of medial plantar nerve (>1840)*** to medial part of third toe; in the original Latin, *ramulus plantaris digitalis digiti tertii internus*, p. 37.
15. *external plantar digital twig of third toe (Fischer, 1791)*
Macrodissected adult human ***proper plantar digital nerve of medial plantar nerve (>1840)*** to lateral part of third toe; in the original Latin, *ramulus plantaris digitalis digiti tertii externus*, p. 37.
16. *internal plantar digital twig of fourth toe (Fischer, 1791)*
Macrodissected adult human ***proper plantar digital nerve of medial plantar nerve (>1840)*** to medial part of fourth toe; in the original Latin, *ramulus plantaris digitalis digiti quarti internus*, p. 37.
17. *external plantar digital twig of fourth toe (Fischer, 1791)*
Macrodissected adult human ***proper plantar digital nerve of medial plantar nerve (>1840)*** to lateral part of fourth toe; in the original Latin, *ramulus plantaris digitalis quarti externus*, p. 37.
18. *internal plantar digital twig of fifth toe (Fischer, 1791)*
Macrodissected adult human ***proper plantar digital nerve of medial plantar nerve (>1840)*** to medial part of fifth (little) toe; in the original Latin, *ramulus plantaris digitalis digiti quinti internus*, p. 37.
19. *internal plantar nerve of big toe (Mayer, 1794)*
Macrodissected adult human ***proper plantar digital nerve of medial plantar nerve (>1840)*** to medial part of big toe; in the original Latin, *nervus plantaris internus pollicis pedis*; Part 5, Table VI-*36* (p. 38). Bock (1827; Tab. VI, Fig. 4-*7*) used the clearer *nerv. plantaris internus halucis*.
20. *external plantar nerve of big toe (Mayer, 1794)*
Macrodissected adult human ***proper plantar digital nerve of medial plantar nerve (>1840)*** to lateral part of big toe; in the original Latin, *nervus plantaris externus pollicis pedis*; Part 5, Table VI-*38* (p. 38). Bock (1827; Tab. VI, Fig. 4-*13*) used the clearer *nerv. plantaris externus halucis*.
21. *internal plantar nerve of first small toe (Mayer, 1794)*
Macrodissected adult human ***proper plantar digital nerve of medial plantar nerve (>1840)*** to medial part of second toe; in the original Latin, *nervus plantaris internus digiti primi minoris pedis*; Part 5, Table VI-*39* (p. 38).
22. *external plantar nerve of first small toe (Mayer, 1794)*
Macrodissected adult human ***proper plantar digital nerve of medial plantar nerve (>1840)*** to lateral part of second toe; in the original Latin, *nervus plantaris*

externus digiti primi minoris pedis; Part 5, Table VI-*41* (p. 38).

23. *internal plantar nerve of second small toe (Mayer, 1794)*
Macrodissected adult human ***proper plantar digital nerve of medial plantar nerve (>1840)*** to medial part of third toe; in the original Latin, *nervus plantaris internus digiti secundi minoris pedis*; Part 5, Table VI-*42* (p. 38).
24. *external plantar nerve of second small toe (Mayer, 1794)*
Macrodissected adult human ***proper plantar digital nerve of medial plantar nerve (>1840)*** to lateral part of third toe; in the original Latin, *nervus plantaris externus digiti secundi minoris pedis*; Part 5, Table VI-*43* (p. 38).
25. *internal plantar nerve of third small toe (Mayer, 1794)*
Macrodissected adult human ***proper plantar digital nerve of medial plantar nerve (>1840)*** to medial part of fourth toe; in the original Latin, *nervus plantaris internus digiti tertii minoris pedis*; Part 5, Table VI-*44* (p. 38).
26. *tibio-plantar nerve (Meckel, 1817)*
Synonym for *internal nerve of great toe (Meckel, 1817)*; see translation (1832, Vol. 3, p. 20).
27. *internal nerve of great toe (Meckel, 1817)*
Terminal end of *first plantar nerve of toes (Meckel, 1817)* corresponding to medial ***proper plantar digital nerve of medial plantar nerve (>1840)*** for macrodissected adult human big toe; see translation (1832, Vol. 3, p. 20).
28. *nervus plantaris internus (Meckel, 1817)*
Synonym for *internal nerve of great toe (Meckel, 1817)*; see translation (1832, Vol. 3, p. 20).
29. *nervus tibialis hallucis (Meckel, 1817)*
Synonym for *internal nerve of great toe (Meckel, 1817)*; see translation (1832, Vol. 3, p. 20).
30. *external plantar nerve of second toe (Meckel, 1817)*
Macrodissected adult human medial branch of third ***common plantar digital nerve of medial plantar nerve (>1840)*** forming ***proper plantar digital nerve of medial plantar nerve (>1840)*** to lateral part of second toe; see translation (1832, Vol. 3, p. 20) and Durward (1951, Fig. 951).
31. *internal plantar nerve of third toe (Meckel, 1817)*
Macrodissected adult human lateral branch of third ***common plantar digital nerve of medial plantar nerve (>1840)*** forming ***proper plantar digital nerve of medial plantar nerve (>1840)*** to medial part of third toe; see translation (1832, Vol. 3, p. 20) and Durward (1951, Fig. 951).
32. *external plantar nerve of third toe (Meckel, 1817)*
Macrodissected adult human medial branch of fourth ***common plantar digital nerve of medial plantar nerve (>1840)*** forming ***proper plantar digital nerve of medial plantar nerve (>1840)*** to lateral part of third toe; see translation (1832, Vol. 3, p. 20) and Durward (1951, Fig. 951).
33. *internal plantar nerve of fourth toe (Meckel, 1817)*
Macrodissected adult human lateral branch of fourth ***common plantar digital nerve of medial plantar nerve (>1840)*** forming ***proper plantar digital nerve of medial plantar nerve (>1840)*** to medial part of fourth toe; see translation (1832, Vol. 3, p. 20) and Durward (1951, Fig. 951).
34. *internal plantar nerve of second toe (Bock, 1827)*
Macrodissected adult human lateral branch of second ***common plantar digital nerve of medial plantar nerve (>1840)*** forming ***proper plantar digital nerve of medial plantar nerve (>1840)*** to medial part of second toe; in the original Latin, *nerv. plantaris internus digiti secundi*; Table VI, Figure 4-*15*. Also see Durward (1951, Fig. 951).
35. *internal collateral nerve of big toe (Cloquet, 1828)*
Macrodissected adult human ***proper plantar digital nerve of medial plantar nerve (>1840)*** to medial part of big toe; in the original French, *N. collatéral interne du gros orteil*, Plate CLXXIV, Figure 3-*10*.
36. *plantar internal collateral nerve of big toe (Cruveilhier, 1836)*
Macrodissected adult human ***proper plantar digital nerve of medial plantar nerve (>1840)*** to medial part of big toe; in the original French, *nerf collatéral interne plantaire du gros orteil*, p. 872.
37. *dorsal branch of plantar internal collateral nerve of big toe (Cruveilhier, 1836)*
Terminal branch of *plantar internal collateral nerve of big toe (Cruveilhier, 1836)* to dorsomedial parts of big toe; in the original Latin, *rameau dorsal*, p. 873.
38. *unguinal branch of plantar internal collateral nerve of big toe (Cruveilhier, 1836)*
Synonym for *dorsal branch of plantar internal collateral nerve of big toe (Cruveilhier, 1836)*; in the original French, *rameau onguéal*, p. 873.
39. *plantar branch of plantar internal collateral nerve of big toe (Cruveilhier, 1836)*
Terminal branch of *plantar internal collateral nerve of big toe (Cruveilhier, 1836)* to ventromedial parts of big toe; in the original Latin, *rameau plantaire*, p. 873.
40. *external collateral nerve of big toe (Cruveilhier, 1836)*
Macrodissected adult human ***proper plantar digital nerve of medial plantar nerve (>1840)*** to lateral part of big toe; in the original French, *nerf collatéral externe du gros orteil*, p. 873.
41. *external plantar collateral nerve of second toe (Cruveilhier, 1836)*
Macrodissected adult human ***proper plantar digital nerve of medial plantar nerve (>1840)*** to lateral part of second toe; in the original French, *nerf collatéral plantaire externe du second orteil*, p. 874.
42. *internal plantar collateral nerve of third toe (Cruveilhier, 1836)*
Macrodissected adult human ***proper plantar digital nerve of medial plantar nerve (>1840)*** to medial part of third toe; in the original French, *nerf collatéral plantaire interne du troisième*, p. 874.
43. *external collateral nerve of third toe (Cruveilhier, 1836)*
Macrodissected adult human ***proper plantar digital nerve of medial plantar nerve (>1840)*** to lateral part of third toe; in the original French, *nerf collatéral externe du troisième*, p. 874.

44. *internal collateral nerve of fourth toe (Cruveilhier, 1836)*
Macrodissected adult human ***proper plantar digital nerve of medial plantar nerve (>1840)*** to medial part of fourth toe; in the original French, *nerf collatéral plantaire interne du quatrième*, p. 874.

prostatic plexus (>1840)

As described for adult human male, it extends from the caudal (lower) part of the ***inferior hypogastric plexus (Tiedemann, 1822)***, where it is partly united with small ***nerves (Herophilus, c335–c280 BC)*** supplying the neck of the bladder, and enters and ramifies in the prostate gland. Minute ***ganglia (Galen, c173)*** are found on the ***nerves (Herophilus, c335–c280 BC)***, which also supply the prostatic urethra and ejaculatory ducts, and terminal ***axons (Kölliker, 1896)*** of the ***plexus (Galen, c192)*** communicate with small branches of the ***pudendal nerves (Camper, 1762)***; together they go on to innervate the penile blood vessels, erectile tissue, urethra, and bulbourethral glands; see Mitchell (1953, p. 307). It corresponds to the female ***uterovaginal plexus (>1840)***; see Durward (1951, p. 1144). It was perhaps first clearly described as the *nerve into glandules prostatae (Willis, 1664)*.

EARLIER REFERENCES:

Earlier synonyms:

1. *nerve into glandules prostatae (Willis, 1664)*
Willis mentioned ***nerves (Herophilus, c335–c280 BC)*** to prostate in macrodissected adult human and other common large mammals—reference to ***prostatic plexus (>1840)***; see Pordage translation (1681, p. 159 and Tab. 11-*g*).
2. *prostatic filaments of horizontal vesical plexus (Cruveilhier, 1836)*
Synonym for macrodissected adult human male ***prostatic plexus (>1840)***; in the original French, *filets prostatiques*, p. 1026.

proximal glossopharyngeal ganglion (>1840)

As described for macrodissected adult human, the smaller of two sensory ***cranial nerve ganglia (>1840)*** of the ***glossopharyngeal nerve (Huber, 1744)*** associated with the proximal part of the ***glossopharyngeal nerve trunk (Wrisberg, 1786; Günther, 1786)*** between ***glossopharyngeal nerve root (>1840)*** and ***distal glossopharyngeal ganglion (>1840)*** in the proximal (upper) part of the jugular foramen. It is often regarded as a detached part of the ***distal glossopharyngeal ganglion (>1840)***; see Williams & Warwick (1980, p. 1075 and Fig. 7.189). Its discovery is usually attributed to Ehrenritter; see ***[proximal glossopharyngeal ganglion (>1840)] (Ehrenritter, 1791)***.

EARLIER REFERENCES:

Described, not named or illustrated:

1. ***[proximal glossopharyngeal ganglion (>1840)] (Ehrenritter, 1791)***
Ehrenritter apparently discovered it, without realizing its exact relationship with ***glossopharyngeal nerve (Huber, 1744)***; see Soemmerring (1798, p. 262), Müller (1838, p. 609), Hovelacque (1927, p. 194).

Earlier synonyms:

1. *Ehrenritter's ganglion (Soemmerring, 1798)*
Eponym for macrodissected adult human ***proximal glossopharyngeal ganglion (>1840)*** without providing citation for Ehrenritter; p. 262, note 5. Also see Arnold (1826b), Müller (1837, p. 275), Todd (1836–1839, p. 495). In his 1798 footnote, Soemmerring went on, "Ganglion describunt Andersch, p. 5. Huber *Epistola ad Wigandum* p. 12-18."
2. *jugular ganglion (Müller, 1834)*
Synonym for macrodissected adult human ***proximal glossopharyngeal ganglion (>1840)***; pp. 588–589. Also see Todd (1836–1839, p. 495).
3. *superior ganglion of glossopharyngeal nerve (Todd, 1836–1839)*
Synonym for macrodissected adult human ***proximal glossopharyngeal ganglion (>1840)***; p. 495. Also see Arnold (1838a, p. 180).

proximal vagal ganglion (>1840)

As described for macrodissected adult human, the smaller of two sensory ***cranial nerve ganglia (>1840)*** of the ***vagus nerve (Galen, c192)*** associated with proximal parts of the ***vagus nerve trunk (Wrisberg, 1786; Günther, 1786)*** just proximal to the ***distal vagal ganglion (>1840)***; see Williams & Warwick (1980, pp. 1076, 1078 and Fig. 7.189). It was probably first identified as the *upper ganglioform infolding of wandring pair (Willis, 1664)*.

EARLIER REFERENCES:

Earlier synonyms:

1. *upper ganglioform infolding of wandring pair (Willis, 1664)*
Synonym for macrodissected adult human ***proximal vagal ganglion (>1840)***; in the original Latin, *plexus ganglioformis superior paris vagi*, see Pordage translation (1681, Tab. 9-*H*). Possible involvement of the ***proximal glossopharyngeal ganglion (1840)*** is not clear.
2. *highest ganglion of vagus nerve (Bischoff, 1832)*
Synonym for macrodissected adult human ***proximal vagal ganglion (>1840)***; in the original Latin, *ganglion supremum nervi Vagi*, Table I, Figure 1-27.
3. *superior vagal ganglion (>1840)*
Synonym for macrodissected adult human ***proximal vagal ganglion (>1840)***; see *Terminologia Anatomica* (1998, p. 136).
4. *jugular ganglion (>1840)*
Synonym for macrodissected adult human ***proximal vagal ganglion (>1840)***; see Williams & Warwick (1980, p. 1078), *Dorland's* (2003, p. 752).

pterygopalatine ganglion (>1840)

As described for macrodissected adult human, a ***terminal ganglion (Gaskell, 1886)*** in the pterygopalatine fossa with the ***nerve of pterygoid canal (>1840)*** and ***pharyngeal nerve (Bock, 1817)*** attached caudally, the ***pterygopalatine nerves (Wrisberg, 1786)*** attached dorsally, and the ***palatine nerves (Schaarschmidt, 1750)*** attached ventrally and rostrally; see Williams & Warwick (1980, pp. 1064–1066 and Figs. 7.177–179, 181). It was discovered and described as the *sphenopalatine ganglion (Meckel, 1751)*.

EARLIER REFERENCES:

Earlier synonyms:

1. *sphenopalatine ganglion (Meckel, 1751)*
   Synonym for macrodissected adult human ***pterygopalatine ganglion (>1840)*** discovered, described, and illustrated by Meckel; in the original French, *le ganglion sphénopalatin*, p. 86 and Figure 1-*n*.
2. *maxillo-pterygoid plexus (Le Cat, 1768)*
   Synonym for macrodissected adult human ***pterygopalatine ganglion (>1840)***; in the original French, *plexus maxillo-pterigoïdien*, Plate VIII, Figure 4-*i*.
3. *maxillo-Vidian plexus (Le Cat, 1768)*
   Synonym for macrodissected adult human ***pterygopalatine ganglion (>1840)***; in the original French, *plexus maxillo-vidien*, Plate VIII, Figure 4-*i*.
4. *sphenomaxillary ganglion (Wrisberg, 1786)*
   Synonym for macrodissected adult human ***pterygopalatine ganglion (>1840)***; in the original Latin, *ganglion sphenomaxillare*, see Wrisberg reprint (1800, p. 373).
5. *spheno-palatin ganglion (Bell, 1803b)*
   Alternate form of *sphenopalatine ganglion (Meckel, 1751)*; Plate 1-*G*.
6. *ganglion of Miekel (Bell & Bell, 1803a)*
   Unusual spelling of eponym for macrodissected adult human ***pterygopalatine ganglion (>1840)***; p. 140.
7. *Meckel's ganglion (Portal, 1803a)*
   Eponym for macrodissected adult human *sphenopalatine ganglion (Meckel, 1751)*; in the original French, *ganglion de Meckel*, p. 162.
8. *sphenoidal ganglion (Burdin, 1803)*
   Synonym for macrodissected adult human ***pterygopalatine ganglion (>1840)***; see translation (1803, Vol. 1, p. 173).
9. *sphenopalatine ganglion of Meckel (Bock, 1817)*
   Eponym for macrodissected adult human *sphenopalatine ganglion (Meckel, 1751)*; in the original Latin, *ganglion sphenopalatinum Meckelii*, p. 26.
10. *rhinal ganglion (Arnold, 1834)*
   Synonym for macrodissected adult human ***pterygopalatine ganglion (>1840)***; in the original Latin, *ganglion rhinicum*, p. 9. Arnold described filaments of ***pterygopalatine ganglion (>1840)*** joining ***optic nerve (Vicq d'Azyr, 1784)***, and sometimes associating with ***ciliary ganglion (Loder, 1778)***; p. 9.
11. *nasal ganglion (Arnold, 1834)*
   Synonym for macrodissected adult human ***pterygopalatine ganglion (>1840)***; in the original Latin, *ganglion nasale*, p. 9.

pterygopalatine nerves (Wrisberg, 1786)

As described for macrodissected adult human, one, usually two, or even three short ***communicating branches (Winslow, 1733)*** between ***maxillary nerve (Meckel, 1753)*** dorsally and ***pterygopalatine ganglion (>1840)*** ventrally, also known as *ganglionic branches of maxillary nerve (>1840)* and *sensory root of pterygopalatine ganglion (>1840)*. Functionally, they contain secretomotor ***axons (Kölliker, 1896)*** for the lacrimal gland and sensory ***dendrites (His, 1889)*** ending in the orbital periosteum and mucus membranes of the nose, palate, and pharynx; see Hamilton (1976, p. 624), Williams & Warwick (1980, p. 1063 and Figs. 7.177–179). For Wrisberg's use in macrodissected adult human, see p. 373. They were probably discovered by Winslow; see ***[pterygopalatine nerves (Wrisberg, 1786)] (Winslow, 1733)***.

EARLIER REFERENCES:

Described, not named or illustrated:

1. ***[pterygopalatine nerves (Wrisberg, 1786)] (Winslow, 1733)***
   Probably alluded to for macrodissected adult human, especially in relation to innervation of auditory (Eustachian) tube by branch of *spheno-palatine ramus of superior maxillary nerve (Winslow, 1733)*; Section VI, p. 65.

Earlier synonyms:

1. *descending branch of superior maxillary nerve (Meckel, 1748)*
   Roughly synonymous with macrodissected adult human ***pterygopalatine nerves (Wrisberg, 1786)***; in the original Latin, *ramus descendens nervi maxillaris superioris*, Figure 1-57. Also see *sphenopalatine ganglion (Meckel, 1751)*. It was nicely illustrated for macrodissected adult human by Le Cat (1768; Pl. VIII, Fig. 5).
2. *sphenopalatine nerve (Schaarschmidt, 1750)*
   Synonym for macrodissected adult human ***pterygopalatine nerves (Wrisberg, 1786)***; in the original Latin, *nervus sphenopalatinus*, p. 19. Also see His (1895, p. 88).

LATER SYNONYMS:

1. *common trunk of pterygoid and palatine nerves (Soemmerring, 1791)*
   Synonym for macrodissected adult human ***pterygopalatine nerves (Wrisberg, 1786)***; in the original Latin, *truncus communis pro Pterygoideo et Palatino*, p. 201.
2. *trunk of pterygopalatine nerve (Meckel, 1817)*
   Synonym for macrodissected adult human ***pterygopalatine nerves (Wrisberg, 1786)***; see translation (1832, Vol. 3, p. 68). Wrisberg (1786) had referred in macrodissected adult human to *trunco pterygoideo*; see Wrisberg reprint (1800, p. 373).
3. *sphenopalatine branch of superior maxillary branch of fifth pair of nerves (Bock, 1817)*
   Synonym for macrodissected adult human ***pterygopalatine nerves (Wrisberg, 1786)***; in the original Latin, *ramus sphenopalatinus*, p. 20.

4. *sphenopalatine ganglion branches from superior maxillary nerve (Langenbeck, 1826–1830)*
   Synonym for macrodissected adult human ***pterygopalatine nerves (Wrisberg, 1786)***; in the original Latin, *ganglii sphenopalatini rami ex nervo maxillari superiori*, Fascicle III, Table XIX-*b*.
5. *ascending branches of spheno-palatine ganglion (Quain, 1828)*
   Synonym for macrodissected adult human ***pterygopalatine nerves (Wrisberg, 1786)***; p. 666.
6. *naso-palatine nerve (Todd, 1836–1839)*
   Todd noted it is sometimes a synonym for ***pterygopalatine nerves (Wrisberg, 1786)*** in "inferior Mammalia" where ***pterygopalatine ganglion (>1840)*** was not identified; p. 287.
7. *superior branches of spheno-palatine ganglion (Quain, 1837)*
   Synonym for macrodissected adult human ***pterygopalatine nerves (Wrisberg, 1786)***; p. 811.
8. *branches of communication of superior maxillary nerve from Meckel's ganglion (Quain & Wilson, 1839)*
   Synonym for macrodissected adult human ***pterygopalatine nerves (Wrisberg, 1786)***; Plate XIII, Figure 2-*o*.
9. *spheno-palatine ganglion ascending branches of communication with superior maxillary nerve (Quain & Wilson, 1839)*
   Synonym for macrodissected adult human ***pterygopalatine nerves (Wrisberg, 1786)***; Plate XXVII-*G,l*.
10. *ganglionic branches to maxillary nerve (>1840)*
   Synonym for macrodissected adult human ***pterygopalatine nerves (Wrisberg, 1786)***; see Durward (1951, p. 1033), Williams & Warwick (1980, p. 1063), *Terminologia Anatomica* (1998, p. 134).
11. *sensory root of pterygopalatine ganglion (>1840)*
   Misleading synonym for macrodissected adult human ***pterygopalatine nerves (Wrisberg, 1786)***; see *Terminologia Anatomica* (1998, p. 134).

PARTLY CORRESPONDS:

1. *anterior root of sphenopalatine ganglion (Meckel, 1751)*
   Rostral (anterior) ***pterygopalatine nerve (Wrisberg, 1786)***; in the original French, *la racine antérieure du ganglion sphénopalatin*, see Figure 1-*l*.
2. *posterior descending branchlet to sphenopalatine ganglion (Meckel, 1751)*
   Caudal (posterior) ***pterygopalatine nerve (Wrisberg, 1786)***; in the original French, *la petit branche postérieure descendente pour le ganglion sphénopalatin*, see Figure 1-*m*.
3. *anterior superior nasal nerves (Soemmerring, 1791)*
   Complementary to ***posterior superior nasal nerves (Soemmerring, 1791)*** for macrodissected adult human component of ***pterygopalatine nerves (Wrisberg, 1786)***; in the original Latin, *nervos nasales superiores anteriores*, p. 201.
4. *nervos nasales priores (Soemmerring, 1798)*
   Synonym for *anterior superior nasal nerves (Soemmerring, 1791)*, p. 223.

pudendal nerve (Camper, 1762)

As described for macrodissected adult human, the major somatic ***nerve (Herophilus, c335–c280 BC)*** of the perineum; see Durward (1951, p. 1144). It commonly arises from the 2nd–4th sacral ***sacral plexus ventral divisions (Paterson, 1887)*** and generates the ***inferior rectal nerves (>1840)*** before dividing into two terminal branches, ***perineal nerve (Camper, 1762)*** and ***dorsal nerve of clitoris (>1840)*** or ***dorsal nerve of penis (Camper, 1762)***; see Durward (1951, pp. 1101–1102, Fig. 943), Williams & Warwick (1980, pp. 1115–1116). For Camper's use in macrodissected adult human, see p. 7. It was known to Galen; see ***[pudendal nerve (Camper, 1762)] (Galen, c173)***.

TRANSLATIONS:

1. *nervus pudendus (Camper, 1762)*
   Original Latin form of ***pudendal nerve (Camper, 1762)***; p. 7.

EARLIER REFERENCES:

Described, not named or illustrated:

1. ***[pudendal nerve (Camper, 1762)] (Galen, c173)***
   Galen clearly described ***nerve (Herophilus, c335–c280 BC)*** to rectum, penis, uterus, and muscles and skin associated with the latter two in macrodissected adult beef, pig, and/or macaque but not human; see May translation (1968, pp. 651, 652), Duckworth translation (1962, pp. 132, 263). Colombo (1559) has been credited with the first modern description for macrodissected adult human; see Crooke (1615, p. 906). Fischer provided extremely detailed account for macrodissected adult human (1791, pp. 20–22).

Illustrated, not named or described:

1. ***[pudendal nerve (Camper, 1762)] (Eustachi, 1552)***
   Illustrated clearly for macrodissected adult human, although origin was not shown; see Albinus edition (1761, Tab. 20/2-φ, p. 120).

Illustrated and described, not named:

1. ***[pudendal nerve (Camper, 1762)] (Vieussens, 1684)***
   Illustrated and described clearly for macrodissected adult human; see Table 29-*N*.

LATER SYNONYMS:

1. *common pudendal nerve (Haase, 1781)*
   Synonym for macrodissected adult human ***pudendal nerve (Camper, 1762)***; in the original Latin, *nervus pudendus communis*, p. 108. It may also refer to trunk of ***pudendal nerve (Camper, 1762)***.
2. *scrotal nerve (Martin, 1781)*
   Synonym for macrodissected adult human ***pudendal nerve (Camper, 1762)***; p. 234.
3. *external pudendal nerve (Mayer, 1794)*
   Synonym for macrodissected adult human ***pudendal nerve (Camper, 1762)***; in the original Latin, *nervus pudendus externus*; see Part 6, Table VI-*178* (p. 40).
4. *nervi pudici (Fyfe, 1800)*
   Synonym for right and left macrodissected adult human ***pudendal nerve (Camper, 1762)***, which Fyfe described as having superior and inferior fasciculi; Vol. 2, p. 325.

5. *ischio-penian nerve (Burdin, 1803)*
Synonym for macrodissected adult human male ***pudendal nerve (Camper, 1762)***; see translation (1803, Vol. 1, p. 203).
6. *ischio-clitorian nerve (Burdin, 1803)*
Synonym for macrodissected adult human female ***pudendal nerve (Camper, 1762)***; see translation (1803, Vol. 1, p. 203).
7. *pudic nerve (Bell & Bell, 1816)*
English form (singular) of macrodissected adult human *nervi pudici (Fyfe, 1800)*; Vol. 2, p. 542.
8. *external common hemorrhoidal nerve (Meckel, 1817)*
Synonym for macrodissected adult human ***pudendal nerve (Camper, 1762)***; see translation (1832, Vol. 3, p. 14).
9. *external common pudendohemorrhoidal nerve (Meckel, 1817)*
Synonym for macrodissected adult human ***pudendal nerve (Camper, 1762)***; in the original Latin, *nervus pudendo-haemorrhoidalis communis externus*, see translation (1832, Vol. 3, p. 14).
10. *inferior pudic nerve (Knox, 1832)*
Synonym for macrodissected adult human ***pudendal nerve (Camper, 1762)***; Plate XI-*133*, in describing Walter (1783, Tab. I, Fig. 2).
11. *long pudic nerve (Knox, 1832)*
Synonym for macrodissected adult human ***pudendal nerve (Camper, 1762)***; Plate XI-*133*, in describing Walter (1783, Tab. I, Fig. 2).
12. *internal pudic nerve (Quain & Wilson, 1839)*
Synonym for macrodissected adult human ***pudendal nerve (Camper, 1762)***; Plate XXII-*C*.

PARTLY CORRESPONDS:
1. *internal pudendal nerve (Cruveilhier, 1836)*
Essentially macrodissected adult human ***perineal nerve (Camper, 1762)*** and ***dorsal nerve of penis (Camper, 1762)*** or ***dorsal nerve of clitoris (>1840)*** considered together; in the original French, *nerf honteux interne*, pp. 851–852.

pulmonary branches of vagus nerve (Cloquet, 1828)

As described for macrodissected adult human, numerous branches derived mostly from parts of the ***vagus nerve trunk (Wrisberg, 1786; Günther, 1786)*** lying dorsal to (behind) the root of the lung, although 3–4 branches depart before the trunk splits into the two ***esophageal branches of vagus nerve (>1840)***, and smaller branches are generated from the short segment of the ***vagus nerve trunk (Wrisberg, 1786; Günther, 1786)*** passing ventral (anterior) to the lung root; see Mitchell (1953, p. 183), Standring (2008, p. 945). Sometimes they are divided into anterior pulmonary (bronchial) branches and posterior pulmonary (bronchial) branches; see Williams & Warwick (1980, p. 1081), Standring (2008, p. 945). They initially course along the trachea and bronchi, as beautifully illustrated by Scarpa (1794, Tab. V). For Cloquet's use in macrodissected adult human, see Plate CLXXVII:*189–195*. They were first described as *branches in thorax to lung from sixth pair of nerves (Galen, c173)*.

TRANSLATIONS:
1. *rameaux pulmonaires du nerf vague (Cloquet, 1828)*
Original French form of ***pulmonary branches of vagus nerve (Cloquet, 1828)***; Plate CLXXVII:*189–195*.

EARLIER REFERENCES:

Earlier synonyms:
1. *branches in thorax to lung from sixth pair of nerves (Galen, c173)*
Synonym for ***pulmonary branches of vagus nerve (Cloquet, 1828)*** in macrodissected beef, pig, and/or macaque but not human; see May translation (1960, pp. 367, 694), Duckworth translation (1962, p. 204). For Galen's clinical observations see Siegel translation (1976, p. 122). Vesalius (1543a) used essentially the same description for macrodissected adult human, which he also illustrated; see Richardson & Carman translation (2002, p. 199).
2. *pneumonic branches of wandring pair (Willis, 1664)*
Synonym for macrodissected adult human ***pulmonary branches of vagus nerve (Cloquet, 1828)***; see Pordage translation (1681, p. 148) where it is spelled *pneumonick*.
3. *pneumonic nerves arising from eighth pair of cerebral nerves (Albinus, 1744)*
Synonym for macrodissected adult human ***pulmonary branches of vagus nerve (Cloquet, 1828)***; in the original Latin, *nervi pneumonici orientes ab octavo pari nervorum cerebri*, Table 18, Figure 2-*δ*.
4. *pulmonary nerves (Walter, 1783)*
Synonym for macrodissected adult human ***pulmonary branches of vagus nerve (Cloquet, 1828)***; Walter enumerated at least seven of them. In the original Latin (singular), *nervus pulmonalis*, Table III:*406–429*.
5. *inferior tracheal nerves (Meckel, 1817)*
Synonym for macrodissected adult human ***pulmonary branches of vagus nerve (Cloquet, 1828)***; see translation (1832, Vol. 3, p. 49).

LATER SYNONYMS:
1. *tracheal branches of vagus nerve (Quain, 1828)*
Synonym for macrodissected adult human ***pulmonary branches of vagus nerve (Cloquet, 1828)***; p. 657.
2. *bronchial branches of vagus nerve (Quain, 1832)*
Synonym for macrodissected adult human ***pulmonary branches of vagus nerve (Cloquet, 1828)***; p. 669.

PARTLY CORRESPONDS:
1. *inferior tracheal nerves proceeding before trachea (Meckel, 1817)*
Macrodissected adult human ventral (anterior) branches of ***pulmonary branches of vagus nerve (Cloquet, 1828)***; see translation (1832, Vol. 3, p. 49).
2. *inferior tracheal nerves proceeding behind trachea (Meckel, 1817)*
Macrodissected adult human dorsal (posterior) branches of ***pulmonary branches of vagus nerve (Cloquet, 1828)***; see translation (1832, Vol. 3, p. 49).

3. *anterior pulmonary branches of pneumogastric nerve (Cruveilhier, 1836)*
   Synonym for macrodissected adult human *inferior tracheal nerves proceeding before trachea (Meckel, 1817)*; in the original French, *rameaux pulmonaires antérieurs*, p. 964.
4. *posterior pulmonary branches of pneumogastric nerve (Cruveilhier, 1836)*
   Synonym for macrodissected adult human *inferior tracheal nerves proceeding behind trachea (Meckel, 1817)*; in the original French, *rameaux pulmonaires postèrieur*, p. 964.
5. *posterior bronchial branches of pneumogastric nerve (Cruveilhier, 1836)*
   Synonym for *inferior tracheal nerves proceeding behind trachea (Meckel, 1817)*; in the original French, *rameaux bronchiques postèrieur*, p. 964.

pulmonary plexus (Winslow, 1733)

As described structurally and functionally for adult human, a mixture of sympathetic and parasympathetic ***axons (Kölliker, 1896)***, parasympathetic ***ganglia (Galen, c173)***, and sensory ***dendrites (His, 1889)***—with branches to vascular and bronchial structures, and the pleura; see Mitchell (1953, p. 256), Williams & Warwick (1980, pp. 1133, 1267). "Communications between the pulmonary, cardiac, aortic, and oesophageal plexuses are always present [Fig. 105]" (Mitchell, 1953, p. 256). It is traditionally divided into ***anterior pulmonary plexus (Haller, 1762)*** and ***posterior pulmonary plexus (Haller, 1762)***. For Winslow's use in macrodissected adult human, see Section VI, pp. 74, 97. It was probably known to Vieussens; see *nerveos plexus pneumonicos (Vieussens, 1684)*.

TRANSLATIONS:

1. *plexus pulmonaris (Winslow, 1733)*
   Original Latin form of ***pulmonary plexus (Winslow, 1733)***; Section VI, pp. 74, 97.

EARLIER REFERENCES:

Earlier synonyms:

1. *nerveos plexus pneumonicos (Vieussens, 1684)*
   Apparently refers to macrodissected adult human ***pulmonary plexus (Winslow, 1733)***; Table 23-13.
2. *plexus pneumonicus (Drake, 1707)*
   Derived from *nerveos plexus pneumonicos (Vieussens, 1684)* for macrodissected adult human; p. 517. Palfijn (1726, Part 2, p. 334) used the French, *plexus pneumonique*.

LATER SYNONYMS:

1. *bronchial plexus (Cruveilhier, 1836)*
   Synonym for macrodissected adult human ***pulmonary plexus (Winslow, 1733)***; in the original French, *plexus bronchiques*, p. 965.

PARTLY CORRESPONDS:

1. *nerves to sheaths of lungs (Galen, c192)*
   Galen reported these branches of ***pulmonary plexus (Winslow, 1733)*** in macrodissected adult beef, pig, and/or macaque but not human; see Duckworth translation (1962, p. 204). Vesalius (1543a) described and illustrated for macrodissected adult human "small branches of the sixth pair; they run into the tunic of the lungs" (Richardson & Carman translation, 2002, p. 172, item q2). Willis described them in more detail for macrodissected adult human; see Pordage translation (1681, p. 148).
2. *nerve of right pulmonary branches (Andersch & Soemmerring, 1792)*
   Branch of *anterior branch of right trunk of right nerve of heart (Andersch & Soemmerring, 1792)* also associated with *right auricular nerve of heart (Andersch & Soemmerring, 1792)* and right ***pulmonary branches of vagus nerve (Cloquet, 1828)***-essentially component of ***pulmonary plexus (Winslow, 1733)***; in the original Latin, *nervum rami pulmonarii dexteri*, p. 196.
3. *nerve to right pulmonary sinus (Andersch & Soemmerring, 1792)*
   Ultimately branch of macrodissected adult human right ***pulmonary plexus (Winslow, 1733)***; in the original Latin, *nervum dextrum sinus pulmonarii*, p. 197.
4. *nerve of right pulmonary artery branches (Andersch, 1797)*
   Synonym for *nerve of right pulmonary branches (Andersch & Soemmerring, 1792)*; in the original Latin, *nervum rami dextri arteriae pulmonariae*, Vol. 1, p. 164.
5. *nerve to left pulmonary sinus (Andersch, 1797)*
   Ultimately branch of macrodissected adult human right ***pulmonary plexus (Winslow, 1733)***; in the original Latin, *nervo sinistro sinus pulmonarii*, Vol. 2, p. 25.
6. *superior superficial nerve to pulmonary arteries (Andersch, 1797)*
   Ultimately branch of macrodissected adult human right ***pulmonary plexus (Winslow, 1733)*** to caudal (inferior) regions of pulmonary artery; in the original Latin, *nervus superficialis superioris arteriae pulmonariae*, Vol. 2, p. 32.
7. *inferior superficial nerve to pulmonary arteries (Andersch, 1797)*
   Ultimately branch of macrodissected adult human right ***pulmonary plexus (Winslow, 1733)*** to rostral (superior) regions of pulmonary artery; in the original Latin, *nervus superficialis inferioris arteriae pulmonariae*, Vol. 2, p. 32.
8. *pulmonary branches of left superior superficial nerve (Andersch, 1797)*
   Pulmonary branches of left *superior superficial nerve to pulmonary arteries (Andersch, 1797)*-essentially component of ***pulmonary plexus (Winslow, 1733)***; in the original Latin, *nervus superficialis superior rami pulmonarii sinistri*, Vol. 2, p. 33.
9. *nerve to left pulmonary sinus of heart (Andersch, 1797)*
   Synonym for *nerve to left pulmonary sinus (Andersch, 1797)*; in the original Latin, *nervum sinistrum sinus pulmonarii cordis*, p. 40.
10. *nerve to right pulmonary sinus of heart (Andersch, 1797)*
   Ultimately branch of macrodissected adult human right ***pulmonary plexus (Winslow, 1733)***; in the original Latin, *nervum dextrum sinus pulmonarii cordis*, p. 40.

11. *pulmonary nerves (Chaussier, 1809)*
    Basically synonym for macrodissected adult human *nerves to sheaths of lungs (Galen, c192)*; in the original French, *nerfs pulmonaires.*

pulvinar (Burdach, 1822)

As described for macrodissected adult human, a large swelling on the caudal end of the ***thalamus (His, 1893a)***, just dorsal to the ***dorsal lateral geniculate nucleus (>1840)***. Based on cellular architecture and connections, the largest component of the human ***lateral thalamic nuclei (>1840)***, although its identification in some nonprimate species is problematic; see Williams & Warwick (1980, p. 960), Jones (1985, Ch. 10), Nieuwenhuys et al. (2008, Figs. 5.9, 5.22, 5.31). For Burdach's use in macrodissected adult human, see p. 117. It was first described as the *posterior thalamic tubercle (Vicq d'Azyr, 1786).*

EARLIER REFERENCES:

Earlier synonyms:

1. *posterior thalamic tubercle (Vicq d'Azyr, 1786)*
   Synonym for macrodissected adult human ***pulvinar (Burdach, 1822)***; Table XX-30. See Burdach (1822, p. 341), Polyak (1957, p. 115), Meyer (1971, p. 23).
2. *corpus geniculatum internum (Ramsay, 1813)*
   Mistakenly used as synonym for macrodissected adult human *posterior thalamic tubercle (Vicq d'Azyr, 1786)*; p. 45.
3. *tuberculum ganglii postici posterius (Meckel, 1817)*
   Synonym for macrodissected adult human ***pulvinar (Burdach, 1822)***; p. 511. See Burdach (1822, p. 341), Polyak (1957, p. 115).
4. *tuberculum ganglii postici posterius superius (Meckel, 1817)*
   Synonym for macrodissected adult human ***pulvinar (Burdach, 1822)***; p. 511. See Burdach (1822, p. 341), Polyak (1957, p. 115).

putamen (Burdach, 1822)

As described for macrodissected adult human, one of two distinct components of the ***caudoputamen (Heimer & Wilson, 1975)***, separated from the other component, ***caudate nucleus (Arnold, 1838b)***, by the ***anterior limb of internal capsule (>1840)***; see Nieuwenhuys et al. (p. 429 and Fig. 5.31). For Burdach's use in macrodissected adult human, see p. 117; also see Meyer (1971, p. 30). It was clearly illustrated by Vesalius; see ***[putamen (Burdach, 1822)] (Vesalius, 1543a).***

EARLIER REFERENCES:

Illustrated, not named or described:

1. ***[putamen (Burdach, 1822)] (Vesalius, 1543a)***
   Clearly illustrated in frontal (horizontal) section of macrodissected adult human; see Singer translation (1952, p. 100).

Earlier synonyms:

1. *external part of superior great cerebral ganglion (Gall & Spurzheim, 1810)*
   Synonym for macrodissected adult human ***putamen (Burdach, 1822)***; in the original French, *partie externe du grand ganglion cérébral supérieur*, p. 234 and Plate V-*L*.

pyloric branches of anterior vagal trunk (>1840)

As described for macrodissected adult human, there are usually two of them going most prominently to the pylorus and upper duodenum, and communicating with the ***hepatic plexus (Rau, 1720)***; see Mitchell (1953, pp. 186–187). They were known to Vesalius; see ***[pyloric branches of anterior vagal trunk (>1840)] (Vesalius, 1543a).***

EARLIER REFERENCES:

Described, not named or illustrated:

1. ***[pyloric branches of anterior vagal trunk (>1840)] (Vesalius, 1543a)***
   Described and illustrated for macrodissected adult human; see Richardson & Carman translation (2002, pp. 199–200; 2007, Fig. 15-*X*, p. 21), and Haller (1762, pp. 236–237).

pyramid (Willis, 1664)

As described for macrodissected adult human, and mammal generally with histological methods for ***axons (Kölliker, 1896)***, the ventral segment of the ***corticospinal tract (>1840)*** on either side of the median plane of the ***medulla (Winslow, 1733)***, between ***longitudinal pontine fibers (Arnold, 1838b)*** rostrally and ***pyramidal decussation (Reil, 1809c)*** caudally; see Nieuwenhuys et al. (2008, Figure 3.12-36, called *pyramid* on surface; and Figures 6.22–6.24, called *pyramidal tract* in cross section). Willis named the ***pyramids (Willis, 1664)*** in macrodissected adult human and other large mammals and indicated they resemble great ***nerves (Herophilus, c335–c280 BC)*** emerging from the caudal border of the ***middle cerebellar peduncle (Rolando, 1819)*** on either side of the ventral surface (base) of the ***medulla (Winslow, 1733)***; see Pordage translation (1681, pp. 68, 124). It was vaguely indicated by Vesalius; see ***[pyramid (Willis, 1664)] (Vesalius, 1543a).***

EARLIER REFERENCES:

Illustrated, not named or described:

1. ***[pyramid (Willis, 1664)] (Vesalius, 1543a)***
   In illustrating ventral surface of macrodissected adult human ***brain (Smith Papyrus, c1700 BC)***, Vesalius vaguely depicted left ***pyramid (Willis, 1664)*** on right side of figure; see Richardson & Carman translation (2002, p. 168). There is no hint of the ***olive (Tiedemann, 1821)***. Eustachi (1552) illustrated ***pyramid (Willis, 1664)*** much more clearly, although his plates (without text) were not published until 1714; see Albinus edition (1744, Plate XVIII), Roberts & Tomlinson (1992, Pl. 46).

Earlier synonyms:

1. *pyramidal body (Willis, 1664)*
   Synonym for ***pyramid (Willis, 1664)***; see Pordage translation (1681, pp. 68, 124).

LATER SYNONYMS:

1. *olivaria (Du Verney, 1683)*
   Synonym for macrodissected adult human ***pyramids (Willis, 1664)***; see translation (1737, Pl. XI, Fig. I-*Y*). Also see Winslow (1733, Sect. X, p. 41).

2. *pyramidal eminence (Garengeot, 1728)*
   Synonym for macrodissected adult human ***pyramid (Willis, 1664)***; in the original French, *éminence piramidale*, p. 485.
3. *corpora olivaria (Winslow, 1733)*
   Following Du Verney, synonym for macrodissected adult human ***pyramids (Willis, 1664)***; Section X, p. 42. See *olivaria (Du Verney, 1683)*; Winslow and Du Verney switched ***pyramid (Willis, 1664)*** and ***olive (Tiedemann, 1821)***.
4. *posterior pyramidal body (Tarin, 1750)*
   Synonym for macrodissected adult human ***pyramid (Willis, 1664)***; in the original Latin (plural), *corpora pyramidalis posteriora*, Table I, Figure 4-S. Clearly a mistake, called inept by Günther (1786, p 22); see *anterior pyramidal body (Tarin, 1750, Tab. II)*. Also see *posterior cerebellar process (Willis, 1664)* and *posterior pyramid (Procháska, 1800)*, both synonyms for roughly macrodissected adult human ***inferior cerebellar peduncle (Günther, 1786)***.
5. *anterior pyramidal body (Tarin, 1750, Tab. II)*
   Synonym for macrodissected adult human ***pyramid (Willis, 1664)***; in the original Latin, *corpus pyramidale anterius*, Table II, Figure 1-*d*.
6. *fasciae medullares (Malacarne, 1776)*
   Synonym for macrodissected adult human ***pyramids (Willis, 1664)***; p. 86, according to Burdach (1822, p. 281). Gordon (1815, p. 177) supplied the French, *bandes medulaires*.
7. *crus cerebri posteriora Tarini (Soemmerring, 1778)*
   Eponym for macrodissected adult human ***pyramid (Willis, 1664)***; Table II-*Z*.
8. *crus cerebri super pontem emergentia (Soemmerring, 1778)*
   Synonym for macrodissected adult human ***pyramid (Willis, 1664)***; Table II-*Z*.
9. *corpora pyramidalia superiora (Mayer, 1779)*
   Synonym for macrodissected adult human ***pyramids (Willis, 1664)***; p. 65, according to Burdach (1822, p. 281).
10. *posterior pyramidal body of Tarin (Vicq d'Azyr, 1786)*
   Eponym for macrodissected adult human ***pyramid (Willis, 1664)***; Plate XVIII-57. Also see *anterior pyramidal body (Tarin, 1750, Tab. II)*.
11. *anterior and internal pyramidal bodies (Günther, 1786)*
   Synonym for macrodissected adult human ***pyramids (Willis, 1664)***; in the original Latin, *corpora pyramidalia, quae anteriora & interna quibusdam audiunt*, p. 22.
12. *corpora pyramidalia interiora (Procháska, 1800)*
   Synonym for macrodissected adult human ***pyramids (Willis, 1664)***; Vol. 1, p. 357, according to Burdach (1822, p. 281), who wrote that Procháska also used *corpora pyramidalia antica*—see *anterior pyramidal body (Haase, 1781)*.
13. *median eminences of spinal bulb (Chaussier, 1807)*
   Synonym for macrodissected adult human ***pyramids (Willis, 1664)***; in the original French, *éminences médianes du bulb rachidien*, p. 122. Burdach (1822, p. 281) gave the Latin form, *eminentias medianas bulbi rachidici*.
14. *oblong eminence (Gordon, 1815)*
   Synonym for macrodissected adult human ***pyramid (Willis, 1664)***; p. 177. Burdach (1822, p. 281) supplied the Latin (plural), *eminentias oblongas*.
15. *pyramidal fasciculus (Tiedemann, 1816)*
   Synonym for ***pyramid (Willis, 1664)*** observed in alcohol-hardened macrodissected fetal human; Tiedemann noted it can be followed uninterrupted through ***pons (Haller, 1747)***; see translation (1826, p. 143).
16. *eminentiae medianae internae (Meckel, 1817)*
   Synonym listed for macrodissected adult human ***pyramids (Willis, 1664)***; see translation (1832, Vol. 2, p. 420).
17. *funiculi pyramidum (Burdach, 1822)*
   Synonym for macrodissected adult human ***pyramids (Willis, 1664)***; p. 31.
18. *inferior pyramids (Desmoulins, 1825)*
   Synonym for macrodissected adult human ***pyramids (Willis, 1664)***; in the original French, *pyramides inférieures*, p. 219.

PARTLY CORRESPONDS:

1. *superior pyramidal body (Mayer, 1794)*
   Rostral part of macrodissected adult human ***pyramid (Willis, 1664)***, toward ***pons (Haller, 1747)***; in the original Latin (plural), *corpora pyramidalia superiora*; Part 5, Table III, Figure 1-*o*.
2. *inferior pyramidal body (Mayer, 1794)*
   Caudal part of macrodissected adult human ***pyramid (Willis, 1664)***, toward ***spinal cord (*****Galen, c162–c166*****)***; in the original Latin (plural), *corpora pyramidalia inferiora*; Part 5, Table III, Figure 1-*q*.

pyramidal decussation (Reil, 1809c)

As described for macrodissected adult human, and mammal generally with histological methods for ***axons (Kölliker, 1896)***, the short segment of the ***corticospinal tract (>1840)*** between ***pyramid (Willis, 1664)*** rostrally and ***crossed corticospinal tract (>1840)*** and ***uncrossed corticospinal tract (>1840)*** caudally. It is usually described as lying at the ventral border or transition between ***medulla (Winslow, 1733)*** and ***spinal cord (Galen, c162–c166)***; see Crosby et al. (1962, pp. 112, 116–118), Nieuwenhuys et al. (2008, p. 69 and Figs. 6.6, 6.21). For Reil's use in macrodissected adult human, see Mayo translation, "decussation of the pyramids" (1823, p. 85). Burdach (1822, p. 31) wrote of the *fibrae decussantes pyramidum*, in contrast to the longitudinal fibers, which he referred to as the *fibrae primitivae pyramidum*. Its first accurate description and illustration were by Pourfour du Petit; see ***[pyramidal decussation (Reil, 1809c)] (Pourfour du Petit, 1710)***.

EARLIER REFERENCES:

Illustrated and described, not named:

1. ***[pyramidal decussation (Reil, 1809c)] (Pourfour du Petit, 1710)***
   Pourfour du Petit clearly described and illustrated it for macrodissected adult human, tracing fibrous *white substance (Vesalius, 1543a)* from ***cerebral cortex***

(>1840) to ***pyramidal decussation (Reil, 1809c)***; see Clarke & O'Malley (1996, pp. 283–284). A year earlier, Mistichelli (1709) described what some have interpreted as the same feature, although the crossing he described is actually associated with fibers in covering ***dura (Galen, c177)*** rather than the *white substance (Vesalius, 1543a)*; see Burdach (1822, pp. 280, 282–283), Thomas (1910), Clarke & O'Malley (1996, pp. 282–283), Bennett & Hacker (2002, p. 18).

LATER SYNONYMS:

1. *decussation of pyramidal bodies (Spurzheim, 1826)*
   Synonym for macrodissected adult mammalian ***pyramidal decussation (Reil, 1809c)***; p. 147. Quain & Wilson (1839, Pl. XII, Fig. 1-C) used *decussation of corpora pyramidalia* for macrodissected adult human.
2. *decussation of anterior pyramids (Spurzheim, 1826)*
   Synonym for macrodissected adult mammalian ***pyramidal decussation (Reil, 1809c)***; p. 231-*1*.

PARTLY CORRESPONDS:

1. *pyramidal commissure (Arnold, 1838b)*
   As described for macrodissected adult human, feature sometimes found just rostral to ***pyramidal decussation (Reil, 1809c)***; in the original Latin, *commissura pyramidum*, Table II, Figure 4-*e*.

pyramis (Malacarne, 1776)

As described for macrodissected adult human, the part of the ***cerebellar vermis (Meckel, 1817)*** between ***tuber vermis (>1840)*** and ***uvula (Malacarne, 1776)***, roughly medial to the right and left ***biventral lobule (>1840)*** of the ***cerebellar hemisphere (Willis, 1664)***; see Angevine et al. (1961, Fig. 24), Larsell & Jansen (1972, Fig. 118), Carpenter (1976, Figs. 2.26, 14.1), Nieuwenhuys et al. (2008, Fig. 3.8-36). The English form *pyramid* is to be avoided because of possible confusion with ***pyramid (Willis, 1664)***; see *Terminologia Anatomica* (1998, p. 119). For Malacarne's discovery and use in macrodissected adult human, see Clarke & O'Malley (1996, p. 645).

EARLIER REFERENCES:

Earlier synonyms:

1. *pyramis laminosa (Malacarne, 1776)*
   Original full Latin form of ***pyramis (Malacarne, 1776)***; see Clarke & O'Malley (1996, p. 645).
2. *laminated pyramid (Malacarne, 1776)*
   English form of *pyramis laminosa (Malacarne, 1776)*; see Clarke & O'Malley (1996, p. 645).

LATER SYNONYMS:

1. *thick part of inferior vermis (Vicq d'Azyr, 1786)*
   Synonym for macrodissected adult human ***pyramis (Malacarne, 1776)***; p. 95. A Latin form is *portio crassa vermis inferioris*, see Burdach (1822, p. 295).
2. *posterior part of inferior vermal process (Gordon, 1815)*
   Synonym for macrodissected adult human ***pyramis (Malacarne, 1776)***; p. 114. A Latin form is *pars posterior vermis inferioris*, see Burdach (1822, p. 295).
3. *central part of inferior vermiform process (Meckel, 1817)*
   Synonym for macrodissected adult human ***pyramis (Malacarne, 1776)***; see translation (1832, Vol. 2, p. 432).

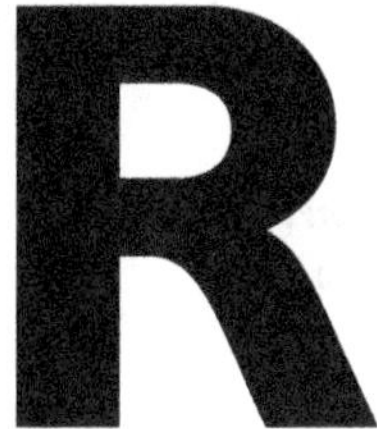

radial nerve (Du Verney, 1697)

As described for macrodissected adult human, it is the largest branch of the ***brachial plexus (Camper, 1760)*** and arises from the ***brachial plexus dorsal cord (Paterson, 1887)***. It is usually now said to have muscular, cutaneous, and articular branches before dividing into two terminal branches, ***superficial branch of radial nerve (Martin, 1781)*** and ***deep branch of radial nerve (Martin, 1781)***; see Durward (1951, Figs. 923, 933) and Williams & Warwick (1980, pp. 1101–1103). According to Winslow (1733, Sect. VI, p. 79), his mentor Du Verney in 1697 named it for macrodissected adult human because it accompanies the radius and radial artery. Klint (1784, pp. 27–32) provided an unusually thorough early account of the macrodissected adult human ***radial nerve (Du Verney, 1697)***. It was first known as the *third nerve from spine to upper arm (Galen, c177)*.

TRANSLATIONS:

1. *nervus radialis (Du Verney, 1697)*
   Original Latin form of ***radial nerve (Du Verney, 1697)***; see Winslow (1733, Sect. VI, p. 79).

EARLIER REFERENCES:

Earlier synonyms:

1. *second nerve entering upper arm from spine (Galen, c177)*
   Apparently same as *third nerve from spine to upper arm (Galen, c177)*; see Singer translation (1999, p. 66). May be inconsistency on Galen's part or mistake by Singer.
2. *third nerve from spine to upper arm (Galen, c177)*
   Synonym for ***radial nerve (Du Verney, 1697)*** in macrodissected adult beef, pig, and/or monkey but not human; see Singer translation (1999, p. 68; also pp. 66, 69–74, 80, 82). Also see May translation (1968, pp. 138, 705), Duckworth translation (1962, p. 252).
3. *fourth nerve entering arm (Vesalius, 1543a)*
   Synonym for macrodissected adult human ***radial nerve (Du Verney, 1697)***; see Richardson & Carman translation (2002, p. 241).
4. *fourth sinew going under arm (Geminus, 1553)*
   Synonym for macrodissected adult human *fourth nerve entering arm (Vesalius, 1543a)*; originally spelled, *fourth synnowe goynge under arme*, see *The table of the figures of sinowes*.
5. *fourth nerve of hand (Bauhin, 1605)*
   Synonym for macrodissected adult human *fourth nerve entering arm (Vesalius, 1543a)*; see Crooke translation (1615, p. 903).
6. *quartus brachium ingrediens nervus (Casseri, 1627)*
   Synonym for macrodissected adult human ***radial nerve (Du Verney, 1697)***; p. 128, see Klint (1784, p. 27).
7. *quartus crassisimus nervus (Diemerbroeck, 1672)*
   Synonym for macrodissected adult human ***radial nerve (Du Verney, 1697)***; p. 128, see Klint (1784, p. 27).
8. *fifth brachial nerve (Vieussens, 1684)*
   Synonym for macrodissected adult human ***radial nerve (Du Verney, 1697)***; in the original Latin, *quintus nervus brachialis*, p. 220-*M*.

LATER SYNONYMS:

1. *muscularis nerve (Cheselden, 1726)*
   Apparently corresponds loosely to macrodissected adult human ***radial nerve (Du Verney, 1697)***; in the original Latin, *nervus muscularis*, p. 265, which was essentially written by Monro *primus* as stated in the Preface. Also see Klint (1784, p. 27).
2. *posterior brachial nerve (Pietro da Cortona, 1741)*
   Synonym for macrodissected adult human ***radial nerve (Du Verney, 1697)***; in the original Latin, *posterior brachialium nervus*, p. 11.
3. *third great brachial nerve (Albinus, 1744)*
   Synonym for macrodissected adult human ***radial nerve (Monro, 1732)***; in the original Latin, *tertium nervus brachialis magnus* (Tab. 19-29), or *nervorum brachium magni tertii* (Tab. 20-29). Also see Camper (1760, p. 12).
4. *brachial nerve (Günther, 1786)*

Synonym listed for macrodissected adult human ***radial nerve (Du Verney, 1697)***; in the original Latin, *nervus brachialis*, p. 78.

5. *brachial muscular nerve (Günther, 1786)*
   Synonym listed for macrodissected adult human ***radial nerve (Du Verney, 1697)***; in the original Latin, *nervus muscularis brachii*, p. 78.
6. *radio-digital nerve (Burdin, 1803)*
   Synonym for macrodissected adult human ***radial nerve (Du Verney, 1697)***; see translation (1803, Vol. 1, p. 192).

PARTLY CORRESPONDS:

1. *muscular spiral nerve (Monro, 1783)*
   Synonym for segment or trunk of macrodissected adult human ***radial nerve (Du Verney, 1697)*** before splitting into two terminal branches, ***superficial branch of radial nerve (Martin, 1781)*** and ***deep branch of radial nerve (Martin, 1781)***; p. 66, also see Foster (1894, p. 2398). Quain & Wilson (1839, Pl. XVII-*F*) spelled it *musculo-spiral nerve* for macrodissected adult human.
2. *spiral muscular nerve (Monro, 1783)*
   Synonym for *muscular spiral nerve (Monro, 1783)*, Table 15-*15*. Monro wrote that this was the name given by his father; see *muscularis nerve (Cheselden, 1726)*.
3. *spiral nerve (Fyfe, 1800)*
   Synonym for macrodissected adult human *muscular spiral nerve (Monro, 1783)*; Vol. 2, p. 309.
4. *terminal branches of radial nerve (Cruveilhier, 1836)*
   Synonym for macrodissected adult human ***deep branch of radial nerve (Martin, 1781)*** and ***superficial branch of radial nerve (Martin, 1781)*** considered together; in the original French, *branches terminales du nerf radial*, p. 817.

radial nerve cord (>1840)

A differentiated linear zone of the ***nerve net (>1840)*** in Echinoderms with periodic small ***ganglia (Galen, c173)*** along its length, and extending into each of the (most commonly five) arms from the ***circumoral nerve ring (Tiedemann, 1815)***. There is no convincing evidence that the Echinoderm ***nervous system (Monro, 1783)*** is divided into ***central nervous system (Carus, 1814)*** and ***peripheral nervous system (Meckel, 1817)***; see Cobb (1995, p. 411). A cord segment between two adjacent ganglia is called a ***longitudinal communicating branch (>1840)***. It was perhaps first pointed out as a *radiating nerve (Tiedemann, 1815)*.

EARLIER REFERENCES:

Earlier synonyms:

1. *radiating nerve (Tiedemann, 1815)*
   Synonym for ***radial nerve cord (>1840)*** of the macrodissected adult starfish viewed with a microscope; in the original German (plural), *ausstrahlenden Nerven*, p. 173.

radiation of corpus callosum (Dejerine & Dejerine-Klumpke, 1895)

As described for macrodissected adult human, ***axons (Kölliker, 1896)*** fanning out from the ***corpus callosum (Galen, c177)*** into all parts of the rest of the ***cerebral cortex white matter (>1840)***. Although containing commissural ***axons (Kölliker, 1896)*** from the ***corpus callosum (Galen, c177)***, the radiation also contains association and projection ***axons (Kölliker, 1896)*** as well. Major named differentiations include ***frontal forceps (>1840)***, ***tapetum (Reil, 1809b)***, and ***occipital forceps (>1840)***; see Williams & Warwick (1980, pp. 1023–1024), *Nomina Anatomica* (1983, pp. A71–A72), *Terminologia Anatomica* (1998, p. 127), *Dorland's* (2003, p. 1561), Nieuwenhuys et al. (2008, p. 596). For Dejerine & Dejerine-Klumpke's use in macrodissected adult human, see pp. 338, 344. Reil (1809b) perhaps first clearly identified all major components.

recurrent laryngeal nerve (Albinus, 1744)

As described for macrodissected adult human, it arises asymmetrically on the right and left sides from the ***vagus nerve trunk (Wrisberg, 1786; Günther, 1786)***, extends caudally (descends) and then rostrally (ascends) to supply all laryngeal muscles except cricothyroid, as well as somatic sensory and proprioceptive ***dendrites (His, 1889)*** to parts of the larynx; for details on these and other, smaller, branches see Williams & Warwick (1980, pp. 1080–1081), Durward (1951, Fig. 907). For Albinus's use in macrodissected adult human, see Table 18, Figure 2-*p*. It was discovered by Marinus of Pergamum; see ***[recurrent laryngeal nerve (Albinus, 1744)] (Marinus of Pergamum, fl. c75)***.

EARLIER REFERENCES:

Described, not named or illustrated:

1. ***[recurrent laryngeal nerve (Albinus, 1744)] (Marinus of Pergamum, fl. c75)***
   Galen mentioned that one of his forerunners, Marinus of Pergamum, discovered the ***nerves (Herophilus, c335–c280 BC)*** responsible for voice; see Singer (1999, p. 211 note *10*).
2. ***[recurrent laryngeal nerve (Albinus, 1744)] (Rufus of Ephesus, fl. c90–120)***
   Rufus of Ephesus has been credited with listing it; see Rasmussen (1947, p. 2). May (1968, p. 30) disputed this claim.

Earlier synonyms:

1. *recurrent nerve (Galen, c173)*
   Galen provided a brilliant description of the course taken by ***recurrent laryngeal nerve (Albinus, 1744)***, and an experimental analysis of its function—perhaps his single greatest discovery. He described it for macrodissected adult macaque, beef, pig, bear, lion, goat, dog, "and other such animals," birds with long necks (cranes, swans, and ostriches), and two humans during surgery; see May translation (1968, pp. 42, 63, 352 note *31*, 362–371, 691–694; name on p. 693), Duckworth translation (1962, pp. 205–217); also see Walsh (1937, p. 51 ff.). Vesalius (1543a) provided two illustrations of it for macrodissected adult human (see Richardson & Carman translation, 2002, pp. 169, 196), and Casseri ([1601], tractus primo) provided superb illustrations of it in macrodissected adult

human (Tabs. XII, Fig. 1 and XV, Figs. 1 & 2), pig (Tab. XVI, Figs. 1 & 2), and rat (Tab. VII, Fig. 9-O).

2. *upwardly recurrent nerve (Galen, c192)*
   Synonym for *recurrent nerve (Galen, c173)*; see Duckworth translation (1962, p. 205).
3. *vocal nerve (Galen, c192)*
   Synonym for *recurrent nerve (Galen, c173)*; see Duckworth translation (1962, p. 207).
4. *nervi motivi (Copho, c1070–c1100)*
   Apparently synonym for macrodissected adult pig *recurrent nerve (Galen, c173)*; see Corner translation (1927, p. 51).
5. *recursive nerve (Massa, 1536)*
   Synonym for macrodissected adult human *recurrent nerve (Galen, c173)*; in the original Latin (plural), *reversivi nervi*, see Lind translation (1975, p. 219).
6. *returning sinew (Geminus, 1553)*
   Synonym for macrodissected adult human *recurrent nerve (Galen, c173)*; originally spelled *returnynge synowe*, see *The table of the figure of synowes*.
7. *sinew of voice (Geminus, 1553)*
   Synonym for macrodissected adult human *vocal nerve (Galen, c192)*; originally spelled *synowe of the voyce*, see *The table of the figure of synowes*.
8. *sinew returning back (Geminus, 1553)*
   Synonym for macrodissected adult human *recurrent nerve (Galen, c173)*; originally spelled *sinowe returninge backe*, see *The table of the figures of synowes*.
9. *recurrent branch of sixth conjugation (Paré, 1634)*
   Synonym for macrodissected adult human *recurrent nerve (Galen, c173)*; see Paré (1561, p. cxiii), translated here on p. 152.
10. *returning nerve (Willis, 1664)*
    Synonym for macrodissected adult mammalian *recurrent nerve (Galen, c173)*; see Pordage translation (1681, Tab. IX-*n,L*).
11. *turn-again nerve (Diemerbroeck, 1689)*
    Synonym for macrodissected adult human ***recurrent laryngeal nerve (Albinus, 1744)***; p. 417.

LATER SYNONYMS:

1. *inferior laryngeal nerve (Albinus, 1744)*
   Synonym for macrodissected adult human ***recurrent laryngeal nerve (Albinus, 1744)***; in the original Latin, *nervus laryngaeus inferior*, Table 18, Figure 2-*p*.
2. *recurrent nerve of Galen (Günther, 1786)*
   Eponym for macrodissected adult human ***recurrent laryngeal nerve (Albinus, 1744)***; in the original Latin, *nervus recurrens Galeni*, p. 64.
3. *tracheal nerve (Burdin, 1803)*
   Synonym for macrodissected adult human ***recurrent laryngeal nerve (Albinus, 1744)***; see translation (1803, Vol. 1, p. 183).
4. *inferior laryngeal branch of pneumogastric nerve (Cloquet, 1816)*
   Synonym for macrodissected adult human ***recurrent laryngeal nerve (Albinus, 1744)***; in the original French, *rameaux laryngés inférieurs*, p. 623.
5. *ascending nerve (Meckel, 1817)*
   Listed as synonym for macrodissected adult human ***recurrent laryngeal nerve (Albinus, 1744)***; in the original Latin, *nervus adscendens*, see translation (1832, Vol. 3, p. 48).

PARTLY CORRESPONDS:

1. *nervi recurrentis portio in musculum aperientem (Fabricius ab Aquapendente, 1613)*
   Macrodissected adult human branch of ***recurrent laryngeal nerve (Albinus, 1744)*** to posterior cricoarytenoid muscle, critical for respiration; Chapter X, Figure 38-*a*. See Scarpa (1794, Tab. III).
2. *descending branches of recurrent nerve (Haase, 1781)*
   Branches of macrodissected adult human ***recurrent laryngeal nerve (Albinus, 1744)*** including ***inferior cervical cardiac branches of recurrent laryngeal nerve (>1840)*** and ***tracheal branches of recurrent laryngeal nerve (>1840)***; in the original Latin, *nervi recurrentis rami descendentes*, p. 87.
3. *anastomosis of left recurrent with anterior pulmonary plexus of right pneumogastric nerve (Knox, 1832)*
   Macrodissected adult human ***communicating branch (Winslow, 1733)*** between left ***recurrent laryngeal nerve (Albinus, 1744)*** and ***anterior pulmonary plexus (Haller, 1762)*** from right ***vagus nerve (Galen, c192)***; Plate III-*109*, in Knox's translation of Scarpa (1794).
4. *collateral branches of recurrent nerve (Cruveilhier, 1836)*
   Macrodissected adult human ***inferior cervical cardiac branches of recurrent laryngeal nerve (>1840)***, ***esophageal branches of recurrent laryngeal nerve (Arnold, 1834)***, ***tracheal branches of recurrent laryngeal nerve (>1840)***, and ***pharyngeal branches of recurrent laryngeal nerve (>1840)*** considered together; in the original French, *rameaux collatéraux*, p. 963.

red nucleus (Burdach, 1822)

As described for macrodissected adult human, and for adult mammal in general with cellular architecture and connections, a large roundish ***gray matter region (Swanson & Bota, 2010)*** in the ***tegmentum (Swanson, 2000b)***, ventromedial to the ***midbrain reticular nucleus (>1840)***; see Nieuwenhuys et al. (2008, p. 208). For Burdach's use in macrodissected adult human, see pp. 104, 327. Although Burdach (p. 327) credited Le Boë (1663; Part 4, p. 19), also known as F. Sylvius, with perhaps first mentioning the ***red nucleus (Burdach, 1822)*** or its general region—his *substantia colore subcarneo imbuta*—Meyer (1971, p. 25) doubted this specificity and suggested instead that Le Boë referred to "basal ganglia in general." In contrast, it was quite clearly illustrated by Santorini; see ***[red nucleus (Burdach, 1822)] (Santorini, 1775)***.

TRANSLATIONS:

1. *rothen Kern (Burdach, 1822)*
   Original German form of ***red nucleus (Burdach, 1822)***; pp. 104, 327.

EARLIER REFERENCES:

Illustrated, not named or described:

1. ***[red nucleus (Burdach, 1822)] (Santorini, 1775)***
   Clearly illustrated for macrodissected adult human in transverse section; Table 3, Figure 3-*E*, also see Meyer (1971, Fig. 8). For an essentially identical plane of section, with modern interpretation, see Nieuwenhuys et al. (2008, Fig. 5.8).

Earlier synonyms:

1. *reddish spot (Vicq d'Azyr, 1786)*
   Vicq d'Azyr clearly pointed out, illustrated, and named in cross sections of macrodissected adult human the ***red nucleus (Burdach, 1822)***, along with the surrounding *white substance (Vesalius, 1543a)* "capsule" formed by the ***superior cerebellar peduncle (Procháska, 1800)***; in the original French, *tache rougeâtre*, Plate XXV, Figure III-*a*. Reil (1809c, pp. 493, 508, 512) also rather clearly described, without naming, this feature and its relationship with ***superior cerebellar peduncle (Procháska, 1800)***.

renal branch of lesser splanchnic nerve (>1840)

As defined for macrodissected adult human, one or two terminal filaments of the ***lesser splanchnic nerve (>1840)*** ending in the ***renal plexus (Drake, 1707)***, although they are not always found; see Mitchell (1953, p. 245 and Fig. 110). It was first illustrated by Walter; see ***[renal branch of lesser splanchnic nerve (>1840)] (Walter, 1783)***.

EARLIER REFERENCES:

Described, not named or illustrated:

1. ***[renal branch of lesser splanchnic nerve (>1840)] (Walter, 1783)***
   Illustrated for macrodissected adult human; see Table I-217.

renal ganglia (Walther, 1735)

As described for macrodissected adult human, ***terminal ganglia (Gaskell, 1886)*** associated with the ***renal plexus (Drake, 1707)*** varying considerably in location, number, and size with the largest and most consistent being the ***posterior renal ganglion (Tiedemann, 1822)***; see Mitchell (1953, pp. 288–290 and Figs. 84 and 104, his *posterior renal ganglion*). For Walther's discovery and use in macrodissected adult human, see reprinting in Haller (1747–1751, Vol. 2, p. 937). Walter (1783) illustrated them (at least 7) superbly for macrodissected adult human.

TRANSLATIONS:

1. *ganglia renalia (Walther, 1735)*
   Original Latin form of ***renal ganglia (Walther, 1735)***. It was in the phrase, *Nam, praeter renalia illa ganglia,...* ; see reprinting in Haller (1747–1751, Vol. 2, p. 937).

renal nerves (Haase, 1781)

As described for macrodissected adult human, they supply the ***renal plexus (Drake, 1707)*** and arise from the ***celiac plexus (Winslow, 1733), greater splanchnic nerve (Walter, 1783), lesser splanchnic nerve (Haller, 1762), least splanchnic nerve (>1840)***, rostral (upper) ***lumbar splanchnic nerves (Cruveilhier, 1836)***, rostral (upper) parts of the ***intermesenteric plexus (>1840)***, and caudal (lower) ends of the ***intermesenteric plexus (>1840)*** and/or ***superior hypogastric plexus (Tiedemann, 1822)***; see Mitchell (1953, pp. 284–286), Williams & Warwick (1980, p. 1134). For Haase's use in macrodissected adult human, see p. 125. It was known as long ago as *nerve inserted into kidney (Galen, c173)*.

TRANSLATIONS:

1. *nervi renali (Haase, 1781)*
   Original Latin form of ***renal nerves (Haase, 1781)***; p. 125.

EARLIER REFERENCES:

Earlier synonyms:

1. *nerve inserted into kidney (Galen, c173)*
   Synonym for ***renal nerves (Haase, 1781)*** in macrodissected adult beef, pig, and/or macaque but not human; see May translation (1968, p. 263). Vesalius (1543a) mentioned a ***lumbar splanchnic nerve (Cruveillhier, 1836)*** to kidney in macrodissected adult human; see Richardson & Carman translation (2002, p. 2000). Willis (1664) illustrated for macrodissected adult human and other common large mammals a distinction between ***renal nerves (Haase, 1781), renal plexus (Drake, 1707)***, and ***intrinsic renal nerves (>1840)***; see Table XI-*ν,γ*. This was done considerably better for macrodissected adult human by Vieussens (1684, Tab. 23).
2. *nerve conferred on kidney (Galen, c173)*
   Synonym for ***renal nerves (Haase, 1781)*** in macrodissected adult beef, pig, and/or macaque but not human; see May translation (1968, p. 263).
3. *nerve branch to kidney (Galen, c192)*
   Synonym for ***renal nerves (Haase, 1781)*** in macrodissected adult beef, pig, and/or macaque but not human; see Duckworth translation (1962, p. 222).

renal plexus (Drake, 1707)

As described for macrodissected adult human, a rich, open-meshed ***plexus (Galen, c192)*** supplied by the ***renal nerves (Haase, 1781)*** containing variable numbers of small ***renal ganglia (Walther, 1735)*** and in turn generating the ***intrinsic renal nerves (>1840)***, and contributing to the ***superior ureteric nerves (Walter, 1783)*** and the ***superior testicular nerves (>1840)*** or ***superior ovarian nerves (>1840)***; see Mitchell (1953, pp. 284–296 and Figs. 104, 120), Williams & Warwick (1980, p. 1134). For Drake's use in macrodissected adult human, see pp. 519, 520. It was known to Willis; see ***[renal plexus (Drake, 1707)] (Willis, 1664)***.

TRANSLATIONS:

1. *plexus renalis (Drake, 1707)*
   Original Latin form of ***renal plexus (Drake, 1707)***, though Drake used plural; p. 519.

EARLIER REFERENCES:

Illustrated, not named or described:

1. ***[renal plexus (Drake, 1707)] (Willis, 1664)***
   Willis (1664) illustrated for macrodissected adult human and other common large mammals a distinction between ***renal nerves (Haase, 1781)***, ***renal plexus (Drake, 1707)***, and ***intrinsic renal nerves (>1840)***; see Table XI-*v,y*.

Earlier synonyms:

1. *nerveo plexui renali (Vieussens, 1684)*
   Synonym for macrodissected adult human ***renal plexus (Drake, 1707)***; Table 23-67.
2. *nerveum plexum renalem (Vieussens, 1684)*
   Alternate form of *nerveo plexui renali (Vieussens, 1684)*; Table 23-69.
3. *nerveus plexus renalis (Vieussens, 1684)*
   Alternate form of *nerveo plexui renali (Vieussens, 1684)*; Table 23-70.

LATER SYNONYMS:

1. *emulgent plexus (Cloquet, 1816)*
   Synonym listed for macrodissected adult human ***renal plexus (Drake, 1707)***; in the original French, *plexus émulgens*, p. 709.

PARTLY CORRESPONDS:

1. *spermatic plexus (Mayer, 1794)*
   Region of macrodissected adult human ***renal plexus (Drake, 1707)*** associated with origin of ***superior testicular nerves (>1840)***; in the original Latin, *plexus spermaticus*; Part 6, Table 6, p. 43.
2. *plexus nervorum renum ganglioformis dexter (Soemmerring, 1798)*
   Basically right macrodissected adult human ***renal plexus (Drake, 1707)***; p. 359.
3. *plexus nervorum renum ganglioformis sinister (Soemmerring, 1798)*
   Basically left macrodissected adult human ***renal plexus (Drake, 1707)***; p. 359.

rete mirabile (Herophilus, c335–c280 BC)

The "marvelous net" is a component of the ***circulatory system***; an elaboration of the carotid arteries near the base of the ***hypothalamus (Kuhlenbeck, 1927)***, much reduced in human but extensive in, for example, ungulate. It was discovered and named (in Greek) by Herophilus, as related by Galen; see Singer (1952, p. 79 note 49), May translation (1968, pp. 25, 430–434), von Staden (1989, pp. 179, 223). Berengario da Carpi (1522) did not observe it in human (see Lind translation, 1959, p. 147), which was confirmed in 1543 by Vesalius (see Singer translation, 1952, p. 10) who illustrated and compared what he observed in human and in sheep and oxen, in contrast to what Galen reported; see Singer translation (1952, Figs. 16, 17-*B*, and Fig. 17-*A*, respectively). Burdach provided an interesting early history (1822, p. 399).

TRANSLATIONS:

1. *wonderful net (Crooke, 1615)*
   English form of ***rete mirabile (Herophilus, c335–c280 BC)*** for macrodissected adult human; see p. 469. Pordage (1681, p. 71) also used it in translating Willis (1664), who noted it is absent in some animals like human and horse, but extensive in others.

LATER SYNONYMS:

1. *retiform plexus (Galen, c173)*
   The ***rete mirabile (Herophilus, c335–c280 BC)***, probably in macrodissected adult pig; see May translation (1968, pp. 430–432). Vesalius (1543a) used the Latin form, *plexus reticularis*, translating Galen's *diktyoeides plegma*; see Richardson and Carman (2009, p. 218 first note).
2. *mirabilis plexus reticularis (Vesalius, 1543a)*
   Synonym for ***rete mirabile (Herophilus, c335–c280 BC)***; Book 7, Ch. 12. The marvelous netlike plexus.
3. *netlike plexus (Vesalius, 1543a)*
   English form of *retiform plexus (Galen, c173)*, see Richardson & Carman translation (2009, p. 217).
4. *retiformis (Geminus, 1553)*
   Geminus stated that this Latin term is synonymous with ***rete mirabile (Herophilus, c335–c280 BC)***, which he spelled *rethe mirabile*, f. BII; or *rete mirabile*, f. BII.
5. *plexus vasorum et fibrarum usus incogniti (Heister, 1717)*
   Synonym for macrodissected adult human ***rete mirabile (Herophilus, c335–c280 BC)***, p. 81; see Monro (1783, p. 2).

reticular part of substantia nigra (>1840)

One of two major ***gray matter regions (Swanson & Bota, 2010)*** of the mammalian ***substantia nigra (Soemmerring, 1791)***, lying generally ventrolateral to the ***compact part of substantia nigra (>1840)*** and characterized in adult human by unpigmented ***neurons (Waldeyer, 1891)*** that in all mammals utilize GABA as a neurotransmitter; see Nieuwenhuys et al. (2008, pp. 438–439). It was first illustrated clearly by Vicq d'Azyr; see ***[reticular part of substantia nigra (>1840)] (Vicq d'Azyr, 1786)***.

EARLIER REFERENCES:

Illustrated, not named or described:

1. ***[reticular part of substantia nigra (>1840)] (Vicq d'Azyr, 1786)***
   Its location in macrodissected adult human was illustrated schematically in cross section between ventrolaterally directed rays of ***compact part of substantia nigra (>1840)***. Vicq d'Azyr did not specifically describe presence of ***gray matter region (Swanson & Bota, 2010)*** between rays, which would have identified unambiguously ***reticular part of substantia nigra (>1840)***; Plate XXI, Figure 1-*41*.

reticular thalamic nucleus (>1840)

As described for macrodissected adult human, and based on cellular architecture and connections in mammal, the middle part of the ***ventral part of thalamus (Herrick, 1910)*** lying between ***zona incerta (>1840)*** ventromedially and ***ventral lateral geniculate nucleus (>1840)*** dorsolaterally; see Jones (1985, Ch. 15.2), Nieuwenhuys et al. (2008, Fig. 5.8-*18*). It was first delineated by Vieussens; see ***[reticular thalamic nucleus (>1840)] (Vieussens, 1684)***.

EARLIER REFERENCES:

Described, not named or illustrated:

1. ***[reticular thalamic nucleus (>1840)] (Vieussens, 1684)***
   Observed in macrodissected adult human; see Meyer (1971, p. 44).

Earlier synonyms:

1. *lamina cornea (Vicq d'Azyr, 1786)*
   Roughly synonymous with macrodissected adult human ***reticular thalamic nucleus (>1840)***, including its combination of *gray substance (Vesalius, 1543a)* and *white substance (Vesalius, 1543a)*; pp. 7, 16. Also see Burdach (1822, p. 122), Meyer (1971, p. 31). Burdach (1822, p. 345) suggested it is one of two *entrelacemens transversau* described and illustrated by Gall & Spurzheim (1810). Rolando (1825a; Tab. VIII, Fig. 1-*y*) illustrated it clearly in transverse section of macrodissected adult beef.

retina (Herophilus, c335–c280 BC)

The main peripheral sensory organ of sight, distal to the ***optic nerve (Vicq d'Azyr, 1786)***. During early mammalian development the optic stalk evaginates from the wall of the ***hypothalamus (Kuhlenbeck, 1927)*** in a region just caudal to what will become the *preoptic level of hypothalamus (>1840)*, and the optic stalk goes on to generate the ***retina (Herophilus, c335–c280 BC)*** from the optic cup; see Alvarez-Bolado & Swanson (1996, pp. 22–23), Dowling (2012). According to Rufus of Ephesus (c90–120) the term originated with Herophilus, who dissected human cadavers; see May (1968, p. 25), Lloyd (1975, p. 120), Longrigg (1993, 193). "Retina" is a Latin form of the Arabic word "alshabakiyya" (the netlike tunic), which according to Polyak (1957, p. 43) was translated from the Greek name "amphiblestroëides hitón". The ***retina (Herophilus, c335–c280 BC)*** reminded Herophilus of a folded fishing net, and Galen regarded it (correctly) as an extension of the ***brain (Smith Papyrus, c1700 BC)***; see May translation (1968, pp. 402, 465–467). According to Vesalius (1543a; see Richardson & Carman translation, 2002, p. 183), the Greeks applied to the term ***retina (Herophilus,c335–c280 BC)*** the adjective *amphiblestroeides* ("netlike"). Zinn (1755, pp. 103–109) provided a thorough review of the earlier literature and Polyak (1941, pp. 145–147) provided a thorough list of synonyms in various languages. Apparently, Briggs (1685) first illustrated the fibrous nature of the ***retina (Herophilus, c335–c280 BC)***; see Polyak (1941, p. 151). Leeuwenhoek (1684, published in 1722) first mentioned oblong elements that may have been rods and cones (see Polyak, 1941, pp. 149–150).

EARLIER REFERENCES:

Earlier synonyms:

1. *arachnoid (Rufus of Ephesus, c90–120)*
   According to Rufus of Ephesus it was in use before ***retina (Herophilus, c335–c280 BC)*** was introduced; see Polyak (1941, pp. 96–100), May (1968, p. 25). Listed as *arachnoeides* by Hall (1565, p. 47).

LATER SYNONYMS:

1. *retiform tunic (Galen, c173)*
   According to Galen, synonym used by some people for ***retina (Herophilus, c335–c280 BC)***; see May translation (1968, p. 465).
2. *netlike body (Galen, c173)*
   Synonym for ***retina (Herophilus, c335–c280 BC)***; see May translation (1968, p. 466).
3. *tunic of eye (Vesalius, 1543a)*
   Synonym for macrodissected adult human ***retina (Herophilus, c335–c280 BC)***; in the original Latin, *oculi tunica*, see Richardson & Carman translation (2002, p. 170). The full description was, *tunic of the eye, into which the optic nerve expands and transforms.*
4. *coat of eye (Geminus, 1553)*
   Synonym for macrodissected adult human *tunic of eye (Vesalius, 1543a)*; the original spelling was, *cote of the eye*, see *The table of the figure of synowes.*

retrohippocampal region (Swanson et al., 1987)

As described with cellular architecture and connections in mammal, it corresponds to the macrodissected adult human ***parahippocampal gyrus (>1840)*** and is subdivided into ***subicular complex (Swanson, et al., 1987)*** medially and ***entorhinal area (Brodmann, 1909)*** laterally; see Swanson (2004, Table B, p. 169). It was not identified as thus defined by 1840.

retrolentiform part of internal capsule (>1840)

As commonly described for macrodissected adult human, a ventral differentiation of the ***posterior limb of internal capsule (>1840)*** with partly segregated ***axons (Kölliker, 1896)*** associated with ***interbrain corticospinal tract (>1840)*** and ***posterior thalamic radiation (>1840)***; see Crosby et al. (1962, p. 394, Fig. 272, called *postlenticular part*), Nieuwenhuys et al. (2008, Fig. 5.32-*11*). It was perhaps first clearly distinguished as the *posterior part of base of corona radiata (Arnold, 1838b)*.

EARLIER REFERENCES:

Earlier synonyms:

1. *meditulli albi pars posterior (Arnold, 1838b)*
   Synonym for macrodissected adult human ***retrolentiform part of internal capsule (>1840)***; Table IV, Figure 4-α.
2. *posterior part of base of corona radiata (Arnold, 1838b)*
   Synonym for *meditulli albi pars posterior (Arnold, 1838b)*; in the original Latin, *pars posterior basis corona radiata*, Table X, Figures 1-*h*, 2-*d*.

retrosplenial region (>1840)

As described with cellular architecture in adult mammal, the most caudal subdivision of the ***cingulate region***

(>1840), further subdivided in adult human into a dorsal or outer ***agranular retrosplenial area (>1840)***, or *area 30 (Brodmann, 1909)*, and a ventral or inner ***granular retrosplenial area (>1840)***, or *area 29 (Brodmann, 1909)*; see Nieuwenhuys et al. (2008, Fig. 12.13). It was not identified by 1840.

rhinal sulcus (>1840)

As described for macrodissected adult mammal, a longitudinal groove starting rostrally between ***olfactory region (>1840)*** ventrally and ***frontal region (Vicq d'Azyr, 1786)*** dorsally, extending caudally in ventral parts of the ***insular region (Brodmann, 1909)***, and ending between ***hippocampal formation (Swanson & Cowan, 1977)*** ventrally and ***temporal region (>1840)*** dorsally; see Swanson (2004, Atlas Levels 6–45). It was first identified by Vicq d'Azyr; see ***[rhinal sulcus (>1840)] (Vicq d'Azyr, 1784)***.

EARLIER REFERENCES:

Described, not named or illustrated:

1. ***[rhinal sulcus (>1840)] (Vicq d'Azyr, 1784)***
   Described for macrodissected adult human as *sillon longitudinal* extending essentially along length of ***lateral olfactory tract (>1840)***; p. 549.

Earlier synonyms:

1. *fissure dividing external root of olfactory nerve from superincumbent hemisphere (Owen, 1837)*
   Synonym for macrodissected adult mammalian, including wombat where it is very distinct, ***rhinal sulcus (>1840)***; p. 95 and Plate V, Figure 8-*i*.

rhombic lip (>1840)

A thin layer of neural tissue extending dorsomedially from the developing ***rhombicbrain (His, 1893b)*** to cover part of the early ***fourth ventricle (Galen, c192)***. It is neurogenic and generates much of the ***cerebellum (Aristotle)*** and a number of other ***gray matter regions (Swanson & Bota, 2010)*** including the ***inferior olivary complex (>1840)*** and ***pontine nuclei (Jacobsohn, 1909)***; see Nieuwenhuys et al. (2008, pp. 30–32). Tiedemann probably first pointed it out; see *narrow plate arising from margin of spinal marrow (Tiedemann, 1816)*.

EARLIER REFERENCES:

Earlier synonyms:

1. *narrow plate arising from margin of spinal marrow (Tiedemann, 1816)*
   Roughly synonymous with ***rhombic lip (>1840)*** in macrodissected developing human during the second and third months; see translation (1826, pp. 21, 30, 33, 154 ff.).

rhombicbrain (His, 1893b)

The most caudal of the three main topographic divisions of the adult ***vertebrate brain (Cuvier, 1800)***. The three main topographic divisions of the ***rhombicbrain (His, 1893b)*** are ***cerebellum (Aristotle)*** and ***pons (Haller, 1747)***, considered together as the ***hindbrain (Baer, 1837)***, and caudal to it the ***medulla (Winslow, 1733)*** or equally acceptable synonym, ***afterbrain (Baer, 1837)***. The ***rhombicbrain (His, 1893)*** is bordered rostrally by the ***midbrain (Baer, 1837)*** and caudally by the ***spinal cord (Galen, c162–c166)***. For these precise definitions, based on the comparative embryological work of Baer and ***primary hindbrain vesicle (Baer, 1837)***, see Swanson & Bota (2010). It was described long ago in rough outline as the *cerebellum (Galen, c173)*. For His's introduction of the term see p. 173; also see Sharpey et al. (1867, p. 577).

TRANSLATIONS:

1. *Rautenhirn (His, 1893b)*
   Original German form of ***rhombicbrain (His, 1893)***; p. 173.
2. *rhombencephalon (His, 1893b)*
   Original Latin form of ***rhombicbrain (His, 1893)***; p. 173.

EARLIER REFERENCES:

Earlier synonyms:

1. *cerebellum (Galen, c173)*
   Galen was not always consistent in his use of the term *cerebellum* or *parencephalis*. Sometimes he meant ***cerebellum (Aristotle)*** proper, and sometimes he used the term to include ***cerebellum (Aristotle)***, ***pons (Haller, 1747)***, and ***medulla (Winslow, 1733)*** considered together, the ***rhombicbrain (His, 1893b)***—leading to some confusion; see May translation (1968, pp. 398, 413, 417–418, 444). However, in at least one place, in *On the Usefulness of the Parts*, he did refer to the base of the *parencephalis*, or *base of cerebellum (Galen, 173)*, which can only refer roughly to ***pons (Haller, 1747)*** and ***medulla (Winslow, 1733)*** considered together; see May translation (1968, pp. 718–719). Thus, when Galen referred to hard (motor) nerves (for example, May translation, 1968, p. 398), or to spinal cord (for example, May translation, 1968, p. 417) as arising from the parencephalis, he was referring to them as arising from *base of parencephalis (Galen, c173)* or *base of cerebellum (Galen, c173)*. This interpretation was followed, for example, by Haly Abbas (Wiberg translation, 1914, p. 31), Constantine the African (see Manzoni, 1998, pp. 122–123), and Mondino (Singer translation, 1925, pp. 92–93). Aristotle's exact definition of cerebellum is of course not known; see ***cerebellum (Aristotle)***.
2. *poop (Constantine the African, c1017–1087)*
   Constantine the African used it (meaning enclosure on main deck at stern of a ship) for *cerebellum (Galen, c173)*, that is, ***cerebellum (Aristotle)***, ***pons (Haller, 1747)***, and ***medulla (Winslow, 1733)*** considered together, because he wrote that ***nerves (Herophilus, c335–c280 BC)*** for voluntary movement arise from *poop*; see Manzoni (1998, p. 122).
3. *posterior belly of brain (William of Saliceto, 1275)*
   Basically macrodissected adult human ***rhombicbrain (His, 1893b)***; see Rosenman translation (1998, p. 181).

4. *hind brain (Mondino, 1316)*
   In *Anathomia*, Mondino referred to macrodissected adult human *hind brain* in the sense of *cerebellum (Galen, c173)*, that is, ***rhombicbrain (His, 1893b)***, because he wrote that *nucha (Constantine the African, c1017–1087)*, or ***spinal cord (Galen, c162–c166)***, arises from *hind brain*; see Singer translation (1925, pp. 92–93).

PARTLY CORRESPONDS:

1. *base of cerebellum (Galen, c173)*
   In *On the Usefulness of the Parts*, Galen referred to base of *parencephalis (Galen, c173)*, or *base of cerebellum*; see May translation (1968, pp. 718–719). This can only refer roughly to ***pons (Haller, 1747)*** and ***medulla (Winslow, 1733)*** considered together, because Galen wrote in some places that hard (motor) nerves arise from *parencephalis*, and in some places he also seemed to use "parencephalis" in two ways: as ***cerebellum (Aristotle)***, or as ***cerebellum (Aristotle)*** along with underlying ***brainstem (Schwalbe, 1881)***; see May translation (1968, pp. 398, 413, 417–418, 444). Because the region associated with Galen's *nates (Galen, c177)* and *testes (Galen, c177)*, the ***tectum (Baer, 1837)***, is also associated with channel to *parencephalis* or *cerebellum* [see *passage or canal extending from middle to posterior ventricle (Galen, c173, c177)*], it corresponds roughly to ***midbrain (Baer, 1837)***, leaving *base of cerebellum (Galen, c173)* to encompass roughly ***pons (Haller, 1747)*** and ***medulla (Winslow, 1733)*** considered together. In the same passage Galen also referred to *entire base of encephalon (Galen, c173)* or *entire base of brain (Galen, c173)*; see May translation (1968, p. 719). Galen macrodissected a variety of adult mammals but not human.
2. *base of parencephalis (Galen, c173)*
   Alternate form of *base of cerebellum (Galen, c173)*.
3. *origin of dorsal medulla (Vesalius, 1543a)*
   Vesalius included ***pons (Haller, 1747)*** and ***medulla (Winslow, 1733)*** considered together in macrodissected adult human *spinal cord (Vesalius, 1543a)*, which he also called *dorsal medulla (Vesalius, 1543a)* because large paired ***nerves (Herophilus, c335–c280 BC)*** arise from it. He referred to part of *dorsal medulla (Vesalius, 1543a)* within skull, beginning just caudal to ***tectum (Baer, 1837)***, as *origin of dorsal medulla*; see Singer translation (1952, pp. 21, 22, 27, 36, 46–47).
4. *origin of spinal marrow (Vesalius, 1543a)*
   Alternate form of *origin of dorsal medulla (Vesalius, 1543a)*; see Richardson & Carman translation (2002, p. 176).
5. *first part of spinal marrow (Vesalius, 1543a)*
   Synonym for *origin of dorsal medulla (Vesalius, 1543a)*; see Richardson & Carman translation (2002, p. 177).
6. *hinder region of oblong marrow (Willis, 1664)*
   Refers roughly to ***pons (Haller, 1747)*** and ***medulla (Winslow, 1733)*** considered together, though without ***middle cerebellar peduncle (Rolando, 1819)***, in macrodissected adult human and other large mammals; in the original Latin, *posticae medullae oblongatae regionis*, see Pordage translation (1681, pp. 61, 67).
7. *tail of oblong marrow (Willis, 1664)*
   Roughly synonymous with *hinder regions of oblong marrow (Willis, 1664)*. Whether it included any of the ***midbrain (Baer, 1837)*** is unclear; see Pordage translation (1681, p. 61).
8. *hinder part of medulla oblongata (Gibson, 1684)*
   Synonym for *hinder region of oblong marrow (Willis, 1664)*; pp. 350, 366.
9. *lower-middle-white portion of brain (Haller, 1747)*
   Synonym for macrodissected adult human *origin of spinal marrow (Vesalius, 1543a)*; see Mihles translation (1754b, p. 287).
10. *basin of fourth ventricle (Reil, 1809c)*
    Part of Reil's description of what roughly corresponds to macrodissected adult human *gray substance (Vesalius, 1543a)* lying ventral to ***fourth ventricle (Galen, c192)***, in ***medulla (Winslow, 1733)*** and in part of ***pons (Haller, 1747)*** dorsal to **pontine nuclei (Jacobsohn, 1909)**; see Mayo translation (1823, p. 86).
11. *chamber of fourth ventricle (Reil, 1809c)*
    Another way Reil referred to *basin of fourth ventricle (Reil, 1809c)*, where he postulated ***trigeminal nerve (Winslow, 1733)***, ***intermediofacial nerve (Strong & Elwyn, 1943)***, and ***vestibulocochlear nerve (>1840)*** arise; see Mayo translation (1823, p. 87).
12. *medulla oblongata (Meckel, 1817)*
    Macrodissected adult human ***medulla (Winslow, 1733)*** and ***pons (1747)*** considered together, so that ***brain (Smith Papyrus, c1700 BC)*** is divided into *medulla oblongata (Meckel, 1817)*, *cerebrum (Vesalius, 1543a)*, and ***cerebellum (Aristotle)***; see translation (1832, Vol. 2, p. 419). Recently, Ariëns Kappers et al. (1936, Vol. 1, p. 355) used the term for vertebrates in general, as did Kuhlenbeck (1975a, p. 288) in *medulla oblongata sensu latiori* and *oblongata*.
13. *medulla elongata (Meckel, 1817)*
    Alternate form of *medulla oblongata (Meckel, 1817)*; see translation (1832, Vol. 2, p. 458).
14. *lobe of fourth ventricle (Desmoulins, 1825)*
    Macrodissected adult human ***pons (Haller, 1747)*** and ***medulla (Winslow, 1733)*** considered together; Plate XIII, Figure 1. For other vertebrates Desmoulins's description often indicated he was simply referring to ***medulla (Winslow, 1733)*** but descriptions may have been unclear; in the original French, *lobe du quatrième ventricule*, pp. 242, 246, 261.

right colic plexus (>1840)

As described for macrodissected adult human, it extends from the ***superior mesenteric plexus (Rau, 1720)*** along the right colic artery to supply it and the ascending colon; see Mitchell (1953, p. 283). It was known to Vesalius; see ***[right colic plexus (>1840)] (Vesalius, 1543a)***.

EARLIER REFERENCES:

Described, not named or illustrated:

1. ***[right colic plexus (>1840)] (Vesalius, 1543a)***
Mentioned and vaguely illustrated for macrodissected adult human, in combination with ***middle colic plexus (>1840)***; see Richardson & Carman translation (2002, p. 200 and Fig. on p. 169, part κ).

right coronary plexus (Scarpa, 1794)

As described for macrodissected adult human, the smaller of the two ***coronary plexuses (Meckel, 1817)***, accompanying the right coronary artery, and supplying the right atrium and ventricle; see Williams & Warwick (1980, p. 1132). For Scarpa's use in macrodissected adult human, see Table III-*124*; also see Mitchell (1953, p. 253). It was distinguished by Neubauer; see ***[right coronary plexus (Scarpa, 1794)] (Neubauer, 1772)***.

TRANSLATIONS:

1. *plexus coronarius dexter (Scarpa, 1794)*
Original Latin form of ***right coronary plexus (Scarpa, 1794)***; Table III-*124*.

EARLIER REFERENCES:

Illustrated and described, not named:

1. ***[right coronary plexus (Scarpa, 1794)] (Neubauer, 1772)***
Presence indicated in macrodissected adult human; p. 186-*112*.

LATER SYNONYMS:

1. *anterior coronary plexus (Scarpa, 1794)*
Synonym for macrodissected adult human ***right coronary plexus (Scarpa, 1794)***; in the original Latin, *plexus coronarius anterior*, Table III-*124*, also see Mitchell (1953, p. 253).
2. *superficial nerve of right artery of septum of heart (Andersch, 1797)*
Essentially macrodissected adult human ***right coronary plexus (Scarpa, 1794)*** arising from *middle trunk of superficial nerve of nerve layers of septum of heart (Andersch, 1797)*; in the original Latin, *nervum superficialem sinistrum arteriae septi cordis*, Vol. 2, p. 60. It was first printed c1751–c1755.

right gastric plexus (>1840)

As described for macrodissected adult human, a very thin extension of the ***hepatic plexus (Rau, 1720)*** extending along the right gastric artery, and distributing to rostral (upper) parts of the pyloric region and right end of the stomach's lesser curvature; distally it joins the end of the ***left gastric plexus (>1840)***; see Mitchell (1953, Fig. 119 and p. 280). It was first clearly distinguished by Willis; see ***[right gastric plexus (>1840)] (Willis, 1664)***.

EARLIER REFERENCES:

Illustrated and described, not named:

1. ***[right gastric plexus (>1840)] (Willis, 1664)***
Clearly described and illustrated for macrodissected adult human and other common large mammals; see Pordage translation (1681, pp. 158–159 and Tab. 11-*a*).

Earlier synonyms:

1. *great gastric plexus (Langenbeck, 1826–1830)*
Probably synonym for macrodissected adult human ***right gastric plexus (>1840)***; in the original Latin, *plexus gastricus magnus*, Fascicle III, Table III-*15*.
2. *superior posterior gastric plexus (Langenbeck, 1826–1830)*
Synonym for *great gastric plexus (Langenbeck, 1826–1830)*; in the original Latin, *plexus gastricus posterior superior*, Fascicle III, Table III-*15*.

PARTLY CORRESPONDS:

1. *pyloric nerves (Walter, 1783)*
Differentiations of macrodissected adult human ***right gastric plexus (>1840)***. Walter described posterior and inferior *pyloric nerves (Walter, 1783)*; in the original Latin, *nervi pylorici posteriores et inferiores*, Table IV-*144,145*.
2. *right superior gastric nerves (Mayer, 1794)*
Macrodissected adult human branches of ***right gastric plexus (>1840)*** ending in pyloric region of stomach; in the original Latin, *nervi gastrici superiores dextri*; Part 6, Table IV-*III* (p. 26).

right gastroepiploic plexus (Wrisberg, 1800)

As described for macrodissected adult human, an extension of the ***gastroduodenal plexus (>1840)*** accompanying the right gastroepiploic artery along the right two-thirds of the greater curvature of the stomach, extending branches onto the greater omentum, and meeting distally the ***left gastroepiploic plexus (>1840)***; see Mitchell (1953, pp. 280–282, Figs. 119, 122). For Wrisberg's use in macrodissected adult human, see p. 568. It was first correctly identified as the *right gastroepiploic nerves (Walter, 1783)*.

TRANSLATIONS:

1. *plexus gastro-epiploicus dexter (Wrisberg, 1800)*
Original Latin form of ***right gastroepiploic plexus (Wrisberg, 1800)***; p. 568.

EARLIER REFERENCES:

Earlier synonyms:

1. *right gastroepiploic nerves (Walter, 1783)*
Synonym for macrodissected adult human ***right gastroepiploic plexus (Wrisberg, 1800)***; in the original Latin, *nervi gastro-epiploici dextri*; Table IV:*132–143*.
2. *plexus nervorum iecoris dexter (Soemmerring, 1798)*
Synonym for macrodissected adult human ***right gastroepiploic nerves (Walter, 1783)***; p. 357, also see Soemmerring (1791, p. 337).

PARTLY CORRESPONDS:

1. *omental nerve (Walter, 1783)*
Walter described five such branches of macrodissected adult human ***right gastroepiploic plexus (>1840)*** extending radially away from stomach in greater omentum; in the original Latin, *nervus omentalis*, Table IV:*147-151*.
2. *right gastroepiploic nerve (Mayer, 1794)*
As described for macrodissected adult human, single ***nerve (Herophilus, c335–c280 BC)*** stretching along distal half of lesser curvature of stomach and generating *right*

inferior gastric nerves (Mayer, 1794) and *right omental nerves (Mayer, 1794)*; in the original Latin, *nervus gastroepiploicus dexter*; Part 6, Table IV-*IV* (p. 27). A component of ***right gastroepiploic plexus (Wrisberg, 1800)***.

3. *right inferior gastric nerves (Mayer, 1794)*
Macrodissected adult human branches of *right gastroepiploic nerve (Mayer, 1794)* to lesser curvature of stomach; in the original Latin, *nervi gastrici inferiores dextri*; Part 6, Table IV-27 (p. 27).
4. *right omental nerves (Mayer, 1794)*
Macrodissected adult human branches of *right gastroepiploic nerve (Mayer, 1794)* extending transversely across stomach in greater omentum; in the original Latin, *nervi omentales dextri*; Part 6, Table IV-28 (p. 27).
5. *epiploic nerves (Cloquet, 1828)*
Synonym for macrodissected adult human *omental nerves (Walter, 1783)*; in the original French, *nerfs de l'épiploon*, Plate CLXXVIII-60.

roof of fourth ventricle (Vesalius, 1543a)

Developmentally in mammal, a combination of the thin ***ependymal roof plate (>1840)*** associated with the ***rhombicbrain (His, 1893b)***, the overlying ***pia (Galen, c192)***, and variable amounts of ***central nervous system white matter tracts (>1840)*** extending between the two; see Hamilton & Mossman (1972, Figs. 437, 439). As described for macrodissected adult human, the thin dorsal covering of the ***fourth ventricle (Galen, c192)*** that is triangular when viewed laterally, with the apex, or ***fastigium of fourth ventricle (Burdach, 1822)***, lying dorsally. The part rostral to the apex is formed by the ***rostral medullary velum (>1840)***, whereas the part caudal to the apex is formed by the ***caudal medullary velum (>1840)*** laterally on the right and left, and the combined ***choroid membrane of fourth ventricle (>1840)*** and underlying ***choroid epithelium of fourth ventricle (>1840)*** with their invaginated ***choroid plexus of fourth ventricle (Vieussens, 1684)*** medially; see Millen & Woollam (1962, p. 66 ff. & Figs. 19, 26, 30), Carpenter (1976, p. 132 ff.), Williams & Warwick (1980, pp. 914, 932), *Terminologia Anatomica* (1998, p. 115). For Vesalius's use of *roof* in macrodissected adult human, see Singer translation (1952, p. 37); in Latin, *ventriculum obvolvit*.

TRANSLATIONS:

1. *tectum ventriculi quarti (Burdach, 1822)*
Specific Latin term for macrodissected adult human ***roof of fourth ventricle (Vesalius, 1543a)***; pp. 79, 306.
2. *tegmen ventriculi quarti (>1840)*
Current preferred Latin form of ***roof of fourth ventricle (Vesalius, 1543a)***; see *Dorland's* (2003, p. 1860).

LATER SYNONYMS:

1. *cistern of fourth ventricle (Diemerbroeck, 1689)*
Diemerbroeck indicated it is a term some use for dorsal or top part of ***fourth ventricle (Galen, c192)***, near ***cerebellum (Aristotle)*** and away from ***floor of fourth ventricle (Reil, 1807–1808a)***—essentially macrodissected adult human ***roof of fourth ventricle (Vesalius, 1543a)***; p. 403.
2. *posterior face of cerebellar ventricle (Chaussier, 1807)*
Synonym for macrodissected adult human ***roof of fourth ventricle (Vesalius, 1543a)***; in the original French, *la face postérieure de la ventricule du cervelet*, pp. 99–100.
3. *tent (Reil, 1807–1808a)*
Synonym for macrodissected adult human ***roof of fourth ventricle (Vesalius, 1543a)***; in the original German, *das Zelt*, pp. 39, 50.
4. *vault of fourth ventricle (Tiedemann, 1816)*
Synonym for macrodissected fetal human *tent (Reil, 1807–1808a)*; see translation (1826, p. 33).

roof of third ventricle (>1840)

As described for macrodissected adult mammal, the free ***ependymal roof plate (>1840)*** of the ***third ventricle (Galen, c173)***—called in adult ***choroid epithelium of third ventricle (>1840)***—stretching between the ***choroid lines of thalamus (>1840)***, along with its covering ***choroid membrane of third ventricle (>1840)*** and the associated ***choroid plexus of third ventricle (Vicq d'Azyr, 1784)***; see Carpenter (1976, p. 132 ff.), Williams & Warwick (1980, p. 981), *Dorland's* (2003, p. 1641). It was probably first indicated by Steno; see ***[roof of third ventricle (>1840)] (Steno, 1669)***.

EARLIER REFERENCES:

Illustrated, not named or described:

1. ***[roof of third ventricle (>1840)] (Steno, 1669)***
Steno may have indicated it crudely in the outline drawing of a transverse section of a macrodissected adult human; Table III (top).

roof plate (>1840)

As described for developing vertebrate, the thin dorsal region in the median plane of the ***neural tube (Baer, 1837)*** that does not generate neural tissue; see Alvarez-Bolado & Swanson (1996, p. 13 ff.). Not described clearly by 1840.

rostral fovea (>1840)

As described for macrodissected adult human, a slight depression in the ***floor of fourth ventricle (Reil, 1807–1808a)*** in the region where the rostral edges of the ***facial colliculus (>1840)*** and ***vestibular area of fourth ventricle (>1840)*** meet, along the ***limiting sulcus of fourth ventricle (>1840)***; see Crosby et al. (1962, Fig. 97), *Nomina Anatomica* (1983, p. A66). It was perhaps first described as the *anterior fovea (Arnold, 1838a)*.

EARLIER REFERENCES:

Earlier synonyms:

1. *anterior fovea (Arnold, 1838a)*
Synonym for macrodissected adult human ***rostral fovea (>1840)***; in the original Latin, *fovea anterior*, p. 26.

rostral medullary velum (>1840)

As described for macrodissected adult human, a thin ***central nervous system white matter tract (>1840)*** extending from the ***arbor vitae (Winslow, 1733)*** and stretching between the right and left ***superior cerebellar peduncle (Procháska, 1800)***. It forms the rostral part of the ***roof of fourth ventricle (Vesalius, 1543a)*** associated with the ***pons (Haller, 1747)***, with its ventral or ventricular surface formed by a layer of ***ependyma (>1840)*** and much of its dorsal or outer surface lined by the ***lingula (Malacarne, 1776)***; see Williams & Warwick (1980, p. 914, Fig. 7.88), *Dorland's* (2003, p. 2020), Nieuwenhuys et al. (2008, Fig. 3.8). It may have been seen as early as Galen; see ***[rostral medullary velum (>1840)] (Galen, c173)***.

TRANSLATIONS:

1. *velum medullare rostralis (>1840)*
   Latin form of ***rostral medullary velum (>1840)***; see *Dorland's* (2003, p. 2020).

EARLIER REFERENCES:

Described, not named or illustrated:

1. ***[rostral medullary velum (>1840)] (Galen, c173)***
   In *On the Usefulness of the Parts* (May, 1968, p. 420 note 76) and *On Anatomical Procedures* (Burdach, 1822, p. 323; Wiberg, 1914, p. 29), Galen may deal briefly with it in macrodissected adult beef, pig, and/or macaque but not human explicitly.
2. ***[rostral medullary velum (>1840)] (Vesalius, 1543a)***
   Apparently referred vaguely to in macrodissected adult human; see Singer translation (1952, p. 37).

Earlier synonyms:

1. *restraining membrane (Willis, 1664)*
   Synonym for macrodissected adult human and other common large mammalian ***rostral medullary velum (>1840)***; see Pordage translation (1681, p. 123).Willis also provided a good description and illustrations; see Pordage translation (1681, pp. 65, 110, Figs. VII, VIII).
2. *transverse medullary process (Willis, 1664, p. 65)*
   Synonym for macrodissected adult human and other common large mammalian ***rostral medullary velum (>1840)***, as well as simply *transverse process*, which Willis described as medullary or fibrous; see Pordage translation (1681, p. 65). He also used the term *transverse medullary process (Willis, 1664, p. 61)* with reference to ***terminal stria (Wenzel & Wenzel, 1812)***.
3. *commissura processuum e testibus in cerebelli meditullia protensorum (Willis, 1664)*
   Synonym for macrodissected adult human and other large mammalian ***rostral medullary velum (>1840)***; Chs. 3 and 10, Figures IV-*K* and VII-*R*, according to Burdach (1822, p. 326).
4. *velum apophysi vermiformi obtentum (Drelincourt, 1672)*
   Synonym for macrodissected adult human ***rostral medullary velum (>1840)***; p. 47; see Schreger (1803, p. 327), Burdach (1822, p. 325).
5. *incrementa fibrosa (Drelincourt, 1672)*
   Synonym for macrodissected adult human ***rostral medullary velum (>1840)***; p. 47, see Burdach (1822, p. 326).
6. *valvula major cerebri (Vieussens, 1684)*
   Synonym for macrodissected adult human ***rostral medullary velum (>1840)***. It was supposed to be a valve between caudal end of ***cerebral aqueduct (>1840)*** and rostral end of ***fourth ventricle (Galen, c192)***; p. 76; also see Ridley (1695, p. 128), Winslow (1733, Sect. X, p. 40), Clarke & O'Malley (1996, pp. 641–642). Vieussens also used the forms *valvula cerebri major* (Tab. VIII-*I*), *valvulam cerebri majorem* (p. 76), and *valvulae majoris cerebri* (Tab. XI-*i*).
7. *valvular lamina (Winslow, 1733)*
   Synonym for macrodissected adult human ***rostral medullary velum (>1840)***; Section X, p. 40.
8. *valviform expansion (Winslow, 1733)*
   Synonym for macrodissected adult human ***rostral medullary velum (>1840)***; Section X, p. 47.
9. *valve of Vieussens (Lieutaud, 1742)*
   Eponym for macrodissected adult human ***rostral medullary velum (>1840)***, first described by Galen; p. 397.
10. *valvula major cerebri Vieussenii (Tarin, 1753)*
    Eponymous form of *valvula major cerebri (Vieussens, 1684)*; p. 25.
11. *velum interjectum (Haller, 1762)*
    Synonym for macrodissected adult human ***rostral medullary velum (>1840)***; p. 74, see Vicq d'Azyr (1786, p. 93). Burdach (1822, p. 325) gave the full term as *velum processibus a cerebello ad testes interjectum*.
12. *valvulam magnam cerebri (Haller, 1762)*
    Haller's variation on *valvula major cerebri (Vieussens, 1684)*; p. 75.
13. *medullary velum (Malacarne, 1776)*
    Synonym for macrodissected adult human ***rostral medullary velum (>1840)***; see p. 9 from 1780 reprint. Vicq d'Azyr (1784, p. 580) supplied the Latin, *velum medullare*.
14. *lacunar ventriculi quarti (Soemmerring, 1778)*
    Synonym for macrodissected adult human ***rostral medullary velum (>1840)***; p. 109, see Burdach (1822, p. 325).
15. *cerebral valve (Vicq d'Azyr, 1784)*
    Synonym for macrodissected adult human ***rostral medullary velum (>1840)***; in the original French, *valvule du cerveau*; pp. 557, 577; and Vicq d'Azyr (1786, Pl. XVII, Fig. I-45).
16. *middle medullary lamina of cerebellum (Vicq d'Azyr, 1784)*
    Synonym for macrodissected adult human ***rostral medullary velum (>1840)***; in the original French, *lame médullaire moyenne du cervelet*, p. 580. Burdach (1822, p. 325) gave the Latin form, *lamina medullaris media cerebelli*.
17. *valvula magna cerebelli (Günther, 1786)*
    Synonym for macrodissected adult human ***rostral medullary velum (>1840)***; p. 20.
18. *valvula magna cerebri (Günther, 1786)*
    According to Günther, inept name for macrodissected adult human ***rostral medullary velum (>1840)***; p. 20.
19. *valvula ovalis (Günther, 1786)*
    Synonym for macrodissected adult human ***rostral medullary velum (>1840)***; p. 20.

20. *valvula Galeni (Günther, 1786)*
Eponym for macrodissected adult human ***rostral medullary velum (>1840)***; p. 46.
21. *medullary lamina of cerebellum (Burdin, 1803)*
Synonym for macrodissected adult human ***rostral medullary velum (>1840)***; see translation (1803, Vol. 1, p. 163).
22. *anterior medullary velum (Reil, 1807–1808a)*
Synonym for macrodissected adult human ***rostral medullary velum (>1840)***; in the original German, *vördere Marksegel*, see Mayo translation (1822, p. 25). Burdach (1822, p. 326) gave Meckel's (1817, Vol. I, p. 470) variations on this in Latin as *velum medullare anticum* and *pars anterior veli medullaris.*
23. *processus cerebelli ad testes (Bell & Bell, 1816)*
Synonym for macrodissected adult human ***rostral medullary velum (>1840)***; Vol. 2, p. 462.
24. *Vieussenian valve (Gordon, 1817)*
Eponym for macrodissected adult human ***rostral medullary vellum (>1840)***; p. 166.
25. *valve of Aqueduct of Sylvius (Gordon, 1817)*
Synonym listed for macrodissected adult human ***rostral medullary vellum (>1840)***; in the original French, *valvule de l'Aqueduc de Sylvius*, p. 110.
26. *velum Vieussenii (Gordon, 1817)*
Eponym for macrodissected adult human ***rostral medullary vellum (>1840)***; p. 166.
27. *trabecula medullaris cerebelli (Bock, 1820)*
Synonym for macrodissected adult human *incrementa fibrosa (Drelincourt, 1672)* according to Foster (1892, p. 2945); p. 263. Also see Burdach (1822, p. 326).
28. *superior medullary velum (Tiedemann, 1821)*
Synonym for macrodissected adult monkey ***rostral medullary velum (>1840)***; in the original Latin, *veli medullaris superioris*, Table II, Figure 2-*k*.
29. *anterior valve (Burdach, 1822)*
Synonym for macrodissected adult human ***rostral medullary vellum (>1840)***; in the original German, *vordere Klappe*, p. 50.
30. *medullary curtain of cerebellum (Knox, 1832)*
Synonym for macrodissected adult human ***rostral medullary vellum (>1840)***; Supplemental Plate III-22.

PARTLY CORRESPONDS:

1. *tractus medullaris transversus (Vieussens, 1684)*
A tract Vieussens described in macrodissected adult human as forming caudal end of ***rostral medullary velum (>1840)*** giving rise to ***trochlear nerves (Molinetti, 1669)***; its existence is doubtful; p. 69 and Table IX-*g,h*. Also see Burdach (1822, p. 326) and *transverse medullary process (Willis, 1664, p. 65)*.
2. *transverse cerebral stria (Günther, 1786)*
Perhaps synonym for macrodissected adult human *tractus medullaris transversus (Vieussens, 1684)*; in the original Latin, *stria cerebri transversalis*, p. 14.
3. *lyra veli anterioris (Bergmann, 1831)*
Markings or slight grooves Bergmann reported on ventral (under) side of macrodissected adult human ***rostral medullary vellum (>1840)***; p. 64, also see Arnold (1838a, p. 41).
4. *transverse medullary lamina (Arnold, 1838b)*
Synonym for macrodissected adult human *tractus medullaris transversus (Vieussens, 1684)*; in the original Latin, *lamina medullaris transversa*, Table IV, Figure 2-*w*. See Henle (1871, p. 125).

rostral part of vestibular nerve (>1840)

As described for macrodissected adult human, a branch from middle regions of the ***vestibulocochlear nerve trunk (>1840)*** generating the ***utriculoampullary nerve (>1840)*** and ***anterior ampullary nerve (>1840)***; see *Nomina Anatomica* (1983, p. A75). It was first clearly delineated as the *superior and anterior fascicle of soft nerve (Cotugno, 1760)* and is commonly known as the *superior part of vestibular nerve (>1840)*.

EARLIER REFERENCES:

Earlier synonyms:

1. *superior and anterior fascicle of soft nerve (Cotugno, 1760)*
Synonym for macrodissected adult human ***rostral part of vestibular nerve (>1840)***; in the original Latin, *fasciculus superior, & anterior*, p. 408, Table II-*g1*.
2. *superior fascicle of soft nerve (Cotugno, 1760)*
Synonym for *superior and anterior fascicle of soft nerve (Cotugno, 1760)*; p. 408.
3. *superior anterior branch of auditory nerve proper (Günther, 1786)*
Synonym for macrodissected adult human ***rostral part of vestibular nerve (>1840)***; in the original Latin, *nervus auditorius proprius ramus anterior superior*, p. 60.
4. *major branch of anterior fascicles of acoustic nerve (Scarpa, 1789)*
Description and illustration of macrodissected adult human ***rostral part of vestibular nerve (>1840)***; Table 8, Figure 2-*i*.
5. *major twig of posterior branch of auditory nerve (Soemmerring, 1791)*
Synonym for macrodissected adult human *major branch of anterior fascicles of acoustic nerve (Scarpa, 1789)*; p. 226, also see Soemmerring (1798, p. 259).
6. *posterior twig of posterior branch of auditory nerve (Soemmerring, 1791)*
Synonym for macrodissected adult human *major branch of anterior fascicles of acoustic nerve (Scarpa, 1789)*; p. 226, also see Soemmerring (1798, p. 259).
7. *major anterior vestibular nerve (Langenbeck, 1826–1830)*
Synonym for macrodissected adult human ***rostral part of vestibular nerve (>1840)***; in the original Latin, *nervi vestibuli anterior—major*, Fascicle III, Table XXIX-7.
8. *major branch of posterior branch of acoustic nerve (Cloquet, 1828)*
Synonym for macrodissected adult human ***rostral part of vestibular nerve (>1840)***; in the original

French, *grand rameau de la branche postérieure du nerf acoustique*, Table CXXX, Figure 9-20.
9. *nervus ampullarum externarum canalis semicircularis superioris atque externi (Arnold, 1834)*
Synonym for macrodissected adult human ***rostral part of vestibular nerve (>1840)***; p. 12, Table III-40.
10. *superior part of vestibular nerve (>1840)*
Synonym for macrodissected adult human ***rostral part of vestibular nerve (>1840)***; see Streeter (1907, p. 155), Durward (1951, Fig. 904), Williams & Warwick (1980, pp. 1213), *Terminologia Anatomica* (1998, p. 135).

rostrum of corpus callosum (Reil, 1809b)

As described for macrodissected adult human, the thin extension of the ***corpus callosum (Galen, c177)*** ventral to the ***genu of corpus callosum (Reil, 1809b)*** becoming even thinner as it approaches the ***anterior commissure (Lieutaud, 1742)*** near the ***terminal lamina (Burdach, 1822)***, where it is sometimes called the *copula (>1840)*; see Mettler (1948, pp. 100–102, Fig. 68), Williams & Warwick (1980, p. 1024). For Reil's use in macrodissected adult human, see Table XIII-*d*, where the original German was *das Schnabel*. For Latin form, *corpus callosum rostrum*, see Foster (1894, p. 2727); also see Burdach (1822, p. 367). It was first identified by Steno; see ***[rostrum of corpus callosum (Reil, 1809b)] (Steno, 1669)***.

TRANSLATIONS:

1. *extremity of genu of corpus callosum (Reil, 1809b)*
English form of ***rostrum of corpus callosum (Reil, 1809b)***; see Mayo translation (1823, pp. 52, 120), also see ***genu of corpus callosum (Reil, 1809b)***.
2. *beak of corpus callosum (Reil, 1809b)*
English form of ***rostrum of corpus callosum (Reil, 1809b)***; see Meckel translation (1832, Vol. 2, p. 448).

EARLIER REFERENCES:

Illustrated, not named or described:

1. ***[rostrum of corpus callosum (Reil, 1809b)] (Steno, 1669)***
Clearly illustrated in first accurate midsagittal view of macrodissected adult human ***brain (Smith Papyrus, c1700 BC)***; Plate I. Malacarne (1780; see Burdach, 1822, p. 366) and Vicq d'Azyr (1784, pp. 545–546) described it further.

LATER SYNONYMS:

1. *lamina genu corpus callosi (Burdach, 1822)*
Probably synonym for macrodissected adult human ***rostrum of corpus callosum (Reil, 1809b)***; in the original German, *ausbreitung das Knieblatt*, p. 146. Also see Reichert (1859, Table X).

PARTLY CORRESPONDS:

1. *taeniolae corporis callosi (Reil, 1812c)*
Apparently, thin distal end of macrodissected adult human ***rostrum of corpus callosum (Reil, 1809b)*** extending toward *anterior perforated substance (Vicq d'Azyr, 1784)*; in the original German, *Balkenleistchen*, Table XIII-*e*. Burdach (1822, p. 147) gave the Latin form, *taeniolae corporis callosi*. Also see Foster (1894, p. 2901) and *Dorland's* (2003, p. 1852), where it is linked eponymously with Reil and said to be synonym for *lamina rostralis (>1840)*.
2. *lamina rostralis (>1840)*
Synonym for macrodissected adult human *copula (>1840)*; see Mettler (1948, p. 100). In English, *rostral lamina*.
3. *copula (>1840)*
Thin distal segment of macrodissected adult human ***rostrum of corpus callosum (Reil, 1809b)*** as it approaches ***anterior commissure (Lieutaud, 1742)*** near ***terminal lamina (Burdach, 1822)***; see Mettler (1948, p. 100).

rubrospinal tract (>1840)

As described in macrodissected adult human, and mammal generally with experimental histological methods for ***axons (Kölliker, 1896)***, the longitudinal, caudally directed extension of the ***ventral tegmental decussation (>1840)*** reaching intermediate and medial regions of the ***lateral funiculus (Burdach, 1822)*** of the ***spinal cord (Galen, c162–c166)***. Along the way there are major branches to ***cerebellum (Aristotle)*** and ***medulla (Winslow, 1733)***; see Carpenter (1976, pp. 261–263 and Fig. 10.17). For topographic description there are ***tegmental rubrospinal tract (>1840)***, ***pontine rubrospinal tract (>1840)***, ***medullary rubrospinal tract (>1840)***, and ***spinal rubrospinal tract (>1840)*** segments. In the ***brain (Smith Papyrus, c1700 BC)*** it lies within the ***ventrolateral fascicle (>1840)***. It was not delineated clearly by 1840.

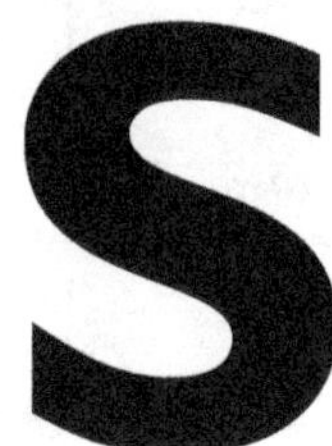

saccular nerve (>1840)

As described for macrodissected adult human, a terminal branch of the ***caudal part of vestibular nerve (>1840)*** to the macula of the saccule that is commonly the major, rostral supply of the saccule; see Durward (1951, p. 1035 and Fig. 904), *Terminologia Anatomica* (1998, p. 136). It was probably first clearly delineated as the *third branch of anterior fascicles of acoustic nerve (Scarpa, 1789).*

EARLIER REFERENCES:

Earlier synonyms:

1. *third branch of anterior fascicles of acoustic nerve (Scarpa, 1789)*
   Probably description and illustration of macrodissected adult human ***saccular nerve (>1840)***; Table 8, Figure 2.
2. *middle twig of posterior branch of auditory nerve (Soemmerring, 1791)*
   Synonym for *third branch of anterior fascicles of acoustic nerve (Scarpa, 1789)*; p. 226 and Soemmerring (1798, p. 259).
3. *middle branch of posterior branch of acoustic nerve (Cloquet, 1828)*
   Synonym for macrodissected adult human ***saccular nerve (>1840)***; in the original French, *rameau moyen de la branche postérieure du nerf acoustique*, Table CXXX, Figure 9-21.
4. *middle branch of vestibular nerve (Arnold, 1839)*
   Probably synonym for macrodissected adult human ***saccular nerve (>1840)***; in the original Latin, *ramus medius nervi vestubli*, Table VII, Figure 9-*t*.

sacral nerves (Camper, 1760)

As described for macrodissected adult human, the five pairs of ***spinal nerves (Camper, 1760–1762)*** associated with the ***sacral part of spinal cord (>1840)***; see Carpenter (1976, pp. 213–216). For Camper's use in macrodissected adult human, see p. 8. The first accurate description for macrodissected adult human was *nerves proceeding from pith of os sacrum (Diemerbroeck, 1689)*; Galen's descriptions were unclear, see *sacral nerves (Galen, c173).*

EARLIER REFERENCES:

Earlier synonyms:

1. *nerves proceeding from pith of os sacrum (Diemerbroeck, 1689)*
   Synonym for macrodissected adult human ***sacral nerves (Camper, 1760)***; p. 561.
2. *nerves of spinal marrow of os sacrum (Heister, 1717)*
   Synonym for macrodissected adult human ***sacral nerves (Camper, 1760)***; for translation see Heister (1721, p. 250).

LATER SYNONYMS:

1. *pelvian pairs of nerves (Burdin, 1803)*
   Synonym for macrodissected adult mammalian ***sacral nerves (Camper, 1760)***; see translation (1803, Vol. 3, p. 150).

PARTLY CORRESPONDS:

1. *sacral nerves (Galen, c173)*
   In *On the Usefulness of the Parts*, Galen described and named four pairs of *sacral nerves (Galen, c173)* emerging from the bone (his "sacred bone" or *os sacrum*) associated with them in adult human, although his dissections apparently were confined to other common large mammals; see May translation (1968, pp. 602–603), and ***sacral nerves (Camper, 1760)***. In *De Ossibus ad Tirones* he mentioned three *sacral nerves* (see Kühn translation, 1821, Vol. 2, p. 762), which is true in some mammals but not human (see de Koning, 1903, pp. 33–37, 487). He noted that "Nature has created the so-called broad bone, to which some have given the name 'sacrum.'" (May translation, 1968, p. 602). Elsewhere he wrote that, "The 'wide bone' is also, as I have said previously, called the 'greatest bone', that is, the 'cross.'" (Duckworth translation, 1962, p. 261). According to Foster (1894, p. 2736) it got the name *sacrum* (from *sacer* or "sacred" in Latin) from an ancient belief that it is indestructible.

2. *nervi sacrales (Galen, c173)*
   Latin form of *sacral nerves (Galen, c173)*; e.g., Haase (1781, p. 42).
3. *nervi sacri (Galen, c173)*
   Latin form of *sacral nerves (Galen, c173)*; e.g., Haase (1781, p. 42).
4. *pairs of nerves associated with sacral bone (Razi, c910)*
   Razi counted three such pairs in his account of human anatomy, apparently based on Galen's description of the sacrum in *De Ossibus ad Tirones*, where he mentioned three *sacral nerves (Galen, c173)*; see Kühn translation (1821, Vol. 2, p. 762). This is true in some mammals but not human; see de Koning (1903, pp. 33–37, 487).
5. *nerves from medulla of alhovius (Achillini, 1520)*
   Synonym for *pairs of nerves associated with sacral bone (Razi, c910)*; see Lind translation (1975, pp. 62, 63).
6. *nerves of nape alhovius (Berengario da Carpi, 1523)*
   Synonym for *pairs of nerves associated with sacral bone (Razi, c910)*; see Lind translation (1959, p. 160).

sacral part of spinal cord (>1840)

As described for macrodissected adult vertebrate, the longitudinal ***spinal cord part (>1840)*** generating the *sacral nerves*; see Carpenter (1976, pp. 213–216). As described for macrodissected adult human, the longitudinal ***spinal cord part (>1840)*** generating the five ***sacral nerves (Camper, 1760)***; see *Nomina Anatomica* (1983, p. A64), *Terminologia Anatomica* (1998, p. 105). It was first delineated by Galen; see ***[sacral part of spinal cord (>1840)] (Galen, c173)***.

EARLIER REFERENCES:

Described, not named or illustrated:

1. ***[sacral part of spinal cord (>1840)] (Galen, c173)***
   In *On the Usefulness of the Parts*, Galen described *sacral nerves (Galen, c173)*, without applying specific name to ***spinal cord part (>1840)*** associated with his sacred bone (*os sacrum*) from which they arise; see May translation (1968, pp. 602–603). He did refer specifically to *cervical spinal medulla (Galen, c173)*, *thoracic spinal medulla (c173)*, and *lumbar spinal medulla (Galen, c173)* in a variety of macrodissected adult mammals, but not human specifically.

Earlier synonyms:

1. *medulla of alhovius (Achillini, 1520)*
   Achillini used this synonym for ***sacral part of spinal cord (>1840)***, implying it was derived from first book of Razi's *Almansor*; see Lind translation (1975, pp. 62–63).
2. *nape alhovius (Berengario da Carpi, 1523)*
   Synonym for macrodissected adult human ***sacral part of spinal cord (>1840)***; see Lind translation (1959, p. 160).

sacral plexus (Vesalius, 1543a)

As described for macrodissected adult human, commonly formed by the ***spinal nerve ventral branches (>1840)*** of part of the fourth and all of the fifth ***lumbar nerves (Diemerbroeck, 1672)*** and the first three, and part of the fourth ***sacral nerves (Camper, 1760)***; see ***lumbosacral plexus (Vesalius, 1543a)***, ***lumbosacral trunk (Cruveilhier, 1836)***, and Durward (1951, p. 1099), Williams & Warwick (1980, pp. 1110–1011). The ***sacral plexus (Vesalius, 1543a)*** itself consists of ***sacral plexus dorsal divisions (Paterson, 1887)*** and ***sacral plexus ventral divisions (Paterson, 1887)*** formed by the proximal ***sacral plexus ventral branches (>1840)***. The distal branches or ***nerves (Herophilus, c335–c280 BC)*** of the ***sacral plexus (Vesalius, 1543a)*** may arise from just ***sacral plexus dorsal divisions (Paterson, 1887)*** or ***sacral plexus ventral divisions (Paterson, 1887)***, or from both—as for the ***sciatic nerve (Keill, 1698)*** and ***posterior cutaneous nerve of thigh (Günther, 1786)***; see Durward (1951, Fig. 937), Williams & Warwick (1980, Fig. 7.213). The term has its origins in the passage quoted under ***lumbosacral plexus (Vesalius, 1543a)***; also see Richardson & Carman translation (2002, pp. 255, 257). It was known to Galen; see ***[sacral plexus (Vesalius, 1543a)] (Galen, c173)***.

EARLIER REFERENCES:

Described, not named or illustrated:

1. ***[sacral plexus (Vesalius, 1543a)] (Galen, c173)***
   Galen referred to ***nerves (Herophilus, c335–c280 BC)*** of ***sacral plexus (Vesalius, 1543a)***, including ***lumbosacral plexus (Vesalius, 1543a)***, without using specific terms, in *On the Usefulness of the Parts* and *On Anatomy of Nerves*; see May translation (1969, pp. 602–603, 703) and Goss (1966, p. 334), respectively.

LATER SYNONYMS:

1. *intertexture of nervi sacri (Winslow, 1733)*
   Synonym for macrodissected adult human ***sacral plexus (Vesalius, 1543a)***; Section VI, p. 89.
2. *plexus of all nervi sacri (Winslow, 1733)*
   Synonym for macrodissected adult human ***sacral plexus (Vesalius, 1543a)***; Section VI, p. 89.
3. *sacral part of crural plexus (Chaussier, 1809)*
   Synonym for macrodissected adult human ***sacral plexus (Vesalius, 1543a)***.
4. *sciatic plexus (Cloquet, 1816)*
   Synonym for macrodissected adult human ***sacral plexus (Vesalius, 1543a)***; in the original French, *plexus sciatique*, p. 669. Quain (1828, p. 290) used the Latin form, *plexus ischiadicus*.
5. *crural plexus (Cruveilhier, 1836)*
   Synonym for macrodissected adult human ***sacral plexus (Vesalius, 1543a)***; in the original French, *plexus crural*, p. 778.

PARTLY CORRESPONDS:

1. *plexum ischiadicum (Camper, 1762)*
   Sacral plexus (Vesalius, 1543a) parts leading directly to formation of ***sciatic nerve (Keill, 1698)*** in macrodissected adult human, that is, roots of ***sciatic nerve (Keill, 1698)***; p. 7 and Table 1, Figure 2-22,23.
2. *major pudendal nerve (Günther, 1786)*
   Rare feature of macrodissected adult human described by Günther as generating ***superior gluteal nerve***

(Martin, 1781) and ***nerve to obturator internus (>1840)***; in the original Latin, *pudendalis major*, p. 86.

3. *small femoro-poplitean nerve (Burdin, 1803)*
   Synonym for macrodissected adult human *lesser sciatic nerve (Chaussier, 1809)*; see translation (1803, Vol. 1, p. 204).
4. *ischio-trochanterian branches of small femoro-poplitean nerve (Burdin, 1803)*
   Vaguely described branches of ***sacral plexus (Vesalius, 1543a)*** to "the muscles surrounding the ischium and the trochanter" (translation, 1803, Vol. 1, p. 204). Also see *fessiers nerve (Burdin, 1803)*.
5. *lesser sciatic nerve (Chaussier, 1809)*
   Apparently, roughly macrodissected adult human ***nerve to quadratus femoris (>1840)***, ***nerve to obturator internus (>1840)***, ***posterior cutaneous nerve of thigh (Günther, 1786)***, and other branches to muscles surrounding ischium and trochanter, considered together; in the original French, *nerf petit sciatique*. Cruveilhier (1836, p. 857) attributed without citation the term to Boyer. Quain (1828, p. 291) used this form in English.
6. *sciatic plexus posterior branches (Cloquet, 1816)*
   Essentially macrodissected adult human ***posterior cutaneous nerve of thigh (Günther, 1786)***, ***inferior gluteal nerve (Martin, 1781)***, and ***dorsal nerve of penis (Camper, 1762)*** or ***dorsal nerve of clitoris (>1840)*** considered together; in the original French, *branches et rameaux postérieurs du plexus sciatique*, pp. 670–672.
7. *inferior gluteal nerve (Cloquet, 1816)*
   Essentially macrodissected adult human ***posterior cutaneous nerve of thigh (Günther, 1786)*** and ***inferior gluteal nerve (Martin, 1781)*** considered together; in the original French, *nerf fessier inférieur*, p. 670. Cruveilhier (1836, p. 857) attributed without citation the term to Bichat.
8. *pudendal plexus (Bock, 1827)*
   Part of macrodissected adult human ***sacral plexus (Vesalius, 1543a)*** shown generating ***pudendal nerve (Camper, 1762)***, ***inferior rectal nerves (>1840)***, and ***posterior cutaneous nerve of thigh (Günther, 1786)***; in the original Latin, *plex. pudendus*, Table VI, Figure 1–34.
9. *external pudendal plexus (Bock, 1827)*
   Synonym for *pudendal plexus (Bock, 1827)*; in the original Latin, *plexus pudendalis externus*, Table VII, Figure 2–46.
10. *small sciatic nerve (Quain, 1832)*
   Similar to macrodissected adult human *lesser sciatic nerve (Chaussier, 1809)* but including ***inferior gluteal nerve (Martin, 1781)***; in the original Latin, *nervus ischiadicus minor*, p. 794.
11. *inferior gluteal nerve (Quain, 1832)*
   Synonym for *small sciatic nerve (Quain, 1832)*; in the original Latin, *nervus gluteus inferior*, p. 702.
12. *collateral branches of sacral plexus (Cruveilhier, 1836)*
   All branches of macrodissected adult human ***sacral plexus (Vesalius, 1543a)*** arising proximal to ***sciatic nerve (Keill, 1698)***, which Cruveilhier considered the sole *terminal branch of sacral plexus (Cruveilhier, 1836)*; he described four anterior collateral branches and five posterior collateral branches; in the original French, *branches collatérales du plexus sacré*, p. 851.

sacral plexus dorsal divisions (Paterson, 1887)

In mammals the ***sacral plexus ventral branches (>1840)*** divide into ***sacral plexus dorsal divisions (Paterson, 1887)*** and ***sacral plexus ventral divisions (Paterson, 1887)*** related evolutionarily and developmentally (rather loosely in adult) to the dorsal (extensor) and ventral (flexor) musculature of the leg—except probably the fourth ***sacral plexus ventral branch (>1840)*** with no ***sacral plexus dorsal division (Paterson, 1887)***; see Durward (1951, p. 1115 and Fig. 937), Williams & Warwick (1980, p. 1119 and Fig. 7.213). Branches or ***nerves (Herophilus, c335-c280 BC)*** of the ***sacral plexus (Vesalius, 1543a)*** may arise from just ***sacral plexus dorsal divisions (Paterson, 1887)*** or ***sacral plexus ventral divisions (Paterson, 1887)***, or from both—as for the ***sciatic nerve (Keill, 1698)*** and ***posterior cutaneous nerve of thigh (Günther, 1786)***; see Durward (1951, Fig. 937), Williams & Warwick (1980, Fig. 7.213). For Paterson's use in macrodissected adult mammal, see p. 621. They were not accurately delineated by 1840.

PARTLY CORRESPONDS:

1. *gluteal nerves (Fyfe, 1800)*
   Macrodissected adult human ***superior gluteal nerve (Martin, 1781)*** and ***inferior gluteal nerve (Martin, 1781)*** considered together; Vol. 2, p. 329.

sacral plexus ventral branches (>1840)

As described for macrodissected adult human, the ***spinal nerve ventral branches (>1840)*** for ***lumbar nerves (Diemerbroeck, 1672)*** and ***sacral nerves (Camper, 1760)*** involved in forming the ***sacral plexus (Vesalius, 1543a)***; see Durward (1951, Fig. 937), Williams & Warwick (1980, pp. 1110–1111). They were first delineated by Eustachi; see ***[sacral plexus ventral branches (>1840)] (Eustachi, 1552)***.

EARLIER REFERENCES:

Illustrated, not named or described:

1. *[sacral plexus ventral branches (>1840)] (Eustachi, 1552)*
   Illustrated relatively accurately for macrodissected adult human; see Albinus edition (1761, Tabs. 28 and 19).

Earlier synonyms:

1. *sacral plexus anterior branches (Meckel, 1817)*
   Synonym for macrodissected adult human ***sacral plexus ventral branches (>1840)***; see translation (1832, Vol. 3, pp. 12–13).

sacral plexus ventral divisions (Paterson, 1887)

In mammals the ***sacral plexus ventral branches (>1840)*** divide into ***sacral plexus dorsal divisions (Paterson, 1887)*** and ***sacral plexus ventral divisions (Paterson, 1887)*** related evolutionarily and developmentally (rather loosely in adult) to the dorsal (extensor) and ventral (flexor) musculature of the leg—except probably the fourth sacral ***sacral plexus ventral branch (>1840)*** with no ***sacral plexus dorsal division (Paterson, 1887)***; see Durward (1951, p. 1115 and Fig. 937), Williams & Warwick (1980, p. 1119 and Fig. 7.213). Distal branches or ***nerves (Herophilus, c335–c280 BC)*** of the ***sacral plexus (Vesalius, 1543a)*** may arise from just ***sacral plexus dorsal divisions (Paterson, 1887)*** or ***sacral plexus ventral divisions (Paterson, 1887)***, or from both—as for the ***sciatic nerve (Keill, 1698)*** and ***posterior cutaneous nerve of thigh (Günther, 1786)***; see Durward (1951, Fig. 937), Williams & Warwick (1980, Fig. 7.213). For Paterson's use in macrodissected adult mammal see p. 621. They were not clearly delineated by 1840.

PARTLY CORRESPONDS:

1. *uterine nerve (Fischer, 1791)*
   Described as 18th branch of third pair of macrodissected adult human ***sacral nerves (Camper, 1760)***, thus arising near distal end of ***sacral plexus ventral divisions (Paterson, 1887)***; in the original Latin, *nervus uterinus*, p. 20. Not usually recognized now.
2. *nerve to superior and inferior gemellus muscles (Fischer, 1791)*
   Apparently branch of macrodissected adult human ***sacral plexus ventral divisions (Paterson, 1887)***; in the original Latin, *nervum musculi gemini superioris et inferioris*, p. 29.
3. *deep femoral branch from sacral plexus (Mayer, 1794)*
   As described for macrodissected adult human, trunk from ***sacral plexus ventral divisions (Paterson, 1887)*** supplying branches to superior and inferior gemellus, obturator internus, quadratus femoris, and adductor magnus muscles; in the original Latin, *ramus profundus femoris ex plexus sacrali ortius*; Part 5, Table VI, Figure 3-*η*.
4. *fessiers nerve (Burdin, 1803)*
   Apparently macrodissected adult human ***nerve to quadratus femoris (>1840)*** and ***nerve to obturator internus (>1840)***, arising from common trunk; see translation (1803, Vol. 1, p. 204).
5. *sciatic plexus anterior branches (Cloquet, 1816)*
   Essentially macrodissected adult human ***inferior rectal nerves (>1840)*** and ***pelvic splanchnic nerves (Gaskell, 1886)*** considered together; in the original French, *branches et rameaux antérieurs du plexus sciatique*, pp. 669–670.
6. *vesicle nerves (Cloquet, 1816)*
   Branches of *sciatic plexus anterior branches (Cloquet, 1816)* to base of urinary bladder, prostate, and seminal vesicles in men, and to base of urinary bladder and walls of uterus in women; in the original French, *nerfs vésicaux*, p. 669.
7. *uterine and vaginal nerves (Cloquet, 1816)*
   Branches of *sciatic plexus anterior branches (Cloquet, 1816)* to wall of uterus and to vagina; in the original French, *nerfs utérins et vaginaux*, p. 670.

sacral spinal ganglia (>1840)

As described for macrodissected adult human, there is one ***spinal nerve ganglion (Burdach, 1819)*** for each ***dorsal root (Spurzheim, 1826)*** of the five pairs of ***sacral nerves (Camper, 1760)***. They are numbered sequentially from rostral to caudal; see Williams & Warwick (1980, p. 1086). They were discovered by Coiter; see ***[sacral spinal ganglia (>1840)] (Coiter, 1572)***.

EARLIER REFERENCES:

Described, not named or illustrated:

1. *[sacral spinal ganglia (>1840)] (Coiter, 1572)*
   Coiter stated there is a *knot (Coiter, 1572)*, or ***spinal nerve ganglion (Burdach, 1819)***, for each *spinal nerve (Vesalius, 1543a)* in macrodissected adult human; see translation (1955, p. 115).

sacral splanchnic nerves (>1840)

As described for macrodissected adult human, these relatively sparse visceral branches of the ***sacral sympathetic ganglia (>1840)*** extend medially and communicate ventral to (in front of) the sacrum with corresponding branches from the other side, in the ***hypogastric nerve (Walter, 1783)*** and its lower continuation, the ***inferior hypogastric plexus (Tiedemann, 1822)***, and yet other branches form a ***plexus (Galen, c192)*** on the median (middle) sacral artery; see Durward (1951, p. 1137 and Fig. 967), Mitchell (1953, p. 298 and Fig. 131), Williams & Warwick (1980, p. 1132). Also see ***pelvic splanchnic nerves (Gaskell, 1886)***. They were perhaps first distinguished clearly by Willis; see ***[sacral splanchnic nerves (>1840)] (Willis, 1664)***.

EARLIER REFERENCES:

Described, not named or illustrated:

1. *[sacral splanchnic nerves (>1840)] (Willis, 1664)*
   Several alluded to and illustrated for macrodissected adult human and other common large mammals; see Pordage translation (1681, p. 159 and Tab. 11-*q,r,s*). Vieussens illustrated them clearly for macrodissected adult human; Table 23-*84,85*.

Earlier synonyms:

1. *visceral branches of sacral ganglia of sympathetic (Quain & Wilson, 1839)*
   Synonym for macrodissected adult human ***sacral splanchnic nerves (>1840)***; Plate XXI-*c**.

sacral sympathetic ganglia (>1840)

As described for macrodissected adult human, ***sympathetic trunk ganglia (Winslow, 1733)*** having one or more ***gray communicating branches (>1840)*** between all ***sacral nerves (Camper, 1760)***. There are commonly 4–5 ***sacral sympathetic ganglia (>1840)***, numbered sequentially from rostral (superior) to caudal (inferior); see Mitchell (1953, Ch. 18), Williams & Warwick (1980, p. 1132). The first accurate full account was probably given for the *sacral ganglia (Walter, 1783)*.

EARLIER REFERENCES:

Earlier synonyms:

1. *sacral ganglion (Walter, 1783)*
   Carefully described, and illustrated three, macrodissected adult human ***sacral sympathetic ganglia (>1840)***; in the original Latin, *ganglion sacrale*, Table I-*158,164*.

2. *sacral ganglia of intercostal nerve (Günther, 1786)*
   Five macrodissected adult human ***sacral sympathetic ganglia (>1840)*** described; in the original Latin, *ganglia sacralia nervus intercostalis*, p. 96 (and p. 92). Soemmerring (1791, p. 331) also described five.

saphenous nerve (Haase, 1781)

As described for macrodissected adult human, the largest and longest cutaneous branch of the ***femoral nerve (Haller, 1762)***, supplying skin and fascia on the medial side of the leg and foot; see Durward (1951, p. 1098 and Fig. 941). For Haase's use in macrodissected adult human, see p. 107. Styx (1782, pp. 19–22) and Fischer (1791, Tab. IV, Fig. 1) provided detailed descriptions and illustrations for macrodissected adult human, and Bell (1803b, p. 199) noted it can be regarded as a branch of the *long nerve to vastus internus muscle (Styx, 1782)*; see Hamilton (1976, Fig. 830B). It was known to Galen; see ***[saphenous nerve (Haase, 1781)] (Galen, c173)***.

ALTERNATE SPELLINGS:

1. *saphene nerve (Burdin, 1803)*
   Alternate spelling of ***saphenous nerve (Haase, 1781)***; see translation (1803, Vol. 1, p. 202).

TRANSLATIONS:

1. *nervus saphenus (Haase, 1781)*
   Original Latin form of ***saphenous nerve (Haase, 1781)***; p. 107.

EARLIER REFERENCES:

Described, not named or illustrated:

1. ***[saphenous nerve (Haase, 1781)] (Galen, c173)***
   Clearly described for macrodissected adult beef, pig, and/or macaque but not human; see May translation (1968, p. 707), Singer translation (1999, pp. 83, 84, 87). Vesalius (1543a) described it for macrodissected adult human; see Richardson & Carman translation (2002, pp. 258–259).

LATER SYNONYMS:

1. *inferior cutaneous branch of crural nerve (Martin, 1781)*
   Synonym for macrodissected adult human ***saphenous nerve (Haase, 1781)***; in the original Latin, *nervus cruralis ramus cutaneus inferior*, p. 233 and Table X.
2. *long cutaneous nerve of foot (Günther, 1786)*
   Synonym for macrodissected adult human ***saphenous nerve (Haase, 1781)***; in the original Latin, *nervus cutaneus longus pedis*, p. 83.
3. *inferior cutaneous nerve of foot (Günther, 1786)*
   Synonym for macrodissected adult human ***saphenous nerve (Haase, 1781)***; in the original Latin, *nervus cutaneus pedis inferior*, p. 83.
4. *inferior cutaneous nerve (Fischer, 1791)*
   Synonym for macrodissected adult human *inferior cutaneous branch of crural nerve (Martin, 1781)*; in the original Latin, *nervum cutaneum inferiorem*, p. 7.
5. *great internal cutaneous nerve (Mayer, 1794)*
   Synonym for macrodissected adult human ***saphenous nerve (Haase, 1781)***; in the original Latin, *nervus cutaneus internus major s. inferior pedis*; Part 5, Table V, Figure 1-*14,15* (p. 25).
6. *inferior nerve of foot (Mayer, 1794)*
   Synonym for *great internal cutaneous nerve (Mayer, 1794)*; in the original Latin, *nervus inferior pedis*; Part 5, Table V, Figure 1-*14* (p. 25).
7. *great internal cutaneous nerve of leg (Mayer, 1794)*
   Synonym for macrodissected adult human ***saphenous nerve (Haase, 1781)***; in the original Latin, *nervus cutaneus internus major of foot*; Part 5, Table V, Figure 1-*14* (p. 27).
8. *inferior internal cutaneous nerve of foot (Mayer, 1794)*
   Apparently synonym for *great internal cutaneous nerve of leg (Mayer, 1794)*; in the original Latin, *nervus cutaneus internus inferior pedis*; Part 5, Table VI-*τ* (p. 38).
9. *major inferior cutaneous branch of anterior femoral nerve (Soemmerring, 1798)*
   Synonym for macrodissected adult human ***saphenous nerve (Haase, 1781)***; p. 318.
10. *long cutaneous nerve (Bell, 1803a)*
    Synonym for macrodissected adult human ***saphenous nerve (Haase, 1781)***; Latin given as *nervus cutaneus longus*, Plate VII-*7,8*.
11. *great saphenous nerve (Bell, 1803a)*
    Synonym for macrodissected adult human ***saphenous nerve (Haase, 1781)***; Plate VIII-*12*.
12. *tibio-cutaneous nerve (Burdin, 1803)*
    Synonym for macrodissected adult human ***saphenous nerve (Haase, 1781)***; see translation (1803, Vol. 1, p. 202).
13. *internal saphenous nerve (Cloquet, 1816)*
    Synonym for macrodissected adult human ***saphenous nerve (Haase, 1781)***; in the original French, *nerf saphène interne*, p. 665. The translation of Meckel (1832, Vol. 3, p. 16) spelled it *internal saphena nerve*, giving the Latin, *nervus saphenus internus*.
14. *great internal saphenous nerve (Bock, 1827)*
    Synonym for macrodissected adult human ***saphenous nerve (Haase, 1781)***; in the original Latin, *nerv. saphenus internus major*, Table I, Figure 2-*80*.
15. *long saphenous nerve (Quain & Wilson, 1839)*
    Synonym for macrodissected adult human ***saphenous nerve (Haase, 1781)***; Plate XXIII-*f*.

PARTLY CORRESPONDS:

1. *lesser saphenous nerve (Fischer, 1791)*
   Lateral or external branch of macrodissected adult human ***saphenous nerve (Haase, 1781)***; in the original Latin, *nervi sapheni minoris*, Table III, Figure 1-*337*. In some cadavers it might correspond to *short saphenous nerve (Quain & Wilson, 1839)*.
2. *second saphenous nerve (Fischer, 1791)*
   Synonym for *lesser saphenous nerve (Fischer, 1791)*; in the original Latin, *nervi sapheni secundi*, Table III, Figure 1-*337*.
3. *internal dorsal nerve of big toe (Mayer, 1794, p. 26)*
   Terminal branch of macrodissected adult human ***saphenous nerve (Haase, 1781)*** supplying dorsal and medial regions of big toe; in the original Latin, *nervus internus dorsalis pollicis*; Part 5, Table V, Figure 1-*16* (p. 26).
4. *collateral branches of internal saphenous nerve (Cruveilhier, 1836)*

Three described for macrodissected adult human: *femoral cutaneous branch of internal saphenous nerve (Cruveilhier, 1836)*, *tibial cutaneous branch of internal saphenous nerve (Cruveilhier, 1836)*, and *articular filament of internal saphenous nerve (Cruveilhier, 1836)*; in the original French, *branches collatérales*, p. 846.

5. *femoral cutaneous branch of internal saphenous nerve (Cruveilhier, 1836)*
   First *collateral branch of internal saphenous nerve (Cruveilhier, 1836)*; in the original French, *rameau cutané fémoral*, p. 846.
6. *tibial cutaneous branch of internal saphenous nerve (Cruveilhier, 1836)*
   Second *collateral branch of internal saphenous nerve (Cruveilhier, 1836)*; in the original French, *rameau cutané tibial*, p. 846.
7. *articular filament of internal saphenous nerve (Cruveilhier, 1836)*
   Third *collateral branch of internal saphenous nerve (Cruveilhier, 1836)*, to knee joint; in the original French, *filet articulaire*, p. 846.
8. *terminal branches of internal saphenous nerve (Cruveilhier, 1836)*
   Two described for macrodissected adult human: *anterior terminal branch of internal saphenous nerve (Cruveilhier, 1836)* and *posterior terminal branch of internal saphenous nerve (Cruveilhier, 1836)*; in the original French, *branches terminales*, p. 846.
9. *posterior terminal branch of internal saphenous nerve (Cruveilhier, 1836)*
   Macrodissected adult human continuation of ***saphenous nerve (Haase, 1781)*** distal to origin of ***infrapatellar branch of saphenous nerve (>1840)***; in the original French, *branche postérieure*, p. 847. Cruveilhier further described internal and external branches of this branch; p. 848.
10. *direct terminal branch of internal saphenous nerve (Cruveilhier, 1836)*
    Synonym for *posterior terminal branch of internal saphenous nerve (Cruveilhier, 1836)*; in the original French, *branche directe*, p. 847.
11. *posterior branch of posterior terminal branch of internal saphenous nerve (Cruveilhier, 1836)*
    Dorsal branch of *posterior terminal branch of internal saphenous nerve (Cruveilhier, 1836)*; in the original French, *rameau postérieur*, p. 847.
12. *anterior branch of posterior terminal branch of internal saphenous nerve (Cruveilhier, 1836)*
    Ventral branch of *posterior terminal branch of internal saphenous nerve (Cruveilhier, 1836)*; in the original French, *rameau antérieur*, p. 847.
13. *articular filaments of posterior terminal branch of internal saphenous nerve (Cruveilhier, 1836)*
    Small branches of *posterior terminal branch of internal saphenous nerve (Cruveilhier, 1836)* to tibiotalar joint; in the original French, *filets articulaires*, p. 847.
14. *branches of internal saphenous nerve to knee-joint (Quain & Wilson, 1839)*
    Macrodissected adult human branches of ***saphenous nerve (Haase, 1781)*** to knee joint; Plate XXIII-*h*.

sciatic nerve (Keill, 1698)

As described for macrodissected adult human, the thickest ***nerve (Herophilus, c335–c280 BC)*** in the body and the common trunk of the smaller ***common fibular nerve (>1840)*** and larger ***tibial nerve (Haase, 1781)***, stretching from the distal end of the ***sacral plexus (Vesalius, 1543a)*** to about the distal third of the thigh, where its two divisions separate into spatially distinct ***nerves (Herophilus, c335–c280 BC)***. It is formed by ***sacral plexus dorsal divisions (Paterson, 1887)*** as well as ***sacral plexus ventral divisions (Paterson, 1887)***, and the two ***nerves (Herophilus, c335–c280 BC)*** are bound together by an investing sheath; see Durward (1951, Figs. 946, 947), Williams & Warwick (1980, Figs. 7.213, 216, 217). "In many cases these two nerves are distinct at their origin, and are separated sometimes by fibres of the piriformis muscle. In all cases, on removal of the sheath investing the sciatic nerve, the two divisions can be traced up to the plexus, from which they invariably take origin by distinct and separate roots." (Durward, 1951, p. 1099; also see Meckel, 1832, Vol. 3, pp. 17–18). For Keill's use in macrodissected adult human, see pp. 300–301. It was first described as the *fourth deep nerve of thigh (Galen, c177)*. According to the *Oxford English Dictionary* (Online) in Latin *sciatic-us* is a corrupt form of *ischiadic-us*; also see Cotugno (1760, p. 3 ff.) and Haase (1781, p. 108).

TRANSLATIONS:

1. *nervus sciaticus (Keill, 1698)*
   Original Latin form of ***sciatic nerve (Keill, 1698)***; pp. 300–301.
2. *nervus ischiadicum (Heister, 1717)*
   Latin form of ***sciatic nerve (Keill, 1698)***; p. 95.
3. *nervus ischiadicus (Heister, 1721)*
   Latin form of ***sciatic nerve (Keill, 1698)***; p. 249. Used by *Basel Nomina Anatomica* (His, 1895, p. 92) and *Terminologia Anatomica* (1998, p. 140).

EARLIER REFERENCES:

Earlier synonyms:

1. *fourth deep nerve of thigh (Galen, c177)*
   Synonym for ***sciatic nerve Keill, 1698)*** in macrodissected adult beef, pig, and/or macaque but not human, where Galen emphasized it belongs to two large ***nerves (Herophilus, c335–c280 BC)*** descending through leg, ***tibial nerve (Haase, 1781)*** and ***common fibular nerve (>1840)***; see Singer translation (1999, pp. 85–87), Duckworth translation (1962, p. 263).
2. *fourth nerve traveling to thigh (Vesalius, 1543a)*
   Synonym for *fourth nerve entering leg (Vesalius, 1543a)*; see Richardson & Carman translation (2002, p. 215).
3. *fourth nerve entering leg (Vesalius, 1543a)*
   Variation on *fourth deep nerve of thigh (Galen, c177)*, where Vesalius distinguished 18 components; see Richardson & Carman (2002, pp. 258–261).

4. *fourth sinew going into thigh (Geminus, 1553)*
Synonym for macrodissected adult human *fourth nerve traveling to thigh (Vesalius, 1543a)*; the original phrase was spelled *fourth... synowe of them which doe goe into the thigh*, see *The table of the figures of synowes*.
5. *fourth sinew going into leg (Geminus, 1553)*
Synonym for macrodissected adult human *fourth nerve entering leg (Vesalius, 1543a)*; originally spelled *fourth synowe goynge into legge*, see *The table of the figures of sinowes*.
6. *fourth crural nerve (Crooke, 1615)*
Synonym for macrodissected adult human *fourth nerve entering leg (Vesalius, 1543a)*; in the original text referred to as "the 4. crurall nerve" (p. 492). Essentially direct translation from Bauhin (1605).
7. *posterior crural nerve (Vieussens, 1684)*
Synonym for macrodissected adult human ***sciatic nerve (Keill, 1698)***; in the original Latin, *nervus cruralis posticus*, Table XXIX-*M,O*.
8. *crural trunk (Verheyen, 1693)*
Synonym for macrodissected adult human ***sciatic nerve (Keill, 1698)***; in the original Latin, *truncum cruralem, truncus cruralis*, see Plate 29-*H,I*.

LATER SYNONYMS:

1. *crural nerve proper (Salmon, 1714)*
Synonym for macrodissected adult human ***sciatic nerve (Keill, 1698)***, "The fourth Nerve, which is the proper Crural Nerve." (p. 131).
2. *ischiatic nerve (Cheselden, 1726)*
Synonym for macrodissected adult human ***sciatic nerve (Keill, 1698)***; p. 268, which was essentially written by Monro *primus* as stated in the Preface.
3. *cruralis magnus nervus (Pietro da Cortona, 1741)*
Synonym for macrodissected adult human ***sciatic nerve (Keill, 1698)***; p. 52.
4. *sciatic nerve trunk (Günther, 1786)*
Synonym for macrodissected adult human ***sciatic nerve (Keill, 1698)***, in most common situation where ***tibial nerve (Haase, 1781)*** and ***common fibular nerve (>1840)*** course together before splitting into spatially separated ***nerves (Herophilus, c335–c280 BC)***; in the original Latin, *truncus ischiatici nervi*, p. 86.
5. *common sciatic nerve trunk (Jördens, 1788)*
Synonym for macrodissected adult human *sciatic nerve trunk (Günther, 1786)*; in the original Latin, *truncum nervi ischiadici communem*, p. 1.
6. *sciatic trunk (Fischer, 1791)*
Synonym for macrodissected adult human *crural trunk (Verheyen, 1693)*; in the original Latin, *truncus ischiadicus*, p. 23.
7. *posterior femoral nerve (Fischer, 1791)*
Synonym for macrodissected adult human ***sciatic nerve (Keill, 1698)***; in the original Latin, *nervus femoralis posterior*, Table IV, Figure 2-*91*.
8. *great ischiatic nerve (Bell, 1803a)*
Synonym for macrodissected adult human ***sciatic nerve (Keill, 1698)***; Plate III-22.
9. *body of ischiatic nerve (Bell, 1803b)*
Synonym for macrodissected adult human *sciatic trunk (Fischer, 1791)*; p. 203.
10. *great femoro-poplitean nerve (Burdin, 1803)*
Synonym for macrodissected adult human ***sciatic nerve (Keill, 1698)***; see translation (1803, Vol. 1, p. 204).
11. *greater sciatic nerve (Chaussier, 1809)*
Synonym for macrodissected adult human *great femoro-poplitean nerve (Burdin, 1803)*; in the original French, *nerf grand sciatique*. In contrast to *lesser sciatic nerve (Chaussier, 1809)*. Knox (1832, Pl. XI-*133*) used the term as such in English.
12. *great sciatic nerve (Knox, 1832)*
English form of *greater sciatic nerve (Chaussier, 1809)*; Plate XI-*133*.
13. *terminal branch of sacral plexus (Cruveilhier, 1836)*
Synonym for macrodissected adult human ***sciatic nerve (Keill, 1698)***; in the original French, *branche terminale du plexus sacré*, p. 851.

PARTLY CORRESPONDS:

1. *nervus sciatico-cruralis (Winslow, 1733)*
Segment of ***sciatic nerve (Keill, 1698)*** distal to greater trochanter; Section VI, no. 323, p. 91. Also see Haymaker & Woodhall (1953, Figs. 248, 250).
2. *nervus popliteus (Winslow, 1733)*
According to Winslow, name commonly given to macrodissected adult human distal part of ***sciatic nerve (Keill, 1698)*** just before branching to form ***tibial nerve (Haase, 1781)*** and ***common fibular nerve (>1840)***; Section VI, no. 324, p. 91. Soemmerring (1798, p. 329) used the Latin form, *nervum popliteum*. In English, *popliteal nerve*.
3. *nervi sciatico-tibiales (Winslow, 1733)*
Synonym for two large branches of ***sciatic nerve (Keill, 1698)*** in macrodissected adult human leg, ***tibial nerve (Haase, 1781)*** and ***common fibular nerve (>1840)***; Section VI, no. 325, p. 91.
4. *inferior internal cutaneous nerve (Fischer, 1791)*
Branch of macrodissected adult human trunk of ***sciatic nerve (Keill, 1698)*** arising just distal to origin of ***posterior cutaneous nerve of thigh (Günther, 1786)*** and infrequently recognized now; in the original Latin, *nervus cutaneus internus inferior*, p. 29. Fischer described three branches, internal, middle, and external.
5. *first root of sciatic nerves (Mayer, 1794)*
Described for macrodissected adult human as arising from fourth ***lumbar nerve (Diemerbroeck, 1672)***; in the original Latin, *radix prima nervi ischiadici*; Part 6, Table VI-*112* (p. 39).
6. *lower internal cutaneous nerve (Bell, 1803a)*
Probably synonym for macrodissected adult human *inferior internal cutaneous nerve (Fischer, 1791)*; Plate IX-9.
7. *dorsal digital nerves of foot (Bock, 1827)*
Macrodissected adult human ***dorsal digital nerves of deep fibular nerve (>1840), dorsal digital nerves of intermediate dorsal cutaneous nerve (>1840), dorsal digital nerves of lateral dorsal cutaneous nerve (>1840)***, and ***dorsal digital nerves of medial dorsal cutaneous***

nerve (>1840) considered together; in the original Latin, *nervi digitales dorsales pedis*, Table I, Figure 2-95.

8. *internal inferior cutaneous nerve (Knox, 1832)*
   Knox's form of *inferior internal cutaneous nerve (Fischer, 1791)*; Plate XVI-*136*.
9. *muscular branches of sciatic nerve (Cruveilhier, 1836)*
   Macrodissected adult human ***nerve to hamstring muscles (>1840)*** and ***nerve to short head of biceps femoris (>1840)*** considered together; see Durward (1951, pp. 1105–1106), Williams & Warwick (1980, p. 1112). For Cruveilhier's use in macrodissected adult human, see p. 860.

secondary brain vesicles (>1840)

The linearly arranged ***brain vesicles (Malpighi, 1673)*** derived from the three ***primary brain vesicles (Baer, 1837)*** that in all vertebrates form the *five morphological elements of brain (Baer, 1837)* during Baer's (1837) second stage of ***neural tube (Baer, 1837)*** development; p. 107. They are, from rostral (superior) to caudal (inferior), the ***endbrain vesicle (Kuhlenbeck, 1927)***, which is paired, ***interbrain vesicle (Baer, 1837)***, ***midbrain vesicle (Baer, 1837)***, ***hindbrain vesicle (Baer, 1837)***, and ***afterbrain vesicle (Baer, 1837)***; see Nieuwenhuys et al. (2008, pp. 9–16). They were clearly illustrated by Malpighi; see *five cerebral vesicles (Malpighi, 1673)*.

EARLIER REFERENCES:

Earlier synonyms:

1. *five cerebral vesicles (Malpighi, 1673)*
   Synonym for ***secondary brain vesicles (>1840)*** in the 3-day chick embryo; in the original Latin, *cerebri quinque vesiculae*, p. 16.
2. *five vesicles (Baer, 1837)*
   Synonym for vertebrate ***secondary brain vesicles (>1840)***; in the original German, *fünf Bläschen*, p. 107.
3. *five morphological elements of brain (Baer, 1837)*
   Synonym for *five vesicles (Baer, 1837)*; in the original German, *fünf morphologische Elemente des Hirnes*, p. 107.

secondary fissure (Bolk, 1906)

As described for macrodissected adult human, the groove between ***biventral lobule (>1840)*** and ***tonsil (Malacarne, 1776)*** of the ***cerebellar cortex (Willis, 1664)*** continuing across the median plane between ***pyramis (Malacarne, 1776)*** and ***uvula (Malacarne, 1776)*** of the ***cerebellar vermis (Meckel, 1817)***; see Angevine et al. (1961, p. 20 and Figs. 10, 13, 15, 16,19, 24), *Terminologia Anatomica* (1998, p. 119). Smith (1902, p. 381) used the term only for the vermal segment of the ***secondary fissure (Bolk, 1906)***; see Angevine et al. (1961, Fig. 8). It was perhaps first clearly recognized by Salmon; see ***[secondary fissure (Bolk, 1906)] (Salmon, 1714)***.

EARLIER REFERENCES:

Illustrated, not named or described:

1. ***[secondary fissure (Bolk, 1906)] (Salmon, 1714)***
   Clearly illustrated for macrodissected adult human; Table 20, compare with Nieuwenhuys et al. (2008, Fig. 3.13).

sellar diaphragm (>1840)

As described for macrodissected adult human, "a horizontal fold of the meningeal layer of dura mater attached to the anterior and posterior clinoid processes, where it is continuous with the free and attached borders respectively of the tentorium cerebelli. It is reflected around the infundibulum to form an investment for the hypophysis cerebri." (Millen & Woollam, 1962, p. 128). Also see *Terminologia Anatomica* (1998, p. 104). It was known to Winslow; see ***[sellar diaphragm (>1840)] (Winslow, 1733)***.

TRANSLATIONS:

1. *diaphragma sellae (>1840)*
   Current Latin form of ***sellar diaphragm (>1840)***; see *Terminologia Anatomica* (1998, p. 104).

EARLIER REFERENCES:

Described, not named or illustrated:

1. ***[sellar diaphragm (>1840)] (Winslow, 1733)***
   Very clearly described for macrodissected adult human; Section X, pp. 26–27.

semilunar gyrus (>1840)

As described for macrodissected adult human, the caudal topographic subdivision of the ***olfactory region (>1840)*** between ***ambient gyrus (>1840)*** rostrally and ***parahippocampal gyrus (>1840)*** caudally. Based on cellular architecture and connections in mammal it corresponds generally to the ***cortical amygdalar complex (>1840)***; see Nauta & Haymaker (1969, Fig. 4.10-*GS*). It was probably first delineated by Burdach; see ***[semilunar gyrus (>1840)] (Burdach, 1822)***.

TRANSLATIONS:

1. *gyrus semilunaris (>1840)*
   Latin form of *semilunar gyrus (>1840)*; see Nauta & Haymaker (1969, Fig. 4.10).

EARLIER REFERENCES:

Illustrated, not named or described:

1. ***[semilunar gyrus (>1840)] (Burdach, 1822)***
   Probably illustrated for macrodissected adult human; Table III-*γ* just medial to *amygdaloid nucleus (Burdach, 1822)* indicated at *δ*; also see Nauta & Haymaker (1969, Fig. 4.10), Nieuwenhuys et al. (2008, Figs. 3.6-3.7).

seminal vesicle nerves (Bock, 1827)

As described for macrodissected adult human, they are derived from the ***inferior hypogastric plexus (Tiedemann, 1822)*** and ***ureteric plexus (>1840)*** and are thin and short before entering the seminal vesicles. They are associated with thin ***nerves (Herophilus, c335–c280 BC)*** supplying the base of the bladder and help supply the ejaculatory ducts, and sometimes the vas deferens; see Mitchell (1953, pp. 306-307). For Bock's use in macrodissected adult human, see Table VI, Figure 1-*28*. They were alluded to earlier by Meckel; see ***[seminal vesicle nerves (Bock, 1827)] (Meckel, 1817)***.

TRANSLATIONS:

1. *nervi vesiculae seminalis (Bock, 1827)*
   Original Latin form of ***seminal vesicle nerves (Bock, 1827)***; Table VI, Figure 1-*28*.

EARLIER REFERENCES:

Described, not named or illustrated:

1. ***[seminal vesicle nerves (Bock, 1827)] (Meckel, 1817)***
Alluded to in macrodissected adult human; see translation (1832, Vol. 3, p. 88).

LATER SYNONYMS:

1. *seminal vesicle plexus (Cruveilhier, 1836)*
Synonym for macrodissected adult male human ***seminal vesicle nerves (Bock, 1827)***; in the original French (plural), *plexus des vésicules séminales*, p. 1027.

septal fissure (Burdach, 1822)

As described for macrodissected adult human, the ***subarachnoid space (Magendie, 1827)*** in the median plane between right and left *septum (Galen, c177)* that is a rostromedial remnant of the embryonic evagination of right and left ***endbrain vesicle (Kuhlenbeck, 1927)***. Tiedemann (1816) claimed incorrectly that in the developing human fetus, and some adults, this region communicates directly with the ***third ventricle (Galen, c173)***, unaware of the intervening ***terminal lamina (Burdach, 1822)***; see translation (1826, p. 278). For Burdach's use in macrodissected adult human, see p. 135. It was clearly described long ago by Le Boë, see ***[septal fissure (Burdach, 1822)] (Le Boë, 1663)***.

TRANSLATIONS:

incisura septi (Burdach, 1822)
Original Latin form of ***septal fissure (Burdach, 1822)***; p. 135.

EARLIER REFERENCES:

Described, not named or illustrated:

1. ***[septal fissure (Burdach, 1822)] (Le Boë, 1663)***
An indirect reference to it in macrodissected adult human, between two layers, "To our surprise we chanced to observe last year that there is a *hiatus* where the corpus callosum begins to thin out into the septum pellucidum. Although the septum is very thin it is divided into two layers." (see Baker, 1909, p. 224). Also see Diemerbroeck (1689, p. 397), Burdach (1822, p. 353), and *fossa Sylvii (Vicq d'Azyr, 1786)*. Frans de Le Boë was also known as Franciscus Sylvius.

Earlier synonyms:

1. *cavitas (Vieussens, 1684)*
Illustrated and labeled as *cavitas* [of right and left *septum lucidum (Galen, c177)*], the ***septal fissure (Burdach, 1822)*** in macrodissected adult human; Table VI-*c*, also see ***[septal fissure (Burdach, 1822)] (Le Boë, 1663)***.
2. *canal below corpus callosum (Pourfour du Petit, 1710)*
Synonym for macrodissected adult human ***septal fissure (Burdach, 1822)***; in the original French, *Canal situé dessous le corps calleux*, p. 13.
3. *medullary cavity (Winslow, 1733)*
Synonym for macrodissected adult human ***septal fissure (Burdach, 1822)***, which in some cases, Winslow suggested, might communicate with ***third ventricle (Galen, c173)***; Section X, p. 35.
4. *cavitas Vieussenii (Stumphius, 1736)*
Eponym for macrodissected adult human ***septal fissure (Burdach, 1822)***, from *cavitas (Vieussens, 1684)*; p. 27, see Burdach (1822, p. 353).
5. *anonymous cavity (Haller, 1747)*
Synonym for macrodissected adult human ***septal fissure (Burdach, 1822)***; see Mihles translation (1754b, p. 291).
6. *ventricle of septum lucidum (Meckel, 1767)*
Synonym for macrodissected adult human ***septal fissure (Burdach, 1822)***; in the original Latin, *ventriculus septi lucidi*, p. 96. For use of the term in English see Mayo (1823, p. 69). Meckel (1832, Vol. 2, p. 450) referred simply to *ventricle of septum*.
7. *cavity of septum lucidum (Sabatier, 1775)*
Synonym for macrodissected adult human ***septal fissure (Burdach, 1822)***; in the original French, *cavité du* septum lucidum, Vol. 2, p. 36. Also see Burdach (1822, p. 353), who gave the Latin form, *ventriculus septi lucidi*.
8. *sinus of septum lucidum (Vicq d'Azyr, 1784)*
Synonym for macrodissected adult human ***septal fissure (Burdach, 1822)***; p. 7, Plate V-6.
9. *Sylvian fossa (Vicq d'Azyr, 1786)*
Eponym for ***septal fissure (Burdach, 1822)***; in the original Latin, *fossa Sylvii*, p. 7, Plate V-6; see ***[septal fissure (Burdach, 1822)] (Le Boë, 1663)***. In English it can also be translated *fossa of Sylvius*; see Meckel (1832, Vol. II, p. 450).
10. *fifth ventricle (Soemmerring, 1791)*
Synonym for macrodissected adult human ***septal fissure (Burdach, 1822)***; in the original German, *fünfte Hirnhöle*, p. 48.
11. *fissure of Sylvius (Fyfe, 1800)*
Eponym for macrodissected adult human ***septal fissure (Burdach, 1822)***; Vol. 2, p. 19.
12. *ventricle of septum (Burdin, 1803)*
Synonym for macrodissected adult human ***septal fissure (Burdach, 1822)***; see translation (1803, Vol. 1, p. 158). Arnold (1838b, Tab. IV, Fig. 5-*z*) gave the Latin, *ventriculus septi*, which could also be translated *septal ventricle*.
13. *ventricle of Sylvius (Gall & Spurzheim, 1810)*
Eponym for macrodissected adult human ***septal fissure (Burdach, 1822)***; p. 293; see Burdach (1822, p. 354).
14. *first ventricle (Wenzel & Wenzel, 1812)*
Synonym for ***septal fissure (Burdach, 1822)***; in the original Latin, *ventriculus primus*, p. 69.
15. *ventriculus septi cerebri medii (Wenzel & Wenzel, 1812)*
Synonym for ***septal fissure (Burdach, 1822)***; p. 69.

LATER SYNONYMS:

1. *sinus of median system (Cruveilhier, 1836)*
Synonym for macrodissected adult human ***septal fissure (Burdach, 1822)*** attributed to Chaussier without citation; in the original French, *sinus du système médian*, p. 676.

PARTLY CORRESPONDS:

1. *fovea triangularis infra septi lucidi partem inferiorem obvia (Tarin, 1750)*
   Apparently refers to opening of macrodissected adult human ***septal fissure (Burdach, 1822)*** near ***rostrum of corpus callosum (Reil, 1809b)***; Table I, Figures 4 and 5, part *o*. Also see *fossa of base of septum lucidum (Vicq d'Azyr, 1786)*.
2. *triangular cavity of septum lucidum (Vicq d'Azyr, 1784)*
   Apparently variation on *fovea triangularis infra septi lucidi partem inferiorem obvia (Tarin, 1750)*; in the original French, *la cavitè triangulaire du septum lucidum*, p. 549.
3. *fossa of base of septum lucidum (Vicq d'Azyr, 1786)*
   Synonym for macrodissected adult human *fovea triangularis infra septi lucidi partem inferiorem obvia (Tarin, 1750)*, apparently opening of ***septal fissure (Burdach, 1822)*** at ***rostrum of corpus callosum (Reil, 1809b)***, dorsal to ***anterior commissure (Lieutaud, 1742)***; in the original French, *fossa de la base du septum lucidum*; Plates XXI, Figure I-*4/5*; XXV, Figure I-*31,s*.

septal postcommissural fornix (>1840)

As described in macrodissected adult human, and mammal generally with histological methods for ***axons (Kölliker, 1896)***, the dorsal segment of the ***postcommissural fornix (Loo, 1931)*** in the *septal region (Swanson & Cowan, 1979)* of the ***cerebral nuclei (Swanson, 2000a)***, between the level of the ***subfornical organ (>1840)*** dorsally and the ***anterior commissure (Lieutaud, 1742)*** ventrally; that is, between the rostral end of the ***fimbria (Honegger, 1890)*** dorsally and the ***hypothalamic postcommissural fornix (>1840)*** segment ventrally. It was known to Galen; see ***[postcommissural fornix (Loo, 1931)] (Galen, c177)***.

EARLIER REFERENCES:

Earlier synonyms:

1. *basis of fornix (Willis, 1664)*
   Refers to rostral quarter or so of *body of fornix (Vesalius, 1543a)* in macrodissected adult sheep, perhaps corresponding roughly to ***septal postcommissural fornix (>1840)*** just before splitting into *twofold root of fornix (Willis, 1664)*; Figures 7-*E*, 8-*D*.
2. *base of fornix (Willis, 1664)*
   Form of *basis of fornix (Willis, 1664)*.
3. *basis of roof of ventricles (Poupart, 1712)*
   Probably synonym for *basis of fornix (Willis, 1664)*; pp. 642, 647.
4. *small column of fornix (Soemmerring, 1791)*
   Soemmerring referred in German (plural) to macrodissected adult human *Säulchen des Bogens* [small columns or pillars of fornix], which apparently correspond to right and left ***septal postcommissural fornix (>1840)***; pp. 32–34, see Burdach (1822, p. 357).
5. *fornix column (Burdach, 1822)*
   Basically synonym for macrodissected adult human ***septal postcommissural fornix (>1840)***; in the original Latin (plural), *columnae fornicis* (p. 138, Table VII-*h*); in the original German (plural), *Säulen* (p. 138). See *small column of fornix (Soemmerring, 1791)*, Soemmerring (1800, pp. 36, 39).
6. *free part of fornix column (His, 1895)*
   Essentially synonym for macrodissected adult human ***septal postcommissural fornix (>1840)***; in the original Latin, *pars libera columnae fornicis*, p. 86. For English form see Ranson (1920, p. 272).

PARTLY CORRESPONDS:

1. *base of anterior pillar of fornix (Winslow, 1733)*
   Apparently rostral end of macrodissected adult human *anterior pillar of fornix (Winslow, 1733)* near ***anterior commissure (Lieutaud, 1742)***, and thus rostroventral part or end of ***septal postcommissural fornix (>1840)***; Section X, p. 35.
2. *initial part of fornix (Cajal, 1904)*
   Short dorsal and caudal initial segment of ***septal postcommissural fornix (>1840)*** just rostral to ***fimbria (Honegger, 1890)***, near level of ***subfornical organ (>1840)***, possibly related to *fornix obliquus (Honegger, 1890)*; in the original Spanish, *porción inicial del fornix*, pp. 1004–1005.
3. *fimbrial part of fornix (Cajal, 1904)*
   Synonym for *initial part of fornix (Cajal, 1904)*, described as segment of *anterior column of trigone (Dejerine & Dejerine-Klumpke, 1901)*; in the original Spanish, *porción fimbrial del fornix*, pp. 1004–1005.
4. *descending part of fornix (Cajal, 1904)*
   Long distal segment of ***septal postcommissural fornix (>1840)***, between *ascending part of fornix (Cajal, 1904)* and ***hypothalamic postcommissural fornix (>1840)***; in the original Spanish, *porción descendente*, pp. 1004–1005. Also called *descending segment* (*segmento descendente* in the original Spanish) on p. 1045.
5. *septal segment of fornix (Cajal, 1904)*
   Synonym for *descending part of fornix (Cajal, 1904)*; in the original Spanish, *segmento septal del fimbria*, pp. 1004–1005.

short ciliary nerves (>1840)

As described for macrodissected adult human, there are usually 8–10 of them leaving the rostral end (front) of the ***ciliary ganglion (Loder, 1778)***, piercing the sclera, and supplying the sphincter pupillae and sphincter ciliaris muscles, as well as the choroidal and iridial blood vessels of the eye; see Williams & Warwick (1980, p. 1058 and Figs. 7.173, 176). Zinn (1755, p. 205 ff. and Tab. 6, Figs. 1 and 2) provided an illustration clearly distinguishing ***long ciliary nerves (Soemmerring, 1801)*** and ***short ciliary nerves (>1840)***, and even showed a ***communicating branch (Winslow, 1733)*** between them. They were perhaps first clearly delineated as *lesser nerves out of infolding of third pair (Willis, 1664)*.

EARLIER REFERENCES:

Earlier synonyms:

1. *lesser nerves out of infolding of third pair (Willis, 1664)*
   Synonym for macrodissected adult (presumably human) ***short ciliary nerves (>1840)***; see Pordage translation (1681, p. 145, Fig. 2-*g*).

2. *ciliary nerves (Ruysch, 1702)*
   Apparently applied to ***short ciliary nerves (>1840)*** of macrodissected adult human, although it is difficult to know whether ***long ciliary nerves (Soemmerring, 1801)*** were also involved; Vol. 2, p. 4. According to Pourfour du Petit, "Voilà les nerfs ciliares de Ruisch." (1729, p. 11); also see *pupillary nerves (Pourfour du Petit, 1729)*.
3. *ciliary nerves (Albinus, 1744)*
   Used in describing some unknown combination of ***short ciliary nerves (>1840)*** and ***[long ciliary nerves (Soemmerring, 1801)](Eustachi, 1552)***, although the former were involved and the latter may not have been, see *pupillary nerves (Pourfour du Petit, 1729)*, *ciliary nerves (Meckel, 1748)*; Table 18, Figure 5-*t*.
4. *ciliary nerves (Meckel, 1748)*
   Apparently correspond to ***short ciliary nerves (>1840)*** for macrodissected adult human; divided into *exterior superior*, *exterior inferior*, *interior inferior*, and *interior superior* groups forming *plexum ciliarem* with ***long ciliary nerves (Soemmerring, 1801)***; pp. 39–41, also see Haller (1743, p. 46 note *31*). Arnold (1834, p. 8) simply distinguished superior and inferior fasciculi.
5. *irian nerves (Burdin, 1803)*
   Synonym for macrodissected adult human ***short ciliary nerves (>1840)***; see translation (1803, Vol. 1, p. 223).
6. *ciliary branches of ophthalmic ganglion (Quain & Wilson, 1839)*
   Synonym for macrodissected adult human ***short ciliary nerves (>1840)***; Plate XIII, Figure 2-*i*.

PARTLY CORRESPONDS:

1. *central nerve of retina (Langenbeck, 1826–1830)*
   Macrodissected adult human extensions of ***short ciliary nerves (>1840)*** into eyeball; in the original Latin, *nervus centralis retinae*, Fascicle III, Table XVII, Figure 2.
2. *superior ciliary filaments (Todd, 1836–1839)*
   Macrodissected adult human ***short ciliary nerves (>1840)*** attached to dorsal (superior) and rostral (anterior) angle of ***ciliary ganglion (Loder, 1778)***; p. 282.
3. *inferior ciliary filaments (Todd, 1836–1839)*
   Macrodissected adult human ***short ciliary nerves (>1840)*** attached to ventral (inferior) and rostral (anterior) angle of ***ciliary ganglion (Loder, 1778)***; p. 282.

short gyri of insula (Gall & Spurzheim, 1810)

As described for macrodissected adult human, the rostral 3–4 *cerebral gyri (Vesalius, 1543a)* of the ***insular region (Brodmann, 1909)***, separated from the more caudal ***long gyrus of insula (Valentin, 1841)*** by the ***central sulcus of insula (>1840)***; see Burdach (1822, p. 387), Crosby et al. (1962, pp. 476–477, Fig. 319), Williams & Warwick (1980, pp. 987, 988), *Terminologia Anatomica* (1998, p. 125), Nieuwenhuys et al. (2008, p. 649 ff.). Reil (1809b) wrote about the short gyri of the ***insular region (Brodmann, 1909)*** in general, without distinguishing long and short; see Meyer (1971, pp. 127–128, note *8*).

LATER SYNONYMS:

1. *shorter circumvolutions of island of Sylvian fissure (Meckel, 1817)*
   Synonym for macrodissected adult human ***short gyri of insula (Gall & Spurzheim, 1810)***; see translation (1832, Vol. 2, p. 442).

simple lobule (Jansen & Brodal, 1954)

As described for macrodissected adult human, the part of the ***cerebellar hemisphere (Willis, 1664)*** between ***culmen (Stroud, 1895)*** and ***ansiform lobule crus 1 (Bock, 1906)***, and lateral to the ***declive (1840)*** of the ***cerebellar vermis (Meckel, 1817)***; see Angevine et al. (1961, Fig. 24), Larsell & Jansen (1972, Fig. 118), Carpenter (1976, Fig. 14.1), Williams & Warwick (1980, Fig. 7.74), *Terminologia Anatomica* (1998, p. 119). It was not recognized as such by 1840.

spermatic ganglia (Walter, 1783)

As described for macrodissected adult human, typically two small ***prevertebral ganglia (Quain, 1832)*** on each lateral side of the descending aorta, associated with the ***intermesenteric plexus (>1840)*** and proximal ends of the ***superior ovarian nerves (>1840)*** or ***superior testicular nerves (>1840)***; see Hovelacque (1927, p. 761). Walter discovered and described at least three ***spermatic ganglia (Walter, 1783)***, which he called first, second, and third, on either side of macrodissected adult human; see Tables I-*292*,*293*, II-*306*.

spinal central gray (>1840)

As described for macrodissected adult human, and for adult mammal in general with cellular architecture and connections, the small unpaired ***gray matter region (Swanson & Bota, 2010)*** of the ***intermediate spinal zone (>1840)*** surrounding the ***central canal of spinal cord (>1840)***; see Rexed (1952, pp. 450–452, where it is called *10th region of spinal gray matter, X*), Nahin et al. (1983). It was first observed by Blasius; see ***[spinal central gray (>1840)] (Blasius, 1666)***.

EARLIER REFERENCES:

Illustrated and described, not named:

1. ***[spinal central gray (>1840)] (Blasius, 1666)***
   Discovered and illustrated for macrodissected adult human; see Schulte & Endtz (1977, p. 13).

Earlier synonyms:

1. *middle part of spinal cord ash-colored substance (Vicq d'Azyr, 1784)*
   Roughly synonymous with macrodissected adult human ***spinal central gray (>1840)***, although Vicq d'Azyr's description was understandably vague; pp. 600–601, see Clarke & O'Malley translation (1996, p. 269). He wrote that *ash-colored substance (Winslow, 1733)* or *cortical substance (Willis, 1664)* of ***spinal cord (Galen, c162–c166)*** may be divided into middle and two lateral parts, with middle part being

transverse and thus comparable to middle of letter ***H***. Contemporaneously, Monro wrote that ***spinal cord (Galen, c162–c166)*** is "composed of two cords, joined together at their middle or deepest parts by a lamella, which consists chiefly of red vessels and cineritious matter" (1783, p. 28 and Tab. VII, Fig. 2-*E*); see *cords of spinal marrow (Monro, 1783)*. Bellingeri (1823, see p. 24) used the Latin form, *centro substantiae cinereae.*

2. *transverse part of spinal cord ash-colored substance (Vicq d'Azyr, 1784)*
   Synonym for *middle part of spinal cord ash-colored substance (Vicq d'Azyr, 1784)*; pp. 600–601, see Clarke & O'Malley translation (1996, p. 269).
3. *gray transverse lamina (Keuffel, 1810)*
   Synonym for *transverse lamina of gray substance (Keuffel, 1810)*; in the original Latin, *lamina transversa cinerea*, p. 41.
4. *transverse lamina of gray substance (Keuffel, 1810)*
   Roughly synonymous with macrodissected adult human ***spinal central gray (>1840)***; in the original Latin, *lamina transversa substantiae cinereae*, Figure 2-*c*.
5. *median commissure of spinal marrow (Meckel, 1817)*
   Roughly synonymous with macrodissected adult human ***spinal central gray (>1840)***; see translation (1832, Vol. 2, p. 415).
6. *cortical commissure of spinal marrow (Meckel, 1817)*
   Synonym for *median commissure of spinal marrow (Meckel, 1817)*; see translation (1832, Vol. 2, p. 415).
7. *connecting layer for gray fascicles (Desmoulins, 1825)*
   Roughly synonymous with macrodissected adult human ***spinal central gray (>1840)***; in the original French, *lame de réunion des faisceaux gris*, Plate 13, Figure 5-*o*.
8. *gray commissure (Cruveilhier, 1836)*
   Roughly synonymous with macrodissected adult human ***spinal central gray (>1840)***; in the original French, *commissure grise*, p. 577. Arnold (1838b, Tab. II, Fig. 2-*c*) provided the Latin, *commissura cinerea.*
9. *spinal medulla central gray (Arnold, 1838b)*
   Synonym for macrodissected adult human *gray commissure (Cruveilhier, 1836)*; in the original Latin, *centrum cinereum*, Table II, Figure 2-*c*.
10. *spinal medulla middle gray (Arnold, 1838b)*
    Synonym for *spinal medulla central gray (Arnold, 1838b)*; in the original Latin, *medium cinereum*, Plate III, Figure 1-*b*.
11. *inner gray fascicle (Wagner, 1839)*
    Roughly synonymous with macrodissected adult human ***spinal central gray (>1840)***; in the original Latin, *fasciculus cinereus intimus*, Table XXVII, Figure 10-*9*.

spinal cord (Galen, c162–c166)

The caudal topographic division of the vertebrate ***cerebrospinal axis (Meckel, 1817)***; the rostral topographic division is the ***vertebrate brain (Cuvier, 1800)***. For this definition see Swanson & Bota (2010). The usual convention for distinguishing the two divisions in the adult is that the ***vertebrate brain (Cuvier, 1800)*** lies within the skull, whereas the ***spinal cord (Galen, c162–c166)*** lies within the spinal (vertebral) column, although this is a difficult problem in practice. Galen appears to have used this specific term (in Greek) for the first time in writings that have survived, for example, in *On the Doctrines of Hippocrates and Plato* and *On Anatomical Procedures*; see De Lacy (1978, p. 85) and Duckworth translation (1962, p. 223), also see ***[spinal cord (Galen, c162–c166)] (Smith Papyrus, c1700 BC)***, *spinal marrow (Hippocrates)*. In *On the Usefulness of the Parts*, Galen wrote that the spinal cord, which was explicitly mentioned earlier—*spinal medulla (Hippocrates)*—is like a second *encephalon (Homer, c9th century BC)*, or ***brain (Smith Papyrus, c1700 BC)***, for parts below the head; see May translation (1968, pp. 573, 579). Most or all of Galen's neuroanatomy was done on macrodissected adult beef, pig, and/or macaque; see Woollam (1958, p. 15). He referred back to knowledge obtained from human dissection in Alexandria, mostly by Herophilus and Erasistratus (see von Staden, 1989)—and he probably also learned something of human anatomy as physician to the gladiators. The first clear distinction between *gray substance (Vesalius, 1543a)* and *white substance (Vesalius, 1543a)* in the ***spinal cord (Galen, c162–c166)*** was made by Coiter (1572, translation p. 113), who noted that the former is inner and the latter is outer. Pourfour du Petit (1710, p. 15, Figs. 2, 3) recognized in the macrodissected adult human ***spinal cord (Galen, c162–c166)*** dorsal and ventral (posterior and anterior) divisions indicated by transverse fibers, but denied that the ***spinal cord (Galen, c162–c166)*** contains *gray substance (Vesalius, 1543a)*. For an early history of the rostral end of the ***spinal cord (Galen, c162–c166)*** see Meckel (1832, Vol. 2, p. 410). According to Mettler (1948, pp. 34–35), "The student may experience some difficulty in determining, by superficial examination, the exact cephalic limit of the [human] spinal cord. Several arbitrary standards are used for this differentiation. The most reliable of these is that the upper root filaments [***dorsal rootlets (>1840)***] of the first cervical nerve mark the upper limit of the cord. This falls just below the level of the foramen magnum. Another method of differentiation consists in following the ventral median fissure orad. It will be found that, just above the level of the uppermost root filaments of the first cervical nerve, the fissure is obliterated for a space of about half a centimeter, and a smooth area takes its place... This is the locus of the decussation of the pyramids... the lower border of which forms the caudal limit of the medulla." For a more detailed consideration see Crosby et al. (1962, pp. 112–120).

TRANSLATIONS:

1. *chorda spinalis (Quain, 1837)*
   Latin form of ***spinal cord (Galen, c162–c166)***; p. 718. It is also spelled *corda spinalis*; see *Oxford Latin Dictionary* (1982).

EARLIER REFERENCES:

Described, not named or illustrated:

1. ***[spinal cord (Galen, c162–c166)] (Smith Papyrus, c1700 BC)***
   It has been claimed that ancient Egyptians may have known about soft tissue in human vertebral column's lumen, as judged by symptoms of cervical vertebra dislocations described in Edwin Smith Surgical Papyrus, a c1700 BC copy of a manuscript composed c3200 BC; see Breasted (1930, pp. 12–13, 66–67, 325, 425), Clarke & O'Malley (1996, p. 260), Nunn (2002, pp. 55, 180). This, however, seems very unlikely (Allen, 2005, pp. 91–93). The ***spinal cord (Galen, c162–c166)*** was not illustrated realistically in print until Vesalius (1543a).

Earlier synonyms:

1. *spinal marrow (Hippocrates)*
   This term (in Greek) for ***spinal cord (Galen, c162–c166)*** is found, for example, in *On the Articulations*, where it was used in describing the condition of human patients; see May (1968, p. 575), Adams (1972, p. 234). In a somewhat obscure passage in *Fleshes*, the Hippocratic Corpus seemed to refer to *spinal marrow* as an example of a cord, "The marrow called spinal extends down from the brain, and it, just like the brain, has little fat [is mostly gluey material]. Thus, it does not rightly bear the name 'marrow', since it is not like the other marrow in the bones, it alone having a membrane, and they none. Proof of this difference would be obvious if you were to burn such cords, then something gluey, and then anything else. Whereas anything else is rapidly burnt through, the cords and whatever is gluey refuse to be burnt through because they have so little fat. And fat and what is very rich are quickest to burn." (Potter, 1995, p. 139). Also see *Aphorisms* (Adams, 1972, p. 309). In English, Brunschwig (1525, p. [10]) referred to "ridge bone [spinal] mary", Bannister (1578, f. 106v) spelled it "spinall marey", Crooke (1615, p. 479) spelled it "spinall marrow", Nemesius (see Wither's translation, 1636, p. 426) spelled it "spinall-marrow", and Riolan (Culpeper's 1657 translation, pp. 126–128) spelled it "spinal marrow".
2. *medulla spinalis (Hippocrates)*
   Latin form of *spinal marrow (Hippocrates).*
3. *spinalis medullae (Hippocrates)*
   Latin form of *spinal marrow (Hippocrates).*
4. *spinal medulla (Hippocrates)*
   English-Latin form of *spinal marrow (Hippocrates).*
5. *dorsal marrow (Hippocrates)*
   Alternate translation for *spinal marrow (Hippocrates).* The relevant passage in *Fleshes* has been translated from Greek into English as "The marrow called spinal extends down from the brain…" (Potter, 1995, p. 139), whereas Littré's translation from Greek to French has been translated into English as "…the marrow called dorsal arises from the brain" (Clarke & O'Malley, 1996, p. 261); also see Crooke (1615, pp. 479–480) and Diemerbroeck (1689, p. 404). In Estienne (1545, p. 338) *spinal marrow* is referred to in Latin as *spinalis medullae*, whereas in the French edition (1546, p. 366) it is referred to as *la moelle du dors.*
6. *medulla dorsalis (Hippocrates)*
   Latin form of *dorsal marrow (Hippocrates).*
7. *dorsal medulla (Hippocrates)*
   English-Latin form of *dorsal marrow (Hippocrates).*
8. *marrow in neck and back (Plato)*
   Used in *Timaeus* referring to ***spinal cord (Galen, c162–c166)***; p. 103.
9. *vertebral marrow (Plato)*
   According to Galen, Plato used it (in Greek) for ***spinal cord (Galen, c162–c166)***; see Duckworth translation (1962, p. 223) and *marrow in neck and back (Plato).*
10. *silver cord (Ecclesiastes, 3rd century BC?)*
    Early synonym from Old Testament for ***spinal cord (Galen, c162–c166)***; XII, 6. See Bauhin (1605, p. 628), Crooke (1615, p. 479), and Schiller (1969, p. 77).
11. *trunk (Galen, c173)*
    Used (in Greek) for describing ***spinal cord (Galen, c162–c166)*** in *On the Usefulness of the Parts* (see May translation, 1968, p. 554), "Now the source of the nerves is the encephalon [***brain (Smith Papyrus, c1700 BC)***], the rational soul being sowed in it as in a fertile field. The outgrowth from it of the spinal medulla, like a trunk stretching up into a great tree, a trunk that extends the whole length of the spine, gives off a very large number of nerves like branches dividing into countless offshoots, and so the whole body receives through these first and foremost its share of motion and afterward its share of sensation." Also see pp. 572, 683.
12. *second encephalon (Galen, c173)*
    Galen referred thus to ***spinal cord (Galen, c162–c166)***, "Since the spinal medulla was formed to be like a second encephalon [***brain (Smith Papyrus, c1700 BC)***] for the parts below the head, since, like the encephalon, it had to be protected by a hard enclosure resistant to injury, and since this enclosure had to be made and put somewhere, was it not better to scoop out the keel, so to speak, which underlies the body of the animal as a foundation and is of course entirely bony, and to make its center hollow so as to form a pathway and at the same time a safeguard for the spinal medulla?" (May translation, 1968, p. 573, also see p. 579).
13. *dorsal cord (Galen, c170–c180)*
    Synonym (in Greek) for ***spinal cord (Galen, c162–c166)*** in *The Sites of Diseases III*; see Bennett & Hacker (2002).
14. *dorsal medulla (Galen, c192)*
    Apparently used (in Greek) for ***spinal cord (Galen, c162–c166)*** in later books of *On Anatomical Procedures*; see Duckworth translation (1962, p. 202). Marrow is an English translation of the Latin, *medulla*; see *dorsal marrow (Hippocrates).*

LATER SYNONYMS:

1. *nucha (Constantine the African, c1017–1087)*
Term of Arabic origin meaning *spinal medulla (Hippocrates)*, or more literally, *marrow*; see O'Malley & Saunders (1982, p. 334), Singer (1957, p. 79), and ***spinal cord (Galen, c162–c166)***. Later it was called *nape* in English; see *nape (Berengario da Carpi, 1523)*.
2. *vicar of brain (Albertus Magnus, 13th century)*
Synonym for ***spinal cord (Galen, c162–c166)***; see Kitchell & Resnick (1999, p. 179).
3. *base of brain (Benedetti, 1502)*
Benedetti wrote in his book on human anatomy that the Greeks used it for ***spinal cord (Galen, c162–c166)***; see Lind translation (1975, p. 116).
4. *paracephalus (Benedetti, 1502)*
Benedetti wrote in his book on human anatomy that the Greeks used it for ***spinal cord (Galen, c162–c166)***; see Lind translation (1975, p. 116).
5. *epicranis (Benedetti, 1502)*
Benedetti wrote in his book on human anatomy that the Greeks used it for ***spinal cord (Galen, c162–c166)***; see Lind translation (1975, p. 116).
6. *long brain (Benedetti, 1502)*
Benedetti wrote in his book on human anatomy that physicians use it [in Latin] for ***spinal cord (Galen, c162–c166)***, and seemed to imply that it is vaguely divided into right and left halves; see Lind translation (1975, p. 116). According to Diemerbroeck (1689, p. 405) the term originated with Theophilos Protospatharios (7th century).
7. *longum cerebrum (Benedetti, 1502)*
Latin form of *long brain (Benedetti, 1502)*; see edition translated by G. Ferrari (1998, p. 320).
8. *smooth medulla (Benedetti, 1502)*
Benedetti used it for macrodissected adult human ***spinal cord (Galen, c162–c166)***, and wrote that it acts as something of a substitute or proxy for ***brain (Smith Papyrus, c1700 BC)*** down the length of the spine; see Lind translation (1975, p. 112).
9. *sixth pair of nerves from brain (Benedetti, 1502)*
Synonym for macrodissected adult human ***spinal cord (Galen, c162–c166)***; see Lind translation (1975, pp. 117, 118).
10. *nape (Berengario da Carpi, 1523)*
Lind (1959, pp. 146, 156, 159) translation of Berengario's term *nucha* (or *nuca*) for ***spinal cord (Galen, c162–c166)***; also see *nucha (Constantine the African, c1017–1087)*.
11. *nuca (Berengario da Carpi, 1523)*
Alternate form of *nucha (Constantine the African, c1017–1087)*; see Lind translation (1959, p. 158); also see Vicary (1548, p. 74).
12. *ridge bone mary (Brunschwig, 1525)*
Synonym for macrodissected adult human ***spinal cord (Galen, c162–c166)***, or *spinal marrow (Hippocrates)*, in first account of anatomy in English: "nucha or ridge bone mary groweth of the last part of the brayne" (p. [8]). The first definition of *ridge* in the *Oxford English Dictionary* (Online) is *spine* or back, and *mary* is an early variant spelling of *marrow*. Hall (1565, p. 6) used *marow of ridge*.
13. *back mary (Brunschwig, 1525)*
Alternate form of *ridge bone mary (Brunschwig, 1525)*; p. [10]. Presented as *mary of the backe* in Geminus (1553, *The table of the figures of sinowes*), *marrowe of the backe* in Hall (1565, p. 6), and *marrow of the back* in Nemesius (1636, pp. 426–427).
14. *proxy of brain (Massa, 1536)*
Synonym for macrodissected adult human ***spinal cord (Galen, c162–c166)***; see Lind translation (1975, p. 249).
15. *spinal marrow proper (Vesalius, 1543a)*
Vesalius regarded macrodissected adult human *spinal marrow (Vesalius, 1543a)* as consisting of ***spinal cord (Galen, c162–c166)***, ***medulla (Winslow, 1733)***, and ***pons (Haller, 1747)***. However, he did recognize that part of *spinal marrow (Vesalius, 1543a)* beginning in first cervical vertebra should be called *spinal marrow proper* (see Richardson & Carman translation, 2002, p. 168), in contrast to *origin of spinal marrow (Vesalius, 1543a)*, the ***medulla (Winslow, 1733)*** and ***pons (Haller, 1747)*** considered together. He counted 30 pairs of *spinal nerves (Vesalius, 1543a)* in macrodissected adult human, and about *spinal marrow proper* he wrote, "In this area the spinal marrow is no longer single as it advances downward but rather resembles many threads joined together and proceeding in a straight line." (Richardson & Carman translation, 2002, p. 205, part *B* of the figure).
16. *spinal marrow in backbone (Vesalius, 1543a)*
Synonym for macrodissected adult human ***spinal cord (Galen, c162–c166)***; see Richardson & Carman translation (2002, figure following p. 263).
17. *marrow of spondles (Vicary, 1548)*
Apparently synonym for macrodissected adult human ***spinal cord (Galen, c162–c166)***; p. 31. *Spondles* is synonym for vertebrae.
18. *mynuca (Vicary, 1548)*
Alternate form of *nucha (Constantine the African, c1017–1087)*, apparently synonym for ***spinal cord (Galen, c162–c166)***; p. 31.
19. *minuca (Vicary, 1548)*
Variant form of *mynuca (Vicary, 1748)*.
20. *pith of back (Hall, 1565)*
Synonym for macrodissected adult human ***spinal cord (Galen, c162–c166)***; p. 54.
21. *stem of brain (Coiter, 1572)*
Coiter wrote that many, on good grounds, use it for ***spinal cord (Galen, c162–c166)***; see translation p. 113.
22. *process of brain (Coiter, 1572)*
Coiter wrote that many, on good grounds, use it for ***spinal cord (Galen, c162–c166)***; see translation p. 113.
23. *outgrowth of brain (Coiter, 1572)*
Coiter wrote that many, on good grounds, use it for ***spinal cord (Galen, c162–c166)***; see translation p. 113.
24. *spinal medulla oblongata (Piccolomini, 1586)*
Bauhin explained (pp. 625–628; see Crooke translation, 1615, p. 479) that *medulla oblongata (Piccolomini, 1586)* has a spinal part, ***spinal cord (Galen, c162–c166)*** or *spinal marrow proper (Vesalius, 1543a)*, and an intracranial

part, ***medulla (Winslow, 1733)*** or *intracranial medulla oblongata (Piccolomini, 1586)*. Piccolomini indicated (at *F*) the *spinal medulla oblongata* in his schematic mid-sagittal drawing of macrodissected adult human ***brain (Smith Papyrus, c1700 BC)***; see Clarke and Dewhurst (1996, Fig. 88).

25. *true spinal marrow proper (Bauhin, 1605)*
Translation of more exact term *medulla vero spinalis proprie dicta (Bauhin, 1605)* Bauhin used for *spinal marrow (Hippocrates)*; p. 628.
26. *medulla vero spinalis proprie dicta (Bauhin, 1605)*
Latin form of *true spinal marrow proper (Bauhin, 1605)*.
27. *marrow of chine (Nemesius, 1636)*
Synonym for *spinal marrow (Hippocrates)*; pp. 421, 427.
28. *chine-marrow (Nemesius, 1636)*
Synonym for *spinal marrow (Hippocrates)*; p. 427. In one amazing sentence the translator, Geo. Wither, used four synonyms for ***spinal cord (Galen, c162–c166)***, "Among these [***nerves (Herophilus, c335–c280 BC)***], those are the harder which come from the *spinall-marrow*: and of them, those are the hardest of all, which proceed from the lowest parts of the *marrow of the back*: For by how much farther the marrow of the *chine* descendeth from the braine; so much the more hard is the *chine-marrow* of it selfe, and the sinews [***nerves (Herophilus, c335–c280 BC)***] also which doe spring from the same." (pp. 426–427, italics added).
29. *part within backbone of medulla oblongata (Bartholin, 1662)*
Translation of *spinal medulla oblongata (Piccolomini, 1586)*; p. 322, also see *medulla oblongata (Bartholin, 1651)*.
30. *corpus in toto tractu bifidum (Willis, 1664)*
Term or description Willis used for macrodissected adult mammalian ***spinal cord (Galen, c162–c166)***; p. 232, see Burdach (1819, p. 258). As he wrote, "The figure, situation, as also the body of this, in its whole tract, are known generally to be cloven in two, not only by Anatomists, but also by every Butcher." (Pordage translation, 1681, p. 124).
31. *spinal pith (Diemerbroeck, 1689)*
Synonym favored in England for macrodissected adult human *spinal marrow (Hippocrates)*; p. 405.
32. *pith of spine (Diemerbroeck, 1689)*
Variation on *spinal pith (Diemerbroeck, 1689)*; p. 557.
33. *apophysis (Diemerbroeck, 1689)*
Synonym listed for macrodissected adult human ***spinal cord (Galen, c162–c166)***; p. 406.
34. *posterior part of tail of medulla oblongata (Pourfour du Petit, 1710)*
Synonym for macrodissected adult human ***spinal cord (Galen, c162–c166)***; in the original French, *la queuë de la moelle allongée, partie posterieure*, p. 14.
35. *pith of back-bone (Salmon, 1714)*
Synonym for macrodissected adult human ***spinal cord (Galen, c162–c166)***; p. 405.
36. *body of spinal medulla (Günther, 1786)*
Synonym for macrodissected adult human ***spinal cord (Galen, c162–c166)***; in the original Latin, *medulla spinalis corpus*, p. 32. As Günther explained, it is the medulla strictly speaking, as opposed to the ***cauda equina (Anatomia Magistri Nicolai physici, early 12th century)***.
37. *fistula sacra (Schreger, 1803)*
Synonym for macrodissected adult human ***spinal cord (Galen, c162–c166)***; p. 327.
38. *neural mass of vertebral column (Gall & Spurzheim, 1810)*
Synonym for macrodissected adult human ***spinal cord (Galen, c162–c166)***; in the original French, *la masse nerveuse de la colonne vertébrale*, p. 328.
39. *dorsal portion of cord (Gordon, 1815)*
All of *spinal cord (Gordon, 1815)* caudal to *cervical portion of cord (Gordon, 1815)*; p. 176.
40. *caudex dorsalis (Burdach, 1819)*
Synonym provided without reference for macrodissected adult human ***spinal cord (Galen, c162–c166)***; p. 229.
41. *body of vertebral medulla (Cloquet, 1828)*
Synonym for macrodissected adult human *body of spinal medulla (Günther, 1786)*; in the original French, *corps de la moëlle vertébrale*, p. 385.

PARTLY CORRESPONDS:

1. *columns of spinal marrow (Heister, 1717)*
Synonym for right and left halves of macrodissected adult human ***spinal cord (Galen, c162–c166)***; p. 80.
2. *sectors of spinal marrow (Huber, 1741)*
For descriptive purposes in transverse sections Huber divided macrodissected adult human ***spinal cord (Galen, c162–c166)*** into four equal sectors, regions, or sections with perpendicular lines through the center, that is, into right and left dorsal and ventral sectors; pp. 2–5, see translation in Clarke & O'Malley (1996, p. 267).
3. *duobus tuberculis (Haller, 1762)*
Apparently synonym for ***cervical enlargement (Arnold, 1838b)*** and ***lumbosacral enlargement (>1840)*** of macrodissected adult human ***spinal cord (Galen, c162–c166)*** considered together; p. 83.
4. *cords of spinal marrow (Monro, 1783)*
Term Monro used for right and left halves of macrodissected adult human ***spinal cord (Galen, c162-c166)***; they are "joined together at their middle or deepest parts by a lamella, which consists chiefly of red vessels and cineritious matter. Nay, when either of these two cords is accurately examined, it will be found to be subdivided by a slight furrow [***dorsal horn (>1840)***?], into a small posterior cord and large anterior cord. In the former, fasciculi of longitudinal fibres readily appear; in the latter, the disposition of the medullary fibres is much less evident... When we cut the spinal marrow transversely, the internal cineritious substance makes a cruciform appearance, or consists of four portions, one corresponding to each of the four cords of which I have observed it consists [Tab. VII, Fig. 2]" (pp. 28–29). Writing contemporaneously, Vicq d'Azyr (1784, p. 602) also referred to right and left cords of ***spinal cord (Galen, c162–c166)***; see translation by Clarke & O'Malley (1996, p. 270).
5. *posterior cord of spinal marrow (Monro, 1783)*

Vague description apparently referred to roughly dorsal half of macrodissected adult human ***spinal cord (Galen, c162–c166)***, including ***dorsal funiculus (>1840)***, ***dorsal horn (>1840)***, and adjacent dorsal regions of ***lateral funiculus (Burdach, 1822)***; pp. 28–29, see *cords of spinal marrow (Monro, 1783)*.

6. *anterior cord of spinal marrow (Monro, 1783)*
   Vague description apparently referred to roughly ventral half of macrodissected adult human ***spinal cord (Galen, c162–c166)***, including ***ventral funiculus (>1840)***, ***ventral horn (>1840)***, and adjacent ventral regions of ***lateral funiculus (Burdach, 1822)***; pp. 28–29, see *cords of spinal marrow (Monro, 1783)*.
7. *lateral cords of spinal marrow (Fyfe, 1800)*
   Synonym for macrodissected adult human *cords of spinal marrow (Monro, 1783)*; Vol. 2, p. 301.
8. *lateral portions of spinal marrow (Fyfe, 1800)*
   Synonym for macrodissected adult human *cords of spinal marrow (Monro, 1783)*; Vol. 2, p. 301.
9. *body of spinal prolongation (Chaussier, 1807)*
   As described for macrodissected adult human, ***spinal cord (Galen, c162–c166)*** excluding caudal end or ***medullary cone (Bock, 1827)***; in the original French, *corps du prolongement rachidien*, p. 120 and Plate V, Figure 1-*B,C*.
10. *middle primary part of spinal prolongation (Chaussier, 1807)*
    Synonym for *body of spinal prolongation (Chaussier, 1807)*; in the original French, *partie moyenne et principale du prolongement rachidien*, p. 120.
11. *columns of spinal medulla (Chaussier, 1807)*
    Synonym for macrodissected adult human *cords of spinal marrow (Monro, 1783)*; in the original Latin, *columnae aut virgae medullae spinalis*, p. 144.
12. *nucleus of spinal cord (Meckel, 1817)*
    Refers to ***central nervous system gray matter regions (>1840)*** of macrodissected adult human ***spinal cord (Galen, c162–c166)***; see translation (1832, Vol. 2, p. 413).
13. *anterior half of spinal medulla (Meckel, 1817)*
    Refers in macrodissected adult human ***spinal cord (Galen, c162–c166)*** basically to larger part ventral to ***dorsal roots (Spurzheim, 1826)*** and ***dorsal horn (>1840)***; see translation (1832, Vol. 2, p. 414).
14. *anterior gray substance (Rolando, 1824)*
    For macrodissected adult human viewed at a transverse cut, ***central nervous system gray matter regions (>1840)*** of ***spinal cord (Galen, c162–c166)*** ventral to ***substantia gelatinosa (>1840)*** that Rolando described as spongy and vascular, in distinction to *posterior gray substance darker and almost gelatinous (Rolando, 1824)*; in the original Italian, *sostanza cinericcia anteriore*, p. 55 and Table III, Figure 3-*s*.
15. *central gray substance of spinal medulla (Rolando, 1825a)*
    Central nervous system gray matter region (>1840) of ***spinal cord (Galen, c162–c166)***, here for macrodissected calf; Table VII, Figure 1-*y*. Rolando also referred to macrodissected calf *central gray of medulla oblongata (Arnold, 1838b)*, also in the shape of the *central gray substance of spinal medulla (Rolando, 1825a)*; Table IV, Figure 7-*s.c.* & Table V, Figure 10. For macrodissected adult human, see Rolando (1831, Fig. 10-39), in the original Italian, *sostanza cinericcia centrale del midollo spinale*.
16. *lateral gray column of spinal medulla (Desmoulins, 1825)*
    In macrodissected adult human, ***dorsal horn (>1840)***, ***intermediate gray of spinal cord (>1840)***, and ***ventral horn (>1840)***, excluding ***spinal central gray (>1840)***; in the original French, *faisceaux gris latéraux de la moelle*, Plate XIII, Figure 11-*c.g*.
17. *superior swelling of spinal cord (Quain & Wilson, 1839)*
    In macrodissected adult human, slight enlargement of ***spinal cord (Galen, c162–c166)*** in rostral (upper) ***cervical part of spinal cord (>1840)***, presumably associated with ***cervical plexus (Molinetti, 1675)***; Plate I, Figure 2-*10*.

spinal cord differentiations (>1840)

The vertebrate ***spinal cord (Galen, c162–c166)*** is divided into longitudinal topographic differentiations based on diameter and correlated with the size of related ***spinal nerves (Camper, 1760–1762)***; see Ariëns Kappers et al. (1936), Nieuwenhuys et al. (1998). The macrodissected adult human ***spinal cord differentiations (>1840)*** include, from rostral to caudal, ***cervical enlargement (Arnold, 1838b)*** associated primarily with innervation of the arms, ***lumbosacral enlargement (>1840)*** associated primarily with innervation of the legs, ***medullary cone (Bock, 1827)***, and ***terminal filament (Tiedemann, 1821)***; see Carpenter (1996, pp. 213–216), Nieuwenhuys et al. (2008, Fig. 3.15). Most of these basic features of the macrodissected adult human ***spinal cord (Galen, c162–c166)*** were distinguished by Estienne (1545); see entry for each differentiation.

spinal cord part of neural tube (>1840)

As described for vertebrate, the segment of the ***neural tube (Baer, 1837)*** caudal to the ***brain vesicles (Malpighi, 1673)***, generating the adult ***spinal cord (Galen, c162–c166)***. It was clearly differentiated early on by Malpighi; see ***[spinal cord part of neural tube (>1840)] (Malpighi, 1673)***.

EARLIER REFERENCES:

Illustrated and described, not named:

1. ***[spinal cord part of neural tube (>1840)] (Malpighi, 1673)***
   Clearly differentiated for chick embryo at 40 hours of incubation; Figure XI.

Earlier synonyms:

1. *spinal medulla division of neural tube (Baer, 1837)*
   Synonym for vertebrate ***spinal cord part of neural tube (>1840)***; from a passage on p. 104.

spinal cord parts (>1840)

The vertebrate ***spinal cord (Galen, c162–c166)*** is divided into topographic parts defined by corresponding ***spinal nerve groups (Durward, 1951)***; see Carpenter (1976, pp. 213–216). The macrodissected adult human ***spinal cord (Galen, c162–c166)*** is divided, from rostral to caudal, into ***cervical part of spinal cord (>1840)*** corresponding to the eight ***cervical nerves (Galen, c173)***, ***thoracic part of spinal cord (>1840)*** corresponding to the twelve ***thoracic nerves (Diemerbroeck, 1672)***, ***lumbar part of spinal cord (>1840)*** corresponding to the five ***lumbar nerves (Diemerbroeck, 1672)***, ***sacral part of spinal cord (>1840)*** corresponding to the five ***sacral nerves (Camper, 1760)***, and ***coccygeal part of spinal cord (>1840)*** corresponding to the one to three ***coccygeal nerves (Camper, 1762)***; see *Nomina Anatomica* (1983, p. A64), *Terminologia Anatomica* (1998, p. 105), Nieuwenhuys et al. (2008, Fig. 3.14). All but the ***coccygeal part of spinal cord (>1840)*** were delineated by Galen (c173) in macrodissected adult mammals, but not human; see entry for each part.

spinal cuneate fascicle (>1840)

As described in macrodissected adult human, the caudal topographic segment of the ***cuneate fascicle (Müller, 1834)*** in the ***spinal cord (Galen, c162–c166)***, caudal to the ***medullary cuneate fascicle (>1840)*** segment; see Williams & Warwick (1980, p. 881 and Fig. 7.35A), Nieuwenhuys et al. (2008, Fig. 3.10-21). It was known to Santorini; see ***[spinal cuneate fascicle (>1840)] (Santorini, 1775)***.

EARLIER REFERENCES:

Illustrated, not named or described:

1. ***[spinal cuneate fascicle (>1840)] (Santorini, 1775)***
   Clearly illustrated for macrodissected adult human; Table III, Figure 2.

spinal dorsal spinocerebellar tract (>1840)

As described in macrodissected adult human, and mammal generally with histological methods for ***axons (Kölliker, 1896)***, the caudal topographic segment of the ***dorsal spinocerebellar tract (>1840)*** in the ***spinal cord (Galen, c162–c166)***, caudal to the ***medullary dorsal spinocerebellar tract (>1840)*** segment and centered in outer dorsal parts of the ***lateral funiculus (Burdach, 1822)***; see Williams & Warwick (1980, Fig. 7.43), Nieuwenhuys et al. (2008, Fig. 6.1-19). It was not known by 1840.

spinal gracile fascicle (>1840)

As described in macrodissected adult human, the caudal topographic segment of the ***gracile fascicle (Müller, 1834)*** in the ***spinal cord (Galen, c162–c166)***, caudal to the ***medullary gracile fascicle (>1840)*** segment; see Williams & Warwick (1980, p. 881 and Fig. 7.35A), Nieuwenhuys et al. (2008, Fig. 3.10-23). It was known to Santorini; see ***[spinal gracile fascicle (>1840)] (Santorini, 1775)***.

EARLIER REFERENCES:

Illustrated, not named or described:

1. ***[spinal gracile fascicle (>1840)] (Santorini, 1775)***
   Clearly illustrated for macrodissected adult human; Table III, Figure 2.

spinal lateral reticulospinal tract (>1840)

As described in adult human, especially with experimental pathway tracing methods, the caudal topographic segment of the ***lateral reticulospinal tract (>1840)***, caudal to the ***medullary lateral reticulospinal tract (>1840)*** segment and apparently centered in deep intermediate parts of the ***lateral funiculus (Burdach, 1822)***; see Mettler (1948, p. 238), Crosby et al. (1962, p. 105 and Figs. 85, 86), Williams & Warwick (1980, pp. 875–876 and Fig. 7.44). It was not identified by 1840.

spinal lateral vestibulospinal tract (>1840)

As described in adult human, especially with experimental methods for pathway tracing, the caudal topographic segment of the ***lateral vestibulospinal tract (>1840)*** in the ***spinal cord (Galen, c162–c166)***, caudal to the ***medullary lateral vestibulospinal tract (>1840)*** segment and centered in lateral parts of the ***ventral funiculus (>1840)***; see Carpenter (1976, p. 342 and Fig. 10.21), called simply *vestibulospinal tract* (>1840); Williams & Warwick (1980, p. 875 and Figs. 7.43–44); Nieuwenhuys et al. (2008, p. 725 and Fig. 17.6). It was not clearly delineated by 1840.

spinal medial forebrain bundle (>1840)

As described in mammal generally with experimental histological methods for ***axons (Kölliker, 1896)***, the caudal topographic segment of the ***medial forebrain bundle (Edinger, 1893)*** in the ***spinal cord (Galen, c162–c166)***, caudal to the ***medullary medial forebrain bundle (>1840)*** segment and centered in intermediate to dorsal parts of the ***lateral funiculus (Burdach, 1822)*** with major branches to ***intermediolateral nucleus (>1840)***, ***spinal central gray (>1840)***, and ***marginal zone of spinal cord (Waldeyer, 1889)***; see Saper et al. (1976), Swanson & McKellar (1979). In contrast to the ***corticospinal tract (>1840)***, it is mostly uncrossed. It was not known by 1840.

spinal medial longitudinal fascicle (>1840)

As described in adult human, especially with experimental pathway tracing methods, the caudal topographic segment of the ***medial longitudinal fascicle (>1840)*** in the ***spinal cord (>Galen, c162–c166)***, caudal to the ***medullary medial longitudinal fascicle (>1840)*** segment and centered in the ***ventral funiculus (>1840)*** just lateral to the ***uncrossed corticospinal tract (>1840)***; see Williams & Warwick (1980, Fig. 7.44A), Nieuwenhuys et al. (2008, Fig. 6.1-32, 6.7-17). It was perhaps first indicated as the *fasciculus siliqualis internus (Wagner, 1839)*.

EARLIER REFERENCES:

Earlier synonyms:

1. *fasciculus siliqualis internus (Wagner, 1839)*
   Lateral part of macrodissected adult human ***ventral funiculus (>1840)*** in rostral (upper) ***cervical part of spinal cord (>1840)***, essentially indicating ***spinal medial longitudinal fascicle (>1840)***; Table XXVII, Figure 10-6. See Nieuwenhuys et al. (2008, Fig. 6.7-17).

spinal medial reticulospinal tract (>1840)

As described in adult human, especially with experimental methods for pathway tracing, the caudal topographic segment of the ***medial reticulospinal tract (>1840)*** in the ***spinal cord (Galen, c162–c166)***, caudal to the ***medullary medial reticulospinal tract (>1840)*** segment and centered in deep medial parts of the ***ventral funiculus (>1840)***; see Carpenter (1976, Fig. 10.21), called *pontine reticulospinal tract (>1840)*, and Williams & Warwick (1980, Fig. 7.44A). It was not described by 1840.

spinal nerve dorsal branch (Meckel, 1817)

As described for macrodissected adult human, the typically smaller of the two ***spinal nerve primary branches (>1840)*** extending dorsally from the ***spinal nerve trunk (Frotscher, 1788)***; see Durward (1951, Figs. 913, 936). For Meckel's use in macrodissected adult human, see translation (1832, Vol. 3, p. 12); he used *spinal nerve* and *nerve of spinal marrow*, and posterior and dorsal, synonymously. It was clearly described by Galen; see ***[spinal nerve dorsal branch (Meckel, 1817)] (Galen, c173)***.

TRANSLATIONS:

1. *rami dorsalis nervi spinalis (Meckel, 1817)*
   Current Latin form (plural) of ***spinal nerve dorsal branch (Meckel, 1817)***; see *Dorland's* (2003, p. 1573).

EARLIER REFERENCES:

Described, not named or illustrated:

1. ***[spinal nerve dorsal branch (Meckel, 1817)] (Galen, c173)***
   Clearly described for ***cervical nerves (Galen, c173)***—see May translation (1968, pp. 597–599), and Duckworth translation (1962, pp. 230–231, 238, 257, 262)—and ***thoracic nerves (Diemerbroeck, 1672)***—see Duckworth translation (1962, p. 257)—in macrodissected adult beef, pig, and/or macaque but not human.

Earlier synonyms:

1. *posterior branch of nerve from spinal medulla (Vesalius,1543a)*
   Modern description provided for all ***spinal nerve dorsal branch (Meckel, 1817)*** in macrodissected adult human; see Richardson & Carman translation (2002, pp. 225–255).
2. *external branch of conjugations of nerves from loynes and holy bone (Paré, 1561)*
   Synonym for macrodissected adult human lumbar and sacral ***spinal nerve dorsal branch (Meckel, 1817)***; p. ccxxix, see translation (1634, pp. 226–227).
3. *backward branches of conjugations of neck, chest, loynes, and sacral bone (Crooke, 1615)*
   Synonym for macrodissected adult human ***spinal nerve dorsal branches (Meckel, 1817)***; pp. 488–489. Crook's description is a translation of Bauhin (1605).
4. *lesser branches of conjugations of neck, chest, loynes, and sacral bone (Crooke, 1615)*
   Synonym for macrodissected adult human ***spinal nerve dorsal branches (Meckel, 1817)***; pp. 488–489. Crook's description is a translation of Bauhin (1605).
5. *hindermost branch of pairs of sinews or nerves from neck, back, loins, and os sacrum (Read, 1638)*
   Synonym for macrodissected adult human ***spinal nerve dorsal branch (Meckel, 1817)***; pp. 496–502. Also referred to simply as *hinder branches of nerves from marrow*, for example; see Gibson (1682, pp. 345–353).
6. *hinder nerves of pairs of nerves of medulla spinalis (Salmon, 1714)*
   Synonym for macrodissected adult human ***spinal nerve dorsal branches (Meckel, 1817)***; p. 121 ff. combined with p. 112.
7. *hindermore nerves of pairs of nerves of medulla spinalis (Salmon, 1714)*
   Synonym for macrodissected adult human ***spinal nerve dorsal branches (Meckel, 1817)***; p. 123 ff. combined with p. 112.
8. *spinal nerve posterior branch (Haase, 1781)*
   Synonym for macrodissected adult human ***spinal nerve dorsal branch (Meckel, 1817)***; in the original Latin, *nervi spinales ramus posterior*, p. 191 ff.
9. *spinal nerve inferior branch (Günther, 1786)*
   Synonym for macrodissected adult human ***spinal nerve dorsal branch (Meckel, 1817)***; in the original Latin, *n. spinalium ramus inferior*, p. 69.

LATER SYNONYMS:

1. *nerve of spinal marrow dorsal branch (Meckel, 1817)*
   Synonym for ***spinal nerve dorsal branch (Meckel, 1817)***; see translation (1832, Vol. 3, pp. 5–9).
2. *nerve of spinal marrow posterior branch (Meckel, 1817)*
   Synonym for ***spinal nerve dorsal branch (Meckel, 1817)***; see translation (1832, Vol. 3, pp. 5–9).
3. *posterior trunk of spinal nerves (Swan, 1830)*
   Synonym for macrodissected adult human ***spinal nerve dorsal branch (Meckel, 1817)***; pp. 23, 24.
4. *posterior spinal branches (Cruveilhier, 1836)*
   Synonym for macrodissected adult human ***spinal nerve dorsal branches (Meckel, 1817)***; in the original French, *branches spinales postérieures*, p. 765.

PARTLY CORRESPONDS:

1. *dorsal branches of dorsal nerves (Cloquet, 1816)*
   Macrodissected adult human ***spinal nerve dorsal branches (Meckel, 1817)*** for ***thoracic nerves (Diemerbroeck, 1672)***; in the original French, *branches dorsales*, p. 655.
2. *lumbar branches of lumbar nerves (Meckel, 1817)*
   Macrodissected adult human ***spinal nerve dorsal branches (Meckel, 1817)*** of ***lumbar nerves (Diemerbroeck, 1672)***; see translation (1832, Vol. 3, p. 13).
3. *superior gluteal subcutaneous nerves (Bock, 1827)*
   Macrodissected adult human ***spinal nerve dorsal branches (Meckel, 1817)*** of first three ***lumbar nerves (Diemerbroeck, 1672)***, see Hamilton (1976, Fig. 813); in the original Latin, *nervi subcutanei glutaei superiores*, Table I, Figure 2-61.
4. *lumbal nerve of lumbar nerve (Bock, 1827)*
   Synonym (singular) for macrodissected adult human *lumbar branches of lumbar nerves (Meckel, 1817)*; in the original Latin, *lumbalis nervi lumbaris*, Table IV-57.

5. *superior gluteal cutaneous nerves (Bock, 1827)*
   Synonym for *superior gluteal subcutaneous nerves (Bock, 1827)*; in the original Latin, *nervi cutanei glutaei superiores*, Table IV-59.
6. *lumbal branch of lumbar nerve (Bock, 1827)*
   Synonym for *lumbal nerve of lumbar nerve (Bock, 1827)*; in the original Latin, *ram. lumbalis*, Table VII, Figure 1-3.
7. *lumbal branch of abdominal nerve (Bock, 1827)*
   Synonym for *lumbal branch of lumbar nerve (Bock, 1827)*; in the original Latin, *ram. lumbalis nervi lumbaris*, Table VII, Figure 2-5.
8. *posterior cervical plexus (Cruveilhier, 1836)*
   In macrodissected adult human, carefully described ***plexus (Galen, c192)*** formed by ***communicating branches (Winslow, 1733)*** of ***spinal nerve dorsal branches (Meckel, 1817)*** of first three ***cervical nerves (Galen, c173)***; in the original French, *plexus cervical postérieur*, pp. 771–773.
9. *dorsal branches of intercostal nerves (Quain & Wilson, 1839)*
   Macrodissected adult human ***spinal nerve dorsal branches (Meckel, 1817)*** for ***thoracic nerves (Diemerbroeck, 1672)***; in the original Latin, *rami dorsales*, Plate XX, Figure 1-*c*.
10. *cutaneous branches of dorsal branches of intercostal nerves (Quain & Wilson, 1839)*
   Macrodissected adult human cutaneous branches of ***spinal nerve dorsal branches (Meckel, 1817)*** for ***thoracic nerves (Diemerbroeck, 1672)***; Plate XX, Figure 2-*c*. See Williams & Warwick (1980, Fig. 7.196).

spinal nerve ganglia (Burdach, 1819)

Sensory ***ganglia (Galen, c173)*** associated with vertebrate ***dorsal roots (Spurzheim, 1826)***, hence the most common synonym, *dorsal root ganglia (>1840)*—although an earlier synonym, *intervertebral ganglia (Serres, 1824–1826)*, is more consistent with the sequentially more lateral ***paravertebral ganglia (Durward, 1951)*** and ***prevertebral ganglia (Quain, 1837)***. ***Spinal nerve ganglia (Burdach, 1819)*** are now commonly described sequentially from rostral (superior) to caudal (inferior) and are grouped into ***cervical spinal ganglia (>1840)***, ***thoracic spinal ganglia (>1840)***, ***lumbar spinal ganglia (>1840)***, ***sacral spinal ganglia (>1840)***, and ***coccygeal spinal ganglia (>1840)***; see Williams & Warwick (1980, pp. 1086–1087). For Burdach's use in macrodissected adult human, see p.136. They were discovered by Coiter; see ***knots (Coiter, 1572)***. Haase (1772, p. 87) associated them specifically with ***dorsal roots (Spurzheim, 1826)***, and not ***ventral roots (>1840)***; see Meckel (1832, Vol. 1, p. 170 note *1*).

TRANSLATIONS:

1. *Ganglia der Rückenmarknerven (Burdach, 1819)*
   Original German form of ***spinal nerve ganglia (Burdach, 1819)***; p. 136.

EARLIER REFERENCES:

Earlier synonyms:

1. *knots (Coiter, 1572)*
   Synonym for macrodissected adult human ***spinal nerve ganglia (Burdach, 1819)***; Coiter discovered them and observed there is one for each ***spinal nerve (Camper, 1760–1762)***, and that they are gland-like, hard, and made of a thick substance; see translation p. 115.
2. *plexus ganglioformes nervorum spinalem (Vieussens, 1684)*
   Synonym for macrodissected adult human ***spinal nerve ganglia (Burdach, 1819)***; Table 23-*88*.
3. *ganglions of medulla spinalis (Winslow, 1733)*
   Synonym for macrodissected adult human ***spinal nerve ganglia (Burdach, 1819)***; Section VI, no. 363, p. 94.
4. *posterior bundle ganglia (Monro, 1783)*
   Synonym for macrodissected adult human ***spinal nerve ganglia (Burdach, 1819)***, which Monro demonstrated are associated only with ***dorsal roots (Spurzheim, 1826)***; pp. 30, 50; Table XI-*P*. However, this discovery was made a decade earlier by Haase (1772, p. 87); see Meckel (1832, Vol. 1, p. 170 note *1*).
5. *ganglion in posterior fasciculus of spinal nerves (Monro, 1783)*
   Synonym for *posterior bundle ganglia (Monro, 1783)*; p. 51.
6. *vertebral ganglia (Bichat, 1801)*
   Synonym for ***spinal nerve ganglia (Burdach, 1819)***; in the original French, *ganglions vertébraux*, p. 232.
7. *spinal ganglia (Racchetti, 1816)*
   Synonym for macrodissected adult human ***spinal nerve ganglia (Burdach, 1819)***; in the original Italian, *gangli spinali*, p. 178.
8. *spinal system ganglia (Wutzer, 1817)*
   Synonym for ***spinal nerve ganglia (Burdach, 1819)***; in the original Latin, *ganglia systematis spinalis*, p. 52.
9. *spinal ganglia proper (Wutzer, 1817)*
   Synonym for macrodissected adult human ***spinal nerve ganglia (Burdach, 1819)***; in the original Latin, *ganglia spinalia proprie sic dicta*, p. 92.
10. *intervertebral ganglia (Serres, 1824–1826)*
   Synonym for macrodissected adult ***spinal nerve ganglia (Burdach, 1819)***; in the original French, *ganglions intervertébraux*, Vol. 2, p. 45.

PARTLY CORRESPONDS:

1. *plexus ganglioformes nervorum dorsalium (Vieussens, 1684)*
   Vieussens described and illustrated for macrodissected adult human a ***spinal nerve ganglion (Burdach, 1819)*** for each of the 12 *thoracic nerves (Vesalius, 1543a)* corresponding to eighth ***cervical nerve (Galen, c173)*** through 11th ***thoracic nerve (Diemerbroeck, 1672)***; see Tables 24-*b* and 27-*C*.
2. *plexus ganglioformes nervorum lumbarium (Vieussens, 1684)*
   Vieussens described and illustrated for macrodissected adult human a ***spinal nerve ganglion (Burdach, 1819)*** for each of the five *lumbar nerves (Vesalius, 1543a)* corresponding to 12th ***thoracic nerve (Diemerbroeck, 1672)*** through fourth ***lumbar nerve (Diemerbroeck, 1672)***; see Table 28-*a*.

3. *plexus ganglioformes nervorum ossis sacri (Vieussens, 1684)*
   Vieussens described and illustrated for macrodissected adult human a ***spinal nerve ganglion (Burdach, 1819)*** for the first three of six *sacral nerves (Vesalius, 1543a)* corresponding to fifth ***lumbar nerve (Diemerbroeck, 1672)*** through fifth ***sacral nerve (Camper, 1760)***; see Table 29-*K*.

spinal nerve groups (Durward, 1951)

As described for macrodissected adult human, the ***spinal nerves (Camper, 1760–1762)*** are divided based on their relationship to the bones of the spinal (vertebral) column into the following groups, arranged from rostral to caudal: ***cervical nerves (Galen, c173)***, ***thoracic nerves (Diemerbroeck, 1672)***, ***lumbar nerves (Diemerbroeck, 1672)***, ***sacral nerves (Camper, 1760)***, and ***coccygeal nerves (Camper, 1762)***; p. 1050. The terms are defined specifically for other vertebrate species, where the number of ***spinal nerves (Camper, 1760–1762)*** in a particular ***spinal nerve group (Durward, 1951)*** may vary. They were recognized in outline for mammal by Galen (c173); see entry for each group.

EARLIER REFERENCES:

Earlier synonyms:

1. *nerves of spinal marrow sections (Meckel, 1817)*
   Synonym for macrodissected adult human ***spinal nerve groups (Durward, 1951)***; see translation (1832, Vol. 3, p. 6).
2. *spinal nerve sections (Meckel, 1817)*
   Because Meckel used *spinal nerve* and *nerves of spinal marrow* synonymously (see translation, 1832, Vol. 3, p. 5) this term for ***spinal nerve groups (Durward, 1951)*** is derived from his writing; synonymous with *nerves of spinal marrow sections (Meckel, 1817)*.

spinal nerve parts (>1840)

As described for macrodissected adult mammal, the three main general divisions (parts) of a ***spinal nerve (Camper, 1760–1762)*** are ***spinal nerve roots (Tiedemann, 1816)***, ***spinal nerve trunk (Frotscher, 1788)***, and ***spinal nerve primary branches (>1840)***; see Durward (1951, pp. 1050–1053, Fig. 913). This arrangement was perhaps first clearly delineated and articulated by Winslow; see ***[spinal nerve parts (>1840)] (Winslow, 1733)***.

EARLIER REFERENCES:

Described, not named or illustrated:

1. ***[spinal nerve parts (>1840)] (Winslow, 1733)***
   All components were clearly understood and described for macrodissected adult human; Section VII, p. 76 ff.

spinal nerve primary branches (>1840)

Each ***spinal nerve trunk (Frotscher, 1788)*** divides distally into a ***spinal nerve ventral branch (Meckel, 1817)*** and a ***spinal nerve dorsal branch (>1840)***; see Durward (1951, p. 1052 and Fig. 913). They were clearly described long ago by Galen; see ***[spinal nerve primary branches (>1840)] (Galen, c173)***.

EARLIER REFERENCES:

Described, not named or illustrated:

1. ***[spinal nerve primary branches (>1840)] (Galen, c173)***
   Clearly described for ***cervical nerves (Galen, c173)***—see May translation (1968, pp. 597–599) and Duckworth translation (1962, p. 229 ff.)—and ***thoracic nerves (Diemerbroeck, 1672)***—see Duckworth translation (1962, p. 257)—in macrodissected adult beef, pig, and/or macaque but not human. Vesalius (1543a) provided modern description for all of them in macrodissected adult human; see Richardson & Carman translation (2002, pp. 225–255).

spinal nerve roots (Tiedemann, 1816)

As described for macrodissected adult human, each of the ***spinal nerves (Camper, 1760–1762)*** commonly has a ***ventral root (>1840)*** and a ***dorsal root (Spurzheim, 1826)*** between the surface of the ***spinal cord (Galen, c162–c166)*** and the plane where they merge into a composite ***spinal nerve trunk (Frotscher, 1788)***; see Carpenter (1976, Fig. 7.1). Tiedemann used the term for 2- to 3-month-old macrodissected human fetuses; see translation, where they were called *roots of spinal nerves* (1826, p. 126). They were discovered by Coiter; see ***[spinal nerve roots (Tiedemann, 1816)] (Coiter, 1572)***.

EARLIER REFERENCES:

Described, not named or illustrated:

1. ***[spinal nerve roots (Tiedemann, 1816)] (Coiter, 1572)***
   Clearly described for macrodissected adult human; see translation p. 115.

PARTLY CORRESPONDS:

1. *roots of nerves from spinal marrow (Vesalius, 1543a)*
   Refers very generally to proximal end of macrodissected adult human *spinal nerves (Vesalius, 1543a)* as they emerge from *spinal marrow proper (Vesalius, 1543a)*; Vesalius did not distinguish between ***ventral roots (>1840)*** and ***dorsal roots (Spurzheim, 1826)***; see Richardson & Carman translation (2002, p. 205) and ***[ventral rootlets (>1840)] (Vesalius, 1543a)***.
2. *roots of sinews of marrow of back (Geminus, 1553)*
   Synonym for *roots of nerves from spinal marrow (Vesalius, 1543a)*; originally spelled, *rootes of sinowes of mary of backe*, see *The table of the figures of sinowe*.

spinal nerve trunk (Frotscher, 1788)

The short segment of a ***spinal nerve (Camper, 1760–1762)*** between the junction of the ***dorsal root (Spurzheim, 1826)*** and ***ventral root (>1840)*** proximally, and the origin of the ***spinal nerve dorsal branch (Meckel, 1817)*** and ***spinal nerve ventral branch (>1840)*** distally; see Durward (1951, Fig. 913). For Frotscher's use in macrodissected adult human, see Section XII, p. 83, 1798 reprint; it was clearly described as the *vertebral nerve original trunk (Winslow, 1733)*.

EARLIER REFERENCES:

Earlier synonyms:

1. *vertebral nerve original trunk (Winslow, 1733)*
   Synonym for macrodissected adult human ***spinal nerve trunk (Frotscher, 1788)***; Section VI, p. 76.
2. *vertebral nerve trunk (Winslow, 1733)*
   Synonym for macrodissected adult human ***spinal nerve trunk (Frotscher, 1788)***; Section VI, p. 76.

LATER SYNONYMS:

1. *compound spinal nerve (Grant, 1834c)*
   Synonym for macrodissected adult vertebrate human ***spinal nerve trunk (Frotscher, 1788)***; p. 546.
2. *compound nerve (Grainger, 1837)*
   Synonym for macrodissected adult human ***spinal nerve trunk (Frotscher, 1788)***; p. 31.

spinal nerve ventral branch (>1840)

As described for macrodissected adult human, the typically larger of the two ***spinal nerve primary branches (>1840)*** extending laterally and ventrally from ***spinal nerve trunk (Frotscher, 1788)***; see Durward (1951, Fig. 913). It was clearly described by Galen; see ***[spinal nerve ventral branch (>1840)] (Galen, c173)***.

TRANSLATIONS:

1. *rami ventrales nervi spinales (>1840)*
   Current Latin form (plural) of ***spinal nerve ventral branch (>1840)***; see *Dorland's* (2003, p. 1582).

EARLIER REFERENCES:

Described, not named or illustrated:

1. ***[spinal nerve ventral branch (>1840)] (Galen, c173)***
   Clearly described for ***cervical nerves (Galen, c173)***—see May translation (1968, pp. 597–599), and Duckworth translation (1962, pp. 230–231, 238, 257, 262)—and ***thoracic nerves (Diemerbroeck, 1672)***—see Duckworth translation (1962, p. 257)—in macrodissected adult beef, pig, and/or macaque but not human.

Earlier synonyms:

1. *anterior branch of nerve from spinal medulla (Vesalius, 1543a)*
   Modern description of all macrodissected adult human ***spinal nerve ventral branches (>1840)***; see Richardson & Carman translation (2002, pp. 225–255).
2. *internal branch of conjugations of nerves from loynes and holy bone (Paré, 1561)*
   Synonym for macrodissected adult human lumbar and sacral ***spinal nerve ventral branches (>1840)***; p. ccxxix, see translation (1634, pp. 226–227).
3. *forward branches of conjugations of neck, chest, loynes, and sacral bone (Crooke, 1615)*
   Synonym for macrodissected adult human ***spinal nerve ventral branches (>1840)***; pp. 488–489. Crook's description is a translation of Bauhin (1605). They were also referred to simply as *fore (or foremore) branches of nerves from marrow*; for example, see Gibson (1682, pp. 345–353).
4. *greater branches of conjugations of neck, chest, loynes, and sacral bone (Crooke, 1615)*
   Synonym for macrodissected adult human ***spinal nerve ventral branches (>1840)***; pp. 488–489. Crook's description is a translation of Bauhin (1605).
5. *foremost branch of pairs of sinews or nerves from neck, back, loins, and os sacrum (Read, 1638)*
   Synonym for macrodissected adult human ***spinal nerve ventral branch (>1840)***; pp. 496–502.
6. *fore nerves of pairs of nerves of medulla spinalis (Salmon, 1714)*
   Synonym for macrodissected adult human ***spinal nerve ventral branches (>1840)***; p. 121 ff. combined with p. 112.
7. *foremore nerves of pairs of nerves of medulla spinalis (Salmon, 1714)*
   Synonym for macrodissected adult human ***spinal nerve ventral branches (>1840)***; p. 123 ff. combined with p. 112.
8. *spinal nerve anterior branch (Haase, 1781)*
   Synonym for macrodissected adult human ***spinal nerve ventral branch (>1840)***; in the original Latin, *nervi spinales ramus anterior*, p. 191 ff.
9. *subvertebral nerves (Monro, 1783)*
   Synonym for macrodissected newborn and adult human ***spinal nerve ventral branches (>1840)***; see Table 8, Figure 3:*1-8* and Table 15:3-*7*.
10. *spinal nerve superior branch (Günther, 1786)*
    Synonym for macrodissected adult human ***spinal nerve ventral branch (>1840)***; in the original Latin, *n. spinalium ramus superior*, p. 69.
11. *nerve of spinal marrow anterior branch (Meckel, 1817)*
    Synonym for macrodissected adult human ***spinal nerve ventral branch (>1840)***; see translation (1832, Vol. 3, p. 5 ff.).
12. *ascending trunk of spinal nerves (Swan, 1830)*
    Synonym for macrodissected adult human ***spinal nerve ventral branch (>1840)***; pp. 23, 24.
13. *anterior spinal branches (Cruveilhier, 1836)*
    Synonym for macrodissected adult human ***spinal nerve ventral branches (>1840)***; in the original French, *branches spinales antérieures*, p. 765.

PARTLY CORRESPONDS:

1. *subcervical nerves (Monro, 1783)*
   Cervical ***spinal nerve ventral branches (>1840)*** for macrodissected adult human; see Table 15:3-*8*. Monro followed *cervical nerves (Vesalius, 1543a)*.
2. *subdorsal nerves (Monro, 1783)*
   Thoracic ***spinal nerve ventral branches (>1840)*** for macrodissected adult human; see Table 15:3-*8*.
3. *anterior thoracic nerves (Günther, 1786)*
   Macrodissected adult human ***anterior cutaneous branch of intercostal nerves (>1840), lateral pectoral nerve (>1840)***, and ***medial pectoral nerve (>1840)*** considered together; in the original Latin, *nervi thoracici anteriores*, p. 72.
4. *thoracic plexus (Günther, 1786)*
   Anterior thoracic nerves (Günther, 1786) and *posterior thoracic nerves (Günther, 1786)* considered together; in the original Latin, *plexus thoracici*, p. 72.

5. *thoracic nerves (Günther, 1786)*
Anterior *thoracic nerves (Günther, 1786)* and *posterior thoracic nerves (Günther, 1786)* considered together; in the original Latin, *nervi thoracici*, p. 72.
6. *superior branch of second cervical nerve (Bell, 1803b)*
Macrodissected adult human ***spinal nerve ventral branch (>1840)*** of second ***cervical nerve (Galen, c173)*** forming ***communicating branch (Winslow, 1733)*** of ***cervical plexus (Molinetti, 1675)*** with ***spinal nerve ventral branch (>1840)*** of first ***cervical nerve (Galen, c173)***; p. 164.
7. *abdominal branch of lumbar nerves (Bock, 1827)*
Synonym for macrodissected adult human ***spinal nerve ventral branch (>1840)*** of ***lumbar nerves (Diemerbroeck, 1672)***; in the original Latin, *Ram. abdominalis nervi lumbaris*, Table I, Figure 2-57,62.
8. *cervico-brachial plexus (Cruveilhier, 1836)*
Macrodissected adult human ***cervical plexus (Molinetti, 1675)*** and ***brachial plexus (Camper, 1760)*** considered together; in the original French, *plexus cervico-brachial*, p. 777.

spinal nerves (Camper, 1760–1762)

The caudal topographic division of the amniote ***craniospinal nerves (Herrick, 1915)***, the rostral division being the ***cranial nerves (Soemmerring, 1791)***. They are also distinguished from ***autonomic nerves (Langley, 1898)***, and are now enumerated from rostral to caudal. For macrodissected adult human, Camper was probably the first to use the current enumeration of (most commonly) 31 pairs of ***spinal nerves (Camper, 1760–1762)*** arising from the ***spinal cord (Galen, c162–c166)***, with the following ***spinal nerve groups (Durward, 1951)*** identified in current terminology: eight ***cervical nerves (Galen, c173)***, twelve ***thoracic nerves (Diemerbroeck, 1672)***, five ***lumbar nerves (Diemerbroeck, 1672)***, five ***sacral nerves (Camper, 1760)***, and one ***coccygeal nerve (Camper, 1762)***; pp. 9 and 18 of 1760, 7 and 8 of 1762. Most of them were known long ago to Herophilus; see ***[spinal nerves (Camper, 1760–1762)] (Herophilus, c335–c280 BC)***.

TRANSLATIONS:

1. *nervos spinali (Camper, 1760–1762)*
Original Latin form of ***spinal nerves (Camper, 1760)***; p. 9.

EARLIER REFERENCES:

Described, not named or illustrated:

1. ***[spinal nerves (Camper, 1760–1762)] (Herophilus, c335–c280 BC)***
The founder of human anatomy is credited with discovering ***nerves (Herophilus, c335–c280 BC)***, including most ***cranial nerves (Soemmerring, 1791)*** and ***spinal nerves (Camper, 1760–1762)***; see Solmsen (1961), von Staden (1969), Longrigg (1993), Clarke & O'Malley (1996, p. 261). Herophilus dissected animals and human cadavers.

LATER SYNONYMS:

1. *medullary nerves (Bock, 1827)*
Synonym for macrodissected adult human ***spinal nerves (Camper, 1760–1762)***; in the original Latin, *nervorum medullarum*, see Table I, Figure 1, p. 3.
2. *vertebral nerves (Bock, 1827)*
Synonym for macrodissected adult human ***spinal nerves (Camper, 1760–1762)***; in the original Latin, *nervorum vertebrarum*, see Table I, Figure 1, p. 3.
3. *common nerves (Bell, 1829)*
Synonym for ***spinal nerves (Camper, 1760–1762)*** in "all classes of animals"; p. 318.

PARTLY CORRESPONDS:

1. *pairs of nerves from spinal medulla (Galen, c162–c166)*
Synonym for *pairs of nerves arising from spinal cord (Galen, c192)*. Galen here reported 30 in human; see De Lacy translation (1980, p. 477).
2. *pairs of nerves from spinal cord (Galen, c192)*
Galen here erroneously reported 29 pairs of macrodissected adult human ***spinal nerves (Camper, 1760–1762)***; see Duckworth translation (1962, pp. 223–264); also see De Lacy translation (1980, p. 477), May translation (1968, p. 578). He also referred to their roots, without distinguishing ***dorsal roots (Spurzheim, 1826)*** from ***ventral roots (>1840)***; see Duckworth translation (1962, p. 21). In *On the Usefulness of the Parts*, he reported for human eight cervical, twelve thoracic (dorsal), five lumbar, and four sacral pairs, and also mentioned the coccyx, but not a pair of ***coccygeal nerves (Camper, 1762)***; see May translation (1968, pp. 597–603), also see Duckworth translation (1962, p. 226). He claimed that each *pair of nerves from spinal cord (Galen, c192)* has a voluntary motor and a sensory (for touch) part, see May translation (1968, pp. 684–685), and that ultimately they arise from ***brain (Smith Papyrus, c1700 BC)***; see May translation (1968, pp. 682–683). In *De Ossibus ad Tirones*, he indicated that there are three ***nerves (Herophilus, c335–c280 BC)*** associated with sacrum and three with coccyx, which may be true in some mammals but not human; see Kühn (1821, Vol. 2, p. 762), Koning (1903, pp. 33–37, 487). In this case the total would be 31 pairs of ***spinal nerves (Camper, 1760–1762)***, as counted now; also see *pairs of nerves from spinal medulla (Razi, c910)*.
3. *pairs of nerves from spinal medulla (Razi, c910)*
Razi counted for macrodissected adult human 31 pairs of ***spinal nerves (Camper, 1760–1762)***: eight ***cervical nerves (Galen, c173)***, twelve ***thoracic nerves (Diemerbroeck, 1672)***, five ***lumbar nerves (Diemerbroeck, 1672)***, three ***sacral nerves (Camper, 1760)***, and three ***coccygeal nerves (Camper, 1762)***; this apparently was based on Galen's account of the sacrum and coccyx in *De Ossibus ad Tirones*, where he indicated three ***nerves (Herophilus, c335–c280 BC)*** associated with each, which is true in some mammals but not human; see Kühn (1821, Vol. 2, p. 762), Koning (1903, pp. 33–37, 487), and *pairs of nerves from spinal cord (Galen, c192)*.
4. *spinal nerves (Benedetti, 1502)*
Benedetti referred (in Latin) to "nerves from the spine" in Lind's translation (1975, p. 131), which also translates *spinal nerves*. Benedetti counted 31 pairs of *spinal nerves (Benedetti, 1502)* in macrodissected adult human, almost exactly as now for ***spinal nerves (Camper, 1760–1762)***,

although he had six sacral, rather than five sacral and one coccygeal, and wrote that they provide the ability to feel and move; Lind translation (1975, pp. 130–133).

5. *sacral nerves (Benedetti, 1502)*
Benedetti counted six pairs in adult human, and must have begun with pair emerging from first sacral foramen (see Lind translation, 1975, p. 133), without distinguishing the last as ***coccygeal nerve (Camper, 1762)***.
6. *spinal nerves (Vesalius, 1543a)*
Vesalius's use of it for macrodissected adult human is in legend to first illustration accompanying Chapter IV (parts *G* and *30*; see Richardson and Carman translation, 2002, p. 205). There were 30 *spinal nerves (Vesalius, 1543a)*: seven cervical [1st through 7th ***cervical nerves (Galen, c173)***], twelve thoracic [8th ***cervical nerve (Galen, c173)*** through 11th ***thoracic nerve (Diemerbroeck, 1672)***], five lumbar [12th ***thoracic nerve (Diemerbroeck, 1672)*** through fourth ***lumbar nerve (Diemerbroeck, 1672)***], and six sacral [5th ***lumbar nerve (Diemerbroeck, 1672)*** through fifth ***sacral nerve (Camper, 1760)***]; apparently he did not identify ***coccygeal nerve (Camper, 1762)***; see Richardson and Carman translation (2002, Chapter IV).
7. *thoracic nerves (Vesalius, 1543a)*
The 12 pairs of ***nerves (Herophilus, c335–c280 BC)*** associated with thoracic vertebrae in macrodissected adult human. However, enumeration started between the seventh cervical and first thoracic vertebrae (Richardson & Carman translation, 2002, p. 233), unlike the current convention of beginning between the first and second thoracic vertebrae, which generates the first ***thoracic nerve (Diemerbroeck, 1672)***; see ***[thoracic nerves (Diemerbroeck, 1672)] (Galen, c173)*** and ***thoracic nerves (Diemerbroeck, 1672)***; thus, the twelve *thoracic nerves (Vesalius, 1543a)* correspond to the current 8th ***cervical nerve (Galen, c173)*** through 11th ***thoracic nerve (Diemerbroeck, 1672)***.
8. *lumbar nerves (Vesalius, 1543a)*
The five pairs of ***nerves (Herophilus, c335–c280 BC)*** associated with lumbar vertebrae in macrodissected adult human; see Richardson & Carman translation (2002, p. 257). However, in this enumeration the first lumbar nerve emerges between the last thoracic and first lumbar vertebrae, rather than the current convention, which goes back to Galen, ***[lumbar nerves (Diemerbroeck, 1672)] (Galen, c173)***. Thus, *lumbar nerves (Vesalius, 1543a)* correspond to the current 12th ***thoracic nerve (Diemerbroeck, 1672)*** through fourth ***lumbar nerve (Diemerbroeck, 1672)***.
9. *sacral nerves (Vesalius, 1543a)*
Vesalius counted six pairs in macrodissected adult human, but began with pair emerging between last thoracic vertebra and sacrum, that is, current fifth ***lumbar nerve (Diemerbroeck, 1672)***, and then included current five ***sacral nerves (Camper, 1760)***; see Richardson & Carman translation (2002, p. 254).
10. *thirty pair of motive sinews from spinal marrow (Geminus, 1553)*
Synonym for macrodissected adult human *pairs of nerves from spinal cord (Galen, c192)*; originally spelled *thyrtye payre of Synowes motive frome the Marey of the Backe*, f. BII. Geminus qualified the term by writing that "all these Synowes have both selyinge [sensing] and movynge, althoughe in some more and in some lesse" (f. Bvi).
11. *dorsal nerves (Coiter, 1572)*
Synonym for 30 macrodissected adult human *spinal nerves (Vesalius, 1543a)*; in the original Latin, *dorsi nervorum*, p. 124.
12. *nerves of spinall marey of brest (Bannister, 1578)*
Apparently synonym for macrodissected adult human *thoracic nerves (Vesalius, 1543a)*; f. 109v. A modern spelling is *nerves of spinal marrow of breast.*
13. *nerves of spinall marey of loynes (Bannister, 1578)*
Probably synonym for macrodissected adult human *lumbar nerves (Vesalius, 1543a)*; f. 109v. A modern spelling is *nerves of spinal marrow of loins.*
14. *nerves of chest (Crooke, 1615)*
Synonym for macrodissected adult human *thoracic nerves (Vesalius, 1543a)*; pp. 488, 897.
15. *nerves from marrow of thorax or chest (Crooke, 1615)*
Synonym for macrodissected adult human *thoracic nerves (Vesalius, 1543a)*; p. 488.
16. *nerves of loynes (Crooke, 1615)*
Shortened form of *nerves of spinall marey of loynes (Bannister, 1578)*; pp. 489, 898.
17. *nerves of os sacrum (Crooke, 1615)*
Synonym for macrodissected adult human *sacral nerves (Vesalius, 1543a)*; p. 489.
18. *nerves of holy bone (Crooke, 1615)*
Synonym for *nerves of os sacrum (Crooke, 1615)*; p. 899 and Table XXIII-*E*.
19. *nerves of chest or back (Bartholin, 1662)*
While following *thoracic nerves (Vesalius, 1543a)*, Bartholin noted that some (unnamed) anatomists refer to 11 thoracic nerves (pp. 323, 329), in today's enumeration, 1st–11th ***thoracic nerves (Diemerbroeck, 1672)***.
20. *nerves of loyns (Bartholin, 1662)*
While following *lumbar nerves (Vesalius, 1543a)*, Bartholin noted without further explanation that there are sometimes five of them and sometimes only four; pp. 323, 329.
21. *vertebral nerves (Willis, 1664)*
Synonym for *spinal nerves (Vesalius, 1543a)* in macrodissected adult human and other large mammal; see Pordage translation (1681, p. 158 and Fig. 9-ω).
22. *nerves of spinal marrow (Heister, 1717)*
Heister's account is the same as *spinal nerves (Benedetti, 1502)*, except he stated, as done now, that there are five *nerves of spinal marrow of os sacrum (Heister, 1717)*, rather than 6; see translation in Heister (1721, pp. 248–250).
23. *nerves of medulla spinalis (Winslow, 1733)*
Winslow's account of macrodissected adult human ***nerves (Herophilus, c335–c280 BC)*** associated with ***spinal cord (Galen, c162–c166)***; Section VI, p. 60. He enumerated 30 pairs, beginning with seven ***cervical nerves (Winslow,***

1733) corresponding to 2nd–8th ***cervical nerves (Galen, c173)***, twelve ***thoracic nerves (Diemerbroeck, 1672)***, five ***lumbar nerves (Diemerbroeck, 1672)***, and six *sacral nerves (Benedetti, 1502)*—though he said that occasionally only five sacral are present, for a total then of 29; Section VI, p. 76. His consistent convention was to name ***nerves (Herophilus, c335–c280 BC)***, beginning with the one emerging between the first and second corresponding vertebrae (cervical, thoracic, lumbar) or foramina in the sacrum.

24. *vertebral nerves (Winslow, 1733)*
Synonym for *nerves of medulla spinalis (Winslow, 1733)*; Winslow also provided the Latin, *nervi vertebrales*, Section X, p. 49.

25. *sacral nerves (Winslow, 1733)*
Synonym for macrodissected adult human *sacral nerves (Vesalius, 1543a)*, although Winslow stated that the number can be variable with one pair more (6; 1733; Sect. VI, p. 88) or less (5; Sect. VI, p. 76), where the latter would be missing the fifth ***sacral nerve (Camper, 1760)***. Winslow's account was similar to the briefer description of Monro (1732, p. 8), which he had presented earlier in the 3rd edition of Cheselden's *Anatomy* (1726; see Preface).

26. *nerves of spinal medulla (Lieutaud, 1742)*
Lieutaud enumerated for macrodissected adult human 29, or sometimes 28, pairs, using a mixture of seven *cervical nerves (Winslow, 1733)*; eleven nerves of chest or *nerves of back (Bartholin, 1662)*, the 1st–11th ***thoracic nerves (Diemerbroeck, 1672)***; five *lumbar nerves (Vesalius, 1543a)*, the 12th ***thoracic nerve (Diemerbroeck, 1672)*** through fourth ***lumbar nerve (Diemerbroeck, 1672)***; and either five or six *sacral nerves (Winslow, 1733)*; see p. 451 ff.

27. *intervertebral nerves (Schaarschmidt, 1750)*
Synonym for macrodissected adult human *spinal nerves (Vesalius, 1543a)*; in the original Latin, *nervi intervertebralis*, p. 60.

28. *lumbar nerves (Haller, 1762)*
For macrodissected adult human Haller counted six rather than the now accepted five ***lumbar nerves (Diemerbroeck, 1672)***. For this, he counted 12th ***thoracic nerve (Diemerbroeck, 1672)*** as first *lumbar nerve (Haller, 1762)*; p. 249.

29. *pelvic nerves (Andersch, 1797)*
Not clear but probably synonym for macrodissected adult human *sacral nerves (Benedetti, 1502)*; in the original Latin, *nervi pelvis*, p. 2.

spinal nucleus of trigeminal nerve (>1840)

As described for macrodissected adult human, and for adult mammal in general with cellular architecture and connections, a longitudinal ***gray matter region (Swanson & Bota, 2010)*** centered along the lateral edge of the entire ***medulla (Winslow, 1733)*** but extending from the caudal end of the ***principal sensory nucleus of trigeminal nerve (>1840)*** rostrally, to the ***dorsal horn (>1840)*** near the caudal end of the first level of the ***cervical part of spinal cord (>1840)***. The ***spinal nucleus of trigeminal nerve (>1840)*** is coextensive with the length of the ***spinal tract of trigeminal nerve (>1840)***, its major input tract; see Williams & Warwick (1980, p. 1060), Nieuwenhuys et al. (2008, Figs. 6.6, 6.21–25). It was probably first identified by Rolando; see ***[spinal nucleus of trigeminal nerve (>1840)] (Rolando, 1825a)***.

EARLIER REFERENCES:

Illustrated and described, not named:

1. ***[spinal nucleus of trigeminal nerve (>1840)] (Rolando, 1825a)***
Roughly illustrated and briefly described in transverse section of macrodissected adult human; Table IX, Figures 1–4, indicated by * and legend for *r.5*.

Earlier synonyms:

1. *gray tubercle (Cloquet, 1828)*
Synonym for macrodissected adult human *gray nucleus of medulla oblongata (Arnold, 1838a)*; in the original French (plural), *tubercules cendrés*, Plate CXLV, Figure 6-*16*.
2. *gray nucleus of medulla oblongata (Arnold, 1838a)*
Roughly indicates region of ***spinal nucleus of trigeminal nerve (>1840)*** in section through ***medulla (Winslow, 1733)*** of macrodissected adult human; in the original Latin (plural), *nuclei cinerei medullae oblongatae*, p. 20.
3. *gray body of medulla oblongata (Arnold, 1838a)*
Synonym for *gray nucleus of medulla oblongata (Arnold, 1838a)*; in the original Latin (plural), *corpora cinerea medullae oblongatae*, p. 20. Arnold (1838b, Tab. II, Fig. 6-*e*) gave the singular, *corpus cinereum*.

PARTLY CORRESPONDS:

1. *pons mammillaris (Haller, 1762)*
Synonym for macrodissected adult fish *ganglion of trifacial nerve (Leuret, 1839)*; pp. 594, 695.
2. *ganglion of trifacial nerve (Leuret, 1839)*
Macrodissected adult fish swelling on outer dorsal part of ***pons (Haller, 1747)*** and/or ***medulla (Winslow, 1833)*** associated with ***trigeminal nerve (Winslow, 1733)***, and thus presumably at least part of ***spinal nucleus of trigeminal nerve (>1840)***; in the original French (plural), *ganglions du nerf trifacial*, p. 142. Leuret equated it without citation to *lobus posterior, pons mamilllaris* of Haller.
3. *lobus posterior (Leuret, 1839)*
Synonym for *ganglion of trifacial nerve (Leuret, 1839)*; p. 142.

spinal root of accessory nerve (>1840)

As described for macrodissected adult human, it has two parts: a series of ***spinal root of accessory nerve rootlets (>1840)*** joining at regular intervals and forming a longitudinal, rostrally directed ***spinal root of accessory nerve trunk (>1840)*** in turn merging distally with the ***cranial root of accessory nerve trunks (>1840)*** to form the ***accessory nerve trunk (Wrisberg, 1786)***. The ***spinal root of accessory nerve (>1840)*** eventually supplies two muscles, the trapezius and sternocleidomastoid, with axons from motor ***neurons (Waldeyer, 1891)*** in the ***spinal accessory nucleus (>1840)*** of the rostral (upper) 5–6 levels of the ***cervical part of spinal cord (>1840)***; see Durward (1951, p. 1044 and Fig. 908), Williams & Warwick (1980, p. 1082 and Fig. 7.189). It was known to Galen; see ***[spinal root of accessory nerve (>1840)] (Galen, c192)***.

EARLIER REFERENCES:

Described, not named or illustrated:

1. ***[spinal root of accessory nerve (>1840)] (Galen, c192)***
   Clearly described distribution to trapezius and sternocleidomastoid muscles of macrodissected adult beef, pig, and/or macaque but not human; see Duckworth translation (1962, p. 202).

Illustrated, not named or described:

1. ***[spinal root of accessory nerve (>1840)] (Eustachi, 1552)***
   Only part of ***accessory nerve (Vieussens, 1684)*** illustrated for macrodissected adult human; see Albinus edition (1744, Tab. 18, Figs. 1, 3).

Illustrated and described, not named:

1. ***[spinal root of accessory nerve (>1840)] (Du Verney, 1683)***
   Clearly distinguished between it and ***cranial root of accessory nerve (>1840)*** in macrodissected adult human; see Plate IX, Figure I-Q. It was progressively more clearly illustrated and described by Lobstein (1760, Tab. Va, Fig. I-*d*), Soemmerring (1778, Tab. II), Vicq d'Azyr (1786, Pl. XVIII-39).

Earlier synonyms:

1. *ascending trunk of accessory spinal nerve (Willis, 1664)*
   Basically synonymous with macrodissected adult human ***spinal root of accessory nerve (>1840)***; see Pordage translation (1681, Tab. 9- ♃, ♀, ♂).
2. *spinal part of accessory nerve (Arnold, 1838b)*
   Synonym for macrodissected adult human ***spinal root of accessory nerve (>1840)***; in the original Latin, *pars spinalis nervi accessorii*, Table I, Figure 2-6.

spinal root of accessory nerve rootlets (>1840)

As described for macrodissected adult human, there are typically on the order of seven distinct *nerve fiber (Ehrenberg, 1833)* bundles (rootlets or fascicles) joining at regular intervals and forming a longitudinal, rostrally directed ***spinal root of accessory nerve trunk (>1840)***. The ***spinal root of accessory nerve rootlets (>1840)*** are attached to the outer surface of the rostral (upper) 5–6 levels of the ***cervical part of spinal cord (>1840)***, along a longitudinal line caudal to the ***cranial root of accessory nerve rootlets (>1840)*** and midway between the ***dorsal rootlets (>1840)*** and ***ventral rootlets (>1840)***; see ***spinal root of accessory nerve (>1840)***. They were described specifically as *rootlets* by Durward (1951, p. 1042), Carpenter (1976, p. 308), Williams & Warwick (1980, p. 1082; see Fig. 7.189). At least some of them were clearly illustrated by Eustachi; see ***[spinal root of accessory nerve rootlets (>1840)] (Eustachi, 1552)***.

EARLIER REFERENCES:

Illustrated, not named or described:

1. ***[spinal root of accessory nerve rootlets (>1840)] (Eustachi, 1552)***
   Clearly illustrated rostral three of them for macrodissected adult human; see Albinus edition (1744, Tab. 18, Figs. 1, 2). Willis noted that ***accessory nerve (Vieussens, 1684)*** is "radicated [rooted]" for most of its length along the ***spinal cord (Galen, c162–c166)***, see Pordage translation (1681, p. 174), and that in macrodissected adult human it is first noted at the level of the sixth or seventh cervical vertebra, see Pordage translation (1681, p. 173 and Tab. 9-♀).

Earlier synonyms:

1. *filaments of nervi accessorii of eighth pair (Winslow, 1733)*
   Synonym for macrodissected adult human ***spinal roots of accessory nerve rootlets (>1840)***; Section VI, p. 74.
2. *spinal roots of accessory nerve of Willis (Günther, 1786)*
   Synonym for macrodissected adult human ***spinal roots of accessory nerve rootlets (>1840)***; in the original Latin, *radicibus spinalibus*, p. 89.
3. *roots of accessory nerve from spinal medulla (Frotscher, 1788)*
   Synonym for macrodissected adult human ***spinal roots of accessory nerve rootlets (>1840)***; in the original Latin, *nervi accessorii radiculae ex medulla spinali*, Figure I-*g*.
4. *apparent origin of accessory nerve of Willis (Cruveilhier, 1836)*
   Synonym for macrodissected adult human ***spinal roots of accessory nerve rootlets (>1840)***; in the original French, *origine apparente de l'accessoires de Willis*, p. 899.

spinal root of accessory nerve trunk (>1840)

As described for macrodissected adult human, the part of the ***spinal root of accessory nerve (>1840)*** lying between ***spinal root of accessory nerve rootlets (>1840)*** proximally and ***accessory nerve trunk (Wrisberg, 1786)*** distally. It was described specifically as a trunk by Durward (1951, p. 1042), Carpenter (1976, p. 308), Williams & Warwick (1980, p. 1082; see Fig. 7.189). It was clearly delineated by Eustachi; see ***[spinal root of accessory nerve trunk (>1840)] (Eustachi, 1552)***.

EARLIER REFERENCES:

Illustrated, not named or described:

1. ***[spinal root of accessory nerve trunk (>1840)] (Eustachi, 1552)***
   Clearly illustrated rostral end for macrodissected adult human; see Albinus edition (1744, Tab. 18, Figs. 1, 2).

Earlier synonyms:

1. *nervus spinalis ad par vagum accessorius (Vieussens, 1684)*
   Synonym for macrodissected adult human ***spinal root of accessory nerve trunk (>1840)***; Table 23-*b*.

2. *accessory nerve trunk (Frotscher, 1788)*
   Synonym for macrodissected adult human ***spinal root of accessory nerve trunk (>1840)***; in the original Latin, *trunci nervi accessorii*, Figure I-*e*.

spinal rubrospinal tract (>1840)

As described in adult human with experimental methods for tracing pathways, the caudal topographic segment of the ***rubrospinal tract (>1840)***, in the ***spinal cord (Galen, c162–c166)*** caudal to the ***medullary rubrospinal tract (>1840)*** segment and centered roughly in intermediate parts of the ***lateral funiculus (Burdach, 1822)***, partly overlapping with and ventral to the ***crossed corticospinal tract (>1840)***; see Mettler (1948, Fig. 172), Carpenter (1976, Fig. 10.21), Williams & Warwick (1980, Figs. 7.43–44). It was not known by 1840.

spinal segment of spinal tract of trigeminal nerve (>1840)

As described in macrodissected adult human, and mammal generally with histological methods for ***axons (Kölliker, 1896)***, the short caudal topographic segment of the ***spinal tract of trigeminal nerve (>1840)*** in the ***spinal cord (Galen, c162–c166)***, caudal to the ***medullary segment of spinal tract of trigeminal nerve (>1840)*** and extending in the ***dorsolateral tract (>1840)*** only as far as about the caudal end of the first level of the ***cervical part of spinal cord (>1840)***; see Carpenter (1976, Fig. 12.20), Nieuwenhuys et al. (2008, Figs. 6.6, 16.8). It was probably first identified by Bell; see ***[spinal segment of spinal tract of trigeminal nerve (>1840)] (Bell, 1834)***.

EARLIER REFERENCES:

Described, not named or illustrated:

1. ***[spinal segment of spinal tract of trigeminal nerve (>1840)] (Bell, 1834)***
   Probably identified in macrodissected adult human; p. 479. For other vertebrate classes see Todd (1836–1839, pp. 274–277, Figs. 142–145).

spinal tectospinal tract (>1840)

As described in adult human, especially with experimental pathway tracing methods, the caudal topographic segment of the ***tectospinal tract (>1840)***, in the ***spinal cord (Galen, c1620–c166)*** caudal to the ***medullary tectospinal tract (>1840)*** segment and centered in the ***ventral funiculus (>1840)*** just lateral to the ***uncrossed corticospinal tract (>1840)***; see Carpenter (1976, Fig. 10.21) and Williams & Warwick (1980, Fig. 744A), called *medial tectospinal tract (>1840)*. It was not known by 1840.

spinal tract of trigeminal nerve (>1840)

As described for macrodissected adult human, and for mammal generally with normal and experimental pathway tracing methods, the caudally directed longitudinal branch of the ***trigeminal nerve central sensory root (>1840)*** supplying the ***spinal nucleus of trigeminal nerve (>1840)*** from its convex lateral border. For topographic description it has three segments, ***pontine segment of spinal tract of trigeminal nerve (>1840)*** lateral to the ***principal sensory nucleus of trigeminal nerve (>1840)***, ***medullary segment of spinal tract of trigeminal nerve (>1840)***, and ***spinal segment of spinal tract of trigeminal nerve (>1840)*** only extending in the ***dorsolateral tract (>1840)*** as far as about the caudal end of the first level of the ***cervical part of spinal cord (>1840)***. See Williams & Warwick (1980, p. 1060), Nieuwenhuys et al. (2008, p. 194, Figs. 6.6, 6.21–25). It was probably first observed as the *root of fifth pair of nerves (Rolando, 1825a)*.

EARLIER REFERENCES:

Earlier synonyms:

1. *root of fifth pair of nerves (Rolando, 1825a)*
   Synonym for macrodissected adult beef or human ***spinal tract of trigeminal nerve (>1840)***; Table IV, Figure 1-*r.5*. Also see Desmoulins (1825, Pl. XIII, Figs. 7, 8, 10, part *r.V*) for clear illustration by Rolando in transverse sections of macrodissected adult human, and description in Bell (1834, p. 479). It was clearly described, illustrated, and discussed for other vertebrate classes by Todd (1836–1839, pp. 274–277, Figs. 142–145).

spinal ventral spinocerebellar tract (>1840)

As described in macrodissected adult human, and mammal generally with experimental methods for pathway tracing, the caudal topographic segment of the ***ventral spinocerebellar tract (>1840)*** in the ***spinal cord (Galen, c162–c166)***, caudal to the ***medullary ventral spinocerebellar tract (>1840)*** segment and centered in outer, ventral parts of the ***lateral funiculus (Burdach, 1822)***; see Williams & Warwick (1980, Fig. 7.43), Nieuwenhuys et al. (2008, Fig. 6.1-25). Not clearly delineated by 1840.

spinothalamic tract (>1840)

As described primarily with histological methods for ***axons (Kölliker, 1896)*** and experimental pathway tracing in human and other adult mammals, a longitudinal ***central nervous system white matter tract (>1840)*** extending from the ***ventral white commissure (>1840)*** of the ***spinal cord (Galen, c162–c166)*** caudally to the ***forebrain (Goette, 1873)*** rostrally. In the ***spinal cord (Galen, c162–c166)*** it is divided for clinical and descriptive purposes into ***lateral spinothalamic tract (>1840)*** and ***ventral spinothalamic tract (>1840)*** components and in the ***brain (Smith Papyrus, c1700 BC)*** it extends rostrally as a component of the ***ventrolateral fascicle (>1840)*** where the lateral and ventral parts are not distinct and where it is divided for topographic description into ***medullary spinothalamic tract (>1840)***, ***pontine spinothalamic tract (>1840)***, ***tegmental spinothalamic tract (>1840)***, and ***thalamic spinothalamic tract (>1840)*** segments. The ***spinothalamic tract (>1840)*** has substantial branches to the ***medulla (Winslow, 1733)***, ***pons (Haller, 1747)***, and ***midbrain (Baer, 1837)*** including parts of the ***tectum (Baer, 1837)*** and ***tegmentum (Swanson, 2000b)***, as well as sparser extensions to the ***hypothalamus (Kuhlenbeck, 1927)***, ***cerebral nuclei***

(Swanson, 2000a), and even ***cerebral cortex (>1840)*** from the conventional "end" of the ***spinothalamic tract (>1840)***, the ***thalamic spinothalamic tract (>1840)*** segment; see Crosby et al. (1962, p. 99), Carpenter (1976, pp. 242–249 and Figs. 10.7–8), Williams & Warwick (1980, pp. 876–877, 880), *Terminologia Anatomica* (1998, p. 107), Nieuwenhuys et al. (2008, pp. 697–701). Thus, ***spinothalamic tract (>1840)*** incorporates terms like *spinocortical tract (>1840)*, *spinohypothalamic fibers (>1840)*, *spinotectal tract (>1840)* with additional inputs to the ***periaqueductal gray (>1840)***, *spinopontine fibers (>1840)*, *spinoreticular fibers (>1840)*, and *spino-olivary tract (>1840)*. The ***corticospinal tract (>1840)*** is a topographically separate, caudally directed, longitudinal ***central nervous system white matter tract (>1840)*** originating in the ***cerebral cortex (>1840)*** and extending all the way to the ***spinal cord (Galen, c162–c166)***. The ***spinothalamic tract (>1840)*** was not clearly delineated by 1840, except for the ***thalamic spinothalamic tract (>1840)*** and rostral part of the ***tegmental spinothalamic tract (>1840)***; see ***ventrolateral fascicle (>1840)***.

splanchnic ganglion (>1840)

As sometimes observed in macrodissected adult human, a ***prevertebral ganglion (Quain, 1832)*** associated with the ***greater splanchnic nerve (Walter, 1783)*** at about the level of the 12th thoracic vertebra, although microscopic evidence of ganglion cells is usually found; see Mitchell (1953, p. 243), Williams & Warwick (1980, p. 1131). It was first delineated by Lobstein; see ***[splanchnic ganglion (>1840)] (Lobstein, 1823)***.

EARLIER REFERENCES:

Described, not named or illustrated:

1. ***[splanchnic ganglion (>1840)] (Lobstein, 1823)***
   Lobstein described in two macrodissected adult human cadavers its arrangement on the ***greater splanchnic nerve (Lobstein, 1823)***; see translation (1831, pp. 24–25).

splenic plexus (Palfijn, 1726)

As described for macrodissected adult human, a ***terminal plexus (Swanson & Bota, 2010)*** extending from the ***celiac plexus (Winslow, 1733)*** along the splenic artery and joined by branches from the ***celiac ganglion (Walter, 1783)*** and right ***vagus nerve (Galen, c192)***. It supplies branches to the spleen, pancreas, and stomach; see Durward (1951, p. 1142), Mitchell (1953, p. 188), Williams & Warwick (1980, p. 1134). For Palfijn's use in macrodissected adult human, see Part 2, p. 336. It was first identified as *nerve conferred on spleen (Galen, c173)*.

TRANSLATIONS:

1. *plexus splenique (Palfijn, 1726)*
   Original French form of ***splenic plexus (Palfijn, 1726)***; Part 2, p. 336.
2. *plexus splenicus (Winslow, 1733)*
   Latin form of ***splenic plexus (Palfijn, 1726)***; Section VI, no. 408, p. 98.

EARLIER REFERENCES:

Earlier synonyms:

1. *nerve conferred on spleen (Galen, c173)*
   Synonym for ***splenic plexus (Palfijn, 1726)*** as mentioned for macrodissected adult beef, pig, and/or macaque but not human; see May translation (1968, p. 263).
2. *nerve branch to spleen (Galen, c192)*
   Synonym for ***splenic plexus (Palfijn, 1726)*** as mentioned for macrodissected adult beef, pig, and/or macaque but not human; see Duckworth translation (1962, p. 222). Similarly, Vesalius (1543a) referred to and illustrated a *nerve into spleen* for macrodissected adult human; see Richardson & Carman translation (2007, legend to Fig. 4, p. 9; also see p. 8-*ß*). Willis (1664) described and illustrated it much more clearly for macrodissected adult human and other common large mammals; see Pordage translation (pp. 158, 167 and Tab. XI-*ζ*).
3. *splenic infolding (Willis, 1664)*
   Apparently synonym for part or all of ***splenic plexus (Palfijn, 1726)*** in macrodissected adult human and other common large mammals; see Pordage translation (1681, Tab. XII-*G*).
4. *splenetick nerves (Willis, 1664)*
   Synonym for part or all of ***splenic plexus (Palfijn, 1726)*** in macrodissected adult human and other common large mammals; see Pordage translation (1681, pp. 158, 167 and Tab. XI-*ζ*).
5. *nerveum plexum lienarem (Vieussens, 1684)*
   Synonym for macrodissected adult human ***splenic plexus (Palfijn, 1726)***; Table 23-*64*.

LATER SYNONYMS:

1. *pancreatico-splenic plexus (Wrisberg, 1800)*
   Synonym for macrodissected adult human ***splenic plexus (Palfijn, 1726)***; in the original Latin, *plexus lienalis et pancreaticis* and *plexus pancreatico-lienalis*, p. 559.

PARTLY CORRESPONDS:

1. *splenic plexus (Walter, 1783)*
   Part of macrodissected adult human ***splenic plexus (Palfijn, 1726)*** on proximal parts of splenic artery receiving *splenic plexus roots (Walter, 1783)* and generating *splenic nerves (Walter, 1783)*; in the original Latin, *plexus lienalis*, Table III-*after 285*; *plexum lienalem*, Table III-*286*.
2. *splenic plexus roots (Walter, 1783)*
   Most proximal part of macrodissected adult human ***splenic plexus (Palfijn, 1726)*** arising from ***celiac plexus (Winslow, 1733)*** and forming *splenic plexus (Walter, 1783)*; in the original Latin (singular), *radix plexus lienalis*, Table III:*286–293*.
3. *splenic nerves (Walter, 1783)*
   Part of macrodissected adult human ***splenic plexus (Palfijn, 1726)*** between *splenic plexus (Walter, 1783)* and terminal *splenic nerve plexus (Walter, 1783)*; in the original Latin, *nervi lienales*, Table III:*300–313*; *nervorum lienalium*, Table III:*315–320*.
4. *splenic nerve plexus (Walter, 1783)*
   Most distal part of macrodissected adult human ***splenic plexus (Palfijn, 1726)***, formed by branches of *splenic*

nerves (Walter, 1783); in the original Latin, *nervi plexus lienalis*, Table III:*321–337*.

5. *branch of splenic plexus to pancreas and spleen (Günther, 1786)*
As term indicates, for macrodissected adult human; in the original Latin, *plexus splenicus, unde r. ad pancreas & lien*, p. 95.
6. *short gastric nerves (Mayer, 1794)*
Probably synonym for macrodissected adult human *small inferior plexus of stomach (Meckel, 1817)*; in the original Latin, *nervi gastrici breves*; Part 6, Table IV-*VI* (p. 27).
7. *middle splenic nerves (Mayer, 1794)*
Macrodissected adult human components of ***splenic plexus (Palfijn, 1726)*** extending toward middle of spleen; in the original Latin, nervi *splenici s. lienales medii*; Part 6, Table IV-*41* (p. 27).
8. *superior splenic nerves (Mayer, 1794)*
Macrodissected adult human components of ***splenic plexus (Palfijn, 1726)*** extending toward rostral (upper) part of spleen; in the original Latin, nervi *splenici s. lienales superiores*; Part 6, Table IV-*42* (p. 27).
9. *inferior splenic nerves (Mayer, 1794)*
Macrodissected adult human components of ***splenic plexus (Palfijn, 1726)*** extending toward caudal (lower) part of spleen; in the original Latin, *nervi splenici s. lienales inferiores*; Part 6, Table IV-*43* (p. 27).
10. *small inferior plexus of stomach (Meckel, 1817)*
Described as formed by branches of macrodissected adult human ***splenic plexus (Palfijn, 1726)*** to large cul-de-sac of stomach; in the original Latin, *plexus ventriculi inferior et minor*, see translation (1832, Vol. 3, p. 87).
11. *splenic ganglia (Wutzer, 1817)*
Wutzer did not elaborate for macrodissected adult human; they are not recognized today; in the original Latin, *ganglia lienalia*, p. 110.

splenium of corpus callosum (Burdach, 1822)

As described for macrodissected adult human, the caudal end of the ***corpus callosum (Galen, c177)***, caudal to the ***body of corpus callosum (>1840)*** and dorsal to the ***pineal gland (Galen, c192)***; see Mettler (1948, p. 100, Fig. 68). Burdach described, illustrated, and reviewed its history for macrodissected adult human; pp. 147, 368. It was first clearly delineated as the *brim of corpus callosum (Willis, 1664)*.

TRANSLATIONS:

1. *glove of corpus callosum (Reil, 1809b)*
English form of ***splenium of corpus callosum (Burdach, 1822)***; see Meckel (1832, Vol. 2, p. 448). It is now most commonly translated as a band-like structure; see *Dorland's* (2003, p. 1740).

EARLIER REFERENCES:

Earlier synonyms:

1. *brim of corpus callosum (Willis, 1664)*
Synonym for ***splenium of corpus callosum (Burdach, 1822)*** in macrodissected adult human and other large mammals; see Pordage translation (1681, Tabs. III-*B*, IV-*B*).
2. *corpus transversale (Tyson, 1699)*
Synonym for macrodissected infant chimpanzee ***splenium of corpus callosum (Burdach, 1822)***; Figure 14-*D*.
3. *bourrelet postérieur du corps calleux (Vicq d'Azyr, 1786)*
Synonym for macrodissected adult human ***splenium of corpus callosum (Burdach, 1822)***; Plate XX-57.
4. *superimposed bulge (Soemmerring, 1788)*
Synonym for macrodissected adult human ***splenium of corpus callosum (Burdach, 1822)***; in the original German, *die aufgesetzte Wulst*. Also used by Reil (1809b); see Mayo translation (1823, p. 52) and Meyer (1971, p. 94 note 9). Also see *posterior fold of corpus callosum (Reil, 1809b)*.
5. *posterior fold of corpus callosum (Reil, 1809b)*
Synonym for macrodissected adult human ***splenium of corpus callosum (Burdach, 1822)***; Mayo's (1823, p. 52) English form of the original German, *die aufgesetzte Wulst*. Also see *superimposed bulge (Soemmerring, 1788)*.

LATER SYNONYMS:

1. *Wulst (Burdach, 1822)*
German term (*die Wulst*) for macrodissected adult human ***splenium of corpus callosum (Burdach, 1822)***; p. 147, where he also used the full term, *die Balkenwulst*. Also see *posterior fold of corpus callosum (Reil, 1809b)*.
2. *bourelet di Vicq-d'Azir (Rolando, 1831)*
Eponym for macrodissected adult human ***splenium of corpus callosum (Burdach, 1822)***, referring to *bourrelet postérieur du corps calleux (Vicq d'Azyr, 1786)*; Figure 8-*d*.
3. *tuber of corpus callosum (Arnold, 1834)*
Synonym for macrodissected adult human ***splenium of corpus callosum (Burdach, 1822)***; in the original Latin, *corpus callosum tuber*, Table VI:*M-ζ*.
4. *splenium of great commissure (Arnold, 1838b)*
Synonym for macrodissected adult human ***splenium of corpus callosum (Burdach, 1822)***; in the original Latin, *splenium commissurae maximae*, Table VII, Figure 2-*l*.

stapedial nerve (>1840)

As described for macrodissected adult human, small branch of ***intermediofacial nerve trunk (>1840)*** to stapedial muscle; see *Terminologia Anatomica* (1998, p. 135, as *nerve to stapedius*), *Dorland's* (2003, p. 1236). It was perhaps first delineated by Valsalva; see ***[stapedial nerve (>1840)] (Valsalva, 1704)***.

EARLIER REFERENCES:

Illustrated and described, not named:

1. ***[stapedial nerve (>1840)] (Valsalva, 1704)***
Described and illustrated for macrodissected adult human; Table 7, Figure 3-*i*.

Earlier synonyms:

1. *branch of hard nerve to stapedial muscle (Günther, 1786)*
Synonym for macrodissected adult human ***stapedial nerve (>1840)***; in the original Latin, *nervus durus ramus ad m. stapedis*, p. 56.

2. *nervus communicans faciei ramus ad musculus stapedis (Günther, 1786)*
   Synonym for *branch of hard nerve to stapedial muscle (Günther, 1786)*; p. 56.
3. *stapedial filament of portio major and minor of facial nerve (Bellingeri, 1818)*
   Synonym for macrodissected adult human ***stapedial nerve (>1840)***; in the original Latin, *filamentum stapedis*, see Table II.
4. *branches of facial nerve to stapedial muscle (Langenbeck, 1826–1830)*
   Synonym for macrodissected adult human ***stapedial nerve (>1840)***; in the original Latin, *rami nervi facialis ad musculum stapedium*, Fascicle III, Table XXV-*p*. Also called a twig (*surculus*); Fascicle III, Table XVII-*.

stem of lateral cerebral sulcus (>1840)

As described for macrodissected adult human, the middle segment of the ***lateral cerebral sulcus (>1840)***, with the ***anterior branch of lateral cerebral sulcus (>1840)*** and ***ascending branch of lateral cerebral sulcus (>1840)*** extending rostrally and the ***posterior branch of lateral cerebral sulcus (>1840)*** extending caudally; see Williams & Warwick (1980, p. 984 and Fig. 7.111A). It was distinguished and named as the *stem of Sylvian fissure (Vicq d'Azyr, 1784)*.

EARLIER REFERENCES:

Earlier synonyms:

1. *stem of Sylvian fissure (Vicq d'Azyr, 1784)*
   Synonym for macrodissected adult human ***stem of lateral cerebral sulcus (>1840)***. According to Vicq d'Azyr's description, a rostral and deep *stem* divides on the surface into a *posterior branch* and an *anterior vertical branch*, now called ***posterior branch of lateral cerebral sulcus (>1840)*** and ***ascending branch of lateral cerebral sulcus (>1840)***, respectively; in the original French, *le Tronc*, p. 506.

straight gyrus (Valentin, 1841)

As described for macrodissected adult human, the medial topographic subdivision of the ***orbital region (Rolando, 1831)*** of the ***frontal region (Vicq d'Azyr, 1786)***, the lateral subdivision being the ***orbital gyri (>1840)***. The lateral border of the ***straight gyrus (Valentin, 1841)*** is formed by the ***olfactory sulcus (Quain, 1834)*** and then the ***medial orbital gyrus (>1840)***, and its medial border is formed by the ventral edge of the ***orbital part of inferior frontal gyrus (>1840)***; see Williams & Warwick (1980; Fig. 7.111A, unlabeled below hashed line for *pars orbitalis*; Fig. 7.116, called *gyrus rectus*). For Valentin's use in macrodissected adult human, see Meyer (1971, p. 134). It was first clearly delineated by Soemmerring; see ***[straight gyrus (Valentin, 1841)] (Soemmerring, 1778)***.

TRANSLATIONS:

1. *gyrus rectus (Valentin, 1841)*
   Original Latin form of ***straight gyrus (Valentin, 1841)***; see Meyer (1971, p. 134).

EARLIER REFERENCES:

Illustrated and described, not named:

1. ***[straight gyrus (Valentin, 1841)] (Soemmerring, 1778)***
   Clearly illustrated for macrodissected adult human; Tables I-III.

Earlier synonyms:

1. *internal olfactory convolution (Gerdy, 1838)*
   Synonym for macrodissected adult human ***straight gyrus (Valentin, 1841)***; in the original French, *circonvolution olfactive interne*, p. 259.

striatum (Swanson, 2000a)

Based on histology and development, a ***gray matter region (Swanson & Bota, 2010)*** forming the dorsal of two major divisions of the mammalian ***cerebral nuclei (Swanson, 2000a)***, with the more ventral division being the ***pallidum (Swanson, 2000a)***. The major components are ***caudoputamen (Heimer & Wilson, 1975), accumbens nucleus (Ziehen, 1897–1901), olfactory tubercle (Calleja, 1893), lateral septal complex (Risold & Swanson, 1997), medial amygdalar nucleus (Johnston, 1923)***, and ***central amygdalar nucleus (Johnston, 1923)***; see Swanson (2004, Table B) for detailed list in rat. For Swanson's original use in rat, generalized to all mammals, see pp. 127–130, Figure 19. It was not recognized as such by 1840.

stylohyoid nerve (Meckel, 1753)

As described for macrodissected adult human, a long thin branch of the ***facial nerve trunk (>1840)*** entering the middle part of the stylohyoid muscle, often having other small branches, and often arising from a common trunk with the ***digastric nerve (Meckel, 1753)***; see Durward (1951, Figs. 901, 902), Williams & Warwick (1980, p. 1072), *internal deep nerve of hard nerve (Meckel, 1753)*. For Meckel's use in macrodissected adult human, see p. 72. He described three branches, an anterior branch to the external carotid artery, a second branch to the stylohyoid muscle, and a third branch to the neck. It was probably first delineated by Willis; see ***[stylohyoid nerve (Meckel, 1753)] (Willis, 1664)***.

TRANSLATIONS:

1. *nerf stylohyoïde (Meckel, 1753)*
   Original French form of ***stylohyoid nerve (Meckel, 1753)***; p. 72.

EARLIER REFERENCES:

Illustrated and described, not named:

1. ***[stylohyoid nerve (Meckel, 1753)] (Willis, 1664)***
   Probably mentioned and illustrated for macrodissected adult human; see Pordage translation (1681, p. 144 and Tab. IX-*1*). Winslow clearly mentioned it (1733, Sect. VI, p. 68).

LATER SYNONYMS:

1. *anterior branch of internal deep nerve of hard nerve (Meckel, 1753)*
   Synonym for ***stylohyoid nerve (Meckel, 1753)***; in the original French, *rameau antérieur du le rameau profond intérieur du nerf dur*, Table 1:*124–128*.

2. *portionis durae nervi acustici ramulus stylohyoideus (Neubauer, 1772)*
   Synonym for macrodissected adult human ***stylohyoid nerve (Meckel, 1753)***; Table 2-*71*. It roughly translates "stylohyoid branchlet of hard part of acoustic nerve."
3. *styloglossus nerve (Loder, 1778)*
   Synonym for macrodissected adult human ***stylohyoid nerve (Meckel, 1753)***; in the original Latin, *nervus styloglossus*, p. 25.
4. *par septimum portionis durae ramus stylohyoideus (Haase, 1781)*
   Synonym for macrodissected adult human ***stylohyoid nerve (Meckel, 1753)***; see Index section 180. It roughly translates "stylohyoid branch of hard part of seventh pair."
5. *nerve to stylohyoid muscle (Peipers, 1793)*
   Synonym for macrodissected adult human ***stylohyoid nerve (Meckel, 1753)***; in the original Latin, *nervus musculi stylo-hyoidei*, p. 35.
6. *styloid nerve (Mayer, 1794)*
   Synonym for macrodissected adult human ***stylohyoid nerve (Meckel, 1753)***; in the original Latin, *nervus styloideus*; Part 5, Table VII-*87* (p. 47).
7. *stylohyoid branch of facial nerve (Chaussier, 1809)*
   Synonym for macrodissected adult human ***stylohyoid nerve (Meckel, 1753)***; in the original French, *R. stylo-hyoïdien*, see left column, § VII.

PARTLY CORRESPONDS:

1. *anastomotic filament of stylo-hyoid branch (Bellingeri, 1818)*
   Macrodissected adult human ***communicating branch (Winslow, 1733)*** of ***stylohyoid nerve (Meckel, 1753)***, probably with ***external carotid plexus (>1840)***; in the original Latin, *filamentum anastomoticum*, see Table II. Also see *anastomotic filament of portio major and minor of facial nerve (Bellingeri, 1818)*.
2. *stylo-hyoid surculus proper of stylo-hyoid branch (Bellingeri, 1818)*
   Macrodissected adult human branch of ***stylohyoid nerve (Meckel, 1753)*** to stylohyoid muscle; in the original Latin, *surculus stylo-hyoïdeus proprius*, see Table II.
3. *mylo-hyoid surculus of stylo-hyoid branch (Bellingeri 1818)*
   Macrodissected adult human branch of ***stylohyoid nerve (Meckel, 1753)*** to mylohyoid muscle and skin of neck; in the original Latin, *surculus stylo-hyoïdeus proprius*, see Table II.

stylopharyngeal branch of glossopharyngeal nerve (>1840)

As described for macrodissected adult human, a branch of the ***glossopharyngeal nerve trunk (Wrisberg, 1786; Günther, 1786)*** to the stylopharyngeal muscle; see Hamilton (1976, Fig. 802), Williams & Warwick (1980, p. 1076), *Terminologia Anatomica* (1998, p. 136). It was known to Galen; see ***[stylopharyngeal branch of glossopharyngeal nerve (>1840)] (Galen, c192)***.

EARLIER REFERENCES:

Described, not named or illustrated:

1. ***[stylopharyngeal branch of glossopharyngeal nerve (>1840)] (Galen, c192)***
   Fine twigs branching off ***glossopharyngeal nerve (Huber, 1744)*** and running to "muscle of the pharynx" described in macrodissected adult beef, pig, and/or macaque but not human; see Duckworth translation (1962, p. 201). Haller (1762, p. 233) described it for macrodissected adult human.

Illustrated and described, not named:

1. ***[stylopharyngeal branch of glossopharyngeal nerve (>1840)] (Neubauer, 1772)***
   Carefully illustrated for macrodissected adult human; Table 2:*85–88*.

Earlier synonyms:

1. *second branch of glossopharyngeal nerve (Wrisberg, 1786)*
   Synonym for macrodissected adult human ***stylopharyngeal branch of glossopharyngeal nerve (>1840)***; in the original Latin, *secundus glossopharyngaei ramus*, see Wrisberg reprint (1800, p. 417).
2. *muscular branch of glossopharyngeal nerve (Wrisberg, 1786)*
   Synonym for macrodissected adult human ***stylopharyngeal branch of glossopharyngeal nerve (>1840)***; in the original Latin, *glossopharyngaei ramus muscularis*, see Wrisberg reprint (1800, p. 417), Williams & Warwick (1980, p. 1076).
3. *glossopharyngeal branches to stylopharyngeal muscle (Scarpa, 1788)*
   Synonym for macrodissected adult human ***stylopharyngeal branch of glossopharyngeal nerve (>1840)***; in the original Latin, *glosso-pharyngei rami ad musculum stylo-pharyngeum*, Table X, Figure 1-*34*.
4. *nerve to stylopharyngeal muscle (Andersch & Soemmerring, 1792)*
   Synonym for macrodissected adult human ***stylopharyngeal branch of glossopharyngeal nerve (>1840)***; in the original Latin, *nervus musculi stylopharyngei* and *nervum musculi stylopharyngei*, pp. 116, 118.
5. *nerves of stylopharyngeal muscle proper (Scarpa, 1794)*
   Essentially macrodissected adult human ***stylopharyngeal branch of glossopharyngeal nerve (>1840)***; in the original Latin, *nervi stylo-pharyngaei musculi proprii*, Table II-*17*.
6. *stylopharyngeal muscle branch of glossopharyngeal nerve (Wutzer, 1817)*
   Synonym for macrodissected adult human ***stylopharyngeal branch of glossopharyngeal nerve (>1840)***; in the original Latin, *ramus musculo stylo-pharyngeo*, Figure VII-*p*.
7. *stylopharyngeal muscle branches of glossopharyngeal nerve (Arnold, 1837)*
   Synonym for macrodissected adult human ***stylopharyngeal branch of glossopharyngeal nerve (>1840)***;

in the original Latin, *nervus glossopharyngeus rami musculi stylopharyngei*, p. 13 & Table VI-57.

PARTLY CORRESPONDS:

1. *circumflex nerves of stylopharyngeal muscle (Andersch & Soemmerring, 1792)*
Three short branches of macrodissected adult human ***glossopharyngeal nerve (Haller, 1762)*** contributing to ***stylopharyngeal branch of glossopharyngeal nerve (>1840)***; in the original Latin, *primi nervi circumflexi, secundus nervus circumflexus, tertium nervum circumflexum musculi stylopharyngei*, pp. 16–17.
2. *circumflex stylopharyngeal nerves (Andersch, 1797)*
Synonym for *circumflex nerves of stylopharyngeal muscle (Andersch & Soemmerring, 1792)*; in the original Latin, *primi nervi circumflexi, secundus nervus circumflexus, tertium nervum circumflexum stylopharyngeum*; pp. 9–10.

subarachnoid space (Magendie, 1827)

The region filled with ***cerebrospinal fluid (Magendie, 1827)*** between the outer ***arachnoid (Blasius, 1666)*** and inner ***pia (Galen, c192)***, also traversed by ***arachnoid trabeculae (>1840)*** and their condensation near ***pia (Galen, c192)***, the vascular ***epipial layer (>1840)***; see Key & Retzius (1875–1876), Millen & Woollam (1961). Embryologically, the ***subarachnoid space (Magendie, 1827)*** forms out of a single layer of connective tissue eventually splitting into ***pia (Galen, c192)*** and ***arachnoid (Blasius, 1666)***; see Woolley & Millen (1962), Williams & Warwick (1980, p. 175). In macrodissected adult human a number of differentiations called *subarachnoid cisterns* are named; see Millen & Woollam (1962, pp. 107–109), Carpenter (1976, pp. 10–11), Williams & Warwick (1980, p. 1049). It was known to Galen; see ***[subarachnoid space (Magendie, 1827)] (Galen, c177)***. For Magendie's use see pp. 21, 25, also see excellent history in Millen & Woollam (1962).

TRANSLATIONS:

1. *cavité sous-arachnoïdienne (Magendie, 1827)*
Original French form of ***subarachnoid space (Magendie, 1827)***; see pp. 21, 25.

EARLIER REFERENCES:

Described, not named or illustrated:

1. ***[subarachnoid space (Magendie, 1827)] (Galen, c177)***
Galen clearly described it for macrodissected adult beef, pig, and/or monkey but not human, implied it is empty, and even showed how to expand it by blowing into it with a narrow tube; see Singer translation (1999, p. 230).
2. ***[subarachnoid space (Magendie, 1827)] (Vesalius, 1543a)***
Vesalius clearly described it for macrodissected adult human and claimed it contains "a sort of aqueous liquid"; see Richardson & Carman translation (2009, p. 177; also see p. 171).

Earlier synonyms:

1. *arachnoid cavity (Magendie, 1825)*
Synonym for ***subarachnoid space (Magendie, 1827)***. Magendie described fluid as within the *arachnoid cavity*, "*à l'intérieur de la cavité arachnlïdienne*" of all mammals at all ages; p. 37.

PARTLY CORRESPONDS:

1. *spatium triangulare inter crura (Tarin, 1750)*
Synonym in macrodissected adult human for part of ***subarachnoid space (Magendie, 1827)*** called *interpeduncular cistern (>1840)*, a *subarachnoid cistern (>1840)*; Table I, Figure 4-*H*; also see Meyer (1971, p. 23). For *interpeduncular cistern (>1840)* see Williams & Warwick (1980, p. 1049), *Dorland's* (2003, p. 370).

subclavian nerve (>1840)

As described for macrodissected adult human, a branch of the ***brachial plexus upper trunk (>1840)*** innervating the subclavius muscle (between the 1st rib and clavicle) and usually supplying one or more small branches to the ***phrenic nerve (Galen, c173)***; see Williams & Warwick (1980, p. 1096 and Fig. 7.200), *Terminologia Anatomica* (1998, p. 138). It was known to Galen; see ***[subclavian nerve (>1840)] (Galen, c173)***.

EARLIER REFERENCES:

Described, not named or illustrated:

1. ***[subclavian nerve (>1840)] (Galen, c173)***
Galen alluded to it for macrodissected adult beef, pig, and/or macaque but not human, and referred to branches contributing to ***phrenic nerve (Galen, c173)***; see May translation (1968, p. 599). Later, he described it explicitly; see Duckworth translation (1962, p. 255). Vesalius (1543a) mentioned it for macrodissected adult human; see Richardson & Carman translation (2002, p. 232).

Earlier synonyms:

1. *subclavian branch of brachial plexus (Cruveilhier, 1836)*
Synonym for macrodissected adult human ***subclavian nerve (>1840)***; in the original French, *branche du sous-clavier du plexus brachial*, p. 792.

subclavian plexus (>1840)

As described for macrodissected adult human, a ***plexus (Galen, c192)*** arising predominantly from the ***inferior cervical ganglion (Vieussens, 1684)*** or *cervicothoracic ganglion (>1840)*, the ***ansa subclavia (>1840)***, and occasionally the ***vertebral ganglion (>1840)***. It surrounds the subclavian artery and its branches as least as far as the first part of the axillary artery, and the ***plexus (Galen, c192)*** receives variable branches from multiple other sources as well; see Mitchell (1953, p. 232), Williams & Warwick (1980, p. 1129). It was described at least partly by Neubauer; see ***[subclavian plexus (>1840)] (Neubauer, 1772)***.

EARLIER REFERENCES:

Described, not named or illustrated:

1. ***[subclavian plexus (>1840)] (Neubauer, 1772)***
Partly described but not named for macrodissected adult human; see pp. 129–136.

Earlier synonyms:

1. *subclavian nerve (Andersch, 1797)*
Probably refers to macrodissected adult human ***subclavian plexus (>1840)*** or an obvious feature within

it; in the original Latin, *nervus subclavius*; see pp. 20, 34; and Mitchell (1953, p. 232).

2. *plexus surrounding subclavian artery (Swan, 1830)*
Synonym for macrodissected adult human ***subclavian plexus (>1840)***; Plate III-*1*.

subcostal nerve (>1840)

As described for macrodissected adult human, the ***spinal nerve ventral branch (>1840)*** for the most caudal (last or 12th) ***thoracic nerve (Diemerbroeck, 1672)***, and although larger has essentially the same distribution as the ***intercostal nerves (Vesalius, 1543a)*** rostral to it; see Williams & Warwick (1980, pp. 1104–1105). Quain (1837, p. 783) noted that "The anterior [ventral] branch of the twelfth dorsal [thoracic] nerve passing below the last rib, cannot be named intercostal." It was perhaps first clearly delineated by Eustachi; see ***[subcostal nerve (>1840)] (Eustachi, 1552)***.

EARLIER REFERENCES:

Illustrated, not named or described:

1. ***[subcostal nerve (>1840)] (Eustachi, 1552)***
Illustrated clearly for macrodissected adult human; see Albinus edition (1761, Tab. 19/2-***β***). Earlier illustrated by Vesalius (1543a) in a confused way; see Richardson and Carman translation (2002, p. 206).

Earlier synonyms:

1. *anterior branch of first lumbar nerve (Haller, 1762)*
Synonym for macrodissected adult human ***subcostal nerve (>1840)***; see pp. 249–250. Also see *lumbar nerves (Vesalius, 1543a), lumbar nerves (Haller, 1762)*.
2. *anterior branch of twelfth thoracic nerve (Meckel, 1817)*
Accurate synonym for macrodissected adult human ***subcostal nerve (>1840)***; see translation (1832, Vol. 3, pp. 10–11).
3. *subcostal branch of twelfth thoracic nerve (Bock, 1827)*
Synonym for macrodissected adult human ***subcostal nerve (>1840)***; in the original Latin, *ram. subcostalis nervi thoracici duodecimi*, Table IV-*51*.

PARTLY CORRESPONDS:

1. *anterior gluteal cutaneous nerve (Bock, 1827)*
Macrodissected adult human distal branches of *anterior branch of lateral abdominal cutaneous nerve (Bock, 1827)* for ***subcostal nerve (>1840)***; in the original Latin, *nerv. cutaneus glutaeus anterior*, Table III-*38*.
2. *cutaneous branch of subcostal branch of twelfth thoracic nerve (Bock, 1827)*
Macrodissected adult human *lateral abdominal cutaneous nerve (Bock, 1827)* for ***subcostal nerve (>1840)***; in the original Latin, *ram. cutaneus ram. subcostalis nervi thoracici duodecimi*, Table IV-*51,52*.
3. *lateral branch of subcostal branch of twelfth thoracic nerve (Bock, 1827)*
Synonym for *cutaneous branch of subcostal branch of twelfth thoracic nerve (Bock, 1827)*; in the original Latin, *ram. lateralis ram. subcostalis nervi thoracici duodecimi*, Table IV-*51,52*.

subependymal zone (>1840)

As described in adult mammal with histological methods, a differentiation associated with the ***lateral ventricle (Vesalius, 1543a)***, lying just deep to the ***ependyma (>1840)***, and containing stem cells for ***glia (Virchow, 1846)*** and ***neurons (Waldeyer, 1891)***; see Privat & LeBlond (1972), Swanson (2004, Atlas Levels 1-24), Ortega et al. (2013). It is sometimes considered the part of the *subventricular layer (>1840)* deep to the ***ependyma (>1840)***. It was not identified by 1840.

subicular complex (Swanson & Cowan, 1977)

As described with cellular architecture and connections in mammal, the developmentally and topologically medial division of the ***retrohippocampal region (Swanson et al., 1987)***, including from medial to lateral the ***subiculum (>1840), presubiculum (>1840)*** with its ***postsubiculum (Swanson & Cowan, 1977)*** dorsally, and ***parasubiculum (>1840)***. For Swanson & Cowan's original use based on cytoarchitecture and connections in rat see Table I; for human, see Nieuwenhuys et al (2008, p. 363). The origins of the term go back to *subiculum of Ammon's horn (Burdach, 1822)*. It was not recognized as such by 1840.

subiculothalamic tract (Swanson et al., 1987)

As described in adult mammal with histological methods for ***axons (Kölliker, 1896)***, a dorsal branch of the rostrodorsal ***hypothalamic postcommissural fornix (>1840)*** to mainly the ***anterior thalamic nuclei (>1840)*** and ***midline thalamic nuclei (>1840)***. For use by Swanson et al. based on connectional data mostly in rat see pp. 235–236. It was not known by 1840.

subiculum (>1840)

As described with cellular architecture and connections in mammal, the topologically and developmentally medial division of the ***subicular complex (Swanson & Cowan, 1977)*** lying between ***field CA1 (Lorente de Nó, 1934)*** medially and ***presubiculum (>1840)*** laterally; see Swanson et al. (1987), Nieuwenhuys et al. (2008, p. 372 and Fig. 12.5). ***Subiculum (>1840)*** was used, for example, by Brodmann (1909, p. 149 and Figs. 34, 35). It was not recognized as such by 1840.

sublentiform part of internal capsule (>1840)

As commonly described for macrodissected adult human, a ventral differentiation of the ***posterior limb of internal capsule (>1840)*** with a predominance of ***axons (Kölliker, 1896)*** associated with the ***posterior thalamic radiation (>1840)*** and continuing on in the ***cerebral cortex white matter (>1840)*** as the ***optic radiation (>1840)*** and ***auditory radiation (>1840)***; see Crosby et al. (1962, p. 394, Fig. 272, called *sublenticular part*), Nieuwenhuys et al. (2008, Fig. 5.8-*31*). It was probably first recognized by Reil; see ***[sublentiform part of internal capsule (>1840)] (Reil, 1809b)***.

EARLIER REFERENCES:

Illustrated and described, not named:

1. ***[sublentiform part of internal capsule (>1840)] (Reil, 1809b)***
Clearly illustrated but not distinguished or named for macrodissected adult human; see Mayo translation (1823, p. 65 and Tab. IX, part of groove between *K* and *t*).

sublingual nerve (Henle, 1871)

As described for macrodissected human, one or more branches of the ***lingual nerve (Vesalius, 1543a)*** innervating the sublingual gland and overlying mucous membrane; see *Terminologia Anatomica* (1998, p. 135), *Dorland's* (2003, p. 1242). For Henle's use in macrodissected adult human, see p. 390 and Figure 247-*s*. Todd (1836–1839, p. 371) mentioned a sublingual nerve, based on the work of Mayer, but no citation was provided for Mayer and its identify is unclear. It was perhaps first clearly delineated by Winslow; see ***[sublingual nerve (Henle, 1871)] (Winslow, 1733)***.

EARLIER REFERENCES:

Described, not named or illustrated:

1. ***[sublingual nerve (Henle, 1871)] (Winslow, 1733)***
Branch of *inferior maxillary nerve (Heister, 1717)* to sublingual gland described in macrodissected adult human; Section VI, p. 67.

Earlier synonyms:

1. *branchlets of lingual nerve in sublingual gland (Meckel, 1748)*
Two described and illustrated for macrodissected adult human, corresponding to ***sublingual nerve (Henle, 1871)***; in the original Latin, *ramuli nervi lingualis in glandulam sublingualem*, p. 96 note *a*, and Figure 1-*77*.
2. *sublingual fascicles of lingual surculus with chorda tympani (Bellingeri, 1818)*
Synonym for macrodissected adult human ***sublingual nerve (Henle, 1871)***, described as consisting of two fascicles; in the original Latin, *(duo) fasciculi sublinguales*, see Table I.

PARTLY CORRESPONDS:

1. *buccal branch of lingual nerve (Arnold, 1834)*
Probably branch of macrodissected adult human ***sublingual nerve (Henle, 1871)***; in the original Latin, *nervus lingualis, ramus buccalis*, p. 11.
2. *buccal branch of gustatory nerve (Arnold, 1834)*
Probably branch of macrodissected adult human ***sublingual nerve (Henle, 1871)***; in the original Latin, *nervus gustatorius, ramus buccalis*, p. 11.
3. *lingual nerve branch to oral mucous membrane (Arnold, 1834)*
Branch of macrodissected adult human ***sublingual nerve (Henle, 1871)***; in the original Latin, *ramus nervi lingualis ad membranam oris mucosam tendens*, Table VII:*V-44*.
4. *sublingual ganglion of Mayer (>1840)*
Todd (1836–1839, p. 371) noted, "Mayer [no citation provided] has discovered a minute posterior root of the sublingual nerve, with a ganglion on it, in some mammalia (ox, dog, and pig), and *in one instance in man*."

submandibular ganglion (>1840)

As described for macrodissected adult human, a ***terminal ganglion (Gaskell, 1886)*** lying on the dorsal (upper) surface of the hyoglossus muscle. It is attached to the ***lingual nerve (Vesalius, 1543a)*** by ***communicating branches of lingual nerve with submandibular ganglion (>1840)*** and also receives the ***sympathetic root of submandibular ganglion (>1840)***; see Durward (1951, p. 1028), Williams & Warwick (1980, Fig. 7.177), *Terminologia Anatomica* (1998, p. 142). It was discovered and described as the *maxillary ganglion (Meckel, 1748)*.

EARLIER REFERENCES:

Earlier synonyms:

1. *maxillary ganglion (Meckel, 1748)*
Synonym for macrodissected adult human ***submandibular ganglion (>1840)***; in the original Latin, *ganglion maxillare*, pp. 95, 131.
2. *small maxillary ganglion (Meckel, 1748)*
Synonym for *maxillary ganglion (Meckel, 1748)*; in the original Latin, *gangliolum maxillare*, p. 131.
3. *small maxillary ganglion of superior lingual nerve (Andersch, 1797)*
Synonym for macrodissected adult human *small maxillary ganglion (Meckel, 1748)*; in the original Latin, *gangliolum maxillare nervi lingualis superioris*, Vol. 2, p. 129.
4. *sub-maxillary ganglion (Burdin, 1803)*
Synonym for macrodissected adult human ***submandibular ganglion (>1840)***; see translation (1803, Vol. 1, p. 176). Quain & Wilson (1839, Pl. XXVII-*H*) spelled it *submaxillary ganglion*.
5. *maxillary ganglion of Meckel (Wutzer, 1817; Bock, 1817)*
Eponym for macrodissected adult human ***submandibular ganglion (>1840)***; in the original Latin, *ganglion maxillare Meckelii*, p. 85 for Wutzer and p. 52 for Bock.
6. *glottic ganglion (Arnold, 1834)*
Synonym for macrodissected adult human ***submandibular ganglion (>1840)***; in the original Latin, *ganglion glotticum*, p. 10.
7. *lingual ganglion (Arnold, 1834)*
Synonym for macrodissected adult human ***submandibular ganglion (>1840)***, in the original Latin, *ganglion linguale*, p. 10.
8. *sublingual ganglion (>1840)*
Synonym for macrodissected adult human ***submandibular ganglion (>1840)***; see Henle (1871, p. 391), where there is an excellent review.

PARTLY CORRESPONDS:

1. *branches of maxillary ganglion to Wharton's duct (Arnold, 1834)*
Macrodissected adult human branches of ***submandibular ganglion (>1840)*** to submandibular duct;

in the original Latin, *rami ganglion maxillare ductui Whartoniano destinati*, Table VII:*V-42*.

2. *Langley's ganglion (>1840)*
According to Crosby et al. (1962, p. 532), "The preganglionic fibers for the submandibular gland end along the main ducts of the gland on scattered postganglionic neurons that collectively are known as Langley's ganglion". See Langley (1878).

suboccipital nerve (Winslow, 1733)

As described for macrodissected adult human, the first pair of ***cervical nerves (Galen, c173)***; "There may be no dorsal root and no spinal ganglion on either one or both of the first cervical nerves" (Crosby et al., 1962, p. 58). According to Bartholin (1668, p. 328), "*Joh. Leonicenus* of *Padua*, a dextrous Anatomist in taking out of the Nerves, denied that there was any such pare as this, because he could neither see it, nor can it come out of the first Vertebra having no hole..." For Winslow's use in macrodissected adult human, see Section VI, p. 75, where he described a ***ganglion (Galen, c173)*** associated with the ***nerve (Herophilus, c335–c280 BC)***—but a ***ventral root (>1840)*** and no ***dorsal root (Spurzheim, 1826)***. A complete history of earlier literature on the ***suboccipital nerve (Winslow, 1733)***, along with a detailed description for macrodissected adult human, was provided by Asch (1750); also see Haller (1762, pp. 240–242) and Bang (1770, Fig. I-*I*), where the ***spinal nerve dorsal branch (Meckel, 1817)*** and ***spinal nerve ventral branch (>1840)*** and their various muscular branches and ***communicating branches (Winslow, 1733)*** with the ***cervical plexus (Molinetti, 1675)*** are brilliantly illustrated and described. It was first clearly described by Galen; see ***[suboccipital nerve (Winslow, 1733)] (Galen, c173)***.

TRANSLATIONS:

1. *nervus sub-occipitalis (Winslow, 1733)*
Latin form of ***suboccipital nerve (Winslow, 1733)***; Section VI, p. 60 where the plural, *nervi sub-occipitales*, is given.

EARLIER REFERENCES:

Described, not named or illustrated:

1. ***[suboccipital nerve (Winslow, 1733)] (Galen, c173)***
Clearly described in macrodissected adult beef, pig, lion, other large mammals, including macaque, but not human; see May translation (1968, pp. 597, 701) and Duckworth translation (1962, p. 229). Vesalius (1543a) described and crudely illustrated only dorsally directed muscular branches for macrodissected adult human; see Richardson & Carman translation (2002, p. 224).

Earlier synonyms:

1. *occipital nerve (Bidloo, 1685)*
Synonym for macrodissected adult human ***suboccipital nerve (Winslow, 1733)***; Table 9-*k*. Also see Huber (1741, p. 30).
2. *motor cervical nerve (Hoffmann, 1703)*
Synonym for macrodissected adult human ***suboccipital nerve (Winslow, 1733)***; in the original Latin, *nervus cervicis motorium*, p. 262.
3. *motor occipital nerve (Hoffmann, 1703)*
Synonym for macrodissected adult human ***suboccipital nerve (Winslow, 1733)***; in the original Latin, *nervus cervicis motorium*, p. 262.

LATER SYNONYMS:

1. *tenth pair of nerves of medulla oblongata (Winslow, 1733)*
Winslow counted ***suboccipital nerves (Winslow, 1733)*** as last of ten *pairs of nerves of medulla oblongata (Winslow, 1733)*; Section X, p. 48, also see *tenth pair of nerves arising within skull (Willis, 1664)*.
2. *infraoccipital nerve (Schaarschmidt, 1750)*
Synonym for macrodissected adult human ***suboccipital nerve (Winslow, 1733)***; in the original Latin, *nervis infraoccipitalibus*, p. 46. Haas (1781, p. 91) claimed it was Winslow's term for *nervus sub-occipitalis (Winslow, 1733)*.
3. *tenth cerebral pair of Willis (Bang, 1770)*
Eponym for macrodissected adult human ***suboccipital nerves (Winslow, 1733)***; in the original Latin, *decimum par Willisii cerebrale*, Figure I-*I* (see 1791 reprint). Compare with *tenth pair of nerves arising within skull (Willis, 1664)*.
4. *infraorbital nerve (Bang, 1770)*
Synonym for macrodissected adult human ***suboccipital nerve (Winslow, 1733)***; in the original Latin, *nervus infraorbitalis*, Figure I-*I* (see 1791 reprint).
5. *infraspinal nerve (Bang, 1770)*
Synonym for macrodissected adult human ***suboccipital nerve (Winslow, 1733)***; in the original Latin, *nervus infraspinalis*, Figure I-*I* (see 1791 reprint).
6. *seventeenth pair of nerves (Malacarne, 1791)*
Synonym for macrodissected adult human ***suboccipital nerves (Winslow, 1733)*** counted as last of 17 *cerebral nerves (Malacarne, 1791)*; pp. 193–195, 340–341.
7. *tenth pair of head (Fyfe, 1800)*
Synonym for macrodissected adult human ***suboccipital nerves (Winslow, 1733)***; Vol. 2, p. 305.
8. *first pair of neck (Fyfe, 1800)*
Synonym for macrodissected adult human ***suboccipital nerves (Winslow, 1733)***; Vol. 2, p. 305.
9. *tenth pair of scull (Bell, 1803b)*
Synonym for macrodissected adult human ***suboccipital nerves (Winslow, 1733)***; p. 163.

PARTLY CORRESPONDS:

1. *roots of suboccipital nerve (Malacarne, 1791)*
Macrodissected adult human ***dorsal rootlets (>1840)*** of ***suboccipital nerve (Winslow, 1733)***; pp. 227, 340–341.
2. *anterior trunk of sub-occipital nerve (Swan, 1830)*
Macrodissected adult human ***spinal nerve ventral branch (>1840)*** of ***suboccipital nerve (Winslow, 1733)***; Plate XXIII, Figure 2-*1*.
3. *posterior trunk of sub-occipital nerve (Swan, 1830)*
Macrodissected adult human ***spinal nerve dorsal branch (Meckel, 1817)*** of ***suboccipital nerve (Winslow, 1733)***; Plate XXIII, Figure 2-*2*.
4. *suboccipital nerve (>1840)*
Macrodissected adult human ***spinal nerve dorsal branch (Meckel, 1817)*** of ***suboccipital nerve (Winslow, 1733)***; see

Williams & Warwick (1980, p. 1089), *Dorland's* (2003, pp. 1236, 1242).

subparietal sulcus (>1840)

As described for macrodissected adult human, a groove between ***precuneus (Burdach, 1822)*** dorsally and ***cingulate region (Brodmann, 1909)*** ventrally; see Williams & Warwick (1980, Fig. 7.114A, unlabeled), *Terminologia Anatomica* (1998, p. 126), *Dorland's* (2003, p. 1789). It was first delineated clearly by Vicq d'Azyr; see ***[subparietal sulcus (>1840)] (Vicq d'Azyr, 1786)***.

EARLIER REFERENCES:

Illustrated, not named or described:

1. ***[subparietal sulcus (>1840)] (Vicq d'Azyr, 1786)***
   Illustrated clearly for macrodissected adult human; Table III.

subsartorial plexus (>1840)

As described for macrodissected adult human, it receives contributions from the ***anterior branch of obturator nerve (Haase, 1781; Martin, 1781)***, ***saphenous nerve (Haase, 1781)***, and ***medial cutaneous nerve of thigh (>1840)*** and supplies branches to skin of the medial side of the thigh; see Williams & Warwick (1980, p. 1108). It was perhaps first clearly identified by Meckel; see ***[subsartorial plexus (>1840)] (Meckel, 1817)***.

EARLIER REFERENCES:

Described, not named or illustrated:

1. ***[subsartorial plexus (>1840)] (Meckel, 1817)***
   Meckel partly described without naming for macrodissected adult human, indicating ***communicating branches (Winslow, 1733)*** between ***anterior branch of obturator nerve (Haase, 1781; Martin, 1781)*** and ***saphenous nerve (Haase, 1781)***; see translation (1832, Vol. 3, p. 16).

substantia innominata (Meynert, 1872)

As described for macrodissected adult human, and with cellular architecture and connections for all mammals, a component of the ***pallidum (Swanson, 2000a)*** lying ventral to the ***globus pallidus (Burdach, 1822)***, dorsolateral to the ***medial septal complex (Swanson et al., 1987)***, and lateral to the ***bed nuclei of terminal stria (Gurdjian, 1925)***; the major ***white matter tract (Bell & Bell, 1826)*** associated with it is the ***peduncular loop (Gratiolet, 1857)***. For Meynert's use in unstained histological sections of macrodissected adult human, see Figure 268; for Schwalbe's use in histological sections of adult human, see pp. 748–749. Nauta & Haymaker (1969, pp. 153–156) gave a good modern perspective. It was first illustrated by Steno; see ***[substantia innominata (Meynert, 1872)] (Steno, 1669)***.

EARLIER REFERENCES:

Illustrated, not named or described:

1. ***[substantia innominata (Meynert, 1872)] (Steno, 1669)***
   General location illustrated rather clearly in transverse section of macrodissected adult human; Plate IV, especially on right.

Earlier synonyms:

1. *medulla incognita (Reil, 1809b)*
   Roughly synonymous with macrodissected adult human ***substantia innominata (Meynert, 1872)***; p. 199. Also see Mayo translation (1823, pp. 51, 59) including his Latin translation of Reil's German, *ungennante Marksubstanz*, and Burdach (1822, p. 388). Reil noted that *medulla incognita (Reil, 1809b)* is unusual in that it appears to be neither *gray substance (Vesalius, 1543a)* nor *white substance (Vesalius, 1543a)*; 1812c, see Mayo translation (1823, p. 124).
2. *unnamed medullary substance (Reil, 1809b)*
   English form of Reil's term (in the original German, *ungennante Marksubstanz*) for roughly macrodissected adult human ***substantia innominata (Meynert, 1872)***; see *medulla incognita (Reil, 1809b)*.

LATER SYNONYMS:

1. *substantia innominata of Reil (Meynert, 1872)*
   Eponym for ***substantia innominata (Meynert, 1872)***; see translation (1872, pp. 686, 689).

substantia nigra (Soemmerring, 1791)

As described for macrodissected adult human, a ***gray matter region (Swanson & Bota, 2010)*** in the ventrolateral ***tegmentum (Swanson, 2000b)*** of the ***midbrain (Baer, 1837)***. Based on cellular architecture and connections it has two basic divisions, ***compact part of substantia nigra (>1840)*** characterized in adult human by darkly pigmented ***neurons (Waldeyer, 1891)*** that in all mammals use dopamine as a neurotransmitter, and ***reticular part of substantia nigra (>1840)*** characterized in adult human by unpigmented ***neurons (Waldeyer, 1891)*** that in all mammals use GABA as a neurotransmitter; see Nieuwenhuys et al. (2008, pp. 438–439). Soemmerring (1791) specifically referred to the *blackish substance (Vicq d'Azyr, 1784)*, in German as *eine Vierte Schwarze Substance* (p. 27) or *Schwarzer Substance* (p. 37)—in English, *black substance*, and in Latin, *substantia nigra*. It was perhaps first distinguished clearly as the *brown substance (Vicq d'Azyr, 1784)*, *blackish substance (Vicq d'Azyr, 1784)*, or *locus niger crurum cerebri (Vicq d'Azyr, 1784)*.

EARLIER REFERENCES:

Earlier synonyms:

1. *brown substance (Vicq d'Azyr, 1784)*
   Synonym for *locus niger crurum cerebri (Vicq d'Azyr, 1784)*; in the original French, *substance brune*, p. 556. Vicq d'Azyr (p. 556) noted that Santorini (1775, p. 14) first mentioned irregular brown substance associated with *cerebral peduncles (Vicq d'Azyr, 1784)*.
2. *blackish substance (Vicq d'Azyr, 1784)*
   Synonym for *locus niger crurum cerebri (Vicq d'Azyr, 1784)*; in the original French, *substance noirâtre*, p. 556.
3. *brown region (Vicq d'Azyr, 1784)*
   Synonym for *locus niger crurum cerebri (Vicq d'Azyr, 1786)*; in the original French, *tache brune*; p. 556, also see Vicq d'Azyr (1786, Pl. XXXI, Fig. II-*a*).

4. *locus niger crurum cerebri (Vicq d'Azyr, 1784)*
   Synonym for macrodissected adult human ***substantia nigra (Soemmerring, 1791)***. For Vicq d'Azyr it was component of *cerebral peduncle (Vicq d'Azyr, 1784)*; p. 556, and Vicq d'Azyr (1786, Pl. XV-*16*). See Meyer (1971, p. 25).
5. *black region (Vicq d'Azyr, 1784)*
   Synonym for *locus niger crurum cerebri (Vicq d'Azyr, 1786)*; in the original French, *tache noire*, p. 556, also see Vicq d'Azyr (1786, Pl. XV-*16*).
6. *blackish body (Vicq d'Azyr, 1784)*
   Synonym for *locus niger crurum cerebri (Vicq d'Azyr, 1786)*; in the original French, *corps noirâtre*, p. 556, and Vicq d'Azyr (1786, Pl. XXI-*41*).
7. *blackish segment (Vicq d'Azyr, 1786)*
   Synonym for *locus niger crurum cerebri (Vicq d'Azyr, 1786)*; in the original French, *segment noirâtre*, Plate XXI-*41*.

LATER SYNONYMS:

1. *stratum nigrum (Burdach, 1822)*
   Synonym for macrodissected adult human ***substantia nigra (Soemmerring, 1791)***; p. 101, see Henle (1871, p. 89).
2. *black substance in peduncles of brain (Spurzheim, 1826)*
   Synonym for macrodissected adult human ***substantia nigra (Soemmerring, 1791)***; p. 232-*30*.
3. *corpus nigrum (Bell & Bell, 1829)*
   Latin synonym for ***substantia nigra (Soemmerring, 1791)***; Vol. 2, p. 383.
4. *substantia nigra of Soemmerring (Kölliker, 1896)*
   Eponym for ***substantia nigra (Soemmerring, 1791)***, although Soemmerring's description was not until 1791, where he acknowledged Vicq d'Azyr's discovery; see Schiller (1967, p. 531).

sulcus of corpus callosum (>1840)

As described for macrodissected adult human, the tiny longitudinal groove separating ***indusium griseum (Valentin, 1841)*** ventrally from ***cingulate region (Brodmann, 1909)*** dorsally, and extending caudally and ventrally as the ***hippocampal sulcus (Gratiolet, 1854)***; see Carpenter (1976, p. 27, referred to as *callosal sulcus*), *Terminologia Anatomica* (1998, p. 126), Nieuwenhuys et al. (2008, Figs. 5.4–11). It was first noted by Vesalius; see ***[sulcus of corpus callosum (>1840)] (Vesalius, 1543a)***.

EARLIER REFERENCES:

Described, not named or illustrated:

1. ***[sulcus of corpus callosum (>1840)] (Vesalius, 1543a)***
   Briefly mentioned for macrodissected adult human; see Singer translation (1952, pp. 32, 65 and Fig. 3-*M*).

Illustrated, not named or described:

1. ***[sulcus of corpus callosum (>1840)] (Vicq d'Azyr, 1786)***
   Clearly illustrated for macrodissected adult human; see Tables VI, IX-XI.

Earlier synonyms:

1. *ventricle of corpus callosum (Cruveilhier, 1836)*
   Cruveilhier noted it is inaccurate for macrodissected adult human and refers simply to ***sulcus of corpus callosum (>1840)***; in the original French, *ventricule du corps calleux*, p. 672.
2. *callosal sulcus (>1840)*
   Synonym for macrodissected adult human ***sulcus of corpus callosum (>1840)***; see Carpenter (1976, p. 27), Williams & Warwick (1980, p. 998).

superficial branch of lateral plantar nerve (>1840)

As described for macrodissected adult human, one of two terminal branches of the ***lateral plantar nerve (>1840)***, along with the ***deep branch of lateral plantar nerve (>1840)***. The superficial branch in turn divides into two ***common plantar digital nerves of lateral plantar nerve (>1840)***. Before dividing, the trunk supplies collateral branches to the flexor digitorum accessorius (quadratus plantae) and abductor digiti minimi of foot muscles; see Durward (1951, p. 1112 and Figs. 951, 952), *Terminologia Anatomica* (1998, p. 141). It was probably first clearly delineated by Eustachi; see ***[superficial branch of lateral plantar nerve (>1840)] (Eustachi, 1552)***.

EARLIER REFERENCES:

Illustrated, not named or described:

1. ***[superficial branch of lateral plantar nerve (>1840)] (Eustachi, 1552)***
   Course illustrated for macrodissected adult human; see Albinus edition (1761, Tab. 20).

Illustrated and described, not named:

1. ***[superficial branch of lateral plantar nerve (>1840)] (Vieussens, 1684)***
   Accurately described and illustrated for macrodissected adult human; see Table 30-*S*.

Earlier synonyms:

1. *superficial branch of external plantar branch of tibial nerve (Martin, 1781)*
   Synonym for macrodissected adult human ***superficial branch of lateral plantar nerve (>1840)***; in the original Latin, *nervus tibialis ramus exterior ramus superficialis*, p. 244.
2. *digital branch of external plantar branch of tibial nerve (Martin, 1781)*
   Synonym for macrodissected adult human ***superficial branch of lateral plantar nerve (>1840)***; in the original Latin, *nervus tibialis ramus exterior ramus digitalis*, p. 244.
3. *cutaneous branch of external plantar nerve (Günther, 1786)*
   Synonym for macrodissected adult human ***superficial branch of lateral plantar nerve (>1840)***; in the original Latin, *r. cutaneus*, p. 88.
4. *superficial branch of external plantar nerve (Günther, 1786)*
   Synonym for macrodissected adult human ***superficial branch of lateral plantar nerve (>1840)***; in the original Latin, *r. superficiales*, p. 88.
5. *external branch of external plantar nerve (Jördens, 1788)*
   Synonym for macrodissected adult human ***superficial branch of lateral plantar nerve (>1840)***; in the

original Latin, *ramus externus nervi plantaris externi*, p. 12 and Table III-*218*.

6. *middle branch of external plantar nerve (Fischer, 1791)* Synonym for macrodissected adult human ***superficial branch of lateral plantar nerve (>1840)***; in the original Latin, *ramus medius nervus plantaris externus*, p. 38.
7. *superficial digital branch of external plantar nerve (Soemmerring, 1798)* Synonym for macrodissected adult human ***superficial branch of lateral plantar nerve (>1840)***; in the original Latin, *nervus plantaris externus...ramum superficialem digitalem*, p. 331; also see Soemmerring (1791, p. 310).
8. *superficial branch of exterior branch of tibial nerve (Burdin, 1803)* Synonym for macrodissected adult human ***superficial branch of lateral plantar nerve (>1840)***; see translation (1803, Vol. 1, pp. 207–208).
9. *superficial terminal branch of external plantar nerve (Cruveilhier, 1836)* Synonym for macrodissected adult human ***superficial branch of lateral plantar nerve (>1840)***; in the original French, *branche terminale superficielle*, p. 875.

PARTLY CORRESPONDS:

1. *dorsal twig of foot of superficial branch of external plantar nerve (Jördens, 1788)* Macrodissected adult human branch of ***superficial branch of lateral plantar nerve (>1840)*** stretching along dorsal and lateral parts of fifth (little) toe; in the original Latin, *ramulus dorsalis pedis rami superficialis nervi plantaris externi*, p. 12 and Table III-*221*.
2. *cutaneous twig of middle branch of external plantar nerve (Fischer, 1791)* Synonym for macrodissected adult human *dorsal twig of foot of superficial branch of external plantar nerve (Jördens, 1788)*; in the original Latin, *ramulus cutaneus*, p. 38.

superficial branch of radial nerve (Martin, 1781)

As described for macrodissected adult human, a terminal branch of the ***radial nerve (Du Verney, 1697)*** eventually dividing into five, or less frequently four, ***dorsal digital nerves of radial nerve (>1840)***; see Williams & Warwick (1980, p. 1101). For Martin's use in macrodissected adult human, see p. 220. It was first clearly delineated as the *higher branch of fourth nerve entering arm (Vesalius, 1543a)*.

TRANSLATIONS:

1. *nervus radialis ramus superficialis (Martin, 1781)* Original Latin form of ***superficial branch of radial nerve (Martin, 1781)***; p. 220.

EARLIER REFERENCES:

Earlier synonyms:

1. *higher branch of fourth nerve entering arm (Vesalius, 1543a)* Synonym for ***superficial branch of radial nerve (Martin, 1781)*** in macrodissected adult human; see Richardson & Carman translation (2002, p. 242).
2. *external branch of radial nerve (Haase, 1781)* Synonym for macrodissected adult human ***superficial branch of radial nerve (Martin, 1781)***; in the original Latin, *nervus radialis ramus externus*, pp. 101–102.

LATER SYNONYMS:

1. *anterior branch of radial nerve (Caldani, 1813, 1814)* Synonym for macrodissected adult human ***superficial branch of radial nerve (Martin, 1781)***; in the original Latin, *ramus anterior nervi radialis*, Table CCLIX, Figure 2-39.
2. *superficial nerve of muscular spiral nerve (Bell & Bell, 1816)* Synonym for macrodissected adult human ***superficial branch of radial nerve (Martin, 1781)***; in the original Latin, *nervus superficialis*, Vol. 2, p. 538.
3. *radial branch of muscular spiral nerve (Bell & Bell, 1816)* Synonym for macrodissected adult human ***superficial branch of radial nerve (Martin, 1781)***; Vol. 2, p. 539.
4. *great superficial division of muscular spiral nerve (Bell & Bell, 1816)* Synonym for macrodissected adult human ***superficial branch of radial nerve (Martin, 1781)***; Vol. 2, p. 539.
5. *cutaneous branch of radial nerve (Meckel, 1817)* Synonym for macrodissected adult human ***superficial branch of radial nerve (Martin, 1781)***; see translation (1832, Vol. 3, pp. 25–26).
6. *superficial dorsal branch of radial nerve (Meckel, 1817)* Synonym for macrodissected adult human ***superficial branch of radial nerve (Martin, 1781)***; in the original Latin, *nervus radialis ramus superficialis dorsalis*, see translation (1832, Vol. 3, p. 25).
7. *dorsal radial nerve (Bock, 1824)* Synonym for macrodissected adult human ***superficial branch of radial nerve (Martin, 1781)***; in the original Latin, *nervi radialis dorsalis*, Table XV, Figure 13-3.
8. *dorsal branch of radial nerve (Bock, 1827)* Synonym for *dorsal radial nerve (Bock, 1824)*; in the original Latin, *ramus dorsalis nervi radialis*, Table I, Figure 2-42; Table II-57.
9. *radial branch of spinal nerve (Swan, 1830)* Synonym for macrodissected adult human ***superficial branch of radial nerve (Martin, 1781)***; Plate XXII-4.
10. *radial nerve (Swan, 1830)* Synonym for *radial branch of spinal nerve (Swan, 1830)*; Plate XXII-5.
11. *anterior branch of musculo-spiral nerve (Quain, 1832)* Synonym for macrodissected adult human ***superficial branch of radial nerve (Martin, 1781)***; p. 689.
12. *external dorsal branch of hand of radial nerve (Cruveilhier, 1836)* Synonym for macrodissected adult human ***superficial branch of radial nerve (Martin, 1781)***; in the original French, *branche dorsale externe de la main*, p. 818.

PARTLY CORRESPONDS:

1. *volar superficial branch of radial nerve (Günther, 1786)* Extends to volar (palmar) aspect of macrodissected adult human hand and communicates with branches of

ulnar nerve (Cheselden, 1726) and ***median nerve (Du Verney, 1697)***; in the original Latin, *r. superficialem volarem*, p. 79.

2. *dorsal superficial branch of radial nerve (Günther, 1786)*
Main trunk of macrodissected adult human ***superficial branch of radial nerve (Martin, 1781)***; in the original Latin, *r. superficialem dorsalem*, p. 79.
3. *volar branch of radial nerve (Mayer, 1794)*
Most lateral of two major branches of macrodissected adult human ***superficial branch of radial nerve (Martin, 1781)***; in the original Latin, *ramus volaris nervi radialis*; Part 5, Table VI-*11* (p. 35).
4. *volar branch of superficial branch of radial nerve (Soemmerring, 1798)*
Synonym for macrodissected adult human *volar superficial branch of radial nerve (Günther, 1786)*; p. 304.
5. *anterior branch of radial nerve (Loder, 1803)*
Synonym for macrodissected adult human *volar superficial branch of radial nerve (Günther, 1786)*; in the original Latin, *nervi radialis ramus anterior*, Table CLXXVIII, Figure 2-*51*.
6. *dorsal branch of radial nerve (Loder, 1803)*
Synonym for macrodissected adult human *dorsal superficial branch of radial nerve (Günther, 1786)*; in the original Latin, *nervi radialis ramus dorsalis*, Table CLXXVIII, Figure 2-*56*.
7. *posterior branch of radial nerve (Loder, 1803)*
Synonym for *dorsal branch of radial nerve (Loder, 1803)*; in the original Latin, *nervi radialis ramus posterior*, Table CLXXVIII, Figure 2-*56*.
8. *anterior branch of dorsal branch of radial nerve (Loder, 1803)*
Main branch of macrodissected adult human *dorsal branch of radial nerve (Loder, 1803)*; in the original Latin, *ramus anterior rami dorsalis nervi radialis*, Table CLXXVIII, Figure 2-*62*.
9. *divided branch of dorsal branch of radial nerve (Loder, 1803)*
Main branch of macrodissected adult human *dorsal branch of radial nerve (Loder, 1803)*; in the original Latin, *ramus multifidus rami dorsalis nervi radialis*, Table CLXXVIII, Figure 2-*62*.
10. *internal branches of dorsal radial nerve (Bock, 1824)*
Two medial branches of macrodissected adult human ***superficial branch of radial nerve (Martin, 1781)***; in the original Latin, *Ram. internus Nervi radialis dorsalis*, Table XV, Figure 13-*5,8*.
11. *dorsal branch of superficial branch of radial nerve (Langenbeck, 1826–1830)*
Synonym for macrodissected adult human *internal branches of dorsal radial nerve (Bock, 1824)*; in the original Latin, *ramus dorsalis rami superficialis nervi radialis*; Fascicle III, Table III, Figure 1-*18*.
12. *posterior branch of dorsal branch of radial nerve (Bock, 1827)*
Synonym for macrodissected adult human *posterior branch of radial nerve (Loder, 1803)*; in the original Latin, *ram. posterior*, Table V, Figure 3-*9*.
13. *external branch of dorsal branch of radial nerve (Bock, 1827)*
Synonym for *posterior branch of dorsal branch of radial nerve (Bock, 1827)*; in the original Latin, *ram. externus*, Table V, Figure 3-*9*.
14. *articular branch of anterior branch of dorsal branch of radial nerve (Bock, 1827)*
Macrodissected adult human branch of *anterior branch of dorsal branch of radial nerve (Loder, 1803)* to wrist; in the original Latin, *ram. articularis*, Table V, Figure 4-*7*.
15. *anterior branch of radial nerve (Cloquet, 1828)*
Synonym for macrodissected adult human *anterior branch of dorsal branch of radial nerve (Cloquet, 1828)*; in the original French, *rameau antérieur du nerf radial*, Plate CLXVII, Figure 2-*30*.
16. *posterior branch of radial nerve (Cloquet, 1828)*
Synonym for *posterior branch of dorsal branch of radial nerve (Cloquet, 1828)*; in the original French, *rameau postérieur du nerf radial*, Plate CLXVII, Figure 2-*33*.
17. *anterior branch of dorsal branch of radial nerve (Cloquet, 1828)*
One of two branches of macrodissected adult human *dorsal branch of radial nerve (Bock, 1827)* extending to supply skin on dorsal surface of index finger and thumb; in the original French, *rameau antérieur de la branche dorsale du nerf radial*, Plate CLXVII, Figure 2-*35*.
18. *posterior branch of dorsal branch of radial nerve (Cloquet, 1828)*
One of two branches of macrodissected adult human *dorsal branch of radial nerve (Bock, 1827)* extending to supply skin on dorsal surface of hand; in the original French, *rameau postérieur de la branche dorsale du nerf radial*, Plate CLXVII, Figure 2-*37*.
19. *dorsal branch of radial nerve (Cloquet, 1828)*
Synonym for *anterior branch of dorsal branch of radial nerve (Cloquet, 1828)*; in the original French, *rameau dorsal du nerf radial*, Plate CLXVIII, Figure 1-*14*.
20. *palmar branch of radial nerve (Cloquet, 1828)*
Synonym for *posterior branch of dorsal branch of radial nerve (Cloquet, 1828)*; in the original French, *rameau palmaire du nerf radial*, Plate CLXVIII, Figure 1-*15*.
21. *radial volar nerve (Knox, 1832)*
Synonym for macrodissected adult human *volar branch of radial nerve (Mayer, 1794)*; Plate 20, Figure 2.
22. *branch of first metacarpal space of radial nerve (Quain & Wilson, 1839)*
Macrodissected adult human lateral branch of ***superficial branch of radial nerve (Martin, 1781)*** generating ***dorsal digital nerves of radial nerve (>1840)*** to medial side of thumb and lateral side of index finger; Plate XIX, Figure 1-*i*.
23. *branch of second metacarpal space of radial nerve (Quain & Wilson, 1839)*
Macrodissected adult human medial branch of ***superficial branch of radial nerve (Martin, 1781)*** generating ***dorsal digital nerves of radial nerve (>1840)*** to medial side of index finger and lateral side of middle finger; Plate XIX, Figure 1-*k*.

superficial branch of ulnar nerve (Fyfe, 1800)

As described for macrodissected adult human, a terminal branch supplying the palmaris brevis muscle and skin on the medial side of the hand and then dividing into ***common palmar digital nerves of ulnar nerve (>1840)***; see Hamilton (1976, Fig. 820), Williams & Warwick (1980, p. 1100). For Fyfe's use in macrodissected adult human, see Vol. 2, p. 313. It was known to Galen; see ***[superficial branch of ulnar nerve (Fyfe, 1800)] (Galen, c177)***.

EARLIER REFERENCES:

Described, not named or illustrated:

1. ***[superficial branch of ulnar nerve (Fyfe, 1800)] (Galen, c177)***
   Briefly described for macrodissected adult macaque but not human; see Singer translation (1999, p. 74).

Illustrated, not named or described:

1. ***[superficial branch of ulnar nerve (Fyfe, 1800)] (Eustachi, 1552)***
   Clearly illustrated for macrodissected adult human; see Albinus edition (1761, Tab. 19, just proximal to 52).

Earlier synonyms:

1. *external branch of cubital nerve (Haase, 1781)*
   Synonym for macrodissected adult human ***superficial branch of ulnar nerve (Fyfe, 1800)***; in the original Latin, *nervus cubitalis ramus externus*, pp. 99–100.
2. *ramus superficialis volaris ramus volaris nervus cubitalis (Martin, 1781)*
   Latin form of macrodissected adult human *superficial branch of palmar branch of ulnar nerve (Meckel, 1817)*; p. 216. Frotscher (1788, p. 92) referred to *ramum sublimem*.
3. *volar superficial branch of ulnar nerve (Günther, 1786)*
   Synonym for macrodissected adult human ***superficial branch of ulnar nerve (Fyfe, 1800)***; in the original Latin, *r. superficialem volarem*, p. 75.

LATER SYNONYMS:

1. *superficial palmar nerve (Fyfe, 1800)*
   Synonym for macrodissected adult human ***superficial branch of ulnar nerve (Fyfe, 1800)***; Vol. 2, p. 313.
2. *volar branch of cubital nerve trunk (Loder, 1803)*
   Synonym for macrodissected adult human ***superficial branch of ulnar nerve (Fyfe, 1800)***; in the original Latin, *ramus volaris*, Table CLXXX, Figure 1-*93*.
3. *major branch of cubital nerve trunk (Loder, 1803)*
   Synonym for macrodissected adult human ***superficial branch of ulnar nerve (Fyfe, 1800)***; in the original Latin, *ramus major*, Table CLXXX, Figure 1-*93*.
4. *superficial branch of cubital nerve (Cloquet, 1816)*
   Synonym for macrodissected adult human ***superficial branch of ulnar nerve (Fyfe, 1800)***; p. 651.
5. *superficial branch of palmar branch of ulnar nerve (Meckel, 1817)*
   Synonym for macrodissected adult human ***superficial branch of ulnar nerve (Fyfe, 1800)***; see translation (1832, Vol. 3, p. 28) and *palmar branch of ulnar nerve (Meckel, 1817)*.
6. *cutaneous branch of palmar branch of ulnar nerve (Meckel, 1817)*
   Synonym for macrodissected adult human ***superficial branch of ulnar nerve (Fyfe, 1800)***; see translation (1832, Vol. 3, p. 28) and *palmar branch of ulnar nerve (Meckel, 1817)*.
7. *volar branch of ulnar nerve (Bock, 1827)*
   Synonym for macrodissected adult human ***superficial branch of ulnar nerve (Fyfe, 1800)***; in the original Latin, *Ram. volaris ulnaris*, Table I, Figure 2-*35*. Langenbeck (1826–1830; Fasc. III, Tab. XIV-*11*) used same term for macrodissected adult human but Fascicle III was published in 1830.
8. *palmar branch of cubital nerve (Cloquet, 1828)*
   Synonym for macrodissected adult human ***superficial branch of ulnar nerve (Fyfe, 1800)***; in the original French, *branche palmaire du nerf cubital*, Plate CLXIX, Figure 1-*69*.
9. *superficial terminal branch of cubital nerve (Cruveilhier, 1836)*
   Synonym for macrodissected adult human ***superficial branch of ulnar nerve (Fyfe, 1800)***; in the original French, *branche terminale superficielle*, p. 812.
10. *cubital nerve branch of palmar collateral nerves of fingers (Cruveilhier, 1836)*
    Synonym for *superficial terminal branch of cubital nerve (Cruveilhier, 1836)*; in the original French, *branche des nerfs collatéraux palmaires des doigts*, p. 812.
11. *cutaneous palmar branch of cubital nerve (Cruveilhier, 1836)*
    Synonym for *superficial terminal branch of cubital nerve (Cruveilhier, 1836)*; in the original French, *branche palmaire cutanée*, p. 814.
12. *superficial palmar branch of ulnar nerve (Quain & Wilson, 1839)*
    Synonym for macrodissected adult human ***superficial branch of ulnar nerve (Fyfe, 1800)***; Plate XVIII, Figure 2-*q*.

PARTLY CORRESPONDS:

1. *lesser volar branch of cubital nerve (Loder, 1803)*
   Smaller of two branches forming macrodissected adult human ***superficial branch of ulnar nerve (Fyfe, 1800)***; in the original Latin, *ramus volaris minor nervi cubitalis*, Table CLXXIX, Figure 2-*191*.
2. *greater volar branch of cubital nerve (Loder, 1803)*
   Larger of two branches forming macrodissected adult human ***superficial branch of ulnar nerve (Fyfe, 1800)***; in the original Latin, *ramus volaris major nervi cubitalis*, Table CLXXIX, Figure 2-*193*.
3. *deep branch of volar branch of ulnar nerve (Langenbeck, 1826–1830)*
   Macrodissected adult human muscular branch of ***superficial branch of ulnar nerve (Fyfe, 1800)***; in the original Latin, *ramus profundus rami volaris nervi ulnaris*, Fascicle III, Table XIV-*14*.
4. *twigs of deep branch of volar branch of ulnar nerve to adductor pollicis muscle (Langenbeck, 1826–1830)*

Macrodissected adult human small branches of *deep branch of volar branch of ulnar nerve (Langenbeck, 1826–1830)* to adductor pollicis muscle; in the original Latin, *surculi ad musculum adductorem pollicis*, Fascicle III, Table XIV-*15*.

5. *twigs of deep branch of volar branch of ulnar nerve to interosseous muscles (Langenbeck, 1826–1830)*
 Macrodissected adult human small branches of *deep branch of volar branch of ulnar nerve (Langenbeck, 1826–1830)* to palmar interossei muscles; in the original Latin, *surculi ad musculos interosseos*, Fascicle III, Table XIV-*16*.
6. *cutaneous branches of volar superficial nerve of ulnar nerve (Bock, 1827)*
 Macrodissected adult human branches of ***superficial branch of ulnar nerve (Fyfe, 1800)*** to skin on medial side of hand; in the original Latin, *rami cutanei nervi superficialis volaris ulnaris*, Table V, Figure 4-*21*.

superficial fibular nerve (Fyfe, 1800)

As described for macrodissected adult human, a terminal branch of the ***common fibular nerve (>1840)*** in turn generating ***muscular branches of superficial fibular nerve (>1840)***, the ***medial dorsal cutaneous nerve (>1840)***, and the ***intermediate dorsal cutaneous nerve (1840)***; see Durward (1951, p. 1108 and Figs. 948, 949; referred to as *musculo-cutaneous nerve*). For Fyfe's use in macrodissected adult human, see Vol. 2, p. 331. It was known to Galen; see ***[superficial fibular nerve (Fyfe, 1800)] (Galen, c173)***.

EARLIER REFERENCES:

Described, not named or illustrated:

1. *[superficial fibular nerve (Fyfe, 1800)] (Galen, c173)*
 Alluded to for macrodissected adult beef, pig, and/or macaque but not human; see May translation (1968, p. 706).

Illustrated and described, not named:

1. *[superficial fibular nerve (Fyfe, 1800)] (Vesalius, 1543a)*
 Described and illustrated for macrodissected adult human; see Richardson & Carman translation (2002, pp. 260–261).

Earlier synonyms:

1. *external anterior branch of small sciatic branch (Winslow, 1733)*
 Synonym for macrodissected adult human ***superficial fibular nerve (Fyfe, 1800)***; Section VI, p. 93.
2. *superficial branch of peroneal nerve (Haase, 1781)*
 Synonym for macrodissected adult human ***superficial fibular nerve (Fyfe, 1800)***; in the original Latin, *ramus nervus peroneus superficiales*, p. 113.
3. *anterior dorsal cutaneous nerve of foot (Martin, 1781)*
 Synonym for macrodissected adult human ***superficial fibular nerve (Fyfe, 1800)***; in the original Latin, *nervus cutaneus dorsi pedis anterior*, p. 247.
4. *cutaneous nerve of foot (Martin, 1781)*
 Synonym for macrodissected adult human ***superficial fibular nerve (Fyfe, 1800)***; in the original Latin, *nervus pedalis cutaneus*, p. 247.
5. *superficial peroneal nerve (Günther, 1786)*
 Synonym for macrodissected adult human ***superficial fibular nerve (Fyfe, 1800)***; in the original Latin, *nervus peroneum superficialem*, p. 89.
6. *anterior cutaneous nerve of foot (Soemmerring, 1791)*
 Synonym for macrodissected adult human ***superficial fibular nerve (Fyfe, 1800)***; in the original Latin, *nervus cutaneus pedalis anterior*, p. 311.
7. *anterior superficial branch of peroneal nerve (Mayer, 1794)*
 Synonym for macrodissected adult human ***superficial fibular nerve (Fyfe, 1800)***; in the original Latin, *ramus superficialis anterior nervi peronei*; Part 5, Table V, Figure 1-*F* (p. 27).

LATER SYNONYMS:

1. *dorsal branch of deeper seated branch of fibular nerve (Bell, 1803b)*
 Synonym listed for macrodissected adult human ***superficial fibular nerve (Fyfe, 1800)***; in the original Latin, *ramus dorsalis*, pp. 208–209.
2. *deep branch of foot of deeper seated branch of fibular nerve (Bell, 1803b)*
 Synonym listed for macrodissected adult human ***superficial fibular nerve (Fyfe, 1800)***; in the original Latin, *ramus pedis profundus*, pp. 208–209.
3. *praetibio-digital nerve (Burdin, 1803)*
 Synonym for macrodissected adult human ***superficial fibular nerve (Fyfe, 1800)***; see translation (1803, Vol. 1, p. 205).
4. *great superficial division of fibular nerve (Bell & Bell, 1816)*
 Synonym for macrodissected adult human ***superficial fibular nerve (Fyfe, 1800)***; Vol. 1, p. 551.
5. *musculocutaneous branch of external popliteal nerve (Cloquet, 1816)*
 Synonym for macrodissected adult human ***superficial fibular nerve (Fyfe, 1800)***; in the original French, *branche musculo-cutanée*, p. 674.
6. *muscular cutaneous nerve (Meckel, 1817)*
 Synonym for macrodissected adult human ***superficial fibular nerve (Fyfe, 1800)***; see translation (1832, Vol. 3, p. 18).
7. *cutaneous peroneal nerve (Bock, 1827)*
 Synonym for macrodissected adult human ***superficial fibular nerve (Fyfe, 1800)***; in the original Latin, *nerv. peroneus cutaneus*, Table III-*57*.
8. *dorsal branch of peroneal nerve (Swan, 1830)*
 Apparently synonym for macrodissected adult human ***superficial fibular nerve (Fyfe, 1800)***; Plate XXIII, Figure 4-*9*.
9. *musculo-cutaneous branch of fibular nerve (Quain, 1832)*
 Synonym for macrodissected adult human ***superficial fibular nerve (Fyfe, 1800)***; p. 707.
10. *musculo-cutaneous branch of peroneal nerve (Quain, 1832)*
 Synonym for *musculo-cutaneous branch of fibular nerve (Quain, 1832)*; p. 707.
11. *external peroneal branch of external popliteal sciatic nerve (Cruveilhier, 1836)*

Synonym for macrodissected adult human ***superficial fibular nerve (Fyfe, 1800)***; in the original French, *branche péronière externe*, p. 864.

12. *musculo-cutaneous nerve (Quain & Wilson, 1839)*
Synonym for macrodissected adult human ***superficial fibular nerve (Fyfe, 1800)***; Plate XXIV, Figure 1-*B*. See Durward (1951, p. 1108), and Williams & Warwick (1980, p. 1115) where it is spelled *musculocutaneous nerve*.

PARTLY CORRESPONDS:

1. *branch of superficial peroneal nerve to small peroneal muscle (Günther, 1786)*
Basically combination of macrodissected adult human ***muscular branches of superficial fibular nerve (>1840)***, ***medial dorsal cutaneous nerve (>1840)***, and ***intermediate dorsal cutaneous nerve (>1840)***; in the original Latin, *r. ad m. peroneum parvum*, p. 89.
2. *digital branches of superficial peroneal nerve (Günther, 1786)*
Basically combination of macrodissected adult human ***dorsal digital nerves of medial dorsal cutaneous nerve (>1840)*** and ***dorsal digital nerves of intermediate dorsal cutaneous nerve (>1840)***; in the original Latin, *r. digitales*, p. 89.
3. *metatarsal nerves (Bell, 1803b)*
Macrodissected adult human ***superficial fibular nerve (Fyfe, 1800)*** segment generating ***medial dorsal cutaneous nerve (>1840)*** and ***intermediate dorsal cutaneous nerve (>1840)***; p. 210.
4. *dorsal branches of foot (Bell, 1803b)*
Synonym for *metatarsal nerves (Bell, 1803b)*; in the original Latin, *rami dorsales pedis*, p. 210.
5. *dorsal digital nerves of anterior cutaneous branch of peroneal nerve (Langenbeck, 1826–1830)*
Macrodissected adult human ***dorsal digital nerves of medial dorsal cutaneous nerve (>1840)*** and ***dorsal digital nerves of intermediate dorsal cutaneous nerve (>1840)*** considered together; in the original Latin, *nervi digitales dorsales, ramus cutaneus anterior nervi peronei*; Fascicle III, Table VII, Figure 2.
6. *metatarsal branch of external dorsal branch of superficial peroneal nerve (Cloquet, 1828)*
Branch with two roots from macrodissected adult human ***medial dorsal cutaneous nerve (>1840)*** and ***intermediate dorsal cutaneous nerve (>1840)***, in turn generating dorsal digital nerves to second and third toes; in the original French, *rameau métatarsien du rameau dorsal externe du N. péronier superficiel*, Plate CLXXIII, Figure 1-*81*.
7. *terminal branches of musculocutaneous nerve (Cruveilhier, 1836)*
Macrodissected adult human ***medial dorsal cutaneous nerve (>1840)*** and ***intermediate dorsal cutaneous nerve (>1840)*** considered together; in the original French, *rameaux qui terminent le nerf musculo-cutané*, p. 865. Cruveilhier there enumerated four branches, with the first being internal, and the fourth also called internal (though this was probably an error, external likely correct).
8. *dorsal collateral nerves of musculocutaneous nerve (Cruveilhier, 1836)*
Synonym for macrodissected adult human *digital branches of superficial peroneal nerve (Günther, 1786)*; in the original French, *nerfs collatéraux dorsaux*, p. 866.

superficial medullary lamina of subiculum (Dejerine & Dejerine-Klumpke, 1895)

As described for macrodissected adult human, a conspicuous and unique layer of tangential ***axons (Kölliker, 1896)*** thickest in layer 1 of the ***subiculum (>1840)*** but spreading out also in layer 1 of the adjacent ***presubiculum (>1840)*** and ***parasubiculum (>1840)***, and perhaps into adjacent parts of the ***entorhinal area (Brodmann, 1909)*** as well. Thus, it is a characteristic feature of the ***parahippocampal gyrus (>1840)***; see Dejerine & Dejerine-Klumpke (1895, p. 703, Figs. 350–351). It was probably first described as the *columna externa anonyma (Haller, 1762)*.

EARLIER REFERENCES:

Earlier synonyms:

1. *columna externa anonyma (Haller, 1762)*
Probably synonym for macrodissected adult human *columna anonyma (Haller, 1762)*; p. 37, also see Burdach (1822, p. 375).
2. *columna anonyma (Haller, 1762)*
Probably synonym for macrodissected adult human ***superficial medullary lamina of subiculum (Dejerine & Dejerine-Klumpke, 1895)***; p. 42.
3. *erta della corna d' Ammone (Malacarne, 1780)*
Synonym for macrodissected adult human ***superficial medullary lamina of subiculum (Dejerine & Dejerine-Klumpke, 1895)***; a translation of the Italian is *steep slope or ramp of Ammon's horn*; Part 2, p. 69.
4. *lamina medullaris (Burdach, 1822)*
Synonym for macrodissected adult human ***superficial medullary lamina of subiculum (Dejerine & Dejerine-Klumpke, 1895)***; p. 157, also see p. 375 and Foster (1892, p. 1100).
5. *reticular white substance (Arnold, 1838a)*
Apparently synonym for macrodissected adult human *lamina medullaris (Burdach, 1822)*; in the original Latin, *substantia alba reticularis*, p. 88. Also see Arnold (1838b, Tab. III, Fig. 1-*f* and Tab. VII, Fig. 3-*h*).

LATER SYNONYMS:

1. *superficial fiber plexus of subiculum (Cajal, 1904)*
Synonym for macrodissected adult human ***superficial medullary lamina of subiculum (Dejerine & Dejerine-Klumpke, 1895)***; in the original Spanish, *plexo de fibras superficiales del subiculo*, see Figure 750-*b* for excellent illustration.
2. *reticular layer of Arnold (>1840)*
Eponym for macrodissected adult human ***superficial medullary lamina of subiculum (Dejerine & Dejerine-Klumpke, 1895)***; see Mettler (1948, Fig. 319), *reticular white substance (Arnold, 1838a)*.

superficial temporal branches of auriculotemporal nerve (>1840)

As described for macrodissected adult human, branches of the ***auriculotemporal nerve (Haller, 1762)*** accompanying the superficial temporal artery with terminal branches supplying skin of the temporal region and communicating with ***temporal branches of facial nerve (Swan, 1830)*** and the ***zygomaticotemporal nerve (>1840)***; see Williams & Warwick (1980, p. 1067), *Terminologia Anatomica* (2012, p. 135). They were known to Galen; see ***[superficial temporal branches of auriculotemporal nerve (>1840)] (Galen, c173)***.

EARLIER REFERENCES:

Described, not named or illustrated:

1. ***[superficial temporal branches of auriculotemporal nerve (>1840)] (Galen, c173)***
Described without naming for macrodissected adult pig, beef, and/or macaque but not human; see May translation (1968, pp. 444, 449, 451, 453, 507). Falloppio (1561, p. 453) described them for macrodissected adult human; see Meckel (1748, p. 103 note *y*).

Earlier synonyms:

1. *anterior branch of superficial temporal branch (Loder, 1778)*
Synonym for macrodissected adult human ***superficial temporal branches of auriculotemporal nerve (>1840)***; p. 21.
2. *cutaneous temporal branches of superficial temporal nerve (Günther, 1786)*
Synonym for macrodissected adult human ***superficial temporal branches of auriculotemporal nerve (>1840)***; pp. 53–54.
3. *major anterior branches of auricular nerve (Soemmerring, 1791)*
Synonym for macrodissected adult human ***superficial temporal branches of auriculotemporal nerve (>1840)***; p. 216. In the original Latin, *ramum priorem maiorem*, see Soemmerring (1798, p. 237).
4. *temporal fascicles proper of cutaneous temporal surculus of inferior maxillary branch (Bellingeri, 1818)*
Synonym for macrodissected adult human ***superficial temporal branches of auriculotemporal nerve (>1840)***; in the original Latin, *fasciculi temporalis proprius*, see Table I.
5. *superficial temporal branches of superficial temporal nerve (Arnold, 1834)*
Synonym for macrodissected adult human ***superficial temporal branches of auriculotemporal nerve (>1840)***; in the original Latin, *nervus temporalis superficialis, rami temporales superficiales*, p. 11.
6. *superficial temporal branches of anterior auricular nerve (Arnold, 1834)*
Synonym for macrodissected adult human ***superficial temporal branches of auriculotemporal nerve (>1840)***; in the original Latin, *nervus auricularis anterior, rami temporales superficiales*, p. 11.
7. *ascending branch of auriculotemporal nerve (Cruveilhier, 1836)*
Synonym for macrodissected adult human ***superficial temporal branches of auriculotemporal nerve (>1840)***; in the original French, *branche ascendante*, p. 932.
8. *superior branch of auriculotemporal nerve (Cruveilhier, 1836)*
Synonym for macrodissected adult human ***superficial temporal branches of auriculotemporal nerve (>1840)***; in the original French, *branche supérieure*, p. 932.
9. *temporal branch of auriculotemporal nerve (Cruveilhier, 1836)*
Synonym for macrodissected adult human ***superficial temporal branches of auriculotemporal nerve (>1840)***; in the original French, *branche temporale*, p. 932.

superior branches of transverse nerve of neck (>1840)

As described for macrodissected adult human, they form a ***plexus (Galen, c192)*** with the ***cervical branch of facial nerve (>1840)*** and distribute to skin of the rostral (upper) and ventral (front) parts of the neck; see Hamilton (1976, Fig. 798), Williams & Warwick (1980, p. 1092), *Terminologia Anatomica* (1998, p. 137). They were perhaps first clearly described as *superior branch of subcutaneous nerve of neck (Meckel, 1753)*.

EARLIER REFERENCES:

Earlier synonyms:

1. *superior branch of subcutaneous nerve of neck (Meckel, 1753)*
Synonym for macrodissected adult human ***superior branches of transverse nerve of neck (>1840)***; in the original French, *le rameau supérieur du nerf sous-cutané du cou*, p. 97.
2. *middle cutaneous nerve of neck (Meckel, 1753)*
Synonym for *superior branch of subcutaneous nerve of neck (Meckel)*; Table 1-Ω.
3. *superior branch of superficial nerve of neck (Bang, 1770)*
Synonym for macrodissected adult human ***superior branches of transverse nerve of neck (>1840)***; in the original Latin, *superior ramus*, Figure I-41.
4. *middle superficial branch of superficial nerve of neck (Bang, 1770)*
Synonym for macrodissected adult human ***superior branches of transverse nerve of neck (>1840)***; in the original Latin, *superficialis medius ramus*, Figure I-41.
5. *superior cutaneous nerve of neck (Neubauer, 1772)*
Synonym for ***superior branches of transverse nerve of neck (>1840)***; in the original Latin, *nervum superiorem cutaneum colli*, Table 2-42.
6. *superior branch of middle cutaneous nerve of neck (Peipers, 1793)*
Roughly synonymous with ***superior branches of transverse nerve of neck (>1840)***; in the original Latin, *ramus superior subcutanei colli medii*, p. 34.

7. *superior subcutaneous cervical nerves (Meckel, 1817)* Synonym for ***superior branches of transverse nerve of neck (>1840)***; in the original Latin, *nervi subcutanei colli superiores*, see translation (1832, Vol. 3, p. 32).
8. *middle subcutaneous nerve of neck (Bock, 1817)* Synonym for macrodissected adult human *middle cutaneous nerve of neck (Meckel, 1754)*; in the original Latin, *nerv. subcutaneus colli medius*, Table IV-*6*.
9. *ascending branch of superficial cervical branch of cervical plexus (Cruveilhier, 1836)* Synonym for ***superior branches of transverse nerve of neck (>1840)***; in the original French, *rameau ascendant*, p. 782.

PARTLY CORRESPONDS:

1. *greater superior branch of middle cutaneous nerve of neck (Peipers, 1793)* Major macrodissected adult human ***superior branch of transverse nerve of neck (>1840)*** to region caudal (below) and ventral (anterior) to ear supplied by two main branches; in the original Latin, *ramus superior cutanei colli medii majoris*, p. 34.
2. *auriculofacial branch of middle cutaneous nerve of neck (Peipers, 1793)* Major macrodissected adult human ***superior branch of transverse nerve of neck (>1840)*** to region caudal (below) and ventral (anterior) to ear; in the original Latin, *auriculari facialis*, p. 34.
3. *mental subcutaneous nerve (Peipers, 1793)* Macrodissected adult human ***superior branch of transverse nerve of neck (>1840)*** extending under chin; in the original Latin, *subcutaneus menti*, p. 34.
4. *inferior cutaneous nerve of face (Mayer, 1794)* Major macrodissected adult human ***superior branch of transverse nerve of neck (>1840)***; in the original Latin, *nervus cutaneus faciei inferior*; Part 5, Table VII-*204* (p. 53).
5. *superior branch of middle subcutaneous nerve of neck (Bock, 1827)* More caudal (upper) branch of macrodissected adult human ***superior branches of transverse nerve of neck (>1840)***; in the original Latin, *ram. superior nerv. subcutaneus colli medius*, Table 5, Figure 1-*31*.
6. *inferior branch of middle subcutaneous nerve of neck (Bock, 1827)* More rostral (lower) branch of macrodissected adult human ***superior branches of transverse nerve of neck (>1840)***; in the original Latin, *ram. inferior nerv. subcutaneus colli medius*, Table V, Figure 1-*32*.

superior cardiac nerve (Neubauer, 1772)

As described for macrodissected adult human, it arises as two or more roots from the caudal (lower) aspect of the ***superior cervical ganglion (Vieussens, 1684)***, as well as sometimes by a root from a ***communicating branch of superior and middle cervical ganglia (Cruveilhier, 1836)***. The right and left ***superior cardiac nerves (Neubauer, 1772)*** have somewhat different origins, courses, and complex branching patterns, and both end in the ***cardiac plexus (Keill, 1698)***; see Mitchell (1953, pp. 247–249 and Fig. 94), Williams & Warwick (1980, p. 1128). For Neubauer's use and detailed description for macrodissected adult human, see pp. 93, 194. It was the term adopted by the *Basel Nomina Anatomica* (His, 1895, p. 93) and used by Williams & Warwick (1980, p. 1128). It was clearly identified long ago by Vieussens; see ***[superior cardiac nerve (Neubauer, 1772)] (Vieussens, 1684)***.

TRANSLATIONS:

1. *nervum cardiacum superiorem (Neubauer, 1772)* Original Latin form of ***superior cardiac nerve (Neubauer, 1772)***; p. 93.
2. *nervus cardiacus superior (Meckel, 1817)* Latin form of ***superior cardiac nerve (Neubauer, 1772)*** used by Meckel; see translation (1832, Vol. 3, p. 92).

EARLIER REFERENCES:

Illustrated and described, not named:

1. ***[superior cardiac nerve (Neubauer, 1772)] (Vieussens, 1684)*** Vieussens clearly identified left ***superior cardiac nerve (Neubauer, 1772)*** for macrodissected adult human; see Table 23-*Δ* and Scarpa (1794, Tab. III).

Earlier synonyms:

1. *superior cardiac branch (Haller, 1762)* Apparently refers to macrodissected adult human ***superior cardiac nerve (Neubauer, 1772)***; p. 257.

LATER SYNONYMS:

1. *superficial cardiac nerve (Neubauer, 1772)* Synonym for macrodissected adult human ***superior cardiac nerve (Neubauer, 1772)***; in the original Latin, *nervus cardiacum superficialem*, p. 93 and Table 1-*10*.
2. *highest cardiac nerve (Neubauer, 1772; Haller, 1772)* Synonym for macrodissected adult human ***superior cardiac nerve (Neubauer, 1772)***; in the original Latin, *nervum cardiacum supremum*, p. 93. Scarpa (1794, Tab. III-*84*) ascribed the term to Haller without providing a citation; it was (1772, p. 8-*k,m*).
3. *most superficial of cardiac nerves (Chaussier, 1789)* Synonym for macrodissected adult human ***superior cardiac nerve (Neubauer, 1772)***; in the original French, *le plus superficiel des nerfs cardiaques*, see *Table synoptique du nerf tri-splanchnic*.
4. *superficial nerve of heart (Scarpa, 1794)* Synonym for macrodissected adult human ***superior cardiac nerve (Neubauer, 1772)***; in the original Latin, *nervis superficialis cordis*, Table III-*84*.
5. *cardiac branches of superior cervical ganglion (Cruveilhier, 1836)* Synonym for macrodissected adult human ***superior cardiac nerve (Neubauer, 1772)***; in the original French, *rameaux cardiaques*, p. 994.

PARTLY CORRESPONDS:

1. *superior cardiac nerves (Haase, 1781)* Haase apparently divided ***superior cardiac nerve (Neubauer, 1772)*** into two *superior cardiac nerves (Haase, 1781)* and one *inferior cardiac nerve (Haase,*

1781), the third and fourth, and fifth, of his account of the *soft nerves (Haller, 1762)*, respectively; in the original Latin, *nervus cardiacus superior*, see pp. 119–120, note *d*.

2. *highest superficial cardiac nerve (Soemmerring, 1791)*
Synonym for most rostral of *superior cardiac nerves (Haase, 1781)*; in the original Latin, *nervus cardiacus superficialis supremus*, p. 317.
3. *trunk of superficial cardiac nerve (Scarpa, 1794)*
Unitary segment of macrodissected adult human ***superior cardiac nerve (Neubauer, 1772)*** after its roots coalesce; in the original Latin, *cardiaci nervi superficialis truncus*, Table IV-*18*.
4. *soft nerves (Cloquet, 1816)*
Term sometimes used to describe macrodissected adult human ***communicating branches (Winslow, 1733)*** of ***superior cardiac nerve (Neubauer, 1772)*** with ***recurrent laryngeal nerve (Albinus, 1744)*** and ***vagus nerve trunk (Wrisberg, 1786; Günther, 1786)***; in the original French, *nerfs mous*, p. 697.
5. *anterior branch of right superior cardiac nerve (Cruveilhier, 1836)*
In some macrodissected adult humans the right ***superior cardiac nerve (Neubauer, 1772)*** divides, with this branch passing ventral to (in front of) inferior thyroid artery; in the original French, *rameau antérieur*, p. 1001.
6. *posterior branch of right superior cardiac nerve (Cruveilhier, 1836)*
In some macrodissected adult humans the right ***superior cardiac nerve (Neubauer, 1772)*** divides, with this branch joining ***recurrent laryngeal nerve (Albinus, 1744)***; in the original French, *rameau postérieur*, p. 1001.

superior caroticotympanic nerve (>1840)

As described for macrodissected adult human, one of the two ***caroticotympanic nerves (>1840)*** extending from the ***internal carotid plexus (>1840)***; see Durward (1951, Figs. 901, 905), Williams & Warwick (1980, p. 1200, Fig. 7.184). Jacobson first described it; see ***[superior caroticotympanic nerve (>1840)] (Jacobson, 1818)***.

EARLIER REFERENCES:

Described, not named or illustrated:

1. ***[superior caroticotympanic nerve (>1840)] (Jacobson, 1818)***
Clearly described for macrodissected adult human; see Lobstein translation (1831, p. 36).

superior cerebellar peduncle (Procháska, 1800)

As described in macrodissected adult human, and mammal generally with histological methods for ***axons (Kölliker, 1896)***,[1] a longitudinal extension of the ***arbor vitae (Winslow, 1733)***. Its largest component, from the ***cerebellar nuclei (>1840)***, courses rostrally through the ***pons (Haller, 1747)***, crosses the median plane of the ***midbrain (Baer, 1837)*** as the ***superior cerebellar peduncle decussation (>1840)***, and continues on to supply the ***red nucleus (Burdach, 1822)*** and certain ***gray matter regions (Swanson & Bota, 2010)*** in the ***dorsal part of thalamus (Herrick, 1910)***. For topographic description it has ***pontine superior cerebellar peduncle (>1840)*** and ***tegmental superior cerebellar peduncle (>1840)*** segments. Other smaller components from the ***cerebellar nuclei (>1840)***, cross and extend caudally, or remain uncrossed and extend either rostrally or caudally. Crossed and uncrossed outputs of the ***fastigial nucleus (>1840)*** form a relatively discrete component of the ***superior cerebellar peduncle (Procháska, 1800)*** called the *uncinate fasciculus of cerebellum (>1840)*, or hook bundle, of Russell (1897). Finally, the ***ventral spinocerebellar tract (>1840)*** joins the ***superior cerebellar peduncle (Procháska, 1800)*** in gaining final access to the ***cerebellum (Aristotle)***; see Williams & Warwick (1980, pp. 917–918). For Procháska's use in macrodissected adult human, see Vol. I, p. 382; also see Burdach (1822, p. 324). It was known to Galen; see ***[superior cerebellar peduncle (Procháska, 1800)] (Galen, c177)***.

EARLIER REFERENCES:

Described, not named or illustrated:

1. ***[superior cerebellar peduncle (Procháska, 1800)] (Galen, c177)***
In *On Anatomical Procedures*, Galen described a "tendon" between *nates (Galen, c173, definition 1)*, or ***tectum (Baer, 1837)***, and *vermiform process (Galen, c177)*, or ***cerebellar vermis (Meckel, 1817)***, almost certainly referring to ***superior cerebellar peduncle (Procháska, 1800)***; see Wiberg (1914, p. 29), Singer (1999, p. 237). Vesalius (1543a) pointed out it is not a tendon, but instead is associated with the *tenuous meninx (Aristotle)* or ***pia (Galen, c192)***; see Singer translation (1952, p. 50).

Earlier synonyms:

1. *anterior cerebellar process (Willis, 1664)*
Synonym for macrodissected adult human and other large mammalian ***superior cerebellar peduncle (Procháska, 1800)***; see Pordage translation (1681, p. 113, Figs. VII-Q, VIII-*P*).
2. *processus e testibus in cerebelli meditullia protensi (Willis, 1664)*
Latin synonym for macrodissected adult human and other large mammalian ***superior cerebellar peduncle (Procháska, 1800)***; Ch. 10, p. 53. See Burdach (1822, p. 324), Dejerine & Dejerine-Klumpke (1901, p. 520).
3. *processus a testibus in cerebellum adscendentes (Willis, 1664)*
Latin synonym for macrodissected adult human and other large mammalian ***superior cerebellar peduncle (Procháska, 1800)***; Ch. 10, p. 53. See Burdach (1822, p. 324).
4. *incrementa fibrosa a cerebro ad cerebellum obliqua (Drelincourt, 1672)*
Synonym for macrodissected adult human ***superior cerebellar peduncle (Procháska, 1800)***; p. 85. See Schreger (1803, p. 326), Burdach (1822, p. 324).
5. *processus medullares è cerebello ad testes (Vieussens, 1684)*

Synonym for macrodissected adult human ***superior cerebellar peduncle (Prochåska, 1800)***; Table XIII-*R*.

6. *processus à cerebello ad testes (Vieussens, 1684)*
   Synonym for macrodissected adult human ***superior cerebellar peduncle (Prochåska, 1800)***; p. 79.
7. *superior cerebellar process (Vieussens, 1684)*
   Synonym for macrodissected adult human ***superior cerebellar peduncle (Prochåska, 1800)***; in the original Latin, *processus cerebelli superiores*, p. 78 ff.
8. *first process of cerebellum (Ridley, 1695)*
   Synonym for macrodissected adult human ***superior cerebellar peduncle (Prochåska, 1800)***; Figure VII-*g*.
9. *first or second medullary process of cerebellum (Cowper, 1698)*
   Synonym for macrodissected adult human ***superior cerebellar peduncle (Prochåska, 1800)***; Table 10, Figure 1-*S*; Appendix Figure 28-*s*.
10. *processus ad testes (Pourfour du Petit, 1710)*
    Synonym for macrodissected adult human *processus medullares è cerebello ad testes (Vieussens, 1684)*; p. 14. Also see Vicq d'Azyr (1786, Pl. VIII, Fig. I-*28*).
11. *truncorum medullae cerebelli partes, quae pertinent ad medullae oblongatae partem priorem (Albinus, 1744)*
    Synonym for macrodissected adult human ***superior cerebellar peduncle (Prochåska, 1800)*** in describing the Eustachian plates; Table 17, Figure 2-*E*. Also see Burdach (1822, p. 324).
12. *processus a cerebello ad nates (Haller, 1754a)*
    Synonym for macrodissected adult human ***superior cerebellar peduncle (Prochåska, 1800)***; Table III-*X*.
13. *pedunculos a cerebello ad nates & testes (Zinn, 1755)*
    Synonym for macrodissected adult human ***superior cerebellar peduncle (Prochåska, 1800)***; p. 198.
14. *process from cerebellum to testes (Haller, 1762)*
    Synonym for macrodissected adult human *processus medullares è cerebello ad testes (Vieussens, 1684)*; in the original Latin, *processus è cerebello ad testes*, p. 74. For English form see Swan (1830, Tab. X, Fig. 5-*D*).
15. *crura cerebelli adscendentia (Haller, 1762)*
    Synonym (plural) for macrodissected adult human ***superior cerebellar peduncle (Prochåska, 1800)***; p. 75. See Burdach (1822, p. 324).
16. *pedunculi cerebelli in superiora producti (Santorini, 1775)*
    Synonym (plural) for macrodissected adult human ***superior cerebellar peduncle (Prochåska, 1800)***; p. 42.
17. *ascending part of cerebellar brachia (Malacarne, 1776)*
    Synonym for macrodissected adult human ***superior cerebellar peduncle (Prochåska, 1800)***; in the original Italian, *le porzioni ascendenti delle braccia del cervelletto*, p. 102. For Latin form, *portio adscendens brachiorum cerebelli*, see Burdach (1822, p. 324).
18. *processus cerebelli ad corpora quadrigemina (Soemmerring, 1778)*
    Synonym for macrodissected adult human ***superior cerebellar peduncle (Prochåska, 1800)***; p. 63.
19. *crura cerebelli superiora (Mayer, 1779)*
    Synonym (plural) for macrodissected adult human ***superior cerebellar peduncle (Prochåska, 1800)***; p. 19.
20. *ascending crura of cerebellum (Palletta, 1784)*
    Synonym (plural) for macrodissected adult human ***superior cerebellar peduncle (Prochåska, 1800)***; in the original Latin, *crura ascendentia cerebelli*, see Schreger (1803, p. 326).
21. *column of valve of Vieussens (Vicq d'Azyr, 1786)*
    Synonym for macrodissected adult human ***superior cerebellar peduncle (Prochåska, 1800)*** on edge of ***rostral medullary velum (>1840)***; Plate VIII, Figure I-*28*.
22. *column of cerebellar medullary velum (Vicq d'Azyr, 1786)*
    Synonym for macrodissected adult human ***superior cerebellar peduncle (Prochåska, 1800)***; in the original French and plural, *colonnes de la lame médullaire du cervelet*; Plate XXX, Figure I-*4*.
23. *columnae veli medullaris cerebelli (Vicq d'Azyr, 1786)*
    Latin form of *column of cerebellar medullary velum (Vicq d'Azyr, 1786)*; Plate VIII, Figure I-*28*.
24. *peduncle of cerebellar medullary velum (Vicq d'Azyr, 1786)*
    Synonym for macrodissected adult human ***superior cerebellar peduncle (Prochåska, 1800)***; in the original French and plural, *pédoncules de la lame médullaire du cervelet*; Plate XXX, Figure I-*4*.
25. *processus cerebelli interiores (Günther, 1786)*
    Synonym listed for macrodissected adult human ***superior cerebellar peduncle (Prochåska, 1800)***; p. 19.
26. *pedunculus ad corpora quadrigemina (Soemmerring, 1791)*
    Synonym for macrodissected adult human ***superior cerebellar peduncle (Prochåska, 1800)***; p. 55.
27. *crus ad corpora quadrigemina (Soemmerring, 1791)*
    Synonym for macrodissected adult human ***superior cerebellar peduncle (Prochåska, 1800)***; p. 55.

LATER SYNONYMS:

1. *first cerebellar peduncle (Prochåska, 1800)*
   Synonym for macrodissected adult human ***superior cerebellar peduncle (Prochåska, 1800)***; Vol. 1, p. 371. For Latin (plural) form, *pedunculi cerebelli primi*, see Burdach (1822, p. 324).
2. *anterior cerebellar peduncle (Prochåska, 1800, p. 371)*
   Synonym for macrodissected adult human ***superior cerebellar peduncle (Prochåska, 1800)***; Vol. 1, p. 371. For Latin (plural) form, *pedunculi cerebelli anteriores*, see Burdach (1822, p. 324).
3. *pedunculi cerebelli valvula magna cerebri (Prochåska, 1800)*
   Synonym (plural) for macrodissected adult human ***superior cerebellar peduncle (Prochåska, 1800)***; Vol. 1, p. 371.
4. *superior prolongation of cerebellum (Burdin, 1803)*
   Synonym for macrodissected adult human ***superior cerebellar peduncle (Prochåska, 1800)***; see translation (1803, Vol. 3, p. 165).

5. *crura ad testes (Schreger, 1803)*
Synonym (plural) for macrodissected adult human ***superior cerebellar peduncle (Prochâska, 1800)***; p. 326.

6. *pillar of Vieussenian valve (Reil, 1807–1808a)*
Synonym for macrodissected adult human ***superior cerebellar peduncle (Prochâska, 1800)***, obvious variation on *column of valve of Vieussens (Vicq d'Azyr, 1786)*; see Mayo translation (1822, p. 19). Mayo (1827; Pl. II, Fig. 4-*h*) used *pillar of valve of Vieussens.*

7. *brachium of tubercula quadrigemina (Reil, 1807–1808a)*
Synonym for macrodissected adult human ***superior cerebellar peduncle (Prochâska, 1800)***; in the original German, *arme zu den Vierhugeln*, see Mayo translation (1822, p. 24).

8. *crura cerebelli ad eminentiam quadrigeminam (Meckel, 1817)*
Synonym (plural) for macrodissected adult human ***superior cerebellar peduncle (Prochâska, 1800)***; p. 477.

9. *superior ascending prolongation of cerebellum (Meckel, 1817)*
Synonym for macrodissected adult human ***superior cerebellar peduncle (Prochâska, 1800)***; see translation (1832, Vol. 2, p. 434).

10. *brachium copulativum (Burdach, 1822)*
Synonym for macrodissected adult human ***superior cerebellar peduncle (Prochâska, 1800)***; p. 102.

11. *crura cerebelli ad cerebrum (Burdach, 1822)*
Listed as synonym (plural) some authors use for macrodissected adult human ***superior cerebellar peduncle (Prochâska, 1800)***; p. 324.

12. *upper pedicle of cerebellum (Mayo, 1827)*
Synonym for macrodissected adult human ***superior cerebellar peduncle (Prochâska, 1800)***; Plate II, Figure 4-*h*.

13. *superior pedicle of cerebellum (Mayo, 1827)*
Synonym for macrodissected adult human ***superior cerebellar peduncle (Prochâska, 1800)***; Plate II, Figure 6-*h*.

14. *pillars of medullary velum of cerebellum (Knox, 1832)*
Synonym (plural) for macrodissected adult human *column of cerebellar medullary velum (Vicq d'Azyr, 1786)*; Supplemental Plate III-23.

15. *crus cerebelli ad corpora quadrigemina (Arnold, 1834)*
Synonym for macrodissected adult human ***superior cerebellar peduncle (Prochâska, 1800)***; Table VI-*zz*.

16. *oblique commissure (Solly, 1836)*
Synonym for macrodissected adult human ***superior cerebellar peduncle (Prochâska, 1800)***; pp. 81, 178, 191. Solly divided it into three parts; p. 192.

17. *intercerebral commissure (Solly, 1836)*
Synonym for macrodissected adult human ***superior cerebellar peduncle (Prochâska, 1800)***; pp. 81, 178, 191.

18. *commissure of cerebellum with cerebrum (Arnold, 1838a)*
Synonym for macrodissected adult human ***superior cerebellar peduncle (Prochâska, 1800)***; in the original Latin (plural), *commissurae cerebelli cum cerebro* (p. 35) and German (plural), *Commissuren des kleinen Hirns mit dem grossen* (p. 40).

19. *brachium conjunctivum (>1840)*
Synonym for macrodissected adult human ***superior cerebellar peduncle (Prochâska, 1800)***; see Nieuwenhuys et al. (2008, p. 70). Also see *brachium copulativum (Burdach, 1822)*.

PARTLY CORRESPONDS:

1. *ansa of superior cerebellar peduncle (Reil, 1809c)*
Corresponds to initial part of crossed descending fibers (see Williams & Warwick, 1980, p. 917) of ***superior cerebellar peduncle (Prochâska, 1800)*** in macrodissected adult human; see Mayo translation (1823, pp. 87, 98–100).

2. *body of superior cerebellar peduncle (Reil, 1809c)*
Initial dorsal "exposed" segment of macrodissected adult human and sheep ***superior cerebellar peduncle (Prochâska, 1800)***, with rostral end extending into ***midbrain (Baer, 1837)*** and caudal end extending into ***arbor vitae (Winslow, 1733)***; see Mayo translation (1823, pp. 96–100).

3. *chordae volubiles (Bergmann, 1831)*
Probably superficial aspect of right and left macrodissected adult human ***superior cerebellar peduncle (Prochâska, 1800)*** along rostral wall of ***fourth ventricle (Galen, c192)***; p. 45, Table V-*e*.

4. *chordae tortuosae (Bergmann, 1831)*
Synonym for *chordae volubiles (Bergmann, 1831)*; p. 45.

5. *chordae sinuosae (Bergmann, 1831)*
Synonym for *chordae volubiles (Bergmann, 1831)*; p. 45.

6. *chordae serpentinae (Bergmann, 1831)*
Synonym for *chordae volubiles (Bergmann, 1831)*; p. 45.

7. *uncinate fasciculus of cerebellum (Lewandowsky, 1903)*
Relatively distinct component of adult human ***superior cerebellar peduncle (Prochâska, 1800)*** observed with histological methods for ***axons (Kölliker, 1896)***, formed by crossed and uncrossed outputs of ***fastigial nucleus (>1840)***; see Rasmussen (1933), Carpenter (1976, pp. 421–425), Williams & Warwick (1980, pp. 917–918). Alternate form, *uncinate fascicle of cerebellum (Lewandowsky, 1903)*.

8. *fasciculus uncinatus cerebelli (>1840)*
Current Latin form of *uncinate fasciculus of cerebellum (Lewandowsky, 1903)*; see *Terminologia Anatomica* (1998, p. 120).

9. *uncinate fasciculus of Russell (>1840)*
Eponym for adult human *uncinate fasciculus of cerebellum (>1840)*; see Rasmussen (1933, pp. 166–167), Carpenter (1976, pp. 421–425). It is occasionally called the *hook bundle of Russell*. Also see Russell (1897).

superior cerebellar peduncle decussation (>1840)

As described in macrodissected adult human, and mammal generally with histological methods for ***axons (Kölliker, 1896)***, a transverse ***central nervous system white matter tract (>1840)*** in the median plane of the ***tegmentum (Swanson, 2000b)***, caudal to the ***red nucleus (Burdach, 1822)*** and formed by the right and left ***tegmental superior cerebellar peduncle (>1840)***. Part of it ends in the nearby left and right ***red nucleus (Burdach, 1822)***, and part of it extends rostrally to the left and right ***dorsal part of thalamus (Herrick, 1910)***; see Carpenter (1976, p. 420 and Fig. 14.16), *Terminologia*

Anatomica (1998, p. 116), Nieuwenhuys et al. (p. 202 and Fig. 6.30-24). It was known to Willis; see ***[superior cerebellar peduncle decussation (>1840)] (Willis, 1664)***.

EARLIER REFERENCES:

Illustrated and described, not named:

1. ***[superior cerebellar peduncle decussation (>1840)] (Willis, 1664)***
   Willis mentioned and illustrated crossing of *anterior cerebellar processes (Willis, 1664)*, or ***superior cerebellar peduncle (Procháska, 1800)***, on either side of macrodissected adult human and other large mammals; pp. 65, 109 and Figures III-*K*, VII-*R*, VIII-*M*.

Earlier synonyms:

1. *commissure of medullary process of cerebellum and testes (Tyson, 1699)*
   Synonym for ***superior cerebellar peduncle decussation (>1840)***, illustrated for macrodissected infant chimpanzee; Figure 14-*o*. Also see ***[superior cerebellar peduncle decussation (>1840)] (Willis, 1664)*** and *processus e testibus in cerebelli meditullia protensi (Willis, 1664)*.

superior cervical cardiac branches of vagus nerve (>1840)

As described for macrodissected adult human, usually 2–3 thin branches leaving the ***vagus nerve trunk (Wrisberg, 1786; Günther, 1786)*** in the rostral (upper) half of the neck and soon thereafter joining the ***superior cardiac nerve (Neubauer, 1772)*** to reach eventually the ***cardiac plexus (Keill, 1698)***; see Durward (1951, Fig. 907-*Ca*[1]), Mitchell (1953, p. 181, called *superior group*), *Terminologia Anatomica* (1998, p. 136). They were probably discovered by Falloppio; see ***[superior cervical cardiac branches of vagus nerve (>1840)] (Falloppio, 1561)***.

EARLIER REFERENCES:

Described, not named or illustrated:

1. ***[superior cervical cardiac branches of vagus nerve (>1840)] (Falloppio, 1561)***
   Probably described for macrodissected adult human; see Diemerbroeck (1689, p. 418).

Earlier synonyms:

1. *cardiac nerve of eighth pair (Haase, 1781)*
   Synonym for macrodissected adult human ***superior cervical cardiac branches of vagus nerve (>1840)***; in the original Latin, *nervus cardiacus paris octavi*, p. 86.
2. *cardiac nerve of vagal pair (Haase, 1781)*
   Synonym for *cardiac nerve of eighth pair (Haase, 1781)*; in the original Latin, *paris vagi nervus cardiacus*, p. 86.
3. *cardiac communicating branch (Andersch & Soemmerring, 1792)*
   Synonym for macrodissected adult human ***superior cervical cardiac branches of vagus nerve (>1840)***; in the original Latin, *ramum communicatorium cardiacum*, p. 134.
4. *superior cardiac branch of vagus nerves (Mayer, 1794)*
   Synonym for macrodissected adult human ***superior cervical cardiac branches of vagus nerve (>1840)***; in the original Latin, *ramus cardiacus superior nervi vagi*; Part 6, Table II, Figure 1-70 (p. 11).
5. *cardiac branch of vagus nerve (Loder, 1803)*
   Synonym for macrodissected adult human ***superior cervical cardiac branches of vagus nerve (>1840)***; in the original Latin, *ramus cardiacus*, Table CLXXVII-*68*. Quain (1828, p. 657) referred to *cardiac branches*.
6. *cardiac nerves from pneumogastric nerve (Meckel, 1817)*
   Synonym for macrodissected adult human ***superior cervical cardiac branches of vagus nerve (>1840)***; see translation (1832, Vol. 3, pp. 47, 48).
7. *cardiac branches of cervical part of tenth pair (Arnold, 1834)*
   Synonym for macrodissected adult human ***superior cervical cardiac branches of vagus nerve (>1840)***; in the original Latin, *par decimum, pars cervicalis, rami cardiaci*, pp. 13, 14.
8. *cardiac branches of cervical part of pneumogastric nerve (Arnold, 1834)*
   Synonym for macrodissected adult human ***superior cervical cardiac branches of vagus nerve (>1840)***; in the original Latin, *nervus pneumogastricus, pars cervicalis, rami cardiaci*, pp. 13, 14.
9. *cardiac branches of cervical part of vagus nerve (Arnold, 1834)*
   Synonym for macrodissected adult human ***superior cervical cardiac branches of vagus nerve (>1840)***; in the original Latin, *nervus vagus, pars cervicalis, rami cardiaci*, pp. 13, 14. Cruveilhier (1836, p. 961) used the French, *rameaux cardiaques cervicaux du pneumo-gastrique*.
10. *cardiac branches of pneumo-gastric nerve (Quain & Wilson, 1839)*
    Synonym for macrodissected adult human ***superior cervical cardiac branches of vagus nerve (>1840)***; Plate XV-*q*.

PARTLY CORRESPONDS:

1. *communicating branch of ninth nerves of head and right cardiac nerves (Andersch & Soemmerring, 1792)*
   Probably a macrodissected adult human ***superior cervical cardiac branch of vagus nerve (>1840)***; in the original Latin, *ramus communicatorius noni (vagi) nervi capitis et nervi cardiaci dextri*, p. 135. Also see *right nerve of heart (Andersch & Soemmerring, 1792)*.
2. *superficial cardiac branch of vagus (Scarpa, 1794)*
   A macrodissected adult human ***superior cervical cardiac branch of vagus nerve (>1840)***; in the original Latin, *vagi ramus cardiacus superficialis*, Table III-2. Scarpa described several.
3. *superficial cardiac branch of eight (Scarpa, 1794)*
   Synonym for *superficial cardiac branch of vagus (Scarpa, 1794)*; in the original Latin, *octavi ramus cardiacus superficialis*, Table III-3.
4. *communicating branch of tenth nerves of head and right nerves of heart (Andersch, 1797)*
   Synonym for macrodissected adult human *communicating branch of ninth nerves of head and right cardiac nerves*

(Andersch & Soemmerring, 1792); in the original Latin, *ramus communicatorius decimi nervi capitis et nervi dextri cordis*, p. 43.
5. *superficial cardiac branch of pneumogastric (Knox, 1832)* Synonym for *superficial cardiac branch of vagus (Scarpa, 1794)*; Plate III-*78*, in Knox's translation of Scarpa.

superior cervical ganglion (Vieussens, 1684)

As described for macrodissected adult human, the largest, most constant, and most rostral of the three ***cervical sympathetic ganglia (>1840)*** associated with the ***sympathetic trunk (Winslow, 1733)***; see Henle (1871, Fig. 302), Mettler (1948, Fig. 62), Williams & Warwick (1998, pp. 1127–1128). Vieussens essentially used a longer form of this term in his description of the macrodissected adult human ***sympathetic trunk (Winslow, 1733)***; Table 23. In Vieussens's original Latin, *plexus ganglioformis cervicalis superior nervi intercostalis* ("superior cervical ganglionic infolding of the intercostal nerve"); later shortened to *ganglion cervicale superius*, for example, by Haller (1762, p. 254). It was known to Galen; see ***[superior cervical ganglion (Vieussens, 1684)] (Galen c173)***. The first detailed macrodissections were illustrated by Lancisi (1728, Tab. 6).

EARLIER REFERENCES:

Described, not named or illustrated:

1. ***[superior cervical ganglion (Vieussens, 1684)] (Galen, c173)***
Galen described without naming the ***superior cervical ganglion (Vieussens, 1684)*** and some of the ***nerve (Herophilus, c335–c280 BC)*** branches associated with it; see May translation (1968, pp. 395–396), Duckworth translation (1962, pp. 217–218), Savage-Smith (1971, pp. 179–181). It has been suggested that he included one or both of the ***ganglia (Galen, c173)*** associated with the ***vagus nerve (Galen, c192)*** in his account; for example, Sheehan (1936, p. 1083). Galen explicitly acknowledged dissecting a variety of adult mammals but not human. Falloppio (1561, f. 152v) referred to it as a plexus on the sixth nerve in macrodissected adult human; see Haller (1762, p. 254 note *n*), Schreger (1803, p. 357).

Earlier synonyms:

1. *upper ganglioform infolding of intercostal nerve (Willis, 1664)*
Synonym for macrodissected adult human ***superior cervical ganglion (Vieussens, 1684)***; in the original Latin, *plexus ganglioformis nervi intercostalis superior*, Table IX-*G*. Palfijn (1726, Part 2, p. 333) gave the French, *plexus gangliforme superieur de l'intercostal*.
2. *highest ganglioform infolding of intercostal nerve (Willis, 1664)*
Synonym for macrodissected adult human ***superior cervical ganglion (Vieussens, 1684)***; see Pordage translation (1681, Tab. 9-*D*).
3. *highest knot of intercostal nerve (Willis, 1664)*
Synonym for macrodissected adult human ***superior cervical ganglion (Vieussens, 1684)***; see Pordage translation (1681, Tab. 9-*D*).

LATER SYNONYMS:

1. *cervical fold (Diemerbroeck, 1689)*
Probably synonym for macrodissected adult human ***superior cervical ganglion (Vieussens, 1684)***; p. 418.
2. *cervical plexus (Keill, 1698)*
Probably synonym for macrodissected adult human ***superior cervical ganglion (Vieussens, 1684)***; in the original Latin, *plexus cervicalis*, p. 292.
3. *first cervical ganglion (Winslow, 1733)*
Synonym for macrodissected adult human ***superior cervical ganglion (Vieussens, 1684)***; Section VI, p. 95. For Latin form, *ganglion cervicale primum*, see Soemmerring (1791, p. 314).
4. *long cervical ganglion of intercostal nerve (Meckel, 1751)*
Synonym for macrodissected adult human ***superior cervical ganglion (Vieussens, 1684)***; in the original French, *le ganglion cervical long du nerf intercostal*, see Figure 1-*v*.
5. *ganglion cervicale supremum (Haller, 1762)*
Synonym for macrodissected adult human ***superior cervical ganglion (Vieussens, 1684)***; p. 254.
6. *great cervical ganglion (Neubauer, 1772)*
Synonym for macrodissected adult human ***superior cervical ganglion (Vieussens, 1684)***; in the original Latin, *ganglion cervicale magnum*, p. 44.
7. *uppermost cervical ganglion (Monro, 1783)*
Synonym for macrodissected adult human ***superior cervical ganglion (Vieussens, 1684)***; Table XXI, Figures 1, 2.
8. *first ganglion of neck (Andersch & Soemmerring, 1792)*
Synonym for macrodissected adult human ***superior cervical ganglion (Vieussens, 1684)***; in the original Latin, *primum ganglium colli*, p. 166. An alternate form, *primi ganglii colli*, given on p. 165 in Soemmerring's headline.
9. *olivary ganglion (Mayer, 1794)*
Synonym listed for macrodissected adult human ***superior cervical ganglion (Vieussens, 1684)***; in the original Latin, *ganglion olivare*; Part 6, Table II, Figure 1-*1* (p. 10).
10. *fusiform ganglion (Portal, 1803a)*
Synonym for macrodissected adult human ***superior cervical ganglion (Vieussens, 1684)***; in the original French, *le ganglion fusiforme*, p. 163.
11. *upper cervical ganglion (Lobstein, 1831)*
English form of macrodissected adult human ***superior cervical ganglion (Vieussens, 1684)***; p. 11.

superior clunial nerves (>1840)

As described for macrodissected adult human, branches of the ***lateral branches of spinal nerve dorsal branches (>1840)*** arising from the 1st–3rd ***lumbar nerves (Diemerbroeck, 1672)*** and innervating skin rostrally (superiorly) and laterally in the gluteal region; see Williams & Warwick (1980, Fig. 7.196), *Terminologia Anatomica* (1998, p. 139). They were clearly distinguished by Eustachi; see ***[superior clunial nerves (>1840)] (Eustachi, 1552)***.

EARLIER REFERENCES:

Illustrated, not named or described:

1. ***[superior clunial nerves (>1840)] (Eustachi, 1552)***

Clearly illustrated for macrodissected adult human; see Albinus edition (1761, Tab. 23/2:*L–P*).

Described, not named or illustrated:

1. ***[superior clunial nerves (>1840)] (Winslow, 1733)*** Briefly mentioned for macrodissected adult human, at least from first ***lumbar nerve (Diemerbroeck, 1672)***; Sect, VI, no. 270, p. 86. Also see Meckel (1817; and 1832 translation, Vol. 3, p. 13).

superior colliculus (Haller, 1762)

As described for adult mammal with gross dissection, and with cellular architecture and connections, a ***gray matter region (Swanson & Bota, 2010)*** in the rostral part of the right and left ***tectum (Baer, 1837)***, separated by the transverse arm of the ***cruciform sulcus (>1840)*** from the caudal part, the right and left ***inferior colliculus (Haller, 1762)***; see Nieuwenhuys et al. (2008, p. 206 and Fig. 3.10). For Haller's use in macrodissected adult human, see p. 63, *horum colliculorum par superius*, and p. 64, *superius his colliculis velum imponitur*. It was first described as the *little testicle (Galen, c173, definition 2)*.

EARLIER REFERENCES:

Earlier synonyms:

1. *little testicles (Galen c173, definition 2)* In *On the Usefulness of the Parts*, Galen clearly explained that some people call the ***superior colliculi (Haller, 1762)*** the *didymia (Galen, c173, definition 2)* or little testicles, whereas others refer to the entire ***tectum (Baer, 1837)*** as the *didymia (Galen, c173, definition 1)*; see May translation (1968, p. 420). Galen dissected mostly beef, pig, and/or macaque not human cadavers explicitly. Willis (1672) first reported they consist partly of *gray substance (Vesalius, 1543a)* in some species like sheep and goat, although he found none in others like human, dog, and fox; see Pordage translation (1683, p. 26, Tab. VII-*A*).
2. *didymia (Galen, c173, definition 2)* Greek for *twins (Galen, c173, definition 2)*, synonym for ***superior colliculi (Haller, 1762)***; see May translation (1968, p. 420), Singer translation (1999, p. 236). Another form is *didymoi*.
3. *twins (Galen, c173, definition 2)* English form of *didymia (Galen, c173, definition 2)*. In *On Anatomical Procedures*, Galen wrote that some people use it as a more seemly way to refer to *little testicles (Galen c173, definition 2)* or ***superior colliculi (Haller, 1762)***; see Singer translation (1999, p. 236).
4. *testicles (Galen, c173, definition 2)* Synonym for *little testicles (Galen, c173, definition 2)*; see May translation (1962, p. 420).
5. *testes (Galen, c173, definition 2)* Alternate translation for *testicles (Galen, c173, definition 2)*; see Wiberg (1914, p. 28).
6. *orcheis (Galen, c177)* Greek term for *testicles (Galen, c173, definition 2)*; see Singer translation (1999, p. 236). Another form is *orchis*.
7. *didymos (Vesalius, 1543a)* Form of *didymia (Galen, c173, definition 2)*; see Singer translation (1952, p. 47).
8. *cerebral testicle (Vesalius, 1543a)* Synonym for macrodissected adult human ***superior colliculus (Haller, 1762)***; see Richardson & Carman translation (2009, p. 204).
9. *gemelli (Vesalius, 1543a)* Latin for *twins (Galen, c173, definition 2)*, mentioned by Vesalius as term for ***superior colliculi (Haller, 1762)***; see Singer translation (1952, p. 47).
10. *eminentias superiores (Guidi, 1611)* Synonym for macrodissected adult human ***superior colliculi (Haller, 1762)***; see Burdach (1822, p. 334).
11. *buttocks (Crooke, 1615)* Crooke referred to *testicles (Galen, c173, definition 2)*, the ***superior colliculi (Haller, 1762)***, as *buttocks* (pp. 431–432), as well as *testicles* (Tab. XII, Fig. 10-*D,E*), and discussed the nomenclature confusion (p. 468). Crooke's text was a rough translation of Bauhin (1605).
12. *nates (Read, 1638)* Synonym for macrodissected adult mammalian ***superior colliculi (Haller, 1762)***; p. 407. Read noted that *optic nerves (Galen c173)* spring from them; p. 411. Also see *buttocks (Crooke, 1615)*.
13. *natiform processes (Willis, 1664)* Synonym for macrodissected adult mammalian *nates (Read, 1638)*; see Pordage translation (1681, Fig. III-*G*).
14. *orbicular prominence (Willis, 1664)* Synonym for macrodissected adult mammalian ***superior colliculus (Haller, 1762)***; see Pordage translation (1681, p. 64, Figs. III-*G*, VIII-*K*).
15. *corpora duo subrotunda (Vieussens, 1684)* Latin synonym for macrodissected adult human ***superior colliculi (Haller, 1762)***; Table VIII-*F*.
16. *greater orbicular prominences (Palfijn, 1726)* Synonym for macrodissected adult human ***superior colliculi (Haller, 1762)***; in the original French, *protuberances orbiculaires majeures*, Part 2, p. 27.
17. *anterior tubercle (Winslow, 1733)* Synonym for macrodissected adult human ***superior colliculus (Haller, 1762)***; Section X, p. 37. A Latin form is *tuberculis anterioribus*; see Soemmerring (1778, p. 97).
18. *corpora quadrigemina anteriora (Soemmerring, 1778)* Synonym for macrodissected adult human ***superior colliculi (Haller, 1762)***; Table III-*w*.
19. *superior quadrigeminal tubercle (Vicq d'Azyr, 1786)* Synonym for macrodissected adult human ***superior colliculus (Haller, 1762)***; Plate VIII, Figure I-20, p. 23.
20. *superior quadrigeminal eminence (Günther, 1786)* Synonym for macrodissected adult human ***superior colliculus (Haller, 1762)***; in the original Latin, *eminentia quadrigemina superioribus*, p. 14.
21. *superior midbrain tubercles (Chaussier, 1807)* Synonym for macrodissected adult human ***superior colliculi (Haller, 1762)***; in the original French, *les tubercules supérieurs du mésocéphale*, pp. 110–111.

22. *ganglion of optic nerve (Gall & Spurzheim, 1810)*
Synonym for macrodissected adult human ***superior colliculus (Haller, 1762)***; p. 87.
23. *superior quadrigeminal body (Wenzel & Wenzel, 1812)*
Synonym for macrodissected adult human ***superior colliculus (Haller, 1762)***; in the original Latin (plural), *superiora corpora quadrigemina*, Table I, Figure 4-*g*.
24. *anterior eminence (Ramsay, 1813)*
Synonym for macrodissected adult human ***superior colliculus (Haller, 1762)***; p. 46.
25. *ganglia for optic nerves (Carus, 1814)*
Synonym (plural) for *optic tubercle (Carus, 1814, p. 268)*; in the original German, *Ganglien für die Sehnerven*, p. 268.
26. *optic tubercle (Carus, 1814, p. 268)*
Synonym for macrodissected adult mammalian ***superior colliculus (Haller, 1762)***; in the original German, *Sehhügel (vorderes Paar der Vierhügen)*, p. 268. Also see *optic tubercle (Carus, 1814, p. 176)*, *optic tubercle (Carus, 1818)*.
27. *true optic tubercle (Carus, 1814)*
Synonym for macrodissected adult human ***superior colliculus (Haller, 1762)***; in the original German, *eigentliche Sehhügel*, Table VI-*s*.
28. *superior corpora bigemina (Gordon, 1815)*
Synonym for macrodissected adult human ***superior colliculi (Haller, 1762)***; p. 91. Mayo (1827, Pl. IV, p. 10) supplied the Latin, *corpora bigeminum superius*.
29. *upper corpora bigemina (Gordon, 1815)*
Synonym for *superior corpora bigemina (Gordon, 1815)*; p. 91.
30. *optic tubercle (Carus, 1818)*
Synonym for macrodissected adult fish and bird ***superior colliculus (Haller, 1762)***; in the original German, *Sehhügel (d. i., vordere Vierhügel)*; for example, Table XV, Figure 1-*c*; Table XIX, Figure 2-*b*. Also see *optic tubercle (Carus, 1814, p. 176)*, *optic tubercle (Carus, 1814, p. 268)*.
31. *anterior quadrigeminal bodies (Tiedemann, 1821)*
Synonym for macrodissected adult monkey ***superior colliculi (Haller, 1762)***; in the original Latin, *corpora quadrigemina antica*, Table II, Figure 2-*g*.
32. *natiform eminences (Cruveilhier, 1836)*
Synonym for macrodissected adult human ***superior colliculi (Haller, 1762)***; in the original French, *eminentiae natiformes*, p. 608.
33. *anterior bigeminal bodies (Owen, 1837)*
Synonym for macrodissected adult marsupial ***superior colliculi (Haller, 1762)***; Plate VI-6.

PARTLY CORRESPONDS:
1. *connecting plate of upper corpora bigemina (Gordon, 1815)*
Thin lamina of *white substance (Vesalius, 1543a)* between right and left ***superior colliculus (Haller, 1762)*** of macrodissected adult human, upon which ***pineal gland (Galen, c192)*** lies; pp. 97–98.
2. *superficial white substance of quadrigeminal body (Arnold, 1838a)*
Clearly identified ***superior colliculus zonal layer (>1840)*** for macrodissected adult human; in the original Latin, *substantia alba superficialis corporum quadrigeminorum*, Table II, Figure 8-*i*. See Nieuwenhuys et al. (2008, Fig. 6.32-*16*).
3. *deep white substance of quadrigeminal body (Arnold, 1838a)*
Clearly identified ***superior colliculus deep white layer (>1840)*** for macrodissected adult human; in the original Latin, *substantia alba profunda corporum quadrigeminorum*, Table II, Figure 8-*h*. See Nieuwenhuys et al. (2008, Fig. 6.32-*19*).

superior colliculus commissure (>1840)

As described for macrodissected adult human, and mammal generally with histological methods for ***axons (Kölliker, 1896)***, a short transverse ***central nervous system white matter tract (>1840)*** crossing the median plane between right and left ***superior colliculus (Haller, 1762)***, beginning rostrally at the caudal end of the ***posterior commissure (Winslow, 1733)***; see Mettler (1948, p. 339 and Figs. 329–332), Crosby et al. (1962, p. 229 and Figs. 175, 177, 179), Swanson (2004, Atlas Levels 37–39). It was known to Reil; see ***[superior colliculus commissure (>1840)] (Reil, 1809c)***.

EARLIER REFERENCES:

Described, not named or illustrated:
1. ***[superior colliculus commissure (>1840)] (Reil, 1809c)***
Clearly described for macrodissected adult human as caudal component of ***posterior commissure (Winslow, 1733)***, "Another process of the posterior commissure passes transversely across the lateral processes of the anterior tubercles [***superior colliculi (Haller, 1762)***]." (Mayo translation, 1823, p. 102).

Earlier synonyms:
1. *radiating commissure of optic lobes (Serres, 1824–1826)*
Synonym for *commussure of optic lobes (Serres, 1824–1826)*; in the original French, *commissure rayonnée des lobes optiques*; Plate IV, Figure 90-3 for European Honey Buzzard, and Plate IV, Figure 100-4 for Common House Martin.
2. *commissure of optic lobes (Serres, 1824–1826)*
In macrodissected wren (and other birds) ***central nervous system white matter tract (>1840)*** between *optic lobes (Serres, 1824–1826)*, described by Serres as analogous to *superior commissure of quadrigeminal tubercles (Serres, 1824–1826)*; in the original French, *commissure des lobes optiques*, Plate IV, Figure 102-4.
3. *superior commissure of quadrigeminal tubercles (Serres, 1824–1826)*
Synonym for macrodissected adult armadillo ***superior colliculus commissure (>1840)***; in the original French, *commissure supérieure des tubercules quadrijumenaux*, Plate XIII, Figure 245-16.
4. *commissure of natiform eminences (Rolando, 1825)*
Synonym for macrodissected adult beef ***superior colliculus commissure (>1840)*** illustrated clearly

and described in transverse section; in the original French, *commissure des éminences nates*, Table VIII, Figure 5-*c*.

5. *commissure of anterior quadrigeminal bodies (Desmoulins, 1825)*
Synonym for macrodissected adult human ***superior colliculus commissure (>1840)***; in the original French, *commissure aux tubercules quadri-jumeaux antérieurs*, Plate XIII, Figure 5-+.
6. *commissure of quadrigeminal bodies (Spurzheim, 1826)*
Synonym for macrodissected adult human ***superior colliculus commissure (>1840)***; p. 230-*x*.
7. *commissure of optic ganglions (Spurzheim, 1826)*
Synonym for macrodissected adult bird *commissure of optic lobes (Serres, 1824–1826)*; Table 3, Figure 6.

superior dental branches of superior dental plexus (>1840)

As described for macrodissected adult human, they extend ventrally (descend) from the ***superior dental plexus (>1840)*** to supply teeth of the upper jaw; see Williams & Warwick (1980, Fig. 7.177, unlabeled), *Terminologia Anatomica* (1998, p. 134), *Dorland's* (2003, p. 1572). They were known to Galen; see ***[superior dental branches of superior dental plexus (>1840)] (Galen, c173)***.

EARLIER REFERENCES:

Described, not named or illustrated:

1. ***[superior dental branches of superior dental plexus (>1840)] (Galen, c173)***
Alluded to without naming for macrodissected adult beef, pig, and/or macaque but not human; see May translation (1968, p. 455), Duckworth translation (1962, p. 194). Vesalius (1543a) mentioned them for macrodissected adult human; see Richardson & Carman translation (2002, p. 189).

PARTLY CORRESPONDS:

1. *dental threads of internal dental fascicles (Bellingeri, 1818)*
Four macrodissected adult human ***superior dental branches of superior dental plexus (>1840)*** to maxillary sinus and molar teeth supposedly derived from ***posterior superior dental nerve (Haller, 1762)***; in the original Latin, *surculus dentalis internus stamina dentales*, see Table I.

superior dental plexus (>1840)

As described for macrodissected adult human, a network of ***communicating branches (Winslow, 1733)*** from the ***posterior superior dental nerve (Haller, 1762)***, ***middle superior dental nerve (Henle, 1871)***, and ***anterior superior dental nerve (Haller, 1762)*** in turn generating descending ***superior dental branches of superior dental plexus (>1840)*** and descending ***superior gingival branches of superior dental plexus (>1840)***; see Hamilton (1976, p. 623 and Fig. 793), Williams & Warwick (1980, Fig. 7.177, unlabeled), *Terminologia Anatomica* (1998, p. 134). It was first described by Meckel; see ***[superior dental plexus (>1840)] (Meckel, 1748)***.

EARLIER REFERENCES:

Described, not named or illustrated:

1. ***[superior dental plexus (>1840)] (Meckel, 1748)***
Briefly described for macrodissected adult human (p. 69) and communication (anastomosis) between ***posterior superior dental nerve (Haller, 1762)*** and ***anterior superior dental nerve (Haller, 1762)*** illustrated; see Figure 1–ψ,*c* and p. 115.

Earlier synonyms:

1. *anastomotic threads of internal dental fascicle with anterior dental fascicle (Bellingeri, 1818)*
Synonym for macrodissected adult human ***superior dental plexus (>1840)***; in the original Latin, *stamina anastomoticus fasciculus dentalis internus cum fasciculi dentalis anterior*, see Table I.
2. *dental nerve anastomosis (Arnold, 1834)*
Synonym for macrodissected adult human ***superior dental plexus (>1840)***; in the original Latin, *anastomosis nervorum dentalium*, Table VIII-*36*.

superior fascicle of accessory optic system (Hayhow et al., 1960)

As described for adult mammal with axonal transport pathway tracing methods, a ventrally directed branch of the ***pretectal brachium of superior colliculus (>1840)*** ending in the nearby ***dorsal terminal nucleus of accessory optic system (Hayhow et al., 1960)*** and ***lateral terminal nucleus of accessory optic system (Hayhow et al., 1960)*** and also generating longer inputs to the ***medial terminal nucleus of accessory optic system (Hayhow et al., 1960)*** by coursing around the outside of the ***cerebral peduncle (Tarin, 1753)***, with the main bundle called the ***transverse peduncular tract (Gudden, 1870)***; see Nieuwenhuys et al. (2008, p. 781 and Fig. 19.13). For original use in rat by Hayhow et al. (1960), see p. 198 and Figure 2, where *fasciculus* not *fascicle* was used and the earlier literature was reviewed. Its main identifiable part in macrodissected adult human, the ***transverse peduncular tract (Gudden, 1870)***, was probably first described as the *nervi accessorii de' Motori comuni (Malacarne, 1791)*.

superior frontal gyrus (>1840)

As described for macrodissected adult human, a topographic subdivision of the ***frontal region (Vicq d'Azyr, 1786)*** lying between ***medial frontal gyrus (>1840)*** dorsally and ***middle frontal gyrus (>1840)*** ventrally; see Williams & Warwick (1980, Fig. 7.111A), *Terminologia Anatomica* (1998, p. 125). It was clearly delineated by Vicq d'Azyr; see ***[superior frontal gyrus (>1840)] (Vicq d'Azyr, 1786)***.

EARLIER REFERENCES:

Illustrated, not named or described:

1. ***[superior frontal gyrus (>1840)] (Vicq d'Azyr, 1786)***
Illustrated as clearly for macrodissected adult human as modern attempts; Plate III, where ***lateral cerebral fissure (>1840)*** is not quite exposed.

superior frontal sulcus (>1840)

As described for macrodissected adult human, the groove between ***superior frontal gyrus (>1840)*** dorsally and ***middle frontal gyrus (>1840)*** ventrally; see Williams & Warwick (1980, Fig. 7.111A), *Terminologia Anatomica* (1998, p. 125). It was first delineated clearly by Vicq d'Azyr; see ***[superior frontal gyrus (>1840)] (Vicq d'Azyr, 1786)***.

EARLIER REFERENCES:

Illustrated, not named or described:

1. ***[superior frontal gyrus (>1840)] (Vicq d'Azyr, 1786)***
Illustrated as clearly for macrodissected adult human as modern attempts; Plate III, where ***lateral cerebral fissure (>1840)*** was not quite exposed.

superior gingival branches of superior dental plexus (>1840)

As described for macrodissected adult human, they extend ventrally (descend) from the ***superior dental plexus (>1840)*** to supply gums of the upper jaw; see *Terminologia Anatomica* (1998, p. 134), *Dorland's* (2003, p. 1574). They were known to Galen; see ***[superior gingival branches of superior dental plexus (>1840)] (Galen, c173)***.

EARLIER REFERENCES:

Described, not named or illustrated:

1. ***[superior gingival branches of superior dental plexus (>1840)] (Galen, c173)***
Alluded to without naming for macrodissected adult beef, pig, and/or macaque but not human; see May translation (1968, p. 455). Vesalius (1543a) mentioned them for macrodissected adult human; see Richardson & Carman translation (2002, p. 189).

Earlier synonyms:

1. *first branch of lower branch of second division of fifth pair of nerves arising within skull (Willis, 1664)*
Synonym for macrodissected adult, presumably human, ***superior gingival branches of superior dental plexus (>1840)***; see Pordage translation (1681, p. 145, Fig. 1-*F,h*).
2. *first branch of fourth branch of second division of fifth pair of nerves arising within skull (Willis, 1664)*
Synonym for macrodissected adult, presumably human, ***superior gingival branches of superior dental plexus (>1840)***; see Pordage translation (1681, p. 145, Fig. 1-*F,h*).

superior gluteal nerve (Martin, 1781)

As described for macrodissected adult human, it arises from the fourth and fifth lumbar and first sacral ***sacral plexus dorsal divisions (Patterson, 1887)***, supplies the gluteus medius and gluteus minimus muscles, and ends in the tensor fasciae latae muscle; see Williams & Warwick (1980, p. 1111). For Martin's description in macrodissected adult human, see p. 236. It was known to Galen; see ***[superior gluteal nerve (Martin, 1781)] (Galen, c177)***.

TRANSLATIONS:

1. *nervus gluteus superior (Martin, 1781)*
Original Latin form of ***superior gluteal nerve (Martin, 1781)***; p. 236.

EARLIER REFERENCES:

Described, not named or illustrated:

1. ***[superior gluteal nerve (Martin, 1781)] (Galen, c177)***
Described for macrodissected adult beef, pig, and/or macaque but not human; see Singer translation (1999, pp. 85–86). Vesalius (1543a) noted it in macrodissected adult human; see Richardson & Carman translation (2002, p. 255).

LATER SYNONYMS:

1. *gluteal nerve (Cloquet, 1816)*
Synonym for macrodissected adult human ***superior gluteal nerve (Martin, 1781)***; in the original French, *nerf fessier*, p. 666.

PARTLY CORRESPONDS:

1. *nerve to fascial muscle (Fischer, 1791)*
Vieussens (1684) apparently misidentified this branch of macrodissected adult human ***superior gluteal nerve (Martin, 1781)*** to tensor fasciae latae muscle as arising from ***femoral nerve (Haller, 1762)***. It was correctly delineated and thus named by Fischer; in the original Latin, *nervus musculi fascialis*, p. 6.
2. *tensor fasciae latae nerve (Fischer, 1791)*
Synonym for *nerve to fascial muscle (Fischer, 1791)*; in the original Latin, *nervus tensoris fasciae latae*, p. 6.
3. *superior part of gluteal plexus (Swan, 1830)*
Macrodissected adult human roots from fourth and fifth lumbar and first sacral ***sacral plexus dorsal divisions (Patterson, 1887)*** joining distally to form ***superior gluteal nerve (Martin, 1781)***; Plate XVIII-33.
4. *ascending branch of superior gluteal nerve (Cruveilhier, 1836)*
Macrodissected adult human rostrally directed (ascending) branch of ***superior gluteal nerve (Martin, 1781)***; in the original French, *rameau ascendant*, p. 856.
5. *descending branch of superior gluteal nerve (Cruveilhier, 1836)*
Macrodissected adult human caudally directed (descending) branch of ***superior gluteal nerve (Martin, 1781)***; in the original French, *rameau descendant*, p. 856.

superior hypogastric plexus (Tiedemann, 1822)

As described for macrodissected adult human, an unpaired part in the median plane of the ***prevertebral plexuses (Quain, 1832)*** lying ventral to (in front of) the bifurcation of the abdominal aorta, between ***inferior mesenteric plexus (Rau, 1720)*** rostrally and ***hypogastric nerve (Walter, 1783)*** caudally, and commonly receiving inputs from the third and fourth ***lumbar splanchnic nerves (Cruveillhier, 1836)***; see Mitchell (1953, pp. 275–277 and Figs. 120, 131), Williams & Warwick (1980, p. 1135). For Tiedemann's use in macrodissected adult human female see Table II-3,7. It was first identified as the *lowest infolding of mesentery (Willis, 1664)*.

TRANSLATIONS:

1. *plexum hypogastricum superiorem (Tiedemann, 1822)*
   Original Latin form of ***superior hypogastric plexus (Tiedemann, 1822)***; Table II-3,7.

EARLIER REFERENCES:

Earlier synonyms:

1. *lowest infolding of mesentery (Willis, 1664)*
   Willis probably used it for macrodissected adult human and common large quadruped ***superior hypogastric plexus (Tiedemann, 1822)***; in Latin, *plexus mesenterii infimus*; see Pordage translation (1681, Tab. XI-☾).
2. *lowest infolding of abdomen (Willis, 1664)*
   Synonym for *lowest infolding of mesentery (Willis, 1664)*; see Pordage translation (1681, p. 159).

LATER SYNONYMS:

1. *great common uterine plexus (Tiedemann, 1822)*
   Synonym for macrodissected adult human female ***superior hypogastric plexus (Tiedemann, 1822)*** extending along uterine artery; in the original Latin, *plexus uterinus communis magnus*, Table I-27; also see Table II-3.
2. *common uterine plexus (Tiedemann, 1822)*
   Synonym for *great common uterine plexus (Tiedemann, 1822)*; in the original Latin, *plexum uterinum communem*, Table II-3,7.
3. *iliohypogastric plexus (Bock, 1827)*
   Synonym for macrodissected adult human ***superior hypogastric plexus (Tiedemann, 1822)***; in the original Latin, *plex. ilio-hypogastricus*; Table VI, Figure 1-9.
4. *hypogastric plexus (Mitchell, 1953)*
   Synonym for macrodissected adult human ***superior hypogastric plexus (Tiedemann, 1822)***; p. 275.

superior labial branches of infraorbital nerve (Meckel, 1748)

As described for macrodissected adult human, these large and numerous branches supply skin of the rostral (anterior) part of the cheek and upper lip, mucous membrane of the mouth, and labial glands; see Williams & Warwick (1980, p. 1064), who also indicated they communicate with branches of the ***facial nerve trunk (>1840)*** to form the *infraorbital plexus (Meckel, 1753)*. For Meckel's use in macrodissected adult human, and his illustration of the *infraorbital plexus (Meckel, 1753)*, see pp. 75–77 and Figure 1-*i,m,w*. They were known to Galen; see ***[superior labial branches of infraorbital nerve (Meckel, 1748)] (Galen, c173)***.

TRANSLATIONS:

1. *rami nervus infraorbitalis labiales superiores (Meckel, 1748)*
   Original Latin form of ***superior labial branches of infraorbital nerve (Meckel, 1748)***; p. 75.

EARLIER REFERENCES:

Described, not named or illustrated:

1. ***[superior labial branches of infraorbital nerve (Meckel, 1748)] (Galen, c173)***
   Alluded to for macrodissected adult beef, pig, and/or macaque but not human; see May translation (1968, p. 537), Duckworth translation (1962, p. 194).

Illustrated and described, not named:

1. ***[superior labial branches of infraorbital nerve (Meckel, 1748)] (Willis, 1664)***
   Illustrated for macrodissected adult, presumably human; see Pordage translation (1681, p. 145, Fig. 1-*ggg*).

LATER SYNONYMS:

1. *superior labial nerves (Schaarschmidt, 1750)*
   Convenient synonym for macrodissected adult human ***superior labial branches of infraorbital nerve (Meckel, 1748)***; in the original Latin, *nervi labiales superiores*, p. 25.
2. *labial branches of facial branches of second division of fifth pair of nerves (Todd, 1836–1839)*
   Synonym for macrodissected adult human ***superior labial branches of infraorbital nerve (Meckel, 1748)***; p. 289. Todd also referred to them as descending branches.
3. *descending filaments of superior maxillary nerve (Cruveilhier, 1836)*
   Synonym for macrodissected adult human ***superior labial branches of infraorbital nerve (Meckel, 1748)***; in the original French, *filets descendans*, p. 928.
4. *labial filaments of superior maxillary nerve (Cruveilhier, 1836)*
   Synonym for macrodissected adult human ***superior labial branches of infraorbital nerve (Meckel, 1748)***; in the original French, *filets labiaux*, p. 928.

PARTLY CORRESPONDS:

1. *internal superior labial nerve (Mayer, 1794)*
   A ***superior labial branch of infraorbital nerve (Meckel, 1748)*** to medial regions of macrodissected adult human upper lip; in the original Latin, *nervus labii superioris internus*; Part 5, Table VII-32 (p. 44).
2. *second and third superior labial nerves (Mayer, 1794)*
   Two ***superior labial branches of infraorbital nerve (Meckel, 1748)*** to middle regions of macrodissected adult human upper lip; in the original Latin, *nervus labii superioris secundus* and *nervus labii superioris secundus*; Part 5, Table VII-35,37 (p. 44).
3. *external superior labial nerve (Mayer, 1794)*
   A ***superior labial branch of infraorbital nerve (Meckel, 1748)*** to lateral regions of macrodissected adult human upper lip; in the original Latin, *nervus labii superioris externus*; Part 5, Table VII-39 (p. 44). Here it would correspond to a fourth *superior labial nerve (Schaarschmidt, 1750)*; in Table VIII-*s* (p. 60) referred to as *third superior labial nerve*, perhaps reflecting arrangement in different cadaver.
4. *first superior labial nerve (Mayer, 1794)*
   Synonym for *anterior superior labial nerve (Mayer, 1794)*; in the original Latin, *nervus labii superioris primus*; Part 5, Table VIII-*l* (p. 59).
5. *anterior superior labial nerve (Mayer, 1794)*
   A ***superior labial branch of infraorbital nerve (Meckel, 1748)*** to middle regions of macrodissected adult human upper lip; in the original Latin, *nervus labii superioris anterior*; Part 5, Table VIII-*l* (p. 59).
6. *middle superior labial nerve (Mayer, 1794)*
   A ***superior labial branch of infraorbital nerve (Meckel, 1748)*** to middle regions of macrodissected adult human

upper lip, referred to here as *second superior labial nerve*; in the original Latin, *nervus labii superioris anterior*; Part 5, Table VIII-*l* (p. 59). Also see *second and third superior labial nerves (Mayer, 1794)* and *external superior labial nerve (Mayer, 1794)*.

7. *internal labial branch of infraorbital nerve (Bock, 1817)*
Synonym for macrodissected adult human *internal superior labial nerve (Mayer, 1794)*; in the original Latin, *ramus labialis internus*, p. 37.
8. *first labial branch of infraorbital nerve (Bock, 1817)*
Synonym for macrodissected adult human *first superior labial nerve (Mayer, 1794)*; in the original Latin, *ramus labialis primus*, p. 37.
9. *middle labial branch of infraorbital nerve (Bock, 1817)*
Synonym for macrodissected adult human *middle superior labial nerve (Mayer, 1794)*; in the original Latin, *ramus labialis medius*, p. 37.
10. *second labial branch of infraorbital nerve (Bock, 1817)*
Synonym for macrodissected adult human *second superior labial nerve (Mayer, 1794)*; in the original Latin, *ramus labialis secundus*, p. 37.
11. *external labial branch of infraorbital nerve (Bock, 1817)*
Synonym for macrodissected adult human *external superior labial nerve (Mayer, 1794)*; in the original Latin, *ramus labialis externus*, p. 38.
12. *third labial branch of infraorbital nerve (Bock, 1817)*
Synonym for macrodissected adult human corresponding part of *second and third superior labial nerves (Mayer, 1794)*; in the original Latin, *ramus labialis tertius*, p. 38.
13. *internal superior labial fascicle of infraorbital surculus (Bellingeri, 1818)*
Synonym for macrodissected adult human *internal superior labial nerve (Mayer, 1794)*; in the original Latin, *labialis super. inter.*, see Table I.
14. *middle inferior palpebral thread of internal superior labial fascicle of infraorbital surculus (Bellingeri, 1818)*
Branch of *internal superior labial fascicle of infraorbital surculus (Bellingeri, 1818)* to intermediate regions of lower eyelid; in the original Latin, *palpebralis infer. medius*, see Table I.
15. *labial threads of internal superior labial fascicle of infraorbital surculus (Bellingeri, 1818)*
Branches of *internal superior labial fascicle of infraorbital surculus (Bellingeri, 1818)* to medial regions of upper lip; in the original Latin, *stamina labialia*, see Table I.
16. *middle superior labial fascicle of infraorbital surculus (Bellingeri, 1818)*
Synonym for macrodissected adult human *middle superior labial nerve (Mayer, 1794)*; in the original Latin, *labialis super. med.*, see Table I.
17. *external superior labial fascicle of infraorbital surculus (Bellingeri, 1818)*
Synonym for third of macrodissected adult human *second and third superior labial nerves (Mayer, 1794)*; in the original Latin, *labialis super. exter.*, see Table I.
18. *outermost superior labial fascicle of infraorbital surculus (Bellingeri, 1818)*
Synonym for macrodissected adult human *external superior labial nerve (Mayer, 1794)*; in the original Latin, *labialis super. extim[us].*, see Table I.
19. *external inferior palpebral threads of outermost superior labial fascicle of infraorbital surculus (Bellingeri, 1818)*
Branch of *outermost superior labial fascicle of infraorbital surculus (Bellingeri, 1818)* to ventral part of orbicularis oculi muscle and other parts of lower eyelid; in the original Latin, *palpebralis infer. externus*, see Table I.
20. *palpebral threads proper of outermost superior labial fascicle of infraorbital surculus (Bellingeri, 1818)*
Branches of *outermost superior labial fascicle of infraorbital surculus (Bellingeri, 1818)* to upper lip; in the original Latin, *labiales proprii*, see Table I.

superior laryngeal nerve (Loder, 1778)

As described for macrodissected adult human, a branch of the ***vagus nerve trunk (Wrisberg, 1786; Günther, 1786)*** appearing to leave from the ***distal vagal ganglion (>1840)*** and extend caudally (descend). It receives a branch from the ***superior cervical ganglion (Vieussens, 1684)*** and finally divides into ***external branch of superior laryngeal nerve (Fyfe, 1800)*** and ***internal branch of superior laryngeal nerve (Fyfe, 1800)***; see Williams & Warwick (1980, pp. 1079–1080). For Loder's use in macrodissected adult human, see p. 30. It was known to Galen; see ***[superior laryngeal nerve (Loder, 1778)] (Galen, c173)***.

TRANSLATIONS:

1. *nervum laryngeum superiorem (Loder, 1778)*
Original Latin form of ***superior laryngeal nerve (Loder, 1778)***; p. 30.

EARLIER REFERENCES:

Described, not named or illustrated:

1. ***[superior laryngeal nerve (Loder, 1778)] (Galen, c173)***
Described for macrodissected adult beef, pig, and/or macaque but not human; see May translation (1968, pp. 371, 689, 690 note *11*). Vesalius (1543a) mentioned it for macrodissected adult human; see Richardson & Carman translation (2002, p. 195).

Earlier synonyms:

1. *superior branches of vagus supply larynx (Cheselden, 1726)*
Synonym derived from description of macrodissected adult human ***superior laryngeal nerve (Loder, 1778)***; p. 259, in a chapter largely written by Monro *primus*.
2. *superior laryngeal branches of eighth pair of cerebral nerves (Albinus, 1744)*
Synonym for macrodissected adult human ***superior laryngeal nerve (Loder, 1778)***; in the original Latin, *octavi paris nervorum cerebri rami laryngaei superiores*, Table 18, Figure 2-*n*.
3. *laryngeal nerve from eighth pair (Asch, 1750)*
Synonym for macrodissected infant and adult human ***superior laryngeal nerve (Loder, 1778)***; in the original Latin, *laryngeus nervus ex octavo*, see Figure 3-*16*.

LATER SYNONYMS:

1. *laryngeal nerve (Haase, 1781)*
Synonym for macrodissected adult human ***superior laryngeal nerve (Loder, 1778)***; in the original Latin, *nervus laryngeus*, p. 85.
2. *laryngeal branch of vagus nerve (Mayer, 1794)*
Synonym for macrodissected adult human ***superior laryngeal nerve (Loder, 1778)***; in the original Latin, *ramus laryngeus nervi vagi*; Part 5, Table VIII-96 (p. 61).
3. *laryngeal branch of pneumogastric nerve (Chaussier, 1809)*
Synonym for macrodissected adult human ***superior laryngeal nerve (Loder, 1778)***; in the original French, *R. laryngien*.
4. *descending laryngeal nerve (Quain, 1827)*
Synonym for macrodissected adult human ***superior laryngeal nerve (Loder, 1778)***; p. 657.
5. *superior laryngeal branch of vagus nerve (Bischoff, 1832)*
Synonym for macrodissected adult human ***superior laryngeal nerve (Loder, 1778)***; in the original Latin, *ramus Laryngeus superior nervi Vagi*, Table I, Figure 1-39.
6. *superior laryngeal branch of pneumo-gastric nerve (Quain & Wilson, 1839)*
Synonym for macrodissected adult human ***superior laryngeal nerve (Loder, 1778)***; Plate XV-*m*.

PARTLY CORRESPONDS:

1. *branches of superior laryngeal branch of pneumo-gastric nerve to pharyngeal plexus (Quain & Wilson, 1839)*
For macrodissected adult human they arise from trunk of ***superior laryngeal nerve (Loder, 1778)*** before dividing into ***external branch of superior laryngeal nerve (Fyfe, 1800)*** and ***internal branch of superior laryngeal nerve (Fyfe, 1800)***, and extending to ***pharyngeal plexus (Neubauer, 1772)***; Plate XV-*n*.

superior lateral cutaneous nerve of arm (>1840)

As described for macrodissected adult human, a branch of the ***axillary nerve (Winslow, 1733)*** supplying skin over the caudal (lower) part of the deltoid muscle and proximal (upper) part of the long head of the triceps muscle; see Williams & Warwick (1980, p. 1097), *Terminologia Anatomica* (1998, p. 139). It was known to Galen; see ***[superior lateral cutaneous nerve of arm (>1840)] (Galen, c177)***.

EARLIER REFERENCES:

Described, not named or illustrated:

1. ***[superior lateral cutaneous nerve of arm (>1840)] (Galen, c177)***
Clearly described for macrodissected adult beef, pig, and/or macaque but not human; see Singer translation (1999, pp. 65–66), Duckworth translation (1962, p. 247). Vesalius (1543a) mentioned it for macrodissected adult human; see Richardson & Carman translation (2002, pp. 228, 238).

Earlier synonyms:

1. *superior external humeral cutaneous branch of circumflex nerve (Martin, 1781)*
Synonym for macrodissected adult human ***superior lateral cutaneous nerve of arm (>1840)***; in the original Latin, *ramus cutaneus humeri externus superior*, p. 221.
2. *superior external cutaneous nerve (Günther, 1786)*
Synonym for macrodissected adult human ***superior lateral cutaneous nerve of arm (>1840)***; in the original Latin, *nervus cutaneum externum superiorem*, p. 79.
3. *external humeral cutaneous nerve (Frotscher, 1788)*
Synonym for macrodissected adult human ***superior lateral cutaneous nerve of arm (>1840)***; in the original Latin, *nervus cutaneus humeri externus*, p. 91 of 1795 reprint.
4. *cutaneous nerve of shoulder (Meckel, 1817)*
Synonym for macrodissected adult human ***superior lateral cutaneous nerve of arm (>1840)***; in the original Latin, *nervus cutaneus humeri*, see translation (1832, Vol. 3, p. 24).
5. *cutaneous branches of axillary nerve (Bock, 1827)*
Synonym for macrodissected adult human ***superior lateral cutaneous nerve of arm (>1840)***; in the original Latin, *rami cutanei nervi axillaris*, Table II-40. Cloquet (1828, Pl. CLXVII, Fig. 2-8,9) described for macrodissected adult human superior and inferior divisions of the branch.
6. *cutaneous branch of circumflex nerve (Swan, 1830)*
Synonym for macrodissected adult human ***superior lateral cutaneous nerve of arm (>1840)***; Plate XXIII, Figure 1-8.
7. *cutaneous branch of shoulder of axillary nerve (Cruveilhier, 1836)*
Synonym for macrodissected adult human ***superior lateral cutaneous nerve of arm (>1840)***; in the original French, *rameau cutané de l'épaule du plexus brachial*, p. 796.

PARTLY CORRESPONDS:

1. *superior cutaneous nerve of arm (Cloquet, 1828)*
Its identity is unclear for macrodissected adult human but may be branch of ***superior lateral cutaneous nerve of arm (>1840)***, shown extending more distally than usually described; in the original French, *nerf cutané supérieur du bras*, Plate CLXVII, Figure 2-6.
2. *cutaneous nerve of shoulder (Cruveilhier, 1836)*
Terminal branch, or sometimes branches, of *cutaneous branch of shoulder of axillary nerve (Cruveilhier, 1836)*; in the original French, *nerf cutané de l'épaule*, p. 796.

superior longitudinal fascicle (>1840)

As described for macrodissected adult human, a prominent arched, longitudinally oriented system of long ***association fibers of cerebral cortex (>1840)*** whose main trunk lies dorsal to the ***corpus callosum (Galen, c177)*** and interconnects ***frontal region (Vicq d'Azyr, 1786)***, ***parietal region (>1840)***, ***occipital region (Vesalius, 1543a)***, and ***temporal region (>1840)***. It is often referred to as the *arcuate fascicle (Burdach, 1822)*, as is just the descending caudal segment, *arcuate fascicle (>1840)*; see Crosby et al. (1962, p. 407), Williams & Warwick (1980,

p. 1039, Fig. 7.148), *Nomina Anatomica* (1983, p. A72), *Terminologia Anatomica* (1998, p. 131), *Dorland's* (2003, p. 676). It was first clearly delineated as the *intermediate white matter (Reil, 1809b)*.

EARLIER REFERENCES:

Earlier synonyms:

1. *intermediate white matter (Reil, 1809b)*
   First description of macrodissected adult human ***superior longitudinal fascicle (>1840)***; in the original German, *intermediäre Marksubstanz*, p. 202.
2. *arcuate fascicle (Burdach, 1822)*
   Synonym for macrodissected adult human ***superior longitudinal fascicle (>1840)***; in the original Latin, *fasciculus arcuatus*; p. 153; Table IX, Figure 2-*f,k*. Also see Polyak (1957, p. 135), Meyer (1971, p. 29).
3. *longitudinal striae of Reil (Rolando, 1831)*
   Probably eponym (plural) for macrodissected adult human *superior longitudinal fascicle (>1840)*; in the original Latin, *striae longitudinales Reil*, Figure 10-20.
4. *lateral longitudinal striae (Rolando, 1831)*
   Synonym (plural) for macrodissected adult human ***superior longitudinal fascicle (>1840)*** attributed by Rolando to Reil; in the original Latin, *striae longitudinales laterales*, p. 126.
5. *superior longitudinal commissure (Solly, 1836)*
   Probably synonym for macrodissected adult human ***superior longitudinal fascicle (>1840)***; p. 189 and Plate X-*D*.
6. *longitudinal fascicle of corona radiata (Arnold, 1838b)*
   Probably synonym for macrodissected adult human ***superior longitudinal fascicle (>1840)***; in the original Latin, *coronae radiatae fasciculum longitudinalem*, Table X, Figure 1-*l*.

PARTLY CORRESPONDS:

1. *arcuate fascicle (>1840)*
   Caudal, ventrally directed (descending), arched segment of macrodissected adult human ***superior longitudinal fascicle (>1840)***; see Carpenter (1976, Fig. 2.11).

superior mesenteric ganglion (>1840)

As described for macrodissected adult human, a ***prevertebral ganglion (Quain, 1832)*** that is not always present, and when present is often single rather than paired. It lies just rostral to (above), or sometimes just caudal to (below), the root of the superior mesenteric artery and also lies within the ***superior mesenteric plexus (Rau, 1720)***; see Mitchell (1953, p. 273), *Terminologia Anatomica* (1998, p. 143). It was perhaps first described accurately, if vaguely, by Meckel; see ***[superior mesenteric ganglion (>1840)] (Meckel, 1817)***.

EARLIER REFERENCES:

Described, not named or illustrated:

1. ***[superior mesenteric ganglion (>1840)] (Meckel, 1817)***
   Probably referred to vaguely in macrodissected adult human, "We usually observe between the two principal ganglions [***celiac ganglia (Walter, 1783)***], particularly between their lower extremities in the space between the coeliac and superior mesenteric arteries, two or three which are smaller" (translation, 1832, Vol. 3, p. 86). The third probably corresponds to ***superior mesenteric ganglion (>1840)***.

superior mesenteric plexus (Rau, 1720)

As described for macrodissected adult human, a large extension of the caudal (lower) part of the ***celiac plexus (Winslow, 1733)*** receiving a branch from the right ***vagus nerve (Galen, c192)***, surrounding the superior mesenteric artery, and accompanying it into the mesentery where its main branches include ***pancreatic branches of superior mesenteric plexus (>1840)***, ***jejunal and ileal plexuses (>1840)***, ***right colic plexus (>1840)***, and ***middle colic plexus (>1840)***; see Mitchell (1953, pp. 282–283), Williams & Warwick (1980, p. 1134). For Rau's use in macrodissected adult human, see p. 110. It was known to Galen; see ***[superior mesenteric plexus (Rau, 1720)] (Galen, c173)***.

TRANSLATIONS:

1. *plexus mesentericus superior (Rau, 1720)*
   Original Latin form of ***superior mesenteric plexus (Rau, 1720)***; p. 110.

EARLIER REFERENCES:

Described, not named or illustrated:

1. ***[superior mesenteric plexus (Rau, 1720)] (Galen, c173)***
   Mentioned for macrodissected adult beef, pig, and/or macaque but not human; see May translation (1968, pp. 246, 711).

Illustrated and described, not named:

1. ***[superior mesenteric plexus (Rau, 1720)] (Vesalius, 1543a)***
   Apparently mentioned and vaguely illustrated for macrodissected adult human; see Richardson & Carman translation (2002, p. 200). It was more thoroughly treated by Willis (1664); see Pordage translation (1681, p. 159 and Tab. 9).

LATER SYNONYMS:

1. *plexus mesaraicus superior (Schaarschmidt, 1750)*
   Synonym for macrodissected adult human ***superior mesenteric plexus (Rau, 1720)***; in the original Latin, *plexus mesaraicul superior*, p. 54. Mayer (1794, Part 6, Tab. V, p. 30) gave it as *plexus mesaraicus superior*.
2. *upper mesenteric plexus (Haller, 1762)*
   Synonym for macrodissected adult human ***superior mesenteric plexus (Rau, 1720)***; in the original Latin, *plexus mesentericus supremus*, p. 264.
3. *mesenteric plexus (Chaussier, 1789)*
   Synonym for macrodissected adult human ***superior mesenteric plexus (Rau, 1720)***; in the original French, *mésenterique*, see *Table synoptique du nerf tri-splanchnique*.

PARTLY CORRESPONDS:

1. *[filaments from superior mesenteric plexus to large intestine (Meckel, 1817)] (Vesalius, 1543a)*
   Apparently alluded to (without naming) in macrodissected adult human; see Richardson & Carman translation (2002, p. 200).

2. *filaments from superior mesenteric plexus to large intestine (Meckel, 1817)*
Macrodissected adult human ***right colic plexus (>1840)*** and ***middle colic plexus (>1840)*** considered together; see translation (1832, Vol. 3, p. 87).

superior occipital gyri (>1840)

As described for macrodissected adult human, a topographic subdivision on the dorsolateral face of the ***occipital region (Vesalius, 1543a)*** lying dorsal to the ***lateral occipital sulcus (>1840)*** and ventral to the ***transverse occipital sulcus (>1840)***; see Williams & Warwick (1980, p. 986, Fig. 7.111A). They were perhaps first clearly delineated by Gall & Spurzheim; see ***[superior occipital gyri (>1840)] (Gall & Spurzheim, 1810)***.

EARLIER REFERENCES:

Illustrated, not named or described:

1. ***[superior occipital gyri (>1840)] (Gall & Spurzheim, 1810)***
Clearly illustrated for macrodissected adult human; Table VIII.

superior olivary complex (>1840)

As described for macrodissected adult human, and for adult mammal in general based on cellular architecture and connections, a highly differentiated ***gray matter region (Swanson & Bota, 2010)*** in the ventromedial ***medulla (Winslow, 1733)***, rostral to the ***inferior olivary complex (>1840)***, receiving a massive input from the ***cochlear nuclei (>1840)*** via the **trapezoid body** (>1840) as does the nearby ***nucleus of trapezoid body (>1840)***. It has three parts, ***medial part of superior olivary complex (>1840)***, ***lateral part of superior olivary complex (>1840)***, and ***periolivary region (>1840)***; see Fay-Lund (1986), Nieuwenhuys et al. (2008, pp. 736–739). It was not clearly identified by 1840.

superior ovarian nerves (>1840)

As described for adult human female, they arise as two or more rootlets from the caudal (lower) end of the ***renal plexus (Drake, 1707)*** and ***intermesenteric plexus (>1840)***, often receive additional branchlets from the second or third ***lumbar splanchnic nerves (Cruveilhier, 1836)***, and sometimes receive branchlets from the caudal (lower) part of the ***celiac ganglion (Walter, 1783)*** or origin of the ***superior mesenteric plexus (Rau, 1720)***. They communicate with the ***superior ureteric nerves (Walter, 1783)*** or share common rootlets of origin and the rootlets coalesce into several ***nerves (Herophilus, c335–c280 BC)*** descending along the ovarian artery and supplying the artery and ovary and outer parts of the uterine tubes; see Mitchell (1953, pp. 293–295). They were known to Willis; see ***[superior ovarian nerves (>1840)] (Willis, 1664)***.

EARLIER REFERENCES:

Described, not named or illustrated:

1. ***[superior ovarian nerves (>1840)] (Willis, 1664)***
Briefly described and illustrated for macrodissected adult human and other common large mammalian females; see Pordage translation (1681, p. 159 and Tab. 11-ν,χ).

Earlier synonyms:

1. *superior spermatic nerves (Walter, 1783)*
Synonym for macrodissected adult human female ***superior ovarian nerves (>1783)***; in the original Latin, *nervi spermatici superioris Spermaticus est stricte sic dictus*, Table I-275.

PARTLY CORRESPONDS:

1. *superior internal spermatic nerve (Walter, 1783)*
Term for root or origin of *superior spermatic nerves (Walter, 1783)* from ***renal plexus (Drake, 1707)***; in the original Latin, *nervum spermaticum internum superiorem*, Table I-269.
2. *ansa spermaticae (Walter, 1783)*
Consists of ***communicating branches (Winslow, 1733)*** between ***renal ganglia (Walther, 1735)*** and ***spermatic ganglia (Walter, 1783)*** surrounding origin of inferior root of testicular artery. Described and illustrated for a macrodissected adult human female; Table I-295,296.
3. *first inferior internal spermatic nerve (Walter, 1783)*
Emerges from second ***spermatic ganglion (Walter, 1783)*** and joins *superior spermatic nerves (Walter, 1783)*, so probably a ***superior ovarian nerve (>1840)*** in macrodissected adult human female; in the original Latin, *nervum spermaticus internus inferior primus*, Table I-304.
4. *second inferior internal spermatic nerve (Walter, 1783)*
Emerges from second ***spermatic ganglion (Walter, 1783)*** and courses along Walter's internal spermatic artery to uterus, so probably a ***superior ovarian nerve (>1840)*** in macrodissected adult human female; in the original Latin, *nervum spermaticus internus inferior secundus*, Table I-305.
5. *spermatic nerves (Walter, 1783)*
Apparently roots of macrodissected adult human *superior spermatic nerves (Walter, 1783)* arising from region of ***intermesenteric plexus (>1840)***; in the original Latin, *nervus spermaticus* (Walter identified at least 3 of them); Table II:135-137.
6. *trunk of internal superior spermatic nerve (Walter, 1783)*
Essentially synonymous with *superior internal spermatic nerve (Walter, 1783)*; in the original Latin, *truncus nervi spermatici superioris interni*, Table II-269.

superior parietal lobule (>1840)

As described for macrodissected adult human, a topographic subdivision of the ***parietal region (>1840)*** lying dorsal to the ***intraparietal sulcus (>1840)*** and caudal to the ***postcentral gyrus (>1840)***; see Williams & Warwick (1980, Fig. 7.111A). It was perhaps first clearly delineated by Vicq d'Azyr (1786); see ***[superior parietal lobule (>1840)] (Vicq d'Azyr, 1786)***.

EARLIER REFERENCES:

Illustrated and described, not named:

1. ***[superior parietal lobule (>1840)] (Vicq d'Azyr, 1786)***
Clearly illustrated for macrodissected adult human; Plate III-*k,m*.

superior rectal plexus (>1840)

As described for macrodissected adult human, an extension of the ***inferior mesenteric plexus (Rau, 1720)*** accompanying the superior rectal artery to supply the proximal (upper) part of the rectum; see Mitchell (1953, p. 284), Williams & Warwick (1980, p. 1134). It was known to Willis; see ***[superior rectal plexus (>1840)] (Willis, 1664)***.

EARLIER REFERENCES:

Illustrated and described, not named:

1. ***[superior rectal plexus (>1840)] (Willis, 1664)***
Mentioned and illustrated for macrodissected adult human and other common large mammals; see Pordage translation (1681, p. 159, Tab. 11-*a,b*).

Earlier synonyms:

1. *hemorrhoidal plexus (Cruveilhier, 1836)*
Synonym for macrodissected adult human ***superior rectal plexus (>1840)***; in the original French, *plexus hémorrhoïdal*, p. 1020.
2. *superior hemorrhoidal plexus (Cruveilhier, 1836)*
Synonym for macrodissected adult human ***superior rectal plexus (>1840)***; in the original French, *plexus hémorrhoïdaux supérieurs*, p. 1026.

superior root of ansa cervicalis (>1840)

As described for macrodissected adult human, it splits off from the ***hypoglossal nerve Winslow, 1733)*** and, along with the *inferior root of ansa cervicalis (>1840)*, forms a distal loop, the ansa cervicalis proper. Histologically, the ***superior root of ansa cervicalis (>1840)*** is the continuation of a ***communicating branch of cervical plexus (>1840)*** from the first or sometimes second cervical ***spinal nerve ventral branch (>1840)*** traveling a short distance to and then with the ***hypoglossal nerve (Winslow, 1733)*** before splitting off again as the ***superior root of ansa cervicalis (>1840)*** to form a distal loop, the ansa cervicalis proper; see Williams & Warwick (1980, pp. 1083, 1092 and Figs. 7.193, 197), *Nomina Anatomica* (1983, p. A76), *Terminologia Anatomica* (1998, p. 137). It was first identified as the *parva particula septimae conjugationis (Galen, c180)*.

EARLIER REFERENCES:

Earlier synonyms:

1. *parva particula septimae conjugationis (Galen, c180)*
Synonym for ***superior root of ansa cervicalis (>1840)*** in macrodissected adult beef, pig, and/or macaque but not human in *On Anatomy of Nerves* (Ch. 8) according to Scarpa (1794, Tab. I-*50*); see Goss (1966). Also see Duckworth translation (1962, p. 201) of Galen (c192). Eustachi (1552, Tab. XVIII-*12*) illustrated it for macrodissected adult human, see Scarpa (1794, Tab. I-*10*), as did Vieussens (1684, Tab. 23-*k*), who wrongly had it joining the ***lingual nerve (Vesalius, 1543a)***.
2. *descending branch of ninth pair of nerves of head (Asch, 1750)*
Synonym for macrodissected infant and adult human ***superior root of ansa cervicalis (>1840)***, with *ninth pair* referring to ***hypoglossal nerve (Winslow, 1733)***; in the original Latin, *noni paris capitis ramo descendente*, see Figure 4-5,*10,11*. Neubauer simply used *ramus descendens noni paris* (1772, Tab. 3, Fig. 3-*ω*).
3. *descending branch of hypoglossal nerve (Günther, 1786)*
Synonym for macrodissected adult human ***superior root of ansa cervicalis (>1840)***; in the original Latin, *r. descendentem* (p. 67) and *nervus hypoglossus* (p. 66). See His (1895, p. 90), Durward (1951, Fig. 919), Hamilton (1976, Fig. 816).
4. *descending neck branch of hypoglossal nerve (Soemmerring, 1791)*
Synonym for macrodissected adult human *descending branch of ninth pair of nerves of head (Asch, 1750)*; p. 260. Also see Soemmerring (1798, p. 279).
5. *internal descending nerve of neck (Andersch & Soemmerring, 1792)*
Synonym for macrodissected adult human *descending branch of ninth pair of nerves of head (Asch, 1750)*; in the original Latin, *nervus hypoglossus ramum... descendentem colli interiorem*, p. 260. Also see Soemmerring (1798, p. 279).
6. *ascending part of tenth nerves of head (Andersch & Soemmerring, 1792)*
Apparently synonym for macrodissected adult human ***superior root of ansa cervicalis (>1840)***; in the original Latin, *decimi nervi capitis partis ascendentis*, p. 149.
7. *ascending part of eleventh nerves of head (Andersch & Soemmerring, 1792)*
Apparently synonym for macrodissected adult human ***superior root of ansa cervicalis (>1840)***; in the original Latin, *undecimi nervi capitis partis ascendentis*, p. 72.
8. *radix prior ansae rami e nervo hypoglosso descendentis (Peipers, 1793)*
Synonym for macrodissected adult human ***superior root of ansa cervicalis (>1840)***; p. 33.
9. *internal descending neck branch of ninth nerve (Scarpa, 1794)*
Synonym for macrodissected adult human *descending branch of ninth pair of nerves of head (Asch, 1750)*; in the original Latin, *descendentem colli internum*, Table I-2.
10. *nervo musculos colli movente interno (Andersch, 1797)*
Synonym for *internal descending nerve of neck (Andersch & Soemmerring, 1792)*; p. 91.
11. *nonus descendens nerve (Quain & Wilson, 1839)*
Synonym for macrodissected adult human ***superior root of ansa cervicalis (>1840)***; Plate XVI-*c*.

PARTLY CORRESPONDS:

1. *small muscular branch of infrahyoid region from hypoglossal nerve (Cruveilhier, 1836)*
Macrodissected adult human accessory of ***superior root of ansa cervicalis (>1840)*** supplying infrahyoid muscles; in the original French, *petit rameau musculaire de la région sous-hyoïdienne*, p. 977.

superior salivatory nucleus (>1840)

As described for adult mammal based on cellular architecture and connections, a relatively indistinct ***gray matter region (Swanson & Bota, 2010)*** in ventral parts of the ***medulla (Winslow, 1733)*** lying roughly between ***facial nucleus (>1840)*** rostrally and ***inferior salivatory nucleus (>1840)*** caudally, and generating the motor component of the ***intermediate nerve (>1840)***. Functionally, the ***superior salivatory nucleus (>1840)*** contains preganglionic parasympathetic ***neurons (Waldeyer, 1891)*** preferentially influencing secretions of the lacrimal gland and the submandibular and sublingual salivary glands; see Williams & Warwick (1980, pp. 1070, 1123), Tóth et al. (1999), Nieuwenhuys et al. (2008, pp. 191, 203). It was not delineated by 1840.

superior temporal gyrus (>1840)

As described for macrodissected adult human, a topographic subdivision of the ***temporal region (>1840)*** lying between ***transverse temporal gyri (>1840)*** dorsomedially and ***superior temporal sulcus (>1840)*** ventrally; see Williams & Warwick (1980, Figs. 7.111A, 7.112). It was clearly delineated by Gall & Spurzheim, 1810); see ***[superior temporal gyrus (>1840)] (Gall & Spurzheim, 1810)***.

EARLIER REFERENCES:

Illustrated, not named or described:

1. ***[superior temporal gyrus (>1840)] (Gall & Spurzheim, 1810)***
   As clearly illustrated for macrodissected adult human as modern attempts; Plate VIII; also see Rolando (1831, Fig. 1-4,5).

Earlier synonyms:

1. *superior enteroid processes of middle lobe (Rolando, 1831)*
   Synonym for macrodissected adult human ***superior temporal gyrus (>1840)***; in the original Italian, *processo enteroideo superiore del lobo mezzano*, Figure 1:3-5. Region labeled 3 is now included in ***supramarginal gyrus (>1840)***.

PARTLY CORRESPONDS:

1. *area temporalis superior (Brodmann, 1909)*
   Original Latin form of *superior temporal area (Brodmann, 1909)*; p. 144.
2. *superior temporal area (Brodmann, 1909)*
   Based on cellular architecture in adult human, roughly caudal (posterior) three-quarters of ***superior temporal gyrus (>1840)***; see Garey translation (1994, p. 124 and Fig. 85).
3. *area 22 (Brodmann, 1909)*
   Synonym for adult human *superior temporal area (Brodmann, 1909)*; in the original German, *Feld* 22, p. 144.

superior temporal sulcus (>1840)

As described for macrodissected adult human, a groove lying between ***superior temporal gyrus (>1840)*** and ***middle temporal gyrus (>1840)*** and extending dorsally and caudally into the ***parietal region (>1840)*** where it is surrounded by the ***angular gyrus (>1840)***; see Williams & Warwick (1980, Fig. 7.111A). It was first clearly described by Reil; see ***[superior temporal sulcus (>1840)] (Reil, 1809b)***.

EARLIER REFERENCES:

Described, not named or illustrated:

1. ***[superior temporal sulcus (>1840)] (Reil, 1809b)***
   Clearly described for macrodissected adult human; see Mayo translation (1823, pp. 78–79).

Illustrated, not named or described:

1. ***[superior temporal sulcus (>1840)] (Gall & Spurzheim, 1810)***
   As clearly illustrated for macrodissected adult human as modern attempts; Plate VIII.

superior testicular nerves (>1840)

As described for macrodissected adult human male, they arise as two or more rootlets from the caudal (lower) end of the ***renal plexus (Drake, 1707)*** and ***intermesenteric plexus (>1840)***, often receive additional branchlets from the second or third ***lumbar splanchnic nerves (Cruveilhier, 1836)***, and sometimes receive branchlets from the caudal (lower) part of the ***celiac ganglion (Walter, 1783)*** and/or origin of the ***superior mesenteric plexus (Rau, 1720)***. They communicate with the ***superior ureteric nerves (Walter, 1783)*** or share common rootlets of origin, and the rootlets coalesce into several ***nerves (Herophilus, c335–c280 BC)*** descending along the testicular artery and supplying the artery and testes, but not the epididymis to any great extent; see Mitchell (1953, pp. 293–295). They were known in outline to Haller; see ***[superior testicular nerves (>1840)] (Haller, 1762)***.

EARLIER REFERENCES:

Described, not named or illustrated:

1. ***[superior testicular nerves (>1840)] (Haller, 1762)***
   Vaguely described for macrodissected adult human male; p. 265. Vesalius described ***nerves (Herophilus, c335–c280 BC)*** to testes as a group for macrodissected adult human; see *branch of sixth pair stretching along roots of ribs offshoots to testes (Vesalius, 1543a)*.

Earlier synonyms:

1. *spermatic plexus (Soemmerring, 1791)*
   Probably synonym for macrodissected adult human ***superior testicular nerves (>1840)***; in the original Latin, *plexus spermaticus*, p. 340.
2. *internal spermatic nerve (Mayer, 1794)*
   Probably synonym for macrodissected adult human ***superior testicular nerves (>1840)***; in the original Latin, *nervus spermaticus internus*; Part 6, Table VI-248 (p. 43).
3. *superior branches of spermatic nerve (Fyfe, 1800)*
   Synonym for macrodissected adult human ***superior testicular nerves (>1840)***; Vol. 2, p. 325.
4. *internal branches of spermatic nerve (Fyfe, 1800)*
   Synonym for macrodissected adult human ***superior testicular nerves (>1840)***; Vol. 2, p. 325.

PARTLY CORRESPONDS:

1. *interior superior spermatic plexus (Soemmerring, 1798)*
   Equivalent for macrodissected adult human male of *superior internal spermatic nerve (Walter, 1783)*, which

applied to female; in the original Latin, *plexus spermaticus superior interior*, p. 360; also see Soemmerring (1791, p. 340).

2. *plexum spermaticum inferiorem interiorem (Soemmerring, 1798)*
As described for macrodissected adult human male, probably a ***superior testicular nerve (>1840)***; p. 360.

superior thoracic ganglion (Lieutaud, 1742)

As described for macrodissected adult human, when present the most rostral (superior) of the ***thoracic sympathetic ganglia (>1840)***. In about three-quarters of macrodissected adult humans it is fused with the ***inferior cervical ganglion (Vieussens, 1684)*** forming the *cervicothoracic ganglion (>1840)*; see Mitchell (1953, pp. 227–238), Williams & Warwick (1980, pp. 1130–1131). For Lieutaud's use in macrodissected adult human, see p. 438, where he noted it is often fused with the ***inferior cervical ganglion (Vieussens, 1684)***. It was discovered and described as the *plexus ganglioformis thoracicus nervi intercostalis (Vieussens, 1684)*.

EARLIER REFERENCES:

Earlier synonyms:

1. *plexus ganglioformis thoracicus nervi intercostalis (Vieussens, 1684)*
Synonym for macrodissected adult human ***superior thoracic ganglion (Lieutaud, 1742)***; loosely translated "thoracic ganglionic infolding of intercostal nerve". Palfijn (1726, Part 2, p. 334) gave the French, *plexus gangliforme thorachique de l'intercostal*.
2. *intercostal plexus (Drake, 1707)*
Roughly synonymous with macrodissected adult human ***superior thoracic ganglion (Lieutaud, 1742)***, although perhaps more accurately with *cervicothoracic ganglion (>1840)*; in the original Latin, *plexus intercostalis*, p. 519.
3. *first thoracic ganglion (Winslow, 1733)*
Synonym for macrodissected adult human ***superior thoracic ganglion (Lieutaud, 1742)***; Section VI, p. 96. Soemmerring (1791, p. 325) provided the Latin form, *ganglion thoracicum primus*.
4. *first dorsal ganglion (Winslow, 1733)*
Synonym for macrodissected adult human *first thoracic ganglion (Winslow, 1733)*; Section VI, p. 96. Soemmerring (1791, p. 325) provided the Latin form, *ganglion dorsale primum*.

LATER SYNONYMS:

1. *ganglio dorsali magno (Camper, 1760–1762)*
Synonym for macrodissected adult human ***superior thoracic ganglion (Lieutaud, 1742)***; legend for Table 1, Figure 1-*7,10*. The form, *ganglion dorsale magnum*, listed by Soemmerring (1791, p. 325).
2. *ganglion dorsale superius (Camper, 1760–1762)*
Synonym for macrodissected adult human ***superior thoracic ganglion (Lieutaud, 1742)***; p. 10 and legend for Table 1, Figure 1:*7,10–13*.
3. *second dorsal ganglion (Neubauer, 1772)*
Unfortunate synonym for ***superior thoracic ganglion (Lieutaud, 1742)***; in the original Latin, *ganglion dorsale secundum*, Table I-*88*. Also see Scarpa (1794, Tab. III-*100*).
4. *first pectoral ganglion (Schreger, 1803)*
Synonym listed for macrodissected adult human ***superior thoracic ganglion (Lieutaud, 1742)***; in the original Latin, *g. pectoris primum*, p. 358.
5. *superior pectoral ganglion (Schreger, 1803)*
Synonym listed for macrodissected adult human ***superior thoracic ganglion (Lieutaud, 1742)***; in the original Latin, *g. pectoris supremum*, p. 358.
6. *great pectoral ganglion (Schreger, 1803)*
Synonym listed for macrodissected adult human ***superior thoracic ganglion (Lieutaud, 1742)***; in the original Latin, *g. pectoris magnum*, p. 358.
7. *ganglion thoracicum supremum (Meckel, 1817)*
Latin form of ***superior thoracic ganglion (Lieutaud, 1742)***; see translation (1832, Vol. 3, p. 96).
8. *great thoracic ganglion (Lobstein, 1823)*
Synonym for macrodissected adult human *ganglium dorsale superius (Camper, 1760–1762)*; see translation (1831, p. 12).

superior ureteric nerves (Walter, 1783)

As described for macrodissected adult human, they arise from caudal (lower) parts of the ***renal plexus (Drake, 1707)*** and run caudally (downward) along rostral (upper) parts of the ureter to form rostral (upper) parts of the ***ureteric plexus (>1840)***; see Mitchell (1953, p. 293). For Walter's use in macrodissected adult human, probably its first clear delineation, see Table 1-*281*.

TRANSLATIONS:

1. *nervos uretiricos superiores (Walter, 1783)*
Original Latin form of ***superior ureteric nerves (Walter, 1783)***; Table I-*281*.

LATER SYNONYMS:

1. *ureteric nerves (Tiedemann, 1822)*
Synonym for macrodissected adult human female ***superior ureteric nerves (Walter, 1783)***; Table I-55.

supraclavicular nerves (Meckel, 1817)

As described for macrodissected adult human, they arise from the ***descending superficial branches of cervical plexus (Quain, 1828)*** and divide into three branches—***medial supraclavicular nerves (>1840)***, ***intermediate supraclavicular nerves (>1840)***, and ***lateral supraclavicular nerves (>1840)***—distributing to skin and fascia of the caudal (inferior) part of the side of the neck, ventral side (front) of the chest, and shoulder; see Durward (1951, pp. 1063–1064 and Figs. 919, 921), Williams & Warwick (1980, p. 1092). For Meckel's use in macrodissected adult human, see translation (1832, Vol. 3, p. 31). They were known to Galen; see ***[supraclavicular nerves (Meckel, 1817)] (Galen, c173)***.

EARLIER REFERENCES:

Described, not named or illustrated:

1. ***[supraclavicular nerves (Meckel, 1817)] (Galen, c173)***

Alluded to for macrodissected adult beef, pig, and/or macaque but not human; see May translation (1968, p. 598), and Duckworth translation (1962, p. 238).

Illustrated and described, not named:

1. ***[supraclavicular nerves (Meckel, 1817)] (Vesalius, 1543a)***
Alluded to in macrodissected adult human, although common trunk arose from fifth ***cervical nerve (Galen, c173)***; see Richardson & Carman translation (2002, p. 228). Eustachi illustrated their distribution beautifully for macrodissected adult human; see Albinus edition (1761, Tab. 21-*i*).

Earlier synonyms:

1. *subcutaneous thoracic nerves (Neubauer, 1772)*
Synonym for macrodissected adult human ***supraclavicular nerves (Meckel, 1817)***, with three branches; in the original Latin, *nervi subcutanei throracis*, Table 1-*211*.
2. *nervi summi humeri (Neubauer, 1772)*
Synonym for macrodissected adult human *subcutaneous thoracic nerves (Neubauer, 1772)*; Tables 1-*209*, 2:*56–58*.
3. *superclavicular nerves (Bell & Bell, 1816)*
Synonym for macrodissected adult human ***supraclavicular nerves (Meckel, 1817)***; in the original Latin, *superclaviculares*, Vol. 2, p. 514. Bell & Bell attributed without citation the term to Soemmerring.

LATER SYNONYMS:

1. *supraclavicular branches of cervical plexus (Cruveilhier, 1836)*
Synonym for macrodissected adult human ***supraclavicular nerves (Meckel, 1817)***; in the original French, *branches sus-claviculaires du plexus cervical*, p. 785.

PARTLY CORRESPONDS:

1. *trunk of supraclavicular nerves (Peipers, 1793)*
Single macrodissected adult human ***nerve (Herophilus, c335–c280 BC)*** formed by two roots from third and fourth cervical ***spinal nerve ventral branches (>1840)*** of ***cervical plexus (Molinetti, 1675)*** and dividing distally into three branches corresponding to ***medial supraclavicular nerves (>1840)***, ***intermediate supraclavicular nerves (>1840)***, and ***lateral supraclavicular nerves (>1840)***; in the original Latin, *truncus nervorum supraclavicularium*, p. 35.
2. *supraclavicular branches of cervical plexus (Cloquet, 1816)*
Roughly the ***medial supraclavicular nerves (>1840)*** and ***intermediate supraclavicular nerves (>1840)*** considered together; in the original French, *rameaux sus-claviculaires*, p. 639. See Williams & Warwick (1980, Fig. 7.198).
3. *clavicular branches of descending superficial branches of cervical plexus (Quain, 1828)*
Synonym for macrodissected adult human *supraclavicular branches of cervical plexus (Cloquet, 1816)*; in the original Latin, *claviculares*, p. 490. Quain also described two deeper branches to underlying muscles.
4. *clavicular nerve (Quain, 1828)*
Synonym for *clavicular branches of descending superficial branches of cervical plexus (Quain, 1828)*; p. 681.
5. *supraclavicular nerves (Cruveilhier, 1836)*
Synonym for macrodissected adult human *supraclavicular branches of cervical plexus (Cloquet, 1816)*; in the original French, *nerfs sus-claviculaires*, p. 780.
6. *supraclavicular branch proper of cervical plexus (Cruveilhier, 1836)*
Synonym for *supraclavicular nerves (Cloquet, 1816)*; in the original French, *branche sus-claviculaire proprement dire*, p. 785.

supraesophageal ganglion (Grant, 1834a)

Invertebrate brain (>1840) lying dorsal to the digestive system in annelids and arthropods. One or more ***supraesophageal ganglia (Grant, 1834a)*** may be involved, depending on how many ***central nerve cords (Serres, 1824–1826)*** exist in a species and how much fusion occurs; see Bullock & Horridge (1965, pp. 662, 1609), Reisinger (1972), ***ventral ganglia (Anderson, 1837)***. For Grant's use see pp. 485–486; it was first recognized by Swammerdam, see ***[supraesophageal ganglion (Grant, 1834a)] (Swammerdam, c1675)***.

ALTERNATE SPELLINGS:

1. *supra-oesophageal ganglion (Grant, 1834a)*
Original spelling of ***supraesophageal ganglion (Grant, 1834a)***; p. 485.

EARLIER REFERENCES:

Illustrated and described, not named:

1. ***[supraesophageal ganglion (Grant, 1834a)] (Swammerdam, c1675)***
Swammerdam clearly described the *brain (Aristotle)* of arthropods and annelids as being behind (dorsal to) the digestive system in dissections viewed under the microscope; see translation (1758; e.g., p. 138, Tab. XXII, Fig. 6).

Earlier synonyms:

1. *supraesophageal brain (Cuvier, 1800)*
Synonym for ***supraesophageal ganglion (Grant, 1834a)*** applied to molluscs; in the original French, *cerveau placé sur l'esophage*, p. 313.
2. *ganglion before esophagus (Serres, 1824–1826)*
Synonym for ***supraesophageal ganglion (Grant, 1834a)*** applied to molluscs and other invertebrates; in the original French (plural), *ganglions pro-oesophagiens*, Vol. 2, p. 13.
3. *central commissure (Owen, 1832)*
Synonym for ***supraesophageal ganglion Grant, 1834a)*** applied to pearly nautilus; p. 37 & Plate VII, Figure 3-*1*.
4. *general commissure (Owen, 1832)*
Synonym for ***supraesophageal ganglion (Grant, 1834a)*** applied to pearly nautilus; p. 38.
5. *cerebral lobes (Newport, 1832)*
Synonym for ***supraesophageal ganglion (Grant, 1834a)*** applied to hawkmoth, *Sphinx ligustri*; pp. 384–385.
6. *cerebral ganglia (Newport, 1834)*
Synonym for ***supraesophageal ganglion (Grant, 1834a)*** applied to hawkmoth, *Sphinx ligustri*; p. 389.

7. *brain (Solly, 1836)*
   Synonym for ***supraesophageal ganglion (Grant, 1834a)***; p. 42.
8. *superior ganglion of primary nervous ring (Anderson, 1837)*
   Synonym for ***supraesophageal ganglion (Grant, 1834a)*** applied, e.g., to crustaceans, arachnoids, and insects; p. 15.

supramammillary decussation (>1840)

As described for adult mammal with normal and experimental histological pathway tracing methods, a poorly understood ***central nervous system white matter tract (>1840)*** crossing the median plane in the caudal ***hypothalamus (Kuhlenbeck, 1927)***, centered between ***supramammillary nucleus (>1840)*** ventrally and ***posterior hypothalamic nucleus (>1840)*** dorsally; see Nauta & Haymaker (1969, pp. 148–149), Swanson (2004, Atlas Levels 34–35 and p. 178 note *123*). It was not discovered by 1840.

EARLIER REFERENCES:

Earlier synonyms:

1. *posterior subthalamic decussation (Honegger, 1890)*
   Synonym for ***supramammillary decussation (>1840)*** in adult human and other mammals with histological methods for ***axons (Kölliker, 1896)***; in the original Latin, *decussatio subthalamica posterior*, pp. 353–367.

supramarginal gyrus (>1840)

As described for macrodissected adult human, the rostral (anterior) topographic subdivision of the ***inferior parietal lobule (>1840)***, surrounding the ***posterior branch of lateral cerebral sulcus (>1840)***; see Williams & Warwick (1980, p. 986, Fig. 7.111A), *Terminologia Anatomica* (1998, p. 125). It was clearly delineated by Rolando; see ***[supramarginal gyrus (>1840)] (Rolando, 1831)***.

EARLIER REFERENCES:

Illustrated, not named or described:

1. ***[supramarginal gyrus (>1840)] (Rolando, 1831)***
   Clearly illustrated for macrodissected adult human; Figure 1-3,27,15.

Earlier synonyms:

1. *area supramarginalis (Brodmann, 1909)*
   Original Latin form of *supramarginal area (Brodmann, 1909)*; p. 140.
2. *supramarginal area (Brodmann, 1909)*
   Based on cellular architecture in adult human, corresponds roughly with ***supramarginal gyrus (>1840)***; see Garey translation (1994, p. 119 and Fig. 85).
3. *area 40 (Brodmann, 1909)*
   Synonym for adult human *supramarginal area (Brodmann, 1909)*; in the original German, *Feld 40*, p. 140.

supraoptic decussations (>1840)

As described for macrodissected adult human, a set of complex, poorly understood ***central nervous system white matter tracts (>1840)*** crossing the median plane of the ***hypothalamus (Kuhlenbeck, 1927)*** just dorsal and caudal to the ***optic chiasm (Galen, c173)***. They are commonly divided into the ***ventral supraoptic decussation (>1840)***, often called *Gudden's commissure (>1840)*, and the ***dorsal supraoptic decussation (>1840)***, often divided into dorsal and ventral parts called *Ganser's decussation (>1840)* and *Meynert's decussation (>1840)*, respectively; see Nauta & Haymaker (1969, pp. 189–190), *Nomina Anatomica* (1983, p. A70 note *148*). They were probably first identified, however vaguely, by Willis; see ***[supraoptic decussations (>1840)] (Willis, 1672)***.

EARLIER REFERENCES:

Illustrated, not named or described:

1. ***[supraoptic decussations (>1840)] (Willis, 1672)***
   Willis dissected and illustrated a *transverse medullary tract* crossing the median plane of the sheep ***brain (Smith Papyrus, c1700 BC)***, just caudal to the ***optic tracts (Vicq d'Azyr, 1786)*** and rostral to the *pituitary gland (Galen, c192)*; it seems likely he identified the ***supraoptic decussations (>1840)***; see Pordage translation (1683, Tab. VI-*I*). He also labeled a "tract leading to the tunnel [*infundibulum (Rufus of Ephesus, fl. c90–120)*] of the Brain" in the median plane between this transverse medullary tract and the *pituitary gland (Galen, c192)*; see Pordage translation (1683, Tab. VI-*E*). Its identity is unclear.

Described, not named or illustrated:

1. ***[supraoptic decussations (>1840)] (Monro, 1783)***
   Monro illustrated surface of right and left adult human *tuber cinereum (Soemmerring, 1778)*, between ***infundibulum (Rioch et al., 1940)*** caudally and ***optic chiasm (Galen, c173)*** rostrally, and in the legend described them as, "Cineritious [gray] substances intimately connected to the optic nerves, and furnishing some part of their medullary substance..." (Tab. V-*I*). This was confirmed by Meckel (1817); see translation (1832, Vol. 3, p. 78). Solly (1836, p. 244) clearly described them for macrodissected adult human tissue hardened in spirits, and in the mole where ***optic nerves (Vicq d'Azyr, 1786)*** are essentially lacking; he credited Mr. Mayo for pointing out the feature to him.

Earlier synonyms:

1. *transverse band under optic nerve (Spurzheim, 1826)*
   Possibly refers to macrodissected adult human ***supraoptic decussations (>1840)***; p. 232-35 and Plate VIII, Figure 1-*A*.
2. *supraoptic commissures (>1840)*
   Synonym for macrodissected adult human ***supraoptic decussations (>1840)***; see *Nomina Anatomica* (1983, p. A70 note *148*).

supraorbital nerve (Meckel, 1753)

As described for macrodissected adult human, a lateral branch of the ***frontal nerve (Cheselden, 1726)*** supplying palpebral branches to the upper eyelid and conjunctiva and then dividing into a ***medial branch of supraorbital***

nerve (>1840) and ***lateral branch of supraorbital nerve (>1840)*** supplying skin of the scalp, and reaching nearly as far dorsally (back) as the lambdoid suture; in addition the undivided trunk and both branches supply smaller branches to mucous membrane of the frontal sinus and the pericranium; see Hamilton (1976, Figs. 791, 798), Williams & Warwick (1980, p. 1061). For Meckel's use in macrodissected adult human, see p. 42. It was originally described as the *first offshoot of thinner root of third pair (Vesalius, 1543a).*

EARLIER REFERENCES:

Earlier synonyms:

1. *first offshoot of thinner root of third pair (Vesalius, 1543a)*
 Synonym for ***supraorbital nerve (Meckel, 1753),*** partly described and illustrated for macrodissected adult human; see Richardson & Carman translation (2002, p. 188).
2. *first branch of third conjugation of nerves of brain (Crooke, 1615)*
 Synonym for macrodissected adult human ***supraorbital nerve (Meckel, 1753)***; p. 486. Crooke's description was translation of Bauhin (1605), where it was pointed out that Falloppio (1561) regarded this branch as purely motor; see Crooke (1615, p. 889).
3. *exterior twig of superior branch of first branch of fifth pair (Haller, 1743)*
 Synonym for macrodissected adult human ***supraorbital nerve (Meckel, 1753)***; in the original Latin, *primi rami quinti paris ramus superior surculus exterior,* p. 45 note 21.

LATER SYNONYMS:

1. *greater frontal nerve (Meckel, 1753)*
 Synonym for macrodissected adult human ***supraorbital nerve (Meckel, 1753)***; in the original French, *le grand nerf frontal (du premier rameau de la cinquième paire),* p. 40, Table 1-*I*. Günther provided the Latin, *nervis frontalis major,* p. 42.
2. *supraorbital branch of first branch of fifth pair of nerves (Meckel, 1753)*
 Synonym for macrodissected adult human ***supraorbital nerve (Meckel, 1753)***; in the original French, *le rameau sous-orbital (du premier rameau de la cinquième paire),* p. 40.
3. *frontal nerve proper (Meckel, 1817)*
 Synonym for ***supraorbital nerve (Meckel, 1753)***; see translation (1832, Vol. 3, p. 64). Bell & Bell (1829, p. 490) called it *proper frontal nerve.*
4. *external branch of frontal nerve (Quain, 1828)*
 Synonym for macrodissected adult human ***supraorbital nerve (Meckel, 1753)***; p. 648.
5. *supra-orbital branch of first trunk of fifth nerve (Swan, 1830)*
 Synonym for macrodissected adult human ***supraorbital nerve (Meckel, 1753)***; Plate XII, Figure 6-7.
6. *supraorbital branch of frontal nerve (Arnold, 1834)*
 Synonym for macrodissected adult human ***supraorbital nerve (Meckel, 1753)***; in the original Latin, *nervus frontalis, ramus supraorbitalis,* p. 7.
7. *external frontal nerve (Cruveilhier, 1836; Todd, 1836–1839)*
 Synonym for macrodissected adult human ***supraorbital nerve (Meckel, 1753)***; Cruveilhier, p. 912; Todd, p. 279.

PARTLY CORRESPONDS:

1. *anastomotic branch of greater frontal nerve (Meckel, 1753)*
 A third branch of macrodissected adult human ***supraorbital nerve (Meckel, 1753),*** communicating with ***temporal branches of facial nerve (Swan, 1830)***; in the original French, *le rameau anastomotique du grand nerf frontal,* Table 1-3. Also see Hamilton (1976, Fig. 798).
2. *external superior palpebral nerve (Meckel, 1753)*
 Branch of *anastomotic branch of greater frontal nerve (Meckel, 1753)* for macrodissected adult human; in the original French, *le nerf palpébral supérieur (de le rameau anastomotique du grand nerf frontal),* Table 1-4.
3. *superficial frontal thread of supraorbital fascicle (Bellingeri, 1818)*
 Branch of macrodissected adult human ***supraorbital nerve (Meckel, 1753)*** for which Bellingeri described and named three finer branches; in the original Latin, *frontalis superficialis,* see Table I.
4. *palpebro-frontal filament of superficial frontal thread of supraorbital fascicle (Bellingeri, 1818)*
 Branch of macrodissected adult human ***supraorbital nerve (Meckel, 1753)*** to upper eyelid; in the original Latin, *filament palpebro-frontalis,* see Table I.
5. *external anastomotic filament of superficial frontal thread of supraorbital fascicle (Bellingeri, 1818)*
 Macrodissected adult human ***communicating branch (Winslow, 1733)*** of ***supraorbital nerve (Meckel, 1753)*** with ***zygomatic branches of facial nerve (>1840)***; in the original Latin, *stamen anastomoticus externus,* see Table I.
6. *internal anastomotic filament of superficial frontal thread of supraorbital fascicle (Bellingeri, 1818)*
 Macrodissected adult human ***communicating branch (Winslow, 1733)*** of ***supraorbital nerve (Meckel, 1753)*** with ***zygomatic branches of facial nerve (>1840)*** and ***supratrochlear nerve (Schaarschmidt, 1750)***; in the original Latin, *stamen anastomoticus internus,* see Table I.
7. *deep frontal thread of supraorbital fascicle (Bellingeri, 1818)*
 Branch of macrodissected adult human ***supraorbital nerve (Meckel, 1753)*** for which Bellingeri described and named two finer branches; in the original Latin, *frontalis profundus,* see Table I.
8. *external subcutaneous filament of deep frontal thread of supraorbital fascicle (Bellingeri, 1818)*
 Lateral cutaneous branch of *deep frontal thread of supraorbital fascicle (Bellingeri, 1818)* for which Bellingeri described and named three even smaller branches; in the original German, *subcutaneus externus,* see Table I.
9. *anastomotic fibril of external subcutaneous filament of deep frontal thread of supraorbital fascicle (Bellingeri, 1818)*
 Communicating branch (Winslow, 1733) of *external subcutaneous filament of deep frontal thread of supraorbital fascicle (Bellingeri, 1818)* with frontal threads of ***supratrochlear nerve (Schaarschmidt, 1750)***; in the original Latin, *fibril anastomoticus,* see Table I.

10. *orbicular fibril of external subcutaneous filament of deep frontal thread of supraorbital fascicle (Bellingeri, 1818)*
Branch of *external subcutaneous filament of deep frontal thread of supraorbital fascicle (Bellingeri, 1818)* communicating with ***zygomatic branches of facial nerve (>1840)*** and supplying orbicularis oculi muscle; in the original Latin, *fibril anastomoticus*, see Table I.
11. *subcutaneous fibrils of external subcutaneous filament of deep frontal thread of supraorbital fascicle (Bellingeri, 1818)*
Cutaneous branches of *external subcutaneous filament of deep frontal thread of supraorbital fascicle (Bellingeri, 1818)*; in the original Latin, *fibrillae anastomoticus*, see Table I.
12. *palpebral branches of external frontal nerve (Cruveilhier, 1836; Todd, 1836–1839)*
Synonym for macrodissected adult human *palpebral branches of supraorbital nerve (Cruveilhier, 1836)*; Cruveilhier, p. 912; Todd, p. 280.
13. *palpebral branches of supraorbital nerve (Cruveilhier, 1836)*
Macrodissected adult human branches of ***supraorbital nerve (Meckel, 1753)*** to upper eyelid; in the original French, *rameaux palpébraux*, p. 912.
14. *descending branches of external frontal nerve (Cruveilhier, 1836)*
Synonym for *palpebral branches of supraorbital nerve (Cruveilhier, 1836)*; in the original French, *rameaux descendans*, p. 912.
15. *descending branches of supraorbital nerve (Cruveilhier, 1836)*
Synonym for *palpebral branches of supraorbital nerve (Cruveilhier, 1836)*; in the original French, *rameaux descendans*, p. 912.
16. *ascending branches of external frontal nerve (Cruveilhier, 1836)*
Synonym for *ascending branches of supraorbital nerve (Cruveilhier, 1836)*; in the original French, *rameaux ascendans*, p. 912.
17. *ascending branches of supraorbital nerve (Cruveilhier, 1836)*
Macrodissected adult human ***medial branch of supraorbital nerve (>1840)*** and ***lateral branch of supraorbital nerve (1840)*** considered together; in the original French, *rameaux ascendans*, p. 912.
18. *frontal branches of external frontal nerve (Cruveilhier, 1836)*
Synonym for *ascending branches of supraorbital nerve (Cruveilhier, 1836)*; in the original French, *rameaux frontaux*, p. 912.
19. *frontal branches of supraorbital nerve (Cruveilhier, 1836)*
Synonym for *ascending branches of supraorbital nerve (Cruveilhier, 1836)*; in the original French, *rameaux frontaux*, p. 912.
20. *osseous frontal branch of external frontal nerve (Cruveilhier, 1836)*
Synonym for *osseous frontal branch of supraorbital nerve (Cruveilhier, 1836)*; p. 913.
21. *osseous frontal branch of supraorbital nerve (Cruveilhier, 1836)*
For some macrodissected adult humans, branch of ***supraorbital nerve (Meckel, 1753)*** giving off periosteal filaments in a canal of the frontal bone and then becoming subcutaneous; in the original French, *rameau frontal osseux*, p. 913.

suprapineal recess (>1840)

As described for macrodissected adult human, a small extension of the **roof of third ventricle (>1840)** just rostral and then dorsal to the **pineal stalk (Burdach, 1822)**; see Williams & Warwick (1980, p. 981). It was not described by 1840.

suprascapular nerve (Bang, 1770)

As described for macrodissected adult human, it arises from the ***brachial plexus upper trunk (>1840)***, courses through the suprascapular notch, and distributes to the supraspinatus and infraspinatus muscles, and to the shoulder and acromioclavicular joints. See Durward (1951, p. 1070), Williams & Warwick (1980, p. 1096). For Bang's description in macrodissected adult human, see Figure I-70. It was known to Galen; see ***[suprascapular nerve (Bang, 1770)] (Galen, c192)***.

TRANSLATIONS:

1. *nervus suprascapularem (Bang, 1770)*
Original Latin form of ***suprascapular nerve (Bang, 1770)***; Figure I-70.

EARLIER REFERENCES:

Described, not named or illustrated:

1. ***[suprascapular nerve (Bang, 1770)] (Galen, c192)***
Clearly described for macrodissected adult beef, pig, and/or macaque but not human; see Duckworth translation (1962, pp. 245–247, 253–254, 256).

Earlier synonyms:

1. *first nerve entering arm (Vesalius, 1543a)*
Synonym for macrodissected adult human ***suprascapular nerve (Bang, 1770)***; see Richardson & Carman translation (2002, p. 238).
2. *first sinew coming to arm (Geminus, 1553)*
Synonym for macrodissected adult human *first nerve entering arm (Vesalius, 1543a)*; originally spelled *fyrste sinowe commynge to arme*, see *The table of the figures of sinewes*.
3. *first nerve of hand (Bauhin, 1605)*
Synonym for macrodissected adult human *first nerve entering arm (Vesalius, 1543a)*; see Crooke translation (1615, p. 901).
4. *scapular nerve (Monro, 1732)*
Synonym for macrodissected adult human ***suprascapular nerve (Bang, 1770)***, which Monro wrote becomes lost in the "supra and infra spinati muscles" (p. 28); in Latin, *nervus scapularis, scapularem*, see Haase (1781, pp. 96, 98).
5. *superscapular nerve (Haller, 1747)*
Synonym for macrodissected adult human ***suprascapular nerve (Bang, 1770)***; for Latin form, *nervus superscapularis*, see Haase (1781, p. 98). Spelled *superscapulary nerve* in translation of Burdin (1803, Vol. 1, p. 190).

6. *superior posterior scapular nerve (Monro, 1783)*
   Synonym for macrodissected adult human ***suprascapular nerve (Bang, 1770)***; Table 15-*11*.
7. *posterior scapular nerve (Monro, 1783)*
   Synonym for *superior posterior scapular nerve (Monro, 1783)*; Table 16-*15*.
8. *external scapular nerve (Günther, 1786)*
   Synonym for macrodissected adult human ***suprascapular nerve (Bang, 1770)***; in the original Latin, *nervus scapularis externus*, p. 73.
9. *exterior scapular nerve (Mayer, 1794)*
   Synonym for macrodissected adult human ***suprascapular nerve (Bang, 1770)***; in the original Latin, *nervus scapularis exterior*; Part 5, Table VI-α (p. 34).
10. *nervus supraspinatus scapulae (Scarpa, 1794)*
    Synonym for macrodissected adult human ***suprascapular nerve (Bang, 1770)***; Table III-*175*.
11. *suprascapular branch of brachial plexus (Cloquet, 1816)*
    Synonym for macrodissected adult human ***suprascapular nerve (Bang, 1770)***; in the original Latin, *branche sus-scapulaire*, p. 643.
12. *superior scapular nerve (Swan, 1830)*
    Synonym for macrodissected adult human ***suprascapular nerve (Bang, 1770)***; p. 26. Swan described all of its main branches.
13. *nerve of supraspinatus and infraspinatus muscles (Cruveilhier, 1836)*
    Synonym for macrodissected adult human ***suprascapular nerve (Bang, 1770)***; in the original French, *nerf des muscles sus et sous-épineux*, p. 793.

PARTLY CORRESPONDS:

1. *branch to supraspinatus muscle (Bock, 1827)*
   Branch of macrodissected adult human ***suprascapular nerve (Bang, 1770)***; in the original Latin, *ramus musculi supraspinati*, Table V, Figure 2-*46*.
2. *branch to infraspinatus muscle (Bock, 1827)*
   Branch of macrodissected adult human ***suprascapular nerve (Bang, 1770)***; in the original Latin, *ramus musculi infraspinati*, Table V, Figure 2-*47*.
3. *branch of superior scapular nerve to superior spinous muscle (Swan, 1830)*
   Branch from macrodissected adult human ***suprascapular nerve (Bang, 1770)*** to supraspinatus muscle; Plate XXIII, Figure 1-2.
4. *branch of superior scapular nerve to capsular ligament of shoulder joint (Swan, 1830)*
   Branch from macrodissected adult human ***suprascapular nerve (Bang, 1770)*** to shoulder joint; Plate XXIII, Figure 1-*4*.

supratrochlear nerve (Schaarschmidt, 1750)

As described for macrodissected adult human, a branch of the ***frontal nerve (Cheselden, 1726)*** sending smaller branches to conjunctiva and skin of the upper eyelid and then generating branches to skin of the lower part of the forehead near the median plane; see Williams & Warwick (1980, p. 1061), Hamilton (1976, Fig. 791). For Schaarschmidt's use in macrodissected adult human, see p. 15. It was first clearly delineated by Eustachi; see ***[supratrochlear nerve (Schaarschmidt, 1750)] (Eustachi, 1552)***.

TRANSLATIONS:

1. *nervus supratrochlearis (Schaarschmidt, 1750)*
   Original Latin form of ***supratrochlear nerve (Schaarschmidt, 1750)***; p. 15.

EARLIER REFERENCES:

Illustrated, not named or described:

1. ***[supratrochlear nerve (Schaarschmidt, 1750)] (Eustachi, 1552)***
   Illustrated for macrodissected adult human; see Albinus edition (1761, Tab. 18, Figs. 1, 3, 5-*Z*) and Meckel (1748, p. 31 note *a*).

Earlier synonyms:

1. *interior twig of superior branch of first branch of fifth pair (Haller, 1743)*
   Synonym for macrodissected adult human ***supratrochlear nerve (Schaarschmidt, 1750)***; in the original Latin, *primi rami quinti paris ramus superior surculus interior*, Fascicle 1, p. 45-*22*.
2. *supratrochlear branch of frontal nerve (Meckel, 1748)*
   Synonym for macrodissected adult human ***supratrochlear nerve (Schaarschmidt, 1750)***; in the original Latin, *supratrochlearem ramum frontalis nervi*, p. 31.

LATER SYNONYMS:

1. *lesser frontal nerve (Meckel, 1753)*
   Synonym for macrodissected adult human ***supratrochlear nerve (Schaarschmidt, 1750)***; in the original French, *le frontal moindre*, p. 44; *le petit nerf frontal*, Table 1-*13,20*. Günther (1786, p. 43) used Latin form, *nervis frontalis minor*, p. 43.
2. *internal frontal nerve (Meckel, 1753)*
   Synonym for macrodissected adult human ***supratrochlear nerve (Schaarschmidt, 1750)***; in the original French, *le nerf frontal intérieur*, p. 44.
3. *external lesser frontal nerve (Meckel, 1753)*
   Synonym for macrodissected adult human ***supratrochlear nerve (Schaarschmidt, 1750)***; in the original French, *le petit nerf frontal extérieur*, Table 1-*14*.
4. *super trochlearis (Bell & Bell, 1816)*
   Synonym for macrodissected adult human ***supratrochlear nerve (Schaarschmidt, 1750)***; Vol. 2, p. 489.
5. *internal branch of frontal nerve (Quain, 1828)*
   Synonym for macrodissected adult human ***supratrochlear nerve (Schaarschmidt, 1750)***; p. 648.
6. *supertrochlear branch of frontal nerve (Quain, 1828)*
   Synonym for macrodissected adult human ***supratrochlear nerve (Schaarschmidt, 1750)***; p. 648.

PARTLY CORRESPONDS:

1. *middle superior palpebral nerve (Meckel, 1753)*
   Apparently branch of macrodissected adult human ***supratrochlear nerve (Schaarschmidt, 1750)***; in the original French, *le nerf palpébral supérieur moyen*, Table 1-*15*.

2. *frontal branch of supratrochlear nerve (Meckel, 1753)*
   Described for macrodissected adult human ***supratrochlear nerve (Schaarschmidt, 1750)***; in the original French, *le rameau frontal du nerf supra-trochleaire*, Table 1-21.
3. *anastomotic threads of supratrochlear fascicle (Bellingeri, 1818)*
   Two macrodissected adult human ***communicating branches (Winslow, 1733)*** of ***supratrochlear nerve (Schaarschmidt, 1750)*** with ***infratrochlear nerve (Schaarschmidt, 1750)*** were described (1st and 4th *stamina*); in the original Latin, *stamina anastomoticus*, see Table I.
4. *internal superior palpebral thread of supratrochlear fascicle (Bellingeri, 1818)*
   Macrodissected adult human branch of ***supratrochlear nerve (Schaarschmidt, 1750)*** to medial part of upper eyelid; in the original Latin, *stamen palpebris superior internus*, see Table I.
5. *muscular threads of supratrochlear fascicle (Bellingeri, 1818)*
   Macrodissected adult human branches of ***supratrochlear nerve (Schaarschmidt, 1750)*** to orbicularis oculi muscle and "musculum supraciliarem"; in the original Latin, *stamina musculares*, see Table I.
6. *internal frontal thread of supratrochlear fascicle (Bellingeri, 1818)*
   Macrodissected adult human branch of ***supratrochlear nerve (Schaarschmidt, 1750)*** to lateral part of frontalis muscle; in the original Latin, *stamen frontalis internus*, see Table I.
7. *middle frontal threads of supratrochlear fascicle (Bellingeri, 1818)*
   Macrodissected adult human branch of ***supratrochlear nerve (Schaarschmidt, 1750)*** to lateral part of frontalis muscle, "musculum supraciliarem", and skin of forehead; in the original Latin, *stamina frontalis medius*, see Table I.
8. *external frontal thread of supratrochlear fascicle (Bellingeri, 1818)*
   Macrodissected adult human branch of ***supratrochlear nerve (Schaarschmidt, 1750)*** to lateral part of orbicularis oculi muscle; in the original Latin, *stamen frontalis externus*, see Table I.
9. *anastomotic thread of supratrochlear fascicle (Bellingeri, 1818)*
   Macrodissected adult human ***communicating branch (Winslow, 1733)*** of ***supratrochlear nerve (Schaarschmidt, 1750)*** with ***supraorbital nerve (Meckel, 1753)***; in the original Latin, *stamen anastomoticus*, see Table I.
10. *superior frontal threads of supratrochlear fascicle (Bellingeri, 1818)*
   Two macrodissected adult human branches of ***supratrochlear nerve (Schaarschmidt, 1750)*** to upper parts of frontalis muscle and overlying skin; in the original Latin, *stamina frontalis superior*, see Table I.
11. *anastomosis between supratrochlear nerve and infratrochlear (Langenbeck, 1826–1830)*
   Macrodissected adult human ***communicating branch (Winslow, 1733)*** between ***supratrochlear nerve (Schaarschmidt, 1750)*** and ***infratrochlear nerve (Schaarschmidt, 1750)***; in the original Latin, *anastomosis inter nervum supratrochlearem et infratrochlearem*, Fascicle III, Table XVII-25.
12. *ascending filaments of internal frontal nerve (Cruveilhier, 1836)*
   Synonym for *ascending filaments of supratrochlear nerve (Cruveilhier, 1836)*; p. 913.
13. *ascending filaments of supratrochlear nerve (Cruveilhier, 1836)*
   Macrodissected adult human small branches of ***supratrochlear nerve (Schaarschmidt, 1750)*** to forehead; in the original French, *filets ascendans*, p. 913.
14. *frontal filaments of internal frontal nerve (Cruveilhier, 1836)*
   Synonym for *ascending filaments of supratrochlear nerve (Cruveilhier, 1836)*; p. 913.
15. *frontal filaments of supratrochlear nerve (Cruveilhier, 1836)*
   Synonym for *ascending filaments of supratrochlear nerve (Cruveilhier, 1836)*; in the original French, *filets frontaux*, p. 913.
16. *descending filaments of internal frontal nerve (Cruveilhier, 1836)*
   Synonym for *descending filaments of supratrochlear nerve (Cruveilhier, 1836)*; p. 913.
17. *descending filaments of supratrochlear nerve (Cruveilhier, 1836)*
   Macrodissected adult human small branches of ***supratrochlear nerve (Schaarschmidt, 1750)*** to upper eyelid and ridge (dorsum) of nose; in the original French, *filets descendans*, p. 913.
18. *palpebral and nasal filaments of internal frontal nerve (Cruveilhier, 1836)*
   Synonym for *descending filaments of supratrochlear nerve (Cruveilhier, 1836)*; p. 913.
19. *palpebral and nasal filaments of supratrochlear nerve (Cruveilhier, 1836)*
   Synonym for *descending filaments of supratrochlear nerve (Cruveilhier, 1836)*; in the original French, *filets palpébraux et nasaux*, p. 913.
20. *palpebral branch of supra-trochlear nerve (Todd, 1836–1839)*
   Described for macrodissected adult human ***supratrochlear nerve (Schaarschmidt, 1750)***; p. 280.

sural communicating branch of common fibular nerve (>1840)

As described for macrodissected adult human, it arises near the head of the fibula from the ***common fibular nerve (>1840)*** and usually descends obliquely across the lateral head of the gastrocnemius muscle before joining in the middle of the leg the ***tibial root of sural nerve (>1840)*** of the ***medial cutaneous nerve of thigh (>1840)*** to form the ***sural nerve (Pietro da Cortona,***

1741), although sometimes it descends as a separate branch as far as the heel; see Cruveilhier (1836, p. 862), Williams & Warwick (1980, p. 1115 and Figs. 7.215, 216), *Terminologia Anatomica* (1998, p. 140). It was probably known to Galen; see ***[sural communicating branch of common fibular nerve (>1840)] (Galen, c177)***.

EARLIER REFERENCES:

Described, not named or illustrated:

1. ***[sural communicating branch of common fibular nerve (>1840)] (Galen, c177)***
   Probably alluded to in macrodissected adult beef, pig, and/or macaque but not human; see Singer translation (1999, p. 86, where Singer probably misidentified it as a nonhuman feature). Vesalius (1543a) clearly described and illustrated it for macrodissected adult human; see Richardson & Carman translation (2002, p. 260).

Earlier synonyms:

1. *peroneal communicating branch (Jördens, 1788)*
   Synonym for macrodissected adult human ***sural communicating branch of common fibular nerve (>1840)***; in the original Latin, *ramus* est *communicans peronei*, p. 3. Also see *tibial communicating nerve (Jördens, 1788)*.
2. *peroneal communicating nerve (Fischer, 1791)*
   Synonym for macrodissected adult human ***sural communicating branch of common fibular nerve (>1840)***; in the original Latin, *nervi communicantis peronei*, p. 31.
3. *fibular communicating branch (Bock, 1827)*
   Synonym for macrodissected adult human ***sural communicating branch of common fibular nerve (>1840)***; in the original Latin, *ram. communicans fibularis*, Table III-53. Spelled *communicans fibulae* by Quain & Wilson (1839, Pl. XXV, Fig. 1-*c*). Used by *Nomina Anatomica* (1983, p. A78), *Terminologia Anatomica* (1998, p. 140).
4. *communicating tibial branch from sciatic nerve (Swan, 1830)*
   Probably synonym for macrodissected adult human ***sural communicating branch of common fibular nerve (>1840)***; Plate XXV, Figure 2-20.
5. *peroneal saphenous nerve (Cruveilhier, 1836)*
   Synonym for macrodissected adult human ***sural communicating branch of common fibular nerve (>1840)***; in the original French, *nerf saphène péronier*, p. 862. Cruveilhier pointed out that no ***nerve (Herophilus, c335–c280 BC)*** shows more variability, especially for extent of its communication with ***tibial root of sural nerve (>1840)***.

PARTLY CORRESPONDS:

1. *common trunk for peroneal communicating and sural nerves (Fischer, 1791)*
   Probably segment of macrodissected adult human ***sural communicating branch of common fibular nerve (>1840)***; in the original Latin, *trunculum communem nervi communicantis peronei et suralis*, p. 31.
2. *communicating nerve of peroneal and posterior inferior cutaneous nerve (Knox, 1832)*
   Synonym for *common trunk for peroneal communicating and sural nerves (Fischer, 1791)*; Plate XVI-235.
3. *anastomotic branch of peroneal saphenous nerve with tibial saphenous nerve (Cruveilhier, 1836)*
   Macrodissected adult human ***communicating branch (Winslow, 1733)*** between *peroneal saphenous nerve (Cruveilhier, 1836)* and *tibial saphenous nerve (Cruveilhier, 1836)*; in the original French, *rameau anastomotique avec le saphène tibial*, p. 863.
4. *calcaneal branches of peroneal saphenous nerve (Cruveilhier, 1836)*
   Macrodissected adult human branches of *peroneal saphenous nerve (Cruveilhier, 1836)* to skin near heel; in the original French, *rameaux calcaniens*, p. 863.
5. *maleolar branch of peroneal saphenous nerve (Cruveilhier, 1836)*
   Macrodissected adult human branch of *peroneal saphenous nerve (Cruveilhier, 1836)* to skin near lateral malleolus; in the original French, *rameaux malléolaire*, p. 863.

sural nerve (Pietro da Cortona, 1741)

As described for macrodissected adult human, it most commonly arises in the popliteal fossa from the junction of the ***tibial root of sural nerve (>1840)*** and ***sural communicating branch of common fibular nerve (>1840)*** and then extends distally to supply cutaneous branches to the lateral and dorsal (back) sides of the distal third of the leg, ankle and heel, and lateral border of the foot, as well as articular branches to the ankle joint and tarsal joints; see Williams & Warwick (1980, Fig. 7.215) where the ***tibial root of sural nerve (>1840)*** is unlabeled proximal to (above) the junction, and the ***sural nerve ((Pietro da Cortona, 1741)*** is labeled distal to (below) the junction. In some textbooks the ***sural nerve (Pietro da Cortona, 1741)*** is shown arising directly from the ***tibial nerve (Haase, 1781)*** without considering the ***medial cutaneous nerve of calf (>1840)*** and its proximal ***tibial root of sural nerve (>1840)***; this is probably a less common way the ***sural nerve (Pietro da Cortona, 1741)*** arises in human. The ***sural nerve (Pietro da Cortona, 1741)*** was first clearly described by Galen; see ***[sural nerve (Pietro da Cortona, 1741)] (Galen, c177)***.

TRANSLATIONS:

1. *suralem nervum (Pietro da Cortona, 1741)*
   Original Latin form of ***sural nerve (Pietro da Cortona, 1741)***; p. 18.

EARLIER REFERENCES:

Described, not named or illustrated:

1. ***[sural nerve (Pietro da Cortona, 1741)] (Galen, c177)***
   Clearly described for macrodissected adult beef, pig, and/or macaque but not human; see Singer translation (1999, p. 87).

Illustrated and described, not named:

1. ***[sural nerve (Pietro da Cortona, 1741)] (Vesalius, 1543a)***

Described and illustrated for macrodissected adult human; see Richardson & Carman translation (2002, p. 261).

LATER SYNONYMS:

1. *posterior long cutaneous nerve of tibia (Martin, 1781)*
Synonym for macrodissected adult human ***sural nerve (Pietro da Cortona, 1741)***; in the original Latin, *nervus cutaneus longus posterior tibiae*, p. 241.
2. *external cutaneous nerve of foot (Günther, 1786)*
Synonym for macrodissected adult human ***sural nerve (Pietro da Cortona, 1741)***; in the original Latin, *nervus cutaneus externus pedis*, p. 87.
3. *long cutaneous nerve (Günther, 1786)*
Synonym for *external cutaneous nerve of foot (Günther, 1786)*; in the original Latin, *nervus cutaneus longus*, p. 87.
4. *exterior dorsal nerve (Günther, 1786)*
Synonym for *external cutaneous nerve of foot (Günther, 1786)*; in the original Latin, *nervus dorsalis exterior*, p. 87.
5. *first external inferior posterior cutaneous nerve (Fischer, 1791)*
Synonym for macrodissected adult human ***sural nerve (Pietro da Cortona, 1741)***; in the original Latin, *nervi cutanei posterioris inferioris externi primi*, p. 31.
6. *superior external subsural cutaneous nerve (Fischer, 1791)*
Synonym for macrodissected adult human ***sural nerve (Pietro da Cortona, 1741)***; in the original Latin, *nervi cutanei subsuralis externi superioris*, Table II, Figure 2-*238*.
7. *posterior long cutaneous nerve of leg (Mayer, 1794)*
Synonym for macrodissected adult human ***sural nerve (Pietro da Cortona, 1741)***; in the original Latin, *nervus cutaneus longus posterior cruris*; Part 5, Table VI-*18* (p. 37).
8. *long posterior cutaneous nerve of foot and leg (Meckel, 1817)*
Synonym for macrodissected adult human ***sural nerve (Pietro da Cortona, 1741)***; in the original Latin, *nervus cutaneus longus posterior tibiae*, see translation (1832, Vol. 3, p. 19).
9. *external cutaneous tibial nerve of foot (Meckel, 1817)*
Synonym for macrodissected adult human ***sural nerve (Pietro da Cortona, 1741)***; in the original Latin, *nervus cutaneus pedis externus tibiae*, see translation (1832, Vol. 3, p. 19).
10. *long cutaneous nerve of leg (Bock, 1827)*
Synonym for macrodissected adult human ***sural nerve (Pietro da Cortona, 1741)***; in the original Latin, *nerv. longus cutaneus cruris*, Table IV-*95*.
11. *long cutaneous branch of leg (Bock, 1827)*
Synonym for macrodissected adult human ***sural nerve (Pietro da Cortona, 1741)***; in the original Latin, *ram. longus cutaneus cruris*, Table IV-*95*.
12. *posterior long cutaneous nerve (Quain, 1828)*
Synonym for macrodissected adult human ***sural nerve (Pietro da Cortona, 1741)***; p. 274.
13. *external inferior posterior cutaneous nerve (Cloquet, 1828)*
Synonym for macrodissected adult human ***sural nerve (Pietro da Cortona, 1741)***; in the original French, *nerf cutané postérieur inférieur externe*, Plate CLXXI, Figure 2-*31*.
14. *first posterior inferior external cutaneous nerve (Knox, 1832)*
Knox's translation of *first external inferior posterior cutaneous nerve (Fischer, 1791)*; Plate XIV-*238*.
15. *external superior subsural cutaneous nerve (Knox, 1832)*
Knox's translation of *superior external subsural cutaneous nerve (Fischer, 1791)*; Plate XIV-*238*.
16. *first external posterior inferior cutaneous nerve (Knox, 1832)*
Knox's translation of *first external inferior posterior cutaneous nerve (Fischer, 1791)*; Plate XVI-*238*.

PARTLY CORRESPONDS:

1. *external saphenous nerve (Cloquet, 1816)*
Basically macrodissected adult human ***sural nerve (Pietro da Cortona, 1741)*** distal to ***tibial root of sural nerve (>1840)***; in the original French, *nerf saphène externe*, p. 677.
2. *tibial saphenous nerve (Cruveilhier, 1836)*
Synonym for macrodissected adult human *external saphenous nerve (Cloquet, 1816)*; in the original French, *nerf saphène tibial*, p. 868.
3. *external saphenous nerve branch of communication with external branch of musculo-cutaneous (Quain & Wilson, 1839)*
Macrodissected adult human ***communicating branch (Winslow, 1733)*** between ***sural nerve (Pietro da Cortona, 1741)*** and ***intermediate dorsal cutaneous nerve (>1840)***; Plate XXIV, Figure 1-*h*.

sympathetic cord (>1840)

As described for macrodissected adult mammal, a topographic division of the ***peripheral nervous system (Meckel, 1817)*** including the ***sympathetic trunk (Winslow, 1733)*** and ***sympathetic trunk ganglia (>1840)*** considered together; for description of human, see Mitchell (1953, pp. 29–31, 207–209). Gaskell called it the *sympathetic chain* in macrodissected dog (1886, p. 2), Herrick called it the *ganglionated cord* in macrodissected adult human (1915, Fig. 41), and Ranson called it the *sympathetic trunk* in macrodissected adult human (1920, p. 335). It was discovered by Galen; see ***[sympathetic cord (>1840)] (Galen, c173)***.

EARLIER REFERENCES:

Described, not named or illustrated:

1. ***[sympathetic cord (>1840)] (Galen, c173)***
Discovered in macrodissected adult beef, pig, and/or macaque but not human. Thus, Galen described ***sympathetic trunk (Winslow, 1733)***, which he called *nerve extending along roots of ribs (Galen, c173)*, and at least one ***sympathetic trunk ganglion (>1840)***, which he did not name but corresponds to ***superior cervical ganglion (Vieussens, 1684)***, see ***[superior cervical ganglion (Vieussens, 1684)] (Galen, c173)***.

Earlier synonyms:

1. *tri-splanchnic nerve (Chaussier, 1789)*
Synonym for macrodissected adult human ***sympathetic cord (>1840)***; in the original French, *nerf tri-splanchnique*, see *Table synoptique du nerf*

tri-splanchnic. It spans three of Chaussier's splanchnic compartments, tracheal, thoracic, and abdominal. Also see Burdin translation (1803, Vol. 1, p. 208).

2. *accessory great sympathetic nerve (Schmidt, 1794)*
   Apparently synonym for macrodissected adult human ***sympathetic cord (>1840)***; in the original Latin, *nervum sympathicum magnum accessorii*, see Table II:*7-18*.
3. *limiting cord (Meckel, 1817)*
   Synonym for macrodissected adult human ***sympathetic cord (>1840)***, and its full expression was limiting cord of *ganglionnary nerve (Meckel, 1817)*; see translation (1832, Vol. 3, p. 88). Meckel also mentioned *limiting cord trunk (Meckel, 1817)*, synonymous with ***sympathetic trunk (Winslow, 1733)***.
4. *external ganglionnary cord (Meckel, 1817)*
   Synonym for *limiting cord (Meckel, 1817)*, with *external* meaning *lateral*; see translation (1832, Vol. 3, p. 98).
5. *intercostal nerve (Lobstein, 1823)*
   Clearly used as synonym for macrodissected adult human ***sympathetic cord (>1840)***; see translation (1831, p. 54).
6. *sympathetic nerve (Lobstein, 1823)*
   Clearly used as synonym for macrodissected adult human ***sympathetic cord (>1840)***; see translation (1831, p. 55).
7. *ganglionated nerve (Bock, 1827)*
   Synonym for macrodissected adult human ***sympathetic cord (>1840)***; in the original Latin (plural), *nervi gangliosi*, Table I, Figure 1-*o,1*.
8. *sympathetic chain (Gaskell, 1886)*
   Synonym for macrodissected adult dog ***sympathetic cord (>1840)***, as nicely illustrated (with different nomenclature) for macrodissected adult human by Herrick (1915, Fig. 41); p. 2.

sympathetic root of ciliary ganglion (>1840)

As described for macrodissected adult human, a common but not invariant branch of the ***internal carotid plexus (>1840)*** going either directly to the ***ciliary ganglion (Loder, 1778)*** or indirectly via the ***nasociliary nerve (Meckel, 1817, Wutzer, 1817)*** and ***communicating branch of nasociliary nerve with ciliary ganglion (>1840)***; or sometimes even bypassing the ***ciliary ganglion (Loder, 1778)*** altogether and coursing through the ***long ciliary nerves (Soemmerring, 1801)*** directly to the eye; see Mitchell (1953, pp. 203–204, 217). For a history of ***nasociliary nerve (Meckel, 1817, Wutzer, 1817)*** involvement see Todd (1836–1839, p. 281). It was described at least as early as ***[sympathetic root of ciliary ganglion (>1840)] (Burdin, 1803)***.

EARLIER REFERENCES:

Described, not named or illustrated:

1. ***[sympathetic root of ciliary ganglion (>1840)] (Burdin, 1803)***
   Described for macrodissected adult human; see translation (1803, Vol. 1, p. 209). Also see Ribes (1811, p. 97), Lobstein (1831, pp. 34–35), Meckel (1832, Vol. 3, pp. 91–92). According to Cruveilhier (1836, p. 988), who provided no citation, Le Cat first described and illustrated it.

Earlier synonyms:

1. *middle root of ophthalmic ganglion (Arnold, 1834)*
   Synonym for macrodissected adult human ***sympathetic root of ciliary ganglion (>1840)***; in the original Latin, *ganglion ophthalmicum, radix media*, p. 8.
2. *middle root of ciliary ganglion (Arnold, 1834)*
   Synonym for macrodissected adult human ***sympathetic root of ciliary ganglion (>1840)***; in the original Latin, *ganglion ciliare, radix media*, p. 8.
3. *connection of cavernous sinus with ophthalmic ganglion (Arnold, 1834)*
   Synonym for macrodissected adult human ***sympathetic root of ciliary ganglion (>1840)***; in the original Latin, *conjunctio plexus cavernosus cum ganglio ophthalmico*, p. 18.
4. *connection of ophthalmic ganglion with sympathetic nerve (Arnold, 1834)*
   Synonym for macrodissected adult human ***sympathetic root of ciliary ganglion (>1840)***; in the original Latin, *conjunctio ganglion ophthalmicum cum nervo sympathico*; Table VIII-*21*.
5. *soft root of ophthalmic ganglion (Cruveilhier, 1836)*
   Synonym for macrodissected adult human ***sympathetic root of ciliary ganglion (>1840)***; in the original French, *racine molle*, p. 917.
6. *ganglionic root of ophthalmic ganglion (Cruveilhier, 1836)*
   Synonym for macrodissected adult human ***sympathetic root of ciliary ganglion (>1840)***; in the original French, *racine ganglionnaire*, p. 917.
7. *communicating filament between ophthalmic ganglion and superior cervical ganglion (Cruveilhier, 1836)*
   Synonym for macrodissected adult human ***sympathetic root of ciliary ganglion (>1840)***; in the original French, *filet de communication entre ce ganglion et le ganglion cervical supérieur*, p. 917.
8. *communicating filament of cavernous plexus with ophthalmic ganglion (Cruveilhier, 1836)*
   Synonym for macrodissected adult human ***sympathetic root of ciliary ganglion (>1840)***; in the original French, *filet de communication avec le ganglion ophthalmique*, p. 988.
9. *filament from carotid plexus to ciliary ganglion (Todd, 1836–1839)*
   Essentially synonym for macrodissected adult human ***sympathetic root of ciliary ganglion (>1840)***; p. 281.
10. *filament from cavernous ganglion to ciliary ganglion (Todd, 1836–1839)*
    Essentially synonym for macrodissected adult human ***sympathetic root of ciliary ganglion (>1840)***; p. 281.
11. *ciliary ganglion branch of communication to carotid plexus (Quain & Wilson, 1839)*
    Synonym for macrodissected adult human ***sympathetic root of ciliary ganglion (>1840)***; Plate XXVII-*E,i*.

12. *lenticular ganglion branch of communication to carotid plexus (Quain & Wilson, 1839)*
Synonym for macrodissected adult human ***sympathetic root of ciliary ganglion (>1840)***; Plate XXVII-*E,i*.

sympathetic root of otic ganglion (>1840)

As described for macrodissected adult human, extensions of the ***external carotid plexus (>1840)***, usually associated with the maxillary and middle meningeal arteries, to the ***otic ganglion (Arnold, 1828)***; see Mitchell (1953, p. 221). First described as the *soft root of otic ganglion (Arnold, 1834)*.

EARLIER REFERENCES:

Earlier synonyms:

1. *soft root of otic ganglion (Arnold, 1834)*
Synonym for macrodissected adult human ***sympathetic root of otic ganglion (>1840)***; in the original Latin, *ganglion oticum, radix mollis*, p. 10.
2. *soft root of auricular ganglion (Arnold, 1834)*
Synonym for macrodissected adult human ***sympathetic root of otic ganglion (>1840)***; in the original Latin, *ganglion auriculare, radix mollis*, p. 10.
3. *connection of soft nerves with otic ganglion (Arnold, 1834)*
Synonym for macrodissected adult human ***sympathetic root of otic ganglion (>1840)***; in the original Latin, *conjunctio nervi molles cum ganglio otico*, p. 18.
4. *connection of otic ganglion with supreme cervical ganglion* (Arnold, 1834)
Synonym for macrodissected adult human ***sympathetic root of otic ganglion (>1840)***; in the original Latin, *conjunctio ganglii otici cum ganglio cervicali supremo*, Table VII:*V-30*.
5. *soft nerves to otic ganglion from superior cervical ganglion (Quain & Wilson, 1839)*
Synonym for macrodissected adult human ***sympathetic root of otic ganglion (>1840)***; Plate XIII, Figure 1-*o*.

sympathetic root of submandibular ganglion (>1840)

As described for macrodissected adult human, the sympathetic rootlet(s) to the ***submandibular ganglion (>1840)*** are derived from an extension of the ***internal carotid plexus (>1840)*** along the facial artery or its submental branch; after passing through the ***submandibular ganglion (>1840)*** they extend into the submandibular and sublingual glands in the ***glandular branches of submandibular ganglion (>1840)*** along with postganglionic parasympathetic ***axons (Kölliker, 1896)***; see Mitchell (1953, p. 165), Williams & Warwick (1980, p. 1072), *Terminologia Anatomica* (1998, p. 142). It was first described by Scarpa; see ***[sympathetic root of submandibular ganglion (>1840)] (Scarpa, 1794)***.

EARLIER REFERENCES:

Illustrated and described, not named:

1. ***[sympathetic root of submandibular ganglion (>1840)] (Scarpa, 1794)***
Clearly described and illustrated for macrodissected adult human; in the original Latin, *mollia ganglii cervicalis superioris nervi intercostalis fila maxillarem glandulam subeuntia*, Table III-*69,70*.

Earlier synonyms:

1. *soft root of glottic ganglion (Arnold, 1834)*
Synonym for macrodissected adult human ***sympathetic root of submandibular ganglion (>1840)***; in the original Latin, *ganglion glotticum, radix mollis*, p. 11.
2. *soft root of lingual ganglion (Arnold, 1834)*
Synonym for macrodissected adult human *soft root of glottic ganglion (Arnold, 1834)*; in the original Latin, *ganglion linguale, radix mollis*, p. 11.
3. *soft root of maxillary ganglion (Arnold, 1834)*
Synonym for macrodissected adult human *soft root of glottic ganglion (Arnold, 1834)*; in the original Latin, *ganglion maxillare, radix mollis*, p. 11.
4. *soft root of Meckel's ganglion (Arnold, 1834)*
Synonym for macrodissected adult human *soft root of glottic ganglion (Arnold, 1834)*; in the original Latin, *ganglion Meckelii, radix mollis*, p. 11.
5. *connection of soft nerves with maxillary ganglion (Arnold, 1834)*
Synonym for macrodissected adult human *soft root of glottic ganglion (Arnold, 1834)*; in the original Latin, *conjunctio nervi molles cum ganglio maxillari*, p. 18.
6. *connection of maxillary ganglion with sympathetic nerve (Arnold, 1834)*
Synonym for macrodissected adult human *soft root of glottic ganglion (Arnold, 1834)*; in the original Latin, *conjunctio ganglion maxillare cum nervo sympathico*, Table VII:*V-41*.
7. *third root of maxillary ganglion (Arnold, 1834)*
Synonym for macrodissected adult human *soft root of glottic ganglion (Arnold, 1834)*; in the original Latin, *ganglion maxillare radix tertia*, Table VII:*V-41*.

sympathetic trunk (Winslow, 1733)

The ***nerve (Herophilus, c335–c280 BC)*** or ***white matter tract (Bell & Bell, 1826)*** part of the ***sympathetic cord (>1840)***. The ***sympathetic trunk ganglia (Winslow, 1733)*** are distributed along it, and it includes a rostral branch or extension, the ***internal carotid nerve (>1840)***. *Sympathetic trunk* is a synonym Winslow used (Sect. VI, p. 100) in macrodissected adult human for *great sympathetic nerve (Winslow, 1733)*, a feature known to Galen; see *nerve extending along roots of ribs (Galen, c173)*. Just before Winslow's description, Pourfour du Petit (1729) was the first clearly to separate its true origin from the ***cranial nerves (Soemmerring, 1791)***; see Best (1969). Winslow wrote that, "The Situation of these two Nerves in general, is on the lateral parts of the whole twenty-four Vertebrae, immediately before the Roots of the transverse Apophyses, and likewise on the lateral Parts of the inside of the Os Sacrum.

Through this large extent, they appear like two Ropes divided, in a manner intersected at different distances, by a great number of ganglioform tubercles, by means of which they communicate backward with the Ganglions of the Medulla Spinalis, by short collateral Filaments; and produce forward, all their particular Ramifications." (1733, Sect. VI, p. 94). He basically regarded the *sympathetic trunk (Winslow, 1733)* as a ***nerve (Herophilus, c335–c280 BC)*** that forms ***ganglia (Galen, c173)***, for example: "In its passage, each Trunk receives commonly two Filaments from each Ganglion of the Nervi Lumbares and Sacri, and likewise forms small Ganglions between each Vertebra, which send some Filaments to the neighbouring parts, and others which communicate with the Fasciculi of the Plexus Mesenterici." (1733, Sect. VI, p. 100). Earlier he wrote, "These Ganglions differ more or less from each other in Size, Colour and Consistence; and may be look'd upon as so many Origins or Germina dispersed through this great Pair of Nerves, and consequently as so many little Brains." (1733, Sect. VI, p. 94). They are now often classified as ***paravertebral ganglia (Durward, 1951)***. The ***sympathetic trunk (Winslow, 1733)*** was masterfully illustrated in Henle (1871, Fig. 299). This distinction between ***sympathetic trunk (Winslow, 1733)*** and ***sympathetic cord (>1840)*** is frequently not made, but has long been recognized by authorities like Willis [*trunk of intercostal nerve (Willis, 1664)*], Winslow, Meckel [*limiting cord trunk (Meckel, 1817)*], Herrick (1915, Fig. 41), and *Dorland's* (2003, p. 1956): "sympathetic trunk: two long nerve strands, one on each side of the vertebral column, extending from the base of the skull to the coccyx. Interconnected by nerve strands, each has cervical, thoracic, lumbar, and sacral sympathetic ganglia." A hint of the complex fiber organization of the ***sympathetic trunk (Winslow, 1733)*** is provided in illustrations by Strong & Elwyn (1943, Fig. 166, called *Sympathetic trunk*) and Williams & Warwick (1980, Fig. 7.224). Segments of the ***sympathetic trunk (Winslow, 1733)*** between successive ***sympathetic trunk ganglia (Winslow, 1733)*** are ***communicating branches of sympathetic trunk (>1840)***.

EARLIER REFERENCES:

Earlier synonyms:

1. *nerve extending along roots of ribs (Galen, c173)*
Galen discovered, described, and named the ***sympathetic trunk (Winslow, 1733)***; see May translation (1968, pp. 367, 695). He had it arise in some passages from the ***trigeminal nerve (Winslow, 1733)*** [his *third pair of nerves from brain (Galen, c192)* and *fourth pair of nerves from brain (Galen, c192)*; see Duckworth translation (1962, pp. 178, 192) and Savage-Smith (1971, pp. 178–179)] near the carotid canal, and then passing caudally (downward) through the canal; see Duckworth translation (1962, p. 198). In other passages he implied that it departs from the ***vagus nerve (Galen, c192)*** [part of *sixth pair of nerves from brain (Galen, c192)*; see May translation (1968, pp. 367, 694–696)] near its entry into the thorax, although he did note that the ***vagus nerve (Galen, c192)*** and *nerve extending along roots of ribs (Galen, c173)* travel together in a common sheath for some distance; see Duckworth translation (1962, pp. 198–199, 217). He also described, without naming, the ***superior cervical ganglion (Vieussens, 1684)***, *cervicothoracic ganglion (>1840)*, and perhaps ***celiac ganglion (Walter, 1783)***; see Mitchell (1953, p. 1), Duckworth translation (1962, p. 192), May translation (1968, pp. 695–696), Savage-Smith (1971, pp. 178–180), and Clarke & Jacyna (1987, p. 311). He dissected common large adult mammals but did not openly describe the results of human dissection. In a vague description, Achillini (1520; see Lind translation, 1975, pp. 59–60) had it arising from the *fourth pair of nerves arising from brain (Galen, c192)*—roughly ***trigeminal nerve motor root (Bell, 1829)***; see Burdach (1819, p. 213).
2. *nerve traversing canal in petrosal bone (Galen, c192)*
Synonym for *nerve extending along roots of ribs (Galen, c173)*, referring to carotid canal; see Duckworth translation (1962, p. 198).
3. *nerve emerging from petrosal bone (Galen, c192)*
Synonym for *nerve extending along roots of ribs (Galen, c173)*; see Duckworth translation (1962, p. 199).
4. *intercostal nerve (Willis, 1664)*
Synonym for ***sympathetic trunk (Winslow, 1733)***, regarded as branch of both ***trigeminal nerve (Winslow, 1733)*** and ***abducens nerve (Heister, 1717)***; see Pordage translation (1681, pp. 58, 115–116, 157 ff.), also see Best (1969, p. 159 ff.). In his unpublished plates finished around 1552, Eustachi illustrated branch from ***abducens nerve (Heister, 1717)*** to *intercostal nerve (Willis, 1664)*; see Best (1969, p. 160).
5. *trunk of intercostal nerve (Willis, 1664)*
Synonym for ***sympathetic trunk (Winslow, 1733)***; in the original Latin (plural), *nervi intercostalis truncus*, see Pordage translation (1681, pp. 116, 157 ff., and Tab. IX-D). Willis wrote, "The beginning of the Intercostal nerve are two or three shoots reflected or turned back from the Nerves of the fifth and sixth pair, and united into the same Trunk, *Figure 9. D. a.a.b.* Here we may wonder at the birth of this Nerve, as it were borrowed; for it grows as a shrub upon another tree or shrub; and therefore dispenses the common virtues and influences of either with a double branching, *viz.*, both its own and that of its parent: by which ramification or branching it comes to pass, that there are very quick commerces and consent between the conceptions of the Brain and the affections of the *Praecordia*, also between the Actions and Passions almost of all the parts of the whole body, which belong to the involuntary Function…
The intercostal Nerve being slid out of the Skull, presently constitutes the Ganglioform infolding [***superior cervical ganglion (Vieussens, 1684)***], Fig. 9.G. it being after the same manner in the Trunk of the wandring pair." (Pordage translation, 1681, p. 16). So basically, he thought of *intercostal nerve*

(Willis, 1664) as arising from roots associated with ***trigeminal nerve (Winslow, 1733)*** and ***abducens nerve (Heister, 1717)*** joining to form *trunk of intercostal nerve (Willis, 1664)*, which has ***ganglia (Galen, c173)*** associated with it, just as ***vagus nerve trunk (Wrisberg, 1786; Günther, 1786)*** has ***ganglia (Galen, c173)*** associated with it. And his hypothesis was that ultimately ***trigeminal nerve (Winslow, 1733)*** and ***abducens nerve (Heister, 1717)*** arise in ***cerebellum (Aristotle)***, the origins of instinctive and involuntary behaviors; see Pordage translation (1681, pp. 115–117).

6. *intercostal trunk (Willis, 1664)*
   Synonym for *trunk of intercostal nerve (Willis, 1664)*; see Pordage translation (1681, p. 157).
7. *little rope (Willis, 1664)*
   Synonym for *trunk of intercostal nerve (Willis, 1664)*; see Pordage translation (1681, p. 161).
8. *ninth pair of nerves arising within skull (Gibson, 1682)*
   Synonym for macrodissected adult human ***sympathetic trunk (Winslow, 1733)***; p. 339, also see *pairs of nerves arising within skull (Gibson, 1682)*.
9. *fibrous nerve (Salmon, 1714)*
   Synonym for macrodissected adult human *intercostal nerve (Willis, 1664)*, counting it as ninth pair of nerves from brain; p. 400. Also see *ninth pair of nerves arising within skull (Gibson, 1682)*.

LATER SYNONYMS:

1. *great sympathetic nerve (Winslow, 1733)*
   Synonym for macrodissected adult human ***sympathetic trunk (Winslow, 1733)***; Section VI, p. 93 and Section X, pp. 48, 51; also see Clarke & Jacyna (1987, p. 314). Winslow claimed to have concluded independently of Pourfour du Petit (1729) that it does not arise from the *pairs of nerves of medulla oblongata (Winslow, 1733)*; Section VI, p. 94. Winslow wrote, "These nerves, as I have said, are commonly called Intercostales, tho' this Name does not agree either with their Situation, or with the Extent of their Course, as we shall presently see; and therefore I believe the name of Sympathetici Majores, or Maximi, will be more proper, because of their frequent Communications with almost all the other principal Nerves of the Body." (1733, Sect. VI, p. 94). Neubauer (1772, p. 13) gave the Latin, *nervum sympatheticum magnum*.
2. *nervi sympathetici majores (Winslow, 1733)*
   Latin form of right and left *great sympathetic nerve (Winslow, 1733)*; Section VI, p. 94.
3. *nervi sympathetici maximi (Winslow, 1733)*
   Latin form of right and left *great sympathetic nerve (Winslow, 1733)*; Section VI, p. 94.
4. *vertebral nerve (Lieutaud, 1742)*
   Synonym for macrodissected adult human ***sympathetic trunk (Winslow, 1733)***; p. 435. Burdach (1819, p. 214) gave the Latin, *nervus vertebralis*.
5. *spinal nerve (Haller, 1747)*
   Synonym for macrodissected adult human ***sympathetic trunk (Winslow, 1733)***; see Mihles translation (1754b, p. 303).
6. *consensual nerve (Mayer, 1779)*
   Synonym for macrodissected adult human ***sympathetic trunk (Winslow, 1733)***; in the original Latin, *nervus consensualis*, according to Burdach (1819, p. 214).
7. *posterior intercostal nerve (Haase, 1781)*
   Synonym for macrodissected adult human ***sympathetic trunk (Winslow, 1733)***, at least at thoracic levels; in the original Latin, *nervus intercostalem posteriorem*, p. 123.
8. *trunk of great sympathetic nerve (Walter, 1783, Tab. 1)*
   Synonym for macrodissected adult human ***sympathetic trunk (Winslow, 1733)***, specifically without its branches; in the original Latin, *truncus nervi sympatheci magni*, see Tables 1-36, 3-346,347.
9. *sympathetic nerve (Soemmerring, 1791)*
   Synonym for macrodissected adult human ***sympathetic trunk (Winslow, 1733)***; in the original Latin, *nervus sympathicus* or *nervus sympatheticus*, p. 313. Müller (1828a,b) provided a detailed history and analysis of the invertebrate analog.
10. *forty-fourth nerve (Soemmerring, 1791)*
    Synonym for *sympathetic nerve (Soemmerring, 1791)*; in the original Latin, *quadragesimus quartus nervus*, p. 313.
11. *trunk of sympathetic nerve (Soemmerring, 1791)*
    Synonym for macrodissected adult human ***sympathetic trunk (Winslow, 1733)***; p. 323, also see Soemmerring (1798, p. 344) for the Latin, *nervi sympathici truncus*. See Lobstein translation (1831, p. 11) for term in English.
12. *eleventh pair of nerves (Malacarne, 1791)*
    Malacarne counted ***sympathetic trunk (Winslow, 1733)*** as 11th of 17 pairs of *cranial nerves (Malacarne, 1791)*; p. 227 ff.
13. *forty-fourth nerve of body (Andersch & Soemmerring, 1792)*
    Synonym for macrodissected adult human ***sympathetic trunk (Winslow, 1733)***; in the original Latin, *quadragesimus quartus nervus corporis*, p. 163.
14. *great nerve of body (Andersch, 1797)*
    Synonym for macrodissected adult human ***sympathetic trunk (Winslow, 1733)***; in the original Latin, *magno nervo corporis*, Vol. 1, p. 102.
15. *great harmonic nerve of body (Andersch, 1797)*
    Synonym for macrodissected adult human ***sympathetic trunk (Winslow, 1733)***; in the original Latin, *magno nervo harmonico corporis*, Vol. 1, p. 102.
16. *first nerve of body (Andersch, 1797)*
    Synonym for macrodissected adult human ***sympathetic trunk (Winslow, 1733)***; in the original Latin, *primum nervum corporis*, Vol. 1, p. 102. Later given as *primus nervus corporis*; Vol. 1, p. 105.
17. *forty-fifth nerve of body (Andersch, 1797)*
    Synonym for macrodissected adult human ***sympathetic trunk (Winslow, 1733)***; in the original Latin, *quadragesimus quintus nervus corporis*, Vol. 1, p. 102.
18. *first nerve of trunk (Andersch, 1797)*
    Almost certainly synonym for macrodissected adult human ***sympathetic trunk (Winslow, 1733)***; in the original Latin, *primus nervus trunci*, Vol. 2, p. 4.

19. *great intercostal nerve (Cuvier, 1800)*
Synonym for macrodissected adult human ***sympathetic trunk (Winslow, 1733)***; in the original French, *nerf grand intercostal*, Vol. 2, p. 285.
20. *limiting cord trunk (Meckel, 1817)*
Synonym for macrodissected adult human ***sympathetic trunk (Winslow, 1733)***; see translation (1832, Vol. 3, p. 93).
21. *ganglionated trunk (Burdach, 1819)*
Synonym for macrodissected adult human ***sympathetic trunk (Winslow, 1733)***; in the original German, *Ganglienstämme*, p. 78.
22. *Rumpfnerve (Burdach, 1819)*
German synonym for macrodissected adult human ***sympathetic trunk (Winslow, 1733)***; p. 213.
23. *trunk nerve (Burdach, 1819)*
English form of *Rumpfnerve (Burdach, 1819)*.
24. *harmonic nerve (Burdach, 1819)*
Synonym for macrodissected adult human ***sympathetic trunk (Winslow, 1733)***; in the original Latin, *nervus harmonicus*, according to Burdach (1819, pp. 213–214), who mistakenly attributed this exact term to Andersch; see *great harmonic nerve of body (Andersch, 1797)*.
25. *vascular nerve (Lobstein, 1823)*
Synonym for macrodissected adult human ***sympathetic trunk (Winslow, 1733)***; "...some very distinguished men have believed, that the sympathetic nerve is fabricated for the use of the arteries, and have designated it by the name of *vascular nerve*" (1831 translation, p. 44).
26. *trunk of ganglionated nerves (Bock, 1827)*
Synonym for macrodissected adult human ***sympathetic trunk (Winslow, 1733)***; in the original Latin, *truncus nervi gangliosi*; Table I, Figure 1-*o*.
27. *forty-third pair of nerves (Cloquet, 1828)*
Synonym for macrodissected adult human right and left ***sympathetic trunk (Winslow, 1733)***; in the original French, *quarante-troisième paire*, p. 326.
28. *vasomotor nerve (Stilling, 1840)*
Synonym for macrodissected adult human ***sympathetic trunk (Winslow, 1733)***; see Schiller (1969, pp. 76–77).

PARTLY CORRESPONDS:

1. *branch of sixth pair stretching along roots of ribs (Vesalius, 1543a)*
Vesalius clearly had ***sympathetic trunk (Winslow, 1733)*** arising as branch at rostral part (top) of thorax from ***vagus nerve (Galen, c192)***, and described and illustrated right and left "branches" separately because they are asymmetrical; see Richardson & Carman translation (2002, pp. 199–200; also see pp. 195, 252).
2. *branch of sixth pair of sinews stretched to roots of ribs (Geminus, 1553)*
Synonym for macrodissected adult human *branch of sixth pair stretching along roots of ribs (Vesalius, 1543a)*; originally spelled, *braunche of the syxth payre of synowes stretched to rootes of rybbes*, see *The table of the figure of synowes*.
3. *costal nerve (Paré, 1561)*
Probably first technical term for at least part of macrodissected adult human ***sympathetic trunk (Winslow, 1733)***, which Paré regarded, following *branch of sixth pair stretching along roots of ribs (Vesalius, 1543a)*, as branch of ***vagus nerve (Galen, c192)***; in the original French, *nerf costal*; p. cxiii.
4. *intercostal nerve (Bauhin, 1605)*
Apparently synonym for macrodissected adult human *costal nerve (Paré, 1561)*; in the original Latin, *intercostalem nervum*, p. 676. For English translation see Crooke (1615, Tab. XXIIII-*rr*).
5. *inner branch of sixth pair of nerves (Crooke, 1615)*
Synonym for *branch of sixth pair stretching along roots of ribs (Vesalius, 1543a)*; p. 365, Table VIII, Figure 1-*i* of Book 6, Ch. 10—where it is also called *inward branch*.
6. *rib nerve (Crooke, 1615)*
Synonym for macrodissected adult human *costal nerve (Bauhin, 1605)*; p. 367.
7. *costall branch of sixth conjugation (Paré, 1634)*
English form of *costal nerve (Paré, 1561)*, accompanied by Latin form, *ramus costalis*; p. 152.
8. *costal branch of sixth pair of nerves (Vesling, 1647)*
Presumably synonym for macrodissected adult human *branch of sixth pair stretching along roots of ribs (Vesalius, 1543a)*; see translation (1653, Tab. 3, Fig. 8-*B*).
9. *inferior rope of intercostal nerve (Winslow, 1733)*
Winslow stated it commonly refers to segment of ***sympathetic trunk (Winslow, 1733)*** adjacent to first two lumbar vertebrae; Section VI, no. 412, p. 99.
10. *cerebral roots of great intercostal nerve (Günther, 1786)*
For macrodissected adult human, Günther listed three "cerebral roots" of ***sympathetic trunk (Winslow, 1733)***, from ***maxillary nerve (Meckel, 1753)***, ***deep petrosal nerve (Meckel, 1817)***, and ***abducens nerve (Heister, 1717)***; in the original Latin, *radicibus cerebralibus*, p. 92.

sympathetic trunk ganglia (Winslow, 1733)

As described for macrodissected adult mammal, the ***paravertebral ganglia (Durward, 1951)*** distributed along the ***sympathetic trunk (Winslow, 1733)*** and currently described from rostral (superior) to caudal (inferior); see Williams & Warwick (1980, pp. 1124–1132). The ***sympathetic trunk ganglia (Winslow, 1733)*** and ***sympathetic trunk (Winslow, 1733)*** together form the ***sympathetic cord (>1840)***. Winslow used in English the terms ***sympathetic trunk (Winslow, 1733)*** and *ganglions of trunk (Winslow, 1733)*, which together reasonably form the term ***sympathetic trunk ganglia (Winslow, 1733)***. Galen identified the first major component; see ***[sympathetic trunk ganglia (Winslow, 1733)] (Galen, c173)***.

EARLIER REFERENCES:

Described, not named or illustrated:

1. ***[sympathetic trunk ganglia (Winslow, 1733)] (Galen, c173)***
Galen identified the first major component in macrodissected adult beef, pig, and/or macaque but not human, the *cervicothoracic ganglion (>1840)*; see May translation (1968, pp. 695–696), Duckworth translation (1962, p. 227), Savage-Smith (1971, pp. 179–181).

LATER SYNONYMS:

1. *ganglions of trunk (Winslow, 1733)*
   Synonym for ***sympathetic trunk ganglia (Winslow, 1733)***; Section VI, p. 100.
2. *intercostal nerve ganglia (Günther, 1786)*
   Synonym for macrodissected adult human ***sympathetic trunk ganglia (Winslow, 1733)***; in the original Latin, *gangliorum n. intercostalis*, p. 92.
3. *sympathetic nerve ganglia (Carus, 1814)*
   Synonym for ***sympathetic trunk ganglia (Winslow, 1733)*** in unspecified species; in the original German, *den Ganglien des sympathischen Nerven*, p. 66.

PARTLY CORRESPONDS:

1. *intercostal infolding (Willis, 1664)*
   From description and illustration, synonym for macrodissected adult human *cervicothoracic ganglion (>1840)*; see Pordage translation (1681, p. 158 and Fig. 9-Θ).
2. *lower infolding of intercostal nerve (Willis, 1664)*
   Synonym for *intercostal infolding (Willis, 1664)*; see Pordage translation (1681, Fig. 9-Θ).
3. *thoracical infolding (Willis, 1664)*
   Synonym for *intercostal infolding (Willis, 1664)*; see Pordage translation (1681, Fig. 9-Θ).
4. *plexus ganglioformis hordeiformes (Vieussens, 1684)*
   Macrodissected adult human ***lumbar sympathetic ganglia (>1840)*** and ***sacral sympathetic ganglia (>1840)*** considered together; Table 23-82.
5. *lateral cervical ganglia (Neubauer, 1772)*
   Ganglia (Galen, c173) associated with ***ansa subclavia (Neubauer, 1772)*** of macrodissected adult human described; in the original Latin, *gangliis cervicalibus lateralibus*, p. 144 and Table 1-53,54.
6. *posterior cervical ganglia (Neubauer, 1772)*
   Synonym for *lateral cervical ganglia (Neubauer, 1772)*; p. 144.
7. *abdominal ganglions of limiting cord (Meckel, 1817)*
   Macrodissected adult human *lumbar ganglions of limiting cord (Meckel, 1817)* and *pelvic ganglions of limiting cord (Meckel, 1817)* considered together; see translation (1832, Vol. 3, pp. 97–98).
8. *pelvic ganglions of limiting cord (Meckel, 1817)*
   Macrodissected adult human ***sacral sympathetic ganglia (>1840)*** and ***ganglion impar (Quain & Wilson, 1839)*** considered together; see translation (1832, Vol. 3, p. 98).
9. *stellate ganglion (>1840)*
   Synonym for *cervicothoracic ganglion (>1840)*; see Williams & Warwick (1980, p. 1129), *Dorland's* (2003, p. 753).
10. *cervicothoracic ganglion (>1840)*
    Macrodissected adult human fusion product of ***inferior cervical ganglion (Vieussens, 1684)*** and ***superior thoracic ganglion (Lieutaud, 1742)***; see Mitchell (1953, pp. 227–229), *Terminologia Anatomica* (1998, p. 141). Lieutaud (1742, p. 438) noted that ***inferior cervical ganglion (Vieussens, 1684)*** and ***superior thoracic ganglion (Lieutaud, 1742)*** are sometimes fused in macrodissected adult human; also see Haller (1762, p. 259 note *u*). It is usually stated now that fusion occurs in about three-quarters of individuals; see Mitchell (1953, p. 227), Williams & Warwick (1980, p. 1129).

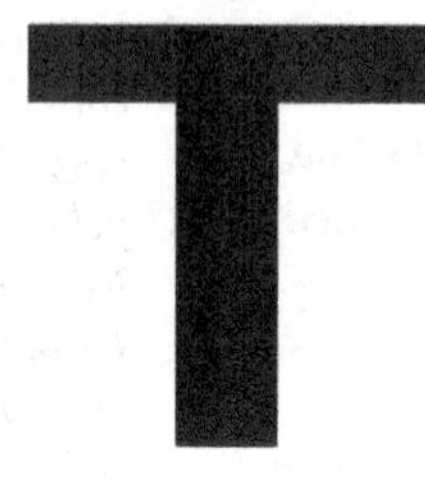

tail of caudate nucleus (Arnold, 1838b)

As defined arbitrarily for macrodissected adult human, the thin, long part of the ***caudate nucleus (Arnold, 1838b)*** curving concavely caudally and ventrally between the ***body of caudate nucleus (>1840)*** and ***central amygdalar nucleus (Johnston, 1923)***; see Carpenter (1976, p. 497, Fig. 17.4). For Arnold's original use in macrodissected adult human, see Table IV, Figure 5-*s*. It was clearly illustrated by Vieussens; see ***[tail of caudate nucleus (Arnold, 1838b)] (Vieussens, 1684)***.

TRANSLATIONS:

1. *cauda nucleus caudatus (Arnold, 1838b)*
   Original Latin form of ***tail of caudate nucleus (Arnold, 1838b)***; Table IV, Figure 5-*s* where the plural, *caudae nuclei caudati*, was used. Arnold recognized in *cauda nucleus caudatus (Arnold, 1838b)* a posterior part (*pars posterior*; Tab. IV, Fig. 5-*s*), which was quite ventral. See Nieuwenhuys et al. (2008, Fig. 5.31).

EARLIER REFERENCES:

Illustrated and described, not named:

1. ***[tail of caudate nucleus (Arnold, 1838b)] (Vieussens, 1684)***
   Clearly illustrated for macrodissected adult human; part of *striata corpora superna anteriora (Vieussens, 1684)* just above *E* in Table XIII.

tapetum (Reil, 1809b)

As described for macrodissected adult human, the extension of ***body of corpus callosum (Arnold, 1838a) axons (Kölliker, 1896)*** over the dorsolateral wall of the ***posterior horn of lateral ventricle (Haller, 1747)*** and subjacent lateral wall of the ***inferior horn of lateral ventricle (Bell, 1802)***, and thus a ***radiation of corpus callosum (Dejerine & Dejerine-Klumpke, 1895)*** in the ***cerebral cortex white matter (>1840)***; see Charpy (1889, Fig. 89), Carpenter (1976, Fig. 2.16), Williams & Warwick (1980, pp. 1024, 1029, 1031), Nieuwenhuys et al. (2008, Fig. 5.30-*11*). Clearly, it has ***axons (Kölliker, 1896)*** other than those associated with the ***corpus callosum (Galen, c177)***; see Obersteiner & Hill (1900, pp. 431–432). For Reil's discovery and use in macrodissected adult human, see Mayo translation (1823, pp. 53, 58); in Latin, *tapetum* means "carpet".

TRANSLATIONS:

1. *Tapete (Reil, 1809b)*
   Original German form of ***tapetum (Reil, 1809b)***; see Mayo translation (1823, p. 53).

tectospinal tract (>1840)

As described in macrodissected adult human, and mammal generally with histological methods for ***axons (Kölliker, 1896)***, the longitudinal ***central nervous system white matter tract (>1840)*** extending ventromedially from the ***superior colliculus (Haller, 1762)*** to cross the median plane of the ***midbrain (>1840)*** in the ***dorsal tegmental decussation (>1840)*** before extending caudally as far as the ***spinal cord (Galen, c162–c166)*** where it lies in ventral regions of the ***ventral funiculus (>1840)***. It has branches along the way to sites in the ***tegmentum (Swanson, 2000b)***, ***pons (Haller, 1747)***, and ***medulla (Winslow, 1733)***; see Carpenter (1976, p. 261 and Fig. 10.17). For topographic description it has ***tegmental tectospinal tract (>1840)***, ***pontine tectospinal tract (>1840)***, ***medullary tectospinal tract (>1840)***, and ***spinal tectospinal tract (>1840)*** segments. It was not clearly delineated by 1840.

EARLIER REFERENCES:

Earlier synonyms:

1. *predorsal bundle (>1840)*
   Earlier synonym for macrodissected adult human ***tectospinal tract (>1840)***; see Carpenter (1976, p. 261), Harting (1977, p. 583).

2. *medial tectospinal tract (>1840)*
Synonym for macrodissected adult human ***tectospinal tract (>1840)***; see Crosby et al. (1962, p. 102).

tectum (Baer, 1837)

The dorsal topographic division of the vertebrate ***midbrain (Baer, 1837)***, essentially dorsal to the ***cerebral aqueduct (>1840)*** and formed in mammals by the paired ***superior colliculi (Haller, 1762)*** and ***inferior colliculi (Haller, 1762)***, and contrasting with the ventral topographic division or ***tegmentum (Swanson, 2000b)***; for this definition see Swanson & Bota (2010). It was identified and named long ago, *little buttocks (Galen, c173, definition 1)*, and Vesalius (1543a) first pointed out that it consists of *gray substance (Vesalius, 1543)*; see Richardson & Carman translation (2009, p. 207). Baer (1837, p. 111), like Schwalbe (1881, p. 454), called it the "roof of the midbrain", *decke des Mittelhirns* in German (p. 454). Cajal (1904, Vol. 2, pt. 1, p. 449) referred to it in Spanish as *el techo, la porción tectal.*

EARLIER REFERENCES:

Earlier synonyms:

1. *little buttocks (Galen, c173, definition 1)*
In *On the Usefulness of the Parts*, Galen wrote there are two uses of this term. One refers to ***inferior colliculi (Haller, 1762)***, and the other (here) refers to ***superior colliculi (Haller, 1762)*** together with ***inferior colliculi (Haller, 1762)***—that is, the ***tectum (Baer, 1837)***. The colliculi are described as "delicate, elongate eminences of the encephalon" on either side of canal between ***third ventricle (Galen, c173)*** and ***fourth ventricle (Galen, c192)*** in macrodissected adult large mammal but not human; see May translation (1968, p. 420). They have nothing in common with *buttocks (Mondino, 1316)*.
2. *gloutia (Galen, c173, definition 1)*
Greek form of *little buttocks (Galen, c173, definition 1)*; see May translation (1962, p. 420). Spelled *gloutiae* by Hall (1565).
3. *buttocks (Galen, c173, definition 1)*
Alternate translation of *little buttocks (Galen, c173, definition 1)*; see Singer (1999, p. 236).
4. *nates (Galen, c173, definition 1)*
Alternate translation of *buttocks (Galen, c173, definition 1)*; see Singer (1999, p. 236).
5. *little testicles (Galen, c173, definition 1)*
Synonym for *little buttocks (Galen, c173, definition 1)*; see May translation (1962, p. 420).
6. *testicles (Galen, c173, definition 1)*
Alternate translation of *little testicles (Galen, c173, definition 1)*; see May (1962, p. 420).
7. *testes (Galen, c173, definition 1)*
Alternate translation of *testicles (Galen, c173, definition 1)*; see Wiberg (1914, p. 28).
8. *didymia (Galen, c173, definition 1)*
Greek form of *little testicles (Galen, c173, definition 1)*; see May translation (1968, p. 420).
9. *twins (Galen, c173, definition 1)*
English form of *didymia (Galen, c173, definition 1)*; see Singer (1999, p. 236).
10. *testes and nates (Vesalius, 1543a)*
Vesalius wrote that "This portion, by reason of its function and albeit named by a plural word, is not really divided into several or disjointed parts, but is a unity..." in referring to macrodissected adult human ***tectum (Baer, 1837)***, which he included in *cerebrum (Vesalius, 1543a)*, as opposed to ***cerebellum (Aristotle)*** and *spinal marrow (Vesalius, 1543a)*; see Singer translation (1952, pp. 46–47, 102).
11. *naticulae (Hall, 1565)*
Synonym for macrodissected adult human *gloutia (Galen, c173, definition 1)*; p. 38.
12. *anceformes (Hall, 1565)*
According to Hall, a recent synonym for macrodissected adult human *gloutia (Galen, c173, definition 1)*; p. 38.
13. *corpuscula quatuor eminentia (Bauhin, 1605)*
Synonym for macrodissected adult human ***tectum (Baer, 1837)***, according to Burdach (1822, pp. 334–335).
14. *circumjacent eminences (Riolan, 1649)*
Synonym for macrodissected adult human ***tectum (Baer, 1837)***; see translation of *eminentiae circumiectae (Riolan 1649, p. 247)* in Riolan (1657, p. 123).
15. *pons testibut et natibus (in quatuor ipsius extremis eminentibus) ornatus (Le Böe, 1663)*
Synonym for macrodissected adult human ***tectum (Baer, 1837)***, according to Burdach (1822, p. 335).
16. *protuberantiae orbiculares (Willis, 1664)*
Latin form of *orbicular prominences (Willis, 1664)*; see Tyson (1699, p. 56).
17. *orbicular prominences (Willis, 1664)*
Synonym for ***tectum (Baer, 1837)*** in macrodissected adult human and other large mammal; see Pordage translation (1681, p. 106, Tabs. 7-*T*, 8-*N*). Willis wrote (1664, p. 64) that they are distinct part of *oblong marrow (Willis, 1664)*, not *cerebrum (Willis, 1664)* or ***cerebellum (Aristotle)***.
18. *four protuberances of oblong marrow (Willis, 1664)*
Synonym for *orbicular prominences (Willis, 1664)*; see Pordage translation (1681, p. 64).
19. *superior protuberances (Willis, 1664)*
Synonym for ***tectum (Baer, 1837)*** in macrodissected adult human and other large mammal; see Pordage translation (1681, pp. 64–65).
20. *superior prominences (Willis, 1664)*
Synonym for *superior protuberances (Willis, 1664)*; see Pordage translation (1681, pp. 64–65).
21. *hollow medullary prominences (Willis, 1664)*
Willis wrote that macrodissected adult birds and fish seem to have *hollow medullary prominences* instead of *orbicular prominences (Willis, 1664)*, the ***tectum (Baer, 1837)***; see Pordage translation (1681, pp. 76–77).
22. *four mole hills (Willis, 1664)*
Synonym for *orbicular prominences (Willis, 1664)*; see Pordage translation (1681, p. 107).

23. *quatuor moleculas (Willis, 1664)*
Original Latin for *four mole hills (Willis, 1664)*.
24. *anterior appendix of cerebellum (Willis, 1664)*
Synonym for *orbicular prominences (Willis, 1664)*; see Pordage translation (1681, p. 121).
25. *third pair of tubercles (Steno, 1669)*
Synonym for macrodissected adult human **tectum** ***(Baer, 1837)***; see translation, pp. 130, 134.
26. *two posterior pairs of tubercles (Steno, 1669)*
Synonym for macrodissected adult human **tectum** ***(Baer, 1837)***; see translation, p. 137.
27. *isthmus (Ridley, 1695)*
Synonym for macrodissected adult human **tectum** ***(Baer, 1837)***, "...being placed upon the upper part of the *Medulla Oblongata*, made a sort of an *Isthmus* betwixt the *Cerebrum* and *Cerebellum*" (p. 9), and then later, "...in the *Isthmus* or space betwixt the *Cerebrum* and *Cerebellum*" (p. 13, his italics). Ridley also mentioned without reference (p. 126) earlier use of *isthmus* in this way. Meyer (1971, p. 29) suggested Ridley may also refer to ***tegmentum (Swanson, 2000b)***, but this is a stretch and not what Ridley actually wrote, unless his view of *tectum* at the time included the whole ***midbrain (Baer, 1837)***.
28. *tubercula quadrigemina (Winslow, 1733)*
Synonym for macrodissected adult human **tectum** ***(Baer, 1837)***; Section X, p. 37.
29. *quadrigeminal tubercles (Winslow, 1733)*
English form of *tubercula quadrigemina (Winslow, 1733)*.
30. *quadrigeminal eminences (Haller, 1762)*
Synonym for macrodissected adult human **tectum** ***(Baer, 1837)***; in the original Latin, *eminentiae quadrigeminae*, pp. 62, 63.
31. *quadrigeminal protuberances (Soemmerring, 1778)*
Synonym for macrodissected adult human **tectum** ***(Baer, 1837)***; in the original Latin, *prominentiarum quadrigeminarum*, pp. 96–97.
32. *processus anceformes (Soemmerring, 1778)*
Synonym for macrodissected adult human **tectum** ***(Baer, 1837)***; p. 78, according to Burdach (1822, p. 335).
33. *gray rounded spaces (Vicq d'Azyr, 1786)*
Synonym for macrodissected adult human ***tectum (Baer, 1837)*** when viewed in transverse section with the naked eye; Plate XV-*18*. The relevant illustration is of a section through ***superior colliculi (Haller, 1762)***.
34. *globose tubercles (Günther, 1786)*
The two ***superior colliculi (Haller, 1762)*** and two ***inferior colliculi (Haller, 1762)*** of macrodissected adult human ***tectum (Baer, 1837)***, each with gray interior and white plate superficially; in the original Latin, *tuberculis globosis*, p. 14.
35. *corpora bigemina (Soemmerring, 1798)*
Synonym for macrodissected adult human **tectum** ***(Baer, 1837)***; pp. 61–62.
36. *tubercles of mesencephalon (Burdin, 1803)*
Synonym for macrodissected adult human **tectum** ***(Baer, 1837)***; see translation (1803, Vol. 3, p. 162). Also see *midbrain (Burdin, 1803)*.
37. *monticuli (Schreger, 1803)*
Synonym for macrodissected the adult human ***tectum (Baer, 1837)***; p. 321.
38. *bigeminal prominences (Rolando, 1809)*
Synonym for macrodissected adult human **tectum** ***(Baer, 1837)***; in the original Italian, *prominenze bigemine*, p. 10. Burdach (1822, p. 335) gave the Latin, *prominentiae bigeminae*.
39. *corpus bigeminum (Wenzel & Wenzel, 1812)*
Singular of *corpora bigemina (Soemmerring, 1798)* for macrodissected adult human; p. 203.
40. *corpora quadrigemina (Wenzel & Wenzel, 1812)*
Synonym for macrodissected adult human **tectum** ***(Baer, 1837)***; p. 313.
41. *quadrigeminal bodies (Wenzel & Wenzel, 1812)*
English form of *corpora quadrigemina (Wenzel & Wenzel, 1812)*.
42. *eminentia bigemina (Meckel, 1817)*
Synonym for macrodissected adult human **tectum** ***(Baer, 1837)***; see translation (1832, Vol. 2, p. 444).
43. *pair of ophthalmic tubercles (Bojanus, 1819–1821)*
Synonym for macrodissected adult turtle *quadrigeminal bodies (Wenzel & Wenzel, 1812)*; in the original Latin, *tubera ophthalmica bina*, Figure 83-*b*.
44. *optic lobes (Serres, 1824–1826)*
Macrodissected adult bird ***tectum (Baer, 1837)***; see Vol. 2, p. 795. Serres described them as consisting of four alternating gray and white layers, beginning with a white layer on surface; Vol. 1, pp. 277–278.
45. *pons of Sylvius (Bock, 1824)*
Eponym for macrodissected adult human **tectum** ***(Baer, 1837)***; p. 120.
46. *bigeminal bodies (Spurzheim, 1826)*
Apparently synonym for *optic lobes (Serres, 1824–1826)* in macrodissected nonmammalian vertebrate; p. 76.
47. *optic ganglions (Spurzheim, 1826)*
Synonym for macrodissected adult bird *optic lobes (Serres, 1824–1826)*; Table 3, Figure 6.
48. *optic tubercles (Solly, 1836)*
Synonym for macrodissected adult fish, amphibian, bird, and mammalian *optic lobes (Serres, 1824–1826)*; pp. 74–75, 81, 86, 87, 178.
49. *second cerebral mass (Anderson, 1837)*
Synonym for macrodissected vertebrate **tectum** ***(Baer, 1837)***; p. 16 ff.

LATER SYNONYMS:

1. *quadrigeminal colliculi (Arnold, 1838a)*
Synonym for macrodissected adult human ***tectum (Baer, 1837)***; in the original Latin, *colliculi quadrigemini*, p. 56.

PARTLY CORRESPONDS:

1. *middle commissure of quadrigeminal bodies (Bojanus, 1819–1821)*
In macrodissected adult turtle, region near median plane of ***tectum (Baer, 1837)***; in the original Latin, *corporum quadrigeminorum media commissura*, Figure 89-*b*.

tegmental central tegmental tract (>1840)

As described in macrodissected adult human, and mammal generally with histological methods for ***axons (Kölliker, 1896)***, the most rostral topographic segment of the ***central tegmental tract (Bechterew, 1889)***, from parts of the ***midbrain reticular nucleus (>1840)*** dorsomedial to the ***red nucleus (Burdach, 1822)*** rostrally to the rostral end of the ***pontine tegmental central tegmental tract (>1840)*** segment caudally; see Riley (1943, pp. 693–694), Crosby et al. (1962, pp. 256–257), Nieuwenhuys et al. (2008, Figs. 6.29–33). It was not clearly described by 1840.

tegmental dorsal longitudinal fascicle (>1840)

As described in adult human with histological methods for ***axons (Kölliker, 1896)***, the rostral topographic segment of the ***dorsal longitudinal fascicle (Schütz, 1891)*** in the ***tegmentum (Swanson, 2000b)***, between the caudal ends of the ***periventricular bundle of hypothalamus (>1840)***, ***periventricular bundle of thalamus (>1840)***, and ***hypothalamic medial forebrain bundle (>1840)*** rostrally and the ***pontine dorsal longitudinal fascicle (>1840)*** segment caudally, and centered in the ***periaqueductal gray (>1840)***; see Mettler (1948, Figs. 242, 244), Crosby et al. (1962, Figs. 174, 179), Nieuwenhuys et al. (2008, Figs. 6.29–33). It was not recognized by 1840.

tegmental habenulo-interpeduncular tract (>1840)

As described in macrodissected adult human, and mammal generally with histological methods for ***axons (Kölliker, 1896)***, the dorsoventrally oriented segment of the ***habenulo-interpeduncular tract (>1840)*** in the ***tegmentum (Swanson, 2000b)***, between ***thalamic habenulo-interpeduncular tract (>1840)*** segment rostrally and dorsally, and ***interpeduncular nucleus (>1840)*** ventrally. It was known to Cruveilhier; see ***[tegmental habenulo-interpeduncular tract (>1840)] (Cruveilhier, 1836)***.

EARLIER REFERENCES:

Described, not named or illustrated:

1. *[tegmental habenulo-interpeduncular tract (>1840)] (Cruveilhier, 1836)*
   Described but not explicitly distinguished from ***thalamic habenulo-interpeduncular tract (>1840)***; see *inferior peduncles of pineal body (Cruveilhier, 1836)*.

tegmental mammillotegmental tract (>1840)

As described in macrodissected adult human, and mammal generally with histological methods for ***axons (Kölliker, 1896)***, the caudal topographic segment of the ***mammillotegmental tract (>1840)*** in the ***tegmentum (Swanson, 200b)***, caudal to the ***hypothalamic mammillotegmental tract (>1840)*** segment. It was first clearly delineated by Vicq d'Azyr; see ***[tegmental mammillotegmental tract (>1840)] (Vicq d'Azyr, 1786)***.

EARLIER REFERENCES:

Illustrated and described, not named:

1. *[tegmental mammillotegmental tract (>1840)] (Vicq d'Azyr, 1786)*
   Described and illustrated clearly in macrodissected adult human, though without a separate name; Plate XXV, Figure II-*41*.

tegmental medial forebrain bundle (>1840)

As described in mammal generally with experimental histological methods for ***axons (Kölliker, 1896)***, the topographic segment of the ***medial forebrain bundle (Edinger, 1893)*** in the ***tegmentum (Swanson, 2000b)***, between ***hypothalamic medial forebrain bundle (>1840)*** segment rostrally and ***pontine medial forebrain bundle (>1840)*** segment caudally. It is centered in and around the ***ventral tegmental area (Tsai, 1925)*** and has a major dorsally directed branch to the ***periaqueductal gray (>1840)*** at the level of the ***trochlear nucleus (>1840)***; see Saper et al. (1976). It was not known by 1840.

tegmental medial lemniscus (>1840)

As described in macrodissected adult human, and mammal generally with histological methods for ***axons (Kölliker, 1896)***, the topographic segment of the ***medial lemniscus (>1840)*** in the ***tegmentum (Swanson, 2000b)***, between ***thalamic medial lemniscus (>1840)*** segment rostrally and ***pontine medial lemniscus (>1840)*** segment caudally; see Nieuwenhuys et al. (2008, Figs. 6.17–18). It was known to Reil; see ***[tegmental medial lemniscus (>1840)] (Reil, 1809c)***.

EARLIER REFERENCES:

Described, not named or illustrated:

1. *[tegmental medial lemniscus (>1840)] (Reil, 1809c)*
   Segment of *external part of lemniscus (Reil, 1809c)* in ***tegmentum (Swanson, 2000b)***, vaguely described; see Mayo translation (1823, p. 95).

tegmental medial longitudinal fascicle (>1840)

As described in macrodissected adult human, and mammal generally with histological methods for ***axons (Kölliker, 1896)***, the rostral topographic segment of the ***medial longitudinal fascicle (>1840)*** in the ***tegmentum (Swanson, 2000b)***, rostral to the ***pontine medial longitudinal fascicle (>1840)*** segment. It was probably known to Vicq d'Azyr; see ***[tegmental medial longitudinal fascicle (>1840)] (Vicq d'Azyr, 1786)***.

EARLIER REFERENCES:

Illustrated, not named or described:

1. *[tegmental medial longitudinal fascicle (>1840)] (Vicq d'Azyr, 1786)*
   Apparently illustrated for macrodissected adult human; Plate XXXI, Figure II-2 toward *6*.

tegmental rubrospinal tract (>1840)

As described in adult human and other mammals most clearly with experimental pathway tracing methods, the rostral topographic segment of the ***rubrospinal tract (>1840)*** extending caudally in the ***tegmental ventrolateral fascicle (>1840)***, between ***ventral tegmental decussation (>1840)*** rostrally and ***pontine rubrospinal tract (>10840)*** segment caudally. See Mettler (1948, Figs. 242,

244, 246, 248, 254, 256, 259), Swanson (2004, Atlas Levels 40–42). It was not identified by 1840.

tegmental segment of midbrain tract of trigeminal nerve (>1840)

As described in macrodissected adult human, and mammal generally with histological methods for ***axons (Kölliker, 1896)***, the rostral segment of the ***midbrain tract of trigeminal nerve (>1840)***, rostral to the ***pontine segment of midbrain tract of trigeminal nerve (>1840)*** and lying on the lateral edge of the caudal half of the ***periaqueductal gray (>1840)*** just lateral to the ***midbrain nucleus of trigeminal nerve (>1840)***; see Nieuwenhuys et al. (2008, Figs. 6.29–32). It was not known by 1840.

tegmental spinothalamic tract (>1840)

As described for adult human and other mammals most clearly with experimental pathway tracing methods, a topographic segment of the ***spinothalamic tract (>1840)*** in the ***tegmentum (Swanson, 2000b)***, extending rostrally between ***thalamic spinothalamic tract (>1840)*** segment rostrally and ***pontine spinothalamic tract (>1840)*** segment caudally; it lies within the ***tegmental ventrolateral fascicle (>1840)*** and its largest branches are to the ***tectum (Baer, 1837)*** and underlying ***periaqueductal gray (>1840)***; see Nieuwenhuys et al. (2008, Figures 6.17–18, called *anterolateral fasciculus*). It was identified at least partly by Rolando; see ***[tegmental spinothalamic tract (>1840)] (Rolando, 1825a)***.

EARLIER REFERENCES:

Illustrated and described, not named:

1. ***[tegmental spinothalamic tract (>1840)] (Rolando, 1825a)***
   Rolando traced *anterolateral cord of oblong medulla (Rolando, 1825a)* or ***ventrolateral fascicle (>1840)*** into ***thalamus (His, 1893a)***, so he observed at least rostral part of ***tegmental spinothalamic tract (>1840)*** after its last branches to ***tectum (Baer, 1837)*** and ***periaqueductal gray (>1840)*** and its rostral extension as ***thalamic spinothalamic tract (>1840)***; see Table VIII, Figure 1-*z*.

tegmental superior cerebellar peduncle (>1840)

As described in macrodissected adult human, and mammal generally with histological methods for ***axons (Kölliker, 1896)***, the topographic segment of the ***superior cerebellar peduncle (Procháska, 1800)*** in the ***tegmentum (Swanson, 2000b)***, between ***pontine superior cerebellar peduncle (>1840)*** segment caudally and ***superior cerebellar peduncle decussation (>1840)*** rostrally; see Carpenter (1976, p. 420 and Fig. 14.16). It was known to Willis; see ***[tegmental superior cerebellar peduncle (>1840)] (Willis, 1664)***.

EARLIER REFERENCES:

Illustrated and described, not named:

1. ***[tegmental superior cerebellar peduncle (>1840)] (Willis, 1664)***
   Willis mentioned and illustrated it for macrodissected adult human and other large mammals, tracing ***superior cerebellar peduncle (Procháska, 1800)*** into ***superior cerebellar peduncle decussation (>1840)***; see pp. 65, 109, Figures III-*K*, VII-*R*, VIII-*M*.

tegmental tectospinal tract (>1840)

As described in macrodissected adult human, and mammal generally with histological methods for ***axons (Kölliker, 1896)***, there are two segments of the ***tectospinal tract (>1840)*** in the ***tegmentum (Swanson, 2000b)***. A transverse segment extends from the ***superior colliculus (Haller, 1762)*** dorsally to the ***dorsal tegmental decussation (>1840)*** ventromedially, and a short longitudinal segment extends from the contralateral side of the ***dorsal tegmental decussation (>1840)*** to the rostral end of the ***pontine tectospinal tract (>1840)*** segment; see Carpenter (1976, p. 261), Harting (1977, p. 583). It was not recognized by 1840.

tegmental ventrolateral fascicle (>1840)

As described for macrodissected adult human, the rostral topographic segment of the ***ventrolateral fascicle (>1840)*** in the ***tegmentum (Swanson, 2000b)***, between the ***thalamic spinothalamic tract (>1840)*** or *thalamic ventrolateral fascicle (>1840)* segment rostrally and the ***pontine ventrolateral fascicle (>1840)*** segment caudally; with two main components, ***tegmental spinothalamic tract (>1840)*** and ***tegmental rubrospinal tract (>1840)***; see Nieuwenhuys et al. (2008, Figs. 6.17–18, called *anterolateral fasciculus*). It was observed but not separately named by Rolando; see ***[tegmental ventrolateral fascicle (>1840)] (Rolando, 1825a)***.

EARLIER REFERENCES:

Illustrated and described, not named:

1. ***[tegmental ventrolateral fascicle (>1840)] (Rolando, 1825a)***
   Rolando observed *anterolateral cord of oblong medulla (Rolando, 1825a)* or ***ventrolateral fascicle (>1840)*** in ***tegmentum (Swanson, 2000b)*** without separately naming it; see Table VIII, Figure 1-*z*.

tegmentum (Swanson, 2000b)

The ventral topographic division of the vertebrate ***midbrain (Baer, 1837)***, including the ***pretectal region (Scalia, 1972)***; the dorsal topographic division is the ***tectum (Baer, 1837)***. For this definition see Swanson & Bota (2010) and for Swanson's original use in mammals, see pp. 522, 526 and Figure 2. It was originally identified as the *cerebral peduncle (Vicq d'Azyr, 1784)*. Use of the term tegmentum is very complex, inconsistent, and illogical. For example, Crosby et. al. (1962, pp. 221, 260, 262) defined *tegmentum* as the ***midbrain (Baer, 1837)*** region between ***tectum (Baer, 1837)*** and basis pedunculi (cerebral peduncle, the pes pedunculi, and substantia nigra); Carpenter (1976, p. 367 ff.) wrote that the ***midbrain (Baer, 1837)*** has three parts: tectum, crura cerebri, and tegmentum; the term cerebral peduncle, according to accepted nomenclature, has two parts: a dorsal tegmentum and a ventral crus cerebri, separated by the ***substantia nigra (Soemmerring, 1791)*** [the latter must be a part of the tegmentum as defined by Carpenter]. Williams & Warwick (1980, p. 935 ff.) wrote that the ***midbrain (Baer, 1837)*** is divided for descriptive purposes into right and left halves—the cerebral peduncles, each of which is further subdivided by the ***substantia nigra (Soemmerring, 1791)*** into a ventral part, the crus cerebri, and a dorsal part, the tegmentum; the part of the tegmentum dorsal to the cerebral aqueduct is called the tectum [apparently the substantia nigra here is neither crus nor tegmentum]. In Latin, tegmentum means a covering, so its use here is literally illogical, but no better term currently exists.

EARLIER REFERENCES:

Earlier synonyms:

1. *cerebral peduncle (Vicq d'Azyr, 1784)*
   Synonym for macrodissected adult human ***tegmentum (Swanson, 2000b)***; pp. 555–556. Also see Vicq d'Azyr (1786, Pl. XXVI, Fig. I-*18,24,26,27*) and *crus cerebri magna (Meckel, 1817)*. This was the usage in Arnold (1838b, Pl. III, Fig. 1-*h*), where the Latin *pedunculus cerebri* was given, and in the *Basel Nomina Anatomica* (His, 1895, p. 158). Herrick (1915, p. 160) and Strong & Elwyn (1943, p. 17) also referred to this usage.
2. *crus cerebri (Vicq d'Azyr, 1784)*
   Synonym for *cerebral peduncle (Vicq d'Azyr, 1784)*; in the original French, *jambe du cerveau*; *crus* in Latin means *leg* in English; Vicq d'Azyr used the French form. Haase (1781, p. 25) also used the Latin form although what he meant by it was not clear. Solly (1836, pp. 226, 230) described it as consisting of an upper layer of sensory tracts separated from a lower layer of motor tracts [the ***cerebral peduncle (Tarin, 1753)***] by the *locus niger crurum cerebri (Vicq d'Azyr, 1784)*, based on the work of Charles Bell.
3. *crus cerebri magna (Meckel, 1817)*
   Listed as synonym for *cerebral peduncle (Vicq d'Azyr, 1784)*; see translation (1832, Vol. 2, p. 436). Meckel described it clearly as having a *base*, the ***cerebral peduncle (Tarin, 1753)***, and a *cap* or *tegmentum (Meckel, 1817)*, also with two parts, ***substantia nigra (Soemmerring, 1791)***, and the region between it and ***tectum (Baer, 1837)***; see translation (1832, Vol. 2, p. 467).

PARTLY CORRESPONDS:

1. *crus cerebri (Bell, 1803b)*
   Probably synonym for *basis pedunculi (Henle, 1871)*, although Bell may have included *perforated substance of Vicq d'Azyr (Bell, 1803b)*; pp. 106–107, where the plural, *crura cerebri*, was used.
2. *tegmentum (Meckel, 1817)*
   Apparently macrodissected adult human ***tegmentum (Swanson, 2000b)***, excluding right and left ***cerebral peduncle (Tarin, 1753)*** ventrally; see translation (1832, Vol. 2, p. 467). Gordon (1815, p. 133) described, without naming, *gray substance (Vesalius, 1543a)* in this region of macrodissected adult human two years earlier. Burdach (1822, p. 101), whose full term in Latin was *tegmentum caudicis cerebri*, used the same definition for macrodissected adult human. See ***tegmentum (Swanson, 2000b)***.
3. *cap of cerebral peduncle (Meckel, 1817)*
   Full English form of *tegmentum of cerebral peduncle (Meckel, 1817)*; see translation (1832, Vol. 2, p. 467). The original word in German for *tegmentum* was *Haube*.
4. *tegmentum of cerebral peduncle (Meckel, 1817)*
   Synonym for *cap of cerebral peduncle (Meckel, 1817)*; see translation (1832, Vol. 2, p. 467).
5. *commissure of quadrigeminal bodies (Bojanus, 1819–1821)*
   For macrodissected adult turtle, apparently roughly *tegmentum (Meckel, 1817)*; in the original Latin, *commissura corporum quadrigeminerum*, Figure 89-*p*.
6. *tegmentum caudicis cerebri (Burdach, 1822)*
   Full Latin term Burdach provided for macrodissected adult human *tegmentum (Meckel, 1817)*; p. 101.
7. *crus cerebri (Quain, 1832)*
   For macrodissected adult human, refinement of *crus cerebri (Haller, 1747)*, including just ***cerebral peduncle (Tarin, 1753)*** and ***substantia nigra (Soemmerring, 1791)***; p. 642; Quain used the plural, *crura cerebri*.
8. *integumentum (Arnold, 1838a)*
   Synonym for macrodissected adult human *tegmentum (Arnold, 1838b)*; p. 30.
9. *tegmentum cruris (Arnold, 1838a)*
   Synonym for macrodissected adult human *tegmentum (Arnold, 1838b)*; p. 30.
10. *tegmentum of cerebral peduncle (Arnold, 1838b)*
    Synonym for macrodissected adult human *tegmentum (Arnold, 1838b)*; in the original Latin (plural), *tegmenti pedunculorum cerebri*, Table II, Figure 9-*c*.
11. *tegmentum (Arnold, 1838b)*
    Macrodissected adult human ***tegmentum (Swanson, 2000b)*** excluding ***cerebral peduncle (Tarin, 1753)*** and ***substantia nigra (Soemmerring, 1791)***; see Plate III, Figure 1-*l* and Plate IX, Figure 4-*i*.
12. *posterior part of cerebral peduncle (Arnold, 1838b)*
    Synonym for macrodissected adult human *tegmentum (Arnold, 1838b)*; in the original Latin, *pedunculus cerebri pars posterior*, Table X, Figure 1-*c*.
13. *peduncular tegmentum (Arnold, 1838b)*
    Synonym for macrodissected adult human *tegmentum (Arnold, 1838b)*; in the original Latin, *tegmentum pedunculi*, Table X, Figure 1-*c*.
14. *basis pedunculi (Henle 1871)*
    Macrodissected adult human ***cerebral peduncle (Tarin, 1753)*** and ***substantia nigra (Soemmerring, 1791)*** considered together; p. 244. Also used thus by Strong & Elwyn (1943, p. 228), Crosby et al. (1962, pp. 221, 260). Called *pars peduncularis* by Kappers et al. (1936, Vol. 2, p. 1091).

temporal branches of facial nerve (Swan, 1830)

As described for macrodissected adult human, the most dorsal terminal branches of the ***facial nerve trunk***

(>1840) innervating mainly the anterior and superior auricular muscles, frontal belly of occipitofrontalis (frontalis) muscle, and orbicularis oculi and corrugator muscles; see Williams & Warwick (1980, p. 1072 and Fig. 7.186), *Terminologia Anatomica* (1998, p. 135). For Swan's use in macrodissected adult human, see Plate XV, Figure 6-9. They were first described by Galen; see ***[temporal branches of facial nerve (Swan, 1830)] (Galen, c173)***.

EARLIER REFERENCES:

Described, not named or illustrated:

1. ***[temporal branches of facial nerve (Swan, 1830)] (Galen, c173)***
   Described for macrodissected adult beef, pig, and/or macaque but not human; see May translation (1968, pp. 451–452, 455–456, 686), Duckworth translation (1962, p. 196).

Illustrated, not named or described:

1. ***[temporal branches of facial nerve (Swan, 1830)] (Eustachi, 1552)***
   Illustrated for macrodissected adult human; see Albinus edition (1761, Tab. 21/2-branch above *e*).

Illustrated and described, not named:

1. ***[temporal branches of facial nerve (Swan, 1830)] (Willis, 1664)***
   Mentioned and illustrated for macrodissected adult human; see Pordage translation (1681, p. 144 and Tab. IX-4).

Earlier synonyms:

1. *temporal branch of superior branch of anterior branch of hard nerve (Loder, 1778)*
   Roughly synonymous with macrodissected adult human ***temporal branches of facial nerve (Swan, 1830)***; in the original Latin, *ramus temporalis*, p. 26.
2. *suprazygomatic branch of superior branch of anterior branch of hard nerve (Loder, 1778)*
   Synonym for *temporal branch of hard nerve (Loder, 1778)*; in the original Latin, *ramus suprazygomaticum*, p. 26.
3. *suprajugal branches of ascending branch of superficial branch of hard nerve (Günther, 1786)*
   Basically synonym for macrodissected adult human ***temporal branches of facial nerve (Swan, 1830)***; in the original Latin, *rami suprajugales*, p. 58. *Jugum* is zygomatic process; see Bell (1803b, p. 150).
4. *zygomatic branches of ascending branch of superficial branch of hard nerve (Günther, 1786)*
   Basically synonym for macrodissected adult human ***temporal branches of facial nerve (Swan, 1830)***; in the original Latin, *rami zygomaticos*, p. 58.
5. *super-orbitar branches of facial nerve (Burdin, 1803)*
   Basically synonym for macrodissected adult human ***temporal branches of facial nerve (Swan, 1830)***; see translation (1803, Vol. 1, p. 179).
6. *ascending branch of portio dura (Bell & Bell, 1816)*
   Essentially synonym for ***temporal branches of facial nerve (Swan, 1830)***; p. 501.
7. *temporal nerves (Meckel, 1817)*
   Synonym for macrodissected adult human ***temporal branches of facial nerve (Swan, 1830)***; see translation (1832, Vol. 3, p. 55).
8. *temporal surculus of superior branch of portio major and minor of facial nerve (Bellingeri, 1818)*
   Synonym for macrodissected adult human ***temporal branches of facial nerve (Swan, 1830)***; in the original Latin, *surculus temporalis*, see Table II.
9. *temporal surculus of temporo-facial branch of portio major and minor of facial nerve (Bellingeri, 1818)*
   Synonym for macrodissected adult human ***temporal branches of facial nerve (Swan, 1830)***; in the original Latin, *surculus temporalis*, see Table II.
10. *superior facial branch of facial nerve (Cloquet, 1828)*
    Synonym for macrodissected adult human ***temporal branches of facial nerve (>1840)***; in the original French, *rameau facial supérieur*, Plate CLVII-69.

LATER SYNONYMS:

1. *temporal branch of portio dura (Knox, 1832)*
   Synonym for macrodissected adult human ***temporal branches of facial nerve (Swan, 1830)***; Plate II-*105*.
2. *temporal branches of superior branch of facial nerve (Arnold, 1834)*
   Synonym for macrodissected adult human ***temporal branches of facial nerve (Swan, 1830)***; in the original Latin, *ramus superior nervi facialis rami temporales*, p. 12.
3. *temporal branches of temporofacial branch of facial nerve (Cruveilhier, 1836)*
   Synonym for macrodissected adult human ***temporal branches of facial nerve (Swan, 1830)***; in the original French, *rameaux temporaux*, p. 944.

PARTLY CORRESPONDS:

1. *middle temporal nerves (Meckel, 1753)*
   First three (starting caudally or posteriorly) macrodissected adult human ***temporal branches of facial nerve (Swan, 1830)***; in the original French, *les nerfs temporaux moyens*, p. 78.
2. *posterior temporal nerve of hard nerve (Meckel, 1753)*
   Synonym for *posterior zygomatic nerve of superior branch of hard nerve (Meckel, 1753)*; in the original French, *le nerf postérieur du temporal du nerf dur*, p. 79.
3. *posterior zygomatic nerve of superior branch of hard nerve (Meckel, 1753)*
   First of macrodissected adult human *middle temporal nerves (Meckel, 1753)*; in the original French, *le nerf zygomatique postérieur du rameau supérieur du dur*, Table 1-*130*. Though not so named, by extension Meckel's first temporal branch of hard nerve; see *second temporal branch of hard nerve (Meckel, 1753)*.
4. *anterior auricular branches of posterior zygomatic nerve (Meckel, 1753)*
   Branches of *posterior zygomatic nerve of superior branch of hard nerve (Meckel, 1753)*; in the original French, *le rameau auriculaire antérieur du le nerf zygomatique postérieur*, Table 1-*131*.

5. *posterior cutaneous temporal branches of zygomatic nerve (Meckel, 1753)*
Branches of *posterior zygomatic nerve of superior branch of hard nerve (Meckel, 1753)*; in the original French, *le rameau cutané des temples postérieur du nerf zygomatique*, Table 1-*133*.
6. *second zygomatic branch of superior branch of hard nerve (Meckel, 1753)*
Synonym for *second temporal branch of hard nerve (Meckel, 1753)*; in the original French, *le rameau zygomatique second du rameau supérieur du dur*, Table 1-*141*.
7. *second temporal branch of hard nerve (Meckel, 1753)*
Middle of macrodissected adult human *middle temporal nerves (Meckel, 1753)*; in the original French, *le rameau temporal second du dur*, Table 1-*141*.
8. *third temporal branch of hard nerve (Meckel, 1753)*
Third and last of macrodissected adult human *middle temporal nerves (Meckel, 1753)*; in the original French, *le troisième rameau temporal du dur*, Table 1-*149*.
9. *supraorbital branch of temporal branches (Meckel, 1753)*
Synonym for *third temporal branch of hard nerve (Meckel, 1753)*; in the original French, *la branche sur-orbitaire du temporal*, Table 1-*154*.
10. *external temporal branch of zygomatic branch of hard nerve (Meckel, 1753)*
Synonym for *third temporal branch of hard nerve (Meckel, 1753)*; in the original French, "*le troisième rameau des zygomatiques du nerf dur est le temporal extérieur*" (p. 80).
11. *anterior temporal nerve of hard nerve (Meckel, 1753)*
Synonym for *third temporal branch of hard nerve (Meckel, 1753)*; in the original French, *le nerf temporal antérieur du nerf dur*, p. 81.
12. *fourth temporal branch of hard nerve (Meckel, 1753)*
Fourth branch of *superior branch of hard nerve (Meckel, 1753)*, corresponding to most rostral (anterior) of ***temporal branches of facial nerve (Swan, 1830)***; in the original French, *le quatrième rameau temporal du dur*, Table 1-*149,150*.
13. *superior orbital branch of hard nerve (Meckel, 1753)*
Synonym for *fourth temporal branch of hard nerve (Meckel, 1753)*; in the original French, *le rameau orbital supérieur du dur*, Table 1-*150*.
14. *superior orbital nerve (Meckel, 1753)*
Synonym for *fourth temporal branch of hard nerve (Meckel, 1753)*; in the original French, *le nerf orbital supérieur*, p. 82, Table 1-*155*.
15. *supraorbital branch of fourth temporal branch of hard nerve (Meckel, 1753)*
Supraorbital branch of *fourth temporal branch of hard nerve (Meckel, 1753)*, also called *superior orbital nerve (Meckel, 1753)*; in the original French, *la branche sur-orbitale de le quatrième rameau temporal du dur*, Table 1-*157*.
16. *temporal branches of suprajugal branches of ascending branch of superficial branch of hard nerve (Günther, 1786)*
Basically synonym for macrodissected adult human dorsal (upper) branches of ***temporal branches of facial nerve (Swan, 1830)***; in the original Latin, *rami temporales*, p. 58. Günther described further posterior, middle, and anterior divisions of the temporal branches.
17. *temporal branches of zygomatic branches of ascending branch of superficial branch of hard nerve (Günther, 1786)*
Synonym for *temporal branches of suprajugal branches of ascending branch of superficial branch of hard nerve (Günther, 1786)*; in the original Latin, *rami temporales*, p. 58.
18. *orbital branches of suprajugal branches of ascending branch of superficial branch of hard nerve (Günther, 1786)*
Basically synonym for macrodissected adult human ventral (lower) branches of ***temporal branches of facial nerve (Swan, 1830)***; in the original Latin, *rami orbitales*, p. 58. Günther described further superior and inferior divisions of the orbital branches.
19. *orbital branches of zygomatic branches of ascending branch of superficial branch of hard nerve (Günther, 1786)*
Synonym for *orbital branches of suprajugal branches of ascending branch of superficial branch of hard nerve (Günther, 1786)*; in the original Latin, *rami orbitales*, p. 58.
20. *zygomatic nerve (Soemmerring, 1791)*
Synonym for macrodissected adult human *posterior temporal nerve of hard nerve (Meckel, 1753)*; in the original Latin, *nervus zygomaticus*, p. 233.
21. *nervus jugalis primus (Soemmerring, 1791)*
Synonym for macrodissected adult human *posterior temporal nerve of hard nerve (Meckel, 1753)*; p. 233. *Jugum* is zygomatic process; see Bell (1803b, p. 150).
22. *middle temporal nerve (Soemmerring, 1791)*
Synonym for macrodissected adult human *second temporal branch of hard nerve (Meckel, 1753)*; in the original Latin, *nervus temporalis medius*, p. 234.
23. *nervus jugalis secundus (Soemmerring, 1791)*
Synonym for macrodissected adult human *second temporal branch of hard nerve (Meckel, 1753)*; p. 234.
24. *anterior temporal nerve (Soemmerring, 1791)*
Synonym for macrodissected adult human *third temporal branch of hard nerve (Meckel, 1753)*; in the original Latin, *nervus temporalis anterior*, p. 234.
25. *nervus jugalis tertius (Soemmerring, 1791)*
Synonym for macrodissected adult human *third temporal branch of hard nerve (Meckel, 1753)*; p. 234.
26. *nervus jugalis quartus (Soemmerring, 1791)*
Synonym for macrodissected adult human *fourth temporal branch of hard nerve (Meckel, 1753)*; p. 234.
27. *nervus jugalis posterior (Mayer, 1794)*
Synonym for macrodissected adult human *nervus jugalis primus (Soemmerring, 1791)*; Part 5, Table VII-*92* (p. 48).
28. *anterior auricular nerve (Mayer, 1794)*
Synonym for macrodissected adult human *anterior auricular branches of posterior zygomatic nerve (Meckel, 1753)*; in the original Latin, *nervus auricularis anterior*; Part 5, Table VII-*93* (p. 48).
29. *second temporal nerve (Soemmerring, 1798)*
Synonym for macrodissected adult human *second temporal branch of hard nerve (Meckel, 1753)*; in the original Latin, *nervus temporalis secundus*, p. 249.

30. *posterior zygomatic threads of temporal surculus (Bellingeri, 1818)*
    Most caudal macrodissected adult human ***temporal branches of facial nerve (Swan, 1830)*** to pinna and adjacent regions of temporal muscle and overlying skin; in the original Latin, *stamen zygomaticus posterior*, see Table II.
31. *auricular filament of posterior zygomatic threads of temporal surculus (Bellingeri, 1818)*
    Caudal branch of *posterior zygomatic threads of temporal surculus (Bellingeri, 1818)* to pinna; in the original Latin, *filament auricularis*, see Table II.
32. *temporal filaments of posterior zygomatic threads of temporal surculus (Bellingeri, 1818)*
    Rostral branch of *posterior zygomatic threads of temporal surculus (Bellingeri, 1818)* to caudal regions of temporal muscle and accompanying skin; in the original Latin, *filamenta temporalia*, see Table II.
33. *middle zygomatic threads of temporal surculus (Bellingeri, 1818)*
    Intermediate macrodissected adult human ***temporal branches of facial nerve (Swan, 1830)*** to intermediate regions of temporal muscle and overlying skin; in the original Latin, *stamen zygomaticus medius*, see Table II.
34. *anterior zygomatic threads of temporal surculus (Bellingeri, 1818)*
    Rostral macrodissected adult human ***temporal branches of facial nerve (Swan, 1830)*** to rostral regions of temporal muscle and overlying skin; in the original Latin, *stamen zygomaticus anterior*, see Table II.
35. *superior orbital thread of temporal surculus (Bellingeri, 1818)*
    More dorsal macrodissected adult human ***temporal branch of facial nerve (Swan, 1830)*** associated with upper eyelid and dorsal part of orbicularis oculi muscle; in the original Latin, *stamen orbitarius superior*, see Table II. Also see *inferior orbital thread of temporal surculus (Bellingeri, 1818)*.
36. *inferior orbital thread of temporal surculus (Bellingeri, 1818)*
    More ventral macrodissected adult human ***temporal branch of facial nerve (Swan, 1830)*** generating four named smaller branches; in the original Latin, *stamen orbitarius inferior*, see Table II. Also see *superior orbital thread of temporal surculus (Bellingeri, 1818)*.
37. *upper filament of inferior orbital thread of temporal surculus (Bellingeri, 1818)*
    Dorsal branch of *inferior orbital thread of temporal surculus (Bellingeri, 1818)* to some dorsal parts of orbicularis oculi muscle; in the original Latin, *filamentum superius*, see Table II.
38. *middle filament of inferior orbital thread of temporal surculus (Bellingeri, 1818)*
    Intermediate branch of *inferior orbital thread of temporal surculus (Bellingeri, 1818)* to orbicularis oculi muscle and both eyelids; in the original Latin, *filamentum medium*, see Table II.
39. *lower filament of inferior orbital thread of temporal surculus (Bellingeri, 1818)*
    Intermediate branch of *inferior orbital thread of temporal surculus (Bellingeri, 1818)* to lower eyelid and dorsal region of medial angle of eye; in the original Latin, *filamentum inferius*, see Table II.
39. *lowest filament of inferior orbital thread of temporal surculus (Bellingeri, 1818)*
    Ventral branch of *inferior orbital thread of temporal surculus (Bellingeri, 1818)* to lower eyelid and "musculum zygomaticum"; in the original Latin, *filamentum infimum*, see Table II.
40. *temporal branch of facial nerve (Swan, 1830)*
    Branch of macrodissected adult human ***temporal branches of facial nerve (Swan, 1830)*** specifically to frontal belly of occipitofrontalis (frontalis) muscle; Plate XIII-3.

temporal ganglion (Andersch & Soemmerring, 1792)

As described in the older literature for macrodissected adult human, a small ***paravertebral ganglion (Durward, 1951)*** usually associated with the ***external carotid plexus (>1840)*** near the posterior auricular artery, but sometimes found near the parotid gland, and having a ***communicating branch (Winslow, 1733)*** with the ***superior cervical ganglion (Vieussens, 1684)***; see Foster (1892, p. 1678). For Andersch & Soemmerring's use in macrodissected adult human, see p. 173. Andersch completed his thesis work c1751–c1755 but it was not published for distribution until edited by Soemmerring in 1792; also see Andersch (1797). Its relationship to the ***facial ganglion (Lazorthes, 1949)*** is unclear.

TRANSLATIONS:

1. *ganglium temporale (Andersch & Soemmerring, 1792)*
   Original Latin form of ***temporal ganglion (Andersch & Soemmerring, 1792)***; p. 173.

EARLIER REFERENCES:

Earlier synonyms:

1. *temporal small ganglion (Andersch & Soemmerring, 1792)*
   Synonym for ***temporal ganglion (Andersch & Soemmerring, 1792)***; in the original Latin, *gangliolum temporale*, p. 172. A ***communicating branch (Winslow, 1733)*** was also described with *facial nerve (Vicq d'Azyr, 1784)*.
2. *temporal soft small ganglion (Andersch & Soemmerring, 1792)*
   Synonym for ***temporal ganglion (Andersch & Soemmerring, 1792)***; in the original Latin, *gangliolum molle temporale*, p. 172.

LATER SYNONYMS:

1. *ganglion of temporal nervi molles (Knox, 1832)*
   Synonym for macrodissected adult human ***temporal ganglion (Andersch & Soemmerring, 1792)***. It was described as associated with one of the deep temporal arteries; Plate III-*191* in Knox's translation of Scarpa

(1794), who pointed out that Andersch had identified it earlier. Scarpa noted that it has *soft nerve (Haller, 1762)* input and output; see Plate III-*116*.

temporal limb of anterior commissure (>1840)

As described in macrodissected adult human, and mammal generally with histological methods for ***axons (Kölliker, 1896)***, the caudally directed division of the ***anterior commissure (Lieutaud, 1742)*** interconnecting parts of the right and left ***temporal region (>1840)*** and *amygdalar region (>1840)* considered together; see Nieuwenhuys et al. (2008, p. 596). A minor component is the continuation of the ***terminal stria commissure (>1840)*** after it joins near the median plane. It was first identified by Malpighi; see ***[temporal limb of anterior commissure (>1840)] (Malpighi, 1665)***.

EARLIER REFERENCES:

Described, not named or illustrated:

1. ***[temporal limb of anterior commissure (>1840)] (Malpighi, 1665)***
   Malpighi briefly noted it, "A large fibre bundle has been observed—so far a puzzle to the mind—which courses transversally through the anterior part of the spinal medulla [*striate body (Willis, 1664)* or ***cerebral nuclei (Swanson, 2000a)***], to twine itself densely round like a girdle and finally to terminate in two roots, after it had been carried laterally." (Meyer translation, 1967, p. 187). The two roots are ***olfactory limb of anterior commissure (>1840)*** and ***temporal limb of anterior commissure (>1840)***; see Meyer (1971, p. 14). Malpighi dissected a variety of mammals including human, but the species used for this observation is unclear.
2. ***[temporal limb of anterior commissure (>1840)] (Reil, 1809b)***
   Described in macrodissected adult human thus, "The foremost fasciculus [of the *corona radiata (Reil, 1809b)*] attaches itself to the curved central part of the anterior commissure; or the anterior commissure passes between the first fasciculi of the fibrous cone [*corona radiata (Reil, 1809b)*], and then spreads itself out in the under surface of the middle [temporal] lobe." (Mayo translation, 1823, p. 60; also see Meyer, 1971, p. 25).

Earlier synonyms:

1. *posterior branch of anterior commissure (Reil, 1812a)*
   Synonym for macrodissected adult sheep and rabbit ***temporal limb of anterior commissure (>1840)***, distinguishing it clearly from *anterior branch of anterior commissure (Reil, 1812a)*; see Mayo translation (1823, p. 110).
2. *posterior part of anterior commissure (Rolando, 1831)*
   Synonym for macrodissected adult human ***temporal limb of anterior commissure (>1840)***; in the original Italian, *parte posteriore della commessura anteriore*, Figure 9-*15*.

temporal operculum (>1840)

As described for macrodissected adult human, the surface of the ***temporal region (>1840)*** lining the floor of the ***lateral cerebral sulcus (>1840)*** up to the ***circular sulcus (Schwalbe, 1881)***, and including dorsomedial parts of the ***superior temporal gyrus (>1840)***, called the ***temporal plane (>1840)***, and the caudomedially adjacent ***transverse temporal gyri (>1840)***; see Carpenter (1976, Fig. 2.3), Williams & Warwick (1980, Fig. 7.112), *Terminologia Anatomica* (1998, p. 125), *Dorland's* (2003, p. 1316). It was not clearly delineated by 1840.

temporal plane (Heschl, 1878)

As described for macrodissected adult human, the surface of the ***superior temporal gyrus (>1840)*** lying within the ***temporal operculum (>1840)***, and separated from the medially adjacent ***transverse temporal gyri (Heschl, 1878)*** by the ***transverse temporal sulcus (Heschl, 1878)***; see Crosby et al. (1962, Fig. 316), Williams & Warwick (1980, Fig. 7.112 labeled *superior temporal gyrus*), Nieuwenhuys et al. (2008, p. 737 and Fig. 18.1A-*1*), *Terminologia Anatomica* (1998, p. 125). It was first clearly delineated by Gall & Spurzheim; see ***[temporal plane (Heschl, 1878)] (Gall & Spurzheim, 1810)***.

TRANSLATIONS:

1. *Schläfenfläche (Heschl, 1878)*
   Original German form of ***temporal plane (Heschl, 1878)***; p. 5.
2. *planum temporale (>1840)*
   Current Latin form of ***temporal plane (Heschl, 1878)***; see *Terminologia Anatomica* (1998, p. 125).

EARLIER REFERENCES:

Illustrated, not named or described:

1. ***[temporal plane (Heschl, 1878)] (Gall & Spurzheim, 1810)***
   Very clearly illustrated for macrodissected adult human; Plate V, right side.

temporal pole (Broca, 1878a)

As described for macrodissected adult human, the rostral tip of the ***temporal region (>1840)*** of the ***cerebral cortex gray matter (>1840)***; see Williams & Warwick (1980, p. 982), *Terminologia Anatomica* (1998, p. 125). For Broca's use in macrodissected adult human, see p. 209. Attention was perhaps first drawn to it as the *monticulus (Vicq d'Azyr, 1786)*.

EARLIER REFERENCES:

Earlier synonyms:

1. *monticulus (Vicq d'Azyr, 1786)*
   Synonym for macrodissected adult human ***temporal pole (Broca, 1878a)***; p. 50, Plate XVII-*14,19*. Vicq d'Azyr attributed the term used in this way to Vesalius but this is doubtful; see *monticulus (Vesalius, 1555)*.
2. *eminence (Vicq d'Azyr, 1786)*
   Synonym for *monticulus (Vicq d'Azyr, 1786)*; p. 50, Plate XVII-*14*.
3. *sphenoidal horn (Cruveilhier, 1836)*
   Synonym for macrodissected adult human ***temporal pole (>1840)***; in the original French, *corne sphénoïdal*, p. 658.

temporal region (>1840)

As described for macrodissected adult human, a topographic division of the ***cerebral cortex gray matter (>1840)*** lying ventral to the ***insular region (Brodmann, 1909)*** and ***parietal region (>1840)***. Its major topographic subdivisions, from dorsomedial to lateral to ventromedial include sequentially the ***transverse temporal gyri (>1840)***, ***superior temporal gyrus (>1840)***, ***middle temporal gyrus (>1840)***, ***inferior temporal gyrus (>1840)***, ***lateral occipitotemporal gyrus (>1840)***, and ***medial occipitotemporal gyrus (>1840)***. In macrodissected adult human there are no clear surface landmarks between **temporal region (>1840)** and ***occipital region (Vesalius, 1543a)***. For general modern overview see Nieuwenhuys et al. (2008, p. 613 ff.). ***Temporal region (>1840)*** is preferred to *temporal lobe (Rolando, 1831)* because an actual lobe cannot be distinguished and because the term *region* applies to all mammals, whether gyrencephalic or lissencephalic. Its location was first vaguely indicated as the *lower substance of brain (Dryander, 1536)*, whereas it was relatively clearly described and illustrated by Vesalius; see *lower substance of brain (Dryander, 1536)*.

EARLIER REFERENCES:

Earlier synonyms:

1. *lower substance of brain (Dryander, 1536)*
   Dryander indicated location of macrodissected adult human ***temporal region (>1840)*** in dissection illustrated in Figure 7 and its legend; see Lind translation (1975, p. 301). Shortly thereafter, Vesalius very clearly illustrated base of macrodissected adult human ***temporal region (>1840)*** in first published view of base of ***brain (Smith Papyrus, c1700 BC)***; see Richardson and Carman translation (2002, p. 168). However, his lateral view of ***cerebral cortex gray matter (>1840)*** does not indicate ***lateral cerebral sulcus (>1840)***, and thus does not distinguish between ***temporal region (>1840)*** and ***parietal region (>1840)***; see Richardson & Carman translation (2002, p. 169). Vesalius also mentioned ***temporal region (>1840)*** and labeled it; see Richardson & Carman translation (2002, *B* in figure following p. 263). Also see nice description of macrodissected adult human ***temporal region (>1840)*** as related to underlying skull in Richardson & Carman translation (2009, p. 182).
2. *middle cerebral prominence (Varoli, 1573)*
   Varoli recognized part of macrodissected adult human ***cerebral cortex gray matter (>1840)*** lying in middle cranial fossa as *middle cerebral prominence (Varoli, 1573)*, corresponding roughly to ***temporal region (>1840)***. It has also been translated *medial cerebral prominence* and *inferior cerebral prominence*; see Varoli (1573, ff. 5–6, and Fig. I on f. 17v), Meyer (1971, p. 122), Clarke & O'Malley (1996, p. 822).
3. *middle and inferior cerebral prominence (Varoli, 1573)*
   Synonym for *middle cerebral prominence (Varoli, 1573)*; f. 5, see Burdach (1822, p. 389).
4. *middle prominence of brain (Crooke, 1615)*
   English form of macrodissected adult human *middle cerebral prominence (Varoli, 1573)*; pp. 497–498.
5. *middle part of brain (Crooke, 1615)*
   English form of macrodissected adult human *middle cerebral prominence (Varoli, 1573)*; p. 497.
6. *middle lobe of cerebrum (Winslow, 1733)*
   Corresponds roughly to macrodissected adult human ***temporal region (>1840)***, separated from *anterior lobe of cerebrum (Winslow, 1733)* by ***lateral cerebral sulcus (>1840)***. Thus, *middle lobe of cerebrum (Winslow, 1733)* is better defined version of *middle cerebral prominence (Varoli, 1573)*.
7. *temporal cerebral lobule (Chaussier, 1807)*
   Roughly synonymous with macrodissected adult human ***temporal region (>1840)***; p. 37, see Meyer (1971, p. 122).
8. *inferior lobe (Burdach, 1822)*
   Roughly synonymous with macrodissected adult human ***temporal region (>1840)***; in the original Latin, *lobus inferior*, and German, *der Unterlappen*, p. 172.
9. *temporal lobe (Rolando, 1831)*
   Roughly synonymous with macrodissected adult human ***temporal region (>1840)***; in the original Italian, *lobo temporale*, p. 114.

PARTLY CORRESPONDS:

1. *lateral lobe (Fyfe, 1800)*
   Ventral (Inferior) surface or base of macrodissected adult human ***temporal region (>1840)***; p. 15.
2. *middle lobe (Fyfe, 1800)*
   Synonym for *lateral lobe (Fyfe, 1800)*; p. 15.
3. *lateral process (Fyfe, 1800)*
   Synonym for *lateral lobe (Fyfe, 1800)*; p. 15.
4. *middle process (Fyfe, 1800)*
   Synonym for *lateral lobe (Fyfe, 1800)*; p. 15.
5. *sphenoidal lobule (Serres, 1824–1826)*
   Rostral zone of ventral (inferior) ***temporal region (>1840)*** in mammal, roughly bordering greater wing of sphenoid bone; in the original French, *lobule sphénoïdal*, p. 548 ff.
6. *temporal lobe (Arnold, 1838a)*
   Synonym for macrodissected adult human *temporal lobe (Rolando, 1831)* except specifically without ***cerebral cortex gray matter (>1840)*** associated with ***temporal operculum (>1840)***, which Arnold included in *intermediate lobe (Arnold, 1838a)*; in the original Latin, *lobus temporalis*, pp. 51–52.
7. *sphenoidal lobe (Arnold, 1838a)*
   Synonym for *temporal lobe (Arnold, 1838a)*; in the original Latin, *lobus sphenoidalis*, p. 52.
8. *area temporopolaris (Brodmann, 1909)*
   Original Latin form of *temporopolar area (Brodmann, 1909)*; p. 143.
9. *temporopolar area (Brodmann, 1909)*
   Based on cellular architecture in adult human, rostral zone of ***temporal region (>1840)*** coinciding with ***temporal pole (Broca, 1878a)*** and basically including rostral

(anterior) ends of ***superior temporal gyrus (>1840)***, ***middle temporal gyrus (>1840)***, ***inferior temporal gyrus (>1840)***, ***lateral occipitotemporal gyrus (>1840)***, and ***medial occipitotemporal gyrus (>1840)***; see p. 124 and Figures 85, 86. Compare with Williams & Warwick (1980, Figs. 7.111A, 7.114A).

10. *area 38 (Brodmann, 1909)*
 Synonym for adult human *temporopolar area (Brodmann, 1909)*; in the original German, *Feld 38*, p. 143.
11. *area temporalis inferior (Brodmann, 1909)*
 Original Latin form of *inferior temporal area (Brodmann, 1909)*; p. 143.
12. *inferior temporal area (Brodmann, 1909)*
 Based on cellular architecture in adult human, zone of ***temporal region (>1840)*** coinciding roughly with large middle parts of ***inferior temporal gyrus (>1840)*** and adjacent ***lateral occipitotemporal gyrus (>1840)***. The rostral (anterior) parts are occupied by *temporopolar area (Brodmann, 1909)* whereas caudal (posterior) parts are occupied by *occipitotemporal area (Brodmann, 1909)*; see p. 124 and Figures 85, 86. Compare with Williams & Warwick (1980, Figs. 7.111A, 7.114A).
13. *area 20 (Brodmann, 1909)*
 Synonym for adult human *inferior temporal area (Brodmann, 1909)*; in the original German, *Feld 20*, p. 143.
14. *area occipito-temporalis (Brodmann, 1909)*
 Original Latin form of *occipitotemporal area (Brodmann, 1909)*; p. 143.
15. *occipitotemporal area (Brodmann, 1909)*
 Based on cellular architecture in adult human, zone of ***temporal region (>1840)*** coinciding with caudal ends of ***lateral occipitotemporal gyrus (>1840)*** and ***medial occipitotemporal gyrus (>1840)***. It is transitional with ***occipital region (Vesalius, 1543a)***, although Brodmann pointed out that its caudal (posterior) border with *preoccipital area (Brodmann, 1909)* or *area 19 (Brodmann, 1909)* of ***occipital region (Vesalius, 1543a)*** is quite clear histologically if not grossly; see pp. 122, 124 and Figures 85, 86. Compare with Williams & Warwick (1980, Figs. 7.111A, 7.114A).
16. *area 37 (Brodmann, 1909)*
 Synonym for adult human *occipitotemporal area (Brodmann, 1909)*; in the original German, *Feld 37*, p. 143.
17. *fusiform gyrus (>1840)*
 Topographic subdivision of macrodissected adult human ***temporal region (>1840)*** including ***lateral occipitotemporal gyrus (>1840)*** and ***medial occipitotemporal gyrus (>1840)*** considered together; see Williams & Warwick (1980, p. 1020), *Dorland's* (2003, p. 806).

tenia tecta (Swanson, 1992)

As described with cellular architecture for mammal, the tiny rostral segment of the ***hippocampal region (Swanson et al., 1987)***, extending ventral to the rostral end of the ***indusium griseum (Valentin, 1841)*** and ending between the ***anterior olfactory nucleus (Herrick, 1910)*** and ***piriform area (Smith, 1919)***. For Swanson's use in cytoarchitectonic sections of adult rat see (2004, Atlas Levels 5–13, p. 197 note 29); for similar use in human, see Nieuwenhuys et al. (2008, Fig. 12.3, p. 366). In macrodissected adult human it was often described as the *medial olfactory stria (>1840)*, lying between *parolfactory gyrus (>1840)* and *paraterminal gyrus (>1840)*; see Nauta & Haymaker (1969, Fig. 4.10, p. 158), Williams & Warwick (1980, p. 991). It was first clearly delineated by Casseri; see ***[tenia tecta (Swanson, 1992)] (Casseri, 1609)***.

EARLIER REFERENCES:

Illustrated, not named or described:

1. ***[tenia tecta (Swanson, 1992)] (Casseri, 1609)***
 First clear illustration, in macrodissected adult human; see Meyer (1971, p. 77 and Fig. 4-*H*). Compare with Nauta & Haymaker (1969, Fig. 4.10) and *short internal root of olfactory nerve (Vicq d'Azyr, 1786)*.

Earlier synonyms:

1. *short internal root of olfactory nerve (Vicq d'Azyr, 1786)*
 Synonym for macrodissected adult human *medial olfactory stria (>1840)*; Plate XVII, Figure I-22.
2. *gray root of olfactory nerve (Cloquet, 1816)*
 Synonym for macrodissected adult human *short internal root of olfactory nerve (Vicq d'Azyr, 1786)*; in the original French, *racine grise*, p. 585.
3. *internal root of olfactory nerve (Swan, 1830)*
 Synonym for macrodissected adult human *medial olfactory stria (>1840)*; Plate X, Figure 3-*c*. Arnold (1834, Tab. I-3) gave the Latin, *nervus olfactorius radix interna*.
4. *superior root of olfactory nerve (Knox, 1832)*
 Synonym for macrodissected adult human *gray root of olfactory nerve (Cloquet, 1816)*; Supplemental Plate I-*15c*.
5. *cineritious root of olfactory nerve (Knox, 1832)*
 Synonym for macrodissected adult human *gray root of olfactory nerve (Cloquet, 1816)*; Supplemental Plate I-*15c*.
6. *medial olfactory stria (>1840)*
 Can be synonym for macrodissected adult human ***tenia tecta (Swanson, 1992)*** according to Nauta & Haymaker (1969, Fig. 4.10); also see Gurdjian (1925, p. 134).
7. *prehippocampal rudiment (>1840)*
 Can be synonym for macrodissected adult human *medial olfactory stria (>1840)* or ***tenia tecta (Swanson, 1992)***, although how much, if any, of rostral end of ***indusium griseum (Valentin, 1841)*** is included is unclear; see Nauta & Haymaker (1969, Fig. 4.10), Williams & Warwick (1980, p. 988).

tentorial nerve (Arnold, 1838a)

As described for macrodissected adult human, the first (most proximal) branch of the ***ophthalmic nerve (Winslow, 1733)***, arising in the wall of the ***cavernous sinus (Winslow, 1733)*** and turning dorsally and caudally to supply ***dura (Galen, c177)*** of the ***cerebellar tentorium (Winslow, 1733)*** and ***cerebral falx (Vesalius, 1543a)*** with sensory ***dendrites (His, 1889)***; see Durward (1951, p. 1019 and Fig. 999), Williams & Warwick (1980, p. 1061), *Dorland's* (2003, p. 1576). For Arnold's use in macrodissected adult human, see p. 187. It was first identified by Vieussens; see ***[tentorial nerve (Arnold, 1838a)] (Vieussens, 1684)***.

TRANSLATIONS:

1. *nervus tentorii (Arnold, 1838a)*
   Original Latin form of ***tentorial nerve (Arnold, 1838a)***; the full expression was *nervus tentorii primi rami quinti paris*, the *tentorial nerve of first branch of fifth pair*; p. 187.

EARLIER REFERENCES:

Illustrated and described, not named:

1. ***[tentorial nerve (Arnold, 1838a)] (Vieussens, 1684)***
   Briefly described and illustrated for macrodissected adult human; see p. 170 and Figure 22-*a*.

Earlier synonyms:

1. *recurrent nerve (Arnold, 1834)*
   Synonym for macrodissected adult human ***tentorial nerve (Arnold, 1838a)***; in the original Latin, *nervus recurrens*, p. 7. According to Cruveilhier (1836, p. 910) several small branches (filaments) destined for ***cerebellar tentorium (Winslow, 1733)*** arise from ***trigeminal ganglion (>1840)*** itself in macrodissected adult human.

LATER SYNONYMS:

1. *ramus meningeus recurrens nervi ophthalmici (>1840)*
   Current Latin form of ***tentorial nerve (Arnold, 1838a)***; see *Terminologia Anatomica* (1998, p. 133). The *recurrent meningeal branch of ophthalmic nerve.*

tentorial notch (>1840)

As described for macrodissected adult human, the oval space between the free border of the right and left ***cerebellar tentorium (Winslow, 1733)*** occupied by the ***midbrain (Baer, 1837)*** and rostral part of the *superior vermis (>1840)* of the ***cerebellum (Aristotle)***; see Carpenter (1976, p. 1, Figs. 1.2–1.4), Williams & Warwick (p. 1045, Fig. 7.162), *Terminologia Anatomica* (1998, p. 104). It was clearly described and named by Winslow; see *great oval notch (Winslow, 1733)*.

TRANSLATIONS:

1. *incisura tentorii (>1840)*
   Current Latin form of ***tentorial notch (>1840)***; see *Terminologia Anatomica* (1998, p. 104).

EARLIER REFERENCES:

Earlier synonyms:

1. *great oval notch (Winslow, 1733)*
   Synonym for macrodissected adult human ***tentorial notch (>1840)***; Section X, p. 26.

terminal autonomic nerves (Swanson & Bota, 2010)

Autonomic nerves (>1840) appearing macroscopically to arise predominantly from ***terminal ganglia (Gaskell, 1886)*** and/or ***terminal plexuses (Swanson & Bota, 2010)***, and now generally described sequentially from rostral (superior) to caudal (inferior). They were nicely illustrated by Ranson (1920, Fig. 250). The ***short ciliary nerves (>1840)*** or *lesser nerves out of infolding of third pair (Willis, 1664)* were perhaps the first clear example described macroscopically.

terminal filament (Tiedemann, 1821)

As described for macrodissected adult human, a slender ***spinal cord differentiation (>1840)*** extending from the caudal end of the ***medullary cone (Bock, 1827)*** to the base of the coccyx and consisting mostly of connective tissue; see *Dorland's* (2003, p. 702), Standring (2008, p. 749). For Tiedemann's use in macrodissected adult monkey, see Table I, Figure 5-*i*. It was known to Galen; see ***[terminal filament (Tiedemann, 1821)] (Galen, c181)***.

TRANSLATIONS:

1. *filum terminale (Tiedemann, 1821)*
   Original Latin form of ***terminal filament (Tiedemann, 1821)***; Table I, Figure 5-*i*.
2. *filamentum terminale (Arnold, 1838b)*
   Latin form of ***terminal filament (Tiedemann, 1821)***; Table I, Figure 2-*n*.

EARLIER REFERENCES:

Described, not named or illustrated:

1. ***[terminal filament (Tiedemann, 1821)] (Galen, c181)***
   In *On Bones, for Beginners (De Ossibus ad Tirones*, cap. 12) Galen mentioned caudal end of macrodissected adult beef, pig, and/or macaque (but not human) ***spinal cord (Galen, c192)***, "What remains of the spinal cord at the end of the third bone [of the coccyx] emerges alone and unpaired." (Richardson & Carman translation, 2002, p. 255).

Illustrated and described, not named:

1. ***[terminal filament (Tiedemann, 1821)] (Vesalius, 1543a)***
   At least part of it was clearly described and illustrated for macrodissected adult human; see Richardson & Carman translation (2002, p. 222, part *H* of figure on pp. 205, 255, and in figure following p. 263).

Earlier synonyms:

1. *unpaired nerve (Haly Abbas or Ali ibn' ul-Abbas, d. 994)*
   In *The Complete Book of Medical Art, Called the Royal Book*, Haly Abbas or Ali ibn' ul-Abbas referred to ***terminal filament (Tiedemann, 1821)*** as unpaired ***nerve (Herophilus, c335–c280 BC)***, in the French translation, "Quand aux trois paires et au nerf unique, impair qui naissent du coccyx" (second section of first part, Chapter 10; Razi, 1903, p. 169). His predecessor Razi referred to "le nerv unique" in the French translation (Chapter 4 of *al-Mansuri*; Razi, 1903, p. 37), and his successor Avicenna referred to "le nerf impair" in the French translation (first book of the *Canon*; Razi, 1903, p. 602).
2. *nervus sine pari (Hall, 1565)*
   Latin synonym for macrodissected adult human ***terminal filament (Tiedemann, 1821)***; p. 6.
3. *nervum conjuge carentem (Bauhin, 1605)*
   Latin synonym for macrodissected adult human ***terminal filament (Tiedemann, 1821)***; p. 682. Also see *nervum sine conjuge (Crooke, 1615)*.

4. *nervum sine conjuge (Crooke, 1615)*
   Synonym for macrodissected adult human ***terminal filament (Tiedemann, 1821)***, and translated as *nerve without a companion*; p. 900, based on *nervum conjuge carentem (Bauhin, 1605)*.
5. *nervus impar (Haller, 1762)*
   Synonym for macrodissected adult human ***terminal filament (Tiedemann, 1821)***; p. 254.
6. *ligamentum piae matris (Fyfe, 1800)*
   Synonym listed for macrodissected adult human ***terminal filament (Tiedemann, 1821)***; Vol. 2, p. 302.
7. *fortieth pair of nerves (Fyfe, 1800)*
   Synonym listed for macrodissected adult human ***terminal filament (Tiedemann, 1821)***; Vol. 2, p. 302.
8. *nervus imparus sacrus (Fyfe, 1800)*
   Synonym listed for macrodissected adult human ***terminal filament (Tiedemann, 1821)***; Vol. 2, p. 302.

terminal ganglia (Gaskell, 1886)

Based on structure-function criteria in vertebrate, a topographic division of ***autonomic ganglia (Langley, 1900)*** lying on or in the walls of innervated viscera, also known as *parasympathetic ganglia (Kuntz, 1929)*; p. 3, also see Durward (1951, p. 1128), Crosby et al. (1962, p. 524). They may or may not be associated with a ***terminal plexus (Swanson & Bota, 2010)***, and now are commonly described sequentially from rostral (superior) to caudal (inferior). The first two were discovered by Willis; see ***[terminal ganglia (Gaskell, 1886)] (Willis, 1664)***.

EARLIER REFERENCES:

Illustrated and described, not named:

1. ***[terminal ganglia (Gaskell, 1886)] (Willis, 1664)***
   Without providing a general term Willis discovered two in macrodissected adult human and other common large mammals, the *infolding of third pair (Willis, 1664)* or ***ciliary ganglion (Loder, 1778)***, and *cardiac infolding (Willis, 1664)* or ***cardiac ganglion (Neubauer, 1772; Haller, 1772)***.

LATER SYNONYMS:

1. *parasympathetic ganglia (Kuntz, 1929)*
   Functional systems synonym for ***terminal ganglia (Gaskell, 1886)***; see p. 114.

PARTLY CORRESPONDS:

1. *pharyngeal ganglion (Wrisberg, 1786)*
   As described for macrodissected adult human, associated with ***pharyngeal plexus (Neubauer, 1772)***; see Wrisberg (1800, pp. 425–426). Detailed history given in Todd (1836–1839, p. 496), concluding it is probably connective tissue or *pseudoganglion (>1840)*.
2. *ganglioform plexus of pharyngeal nerve (Knox, 1832)*
   Macrodissected adult human synonym for *pharyngeal ganglion (Wrisberg, 1786)*; Plate II-*64* in Knox's translation of Scarpa (1794).

terminal ganglion (>1840)

As described for macrodissected adult human, a ***cranial nerve ganglion (>1840)*** consisting of mostly scattered ***neurons (Waldeyer, 1891)*** along the ***terminal nerve (>1840)***; see Mettler (1948, Fig. 51), Williams & Warwick (1980, p. 1055), *Terminologia Anatomica* (1998, p. 133). It was not identified by 1840.

terminal lamina (Burdach, 1822)

As described for macrodissected developing and adult human, a thin, narrow, unpaired plate of tissue in the median plane with poorly defined borders forming the rostral end of the ***hypothalamic part of third ventricle (Swanson, 2004)***, in the ***periventricular hypothalamic zone (Nauta & Haymaker, 1969)*** stretching between ***optic chiasm (Galen, c173)*** ventrally and ***anterior commissure (Lieutaud, 1742)*** dorsally; see Mettler (1948, p. 102 and Fig. 68), Hamilton & Mossman (1972, p. 456). Based on cellular architecture in mammal generally, its main features are the ***vascular organ of lamina terminalis (>1840)*** in the ventral tip and the ***median preoptic nucleus (>1840)*** more dorsally. For Burdach's use in macrodissected adult human, see p. 108; also see *vulva (Casseri, 1627)* and *gray plate (Meckel, 1817)*. It was first clearly delineated by Steno; see ***[terminal lamina (Burdach, 1822)] (Steno, 1669)***.

TRANSLATIONS:

1. *Endplatte (Burdach, 1822)*
   Original German form of ***terminal lamina (Burdach, 1822)***; p. 108.
2. *lamina terminalis (Burdach, 1822)*
   Original Latin form of ***terminal lamina (Burdach, 1822)***; p. 108.

EARLIER REFERENCES:

Illustrated, not named or described:

1. ***[terminal lamina (Burdach, 1822)] (Steno, 1669)***
   In first realistic midsagittal illustrations of ***brain (Smith Papyrus, c1700 BC)***, for macrodissected adult human, Steno clearly showed its disposition at rostral end of ***hypothalamic part of third ventricle (Swanson, 2004)***, between ***optic chiasm (Galen, c173)*** ventrally and ***anterior commissure (Lieutaud, 1742)*** dorsally; Plates I, II.

Earlier synonyms:

1. *pars infundibuli anterior, pars pellucida (Tarin, 1750)*
   Synonym for macrodissected adult human ***terminal lamina (Burdach, 1822)***; Table I, Figure 5-*X*. Burdach (1822, p. 327) also listed for Tarin the term, *pars infundibuli anterior, peculiari substantia circumscripta*.
2. *gray lamina of optic chiasm (Vicq d'Azyr, 1784)*
   Synonym for macrodissected adult human ***terminal lamina (Burdach, 1822)***; in the original French, *lame grise de la jonction des nerfs optiques*, p. 547. Also see Vicq d'Azyr (1786, p. 72 and Pl. XXI-*8*). Burdach (1822, p. 327) gave the Latin form, *lamina grysea juncturae nervorum opticorum*.
3. *pulpy septum of third ventricle (Vicq d'Azyr, 1784)*
   Synonym for macrodissected adult human ***terminal lamina (Burdach, 1822)***; in the original French, *cloison pulpeuse du troisième ventricule*, p. 547. Also see Vicq d'Azyr (1786, p. 72, Pl. XXI-*8*).

4. *medullary septum of third ventricle (Vicq d'Azyr, 1786)*
Synonym for macrodissected adult human ***terminal lamina (Burdach, 1822)***; in the original French, *cloison médullaire du troisième ventricule*, p. 85.

LATER SYNONYMS:

1. *gray terminal lamina (Burdach, 1822)*
Synonym for ***terminal lamina (Burdach, 1822)***; in the original German, *graue Endplatte*, and in the original Latin, *lamina cinerea terminalis*; pp. 108, 327.
2. *velum commissurae anterioris (Bergmann, 1831)*
Apparently, region in and perhaps around macrodissected adult human ***terminal lamina (Burdach, 1822)*** described and illustrated as having 8–12 transverse bundles, *chordis transversalibus sive pectine*; p. 18, Table I-*f*.
3. *anterior floor of third ventricle (Cruveilhier, 1836)*
Apparently corresponds roughly to macrodissected adult human ***terminal lamina (Burdach, 1822)***; in the original French, *plancher antérieur du troisième ventricule*, p. 654. See Henle (1871, p. 94).

terminal nerve (>1840)

As described for macrodissected adult human, a tiny ***cranial nerve (Soemmerring, 1791)*** extending from the nasal mucosa through the cribriform plate of the ethmoid bone in association with the ***olfactory nerve (Winslow, 1733)*** to end in ventromedial regions of the ***forebrain (Goette, 1873)*** just rostral and caudal to the ***terminal lamina (Burdach, 1822)***; see Williams & Warwick (1980, p. 1055), *Terminologia Anatomica* (1998, p. 133), Kawai et al. (2009). It is sometimes called *cranial nerve 0*. It was not known by 1840.

terminal plexuses (Swanson & Bota, 2010)

More or less discrete networks of small ***autonomic nerve (Langley, 1898)*** fiber bundles in or near the walls of innervated viscera, characterized by parasympathetic ganglion cells that only sometimes condense into macroscopically obvious ***terminal ganglia (Gaskell, 1886)***. The functional composition of this class of *autonomic plexus (Strong & Elwyn, 1943)* is complex histologically and consists of varying mixtures of postganglionic sympathetic ***axons (Kölliker, 1896)***, pre- and postganglionic parasympathetic ***axons (Kölliker, 1896)***, and visceral afferent *nerve fibers (Ehrenberg, 1833)* or more correctly, ***dendrites (His, 1889)***; see Williams & Warwick (1980, pp. 1122–1137). The distinction between ***terminal plexuses (Swanson & Bota, 2010)*** and ***prevertebral plexuses (Quain, 1837)*** was clearly illustrated in Ranson (1920, Fig. 250) and Williams & Warwick (1980, Fig. 7.224). They are now described in a generally rostral (superior) to caudal (inferior) order. Perhaps the first clear suggestion of them was *posterior pulmonoaortic plexus (Andersch, 1797)*.

PARTLY CORRESPONDS:

1. *posterior pulmonoaortic plexus (Andersch, 1797)*
Extension of macrodissected adult human *great double plexus of arteries of heart (Andersch, 1797)* formed by parts of ***cardiac plexus (Keill, 1698)*** and ***pulmonary plexus (Winslow, 1733)***; in the original Latin, *plexum pulmonarioaorticum posteriorem*, p. 67.
2. *enteric nervous system (Langley, 1900)*
"The plexuses of Auerbach and Meissner are peculiar to the gut; they extend from the beginning of the unstriated portion of the oesophagus to the end of the rectum. They have usually been considered to belong to the sympathetic system, but it appears to me preferable to place them in a class by themselves. We may speak of them as forming the enteric nervous system." (p. 668). They are ***terminal plexuses (Swanson & Bota, 2010)***.

terminal stria (Wenzel & Wenzel, 1812)

As described in macrodissected adult human, and mammal generally with histological methods for ***axons (Kölliker, 1896)***, a longitudinal ***central nervous system white matter tract (>1840)*** extending primarily between the *amygdalar region (>1840)* and the rostral end of the ***medial forebrain bundle (Edinger, 1893)***, with major branches along the way to the ***bed nuclei of terminal stria (Gurdjian, 1925)***. It lies in the ***terminal sulcus (>1840)*** stretching between *amygdalar region (>1840)* and ***bed nuclei of terminal stria (Gurdjian, 1925)*** and in the latter also generates the ***terminal stria commissure (>1840)***. At the border between ***cerebral nuclei (Swanson, 2000a)*** and ***hypothalamus (Kuhlenbeck, 1927)*** it mostly joins the ***medial forebrain bundle (Edinger, 1893)*** in the ***lateral preoptic area (>1840)*** before fanning out into many parts of the ***hypothalamus (Kuhlenbeck, 1927)***, and to limited parts of the ***thalamus (His, 1893a)*** as well. For this use in English see *Dorland's* (2003, p. 1773, under *stria terminalis*). For Wenzel & Wenzel's use in macrodissected adult human, see p. 85, and for its association with the *substantia cornea* see p. 82 ff. Also see Meyer (1971, p. 16). It was known to Fabricius ab Aquapendente; see ***[terminal stria (Wenzel & Wenzel, 1812)] (Fabricius ab Aquapendente, c1610)***. It first appeared in print as the *transverse medullary process (Willis, 1664, p. 61)*.

TRANSLATIONS:

1. *stria terminalis (Wenzel & Wenzel, 1812)*
Original Latin form of ***terminal stria (Wenzel & Wenzel, 1812)***; p. 85.

EARLIER REFERENCES:

Illustrated, not named or described:

1. ***[terminal stria (Wenzel & Wenzel, 1812)] (Fabricius ab Aquapendente, c1610)***
Clearly illustrated for macrodissected adult human in a painting commissioned by Fabricius ab Aquapendente (c. 1610), used for teaching but never published, and only rediscovered in 1910; see Zanchin & de Caro (2006, Fig. 2).

Earlier synonyms:

1. *transverse medullary process (Willis, 1664, p. 61)*
Synonym for ***terminal stria (Wenzel & Wenzel, 1812)***, clearly illustrated for macrodissected adult sheep and described for macrodissected adult human

and other large mammals. Willis noted it "looks like a great nerve", linking the right and left *striated body (Willis, 1664)*, and illustrated it crossing the median plane, which is either imaginary (as suggested by Steno, 1669; see translation, p. 135), misidentified as the crossing of the ***anterior commissure (Lieutaud, 1742)***, or possibly the tiny ***terminal stria commissure (>1840)***; in the original Latin, *processus medullaris transversus*, see Pordage translation (1681, pp. 61, 63, 101–102, Tab. 7-*G*). Also see Haller (1762, p. 50), Burdach (1822, p. 361). Willis also used *transverse medullary process (Willis, 1664, p. 65)* for ***rostral medullary velum (>1840)***.

2. *transversus medullaris (Willis, 1664)*
Latin form of *transverse medullary process (Willis, 1664, p. 61)*; also see Bell (1802, p. 43), who did not distinguish between ***anterior commissure (Lieutaud, 1742)*** and ***terminal stria (Wenzel & Wenzel, 1812)***.
3. *processus medullaris (Willis, 1664)*
Synonym for ***terminal stria (Wenzel & Wenzel, 1812)***, according to Soemmerring (1778, p. 97).
4. *posterior limb of corpus striatum (Willis, 1672)*
Probably synonym for ***terminal stria (Wenzel & Wenzel, 1812)***; Ch. 4, p. 39. See Haller (1762, p. 50), Vicq d'Azyr (1786, Pl. 5), Bell (1802), Burdach (1822, p. 345); in Latin, *limbus posterior corporis striati*, or *limbo posteriore corporum striatorum* (see Soemmerring, 1778, p. 97). However, Meyer (1971, p. 13) believed it referred to ***internal capsule (Burdach, 1822)*** as illustrated in Plate VIII-*H*; see posterior *limbus of corpus striatum (Willis, 1672)*.
5. *semicircularis centri pars superior (Vieussens, 1684)*
Synonym for macrodissected adult human ***terminal stria (Wenzel & Wenzel, 1812)***; Table XII-*a*, see Meyer (1971, p. 14).
6. *nerve joining together corpus striatum (Ridley, 1695)*
Synonym for macrodissected adult human *transverse medullary process (Willis, 1664, p. 61)*; pp. 125–126. Burdach (1822, p. 361) gave Latin form, *nervus corpora striata conjugens*.
7. *frenulum novum (Tarin, 1750)*
Synonym for macrodissected adult human ***terminal stria (Wenzel & Wenzel, 1812)***, with a branch going to ***anterior thalamic nuclei (>1840)***, and associated *membrana cornea (Tarin, 1750)*; Table I, Figure 1-*U*. Other Latin forms include *fraenulo novo* (Soemmerring, 1778, p. 97), *frenula nova* or *noua* (Schreger, 1803, p. 320). According to Chaussier (1807, p. 65 note *1*), Tarin also referred to it as *gray layer* (in French, *lame grise*), although Chaussier provided no citation, and it has not been traced in Tarin's work. Interestingly, a small amount of ***gray matter (Meckel, 1817)*** accompanies the ***terminal stria (Wenzel & Wenzel, 1812)*** in many species; see Johnston (1923, p. 381 ff.).
8. *taenia semicircularis (Haller, 1754a)*
Synonym for macrodissected adult human ***terminal stria (Wenzel & Wenzel, 1812)***; p. 18, see Burdach (1822, p. 346). Soemmerring (1778, p. 97) gave Latin form, *taenia semicirculari*.
9. *centrum geminum (Haase, 1781)*
Synonym for macrodissected adult human ***terminal stria (Wenzel & Wenzel, 1812)***; p. 21, see Burdach (1822, p. 346).
10. *centrum semicirculare geminum (Monro, 1783)*
Synonym for macrodissected adult human ***terminal stria (Wenzel & Wenzel, 1812)***; Table III, Figure 1-*B*. Haller (1762, p. 50), Soemmerring (1778, p. 97), Vicq d'Azyr (1786, Pl. 5-*o*), and Burdach (1822, p. 345) claimed Vieussens first used it for ***terminal stria (Wenzel & Wenzel, 1812)***, but this is doubtful; see *geminum centrum semicirculare (Vieussens, 1684)*. Alternate Latin form, *centro gemino semilunari*; Soemmerring (1778, p. 97). Chaussier (1807, p. 64) gave Vieussens's term as *geminum centrum semi-circulare*.
11. *taenia striata (Vicq d'Azyr, 1786)*
Synonym for macrodissected adult human ***terminal stria (Wenzel & Wenzel, 1812)***; Plate V-o. Vicq d'Azyr observed no filaments from ***terminal stria (Wenzel & Wenzel, 1812)*** directly enter ***anterior commissure (Lieutaud, 1742)***, but nearby ***white matter (Meckel, 1817)***, where ***terminal stria (Wenzel & Wenzel, 1812)*** fans out, is shown to communicate with ***anterior commissure (Lieutaud, 1742)***; see Plate XXV, Figure II-*66*. Vicq d'Azyr also reviewed the earlier literature (1784, pp. 530–531).
12. *striated band (Vicq d'Azyr, 1786)*
Synonym for macrodissected adult human ***terminal stria (Wenzel & Wenzel, 1812)***; in the original French, *la bandelette striée*, Plates V-o; XXI-*31*.
13. *taenia fibrosa corporis striati (Vicq d'Azyr, 1786)*
More complete term for *taenia striata (Vicq d'Azyr, 1786)*; see Burdach (1822, p. 346).
14. *centrum semicirculare (Günther, 1786)*
Synonym for macrodissected adult human (plural) *corpora striata superna et posteriora (Vieussens, 1684)*; p. 10.
15. *stria cornea (Soemmerring, 1798)*
Synonym for macrodissected adult human ***terminal stria (Wenzel & Wenzel, 1812)***; see Meyer (1971, p. 16). Burdach (1822, p. 346) cited Soemmerring (1800, p. 45). Chaussier (1807, p. 65) credited Tarin with the term but provided no citation. It has not been traced in Tarin's work, though he did refer to *membranae corneae* in describing *frenulum novum (Tarin, 1750)*; Table I, Figure 1-*U*.
16. *taenia (Fyfe, 1800)*
Synonym for macrodissected adult human ***terminal stria (Wenzel & Wenzel, 1812)***; Vol. 2, p. 18.
17. *small bands of pyriform eminences (Burdin, 1803)*
Synonym for right and left macrodissected adult human ***terminal stria (Wenzel & Wenzel, 1812)***; see translation (1803, Vol. 1, p. 160).
18. *small semicircular bands (Burdin, 1803)*

Synonym for right and left macrodissected adult human ***terminal stria (Wenzel & Wenzel, 1812)***; see translation (1803, Vol. 1, p. 160).

19. *tractus medullaris transversus et nonnihil obliquus (Schreger, 1803)*
Schreger claimed Vieussens (1684, Tab. XIV-*D*) used it for macrodissected adult human ***terminal stria (Wenzel & Wenzel, 1812)***; p. 320.

20. *taenia corporis striati (Chaussier, 1807)*
Slight variation on *taenia striata (Vicq d'Azyr, 1786)* for macrodissected adult human; in the original French, *bandelette du corps strié*, p. 64.

LATER SYNONYMS:

1. *geminum centrum semicirculare (Meckel, 1817)*
Simply alternate form of macrodissected adult human *centrum semicirculare geminum (Monro, 1783)*; see translation (1832, Vol. 2, p. 457). Meckel also described a hard and solid brownish layer appearing as subjects get older or cephalic affections exist, the *lamina cornea (Vicq d'Azyr, 1786)*.
2. *medullary semicircular band (Meckel, 1817)*
English form of *geminum centrum semicirculare (Meckel, 1817)*; see translation (1832, Vol. 2, p. 440).
3. *semicircular tape-worm of Haller (Spurzheim, 1826)*
English eponym for *taenia semicircularis (Haller, 1754a)*; p. 187. *Taenia* is also translated strip, ribbon, string, and so on.

PARTLY CORRESPONDS:

1. *posterior ligament of cerebral hemispheres (Serres, 1824–1826)*
Serres suggested it might be analogous in bird and reptile to mammalian ***terminal stria (Wenzel & Wenzel, 1812)***; in the original French, *ligament postérieur des hémisphères cérébraux*, Vol. 2, p. 461.
2. *penicillus (Bergmann, 1831)*
Fanning out of macrodissected adult human ***terminal stria (Wenzel & Wenzel, 1812)*** in *amygdalar region (>1840)*; Table III, Figure 1-*c,e*.

terminal stria commissure (>1840)

As described in macrodissected adult human, and mammal generally with histological methods for ***axons (Kölliker, 1896)***, a branch of the ***terminal stria (Wenzel & Wenzel, 1812)*** crossing the median plane in and then traveling with the ***temporal limb of anterior commissure (>1840)***; see Johnston (1923, p. 382). It may have been observed by Willis, although this is doubtful; see ***[terminal stria commissure (>1840)] (Willis, 1664)***. It was clearly identified as the *semicircular commissure (Serres, 1824–1826)*.

EARLIER REFERENCES:

Described, not named or illustrated:

1. ***[terminal stria commissure (>1840)] (Willis, 1664)***
Willis may have identified it, but this is not clear; see *transverse medullary process (Willis, 1664, p. 61)*. It may also have been observed by Vicq d'Azyr, but again this is not clear; see *taenia striata (Vicq d'Azyr, 1786)*.

Earlier synonyms:

1. *semicircular commissure (Serres, 1824–1826)*
Synonym for macrodissected adult human and monkey ***terminal stria commissure (>1840)***; in the original French, *commissure demi-circulaire*, Vol. 2, p. 465.
2. *commissural bundle of stria terminalis (Johnston, 1923)*
Synonym for ***terminal stria commissure (>1840)*** described for opossum specifically and for mammal generally, with normal histological methods showing ***axons (Kölliker, 1896)***; p. 382.

terminal sulcus (>1840)

As described for macrodissected adult human, the shallow groove on the surface between ***cerebral nuclei (Swanson, 2000a)*** rostrally and ***thalamus (His, 1893a)*** caudally, where the ***terminal stria (Wenzel & Wenzel, 1812)*** runs; see Mettler (1948, p. 152). It was first delineated by Vesalius; see ***[terminal sulcus (>1840)] (Vesalius, 1543a)***.

EARLIER REFERENCES:

Illustrated and described, not named:

1. ***[terminal sulcus (>1840)] (Vesalius, 1543a)***
Clearly illustrated, and referred to as a "shallow channel" in macrodissected adult human; see Singer translation (1952, p. 98 and Figs. 4–6). Tiedemann (1816, Tab. V, Fig. 3) clearly illustrated it for 5-month human fetus.

terminal ventricle (>1840)

As described for macrodissected adult human, a swelling of the ***central canal of spinal cord (>1840)*** in the ***medullary cone (Bock, 1827)***; see Millen & Woollam (1962, p. 59), *Terminologia Anatomica* (1998, p. 105). It was not described by 1840.

testicular plexus (Cruveilhier, 1836)

As described for macrodissected adult human male, it arises from the ***superior testicular nerves (>1840)***, ***middle testicular nerves (>1840)***, and ***inferior testicular nerves (>1840)*** and supplies the testicles with branches to the epididymis and deferent duct; see Mitchell (1953, pp. 293–295), Williams & Warwick (1980, p. 1134). Willis wrote that "we find scarce any nerve to belong to mens Testicles" (Pordage translation, 1681, p. 169, also passage on p. 172). For Cruveilhier's use in macrodissected adult human male, see pp. 1020–1021. It was perhaps first clearly delineated as the *spermatic plexus (Haller, 1762)*.

TRANSLATIONS:

1. *plexus testiculaire (Cruveilhier, 1836)*
Original French form of ***testicular plexus (Cruveilhier, 1836)***; pp. 1020–1021.

EARLIER REFERENCES:

Earlier synonyms:

1. *spermatic plexus (Haller, 1762)*
Synonym for macrodissected adult human male ***testicular plexus (>1840)***, and Haller also applied it to macrodissected adult human female ***ovarian plexus (>1840)***; p. 265.

thalamic brachium of superior colliculus (>1840)

As described in macrodissected adult human, and mammal generally with histological methods for ***axons* (Kölliker, 1896)**, the short rostral segment of the ***brachium of superior colliculus* (>1840)** in the ***thalamus* (His, 1893a)**, between ***optic tract* (Vicq d'Azyr, 1784)** rostrally and ventrally, and ***pretectal brachium of superior colliculus* (>1840)** segment caudally. It lies adjacent to the ***lateral thalamic nuclei* (>1840)**; see Mettler (1948, p. 161 and Fig. 119), Swanson (2004, Atlas Levels 32–39). It was known to Willis; see ***[thalamic brachium of superior colliculus (>1840)] (Willis, 1664)***.

EARLIER REFERENCES:

Illustrated and described, not named:

1. ***[thalamic brachium of superior colliculus (>1840)] (Willis, 1664)***
   Clearly described and illustrated for macrodissected adult human and sheep although not explicitly distinguished from ***pretectal brachium of superior colliculus* (>1840)** segment; see *appendix of nates (Willis, 1664)*.

thalamic habenulo-interpeduncular tract (>1840)

As described in macrodissected adult human, and mammal generally with histological methods for ***axons* (Kölliker, 1896)**, the short, dorsal, longitudinal segment of the ***habenulo-interpeduncular tract* (>1840)** in the ***thalamus* (His, 1893a)**, between ***habenular nuclei* (>1840)** rostrally and dorsoventrally (transversely) oriented ***tegmental habenulo-interpeduncular tract* (>1840)** segment caudally. It was known to Cruveilhier; see ***[thalamic habenulo-interpeduncular tract (>1840)] (Cruveilhier, 1836)***.

EARLIER REFERENCES:

Described, not named or illustrated:

1. ***[thalamic habenulo-interpeduncular tract (>1840)] (Cruveilhier, 1836)***
   Described but not explicitly distinguished from ***tegmental habenulo-interpeduncular tract* (>1840)** segment; see *inferior peduncles of pineal body (Cruveilhier, 1836)*.

thalamic mammillothalamic tract (>1840)

As described in macrodissected adult human, and mammal generally with histological methods for ***axons* (Kölliker, 1896)**, the dorsal topographic segment of the ***mammillothalamic tract* (>1840)** in the ***thalamus* (His, 1893a)**, dorsal to the ***hypothalamic mammillothalamic tract* (>1840)** segment. It was probably first clearly observed by Pourfour du Petit; see ***[thalamic mammillothalamic tract (1840)] (Pourfour du Petit, 1710)***.

EARLIER REFERENCES:

Described, not named or illustrated:

1. ***[thalamic mammillothalamic tract (1840)] (Pourfour du Petit, 1710)***
   Delineated without separately naming for macrodissected adult human; see ***[mammillothalamic tract (>1840)] (Pourfour du Petit, 1710)***.

thalamic medial lemniscus (>1840)

As described in macrodissected adult human, and mammal generally with histological methods for ***axons* (Kölliker, 1896)**, the most rostral topographic segment of the ***medial lemniscus* (>1840)**, in the ***thalamus* (His, 1893a)**, rostral to the ***tegmental medial lemniscus* (>1840)** segment. It was known to Reil; see ***[thalamic medial lemniscus (>1840)] (Reil, 1809c)***.

EARLIER REFERENCES:

Described, not named or illustrated:

1. ***[thalamic medial lemniscus (>1840)] (Reil, 1809c)***
   Segment of *external part of lemniscus (Reil, 1809c)* in ***thalamus* (His, 1893a)**, vaguely described; see Mayo translation (1823, p. 95).

Earlier synonyms:

1. *fasciculus (Bergmann, 1831)*
   Probably synonym for macrodissected adult human ***thalamic medial lemniscus* (>1840)**; see Table II-*w* and Table III, Figure 2-*b*.

thalamic optic tract (>1840)

As described for macrodissected adult mammal, the dorsal topographic segment of the ***optic tract* (Vicq d'Azyr, 1786)** in the ***thalamus* (His, 1893a)**, between ***hypothalamic optic tract* (>1840)** segment ventrally and ***brachium of superior colliculus* (>1840)** dorsally, a change in name occurring at the level of the ***dorsal lateral geniculate nucleus* (>1840)**. It was known to Galen, who did not name or delineate it separately; see ***[thalamic optic tract (>1840)] (Galen, c173)***.

EARLIER REFERENCES:

Described, not named or illustrated:

1. ***[thalamic optic tract (>1840)] (Galen, c173)***
   Observed as part of *optic nerve (Galen, c173)* in macrodissected adult beef, pig, and/or macaque but not described separately.

thalamic part of third ventricle (Swanson, 2004)

The part of the ***third ventricle* (Galen, c173)** dorsal to the ***hypothalamic sulcus* (>1840)**, in contrast to the ***hypothalamic part of third ventricle* (Swanson, 2004)** ventral to the ***hypothalamic sulcus* (>1840)**; p. 166. It was first distinguished by Peyligk (1499); see ***[thalamic part of third ventricle (Swanson, 2004)] (Peyligk, 1499)***.

EARLIER REFERENCES:

Illustrated, not named or described:

1. ***[thalamic part of third ventricle (Swanson, 2004)] (Peyligk, 1499)***
   Clearly illustrated schematically, and distinguished, presumably for macrodissected adult human; see Clarke and Dewhurst (1996, Fig. 46b).

Earlier synonyms:

1. *superior wall of middle ventricle (Gerdy, 1838)*
   For macrodissected adult human, essentially ***thalamic part of third ventricle* (Swanson, 2004)**; in the original French, *paroi supérieur*, p. 263.

PARTLY CORRESPONDS:

1. ***[thalamic part of third ventricle (Swanson, 2004)] (Galen, c173)***
   Base of third ventricle (Galen, 177) or *infundibulum (Galen, c173)* corresponds roughly to ***hypothalamic part of third ventricle (Swanson, 2004)***—so by exclusion regions of ***third ventricle (Galen, c173)*** dorsally must include ***thalamic part of third ventricle (Swanson, 2004)***. However, Galen certainly did not recognize ependymal ***roof of third ventricle (>1840)***, so it is unclear how much, if any, of ***choroid membrane of third ventricle (>1840)*** he included in ***third ventricle (Galen, c173)***; for references see ***third ventricle (Galen, c173)*** and *passage or canal extending from middle to posterior ventricle (Galen, c173, c177)*. Vesalius (1543a) clearly distinguished between ***thalamic part of third ventricle (Swanson, 2004)*** and ***hypothalamic part of third ventricle (Swanson, 2004)*** in macrodissected adult human; see Richardson & Carman translation (2009, p. 195).

thalamic radiations (Reil, 1809b)

As described for macrodissected adult human, bidirectional ***central nervous system white matter tracts (>1840)*** extending between ***dorsal part of thalamus (Herrick, 1910)*** and ***cerebral cortex white matter (>1840)***. Specifically, they form a continuous fan extending along the whole lateral extent of the ***dorsal part of thalamus (Herrick, 1910)*** as a component of the ***internal capsule (Burdach, 1822)*** before merging into the ***cerebral cortex white matter (>1840)***. Topographically there is a rostral ***cerebral nuclear part of thalamic radiations (>1840)*** associated with the ***anterior limb of internal capsule (>1840)*** and a caudal ***thalamic part of thalamic radiations (>1840)*** associated with the ***posterior limb of internal capsule (>1840)***. For topographic description they are grouped into four subradiations: ***anterior thalamic radiation (>1840)*** or *frontal thalamic peduncle (>1840)*, ***superior thalamic radiation (>1840)*** or *centroparietal thalamic peduncle (>1840)*, ***posterior thalamic radiation (>1840)*** or *occipital thalamic peduncle (>1840)*, and ***inferior thalamic radiation (>1840)*** or *temporal thalamic peduncle (>1840)*, which has two parts, one within the ***internal capsule (Burdach, 1822)*** and the other just medial to it and called the ***inferior thalamic radiation peduncular loop (>1840)***; see Crosby et al. (1962, pp. 395–396 and 301, 370), Nauta & Haymaker (1969, p. 168), Carpenter (1976, p. 462 and Fig. 15.18), Nieuwenhuys et al. (2008, p. 253 and Fig. 8.1). For Reil's use in macrodissected adult human, see Mayo translation (1823, p. 124). Also see Mayo translation (1823, pp. 55, 65) and Reil (1812c).

thalamic spinothalamic tract (>1840)

As described in macrodissected adult human, and mammal generally with histological methods for ***axons (Kölliker, 1896)***, the most rostral topographic segment of the ***spinothalamic tract (>1840)***, in the ***thalamus (His, 1893a)*** rostral to the ***tegmental spinothalamic tract (>1840)*** segment. It has additional sparse extensions to ***hypothalamus (Kuhlenbeck, 1927)***, ***cerebral nuclei (Swanson, 2000a)***, and even ***cerebral cortex (>1840)***; see Crosby et al. (1962, p. 99), Nieuwenhuys et al. (2008, pp. 697–701). It was identified by Rolando; see ***[thalamic spinothalamic tract (>1840)] (Rolando, 1825a)***.

EARLIER REFERENCES:

Illustrated and described, not named:

1. ***[thalamic spinothalamic tract (>1840)] (Rolando, 1825a)***
   Rolando traced *anterolateral cord of oblong medulla (Rolando, 1825a)* or ***ventrolateral fascicle (>1840)*** into ***thalamus (His, 1893a)***; see Table VIII, Figure 1-*z*. The ***thalamic spinothalamic tract (>1840)*** is the only component of the ***ventrolateral fascicle (>1840)*** in the ***thalamus (His, 1893a)***.

Earlier synonyms:

1. *thalamic ventrolateral fascicle (>1840)*
   Synonymous with or corresponds to ***thalamic spinothalamic tract (>1840)*** because ***spinothalamic tract (>1840)*** is only component of ***ventrolateral fascicle (>1840)*** at level of ***thalamus (His, 1893a)***, unlike more caudal levels of ***ventrolateral fascicle (>1840)***.

thalamus (His, 1893a)

The dorsal topographic division of the vertebrate ***interbrain (Baer, 1837)***, the ventral topographic division being the ***hypothalamus (Kuhlenbeck, 1927)***; for this definition see Swanson & Bota (2010). Based on phylogeny, development, cellular architecture, and connections it includes three subdivisions, from ventral to dorsal, ***ventral thalamus (Herrick, 1910)***, ***dorsal thalamus (Herrick, 1910)***, and ***epithalamus (His, 1893b)***, along with the ***thalamic part of third ventricle (Swanson, 2004)*** in the median plane; also see Kuhlenbeck (1927, Ch. 9), Jones (2007, pp. 87–89). For His's use in embryonic and adult human, see pp. 161–162. It was clearly illustrated by Vesalius; see ***[thalamus (His, 1893a)] (Vesalius, 1543a)***.

EARLIER REFERENCES:

Illustrated, not named or described:

1. ***[thalamus (His, 1893a)] (Vesalius, 1543a)***
   Very clearly illustrated for macrodissected adult human, both grossly and in cross section; see Singer translation (1952, Figs. 4–8).

Earlier synonyms:

1. *optic colliculus (Wenzel & Wenzel, 1812)*
   Probably indicates roughly the macrodissected developing and adult human ***thalamus (His, 1893a)***; in the original Latin, *colliculus opticus*, p. 309 ff. & Table IV, Figure 1-*e*. Tiedemann (1821) clearly used it thus for macrodissected adult monkey (Tab. I, Fig. 7-*o*), lion (Tab. III, Fig. 5-*o*), lemur (Tab. IV, Fig. 10-*i*), and guinea pig (Tab. V, Fig. 2-*k*).
2. *optic nerve colliculus (Wenzel & Wenzel, 1812)*
   Synonym for *optic colliculus (Wenzel & Wenzel, 1812)*; in the original Latin (plural), *colliculi nervorum opticorum*, pp. 203, 309.

third occipital nerve (>1840)

As described for macrodissected adult human, a branch of the **medial branch of *spinal nerve dorsal branch (>1840)*** of the third ***cervical nerve (Galen, c173)***; it innervates skin on the caudal (lower) part of the occipital region; see Durward (1951, Fig. 916), Hamilton (1976, Fig. 811), *Terminologia Anatomica* (1998, p. 137). It was perhaps first identified as an unusual feature by Bock; see *posterior cutaneous branch of posterior branches of third cervical nerve (Bock, 1827)*.

EARLIER REFERENCES:

Earlier synonyms:

1. *posterior cutaneous branch of posterior branches of third cervical nerve (Bock, 1827)*
   Synonym for macrodissected adult human ***third occipital nerve (>1840)***, clearly described and illustrated; in the original Latin, *ram. cutaneus posterior rami posterioris nervi cervicalis tertii*, Table V, Figure 1-*48*.

third ventricle (Galen, c173)

The ***ventricle (Hippocrates)*** associated with the ***interbrain vesicle (Baer, 1837)*** of the ***vertebrate neural tube (Baer, 1837)***, both during development and in the adult; it lies between right and left ***lateral ventricle (Vesalius, 1543a)*** rostrally and the ***cerebral aqueduct (>1840)*** caudally. For topographic description it is divided into ***hypothalamic part of third ventricle (Swanson, 2004)*** ventrally and ***thalamic part of third ventricle (Swanson, 2004)*** dorsally, separated by the ***hypothalamic sulcus (>1840)***. Galen used it roughly in the modern sense, based mostly on macrodissected adult beef, pig, and/or macaque but not human; see Woollam (1958), May translation (1968, p. 414), Singer translation (1999, p. 234). Nevertheless, his and other early worker's exact understanding of its limits is not clear, particularly with respect to how much, if any, of the ***choroid membrane of third ventricle (>1840)*** and/or ***cerebral aqueduct (>1840)*** were included; see Steno translation (1669, pp. 137–138). Galen referred to a *passage or canal extending from middle to posterior ventricle (Galen, c173, c177)*, that is, ostensibly from ***third ventricle (Galen, c173)*** to ***fourth ventricle (Galen, c192)***, but it is unclear whether the canal is part of one or the other, or is separate. In contrast, Vesalius clearly included the ***cerebral aqueduct (>1840)*** as part of *third cerebral ventricle (Vesalius, 1543a)*; see *hind passage of third ventricle (Vesalius, 1543a), base of third ventricle (Galen, c177), infundibulum (Galen, c173)*. Colombo (1559) apparently stated that the "third ventricle" stops near the ***pineal gland (Galen, c192)***, excluding the ***cerebral aqueduct (>1840)***; see Bauhin (1605, p. 594; Crooke translation, 1615, p. 462). Aranzi clearly distinguished ***cerebral aqueduct (>1840)*** from ***third ventricle (Galen, c173)***; see *aqueduct (Aranzi, 1587)*. Steno (1669, Plates I–IV) provided the first clear illustrations in midsagittal and transverse drawings of macrodissected adult human ***third ventricle (Galen, c173)***.

ALTERNATE SPELLINGS:

1. *thyrde ventricle (Geminus, 1553)*
   Early English form of ***third ventricle (Galen, c173)***; see *The tables of the brayne*, Figure 6-*A*.

LATER SYNONYMS:

1. *fourth ventricle (Galen, c173)*
   Galen occasionally referred to ***third ventricle (Galen, c173)*** as a fourth ventricle, in addition to right and left *anterior ventricle (Galen, c173)* and *posterior ventricle (Galen, c177)*; see May translation (1968, p. 414). It was also called fourth ventricle by Wenzel & Wenzel (1812), according to Burdach (1822, p. 379).
2. *common cavity (Galen, c173)*
   Synonym for ***third ventricle (Galen, c173)***. Galen noted that, "There are some, however, who call it [the ***third ventricle (Galen, c173)***] the connection between the two [lateral] ventricles and do not grant that it is proper to think of it as another ventricle. I myself think that it does nothing either to help or to hinder the course of our discussion of this question if one wishes to interpret this place as a meeting place of the two [lateral] ventricles or as a third ventricle in addition to these, but I do consider it worth while to know why the anterior [lateral] ventricles come together in one place. The reason for it is the formation of the canal [***cerebral aqueduct (>1840)***] connecting them with the *parencephalis* [**cerebellum (Aristotle)**; that is, with the *fourth ventricle (Galen, c192)* associated with the ***cerebellum (Aristotle)***]..." (May translation, 1968, p. 415). Many years later, according to du Laurens (1600), Varoli (1573) adopted the view that there are only two ventricles, the ***lateral ventricles (Vesalius, 1543a)*** and ***third ventricle (Galen, c173)*** combined, and the ***fourth ventricle (Galen, c192)***—as had certain ancient anatomists alluded to by Galen; see Crooke translation (1615, p. 528).
3. *middle ventricle (Galen, c173)*
   Synonym for ***third ventricle (Galen, c173)***; May translation (1968, p. 418).
4. *cellula logistica or rationalis (Anatomia Magistri Nicolai physici, early 12th century; Guillaume de Conches, c1100–1154)*
   According to the most popular version of the cell theory of ***brain (Smith Papyrus, c1700 BC)*** function, the ***third ventricle (Galen, c173)*** is the "cell of thinking or cognition" (see Corner translation, 1927, p. 71; Manzoni, 1998, p. 125).
5. *venter medius (Berengario da Carpi, 1521)*
   Alternate Latin form of macrodissected adult human *middle ventricle (Galen, c173)*; ff. 438, 444. Also see Berengario da Carpi (1523, bottom figure on f. 56).
6. *sinus medius (Landi, 1542)*
   Synonym for macrodissected adult human ***third ventricle (Galen, c173)***; p. 56, see Burdach (1822, p. 378).
7. *middle cell (Geminus, 1553)*
   Synonym for macrodissected adult human *middle ventricle (Galen, c173)*; f. BII.

8. *hollowness common to right and left ventricles (Geminus, 1553)*
Synonym for macrodissected adult human ***third ventricle (Galen, c173)***; originally spelled *holownes common to the ryghte and the lefte ventricles*, see *The tables of the brayne*, Figure 6-H.
9. *fifth ventricle (Aranzi, 1587)*
Synonym for macrodissected adult human ***third ventricle (Galen, c173)***; p. 46, see Burdach (1822, p. 378, quoting the 1595 edition) and *hippocampal ventricle (Aranzi, 1587)*.
10. *middle pan of braine (Nemesius, 1636)*
Early synonym in English for ***third ventricle (Galen, c173)*** in this translation of Nemesius's 4th-century work *On the Nature of Man*; p. 306.
11. *long chink (Bartholin, 1662)*
Synonym, in English translation, for macrodissected adult human ***third ventricle (Galen, c173)***; p. 141.
12. *ventriculus medius anterior (Haller, 1762)*
Synonym for macrodissected adult human ***third ventricle (Galen, c173)***; p. 55, see Burdach (1822, p. 379).
13. *ventricle of optic thalamus (Vicq d'Azyr, 1786)*
Synonym for macrodissected adult human ***third ventricle (Galen, c173)***; p. 79; Plate XXV, Figure I-59.
14. *intervallum inter ganglia magna inferiora (Gall & Spurzheim, 1810)*
Synonym for macrodissected adult human ***third ventricle (Galen, c173)***, according to Burdach (1822, p. 379).
15. *fissura inter lobulos (Rosenthal, 1815)*
Synonym for macrodissected adult human ***third ventricle (Galen, c173)***; p. 16, see Burdach (1822, p. 379).
16. *vertical prolongation of middle part of central fissure (Gordon, 1815)*
Synonym for macrodissected adult human ***third ventricle (Galen, c173)***; p. 96, also see Burdach (1822, p. 379).
17. *anterior ventricle (Gordon, 1815)*
Synonym listed for macrodissected adult human ***third ventricle (Galen, c173)***; p. 157.
18. *processus perpendicularis fissurae medianae (Meckel, 1817)*
Synonym listed for macrodissected adult human ***third ventricle (Galen, c173)***; Vol. 3, p. 525 and 1832 translation, Vol. 2, p. 461; also see Burdach (1822, p. 379). Derived from *vertical prolongation of middle part of central fissure (Gordon, 1815)*.
19. *ventricle of thalamus (Rolando, 1831)*
Synonym listed for macrodissected adult human ***third ventricle (Galen, c173)***; in the original Italian, *ventricolo dei talami*, Figure 10, p. 144.

thoracic aortic plexus (>1840)

As described for macrodissected adult human, it surrounds the thoracic aorta, is derived from medial branches of the ***thoracic sympathetic ganglia (>1840)*** and from the ***vagus nerves (Galen, c192)***, is most dense around the aortic arch, a region supplied by the rostral (upper) five ***thoracic sympathetic ganglia (>1840)***, and is continuous caudally (below) with the ***celiac plexus (Winslow, 1733)***; see Durward (1951, p. 1136 and Fig. 965), Williams & Warwick (1980, p. 1131). It was first distinguished clearly by Walter; see ***[thoracic aortic plexus (>1840)] (Walter, 1783)***.

EARLIER REFERENCES:

Described, not named or illustrated:

1. ***[thoracic aortic plexus (>1840)] (Walter, 1783)***
Walter illustrated in macrodissected adult human parts of it arising from 7th–10th ***thoracic sympathetic ganglia (>1840)***, Table III:*193–210*, and from ***vagus nerves (Galen, c192)***, Table III:*466–470*. Referred to in the original Latin as *surculi aorticos*.

Earlier synonyms:

1. *aortic plexus (Lobstein, 1823)*
Synonym for macrodissected adult human ***thoracic aortic plexus (>1840)***; see translation (1831, p. 32).

thoracic cardiac branches of vagus nerve (>1840)

As described for macrodissected adult human, branches of the ***vagus nerve trunk (Wrisberg, 1786; Günther, 1786)*** arising in the thorax, proceeding to the ***cardiac plexus (Keill, 1698)***, and communicating in a complex way with other ***nerves (Herophilus, c335–c280 BC)*** to the heart; see Mitchell (1953, pp. 181–182, called *inferior group*), Williams & Warwick (1980, p. 1081), *Terminologia Anatomica* (1998, p. 136). They were probably known to Galen; see *branches in thorax to heart from sixth pair of nerves (Galen, c173)*.

EARLIER REFERENCES:

Earlier synonyms:

1. *branches in thorax to heart from sixth pair of nerves (Galen, c173)*
Apparently synonymous with ***thoracic cardiac branches of vagus nerve (>1840)*** in macrodissected adult beef, pig, and/or macaque but not human; see May translation (1968, pp. 367, 695), Duckworth translation (1962, pp. 204–205). It is not possible to know if Galen included any of the ***thoracic cardiac nerves (>1840)***, which arise from some of the rostral (upper) ***thoracic sympathetic ganglia (>1840)***, in the description because his differentiation of ***vagus nerve (Galen, c173)*** and ***sympathetic trunk (Winslow, 1733)*** was not always clear. He wrote, "On the heart you cannot see any obvious nerve which breaks up in its substance. Only in the bodies of very large animals will you detect there a nerve penetrating slightly towards its cavity." (Duckworth translation, 1962, p. 205).
2. *nerve to heart (Vesalius, 1543a)*
Vague reference to macrodissected adult human ***thoracic cardiac branches of vagus nerve (>1840)***; see Richardson & Carman translation (2002, p. 172 and figure on p. 169, part *r2*; also see pp. 160, 167, 199). Willis (1664, Ch. 23) used the specific Latin (plural) form, *nervorum cardiacorum*.
3. *sinew to heart (Geminus, 1553)*
Synonym for macrodissected adult human *nerve to heart (Vesalius, 1543a)*; original spelling was *synowe of the hearte*, see *Table of the figure of synowes*.

4. *cardiac branch of wandring pair (Willis, 1664)*
   Essentially synonym for macrodissected adult human ***thoracic cardiac branches of vagus nerve (>1840)***; see Table IX-O. Also see Vieussens (1684, Tab. 23).
5. *cardiac branches of eighth pair (Walter, 1783)*
   Synonym for macrodissected adult human ***thoracic cardiac branches of vagus nerve (>1840)***; in the original Latin, *rami cardiaci nervi octavi paris*, Table III:*396–400*.
6. *cardiac branches of vagus nerve (Cloquet, 1828)*
   Synonym for macrodissected adult human ***thoracic cardiac branches of vagus nerve (>1840)***; in the original French, *rameaux cardiaques du N. vague*, Plate CLXXVII-*187*.
7. *thoracic cardiac branches of pneumogastric nerve (Cruveilhier, 1836)*
   Synonym for macrodissected adult human ***thoracic cardiac branches of vagus nerve (>1840)***; in the original French, *rameaux cardiaques thoraciques*, p. 964.

PARTLY CORRESPONDS:

1. *communicating branches of ninth nerves of head and right nerves of heart (Andersch & Soemmerring, 1792)*
   Refers in macrodissected adult human to at least several ***thoracic cardiac branches of vagus nerve (>1840)***; in the original Latin, *rami communicatorii noni nervi capitis et nervi dextri cordis*, p. 191.
2. *communicating branches of tenth nerves of head and right nerves of heart (Andersch, 1797)*
   Synonym for *communicating branches of ninth nerves of head and right nerves of heart (Andersch & Soemmerring, 1792)*; in the original Latin, *rami communicatorii decimi nervi capitis et nervi dextri cordis*, p. 155.
3. *thoracic pericardial branches of pneumogastric nerve (Cruveilhier, 1836)*
   Branches of macrodissected adult human *thoracic cardiac branches of pneumogastric nerve (Cruveilhier, 1836)* to pericardium; in the original French, *rameaux péricardiaques*, p. 964.
4. *thoracic cardiac branches proper of pneumogastric nerve (Cruveilhier, 1836)*
   Branches of macrodissected adult human *thoracic cardiac branches of pneumogastric nerve (Cruveilhier, 1836)* contributing to ***cardiac plexus (Keill, 1698)***; in the original French, *rameaux cardiaques proprement dits*, p. 964.

thoracic cardiac nerves (>1840)

As described for macrodissected adult human, delicate medial branches of the second, third, fourth, and sometimes fifth ***thoracic sympathetic ganglia (>1840)*** extending to the ***cardiac plexus (Keill, 1698)***; see Mitchell (1953, p. 250). Attention was first drawn to them clearly in 1817; see ***[thoracic cardiac nerves (>1840)] (Weber, 1817; Meckel, 1817)***.

EARLIER REFERENCES:

Described, not named or illustrated:

1. ***[thoracic cardiac nerves (>1840)] (Weber, 1817; Meckel, 1817)***
   Weber described and illustrated them for macrodissected calf; pp. 17–19, Table IV; see Mitchell (1953, p. 250). Meckel mentioned them for macrodissected adult human; see translation (1832, Vol. 3, p. 97).

thoracic nerves (Diemerbroeck, 1672)

As described for macrodissected adult human, the 12 pairs of ***spinal nerves (Camper, 1760–1762)*** associated with the ***thoracic part of spinal cord (>1840)***; see Carpenter (1976, pp. 213–216). For Diemerbroeck's use in macrodissected adult human, see p. 872. They were first clearly described by Galen; see ***[thoracic nerves (Diemerbroeck, 1672)] (Galen, c173)***.

EARLIER REFERENCES:

Described, not named or illustrated:

1. ***[thoracic nerves (Diemerbroeck, 1672)] (Galen, c173)***
   In *On the Usefulness of the Parts*, Galen wrote about 12 ***nerves (Herophilus, c335–c280 BC)*** associated with intercostal spaces in adult human; see May translation (1968, pp. 599–602). He used specific terms ***cervical nerves (Galen, c173)*** and *sacral nerves (Galen, c173)*, but apparently not *thoracic nerves*; he did, however, refer to *thoracic spinal medulla (Galen, c173)*. He dissected many mammalian species including monkey, but not explicitly human.

Earlier synonyms:

1. *nerves from medulla of chest (Achillini, 1520)*
   Synonym for macrodissected adult human ***thoracic nerves (Diemerbroeck, 1672)***; see Lind translation (1975, p. 63).
2. *nerves of nape of back (Berengario da Carpi, 1523)*
   Synonym for macrodissected adult human ***thoracic nerves (Diemerbroeck, 1672)***; see Lind translation (1959, p. 160).
3. *nerves of nape of ribs (Berengario da Carpi, 1523)*
   Synonym for macrodissected adult human ***thoracic nerves (Diemerbroeck, 1672)***; see Lind translation (1959, p. 160).

LATER SYNONYMS:

1. *nerves of breast (Diemerbroeck, 1689)*
   Synonym for macrodissected adult human ***thoracic nerves (Diemerbroeck, 1672)***; p. 559.
2. *nerves of back (Diemerbroeck, 1689)*
   Synonym for *nerves of breast (Diemerbroeck, 1689)*; p. 559.
3. *dorsal nerves (Winslow, 1733)*
   Synonym for macrodissected adult human ***thoracic nerves (Diemerbroeck, 1672)***; in the original Latin, *nervi dorsales*, Section X, p. 49.
4. *costal nerves (Winslow, 1733)*
   Synonym for macrodissected adult human ***thoracic nerves (Diemerbroeck, 1672)***; Section X, p. 49.
5. *true intercostal nerves (Winslow, 1733)*
   Synonym for macrodissected adult human ***thoracic nerves (Diemerbroeck, 1672)***; Section X, p. 49.
6. *dorsal intervertebral nerves (Schaarschmidt, 1750)*

Synonym for macrodissected adult human ***thoracic nerves (Diemerbroeck, 1672)***; in the original Latin, *nervi intervertebrales dorsi*, p. 60.

7. *pectoral nerves (Haase, 1781)*
Synonym for macrodissected adult human ***thoracic nerves (Diemerbroeck, 1672)***; in the original Latin, *nervi pectorales*, p. 42. Andersch (1797, p. 2) also used it.
8. *proper dorsal nerves (Monro, 1783)*
Synonym for macrodissected adult ox *true intercostal nerves (Winslow, 1733)*; p. 144.
9. *proper intercostal nerves (Monro, 1783)*
Synonym for macrodissected adult ox *true intercostal nerves (Winslow, 1733)*; p. 144.
10. *intercostal nerves (Bell, 1803b)*
Synonym for macrodissected adult human ***thoracic nerves (Diemerbroeck, 1672)***; pp. 168–169.

PARTLY CORRESPONDS:

1. *dorsal nerves (Haller, 1762)*
Haller enumerated 11 rather than 12 macrodissected adult human ***thoracic nerves (Diemerbroeck, 1672)***, preferring to call 12th the first lumbar nerve, having six rather than five ***lumbar nerves (Diemerbroeck, 1672)***; p. 248.

thoracic part of spinal cord (>1840)

As described for macrodissected adult vertebrate, the longitudinal ***spinal cord part (>1840)*** generating the *thoracic nerves*; see Carpenter (1976, pp. 213–216). As described for macrodissected adult human, the longitudinal ***spinal cord part (>1840)*** generating the 12 ***thoracic nerves (Diemerbroeck, 1672)***; see *Nomina Anatomica* (1983, p. A64), *Terminologia Anatomica* (1998, p. 105). It was first described as the *thoracic spinal medulla (Galen, c173)*.

EARLIER REFERENCES:

Earlier synonyms:

1. *thoracic spinal medulla (Galen, c173)*
In *On the Usefulness of the Parts*, Galen specifically referred thus to macrodissected adult large mammal (but not human) ***thoracic part of spinal cord (>1840)***; see May translation (1968, p. 601).
2. *dorsal spinal medulla (Galen, c173)*
Synonym for *thoracic spinal medulla (Galen, c173)*; see May translation (1968, p. 601).
3. *medulla of chest (Achillini, 1520)*
Synonym for macrodissected adult human ***thoracic part of spinal cord (>1840)***; see Lind translation (1959, p. 63).
4. *nape of back (Berengario da Carpi, 1523)*
Synonym for macrodissected adult human ***thoracic part of spinal cord (>1840)***; see Lind translation (1959, p. 160).
5. *nape of ribs (Berengario da Carpi, 1523)*
Synonym for macrodissected adult human ***thoracic part of spinal cord (>1840)***; see Lind translation (1959, p. 160).
6. *thoracic part of spinal medulla (Tiedemann, 1821)*
Synonym for macrodissected adult monkey ***thoracic part of spinal cord (>1840)*** with 12 ***thoracic nerves (Diemerbroeck, 1672)***; in the original Latin, *pars thoracica medullae spinalis*, Table I, Figure 5-*f*.

thoracic pulmonary nerves (>1840)

As described for macrodissected adult human, delicate medial branches of the 2nd–5th ***thoracic sympathetic ganglia (>1840)*** extending to the ***pulmonary plexus (Winslow, 1733)***; see Mitchell (1953, p. 238), who called them *thoracic pulmonary branches*. The first clear description was probably by Meckel; see ***[thoracic pulmonary nerves (>1840)] (Meckel, 1817)***.

EARLIER REFERENCES:

Described, not named or illustrated:

1. ***[thoracic pulmonary nerves (>1840)] (Meckel, 1817)***
Described for macrodissected adult human; see translation (1832, Vol. 3, p. 97).

thoracic spinal ganglia (>1840)

As described for macrodissected adult human, there is one ***spinal nerve ganglion (Burdach, 1819)*** for each ***dorsal root (Spurzheim, 1826)*** of the 12 pairs of ***thoracic nerves (Diemerbroeck, 1672)***. They are numbered sequentially from rostral to caudal; see Williams & Warwick (1980, p. 1086). They were discovered by Coiter; see ***[thoracic spinal ganglia (>1840)] (Coiter, 1572)***.

EARLIER REFERENCES:

Described, not named or illustrated:

1. ***[thoracic spinal ganglia (>1840)] (Coiter, 1572)***
Coiter stated there is a *knot (Coiter, 1572)*, or ***spinal nerve ganglion (Burdach, 1819)***, for each *spinal nerve (Vesalius, 1543a)* in macrodissected adult human; see translation (1955, p. 115).

Earlier synonyms:

1. *thoracic ganglia of intercostal nerve (Günther, 1786)*
Günther described 11–12 ***thoracic spinal ganglia (>1840)*** for macrodissected adult human; in the original Latin, *ganglia thoracica nervus intercostalis*, p. 93 (and p. 92).

thoracic sympathetic ganglia (>1840)

As described for macrodissected adult human, ***sympathetic trunk ganglia (Winslow, 1733)*** having ***gray communicating branches (>1840)*** and ***white communicating branches (>1840)*** with the ***thoracic nerves (Diemerbroeck, 1672)***. There are typically 11, although there may be 10 or 12, and they are numbered sequentially from rostral (superior) to caudal (inferior); see Mitchell (1953, Ch. 16), Williams & Warwick (1980, pp. 1130–1131). The first accurate full account was probably given for each *thoracic ganglion of greatest sympathetic nerve (Wrisberg, 1780)*.

EARLIER REFERENCES:

Earlier synonyms:

1. *thoracic ganglion of greatest sympathetic nerve (Wrisberg, 1780)*
Wrisberg described in considerable detail 11 ***thoracic sympathetic ganglia (>1840)*** and their branches for

macrodissected adult human; in the original Latin, *ganglion thoracicum nervi sympathici maximus*, see Wrisberg reprint (1800, pp. 262–266).

2. *thoracic ganglion of great sympathetic nerve (Walter, 1783)*
   Walter described 11 ***thoracic sympathetic ganglia (>1840)*** for macrodissected adult human; in the original Latin, *ganglion thoracicum nervi sympathici magni*, Table I:36–55.
3. *thoracic ganglion of intercostal nerve proper (Walter, 1783)*
   Synonym for *thoracic ganglion of great sympathetic nerve (Walter, 1783)*; in the original Latin, *ganglion thoracicum nervi intercostalis stricte sic dicti*, Table I-36.
4. *thoracic ganglion (Walter, 1783)*
   Synonym for *thoracic ganglion of great sympathetic nerve (Walter, 1783)*; in the original Latin, *ganglion thoracicum*, Table I:39–55.
5. *dorsal ganglion (Mayer, 1794)*
   Synonym for macrodissected adult human *thoracic ganglion (Walter, 1783)*. Mayer described 11 of them. In the original Latin, *ganglion dorsale*; Part 6, Table VI-47 (p. 37).
6. *hordeiforme ganglia (Portal, 1803a)*
   Synonym for macrodissected adult human ***thoracic sympathetic ganglia (1840)***; in the original French, *ganglions hordéiformes*, p. 205. Also see Lobstein (1831, pp. 23–24).
7. *thoracic ganglions of limiting cord (Meckel, 1817)*
   Synonym for macrodissected adult human ***thoracic sympathetic ganglia (>1840)***; see translation (1832, Vol. 3, pp. 96–97).

thoracodorsal nerve (>1840)

As described for macrodissected adult human, a branch of the ***brachial plexus dorsal cord (Paterson, 1887)*** innervating primarily the latissimus dorsi muscle; see Williams & Warwick (1980, p. 1096). It was known to Galen; see ***[thoracodorsal nerve (>1840)] (Galen, c173)***.

EARLIER REFERENCES:

Described, not named or illustrated:

1. ***[thoracodorsal nerve (>1840)] (Galen, c173)***
   Clearly alluded to for macrodissected adult beef, pig, and/or macaque but not human; see May translation (1968, pp. 701–703), Duckworth translation (1962, pp. 250–251, 256, 258). Vesalius (1543a) mentioned it for macrodissected adult human; see Richardson & Carman translation (2002, p. 234).

Earlier synonyms:

1. *greater posterior thoracic nerve (Günther, 1786)*
   Synonym for macrodissected adult human ***thoracodorsal nerve (>1840)***; in the original Latin, *nervus thor. post. major*, p. 73.
2. *costothoracic branch of subscapular nerves (Chaussier, 1809)*
   Probably synonym for macrodissected adult human ***thoracodorsal nerve (>1840)***; in the original French, *filet costo-thoracique*.
3. *first subscapular branch of brachial plexus (Cloquet, 1816)*
   Synonym for macrodissected adult human ***thoracodorsal nerve (>1840)***; p. 644.
4. *inferior subscapular nerve (Bock, 1827)*
   Synonym for macrodissected adult human ***thoracodorsal nerve (>1840)***; in the original Latin, *nerv. subscapularis inferior*, Table II-24.
5. *long subscapular nerve (Bock, 1827)*
   Synonym for macrodissected adult human ***thoracodorsal nerve (>1840)***; in the original Latin, *nerv. subscapularis longus*, Table I, Figure 1-15; Table II-24.
6. *nerve of great dorsal muscle (Cruveilhier, 1836)*
   Synonym for macrodissected adult human ***thoracodorsal nerve (>1840)***; in the original French, *nerf du grand dorsal*, p. 797.

PARTLY CORRESPONDS:

1. *nerve to latissimus dorsi muscle (Langenbeck, 1826–1830)*
   Probably greater part of macrodissected adult human ***thoracodorsal nerve (>1840)***; in the original Latin, *nerv. ad musculum latissimum dorsi*, Fascicle III, Table XIII-5.

thyrohyoid branch of hypoglossal nerve (Meckel, 1817)

As described for macrodissected adult human, a branch of the ***hypoglossal nerve trunk (Günther, 1786)*** supplying the thyrohyoid muscle. It is often described as a branch of the ***superior root of ansa cervicalis (>1840)***; see Williams & Warwick (1980, pp. 1083, 1092 and Figs. 7.193, 197), *Terminologia Anatomica* (1998, p. 137). However, motor ***neurons Kölliker, 1896)*** for the thyrohyoid muscle are in the ***hypoglossal nucleus (>1840)*** and caudally adjacent dorsomedial part of the ***ventral horn (>1840)*** of adult cat, based on HRP retrograde tracing; Miyazaki et al. (1981). For Meckel's use in macrodissected adult human, see translation (1832, Vol. 3, p. 41). It was known to Galen; see ***[thyrohyoid branch of hypoglossal nerve (Meckel, 1817)] (Galen, c173)***.

EARLIER REFERENCES:

Described, not named or illustrated:

1. ***[thyrohyoid branch of hypoglossal nerve (Meckel, 1817)] (Galen, c173)***
   Alluded to for macrodissected adult beef, pig, and/or macaque but not human; see May translation (1968, pp. 449, 690), Duckworth translation (1962, p. 204).

Illustrated and described, not named:

1. ***[thyrohyoid branch of hypoglossal nerve (Meckel, 1817)] (Vesalius, 1543a)***
   Alluded to vaguely in macrodissected adult human; see Richardson & Carman translation (2002, p. 204). Also see Haller (1762, p. 238). Neubauer (1772, Tab. 2-*101*) illustrated it clearly for macrodissected adult human.

Earlier synonyms:

1. *thyrohyoid muscle twigs from hypoglossal nerve (Soemmerring, 1791)*
   Synonym for macrodissected adult human ***thyrohyoid branch of hypoglossal nerve (Meckel, 1817)***; pp. 260–261, also see Soemmerring (1798, p. 280).

2. *hyothyroid nerves (Scarpa, 1794)*
   Synonym for macrodissected adult human ***thyrohyoid branch of hypoglossal nerve (Meckel, 1817)***; in the original Latin, *nervi hyo-thyreoidei*, Table I-33,34.
3. *hyo-thyroidian branch of hyoglossal nerve (Burdin, 1803)*
   Synonym for macrodissected adult human ***thyrohyoid branch of hypoglossal nerve (Meckel, 1817)***; see translation (1803, Vol. 1, p. 184).

LATER SYNONYMS:

1. *branch of hypoglossal nerve descending branch to hyothyreoidei muscle (Arnold, 1834)*
   Synonym for macrodissected adult human ***thyrohyoid branch of hypoglossal nerve (Meckel, 1817)***; in the original Latin, *nervus hypoglossus, ramus descendens, ramus musculi hyothyreoidei*, p. 15.

thyroid branches of middle cervical ganglion (>1840)

As described for macrodissected adult human, most of them follow the inferior thyroid artery to form the ***thyroid plexus (Portal, 1803a)***, which innervates the thyroid and parathyroid glands and communicates with the ***superior cardiac nerve (Neubauer, 1772)***, ***external branch of superior laryngeal nerve (Fyfe, 1800)***, and ***recurrent laryngeal nerve (Albinus, 1744)***; see Mitchell (1953, Figs. 94, 95), Williams & Warwick (1980, p. 1128). They were probably known to Haller; see ***[thyroid branches of middle cervical ganglion (>1840)] (Haller, 1762)***.

EARLIER REFERENCES:

Described, not named or illustrated:

1. ***[thyroid branches of middle cervical ganglion (>1840)] (Haller, 1762)***
   Apparently alluded to for macrodissected adult human; pp. 256–257.

Earlier synonyms:

1. *internal branches of middle cervical ganglion (Meckel, 1817)*
   Synonym for macrodissected adult human ***thyroid branches of middle cervical ganglion (>1840)***; see translation (1832, Vol. 3, p. 94).
2. *plexus on inferior thyroidal artery (Swan, 1830)*
   Synonym for macrodissected adult human ***thyroid branches of middle cervical ganglion (>1840)***; Plate II-*k*.

thyroid plexus (Portal, 1803a)

As described for macrodissected adult human, the continuation of the ***thyroid branches of middle cervical ganglion (>1840)*** distributing to the thyroid and parathyroid glands and communicating with the ***superior cardiac nerve (Neubauer, 1772)***, ***external branch of superior laryngeal nerve (Fyfe, 1800)***, and ***recurrent laryngeal nerve (Albinus, 1744)***; see Mitchell (1953, Figs. 94, 95), Williams & Warwick (1980, p. 1128). For Portal's use in macrodissected adult human, see p. 173. It was probably known to Haller; see ***[thyroid plexus (Portal, 1803a)] (Haller, 1762)***.

TRANSLATIONS:

1. *plexus thyroïdien (Portal, 1803a)*
   Original French form of ***thyroid plexus (Portal, 1803a)***; p. 173.

EARLIER REFERENCES:

Described, not named or illustrated:

1. ***[thyroid plexus (Portal, 1803a)] (Haller, 1762)***
   Apparently alluded to for macrodissected adult human; p. 257.

tibial nerve (Haase, 1781)

As described for macrodissected adult human, the larger division of the ***sciatic nerve (Keill, 1698)*** arising from the fourth and fifth lumbar and first–third ***sacral plexus ventral divisions (Paterson, 1887)*** and generating ***muscular branches of tibial nerve (>1840)***, ***articular branches of tibial nerve (>1840)***, ***medial cutaneous nerve of calf (>1840)***, ***medial calcaneal nerve (>1840)***, ***medial plantar nerve (>1840)***, and ***lateral plantar nerve (1840)***. It corresponds to a combination of the ***median nerve (Du Verney, 1697)*** and ***ulnar nerve (Cheselden, 1726)*** of the upper limb; Durward (1951, p. 1106). For Haase's use in macrodissected adult human, see p. 111. It was known to Galen; see ***[tibial nerve (Haase, 1781)] (Galen, c173)***.

TRANSLATIONS:

1. *nervus tibialis (Haase, 1781)*
   Original Latin form of ***tibial nerve (Haase, 1781)***; p. 111.

EARLIER REFERENCES:

Described, not named or illustrated:

1. ***[tibial nerve (Haase, 1781)] (Galen, c173)***
   Clearly described for macrodissected adult beef, pig, and/or macaque but not human; see May translation (1968, p. 706), Singer translation (1999, pp. 85–87).

Earlier synonyms:

1. *inner trunk of fourth nerve entering leg (Vesalius, 1543a)*
   Synonym for macrodissected adult human ***tibial nerve (Haase, 1781)***; see Richardson & Carman translation (2002, p. 260).
2. *greater trunk of fourth nerve of thigh (Vesalius, 1543a)*
   Synonym for *inner trunk of fourth nerve entering leg (Vesalius, 1543a)*; see Richardson & Carman translation (2002, p. 265).
3. *inner and thicker trunk or stock of great division of fourth sinew (Geminus, 1553)*
   Synonym for macrodissected adult human *inner trunk of fourth nerve entering leg (Vesalius, 1543a)*; originally spelled *inner and thicker truncke or stocke of great division of fourth sinowe*, see *The table of the figures of sinowes*.
4. *greater trunk or stock of fourth sinew of thigh (Geminus, 1553)*
   Synonym for *inner and thicker trunk or stock of great division of fourth sinew (Geminus, 1553)*; originally spelled *greater trunke or stocke of fourth sinowe of thigh*, see *The table of the figures of sinowes*, Figure 7.

5. *internal branch of crural trunk (Diemerbroeck, 1672)*
Synonym for macrodissected adult human ***tibial nerve (Haase, 1781)***; pp. 875–876, see translation (1689, p. 563).
6. *internal branch of posterior crural nerve (Vieussens, 1684)*
Synonym for macrodissected adult human ***tibial nerve (Haase, 1781)***; in the original Latin, *nervus cruralis posticus, ramus interior*, Table XXIX-*R*.
7. *internal branch of crural nerve proper (Salmon, 1714)*
Synonym for macrodissected adult human ***tibial nerve (Haase, 1781)***; p. 132.
8. *popliteaus nerve (Monro, 1732)*
Synonym for macrodissected adult human ***tibial nerve (Haase, 1781)***; p. 32. Soemmerring used Latin forms, *nervus popliteus* (1791, p. 309) and *nervum popliteum* (1798, p. 329).
9. *internal crural nerve (Winslow, 1733)*
Synonym for macrodissected adult human *internal sciatic nerve (Winslow, 1733)*; in the original Latin, *nervus cruralis internus*, Section VI, p. 91.
10. *internal popliteal nerve (Winslow, 1733)*
Synonym for macrodissected adult human *internal sciatic nerve (Winslow, 1733)*; in the original Latin, *nervus popliteus internus*, Section VI, p. 91.
11. *large sciatic branch (Winslow, 1733)*
Synonym for macrodissected adult human ***tibial nerve (Haase, 1781)***; Section VI, p. 91. Walter (1783) used Latin form, *ramus nervi ischiatici major*, Table I-*391*.
12. *sciatico-tibialis nerve (Winslow, 1733)*
Synonym for macrodissected adult human *internal sciatic nerve (Winslow, 1733)*; Section VI, p. 91.
13. *internal sciatic nerve (Winslow, 1733)*
Synonym for macrodissected adult human ***tibial nerve (Haase, 1781)***; in the original Latin, *nervus sciaticus internus*, Section VII, p. 114.
14. *posterior tibial nerve (Haller, 1762)*
Synonym for macrodissected adult human ***tibial nerve (Haase, 1781)***; in the original Latin, *nervus tibialis posterior*, p. 251.
15. *internal popliteal sciatic nerve (Sabatier, 1775)*
Synonym for macrodissected adult human ***tibial nerve (Haase, 1781)***; in the original French, *nerf sciatique poplité interne*, pp. 744, 745.

LATER SYNONYMS:

1. *internal branch of sciatic nerve trunk (Günther, 1786)*
Synonym for macrodissected adult human ***tibial nerve (Haase, 1781)***; in the original Latin, *r. interior*, p. 86.
2. *major branch of sciatic nerve trunk (Günther, 1786)*
Synonym for macrodissected adult human ***tibial nerve (Haase, 1781)***; in the original Latin, *r. major*, p. 86.
3. *internal major branch of sciatic nerve trunk (Soemmerring, 1791)*
Synonym for macrodissected adult human ***tibial nerve (Haase, 1781)***; in the original Latin, *nervus ischiadicus ramus major interior*, p. 309, also see Soemmerring (1798, p. 330).
4. *tibial branch of large sciatic nerve (Chaussier, 1809)*
Synonym for macrodissected adult human ***tibial nerve (Haase, 1781)***.
5. *internal or larger division of sciatic nerve (Quain, 1828)*
Synonym for macrodissected adult human ***tibial nerve (Haase, 1781)***; p. 294.
6. *popliteal nerve (Quain, 1828)*
Alternate form of *popliteaus nerve (Monro, 1732)*; p. 294.
7. *medial popliteal nerve (>1840)*
Synonym for macrodissected adult human ***tibial nerve (Haase, 1781)***; see Durward (1951, p. 1109).

PARTLY CORRESPONDS:

1. *[plantar nerve (Haase, 1781)] (Galen, c177)*
In human there is commonly a separate ***medial plantar nerve (>1840)*** and ***lateral plantar nerve (>1840)***, whereas in some other mammals Galen macrodissected (specifically macaque) it is commonly a single ***nerve (Herophilus, c335–c280 BC)***; see Singer translation (1999, p. 87).
2. *plantar nerve (Haase, 1781)*
Common trunk for ***medial plantar nerve (>1840)*** and ***lateral plantar nerve (>1840)***, a somewhat unusual arrangement for macrodissected adult human; in the original Latin, *nervus plantaris*, p. 111. Also see *[plantar nerve (Haase, 1781)] (Galen, c177)*.
3. *plantar cutaneous nerves (Günther, 1786)*
Synonym for macrodissected adult human *plantar nerve (Haase, 1781)*; in the original Latin, *nervi cutanei plantares*, p. 87.
4. *tibial nerve trunk (Jördens, 1788)*
Proximal segment of macrodissected adult human ***tibial nerve (Haase, 1781)*** up to point of division into ***medial plantar nerve (>1840)*** and ***lateral plantar nerve (>1840)***; in the original Latin, *trunci nervi tibiei* (p. 9) or *trunco nervi tibiei* (Tab. II-*150*).
5. *lateral twig of tibial nerve to interosseal ligament (Jördens, 1788)*
Apparently supplement to macrodissected adult human ***interosseal nerve of leg (>1840)***; in the original Latin, *ramulus lateralis nervi tibiei ad ligamentum interosseum*, p. 10 and Table III-*164*. Jördens described two branches of this twig; Table III-*165,165**.
6. *inferior posterior cutaneous nerve (Jördens, 1788)*
Seldom recognized branch of macrodissected adult human *tibial nerve trunk (Jördens, 1788)* innervating skin near calcaneal (Achilles) tendon; in the original Latin, *nervus cutaneus posticus inferior*, p. 10 and Table III-*180*. It has two roots (Tab. III-*179,179*) and generates two identifiable small branches (Tab. III-*181,182*).
7. *first internal inferior posterior cutaneous nerve (Fischer, 1791)*
Probably synonym for macrodissected adult human *inferior posterior cutaneous nerve (Jördens, 1788)* Fischer had arising distal to ***sural nerve (Pietro da Cortona)*** from branch of *common nerve to tibialis posterior, flexor digitorum longus, and flexor longus of big toe muscles and first internal inferior posterior cutaneous nerve (Fischer, 1791)*;

in the original Latin, *nervi cutanei posterioris inferioris interni primi*, p. 35.

8. *superior internal subsural nerve (Fischer, 1791)*
Synonym for *first internal inferior posterior cutaneous nerve (Fischer, 1791)*; in the original Latin, *nervum subsuralem internum superiorem*, p. 35.
9. *superior internal subsural subcutaneous nerve (Fischer, 1791)*
Synonym for *first internal inferior posterior cutaneous nerve (Fischer, 1791)*; in the original Latin, *nervus subcutaneus subsuralis internus superior*, Table III, Figure 2-*466*.
10. *second internal inferior posterior cutaneous nerve (Fischer, 1791)*
Macrodissected adult human small branch of *tibial nerve trunk (Jördens, 1788)* to skin over and proximal to medial malleolus; in the original Latin, *nervus cutaneus posterior inferior internus secundus*, p. 35.
11. *inferior internal subsural nerve (Fischer, 1791)*
Synonym for *second internal inferior posterior cutaneous nerve (Fischer, 1791)*; in the original Latin, *nervus subsuralis internus inferior*, p. 35.
12. *inferior internal subsural cutaneous nerve (Fischer, 1791)*
Synonym for *second internal subsural nerve (Fischer, 1791)*; in the original Latin, *nervus cutaneus subsuralis internus inferior*, Table III, Figure 2-*493*.
13. *second external inferior posterior cutaneous nerve (Fischer, 1791)*
Macrodissected adult human small branch of *tibial nerve trunk (Jördens, 1788)* to skin dorsal (posterior) to medial malleolus; in the original Latin, *nervus cutaneus posterior inferior externus secundus*, p. 35.
14. *inferior external subsural nerve (Fischer, 1791)*
Synonym for *second external inferior posterior cutaneous nerve (Fischer, 1791)*; in the original Latin, *nervus subsuralis externus inferior*, p. 35.
15. *plantar digital nerves (Bock, 1827)*
Macrodissected adult human ***proper plantar digital nerves of medial plantar nerve (>1840)*** and ***proper plantar digital nerves of lateral plantar nerve (>1840)*** considered together; in the original Latin, *nervi digitales plantares*, Table IV-*106,108*. Langenbeck (1826–1830; Fasc. III, Tab. VII, Figure 3) also used the term for macrodissected adult human.
16. *posterior tibial nerve (Quain, 1828)*
Corresponds to macrodissected adult human ***tibial nerve (Haase, 1781)*** after it descends past popliteus muscle; p. 294.
17. *first posterior inferior internal cutaneous nerve (Knox, 1832)*
Knox's form of *first internal inferior posterior cutaneous nerve (Fischer, 1791)*; Plate XIV-*466*.
18. *posterior inferior external cutaneous nerve (Knox, 1832)*
Knox's form of *second external inferior posterior cutaneous nerve (Fischer, 1791)*; Plate XIV-*500*.
19. *inferior subsural external cutaneous nerve (Knox, 1832)*
Knox's form of *inferior external subsural nerve (Fischer, 1791)*; Plate XIV-*500*.
20. *first internal posterior inferior cutaneous nerve (Knox, 1832)*
Synonym for *first posterior inferior internal cutaneous nerve (Knox, 1832)*; Plate XVI-*466*.
21. *internal superior subsural cutaneous nerve (Knox, 1832)*
Form of *superior internal subsural cutaneous nerve (Fischer, 1791)*; Plate XIV-*466*.
22. *second internal posterior inferior cutaneous nerve (Knox, 1832)*
Form of *second internal inferior posterior cutaneous nerve (Fischer, 1791)*; Plate XVI-*493*.
23. *internal subsural cutaneous nerve (Knox, 1832)*
Form of *inferior internal subsural cutaneous nerve (Fischer, 1791)*; Plate XVI-*493*.
24. *posterior inferior cutaneous nerve (Knox, 1832)*
Form of *inferior posterior cutaneous nerve (Jördens, 1788)*; Plate XVIII-*231*.
25. *second posterior inferior internal cutaneous nerve (Knox, 1832)*
Form of *second internal inferior posterior cutaneous nerve (Fischer, 1791)*; Plate XVIII, Figure 2-*493*.
26. *internal inferior subsural cutaneous nerve (Knox, 1832)*
Form of *inferior internal subsural nerve (Fischer, 1791)*; Plate XVIII, Figure 2-*493*.
27. *second posterior inferior external cutaneous nerve (Knox, 1832)*
Form of *second external inferior posterior cutaneous nerve (Fischer, 1791)*; Plate XVIII, Figure 2-*500*.
28. *inferior external subsural cutaneous nerve (Knox, 1832)*
Form of *inferior external subsural nerve (Fischer, 1791)*; Plate 18-*500*.
29. *popliteal nerve (Quain & Wilson, 1839)*
Macrodissected adult human proximal part of ***tibial nerve (Haase, 1781)*** trunk before it passes distal to popliteus muscle; pp. 51–52 and Plate XXV, Figure 2-*A*.

tibial root of sural nerve (>1840)

As described for macrodissected adult human, the major proximal segment of the ***medial cutaneous nerve of calf (>1840)*** joining with the ***sural communicating branch of common fibular nerve (>1840)*** to form the ***sural nerve (Pietro da Cortona, 1741)***; see *Dorland's* (2003, p. 1238, under *nervus cutaneus surae medialis*), and Williams & Warwick (1980, Fig. 7.215) where the ***medial cutaneous nerve of calf (>1840)*** is unlabeled proximal to (above) the junction and the ***sural nerve (Pietro da Cortona, 1741)*** is labeled distal to (below) the junction. Some authors subsume it under the ***sural nerve ((Pietro da Cortona, 1741)***, in which case no ***medial cutaneous nerve of calf (>1840)*** is recognized. The ***tibial root of sural nerve (>1840)*** was first clearly delineated as the *tibial communicating nerve (Jördens, 1788)*.

EARLIER REFERENCES:

Earlier synonyms:

1. *tibial communicating nerve (Jördens, 1788)*
Essentially macrodissected adult human ***tibial root of sural nerve (>1840)***; in the original Latin, *nervum*

communicantem tibiei, p. 3. Jördens described there a short superior and a long inferior anastomotic branch between *tibial communicating nerve (Jördens, 1788)* and *peroneal communicating branch (Jördens, 1788)*. Fischer (1791, Tab. IV, Fig. 2-387) spelled it *nervus communicans tibiei*. Quain (1828, p. 294) ascribed the term to Soemmerring without citation. Quain & Wilson (1839, Pl. XXV, Fig. 1-*b*) spelled it *nervus communicans tibiae*. Also see Quain & Wilson (1839, Pl. XXV, Fig. 1-*c*).

2. *tibial communicating branch (Jördens, 1788)*
   Synonym for *tibial communicating nerve (Jördens, 1788)*; Table 1-*110*.
3. *external saphenous branch of internal popliteal nerve (Cloquet, 1816)*
   Synonym for macrodissected adult human ***tibial root of sural nerve (>1840)***; in the original French, *rameau saphène externe*, p. 677.
4. *communicating branch of tibial nerve (Bock, 1827)*
   Synonym for macrodissected adult human ***tibial root of sural nerve (>1840)***; in the original Latin, *ram. communicans tibialis*, Table IV-*95*.

tonsil (Malacarne, 1776)

As described for macrodissected adult human, the part of the ***cerebellar hemisphere (Willis, 1664)*** between ***biventral lobule (>1840)*** and ***flocculus (Meckel, 1817)***, and lateral to the ***uvula (Malacarne, 1776)*** of the ***cerebellar vermis (Meckel, 1817)***. It has a lateral extension, the ***paraflocculus (Stroud, 1895)***; see Angevine et al. (1961, Figs. 5, 11, 13, 19, 20, 22), Larsell & Jansen (1972, Fig. 118), Carpenter (1976, Fig. 14.1). For Malacarne's use in macrodissected adult human, see pp. 23, 24. Also see Larsell (1967, p. 4), Clarke & O'Malley (1996, p. 645). It was first clearly delineated as the *portiones cerebelli processus vermiformes aemulantes (Ruysch, 1728)*.

TRANSLATIONS:

1. *tonsilla (Malacarne, 1776)*
   Latin form of ***tonsil (Malacarne, 1776)***; see Burdach (1822, p. 296, for the plural, *tonsillae*).
2. *amygdala (Malacarne, 1776)*
   Latin form of ***tonsil (Malacarne, 1776)***; see Vicq d'Azyr (1784, p. 571, spelled *amigdales*), Meckel (1817; see translation, 1832, Vol. 2, p. 432, where the plural was given, *amygdalae*).

EARLIER REFERENCES:

Earlier synonyms:

1. *portiones cerebelli processus vermiformes aemulantes (Ruysch, 1728)*
   Roughly synonymous with ***tonsil (Malacarne, 1776)***, according to Burdach (1822, p. 296); Epist. XII.

LATER SYNONYMS:

1. *particulae segregatae cerebelli posteriores (Soemmerring, 1778)*
   Roughly synonymous with macrodissected adult human ***tonsil (Malacarne, 1776)***; p. 16, see Burdach (1822, p. 296).
2. *lobule of medulla oblongata (Vicq d'Azyr, 1784)*
   Synonym for macrodissected adult human ***tonsil (Malacarne, 1776)***; p. 568, also see Vicq d'Azyr (1786, Pl. XVII, Fig. I-93).
3. *monticulus (Vicq d'Azyr, 1784)*
   Synonym for *lobule of medulla oblongata (1784)*; p. 568.
4. *superior anterior tubercle (Günther, 1786)*
   Apparently synonym for macrodissected adult human ***tonsil (Malacarne, 1776)***; in the original Latin, *tubercula anteriora superiora*, p. 18. Also see *inferior anterior tubercle of Tarin (Günther, 1786)*.
5. *almond-like lobe (Reil, 1807–1808a)*
   Synonym for macrodissected adult human ***tonsil (Malacarne, 1776)***; see Mayo translation (1822, p. 23).
6. *spinal lobule (Gordon, 1815)*
   Synonym for macrodissected adult human ***tonsil (Malacarne, 1776)***; p. 118, see Burdach (1822, p. 296).
7. *inferior internal lobe (Meckel, 1817)*
   Synonym for macrodissected adult human ***tonsil (Malacarne, 1776)***; in the original Latin, *lobus inferior internus*; p. 466, see translation (1832, Vol. 2, p. 429). Also see Burdach (1822, p. 296).

tonsillar branches of glossopharyngeal nerve (Wrisberg, 1786)

As described for macrodissected adult human, terminal branches of the ***glossopharyngeal nerve trunk (Wrisberg, 1786; Günther, 1786)*** forming along with ***tonsillar branches of lateral palatine nerve (>1840)*** a ***plexus (Galen, c192)*** around the palatine tonsil, with branches then extending to the soft palate and region of the fauces; see Hamilton (1976, Fig. 802), Williams & Warwick (1980, p. 1076), *Terminologia Anatomica* (1998, p. 136). For Wrisberg's discovery and first use in print for macrodissected adult human, see Wrisberg reprint (1800, p. 419). Kilian (1822, pp. 104–105) also described them clearly for macrodissected adult human.

LATER SYNONYMS:

1. *fourth branch of glossopharyngeal nerve (Wrisberg, 1786)*
   Synonym for ***tonsillar branches of glossopharyngeal nerve (Wrisberg, 1786)***; see Wrisberg reprint (1800, p. 419).
2. *inferior tonsillar nerve (Andersch & Soemmerring, 1792)*
   Synonym for macrodissected adult human ***tonsillar branches of glossopharyngeal nerve (Wrisberg, 1786)***; in the original Latin, *nervus tonsillaris inferior* and *nervum tonsillarem inferiorem*, pp. 116, 118.
3. *tonsillar nerve (Andersch, 1797)*
   Synonym for macrodissected adult human ***tonsillar branches of glossopharyngeal nerve (Wrisberg, 1786)***; in the original Latin, *nervum tonsillarem*, p. 11. Andersch's thesis was carried out c1751–c1755 but not published unaltered until here.

PARTLY CORRESPONDS:

1. *tonsillar branch of greatest pharyngeal branches of glossopharyngeal nerves (Kilian, 1822)*
   Macrodissected adult human ***tonsillar branches of glossopharyngeal nerve (Wrisberg, 1786)*** from inferior,

greatest, or third ***pharyngeal branch of glossopharyngeal nerve (Neubauer, 1772)***; in the original Latin, *ramus tonsillaris rami pharyngei maximi*, p. 99.

tonsillar branches of lateral palatine nerve (>1840)

As described for macrodissected adult human, a branch of the ***lateral palatine nerve (Henle, 1871)*** to the region of the palatine tonsil; see Durward (1951, p. 1023). It was probably first identified as the *external branch of external least branch of palatine nerve (Meckel, 1748)*.

EARLIER REFERENCES:

Earlier synonyms:

1. *external branch of external least branch of palatine nerve (Meckel, 1748)*
   Synonym for macrodissected adult human ***tonsillar branches of lateral palatine nerve (>1840)***; p. 64.
2. *branch to tonsil from external palatine nerve (Scarpa, 1785)*
   Synonym for macrodissected adult human ***tonsillar branches of lateral palatine nerve (>1840)***; in the original Latin, *ramus ad tonsillam*, Table II, Figure II-33.
3. *exterior branch to tonsils of exterior palatine nerve (Günther, 1786)*
   Synonym for macrodissected adult human ***tonsillar branches of lateral palatine nerve (>1840)***; p. 48.
4. *amygdala input from small palatine nerves (Meckel, 1817)*
   Input to macrodissected adult human palatine tonsils (amygdalae) from ***lesser palatine nerves (Meckel, 1817)***, specifically ***tonsillar branches of lateral palatine nerve (>1840)***; see translation (1832, Vol. 3, p. 69).
5. *tonsillar branches of lesser palatine nerves (>1840)*
   Synonym for macrodissected adult human ***tonsillar branches of lateral palatine nerve (>1840)***; see *Terminologia Anatomica* (1998, p. 134).

tracheal branches of recurrent laryngeal nerve (>1840)

As described for macrodissected adult human, they arise from the rostrally directed (ascending) limb of the ***recurrent laryngeal nerve (Albinus, 1744)*** and supply mucous membrane and muscle fibers of the trachea; see Williams & Warwick (1980, p. 1081), *Terminologia Anatomica* (1998, p. 136). They were first described as *nerve branches to trachea (Galen, c192)*.

EARLIER REFERENCES:

Earlier synonyms:

1. *nerve branches to trachea (Galen, c192)*
   Galen observed ***tracheal branches of recurrent laryngeal nerve (>1840)*** in macrodissected adult beef, pig, and/or macaque but not human, although he could not separate them from intermingled branches from ***vagus nerve trunk (Wrisberg, 1786; Günther, 1786)***; see Duckworth translation (1962, p. 204) and May translation (1968, p. 694, where trachea is called rough artery).
2. *shoots to rough artery [from returning nerve] (Willis, 1664)*
   Synonym for macrodissected adult human ***tracheal branches of recurrent laryngeal nerve (>1840)***; see Pordage translation (1681, p. 148 and Tab. IX-*n*,+). Later Willis indicated shoots to tracheal muscles; see Pordage translation (1681, p. 153).
3. *descending branches of inferior laryngeal nerve (Günther, 1786)*
   As described for macrodissected adult human, basically ***tracheal branches of recurrent laryngeal nerve (>1840)***; in the original Latin, *r. descendentes*, p. 64.
4. *superior tracheal nerves (Meckel, 1817)*
   Synonym for macrodissected adult human ***tracheal branches of recurrent laryngeal nerve (>1840)***; see translation (1832, Vol. 3, p. 48).
5. *bronchial branches of inferior laryngeal nerve (Arnold, 1834)*
   Synonym for macrodissected adult human ***tracheal branches of recurrent laryngeal nerve (>1840)***; in the original Latin, *rami bronchiales nervus laryngeus inferior*, p. 14.
6. *bronchial branches of recurrent laryngeal nerve (Arnold, 1834)*
   Synonym for *bronchial branches of inferior laryngeal nerve (Arnold, 1834)*; in the original Latin, *rami bronchiales nervus recurrens laryngeus*, p. 14.
7. *tracheal branches of recurrent nerve (Cruveilhier, 1836)*
   Synonym for macrodissected adult human ***tracheal branches of recurrent laryngeal nerve (>1840)***; in the original French, *rameaux trachéens*, p. 963.
8. *branches from curve of recurrent nerve to pulmonary plexus (Quain & Wilson, 1839)*
   Synonym for macrodissected adult human ***tracheal branches of recurrent laryngeal nerve (>1840)***; Plate XV-*w*.

transverse cerebellar fissure (Burdach, 1822)

As described for macrodissected adult human, the space between the caudal half of the ***roof of fourth ventricle (Vesalius, 1543a)*** ventrally, and the overlying ventral surface of the ***cerebellum (Aristotle)*** dorsally, occupied by the cerebellomedullary cistern of the ***subarachnoid space (Magendie, 1827)***; see Rasmussen (1932, Fig. 1), Williams & Warwick (1980, p. 1049 and Fig. 7.164), and compare with ***transverse cerebral fissure (>1840)***. For Burdach's use in macrodissected adult human, see pp. 79, 165, 307. It was perhaps first clearly delineated by Steno; see ***[transverse cerebellar fissure (Burdach, 1822)] (Steno, 1669)***.

TRANSLATIONS:

1. *rima transversa cerebelli (Burdach, 1822)*
   Original Latin form of ***transverse cerebellar fissure (Burdach, 1822)***; pp. 79, 165, 307.

EARLIER REFERENCES:

Illustrated, not named or described:

1. ***[transverse cerebellar fissure (Burdach, 1822)] (Steno, 1669)***
   Illustrated for macrodissected adult human in midsagittal view; Plate I.

LATER SYNONYMS:

1. *small transverse fissure (Meckel, 1817)*
   Synonym for macrodissected adult human ***transverse cerebellar fissure (Burdach, 1822)***; see translation (1832, Vol. 2, p. 459).
2. *fissura cerebri transversa parva (Meckel, 1817)*
   Latin form of *small transverse fissure (Meckel, 1817)*; see translation (1832, Vol. 2, p. 459).
3. *small cerebral fissure (Meckel, 1817)*
   Synonym for *fissura cerebri transversa parva (Meckel, 1817)*; see translation (1832, Vol. 2, p. 460).
4. *fissura cerebri transversa cerebelli (Burdach, 1822)*
   Synonym for macrodissected adult human *fissura cerebri transversa parva (Meckel, 1817)*; p. 307.

transverse cerebral fissure (>1840)

As described for macrodissected adult human, it has two continuous parts. The ***inner part of transverse cerebral fissure (>1840)*** occupies the rostrocaudal (horizontal) space between the dorsal surface of the ***thalamus (His, 1893a)*** and ***tectum (Baer, 1837)***, and the ventral surface of the ***fornix (Vesalius, 1543a)***, and contains the ***choroid membrane of third ventricle (>1840)***, filled with ***cerebrospinal fluid (Magendie, 1827)***. The ***outer part of transverse cerebral fissure (>1840)*** continues on between the ventral surface of the ***occipital region (Vesalius, 1543a)*** and the nearby face of the ***cerebellum (Aristotle)*** and is partly occupied by the ***cerebellar tentorium (Winslow, 1733)***; see Carpenter (1976, pp. 9, 65 and Figs. 2.22, 3.13) and illustrated beautifully by Rasmussen (1932, Fig. 1). The part near the ***tectum (Baer, 1837)*** is sometimes called the mouth of the ***transverse cerebral fissure (>1840)***; see Millen & Woollam (1962); compare with ***transverse cerebellar fissure (Burdach, 1822)***. It was first delineated clearly by Steno; see ***[transverse cerebral fissure (>1840)] (Steno, 1669)***.

EARLIER REFERENCES:

Illustrated, not named or described:

1. ***[transverse cerebral fissure (>1840)] (Steno, 1669)***
   Clearly illustrated for macrodissected adult human in midsagittal view; Plate I.

transverse nerve of neck (>1840)

As described for macrodissected adult human, an ***ascending superficial branch of cervical plexus (Quain, 1828)*** commonly arising from the second and third cervical ***spinal nerve ventral branches (>1840)*** and supplying ventrolateral (anterolateral) cutaneous parts of the neck through its ***superior branches of transverse nerve of neck (>1840)*** and ***inferior branches of transverse nerve of neck (>1840)***; see Williams & Warwick (1980, p. 1092 and Figs. 7.198, 199). It was known to Galen; see ***[transverse nerve of neck (>1840)] (Galen, c173)***.

TRANSLATIONS:

1. *nervus transversus colli (>1840)*
   Current Latin form of ***transverse nerve of neck (>1840)***; see *Terminologia Anatomica* (1998, p. 137).

EARLIER REFERENCES:

Described, not named or illustrated:

1. ***[transverse nerve of neck (>1840)] (Galen, c173)***
   Alluded to in macrodissected adult beef, pig, and/or macaque but not human; see May translation (1968, p. 598), and Duckworth translation (1962, p. 238).

Illustrated, not named or described:

1. ***[transverse nerve of neck (>1840)] (Eustachi, 1552)***
   Probably illustrated for macrodissected adult human; see Albinus edition (1761, Tab. 21/2, lowest branch of *h* on left side of body).

Earlier synonyms:

1. *subcutaneous nerve of neck (Meckel, 1753)*
   Synonym for macrodissected adult human ***transverse nerve of neck (>1840)***; in the original French, *le nerf sous-cutané du cou*, p. 97.
2. *cutaneous nerve of neck (Meckel, 1753)*
   Synonym for macrodissected adult human ***transverse nerve of neck (>1840)***; in the original French, *le nerf cutané du col*, Table 1-Ξ. Also see His (1895, p. 91).
3. *superficial nerve of neck (Bang, 1770)*
   Synonym for macrodissected adult human ***transverse nerve of neck (>1840)***; in the original Latin, *nervus superficialis colli*; Figure I-40.
4. *middle subcutaneous nerve of neck (Mayer, 1794)*
   Synonym for macrodissected adult human ***transverse nerve of neck (>1840)***; in the original Latin, *nervus subcutaneus colli medius*; Part 5, Table VII-*IX* (p. 53).
5. *sub-mentonnair branch of cephalic part of trachelo-cutanean plexus (Burdin, 1803)*
   From vague description probably synonym for macrodissected adult human ***transverse nerve of neck (>1840)***; see translation (1803, Vol. 1, p. 188).
6. *superficial cervical branches of cervical plexus (Cloquet, 1816)*
   Apparently synonym for macrodissected adult human ***transverse nerve of neck (>1840)***; in the original French, *branches cervicales superficielles*, p. 640.
7. *internal ascending superficial branch of cervical plexus (Quain, 1828)*
   Synonym for macrodissected adult human ***transverse nerve of neck (>1840)***; p. 489.
8. *superficial branch of neck of superficial branches of cervical plexus (Quain, 1832)*
   Synonym for macrodissected adult human ***transverse nerve of neck (>1840)***; in the original Latin, *r. superficialis colli*, p. 680.
9. *inferior and middle subcutaneous nerve of neck (Arnold, 1834)*
   Synonym for macrodissected adult human ***transverse nerve of neck (>1840)***; in the original Latin, *nervus subcutaneus colli medius et inferior*, p. 17.
10. *internal branch of cervical plexus (Quain & Wilson, 1839)*
    Synonym for macrodissected adult human ***transverse nerve of neck (>1840)***; Plate XIV-*m*.
11. *transverse cervical nerve (>1840)*
    Synonym for macrodissected adult human ***transverse nerve of neck (>1840)***; current Latin form in

Terminologia Anatomica (1998, p. 137), *n. transversus cervicalis.*

PARTLY CORRESPONDS:

1. *lesser superficial branch of middle subcutaneous nerve of neck (Peipers, 1793)*
   Superficial and smaller branch of macrodissected adult human ***transverse nerve of neck (>1840)*** with further ascending and descending branches; in the original Latin, *subcutaneus colli medius superficialis minor*, p. 33.
2. *greater deep branch of middle subcutaneous nerve of neck (Peipers, 1793)*
   Deep and larger branch of ***transverse nerve of neck (>1840)*** with further ascending and descending branches; in the original Latin, *subcutaneus colli medius magnus profundus*, p. 34.
3. *submental branch of cephalic part of tracheosubcutaneous nerves (Chaussier, 1809)*
   Synonym for macrodissected adult human *middle subcutaneous nerve of neck (Meckel, 1817)* according to Meckel (1832, Vol. 3, p. 32).
4. *superficial cervical nerve (Meckel, 1817)*
   Synonym for *middle subcutaneous nerve of neck (Meckel, 1817)*; in the original Latin, *nervus superficialis colli*, see translation (1832, Vol. 3, p. 32).
5. *middle subcutaneous nerve of neck (Meckel, 1817)*
   Trunk of ***transverse nerve of neck (>1840)***, before it branches; in the original Latin, *nervus sub-cutaneus colli medius*, see translation (1832, Vol. 3, p. 32).

transverse occipital sulcus (>1840)

As described for macrodissected adult human, a short diagonal groove on the rostral, dorsal, and lateral surface of the ***occipital region (Vesalius, 1543a)***, just caudal to the dorsolateral tip of the ***parieto-occipital sulcus (>1840)***; see Williams & Warwick (1980, Fig. 7.111A). It was perhaps first clearly delineated by Rolando; see ***[transverse occipital sulcus (>1840)] (Rolando, 1831)***.

EARLIER REFERENCES:

Illustrated, not named or described:

1. ***[transverse occipital sulcus (>1840)] (Rolando, 1831)***
   Clearly illustrated for macrodissected adult human; Figure 1, between *c* and *a*.

transverse peduncular tract (Gudden, 1870)

As described in macrodissected adult human, and mammal generally with axonal transport pathway tracing methods, the main ventrally directed component of the ***superior fascicle of accessory optic system (Hayhow et al., 1960)*** coursing over the outside of the ***cerebral peduncle (Tarin, 1753)*** to end in the ***medial terminal nucleus of accessory optic system (Hayhow et al., 1960)***; see Hayhow et al. (1960), Nieuwenhuys et al. (2008, p. 781 and Fig. 19.13, called *transpeduncular tract*). For original use by Gudden see p. 364. It was probably first delineated as the *nervi accessorii de' Motori comuni (Malacarne, 1791)*.

TRANSLATIONS:

1. *tractus peduncularis transversus (Gudden, 1870)*
   Original Latin form of ***transverse peduncular tract (Gudden, 1870)***; p. 364.

EARLIER REFERENCES:

Earlier synonyms:

1. *nervi accessorii de' Motori comuni (Malacarne, 1791)*
   Probably synonym (plural) for macrodissected adult human ***transverse peduncular tract (Gudden, 1870)***; pp. 171–172. In English, *accessory nerve of common motor nerve.*
2. *entrelacement transversal du gros faisceau fibreux (Gall & Spurzheim, 1810)*
   Probably synonym for macrodissected adult human ***transverse peduncular tract (Gudden, 1870)***; Plate IV-34. In English, *transverse intertwining of great fibrous fascicle.* Also illustrated in Desmoulins (1825, Pl. 13, Fig. 1-z, drawn by Rolando).

transverse pontine fibers (>1840)

As described for macrodissected adult human, and mammal generally with histological methods for ***axons (Kölliker, 1896)***, the transversely oriented ***white matter (Meckel, 1817)*** bundles forming the part of the ***middle cerebellar peduncle (Rolando, 1819)*** associated with the ***pontine nuclei (Jacobsohn, 1909)***, crossing the median plane, and forming the commissure of the ***middle cerebellar peduncle (Rolando, 1819)***; contrasted with the ***longitudinal pontine fibers (Arnold, 1838b)***; see Clark (1951, pp. 898–900), Carpenter (1976, p. 324), Williams & Warwick (1980, p. 907), *Dorland's* (2003, p. 694), *Terminologia Anatomica* (1998, p. 112), Nieuwenhuys et al. (2008, p. 202). They were first delineated as the *transverse medullary tracts of pons Varolii (Ridley, 1695)*.

EARLIER REFERENCES:

Earlier synonyms:

1. *transverse medullary tracts of pons Varolii (Ridley, 1695)*
   Synonym for macrodissected adult human ***transverse pontine fibers (>1840)***; p. 136. Ridley noted (p. 193) that in fact *transverse medullary tracts of pons Varolii (Ridley, 1695)* give the *pons Varolii (Steno, 1669)* a more striated appearance than the *striated body (Willis, 1664)*.
2. *transverse striae of pons Varolii (Ridley, 1695)*
   Synonym for *transverse medullary tracts of pons Varolii (Ridley, 1695)*; Figure 6-*e*.
3. *pontocerebellar fibers (>1840)*
   Synonym for macrodissected adult human ***transverse pontine fibers (>1840)***; see Williams & Warwick (1980, p. 907).
4. *pontocerebellar bundles (>1840)*
   Synonym for macrodissected adult human ***transverse pontine fibers (>1840)***; see Nieuwenhuys et al. (2008, Fig. 6.28-23).

PARTLY CORRESPONDS:

1. *middle medullary tract (Ridley, 1695)*
   Ridley described and illustrated *white substance (Vesalius, 1543a)* in median plane of transversely sliced

macrodissected adult human ***pontine nuclei (Jacobsohn, 1909)***, probably part of ***transverse pontine fibers (>1840)***; p. 193, Figure VI-*e*. See Dejerine & Dejerine-Klumpke (1901, Fig. 395-*r*), Nieuwenhuys et al. (2008, Figs. 6.15–17).

2. *intervening medullary tract (Ridley, 1695)*
   Synonym for *middle medullary tract (Ridley, 1695)*; Figure VI-*e*.
3. *inferior and superior level of annular protuberance (Desmoulins, 1825)*
   Major concentrations of macrodissected adult human ***transverse pontine fibers (>1840)***, which he divided into three fibrous bands, anterior, middle, and posterior [ventral or superficial, middle, and dorsal or deep, respectively]; in the original French, *l'étage inférieur et superficiel du renflement appelé protubérance annulaire*, with *trois bandes fibreuses, antérieure, moyenne, postérieure*; pp. 246–247.
4. *superficial transverse fibres of pons (Bell, 1834)*
   Probably corresponds in macrodissected adult human to component of ***middle cerebellar peduncle (>1840)*** on outer (ventral) surface of ***pontine nuclei (Jacobsohn, 1909)***; that is, to most superficial ***transverse pontine fibers (>1840)***; p. 474.
5. *deeper transverse septum of pons (Bell, 1834)*
   Corresponds in macrodissected adult human to ***transverse pontine fibers (>1840)*** leading into the *superficial transverse fibres of pons (Bell, 1834)*; p. 475. Bell also referred to it as *deep-seated transverse lamina of fibres*, *deep septum*, and *posterior set of transverse fibres*; p. 475.
6. *septum of pons (Bell, 1834)*
   Synonym for *deeper transverse septum of pons (Bell, 1834)*; p. 476.

transverse tectal sulcus (>1840)

As defined for macrodissected adult human, the arm of the ***cruciform sulcus (>1840)*** separating ***superior colliculi (Haller, 1762)*** rostrally from ***inferior colliculi (Haller, 1762)*** caudally; see Williams & Warwick (1980, p. 935). It was known to Galen; see ***[transverse tectal sulcus (>1840)] (Galen, c173)***.

EARLIER REFERENCES:

Described, not named or illustrated:

1. ***[transverse tectal sulcus (>1840)] (Galen, c173)***
   In describing the ***superior colliculi (Haller, 1762)*** and ***inferior colliculi (Haller, 1762)*** of macrodissected adult beef, pig, and/or macaque but not human, Galen must have observed it; see *little buttocks (Galen, c173, definition 1)*.

Illustrated and described, not named:

1. ***[transverse tectal sulcus (>1840)] (Vesalius, 1543a)***
   Clearly illustrated and described as a "*transverse linear impression*" separating ***superior colliculi (Haller, 1762)*** rostrally from ***inferior colliculi (Haller, 1762)*** caudally in macrodissected adult human; see Singer translation (1952, pp. 47, 106 and Fig. 10).

Earlier synonyms:

1. *transverse furrow of corpora bigemina (Gordon, 1815)*
   Synonym for macrodissected adult human ***transverse tectal sulcus (>1840)***; p. 91.
2. *transverse sulcus of quadrigeminal tubercles (Serres, 1824–1826)*
   Synonym for macrodissected embryonic and adult human ***transverse tectal sulcus (>1840)***; in the original French, *sillon transverse des tubercules quadrijumeaux*, Plate II, Figure 71-5 and elsewhere.

transverse temporal gyri (Heschl, 1878)

As described for macrodissected adult human, the most dorsal and medial topographic subdivision of the ***temporal region (>1840)*** lying between ***circular sulcus (Schwalbe, 1881)*** medially and ***transverse temporal sulcus (Heschl, 1878)*** laterally, dorsal (superior) and medial to the ***superior temporal gyrus (>1840)***. They are variable in number, often differing on the right and left sides as well and contain *area 41 (Brodmann, 1909)* and most or all of *area 42 (Brodmann, 1909)*, related to the auditory system; see Heschl (1878), Crosby et al. (1962, Fig. 316), Williams & Warwick (1980, pp. 986, 1021 and Figs. 7.112, 7.138-*AI*), *Terminologia Anatomica* (1998, p. 125), Nieuwenhuys et al. (2008, pp. 742–744 and Fig. 18.3). For Heschl's original use in adult human, see p. 6. They were clearly delineated by Gall & Spurzheim; see ***[transverse temporal gyri (Heschl, 1878)] (Gall & Spurzheim, 1810)***.

TRANSLATIONS:

1. *queren Schläfenwindungen (Heschl, 1878)*
   Original German form of ***transverse temporal gyri (Heschl, 1878)***; see p. 6.

EARLIER REFERENCES:

Illustrated, not named or described:

1. ***[transverse temporal gyri (Heschl, 1878)] (Gall & Spurzheim, 1810)***
   Very clearly illustrated for macrodissected adult human; Plate V, right side.

PARTLY CORRESPONDS:

1. *area parainsularis (Brodmann, 1909)*
   Original Latin form of *parainsular area (Brodmann (1909)*; p. 145.
2. *parainsular area (Brodmann, 1909)*
   Based on cellular architecture in adult human, most medial zone of ***transverse temporal gyri (Heschl, 1878)*** lying between ***insular region (Brodmann, 1909)*** medially and dorsally, and *medial (anterior) transverse temporal area (Brodmann, 1909)* laterally; see Garey translation (1994, p. 125 and Fig. 89).
3. *area 52 (Brodmann, 1909)*
   Synonym for adult human *parainsular area (Brodmann, 1909)*; in the original German, *Feld 52*, p. 145.
4. *area temporalis transversa interna (anterior) (Brodmann, 1909)*
   Original Latin form of *medial (anterior) transverse temporal area (Brodmann (1909)*; p. 145.
5. *medial (anterior) transverse temporal area (Brodmann, 1909)*

Based on cellular architecture in adult human, middle zone of ***transverse temporal gyri (Heschl, 1878)*** lying between *parainsular area (Brodmann, 1909)* medially and *lateral (posterior) transverse temporal area (Brodmann, 1909)* laterally; see Garey translation (1994, p. 125 and Fig. 89). It corresponds to Heschl's (1878) *anterior transverse temporal gyrus*, or in the original German, *vordere quere Schläfenwindung*.

6. *area 41 (Brodmann, 1909)*
   Synonym for adult human *medial (anterior) transverse temporal area (Brodmann, 1909)*; in the original German, *Feld 41*, p. 145. It is also known as the *primary auditory area (>1840)*, in adult primate receiving direct inputs from ***ventral part of medial geniculate complex (>1840)*** and containing three tonotopic maps of the cochlea; see Nieuwenhuys et al. (2008, p. 742 and Fig. 18.3).
7. *area temporalis transversa externa (posterior) (Brodmann, 1909)*
   Original Latin form of *lateral (posterior) transverse temporal area (Brodmann, 1909)*; p. 145.
8. *lateral (posterior) transverse temporal area (Brodmann, 1909)*
   Based on cellular architecture in adult human, lateral zone of ***transverse temporal gyri (Heschl, 1878)*** lying between *medial (anterior) transverse temporal area (Brodmann, 1909)* medially and *superior temporal area (Brodmann, 1909)* laterally; see Garey translation (1994, p. 125 and Fig. 89).
9. *area 42 (Brodmann, 1909)*
   Synonym for adult human *medial (anterior) transverse temporal area (Brodmann, 1909)*; in the original German, *Feld 42*, p. 145.
10. *primary auditory area (>1840)*
    Synonym for *area 41 (Brodmann, 1909)*, in adult primate receiving direct inputs from ***ventral part of medial geniculate complex (>1840)*** and containing three tonotopic maps of the cochlea; see Carpenter (1976, p. 574), Nieuwenhuys et al. (2008, p. 742 and Fig. 18.3).

transverse temporal sulcus (Heschl, 1878)

As described for macrodissected adult human, the gently curving groove between the medial edge of the ***superior temporal gyrus (>1840)*** and lateral parts of the ***transverse temporal gyri (Heschl, 1878)***; see Williams & Warwick (1980, p. 986, Fig. 7.112 unlabeled), *Terminologia Anatomica* (1998, p. 125), *Dorland's* (2003, p. 1789). It was first clearly delineated by Gall & Spurzheim; see ***[transverse temporal sulcus (Heschl, 1878)] (Gall & Spurzheim, 1810)***.

TRANSLATIONS:

1. *Schläfenfurche quer (Heschl, 1878)*
   Original German form of ***transverse temporal sulcus (Heschl, 1878)***; see p. 8.

EARLIER REFERENCES:

Illustrated, not named or described:

1. ***[transverse temporal sulcus (Heschl, 1878)] (Gall & Spurzheim, 1810)***
   Very clearly illustrated for macrodissected adult human; Plate V, right side.

trapezoid body (Treviranus, 1820)

As described for macrodissected adult human, and mammal generally with histological methods for ***axons (Kölliker, 1896)***, the essentially transverse ***central nervous system white matter tract (>1840)*** of the ***medulla (Winslow, 1733)***, beginning in the ***cochlear nuclei (>1840)*** and extending ventrally to cross the median plane to become the rostrally directed ***lateral lemniscus (Bechterew, 1885b)***; see Nieuwenhuys et al. (2008, pp. 737–742). Smaller numbers of ***axons (Kölliker, 1896)*** from the ***cochlear nuclei (>1840)*** cross the median plane more dorsally to enter the contralateral ***superior olivary complex (>1840)*** or ***lateral lemniscus (Bechterew, 1885b)*** through the ***intermediate acoustic stria (>1840)*** or ***dorsal acoustic stria (>1840)***, respectively; see Nieuwenhuys et al. (2008, Fig. 18.2). For Treviranus's use in macrodissected adult human, see p. 12. It was first described as the *lesser annulary protuberance (Willis, 1664)*.

TRANSLATIONS:

1. *corpus trapezoideum (Treviranus, 1820)*
   Original Latin form of ***trapezoid body (Treviranus, 1820)***; p. 12.

EARLIER REFERENCES:

Earlier synonyms:

1. *lesser annulary protuberance (Willis, 1664)*
   Synonym for macrodissected adult large mammal (though not human) ***trapezoid body (Treviranus, 1820)***, which Willis discovered; see Pordage translation (1681, p. 68). Reil (1809b) described crossing of *internal part of lemniscus (Reil, 1809c)* or ***lateral lemniscus (Bechterew, 1885b)*** in macrodissected adult human; see Mayo translation (1823, p. 57).
2. *lesser annulary process (Willis, 1664)*
   Synonym for *lesser annulary protuberance (Willis, 1664)*; see Pordage translation (1681, p. 58).
3. *lesser protuberance of auditory nerve (Willis, 1664)*
   Synonym for *lesser annulary protuberance (Willis, 1664)*; see Pordage translation (1681, p. 68). Also see *auditory nerve (Willis, 1664)*.
4. *lesser ring (Willis, 1664)*
   Synonym for *lesser annulary protuberance (Willis, 1664)*; see Pordage translation (1681, p. 117).
5. *lower ring (Willis, 1664)*
   Synonym for *lesser annulary protuberance (Willis, 1664)*; see Pordage translation (1681, p. 117).
6. *medullary plates (Malacarne, 1795)*
   Synonym for macrodissected adult human ***trapezoid body (Treviranus, 1820)***; in the original Italian, *Lastre medollare*, p. 82. See Tiedemann (1821, Tab. I, Fig. 5-*n*); according to Treviranus (1820) it was on p. 87.
7. *commissure of acoustic nerves (Gall & Spurzheim, 1810)*
   Synonym for macrodissected adult "animal" ***trapezoid body (Treviranus, 1820)***; p. 76.

LATER SYNONYMS:

1. *trapezium (Tiedemann, 1821)*
   Synonym for macrodissected adult mammalian ***trapezoid body (Treviranus, 1820)***; see Table IV, Figure 4-*d*.
2. *trapezium of medulla oblongata (Serres, 1824–1826)*
   Synonym for macrodissected adult mammalian ***trapezoid body (Treviranus, 1820)***; in the original French, *trapèze de la moelle allongée*; Plate VIII, Figure 194-*T*. English forms were provided as *trapezoideum* (Todd, 1845, p. 168) and *trapezium* (Todd, 1845, p. 168).
3. *lesser pons (Serres, 1824–1826)*
   Synonym for macrodissected adult brown bear ***trapezoid body (Treviranus, 1820)***; in the original French, *petit pont*; Plate XI, Figure 251-*T*.
4. *superior level of commissure (Desmoulins, 1825)*
   Synonym for macrodissected adult human ***trapezoid body (Treviranus, 1820)***, which Desmoulins considered deep component of *great cerebellar commissure (Gall & Spurzheim, 1810)*; in the original French, *l'étage supérieur de la commissure*, p. 247.
5. *commissure of auditory nerves (Desmoulins, 1825)*
   Synonym for *commissure of acoustic nerve (Gall & Spurzheim, 1810)*; in the original French, *commissure des nerfs auditifs*, p. 432.
6. *posterior band of cerebral protuberance (Rolando, 1825a)*
   Synonym for macrodissected adult sheep ***trapezoid body (Treviranus, 1820)***; in the original French, *bande postérieure de la protubérance cérébrale*, Table VI, Figure 3-*b.p*.
7. *posterior transverse band (Rolando, 1825a)*
   Synonym for macrodissected large calf ***trapezoid body (Treviranus, 1820)***; in the original French, *bande transversale postérieure*, Table VII, Figure 3-*b.p*.
8. *ponticulus (Arnold, 1828a)*
   Possibly this term, meaning "little bridge," is synonym for macrodissected adult human ***trapezoid body (Treviranus, 1820)***; p. 21 and Arnold (1838b, Tab. 2, Fig. 5-*b*).

triangular part of inferior frontal gyrus (>1840)

As described for macrodissected adult human, a ventral topographic zone of the ***inferior frontal gyrus (>1840)*** between ***anterior branch of lateral cerebral sulcus (>1840)*** and ***ascending branch of lateral cerebral sulcus (>1840)***; see Williams & Warwick (1980, Fig. 7.111A), *Terminologia Anatomica* (1998, p. 125). It was clearly delineated by Rolando; see ***[triangular part of inferior frontal gyrus (>1840)] (Rolando, 1831)***.

EARLIER REFERENCES:

Illustrated, not named or described:

1. ***[triangular part of inferior frontal gyrus (>1840)] (Rolando, 1831)***
   Clearly illustrated for macrodissected adult human; Figure 1-9.

Earlier synonyms:

1. *area triangularis (Brodmann, 1909)*
   Original Latin form of *triangular area (Brodmann, 1909)*; p. 138.
2. *triangular area (Brodmann, 1909)*
   Based on cellular architecture in adult human roughly synonymous with ***triangular part of inferior frontal gyrus (>1840)***; see Garey translation (1994, p. 117 and Fig. 85).
3. *area 45 (Brodmann, 1909)*
   Synonym for adult human *triangular area (Brodmann, 1909)*; in the original German, *Feld 45*, p. 138.

trigeminal ganglion (>1840)

As described for macrodissected adult human, the sensory ***cranial nerve ganglion (>1840)*** of the ***trigeminal nerve (Winslow, 1733)*** associated with the distal end of the ***trigeminal nerve sensory root (>1840)*** and the proximal ends of the three ***trigeminal nerve branches (Winslow, 1733)***; see Williams & Warwick (1980, pp. 1059–1060 and Figs. 7.175–178, 181). Vieussens is credited with discovering it; see *ganglioform plexus (Vieussens, 1684)*.

EARLIER REFERENCES:

Earlier synonyms:

1. *ganglioform plexus (Vieussens, 1684)*
   Synonym for macrodissected adult human ***trigeminal ganglion (>1840)***; in the original Latin, *plexus ganglioformis*; Book III, Chapter 3 and Table 22-*B*. Also see Haller (1762, p. 202 note *q*), Burdach (1822, p. 317), Meckel (1832, Vol. 3, p. 61).
2. *ganglioform tumor (Rau, 1694)*
   Synonym for *ganglioform plexus (Vieussens, 1684)*; in the original Latin, *ganglioformem tumorem*, p. 190.
3. *ganglion of fifth nerve (Ridley, 1695)*
   Clear description and illustration of macrodissected adult human ***trigeminal ganglion (>1840)***, along with three ***trigeminal nerve branches (Winslow, 1733)*** emerging distally; p. 147, Figure 3-*B*.
4. *taenia nervosa (Meckel, 1748)*
   Synonym for macrodissected adult human ***trigeminal ganglion (>1840)***; p. 21, see Burdach (1822, p. 317).
5. *Gasserian ganglion (Hirsch, 1765)*
   Hirsch named ***trigeminal ganglion (>1840)*** after his professor, J.L. Gasser; see Neubauer (1772, p. 22). According to Johnstone (1795, pp. 36–37), Gasser indeed noticed it shortly after Johnstone's 1765 paper appeared, and while Gasser's pupils accepted the originality of the observation, later anatomists did not. The variant eponym, *ganglion of Gasser*, is found in, for example, Lobstein (1831, p. 14).
6. *semilunar ganglion (Neubauer, 1772)*
   Synonym for macrodissected adult human ***trigeminal ganglion (>1840)***; p. 22.
7. *retiform plexus (Santorini, 1775)*
   Synonym for macrodissected adult human ***trigeminal ganglion (>1840)***; in the original Latin, *plexus retiformis*, p. 19. See Meckel (1817; and translation, 1832, Vol. 3, p. 61), Burdach (1822, p. 317).
8. *semilunar intumescence (Wrisberg, 1777)*
   Synonym for macrodissected adult human ***trigeminal ganglion (>1840)***; in the original Latin, *intumescentia semilunaris*, p. 11.

9. *intumescentiam ganglio affinem (Scarpa, 1779)*
Synonym for macrodissected adult human ***trigeminal ganglion (>1840)***; p. 74. See Haase (1781, p. 54 note *f*), Meckel (1832, Vol. 3, p. 61).
10. *ganglion in trunk of fifth pair of nerves (Monro, 1783)*
Synonym for macrodissected adult human ***trigeminal ganglion (>1840)***; Monro illustrated the course of "nervous fibrils" from the trunk through the ***ganglion (Galen, c173)*** and into the three ***trigeminal nerve branches (Winslow, 1733)*** in macrodissected adult human observed with naked eye or simple magnifying glass; Table XX. See p. 51 for method.
11. *zona (Palletta, 1784)*
Synonym for macrodissected adult human ***trigeminal ganglion (>1840)***; p. 119. See Burdach (1822, p. 317).
12. *armilla (Malacarne, 1791)*
Italian synonym for macrodissected adult human ***trigeminal ganglion (>1840)***; p. 190. See Meckel (1817; and translation, 1832, Vol. 3, p. 61), Burdach (1822, p. 317). Bell & Bell (1828, p. 485) ascribed the name without citation to "Paletta".
13. *agger lunatus (Meckel, 1817)*
Synonym for macrodissected adult human ***trigeminal ganglion (>1840)*** attributed to Neubauer without citation; see translation (1832, Vol. 3, p. 61).
14. *ganglion intervertebrale capitis anticum (Arnold, 1834)*
Synonym for macrodissected adult human ***trigeminal ganglion (>1840)***; p. 7. Roughly translated *anterior intervertebral ganglion of head.*
15. *Casserian ganglion (Todd, 1836–1839)*
Erroneous eponym for macrodissected adult human *Gasserian ganglion (Hirsch, 1765)*; p. 496. Also see Quain (1837, p. 760).

trigeminal nerve (Winslow, 1733)

As described for macrodissected adult human, the thickest ***cranial nerve (Soemmerring, 1791)***, and homologous to a ***spinal nerve (Camper, 1760–1762)***. It is attached to the ventrolateral ***pons (Haller, 1747)*** by the ***trigeminal nerve motor root (Bell, 1829)*** and ***trigeminal nerve sensory root (>1840)*** with an expansion, the ***trigeminal ganglion (>1840)*** occupying a corresponding indentation (the trigeminal cave) in the petrous part of the temporal bone. Three primary branches lie distal to the ***trigeminal ganglion (>1840): ophthalmic nerve (Winslow, 1733), maxillary nerve (Meckel, 1753)***, and ***mandibular nerve sensory root (>1840)*** receiving the ***trigeminal nerve motor root (Bell, 1829)*** to form the ***mandibular nerve trunk (>1840)***. See Williams & Warwick (1980, pp. 1059–1061 and Figs. 7.176–181). "Trigeminal" is from the Latin *trigeminus* (*tres*, three, and *geminus*, twin-born), meaning tripartite or threefold (three at origin); see Foster (1894, p. 2959). It is entirely unclear who should get credit for the first description corresponding to modern views of the ***trigeminal nerve (Winslow, 1733)***; for early histories see Meckel (1748, pp. 1–19), Soemmerring (1778, p. 130 ff.), Burdach (1822, p. 314 ff.). For Winslow's use in macrodissected adult human, which is certainly modern, see Section X, p. 47. Despite considerable confusion, the *third pair of nerves from brain (Falloppio, 1561)* was the first broadly accurate, clear description of three main branches, which had been illustrated accurately but not published by Eustachi; see Albinus edition (1761, Tab. 18, Fig. 2-*V*). Willis referred to the *fifth pair of nerves arising within skull (Willis, 1664)* in a description that was also broadly accurate except he had the ***sympathetic trunk (Winslow, 1733)*** as a branch.

TRANSLATIONS:

1. *nervi trigemini (Winslow, 1733)*
Original Latin form of right and left ***trigeminal nerve (Winslow, 1733)***; Section X, p. 47. For singular form, *nervus trigeminus*, see Burdach (1822, p. 86).

EARLIER REFERENCES:

Described, not named or illustrated:

1. ***[trigeminal nerve (Winslow, 1733)] (Herophilus, c335–c280 BC)***
Herophilus, the founder of human anatomy, is credited with discovering most of the ***cranial nerves (Soemmerring, 1791)***. Although his account of the ***trigeminal nerve (Winslow, 1733)*** must have been vague, it has been suggested that he observed in macrodissected adult human and other mammals the ***trigeminal nerve motor root (Bell, 1829)*** and ***trigeminal nerve sensory root (>1840)***, which he apparently did not name; see Solmsen (1961), von Staden (1969), Longrigg (1993), Clarke & O'Malley (1996, p. 261).

Earlier synonyms:

1. *gustatory pair of nerves (Heister, 1717)*
Synonym for macrodissected adult human ***trigeminal nerves (Winslow, 1733)***; in the original Latin, *par gustatorium*, see translation (1721, p. 245).
2. *nervi innominati (Winslow, 1733)*
Synonym for macrodissected adult human ***trigeminal nerves (Winslow, 1733)***, Section X, p. 47. For singular form, *nervus innominatus*, see Burdach (1822, p. 315), who wrote that König used this term, though citation has not been traced.

LATER SYNONYMS:

1. *nervi sympathetici medii (Wrisberg, 1777)*
Synonym for macrodissected adult human ***trigeminal nerves (Winslow, 1733)***; p. 5. In a footnote Wrisberg referred to Andersch for the term used in his "*Nervorum Cordis Opera*, p. 109".
2. *nervum divisum (Günther, 1786)*
Synonym listed for macrodissected adult human ***trigeminal nerve (Winslow, 1733)***; p. 40. Also see Meckel (1832, Vol. 3, p. 59).
3. *nervum trium funiculorum (Günther, 1786)*
Synonym listed for macrodissected adult human ***trigeminal nerve (Winslow, 1733)***; p. 40.
4. *nervum balneare (Günther, 1786)*
Synonym listed for macrodissected adult human ***trigeminal nerve (Winslow, 1733)***; p. 40.
5. *nervum sympatheticum medium Wrisbergii (Günther, 1786)*

Eponym listed for macrodissected adult human ***trigeminal nerve (Winslow, 1733)***; p. 40.

6. *nervorum cerebralium maximum (Günther, 1786)*
Synonym listed for macrodissected adult human ***trigeminal nerve (Winslow, 1733)***; p. 40.
7. *seventh, eighth, and ninth pairs (Malacarne, 1791)*
Synonym for macrodissected adult human ***trigeminal nerves (Winslow, 1733)***; pp. 174–186.
8. *fifth pair of cranial nerves (Soemmerring, 1791)*
Synonym for macrodissected adult human ***trigeminal nerves (Winslow, 1733)***; see ***cranial nerves (Soemmerring, 1791)***.
9. *fifth pair of cerebral nerves (Soemmerring, 1791)*
Synonym for *fifth pair of cranial nerves (Soemmerring, 1791)*; see p. 103 and *cerebral nerves (Soemmerring, 1791)*. For original Latin form, *par quintum nervorum cerebri*, see Soemmerring (1798, p. 125).
10. *nervus consensorius medius capitis (Andersch, 1797)*
Synonym for macrodissected adult human ***trigeminal nerve (Winslow, 1733)***; p. 1, also see Burdach (1822, p. 315). It is a different form of *nervi sympathetici medii (Wrisberg, 1777)*.
11. *trifacial pair of nerves (Burdin, 1803)*
Synonym for macrodissected adult human ***trigeminal nerves (Winslow, 1733)***; see translation (1803, Vol. 1, p. 144). The Latin form, *nervus trifacialis*, was given by Burdach (1822, p. 315), who also wrote that Hebenstreit used the term *nervus trimellus*, though citation has not been traced.
12. *mixed pair (Gall & Spurzheim, 1810)*
Synonym for macrodissected adult human ***trigeminal nerves (Winslow, 1733)***; in the original French, *la paire mixte*, p. 78.
13. *mixed nerve (Gall & Spurzheim, 1810)*
Synonym for *mixed pair (Gall & Spurzheim, 1818)*; see p. 109. Burdach (1822, p. 315) supplied the Latin form, *nervus mixtus*.
14. *manducatory nerve (Bell, 1829)*
Synonym for macrodissected adult mammalian ***trigeminal nerve (Winslow, 1733)***; pp. 324–325.
15. *three-fold nerve (Swan, 1830)*
Synonym for macrodissected adult human ***trigeminal nerve (Winslow, 1733)***; p. 16.

PARTLY CORRESPONDS:

1. *third and fourth pairs of nerves from brain (Galen, c192)*
Together these *pairs of nerves from brain (Galen, c192)* roughly correspond to ***trigeminal nerves (Winslow, 1733)***, but exact relationship is complex and remains uncertain. Galen's description was based largely on macrodissected adult pig, beef, and/or macaque but not explicitly human; see Savage-Smith (1971, p. 173 ff.). He credited Marinus of Pergamum with observing them earlier; see Goss (1966, p. 329). Vesalius (1543a) added little to Galen's basic description; see Richardson & Carman translation (2002, pp. 188–192) and *pairs of nerves from brain (Galen, c192)*.
2. *third pair of nerves from brain (Galen, c192)*
Frequently though misleadingly equated with ***trigeminal nerve sensory root (>1840)***; see for example Duckworth translation (1962, pp. 9, 189, 191) and May (1968, p. 438), based largely on descriptions of macrodissected adult pig, beef, and/or macaque but not human. Also see Savage-Smith (1971, p. 173 ff.), who suggested it is best to consider just the *third and fourth pairs of nerves from brain (Galen, c192)* together. Galen credited Marinus of Pergamum with observing these features earlier; see Goss (1966, p. 329). Also see *pairs of nerves from brain (Galen, c192)*.
3. *roots of third pair of nerves from brain (Galen, c192)*
Refers to texture of proximal part of *third pair of nerves from brain (Galen, c192)*, and not any specific structure recognized today. Galen wrote, "if you grasp it by putting your fingers round it, its parts cleave together and are set in motion. The reason is that this pair has a plurality of roots and not, as has the optic nerve-pair, one single root. Since these roots are loosely attached and connected to one another, when anyone fingers them with a twisting movement, they become supple between his fingers, and on this ground one regards them as softer than those nerves which have an undivided root." (Duckworth translation, 1962, p. 189).
4. *soft pair of nerves (Galen, c192)*
Synonym for *third pair of nerves from brain (Galen, c192)*; see Duckworth translation (1962, p. 195).
5. *fourth pair of nerves from brain (Galen, c192)*
Frequently though misleadingly equated with ***trigeminal nerve motor root (Bell, 1829)***; see, for example, Duckworth translation (1962, pp. 9, 191) and May translation (1968, p. 438), based largely on descriptions of macrodissected adult pig, beef, and/or macaque but not human. Also see Savage-Smith (1971, p. 173 ff.), who suggested it is best to consider just the *third and fourth pairs of nerves from brain (Galen, c192)* together.
6. *fourth and fifth pairs of nerves from brain (Theophilos Protospatharios, fl. 610–641)*
Synonym for *third and fourth pairs of nerves from brain (Galen, c192)*; see *pairs of nerves from brain (Theophilos Protospatharios, fl. 610–641)*.
7. *lesser, thinner, harder root of third pair of nerves (Vesalius, 1543a)*
Obvious from descriptions and illustrations that it referred to major parts of ***trigeminal nerve sensory root (>1840)***, ***ophthalmic nerve (Winslow, 1733)***, and ***maxillary nerve (Meckel, 1753)***—including ***supraorbital nerve (Meckel, 1753)***, ***infraorbital nerve (Schaarschmidt, 1750)***, ***anterior ethmoidal nerve (>1840)***, and ***zygomaticotemporal nerve (>1840)***—in macrodissected adult human; see Richardson and Carman translation (2002, pp. 170, 188). Richardson and Carman (2002, pp. 165, 174) erroneously equated it with ***trochlear nerve (Molinetti, 1669)***; also see Soemmerring (1778, p. 120).
8. *thinner root of third pair of cerebral nerves (Vesalius, 1543a)*
Richardson & Carman (2009, p. 156) equated it with ***trochlear nerve (Molinetti, 1669)*** but this seems clearly erroneous based on extensive descriptions by Vesalius in Book IV; see *lesser, thinner, harder root of third pair of nerves (Vesalius, 1543a)*.

9. *radix gracilis, tenuis, posterior tertii paris (Vesalius, 1543a)*
According to Burdach (1822, p. 389), description on p. 367 of ***trochlear nerve (Molinetti, 1669)*** although this is clearly erroneous—it corresponds to *lesser, thinner, harder root of third pair of nerves (Vesalius, 1543a)*.
10. *third pair of cerebral nerves (Vesalius, 1543a)*
Essentially macrodissected adult human *third pair of nerves from brain (Galen, c192)*; see Richardson & Carman translation (2002, pp. 188–192). Vesalius added little to Galen's description.
11. *root of third pair of cerebral nerves (Vesalius, 1543a)*
Proximal part of *third pair of cerebral nerves (Vesalius, 1543a)*; see Richardson & Carman translation (2002, p. 205, no. 3 in the figure).
12. *third pair of sinews of brain (Geminus, 1553)*
Synonym for macrodissected adult human *third pair of cerebral nerves (Vesalius, 1543a)*; originally spelled *thyrde payre of synowes of b[rayne]*, see *The table of the figure of synowes*, part *L:1,2*.
13. *root of third pair of sinews of brain (Geminus, 1553)*
Synonym for macrodissected adult human *root of third pair of cerebral nerves (Vesalius, 1543a)*; originally spelled *roote of thyrde payre of sinowes of brayne*, see *The table of the figures of sinowes*.
14. *lesser, thinner, harder root of third pair of sinews (Geminus, 1553)*
Synonym for macrodissected adult human *lesser, thinner, harder root of third pair of nerves (Vesalius, 1543a)*; originally spelled *lesser, thynner, harder roote of thyrde payre of synowes of b[rayne]*, see *The table of the figure of synowes*.
15. *slenderer root of third pair of sinews (Geminus, 1553)*
Synonym for macrodissected adult human *lesser, thinner, harder root of third pair of nerves (Vesalius, 1543a)*; originally spelled *slenderer roote of thyrde payre of synowes of brayne*, see *The tables of the brayne*, Figure 14-*H*.
16. *third pair of nerves from brain (Falloppio, 1561)*
In enumerating *pairs of nerves from brain (Falloppio, 1561)*, Falloppio described three trunks arising from this ***nerve (Herophilus, c335–c280 BC)*** pair, corresponding roughly to right and left ***ophthalmic nerve (Winslow, 1733)***, ***mandibular nerve (Meckel, 1753)***, and ***maxillary nerve (>1840)*** according to Harvey (1961, p. 234 note 844) and Crooke (1615, p. 889), where lingering confusion about the complex poorly understood anatomy was mentioned.
17. *third conjugation of nerves of brain (Bauhin, 1605)*
Synonym for macrodissected adult human *thinner root of third pair of nerves (Vesalius, 1543a)*. Bauhin claimed it deserves its own ***nerve (Herophilus, c335–c280 BC)*** number because it arises separately from, and has nothing in common with, the following ***nerve (Herophilus, c335–c280 BC)***, the *fourth conjugation of nerves of brain (Bauhin, 1605)*; see Crooke translation (1615, pp. 486, 889).
18. *fourth conjugation of nerves of brain (Bauhin, 1605)*
Corresponds to combination of *thicker root of third pair of nerves (Vesalius, 1543a)* and *fourth pair of nerves (Vesalius, 1543a)* for macrodissected adult human; see Crooke translation (1615, pp. 486, 890–891). Also see *third conjugation of nerves of brain (Bauhin, 1605)*.
19. *fifth and sixth pairs of nerves from brain (Bartholin, 1641)*
Together correspond roughly to ***trigeminal nerves (Winslow, 1733)***, to which certain components of the *fourth pair of nerves from brain (Bartholin, 1641)* also contribute; see translation in Bartholin (1662, p. 325).
20. *fifth pair of nerves arising within skull (Willis, 1664)*
Overall corresponds quite well to ***trigeminal nerves (Winslow, 1733)***, except Willis, like Galen, had ***sympathetic trunks (Winslow, 1733)*** arising in part from them; pp. 58, 141–143.
21. *trunk of fifth pair of nerves arising within skull (Willis, 1664)*
Synonym for macrodissected adult, presumably human, *trigeminal nerve trunk (Winslow, 1733)*; see Pordage translation (1681, p. 141 and Fig. 1 on p. 302). Vieussens also illustrated for macrodissected adult human *truncus nervi quintae conjugationis*; Table 23-*A*.
22. *greater branch of fifth pair of nerves arising within skull (Willis, 1664)*
Corresponds roughly to macrodissected adult, presumably human, ***maxillary nerve (Meckel, 1753)*** and ***mandibular nerve (>1840)*** considered together; see Pordage translation (1681, p. 142).
23. *superior branch of fifth pair of nerves arising within skull (Willis, 1664)*
Corresponds roughly to macrodissected adult, presumably human, ***maxillary nerve (Meckel, 1753)*** and ***mandibular nerve (>1840)*** considered together; see Pordage translation (1681, p. 142).
24. *upper part of trunk of fifth pair of nerves arising within skull (Willis, 1664)*
Corresponds roughly to macrodissected adult, presumably human, ***maxillary nerve (Meckel, 1753)*** and ***mandibular nerve (>1840)*** considered together; see Pordage translation (1681, p. 142).
25. *second division of fifth pair of nerves arising within skull (Willis, 1664)*
Corresponds roughly to macrodissected adult, presumably human, ***maxillary nerve (Meckel, 1753)*** and ***mandibular nerve (>1840)*** considered together; see Pordage translation (1681, pp. 144–145, Fig. 1-*D,E,F*).
26. *trigeminal nerve trunk (Winslow, 1733)*
Segment of macrodissected adult human ***trigeminal nerve (Winslow, 1733)*** between plane where it meets surface of ***pons (Haller, 1747)*** proximally and ***trigeminal ganglion (>1840)*** distally; Sections. VI, p. 62 and X, p. 47. Early research was reviewed by Hirsch (1765).
27. *palatine ramus of superior maxillary nerve (Winslow, 1733)*
Somewhat vague description corresponds roughly to currently unrecognized combination in macrodissected adult human of ***palatine nerves (Schaarschmidt, 1750)***, ***lateral pterygoid nerve (>1840)***, and ***posterior superior dental nerve (Haller, 1762)***; in the original Latin, *ramus palatinus*, Section VI, p. 65.

28. *spheno-palatine ramus of superior maxillary nerve (Winslow, 1733)*
Somewhat vague description corresponds roughly to currently unrecognized combination in macrodissected adult human of ***medial pterygoid nerve (>1840), posterior superior nasal nerves (Soemmerring, 1791)***, and ***pterygopalatine nerves (Wrisberg, 1786)***; in the original Latin, *ramus spheno-palatinus*, Section VI, p. 65. Meckel (1748, p. 50 note *c*) tried to clarify the situation.
29. *trunk of fifth pair of cerebral nerves (Procháska, 1779)*
Synonym for macrodissected adult human *trigeminal nerve trunk (Winslow, 1733)*; in the original Latin, *truncus quinti paris nervorum cerebri*, Table 2, Figure 4-*a*.
30. *root of fifth pair of nerves (Monro, 1783)*
Synonym for macrodissected adult human *trigeminal nerve trunk (Winslow, 1733)*; Table 8, Figure 1-*L*.
31. *nervus crotaphiticus-nervus buccinatorius (Palletta, 1784)*
Basically macrodissected adult human ***trigeminal nerve motor root (Bell, 1829)*** and its continuation through the ***mandibular nerve motor root (>1840), mandibular nerve trunk (>1840)***, and ***anterior branch of mandibular nerve (>1840)*** to form the ***masseteric nerve (Meckel, 1748), deep temporal nerves (Haase, 1781)***, and ***lateral pterygoid nerve (>1840)***; p. 3 and Figure 2-*m,n*. Also see Bell & Bell (1829, p. 499). Todd (1835–1839, Vol. 2, pp. 270–271) explained that Palletta observed ***trigeminal nerve motor root (Bell, 1829)*** divided into two separate fascicles, superior to temporal muscle he called *nervus crotaphiticus*, and inferior to buccinator muscle he called *nervus buccinatorius*. Todd noted that this separation, which was first noted by Santorini (1724), frequently is not observed in macrodissected adult human; also see *anterior and posterior roots of trigeminal nerve (Meckel, 1817)*.
32. *nervus crotaphito-buccinatorius (Meckel, 1817)*
Alternate form of macrodissected adult human *nervus crotaphiticus-nervus buccinatorius (Palletta, 1784)*; see translation (1832, Vol. 3, p. 62).
33. *trunk of temporo-buccal nerve (Meckel, 1817)*
According to Meckel's description in macrodissected adult human, *two small roots of trigeminal nerve (Meckel, 1817)*, also called *anterior and posterior roots of trigeminal nerve (Meckel, 1817)*, join to form trunk of *temporo-buccal nerve (Meckel, 1832)*, also called *nervus crotaphiticus-nervus buccinatorius (Palletta, 1784)*; see translation (1832, Vol. 3, p. 62).
34. *fourth branch of fifth pair (Desmoulins, 1825)*
Described as most inferior branch of macrodissected adult fish ***trigeminal nerve (Winslow, 1733)***, inferior to *inferior maxillary branch of fifth nerve (La Charrère, 1703)*, in part communicating with first ***cervical nerve (Galen, c173)***; in the original French, *quatrième branche*, p. 363. Desmoulins noted that Weber (no citation provided) misidentified this communication.
35. *fifth branch of fifth pair (Desmoulins, 1825)*
Branch of ***trigeminal nerve (Winslow, 1733)*** described as found only in macrodissected adult bony fish; in the original French, *cinquième branche*, p. 366.
36. *sixth nerve of fifth pair (Desmoulins, 1825)*
Branch of ***trigeminal nerve (Winslow, 1733)*** in macrodissected adult codfish and catfish; in the original French, *sixième nerf de la cinquième paire*, p. 369.
37. *pterygodorsal nerve (Desmoulins, 1825)*
Synonym for *sixth nerve of fifth pair (Desmoulins, 1825)*: in the original French, *nerf ptérigo-dorsal*, p. 369.
38. *temporo-buccal nerve (Meckel, 1832)*
Translation of *nervus crotaphito-buccinatorius (Meckel, 1817)*; Vol. 3, p. 62.
39. *root of fifth nerve (Bell, 1834)*
Apparently macrodissected adult human ***trigeminal nerve sensory root (>1840)*** and ***trigeminal nerve motor root (Bell, 1829)*** considered together; p. 480.
40. *cerebral part of fifth pair (Arnold, 1834)*
Proximal segment of macrodissected adult human *trigeminal nerve trunk (Winslow, 1733)* before piercing ***dura (Galen, c177)***; in the original Latin, *par quintum, pars cerebralis*, p. 7.
41. *cerebral part of trigeminal nerve (Arnold, 1834)*
Synonym for *cerebral part of fifth pair (Arnold, 1834)*; in the original Latin, *nervus trigeminus, pars cerebralis*, p. 7.
42. *trunk of fifth pair (Arnold, 1834)*
Macrodissected adult human distal segment of *trigeminal nerve trunk (Winslow, 1733)*, distal to *cerebral part of fifth pair (Arnold, 1834)* and proximal to ***trigeminal ganglion (>1840)***; in the original Latin, *truncus quinti paris*, p. 7.
43. *apparent origin of trigeminal nerve (Cruveilhier, 1836)*
Large root of trigeminal nerve (Cruveilhier, 1836) and *small root of trigeminal nerve (Cruveilhier, 1836)* considered together; in the original French, *origine apparente*, pp. 893–894.

trigeminal nerve branches (Winslow, 1733)

As described for macrodissected adult human, three primary branches extend distally from the distal end of the ***trigeminal ganglion (>1840): ophthalmic nerve (Winslow, 1733), maxillary nerve (Meckel, 1753)***, and ***mandibular nerve (>1840)***; see Williams & Warwick (1980, Figs. 7.177, 181). For Winslow's use in macrodissected adult human, see Sections VI, p. 63 and X, p. 47. They were first clearly delineated by Eustachi; see ***[trigeminal nerve branches (Winslow, 1733)] (Eustachi, 1552)***.

EARLIER REFERENCES:

Described, not named or illustrated:

1. ***[trigeminal nerve branches (Winslow, 1733)] (Eustachi, 1552)***
Beautifully illustrated for macrodissected adult human; see Albinus edition (1761, Tab. 18, Fig. 2-*W,X,Y*).

Earlier synonyms:

1. *trunks of third pair (Falloppio, 1561)*
Synonym for macrodissected adult human ***trigeminal nerve branches (Winslow, 1733)***; see Meckel (1748, pp. 29 note *r*, 30 note *y*, 46 note *q*) and *third pair of nerves from brain (Falloppio, 1561)*.

2. *branches of third pair (Marchetti, 1652)*
   Synonym for macrodissected adult human ***trigeminal nerve branches (Winslow, 1733)***; see p. 122.
3. *branches of fifth pair (Rau, 1694)*
   Synonym for macrodissected adult human ***trigeminal nerve branches (Winslow, 1733)***; see pp. 190–191.
4. *divisions of fifth pair (Bell, 1803a)*
   Synonym for macrodissected adult human ***trigeminal nerve branches (Winslow, 1733)***; see Plate I-*A,E,N* and *Terminologia Anatomica* (1998, pp. 133–134).
5. *principal branches of fifth pair (Meckel, 1817)*
   Synonym for macrodissected adult human ***trigeminal nerve branches (Winslow, 1733)***; see translation (1832, pp. 65, 71).
6. *external portion of fifth pair of nerves (Todd, 1836–1839)*
   Part of macrodissected adult vertebrate ***trigeminal nerve (Winslow, 1733)*** distal to ***trigeminal ganglion (>1840)***; that is, ***trigeminal nerve branches (Winslow, 1733)***; p. 269.
7. *peripheric portion of fifth pair of nerves (Todd, 1836–1839)*
   Synonym for *external portion of fifth pair of nerves (Todd, 1835–1859)*; p. 269.

trigeminal nerve central motor root (>1840)

As described for macrodissected adult human, and mammal generally with histological methods for ***axons (Kölliker, 1896)***, a ***central nervous system white matter tract (>1840)*** between the ***motor nucleus of trigeminal nerve (>1840)*** dorsally and the surface of the ***pons (Haller, 1747)*** ventrolaterally, where it becomes the peripheral ***trigeminal nerve motor root (Bell, 1829)***; see Carpenter (1976, p. 360 and Fig. 12.22). It was clearly described in outline by Meckel; see ***[trigeminal nerve central motor root (>1840)] (Meckel, 1817)***.

EARLIER REFERENCES:

Described, not named or illustrated:

1. ***[trigeminal nerve central motor root (>1840)] (Meckel, 1817)***
   Described for macrodissected adult human; see translation (1832, Vol. 3, pp. 61–62). Santorini (1742, pp. 65–66) may have observed it earlier; see Meckel (1832, Vol. 3, pp. 61–62). Todd (1836–1839, pp. 271–272) described it quite clearly for macrodissected adult human.

Earlier synonyms:

1. *small root of fifth pair (Cruveilhier, 1836)*
   Synonym for macrodissected adult human ***trigeminal nerve central motor root (>1840)***; in the original French, *petite racine*, p. 895.

trigeminal nerve central sensory root (>1840)

As described for macrodissected adult human, and mammal generally with histological methods for ***axons (Kölliker, 1896)***, the continuation of the peripheral ***trigeminal nerve sensory root (>1840)*** within the ***pons (Haller, 1747)***, from its ventrolateral surface to the region where many of the ***axons (Kölliker, 1896)*** bifurcate, with long branches extending caudally in the ***spinal tract of trigeminal nerve (>1840)***, and much shorter branches extending rostrally into the ***principal sensory nucleus of trigeminal nerve (>1840)***; see Carpenter (1976, p. 354 and Figs. 12.20–22). It was known to Santorini; see ***[trigeminal nerve central sensory root (>1840)] (Santorini, 1724)***.

EARLIER REFERENCES:

Described, not named or illustrated:

1. ***[trigeminal nerve central sensory root (>1840)] (Santorini, 1724)***
   Santorini apparently first traced central distribution of macrodissected adult human ***trigeminal nerve (Winslow, 1733)***, essentially ***trigeminal nerve central sensory root (>1840)***; pp. 65–66, see Meckel (1832, Vol. 3, p. 59), where earlier work was reviewed. Bell (1834, p. 479) described it clearly in macrodissected adult human. Todd (1836–1839, pp. 271–272, Fig. 141) clearly described and illustrated it branching just ventral to (below) ***fourth ventricle (Galen, c192)*** with rostral component he described as cineritious, essentially ***principal sensory nucleus of trigeminal (>1840)***, and descending component, ***spinal tract of trigeminal nerve (>1840)***.

Earlier synonyms:

1. *great root of fifth nerve (Cruveilhier, 1836)*
   Synonym for macrodissected adult human ***trigeminal nerve central sensory root (>1840)***; in the original French, *grosse racine de la 5^e^ paire*, p. 895, see translation (1844, p. 821).

trigeminal nerve motor root (Bell, 1829)

For macrodissected adult human, the smaller of the two roots of the ***trigeminal nerve (Winslow, 1733)***, the larger being the ***trigeminal nerve sensory root (>1840)***. It is a bundle of motor ***axons (Kölliker, 1896)*** extending from the plane where the ***trigeminal nerve central motor root (>1840)*** leaves the ventrolateral surface of the ***pons (Haller, 1747)*** to the region where it joins the ***mandibular nerve sensory root (>1840)*** to form the ***mandibular nerve trunk (>1840)***. Obersteiner and Hill (1900, p. 356) pointed out that it is, more accurately, the *trigeminal nerve peripheral motor root*, a description analogous to that for ***ventral roots (>1840)*** and ***dorsal roots (Spurzheim, 1826)*** of the ***spinal nerves (Camper, 1760–1762)***; see Williams & Warwick (1980, Figs. 7.55, 181) and Meckel (1817; translation, 1832, Vol. 3, p. 62). As noted by Santorini (1724) and Palletta (1784) the ***trigeminal nerve motor root (Bell, 1829)*** may arise as two separate fascicles (superior, posterior or dorsal, and inferior, anterior, or ventral), but as Todd (1835–1839, Vol. 2, pp. 270–271) discussed, this is not always the case; see *anterior and posterior roots of trigeminal nerve (Meckel, 1817)*. Bell's term for macrodissected adult mammal comes from "Of the Motor or Manducatory portion of the Fifth Nerve. The fifth nerve is usually called Trigeminus, from piercing the skull in three grand divisions. But when it has been shown that it is composed of two distinct roots having different functions..." (p. 321; and from Pl. IX, Fig. 1-C). It was apparently known to Herophilus; see ***[trigeminal nerve motor root (Bell, 1829)] (Herophilus, c335–c280 BC)***.

EARLIER REFERENCES:

Described, not named or illustrated:

1. ***[trigeminal nerve motor root (Bell, 1829)] (Herophilus, c335–c280 BC)***
   Herophilus, the founder of human anatomy, is credited with discovering but apparently not naming it for macrodissected adult human and other mammals. See Solmsen (1961), von Staden (1969), Longrigg (1993), Clarke & O'Malley (1996, p. 261), *fourth pair of nerves from brain (Galen, c192)*.

Earlier synonyms:

1. *fourth pair of cerebral nerves (Vesalius, 1543a)*
   Probably corresponds to at least major part of macrodissected adult human ***trigeminal nerve motor root (Bell, 1829)***, whereas *third pair of cerebral nerves (Vesalius, 1543a)* is associated with ***trigeminal nerve sensory root (>1840)***; see Richardson & Carman translation (2002, pp. 188–192). In addition, Vesalius described a *thinner root of fifth pair of cerebral nerves (Vesalius, 1543a)* supplying temporal and medial pterygoid muscles, thus part of ***trigeminal nerve motor root (Bell, 1829)***; see Richardson & Carman translation (2002, p. 193). Meckel (see translation, 1832, Vol. 3, p. 59) credited Santorini (1724, p. 65) with first clearly distinguishing adult human ***trigeminal nerve sensory root (>1840)*** and ***trigeminal nerve motor root (Bell, 1829)***, whereas Vicq d'Azyr (1786, p. 52) credited Neubauer (1772) with this discovery. Finally, Procháska (1779; Tab. 2, Figs. 5-*i*, 6-*f*) has been credited with definitively isolating by dissection of adult human ***pons (Haller, 1747)*** this component of ***trigeminal nerve (Winslow, 1733)***; see Rasmussen (1947, p. 16), also see Vicq d'Azyr (1784, p. 565).
2. *fourth pair of sinews of brain (Geminus, 1553)*
   Synonym for macrodissected adult human *fourth pair of cerebral nerves (Vesalius, 1543a)*; the original spelling was *fourth payre of sinowes of the brayne*, see *The table of the figure of synowes*.
3. *par quintum portio minor (Wrisberg, 1777)*
   Synonym for macrodissected adult human ***trigeminal nerve motor root (Bell, 1829)***; p. 28.
4. *par quintum portio superior et anterior (Wrisberg, 1777)*
   Synonym for macrodissected adult human ***trigeminal nerve motor root (Bell, 1829)***; p. 28.
5. *nervus quintus portio minor of Wrisberg (Soemmerring, 1778)*
   Eponym for macrodissected adult human ***trigeminal nerve motor root (Bell, 1829)***; p. 180.
6. *anterior part of trigeminal nerve (Vicq d'Azyr, 1786; Günther, 1786)*
   Synonym for macrodissected adult human ***trigeminal nerve motor root (Bell, 1829)***; Vicq d'Azyr: Plate XVII, Figure I-47; Günther: p. 41. Also see *posterior part of trigeminal nerve (Vicq d'Azyr, 1786)*, *anterior and posterior roots of trigeminal nerve (Meckel, 1817)*, and Meckel (1832, Vol. 3, pp. 59, 62). Today it would be called *ventral root of trigeminal nerve*.
7. *upper bundle of trigeminal nerve (Gordon, 1815)*
   Synonym for macrodissected adult human ***trigeminal nerve motor root (Bell, 1829)***; p. 209.
8. *muscular nerve of fifth pair (Bell, 1826)*
   Synonym for macrodissected adult human ***trigeminal nerve motor root (Bell, 1829)***; "It [fifth pair] arises in two roots, one of these is the muscular nerve, the other the sensible nerve." (p. 166).
9. *masticatory nerve (Eschricht, 1826)*
   Synonym for macrodissected adult ***trigeminal nerve motor root (Bell, 1829)***; in the original Latin, *masticatorii*, p. 246; also see Durward (1951, p. 1019).

LATER SYNONYMS:

1. *motor portion of fifth nerve (Bell, 1829)*
   Synonym for macrodissected adult mammalian ***trigeminal nerve motor root (Bell, 1829)***; p. 321.
2. *manducatory portion of fifth nerve (Bell, 1829)*
   Synonym for macrodissected adult mammalian ***trigeminal nerve motor root (Bell, 1829)***; p. 321.
3. *anterior root of fifth nerve (Bell, 1829)*
   Synonym for macrodissected adult mammalian ***trigeminal nerve motor root (Bell, 1829)***; Plate IX, Figure 1-C.
4. *anterior portion of three-fold nerve (Swan, 1830)*
   Synonym for macrodissected adult human ***trigeminal nerve motor root (Bell, 1829)***; Plate X, Figure 1-5.
5. *small root of trigeminal nerve (Cruveilhier, 1836)*
   Synonym for macrodissected adult human ***trigeminal nerve motor root (Bell, 1829)***; in the original French, *petite racine*, p. 894.
6. *nonganglionic root of trigeminal nerve (Cruveilhier, 1836)*
   Synonym for macrodissected adult human ***trigeminal nerve motor root (Bell, 1829)***; in the original French, *racine non-ganglionnaire*, p. 894.
7. *smaller portion of fifth pair of nerves (Todd, 1836–1839)*
   Synonym for macrodissected adult mammalian ***trigeminal nerve motor root (Bell, 1829)***; p. 269.
8. *non-ganglionic portion of fifth pair of nerves (Todd, 1836–1839)*
   Synonym for macrodissected adult mammalian ***trigeminal nerve motor root (Bell, 1829)***; p. 269.
9. *voluntary portion of fifth pair of nerves (Todd, 1836–1839)*
   Synonym for macrodissected adult mammalian ***trigeminal nerve motor root (Bell, 1829)***; p. 269.

PARTLY CORRESPONDS:

1. *thinner root of fifth pair of cerebral nerves (Vesalius, 1543a)*
   Briefly described by Vesalius who claimed he was the first to see it; illustrated as supplying macrodissected adult human temporal and medial pterygoid muscles. As such, part of ***trigeminal nerve motor root (>1840)***; see Singer translation (1952, p. 14), Richardson and Carman translation (2002, part *d* in two figures on pp. 168–169, and pp. 177, 193–194). The same ***nerve (Herophilus,***

c335–c280 BC) is illustrated in Figure 14-*L* of Book VII, where Singer (1952, pp. 112–113) probably misidentified as ***intermediate nerve (>1840)***. Also see *anterior and posterior roots of trigeminal nerve (Meckel, 1817)*. Richardson & Carman elsewhere (2002, see *N* in figure following p. 263, and p. 267) ascribed it to ***abducens nerve (Heister, 1717)***. In the end, its identity is ambiguous.

2. *smaller root of fifth pair of cerebral nerves (Vesalius, 1543a)*
   Minor variation on, or different translation of, *thinner root of fifth pair of cerebral nerves (Vesalius, 1543a)*; see Singer translation (1952, Fig. 14-*L*).
3. *root of fourth pair of cerebral nerves (Vesalius, 1543a)*
   Apparently, proximal part of *fourth pair of cerebral nerves (Vesalius, 1543a)*; see Richardson & Carman translation (2002, p. 205, and no. 4 in the figure).
4. *root of fourth pair of sinews of brain (Geminus, 1553)*
   Synonym for macrodissected adult human *root of fourth pair of cerebral nerves (Vesalius, 1543a)*; originally spelled, *roote of the fourth payre of sinowes of the brayne*, see *The table of the figures of sinowes*.
5. *thinner root of fifth pair of sinews of brain (Geminus, 1553)*
   Synonym for macrodissected adult human *thinner root of fifth pair of cerebral nerves (Vesalius, 1543a)*; originally spelled *thynner roote of fyfte payre of synowes of brayne*, see *The table of the figures of sinowes*, Figure 7-*I,N*.
6. *lesser root of fifth pair of sinews of brain (Geminus, 1553)*
   Alternate translation of *smaller root of fifth pair of cerebral nerves (Vesalius, 1543a)* for macrodissected adult human; see *The tables of the brayne*, Figure 14-*L*.
7. *eighth pair of nerves arising from brain (Colombo, 1559)*
   Probably refers basically to *thinner root of fifth pair of nerves (Vesalius, 1543a)*; p. 198. Also see Bannister (1578, f. 106). Bartholin (see 1662, p. 325) mentioned it had been referred to also as *ninth pair*, but source of attribution not identified.
8. *anterior and posterior roots of trigeminal nerve (Meckel, 1817)*
   Meckel perceptively wrote, "These two small roots form the small portion of the fifth pair, which is whiter and harder than the large. Their separation with the ganglion formed by the large portion is extremely curious, as it presents a repetition of the formation peculiar to the nerves of the spinal marrow." (see translation, 1832, p. 62). They join to form *trunk of temporo-buccal nerve (Meckel, 1817)* and thus form proximal part of ***trigeminal nerve motor root (>1840)***, whereas large portion corresponds to ***trigeminal nerve sensory root (>1840)***; see translation (1832, Vol. 3, pp. 59, 62). They may correspond to *fourth pair of cerebral nerves (Vesalius, 1543a)* and *thinner root of fifth pair of cerebral nerve (Vesalius, 1543a)* considered together.
9. *two small roots of trigeminal nerve (Meckel, 1817)*
   Synonym for *anterior and posterior roots of trigeminal nerve (Meckel, 1817)*; see translation (1832, Vol. 3, p. 62).

trigeminal nerve sensory root (>1840)

As described for macrodissected adult human, the larger of the two roots of the ***trigeminal nerve (Winslow, 1733)***, the smaller being the ***trigeminal nerve motor root (Bell, 1929)***. Histologically it is a bundle of ***axons (Kölliker, 1896)*** from the ***trigeminal ganglion (>1840)***, between its origin distally in the ***ganglion (Galen, c173)*** and the plane proximally on the ventrolateral surface of the **pons (Haller, 1747)** where it meets the ***trigeminal nerve central sensory root (>1840)***. Obersteiner and Hill (1900, p. 356) pointed out that it is, more accurately, the *trigeminal nerve peripheral sensory root*, a description analogous to that for ***dorsal roots (Spurzheim, 1826)*** and ***ventral roots (>1840)*** of the ***spinal nerves (Camper, 1760–1762)***; see Williams & Warwick (1980, Figs. 7.55, 181) and Meckel (1817; translation, 1832, Vol. 3, p. 62). It was apparently known to Herophilus; see ***[trigeminal nerve sensory root (>1840)] (Herophilus, c335–c280 BC)***.

EARLIER REFERENCES:

Described, not named or illustrated:

1. ***[trigeminal nerve sensory root (>1840)] (Herophilus, c335–c280 BC)***
   Herophilus, the founder of human anatomy, is credited with discovering but apparently not naming it for macrodissected adult human and other mammals. See Solmsen (1961), von Staden (1969), Longrigg (1993), Clarke & O'Malley (1996, p. 261), *fourth pair of nerves from brain (Galen, c192)*.

Earlier synonyms:

1. *par quintum portio inferior posterior (Wrisberg, 1777)*
   Synonym for macrodissected adult human ***trigeminal nerve sensory root (>1840)***; p. 28.
2. *par quintum portio major (Wrisberg, 1777)*
   Synonym for macrodissected adult human ***trigeminal nerve sensory root (>1840)***; p. 28.
3. *nervus quintus portio major (Soemmerring, 1778)*
   Synonym for macrodissected adult human ***trigeminal nerve sensory root (>1840)***; p. 180.
4. *posterior part of trigeminal nerve (Vicq d'Azyr, 1786; Günther, 1786)*
   Synonym for macrodissected adult human ***trigeminal nerve sensory root (>1840)***; Vicq d'Azyr: Plate XVII, Figure I-46; Günther: p. 41. Also see *anterior part of trigeminal nerve (Vicq d'Azyr, 1786; Günther, 1786)*. Today it would be called *dorsal root of trigeminal nerve*.
5. *lower bundle of trigeminal nerve (Gordon, 1815)*
   Synonym for macrodissected adult human *posterior part of trigeminal nerve (Vicq d'Azyr, 1786; Günther, 1786)*; p. 209.
6. *central root of trigeminal nerve (Meckel, 1817)*
   Synonym for macrodissected adult human ***trigeminal nerve sensory root (>1840)***; see translation (1832, Vol. 3, p. 59).
7. *middle root of trigeminal nerve (Meckel, 1817)*
   Synonym for macrodissected adult human ***trigeminal nerve sensory root (>1840)***; see translation (1832, Vol. 3, p. 59).
8. *principal root of trigeminal nerve (Meckel, 1817)*
   Synonym for macrodissected adult human ***trigeminal nerve sensory root (>1840)***; see translation (1832, Vol. 3, p. 61).

9. *sensible nerve of fifth pair (Bell, 1826)*
Synonym for macrodissected adult human ***trigeminal nerve sensory root (>1840)***; p. 166, see *muscular nerve of fifth pair (Bell, 1826)*.
10. *posterior root of fifth pair (Bell, 1829)*
Synonym for macrodissected adult human ***trigeminal nerve sensory root (>1840)***; Plate IX-A.
11. *sensitive root of fifth pair (Bell, 1829)*
Synonym for macrodissected adult human ***trigeminal nerve sensory root (>1840)***; Plate IX-A.
12. *posterior portion of three-fold nerve (Swan, 1830)*
Synonym for macrodissected adult human ***trigeminal nerve sensory root (>1840)***; Plate X, Figure 1-6.
13. *large root of trigeminal nerve (Cruveilhier, 1836)*
Synonym for macrodissected adult human ***trigeminal nerve sensory root (>1840)***; in the original French, *grosse racine*, p. 894.
14. *ganglionic root of trigeminal nerve (Cruveilhier, 1836)*
Synonym for macrodissected adult human ***trigeminal nerve sensory root (>1840)***; in the original French, *racine ganglionnaire*, p. 894.
15. *larger portion of fifth pair of nerves (Todd, 1836–1839)*
Synonym for macrodissected adult human ***trigeminal nerve sensory root (>1840)***; p. 269.
16 *ganglionic portion of fifth pair of nerves (Todd, 1836–1839)*
Synonym for macrodissected adult human ***trigeminal nerve sensory root (>1840)***; p. 269.
17. *sentient portion of fifth pair of nerves (Todd, 1836–1839)*
Synonym for macrodissected adult human ***trigeminal nerve sensory root (>1840)***; p. 269.

trigeminal tubercle (>1840)

As described for macrodissected adult human, an eminence on the surface of the ***medulla (Winslow, 1733)*** formed by the ***medullary segment of spinal tract of trigeminal nerve (>1840)***, which is in turn partly covered by ***inferior cerebellar peduncle (Günther, 1786)*** dorsally and ***ventrolateral fascicle (>1840)*** ventrally. Basically it lies between ***cuneate tubercle (>1840)*** dorsally and ***olive (Tiedemann, 1821)*** ventrally, with the ***spinal nucleus of trigeminal nerve (>1840)*** lying deep to it; see Crosby et al. (1962, p. 114), Williams & Warwick (1980, p. 899), *Terminologia Anatomica* (1998, p. 109), *Dorland's* (2003, p. 1964). It was perhaps first identified roughly as the *lateral pyramidal body (Tarin, 1750)*.

TRANSLATIONS:

1. *tuberculum trigeminale (>1840)*
Current Latin form of ***trigeminal tubercle (>1840)***; see *Terminologia Anatomica* (1998, p. 109).

EARLIER REFERENCES:

Earlier synonyms:

1. *lateral pyramidal body (Tarin, 1750)*
Roughly synonymous with macrodissected adult human ***trigeminal tubercle (>1840)***; in the original Latin (plural), *corpora pyramidalia lateralia*, Table I, Figure 4-*T*. Tarin also indicated it was sometimes called anterior. Soemmerring clarified the term's use as referring to lateral surface of ***medulla (Winslow, 1733)***, see Table II-**, p. 178. Burdach (1822, p. 288) indicated that Tarin's term refers to or includes ***inferior cerebellar peduncle (Günther, 1786)***, based on a passage in Procháska (1800, Part 1, p. 361), and gave the Latin form, *corpora pyramidalia anteriora s. lateralia*.
2. *anterior pyramidal body (Tarin, 1750, Tab. I)*
Tarin wrote that sometimes *lateral pyramidal body (Tarin, 1750)* is referred to thus; in the original Latin (plural), *corpora pyramidalia anteriora*, Table I, Figure 4-*T*.
3. *lateral tract of medulla oblongata (Vicq d'Azyr, 1784)*
Synonym for macrodissected adult human ***trigeminal tubercle (>1840)***, corresponding to *lateral pyramidal body (Tarin, 1750)* or *anterior pyramidal body (Tarin, 1750, Tab. I)*; p. 590, and Vicq d'Azyr (1786, Pl. XXVII, Fig. I:*48*,*49*).
4. *corpora pyramidalia lateralia vel anteriora Tarini (Vicq d'Azyr, 1786)*
Eponym for right and left macrodissected adult human ***trigeminal tubercle (>1840)***; Plates XVII, Fig. I:*48*,*49*; XVIII-*55x*). Also see *lateral pyramidal body (Tarin, 1750)* and *anterior pyramidal body (Tarin, 1750, Tab. I)*.
5. *lateral pyramid (Vicq d'Azyr, 1786)*
Abbreviated English form of *corpora pyramidalia lateralia vel anteriora Tarini (Vicq d'Azyr, 1786)*; see Foster (1894, p. 2674). Meckel ascribed the term without citation to Tarin; see translation (1832, Vol. 3, p. 422) and *lateral pyramidal body (Tarin, 1750)*.
6. *gray tubercle (Rolando, 1825a)*
First clear account of macrodissected adult human ***trigeminal tubercle (>1840)***; in the original French (plural), *tubercules cendrés*, p. 18; Table I, Figure 1-*t.c*; Table IV, Figure 6-*t.c*.
7. *tubercle of gray substance of medulla oblongata (Rolando, 1825a)*
Synonym for *gray tubercle (Rolando, 1825a)*; in the original French, *tubercule de la substance cendrée de la moelle alongée*, p. 22. It was indicated but not commented on by Gall & Spurzheim (1810, Pl. X).
8. *tuberculum cinereum (Arnold, 1838a)*
Latin form of *gray tubercle (Rolando, 1825a)*; p. 19, where plural, *tubercula cinerea*, was given.
9. *tubercle of Rolando (>1840)*
Eponym for macrodissected adult human ***trigeminal tubercle (>1840)***; see *Dorland's* (2003, p. 1965).

trochlear nerve (Molinetti, 1669)

As described for macrodissected adult human, a ***cranial nerve (Soemmerring, 1791)*** attached to the ***rostral medullary velum (>1840)***, distal to the ***trochlear nerve decussation (>1840)***, and supplying the superior oblique muscle primarily to move the eye downward and laterally; see Crosby et al. (1962, pp. 239–240). According to Meckel (1817) there are normally two roots, anterior and posterior, in adult human, although this is not mentioned in 20th century textbooks; see translation (1832, Vol. 3, p. 75) and *roots of pathetic nerve (Malacarne, 1791)*. For Molinetti's use in macrodissected adult human, see p. 47; also see Soemmerring (1778, p. 122). Credit for its discovery is usually given to Achillini; see ***[trochlear nerve (Molinetti, 1669)] (Achillini, 1520)***. For review of early research on this ***nerve (Herophilus, c335–c280 BC)*** see Zinn (1755, pp. 198–199). Winslow probably first used the term *trochlear nerve* in English; Section X, p. 47.

TRANSLATIONS:

1. *nervus trochlearis (Molinetti, 1669)*
   Original Latin form of ***trochlear nerve (Molinetti, 1669)***; p. 47.

EARLIER REFERENCES:

Described, not named or illustrated:

1. ***[trochlear nerve (Molinetti, 1669)] (Achillini, 1520)***
   Achillini probably discovered it in macrodissected adult human; see Soemmerring (1778, pp. 8, 120), Gall & Spurzheim (1810, p. 79 note *1*), O'Malley (1964, p. 18), Lind (1975, p. 60).

Illustrated, not named or described:

1. ***[trochlear nerve (Molinetti, 1669)] (Eustachi, 1552)***
   Origin in roof of macrodissected adult human ***brainstem (Schwalbe, 1881)*** very clearly illustrated, although plates not published until 1714, and then without Eustachi's text; see Albinus edition (1744, Plate XVII, Fig. II-*M*), Soemmerring (1778, p. 121).

Earlier synonyms:

1. *ninth pair of nerves from brain (Colombo, 1559)*
   Probably synonym for macrodissected adult human ***trochlear nerves (Molinetti, 1669)***, arising near ***tectum (Baer, 1837)*** and ending in an extraocular muscle; p. 198, also see Bannister (1578, f. 106), Crooke (1615, p. 894), Soemmerring (1778, p. 121), Hierons & Meyer (1962, p. 289).
2. *eighth pair of nerves from brain (Falloppio, 1561)*
   Excellent description of macrodissected adult human ***trochlear nerves (Molinetti, 1669)***; f. 155, see Soemmerring (1778, p. 121), Harvey (1961, p. 231 note *828*).
3. *third pair of nerves (Bauhin, 1605)*
   Synonym for macrodissected adult human ***trochlear nerves (Molinetti, 1669)***; see Bartholin (1662, p. 325), Soemmerring (1778, p. 122).
4. *fourth pair of nerves (Bartholin, 1632)*
   First reference to ***trochlear nerves (Molinetti, 1669)*** with their current number for ***cranial nerves (Soemmerring, 1791)***; see Burdach (1822, p. 389), Hierons & Meyer (1962, p. 292).
5. *nerveos funiculos (Le Boë, 1663)*
   According to Collins (1685, pp. 1020–1021), synonym for *pathetic nerve (Willis, 1664)* or ***trochlear nerve (Molinetti, 1669)***; also see *funiculi nervei (Le Boë, 1663)*.
6. *pathetic nerve (Willis, 1664)*
   Synonym for ***trochlear nerve (Molinetti, 1669)*** because, Willis suggested, it moves the eyes in relation to pathos or emotion; see Pordage translation (1681, pp. 56–57, 140–141).

LATER SYNONYMS:

1. *sixth pair (Molinetti, 1669)*
   Synonym for ***trochlear nerves (Molinetti, 1669)***; p. 85.
2. *nervi amatorii (Drake, 1707)*
   Drake noted that some people call the human *fourth pair of nerves (Bartholin, 1632)*—the *pathetic nerves (Willis, 1664)*—*nerves of love* or *amorous nerves*; p. 485.
3. *nerves of love (Drake, 1707)*
   English form of *nervi amatorii (Drake, 1707)*.
4. *nervi musculares obliqui superiores (Winslow, 1733)*
   Synonym for macrodissected adult human ***trochlear nerves (Molinetti, 1669)***; Section X, p. 47. Another form is *nervos musculorum obliquorum superiorum*; see Soemmerring (1778, p. 123).
5. *fifth pair of nerves (Malacarne, 1791)*
   Synonym for macrodissected adult human ***trochlear nerves (Molinetti, 1669)***; p. 172, see Burdach (1822, p. 389).
6. *fourth pair of cranial nerves (Soemmerring, 1791)*
   Synonym for macrodissected adult human ***trochlear nerves (Molinetti, 1669)***; see ***cranial nerves (Soemmerring, 1791)***.
7. *fourth pair of cerebral nerves (Soemmerring, 1791)*
   Synonym for *fourth pair of cranial nerves (Soemmerring, 1791)*; see p. 103 and *cerebral nerves (Soemmerring, 1791)*. In the original Latin, *par quartum nervorum cerebri*, Soemmerring (1798, p. 125).
8. *nervus internus oculi (Andersch, 1797)*
   Synonym for macrodissected adult human ***trochlear nerve (Molinetti, 1669)***; p. 1, see Burdach (1822, p. 389).
9. *interior oculo-muscular pair of nerves (Burdin, 1803)*
   Synonym for macrodissected adult human ***trochlear nerves (Molinetti, 1669)***; see translation (1803, Vol. 1, p. 144). Burdach (1822, p. 389) gave the Latin, *nervus oculo-muscularis internus*. Also see *nervi oculo-musculares externi (Winslow, 1733)*.
10. *nerve of superior oblique muscle of eye (Gall & Spurzheim, 1810)*
    Synonym for macrodissected adult human ***trochlear nerve (Molinetti, 1669)***; in the original French, *nerf du muscle oblique supérieur de l'oeil*, p. 79.
11. *nervus oculomuscularis superior (Meckel, 1817)*
    Synonym listed for macrodissected adult human ***trochlear nerve (Molinetti, 1669)***; p. 739.
12. *nervus oculomuscularis minimus (Meckel, 1817)*
    Synonym listed for macrodissected adult human ***trochlear nerve (Molinetti, 1669)***; p. 739.
13. *superior motor nerve (Meckel, 1817)*
    Synonym listed for macrodissected adult human ***trochlear nerve (Molinetti, 1669)***; see translation (1832, Vol. 3, p. 75).
14. *internal motor nerve (Meckel, 1817)*
    Synonym listed for macrodissected adult human ***trochlear nerve (Molinetti, 1669)***; see translation (1832, Vol. 3, p. 75).

15. *superior oblique nerve (Spurzheim, 1826)*
Sensible synonym for macrodissected adult human ***trochlear nerve (Molinetti, 1669)***; p. 231-13.
16. *superior oblique oculo-muscular nerve (Swan 1830)*
Synonym for macrodissected adult human ***trochlear nerve (Molinetti, 1669)***; p. 15.
17. *inner oculo-muscular nerve (Solly, 1836)*
Synonym for macrodissected adult human ***trochlear nerve (Molinetti, 1669)***; p. 247.
18. *internal superior oculomuscular nerve (Cruveilhier, 1836)*
Synonym listed for macrodissected adult human ***trochlear nerve (Molinetti, 1669)***; in the original French, *nerf oculo-musculaire interne et supérieur*, p. 892.

PARTLY CORRESPONDS:

1. *nervus accessorius ad patheticum (Palletta, 1784)*
Palletta described an "accessory trochlear nerve" in macrodissected adult human (p. 118), as did Malacarne (1791, p. 174), but Burdach (1822, p. 390) did not confirm its existence.
2. *roots of pathetic nerve (Malacarne, 1791)*
Malacarne described several peripheral roots for macrodissected adult human ***trochlear nerve (Molinetti, 1669)*** on emerging from ***rostral medullary velum (>1840)***; pp. 227, 230–231.
3. *cerebral part of fourth pair (Arnold, 1834)*
Macrodissected adult human proximal segment of ***trochlear nerve (Molinetti, 1669)***, from surface of ***rostral medullary velum (>1840)*** to site where it pierces ***dura (Galen, c177)***; in the original Latin, *par quartum, pars cerebralis*, p. 7.
4. *cerebral part of trochlear or pathetic nerve (Arnold, 1834)*
Synonym for *cerebral part of fourth pair (Arnold, 1834)*; in the original Latin, *nervus trochlearis s. patheticus, pars cerebralis*, p. 7.
5. *orbital part of fourth pair (Arnold, 1834)*
Macrodissected adult human middle segment of ***trochlear nerve (Molinetti, 1669)***, between *cerebral part of fourth pair (Arnold, 1834)* and terminal branch to superior oblique muscle; in the original Latin, *par quartum, pars orbitalis*, p. 7.
6. *orbital part of trochlear or pathetic nerve (Arnold, 1834)*
Synonym for *orbital part of fourth pair (Arnold, 1834)*; in the original Latin, *nervus trochlearis s. patheticus, pars orbitalis*, p. 7.
7. *apparent origin of pathetic nerve (Cruveilhier, 1836)*
Macrodissected adult human proximal end of ***trochlear nerve (Molinetti, 1669)*** as it emerges from ***rostral medullary velum (>1840)***; in the original French, *origine apparente*, p. 892. Cruveilhier could not identify a real origin, or ***trochlear nerve central root (>1840)***.
8. *branch of tentorium cerebelli of pathetic nerve (Cruveilhier, 1836)*
For macrodissected adult human, Cruveilhier insisted there is often a branch of ***trochlear nerve (Molinetti, 1669)*** arising in ***cavernous sinus (Winslow, 1733)*** and dividing 2–3 times in substance of ***cerebellar tentorium (Winslow, 1733)***, although it may arise occasionally from ***ophthalmic nerve (Winslow, 1733)***; in the original French, *rameau de la tente du cervelet*, p. 908. Also see Todd (1936–1839, p. 371) and ***tentorial nerve (>1840)***.

trochlear nerve central root (>1840)

As described in macrodissected adult human, and mammal generally with histological methods for ***axons (Kölliker, 1896)***, the ***central nervous system white matter tract (>1840)*** extending from the ***trochlear nucleus (>1840)*** laterally, just ventral to the ***periaqueductal gray (>1840)*** and then ***pontine central gray (>1840)***, to enter the ***rostral medullary velum (>1840)*** and course medially to the ***trochlear nerve decussation (>1840)***; see Williams & Warwick (1980, p. 937), Swanson (2004, Atlas Levels 44–49). It was first identified by Mayo; see ***[trochlear nerve central root (>1840)] (Mayo, 1827)***.

EARLIER REFERENCES:

Illustrated and described, not named:

1. ***[trochlear nerve central root (>1840)] (Mayo, 1827)***
Traced in macrodissected, alcohol-hardened, adult human to region of ***superior cerebellar peduncle (Procháska, 1800)***; Plate VII, Figure 2-*IV*.

Earlier synonyms:

1. *real origin of pathetic nerve (Cruveilhier, 1836)*
Synonym for macrodissected adult human ***trochlear nerve central root (>1840)***. Cruveilhier reviewed earlier views on its origins and stated that he could not identify it; in the original French, *origine réelle*, p. 893.

trochlear nerve decussation (>1840)

As described for macrodissected adult human, and mammal generally with histological methods for ***axons (Kölliker, 1896)***, it lies in the ***rostral medullary velum (>1840)*** between the right and left ***trochlear nerve central root (>1840)*** proximally and the left and right ***trochlear nerve (Molinetti, 1669)*** distally; see Crosby et al. (1962, Fig. 171), Williams & Warwick (1980, p. 1059). It was apparently first identified as the *commissure of fourth pair (Laurencet, 1825)*.

EARLIER REFERENCES:

Earlier synonyms:

1. *commissure of fourth pair (Laurencet, 1825)*
Apparently feature of macrodissected adult human ***rostral medullary vellum (>1840)*** generating right and left ***trochlear nerve (Molinetti, 1669)***; in the original French, *commissure de la quatrième paire*, p. 140. Laurencet did not suggest that ***trochlear nerves (Molinetti, 1669)*** cross the median plane, although he apparently identified ***trochlear nerve decussation (>1840)***. According to Solly (1836, pp. 247–248), "The fourth pair of nerves, at their origin, are connected together by a distinct commissure, represented in Plate XI. fig. 2, and more evident in some [human] brains than others." Cruveilhier (1836, p. 893) made the same observation: the right and left ***trochlear nerves (Molinetti, 1669)*** are often united by some white streaks forming a transverse commissure. Solly

and Cruveilhier did not state directly that the ***trochlear nerves (Molinetti, 1669)*** themselves decussate.

tubal branch of tympanic plexus (>1840)

As described for macrodissected adult human, branch or branches of the ***tympanic plexus (Müller, 1834)*** to mucus membrane lining tympanic cavity, auditory (Eustachian) tube, and mastoid air cells; see Mitchell (1953, p. 169), Williams & Warwick (1980, pp. 1075, 1200), *Terminologia Anatomica* (1998, p. 136). First identified by Jacobson; see ***[tubal branch of tympanic plexus (>1840)] (Jacobson, 1818).***

EARLIER REFERENCES:

Described, not named or illustrated:

1. ***[tubal branch of tympanic plexus (>1840)] (Jacobson, 1818)***
   Jacobson began to describe it for macrodissected adult human; see Lobstein translation (1831, pp. 36–37). Soon thereafter it was described in more detail by Kilian (1822, p. 71 ff.) and Lobstein (1823; see translation, 1831, pp. 38–39).

Earlier synonyms:

1. *tympanic nerve branchlet to Eustachian tube (Arnold, 1834)*
   Synonym for macrodissected adult human ***tubal branch of tympanic plexus (>1840)***; in the original Latin, *nervus tympanicus ramulus ad tubam Eustachianam*, p. 13.

tuber vermis (>1840)

As described for macrodissected adult human, the part of the ***cerebellar vermis (Meckel, 1817)*** between ***folium vermis (>1840)*** and ***pyramis (Malacarne, 1776)***, roughly medial to the right and left ***ansiform lobule crus II (Bolk, 1906)*** and ***gracile lobule (>1840)*** of the ***cerebellar hemisphere (Willis, 1664)***; see Larsell & Jansen (1972, Fig. 118), Carpenter (1976, Figs. 2.26, 14.1), Nieuwenhuys et al. (2008, Fig. 3.8-34). It was first clearly described as the *transverse laminated cords of cerebellum (Malacarne, 1776).*

EARLIER REFERENCES:

Earlier synonyms:

1. *transverse laminated cords of cerebellum (Malacarne, 1776)*
   Synonym for macrodissected adult human ***tuber vermis (>1840)***; see Clarke & O'Malley (1996, p. 645).
2. *transverse laminated commissures of cerebellum (Malacarne, 1776)*
   Synonym for macrodissected adult human ***tuber vermis (>1840)***; see Clarke & O'Malley (1996, p. 645).
3. *long hidden commissure of cerebellum (Reil, 1807–1808a)*
   Synonym for macrodissected adult human ***tuber vermis (>1840)***; see Mayo translation (1822, p. 23). Also see Burdach (1822, p. 295).
4. *tuber valvulae (Burdach, 1822)*
   Synonym for macrodissected adult human ***tuber vermis (>1840)***; p. 61. Meckel (1817) earlier referred to slight prominence in this region; see translation (1832, Vol. 2, pp. 431–432).

tubo-uterine nerve (1840)

As described for macrodissected adult human female, a caudal (inferior) extension of the ***inferior ovarian nerves (>1840)*** coursing rostrally (ascending) with the uterine artery, and also associated with the uterus and inner part of the uterine tube, but not the ovary; see Mitchell (1953, pp. 295–296). It was probably first identified as the *tubal nerves (Cruveilhier, 1836).*

EARLIER REFERENCES:

Earlier synonyms:

1. *tubal nerves (Cruveilhier, 1836)*
   Apparently synonym for macrodissected adult female human ***tubo-uterine nerve (>1840)***; in the original French, *nerfs tubaires*, p. 1027.

tubo-uterine plexus (>1840)

As described for macrodissected adult human female, a delicate intermixing of *uterine nerves (Galen, c173)*—components of the ***uterovaginal plexus (>1840)***—and ***inferior ovarian nerves (>1840)*** ascending between the layers of the broad ligament of the uterus and sometimes having small ***prevertebral ganglia (Quain, 1832)*** associated with it; see Mitchell (1953, pp. 295–296), who may have coined the term. It was perhaps first clearly delineated by Cruveilhier; see ***[tubo-uterine plexus (>1840)] (Cruveilhier, 1836).***

EARLIER REFERENCES:

Described, not named or illustrated:

1. ***[tubo-uterine plexus (>1840)] (Cruveilhier, 1836)***
   Clearly indicated for macrodissected adult human; p. 1027.

tympanic membrane branch of external acoustic meatus nerves (>1840)

As described for macrodissected adult human, one or sometimes two small branches of the dorsal (upper) ***external acoustic meatus nerve (Meckel, 1817)***, derived from the ***auriculotemporal nerve (Haller, 1762)*** and supplying the tympanic membrane; see Williams & Warwick (1980, p. 1066), *Terminologia Anatomica* (1998, p. 134). It was probably first clearly distinguished in 1817; see ***[tympanic membrane branch of external acoustic meatus nerves (>1840)] (Meckel, 1817)***, *tympanic nerve (Bock, 1817).*

EARLIER REFERENCES:

Described, not named or illustrated:

1. ***[tympanic membrane branch of external acoustic meatus nerves (>1840)] (Meckel, 1817)***
   Described without specifically naming for macrodissected adult human; see translation (1832, Vol. 3, p. 73), where Meckel noted that Bock (1817, p. 48) also described a communication of this branch with the ***chorda tympani (Falloppio, 1561)*** via one or two filaments.

Earlier synonyms:

1. *tympanic nerve (Bock, 1817)*
   Sensible synonym for macrodissected adult human ***tympanic membrane branch of external acoustic meatus nerves (>1840)***; in the original Latin, *nervus tympani*, p. 49.

tympanic nerve (Arnold, 1834)

As described for macrodissected adult human, a branch of the ***glossopharyngeal nerve trunk (Wrisberg, 1786; Günther, 1786)*** leaving from the region of the ***distal glossopharyngeal ganglion (>1840)*** and contributing branches to the ***tympanic plexus (Müller, 1834)***, which in turn gives off branches to join the ***greater petrosal nerve (>1840)***, to supply mucous membranes lining the tympanic cavity, auditory (Eustachian) tube, and mastoid air cells, and to join the ***lesser petrosal nerve (>1840)***, which extends to the ***otic ganglion (Arnold, 1828)***, and then the parotid gland; see Williams & Warwick (1980, p. 1075 and Fig. 7.184). For Arnold's use in macrodissected adult human, see p. 13. It was probably discovered as the *auricular branch of petrosal small ganglion (Andersch, 1797)*.

ALTERNATE SPELLINGS:

1. *tympanine nerve (Swan, 1830)*
   Alternate form of ***tympanic nerve (Arnold, 1834)***; p. 22.

TRANSLATIONS:

1. *nervus tympanicus (Arnold, 1834)*
   Original Latin form of ***tympanic nerve (Arnold, 1834)***; p. 13.

EARLIER REFERENCES:

Earlier synonyms:

1. *auricular branch of petrosal small ganglion (Andersch, 1797)*
   Probably macrodissected adult human ***tympanic nerve (Arnold, 1834)*** but not enough description to be certain; in the original Latin, *(ganglioli petrosi) ramum auricularem*, p. 7. Meckel (1817, p. 694) described this macrodissected adult human "filament" of ***glossopharyngeal nerve (Huber, 1744)***, and mentioned two branches difficult now to identify clearly; see translation (1832, Vol. 3, p. 51). It was also described by Jacobson (1818, p. 292) in association with ***tympanic plexus (>1840)***. Also see Bock (1817, pp. 48–49) and detailed accounts of history by Kilian (1822, p. 77 ff.) and Todd (1836–1839, p. 495).
2. *Jacobson's branch (Kilian, 1822)*
   Eponym for macrodissected adult human ***tympanic nerve (Arnold, 1834)***; in the original Latin, *ramus Jacobsii*, p. 77. Kilian referred to Rosenmüller (1819, p. 407).
3. *recurrent branch of glossopharyngeal nerves (Kilian, 1822)*
   Apparently synonym for macrodissected adult human ***tympanic nerve (Arnold, 1834)***; in the original Latin, *ramus recurrens Nervi Glossopharyngei*, p. 84.
4. *petrosal branch of glossopharyngeal nerves (Kilian, 1822)*
   Synonym for *recurrent branch of glossopharyngeal nerves (Kilian, 1822)*; in the original Latin, *ramus petrosus*, p. 84.
5. *Jacobson's nerve (Langenbeck, 1826–1830)*
   Eponym for macrodissected adult human ***tympanic nerve (Arnold, 1834)***; in the original Latin, *nervus Jacobsonii*, Fascicle III, Table XVIII-*1*. Another form is *nerve of Jacobson*.

LATER SYNONYMS:

1. *tympanic branch of glosso-pharyngeal nerve (Todd, 1836–1839)*
   Synonym for *recurrent branch of glossopharyngeal nerves (Kilian, 1822)*; p. 495, with good account of earlier observations.

PARTLY CORRESPONDS:

1. *anastomosis of Jacobson's nerve with Vidian nerve (Langenbeck, 1826–1830)*
   Macrodissected adult human ***communicating branch (Winslow, 1733)*** between ***tympanic nerve (Arnold, 1834)*** and ***nerve of pterygoid canal (>1840)***; in the original Latin, *anastomosis nervi Jacobsonii cum nervo Vidiano*, Fascicle III, Table XVIII-*3*.
2. *conjunction of Jacobson's branch with superficial branch of Vidian nerve (Langenbeck, 1826–1830)*
   Macrodissected adult human ***communicating branch (Winslow, 1733)*** between ***tympanic nerve (Arnold, 1834)*** and ***greater petrosal nerve (>1840)***; in the original Latin, *conjunctio rami Jacobsonii cum ramo superficiali nervi Vidiani*; Fascicle III, Table XVIII-*6*.
3. *connection of tympanic nerve with external carotid nerve (Arnold, 1834)*
   Communicating branch (Winslow, 1733) between macrodissected adult human ***tympanic nerve (Arnold, 1834)*** and ***external carotid plexus (>1840)***; in the original Latin, *nervus tympanicus conjunctio cum nervo carotico externo*, p. 13.
4. *connection of tympanic nerve with Jacobson's nerve (Arnold, 1834)*
   Synonym for *connection of tympanic nerve with external carotid nerve (Arnold, 1834)*; in the original Latin, *nervus Jacobsonii conjunctio cum nervo carotico externo*, p. 13.

tympanic plexus (Müller, 1834)

As described for macrodissected adult human, a ramification of the ***tympanic nerve (Arnold, 1834)*** from the ***glossopharyngeal nerve (Huber, 1744)***, and of the ***caroticotympanic nerves (>1840)***, on the surface of the promontory of the tympanic cavity. It supplies branches to mucus lining of the tympanic cavity, auditory (Eustachian) tube, and mastoid air cells; a ***communicating branch of tympanic plexus with greater petrosal nerve (>1840)***; and the ***lesser petrosal nerve (>1840)***, which can be viewed as a continuation of the ***tympanic nerve (>1840)*** to the ***otic ganglion (Arnold, 1828)*** and then parotid gland; see Cochet (1967), Williams & Warwick (1980, p. 1200, Fig. 7.184). For Müller's use in human material examined microscopically see translation (1838,

p. 671). It was first described by Jacobson; see ***[tympanic plexus (Müller, 1834)] (Jacobson, 1818)***.

EARLIER REFERENCES:

Described, not named or illustrated:

1. ***[tympanic plexus (Müller, 1834)] (Jacobson, 1818)***
   Described clearly as a nervous anastomosis for macrodissected adult human and other animals examined; also see Lobstein translation (1831, pp. 36–37) and Lekakis (2003, p. 30). Jacobson's findings were first reported at a Paris meeting in 1813; see Morton & Norman (1991, p. 243). It was described even more carefully by Kilian (1822, p. 71 ff.) and Lobstein (1823; see translation, 1831, pp. 38–39). It was incompletely described in macrodissected adult human by Cloquet (1816, p. 689).

Earlier synonyms:

1. *Jacobson's anastomosis (Lobstein, 1823)*
   Eponym for macrodissected adult human ***tympanic plexus (Müller, 1834)***; see translation (1831, p. 36).

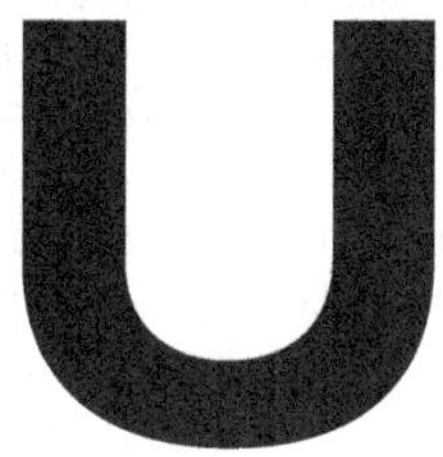

ulnar nerve (Cheselden, 1726)

As described for macrodissected adult human, it arises from the ***brachial plexus medial cord (Schwalbe, 1881)*** and generates ***muscular branches of ulnar nerve (Quain & Wilson, 1839)***, and a ***palmar branch of ulnar nerve (Soemmerring, 1791)***, ***dorsal branch of ulnar nerve (Günther, 1786)***, ***superficial branch of ulnar nerve (Fyfe, 1800)***, and ***deep branch of ulnar nerve (Fyfe, 1800)***; see Williams & Warwick (1980, pp. 1100–1101). In Cheselden's book (p. 265) this name was applied to the macrodissected adult human ***nerve (Herophilus, c335–c280 BC)*** in a chapter essentially written by Monro *primus* as stated in the Preface. It was first described as the *fourth nerve from spine to upper arm (Galen, c177)*.

TRANSLATIONS:

1. *nervus ulnaris (Cheselden, 1726)*
   Original Latin form of ***ulnar nerve (Cheselden, 1726)***; p. 265.

EARLIER REFERENCES:

Earlier synonyms:

1. *fourth nerve from spine to upper arm (Galen, c177)*
   Synonym for ***ulnar nerve (Cheselden, 1726)*** in macrodissected adult beef, pig, and/or macaque but not human; see Singer translation (1999, pp. 69–71, 73–75, 82); also see Duckworth translation (1962, p. 252), May translation (1968, pp. 137, 704–705).
2. *fifth nerve entering arm (Vesalius, 1543a)*
   Synonym for macrodissected adult human ***ulnar nerve (Cheselden, 1726)***; see Richardson & Carman translation (2002, p. 243).
3. *fifth sinew going into arm (Geminus, 1553)*
   Synonym for macrodissected adult human *fifth nerve entering arm (Vesalius, 1543a)*; originally spelled *fifte synowe goynge into arme*, see *The table of the figures of synowes*.
4. *fifth nerve of hand (Bauhin, 1605)*
   Synonym for macrodissected adult human *fifth nerve entering arm (Vesalius, 1543a)*; see Crooke translation (1615, p. 903).
5. *quintus brachium invadens nervus (Casseri, 1627)*
   Synonym for macrodissected adult human ***ulnar nerve (Cheselden, 1726)***; p. 128.
6. *cubital nerve (Du Verney, 1697)*
   Synonym for macrodissected adult human ***ulnar nerve (Cheselden, 1726)***; in the original Latin, *nervus cubitalis*. According to Winslow (1733, Sect. VI, p. 79), his mentor Du Verney gave this name for macrodissected adult human in 1697.
7. *inferior cubital nerve (Cheselden, 1713)*
   In an obscure description of the ***nerves (Herophilus, c335–c280 BC)***, the ***ulnar nerve (Cheselden, 1726)*** may be referred to thus; in the original Latin, *nervus cubitalis inferior*, p. 143.

LATER SYNONYMS:

1. *fourth great brachial nerve (Albinus, 1744)*
   Synonym for macrodissected adult human ***ulnar nerve (Cheselden, 1726)***; in the original Latin, *nervorum brachium magni quarti*, Table 19-30, also see Camper (1760, p. 11).
2. *cubito-digital nerve (Burdin, 1803)*
   Synonym for macrodissected adult human ***ulnar nerve (Cheselden, 1726)***; see translation (1803, V. 1, p. 194).

PARTLY CORRESPONDS:

1. *volar branch of cubital nerve (Martin, 1781)*
   Macrodissected adult human segment of ***ulnar nerve (Cheselden, 1726)*** between ***dorsal branch of ulnar nerve (Günther, 1786)*** and its two terminal branches, ***superficial branch of ulnar nerve (Fyfe, 1800)*** and ***deep branch of ulnar nerve (Fyfe, 1800)***; in the original Latin, *ramus volaris nervus cubitalis*, p. 216.
2. *subcutaneous branch of ulnar nerve (Günther, 1786)*

Branch of macrodissected adult human ***ulnar nerve (Cheselden, 1726)*** arising in arm, proximal to elbow; in the original Latin, *ramus subcutaneum*, p. 75.

3. *elbow joint branch of ulnar nerve (Günther, 1786)*
Branch of macrodissected adult human ***ulnar nerve (Cheselden, 1726)***; in the original Latin, *ramus ad articulationem cubiti*, p. 75.
4. *volar branch of ulnar nerve (Günther, 1786)*
Macrodissected adult human ***superficial branch of ulnar nerve (Fyfe, 1800)*** and ***deep branch of ulnar nerve (Fyfe, 1800)*** considered together; in the original Latin, *r. volarem*, p. 75.
5. *internal branch of ulnar nerve (Günther, 1786)*
Synonym for *volar branch of ulnar nerve (Günther, 1786)*; in the original Latin, *r. internum*, p.75.
6. *subcutaneous branch of cubital nerve (Frotscher, 1788)*
Synonym for *subcutaneous branch of ulnar nerve (Günther, 1786)*; in the original Latin, *ramum subcutaneum ex cubitali*, p. 92; also referred to there as *first branch of cubital nerve*.
7. *posterior branch of cubital nerve (Frotscher, 1788)*
Synonym for macrodissected adult human *volar branch of cubital nerve (Martin, 1781)*; p. 92.
8. *cutaneous branch of cubital nerve (Mayer, 1794)*
Synonym for macrodissected adult human *subcutaneous branch of cubital nerve (Frotscher, 1788)*; in the original Latin, *ramus cutaneus ex nervo cubitali*; Part 5, Table V, Figure 1-2 (p. 22).
9. *palmar branch of ulnar nerve (Meckel, 1817)*
Synonym for macrodissected adult human *volar branch of cubital nerve (Martin, 1781)*; see translation (1832, Vol. 3, p. 28). Also see *long palmar nerve of ulnar nerve (Meckel, 1817)*.
10. *articular filaments of cubital nerve (Cruveilhier, 1836)*
Synonym for macrodissected adult human *elbow joint branch of ulnar nerve (Günther, 1786)*; in the original French, *filets articulaires*, p. 811.
11. *filament of cubital nerve to cubital artery (Cruveilhier, 1836)*
Macrodissected adult human branch of ***ulnar nerve (Cheselden, 1726)*** to ulnar artery; in the original French, *filet de l'artère cubitale*, p. 811.
12. *anastomotic filament of cubital nerve (Cruveilhier, 1836)*
Macrodissected adult human ***communicating branch (Winslow, 1733)*** between ***ulnar nerve (Cheselden, 1726)*** and ***medial cutaneous nerve of arm (>1840)***; in the original French, *filet anastomotique*, p. 811.
13. *cutaneous branch of ulnar nerve (Quain & Wilson, 1839)*
Macrodissected adult human small branch of ***ulnar nerve (Cheselden, 1726)*** generated in forearm, just proximal to ***deep branch of ulnar nerve (Fyfe, 1800)***; Plate XVIII, Figure 2-*n*.

uncinate fascicle (Reil, 1809b)

As described for macrodissected adult human, a thick arching bundle of ***association fibers of cerebral cortex (>1840)*** between ventral (inferior) parts of the ***frontal region (Haller, 1754)*** and rostral (anterior) parts of the ***temporal region (>1840)***; see Crosby et al. (1962, Fig. 281), Williams & Warwick (1980, p. 1030, Fig. 7.148). For Reil's discovery and use in macrodissected adult human, see Mayo translation (1823, pp. 51, 52; Tab. X-*b*).

TRANSLATIONS:

1. *haakenförmige Markbundel (Reil, 1809b)*
Original German form of ***uncinate fascicle (Reil, 1809b)***.
2. *fasciculi unciformes (Burdach, 1822)*
Latin form (plural) of ***uncinate fascicle (Reil, 1809b)***; p. 152.
3. *hamular fasciculus (Mayo, 1823)*
Mayo's English translation of Reil's German, *haakenförmige Markbundel*, for ***uncinate fascicle (Reil, 1809b)***; p. 51.
4. *unciform fascicle (Reil, 1809b)*
English form of *haakenförmige Markbundel (Reil, 1809b)*.
5. *fasciculus uncinatus (>1840)*
Current Latin form of ***uncinate fascicle (Reil, 1809b)***; see *Terminologia Anatomica* (1998, p. 131).

LATER SYNONYMS:

1. *white nucleus of Sylvian fossa (Treviranus & Treviranus, 1816–1821)*
Synonym for macrodissected adult human ***uncinate fascicle (Reil, 1809b)***, according to Burdach (1822, p. 371); in the original German, *den Markkern der fossa Sylvii*, Vol. 3, p. 102.
2. *anteromedial arch (Rolando, 1831)*
Synonym for macrodissected adult human ***uncinate fascicle (Reil, 1809b)***; in the original Italian, *arco anteromedio*, Figure 4:*1-3*.
3. *olfactory arch (Rolando, 1831)*
Synonym for macrodissected adult human ***uncinate fascicle (Reil, 1809b)***; in the original Italian, *arco olfattorio*, Figures 4:*1-3*, 5:*1*.

PARTLY CORRESPONDS:

1. *longitudinal association bundle (>1840)*
As described histologically for nonprimate mammal, probably roughly synonymous with, or part of, macrodissected adult human ***uncinate fascicle (Reil, 1809b)***; see Johnston (1923).

uncrossed corticospinal tract (>1840)

As described for macrodissected adult human, and especially with experimental pathway tracing methods, the ipsilateral (direct) caudal segment of the right or left ***corticospinal tract (>1840)***, caudal to the ***pyramidal decussation (Reil, 1809c)*** and centered in medial regions of the right or left ***ventral funiculus (>1840)***; see Williams & Warwick (1980, p. 875 and Fig. 7.43), called *anterior corticospinal tract (>1840)*, Nieuwenhuys et al. (2008, Fig. 6.1-30). Its size and location can vary greatly between adult individuals and species, like the ***crossed corticospinal tract (>1840)***, although it is typically much smaller than the latter. It was perhaps first clearly described as the *fibrae primitivae pyramidalis (Arnold, 1838b)*.

EARLIER REFERENCES:

Earlier synonyms:

1. *fibrae primitivae pyramidalis (Arnold, 1838b)*
   Synonym for macrodissected adult human ***uncrossed pyramidal tract (>1840)***; Table IX, Figure 7-*a*.
2. *fasciculus siliqualis externus (Wagner, 1839)*
   Medial part of macrodissected adult human ***ventral funiculus (>1840)*** at rostral (upper) levels of ***cervical part of spinal cord (>1840)***, essentially the ***uncrossed pyramidal tract (>1840)*** there; Table XXVII, Figure 10-*6*. Compare with Nieuwenhuys et al. (2008, Fig. 6.7).
3. *anterior corticospinal tract (>1840)*
   Synonym for macrodissected adult human ***uncrossed pyramidal tract (>1840)***; see *Terminologia Anatomica* (1998, p. 107).
4. *ventral corticospinal tract (>1840)*
   Synonym for macrodissected adult human ***uncrossed pyramidal tract (>1840)***; see *Terminologia Anatomica* (1998, p. 107).

upper esophageal branches of vagus nerve (Cloquet, 1828)

As described for macrodissected adult human, branches of the ***vagus nerve trunk (Wrisberg, 1786; Günther, 1786)*** arising rostral to (above) ***pulmonary branches of vagus nerve (Cloquet, 1828)*** and joining the ***esophageal plexus (Haller, 1762)***; see Williams & Warwick (1980, p. 1081). For Cloquet's use in macrodissected adult human, see Plate CLXXVII-*188*. They were first described as *nerve branches to esophagus (Galen, c192)*.

TRANSLATIONS:

1. *rameaux oesophagiens supérieur du nerf vague (Cloquet, 1828)*
   Original French form of ***upper esophageal branches of vagus nerve (Cloquet, 1828)***; Plate CLXXVII-*188*.

EARLIER REFERENCES:

Earlier synonyms:

1. *nerve branches to esophagus (Galen, c192)*
   Synonym for ***upper esophageal branches of vagus nerve (Cloquet, 1828)*** in macrodissected adult beef, pig, and/or macaque but not human. Galen noted their intermingling with ***esophageal branches of recurrent laryngeal nerve (Arnold, 1834)***; see Duckworth translation (1962, p. 204) and May translation (1968, p. 694, where trachea is called rough artery). They were illustrated for macrodissected adult human by Vieussens (1684, Tab. 23-*15*).
2. *esophageal nerves (Loder, 1778)*
   Synonym for macrodissected adult human ***upper esophageal branches of vagus nerve (Cloquet, 1828)***; in the original Latin, *nervos oesophageos*, p. 31.
3. *upper esophageal branches of eighth pair (Walter, 1783)*
   Synonym for macrodissected adult human ***upper esophageal branches of vagus nerve (Cloquet, 1828)***; in the original Latin, *rami oesophagei superiores octavi paris*, Table III:*401–405,433,460*.

PARTLY CORRESPONDS:

1. *small posterior esophageal plexus of pneumogastric (Cloquet, 1828)*
   For macrodissected adult human it is formed on rostral (upper) and dorsal (back) parts of esophagus by ***upper esophageal branches of vagus nerve (Cloquet, 1828)***; in the original French, *petit plexus oesophagien postérieur du pneumo-gastrique*, Plate CLXIII-*34*.

upper subscapular nerve (>1840)

As described for macrodissected adult human, a branch of the ***brachial plexus dorsal cord (Paterson, 1887)*** ending by supplying the rostral (upper) part of the subscapular muscle; see Williams & Warwick (1980, p. 1096). It was known to Galen; see ***[upper subscapular nerve (>1840)] (Galen, c173)***.

EARLIER REFERENCES:

Described, not named or illustrated:

1. ***[upper subscapular nerve (>1840)] (Galen, c173)***
   Clearly described innervation of subscapular muscle in macrodissected adult beef, pig, and/or macaque but not human; see May translation (1968, pp. 598–599), and Duckworth translation (1962, pp. 243, 253, 257). Vesalius (1543a) also mentioned this supply for macrodissected adult human; see Richardson & Carman translation (2002, pp. 228–229, 233).

Earlier synonyms:

1. *second subscapular branch of brachial plexus (Cloquet, 1816)*
   Synonym for macrodissected adult human ***upper subscapular nerve (>1840)***; p. 644.
2. *subscapular nerves (Bock, 1817)*
   Synonym for macrodissected adult human ***upper subscapular nerve (>1840)***; in the original Latin, *nervi subscapulares*, Table I, Figure 2-*14*.
3. *superior subscapular branch of brachial plexus (Cruveilhier, 1836)*
   Synonym for macrodissected adult human ***upper subscapular nerve (>1840)***; in the original French, *branche sous-scapulaire supérieure du plexus brachial*, p. 794.

ureteric plexus (>1840)

As described for macrodissected adult human, it arises from the ***superior ureteric nerves (Walter, 1783), middle ureteric nerves (>1840)***, and ***inferior ureteric nerves (>1840)*** and supplies the ureter; see Mitchell (1953, p. 293), Williams & Warwick (1980, p. 1134). It was known to Willis; see ***[ureteric plexus (>1840)] (Willis, 1664)***.

EARLIER REFERENCES:

Illustrated and described, not named:

1. ***[ureteric plexus (>1840)] (Willis, 1664)***
   Mentioned and illustrated for macrodissected adult human and other common large mammals; see Pordage translation (1681, p. 159 and Table 11-*v[u]*).

urethral branches of inferior hypogastric plexus (>1840)

As described for macrodissected adult human, they arise from the ***inferior hypogastric plexus (Tiedemann, 1822)*** and extend along the urethra; see Mitchell (1953, p. 305, Fig. 131). They were perhaps first clearly described as the *urethral branchlets from hypogastric plexus (Walter, 1783)*.

EARLIER REFERENCES:

Earlier synonyms:

1. *urethral branchlets from hypogastric plexus (Walter, 1783)* Synonym for macrodissected adult human ***urethral branches of inferior hypogastric plexus (>1840)***; in the original Latin, *surculi uretherici ex plexu hypogastrico*, Table II-*463,464*.

PARTLY CORRESPONDS:

1. *ureteric nerve to urethra (Walter, 1783)* A macrodissected adult human ***nerve (Herophilus, c335–c280 BC)*** with several roots corresponding to a ***urethral branch of inferior hypogastric plexus (>1840)***; in the original Latin, *nervus uretericus qui ad uretherem migrat*, Table II-*188*.

uterine cervical ganglion (>1840)

As described for macrodissected adult human female, the largest, most consistent of the ***paracervical ganglia (>1840)***; see Williams & Warwick (1980, p. 1136). It was first described as the *ganglion of uterine plexus (Tiedemann, 1822)*.

EARLIER REFERENCES:

Earlier synonyms:

1. *ganglion of uterine plexus (Tiedemann, 1822)* Synonym for macrodissected adult human female ***uterine cervical ganglion (>1840)***; in the original Latin, *ganglion plexui uterino*, Table I-*60,67*.

uterovaginal plexus (>1840)

As described for macrodissected adult human female, an extension of the ***inferior hypogastric plexus (Tiedemann, 1822)*** lying in the base of the broad ligament. One part of the ***plexus (Galen, c192)*** is formed by what are sometimes called the *uterine nerves (Galen, c173)*. This part passes directly to the uterine cervix as well as extends rostrally (upward) with the uterine arteries to the uterine body. The other part of the ***plexus (Galen, c192)*** is formed partly by the ***vaginal nerves (Walter, 1783)***; this part follows the vaginal arteries and their branches to the walls of the vagina, erectile tissue of the vestibular bulbs and clitoris, urethra, and greater vestibular glands; see Mitchell (1953, pp. 308–310 and Fig. 311), Williams & Warwick (1980, p. 1136). It corresponds to the ***prostatic plexus (>1840)*** in male; see Durward (1951, p. 1144). At least part of it was known to Galen; see *uterine nerves (Galen, c173)*.

PARTLY CORRESPONDS:

1. *uterine nerves (Galen, c173)* As described for macrodissected adult human female, components of ***uterovaginal plexus (>1840)***. Some pass caudally, down the vaginal arteries, while others pass directly to cervix of uterus and ***paracervical ganglia (>1840)***, or pass rostrally, upward with or near uterine arteries in broad ligament, to supply body of uterus and uterine tube, and to communicate with tubal ***nerves (Herophilus, c335–c280 BC)*** from ***inferior hypogastric plexus (Tiedemann, 1822)*** and ***inferior ovarian nerves (>1840)***, forming parasympathetic ***tubo-uterine plexus (>1840)***; see Mitchell (1953, pp. 308–309), Williams & Warwick (1980, pp. 1136, 1431). For Galen's reference to ***nerves (Herophilus, c335–c280 BC)*** to uterus of macrodissected adult beef, pig, and/or macaque but not human, see May translation (1968, p. 651), Duckworth translation (1962, p. 263). Vesalius (1543a) described them briefly for macrodissected adult human female, see Richardson & Carman translation (2002, p. 200), and Walter (1783, Tab. I-*455*) illustrated them clearly for macrodissected adult human.
2. *nerves into womb (Willis, 1664)* Synonym for *uterine nerves (Galen, c173)* as illustrated and described for macrodissected adult human and other common large mammalian females; see Table XI-ε.
3. *superior uterine plexus (Tiedemann, 1822)* In macrodissected adult human female, upper, rostral, or proximal part of ***uterovaginal plexus (>1840)*** on right and left side of uterus; in the original Latin, *plexum uterinum superiorem*, Table I-*34,36*.
4. *superior lateral uterine plexus (Tiedemann, 1822)* Synonym for *superior uterine plexus (Tiedemann, 1822)*; in the original Latin, *plexum uterinum lateralem superiorem*, Table II-*14*.
5. *uterovaginal nerves (Cruveilhier, 1836)* Basically synonym for macrodissected adult human female *uterine nerves (Galen, c173)*; in the original French, *nerfs utéro-vaginaux*, p. 1027.
6. *ascending uterine nerves (Cruveilhier, 1836)* Basically the upper, rostral, or proximal *uterine nerves (Galen, c173)* of macrodissected adult human female; in the original French, *ascendans*, p. 1028.
7. *descending uterine nerves (Cruveilhier, 1836)* Basically the lower, caudal, or distal *uterine nerves (Galen, c173)* of macrodissected adult human female; in the original French, *descendans*, p. 1028.

utricular nerve (>1840)

As described for macrodissected adult human, a terminal branch of the ***utriculoampullary nerve (>1840)*** to the utricle; see Durward (1951, Fig. 904), *Terminologia Anatomica* (1998, p. 135). It was probably first clearly delineated as the *middle branch of vestibular nerve to common utricle (Langenbeck, 1826–1830)*.

EARLIER REFERENCES:

Earlier synonyms:

1. *middle branch of vestibular nerve to common utricle (Langenbeck, 1826–1830)* Synonym for macrodissected adult human ***utricular nerve (>1840)***; in the original Latin, *ramus medius*

nervi vestibuli ad utriculum communem, Fascicle III, Table XXIX-9.

2. *superior branch of vestibular nerve (Arnold, 1839)*
Probably synonym for macrodissected adult human ***utricular nerve (>1840)***; in the original Latin, *ramus superior nervi vestibuli*, Table VII, Fig 9-*w*.

utriculoampullary nerve (>1840)

As described for macrodissected adult human, a branch of the ***rostral part of vestibular nerve (>1840)*** generating in turn the ***utricular nerve (>1840)*** and commonly the ***lateral ampullary nerve (>1840)***; see Durward (1951, Fig. 904, unlabeled), *Nomina Anatomica* (1983, p. A75), *Terminologia Anatomica* (1998, p. 134). It was perhaps first clearly indicated by Langenbeck; see ***[utriculoampullary nerve (>1840)] (Langenbeck, 1826–1830)***.

EARLIER REFERENCES:

Illustrated and described, not named:

1. ***[utriculoampullary nerve (>1840)] (Langenbeck, 1826–1830)***
For macrodissected adult human, Langenbeck described both parts as *branch of anterior branch of vestibular nerve to ampulla of external semicircular canal (Langenbeck, 1826–1830)* and *middle branch of vestibular nerve to common utricle (Langenbeck, 1826–1830)*; Fascicle III, Table XXIX-7.

uvula (Malacarne, 1776)

As described for macrodissected adult human, the part of the ***cerebellar vermis (Meckel, 1817)*** between ***pyramis (Malacarne, 1776)*** and ***nodule (Reil, 1807–1808a)***, roughly medial to the right and left ***tonsil (Malacarne, 1776)*** and ***paraflocculus (Stroud, 1895)*** of the ***cerebellar hemisphere (Willis, 1664)***; see Larsell & Jansen (1972, Fig. 118), Carpenter (1976, Figs. 2.25, 2.26, 14.1), Nieuwenhuys et al. (2008, Fig. 3.8-38). For Malacarne's discovery and naming after resemblance to palatine uvula see Clarke & O'Malley (1996, p. 645).

TRANSLATIONS:

1. *ugola (Malacarne)*
Original Italian form of ***uvula (Malacarne, 1776)***; pp. 23–24.

LATER SYNONYMS:

1. *spigot of cerebellum (Reil, 1807–1808a)*
Synonym for macrodissected adult human ***uvula (Malacarne, 1776)***; see Mayo translation (1822, p. 24).
2. *middle part of inferior vermal process (Gordon, 1815)*
Synonym for macrodissected adult human ***uvula (Malacarne, 1776)***; p. 114. Burdach (1822, p. 296) gave the Latin, *pars media vermis inferioris*.
3. *mamillary eminence of inferior vermis (Cloquet, 1828)*
Synonym for macrodissected adult human ***uvula (Malacarne, 1776)***; in the original French, *éminence mamillaire du vermis inferior*, p. 383.

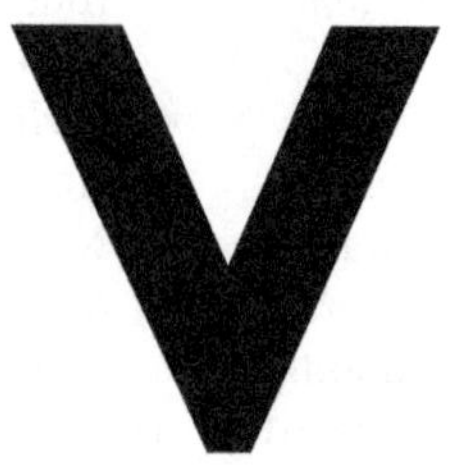

vagal triangle (>1840)

As described for macrodissected adult human, an elevation in the caudal half of the ***floor of fourth ventricle (Reil, 1807–1808a)*** between **hypoglossal triangle (>1840)** medially and ***funiculus separans (>1840)*** laterally and caudally—basically overlying the ***nucleus of solitary tract (>1840)*** and ***dorsal motor nucleus of vagus nerve (>1840)***; see Williams & Warwick (1980, p. 934, Fig. 7.89). It was clearly indicated by Vicq d'Azyr; see ***[vagal triangle (>1840)] (Vicq d'Azyr, 1786)***.

TRANSLATIONS:

1. *trigonum vagale (>1840)*
   Current Latin form of ***vagal triangle (>1840)***; see *Terminologia Anatomica* (1998, p. 115).
2. *vagal trigone (>1840)*
   Current English form of *trigonum vagale (>1840)*; see *Terminologia Anatomica* (1998, p. 115).

EARLIER REFERENCES:

Illustrated and described, not named:

1. ***[vagal triangle (>1840)] (Vicq d'Azyr, 1786)***
   Clearly indicated in macrodissected adult human, although probably not distinguished from ***area postrema (>1840)***; Plate XXX, Figure III-4. Vicq d'Azyr further noted that it, along with ***vestibular area of fourth ventricle (>1840)***, and ***floor of fourth ventricle (Reil, 1807–1808a)*** in general, is associated with a layer of ***gray matter (Meckel, 1817)***; Plate XXX, Figure III-*11*.

Earlier synonyms:

1. *gray substance leaves (Rolando, 1825a)*
   Rolando's illustration for macrodissected large calf generally indicates the ***[vagal triangle (>1840)] (Vicq d'Azyr, 1786)***; in the original French, *feuilles de substance cendrée*, Table VII, Figure 1-*f.c.* (*f* in Figure). Also see *gray lanceolate leaves (Desmoulins, 1825)*.
2. *substantia ochracea (Bergmann, 1831)*
   Synonym for macrodissected adult human ***vagal triangle (>1840)***, which he also referred to as *substantia cinerea*; p. 56, see Arnold (1838a, p. 24).
3. *ala cinerea (Arnold, 1838b)*
   Synonym for macrodissected adult human ***vagal triangle (>1840)***; Table IV, Figure 3-*h*. Also see Arnold (1838a, p. 24).

vaginal nerves (Walter, 1783)

As described for macrodissected adult human female, they extend from the ***uterovaginal plexus (>1840)*** along the vaginal arteries and their branches to the walls of the vagina, erectile tissue of the vestibular bulbs, and the clitoris—the ***cavernous nerves of clitoris (>1840)***, urethra, and greater vestibular glands; see Mitchell (1953, p. 310 and Fig. 131), Williams & Warwick (1980, p. 1136). For Walter's illustration in a macrodissected adult human female cadaver, perhaps its first clear delineation, see Table I:*428–437, 440–442*; also see Tiedemann (1822, Tab. II-*41*).

TRANSLATIONS:

1. *nervi vaginae (Walter, 1783)*
   Original Latin form of ***vaginal nerves (Walter, 1783)***; Table I:*428–437, 440–442*.

LATER SYNONYMS:

1. *vaginal branches of small plexus from first hypogastric plexus (Cloquet, 1828)*
   Synonym for macrodissected adult human ***vaginal nerves (Walter, 1783)***; in the original French, *rameaux vaginaux*, Plate CLXXV-*226*.

vagus nerve (Galen, c192)

As described for macrodissected adult human, a ***cranial nerve (Soemmerring, 1791)*** with a proximal part, the ***vagus nerve root (>1840)*** attached to the outer surface of the ***medulla (Winslow, 1733)*** in a longitudinal line between ***glossopharyngeal nerve root (>1840)*** rostrally and ***cranial root of accessory nerve (>1840)*** caudally, and a distal part, the ***vagus nerve trunk (Wrisberg, 1786; Günther, 1786)*** with a variety of branches; see Mettler (1948, Figs. 57, 61–65), Durward (1951, Fig. 907), Hamilton (1976, Figs. 803–807), Williams & Warwick (1980, Fig. 7.191). Galen provided a brilliant description of the ***vagus nerve (Galen, c192)*** and its branches in macrodissected adult beef, pig and/or macaque but not human; see Savage-Smith (1971, p. 183 ff.). He was especially impressed with the large input to the stomach, which he related to the sensation of hunger (May translation, 1968, pp. 53, 447, 694), and some of his greatest work involved discovery and experimental analysis of the ***recurrent laryngeal nerve (Albinus, 1744)***, which he called the *upwardly recurrent nerve (Galen, c192)*, *recurrent nerve (Galen, c173)*, or *vocal nerve (Galen, c192)*; see Duckworth translation (1962, pp. 207–209), May translation (1968, p. 68). The ***vagus nerve (Galen, c192)***—for the term itself see Duckworth translation (1962, pp. 205, 208)—was a separately named part of the *sixth pair of nerves from brain (Galen, c192)*; see Savage-Smith (1971, p. 183 ff.), Duckworth translation (1962, p. 203 ff.). Galen regarded it as a sensory ***nerve (Herophilus, c335–c280 BC)***; see May translation (1968, p. 685). As noted in the *Anatomia Magistri Nicolai physici* (early 12th century; see Corner translation, 1927, p. 73), "certain other nerves [***vagus nerves (Galen, c192)***]... pass through the whole length of the neck to the heart and surround the sides of the heart; by means of these, animal spirits are carried to the heart to produce the emotions, such as anger, joy, sadness, and the like, for all the operations of the mind and soul originate in the brain and terminate in the heart." Its discovery is usually credited to Herophilus; see ***[vagus nerve (Galen, c192)] (Herophilus, c335–c280 BC)***.

ALTERNATE SPELLINGS:

1. *vagous nerve (Diemerbroeck, 1689)*
   Alternate form of ***vagus nerve (Galen, c192)***; p. 416.
2. *vague nerve (Haller, 1754b)*
   Alternate form of ***vagus nerve (Galen, c192)***; see p. 303.

EARLIER REFERENCES:

Described, not named or illustrated:

1. ***[vagus nerve (Galen, c192)] (Herophilus, c335–c280 BC)***
   Herophilus, the founder of human anatomy, is credited with discovering but not naming ***glossopharyngeal nerve (Huber, 1744)***, ***vagus nerve (Galen, c192)***, and ***accessory nerve (Vieussens, 1684)***, apparently considering the three together; see Solmsen (1961), von Staden (1969), Longrigg (1993), Clarke & O'Malley (1996, p. 261). He dissected adult animals and human cadavers.

LATER SYNONYMS:

1. *great nerve (Galen, c192)*
   Synonym for ***vagus nerve (Galen, c192)***; see Duckworth translation (1962, p. 207).
2. *nervus tornabilis (Second Salernitan Demonstration, c1070–c1100)*
   Apparently synonym for ***vagus nerve (Galen, c192)***; see Corner translation (1927, p. 58; also see pp. 28–29).
3. *apoplectic nerve (Berengario da Carpi, 1522)*
   Ancient synonym for ***vagus nerve (Galen, c192)***, according to Berengario da Carpi; see Lind translation (1959, p. 110).
4. *posterior fibers of vagus nerve pair (Morgagni, 1719)*
   Synonym for macrodissected adult human ***vagus nerve (Galen, c192)***; p. 14. Also see Burdach (1822, p. 311), who used the Latin phrase *fibras posteriores paris octavi*.
5. *second spinal nerve (Soemmerring, 1778)*
   Synonym for macrodissected adult human ***vagus nerve (Galen, c192)***; in the original Latin, *nervus spinalis secundus*, p. 180.
6. *second pair of nerves of medulla oblongata (Haller & Wrisberg, 1780)*
   Synonym for macrodissected adult human ***vagus nerves (Galen, c192)***; see translation (1786, p. 208).
7. *posterior part of eighth pair (Haase, 1781)*
   Synonym listed for macrodissected adult human ***vagus nerves (Galen, c192)***; in the original Latin, *paris octavi portio posterior*, p. 41.
8. *fourteenth pair, intermediate sympathetic (Malacarne, 1791)*
   Synonym listed for macrodissected adult human ***vagus nerves (Galen, c192)***; in the original Latin, *par decimum quartum, sympathicus medius*, p. 193.
9. *tenth pair of cranial nerves (Soemmerring, 1791)*
   Synonym for macrodissected adult human ***vagus nerves (Galen, c192)***; see ***cranial nerves (Soemmerring, 1791)***.
10. *tenth pair of cerebral nerves (Soemmerring, 1791)*
    Synonym for *tenth pair of cranial nerves (Soemmerring, 1791)*; see p. 103 and *cerebral nerves (Soemmerring, 1791)*. In the original Latin, *par decimum nervorum cerebri*, Soemmerring (1798, p. 125).
11. *ninth pair of nerves of head (Andersch & Soemmerring, 1792)*
    Synonym for macrodissected adult human ***vagus nerves (Galen, c192)***; in the original Latin, *nervus nonum nervum*, p. 114.
12. *ninth nerve proper of nerves of head (Andersch & Soemmerring, 1792)*
    Synonym for macrodissected adult human ***vagus nerve (Galen, c192)***; in the original Latin, *proprius nervus noni nervi capitis*, p. 125.
13. *tenth pair of nerves of head (Andersch, 1797)*
    Synonym for macrodissected adult human ***vagus nerves (Galen, c192)***; see p. 1, also see Meckel (1832, Vol. 3, p. 45).
14. *nervus consentiens magnus capitis (Andersch, 1797)*
    Synonym for macrodissected adult human ***vagus nerve (Galen, c192)***; p. 1, also see Burdach (1822, p. 309).
15. *tenth nerves of head (Andersch, 1797)*
    Synonym for *tenth pair of nerves of head (Andersch, 1797)*; in the original Latin, *decimo nervo capitis*, p. 19.
16. *nervo harmonico magno capitis (Andersch, 1797)*
    Synonym for *nervus consentiens magnus capitis (Andersch, 1797)*; p. 19.

17. *tenth nerve proper of nerves of head (Andersch, 1797)*
Synonym for macrodissected adult human ***vagus nerve (Galen, c192)***; in the original Latin, *nervum proprium decimi nervi capitis*, p. 24.
18. *pars vaga of eighth pair (Fyfe, 1800)*
Synonym for macrodissected adult human ***vagus nerve (Galen, c192)***; Vol. 2, p. 315.
19. *pneumo-gastric pair of nerves (Burdin, 1803)*
Synonym for macrodissected adult human ***vagus nerves (Galen, c192)***; see translation (1803, Vol. 1, p. 144). Meckel called it in German, *Lungenmagennerve* (1817, p. 689); see Burdach (1822, p. 310).
20. *pneumo-gastric nerve (Chaussier, 1807)*
Synonym for macrodissected adult human ***vagus nerve (Galen, c192)***; in the original French, *N. pneumo-gastrique*, p. 195. Later it was often unhyphenated.
21. *vocal nerve (Gall & Spurzheim, 1810)*
Synonym for macrodissected adult human ***vagus nerve (Galen, c192)***; in the original French, *nerf vocal*, p. 72.
22. *pulmonary nerve (Bartels, 1813)*
Synonym for ***vagus nerve (Galen, c192)***; p. 210, according to Meckel (1832, Vol. 3, p. 44 note *1*).
23. *gastropulmonary nerve (Gordon, 1815)*
Variation on macrodissected adult human *pneumo-gastric pair of nerves (Burdin, 1803)*; p. 181.
24. *par consensorius magnus capitis sive nonum (Burdach, 1822)*
Burdach's interpretation of Andersch's term for macrodissected adult human ***vagus nerves (Galen, c192)***; p. 309. Also see *ninth pair of nerves of head (Andersch & Soemmerring, 1792)* and *tenth pair of nerves of head (Andersch, 1797)*.
25. *branchiogastric nerve (Solly, 1836)*
Synonym for macrodissected adult fish ***vagus nerve (Galen, c192)***; p. 76.
26. *branchial nerve (Leuret, 1839)*
Synonym for macrodissected adult fish ***vagus nerve (Galen, c192)***; in the original French (plural), *nerfs branchiaux*, p. 149.

PARTLY CORRESPONDS:

1. *stomach nerve (Paré, 1561)*
Paré described and illustrated this part of macrodissected adult human ***vagus nerve (Galen, c192)***, roughly distal to ***pulmonary branches of vagus nerve (Cloquet, 1828)***; in the original French, *nerf stomachique*, p. cxiii and part *C* of figure on p. lxxx-verso. Spiegel (1627, p. 208) gave the Latin form, *nervum stomachicum*.
2. *stomacke branch of sixth conjugation (Paré, 1634)*
Original English form of *stomach nerve (Paré, 1561)*; in the original Latin, *ramus stomachicus*, p. 153.
3. *lower infolding of wandring pair (Willis, 1664)*
Probably a *pseudoganglion (>1840)*—associated with thoracic segment of ***vagus nerve (Galen, c192)*** and "generating" ***thoracic cardiac branches of vagus nerve (>1840)*** and ***recurrent laryngeal nerve (Albinus, 1744)*** in macrodissected adult human and other common large mammals; in the original Latin, *plexus inferior paris vagi*, see Pordage translation (1681, Tab. 9-*K*). Willis may have illustrated it based on his conjecture that *infoldings*—***ganglia (Galen, c173)***—are typically associated with true branch points in ***nerves (Herophilus, c335–c280 BC)***; see Pordage translation (1681, p. 146).
4. *knot of reflection or turning back (Willis, 1664)*
Synonym for *lower infolding of wandring pair (Willis, 1664)*; see Pordage translation (1681, p. 147).
5. *thoracic ganglioform plexus of eighth pair of nerves (Vieussens, 1684)*
Synonym for macrodissected adult human *lower infolding of wandring pair (Willis, 1664)*; in the original Latin, *plexus ganglioformis thoracicus nervi octavi paris*, Table 23-*I*. Vieussens also described two more *pseudoganglia (>1840)* farther down left ***vagus nerve (Galen, c192)***, just distal to level of aortic arch; Table 23-*16*.
6. *communicating branch of vagus nerve with ninth pair of cerebral nerves (Loder, 1778)*
Macrodissected adult human ***communicating branch (Winslow, 1833)*** between ***vagus nerve (Galen, c192)*** and ***hypoglossal nerve (Winslow, 1733)***; in the original Latin, *ramulum communicantem cum nono pare nervorum cerebri*, p. 30. It was first described for macrodissected adult human by Falloppio (1561, p. 155).
7. *left vagus nerve (Mayer, 1794)*
Included distally the macrodissected adult human ***anterior vagal trunk (Wrisberg, 1780)***; in the original Latin, *nervus vagus sinister*; Part 6, Table IV-*I* (p. 25).
8. *right vagus nerve (Mayer, 1794)*
For macrodissected adult human, included distally the ***posterior vagal trunk (Wrisberg, 1780)***; in the original Latin, *nervus vagus sinister*; Part 6, Table IV-*II* (p. 26).
9. *secondary ganglion of vagus nerves (Wutzer, 1817)*
Probably a *pseudoganglion (>1840)*, associated with macrodissected adult human ***vagus nerve (Galen, c192)*** just proximal to origin of ***superior laryngeal nerve (Loder, 1778)***; in the original Latin, *ganglion secundum nervi vagi*, Figure VII-*s*.
10. *nodular plexus of vagus nerves of Meckel (Kilian, 1822)*
Eponym for macrodissected adult human *secondary ganglion of vagus nerve (Wutzer, 1817)*, a *pseudoganglion (>1840)*. Meckel (1817, Vol. 3, p. 687) described it as a "Knotengeflecht" associated with origin of ***pharyngeal branches of vagus nerve (Wrisberg, 1786)***. It was translated as "ganglionary plexus" (Meckel; 1832, Vol. 3, p. 46).
11. *lateral line nerve (Desmoulins, 1825)*
Classed as part of macrodissected adult fish ***vagus nerve (Galen, c192)*** and considered poorly named by Desmoulins; in the original French, *nerf de la ligne latéral*, p. 445 and Atlas p. 4.
12. *ganglioform plexus of vagus nerve (Arnold, 1834)*
Synonym for macrodissected adult human *secondary ganglion of vagus nerve (Wutzer, 1817)*, a *pseudoganglion (>1840)*; in the original Latin, *plexus ganglioformis nervi vagi*, p. 14.

vagus nerve central root (>1840)

As described for macrodissected adult human, and mammal generally with histological methods for ***axons***

(Kölliker, 1896), the central extension of the peripheral ***vagus nerve root (>1840)*** coursing transversely through the ***medullary segment of spinal tract of trigeminal nerve (>1840)*** and medially adjacent ***spinal nucleus of trigeminal nerve (>1840)***, caudal to the **glossopharyngeal nerve central root** (>1840), primarily to parts of the ***ambiguus nucleus (>1840)***, ***dorsal motor nucleus of vagus nerve (>1840)***, and ***nucleus of solitary tract (>1840)***. It is formed by smaller individual fascicles, the ***vagus nerve central rootlets (>1840)***; see Villiger et al. (1951, Figs. 10, 11), Carpenter (1976, pp. 309–312 and Figs. 11.16–18). Mayo perhaps first identified at least part of it; see ***[vagus nerve central root (>1840)] (Mayo, 1827)***.

EARLIER REFERENCES:

Illustrated and described, not named:

1. ***[vagus nerve central root (>1840)] (Mayo, 1827)***
Mayo traced at least part of it to region of macrodissected adult human ***inferior cerebellar peduncle (Günther, 1786)***; Plate VII, Figure 2-*VIII*. Grainger (1837, p. 41) accurately traced at least part of it in macrodissected adult human to "the grey matter placed in the posterior part of the medulla oblongata".

vagus nerve central rootlets (>1840)

As described in macrodissected adult human, and mammal generally with histological methods for ***axons (Kölliker, 1896)***, the central extensions of the peripheral ***vagus nerve rootlets (>1840)***, together forming the ***vagus nerve central root (>1840)***; see Villiger et al. (1951, Figs. 10, 11), Carpenter (1976, pp. 309–312). They were not clearly identified by 1840.

vagus nerve root (>1840)

As described for macrodissected adult human, it is attached to the outer surface of the ***medulla (Winslow, 1733)*** in a longitudinal line between the ***glossopharyngeal nerve root (>1840)*** rostrally and ***cranial root of accessory nerve (>1840)*** caudally. It consists of ***vagus nerve rootlets (>1840)*** coalescing distally into the ***vagus nerve trunk (Wrisberg, 1786; Günther, 1786)*** at the jugular foramen; see Williams & Warwick (1980, Fig. 7.189). Also see ***dorsal root (Spurzheim, 1826)***. It was known to Galen; see ***[vagus nerve root (>1840)] (Galen, c192)***.

EARLIER REFERENCES:

Described, not named or illustrated:

1. ***[vagus nerve root (>1840)] (Galen, c192)***
Galen clearly referred to it as one of three *roots of sixth pair of nerves from brain (Galen, c192)*, described for macrodissected adult beef, pig, and/or macaque but not human; see May translation (1968, p. 445, note 41). Vesalius (1543a) vaguely described and illustrated it for macrodissected adult human, although he did not distinguish the ***glossopharyngeal nerve root (>1840)***; see *root of sixth pair of cerebral nerves (Vesalius, 1543a)*. Eustachi (1552) illustrated more clearly than Vesalius the *root of sixth pair of cerebral nerves (Vesalius, 1543a)*, although he also did not distinguish the ***glossopharyngeal nerve root (>1840)***; see Albinus edition (1761, Tab. 18, Figs. 1, 3, 4-ε and Fig. 2-*d*).

Earlier synonyms:

1. *cerebral part of tenth pair (Arnold, 1834)*
Essentially synonymous with macrodissected adult human ***vagus nerve root (>1840)***; in the original Latin, *par decimum, pars cerebralis*, p. 13.
2. *cerebral part of pneumogastric nerve (Arnold, 1834)*
Synonym for *cerebral part of tenth pair (Arnold, 1834)*; in the original Latin, *nervus pneumogastricus, pars cerebralis*, p. 13.
3. *cerebral part of vagus nerve (Arnold, 1834)*
Synonym for *cerebral part of tenth pair (Arnold, 1834)*; in the original Latin, *nervus vagus, pars cerebralis*, p. 13.

vagus nerve rootlets (>1840)

As described for macrodissected adult human, thin bundles of ***axons (Kölliker, 1896)*** between outer surface of ***medulla (Winslow, 1733)*** proximally and ***vagus nerve trunk (Wrisberg, 1786; Günther, 1786)*** distally, together forming the ***vagus nerve root (>1840)***. They were called rootlets by Durward (1951, p. 1037), and Williams & Warwick (1980, p. 1076) mentioned 8–10 of them for macrodissected adult human. They were first observed as part of the *beginnings and twigs of sixth pair of cerebral nerves (Vesalius, 1543a)*, and clearly distinguished from adjacent rootlets as the *main body of filaments of nerves of eighth pair (Winslow, 1733)*.

EARLIER REFERENCES:

Earlier synonyms:

1. *main body of filaments of nerves of eighth pair (Winslow, 1733)*
Winslow stated that in macrodissected adult human they are separated from the anterior filaments by a thin septum; he was referring to the ***vagus nerve rootlets (>1840)*** and ***glossopharyngeal nerve rootlets (>1840)***, respectively; Section VI, no. 106, p. 70.
2. *vagus nerve roots (Günther, 1786)*
Synonym for macrodissected adult human ***vagus nerve rootlets (>1840)***; pp. 62–63.
3. *pneumogastric nerve filaments (Meckel, 1817)*
Meckel described 10–16 of them for macrodissected adult human, synonymous with ***vagus nerve rootlets (>1840)***; see translation (1832, Vol. 3, p. 45).

vagus nerve trunk (Wrisberg, 1786; Günther, 1786)

As described for macrodissected adult human, the condensed part of the ***vagus nerve (Galen, c192)*** distal to the ***vagus nerve root (>1840)*** and forming in the jugular foramen; see Durward (1951, p. 1037), Mitchell (1953, p. 176). For Wrisberg's use in macrodissected adult human, see p. 423 of 1800 reprinting; for Günther's use in macrodissected adult human, see pp. 62–63. It was perhaps first clearly identified as the *trunk of sixth pair (Vesalius, 1543a)*.

TRANSLATIONS:

1. *truncus nervi vagi (Wrisberg, 1786)*
   Original Latin form of ***vagus nerve trunk (Wrisberg, 1786; Günther, 1786)***; see Wrisberg reprint (1800, p. 423).

EARLIER REFERENCES:

Earlier synonyms:

1. *trunk of sixth pair (Vesalius, 1543a)*
   Synonym for macrodissected adult human ***vagus nerve trunk (Wrisberg, 1786; Günther, 1786)***; see Richardson & Carman translation (2002, p. 195).
2. *stem of sixth pair of cerebral nerves (Vesalius, 1543a)*
   Synonym for *trunk of sixth pair (Vesalius, 1543a)*; see Richardson & Carman translation (2002, p. 196-*N,O*).
3. *stock of sixth pair of nerves of brain (Geminus, 1553)*
   Synonym for macrodissected adult human *stem of sixth pair of cerebral nerves (Vesalius, 1543a)*; originally spelled *stocke of syxte payre of synowes of brayne*, see *The table of the figures of synowes.*
4. *trunk of wandring pair (Willis, 1664)*
   Synonym for macrodissected adult human ***vagus nerve trunk (Wrisberg, 1786; Günther, 1786)***; see Pordage translation (1681, p. 147). Modern spelling is *trunk of wandering pair.*
5. *trunk of eighth pair of nerves (Vieussens, 1684)*
   Synonym for macrodissected adult human ***vagus nerve trunk (Wrisberg, 1786; Günther, 1786)***; Table 23-*E*.
6. *pneumogastric nerve trunk (Meckel, 1817)*
   Synonym for macrodissected adult human ***vagus nerve trunk (Wrisberg, 1786; Günther, 1786)***; see translation (1832, Vol. 3, p. 45).

PARTLY CORRESPONDS:

1. *branches in thorax to esophagus from sixth pair of nerves (Galen, c173)*
   Included ***upper esophageal branches of vagus nerve (Cloquet, 1828)*** and ***esophageal plexus (Haller, 1762)*** in macrodissected adult beef, pig, and/or macaque, but not human; see May translation (1968, pp. 367, 448–449, 694). They were described but not named for macrodissected adult human by Vesalius (1543a); see Richardson & Carman translation (2002, p. 199). Willis (1664) described for macrodissected adult human, "Small shoots sent out of the trunk of the wandring pair which are inserted by a long tract to the Oesophagus" (Pordage translation, 1681, Tab. 9-*r*).
2. *thyroid branch of vagus nerve trunk (Neubauer, 1772)*
   Described for macrodissected infant human as descending and dividing into two branches, one clearly going to thyroid gland; in the original Latin, *truncus paris octavi ramus thyroideus*; Table 3, Figure 3-*o*.
3. *communicating branches of recurrent and internal laryngeal nerves (Andersch & Soemmerring, 1792)*
   Apparently macrodissected adult human ***communicating branches (Winslow, 1733)*** between ***pharyngeal branches of vagus nerve (Wrisberg, 1786)*** and ***internal branch of superior laryngeal nerve (Fyfe, 1800)***; in the original Latin, *rami communicatorii nervi recurrentis et laryngei interni*, p. 139.
4. *communicating branch of recurrent nerves of neck and internal laryngeal nerves (Andersch, 1797)*
   Synonym for *communicating branches of recurrent and internal laryngeal nerves (Andersch & Soemmerring, 1792)*; in the original Latin, *ramum communicatorium nervi recurrentis colli et nervi laryngei internus*, p. 51.
5. *esophageal branches of pneumogastric nerve (Chaussier, 1809)*
   Synonym for macrodissected adult human *branches in thorax to esophagus from sixth pair of nerves (Galen, c173)*; in the original French, *R. aesophagiens.*
6. *anastomotic branch between anterior branch of second cervical nerve and vagus (Langenbeck, 1826–1830)*
   Macrodissected adult human ***communicating branch (Winslow, 1733)*** between ***spinal nerve ventral branch (>1840)*** of second ***cervical nerve (Galen, c173)*** and ***vagus nerve trunk (Wrisberg, 1786; Günther, 1786)***; in the original Latin, *ramus anastomoticus inter ramum anteriorem nervi cervicalis secundi et Vagum*; Fascicle III, Table XV-*n*.
7. *petrous part of tenth pair (Arnold, 1834)*
   Macrodissected adult human proximal segment of ***vagus nerve trunk (Wrisberg, 1786; Günther, 1786)*** within petrous part of temporal bone; in the original Latin, *par decimum, pars petrosa*, p. 13.
8. *petrous part of pneumogastric nerve (Arnold, 1834)*
   Synonym for *petrous part of tenth pair (Arnold, 1834)*; in the original Latin, *nervus pneumogastricus, pars petrosa*, p. 13.
9. *petrous part of vagus nerve (Arnold, 1834)*
   Synonym for *petrous part of tenth pair (Arnold, 1834)*; in the original Latin, *nervus vagus, pars petrosa*, p. 13.
10. *connection of petrous part of vagus nerve with internal branch of accessory nerve (Arnold, 1834)*
    Macrodissected adult human ***communicating branch (Winslow, 1733)*** between *petrous part of vagus nerve (Arnold, 1834)* and ***internal branch of accessory nerve trunk (Meckel, 1817)***; in the original Latin, *nervus vagus, pars petrosa, conjunctio cum ramo interno s. minore nervi accessori*, p. 14 & Table VI-*71*.
11. *cervical part of tenth pair (Arnold, 1834)*
    Macrodissected adult human segment of ***vagus nerve trunk (Wrisberg, 1786; Günther, 1786)*** in neck; in the original Latin, *par decimum pars cervicalis*, pp. 13, 14.
12. *cervical part of pneumogastric nerve (Arnold, 1834)*
    Synonym for *cervical part of tenth pair (Arnold, 1834)*; in the original Latin, *nervus pneumogastricus pars cervicalis*, pp. 13, 14.
13. *cervical part of vagus nerve (Arnold, 1834)*
    Synonym for *cervical part of tenth pair (Arnold, 1834)*; in the original Latin, *nervus vagus pars cervicalis*, pp. 13, 14.
14. *thoracic part of tenth pair (Arnold, 1834)*
    Macrodissected adult human segment of ***vagus nerve trunk (Wrisberg, 1786; Günther, 1786)*** in chest; in the original Latin, *par decimum pars thoracica*, pp. 13, 14.
15. *thoracic part of pneumogastric nerve (Arnold, 1834)*
    Synonym for *thoracic part of tenth pair (Arnold, 1834)*; in the original Latin, *nervus pneumogastricus pars thoracica*, pp. 13, 14.

16. *thoracic part of vagus nerve (Arnold, 1834)*
Synonym for *thoracic part of tenth pair (Arnold, 1834)*; in the original Latin, *nervus vagus pars thoracica*, pp. 13, 14.
17. *abdominal part of tenth pair (Arnold, 1834)*
Macrodissected adult human segment of ***vagus nerve trunk (Wrisberg, 1786; Günther, 1786)*** in abdomen; in the original Latin, *par decimum pars abdominalis*, pp. 13, 14.
18. *abdominal part of pneumogastric nerve (Arnold, 1834)*
Synonym for *abdominal part of tenth pair (Arnold, 1834)*; in the original Latin, *nervus pneumogastricus pars abdominalis*, pp. 13, 14.
19. *abdominal part of vagus nerve (Arnold, 1834)*
Synonym for *abdominal part of tenth pair (Arnold, 1834)*; in the original Latin, *nervus vagus pars abdominalis*, pp. 13, 14.
20. *tracheal branches of thoracic part of pneumogastric nerve (Cruveilhier, 1836)*
Macrodissected adult human branches of *thoracic part of pneumogastric nerve (Arnold, 1834)* mainly to dorsal (back or membranous) part of trachea; in the original French, *rameaux trachéens*, p. 964.

vallecula of cerebellum (Haller, 1762)

As described for macrodissected adult human, a deep longitudinal fossa on the ventral surface of the ***cerebellum (Aristotle)*** in the median plane. Its base is formed by the *inferior vermis (>1840)*, it is continuous with the ***posterior cerebellar notch (Chaussier, 1807)***, and the dorsal part of the ***medulla (Winslow, 1733)*** rests within it; see Carpenter (1976, p. 46 and Fig. 2.24), *Terminologia Anatomica* (1998, p. 118), *Dorland's* (2003, p. 2002). Also see Malacarne (1776; *valetta* in the original Italian, pp. 17, 20), Vicq d'Azyr (1786, p. 95), Burdach (1822, p. 49). It was beautifully illustrated by Vesalius; see ***[vallecula of cerebellum (Haller, 1762)] (Vesalius, 1543a)***.

TRANSLATIONS:

1. *vallecula cerebelli (Haller, 1762)*
Original Latin form of ***vallecula of cerebellum (Haller, 1762)***; p. 71.
2. *valley of cerebellum (Reil, 1807–1808a)*
Translation of *vallecula cerebelli (Haller, 1762)* by Mayo (1822, p. 21).

EARLIER REFERENCES:

Illustrated, not named or described:

1. ***[vallecula of cerebellum (Haller, 1762)] (Vesalius, 1543a)***
Beautifully illustrated for macrodissected adult human; see Singer translation (1952, Fig. 9 at *C, E* on p. 105).

LATER SYNONYMS:

1. *valleculam (Soemmerring, 1778)*
Synonym for macrodissected adult human *vallecula cerebelli (Haller, 1762)*; in the phrase "valleculam lobis interjacentem relinquunt" (p. 61).
2. *vallecula inter lobos cerebri (Soemmerring, 1778)*
Synonym for macrodissected adult human *valleculam (Soemmerring, 1778)*; p. 173, Table I-*E*. Seemingly a typographical error for *vallecula inter lobos cerebelli*.
3. *great median fissure of cerebellum (Cruveilhier, 1836)*
Synonym for macrodissected adult human ***vallecula of cerebellum (Haller, 1762)***; in the original French, *grande scissure médiane du Cervelet*, p. 620.

PARTLY CORRESPONDS:

1. *median fossa (Gordon, 1815)*
Dorsal (posterior) part of macrodissected adult human ***vallecula of cerebellum (Haller, 1762)***; p. 108, see definition in Foster (1892, p. 1634).

ventral anterior cingulate area (Brodmann, 1909)

As described with cellular architecture for adult human, the ventral part of the ***anterior cingulate area (Brodmann, 1909)***; pp. 147–148. It was not identified by 1840.

TRANSLATIONS:

1. *area cingularis anterior ventralis (Brodmann, 1909)*
Original Latin form of ***ventral anterior cingulate area (Brodmann, 1909)***; p. 147.

EARLIER REFERENCES:

Earlier synonyms:

1. *area 24 (Brodmann, 1909)*
Synonym for adult human ***ventral anterior cingulate area (Brodmann, 1909)***; in the original German, *Feld 24*, see pp. 147–148.

ventral cord (Anderson, 1837)

An invertebrate ***central nerve cord (Serres, 1824–1826)***, or the segment of such a cord, lying caudal to the ***supraesophageal ganglion (Grant, 1834a)*** and ventral to the digestive system, and bearing ***ventral ganglia (Anderson, 1837)***. From a systems architecture perspective ***ventral ganglia (Anderson, 1837)*** and ***ventral cord trunk (>1840)*** together form a ***ventral cord (Anderson, 1837)***. The proximal (rostral) end of a ***ventral cord (Anderson, 1837)*** is often formed by a *subesophageal ganglion (Straus Durckheim, 1828)*. See Bullock & Horridge (1965, pp. 662, 802–803). For Anderson's use in macrodissected earthworm see Plate I, Figure 10-*d*. It was first described as a *cord (Malpighi, 1669)* or *spinal medulla (Malpighi, 1669)* in silkworm.

EARLIER REFERENCES:

Earlier synonyms:

1. *spinal medulla (Malpighi, 1669)*
Synonym for silkworm ***ventral cord (Anderson, 1837)*** viewed with a microscope; in the original Latin, *medulla spinalis*, pp. 45–46, Table VI.
2. *cord (Malpighi, 1669)*
Synonym for *spinal medulla (Malpighi, 1669)*; in the original Latin, *chorda*, pp. 45–46. Cuvier (1800, Vol. 2, p. 359) used it generally for invertebrates.
3. *spinal rope (Willis, 1672)*
Synonym for insect *spinal medulla (Malpighi, 1669)*; in the original Latin, *spinali funi*, see Pordage translation (1683, p. 8). *Spinali funi* is also translated *spinal cord*.
4. *spinal medulla (Lyonnet, 1762)*
Clearly synonym for ***ventral cord (Anderson, 1837)*** in goat moth larva. As compared to human where

spinal cord (Galen, c162–c166) descends along the back, "cette moëlle descend, au contraire, le long du ventre" (p. 97); in the original French, *moëlle épinière*.

5. *lower nerve cord (Cuvier, 1800)*
Synonym for ***ventral cord (Anderson, 1837)*** in insect larva; in the original French, *cordon nerveux situé au dessous*, p. 321. Carus (1814, p. 90) used the German, *untere Ganglienkette*, p. 90.
6. *ganglion chain (Carus, 1814)*
Synonym for ***ventral cord (Anderson, 1837)***, viewed with a microscope in annelids; in the original German, *Ganglienkette*, p. 91. Carus noted that it is a characteristic distinction from vertebrates; see *nerve ring around esophagus (Carus, 1814)*.
7. *lower nerve chain (Carus, 1814)*
Synonym for ***ventral cord (Anderson, 1837)***, viewed with a microscope in annelid worms; in the original German, *untere Ganglienkette*, p. 91.
8. *abdominal medulla (Carus, 1818)*
Synonym for ***ventral cord (Anderson, 1837)***, viewed with a microscope in describing earthworm; in the original German, *Bauchmark*, Table V, Figures II-*c*, VI.
9. *ganglionated nervous cord (Müller, 1834)*
Synonym for ***ventral cord (Anderson, 1837)*** in segmented invertebrates; see translation (1838, p. 595).
10. *abdominal chord (Grant, 1834a)*
Synonym for ***ventral cord (Anderson, 1837)*** used first for annelids; p. 487.
11. *abdominal column (Grant, 1834a)*
Synonym for ***ventral cord (Anderson, 1837)*** used first for annelids; p. 487.
12. *ganglionated spinal cord (Grainger, 1837)*
Synonym for macrodissected ***ventral cord (Anderson, 1837)*** of an "articulated animal" (Fig. 4-*A,B*).
13. *abdominal nervous cord (Anderson, 1837)*
Synonym for macrodissected ***ventral cord (Anderson, 1837)*** of animals like leech; p. 10.
14. *ganglionic abdominal cord (Anderson, 1837)*
Synonym for macrodissected ***ventral cord (Anderson, 1837)*** of insects, for example; p. 16.

LATER SYNONYMS:

1. *ventral nervous cord (Anderson, 1837)*
Synonym for ***ventral cord (Anderson, 1837)*** in for example the water stick (*Ranatra linearis*); Plate I, Figure 11.

ventral cord trunk (>1840)

A ***central nervous system white matter tract (>1840)*** for an invertebrate ***ventral cord (Anderson, 1837)***, with ***central ganglia (>1840)*** distributed along its length. Not clearly described by 1840.

ventral external arcuate fibers (>1840)

As described for macrodissected adult human, small bundles of ***axons (Kölliker, 1896)*** arising from the ***arcuate nucleus of medulla (>1840)*** and, after crossing the median plane in the ***ventral median fissure of medulla (>1840)*** extending laterally, caudally, and dorsally to enter the contralateral ***inferior cerebellar peduncle (Günther, 1786)***; see Mettler (1948, Figs. 191, 193, 195), Williams & Warwick (1980, p. 916 and Fig. 7.66), *Terminologia Anatomica* (1998, p. 109), *Dorland's* (2003, p. 693). Dorsal external arcuate fibers correspond to the cuneocerebellar tract; see Mettler (1948, p. 264), Carpenter (1976, p. 296), Williams & Warwick (1980, p. 916), *Dorland's* (2003, p. 693 under *fibrae arcuatae externae dorsales*). The ***ventral external arcuate fibers (>1840)*** were first identified as *processus arciformis (Santorini, 1724)*.

TRANSLATIONS:

1. *fibrae arcuatae externae ventrales (>1840)*
Current Latin form of ***ventral external arcuate fibers (>1840)***; see *Dorland's* (2003, p. 693).

EARLIER REFERENCES:

Earlier synonyms:

1. *processus arciformis (Santorini, 1724)*
Term used for first identification of macrodissected adult human ***ventral external arcuate fibers (>1840)***; p. 62; also see Santorini (1775; Tab. II-*u*) and Meyer (1971, p. 12).
2. *transverse bundles of medullary fibers (Monro, 1783)*
Synonym for macrodissected adult human *processus arciformis (Santorini, 1724)*, on surface of ***pyramids (Willis, 1664)***; Table V-Q.
3. *transverse medullary bundles (Monro, 1783)*
Synonym for *transverse bundles of medullary fibers (Monro, 1783)*; p. 28, Table VI-*T*.
4. *transverse interweaving (Gall & Spurzheim, 1810)*
Synonym for macrodissected adult human *processus arciformis (Santorini, 1724)*; in the original French, *entrelacement transversal*, pp. 276, 314, 350.
5. *transverse band behind olivary ganglion (Gall & Spurzheim, 1810)*
Synonym for macrodissected adult human *processus arciformis (Santorini, 1724)*; in the original French, *bande transversale derrière le ganglion olivaire*, Table XIII-66.
6. *arching fascicles (Serres, 1824–1826)*
Apparently synonym for macrodissected adult human *processus arciformis (Santorini, 1724)*; in the original French, *faisceaux en forme d'arcs*, Plate XVI, Figure 289-2.
7. *arcuate filaments (Rolando, 1825a)*
Synonym for macrodissected adult quadruped *processus arciformis (Santorini, 1724)*; in the original French, *filamens arciformes*; pp. 18, 20; Table I, Figure 1-*f.a.*
8. *arcuate fibers (Rolando, 1825a)*
Synonym for macrodissected adult human *processus arciformis (Santorini, 1724)*; in the original French, *fibres arciformes*; Table VI, Figure 4-*f.a.* Arnold (1838b, Tab. II, Figs. 4-*g*, 6-*f*) gave the Latin, *fibrae arciformes*.
9. *pyramidal commissure (Arnold, 1838a)*
Synonym for macrodissected adult human ***ventral external arcuate fibers (>1840)***; in the original Latin, *commissura pyramidum*, p. 21.

10. *external arcuate fibers (>1840)*
Synonym for macrodissected adult human ***ventral external arcuate fibers (>1840)***; see Nieuwenhuys et al. (2008, p. 198 and Figs. 6.22, 24).

ventral funiculus (>1840)

As described for macrodissected adult human and other mammals, the ventral topographic division of the ***funiculi of spinal cord (Burdach, 1822)***, between the ***ventral median fissure of spinal cord (>1840)*** in the median plane and the ***ventral root central parts (>1840)*** and ***lateral funiculus (Burdach, 1822)*** laterally; see Carpenter (1976, pp. 214–216 and Fig. 9.2), Williams & Warwick (1980, p. 868 and Fig. 7.36), *Terminologia Anatomica* (1998, p. 107). It was first identified in illustration by Blasius; see ***[ventral funiculus (>1840)] (Blasius, 1666)***.

EARLIER REFERENCES:

Illustrated, not named or described:

1. ***[ventral funiculus (>1840)] (Blasius, 1666)***
Clearly illustrated for macrodissected adult human; Figures 10, 11, 18.

Earlier synonyms:

1. *anterior bundle of anterior funiculus (Rosenthal, 1815)*
Synonym for macrodissected adult human ***ventral funiculus (>1840)***; in the original German, *vordern Bündle des vordern Strang(s)*, p. 27; see *anterior funiculus (Rosenthal, 1815)* and Burdach (1822, pp. 31, 34–35).
2. *anterior medullary cord (Meckel, 1817)*
Synonym for macrodissected adult human ***ventral funiculus (>1840)***; see translation (1832, Vol. 2, p. 413).
3. *anterior funiculus (Burdach, 1822)*
Synonym for macrodissected adult human ***ventral funiculus (>1840)***; in the original German, *vordern Strang*, p. 31. Burdach divided it into two parts, *inner* and *outer*. Blasius (1674, p. 59) may have mentioned the anterior funiculus.
4. *fasciculus olivarum (Burdach, 1822)*
Synonym for macrodissected adult human ***ventral funiculus (>1840)***; in the original German, *Olivenbündel*, p. 33 and Table III-*d*.
5. *olivary bundle (Burdach, 1822)*
English form of *fasciculus olivarum (Burdach, 1822)*; *olivary fascicle* is another form.
6. *anterior column of spinal marrow (Bell, 1822)*
Synonym for macrodissected adult human and other mammalian ***ventral funiculus (>1840)***; p. 292.
7. *anterior fascicle of spinal medulla (Bellingeri, 1823)*
Synonym for macrodissected adult human and other mammalian ***ventral funiculus (>1840)***; in the original Latin (plural), *fasciculi anteriores medullae spinalis*, Table 1, Figure 1-*d*.
8. *cerebral fascicle (Bellingeri, 1823)*
Synonym for macrodissected adult human and other mammalian ***ventral funiculus (>1840)***; in the original Latin (plural), *fasciculi cerebrales*, p. 9.
9. *abdominal cord of spinal medulla (Desmoulins, 1825)*
Synonym for macrodissected adult human and other mammalian ***ventral funiculus (>1840)***; in the original French (plural), *cordons abdominaux de la moelle épinière*, for example, p. 221 and Plate XIII, Figure 1-*c.a*.
10. *anterior cord of spinal medulla (Desmoulins, 1825)*
Synonym for macrodissected adult human and other mammalian ***ventral funiculus (>1840)***; in the original French (plural), *cordons antérieurs de la moelle épinière*, for example, p. 221 and Plate XIII, Figure 1-*c.a*.
11. *inferior cord (Desmoulins, 1825)*
Synonym for macrodissected adult human and other mammalian ***ventral funiculus (>1840)***; in the original French (plural), *cordon inférieure*, Plate XIII, Figure 2-*x,y*.
12. *anterior part of white substance of spinal medulla (Arnold, 1838b)*
Synonym for macrodissected adult human ***ventral funiculus (>1840)***; in the original Latin (plural), *substantiae albae pars antica*, Plate II, Figure 16-*c*.

ventral ganglia (Anderson, 1837)

The invertebrate ***central ganglia (>1840)*** lying caudal to the ***supraesophageal ganglion (Grant, 1834a)*** and ventral to the digestive system as part of a ***ventral cord (Anderson, 1837)***; see Bullock & Horridge (1965, pp. 662, 802–803). For Anderson's use in crustaceans, arachnoids, insects, and other invertebrates see p. 12. They were first clearly described by Swammerdam, see ***[ventral ganglia (Anderson, 1837)] (Swammerdam, c1675)***.

EARLIER REFERENCES:

Illustrated and described, not named:

1. ***[ventral ganglia (Anderson, 1837)] (Swammerdam, c1675)***
Swammerdam clearly described them for arthropods and annelids as being in front of (ventral to) the digestive system in dissections viewed under the microscope; see translation (1758; e.g., p. 138, Tab. XXII, Fig. 6).

Earlier synonyms:

1. *ganglia of spinal medulla (Lyonnet, 1762)*
Synonym for ***ventral ganglia (Anderson, 1837)***, viewed with a microscope in goat moth larva; in the original French, *moëlle épinière, ses ganglions*, see pp. 92, 97 and *spinal medulla (Lyonnet, 1762)*. Treviranus (Treviranus & Treviranus, 1816–1821, Vol. 2, p. 17) used the German, *Rückenmarksknoten*, for silverfish.
2. *ganglia of lower nerve cord (Carus, 1814)*
Synonym for ***ventral ganglia (Anderson, 1837)***, viewed with a microscope in insects and crustaceans; in the original German, *die Ganglien des untern Nervenstrangs*, p. 90.
3. *lower ganglia (Carus, 1814)*
Synonym for ***ventral ganglia (Anderson, 1837)***, viewed with a microscope in insects and crustaceans; in the original German, *untern Ganglien*, p. 90.

4. *anterior ganglia (Serres, 1824–1826)*
Synonym for ***ventral ganglia (Anderson, 1837)***, viewed with a microscope in a variety of invertebrates; in the original French, *ganglions antérieurs*, Vol. 2, p. 21.
5. *abdominal ganglia (Grant, 1834a)*
Synonym, at least sometimes, for ***ventral ganglia (Anderson, 1837)***, here for leech; p. 487.
6. *suboesophageal ganglia (Newport, 1834)*
Synonym for ***ventral ganglia (Anderson, 1837)***, originally applied to hawkmoth and lobster, pp. 390, 392, 406.
7. *infraoesophageal ganglia (Anderson, 1837)*
Synonym for *suboesophageal ganglia (Newport, 1834)* in annelids, for example; pp. 10, 13.

PARTLY CORRESPONDS:

1. *first ganglion of neck (Lyonnet, 1762)*
Most rostral of the ***ventral ganglia (Anderson, 1837)***, applied to macrodissected adult caterpillar viewed with magnification; in the original French, *premier ganglion du cou*, p. 523.
2. *lower ganglion of nerve ring (Carus, 1818)*
Most rostral of the ***ventral ganglia (Anderson, 1837)***, applied to bivalves; in the original German, *unteres Ganglion dieses Nervenringes*, Table II, Figure X-*c*.
3. *ganglion after esophagus (Serres, 1824–1826)*
Most rostral of the ***ventral ganglia (Anderson, 1837)***, applied to molluscs and other invertebrates; in the original French (plural), *ganglions méta-oesophagiens*, Vol. 2, p. 13.
4. *suboesophageal ganglia (Straus Durckheim, 1828)*
First or most rostral pair of ***ventral ganglia (Anderson, 1837)***, applied to beetle, *Melolontha*, and certain other invertebrates; in the original French, *ganglions sous-oesophagiens*, pp. 365, 394–395. American spelling is *subesophageal ganglia*.
5. *infra-oesophageal ganglia (Müller, 1834)*
Synonym for *suboesophageal ganglia (Straus Durckheim, 1828)*, first used for mollusc; see translation (1838, Vol. 1, p. 594). Grant (1834b, p. 514) applied it to all segmented invertebrates (articulata).

ventral hippocampal commissure (Craigie, 1925)

As described in macrodissected adult human, and mammal generally with histological methods for ***axons (Kölliker, 1896)***, the rostral differentiation of the ***hippocampal commissures (Johnston, 1913)***, rostral to the ***intermediate hippocampal commissure (>1840)*** and containing commissural ***axons (Kölliker, 1896)*** from the ***hippocampal region (Swanson et al., 1987)***; see Swanson and Cowan (1977), Swanson et al. (1978). A clearer term would be *rostral hippocampal commissure*. For Craigie's use in adult rat with the Weigert myelin method see p. 103 and Plate XXVI. It was perhaps first delineated as the *lyra minima (Bergmann, 1831)*.

EARLIER REFERENCES:

Earlier synonyms:

1. *lyra minima (Bergmann, 1831)*
Possibly macrodissected adult human ***ventral hippocampal commissure (Craigie, 1925)***; pp. 75–77, Table II-*r*.
2. *ventral commissure of Ammon's horn (Kölliker, 1896)*
Synonym for adult human ***ventral hippocampal commissure (Craigie, 1925)*** observed with histological methods for ***axons (Kölliker, 1896)***; in the original German, *ventrale Kommissur der Ammonshörner*, p. 776. Dejerine & Dejerine-Klumpke (1901, pp. 295–296) credited Ganser (1882, p. 659?) with first noting a ventral part of *psalterium (Ganser, 1882)* in mole.

LATER SYNONYMS:

1. *commissure of fimbria (Craigie, 1925)*
Synonym listed for adult rodent ***ventral hippocampal commissure (Craigie, 1925)***; p. 103.

ventral horn (>1840)

As described for macrodissected adult human, and for mammal in general with cellular architecture and connections, the ***gray matter region (Swanson & Bota, 2010)*** of the ***spinal cord (Galen, c162–166)*** lying ventral to the ***intermediate spinal zone (>1840)*** and characterized by pools of large somatic motor ***neurons Waldeyer, 1891)***. For a good comparison of classical ***spinal cord (Galen, c162–166)*** parceling with the laminar scheme proposed by Rexed (1952) see Carpenter (1976, pp. 222–229); also see Cajal (1899–1904, Vol. 1, pp. 225–228), Swanson (1998–1999, pp. 212–213). The ***ventral horn (>1840)*** was first distinguished by Blasius; see ***[ventral horn (>1840)] (Blasius, 1666)***.

EARLIER REFERENCES:

Illustrated and described, not named:

1. *[ventral horn (>1840)] (Blasius, 1666)*
Very clearly illustrated for macrodissected adult human, showing it is thicker or fatter than ***dorsal horn (>1840)***; see Schulte & Endtz (1977, p. 13).

Earlier synonyms:

1. *anterior cineritious substance (Monro, 1783)*
Monro roughly indicated difference in macrodissected adult human between ***ventral horn (>1840)*** and ***dorsal horn (>1840)***, although his account is vague, "...when either of these two cords [halves of ***spinal cord (Galen, c162–c166)***] is accurately examined it will be found to be subdivided by a slight furrow, into a small posterior cord and a large anterior cord. In the former, fasciculi of longitudinal fibres readily appear; in the latter, the disposition of the medullary fibres is much less evident...When we cut the spinal marrow transversely, the internal cineritious substance makes a cruciform appearance [*X*-shaped], or consists of four portions, one corresponding to each of the four cords of which I have observed it consists." (pp. 28–29). In contemporaneous work, Vicq d'Azyr (1784, pp. 600–601) more accurately divided lateral part of spinal *ash-colored substance (Winslow, 1733)* into anterior end, body or central part, and posterior end.
2. *anterior end of lateral part of spinal ash-colored substance (Vicq d'Azyr, 1784)*
Roughly synonymous with macrodissected adult human ***ventral horn (>1840)***; in the original French,

l'extrémité antérieure, p. 601, see Clarke & O'Malley translation (1996, p. 269).

3. *anterior crus of gray substance (Keuffel, 1810)*
Roughly synonymous with macrodissected adult human ***ventral horn (>1840)*** viewed in transverse section; in the original Latin (plural), *crura anteriora substantiae cinereae*, Figure 1-*i,k*.
4. *anterior gray column (Burdach, 1819)*
Roughly synonymous with macrodissected adult human ***ventral horn (>1840)***; in the original German, *vordern graue Strang*, p. 134. Also see Burdach (1822, p. 30).
5. *anterior horn of cineritious substance (Bellingeri, 1823)*
Synonym for ***ventral horn (>1840)*** of macrodissected one-month infant and adult human; in the original Latin (plural), *cornua anteriora substantiae cinereae*, p. 6 and Table I, Figure 25.
6. *inferior gray fascicles of central medulla (Desmoulins, 1825)*
Roughly synonymous with macrodissected adult human ***ventral horn (>1840)***; in the original French, *faisceaux inférieurs gris du centre de la moelle*, p. 244 and Plate XIII, Figure 5.
7. *anterior horn of medulla (Quain, 1828)*
Roughly synonymous with macrodissected adult human ***ventral horn (>1840)***; p. 609.
8. *anterior horn of spinal cord (Quain, 1828)*
Roughly synonymous with macrodissected adult human ***ventral horn (>1840)***; p. 720.
9. *anterior crus of spinal medulla (Arnold, 1838b)*
Roughly synonymous with macrodissected adult human ***ventral horn (>1840)***; in the original Latin (plural), *crura anteriora*, Table II, Figure 2-*d*.
10. *anterior gray fascicle (Wagner, 1839)*
Roughly synonymous with macrodissected adult human ***ventral horn (>1840)***; in the original Latin, *fasciculus cinereus anterior*, Table XXVII, Figure 10-*8*.

ventral intersegmental tract (>1840)

As described in macrodissected adult human, and mammal generally with histological methods for ***axons (Kölliker, 1896)***, a narrow ***central nervous system white matter tract (>1840)*** in the deepest part of the ***ventral funiculus (>1840)***, predominantly but not exclusively formed by ***axons (Kölliker, 1896)*** connecting different ***gray matter regions (Swanson & Bota, 2010)*** within the ***spinal cord (Galen, c162–c166)*** itself; see Mettler (1948, pp. 236–237), Crosby et al. (1962, p. 108), Williams & Warwick (1980, p. 877 and Figs. 7.43–44), called *anterior intersegmental tract (>1840)*, and *Dorland's* (2003, p. 678 under *fasciculus proprius anterior medullae spinalis*). It was not identified by 1840.

EARLIER REFERENCES:

Earlier synonyms:

1. *anterior fasciculus proprius (>1840)*
Synonym for macrodissected adult human ***ventral intersegmental tract (>1840)***; see *Terminologia Anatomica* (1998, p. 107).
2. *ventral fasciculus proprius (>1840)*
Synonym for macrodissected adult human ***ventral intersegmental tract (>1840)***; see Williams & Warwick (1980, Fig. 7.44), *Terminologia Anatomica* (1998, p.107).
3. *anterior intersegmental tract (>1840)*
Synonym for macrodissected adult human ***ventral intersegmental tract (>1840)***; see Williams & Warwick (1980, p. 877).

ventral lateral geniculate nucleus (>1840)

Based on cellular architecture and connections in mammal, the small dorsolateral part of the ***ventral part of thalamus (Herrick, 1910)*** lying dorsal to the bulk of the ***reticular thalamic nucleus (>1840)*** with a massive input from ***retina (Herophilus, c335–c280 BC)*** but no output to ***cerebral cortex (>1840)***; see Jones (1985, Ch. 15.2). Also see ***dorsal lateral geniculate nucleus (>1840)***. Not delineated by 1840.

ventral median fissure of medulla (>1840)

As described for macrodissected adult human, the midsagittal groove between right and left ***pyramid (Willis, 1664)*** visible on the ventral surface of the ***medulla (Winslow, 1733)*** and a rostral extension of the ***ventral median fissure of spinal cord (>1840)*** interrupted near the border between ***medulla (Winslow, 1733)*** and ***spinal cord (Galen, c162–c166)*** by the ***pyramidal decussation (Reil, 1809c)***, and ending rostrally as the ***foramen cecum of medulla (>1840)***; see Williams & Warwick (1980, p. 897, called *anterior median fissure*), *Terminologia Anatomica* (1998, p. 108). It was first identified by Vesalius; see ***[ventral median fissure of medulla (>1840)] (Vesalius, 1543a)***.

EARLIER REFERENCES:

Illustrated, not named or described:

1. ***[ventral median fissure of medulla (>1840)] (Vesalius, 1543a)***
Illustrated without mentioning for macrodissected adult human; see Richardson & Carman translation (2002, p. 168).

Illustrated and described, not named:

1. ***[ventral median fissure of medulla (>1840)] (Santorini, 1724)***
Described for macrodissected adult human; pp. 61–62. Santorini also clearly illustrated it later (1775, Tab. II-*).

Earlier synonyms:

1. *sulcus corpora pyramidalia profunde dividens (Soemmerring, 1778)*
Synonym for macrodissected adult human ***ventral median fissure of medulla (>1840)***; p. 178.
2. *rimula Tarini (Günther, 1786)*
Eponym for macrodissected adult human ***ventral median fissure of medulla (>1840)***; p. 23.
3. *anterior sulcus of medulla oblongata (Vicq d'Azyr, 1786)*
Synonym for macrodissected adult human ***ventral median fissure of medulla (>1840)***; Plate XXXI, Figure I-3,4.

4. *basilar furrow of medulla oblongata (Reil, 1807–1808a)*
   Synonym for macrodissected adult human ***ventral median fissure of medulla (>1840)***; see Mayo translation (1822, p. 41).
5. *anterior median furrow of medulla oblongata (Mayo, 1827)*
   Synonym for macrodissected adult human ***ventral median fissure of medulla (>1840)***; Plate I, Figure 3-*o*.
6. *anterior median sulcus of medulla oblongata (Quain, 1832)*
   Synonym for macrodissected adult human ***ventral median fissure of medulla (>1840)***; p. 636.
7. *median sulcus of bulb (Cruveilhier, 1836)*
   Synonym for macrodissected adult human ***ventral median fissure of medulla (>1840)***; in the original French, *silllon médian du bulbe*, p. 584.
8. *longitudinal fissure of medulla oblongata (Arnold, 1838b)*
   Synonym for macrodissected adult human ***ventral median fissure of medulla (>1840)***; in the original Latin, *fissura longitudinalis medullae oblongatae*, Table II, Figure 4-*h*.
9. *anterior longitudinal fissure (Arnold, 1838b)*
   Synonym for macrodissected adult human ***ventral median fissure of medulla (>1840)***; in the original Latin, *fissura longitudinalis anterior*, Table II, Figure 13-*a*.

ventral median fissure of spinal cord (>1840)

As described for macrodissected adult human, the deep longitudinal groove separating right and left ***ventral funiculus (>1840)*** on the ventral surface of the ***spinal cord (Galen, c162–c166)*** in the median plane, and extending rostrally as the ***ventral median fissure of medulla (>1840)***; see Williams & Warwick (1980, p. 864 and Figure 7.36, *called anterior median fissure*). It was probably first noted by Piccolomini; see ***[ventral median fissure of spinal cord (>1840)] (Piccolomini, 1587)***.

EARLIER REFERENCES:

Described, not named or illustrated:

1. ***[ventral median fissure of spinal cord (>1840)] (Piccolomini, 1587)***
   Apparently described for macrodissected adult human; see Bauhin (1605, p. 632) and Crooke translation (1615, p. 482).

Earlier synonyms:

1. *minor anterior fissure (Blasius, 1666)*
   Synonym for macrodissected adult human ***ventral median fissure of spinal cord (>1840)***; Figure X-*f*, also see Haller (1762, p. 82).
2. *anterior sulcus (Vieussens, 1684)*
   Synonym for macrodissected adult human ***ventral median fissure of spinal cord (>1840)***; p. 601, see translation in Clarke & O'Malley (1996, p. 269).
3. *anterior partition (Pourfour du Petit, 1710)*
   Synonym for macrodissected adult human ***ventral median fissure of spinal cord (>1840)***; in the original French, *la division anterieure*, Letter 1, p. 15, see translation in Clarke & O'Malley (1996, p. 265).
4. *anterior fissure (Vicq d'Azyr, 1784)*
   Synonym for macrodissected adult human ***ventral median fissure of spinal cord (>1840)***; in the original French, *le sillon antérieur*, p. 599.
5. *anterior median fissure of spinal cord (Gall & Spurzheim, 1810)*
   Synonym for macrodissected adult human ***ventral median fissure of spinal cord (>1840)***; in the original French, *fissure médiane antérieure*, see pp. 41, 230.
6. *anterior median fissure of neural mass of spinal column (Gall & Spurzheim, 1810)*
   Synonym for macrodissected adult human ***ventral median fissure of spinal cord (>1840)***; see pp. 41, 230.
7. *anterior longitudinal groove (Tiedemann, 1816)*
   Synonym for macrodissected fetal human ***ventral median fissure of spinal cord (>1840)***; see translation (1826, p. 30).
8. *inferior sulcus of spinal medulla (Bojanus, 1819–1821)*
   Synonym for macrodissected adult turtle ***ventral median fissure of spinal cord (>1840)***; in the original Latin, *sulcus medullae spinalis inferior*, Figures 95–100, part *l*.
9. *anterior median sulcus (Bellingeri, 1823)*
   Synonym for macrodissected adult mammalian, including human, ***ventral median fissure of spinal cord (>1840)***; in the original Latin, *sulcus medius anterior*, Table I, Figure 1-*a*.
10. *anterior median furrow (Mayo, 1823)*
    Synonym for macrodissected adult human ***ventral median fissure of spinal cord (>1840)***; p. 133.
11. *mesial abdominal fissure (Spurzheim, 1826)*
    Synonym for macrodissected adult human ***ventral median fissure of spinal cord (>1840)***; p. 65.
12. *anterior middle furrowed line of spinal cord (Knox, 1832)*
    Knox's version of macrodissected adult human *anterior median fissure of spinal cord (Gall & Spurzheim, 1810)*; Plate XXIII, Figure 1-*c,d*.
13. *longitudinal fissure of spinal medulla (Arnold, 1838b)*
    Synonym for macrodissected adult human ***ventral median fissure of spinal cord (>1840)***; in the original Latin, *fissura longitudinalis medulla spinalis*, Table II, Figure 2-*b*.

ventral part of thalamus (Herrick, 1910)

As described for macrodissected adult human, and based on cellular architecture and development in vertebrate, the most ventral of the three topographic subdivisions of the ***thalamus (His, 1893a)***, lying between ***dorsal part of thalamus (Herrick, 1910)*** dorsally and ***hypothalamus (Kuhlenbeck, 1927)*** ventrally. Based on cellular architecture and connections in mammal it has three main parts, ***zona incerta (>1840)*** ventromedially, ***reticular thalamic nucleus (>1840)*** laterally, and ***ventral lateral geniculate nucleus (>1840)*** dorsolaterally; see Jones (1985, p. 701). For Herrick's use in vertebrate see p. 498, as well as pp. 468–469, 492. It was not distinguished by 1840.

TRANSLATIONS:

1. *pars ventralis thalami (Herrick, 1910)*
 Original Latin form of ***ventral part of thalamus (Herrick, 1910)***; see p. 498.

ventral posterior cingulate area (Brodmann, 1909)

As described with cellular architecture for adult human, the ventral part of the ***posterior cingulate area (Brodmann, 1909)***; p. 147. It was not identified by 1840.

TRANSLATIONS:

1. *area cingularis posterior ventralis (Brodmann, 1909)*
 Original Latin form of ***ventral posterior cingulate area (Brodmann, 1909)***; p. 147.

EARLIER REFERENCES:

Earlier synonyms:

1. *area 23 (Brodmann, 1909)*
 Synonym for adult human ***ventral posterior cingulate area (Brodmann, 1909)***; in the original German, *Feld* 23, see p. 147.

ventral premammillary nucleus (>1840)

Based primarily on cellular architecture and connections in mammal, the component of the ***medial hypothalamic zone (Nauta & Haymaker, 1969)*** surrounded by ***ventromedial hypothalamic nucleus (>1840)*** rostrally, ***dorsal premammillary nucleus (>1840)*** dorsally, and ***mammillary body (Ludwig, 1779)*** caudally; see Swanson (1998, Table B, p. 206). It was not described by 1840.

ventral root (>1840)

As described for macrodissected adult human, a ***spinal nerve trunk (Frotscher, 1788)*** typically has associated with it a proximal bundle of ***ventral rootlets (>1840)*** arranged in two or three irregular rows over a distance of about 3 mm across the ventrolateral aspect of the ***spinal cord (Galen, c162–166)***. Collectively these ***ventral rootlets (>1840)*** form a ***ventral root (>1840)***; see Williams & Warwick (1980, p. 1086 and Figure 7.195A, called there *ventral nerve roots*), *Terminologia Anatomica* (1998, p. 113). They were clearly delineated by Coiter; see ***[ventral root (>1840)] (Coiter, 1572)***.

TRANSLATIONS:

1. *radix ventralis (>1840)*
 Current Latin form of ***ventral root (>1840)***; part of full term, *radix ventralis nervi spinalis*; see *Dorland's* (2003, p. 1566).

EARLIER REFERENCES:

Illustrated, not named or described:

1. ***[ventral root (>1840)] (Vesalius, 1543a)***
 Many clearly indicated in illustration of macrodissected adult human ***spinal cord (Galen, c162–c166)***; see Richardson & Carman translation (2002, p. 205, at *D*, for example). However, Vesalius never indicated distinction between ***dorsal roots (Spurzheim, 1826)*** and ***ventral roots (>1840)***.

Described, not named or illustrated:

1. ***[ventral root (>1840)] (Coiter, 1572)***
 Coiter clearly described ***ventral root (>1840)*** component of macrodissected adult human ***spinal nerves (Camper, 1760–1762)***. He referred to them as a row of *anterior medullar threads (Coiter, 1572)*, *anterior medullar filaments (Coiter, 1572)*, or *anterior medullar fibers (Coiter, 1572)*, more or less of which combine to form a ***nerve (Herophilus, c335–c280 BC)*** of greater or lesser thickness, respectively, and provided evidence that the substance of the ***spinal cord (Galen, c162–c166)*** contributes to them; see translation, pp. 115–117. The medullary threads are ***ventral rootlets (>1840)*** together constituting a ***ventral root (>1840)***. Rasmussen (1947) stated that Galen distinguished ***dorsal root (Spurzheim, 1826)*** and ***ventral root (>1840)***, but Rasmussen's source is unknown and his interpretation is not confirmed elsewhere; see Siegel (1970). More likely, Rasmussen's source confused ***dorsal root (Spurzheim, 1826)*** and ***ventral root (>1840)***, with ***spinal nerve dorsal branch (Meckel, 1817)*** and ***spinal nerve ventral branch (>1840)***, which Galen described extensively; see May (1968).

Earlier synonyms:

1. *anterior fasciculus (Winslow, 1733)*
 Synonym for macrodissected adult human ***ventral root (>1840)***; Section VI, p. 76; Section X, p. 45.
2. *anterior filaments (Huber, 1741)*
 Synonym for macrodissected adult human ***ventral roots (>1840)***; pp. 2–5, see translation in Clarke & O'Malley (1996, p. 267).
3. *anterior root (Asch, 1750)*
 Synonym for macrodissected 2-year-old infant human ***ventral root (>1840)***, which Asch described as made of filaments for ***cervical nerves (Galen, c173)***; in the original Latin, *radix antica*, p. 39 and Figure 1:*a–f*.
4. *anterior bundle (Monro, 1783)*
 Synonym for macrodissected adult human *anterior fasciculus (Winslow, 1733)*; Table 10, Figure 1-*N*.
5. *inferior root (Desmoulins, 1825)*
 Synonym for macrodissected adult vertebrate ***ventral root (>1840)***; in the original French (plural), *racines inférieures*, Plate XIII, Figure 1-*x*.
6. *abdominal root (Desmoulins, 1825)*
 Synonym for macrodissected adult vertebrate ***ventral root (>1840)***; in the original French (plural), *racines abdominales*, Plate XIII, Figure 1-*x*.
7. *motor root (Bell, 1829)*
 Synonym for macrodissected adult human ***ventral root (>1840)***; Plate IX, Figure 2-C.

ventral root central part (>1840)

As described in macrodissected adult human, and mammal generally with histological methods for ***axons (Kölliker, 1896)***, the set of ***ventral rootlets central part (>1840)*** that continues at the ventrolateral surface of the ***spinal cord (Galen, c162–c166)*** as a corresponding peripheral ***ventral root (>1840)***; see Nieuwenhuys et al. (2008, Figs. 6.6–10, unlabeled). Perhaps first clearly delineated by Rolando; see ***[ventral root central part (>1840)] (Rolando, 1825a)***.

EARLIER REFERENCES:

Illustrated and described, not named:

1. ***[ventral root central part (>1840)] (Rolando, 1825a)***
   Identified in macrodissected calf because Rolando delineated the ***ventral rootlets central part (>1840)***, the *very white lines meeting anterior roots of spinal nerves (Rolando, 1825a)*; Table VII, Figure 1-*z*.

ventral rootlets (>1840)

As described for macrodissected adult human, the set of individual filaments together forming a ***ventral root (>1840)***; see Williams & Warwick (1980, p. 1086), *Terminologia Anatomica* (1998, p. 133). They were first distinguished by Vesalius; see ***[ventral rootlets (>1840)] (Vesalius, 1543a)***.

EARLIER REFERENCES:

Illustrated, not named or described:

1. ***[ventral rootlets (>1840)] (Vesalius, 1543a)***
   Illustrated but not described for a number of macrodissected adult human ***spinal nerves (Camper, 1760–1762)***; see Richardson & Carman translation (2002, p. 205 at *C* and *D*, for example).

Earlier synonyms:

1. *anterior medullar threads (Coiter, 1572)*
   Synonym for macrodissected adult human ***ventral rootlets (>1840)***; see translation, p. 115.
2. *anterior medullar filaments (Coiter, 1572)*
   Synonym for macrodissected adult human ***ventral rootlets (>1840)***; see translation, p. 115.
3. *anterior medullar fibers (Coiter, 1572)*
   Synonym for macrodissected adult human ***ventral rootlets (>1840)***; see translation, p. 115.
4. *nervi à parte spinalis medulae anteriore procedents (Blasius, 1666)*
   Synonym for macrodissected adult human ***ventral rootlets (>1840)***; Figure X-*b*.
5. *anterior nervous filaments (Winslow, 1733)*
   Synonym for macrodissected adult human ***ventral rootlets (>1840)***; Section VI, p. 76.
6. *anterior bundles (Swan, 1830)*
   Synonym for macrodissected adult human ***ventral rootlets (>1840)***; Plate X, Figure 6-5.

ventral rootlets central part (>1840)

As described for macrodissected adult human, and mammal generally with histological methods for ***axons (Kölliker, 1896)***, the set of ***axon (Kölliker, 1896)*** bundles exiting the ***ventral horn (>1840)*** and coursing ventrolaterally to the edge of the ***spinal cord (Galen, c162–166)*** where they continue as corresponding peripheral ***ventral rootlets (>1840)***. One set of ***ventral rootlets central part (>1840)*** forms a ***ventral root central part (>1840)*** for a corresponding peripheral ***ventral root (>1840)***; see Nieuwenhuys et al. (2008, Figs. 6.6–10, unlabeled). They were perhaps first clearly delineated as *very white lines meeting anterior roots of spinal nerves (Rolando, 1825a)*.

EARLIER REFERENCES:

Earlier synonyms:

1. *very white lines meeting anterior roots of spinal nerves (Rolando, 1825a)*
   Synonym for macrodissected calf ***ventral rootlets central part (>1840)***; in the original French, *lignes très-blanches que répondent aux racines antérieures des nerfs spinaux*; Table VII, Figure 1-*z*. Rolando noted they are not layers of connective tissue.

ventral spinocerebellar tract (>1840)

As described for macrodissected adult human, a longitudinal **central nervous system white matter tract (>1840)** with a ***spinal ventral spinocerebellar tract (>1840)*** segment centered in the ***ventral funiculus (>1840)***, followed by ***medullary ventral spinocerebellar tract (>1840)*** and ***pontine ventral spinocerebellar tract (>1840)*** segments in the ***ventrolateral fascicle (>1840)***, with the ***pontine ventral spinocerebellar tract (>1840)*** entering the ***superior cerebellar peduncle (Procháska, 1800)***; see Carpenter (1976, pp. 251–252 and Fig. 10.10), *Terminologia Anatomica* (1998, p. 107). It was vaguely described by Reil; see ***[ventral spinocerebellar tract (>1840)] (Reil, 1809c)***.

EARLIER REFERENCES:

Described, not named or illustrated:

1. ***[ventral spinocerebellar tract (>1840)] (Reil, 1809c)***
   Described vaguely in macrodissected adult sheep; see Mayo translation (1823, p. 99).

Earlier synonyms:

1. *anterior spinocerebellar tract (>1840)*
   Synonym for macrodissected adult human ***ventral spinocerebellar tract (>1840)***; see *Terminologia Anatomica* (1998, p. 107).

ventral spinothalamic tract (>1840)

As described for adult human most clearly with experimental pathway tracing methods, two adjacent components of the ***spinothalamic tract (>1840)*** in the ***spinal cord (Galen, c162–c166)*** are distinguished for clinical and descriptive purposes, ***ventral spinothalamic tract (>1840)*** centered in deeper regions of the ***ventral funiculus (>1840)***, and ***lateral spinothalamic tract (>1840)*** centered in deeper regions of the ***lateral funiculus (Burdach, 1840)***; see Williams & Warwick (1980, pp. 876–877, 879–880, and Fig. 7.43), *Terminologia Anatomica* (1998, p. 107), Nieuwenhuys et al. (2008, pp. 697–701). Rostrally, in the ***medulla (Winslow, 1733)***, they merge and become essentially indistinguishable in the ***ventrolateral fascicle (>1840)*** where they form the ***medullary spinothalamic tract (>1840)***. It was not known by 1840.

ventral tegmental decussation (>1840)

As described in macrodissected adult human, and mammal generally with histological methods for ***axons***

(Kölliker, 1896), the crossing in the median plane of the ***tegmentum (Swanson, 2000b)*** of ***axons (Kölliker, 1896)*** from the ***red nucleus (Burdach, 1822)*** then extending caudally as the ***rubrospinal tract (>1840)***; see Carpenter (1976, pp. 261–263 and Fig. 10.17). It was not delineated clearly by 1840.

ventral thalamic nuclei (>1840)

As described for macrodissected adult human, and based on cellular architecture and connections in mammal, a large ventral component of the ***dorsal part of thalamus (Herrick, 1910)***. Its main ***gray matter regions (Swanson & Bota, 2010)*** are the ***ventral posterior nucleus (>1840)***, the ***ventral medial thalamic nucleus (>1840)***, and the ***ventral anterior thalamic nucleus (>1840)*** and ***ventral lateral thalamic nucleus (>1840)***, which in some mammals like rat are difficult to distinguish and are referred to together as the *ventral anterior-lateral thalamic complex (>1840)*; see Jones (1985, Ch. 7), Sawyer et al. (1989), Nieuwenhuys et al. (2008, pp. 262–263 and Figs. 5.7, 5.31, 6.35). It was first roughly distinguished as the *nucleus of optic thalamus (Rolando, 1825a)*.

EARLIER REFERENCES:

Earlier synonyms:

1. *nucleus of optic thalamus (Rolando, 1825a)*
   Very roughly the ***ventral thalamic nuclei (>1840)***, observed in transverse sections of macrodissected adult beef; in the original French, *noyau des couches optiques*, Table VIII, Figures 1-4, indicated by *. See Williams & Warwick (1980, pp. 955–960).
2. *center of optic thalamus (Rolando, 1825a)*
   Synonym for *nucleus of optic thalamus (Rolando, 1825a)*; in the original French, *centre des couches optiques*, Table VIII, Figure 3-*.

PARTLY CORRESPONDS:

1. ***[ventral lateral thalamic nucleus (>1840)] (Reil, 1809c)***
   Identified in macrodissected adult human the general region of the ***ventral anterior thalamic nucleus (>1840)*** and ***ventral lateral thalamic nucleus (>1840)***, "The anterior peduncles [***superior cerebellar peduncles (Procháska, 1800)***] finally radiate forward, and surround a mass of gray substance in the inner and posterior part of the thalamus" (Mayo translation, 1823, p. 99).

ventral white commissure (>1840)

As described for macrodissected adult human, and mammal generally with histological methods for ***axons (Kölliker, 1896)***, a transverse ***central nervous system white matter tract (>1840)*** ventral to the ***central canal of spinal cord (>1840)*** and ***spinal central gray (>1840)***, between the dorsomedial ends of the right and left ***ventral funiculus (>1840)***; see Williams & Warwick (1980, Fig. 7.44A), Nieuwenhuys et al. (2008, p. 178 and Fig. 6.1-12). It was perhaps first clearly described as the *anterior white commissure (Vicq d'Azyr, 1784)*.

EARLIER REFERENCES:

Earlier synonyms:

1. *anterior white commissure (Vicq d'Azyr, 1784)*
   Synonym for macrodissected adult human ***ventral white commissure (>1840)***, "on opening the anterior sulcus a very thin white layer, which is situated like a commissure in front of the gray substance, forms the bottom of the sulcus" (pp. 599–603, see Clarke & O'Malley translation, 1996, p. 270). Also see Rolando (1824, Tab. III, Fig. 3-*z*).
2. *anterior commissure (Vicq d'Azyr, 1784)*
   Shortened form of *anterior white commissure (Vicq d'Azyr, 1784)*; p. 603.
3. *longitudinal commissure (Ollivier, 1824)*
   Useful synonym for macrodissected adult human ***ventral white commissure (>1840)***; in the original French, *commissure longitudinale*, Vol. 1, p. 45. Chaussier used the term, presumably earlier, according to Cruveilhier (1836, p. 574), who provided no citation.
4. *commissure of cord (Solly, 1836)*
   Basically synonym for macrodissected adult human ***ventral white commissure (>1840)***; p. 135.
5. *white commissure (Cruveilhier, 1836)*
   Probably synonym for macrodissected adult human *anterior white commissure (Vicq d'Azyr, 1784)*; in the original French, *commissure blanche*, p. 577.

ventricles (Hippocrates)

The lumen of the vertebrate ***neural tube (Baer, 1837)*** filled with ***cerebrospinal fluid (Magendie, 1827)*** and in the adult lined with a ***glial (Virchow, 1846)*** epithelium, the ***ependyma (>1840)***. In *On the Sacred Disease*, the Hippocratic Corpus (c400 BC) makes passing reference to what has been translated as "the brain and its ventricles" (Adams, 1972, p. 353).

EARLIER REFERENCES:

Described, not named or illustrated:

1. ***[ventricles (Hippocrates)] (Anaxagoras of Athens, c488–c428 BC)***
   Anaxagoras was probably aware of their existence; see Mettler (1947), Rasmussen (1947).
2. ***[ventricles (Hippocrates)] (Herophilus, c335–c280 BC)***
   Herophilus is often credited with distinguishing between parts of the macrodissected adult human ***ventricles (Hippocrates)***, and clearly discovered the ***fourth ventricle (Galen, c192)***; see von Staden (1989, p. 247).
3. ***[ventricles (Hippocrates)] (Erasistratus, c310–c250 BC)***
   In *The Doctrines of Hippocrates and Plato* (c162–c166), Galen quoted from a now lost book of Erasistratus where the macrodissected adult human ***brain (Smith Papyrus, c1700 BC)*** "...had a ventricle placed longitudinally on each side, and these were pierced through into one at the junction of the parts [***interventricular foramen (>1840)***]. This [third] one extended to the so-called cerebellum, where there was another, smaller ventricle..." (Clarke & O'Malley translation,

1996, p. 12). This is the first clear description of all the ***ventricles (Hippocrates)***.

LATER SYNONYMS:

1. *hollow (Aristotle)*
In *The Account of Animals*, Aristotle wrote that the great majority of animals have a small hollow in the center of the ***brain (Smith Papyrus, c1700 BC)***, referring to the ***ventricles (Hippocrates)***; he did not dissect human; see Clarke & O'Malley (1996, p. 9).
2. *cavities (Galen, c173)*
In *On the Usefulness of the Parts*, Galen referred to ***ventricles (Hippocrates)*** as cavities (see May translation, 1968, pp. 401, 416–417), and seemed to indicate ***lateral ventricle (Vesalius, 1543a)*** and ***third ventricle (Galen, c173)***, but not ***fourth ventricle (Galen, c192)***, are lined with ***pia (Galen, c192)***, a mistaken idea originating with Rufus of Ephesus (see Millen & Woollam, 1962, p. 5) and persisting at least as long as Meckel (1817; see translation, 1832, Vol. 2, p. 459).
3. *chambers (Galen, c173)*
Alternate form of *cavities (Galen, c177)*; see Manzoni (1998, p. 120). It was used specifically in the first account of anatomy published in English; see Brunschwig (1525, p. [8]).
4. *cerebral ventricles (Galen, c192)*
In *On Anatomical Procedures*, Galen referred specifically to "cerebral ventricles" with reference to ***ventricles (Hippocrates)***; see Duckworth translation (1962, p. 19). He enumerated four: two anterior, a third, and a fourth; see du Laurens (1599, p. 408), Crooke (1615, p. 528), May (1968, pp. 414–415), Clarke & O'Malley (1996, p. 712), Singer (1999, p. 235). According to du Laurens (1599, p. 408), Avicenna numbered three *cerebral ventricles (Galen, c192)*: upper, middle, and hindmost, counting the upper two [***lateral ventricles (Vesalius, 1543a)***] as single; see Crooke (1615, p. 528). Bartholin (1662, p. 140) wrote that there is really only one ventricle, though some distinctions can be made for doctrine's sake. Thus, for example, Meckel (1817) referred to the *cerebral ventricle* (singular) for the whole ***ventricles (Hippocrates)***; see translation (1832, Vol. 2, p. 458).
5. *cells (Anatomia Magistri Nicolai physici, early 12th century)*
The cell (ventricular) theory of ***brain (Smith Papyrus, c1700 BC)*** function was very influential in the Middle Ages, although the exact history of when the term "cells" was introduced for ***ventricles (Hippocrates)*** has not been traced; see Manzoni (1998, p. 120 ff.). The term was used specifically in the anatomical manuscript cited here (as translated by Corner, 1927, p. 71), it was also used at about the same time by the French philosopher Guillaume de Conches (c1100–1154; see Manzoni, 1998, p. 125), and Burdach (1822, p. 261) cited Averroes (12th century) as having used it in *Colliget* (Book I, Chapter 16, p. 7). It was used specifically in the first account of anatomy published in English (Brunschwig, 1525, p. [8]), the singular form there spelled *celle*—and the ***ventricles (Hippocrates)*** were still referred to as cells by Diemerbroeck (1689, p. 397). Virtually all versions of the cell theory referred to anterior/rostral, middle, and posterior/caudal cells (that is, three; see Manzoni 1998, Table 1), and virtually all early illustrations do as well (see Clarke and Dewhurst 1996, Chapter 3). Also see *cerebral cells (Baer, 1837)*.
6. *caverns (Averroes, 12th century)*
Synonym for macrodissected adult human ***ventricles (Hippocrates)***; in Latin, *cavernae*; cited in Burdach (1822 p. 261) as: collectanea sect. I. c. 20. p. 89.
7. *sinuses (Averroes, 12th century)*
Synonym for macrodissected adult human ***ventricles (Hippocrates)***; in Latin, *sinus*; cited in Burdach (1822, p. 261) as: collectanea sect. I. c. 20. p. 89.
8. *vacuities (Averroes, 12th century)*
Synonym for macrodissected adult human ***ventricles (Hippocrates)***; in Latin, *specus*; cited in Burdach (1822, p. 261) as: collectanea sect. I. c. 20. p. 89.
9. *thalami (Berengario da Carpi, 1521)*
Synonym for macrodissected adult human ***ventricles (Hippocrates)***; f. 434, cited in Burdach (1822, p. 261).
10. *camerae (Berengario da Carpi, 1521)*
Synonym for macrodissected adult human ***ventricles (Hippocrates)***; f. 434, cited in Burdach (1822, p. 261).
11. *brain pans (Nemesius, 1636)*
English synonym for macrodissected adult human ***ventricles (Hippocrates)*** in this translation of Nemesius's 4th-century work *On the Nature of Man* (p. 306); actually spelled *braine-pans*; elsewhere *panns* was used (p. 272).
12. *belly (Willis, 1664)*
Synonym for macrodissected mammalian ***ventricles (Hippocrates)***; see Pordage translation (1681, p. 65).
13. *central fissure (Meckel, 1817)*
Synonym for macrodissected adult human ***ventricles (Hippocrates)***, in the original Latin, *fissura centralis*; see translation (1832, Vol. 2, p. 458).
14. *cerebral cavities (Spurzheim, 1826)*
Synonym for macrodissected adult vertebrate ***ventricles (Hippocrates)***; p. 208.

PARTLY CORRESPONDS:

1. *[third ventricle] (Erasistratus, c310–c250 BC)*
In *The Doctrines of Hippocrates and Plato* (c162–c166), Galen quoted from a now lost book of Erasistratus where the human brain "…had a ventricle placed longitudinally on each side, and these were pierced through into one at the junction of the parts [***interventricular foramen (>1840)***]. This [third] one extended to the so-called cerebellum, where there was another, smaller ventricle…" (Clarke & O'Malley translation, 1996, p. 12). It seems likely that this "third" ventricle of Erasistratus corresponds to combination of ***third ventricle (Galen, c173)*** and ***cerebral aqueduct (>1840)*** considered together, or equally likely the *passage or canal extending from middle to posterior ventricle (Galen, c173, c177)*.
2. *common space (Constantine the African, c1017–1087)*
Apparently synonym for *[third ventricle] (Erasistratus, c310–c250 BC)*; see Manzoni (1998, pp. 122–123).

3. *middle ventricle (Avicenna, c1030)*
   Probably synonym for *[third ventricle] (Erasistratus, c310– c250 BC)*, although it is important to note that Avicenna counted three not four ventricles—upper, the two ***lateral ventricles (Vesalius, 1543a)***, middle, and hindmost, the ***fourth ventricle (Galen, c192)***—so his *middle ventricle* would have been his second ventricle; see Crooke (1615, p. 528). Also see *cerebral ventricles (Galen, c192)* and *cells (Anatomia Magistri Nicolai physici, early 12th century)*.
4. *mid ventricle (Mondino, 1316)*
   Probably synonymous with *middle ventricle (Avicenna, c1030)*. Mondino's description is brief and vague: "...the mid ventricle will be apparent to thee. This is a way and passage, as it were, from the fore to the hind ventricle" (Singer translation, 1925, p. 92). Also see *fore ventricle (Mondino, 1316)* and *hind ventricle (Mondino, 1316)*.
5. *second cell (Brunschwig, 1525)*
   Probably synonymous with macrodissected adult human *middle ventricle (Avicenna, c1030)*; spelled *second celle* in the original text.
6. *meatus inter ventriculos anteriores et posteriorem (Benedetti, 1539)*
   Probably synonym for macrodissected adult human *[third ventricle] (Erasistratus, c310–c250 BC)*; p. 236, see Burdach (1822, p. 378).
7. *middle sinus (Landi, 1542)*
   Probably synonym for *middle ventricle (Avicenna, c1030)*; p. 55, see Burdach (1822, p. 378), who gave the Latin as *sinus medius*.
8. *third cerebral ventricle (Vesalius, 1543a)*
   Apparently synonym for ***third ventricle (Galen, c173)*** and *hind passage of third ventricle (Vesalius, 1543a)* or ***cerebral aqueduct (>1840)***, considered together; see Richardson & Carman translation (2009, p. 211) and *hind passage of third ventricle (Vesalius, 1543a)*.
9. *vulva (Casseri, 1627)*
   Casseri seemed to apply it roughly to rostral end of ***hypothalamic part of third ventricle (Swanson, 2004)*** and adjacent ***interventricular foramen (>1840)*** considered together; Tables VI, Figure 2-*N*; VII, Figure 1-*N*; X-*M*. For a different use see *vulva (Colombo, 1559)*; also see Burdach (1822, pp. 379–380). Casseri was probably referring to appearance imparted to this part of ***ventricles (Hippocrates)*** by right and left ***precommissural fornix (Loo, 1931)*** as they descend caudal to ***anterior commissure (Lieutaud, 1742)***, along with aperture formed by right and left ***interventricular foramen (>1840)***; see *pillar of fornix (Pourfour du Petit, 1710)*. Intriguingly, Burdach (1822, p. 380) wrote that Kulmus reported a "hymen" associated with Casseri's vulva, without citing a reference for Kulmus; conceivably this referred to ***terminal lamina (Burdach, 1822)***. Vesalius clearly described but did not name both a rostral and a caudal channel leading down the median plane of the macrodissected adult human ***third ventricle (Galen, c173)*** toward the *pituitary gland (Galen, c192)*; see Richardson & Carman translation (2009, p. 211).
10. *rima (Willis, 1664)*
   Refers to macrodissected adult sheep *vulva (Casseri, 1627)* in Figure VII-*H*; it is referred to as a *foramen* in Figure VIII-*G*. In Latin, *rima* means crack, cleft, or fissure. In the text, the meaning of *rima* for human is ambiguous; see Pordage translation (1681, p. 65, where it is rendered *chink* in English). Burdach (1822, p. 378) claimed that Willis also used the term in referring to *vulva (Colombo, 1559)*. Later, Willis (1672) referred to these rostral and caudal, respectively, regions of ***third ventricle (Galen, c173)*** as rostral and caudal *hiatus* rather than *rima*, and Pordage translated this as gap or chink (1683, Tab. VIII-*W,X*). The situation was clarified by Ridley some 30 years later; see *rima ad infundibulum (Ridley, 1695)*.
11. *hiatus ad infundibulum (Vieussens, 1684)*
   Rough synonym for macrodissected adult human *vulva (Casseri, 1627)*; see Burdach (1822, p. 380).
12. *womb of Vesling (Diemerbroeck, 1689)*
   English form of and eponym for *vulva (Casseri, 1627)*; p. 400.
13. *iter ad infundibulum (Monro, 1783)*
   Latin synonym for macrodissected adult human *vulva (Casseri, 1627)*; p. 12; also see *iter ad tertium ventriculum (Monro, 1783)*.
14. *iter ad tertium ventriculum (Monro, 1783)*
   Latin synonym for macrodissected adult human *vulva (Casseri, 1627)*; p. 12. A good history of early research on it is provided in Bell (1802, p. 81 ff.) and Burdach (1822, pp. 379–380), who gave the term as *iter ad ventriculum tertium*.
15. *posterior oriface of third ventricle (Schreger, 1803)*
   Synonym for macrodissected adult human *vulva (Casseri, 1627)*; p. 321.
16. *foramen commune anterius (Ramsay, 1813)*
   Synonym for macrodissected adult human *vulva (Casseri, 1627)*; p. 45.
17. *central fissure of brain proper (Gordon, 1815)*
   May refer roughly to macrodissected adult human ***lateral ventricle (Vesalius, 1543a)*** and ***third ventricle (Galen, c173)*** considered together; see pp. 95–107, 157–158.
18. *aditus ad infundibulum (Bock, 1824)*
   Synonym for macrodissected adult human *vulva (Casseri, 1627)*; p. 158.

ventricular-subarachnoid space (Swanson & Bota, 2010)

The continuous cavity associated with the vertebrate ***central nervous system (Carus, 1814)*** that is filled with ***cerebrospinal fluid (Magendie, 1827)***. One part of the cavity is the central lumen of the vertebrate ***central nervous system (Carus, 1814)***; that is, the remnant of the embryonic lumen of the ***neural tube (Baer, 1837)***. It is referred to as the (cerebral) ***ventricles (Hippocrates)***, with walls formed by the thin ***ependyma (>1840)***. The other part is the ***subarachnoid space (Magendie, 1827)*** lying between the inner and outer layers of ***meninges (Smith Papyrus, c1700 BC)***, the ***pia (Galen, c192)*** and ***dura (Galen, c177)***, respectively. The ***ventricles (Hippocrates)*** and ***subarachnoid space (Magendie, 1827)*** are continuous through three holes in the ***roof of fourth ventricle (Vesalius, 1543a)*** associated with the ***medulla (Winslow, 1733)***: two ***lateral apertures of fourth ventricle (>1840)*** and a single ***median aperture of fourth ventricle (>1840)***. The ***cerebrospinal fluid (Magendie, 1827)*** is equivalent to lymph for the vertebrate ***central nervous system (Carus, 1814)*** and eventually drains into the venous part of the circulatory system; see Crosby et al. (1962, pp. 568–579). It was clearly described by Magendie; see ***[ventricular-subarachnoid space (Swanson & Bota, 2010)] (Magendie, 1828)***.

EARLIER REFERENCES:

Described, not named or illustrated:

1. ***[ventricular-subarachnoid space (Swanson & Bota, 2010)] (Magendie, 1828)***
   Magendie provided strong experimental arguments for continuity between ***ventricles (Hippocrates)*** and ***subarachnoid space (Magendie, 1827)***, involving the flow of ***cerebrospinal fluid (Magendie, 1827)***; see ***[median aperture of fourth ventricle (>1840] (Magendie, 1828)***.

ventrolateral fascicle (>1840)

As described for macrodissected adult human, a broadly and somewhat vaguely defined longitudinal ***central nervous system white matter tract (>1840)*** including the partly overlapping ***ventral spinocerebellar tract (>1840)***, ***dorsal spinocerebellar tract (>1840)***, ***spinothalamic tract (>1840)***, and ***rubrospinal tract (>1840)***; see Yoss (1953; pp. 615–616), Carpenter (1996, Fig. 10.17), Nieuwenhuys et al. (2008, pp. 182, 196, 202, 320, 844 and Figures 6.3, 6.13–18; called *anterolateral fasciculus*). For topographic description it has ***tegmental ventrolateral fascicle (>1840)***, ***pontine ventrolateral fascicle (>1840)***, and ***medullary ventrolateral fascicle (>1840)*** segments. *Thalamic ventrolateral fascicle (>1840)* is synonymous with ***thalamic spinothalamic tract (>1840)***. It was probably first indicated by Santorini; see ***[ventrolateral fascicle (>1840)] (Santorini, 1775)***.

EARLIER REFERENCES:

Illustrated, not named or described:

1. ***[ventrolateral fascicle (>1840)] (Santorini, 1775)***
   According to Burdach (1822, p. 286), first indicated for macrodissected adult human; p. 25 and Table II-*u*.

Earlier synonyms:

1. *stratum horizontale (Burdach, 1822)*
   Macrodissected adult human ***central nervous system white matter tract (>1840)*** coursing longitudinally in region visible on surface of ***medulla (Winslow, 1733)*** just dorsal to ***olive (Tiedemann, 1821)***, stretching from ***spinal cord (Galen, c162–c166)*** caudally to about middle of ***pons (Haller, 1747)***; in the original German, *wagerechten Schicht*, p. 38, Table VIII-*a*. It probably corresponds roughly to ***ventrolateral fascicle (>1840)***, and Burdach noted (1822, p. 286) it was first shown by Santorini (1775, p. 25 and Tab. II-*u*) and then at least partly by Monro (1783, p. 28), Meckel (1817, Vol. 3, p. 451), Reil (1809c, p. 493), who called it *senkrecht Schichten* or *vertical layer*, and Gordon (1815, p. 185).
2. *horizontal fibers (Burdach, 1822)*
   Synonym for macrodissected adult human *stratum horizontale (Burdach, 1822)*; in the original German, *wagerechten Fasern*, pp. 38, 286; Table VIII-*a*.
3. *anterior cord of oblong medulla (Rolando, 1825a)*
   Synonym for *anterolateral cord of oblong medulla (Rolando, 1825a)* in macrodissected adult beef viewed in transverse section; in the original French (plural): *cordons antérieurs de la moelle alongée*, Table III-*c.a.*
4. *anterolateral cord of oblong medulla (Rolando, 1825a)*
   In macrodissected adult human and beef viewed in transverse section, ***white matter (Meckel, 1817)*** lying rostrocaudally between *anterior cords of medulla oblongata (Rolando, 1825a)* and *anterior cords of spinal medulla (Rolando, 1825a)*, whereas dorsoventrally between ***inferior cerebellar peduncle (Günther, 1786)*** and ***pyramid (Willis, 1664)***; in the original French (plural), *cordons antéro-latéraux de la moelle alongée*; p. 19; Table IV. Also see Table VIII, Figure 1-*z*, where Rolando traced it to ***thalamus (His, 1893a)***, and cross section figures leading up to it, usually abbreviated *c.a.* It corresponds quite roughly to ***ventrolateral fascicle (>1840)***, although in ***pons (Haller, 1747)*** especially it may have included parts of ***central tegmental tract (Bechterew, 1889)***; see Table III-*c.a.*
5. *anterolateral cord (Rolando, 1825a)*
   Synonym for *anterolateral cord of oblong medulla (Rolando, 1825a)* in macrodissected large calf; in the original French (plural), *condons antéro-latéraux*, Table VII, Figure 3-*c.a.*
6. *anterolateral fasciculus (>1840)*
   Synonym for macrodissected adult human ***ventrolateral fascicle (>1840)***; see Nieuwenhuys et al. (2008, p. 182).

ventrolateral sulcus of medulla (>1840)

As described for macrodissected adult human, the rostral extension of the ***ventrolateral sulcus of spinal cord (>1840)*** lying just dorsolateral to the ***pyramid (Willis, 1664)***, from which the ***hypoglossal nerve central root (>1840)*** issues and continues as the peripheral ***hypoglossal nerve root (>1840)***; see Williams & Warwick (1980, p. 1083 and Fig. 7.189), *Terminologia Anatomica* (1998, p. 108). It was first indicated by Vesalius; see ***[ventrolateral sulcus of medulla (>1840)] (Vesalius, 1543a)***.

EARLIER REFERENCES:

Illustrated, not named or described:

1. ***[ventrolateral sulcus of medulla (>1840)] (Vesalius, 1543a)***
   Left ***ventrolateral sulcus of medulla (>1840)*** vaguely depicted on right side of figure illustrating base of macrodissected adult human ***brain (Smith Papyrus,***

c1700 BC); see Richardson & Carman translation (2002, p. 168). For ***hypoglossal nerve rootlets (>1840)*** see Richardson & Carman translation (2009, pp. 155–156, Fig. 14-O). Eustachi (1552) illustrated it much more clearly, although his plates (without text) were not published until 1714; see Albinus edition (1744, Plate XVIII), Roberts & Tomlinson (1992, Pl. 46).

LATER SYNONYMS:

1. *preolivary sulcus (>1840)*
   Synonym for macrodissected adult human ***ventrolateral sulcus of medulla (>1840)***; see *Terminologia Anatomica* (1998, p. 108), where it was given as *sulcus preolivaris* and *pre-olivary groove*. Some authors may restrict its use to just the segment of the ***ventrolateral sulcus of medulla (>1840)*** ventrally adjacent to ***olive (Tiedemann, 1821)***.

ventrolateral sulcus of spinal cord (>1840)

As described for macrodissected adult human, the longitudinal region associated with the ***ventral root (>1840)*** entry zone not actually forming a clear groove. It indicates the border between ***ventral funiculus (>1840)*** and ***lateral funiculus (Burdach, 1822)*** and extends rostrally as the ***ventrolateral sulcus of medulla (>1840)***; see Carpenter (1976, p. 214, called *anterolateral sulcus*), Williams & Warwick (1980, pp. 865, 897, called *anterolateral sulcus*), *Terminologia Anatomica* (1998, p. 108). It was first indicated by Blasius; see ***[ventrolateral sulcus of spinal cord (>1840)] Blasius (1666)***.

EARLIER REFERENCES:

Illustrated, not named or described:

1. ***[ventrolateral sulcus of spinal cord (>1840)] (Blasius, 1666)***
   Indicated for macrodissected adult human in Figures 10, 11, 18.

Earlier synonyms:

1. *anterior lateral sulcus of spinal marrow (Meckel, 1817)*
   Synonym for macrodissected adult human ***ventrolateral sulcus of spinal cord (>1840)***; see translation (1832, Vol. 2, p. 412).
2. *anterior collateral fissure (Bellingeri, 1823)*
   Synonym for macrodissected adult human ***ventrolateral sulcus of spinal cord (>1840)***; in the original Latin (plural), *scissurae collaterales anteriores*, Table 1, Figure 3-*g*.
3. *supposed anterior lateral sulcus (Rolando, 1824)*
   Discussion of actual appearance of *anterior lateral sulcus of spinal marrow (Meckel, 1817)*; in the original Italian, *supposti solchi laterali anteriori*, p. 42.
4. *anterior lateral furrow of spinal marrow (Mayo, 1827)*
   Synonym for macrodissected adult human ***ventrolateral sulcus of spinal cord (>1840)***; Plate I, Figure 1-*c*.

ventromedial hypothalamic nucleus (>1840)

Based primarily on cellular architecture and connections in mammal, the component of the ***medial hypothalamic zone (Nauta & Haymaker, 1969)*** between the ***anterior hypothalamic nucleus (>1840)*** rostrally and the ***ventral premammillary nucleus (>1840)*** and ***dorsal premammillary nucleus (>1840)*** caudally; see Swanson (1998, Table B, p. 206). It was not described by 1840.

vertebral ganglion (>1840)

As described for macrodissected adult human, a small ***sympathetic trunk ganglion (Winslow, 1733)*** usually but not always found on the ***communicating branch of sympathetic trunk (>1840)*** between ***middle cervical ganglion (Haller, 1762)*** and ***inferior cervical ganglion (Vieussens, 1684)***; see Mitchell (1953, pp. 224–225), *Terminologia Anatomica* (1998, p. 141). It was not clearly described by 1840.

vertebral nerve (Cruveilhier, 1836)

As described for macrodissected adult human, one commonly arises from the ***vertebral ganglion (>1840)*** when present, or else from the ***middle cervical ganglion (Haller, 1762)***, and another usually larger ***vertebral nerve (Cruveilhier, 1836)*** may arise from the ***inferior cervical ganglion (Vieussens, 1684)*** or *cervicothoracic ganglion (>1840)*—or occasionally from the ***ansa subclavia (Neubauer, 1772)*** instead. Both ***vertebral nerves (Cruveilhier, 1836)*** commonly arise from several roots, and they begin to anastomose around the vertebral artery, where they contribute to the ***vertebral plexus (Cloquet, 1816)***; see Mitchell (1953, p. 225). For Cruveilhier's use in macrodissected adult human, see p. 996. Perhaps the earliest clear reference to it was *posterior nerve of vertebral artery (Andersch & Soemmerring, 1792)*.

TRANSLATIONS:

1. *nerf vertébral (Cruveilhier, 1836)*
   Original French form of ***vertebral nerve (Cruveilhier, 1836)***; p. 996.

EARLIER REFERENCES:

Earlier synonyms:

1. *posterior nerve of vertebral artery (Andersch & Soemmerring, 1792)*
   Apparently an early, if not the earliest, description of macrodissected adult human ***vertebral nerve (Cruveilhier, 1836)***; in the original Latin, *nervus posterior arteriae vertebralis*, pp. 183–184. Cloquet (1816) described for macrodissected adult human a number of ***vertebral nerves (Cruveilhier, 1836)*** arising from ***inferior cervical ganglion (Vieussens, 1684)*** but did not name them; see p. 695 and ***vertebral plexus (Cloquet, 1816)***. Vieussens may possibly have described and illustrated it for macrodissected adult human; Table 23-54.

vertebral plexus (Cloquet, 1816)

As described for adult human, it arises mainly from the ***vertebral nerve (Cruveilhier, 1836)*** and then surrounds the vertebral artery and its branches; in the cranium it continues on the vertebral arteries and basilar artery and their various branches. It also supplies branches to the adjacent vertebrae, discs, and meninges; and it supplies deep ***communicating branches (Winslow, 1733)*** to the upper five or six ***cervical nerves (Galen, c173)***. There are small collections of ganglion cells on the ***vertebral plexus (Cloquet, 1816)*** and on the ***vertebral nerve (Cruveilhier, 1836)***; see Mitchell (1953, pp. 225–227). For Cloquet's use in macrodissected adult human, see p. 695. It was first clearly described by Wrisberg; see *plexus around vertebral artery (Wrisberg, 1786)*.

TRANSLATIONS:

1. *plexus vertébral (Cloquet, 1816)*
   Original French form of ***vertebral plexus (Cloquet, 1816)***; p. 695.

EARLIER REFERENCES:

Earlier synonyms:

1. *plexus around vertebral artery (Wrisberg, 1786)*
   Synonym for macrodissected adult human ***vertebral plexus (Cloquet, 1816)***; in the original Latin, *plexus circa arteriam vertebralem*, see Wrisberg reprint (1800, p. 404). Swan (1830, Pl. II-*i*) called it *plexus on vertebral artery*.

LATER SYNONYMS:

1. *soft nerves of vertebral and basilar arteries (Arnold, 1834)*
   Synonym for macrodissected adult human ***vertebral plexus (Cloquet, 1816)***, said to arise from ***superior thoracic ganglion (Lieutaud, 1742)***; in the original Latin, *nervi molles arteriae vertebralis et basilaris*, p. 18.

PARTLY CORRESPONDS:

1. *basilar plexus (Cruveilhier, 1836)*
   In macrodissected adult human, rostral component of each ***vertebral plexus (Cloquet, 1816)*** along basilar artery and its terminal branches; in the original French, *plexus basilaire*, p. 997.

vertebrate brain (Cuvier, 1800)

Brain (Smith Papyrus, c1700 BC) is a general term for the rostral topographic division of the ***central nervous system (Carus, 1814)***. ***Invertebrate brain (>1840)*** and ***vertebrate brain (Cuvier, 1800)*** are distinguished and treated separately because the evolutionary relationship between the two is not clear and because whereas there is a common basic plan for the ***vertebrate brain (Cuvier, 1800)*** based on development, there are multiple basic plans for the ***invertebrate brain (>1840)*** and many invertebrates have nothing resembling a ***brain (Smith Papyrus, c1700 BC)***. The ***vertebrate brain (Cuvier, 1800)*** is the rostral topographic division of the vertebrate ***central nervous system (Carus, 1814)*** or ***cerebrospinal axis (Meckel, 1817)***; the caudal division is the ***spinal cord (Galen, c162–c166)***. For these precise definitions see Swanson & Bota (2010, Thesaurus); for Cuvier's use see Vol. 2, p. 93. The first surviving reference to it was ***brain (Smith Papyrus, c1700 BC)***, a term that can refer to the ***invertebrate brain (>1840)*** and ***vertebrate brain (Cuvier, 1800)***.

EARLIER REFERENCES:

Earlier synonyms:

1. *white marrow (Sophocles, 5th century BC)*
   Synonym for ***vertebrate brain (Cuvier, 1800)***, presumably applied to adult mammal. According to Bauhin (1605, p. 571), "Apollodorus thought that none of the Antients had given any name to the Brain in any of their writings, and that therefore Sophocles called it [Greek], the white marrow" (Crooke translation, 1615, p. 453).
2. *great kernel (Hippocrates)*
   According to Riolan, Hippocrates used it for ***vertebrate brain (Cuvier, 1800)***, presumably in human and/or other mammals; see Culpeper translation (1657, p. 121).
3. *marrow of head (Plato)*
   Synonym in *Timaeus* for ***vertebrate brain (Cuvier, 1800)*** of human; see Plato (1965, p. 101), Clarke & O'Malley (1996, p. 7). Plato did not perform dissections himself, basing his statements primarily on speculation.
4. *medulla of head (Plato)*
   Synonym for *marrow of head (Plato)*. *Marrow* is English form of Latin, *medulla*.
5. *medulla cerebrales (Plato)*
   According to Bauhin (1605, p. 624), Plato used the Greek equivalent of this term for ***vertebrate brain (Cuvier, 1800)***; see Crooke translation (1615, p. 479) of Bauhin, where *medulla cerebrales* is "Marrow of the Braine". Bauhin did not cite the source of Plato's term, but see *medulla of head (Plato)*.
6. *marrow of brain (Plato)*
   English form of *medulla cerebrales (Plato)*; see Crooke (1615, p. 479), referring to ***vertebrate brain (Cuvier, 1800)***.
7. *cranial marrow (Plato)*
   According to Galen, Plato used it for ***vertebrate brain (Cuvier, 1800)***; see Duckworth translation (1962, p. 223).
8. *ploughland (Plato)*
   Synonym Plato used in *Timaeus* for ***vertebrate brain (Cuvier, 1800)*** in human; see Plato (1965). Also see *marrow of head (Plato)*.
9. *whole brain (Aristotle)*
   Mainly in *The Account of Animals* and *On the Parts of Animals*, Aristotle provided the first descriptions with any detail of ***nervous system (Monro, 1873)*** structure (see Clarke & O'Malley, 1996, pp. 7–10), including a tripartite distinction between *large brain (Aristotle)*, anteriorly (rostrally) in the cranium, "para-brain" or *small brain (Aristotle)*—the *parencephalon (Aristotle)* or ***cerebellum (Aristotle)***, posterior (caudally) in the cranium—and *spinal marrow (Hippocrates)* or ***spinal cord (Galen, c162–c166)***. Thus, he used "brain" (in English; *encephalon* in Greek) in two ways: as contents of cranium, and as *large brain (Aristotle)* when compared to *small brain (Aristotle)* or "para-brain." He referred to contents of cranium as ***brain (Smith Papyrus, c1700 BC)*** or *whole brain (Aristotle)*—see Clarke & Stannard (1963), von Staden (1989, p. 197), Clarke & O'Malley (1996, p. 630)—and *large brain (Aristotle)* as *brain* or *brain itself (Aristotle)*; see Clarke & O'Malley (1996, p. 9). As a result, "brain" (and thus cerebrum and encephalon) has two different

meanings; see *cerebrum (Celsus, c30)* and ***cerebrum (Obersteiner & Hill, 1900)***. Aristotle based his statements on dissection of many animal species, but not on human material. For an account of this in English, see Crooke (1615, p. 456). In German, Soemmerring (1791, p. 21) distinguished clearly between *Hirnmasse* (encephalus), *grosse Hirn* (cerebrum), *kleine Hirn (cerebellum)*, and *Rückenmark* (medulla spinalis). In the end, Galen (c173) explained the situation best, "Now these are the names the followers of Herophilus are accustomed to use for these two parts [encephalon and parencephalis], giving the anterior part the same name as the whole because of its size; for although the encephalon is paired, as I have said, each of its parts is far larger than the entire *parencephalis*. The posterior part was named, however, because the anterior part had already appropriated the name of the whole, and it was no longer possible to find any name for the *parencephalis* more suitable than the one it now has. But again, others call it not *parencephalis*, but *encranis* and *encranion*. These men should not be blamed if they invent names to make their meaning clear, seeing that all our lives we name many things for their pre-eminence in point of size, power, virtue, or honor" (May translation, 1968, p. 414).

10. *whole encephalon (Aristotle)*
    Alternate translation of *whole brain (Aristotle)*.
11. *entire brain (Aristotle)*
    Synonym for ***vertebrate brain (Cuvier, 1800)***, used mainly in *The Account of Animals* and *On the Parts of Animals*; see *whole brain (Aristotle)*.
12. *entire encephalon (Aristotle)*
    Synonym for ***vertebrate brain (Cuvier, 1800)***, used mainly in *The Account of Animals* and *On the Parts of Animals*; see *whole brain (Aristotle)*.
13. *encephalic medulla (Galen, c173)*
    Galen wrote that many people refer thus to *encephalon (Homer, c9th century BC)* or ***vertebrate brain (Cuvier, 1800)***, in contrast to *spinal medulla (Hippocrates)*; see May translation (1968, p. 394).
14. *medulla of encephalon (Galen, c173)*
    English form of *encephalic medulla (Galen, 173)*; see May translation (1968, p. 394).
15. *brain marrow (Galen, c173)*
    English form of *encephalic medulla (Galen, c173)*.
16. *great king (Galen, c173)*
    Synonym for ***vertebrate brain (Cuvier, 1800)*** used by Galen in *On the Usefulness of the Parts*; see May translation (1968, p. 387) and Clarke & O'Malley (1996, p. 17).
17. *ruling principle (Galen, c173)*
    Synonym for ***vertebrate brain (Cuvier, 1800)*** used by Galen in *On the Usefulness of the Parts*; see May translation (1968, p. 402).
18. *encephalon itself (Galen, c173)*
    Synonym for ***vertebrate brain (Cuvier, 1800)*** used by Galen in *On the Usefulness of the Parts*; see May translation (1968, p. 398). It is the *whole encephalon (Aristotle)*.
19. *brain itself (Galen, c173)*
    English form of *encephalon itself (Galen, c173)*; see *whole brain (Aristotle)*.
20. *cerebral marrow (Berengario da Carpi, 1521)*
    Translation of *encephalic medulla (Galen, c173)*, added to Mondino's (1316) description of macrodissected adult human; compare Singer translation (1925, p. 91) with Clarke & O'Malley translation (1996, p. 22).
21. *medulla (Berengario da Carpi, 1521)*
    Synonym for macrodissected adult human *medulla of head (Plato)* or *medullary substance (Berengario da Carpi, 1523)*; f. 429v. Also see Berengario da Carpi (1523, top illustration on f. 56).
22. *medullary substance (Berengario da Carpi, 1523)*
    Synonym for macrodissected adult human material of ***vertebrate brain (Cuvier, 1800)*** in general. Berengario da Carpi pointed out it is quite different from medulla or marrow of bones; see Lind translation (1959, p. 142). This usage can be traced as far back as first identifications of ***brain (Smith Papyrus, c1700 BC)***.
23. *brain commonly so called (Bartholin, 1662)*
    Synonym for macrodissected adult human *whole brain (Aristotle)*; p. 133.
24. *appendix of spinal medulla (Malpighi, 1665)*
    Malpighi referred to, and affirmed, ancient belief that ***vertebrate brain (Cuvier, 1800)*** is generated from ***spinal cord (Galen, c162–c166)***; see Meyer (1967, p. 186). Malpighi himself appears to have been referring to *cerebrum (Piccolomini, 1586)*.
25. *brain in general (Gibson, 1682)*
    Synonym for macrodissected adult human *whole brain (Aristotle)*; p. 310.
26. *most noble bowel (Diemerbroeck, 1689)*
    Synonym for macrodissected adult human ***vertebrate brain (Cuvier, 1800)***; p. 373.
27. *appendix of spinal pith (Diemerbroeck, 1689)*
    Diemerbroeck explained that Malpighi viewed ***vertebrate brain (Cuvier, 1800)*** thus, as an elaboration of fibers making up ***spinal cord (Galen, c162–c166)***; p. 406. Also see *appendix of spinal medulla (Malpighi, 1665)*.
28. *organ of organs (Winslow, 1733)*
    Synonym for macrodissected adult human ***vertebrate brain (Cuvier, 1800)***; Section X, p. 24.
29. *cerebral masses (Quain, 1832)*
    Synonym for macrodissected adult human ***vertebrate brain (Cuvier, 1800)***; p. 91.

PARTLY CORRESPONDS:

1. *anterior part of brain (Aristotle)*
   Mainly in *The Account of Animals* and *On the Parts of Animals*, Aristotle distinguished between *small brain (Aristotle)* or *posterior part of brain (Aristotle)*—*parencephalon (Aristotle)* or ***cerebellum (Aristotle)***—and *large brain (Aristotle)*, *anterior part of brain (Aristotle)*,

or *whole brain (Aristotle)*; see Clarke & Stannard (1963), Clarke & O'Malley (1996, pp. 7–10), von Staden (1989, p. 197). The *anterior part of brain (Aristotle)* included ***cerebrum (Obersteiner & Hill, 1900)*** and at least part of ***brainstem (Schwalbe, 1881)***, although whether or not he included any of the ***pons (Haller, 1747)*** and/or ***medulla (Winslow, 1733)*** in ***cerebellum (Aristotle)*** is unknown. Aristotle based his statements on dissection of many animal species, but not on human material. Galen (c173) adopted Aristotle's distinction; see *whole brain (Aristotle)*, and May translation (1968, p. 417), von Staden (1989, p. 197), Clarke & O'Malley (1996, p. 630). In *On the Sacred Disease*, Hippocrates stated that in human, as in all other animals, a thin membrane divides ***brain (Smith Papyrus, c1700 BC)*** down the middle into two parts—***brain (Smith Papyrus, c1700 BC)*** "is double"; see Adams translation (1972, p. 351). This is the first preserved indication that ***cerebrum (Obersteiner & Hill, 1900)*** is paired, with right and left halves.

2. *anterior brain (Aristotle)*
   Alternate translation of *anterior part of brain (Aristotle)*.
3. *large brain (Aristotle)*
   Synonym for *anterior part of brain (Aristotle)*.
4. *brain itself (Aristotle)*
   Probably synonym for *anterior part of brain (Aristotle)*. In *The Account of Animals*, Aristotle wrote, "From the eye there go three ducts to the brain: the largest and the medium-sized to the cerebellum, and the least to the brain itself" (Thompson translation, 1962, 495a 10).
5. *enkephalon (Aristotle)*
   Greek synonym for *anterior part of brain (Aristotle)*.
6. *encephalon (Aristotle)*
   Greek form of *enkephalon (Aristotle)*.
7. *cerebrum (Aristotle)*
   Latin form of *encephalon (Aristotle)*.
8. *fore-brain (Galen, c177)*
   Anterior part of brain (Aristotle) from Galen's *On Anatomical Procedures* has been translated fore-brain; see Wiberg (1914, p. 21). Also see *brain itself (Aristotle)*.
9. *front part of brain (Galen, c177)*
   Translation of *anterior part of brain (Aristotle)* from Galen's *On Anatomical Procedures*; see Singer (1999, pp. 227, 229).
10. *prow of brain (Constantine the African, c1017–1087)*
    Synonym for *anterior part of brain (Aristotle)*; see Manzoni (1998, p. 122). Burdach (1822, p. 319) gave Zerbi's later (1502) use in Latin as *prora cerebri*.
11. *anchae (Mondino, 1316)*
    Some writers (for example, Vicq d'Azyr,1786; Lewy, 1942, pp. 2–3) interpret Mondino's use of the term to indicate part of ***caudate nucleus (Arnold, 1838b)*** forming lateral wall of ***lateral ventricle (Vesalius, 1543a)*** on both sides of macrodissected adult human ***cerebrum (Obersteiner & Hill, 1900)***; others (for example, Rasmussen, 1947, p. 4; Meyer, 1971, p. 13) interpret the term to indicate right and left walls of ***interbrain (Baer, 1827)***, formed by ***third ventricle (Galen, c173)***—or perhaps medial walls of right and left ***caudate nucleus (Arnold, 1838b)*** and of ***interbrain (Baer, 1837)***; Meyer (1971, p. 13). A translation of Mondino's rather obscure passage is in Singer (1925, p. 92). Mondino referred to possibly three *anchae (Mondino, 1316)* between ***lateral ventricles (Vesalius, 1543a)*** and ***third ventricle (Galen, c173)***. They form base of ***lateral ventricle (Vesalius, 1543a)*** and are of the substance of the ***brain (Smith Papyrus, c1700 BC)***. At the sides of the *anchae (Mondino, 1316)*, between ***lateral ventricles (Vesalius, 1543a)*** and ***third ventricle (Galen, c173)***, lie red worms or ***choroid plexus of lateral ventricle (Vicq d'Azyr, 1784)***. The worm can lengthen and close the passage between ***lateral ventricles (Vesalius, 1543a)*** and ***third ventricle (Galen, c173)***. Expanding the *anchae (Mondino, 1316)* opens the passage between ventricles. In the end, it is not possible to know with certainty what *anchae (Mondino, 1316)* correspond to in today's terminology. Berengario da Carpi rather clearly used the term to indicate medial walls of ***interbrain (Baer, 1837)***, see *buttocks (Berengario da Carpi, 1522)*, whereas Massa equally clearly used the term to indicate medial walls of right and left ***caudate nucleus (Arnold, 1838b)***, see *anchae (Massa, 1536)*. Vesalius (1543a) may refer to this controversy, although his description is not clear either; see Singer translation (1952, p. 42 and notes 60 and 62). As Singer admitted, his own tentative identification of the ridge in question as *hippocampus (Aranzi, 1587)* is probably incorrect; more likely it is ***caudate nucleus (Arnold, 1838b)***. For a note on the etymology of this obscure word (singular, *ancha*) see Singer and Rabin (1946, p. 34). It clearly has nothing to do with *gloutia (Galen, c177)*.
12. *buttocks (Mondino, 1316)*
    English form of *anchae (Mondino, 1316)*; see Singer translation (1925, p. 92).
13. *haunches (Mondino, 1316)*
    English form of *anchae (Mondino, 1316)*; see Singer and Rabin (1946, p. 34) and Rasmussen (1947, p. 4).
14. *base of fore ventricle (Mondino, 1316)*
    Synonym for *anchae (Mondino, 1316)*; see Singer translation (1925, p. 92), also see *base of anterior ventricle both right and left (Manfredi, 1490)*.
15. *anterior part of brain (Berengario da Carpi, 1522)*
    Berengario da Carpi clearly stated that for macrodissected adult human, ***spinal cord (Galen, c162–c166)***—*nucha (Constantine the African, c1017–1087)* or *nape (Berengario da Carpi, 1523)*—and ***cerebellum (Aristotle)*** arise from *anterior part of brain (Berengario da Carpi, 1522)*, and that ***fourth ventricle (Galen, c192)*** lies between ***cerebellum (Aristotle)*** and *anterior part of brain (Berengario da Carpi, 1522)*; see Lind translation (1959, pp. 144, 145). This is perhaps the first unambiguous definition of *anterior part of brain (Aristotle)*, ***vertebrate brain (Cuvier, 1800)*** without ***cerebellum (Aristotle)***.
16. *cerebral substance (Dryander, 1536)*
    In *The Anatomy of the Human Head*, Dryander referred in Latin to *substantia cerebra*, which can only refer to

brain (Smith Papyrus, c1700 BC) tissue in general, without distinguishing between *gray substance (Vesalius, 1543a)* and *white substance (Vesalius, 1543a)*; see Figure 4. Lind (1975, p. 300) quite inaccurately translated it as "the brain's gray matter itself" and "the gray matter of the left lobe [hemisphere] of the brain."

17. *cerebrum (Vesalius, 1543a)*
Macrodissected adult human ***forebrain (Goette, 1873)*** and ***midbrain (Baer, 1837)*** considered together; see Singer translation (1952, pp. 36, 46–47) and Richardson & Carman translation (2002, pp. 176–177, 205), *dorsal medulla (Vesalius, 1543a), origin of dorsal medulla (Vesalius, 1543a)*. He divided *cerebrum (Vesalius, 1543a)* into two lobes [see *lobe of cerebrum (Vesalius, 1543a)*] united by a common base [see *base of cerebrum (Vesalius, 1543a)*]; Singer translation (1952, pp. 21, 27)—corresponding roughly to ***cerebral cortex (>1840)***, as opposed to ***cerebral nuclei (Swanson, 2000a)***, ***interbrain (Baer, 1837)***, and ***midbrain (Baer, 1837)*** considered together, respectively.

18. *anterior brain (Vesalius, 1543a)*
Synonym for *cerebrum (Vesalius, 1543a)*; see Richardson & Carman translation (2009, p. 181).

19. *base of cerebrum (Vesalius, 1543a)*
Vesalius divided macrodissected adult human *cerebrum (Vesalius, 1543a)* into two *lobes of cerebrum (Vesalius, 1543a)*, roughly corresponding to ***cerebral cortex gray matter (>1840)***, and a common *base of cerebrum (Vesalius, 1543a)*; see Singer translation (1952, pp. 21, 27), Richardson & Carman translation (2009, p. 180). From this and Figure 7 it is reasonably clear that he included ***cerebral cortex white matter (>1840)***, ***cerebral nuclei (Swanson, 2000a)***, ***thalamus (His, 1893b)***, and ***midbrain (Baer, 1837)*** in *base of cerebrum (Vesalius, 1543a)*. This interpretation is corroborated by two other statements. First, in the *Epitome (Vesalius, 1543b)* he noted that *organ of smell (Hippocrates)* arises from *base of cerebrum (Vesalius, 1543a)*; see Lind translation (1949, p. 69). And second, it is clear that Vesalius had *spinal cord (Vesalius, 1543a)* or *dorsal medulla (Vesalius, 1543a)* arising from caudal border of ***midbrain (Baer, 1837)***. Also see *origin of dorsal medulla (Vesalius, 1543a)*.

20. *root foundation of brain (Geminus, 1553)*
Synonym for macrodissected adult human *base of cerebrum (Vesalius, 1543a)*; the original spelling was *roote of brayne*; see *The table of the figure of synowes*.

21. *foundation of brain (Geminus, 1553)*
Synonym for macrodissected adult human *base of cerebrum (Vesalius, 1543a)*; the original spelling was *foundation of brayne*; see *The table of the figure of synowes*.

22. *ground of brain (Geminus, 1553)*
Synonym for macrodissected adult human *base of cerebrum (Vesalius, 1543a)*; the original spelling was *grounde of brayne*; see *The table of the figure of synowes*.

23. *base of brain (Varoli, 1573)*
Varoli also called *base of brain (Varoli, 1573)* in macrodissected adult human *root of spinal marrow (Varoli, 1573)*. It probably included roughly ***cerebral cortex white matter (>1840)***, ***cerebral nuclei (Swanson, 2000a)***, and ***interbrain (Baer, 1837)***, with *infundibulum (Rufus of Ephesus, fl. c90–120)*; see Clarke & O'Malley (1996, pp. 821–822). Also see *anterior spinal marrow (Varoli, 1573)* and *base of cerebrum (Vesalius, 1543a)*.

24. *root of spinal marrow (Varoli, 1573)*
Synonym for *base of brain (Varoli, 1573)*; see Clarke & O'Malley (1996, p. 822). Burdach (1822, p. 320) noted that Varoli used (p. 127) the Latin terms *principium medullae spinalis* and *ortus medullae spinalis*.

25. *rimae (Varoli, 1573)*
Probably synonym for macrodissected adult human *anchae (Mondino, 1316)*; see Meyer (1971, p. 13).

26. *seat of brain (Bannister, 1578)*
Exact meaning is unclear (f. 106), but used in the sense of *base of cerebrum (Vesalius, 1543a)* and *base of brain (Varoli, 1573)* for macrodissected adult human, so it probably includes ***cerebral cortex white matter (>1840)***, ***cerebral nuclei (Swanson, 2000a)***, and ***interbrain (Baer, 1837)***, with or without ***midbrain (Baer, 1837)***. In the original text it is spelled in the archaic form, *brayne*.

27. *foundation of brain (Bannister, 1578)*
Synonym for *seat of brain (Bannister, 1578)*; f. 106.

28. *medulla globosa (Piccolomini, 1586)*
Probably includes for macrodissected adult human, ***cerebral cortex white matter (>1840)***, or at least ***corpus callosum (Galen, c177)***, along with ***cerebral nuclei (Swanson, 2000a)***, ***interbrain (Baer, 1837)***, ***midbrain (Baer, 1837)***, and ***pons (Haller, 1747)***, all considered together; p. 259 and illustrated in his midsagittal drawing of ***brain (Smith Papyrus, c1700 BC)*** indicated by *DDD*, p. 265; also see Clarke and Dewhurst (1996, Fig. 88). As Bauhin (1605, pp. 625–628) explained (see Crooke translation, 1615, p. 479), "The marrow it selfe [*medulla vero (Bauhin 1605)*] may be said to be double—one Globous or round, the other Long. The Globous part [*medulla globosa (Piccolomini, 1586) or globus marrow (Crooke, 1615)*] which is like the figure of the Scull, is of a great bulke [about the size of a hen's egg, he wrote elsewhere] and therein are ventricles excavated or hollowed. At this and continuall with it hangeth the other called *Cerebellum*... The Long Marrow of the Braine [*medulla vero cerebri oblongata (Bauhin 1605)*] which is like a Pith or staff may bee divided into that part which is contained within the Scull, and that which is yssued out which properly is called the spinall marrow [*medulla vero spinalis proprie dicta (Bauhin, 1605)*]; although some there are that give this name [*spinal marrow, Spinalis medullae*] unto all the Long marrow of the Braine [for example, see *spinal marrow (Vesalius, 1543a), spinal marrow (Colombo, 1559), spinal marrow (Crooke, 1615)*] as well within the Scull as without..." Also see *medulla (Piccolomini, 1586), medulla oblongata (Piccolomini, 1586)*, and *spinal medulla in general (Bauhin, 1605)*.

29. *globosa cerebri medulla (Piccolomini, 1586)*
Synonym for *medulla globosa (Piccolomini, 1586)*; p. 259, also see Bauhin (1605, p. 628).

30. *medulla rotunda (Piccolomini, 1586)*
Synonym for *medulla globosa (Piccolomini, 1586)*; p. 265, figure legend *D*.
31. *base of brain (Piccolomini, 1586)*
Synonym for *medulla globosa (Piccolomini, 1586)*, according to Bauhin (1605, pp. 625–630), see Crooke translation (1615, pp. 479–481).
32. *pars anterior cerebelli (Casseri, 1609)*
Synonym for macrodissected adult human *base of cerebrum (Vesalius, 1543a)*; p. 124, see Burdach (1822, p. 320).
33. *globous marrow (Crooke, 1615)*
Translation of *medulla globosa (Piccolomini, 1586)*; p. 479. *Globous* is a rare spelling of *globose*, common in 16th and early 17th centuries; *Oxford English Dictionary* (Online).
34. *globose marrow (Crooke, 1615)*
Modern spelling of *globous marrow (Crooke, 1615)*.
35. *corpus callosum (Read, 1638)*
Applied for macrodissected adult human to combined *medulla globosa (Piccolomini, 1586)* and *intracranial medulla oblongata (Piccolomini, 1586)*; that is, to ***cerebral cortex white matter (>1840)***, ***cerebral nuclei (Swanson, 2000a)***, and ***brainstem (Schwalbe, 1881)*** considered together; p. 398.
36. *crura medullae spinalis superiora (Wharton, 1656)*
Probably roughly synonymous with macrodissected adult human *root of spinal marrow (Varoli, 1573)*; pp. 154–155, see Burdach (1822, p. 320), who referred to 1671 Wesel edition of Wharton's *Adenographia*.
37. *round part of marrow (Bartholin, 1662)*
Based on macrodissected adult human *medulla globosa (Piccolomini, 1586)*; for Bartholin it included ***lateral ventricles (Vesalius, 1543a)*** and ***third ventricle (Galen, c173)***, and thus probably ***cerebral cortex white matter (>1840)***, ***cerebral nuclei (Swanson, 2000a)*** and at least major (dorsal) part of ***interbrain (Baer, 1837)***; p. 133.
38. *globose part of marrow (Bartholin, 1662)*
Synonym for *round part of marrow (Bartholin, 1662)*, spelled there (p. 133) in the old style, *globous* (*Oxford English Dictionary*, Online); the Latin form, *medulla globosa*, was used in Bartholin (1651, p. 317). Also see *tail of marrow (Bartholin, 1662)* and *medulla oblongata (Bartholin, 1651)*.
39. *head of marrow (Bartholin, 1662)*
Synonym for *round part of marrow (Bartholin, 1662)*; p. 133.
40. *marrow itself (Bartholin, 1662)*
Corresponds to macrodissected adult human ***cerebral cortex white matter (>1840)***, ***cerebral nuclei (Swanson, 2000a)***, and ***brainstem (Schwalbe, 1881)*** considered together; pp. 133–137. Based on Varoli's account, with combination of *root of spinal marrow (Varoli, 1573)* and *anterior spinal marrow (Varoli, 1573)*; and then Piccolomini's combination of *medulla globosa (Piccolomini, 1586)* and *intracranial medulla oblongata (Piccolomini, 1586)*.
41. *internal part of brain (Bartholin, 1662)*
Synonym for *marrow itself (Bartholin, 1662)*, also referred to as internal *substance* of brain, *inmost* part or substance of brain, and *middlemost* part or substance of brain; pp. 133–137, also see *cerebral medulla (Piccolomini, 1586)*.
42. *part within skull of medulla oblongata (Bartholin, 1662)*
Although Bartholin's use was sometimes confusing, most often synonym for macrodissected adult human *marrow itself (Bartholin, 1662)*: ***cerebral cortex white matter (>1840)***, ***cerebral nuclei (Swanson, 2000a)***, and ***brainstem (Schwalbe, 1881)*** considered together; pp. 133, 138, 322–323.
43. *trunk of spinal marrow (Bartholin, 1662)*
Roughly macrodissected adult human ***tegmentum (Swanson, 2000b)***, ***pons (Haller, 1747)***, and ***medulla (Winslow, 1733)*** considered together, but excluding ***cerebellar peduncles (Ridley, 1695)***. Following Varoli's account closely—see *root of spinal marrow (Varoli, 1573)* and *anterior spinal marrow (Varoli, 1573)*—Bartholin described four roots associated with *trunk of spinal marrow (Bartholin, 1662)*: two from ***cerebral cortex gray matter (>1840)*** and two from ***cerebellum (Aristotle)***. Two larger *roots from brain (Bartholin, 1662)*, also called *round trunks (Bartholin, 1662)*, merge at level of ***pineal gland (Galen, c192)*** and just caudal to this are joined by two smaller *roots from brainlet (Bartholin, 1662)*; that is, from ***cerebellum (Aristotle)***. The *roots from brain (Bartholin, 1662)* form ***superior colliculi (Haller, 1762)*** of ***tectum (Baer, 1837)***, whereas *roots from brainlet (Bartholin, 1662)* form ***inferior colliculi (Haller, 1762)*** of ***tectum (Baer, 1837)***, arrangement of four colliculi forming ***cerebral aqueduct (>1840)***. Merger of four roots in ***tegmentum (Swanson, 2000b)***, ***pons (Haller, 1747)***, and ***medulla (Winslow, 1733)*** then extends as ***spinal cord (Galen, c162–c166)***; pp. 137–141, Table 2-*d*. *Trunk of spinal marrow (Bartholin, 1662)* extends about four finger breadths above *foramen magnum*, in its beginning is thicker and larger than elsewhere, and like *brain (Piccolomini, 1586, definition 2)—cerebral cortex (Bauhin, 1605)*—is divided by ***pia (Galen, c192)*** into right and left halves or sides; p. 137.
44. *root of spinal marrow (Bartholin, 1662)*
One of four *roots of spinal marrow (Bartholin, 1662)*; p. 140, Table 2-*d*.
45. *roots of spinal marrow (Bartholin, 1662)*
Refers to two *roots from brain (Bartholin, 1662)* and two *roots from brainlet (Bartholin, 1662)* considered together; pp. 137, 140. According to Burdach (1822, p. 320), Le Boë (1663) also used the Latin term *radices medullae spinalis*, probably in roughly the same way; see Le Boë (1680, p. 18).
46. *roots from brain (Bartholin, 1662)*
Two contributors to macrodissected adult human *trunk of spinal marrow (Bartholin, 1662)* emerging from right and left ***cerebral cortex gray matter (>1840)***; p. 141. The right and left root basically included ***cerebral cortex white matter (>1840)***, ***cerebral nuclei (Swanson, 2000a)***, ***interbrain (Baer, 1837)*** and ***superior colliculus (Haller, 1762)*** considered together. See synonym *round trunk (Bartholin, 1662)* for details.

47. *trunks of spinal marrow (Bartholin, 1662)*
Synonym for *roots of spinal marrow (Bartholin, 1662)*; pp. 137, 141.
48. *trunks of medulla oblongata (Bartholin, 1662)*
Synonym for *trunks of spinal marrow (Bartholin, 1662)*; p. 325.
49. *round trunk (Bartholin, 1662)*
Synonym for right and left *roots from brain (Bartholin, 1662)*. This interpretation is from brief reference to macrodissected adult human *striated body (Willis, 1664)* and *thalami nervorum opticorum (Riolan, 1618)*; that is, ***cerebral cortex white matter (>1840), cerebral nuclei (Swanson, 2000a), interbrain (Baer, 1837)***, and ***superior colliculus (Haller, 1762)*** considered together; p. 114. Essentially following *medulla (Piccolomini, 1586)*, Bartholin wrote of two (right and left) round trunks proceeding out of *brain (Piccolomini, 1586, definition 2)*—***cerebral cortex gray matter (>1840)***. Those round trunks correspond to right and left ***cerebral cortex white matter (>1840)*** and *striated body (Willis, 1664)*. Proceeding farther they are then separated by ***third ventricle (Galen, c173)***, right and left segments corresponding to ***interbrain (Baer, 1837)***. Finally they come together at level of ***pineal gland (Galen, c192)***, roughly at rostral end of ***midbrain (Baer, 1837)***. At this level they form ***superior colliculi (Haller, 1762)*** dorsally, and join with *roots from brainlet (Bartholin, 1662)* ventrally to form *trunk of spinal marrow (Bartholin, 1662)*, which begins rostrally in ***tegmentum (Swanson, 2000b)***.
50. *first trunks of medulla oblongata (Bartholin, 1662)*
Synonym for *roots from brain (Bartholin, 1662)*; p. 325.
51. *oblong marrow (Willis, 1664)*
Willis used it [alternate translations are *oblong medulla (Willis, 1664)* and *medulla oblongata (Willis, 1664)*] for macrodissected adult human, other mammals, birds, and fish in the sense of ***cerebral nuclei (Swanson, 2000a)*** and ***brainstem (Schwalbe, 1881)*** considered together but minus ***tectum (Baer, 1837)***—and he wrote that it is *Y*-shaped with two rostral *shanks of oblong marrow (Willis, 1664)* coming together, side by side, to form one and the same caudal *trunk of oblong marrow (Willis, 1664)*, although the *oblong marrow (Willis, 1664)*, synonymous with *trunk of oblong marrow (Willis, 1664)*, as a whole can also be viewed as being composed of a right and a left *stalk of oblong marrow (Willis, 1664)*; see Pordage translation (1681, pp. 61–62, 101). He wrote that birds and fish have a somewhat similar *oblong marrow*, but the *orbicular prominences (Willis, 1664)*, or ***tectum (Baer, 1837)***, seem to be replaced with *hollow medullary prominences (Willis, 1664)*, and the *striated body (Willis, 1664)*, or ***cerebral nuclei (Swanson, 2000a)***, seems to be replaced by the *streaked membrane (Willis, 1664)* and seems to be in *cerebral hemisphere (Willis, 1664)* rather than *oblong medulla (Willis, 1664)*; pp. 75–77. It is an elaboration on the basic accounts of Varoli (1573) and Piccolomini (1586), as adapted by Bartholin (1662); see *marrow itself (Bartholin, 1662), trunk of spinal marrow (Bartholin, 1662)*, and *part within skull of medulla oblongata (Bartholin, 1662)*.
52. *oblong medulla (Willis, 1664)*
Synonym for *oblong marrow (Willis, 1664)*; alternate form of Latin-based *medulla oblongata (Willis, 1664)*.
53. *medulla oblongata (Willis, 1664)*
Latin form of *oblong medulla (Willis, 1664)* or *oblong marrow (Willis, 1664)*; also *medullae oblongatae*, p. 24.
54. *medullae oblongatae caudex (Willis, 1664)*
Original Latin form, later translated *trunk of oblong marrow (Willis, 1664)*; p. 24.
55. *caudicem (Willis, 1664)*
Latin synonym for *trunk of oblong medulla (Willis, 1664)*; p. 153. Shortened form of *medullae oblongatae caudex (Willis, 1664)*.
56. *stock of oblong marrow (Willis, 1664)*
Apparently synonym for *oblong marrow (Willis, 1664)*; see Pordage translation (1681, p. 62).
57. *stock of long marrow (Willis, 1664)*
Form of *stock of oblong marrow (Willis, 1664)*; see Pordage translation, p. 62, Figure 1-*a*.
58. *trunk of oblong marrow (Willis, 1664)*
Synonym for *stock of oblong marrow (Willis, 1664)*; in the original Latin, *caudicem*, see Pordage translation (1681, p. 62).
59. *long marrow (Willis, 1664)*
Synonym for *oblong medulla (Willis, 1664)*; see Pordage translation (1681, p. 64).
60. *shank of oblong marrow (Willis, 1664)*
Right and left *shanks* form rostral arms of *Y*-shaped *oblong medulla (Willis, 1664)*—corresponding roughly to ***cerebral nuclei (Swanson, 2000a)*** and ***interbrain (Baer, 1837)*** considered together; see Pordage translation (1681; pp. 62, 64; Figs. III-*E*, IV-*E*). In the original Latin, *shank* was *crus* and *shanks* were *crura*.
61. *crus of medulla oblongata (Willis, 1664)*
Latin form of *shank of oblong marrow (Willis, 1664)*.
62. *stem of oblong marrow (Willis, 1664)*
Apparently synonym for *stalk of oblong marrow (Willis, 1644)*; see Pordage translation (1681, pp. 62, 64).
63. *anterior portion of oblong marrow (Willis, 1664)*
Corresponds roughly to ***cerebral nuclei (Swanson, 2000a), interbrain (Baer, 1837)***, and ***midbrain (Baer, 1837)*** considered together; see Pordage translation (1681, p. 67).
64. *common trunk (Willis, 1664)*
Synonym for (bilateral) *oblong medulla (Willis, 1664)*, which forms a *common trunk* for *cerebrum (Willis, 1664)* and ***cerebellum (Aristotle)***; see Pordage translation (1681, p. 90).
65. *trunk of brain (Willis, 1664)*
Synonym for *oblong medulla (Willis, 1664)*; see Pordage translation (1681, p. 101).
66. *stalk of oblong marrow (Willis, 1664)*
Willis wrote that *oblong marrow (Willis, 1664)* as a whole seems to be made of two *stalks*, one right and one left, distinguishable along their length; see Pordage translation (1681, pp. 101).

67. *high road (Willis, 1664)*
Synonym for *oblong medulla (Willis, 1664)*; see Pordage translation (1681, p. 101).
68. *king's highway (Willis, 1664)*
Synonym for *oblong medulla (Willis, 1664)*; see Pordage translation (1681, p. 110).
69. *fore part of medulla oblongata (Gibson, 1684)*
Variation on *anterior oblong marrow (Willis, 1664)*; p. 354.
70. *head of spinal marrow (Gibson, 1684)*
Synonym for *trunk of spinal marrow (Bartholin, 1662)*; p. 366.
71. *basis of brain (Bidloo, 1685)*
Bidloo meant whole part of macrodissected adult human ***vertebrate brain (Cuvier, 1800)*** resting on base of cranium, including ventral surfaces of ***frontal region (Vicq d'Azyr, 1786)*** and ***temporal region (>1840)*** of ***cerebral cortex gray matter (>1840)***, ***cerebral nuclei Swanson, 2000a)***, and ***brainstem (Schwalbe, 1881)***; Table IX, Figure 1-*A*. This was followed by Cowper (1698, Appendix Tab. 6, Fig. 26 legend), who complemented with use of term *basis of cranium*. Cowper italicized *basis*, indicating Latin term in English text; *basis* in English is *base*.
72. *base of brain (Bidloo, 1685)*
Complete English form of *basis of brain (Bidloo, 1685)*.
73. *marrow (Collins, 1685)*
Collins sometimes used *marrow* (or medulla) in the sense of *oblong marrow (Willis, 1664)*, "seated in the Base of the Brain" (p. 1017).
74. *cerebrum proper (Haller, 1747)*
Essentially macrodissected adult human *cerebrum (Vesalius, 1543a)*; in the original Latin, *cerebrum magis proprie vocamus*, p. 178. Soemmerring (1798, p. 42) used *cerebrum stricte dictum*.
75. *brain proper (Haller, 1747)*
English form of *cerebrum proper (Haller, 1747)*; see Mihles translation (1754, p. 287). Whole phrase in English was *brain properly so called*.
76. *encephalon (Soemmerring, 1778)*
For macrodissected adult human, ***vertebrate brain (Cuvier, 1800)*** without ***medulla (Winslow, 1733)***; Book 3.
77. *superior part of spinal marrow (Haase, 1781)*
Synonym for *cephalic part of spinal marrow (Haase, 1781)*; in the original Latin, *superior pars medullae spinalis*, p. 29.
78. *nucleus of cerebrum (Reil, 1809b)*
As described for macrodissected adult human, topographic site including two *central nervous system white matter (Meckel, 1817)* components, transverse *corpus callosum system (Reil, 1809b)* and longitudinal *cerebral peduncle system (Reil, 1809b)*, along with "enclosed" ***lateral ventricles (Vesalius, 1543a)***. Reil compared *nucleus of cerebrum (Reil, 1809b)* to a mushroom (as had Willis; see Pordage translation, 1681, p. 101), with *corpus callosum system (Reil, 1809b)* like the head and *cerebral peduncle system (Reil, 1809b)* like the stalk; p. 146 ff., see Mayo translation (1823, p. 53 ff.). Schiller's (1967, 1969) references to Reil's use of term *nucleus* for specific ***central nervous system gray matter region (>1840)*** are inaccurate. The *nucleus* referred to in Reil's quote was *nucleus of cerebrum (Reil, 1809b)*, as well as a similar arrangement for ***cerebellum (Aristotle)***, *nucleus of cerebellum (Reil, 1809b)*. Schiller (1967, p. 527; 1969, p. 68) quoted, "The brain and cerebellum have the same structural type, a nucleus and organs surrounding the nucleus on all sides." The rest of the quote is, "The convolutions of the brain [*cerebrum (Piccolomini, 1586)*], like the laminae [*folia (Malacarne, 1776)*] of the cerebellum, consist of medullary plates [the nucleus referred to above], as these plates again, of fibres, and their exterior surface is covered with a layer of cortical matter [the organs referred to above]..." Later, however, he did allude to a *gray nucleus* [in German, *kern*; in English, *kernel*], the ***inferior colliculus (Haller, 1762)***; 1812c, see Mayo translation (1823, p. 123, Tab. XI-*i*,*w*).
79. *nucleus of hemisphere (Reil, 1809b)*
Synonym for *nucleus of cerebrum (Reil, 1809b)*; see Mayo translation (1823, p. 48).
80. *cerebral nucleus (Reil, 1809b)*
Alternate form of *nucleus of cerebrum (Reil, 1809b)*.
81. *tegmentum (Reil, 1809b)*
Latin form of Reil's German term, *der Haube*; see Meckel (1817; and translation, 1832, Vol. 2, p. 467), Burdach (1822, p. 323), and Foster (1894, p. 2909). Reil distinguished *gray substance (Vesalius, 1543a)* from *white substance (Vesalius, 1543a)* along course of macrodissected adult human ***internal capsule (Burdach, 1822)*** and ***cerebral peduncle (Tarin, 1753)***, and in the *tegmentum (Reil, 1809b)* he apparently included all ***gray matter (Meckel, 1817)*** of ***midbrain (Baer, 1837)***, including ***tectum (Baer, 1837)***, and ***interbrain (Baer, 1837)***, as well as *inner portion of corpus striatum (Vicq d'Azyr, 1786)* or ***caudate nucleus (Arnold, 1838b)***; p. 151, see Mayo translation (1823, p. 56 ff.). Meyer (1971, p. 29) noted that this description basically divided "brainstem" into *pes* (white matter) and *tegmentum* (gray matter), but this is far from current understanding of ***tegmentum (Swanson, 2000b)***, and a distinction between *gray substance (Vesalius, 1543a)* and *white substance (Vesalius, 1543a)* in the ***interbrain (Baer, 1837)*** and ***midbrain (Baer, 1837)*** had long been made; see *medullary part of crus medulla oblongata (Ridley 1695)*.
82. *cylinder of crus cerebri (Reil, 1809b)*
Mayo (1823, p. 56) translation of Reil's German term, *der Haube*, or Latin form, *tegmentum (Reil, 1809b)*.
83. *nucleus of brain (Reil, 1811c)*
Alternate form of *nucleus of cerebrum (Reil, 1809b)*; see Mayo translation (1823, p. 122).
84. *optic tubercle (Carus, 1814, p. 139)*
Macrodissected adult fish presumed ***cerebral nuclei (Swanson, 2000a)*** and ***interbrain (Baer, 1837)*** considered together; in the original German, *Sehhügel*; see pp. 139, 155, 176. In fish, Carus described *hintern innern*

Ganglien des Sehhügels (Carus, 1814) and *vordern innern Ganglien des Sehhügels (Carus, 1814)*; pp. 139, 155.

85. *cerebrum (Cloquet, 1816)*
For macrodissected adult human, ***forebrain (Goette, 1873)*** and ***tegmentum (Swanson, 2000b)*** considered together; in the original French, *cerveau*, p. 528 ff. Quain (1828, pp. 611–620) also used it thus.
86. *brainstem (Burdach, 1822)*
Corresponds to macrodissected adult human ***cerebral nuclei (Swanson, 2000a)*** and ***brainstem (Schwalbe, 1881)*** considered together, and thus basically synonymous with *trunk of spinal marrow (Bartholin, 1662)* and *oblong marrow (Willis, 1664)*. Burdach divided it into three parts: *cerebral brainstem (Burdach, 1822)*, *pontine brainstem (Burdach, 1822)*, and *medulla oblongata brainstem (Burdach, 1822)*. In German it was *der Hirnstamm*, in Latin, *caudex encephali*; p. 11. *Hirnstamm* was apparently used by Dessort (1820, p. 13) in the same way; it was used undefined by Soemmerring (1792, Vol. 4, p. 379).
87. *caudex encephali (Burdach, 1822)*
Original Latin form of *brainstem (Burdach, 1822)*; p. 11.
88. *cerebral brainstem (Burdach, 1822)*
Corresponds roughly to macrodissected adult human ***cerebral nuclei (Swanson, 2000a)***, ***interbrain (Baer, 1837)***, and ***midbrain (Baer, 1837)*** considered together; in the original German, *Grosshirnstamm*, in Latin, *caudex cerebri* (1822, p. 98 ff.). Thus, it corresponds roughly to *base of cerebrum (Vesalius, 1543a)*. However, Foster (1892, p. 875) claimed it refers specifically to ***cerebral peduncle (Tarin, 1753)*** and *tegmentum (Meckel, 1817)* considered together, but this could well be a definition introduced after Burdach.
89. *caudex cerebri (Burdach, 1822)*
Original Latin form of *cerebral brainstem (Burdach, 1822)*; p. 98.
90. *cerebral stem (Burdach, 1822)*
English form of *caudex cerebri (Burdach, 1822)*.
91. *cerebral trunk (Burdach, 1822)*
English form of *caudex cerebri (Burdach, 1822)*.
92. *systema copulativum (Burdach, 1822)*
Essentially macrodissected adult human site including right and left ***superior cerebellar peduncles (Procháska, 1800)*** laterally, combined with ***rostral medullary vellum (>1840)*** in between; p. 102. Also see *brachium copulativum (Burdach, 1822)*, the ***superior cerebellar peduncle (Procháska, 1800)***.
93. *brain (Quain, 1828)*
Synonym for macrodissected adult human *cerebrum (Cloquet, 1816)*; pp. 611–620.
94. *cerebral ganglia (Arnold, 1838a)*
For macrodissected adult human, ***tectum (Baer, 1837)***, ***interbrain (Baer, 1837)***, and ***cerebral nuclei (Swanson, 2000a)*** considered together; in the original Latin, *ganglia cerebri*, p. 56.
95. *cerebral colliculi (Arnold, 1838a)*
Synonym for *cerebral ganglia (Arnold, 1838a)*; p. 56.

vestibular area of fourth ventricle (>1840)

As described for macrodissected adult human, the triangular, lateral region of the ***floor of fourth ventricle (Reil, 1807–1808a)***, overlying or forming the ventricular surface of the ***vestibular nuclei (>1840)***; see Nieuwenhuys et al. (2008, Fig. 3.10-13). It was illustrated long ago by Ridley; see ***[vestibular area of fourth ventricle (>1840)] (Ridley, 1695)***.

EARLIER REFERENCES:

Illustrated, not named or described:

1. ***[vestibular area of fourth ventricle (>1840)] (Ridley, 1695)***
Illustrated for macrodissected adult human; Figure VII, above *l*. Also see Rolando (1825a, Tab. IV, Fig. 1).

Earlier synonyms:

1. *transverse eminence (Leuret, 1839)*
Synonym for macrodissected adult horse ***vestibular area of fourth ventricle (>1840)***; in the original French (plural), *eminences transverses*, p. 418.

vestibular ganglion (>1840)

As described for macrodissected adult human, the sensory ***cranial nerve ganglion (>1840)*** of the ***vestibular nerve (Cotugno, 1760)*** associated with the internal acoustic meatus and presenting clear superior and inferior parts related to the ***rostral part of vestibular nerve (>1840)*** and ***caudal part of vestibular nerve (>1840)***, respectively; see Stein & Carpenter (1967), Carpenter (1976, p. 337), *Terminologia Anatomica* (1998, p. 135). It was first described as the *gangliformis intumescentia (Scarpa, 1789)*.

EARLIER REFERENCES:

Earlier synonyms:

1. *gangliformis intumescentia (Scarpa, 1789)*
Synonym for macrodissected adult human ***vestibular ganglion (>1840)***; Table VIII, Figure 2-*h*.
2. *Scarpa's ganglion (>1840)*
Eponym for ***vestibular ganglion (>1840)***; see *Dorland's* (2003, p. 753).

vestibular nerve (Cotugno, 1760)

As described for macrodissected adult human, a component of the ***vestibulocochlear nerve (>1840)*** extending from the lateral surface of the ***medulla (Winslow, 1733)*** to the membranous labyrinth with two distal branches, ***rostral part of vestibular nerve (>1840)*** and ***caudal part of vestibular nerve (>1840)***. This account is based on the work of Cannieu (1894), which in turn built on Retzius (1884); see review in Streeter (1907, p. 154 ff.), and Durward (1951, Fig. 904). For Cotugno's use in macrodissected adult human, see p. 408. It was perhaps first clearly delineated by Valsalva; see ***[vestibular nerve (Cotugno, 1760)] (Valsalva, 1704)***.

EARLIER REFERENCES:

Illustrated and described, not named:

1. ***[vestibular nerve (Cotugno, 1760)] (Valsalva, 1704)***
Clearly illustrated splitting of macrodissected adult human ***vestibulocochlear nerve (>1840)*** into one

branch to cochlea and another to vestibule and semicircular canals; Table 8, Figure 3-*d*.

Earlier synonyms:

1. *septum nervosum vestibuli (Cotugno, 1760)*
   Whole Latin phrase related to ***vestibular nerve (Cotugno, 1760)***; p. 408.

LATER SYNONYMS:

1. *vestibular root of auditory nerve (>1840)*
   Can be synonym for **vestibular nerve (Cotugno, 1760)** as a whole; see Cajal (1909–1911; and translation, 1995, Vol. 1, p. 616).

PARTLY CORRESPONDS:

1. ***[vestibular nerve (Cotugno, 1760)] (Du Verney, 1683)***
   Du Verney distinguished in macrodissected adult human three branches of ***vestibulocochlear nerve (>1840)***, one to cochlea, one to semicircular canals, and one to vestibule; the latter two arise from ***vestibular nerve (Cotugno, 1760)*** but their relationship to ***rostral part of vestibular nerve (>1840)*** and ***caudal part of vestibular nerve (>1894)*** is unclear; see 1737 translation, pp. 49, 50. Monro described the latter two branches for fish (1783, p. 33).
2. *vestibular root proper of auditory nerve (>1840)*
   Segment of ***vestibular nerve (Cotugno, 1760)*** between ***vestibular ganglion (>1840)*** distally and outer surface of ***medulla (Winslow, 1733)*** proximally; see Cajal (1909–1911; and translation, 1995, Vol. 2, p. 616). Also see Stein & Carpenter (1967, p. 307).
3. *vestibular root of vestibulocochlear nerve (>1840)*
   Synonym for *vestibular root proper of auditory nerve (>1840)*; see *Dorland's* (2003, p. 1566).

vestibular nerve central root (>1840)

As described for macrodissected adult human, and mammal generally with histological methods for ***axons (Kölliker, 1896)***, the central continuation of the ***vestibular nerve (Cotugno, 1760)*** from the plane where it enters the ***medulla (Winslow, 1733)*** to its termination in the ***cerebellum (Aristotle)*** and ***vestibular nuclei (>1840)***, basically coursing between ***inferior cerebellar peduncle (Günther, 1786)*** and ***medullary segment of spinal tract of trigeminal nerve (>1840)***; see Sabin (1901, p. 76). It was probably first described as the *lower and internal part of auditory nerve (Meckel, 1817)*.

EARLIER REFERENCES:

Earlier synonyms:

1. *lower and internal part of auditory nerve (Meckel, 1817)*
   Probably synonym for macrodissected adult human ***vestibular nerve central root (>1840)***, although Meckel's description is difficult to follow; see translation (1832, Vol. 3, p. 52).

vestibular nuclei (>1840)

As described for macrodissected adult human, and for adult mammal in general with cellular architecture and connections, a ***gray matter region (Swanson & Bota, 2010)*** in the rostral half of the dorsal ***medulla (Winslow, 1733)***, medial to the ***cochlear nuclei (>1840)*** and ventral to the ***cerebellar nuclei (>1840)***. The ***vestibular nerve (Cotugno, 1760)*** and its ***vestibular nerve central root (>1840)*** ends there, and its major divisions include ***medial vestibular nucleus (>1840)***, ***superior vestibular nucleus (>1840)***, ***lateral vestibular nucleus (>1840)***, and ***inferior vestibular nucleus (>1840)***; see Nieuwenhuys et al. (2008, pp. 194, 718 ff. and Figs. 6.23–27). They were probably first identified vaguely by Rolando; see ***[vestibular nuclei (>1840)] (Rolando, 1825a)***. They were clearly delineated as the *gray-medullary appendix of acoustic nerve (Rolando, 1831)*.

EARLIER REFERENCES:

Illustrated and described, not named:

1. ***[vestibular nuclei (>1840)] (Rolando, 1825a)***
   Illustrated and vaguely described in transverse section, presumably of adult beef; Table IX, Figure 4, lateral to *e.l.* Also see *eminentias transversales ventriculi quarti (Procháska, 1800)*.

Earlier synonyms:

1. *gray-medullary appendix of acoustic nerve (Rolando, 1831)*
   Essentially macrodissected adult human ***vestibular nuclei (>1840)***; in the original Italian, *appendice cinereo-midollare del nervo acustico*, Figure 10-33. Also see ***[vestibular nuclei (>1840)] (Rolando, 1825a)***.

vestibulocochlear nerve (>1840)

As described for macrodissected adult mammal, a ***cranial nerve (Soemmerring, 1791)*** consisting of two parts, ***vestibular nerve (Cotugno, 1760)*** and ***cochlear nerve (Cotugno, 1760)***; see Williams & Warwick (1980, p. 1073). It is convenient to distinguish a ***vestibulocochlear nerve trunk (>1840)*** where the two ***nerves (Herophilus, c335–c280 BC)*** lie adjacent to one another, and may intertwine to some extent. The ***vestibulocochlear nerve trunk (>1840)*** stretches from the plane where the two ***nerves (Herophilus, c335–c280 BC)*** together enter the ***medulla (Winslow, 1733)*** to the point distally where the trunk separates into spatially separated ***nerves (Herophilus, c335–c280 BC)*** associated with the labyrinth, the free part of the ***cochlear nerve (Cotugno, 1760)*** and the ***caudal part of vestibular nerve (>1840)***; see Sabin (1901, p. 76), Streeter (1907, p. 158), Durward (1951, p. 1035 and Fig. 904). This account is based on the work of Cannieu (1894), which in turn built on Retzius (1884); see review in Streeter (1907, p. 154 ff.). The specific term *vestibulocochlear nerve* was used, for example, by Carpenter (1976, p. 325) and Williams & Warwick (1980, p. 1073). Its existence was postulated by Alcmaeon; see ***[vestibulocochlear nerve (>1840)] (Alcmaeon, c490–c430 BC)***. It was probably first observed by Herophilus; see ***[vestibulocochlear nerve (>1840)] (Herophilus, c335–c280 BC)***.

EARLIER REFERENCES:

Described, not named or illustrated:

1. ***[vestibulocochlear nerve (>1840)] (Alcmaeon, c490–c430 BC)***
   In *De Sensu*, Aristotle's successor, Theophrastus (c327–c287 BC), wrote that Alcmaeon postulated the

existence of a channel (alternate translations: *passage, duct*) between ear and ***brain (Smith Papyrus, c1700 BC)***; see Solmsen (1961, pp. 151–152), Lloyd (1975). Also see ***[cranial nerves (Soemmerring, 1791)] (Alcmaeon, c490–c430 BC)***.

2. ***[vestibulocochlear nerve (>1840)] (Herophilus, c335–c280 BC)***
Herophilus, the founder of human anatomy, is credited with discovering but not naming it in macrodissected adult mammal, including human cadavers. Also see ***[cranial nerves (Soemmerring, 1791)] (Herophilus, c335–c280 BC)***.

Illustrated, not named or described:

1. ***[vestibulocochlear nerve (>1840)] (Eustachi, 1552)***
Eustachi clearly illustrated for macrodissected adult human its origin as distinct from *facial nerve (Vicq d'Azyr, 1784)*; see Albinus edition (1761, Tab. 18, Figs. 1, 3, 4-γ and Fig. 2-*b*).

Earlier synonyms:

1. *acoustic nerve (Galen, c173)*
Term for one of two components of *fifth pair of nerves from brain (Galen, c192)*, the ***vestibulocochlear nerve (>1840)***; see May translation (1968, p. 404), Savage-Smith (1971, p. 181 ff.). Galen's term was still used in the *Basel Nomina Anatomica* (His, 1895, p. 89). In Latin, *nervus acusticus*; see Soemmerring (1778, p. 155).
2. *auditory nerve (Galen, c192)*
Alternate form of *acoustic nerve (Galen, c173)* in English; see Duckworth translation (1962, p. 196). Latin form, *nervus auditivus*. Falloppio referred to it as *auditorium*; see Soemmerring (1778, p. 155).
3. *nervi postici (Anatomia Magistri Nicolai physici, early 12th century)*
Synonym for ***vestibulocochlear nerves (>1840)***; see Corner (1927, p. 72).
4. *second pair of nerves from brain (Benedetti, 1502)*
Synonym for macrodissected adult human ***vestibulocochlear nerves (>1840), nerves (Herophilus, c335–c280 BC)*** going to ear; Book IV, Chapter 14, p. 1237. See Lind translation (1975, p. 117).
5. *fourth pair of nerves from brain (Estienne, 1545)*
Apparently synonym for macrodissected adult human ***vestibulocochlear nerves (>1840), nerves (Herophilus, c335–c280 BC)*** going to ears; see Vicq d'Azyr (1786, p. 49), Burdach (1822, p. 311).
6. *soft part of fifth pair (Falloppio, 1561)*
Synonym for macrodissected adult human ***vestibulocochlear nerve (>1840)***; in the original Latin, *portio mollis paris quinti*, see Burdach (1822, p. 311).
7. *hearing nerve (Falloppio, 1561)*
English form of Falloppio's Latin term for macrodissected adult human ***vestibulocochlear nerve (>1840)***; Diemerbroeck (1689, p. 416).
8. *nervi audibiles (Hall, 1565)*
Latin synonym for macrodissected adult human ***vestibulocochlear nerves (>1840)***; p. 54.
9. *sinew of hearing (Crooke, 1615)*
Synonym for macrodissected adult human *auditory nerve (Galen, c192)*; p. 487.
10. *auditory nerve proper (Willis, 1664)*
Term for one of two components of *seventh pair of nerves arising within skull (Willis, 1664)*—the sensory or soft ***nerve (Herophilus, c335–c280 BC)*** going to inner ear, the ***vestibulocochlear nerve (>1840)***; see Pordage translation (1681, p. 143). Swan (1830, Pl. X, Fig. 2-6) used *proper auditory nerve*.
11. *soft part of seventh pair of nerves arising within skull (Willis, 1664)*
Synonym for *auditory nerve proper (Willis, 1664)*; see Pordage translation (1681, p. 140 ff).
12. *portio mollis of seventh pair of nerves arising within skull (Willis, 1664)*
Latinized form of *soft part of seventh pair of nerves arising within skull (Willis, 1664)*; see Pordage translation (1681, p. 140 ff.). See *soft part of fifth pair (Falloppio, 1561)*.
13. *portio mollis nervi auditorii (Winslow, 1733)*
Synonym for macrodissected adult human *portio mollis of seventh pair of nerves arising within skull (Willis, 1664)*; Section VI, p. 59.
14. *nervus mollis (Haller, 1762)*
Synonym for macrodissected adult human *portio mollis of seventh pair of nerves arising within skull (Willis, 1664)*; see Burdach (1822, p. 311).
15. *nervus acusticus mollis (Haller, 1762)*
Synonym for macrodissected adult human *portio mollis of seventh pair of nerves arising within skull (Willis, 1664)*; see Burdach (1822, p. 311).
16. *eighth pair of nerves leaving skull (Soemmerring, 1778)*
Soemmerring's enumeration of macrodissected adult human ***vestibulocochlear nerves (>1840)***; Latin form, *par octavum*, given by Burdach (1822, p. 311). Also see *nervorum per ossa capitis egredientium (Soemmerring, 1778)* and *eighth pair of nerves of head (Andersch, 1797)*.
17. *cochlear nerve (Haase, 1781)*
Synonym for macrodissected adult human ***vestibulocochlear nerve (>1840)***, in the original Latin, *nervus cochleae*, p. 78.
18. *second nerve of seventh pair (Vicq d'Azyr, 1784)*
Synonym for macrodissected adult human ***vestibulocochlear nerve (>1840)***; p. 591.
19. *thirteenth pair of nerves (Malacarne, 1791)*
Synonym for macrodissected adult human ***vestibulocochlear nerves (>1840)***, the 13th of 17 pairs of *cranial nerves (Malacarne, 1791)*; p. 193.
20. *eighth pair of cranial nerves (Soemmerring, 1791)*
Synonym for macrodissected adult human ***vestibulocochlear nerves (>1840)***; see ***cranial nerves (Soemmerring, 1791)***.
21. *eighth pair of cerebral nerves (Soemmerring, 1791)*
Synonym for *eighth pair of cranial nerves (Soemmerring, 1791)*; see p. 103 and *cerebral nerves (Soemmerring, 1791)*. In the original Latin, *par octavum nervorum cerebri*, Soemmerring (1798, p. 125).

22. *eighth pair of nerves of head (Andersch, 1797)*
Synonym for macrodissected adult human *eighth pair of nerves leaving skull (Soemmerring, 1778)*; p. 1. Andersch's thesis was published finally in 1797, but was written c1751–c1755.

23. *labyrinthic pair of nerves (Burdin, 1803)*
Synonym for macrodissected adult human ***vestibulocochlear nerves (>1840)***; see translation (1803, Vol. 1, p. 144).

24. *par duodecimum (Burdach, 1822)*
Malacarne's enumeration of ***vestibulocochlear nerves (>1840)*** according to Burdach (1822, p. 311), who mistakenly supplied this Latin form; see *thirteenth pair of nerves (Malacarne, 1791)*.

25. *stato-acoustic nerve (>1840)*
Synonym for macrodissected adult human ***vestibulocochlear nerve (>1840)***; see Brodal (1957a, p. 53).

PARTLY CORRESPONDS:

1. *roots of acoustic nerve (Malacarne, 1791)*
Malacarne alluded to peripheral roots of ***vestibulocochlear nerve (>1840)*** in macrodissected adult human, but their identity is unclear; pp. 227, 237.

vestibulocochlear nerve trunk (>1840)

As described for macrodissected adult human, the part of the ***vestibulocochlear nerve (>1840)*** where the ***vestibular nerve (Cotugno, 1760)*** and ***cochlear nerve (Cotugno, 1760)*** lie adjacent to one another, may intertwine to some extent, and are not physically distinguishable in some regions; see Streeter (1907, p. 158). The trunk stretches from the plane where the two ***nerves (Herophilus, c335–c280 BC)*** together enter the ***medulla (Winslow, 1733)*** to the distal point where the trunk physically diverges near the lateral end of the internal acoustic meatus into two parts: the free part of the ***cochlear nerve (Cotugno, 1760)*** and the ***caudal part of vestibular nerve (>1840)***; see Obersteiner & Hill (1900, Fig. 139), Sabin (1901, p. 76), Durward (1951, p. 1035 and Fig. 904). The ***rostral part of vestibular nerve (>1840)*** branches off more proximally, from middle regions of the ***vestibulocochlear nerve trunk (>1840)***. In short, the trunk consists of adjacent segments of the ***cochlear nerve (Cotugno, 1760)*** and ***vestibular nerve (Cotugno, 1760)***; see Riley (1943, p. 535), Durward (1951, Fig. 904), who both use this term, and Stein & Carpenter (1967). It was probably first clearly described by Monro; see ***[vestibulocochlear nerve trunk (>1840)] (Monro, 1783)***.

EARLIER REFERENCES:

Illustrated and described, not named:

1. ***[vestibulocochlear nerve trunk (>1840)] (Monro, 1783)***
Monro clearly described and illustrated for macrodissected adult human "a thin middle portion, by which these two sides or branches [***vestibular nerve (Cotugno, 1760)*** and ***cochlear nerve (Cotugno, 1760)***] are joined together" (Tab. 30, Fig. 4-*L*).

Earlier synonyms:

1. *acoustic nerve trunk (Scarpa, 1789)*
Synonym for macrodissected adult human ***vestibulocochlear nerve trunk (>1840)***; in the original Latin, *nervi acustici truncus*, Table VIII, Figure 2-*e*.
2. *auditory nerve trunk (Meckel, 1817)*
Synonym for macrodissected adult human ***vestibulocochlear nerve trunk (>1840)***; see translation (1832, Vol. 3, p. 52).

PARTLY CORRESPONDS:

1. *cerebral part of eighth pair (Arnold, 1834)*
Macrodissected adult human proximal segment of ***vestibulocochlear nerve trunk (>1840)***, proximal to petrous part of temporal bone and corresponding *petrous part of eighth pair (Arnold, 1834)*; in the original Latin, *par octavum pars cerebralis*, p. 12.
2. *cerebral part of acoustic nerve (Arnold, 1834)*
Synonym for *cerebral part of eighth pair (Arnold, 1834)*; in the original Latin, *nervus acusticus, pars cerebralis*, p. 12.
3. *cerebral part of auditory nerve (Arnold, 1834)*
Synonym for *cerebral part of eighth pair (Arnold, 1834)*; in the original Latin, *nervus auditorius, pars cerebralis*, p. 12.
4. *cerebral part of soft part of seventh pair (Arnold, 1834)*
Synonym for *cerebral part of eighth pair (Arnold, 1834)*; in the original Latin, *portio mollis septimi paris, pars cerebralis*, p. 12.
5. *petrous part of eighth pair (Arnold, 1834)*
Macrodissected adult human distal segment of ***vestibulocochlear nerve trunk (>1840)***, distal to *cerebral part of eighth pair (Arnold, 1834)* and proximal to the point it physically diverges into two parts; in the original Latin, *par octavum, pars petrosa*, p. 12.
6. *petrous part of acoustic nerve (Arnold, 1834)*
Synonym for *petrous part of eighth pair (Arnold, 1834)*; in the original Latin, *nervus acusticus, pars petrosa*, p. 12.
7. *petrous part of auditory nerve (Arnold, 1834)*
Synonym for *petrous part of eighth pair (Arnold, 1834)*; in the original Latin, *nervus auditorius, pars petrosa*, p. 12.
8. *petrous part of soft part of seventh pair (Arnold, 1834)*
Synonym for *petrous part of eighth pair (Arnold, 1834)*; in the original Latin, *portio mollis septimi paris, pars petrosa*, p. 12.

vomeronasal nerve (>1840)

In many adult non-primate mammals, and submammalian forms, a vomeronasal organ lies on each side of the nasal septum and ***axon (Kölliker, 1896)*** bundles from sensory ***neurons (Waldeyer, 1891)*** in its epithelium course with ventral ***axon (Kölliker, 1896)*** bundles of the ***olfactory nerve (Winslow, 1733)*** before converging to form the ***vomeronasal nerve (>1840)*** trunk ending in the ***accessory olfactory bulb (>1840)***; see Williams & Warwick (1980, p. 994) and Larriva-Sahd (2008). Commonly a vomeronasal organ, ***vomeronasal nerve (>1840)***, and ***accessory olfactory bulb (>1840)*** are found in human embryo but not adult; see Crosby et al. (1962, p. 412). It is a ***cranial nerve (Soemmerring, 1791)*** usually considered along with the ***olfactory nerve (Winslow, 1733)*** and was discovered by Jacobson; see ***[vomeronasal nerve (>1840)] (Jacobson, 1809)***.

EARLIER REFERENCES:

Described, not named or illustrated:

1. ***[vomeronasal nerve (>1840)] (Jacobson, 1809)***
   The vomeronasal organ and a ***nerve (Herophilus, c335–c280 BC)*** entering it, not named but the ***vomeronasal nerve (>1840)***, were both clearly described with macrodissection methods in domestic mammals; p. 214. See facsimile in Stamm (1932, p. 98), and full text in Jacobson (1948, p. 23 ff.).

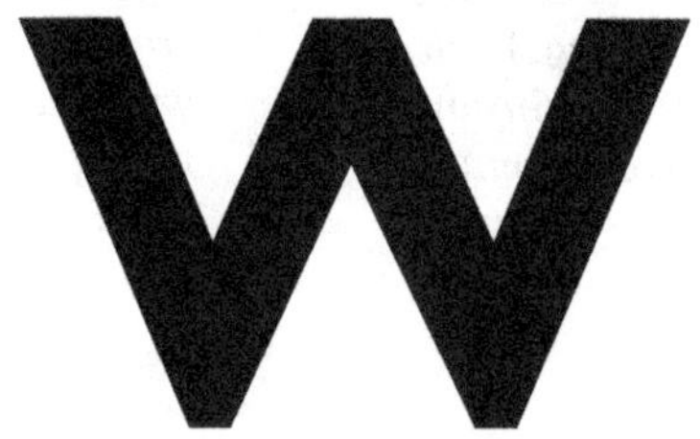

white communicating branch (>1840)

As described for adult human, a ***communicating branch of spinal nerves (Wutzer, 1817)***, specifically of the ***lumbar nerves (Diemerbroeck, 1672)*** and rostral (upper) ***thoracic nerves (Diemerbroeck, 1672)***, which typically have at least one each; see Mitchell (1953, pp. 205–207). ***White communicating branches (>1840)*** typically carry preganglionic sympathetic ***axons (Kölliker, 1896)*** and autonomic sensory ***dendrites (His, 1889)***; see Mitchell (1953, p. 124), Williams & Warwick (1980, pp. 1136–1137). Most often the ***white communicating branch (>1840)*** lies just distal to the ***gray communicating branch (>1840)*** on a ***spinal nerve ventral branch (>1840)***; see Williams & Warwick (1980, pp. 1103, 1125). They were clearly identified by Meckel; see ***[white communicating branch (>1840)] (Meckel, 1751)***.

TRANSLATIONS:

1. *ramus communicans albus (>1840)*

   Current Latin form of ***white communicating branch (1840)***; see *Terminologia Anatomica* (1998, p. 141).

EARLIER REFERENCES:

Described, not named or illustrated:

1. ***[white communicating branch (>1840)] (Meckel, 1751)***

   Meckel distinguished between ***white communicating branch (>1840)*** and ***gray communicating branch (>1840)*** in macrodissected adult human. He wrote that some are white and others reddish [as they are in the fresh state]—later referred to as gray; see Clarke & Jacyna (1987, p. 325).

white matter (Meckel, 1817)

Since the 16th century the entire ***nervous system (Monro, 1783)*** has been divided more and more precisely into ***gray matter (Meckel, 1817)*** and ***white matter (Meckel, 1817)*** based on their appearance in freshly dissected material observed with the naked eye—a systems architecture approach. This began with ***central nervous system white matter tracts (>1840)***. Since the late 1830s this differentiation has also been made at the cellular level. Based on the latter, it is now known that ***white matter (Meckel, 1817)*** is the ***nervous system (Monro, 1783)*** compartment consisting primarily of ***axons (Kölliker, 1896)***. Its name is derived from its appearance in fresh and fixed macroscopically observed material, its whitish color due to the presence of myelinated ***axons (Kölliker, 1896)***. However, ***white matter (Meckel, 1817)*** is often a mixture of myelinated and unmyelinated ***axons (Kölliker, 1896)***, *nerve fibers (Ehrenberg, 1833)*, and entire aggregates of ***axons (Kölliker, 1896)*** can be unmyelinated. Therefore, as defined here ***white matter (Meckel, 1817)*** is a generic term for a ***nervous system (Monro, 1783)*** volume where ***axons (Kölliker, 1896)*** are the predominant neural component, although of course ***glia (Virchow, 1846)*** and parts of the *circulatory system, vascular cells*, are also present. ***White matter (Meckel, 1817)*** can contain scattered ***neurons (Waldeyer, 1891)*** assigned either to an adjacent ***gray matter region (Swanson & Bota, 2010)***, or to a new ***gray matter region (Swanson & Bota, 2010)*** embedded (nested) within the ***white matter (Meckel, 1817)***; assignment depends on differentiable ***neuron types (Bota & Swanson, 2007)*** involved. There is often a fuzzy border of variable width and difficult to measure between ***gray matter (Meckel, 1817)*** and ***white matter (Meckel, 1817)***. ***White matter (Meckel, 1817)*** is parceled into ***white matter tracts (Bell & Bell, 1826)*** based on regional landmarks at the gross anatomical level, and on differences in cellular architecture and connections at a more refined level. This particular definition and description was adapted from Swanson & Bota (2010, Thesaurus). The general term *white matter* found anywhere in the ***nervous system (Monro, 1783)*** was probably introduced by Meckel; see translation (1832, Vol. 2, pp. 152–154), also see Herrick (1915, p. 108). For early history see Clarke & O'Malley

(1996, Ch. 10); for modern histological interpretation see Nauta & Feirtag (1986, pp. 45–46 footnote), Peters et al. (1991), Swanson (2012, pp. 90–103). It was described earlier, however, as *nervous white matter (Gordon, 1815)* and ultimately derives from *white substance (Vesalius, 1543a)*.

EARLIER REFERENCES:

Earlier synonyms:

1. *nervous white matter (Gordon, 1815)*
   Synonym for macrodissected adult human ***white matter (Meckel, 1817)***; p. 120. Gordon described two varieties with slightly different colors, *orange-white white matter (Gordon, 1815)* and *wine-yellow white matter (Gordon, 1815)*; p. 120.

LATER SYNONYMS:

1. *nervous system white matter (Meckel, 1817)*
   Synonym for ***white matter (Meckel, 1817)***. Meckel was the first to use this exact terminology, for macrodissected adult human, distinguishing it from *nervous system gray matter (Meckel, 1817)*; see translation (1832, Vol. 2, pp. 152–154, 166–167).
2. *primary substance (Wutzer, 1817)*
   Synonym for macrodissected adult human ***white matter (Meckel, 1817)***; in the original Latin, *substantia primaria*, p. 53, see Burdach (1819, p. 168).
3. *medullary cerebral matter (Blainville, 1821)*
   Synonym for macrodissected ***white matter (Meckel, 1817)*** in animals generally; in the original French, *matière cérébrale médullaire*, p. 202.
4. *nervous system fibrous substance (Spurzheim, 1826)*
   Synonym for macrodissected ***white matter (Meckel, 1817)*** in animals generally; p. 1.
5. *medullary neurine (Solly, 1836)*
   Synonym for macrodissected ***white matter (Meckel, 1817)*** in animals generally; pp. 6, 119.

PARTLY CORRESPONDS:

1. *orange-white matter (Gordon, 1815)*
   One variety of *nervous white matter (Gordon, 1815)*; p. 120.
2. *wine-yellow matter (Gordon, 1815)*
   One variety of *nervous white matter (Gordon, 1815)*; p. 120.

white matter tracts (Bell & Bell, 1826)

Recognizable volumes of ***white matter (Meckel, 1817)*** in the ***nervous system (Monro, 1783)*** divided topographically into ***central nervous system white matter tracts (>1840)*** and ***peripheral nervous system white matter tracts (>1840)***. All ***white matter tracts (Bell & Bell, 1826)*** are parceled on the basis of differentially segregated connections—a systems architecture approach. In general, ***gray matter regions (Swanson & Bota, 2010)*** are the sites of origin and termination of axonal connections, whereas routes taken by connections are through ***white matter tracts (Bell & Bell, 1826)***, which may range from homogenous to very heterogeneous. For this definition see Swanson & Bota (2010, Fig. 1 and Thesaurus). The term ultimately derives from a passage in Bell & Bell (1826, pp. 375–377). They began to be delineated early on as *medullary substance (Coiter, 1572)*.

EARLIER REFERENCES:

Earlier synonyms:

1. *medullary substance (Coiter, 1572)*
   In describing macrodissected adult human ***spinal cord (Galen, c162–c166)*** Coiter implied its outer region consists at least in part of fibrous *medullar(y) substance* extending into ***nerves (Herophilus, c335–c280 BC)***; see translation pp. 113–117. By Willis's time, *medullary substance* was used synonymously with ***white matter tracts (Bell & Bell, 1826)***; for example, see Willis (1664; and Pordage translation, 1681, pp. 60–61, 93, 101).
2. *medullar substance (Coiter, 1572)*
   Alternate form of *medullary substance (Coiter, 1572)*; see translation pp. 113–117.
3. *tracts (Willis, 1664)*
   General term Willis used for ***white matter tracts (Bell & Bell, 1826)*** in both ***central nervous system (Carus, 1814)*** and ***peripheral nervous system (Meckel, 1817)*** of macrodissected adult mammal; see Pordage translation (1681, pp. 61, 95, 101, 124, Tab. 9-*r*).

PARTLY CORRESPONDS:

1. *optic channel (Herophilus, c335–c280 BC)*
   Probably oldest synonym for *optic nerve (Galen, c173)*. As recounted by Galen, Herophilus called sensory ***nerves (Herophilus, c335–c280 BC)*** between ***brain (Smith Papyrus, c1700 BC)*** and eye "channels" because to him they alone of all ***nerves (Herophilus, c335–c280 BC)*** have a perceptible path for psychic pneuma. Herophilus dissected human cadavers, as well as animals. Thus, Vesalius (1543a) recounted that Greeks called *optic nerves (Galen, c173)* the *poroi optikoi*; see Richardson & Carman translation (2002, pp. 184–185).
2. *poroi optikoi (Herophilus, c335–c280 BC)*
   Greek term (plural) for *optic channel (Herophilus, c335–c280 BC)*; see Richardson & Carman (2002, pp. 184–185).
3. *duct (Aristotle)*
   In *The Account of Animals*, Aristotle referred to perhaps three ***nerves (Herophilus, c335–c280 BC)*** associated with the eye, including *optic channels (Herophilus, c335–c280 BC)*, as ducts (alternate translations of original Greek *poroi*: *passages, channels*), an account almost certainly based on personal dissection of animals; see Lloyd (1975), von Staden (1989, p. 157). This conclusion is strengthened in *On the Generation of Animals* by his description of eye development in animals; see Platt (1958, pp. 743–744). One of these would certainly be the *optic nerve (Galen, c173)*; the description is too vague to even guess about the others.
4. *encephalon extension to crystalline humor (Galen, c173)*
   In *On the Usefulness of the Parts*, Galen described *optic nerve (Galen, c173)* as extension of ***brain (Smith Papyrus, c1700 BC)***; see May translation (1968, p. 402). Crystalline humor refers to lens of eye.
5. *optic nerve (Galen, c173)*
   Galen apparently used it referring to ***optic nerve (Vicq d'Azyr, 1786)***, ***optic chiasm (Galen, c173)***, and ***optic***

tract (Vicq d'Azyr, 1784) considered together, and thus a ***white matter tract (Bell & Bell, 1826)***; see Polyak (1957, p. 77), May translation (1968, pp. 402–403). In *On the Usefulness of the Parts* Galen explained that it is the only ***nerve (Herophilus, c335–c280 BC)*** with a perceptible channel, for transmission of considerable psychic pneuma; see May translation (1968, pp. 399–403, 442). He regarded it as *first pair of nerves from brain (Galen, c173)*; also see *olfactory sense instrument (Galen, c173)*. Galen wrote, "When you have divided the frontal bone so as to reach the deep cavity beneath it, you will be met by the two nerves that go to the eye. If you divide the larger of the two [*optic nerve (Galen, c173)*], then the visual sense of the animal will be impaired. And if you divide the lesser of the two [***oculomotor nerve (Estienne, 1545)***], you will see the eyes immediately remain motionless." (Duckworth translation, 1962, p. 29). In Latin, *opticorum nervorum*; see Soemmerring (1778, p. 95).

6. *first pair of nerves from brain (Galen, c173)*
   Synonym for *optic nerves (Galen, c173)*; see Duckworth translation (1962, p. 8), May translation (1968, p. 444), Savage-Smith (1971, p. 84), also see *olfactory sense instrument (Galen, c173)*. However, Galen acknowledged that some unnamed anatomists regarded *optic nerves (Galen, c173)* as second pair; see *pairs of nerves from skull (Galen, c192)*.
7. *second pair of nerves from brain (Theophilos Protospatharios, fl. 610–641)*
   Synonym for *first pair of nerves from brain (Galen, c173)* in the first real break with Galen's authority on this topic; see 1540 edition, ff. 40v-41 and Meyer (1971, p. 75).
8. *visual nerve (Theophilos Protospatharios, fl. 610–641)*
   Synonym for *optic nerve (Galen, c173)*, also used by Berengario da Carpi in 1522; see Vicq d'Azyr (1786, p. 48), Lind translation (1959, p. 145). As Albertus Magnus explained, "In Greek the nerves are called optic [*optici*], which translates into Latin as 'visual' [*visivi*]" (Kitchell & Resnick translation, 1999, p. 180). In the original Latin, *nervo visorio, nervi visorii* (Theophilos Protospatharios, 1540 edition, ff. 40v-41); *nervus visivus, nervus visorius* (see Soemmerring, 1778, p. 95). According to Burdach (1822, p. 382), Berengario da Carpi (1521) used the plural *nervi visivi*, whereas Vesalius (1543a) used *nervi visorii*. Also see *second pair of nerves from brain (Theophilos Protospatharios, fl. 610–641)*.
9. *concave nerve (William of Saliceto, 1275)*
   Synonym for macrodissected adult human *optic nerve (Galen, c173)*; see Rosenman translation (1998, p. 184).
10. *first pair of nerves from brain (Benedetti, 1502)*
   Benedetti included ***oculomotor nerve (Estienne, 1545)*** or *second pair of nerves from brain (Galen, c173)*, in *first pair of nerves from brain (Galen, c173)*; see Lind (1975, pp. 117–118).
11. *sinowe optico (Brunschwig, 1525)*
   Earliest reference in English to *optic nerve (Galen, c173)*, meaning "optic sinew [***nerve (Herophilus, c335–c280 BC)***]" (p. [8]); spelled *optike sinewes* in Hall (1565, p. 47).
12. *sinew of sight (Geminus, 1553)*
   English form of macrodissected adult human *optic nerve (Galen, c173)*; originally spelled, *synow of syghte*, see *The table of the figure of synowe*, Figure 7-F; or *synowe of sight*, see *The tables of the brain*, Figure 13-N.
13. *seeing nerve (Bartholin, 1662)*
   English form of *optic nerve (Galen, c173)*, originally in Greek; pp. 324–325, also see Burdach (1822, p. 392).
14. *second pair of nerves arising within skull (Willis, 1664)*
   Synonym for macrodissected adult mammalian *first pair of nerves from brain (Galen, c173)*; see Pordage translation (1681, pp. 139–140).
15. *combinatio secunda (Molinetti, 1675)*
   Synonym for *second pair of nerves from brain (Theophilos Protospatharios, fl. 610–641)*; p. 188.
16. *optic pair of cranial nerves (Soemmerring, 1791)*
   Synonym for macrodissected adult human *second pair of cerebral nerves (Arnold, 1834)*; see ***cranial nerves (Soemmerring, 1791)***.
17. *optic pair of cerebral nerves (Soemmerring, 1791)*
   Synonym for *optic pair of cranial nerves (Soemmerring, 1791)*; see p. 103 and *cerebral nerves (Soemmerring, 1791)*. In the original Latin, *par opticum nervorum cerebri*, Soemmerring (1798, p. 125).
18. *ocular pair of nerves (Burdin, 1803)*
   Synonym for macrodissected adult human *optic nerves (Galen, c173)*; see translation (1803, Vol. 1, pp. 143, 168). Burdach (1822, p. 392) gave the Latin, *nervus ocularis*.
19. *second pair of cerebral nerves (Arnold, 1834)*
   Synonym for macrodissected adult human *second pair of nerves from brain (Theophilos Protospatharios, fl. 610–641)*; in the original Latin, *par secundum nervi cerebrales*, p. 6.
20. *central end of common motor nerve of eye (Cruveilhier, 1836)*
   Macrodissected adult human ***white matter tract (Bell & Bell, 1826)*** with both *apparent origin of common motor nerve of eye (Cruveilhier, 1836)* and *real origin of common motor nerve of eye (Cruveilhier, 1836)*; in the original French, *extrémité centrale du nerf moteur oculaire commun*, p. 891.
21. *central end of pathetic nerve (Cruveilhier, 1836)*
   Macrodissected adult human ***white matter tract (Bell & Bell, 1826)*** with both *apparent origin of pathetic nerve (Cruveilhier, 1836)* and *real origin of pathetic nerve (Cruveilhier, 1836)*; in the original French, *extrémité centrale du nerf pathétique*, p. 892.
22. *central end of trigeminal nerves (Cruveilhier, 1836)*
   Macrodissected adult human ***white matter tract (Bell & Bell, 1826)*** with ***trigeminal nerve sensory root (>1840)***, ***trigeminal nerve motor root (Bell, 1829)***, and ***trigeminal nerve central sensory root (>1840)*** considered together; in the original French, *extrémité centrale des nerfs trijumeaux*, p. 893.
23. *central end of external ocular motor nerve (Cruveilhier, 1836)*
   Macrodissected adult human ***white matter tract (Bell & Bell, 1826)*** with both *apparent origin of external ocular motor nerve (Cruveilhier, 1836)* and *real origin of*

external ocular motor nerve (Cruveilhier, 1836); in the original French, *extrémité centrale du nerf moteur oculaire externe*, p. 896.

24. *central end of facial nerve (Cruveilhier, 1836)*
Synonym for *central end of portio dura of seventh pair (Cruveilhier, 1836)*; in the original French, *extrémité central du nerf facial*, p. 897.

25. *central end of portio dura of seventh pair (Cruveilhier, 1836)*
Macrodissected adult human ***white matter tract (Bell & Bell, 1826)*** with both *apparent end of portio dura (Cruveilhier, 1836)* and *real end of portio dura (Cruveilhier, 1836)*; in the original French, *extrémité central du portion dure de la 7e paire*, p. 897.

26. *central end of auditory nerve (Cruveilhier, 1836)*
Basically macrodissected adult human ***medullary striae (Scarpa, 1788)*** and proximal end of ***vestibulocochlear nerve trunk (>1840)*** considered together; in the original French, *extrémité centrale du nerf auditif*, p. 897.

27. *central end of glossopharyngeal and pneumogastric nerves (Cruveilhier, 1836)*
Macrodissected adult human ***white matter tract (Bell & Bell, 1826)*** with ***glossopharyngeal nerve root (>1840)*** and ***vagus nerve root (>1840)***, and what little was known about their extensions into ***medulla (Winslow, 1733)***; in the original French, *extrémité centrale des nerfs glosso-pharyngiens et pneumo-gastrique*, p. 898.

28. *central end of accessory nerve of Willis (Cruveilhier, 1836)*
Macrodissected adult human ***white matter tract (Bell & Bell, 1826)*** with both ***spinal root of accessory nerve rootlets (>1840)*** and what little was known about their extensions into ***spinal cord (Galen, c162–c166)***; in the original French, *extrémité centrale de l'accessoire de Willis*, p. 899.

29. *central end of spinal nerve of Willis (Cruveilhier, 1836)*
Synonym for macrodissected adult human *central end of accessory nerve of Willis (Cruveilhier, 1836)*; in the original French, *extrémité centrale de l'spinal de Willis*, p. 899.

30. *central end of great hypoglossal nerve (Cruveilhier, 1836)*
Macrodissected adult human ***white matter tract (Bell & Bell, 1826)*** with ***hypoglossal nerve central root (>1840)*** and ***hypoglossal nerve rootlets (>1840)*** considered together; in the original French, *extrémité centrale du grand hypoglosse*, p. 901.

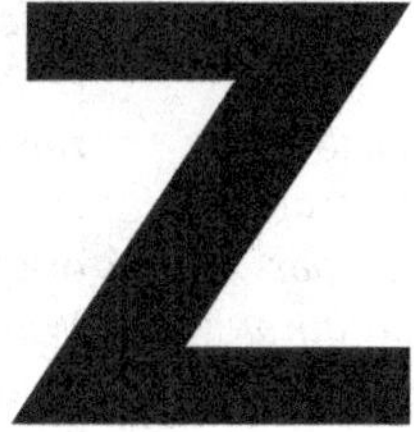

zona incerta (Forel, 1877)

As described for macrodissected adult human, and based on cellular architecture and connections in mammal, the ventromedial part of the ***ventral part of thalamus (Herrick, 1910)*** lying medial to the ***reticular thalamic nucleus (>1840)***; see Jones (1985, Ch. 15.2), Nieuwenhuys et al. (2008, Fig. 5.7-31). For Forel's use in adult human and other mammals with histological methods for ***axons (Kölliker, 1896)***, see pp. 477–478. It was not identified by 1840.

zonal layer of thalamus (Burdach, 1822)

As described for macrodissected adult human, a thin layer of ***white matter (Meckel, 1817)*** on the dorsal surface of the ***dorsal part of thalamus (Herrick, 1910)***; see Williams & Warwick (1980, p. 954), *Dorland's* (2003, p. 1770). For Burdach's use in macrodissected adult human, see p. 119. It was probably first delineated by Ridley; see ***[zonal layer of thalamus (Burdach, 1822)] (Ridley, 1695)***.

TRANSLATIONS:

1. *stratum zonale thalami (Burdach, 1822)*
   Original Latin form of ***zonal layer of thalamus (Burdach, 1822)***; p. 119.

EARLIER REFERENCES:

Described, not named or illustrated:

1. ***[zonal layer of thalamus (Burdach, 1822)] (Ridley, 1695)***
   Probably first noted by Ridley in macrodissected adult human, "The *Thalami Nervorum Opticorum* are two prominent Bodies, more purely medullary on their outward Superficies than within…" (p. 121). It was described somewhat more clearly by Malacarne (1791, p. 36), according to Burdach (1822, p. 343).

Earlier synonyms:

1. *tapetum of thalamus (Reil, 1809b)*
   Synonym for macrodissected adult human ***zonal layer of thalamus (Burdach 1822)***; pp. 343–344, see Mayo translation (1823, p. 70).

zygomatic branches of facial nerve (>1840)

As described for macrodissected adult human, terminal branches of the ***facial nerve trunk (>1840)*** with an *upper set* innervating mainly the orbicularis oculi and zygomatic muscles, and a more extensive *lower set* innervating the same muscles, as well as the buccinator muscle and muscles of the nose and upper lip; see Durward (1951, p. 1032 and Fig. 902). Williams & Warwick (1980, Fig. 7.186) referred to the lower set as the upper buccal branch of facial nerve; also see *Dorland's* (2003, p. 1569). They were first clearly delineated by Eustachi; see ***[zygomatic branches of facial nerve (>1840)] (Eustachi, 1552)***.

EARLIER REFERENCES:

Illustrated, not named or described:

1. ***[zygomatic branches of facial nerve (>1840)] (Eustachi, 1552)***
   Both sets illustrated for macrodissected adult human; see Albinus edition (1744, Tab. 21/2-*e* for lower set, with upper set unlabeled).

Earlier synonyms:

1. *zygomatic branch of portio dura of auditory nerve (Albinus, 1744)*
   Term for ***[zygomatic branches of facial nerve (>1840)] (Eustachi, 1552)***; the original Latin description, *nervorum auditoriorum portio dura, ramus ejus ad zygomaticos*, see Table 21/2-*e*.
2. *zygomatic branch of portio dura of seventh pair of cerebral nerves (Albinus, 1761)*
   Term for ***[zygomatic branches of facial nerve (>1840)] (Eustachi, 1552)***; the original Latin description, *septimi paris nervorum cerebri portio dura, ramus ejus ad zygomaticos*, see Table 21/2-*e*.
3. *great facial branch of superior branch of anterior branch of hard nerve (Loder, 1778)*
   Roughly synonymous with macrodissected adult human ***zygomatic branches of facial nerve (>1840)***; in the original Latin, *ramus facialis maximus*, p. 26.

4. *transverse branch of superior branch of anterior branch of hard nerve (Loder, 1778)*
Synonym for *great facial branch of superior branch of anterior branch of hard nerve (Loder, 1778)*; in the original Latin, *ramus transversus*, p. 26.
5. *middle facial branch of superior branch of anterior branch of hard nerve (Loder, 1778)*
Synonym for *great facial branch of superior branch of anterior branch of hard nerve (Loder, 1778)*; in the original Latin, *ramus facialis medius*, p. 26.
6. *facial branches of ascending branch of superficial branch of hard nerve (Günther, 1786)*
Essentially synonym for macrodissected adult human ***zygomatic branches of facial nerve (>1840)***; in the original Latin, *rami faciales*, p. 59. Günther carefully described superior, middle, and inferior divisions of these branches.
7. *sub-orbitar branches of facial nerve (Burdin, 1803)*
Essentially synonym for macrodissected adult human ***zygomatic branches of facial nerve (>1840)***; see translation (1803, Vol. 1, p. 180).
8. *malar nerves (Meckel, 1817)*
Synonym for macrodissected adult human ***zygomatic branches of facial nerve (>1840)***; see translation (1832, Vol. 3, p. 55).
9. *facial surculus of superior branch of portio major and minor of facial nerve (Bellingeri, 1818)*
Synonym for macrodissected adult human ***zygomatic branches of facial nerve (>1840)***; in the original Latin, *surculus facialis*, see Table II.
10. *facial surculus of temporo-facial branch of portio major and minor of facial nerve (Bellingeri, 1818)*
Synonym for macrodissected adult human ***zygomatic branches of facial nerve (>1840)***; in the original Latin, *surculus facialis*, see Table II.
11. *middle facial branch of facial nerve (Cloquet, 1828)*
Synonym for macrodissected adult human ***zygomatic branches of facial nerve (>1840)***; in the original French, *rameau facial moyen*, Plate CLVII-70.
12. *malar branches of superior branch of facial nerve (Arnold, 1834)*
Synonym for macrodissected adult human ***zygomatic branches of facial nerve (>1840)***; in the original Latin, *ramus superior nervi facialis rami malares*, p. 12.
13. *zygomatic branches of superior branch of facial nerve (Arnold, 1834)*
Synonym for macrodissected adult human ***zygomatic branches of facial nerve (>1840)***; in the original Latin, *ramus superior nervi facialis rami zygomatici*, p. 12.
14. *malar branches of facial nerve (Quain, 1837)*
Synonym for macrodissected adult human *malar nerves (Meckel, 1817)*; in the original Latin, *rami malares*, p. 752.

PARTLY CORRESPONDS:

1. *fifth temporal branch of hard nerve (Meckel, 1753)*
Basically upper set of ***zygomatic branches of facial nerve (>1840)*** in macrodissected adult human; in the original French, *le cinquième rameau temporal du dur*, Table 1-*161*.
2. *inferior orbital nerve of hard nerve (Meckel, 1753)*
Synonym for *fifth temporal branch of hard nerve (Meckel, 1753)*; in the original French, *le nerf orbital inférieur du dur*, p. 83, Table 1-*161*.
3. *malar nerve of hard nerve (Meckel, 1753)*
Synonym for *fifth temporal branch of hard nerve (Meckel, 1753)*; in the original French, *le nerf malaire du dur*, Table 1-*161*.
4. *infraorbital branch of superior facial branch (Meckel, 1753)*
Synonym for *fifth temporal branch of hard nerve (Meckel, 1753)*; in the original French, *la branche infra-orbitaire du rameau facial supérieur [du dur]*, Table 1-*177*.
5. *descending branch of superior branch of hard nerve (Meckel, 1753)*
Second of two major branches of *superior branch of hard nerve (Meckel, 1753)* in macrodissected adult human, consisting of 6th–8th (facial) branches of *superior branch of hard nerve (Meckel, 1753)*, corresponding basically to lower set of ***zygomatic branches of facial nerve (>1840)***; in the original French, *le rameau descendant du supérieur du dur*, p. 76, Table 1-*137*. See *facial branches proper of superior branch of hard nerve (Meckel, 1753)*.
6. *facial branch of hard nerve (Meckel, 1753)*
Synonym for *descending branch of superior branch of hard nerve (Meckel, 1753)*; in the original French, *le rameau des faciaux du nerf dur*, p. 76.
7. *facial branches proper of superior branch of hard nerve (Meckel, 1753)*
Synonym for *descending branch of superior branch of hard nerve (Meckel, 1753)*; in the original French, "*les autres rameaux du rameau supérieur du nerf dur, qui sortent au dessous de ceux-ci de l'arc anastomotique des ses rameaux, s'appellent proprement faciaux...*" (p. 85).
8. *facial nerve (Meckel, 1753)*
Synonym for *descending branch of superior branch of hard nerve (Meckel, 1753)*; in the original French, *le rameau supérieur du nerf facial...*, p. 87.
9. *facial branch of superior branch of hard nerve (Meckel, 1753)*
Synonym for *descending branch of superior branch of hard nerve (Meckel, 1753)*; in the original French, *le rameau facial du supérieur du dur*, Table 1-*137*.
10. *superior facial nerve (Meckel, 1753)*
Synonym for *superior facial branch of superior branch of hard nerve (Meckel, 1753)*; in the original French, *le nerf facial supérieur*, pp. 83, 85; Table 1-*169,171*.
11. *superior facial branch of superior branch of hard nerve (Meckel, 1753)*
First or dorsal (upper) of three facial branches (branches 6–8) of macrodissected adult human *superior branch of hard nerve (Meckel, 1753)*; in the original French, *le rameau facial supérieur*, p. 85, Table 1-*174*.
12. *infraorbital branch of superior facial branch (Meckel, 1753)*
Infraorbital branch of *superior facial branch of superior branch of hard nerve (Meckel, 1753)* in macrodissected adult human; in the original French, *la branche infra-orbitaire du rameau facial supérieur*, Table 1-*177*.

13. *great facial nerve (Meckel, 1753)*
Middle branch of *descending branch of superior branch of hard nerve (Meckel, 1753)*; in the original French, *le grand nerf facial*, p. 87, Table 1-*188*.
14. *middle facial nerve (Meckel, 1753)*
Synonym for *great facial nerve (Meckel, 1753)*; in the original French, *le nerf facial moyen*, p. 87, Table 1-*188*.
15. *middle facial branch of hard nerve (Meckel, 1753)*
Synonym for *middle facial nerve (Meckel, 1753)*; in the original French, *le rameau facial moyen du dur*, Table 1-*175*.
16. *great facial branch of hard nerve (Meckel, 1753)*
Synonym for *great facial nerve (Meckel, 1753)*; in the original French, *le rameau grand facial du dur*, Table 1-*175*.
17. *superior branch of middle facial nerve (Meckel, 1753)*
Dorsal (upper) branch of *middle facial nerve (Meckel, 1753)*; in the original French, *la branche supérieur du facial moyen*, Table 1-*190*.
18. *superior branch of great facial nerve (Meckel, 1753)*
Dorsal (upper) branch of *middle facial nerve (Meckel, 1753)*; in the original French, *la branche supérieur du facial grand*, Table 1-*190*.
19. *superior branch of facial nerve (Meckel, 1753)*
Very confusingly (now), refers to superior branch of *superior branch of middle facial nerve (Meckel, 1753)*; in the original French, *le rameau supérieur du nerf facial*, Table 1-*192*, explained on p. 87. Meckel also described inferior branch of *superior branch of middle facial nerve (Meckel, 1753)*, p. 87, illustrated and referred to in Table 1-*200*.
20. *inferior branch of great facial nerve (Meckel, 1753)*
Second of three branches of *middle facial nerve of hard nerve (Meckel, 1753)*; in the original French, *la branche inférieur du grand nerf facial*, Table 1-*193,194*.
21. *inferior branch of facial nerve (Meckel, 1753)*
Synonym for *inferior branch of great facial nerve (Meckel, 1753)*; in the original French, *le rameau inférieur du nerf facial*, p. 88.
22. *infraorbital cutaneous branch of great facial nerve (Meckel, 1753)*
Third of three branches of *middle facial nerve of hard nerve (Meckel, 1753)*; in the original French, *la branche cutané sous-orbitaire du grand nerf facial*, Table 1-*194*.
23. *third facial nerve of superior branch of hard nerve (Meckel, 1753)*
Eighth and last branch derived from *superior branch of hard nerve (Meckel, 1753)*, and third and last facial branch. It belongs to lower set of ***zygomatic branches of facial nerve (>1840)***; in the original French, *le nerf facial troisième du rameau supérieur du nerf dur*, p. 90, Table 1-*207*. Meckel described superior and inferior branches of this ***nerve (Herophilus, c335–c280 BC)***; p. 90.
24. *lowest facial nerve of superior branch of hard nerve (Meckel, 1753)*
Synonym for *third facial nerve of superior branch of hard nerve (Meckel, 1753)*; in the original French, *le nerf facial le plus bas du rameau supérieur du nerf dur*, p. 90. Mayer (1794; Part 5, Tab. VII-*149*, p. 51) gave the Latin form, *nervus facialis infimus*.
25. *nervus jugalis quintus (Soemmerring, 1791)*
Synonym for macrodissected adult human *fifth temporal branch of hard nerve (Meckel, 1753)*; p. 234. *Jugum* is zygomatic process; see Bell (1803b, p. 150).
26. *third inferior facial nerve (Soemmerring, 1791)*
Synonym for macrodissected adult human *third facial nerve of superior branch of hard nerve (Meckel, 1753)*; in the original Latin, *nervus facialis inferior tertius*, p. 237.
27. *inferior facial nerve (Mayer, 1794)*
Synonym for macrodissected adult human *inferior branch of facial nerve (Meckel, 1753)*; in the original Latin, *nervus facialis inferior*; Part 5, Table VII-*143* (p. 50).
28. *inferior superficial branch of hard nerves (Mayer, 1794)*
Belongs to lower set of macrodissected adult human ***zygomatic branches of facial nerve (>1840)*** lying between *inferior facial nerve (Mayer, 1794)* and *fourth facial nerve (Mayer, 1794)*; in the original Latin, *ramus superficialis inferior nervi duri*; Part 5, Table VII-*VI* (p. 50).
29. *fourth facial nerve (Mayer, 1794)*
Synonym for macrodissected adult human *lowest facial nerve of superior branch of hard nerve (Meckel, 1753)*; in the original Latin, *nervus facialis quartus*; Part 5, Table VII-*149* (p. 51).
30. *superior facial division of portio dura (Bell & Bell, 1816)*
Probably roughly synonymous with upper set of ***zygomatic branches of facial nerve (>1840)***; Vol. 2, p. 501.
31. *middle facial nerve (Bell & Bell, 1816)*
Probably roughly synonymous with upper part of lower set of ***zygomatic branches of facial nerve (>1840)***; Vol. 2, p. 501.
32. *inferior facial nerve (Bell & Bell, 1816)*
Probably roughly synonymous with lower part of lower set of ***zygomatic branches of facial nerve (>1840)***; Vol. 2, p. 501.
33. *superior facial branch of pes anserinus (Bellingeri, 1818)*
Essentially dorsal ***zygomatic branch of facial nerve (>1840)*** with four named smaller branches for macrodissected adult human; in the original Latin, *ramus facialis superior*, see p. 113 and Table II.
34. *anastomotic filament of superior facial branch of pes anserinus (Bellingeri, 1818)*
Communicating branch (Winslow, 1733) of *superior facial branch of pes anserinus (Bellingeri, 1818)* with *middle facial branch of pes anserinus (Bellingeri, 1818)*; in the original Latin, *filament anastomotica*, see Table II.
35. *common anastomotic filament of superior facial branch of pes anserinus (Bellingeri, 1818)*
Communicating branch (Winslow, 1733) of *superior facial branch of pes anserinus (Bellingeri, 1818)* with ***zygomatic nerve (>1840)*** and ***inferior palpebral branches of infraorbital nerve (Meckel, 1748)***; in the original Latin, *filament anastomotica communia*, see Table II.
36. *naso-labial filament of superior facial branch of pes anserinus (Bellingeri, 1818)*

Branch of *superior facial branch of pes anserinus (Bellingeri, 1818)* to "musculum zygomaticum, incisivum, levatorem labii, et alae nasi" (see Tab. II); in the original Latin, *filament naso-labialia.*

37. *naso-frontalis filament of superior facial branch of pes anserinus (Bellingeri, 1818)*
Branch of *superior facial branch of pes anserinus (Bellingeri, 1818)* to roots of nose and beginning of frontalis muscle; in the original Latin, *filament naso-frontalis*, see Table II.

38. *middle facial branch of pes anserinus (Bellingeri, 1818)*
Essentially intermediate ***zygomatic branch of facial nerve (>1840)*** with five named smaller branches for macrodissected adult human; in the original Latin, *ramus facialis medius*, see p. 113 and Table II.

39. *malar filament of middle facial branch of pes anserinus (Bellingeri, 1818)*
Branch of *middle facial branch of pes anserinus (Bellingeri, 1818)* to skin of cheeks; in the original Latin, *filamentum malare*, see Table II.

40. *palpebro-labial filament of middle facial branch of pes anserinus (Bellingeri, 1818)*
Branch of *middle facial branch of pes anserinus (Bellingeri, 1818)* to "musculum caninum, et incisivum" (see Tab. II); in the original Latin, *filamentum palpebro-labialis.*

41. *angle of mouth filament of middle facial branch of pes anserinus (Bellingeri, 1818)*
Branch of *middle facial branch of pes anserinus (Bellingeri, 1818)* to "musculum zygomaticum, et caninum" (see Tab. II); in the original Latin, *filament angularis oris.*

42. *inferior nasal filament of middle facial branch of pes anserinus (Bellingeri, 1818)*
Branch of *middle facial branch of pes anserinus (Bellingeri, 1818)* to upper lip, nasalis muscle, and depressor septi nasi muscle; in the original Latin, *filament nasalia inferiora*, see Table II.

43. *superior nasal filament of middle facial branch of pes anserinus (Bellingeri, 1818)*
Branch of *middle facial branch of pes anserinus (Bellingeri, 1818)* to "musc. elevatorem labii superioris, transversalem, et pyramidalem nasi" (see Tab. II); in the original Latin, *filament nasalia superiora.*

44. *inferior facial branch of pes anserinus (Bellingeri, 1818)*
Essentially ventral ***zygomatic branch of facial nerve (>1840)*** with two named smaller branches for macrodissected adult human; in the original Latin, *ramus facialis inferior*, see p. 113 and Table II.

45. *superior labial filament of inferior facial branch of pes anserinus (Bellingeri, 1818)*
Branch of *inferior facial branch of pes anserinus (Bellingeri, 1818)* to upper lip and angle of mouth; in the original Latin, *filament labiale superius*, see Table II.

46. *bucco-labial filament of inferior facial branch of pes anserinus (Bellingeri, 1818)*
Branch of *inferior facial branch of pes anserinus (Bellingeri, 1818)* to buccinator and depressor anguli oris muscles; in the original Latin, *filament bucco-labialis*, see Table II.

47. *superior facial branch of portio dura (Bell & Bell, 1826)*
Rough synonym for upper set of ***zygomatic branches of facial nerve (>1840)***; Vol. 2, p. 528.

48. *middle facial branch of portio dura (Knox, 1832)*
Rough synonym for lower set of ***zygomatic branches of facial nerve (>1840)***; Plate II-107.

49. *orbital branches of temporofacial branch of facial nerve (Cruveilhier, 1836)*
Synonym for upper set of macrodissected adult human ***zygomatic branches of facial nerve (>1840)***; in the original French, *rameaux orbitaires*, p. 944.

50. *superior palpebral branches of orbital branches of temporofacial branch of facial nerve (Cruveilhier, 1836)*
Macrodissected adult human ***zygomatic branches of facial nerve (>1840)*** described as ending in orbicularis palpebrarum and corrugator supercilii muscles; in the original French, *rameaux palpébraux supérieurs*, p. 944.

51. *middle palpebral branches of orbital branches of temporofacial branch of facial nerve (Cruveilhier, 1836)*
Macrodissected adult human ***zygomatic branches of facial nerve (>1840)*** described as ending in upper and lower eyelids; in the original French, *rameaux palpébraux moyens*, p. 944.

52. *inferior palpebral branches of orbital branches of temporofacial branch of facial nerve (Cruveilhier, 1836)*
Macrodissected adult human ***zygomatic branches of facial nerve (>1840)*** described as ending in lower eyelid; in the original French, *rameaux palpébraux inférieurs*, p. 944.

53. *malar branches of orbital branches of temporofacial branch of facial nerve (Cruveilhier, 1836)*
Synonym for *inferior palpebral branches of orbital branches of temporofacial branch of facial nerve (Cruveilhier, 1836)*; in the original French, *rameaux malaires*, p. 944.

54. *suborbital branches of temporofacial branch of facial nerve (Cruveilhier, 1836)*
Synonym for macrodissected adult human lower set of ***zygomatic branches of facial nerve (>1840)***; in the original French, *rameaux sous-orbitaires*, pp. 944–945.

55. *buccal branches of temporofacial branch of facial nerve (Cruveilhier, 1836)*
Synonym for *suborbital branches of temporofacial branch of facial nerve (Cruveilhier, 1836)*; in the original French, *rameaux buccaux*, p. 944.

56. *superficial branches of suborbital branches of temporofacial branch of facial nerve (Cruveilhier, 1836)*
Branches of *suborbital branches of temporofacial branch of facial nerve (Cruveilhier, 1836)* coursing just beneath the skin; in the original French, *rameaux superficiels*, p. 945.

57. *deep branches of suborbital branches of temporofacial branch of facial nerve (Cruveilhier, 1836)*
Branches of *suborbital branches of temporofacial branch of facial nerve (Cruveilhier, 1836)* described as coursing deep to levator labii superioris muscle; in the original French, *rameaux profonds*, p. 945.

zygomatic nerve (>1840)

As described for macrodissected adult human, a branch of the ***maxillary nerve (Meckel, 1753)*** coursing along the lateral wall of the orbit before dividing into two major branches, ***zygomaticotemporal nerve (>1840)*** and ***zygomaticofacial nerve (>1840)***; see Durward (1951, pp. 1024–1025 and Fig. 898), Hamilton (1976, Figs. 792, 795), Williams & Warwick (1980, p. 1063), *Terminologia Anatomica* (1998, p. 134). It was known to Galen; see ***[zygomatic nerve (>1840)] (Galen, c192)***.

EARLIER REFERENCES:

Described, not named or illustrated:

1. ***[zygomatic nerve (>1840)] (Galen, c192)***
Described briefly for macrodissected adult beef, pig, and/or macaque but not human; see Duckworth translation (1962, p. 194).

Earlier synonyms:

1. *rami minoris inferioris surculus recifus (Vieussens, 1684)*
Synonym for macrodissected adult human ***zygomatic nerve (>1840)***; pp. 171–172, Table 22-*q*.
2. *first branchlet of major branch of fifth pair (Rau, 1694)*
According to Haller (1762, p. 211 note *l*), Rau's synonym for macrodissected adult human *subcutaneous malar nerve (Meckel, 1748)*; in the original Latin, *ramulus primus, quinti paris majori ramo*, p. 191.
3. *subcutaneous malar branch of second branch of fifth pair (Meckel, 1748)*
Synonym for macrodissected adult human ***zygomatic nerve (>1840)***; pp. 35, 47 and Figure 1-56.
4. *subcutaneous malar nerve (Meckel, 1748)*
Synonym for macrodissected adult human ***zygomatic nerve (>1840)***; in the original Latin, *nervus subcutaneus malae*, p. 48.
5. *superficial temporal branch of superior maxillary branch of fifth pair (Haller, 1762)*
Synonym for macrodissected adult human *subcutaneous malar nerve (Meckel, 1748)*; in the original Latin, *ramus temporalis superficialis, paris quinti ramus maxillaris superior*, p. 211.
6. *zygomatic orbital nerve (Le Cat, 1768)*
Synonym for macrodissected adult human ***zygomatic nerve (>1840)***; in the original French, *nerf orbitaire zigomatique*, Plate VIII, Figure 1-23.
7. *orbital branch of submaxillary nerve (Chaussier, 1809)*
Synonym for macrodissected adult human ***zygomatic nerve (>1840)***; in the original French, *R. orbitaire*.
8. *orbital nerve (Quain, 1828)*
Synonym for macrodissected adult human ***zygomatic nerve (>1840)***; p. 649.
9. *malar nerve of second trunk of fifth (Swan, 1830)*
Synonym for macrodissected adult human ***zygomatic nerve (>1840)***; Plate XV, Figure VI-6.
10. *temporo-malar branch of second division of fifth pair of nerves (Todd, 1836–1839)*
Synonym for macrodissected adult human ***zygomatic nerve (>1840)***; p. 284.
11. *orbitar branch of second division of fifth pair of nerves (Todd, 1836–1839)*
Synonym listed for macrodissected adult human ***zygomatic nerve (>1840)*** attributed to the elder Meckel; p. 284, see *orbital branch of submaxillary nerve (Chaussier, 1809)*.
12. *cutaneous malar branch of second division of fifth pair of nerves (Todd, 1836–1839)*
Synonym for macrodissected adult human ***zygomatic nerve (>1840)*** attributed to the elder Meckel; p. 284, see *subcutaneous malar nerve (Meckel, 1748)*.
13. *orbital branch of superior maxillary nerve (Quain & Wilson, 1839)*
Synonym for macrodissected adult human ***zygomatic nerve (>1840)***; Plate XIII, Figure 2-*n*.

PARTLY CORRESPONDS:

1. *nervus facialis quinti (Cheselden, 1726)*
May refer to all or part of macrodissected adult human ***zygomatic nerve (>1840)***, p. 262 (also see p. 254); Alexander Monro *primus* wrote chapter on ***nerves (Herophilus, c335–c280 BC)*** in Cheselden.
2. *ramus subcutaneous malae proprius (Günther, 1786)*
Trunk of macrodissected adult human ***zygomatic nerve (>1840)***, before it divides; p. 46.
3. *lacrimal anastomosis of subcutaneous malar surculus (Bellingeri, 1818)*
Macrodissected adult human ***communicating branch (Winslow, 1733)*** of ***zygomatic nerve (>1840)*** with ***lacrimal nerve (Meckel, 1748; Bonhomme, 1748)***; in the original Latin, *fasciculus anastomot. lacrym.*, see Table I.

zygomaticofacial nerve (>1840)

As described for macrodissected adult human, an occasionally absent branch of the ***zygomatic nerve (>1840)*** supplying skin on the prominence of the cheek; see Hamilton (1976, Figs. 792, 795), Williams & Warwick (1980, p. 1063), *Dorland's* (2003, p. 1236). It was first clearly identified by Meckel; see ***[zygomaticofacial nerve (>1840)] (Meckel, 1748)***.

EARLIER REFERENCES:

Described, not named or illustrated:

1. ***[zygomaticofacial nerve (>1840)] (Meckel, 1748)***
Vaguely described for macrodissected adult human; pp. 48,49—as did his grandson, see Meckel translation (1832, Vol. 3, p. 66).

Earlier synonyms:

1. *subcutaneous nerve of zygomatic bone (Meckel, 1753)*
Synonym for macrodissected adult human ***zygomaticofacial nerve (>1840)***. Meckel distinguished inferior and superior ***nerves (Herophilus, c335–c280 BC)*** (branches of it); in the original French, *le nerf sous-cutané (inférieur, supérieur) de l'os de la pomette*, pp. 56–57.
2. *cutaneous nerve of zygomatic bone (Meckel, 1753)*
Synonym for *subcutaneous nerve of zygomatic bone (Meckel, 1753)*; in the original French, *le nerf cutané (inférieur, supérieur) de l'os de la pomette*, Table 1-66,69.

3. *malo-palpebral fascicle of subcutaneous malar surculus (Bellingeri, 1818)*
   Probably synonym for macrodissected adult human ***zygomaticofacial nerve (>1840)*** though described as entirely forming ***communicating branches (Winslow, 1733)***; in the original Latin, *fasciculus malo-palpebralis*, see Table I.
4. *malar branch of malar nerve (Swan, 1830)*
   Synonym for macrodissected adult human ***zygomaticofacial nerve (>1840)***; Plate XV, Figure 6-7.
5. *inferior branch of subcutaneous malar nerve (Arnold, 1834)*
   Synonym for macrodissected adult human ***zygomaticofacial nerve (>1840)***; in the original Latin, *nervus subcutaneus malae, ramus inferior*, p. 8.
6. *malar branch of temporo-malar branch of second division of fifth pair of nerves (Todd, 1836–1839)*
   Synonym for macrodissected adult human ***zygomaticofacial nerve (>1840)***; p. 284.

PARTLY CORRESPONDS:

1. *inferior subcutaneous malar nerve (Mayer, 1794)*
   Macrodissected adult human inferior or descending (lower) branch or ***nerve (Herophilus, c335–c280 BC)*** of *subcutaneous nerve of zygomatic bone (Meckel, 1753)*; in the original Latin, *nervus subcutaneus malae inferior*; Part 5, Table VII-44 (p. 45).
2. *superior subcutaneous malar nerve (Mayer, 1794)*
   Macrodissected adult human superior or ascending (upper) branch or ***nerve (Herophilus, c335–c280 BC)*** of *subcutaneous nerve of zygomatic bone (Meckel, 1753)*; in the original Latin, *nervus subcutaneus malae superior*; Part 5, Table VII-45 (p. 45).
3. *temporal branch of subcutaneous malar nerve (Bock, 1817)*
   Synonym for macrodissected adult human *superior subcutaneous malar nerve (Mayer, 1794)*; in the original Latin, *ramus temporalis*, p. 24.
4. *lacrimal branch of subcutaneous malar nerve (Bock, 1817)*
   Synonym for macrodissected adult human *superior subcutaneous malar nerve (Mayer, 1794)*; in the original Latin, *ramus lacrymalis*, p. 24.
5. *inferior anastomotic threads of malo-palpebral fascicle of subcutaneous malar surculus (Bellingeri, 1818)*
   Four ventral ***communicating branches (Winslow, 1733)*** of *malo-palpebral fascicle of subcutaneous malar surculus (Bellingeri, 1818)* were named and described; in the original Latin, *stamina anastomoticus inferior*, see Table I.
6. *inferior anastomotic thread of malo-palpebral fascicle of subcutaneous malar surculus with external palpebral thread of infraorbital surculus (Bellingeri, 1818)*
   First ventral ***communicating branch (Winslow, 1733)*** of *malo-palpebral fascicle of subcutaneous malar surculus (Bellingeri, 1818)*; in the original Latin, *stamina anastomoticus inferior cum palpebrali externo infraorbitalis*, see Table I. Also see *external inferior palpebral thread of infraorbital surculus (Bellingeri, 1818)*.
7. *inferior anastomotic thread of malo-palpebral fascicle of subcutaneous malar surculus with superior facial branch of seventh pair (Bellingeri, 1818)*
   Second ventral ***communicating branch (Winslow, 1733)*** of *malo-palpebral fascicle of subcutaneous malar surculus (Bellingeri, 1818)*; in the original Latin, *stamina anastomoticus inferior cum faciali superiori septimi paris*, see Table I. Also see *superior facial branch of seventh pair (Bellingeri, 1818)*.
8. *inferior anastomotic thread of malo-palpebral fascicle of subcutaneous malar surculus with inferior orbital thread of seventh pair (Bellingeri, 1818)*
   Third ventral ***communicating branch (Winslow, 1733)*** of *malo-palpebral fascicle of subcutaneous malar surculus (Bellingeri, 1818)*; in the original Latin, *stamina anastomoticus inferior cum orbitario inferiori septimi paris*, see Table I. Also see *inferior orbital thread of seventh pair (Bellingeri, 1818)*.
9. *inferior anastomotic thread of malo-palpebral fascicle of subcutaneous malar surculus with subcutaneous temporal fascicle (Bellingeri, 1818)*
   Fourth ventral ***communicating branch (Winslow, 1733)*** of *malo-palpebral fascicle of subcutaneous malar surculus (Bellingeri, 1818)*; in the original Latin, *stamina anastomoticus inferior cum temporali subcutaneo*, see Table I. Also see *temporal subcutaneous fascicle of subcutaneous malar surculus (Bellingeri, 1818)*.
10. *superior anastomotic threads of malo-palpebral fascicle of subcutaneous malar surculus (Bellingeri, 1818)*
    Two dorsal branches of *malo-palpebral fascicle of subcutaneous malar surculus (Bellingeri, 1818)* were named and described; in the original Latin, *stamina anastomoticus superior*, see Table I.
11. *external filament of superior anastomotic thread of malo-palpebral fascicle of subcutaneous malar surculus (Bellingeri, 1818)*
    Synonym for *superior anastomotic thread of malo-palpebral fascicle of subcutaneous malar surculus with inferior orbital thread of seventh pair (Bellingeri, 1818)*; in the original Latin, *stamina anastomoticus superior filamentum externum*, see Table I.
12. *superior anastomotic thread of malo-palpebral fascicle of subcutaneous malar surculus with inferior orbital thread of seventh pair (Bellingeri, 1818)*
    Lateral and dorsal ***communicating branch (Winslow, 1733)*** of *malo-palpebral fascicle of subcutaneous malar surculus (Bellingeri, 1818)*; in the original Latin, *stamina anastomoticus superior cum orbitario inferiori septimi paris*, see Table I. Also see *inferior orbital thread of seventh pair (Bellingeri, 1818)*.
13. *internal filament of superior anastomotic thread of malo-palpebral fascicle of subcutaneous malar surculus (Bellingeri, 1818)*
    Medial and dorsal branch of *malo-palpebral fascicle of subcutaneous malar surculus (Bellingeri, 1818)* to upper eyelid; in the original Latin, *stamina anastomoticus superior filamentum internum*, see Table I.

zygomaticotemporal nerve (>1840)

As described for adult human, a branch of the ***zygomatic nerve (>1840)*** supplying a tiny branch carrying parasympathetic postganglionic ***axons (Kölliker, 1896)*** from the ***pterygopalatine ganglion (>1840)*** to the ***lacrimal nerve (Meckel, 1748; Bonhomme, 1748)*** and then lacrimal gland, and finally distributing to skin of rostral (anterior) parts of the temple. It also communicates with ***temporal branches of facial nerve (Swan, 1830)*** and ***auriculotemporal nerve (Haller, 1762)***; see Durward (1951, pp. 1024–1025), Hamilton (1976, Figs. 792, 795), Williams & Warwick (1980, p. 1063 and Fig. 7.179), who used the terms *zygomaticotemporal branch* (for example, p. 1067) and *zygomaticotemporal nerve* (Fig. 7.179-22), *Dorland's* (2003, p. 1236). It was probably first identified as the *fourth offshoot of thinner root of third nerve (Vesalius, 1543a)*.

EARLIER REFERENCES:

Earlier synonyms:

1. *fourth offshoot of thinner root of third nerve (Vesalius, 1543a)*
   Synonym for ***zygomaticotemporal nerve (>1840)***, partly described and illustrated for macrodissected adult human; see Richardson & Carman translation (2002, pp. 188–189).
2. *fourth branch of third conjugation of nerves of brain (Crooke, 1615)*
   Synonym for macrodissected adult human ***zygomaticotemporal nerve (>1840)***; p. 486. Crooke's description is a translation of Bauhin (1605).
3. *anterior cutaneous nerves of temple (Meckel, 1753)*
   Synonym for macrodissected adult human ***zygomaticotemporal nerve (>1840)***; in the original French, *les nerfs cutanés des temples antérieurs*, Table 1:73–81. Meckel recognized three such ***nerves (Herophilus, c335–c280 BC)***.
4. *anterior subcutaneous nerves of temple (Meckel, 1753)*
   Synonym for macrodissected adult human *anterior cutaneous nerves of temple (Meckel, 1753)*; in the original French, *les nerfs sous-cutanés des temples antérieurs*, p. 58.
5. *subcutaneous temporalis nerve (Bell & Bell, 1826)*
   Probably synonym for macrodissected adult human ***zygomaticotemporal nerve (>1840)***; Vol. 2, p. 514.
6. *temporal branch of malar nerve (Swan, 1830)*
   Synonym for macrodissected adult human ***zygomaticotemporal nerve (>1840)***; Plate XV, Figure 6-8.
7. *superior branch of subcutaneous malar nerve (Arnold, 1834)*
   Synonym for macrodissected adult human ***zygomaticotemporal nerve (>1840)***; in the original Latin, *nervus subcutaneus malae, ramus superior*, p. 8.
8. *external temporal branch of temporo-malar branch of second division of fifth pair of nerves (Todd, 1836–1839)*
   Synonym for macrodissected adult human ***zygomaticotemporal nerve (>1840)***; p. 284.

PARTLY CORRESPONDS:

1. *middle cutaneous nerve of temple (Meckel, 1753)*
   Second *anterior cutaneous nerve of temple (Meckel, 1753)*; Table 1-151.

Appendices
Systematic Parts Lists for Nervous System Ontology

The 10 Nomenclature Tables of ***standard parts*** presented individually in the Appendices are organized broadly around terms for the human body that have been under constant formal revision for over a century (His, 1895) and are represented now by the *Nomina Anatomica*, 5th edition (1983) and *Terminologia Anatomica* (1998). The terms for these ***standard parts*** are formatted according to the recently published *Foundational Model of Connectivity* (Swanson & Bota, 2010), with the long-term goal of developing a comparative neuroanatomical nomenclature that applies to animals generally. The tables are organized hierarchically and arranged strictly on topographic, rather than systems, criteria. These ***standard terms*** are used to define all other *nonstandard terms* in the Lexicon—whether alternate spellings, translations, synonyms, or partly corresponding.

Overall, the 10 Nomenclature Tables deal with (1) the topographic architecture of the adult ***nervous system (Monro, 1783)*** in all animals based on ***topographic divisions (Swanson & Bota, 2010)***, (2) the topographic architecture of the developing vertebrate ***nervous system (Monro, 1783)*** based on ***topographic divisions (Swanson & Bota, 2010)***, (3) the systems architecture of the adult human ***nervous system (Monro, 1783)*** based on topographically arranged ***gray matter regions (Swanson & Bota, 2010)*** and ***white matter tracts (Bell & Bell, 1826)***, and (4) the topographic architecture of adult human supporting structures and surface features based on ***topographic divisions (Swanson & Bota, 2010)***. Their relationship to the *Foundational Model of Connectivity* (Swanson & Bota, 2010) is shown in Figure 15.

STANDARD TERMS

These Nomenclature Tables contain only ***standard terms***—main entries in the Lexicon, or in the Lexicon of Swanson & Bota (2010)—with a formal definition and citation for the origin of the term with this definition. All other terms can be defined simply by using these ***standard terms***—they are either defined subdivisions, synonyms, or partly corresponding terms. This approach greatly reduces the number (N) of formal definitions needed, from N^2 to N (Dashti et al., 1997). Terms named after 1840, where the first use of the term has not been traced, are indicated as "Term (>1840)".

EXTENSIONS AND SUBSTITUTIONS

In the future the Nomenclature Tables can be *extended* with lower hierarchy levels without altering their basic organization. For example, separate Tables can be made for each species (and/or taxon) and sex, or specific names can be added for each branch of a ***nerve (Herophilus, c335- c280 BC)*** to a specific muscle, tendon, joint, bone, or blood vessel. Ideally, *substitutions* should be done by an international standing committee or commission operating under a set of written guidelines.

GENERAL PRINCIPLES FOR ORDERING

The general plan follows overall topographic and topological trends in vertebrate ***nervous system (Monro, 1783)*** embryology, first along the longitudinal axis from rostral to caudal and then along the transverse axis from central to peripheral (or proximal to distal). Of the two cardinal transverse planes, medial to lateral is described before ventral to dorsal because the ***neural plate (Stricker, 1860)*** develops before the ***neural tube (Baer, 1837)***. The ***neural plate (Stricker, 1860)***, which lies medially in the ectodermal layer and generates the future ***central nervous system (Carus, 1814)***, differentiates before the ***neural crest (>1840)***, which lies laterally in the ectodermal layer and generates the future ***peripheral nervous system (Meckel, 1817)***—and the ventral part of the ***neural tube (Baer, 1837)***, the ***basal plate (>1840)***, begins differentiation before the dorsal part of the ***neural tube (Baer, 1837)***, the ***alar plate (>1840)***. Overall, then, ordering proceeds from rostral to caudal, central to peripheral, medial to lateral, and ventral to dorsal (Figures 1, 2).

USEFUL BUT PROBLEMATIC TERMS

In any strictly hierarchically ordered set of ***standard terms***, some familiar terms will not appear because they are defined in a different hierarchy scheme. They are generally handled in two ways. First, they may be placed in a general ***standard terms*** category if they can be described accurately by a set of specific ***standard terms***; a good example is ***brainstem (Schwalbe, 1881***) in Appendix 1. And second, they may be defined as partly corresponding to a standard term; good examples include *amygdala (>1840)*, *septal region (Swanson & Cowan, 1979)*, and *lentiform nucleus (Burdach, 1822)* in the Lexicon.

OTHER FUNCTIONAL SYSTEMS

A few terms not fully or partly components of the ***nervous system (Monro, 1783)***, but closely related and useful here for descriptive purposes, are included in the Lexicon. They come from the circulatory system—for example, ***rete mirabile (Herophilus, c335–c280 BC)*** and ***cavernous sinus (Winslow, 1733)***—and endocrine system; for example, ***pituitary gland (>1840)***.

ENGLISH

The ***standard terms*** are primarily in English, following the example of *Terminologia Anatomica (1998)* and Nieuwenhuys et al. (2008).

Appendix I

Basic parts list for adult nervous system in all animals (topographic divisions)

This hierarchical Nomenclature Table provides a general, internally consistent set of ***standard terms*** for describing the larger parts of the ***nervous system (Monro, 1783)*** from a topographic perspective and is based on the *Foundational Model of Connectivity* (FMC; Swanson & Bota, 2010). There are two alternate, orthogonal ways of describing completely ***nervous system (Monro, 1783)*** parts in any animal, whether invertebrate or vertebrate (Figure 15). One grouping or arrangement system is called "topographic architecture" and is based in principle on cutting with a knife or scissors, for example, distinguishing the ***central nervous system (Carus, 1814)*** and ***peripheral nervous system (Meckel, 1817)***, or the ***vertebrate brain (Cuvier, 1800)*** and ***spinal cord (Galen, c162–c166)***. It is essentially gross anatomy carried out with naked eye resolution in animals that are large enough. The other grouping system for the ***nervous system (Monro, 1783)*** is called "systems architecture" and it has come to deal with describing ***nervous system (Monro, 1783)*** network organization or connectivity in terms of differentiable ***gray matter regions (Swanson & Bota, 2010)*** and ***white matter tracts (Bell & Bell, 1826)***, like the ***hypoglossal nucleus (>1840)*** and ***hypoglossal nerve central root (>1840)***. Before the development of effective neurohistological methods in the late 1830s, this was done at the macrodissection or gross anatomy level only; neurohistology then allowed the differentiation of ***gray matter regions (Swanson & Bota, 2010)*** based on the much more precise identification of unique sets of ***neuron types (Swanson & Bota, 2007)*** at the cellular level. This Nomenclature Table is based entirely on macrodissection evidence but is a reliable framework for later subdivisions based on cellular architecture and connections.

GENERAL TERMS

A small number of terms that are very useful, but do not fit precisely into any of the 10 Nomenclature Tables, are included at the top as a special category of "General standard terms" for the sake of clarity and convenience. Examples include ***ganglion (Galen, c173)***, ***plexus (Galen, c192)***, and ***brainstem (Schwalbe, 1881)***.

NERVOUS SYSTEM (MONRO, 1783)

..... General standard terms
.... Brain (Smith Papyrus, c1700 BC)
.... Ganglia (Galen, c173)
.... Gray matter (Meckel, 1817)
.... White matter (Meckel, 1817)
.... Plexus (Galen, c192)
.... Nerve cord (Serres, 1824–1826)
.... Nerve cord trunk (>1840)
.... Communicating branch (Winslow, 1733)
.... Cerebrospinal trunk (>1840)
.... Brainstem (Schwalbe, 1881)
..... Topographic divisions (Swanson & Bota, 2010; also see Figure 15 here, left side)
.... Nerve net (>1840)
.... Nerve ring (Tiedemann, 1815)
.... Circumoral nerve ring (Tiedemann, 1815)
.... Radial nerve cord (>1840)
.... Marginal ganglia (>1840)
.... Central nervous system (Carus, 1814)

....................Central nerve cord (Serres, 1824–1826)
................................Central longitudinal communicating branch (>1840)
....Circumesophageal connective (>1840)
................................Central transverse communicating branch (>1840)
................................Ventral cord (Anderson, 1837)
................................Central ganglia (>1840)
....Invertebrate brain (>1840)
....Supraesophageal ganglion (Grant, 1834a)
....Ventral ganglia (Anderson, 1837)
....................Circumenteric nerve ring (>1840)
....................Cerebrospinal axis (Meckel, 1817) or vertebrate Central nervous system (Carus, 1814)
................................Vertebrate brain (Cuvier, 1800)
....Forebrain (Goette, 1873)
....Endbrain (Kuhlenbeck, 1927) or Cerebrum (Obersteiner & Hill, 1900)
....Cerebral nuclei (Swanson, 2000a)
....Cerebral cortex (>1840)
....Interbrain (Baer, 1837)
....Hypothalamus (Kuhlenbeck, 1927)
....Thalamus (His, 1893a)
....Midbrain (Baer, 1837)
....Tegmentum (Swanson, 2000b)
....Tectum (Baer, 1837)
....Rhombicbrain (His, 1893b)
....Hindbrain (Baer, 1837)
....Pons (Haller, 1747)
....Cerebellum (Aristotle)
....Afterbrain (Baer, 1837) or Medulla (Winslow, 1733)
................................Spinal cord (Galen, c162–c166)
....Spinal cord parts (>1840)
....Cervical part of spinal cord (>1840)
....Thoracic part of spinal cord (1840)
....Lumbar part of spinal cord (>1840)
....Sacral part of spinal cord (>1840)
....Coccygeal part of spinal cord (>1840)
....Spinal cord differentiations (>1840)
....Cervical enlargement (Arnold, 1838b)
....Lumbosacral enlargement (>1840)
....Medullary cone (Bock, 1827)
....Terminal filament (Tiedemann, 1821)
.........Peripheral nervous system (Meckel, 1817)
....................Peripheral nerve cord (Swanson & Bota, 2010)
................................Peripheral longitudinal communicating branch (Swanson & Bota, 2010)
................................Sympathetic cord (>1840)
....................Nerves (Herophilus, c335–c280 BC)
................................Invertebrate nerves (>1840)
................................Craniospinal nerves (Herrick, 1915)
....Cranial nerves (Soemmerring, 1791)
....Spinal nerves (Camper, 1760–1762)
....Spinal nerve roots (Tiedemann, 1816)
....Spinal nerve trunk (Frotscher, 1788)
....Spinal nerve primary branches (>1840)
................................Autonomic nerves (Langley, 1898)
....Communicating branches of spinal nerves (Wutzer, 1817)
....Peripheral nerve cord trunk (Swanson & Bota, 2010)
....Sympathetic trunk (Winslow, 1733)

....Paravertebral nerves (Swanson & Bota, 2010)
....Prevertebral plexuses (Quain, 1837)
....Prevertebral nerves (Swanson & Bota, 2010)
....Terminal plexuses (Swanson & Bota, 2010)
....Terminal autonomic nerves (Swanson & Bota, 2010)
.....................Peripheral ganglia (>1840)
................................Invertebrate peripheral ganglia (Swanson & Bota, 2010)
................................Craniospinal ganglia (>1840)
....Cranial nerve ganglia (>1840)
....Spinal nerve ganglia (Burdach, 1819)
................................Autonomic ganglia (Langley, 1900)
....Paravertebral ganglia (Durward, 1951)
....Prevertebral ganglia (Quain, 1837)
....Terminal ganglia (Gaskell, 1886)

Appendix 2
Vertebrate nervous system development (topographic divisions)

This hierarchical Nomenclature Table provides a general, internally consistent set of ***standard terms*** for describing the larger parts of the embryonic vertebrate ***nervous system (Monro, 1783)*** from a topographic perspective. The parts of the ***neural tube (Baer, 1837)*** generate the ten basic topographic divisions of the ***cerebrospinal axis (Meckel, 1817)*** or vertebrate ***central nervous system (Carus, 1814)*** almost universally recognized today (Figure 15, bottom of left panel), after extensive research beginning in classical antiquity (see Nauta & Feirtag, 1986; Swanson, 2000; Swanson & Bota, 2010).

NERVOUS SYSTEM [VERTEBRATE] (MONRO, 1783)

.....Topographic divisions (Swanson & Bota, 2010; also see Figure 15 here, left side)
.... Development
.... Neural plate (Stricker, 1860)
..............................Neural groove (>1840)
..............................Neural folds (>1840)
.... Neural crest (>1840)
.... Neural placodes (>1840)
.... Neural tube (Baer, 1837)
..............................Brain vesicles (Malpighi, 1673)
....Primary brain vesicles (Baer, 1837)
.... Primary forebrain vesicle (Baer, 1837)
....Infundibulum (>1840)
.... Primary midbrain vesicle (Baer, 1837)
.... Primary hindbrain vesicle (Baer, 1837)
....Rhombic lip (>1840)
....Secondary brain vesicles (>1840)
.... Endbrain vesicle (Kuhlenbeck, 1927)
.... Hemispheric sulcus (Grönberg, 1902)
.... Interbrain vesicle (Baer, 1837)
.... Midbrain vesicle (Baer, 1837)
.... Hindbrain vesicle (Baer, 1837)
.... Afterbrain vesicle (Baer, 1837)
..............................Spinal cord part of neural tube (>1840)
..............................Floor plate (>1840)
..............................Basal plate (>1840)
..............................Limiting sulcus (>1840)
..............................Alar plate (>1840)
..............................Roof plate (>1840)
....Ependymal roof plate (>1840)

Appendix 3
Human CNS gray matter regions (topographic gross anatomy grouping)

This hierarchical Nomenclature Table and the next (Appendix 4) provide sets of ***standard terms*** for describing the ***gray matter regions (Swanson & Bota, 2010)*** and ***white matter tracts (Bell & Bell, 1826)*** of the adult human ***central nervous system (Carus, 1814)*** (CNS) visible to the naked eye or with current MRI imaging techniques (see Figure 15, right side). A distinction between ***gray matter (Meckel, 1817)*** and ***white matter (Meckel, 1817)*** was clear to Vesalius (1543a), and regionalization of both was done more and more precisely with naked-eye observations (resolution on the order of 100 μm) at the gross anatomical or macroscopic level until histological methods began in the late 1830s at the light microscopic level (resolution on the order of 0.1 μm) to provide cellular architecture and connections. Today there is a renaissance of human ***nervous system (Monro, 1783)*** regionalization at the macrolevel with in vivo imaging approaches like MRI (practical resolution on the order of 1 mm).

The organization of the Nomenclature Table is based on a current interpretation of gross anatomical and histological parceling of the ***central nervous system (Carus, 1814)*** as documented in the Lexicon, providing a framework for interpreting and classifying gross anatomical parts described before the introduction of useful histological methods around 1840. This gross anatomical level is nicely illustrated for human in Chapters 3–5 of Nieuwenhuys et al. (2008), with a histological interpretation illustrated in Chapter 6. In many instances, a great deal more is now known about subdivisions of ***gray matter regions (Swanson & Bota, 2010)*** at the bottom of the hierarchy presented here. Some of this information is provided in the Lexicon, but it remains for the future to complete this Nomenclature Table of human ***gray matter regions (Swanson & Bota, 2010)*** to lower hierarchy levels done already for rat; see Swanson (2004, Annotated Nomenclature Table B).

There are multiple ways to group ***gray matter regions (Swanson & Bota, 2010)*** and ***white matter tracts (Bell & Bell, 1826)***. A strictly topographic approach is adopted here, using the broad topographic divisions shown in Figure 15 (left side) for the highest levels of the hierarchy. By definition this approach is done without regard to function. An example of functional grouping of ***gray matter regions (Swanson & Bota, 2010)*** is provided in Annotated Nomenclature Table B of Swanson (2004) for the adult male rat. It remains for the future to develop similar tables for ***gray matter regions (Swanson & Bota, 2010)*** and ***white matter tracts (Bell & Bell, 1826)*** of other species and higher taxa with a ***nervous system (Monro, 1783)***, and to unify the nomenclature as far as possible. In general, controversy and uncertainty about similarities or even homologies between species increases progressively at lower and lower levels of the hierarchy.

It will be necessary to generate a separate Nomenclature Table for the systematic histological resolution of ***gray matter regions (Swanson & Bota, 2010)*** in the ***cerebral cortex (>1840)*** based on the work of Brodmann (1909), Economo & Koskinas (1925), Bailey & von Bonin (1951) and many, many others, considering function as well as structure. As a starting point, correlations with Brodmann's work are given in the Lexicon.

NERVOUS SYSTEM [HUMAN] (MONRO, 1783)

.....Systems architecture (Swanson & Bota, 2010; also see Figure 15 here, right side)
.... Gray matter regions (Swanson & Bota, 2010)
.... Cerebrospinal axis (Meckel, 1817) or Central nervous system (Carus, 1814)
.... Endbrain (Kuhlenbeck, 1927) or Cerebrum (Obersteiner & Hill, 1900)
.... Cerebral nuclei (Swanson, 2000a)
.... Pallidum (Swanson, 2000a)
.... Globus pallidus (Burdach, 1822)
.... Medial globus pallidus (>1840)

- Lateral globus pallidus (>1840)
- Substantia innominata (Schwalbe, 1881)
- Medial septal complex (Swanson et al., 1989)
- Bed nuclei of terminal stria (Gurdjian, 1925)
- Striatum (Swanson, 2000a)
  - Olfactory tubercle (Calleja, 1893)
  - Accumbens nucleus (Ziehen, 1897–1901)
  - Lateral septal complex (Risold & Swanson, 1997)
  - Caudoputamen (Heimer & Wilson, 1975)
    - Putamen (Burdach, 1822)
    - Caudate nucleus (Arnold, 1838b)
      - Head of caudate nucleus (>1840)
      - Body of caudate nucleus (>1840)
      - Tail of caudate nucleus (Arnold, 1838b)
  - Central amygdalar nucleus (Johnston, 1923)
  - Medial amygdalar nucleus (Johnston, 1923)
- Cerebral cortex (>1840)
  - Cerebral cortex gray matter (>1840)
    - Cortical plate (>1840)
      - Limbic region (>1840)
        - Olfactory region (>1840)
          - Olfactory bulb (Weitbrecht, 1751)
            - Main olfactory bulb (>1840)
            - Accessory olfactory bulb (>1840)
          - Olfactory peduncle (Solly, 1836)
          - Ambient gyrus (>1840)
          - Semilunar gyrus (>1840)
        - Hippocampal formation (Swanson & Cowan, 1977)
          - Parahippocampal gyrus (>1840)
          - Hippocampal region (Swanson et al., 1987)
            - Ammon's horn (Vicq d'Azyr, 1784)
            - Dentate gyrus (>1840)
            - Fasciola cinerea (Arnold, 1838b)
            - Indusium griseum (Valentin, 1841)
            - Tenia tecta (Swanson, 1992)
        - Cingulate region (Brodmann, 1909)
          - Isthmus of cingulate region (>1840)
          - Parolfactory gyrus (>1840)
      - Insular region (Brodmann, 1909)
        - Short gyri of insula (Gall & Spurzheim, 1810)
        - Long gyrus of insula (Valentin, 1841)
      - Frontal region (Vicq d'Azyr, 1786)
        - Orbital region (Rolando, 1831)
          - Straight gyrus (Valentin, 1841)
          - Orbital gyri (>1840)
            - Medial orbital gyrus (>1840)
            - Anterior orbital gyrus (>1840)
            - Posterior orbital gyrus (>1840)
            - Lateral orbital gyrus (>1840)
        - Inferior frontal gyrus (>1840)
          - Orbital part of inferior frontal gyrus (>1840)
          - Triangular part of inferior frontal gyrus (>1840)
          - Opercular part of inferior frontal gyrus (>1840)
        - Middle frontal gyrus (>1840)
        - Superior frontal gyrus (>1840)

        - Medial frontal gyrus (>1840)
        - Anterior paracentral gyrus (>1840)
        - Precentral gyrus (>1840)
      - Parietal region (>1840)
        - Postcentral gyrus (>1840)
        - Posterior paracentral gyrus (>1840)
        - Precuneus (Burdach, 1822)
        - Superior parietal lobule (>1840)
        - Inferior parietal lobule (>1840)
          - Supramarginal gyrus (>1840)
          - Angular gyrus (>1840)
      - Temporal region (>1840)
        - Transverse temporal gyri (Heschl, 1878)
        - Superior temporal gyrus (>1840)
        - Middle temporal gyrus (>1840)
        - Inferior temporal gyrus (>1840)
        - Lateral occipitotemporal gyrus (>1840)
        - Medial occipitotemporal gyrus (>1840)
      - Occipital region (Vesalius, 1543a)
        - Lingual gyrus (>1840)
        - Cuneus (Burdach, 1822)
        - Superior occipital gyri (>1840)
        - Inferior occipital gyri (>1840)
    - Cortical subplate (>1840)
      - Basolateral amygdalar complex (>1840)
      - Claustrum (Burdach, 1822)
- Interbrain (Baer, 1837)
  - Hypothalamus (Kuhlenbeck, 1927)
    - Periventricular hypothalamic zone (Nauta & Haymaker, 1969)
      - Terminal lamina (Burdach, 1822)
      - Neurohypophysis (Rioch et al., 1940)
        - Infundibulum (Rioch et al., 1940)
          - Median eminence (Tilney, 1936)
          - Infundibular stem (Hanström, 1966)
        - Posterior lobe of pituitary gland (Haller, 1762)
    - Medial hypothalamic zone (Nauta & Haymaker, 1969)
      - Medial preoptic nucleus (>1840)
      - Anterior hypothalamic nucleus (>1840)
      - Ventromedial hypothalamic nucleus (>1840)
      - Ventral premammillary nucleus (>1840)
      - Dorsal premammillary nucleus (>1840)
      - Mammillary body (Ludwig, 1779)
    - Lateral hypothalamic zone (Nauta & Haymaker, 1969)
    - Retina (Herophilus, 335–263 BC)
  - Thalamus (His, 1893a)
    - Ventral part of thalamus (Herrick, 1910)
      - Zona incerta (Forel, 1877)
      - Reticular thalamic nucleus (>1840)
      - Ventral lateral geniculate nucleus (>1840)
    - Dorsal part of thalamus (Herrick, 1910)
      - Midline thalamic nuclei (>1840)
      - Anterior thalamic nuclei (>1840)
      - Medial thalamic nuclei (>1840)
      - Intralaminar thalamic nuclei (>1840)
      - Ventral thalamic nuclei (>1840)
      - Lateral thalamic nuclei (>1840)
        - Pulvinar (Burdach, 1822)

................Posterior thalamic nuclei (>1840)
................Dorsal lateral geniculate nucleus (>1840)
................Medial geniculate complex (>1840)
............Epithalamus (His, 1893b)
................Habenular nuclei (>1840)
................Pineal gland (Galen, c192)
....................Pineal stalk (Burdach, 1822)
....................Brain sand (Soemmerring & Lisignolo, 1785)
....Midbrain (Baer, 1837)
........Tegmentum (Swanson, 2000b)
............Oculomotor nucleus (>1840)
............Trochlear nucleus (>1840)
............Interpeduncular nucleus (>1840)
............Substantia nigra (Soemmerring, 1791)
................Compact part of substantia nigra (>1840)
................Reticular part of substantia nigra (>1840)
............Red nucleus (Burdach, 1822)
............Midbrain reticular nucleus (>1840)
............Periaqueductal gray (>1840)
............Pretectal region (>1840)
........Tectum (Baer, 1837)
............Superior colliculus (Haller, 1762)
............Inferior colliculus (Haller, 1762)
....Rhombicbrain (His, 1893b)
........Hindbrain (Baer, 1837)
............Pons (Haller, 1747)
................Abducens nucleus (>1840)
................Motor nucleus of trigeminal nerve (>1840)
................Pontine nuclei (Jacobsohn, 1909)
................Pontine raphe nucleus (>1840)
................Pontine reticular nucleus (>1840)
................Pontine central gray (>1840)
....................Locus ceruleus (Wenzel & Wenzel, 1812)
................Parabrachial nucleus (>1840)
................Principal sensory nucleus of trigeminal nerve (>1840)
............Cerebellum (Aristotle)
................Cerebellar nuclei (>1840)
....................Fastigial nucleus (>1840)
....................Interposed nucleus (>1840)
....................Dentate nucleus (>1840)
................Cerebellar cortex (Willis, 1664)
....................Cerebellar vermis (Meckel, 1817)
........................Lingula (Malacarne, 1776)
........................Central lobule (Burdach, 1822)
........................Culmen (Stroud, 1895)
........................Declive (>1840)
........................Folium vermis (>1840)
........................Tuber vermis (>1840)
........................Pyramis (Malacarne, 1776)
........................Uvula (Malacarne, 1776)
........................Nodule (Reil, 1807–1808a)
....................Cerebellar hemisphere (Willis, 1664)
........................Simple lobule (Jansen & Brodal, 1954)
........................Ansiform lobule (Bolk, 1906)
............................Ansiform lobule crus 1 (Bolk, 1906)
............................Ansiform lobule crus 2 (Bolk, 1906)

.... Gracile lobule (>1840)

.... Biventral lobule (>1840)

.... Tonsil (Malacarne, 1776)

..................................Paraflocçulus (Stroud, 1895)

.... Flocculus (Meckel, 1817)

..........................Afterbrain (Baer, 1837) or Medulla (Winslow, 1733)

.... Facial nucleus (>1840)

.... Ambiguus nucleus (>1840

.... Hypoglossal nucleus (>1840)

.... Superior salivatory nucleus (>1840)

.... Inferior salivatory nucleus (>1840)

.... Dorsal motor nucleus of vagus nerve (>1840)

.... Arcuate nucleus of medulla (>1840)

.... Medullary reticular nuclei (>1840)

.... Superior olivary complex (>1840)

.... Inferior olivary complex (>1840)

.... Cochlear nuclei (>1840)

.... Vestibular nuclei (>1840)

.... Nucleus of solitary tract (>1840)

.... Dorsal column nuclei (>1840)

..................................Gracile nucleus (>1840)

..................................Cuneate nucleus (>1840)

..................................Accessory cuneate nucleus (>1840)

.... Spinal nucleus of trigeminal nerve (>1840)

......................Spinal cord (Galen, c162–c166)

..........................Ventral horn (>1840)

..........................Intermediate spinal zone (>1840)

.... Spinal central gray (>1840)

.... Dorsal thoracic nucleus (>1840)

.... Intermediolateral nucleus (>1840)

..........................Dorsal horn (>1840)

Appendix 4
Human CNS white matter tracts (topographic gross anatomy grouping)

This hierarchical Nomenclature Table and its companion (Appendix 3) provide sets of ***standard terms*** for describing the ***gray matter regions (Swanson & Bota, 2010)*** and ***white matter tracts (Bell & Bell, 1826)*** of the adult human ***central nervous system (Carus, 1814)*** (CNS) visible to the naked eye or with current MRI imaging techniques (see Figure 15, right side). There are multiple ways to group ***gray matter regions (Swanson & Bota, 2010)*** and ***white matter tracts (Bell & Bell, 1826)***. A strictly topographic approach is adopted here, using the broad topographic divisions shown in Figure 15 (left side) for the highest levels of the hierarchy. By definition this approach is done without regard to function.

This Nomenclature Table deals with the most confusing aspect of ***central nervous system (Carus, 1814)*** descriptive anatomy: *tracts (Willis, 1664)*, connections, projections, and pathways. These terms are defined clearly in the Foundational Model of Connectivity (Swanson & Bota, 2010; see especially their Figure 5). Briefly, ***white matter tracts (Bell & Bell, 1826)*** are defined macrodivisions of ***white matter (Meckel, 1817)***; connection and projection are synonyms and describe an axonal relationship from one ***gray matter region (Swanson & Bota, 2010)*** to another ***gray matter region (Swanson & Bota, 2010)*** that takes a route through one or more sequential ***white matter tracts (Bell & Bell, 1826)***; and a pathway is the part of a connection revealed in a particular experimental pathway tracing experiment.

There has been no satisfactory systematic account of all ***white matter tracts (Bell & Bell, 1826)*** in any mammalian species. The Nomenclature Table formulated here is somewhat extended from what can be differentiated with the naked eye or with MRI imaging in human, but is minimally necessary to describe the topography of ***white matter tracts (Bell & Bell, 1826)*** followed by ***central nervous system (Carus, 1814)*** connections and their overall circuitry—the routes taken by projections and pathways.

The guiding principles of the scheme presented here are twofold: a topological interpretation of ***central nervous system (Carus, 1814)*** development (Figure 2B, lower part; Appendix 2), and the basic longitudinal-transverse organization of ***nervous systems (Monro, 1783)*** in evolution and comparative anatomy (Figures 1, 2). The general longitudinal-transverse organization of human ***central nervous system white matter tracts (>1840)*** has been emphasized at least since the work of Reil (1809b) and Gall & Spurzheim (1810), and has been documented more recently for ***nervous system (Monro, 1817)*** organization in all bilaterally symmetric animals (for example, Reisinger, 1925, 1972).

In practice, ***central nervous system white matter tracts (>1840)*** in this Table are divided into 4 types: longitudinal, transverse, intrinsic, and central root. They are discussed in Chapter 3 (see Figure 16).

NERVOUS SYSTEM [HUMAN] (MONRO, 1783)

.....Systems architecture (Swanson & Bota, 2010; also see Figure 15 here, right side)
.... White matter tracts (Bell & Bell, 1826)
....................Cerebrospinal axis (Meckel, 1817) or Central nervous system (Carus, 1814)
..............................Central root
....Spinal tract of trigeminal nerve (>1840)
....Gracile fascicle (Müller, 1834)
....Cuneate fascicle (Müller, 1834)
..............................Longitudinal
....Medial longitudinal fascicle (>1840)
....Tectospinal tract (>1840)
....Medial reticulospinal tract (>1840)

............Corticospinal tract (>1840)
............Medial forebrain bundle (Edinger, 1893)
............Lateral vestibulospinal tract (>1840)
............Spinothalamic tract (>1840)
............Ventral spinocerebellar tract (>1840)
............Rubrospinal tract (>1840)
............Lateral reticulospinal tract (>1840)
............Dorsal spinocerebellar tract (>1840)
....Brain (Smith Papyrus, c1700 BC)
........Central root
............Brachium of superior colliculus (>1840)
............Midbrain tract of trigeminal nerve (>1840)
........Longitudinal
............Medial lemniscus (>1840)
............Mammillotegmental tract (Kölliker, 1896)
............Central tegmental tract (Bechterew, 1889)
............Dorsal longitudinal fascicle (Schütz, 1891)
............Ventrolateral fascicle (>1840)
............Habenulo-interpeduncular tract (>1840)
............Cerebellar peduncles (Ridley, 1695)
................Superior cerebellar peduncle (Procháska, 1800)
....Forebrain (Goette, 1873)
........Transverse and longitudinal
............Fornix (Vesalius, 1543a)
........Longitudinal
............Internal capsule (Burdach, 1822)
................Thalamic radiations (Reil, 1809b)
............Postcommissural fornix (Loo, 1931)
....Endbrain (Kuhlenbeck, 1927)
........Transverse
............Precommissural fornix (Loo, 1931)
........Longitudinal
............Lateral septal arcuate fibers (>1840)
............Terminal stria (Wenzel & Wenzel, 1812)
............Peduncular loop (Gratiolet, 1857)
....Cerebral nuclei (Swanson, 2000a)
........Intrinsic
............Medial medullary lamina (>1840)
............Lateral medullary lamina (>1840)
........Transverse
............Terminal stria commissure (>1840)
........Longitudinal
............Anterior limb of internal capsule (>1840)
................Cerebral nuclei corticospinal tract (>1840)
............Genu of internal capsule (>1840)
............Diagonal band (Broca, 1879)
............Septal postcommissural fornix (>1840)
....Cerebral cortex (>1840)
........Central root
............Olfactory nerve layer of main olfactory bulb (>1840)
........Intrinsic
............Lateral olfactory tract (>1840)
............Superficial medullary lamina of subiculum (Dejerine & Dejerine-Klumpke, 1895)
........Transverse
............Cerebral cortex white matter (>1840)
................Anterior commissure (Lieutaud, 1742)

....Olfactory limb of anterior commissure (>1840)
....Temporal limb of anterior commissure (>1840)
....Corpus callosum (Galen, c177)
....Rostrum of corpus callosum (Reil, 1809b)
....Genu of corpus callosum (Reil, 1809b)
....Body of corpus callosum (Arnold, 1838a)
....Splenium of corpus callosum (Burdach, 1822)
....Radiation of corpus callosum (>1840)
....Frontal forceps (>1840)
....Tapetum (Reil, 1809b)
....Occipital forceps (>1840)
....Fimbria (Honegger, 1890)
....Longitudinal striae (>1840)
....Medial longitudinal stria (>1840)
....Lateral longitudinal stria (Arnold, 1838a)
....Alveus (Burdach, 1822)
....Dorsal fornix (Sprague & Meyer, 1950)
....Hippocampal commissures (Johnston, 1913)
....Ventral hippocampal commissure (Craigie, 1925)
....Intermediate hippocampal commissure (>1840)
....Dorsal hippocampal commissure (Craigie, 1925)
....Association fibers of cerebral cortex (>1840)
....Arcuate fibers (Arnold, 1838b)
....Uncinate fascicle (Reil, 1809b)
....Inferior longitudinal fascicle (Burdach, 1822)
....External capsule (Burdach, 1822)
....Superior longitudinal fascicle (>1840)
....Cingulum (Burdach, 1822)
....Optic radiation (>1840)
....Auditory radiation (>1840)
....................Interbrain (Baer, 1837)
................................Central Root
....Optic tract (Vicq d'Azyr, 1784)
................................Transverse
....Medullary stria (Wenzel & Wenzel, 1812)
....Mammillothalamic tract (Kölliker, 1896)
................................Longitudinal
....Posterior limb of internal capsule (1840)
....Sublentiform part of internal capsule (>1840)
....Retrolentiform part of internal capsule (>1840)
....Interbrain corticospinal tract (>1840)
....................Hypothalamus (Kuhlenbeck, 1927)
................................Central Root
....Optic chiasm (Galen, c173)
....Medial retinohypothalamic tract (>1840)
....Hypothalamic optic tract (>1840)
....Lateral retinohypothalamic tract (>1840)
....Inferior fascicle of accessory optic system (Hayhow et al., 1960)
................................Intrinsic
....Periventricular bundle of hypothalamus (>1840)
....Hypothalamohypophysial tract (>1840)
....Principal mammillary tract (Kölliker, 1896)
................................Transverse
....Hypothalamic medullary stria (>1840)
....Hypothalamic mammillothalamic tract (>1840)
................................Longitudinal
....Supraoptic decussations (>1840)

....Hypothalamic mammillotegmental tract (>1840)
....Supramammillary decussation (1840)
....Hypothalamic medial forebrain bundle (>1840)
....Hypothalamic postcommissural fornix (>1840)
....Medial corticohypothalamic tract (Gurdjian, 1927)
......................Thalamus (His, 1893a)
................................Central Root
....Thalamic optic tract (>1840)
....Thalamic brachium of superior colliculus (>1840)
................................Intrinsic
....Periventricular bundle of thalamus (>1840)
....Internal medullary lamina (>1840)
....Middle commissure (>1840)
....External medullary lamina (>1840)
....Zonal layer of thalamus (Burdach, 1822)
................................Transverse
....Epithalamic medullary stria (>1840)
....Habenular commissure (>1840)
....Thalamic mammillothalamic tract (>1840)
................................Longitudinal
....Inferior thalamic radiation peduncular loop (>1840)
....Subiculothalamic tract (Swanson et al., 1987)
....Thalamic spinothalamic tract (>1840)
....Thalamic medial lemniscus (>1840)
....Thalamic habenulo-interpeduncular tract (>1840)
......................Tegmentum (Swanson, 2000b)
................................Central Root
....Oculomotor nerve central root (>1840)
....Oculomotor nerve central rootlets (>1840)
....Pretectal brachium of superior colliculus (>1840)
....Superior fascicle of accessory optic system (Hayhow et al., 1960)
....Transverse peduncular tract (Gudden, 1870)
....Trochlear nerve central root (>1840)
....Trochlear nerve decussation (>1840)
....Tegmental segment of midbrain tract of trigeminal nerve (>1840)
................................Transverse
....Posterior commissure (Winslow, 1733)
....Tegmental habenulo-interpeduncular tract (>1840)
................................Longitudinal
....Tegmental medial longitudinal fascicle (>1840)
....Tegmental tectospinal tract (>1840)
....Dorsal tegmental decussation (>1840)
....Tegmental medial lemniscus (>1840)
....Cerebral peduncle (Tarin, 1753)
....Tegmental medial forebrain bundle (>1840)
....Mammillary peduncle (>1840)
....Tegmental mammillotegmental tract (>1840)
....Tegmental central tegmental tract (>1840)
....Tegmental dorsal longitudinal fascicle (>1840)
....Tegmental ventrolateral fascicle (>1840)
....Tegmental spinothalamic tract (>1840)
....Tegmental rubrospinal tract (>1840)
....Ventral tegmental decussation (>1840)
....Tegmental superior cerebellar peduncle (>1840)
....Superior cerebellar peduncle decussation (>1840)
....Brachium of inferior colliculus (>1840)
......................Tectum (Baer, 1837)

................................Transverse
....Superior colliculus commissure (>1840)
....Inferior colliculus commissure (>1840)
.....................Pons (Haller, 1747)
................................Central Root
....Abducens nerve central root (>1840)
....Abducens nerve central rootlets (>1840)
....Trigeminal nerve central motor root (>1840)
....Pontine segment of midbrain tract of trigeminal nerve (>1840)
....Trigeminal nerve central sensory root (>1840)
....Pontine segment of spinal tract of trigeminal nerve (>1840)
................................Transverse
....Middle cerebellar peduncle (Rolando, 1819)
....Transverse pontine fibers (>1840)
................................Longitudinal
....Pontine medial longitudinal fascicle (>1840)
....Pontine tectospinal tract (>1840)
....Pontine medial reticulospinal tract (>1840)
....Pontine medial lemniscus (>1840)
....Lateral lemniscus (Bechterew, 1885b)
....Longitudinal pontine fibers (Arnold, 1838b)
....Pontine medial forebrain bundle (>1840)
....Pontine central tegmental tract (>1840)
....Pontine dorsal longitudinal fascicle (>1840)
....Pontine ventrolateral fascicle (>1840)
....Pontine spinothalamic tract (>1840)
....Pontine ventral spinocerebellar tract (>1840)
....Pontine rubrospinal tract (>1840)
....Pontine superior cerebellar peduncle (>1840)
.....................Cerebellum (Aristotle)
................................Transverse
....Cerebellar commissure (>1840)
................................Longitudinal
....Arbor vitae (Winslow, 1733)
....Floccular peduncle (Burdach, 1822)
.....................Medulla (Winslow, 1733)
................................Central Root
....Medullary segment of spinal tract of trigeminal nerve (>1840)
....Facial nerve central root (>1840)
....Cochlear nerve central root (>1840)
....Vestibular nerve central root (>1840)
....Glossopharyngeal nerve central root (>1840)
....Glossopharyngeal nerve central rootlets (>1840)
....Vagus nerve central root (>1840)
....Vagus nerve central rootlets (>1840)
....Hypoglossal nerve central root (>1840)
....Hypoglossal nerve central rootlets (>1840)
....Medullary gracile fascicle (>1840)
....Medullary cuneate fascicle (>1840)
................................Transverse
....Trapezoid body (Treviranus, 1820)
....Internal arcuate fibers (>1840)
....Medial lemniscus decussation (>1840)
................................Longitudinal
....Medullary medial longitudinal fascicle (>1840)
....Medullary tectospinal tract (>1840)
....Medullary medial reticulospinal tract (>1840)

....Medullary medial lemniscus (>1840)
....Pyramid (Willis, 1664)
....Pyramidal decussation (Reil, 1809c)
....Medullary medial forebrain bundle (>1840)
....Medullary central tegmental tract (>1840)
....Amiculum of olive (>1840)
....Medullary lateral vestibulospinal tract (>1840)
....Medullary ventrolateral fascicle (>1840)
....Medullary spinothalamic tract (>1840)
....Medullary ventral spinocerebellar tract (>1840)
....Medullary rubrospinal tract (>1840)
....Medullary lateral reticulospinal tract (>1840)
....Medullary dorsal spinocerebellar tract (>1840)
....Inferior cerebellar peduncle (Günther, 1786)
....Ventral external arcuate fibers (>1840)
....Olivocerebellar tract (>1840)
....Medullary striae (Scarpa, 1788)
....................Spinal cord (Galen, c162–c166)
................................Central Root
....Ventral root central part (>1840)
....Ventral rootlets central part (>1840)
....Spinal segment of spinal tract of trigeminal nerve (>1840)
....Dorsal root central part (1840)
....Spinal gracile fascicle (>1840)
....Spinal cuneate fascicle (>1840)
................................Transverse
....Ventral white commissure (>1840)
................................Longitudinal
....Funiculi of spinal cord (Burdach, 1822)
....Ventral funiculus (>1840)
....Ventral intersegmental tract (>1840)
....Spinal medial longitudinal fascicle (>1840)
....Spinal tectospinal tract (>1840)
....Uncrossed corticospinal tract (>1840)
....Spinal lateral vestibulospinal tract (>1840)
....Spinal medial reticulospinal tract (>1840)
....Ventral spinothalamic tract (>1840)
....Lateral funiculus (Burdach, 1822)
....Lateral intersegmental tract (>1840)
....Lateral spinothalamic tract (>1840)
....Spinal ventral spinocerebellar tract (>1840)
....Spinal lateral reticulospinal tract (>1840)
....Spinal rubrospinal tract (>1840)
....Crossed corticospinal tract (>1840)
....Spinal medial forebrain bundle (>1840)
....Spinal dorsal spinocerebellar tract (>1840)
....Dorsolateral tract (>1840)
....Dorsal funiculus (>1840)
....Dorsal intersegmental tract (>1840)

Appendix 5
Human CNS surface features

This hierarchical Nomenclature Table provides a set of ***standard terms*** for describing adult human ***central nervous system surface features (>1840)*** visible with the naked eye and arranged according to basic topographic divisions (see Figure 15, left side under Cerebrospinal axis). Whereas the upper level(s) of the hierarchy generally apply to all vertebrates, lower levels must be tailored for individual species, especially levels related to ***cerebral cortex (>1840)*** and ***cerebellar cortex (Willis, 1664)***.

CEREBROSPINAL AXIS (MECKEL, 1817) OR CENTRAL NERVOUS SYSTEM [HUMAN] (CARUS, 1814)

.....Topographic divisions (Swanson & Bota, 2010; Figure 15 here, left side)
.... Central nervous system surface features (>1840)
.... Brain (Smith Papyrus, c1700 BC)
................................Transverse cerebral fissure (>1840)
....Inner part of transverse cerebral fissure (>1840)
....Outer part of transverse cerebral fissure (>1840)
................................Pontine sulcus (Soemmerring, 1778)
.... Forebrain (Goette, 1873)
................................Terminal sulcus (>1840)
.... Endbrain (Kuhlenbeck, 1927)
................................Longitudinal cerebral fissure (Gordon, 1815)
................................Choroid fissure (>1840)
.... Cerebral nuclei (Swanson, 2000a)
................................Diagonal sulcus (Beccari, 1911)
.... Cerebral cortex (>1840)
................................Frontal pole (>1840)
................................Temporal pole (Broca, 1878a)
................................Occipital pole (Broca, 1878a)
................................Cerebral sulci (Vesalius, 1543a)
....Rhinal sulcus (>1840)
....Fimbriodentate sulcus (>1840)
....Hippocampal sulcus (Gratiolet, 1854)
....Sulcus of corpus callosum (>1840)
....Cingulate sulcus (>1840)
.... Paracentral sulcus (>1840)
.... Marginal sulcus (>1840)
....Subparietal sulcus (>1840)
....Circular sulcus (Schwalbe, 1881)
.... Central sulcus of insula (>1840)
....Olfactory sulcus (Quain, 1834)
....Orbital sulci (>1840)
....Anterior parolfactory sulcus (>1840)
....Posterior parolfactory sulcus (>1840)
....Inferior frontal sulcus (>1840)
....Superior frontal sulcus (>1840)
....Precentral sulcus (>1840)
....Central sulcus (Huschke, 1854)
....Postcentral sulcus (>1840)
....Intraparietal sulcus (>1840)
....Parieto-occipital sulcus (>1840)

....Lateral cerebral sulcus (>1840)
....Anterior branch of lateral cerebral sulcus (>1840)
....Ascending branch of lateral cerebral sulcus (>1840)
....Stem of lateral cerebral sulcus (>1840)
....Posterior branch of lateral cerebral sulcus (>1840)
....Frontal operculum (>1840)
....Parietal operculum (>1840)
....Temporal operculum (>1840)
....Temporal plane (Heschl, 1878)
....Lateral cerebral fossa (>1840)
....Collateral sulcus (1840)
....Occipitotemporal sulcus (>1840)
....Inferior temporal sulcus (>1840)
....Superior temporal sulcus (>1840)
....Transverse temporal sulcus (Heschl, 1878)
....Preoccipital notch (>1840)
....Calcarine sulcus (>1840)
....Lateral occipital sulcus (>1840)
....Lunate sulcus (>1840)
....Transverse occipital sulcus (>1840)
....................Hypothalamus (Kuhlenbeck, 1927)
................................Mammillary sulcus (>1840)
....................Thalamus (His, 1893a)
................................Habenular sulcus (>1840)
................................Habenular trigone (>1840)
....................Tegmentum (Swanson, 2000b)
................................Interpeduncular fossa (>1840)
................................Medial midbrain sulcus (>1840)
................................Lateral midbrain sulcus (>1840)
................................Dorsal midbrain sulcus (>1840)
....................Tectum (Baer, 1837)
................................Cruciform sulcus (>1840)
....Longitudinal tectal sulcus (>1840)
....Transverse tectal sulcus (>1840)
....................Rhombicbrain (His, 1893b)
................................Medullopontine sulcus (>1840)
....Foramen cecum of medulla (>1840)
................................Cerebellopontine angle (>1840)
................................Transverse cerebellar fissure (Burdach, 1822)
....................Pons (Haller, 1747)
................................Basilar sulcus of pons (Gordon, 1815)
....................Cerebellum (Aristotle)
................................Cerebellar cortex (Willis, 1664)
....Anterior cerebellar notch (Chaussier, 1807)
....Vallecula of cerebellum (Haller, 1762)
....Nidus (Reil, 1809c)
....Posterior cerebellar notch (Chaussier, 1807)
....Cerebellar fissures (>1840)
....Paramedian fissure (>1840)
....Precentral fissure (>1840)
....Preculminate fissure (Smith, 1903)
....Primary fissure (Smith, 1902)
....Posterior superior fissure (>1840)
....Horizontal fissure (Malacarne, 1776)
....Ansoparamedian fissure (>1840)
....Prepyramidal fissure (Hayashi, 1924)
....Secondary fissure (Bolk, 1906)

- - - - Posterolateral fissure (Larsell, 1937)
- Medulla (Winslow, 1733)
  - Ventral median fissure of medulla (>1840)
  - Ventrolateral sulcus of medulla (>1840)
  - Olive (Tiedemann, 1821)
  - Dorsolateral sulcus of medulla (>1840)
  - Trigeminal tubercle (>1840)
  - Cuneate tubercle (>1840)
  - Dorsal intermediate sulcus (>1840)
  - Gracile tubercle (>1840)
  - Dorsal median sulcus of medulla (>1840)
- Spinal cord (Galen, c162–c166)
  - Ventral median fissure of spinal cord (>1840)
  - Ventrolateral sulcus of spinal cord (>1840)
  - Dorsolateral sulcus of spinal cord (>1840)
  - Dorsal median sulcus of spinal cord (>1840)
    - Dorsal median septum (>1840)

Appendix 6
Human PNS ganglia (topographic gross anatomy groupings)

This hierarchical Nomenclature Table provides a set of ***standard terms*** for describing the ***gray matter regions (Swanson & Bota, 2010)*** or ***ganglia (Galen, c173)*** of the adult human ***peripheral nervous system (Meckel, 1817)*** (PNS) visible to the naked eye. There are alternate ways to group ***gray matter regions (Swanson & Bota, 2010)***; see Figure 15 (right side). A strictly topographic approach is adopted here, using the broad topographic divisions shown in Figure 15 (left side). Functional grouping is an alternate approach, arranging the same parts in a different hierarchy.

PERIPHERAL GANGLIA [HUMAN] (>1840)

.....Craniospinal ganglia (>1840)
.... Cranial nerve ganglia (>1840)
.....................Terminal ganglion (>1840)
.....................Trigeminal ganglion (>1840)
.....................Geniculate ganglion (Bischoff, 1832)
.....................Cochlear ganglion (>1840)
.....................Vestibular ganglion (>1840)
.....................Proximal glossopharyngeal ganglion (>1840)
.....................Distal glossopharyngeal ganglion (>1840)
.....................Proximal vagal ganglion (>1840)
.....................Distal vagal ganglion (>1840)
.... Spinal nerve ganglia (Burdach, 1819)
.....................Cervical spinal ganglia (>1840)
.....................Thoracic spinal ganglia (>1840)
.....................Lumbar spinal ganglia (>1840)
.....................Sacral spinal ganglia (>1840)
.....................Coccygeal spinal ganglia (>1840)
.....Autonomic ganglia (Langley, 1900)
.... Paravertebral ganglia (Durward, 1951)
.....................Carotid ganglion (Wutzer, 1817; Bock, 1817)
.....................Temporal ganglion (Andersch & Soemmerring, 1792)
.....................Facial ganglion (Lazorthes, 1949)
.....................Sympathetic trunk ganglia (Winslow 1733)
................................Cervical sympathetic ganglia (>1840)
....Superior cervical ganglion (Vieussens, 1684)
....Middle cervical ganglion (Haller, 1762)
....Vertebral ganglion (>1840)
....Inferior cervical ganglion (Vieussens, 1684)
................................Thoracic sympathetic ganglia (>1840)
....Superior thoracic ganglion (Lieutaud, 1742)
................................Lumbar sympathetic ganglia (>1840)
................................Sacral sympathetic ganglia (>1840)
................................Coccygeal sympathetic ganglia (>1840)
....Ganglion impar (>1840)
.....................Intermediate ganglia (>1840)
.... Prevertebral ganglia (Quain, 1832)
.....................Splanchnic ganglion (>1840)
.....................Celiac ganglion (Walter, 1783)
.....................Aorticorenal ganglion (>1840)

.....................Phrenic ganglia (Walter, 1783)
.....................Superior mesenteric ganglion (>1840)
.....................Spermatic ganglia (Walter, 1783)
.....................Inferior mesenteric ganglion (>1840)
.........Terminal ganglia (Gaskell 1886)
.....................Ciliary ganglion (Loder, 1778)
.....................Pterygopalatine ganglion (>1840)
.....................Submandibular ganglion (>1840)
.....................Otic ganglion (>1840)
.....................Cardiac ganglion (Neubauer, 1772; Haller, 1772)
.....................Hepatic ganglia (Walter, 1783)
.....................Renal ganglia (Walther, 1735)
................................Posterior renal ganglion (>1840)
................................Anterior renal ganglion (Tiedemann, 1822)
.....................Pelvic ganglia (>1840)
.....................Paracervical ganglia (>1840)
................................Uterine cervical ganglion (>1840)

Appendix 7

Human PNS cranial nerves (topographic gross anatomy groupings)

This hierarchical Nomenclature Table provides a set of ***standard terms*** for describing the ***cranial nerves (Soemmerring, 1791)***, which are ***white matter tracts (Bell & Bell, 1826)***, of the adult human ***peripheral nervous system (Meckel, 1814)*** (PNS) visible to the naked eye. A strictly topographic approach to grouping is adopted here (Figure 15, right side), using the broad topographic divisions shown in Figure 15 (left side). The naming and arrangement of ***nerves (Herophilus, c335–c280 BC)*** is the most agreed upon part of human ***nervous system (Monro, 1783)*** terminology.

CRANIAL NERVES [HUMAN] (SOEMMERRING, 1791)

.....Terminal nerve (>1840)
.....Vomeronasal nerve (>1840)
.....Olfactory nerve (Winslow, 1733)
.....Optic nerve (Vicq d'Azyr, 1786)
.....Oculomotor nerve (Estienne, 1545)
..........Oculomotor nerve root (>1840)
...............Oculomotor nerve rootlets (>1840)
..........Oculomotor nerve trunk (>1840)
...............Oculomotor nerve superior branch (Winslow, 1733)
...............Oculomotor nerve inferior branch (Haase, 1781)
....................Nerve to medial rectus (>1840)
....................Nerve to inferior rectus (>1840)
....................Nerve to inferior oblique (>1840)
.........................Branch of oculomotor nerve to ciliary ganglion (>1840)
.....Trochlear nerve (Molinetti, 1669)
.....Trigeminal nerve (Winslow, 1733)
..........Trigeminal nerve motor root (Bell, 1829)
..........Trigeminal nerve sensory root (>1840)
..........Trigeminal nerve branches (Winslow, 1733)
...............Ophthalmic nerve (Winslow, 1733)
....................Tentorial nerve (Arnold, 1838a)
....................Nasociliary nerve (Meckel, 1817; Wutzer, 1817)
.........................Communicating branch of nasociliary nerve with ciliary ganglion (>1840)
.........................Long ciliary nerves (Soemmerring, 1801)
.........................Posterior ethmoidal nerve (>1840)
.........................Infratrochlear nerve (Schaarschmidt, 1750)
..............................Palpebral branches of infratrochlear nerve (>1840)
.........................Anterior ethmoidal nerve (>1840)
..............................Nasal branches of anterior ethmoidal nerve (>1840)
...................................Internal nasal branches of anterior ethmoidal nerve (>1840)
....Lateral nasal branches of internal nasal branches of anterior ethmoidal nerve (>1840)
....Medial nasal branches of internal nasal branches of anterior ethmoidal nerve (>1840)
...................................External nasal branch of anterior ethmoidal nerve (>1840)
....................Lacrimal nerve (Meckel 1748; Bonhomme, 1748)
.........................Communicating branch of lacrimal nerve with zygomatic nerve (>1840)
....................Frontal nerve (Cheselden 1726)
.........................Supratrochlear nerve (Schaarschmidt, 1750)

....Supraorbital nerve (Meckel, 1753, p. 42)
....Medial branch of supraorbital nerve (>1840)
....Lateral branch of supraorbital nerve (>1840)
....................Maxillary nerve (Meckel, 1753)
..............................Meningeal branch of maxillary nerve (>1840)
..............................Pterygopalatine nerves (Wrisberg, 1786)
....Orbital branches of pterygopalatine ganglion (>1840)
....Posterior superior nasal nerves (Soemmerring, 1791)
....Lateral posterior superior nasal nerves (>1840)
....Medial posterior superior nasal nerves (>1840)
....Nasopalatine nerve (Scarpa, 1785)
....Pharyngeal nerve (Bock, 1817)
....Palatine nerves (Schaarschmidt, 1750)
....Greater palatine nerve (Cloquet, 1816)
....Posterior inferior nasal nerves (Günther, 1786)
....Lesser palatine nerves (Meckel, 1817)
....Lateral palatine nerve (Henle, 1871)
....Tonsillar branches of lateral palatine nerve (>1840)
....Posterior palatine nerve (Günther, 1786)
..............................Zygomatic nerve (>1840)
....Zygomaticotemporal nerve (>1840)
....Zygomaticofacial nerve (>1840)
..............................Posterior superior dental nerve (Haller, 1762)
..............................Infraorbital nerve (Schaarschmidt, 1750)
....Middle superior dental nerve (Henle, 1871)
....Anterior superior dental nerve (Haller, 1762)
....Nasal branch of anterior superior dental nerve (>1840)
....Inferior palpebral branches of infraorbital nerve (Meckel, 1748)
....External nasal branches of infraorbital nerve (>1840)
....Internal nasal branches of infraorbital nerve (>1840)
....Superior labial branches of infraorbital nerve (Meckel, 1748)
..............................Superior dental plexus (>1840)
....Superior dental branches of superior dental plexus (>1840)
....Superior gingival branches of superior dental plexus (>1840)
....................Mandibular nerve (>1840)
..............................Mandibular nerve sensory root (>1840)
..............................Mandibular nerve trunk (>1840)
....Nervus spinosus (>1840)
....Medial pterygoid nerve (>1840)
....Nerve to tensor veli palatini (>1840)
....Nerve to tensor tympani (Arnold, 1834)
....Anterior branch of mandibular nerve (>1840)
....Masseteric nerve (Meckel, 1748)
....Deep temporal nerves (Haase, 1781)
....Posterior deep temporal nerve (Arnold, 1834)
....Middle deep temporal nerve (>1840)
....Anterior deep temporal nerve (Arnold, 1834)
....Lateral pterygoid nerve (>1840)
....Buccal nerve (Meckel, 1748)
....Posterior branch of mandibular nerve (>1840)
....Auriculotemporal nerve (Haller, 1762)
....Anterior auricular nerves (>1840)
....External acoustic meatus nerves (Meckel, 1817)
....Tympanic membrane branch of external acoustic meatus nerves (>1840)
....Articular branches of auriculotemporal nerve (>1840)
....Parotid branches of auriculotemporal nerve (>1840)

....Communicating branches of auriculotemporal nerve with facial nerve (>1840)
....Superficial temporal branches of auriculotemporal nerve (>1840)
....Lingual nerve (Vesalius, 1543a)
....Isthmus of fauces branches of lingual nerve (>1840)
....Communicating branches of lingual nerve with submandibular ganglion (>1840)
....Sublingual nerve (Henle, 1871)
....Communicating branches of lingual nerve with hypoglossal nerve (>1840)
....Lingual branches of lingual nerve (Arnold, 1834)
....Inferior dental nerve (Meckel, 1817)
....Mylohyoid nerve (Meckel, 1748)
....Inferior dental plexus (>1840)
....Inferior dental branches of inferior dental plexus (>1840)
....Inferior gingival branches of inferior dental plexus (>1840)
....Incisor nerve (>1840)
....Mental nerve (Cheselden, 1726)
....Mental branches of mental nerve (Arnold, 1834)
....Inferior labial branches of mental nerve (Meckel, 1753)
.....Abducens nerve (Heister, 1717)
..........Abducens nerve root (>1840)
....................Abducens nerve rootlets (>1840)
..........Abducens nerve trunk (>1840)
.....Intermediofacial nerve (Strong & Elwyn, 1943)
..........Intermediofacial nerve roots (>1840)
....................Facial nerve root (>1840)
....................Intermediate nerve (>1840)
................................Intermediate nerve root (>1840)
....Intermediate nerve rootlets (>1840)
................................Intermediate nerve trunk (>1840)
..........Intermediofacial nerve trunk (>1840)
....................Greater petrosal nerve (>1840)
................................Nerve of pterygoid canal (>1840)
....................Communicating branch of intermediofacial nerve with tympanic plexus (>1840)
....................Stapedial nerve (>1840)
....................Chorda tympani (Falloppio, 1561)
................................Communicating branch of otic ganglion with chorda tympani (>1840)
....................Communicating branch of intermediofacial nerve with vagus nerve (>1840)
..........Facial nerve trunk (>1840)
....................Posterior auricular nerve (Meckel, 1753)
................................Occipital branch of posterior auricular nerve (Arnold, 1834)
................................Auricular branch of posterior auricular nerve (Arnold, 1834)
....................Digastric nerve (Meckel, 1753)
................................Communicating branch of digastric nerve with glossopharyngeal nerve (>1840)
....................Stylohyoid nerve (Meckel, 1753)
....................Parotid plexus (Meckel, 1817)
....................Temporal branches of facial nerve (Swan, 1830)
....................Zygomatic branches of facial nerve (>1840)
....................Buccal branch of facial nerve (>1840)
....................Marginal mandibular branch of facial nerve (>1840)
....................Cervical branch of facial nerve (>1840)
.....Vestibulocochlear nerve (>1840)
..........Vestibulocochlear nerve trunk (>1840)
....................Vestibular nerve (Cotugno, 1760)
................................Rostral part of vestibular nerve (>1840)
....Utriculoampullary nerve (>1840)

....Utricular nerve (>1840)
....Lateral ampullary nerve (>1840)
....Anterior ampullary nerve (>1840)
..............................Caudal part of vestibular nerve (>1840)
....Posterior ampullary nerve (>1840)
....Saccular nerve (>1840)
....Cochlear communicating branch of vestibular nerve (>1840)
....................Cochlear nerve (Cotugno, 1760)
.....Glossopharyngeal nerve (Huber, 1744)
..........Glossopharyngeal nerve root (>1840)
....................Glossopharyngeal nerve rootlets (>1840)
..........Glossopharyngeal nerve trunk (Wrisberg, 1786; Günther, 1786)
....................Communicating branch of glossopharyngeal nerve with meningeal branch of vagus nerve (>1840)
....................Tympanic nerve (Arnold, 1834)
..............................Tympanic plexus (Müller, 1834)
....Communicating branch of tympanic plexus with greater petrosal nerve (>1840)
....Lesser petrosal nerve (>1840)
....Tubal branch of tympanic plexus (>1840)
....................Communicating branch of glossopharyngeal nerve with auricular branch of vagus nerve (>1840)
....................Carotid branches of glossopharyngeal nerve (Todd, 1836–1839)
....................Pharyngeal branches of glossopharyngeal nerve (Neubauer, 1772)
....................Stylopharyngeal branch of glossopharyngeal nerve (>1840)
..........Tonsillar branches of glossopharyngeal nerve (>1840)
..........Lingual branches of glossopharyngeal nerve (Haller, 1762)
.....Vagus nerve (Galen, c192)
..........Vagus nerve root (>1840)
....................Vagus nerve rootlets (>1840)
..........Vagus nerve trunk (Wrisberg, 1786; Günther, 1786)
....................Meningeal branch of vagus nerve (>1840)
....................Auricular branch of vagus nerve (Arnold, 1834)
....................Communicating branch of vagus nerve with glossopharyngeal nerve (>1840)
....................Pharyngeal branches of vagus nerve (Wrisberg, 1786)
....................Carotid branch of vagus nerve (>1840)
....................Superior laryngeal nerve (Loder, 1778)
..............................External branch of superior laryngeal nerve (Fyfe, 1800)
..............................Internal branch of superior laryngeal nerve (Fyfe, 1800)
....Communicating branch of superior laryngeal nerve with inferior laryngeal nerve (Langenbeck, 1826–1830)
....................Superior cervical cardiac branches of vagus nerve (>1840)
....................Inferior cervical cardiac branches of vagus nerve (>1840)
....................Recurrent laryngeal nerve (Albinus, 1744)
..............................Cardiac branches of recurrent laryngeal nerve (>1840)
..............................Tracheal branches of recurrent laryngeal nerve (>1840)
..............................Esophageal branches of recurrent laryngeal nerve (Arnold, 1834)
..............................Inferior laryngeal nerve (>1840)
..............................Pharyngeal branches of recurrent laryngeal nerve (>1840)
....................Thoracic cardiac branches of vagus nerve (>1840)
....................Upper esophageal branches of vagus nerve (Cloquet, 1828)
....................Pulmonary branches of vagus nerve (Cloquet, 1828)
....................Esophageal plexus (Haller, 1762)
..............................Anterior esophageal plexus (Haller, 1762)
....Anterior vagal trunk (Wrisberg, 1780)
....Gastric branches of anterior vagal trunk (>1840)
....Anterior nerve of lesser curvature (>1840)

.... Pyloric branches of anterior vagal trunk (>1840)
.... Hepatic branches of anterior vagal trunk (>1840)
.... Celiac branches of anterior vagal trunk (>1840)
.... Posterior esophageal plexus (Haller, 1762)
.... Posterior vagal trunk (Wrisberg, 1780)
.... Gastric branches of posterior vagal trunk (>1840)
.... Posterior nerve of lesser curvature (>1840)
.... Hepatic branches of posterior vagal trunk (>1840)
.... Celiac branches of posterior vagal trunk (>1840)
..... Accessory nerve (Vieussens, 1684)
.... Cranial root of accessory nerve (>1840)
.... Cranial root of accessory nerve rootlets (>1840)
.... Cranial root of accessory nerve trunks (>1840)
.... Spinal root of accessory nerve (>1840)
.... Spinal root of accessory nerve rootlets (>1840)
.... Spinal root of accessory nerve trunk (>1840)
.... Accessory nerve trunk (Wrisberg, 1786)
.... Internal branch of accessory nerve trunk (Meckel, 1817)
.... External branch of accessory nerve trunk (Meckel, 1817)
.... Muscular branches of external branch of accessory nerve trunk (>1840)
..... Hypoglossal nerve (Winslow, 1733)
.... Hypoglossal nerve root (>1840)
.... Hypoglossal nerve rootlets (>1840)
.... Hypoglossal nerve trunk (Günther, 1786)
.... Thyrohyoid branch of hypoglossal nerve (Meckel, 1817)
.... Lingual branches of hypoglossal nerve (Cloquet, 1816)

Appendix 8
Human PNS spinal nerves (topographic gross anatomy groupings)

This hierarchical Nomenclature Table provides a set of ***standard terms*** for describing the ***spinal nerves (Camper, 1760–1762)***, which are ***white matter tracts (Bell & Bell, 1826)***, of the adult human ***peripheral nervous system (Meckel, 1814)*** (PNS) visible to the naked eye. A strictly topographic approach to grouping is adopted here (Figure 15, right side), using the broad topographic divisions shown in Figure 15 (left side). The naming and arrangement of ***nerves (Herophilus, c335–c280 BC)*** is the most agreed upon part of human ***nervous system (Monro, 1783)*** terminology.

SPINAL NERVES [HUMAN] (CAMPER, 1760–1762)

.....Spinal nerve groups (Durward, 1951)
..........Cervical nerves (Galen, c173)
....................Suboccipital nerve (Winslow, 1733)
..........Thoracic nerves (Diemerbroeck, 1672)
..........Lumbar nerves (Diemerbroeck, 1672)
..........Sacral nerves (Camper, 1760)
..........Coccygeal nerves (Camper, 1762)
.....Spinal nerve parts (>1840)
..........Spinal nerve roots (Tiedemann, 1816)
....................Ventral root (>1840)
..............................Ventral rootlets (>1840)
....................Dorsal root (Spurzheim, 1826)
..............................Dorsal rootlets (>1840)
....................Cauda equina (Anatomia Magistri Nicolai physici, 12th century)
..........Spinal nerve trunk (Frotscher, 1788)
....................Meningeal branch of spinal nerve trunk (>1840)
..........Spinal nerve primary branches (>1840)
....................Spinal nerve dorsal branch (Meckel, 1817)
..............................Medial branch of spinal nerve dorsal branch (>1840)
....Greater occipital nerve (Haase, 1781)
....Third occipital nerve (>1840)
..............................Lateral branch of spinal nerve dorsal branch (>1840)
....Superior clunial nerves (>1840)
....Medial clunial nerves (>1840)
....................Spinal nerve ventral branch (>1840)
..............................Cervical plexus (Molinetti, 1675)
....Communicating loops of cervical plexus (>1840)
....Communicating branches of cervical plexus (>1840)
....Muscular branches of cervical plexus (Cruveilhier, 1836)
....Ansa cervicalis (>1840)
....Superior root of ansa cervicalis (>1840)
....Inferior root of ansa cervicalis (>1840)
....Phrenic nerve (Galen, c173)
....Pericardial branch of phrenic nerve (>1840)
....Phrenico-abdominal branches of phrenic nerve (Günther, 1786)
....Ascending superficial branches of cervical plexus (Quain, 1828)
....Lesser occipital nerve (Mayer, 1794)
....Great auricular nerve (Haase, 1781)

............Posterior branch of great auricular nerve (Bock, 1827)
............Anterior branch of great auricular nerve (Bock, 1827)
.........Transverse nerve of neck (>1840)
............Superior branches of transverse nerve of neck (>1840)
............Inferior branches of transverse nerve of neck (>1840)
......Descending superficial branches of cervical plexus (Quain, 1828)
.........Supraclavicular nerves (Meckel, 1817)
............Medial supraclavicular nerves (>1840)
............Intermediate supraclavicular nerves (>1840)
............Lateral supraclavicular nerves (>1840)
...Brachial plexus (Camper, 1760)
......Brachial plexus roots (Schwalbe, 1881)
.........Muscular branches of brachial plexus roots (>1840)
.........Dorsal scapular nerve (Bock, 1827)
.........Long thoracic nerve (Quain & Wilson, 1839)
......Brachial plexus trunks (Schwalbe, 1881)
.........Brachial plexus upper trunk (>1840)
............Subclavian nerve (Schwalbe, 1881)
...............Accessory phrenic nerve (>1840)
............Suprascapular nerve (Bang, 1770)
.........Brachial plexus middle trunk (>1840)
.........Brachial plexus lower trunk (>1840)
......Brachial plexus divisions (Paterson, 1887)
.........Brachial plexus ventral divisions (Paterson, 1887)
.........Brachial plexus dorsal divisions (Paterson, 1887)
......Brachial plexus cords (Schwalbe, 1881)
.........Brachial plexus lateral cord (Schwalbe, 1881)
............Lateral pectoral nerve (>1840)
............Musculocutaneous nerve (Du Verney, 1697)
...............Muscular branches of musculocutaneous nerve (Günther, 1786)
...............Lateral cutaneous nerve of forearm (>1840)
............Lateral root of median nerve (>1840)
.........Brachial plexus dorsal cord (Paterson, 1887)
............Upper subscapular nerve (>1840)
............Thoracodorsal nerve (>1840)
............Lower subscapular nerve (>1840)
............Axillary nerve (Winslow, 1733)
...............Muscular branches of axillary nerve (>1840)
...............Superior lateral cutaneous nerve of arm (>1840)
............Radial nerve (Du Verney, 1697)
...............Posterior cutaneous nerve of arm (>1840)
...............Inferior lateral cutaneous nerve of arm (>1840)
...............Posterior cutaneous nerve of forearm (>1840)
...............Muscular branches of radial nerve (>1840)
...............Articular branches of radial nerve (>1840)
...............Deep branch of radial nerve (Martin, 1781)
..................Posterior interosseous nerve (Quain & Wilson, 1839)
...............Superficial branch of radial nerve (Martin, 1781)
..................Communicating branch of radial nerve with ulnar nerve (>1840)
..................Dorsal digital nerves of radial nerve (>1840)
.........Brachial plexus medial cord (Schwalbe, 1881)
............Medial pectoral nerve (>1840)
............Medial cutaneous nerve of arm (>1840)

....................Medial cutaneous nerve of forearm (>1840)
........................Anterior branch of medial cutaneous nerve of forearm (>1840)
........................Posterior branch of medial cutaneous nerve of forearm (>1840)
....................Ulnar nerve (Cheselden, 1726)
........................Muscular branches of ulnar nerve (Quain & Wilson, 1839)
........................Palmar branch of ulnar nerve (Soemmerring, 1791)
........................Dorsal branch of ulnar nerve (Günther, 1786)
............................Dorsal digital nerves of ulnar nerve (>1840)
........................Superficial branch of ulnar nerve (Fyfe, 1800)
............................Common palmar digital nerves of ulnar nerve (>1840)
................................Proper palmar digital nerves of ulnar nerve (>1840)
........................Deep branch of ulnar nerve (Fyfe, 1800)
....................Medial root of median nerve (>1840)
....................Median nerve (Du Verney, 1697)
........................Muscular branches of median nerve (Martin, 1781)
........................Anterior interosseous nerve (Quain, 1832)
........................Palmar branch of median nerve (Bock, 1827)
........................Communicating branch of median nerve with ulnar nerve (Bock, 1827)
........................Common palmar digital nerves of median nerve (>1840)
............................Proper palmar digital nerves of median nerve (>1840)
........Intercostal nerves (Vesalius, 1543a)
............Muscular branches of intercostal nerves (Quain & Wilson, 1839)
............Collateral branch of intercostal nerves (Davies et al., 1931)
................Lateral cutaneous branch of intercostal nerves (>1840)
....................Intercostobrachial nerves (>1840)
....................Anterior branch of lateral cutaneous branch of intercostal nerves (>1840)
........................Lateral mammary branches of intercostal nerves (>1840)
....................Posterior branch of lateral cutaneous branch of intercostal nerves (>1840)
................Anterior cutaneous branch of intercostal nerves (>1840)
....................Medial mammary branches of intercostal nerves (>1840)
........Subcostal nerve (>1840)
........Lumbosacral plexus (Vesalius, 1543a)
............Lumbar plexus (Vesalius, 1543a)
................Lumbar plexus ventral branches (>1840)
....................Muscular branches of lumbar plexus ventral branches (>1840)
................Lumbar plexus dorsal divisions (Paterson, 1887)
....................Lateral cutaneous nerve of thigh (>1840)
....................Femoral nerve (Haller, 1762)
........................Muscular branches of femoral nerve (Quain & Wilson, 1839)
........................Anterior cutaneous branches of femoral nerve (Quain & Wilson, 1839)
........................Medial cutaneous nerve of thigh (>1840)
........................Saphenous nerve (Haase, 1781)
............................Infrapatellar branch of saphenous nerve (>1840)
............................Patellar plexus (>1840)

  - Lumbar plexus ventral divisions (Paterson, 1887)
    - Iliohypogastric nerve (Schmidt, 1794)
      - Lateral cutaneous branch of iliohypogastric nerve (>1840)
      - Anterior cutaneous branch of iliohypogastric nerve (>1840)
    - Ilio-inguinal nerve (Schmidt, 1794)
      - Anterior scrotal nerves (>1840)
      - Anterior labial nerves (>1840)
    - Genitofemoral nerve (>1840)
      - Genital branch of genitofemoral nerve (>1840)
      - Femoral branch of genitofemoral nerve (>1840)
    - Obturator nerve (Cheselden, 1726)
      - Anterior branch of obturator nerve (Haase, 1781; Martin, 1781)
        - Cutaneous branch of obturator nerve (>1840)
          - Subsartorial plexus (>1840)
        - Muscular branches of anterior branch of obturator nerve (>1840)
      - Posterior branch of obturator nerve (Haase, 1781; Martin, 1781)
        - Muscular branches of posterior branch of obturator nerve (>1840)
        - Articular branch of posterior branch of obturator nerve (>1840)
    - Accessory obturator nerve (Schmidt, 1794)
- Sacral plexus (Vesalius, 1543a)
  - Sacral plexus ventral branches (>1840)
    - Lumbosacral trunk (Cruveilhier, 1836)
  - Sacral plexus dorsal divisions (Paterson, 1887)
    - Superior gluteal nerve (Martin, 1781)
    - Inferior gluteal nerve (Martin, 1781)
    - Perforating cutaneous nerve (>1840)
    - Piriformis nerve (>1840)
  - Sacral plexus ventral divisions (Paterson, 1887)
    - Nerve to quadratus femoris (>1840)
      - Articular branch of nerve to quadratus femoris (>1840)
    - Nerve to obturator internus (>1840)
    - Pelvic splanchnic nerves (Gaskell, 1886)
    - Pudendal nerve (Camper, 1762)
      - Inferior rectal nerves (>1840)
      - Perineal nerve (Camper, 1762)
        - Posterior labial nerves (>1840)
        - Posterior scrotal nerves (Mayer, 1794)
        - Muscular branches of perineal nerve (>1840)
      - Dorsal nerve of clitoris (>1840)
      - Dorsal nerve of penis (Camper, 1762)
    - Perineal branch of fourth sacral nerve (>1840)
  - Sciatic nerve (Keill, 1698)
    - Nerve to hamstring muscles (>1840)
    - Common fibular nerve (>1840)
      - Nerve to short head of biceps femoris (>1840)
      - Articular branches of common fibular nerve (>1840)
      - Lateral cutaneous nerve of calf (>1840)
      - Sural communicating branch of common fibular nerve (>1840)

  - Superficial fibular nerve (Fyfe, 1800)
    - Muscular branches of superficial fibular nerve (>1840)
    - Medial dorsal cutaneous nerve (>1840)
      - Dorsal digital nerves of medial dorsal cutaneous nerve (>1840)
    - Intermediate dorsal cutaneous nerve (>1840)
      - Dorsal digital nerves of intermediate dorsal cutaneous nerve (>1840)
  - Deep fibular nerve (Fyfe, 1800)
    - Muscular branches of deep fibular nerve (>1840)
    - Articular branch of deep fibular nerve (>1840)
    - Digital branch of deep fibular nerve (>1840)
      - Dorsal digital nerves of deep fibular nerve (>1840)
- Tibial nerve (Haase, 1781)
  - Muscular branches of tibial nerve (>1840)
    - Nerve to plantaris (>1840)
    - Nerves to gastrocnemius (>1840)
    - Nerve to popliteus (>1840)
      - Nerve to tibialis posterior (Cruveilhier, 1836)
      - Interosseal nerve of leg (>1840)
      - Articular branch of nerve to popliteus (>1840)
      - Medullary branch of nerve to popliteus (>1840)
    - Nerve to soleus (>1840)
    - Nerve to flexor digitorum longus (>1840)
    - Nerve to flexor hallucis longus (>1840)
  - Articular branches of tibial nerve (>1840)
    - Articular branches of tibial nerve to knee joint (>1840)
    - Articular branch of tibial nerve to ankle joint (>1840)
  - Medial cutaneous nerve of calf (>1840)
    - Tibial root of sural nerve (>1840)
      - Sural nerve (Pietro da Cortona, 1741)
        - Lateral dorsal cutaneous nerve (>1840)
          - Dorsal digital nerves of lateral dorsal cutaneous nerve (>1840)
        - Lateral calcaneal branches of sural nerve (>1840)
  - Medial calcaneal nerve (>1840)
  - Medial plantar nerve (>1840)
    - Muscular branches of medial plantar nerve (>1840)
    - Common plantar digital nerves of medial plantar nerve (>1840)
      - Proper plantar digital nerves of medial plantar nerve (>1840)
  - Lateral plantar nerve (>1840)
    - Muscular branches of lateral plantar nerve (>1840)
    - Superficial branch of lateral plantar nerve (>1840)

.... Common plantar digital nerves of lateral plantar nerve (>1840)

.... Proper plantar digital nerves of lateral plantar nerve (>1840)

.... Deep branch of lateral plantar nerve (>1840)

.... Posterior cutaneous nerve of thigh (Günther, 1786)

.... Inferior clunial nerves (>1840)

.... Perineal branches of posterior cutaneous nerve of thigh (>1840)

.... Coccygeal plexus (>1840)

.... Anococcygeal nerves (>1840)

Appendix 9

Human PNS autonomic nerves (topographic gross anatomy groupings)

This hierarchical Nomenclature Table provides a set of ***standard terms*** for describing the ***autonomic nerves (Langley, 1898)***, which are ***white matter tracts (Bell & Bell, 1826)***, of the adult human ***peripheral nervous system (Meckel, 1814)*** (PNS) visible to the naked eye. A strictly topographic approach to grouping is adopted here (Figure 15, right side), using the broad topographic divisions shown in Figure 15 (left side). Another approach involves grouping based on function, for example, using the *autonomic nervous system (Langley, 1898)* concept; see Williams & Warwick (1980, pp. 1121–1132). The functional approach does not lend itself to straightforward topographic description. Naming and arrangement of the very complex ***autonomic nerves (Langley, 1898)*** has always been less satisfactory than for the relatively well understood ***craniospinal nerves (Herrick, 1915)***.

AUTONOMIC NERVES [HUMAN] (LANGLEY, 1898)

.....Communicating branches of spinal nerves (Wutzer, 1817)
..........White communicating branch (>1840)
..........Gray communicating branch (>1840)
.....Peripheral nerve cord trunk (Swanson & Bota, 2010)
..........Sympathetic trunk (Winslow, 1733)
....................Communicating branches of sympathetic trunk (>1840)
..............................Communicating branch of superior and middle cervical ganglia (Cruveilhier, 1836)
....................Ansa subclavia (Neubauer, 1772)
.....Paravertebral nerves (Swanson & Bota, 2010)
..........Internal carotid nerve (>1840)
..........Internal carotid plexus (>1840)
....................Caroticotympanic nerves (>1840)
..............................Superior caroticotympanic nerve (>1840)
..............................Inferior caroticotympanic nerve (>1840)
....................Deep petrosal nerve (Meckel, 1817)
....................Communicating branch from internal carotid plexus to abducens nerve (>1840)
....................Communicating branch from internal carotid plexus to ophthalmic nerve (>1840)
....................Communicating branch from internal carotid plexus to trochlear nerve (>1840)
....................Communicating branch from internal carotid plexus to oculomotor nerve (>1840)
....................Sympathetic root of ciliary ganglion (>1840)
....................Hypophysial plexus (>1840)
....................Middle cerebral artery plexus (>1840)
....................Anterior cerebral artery plexus (Chaussier, 1789)
....................Posterior cerebral artery plexus (Chaussier, 1789)
....................Ophthalmic plexus (>1840)
..........Common carotid plexus (Cloquet, 1816)
..........External carotid plexus (>1840)
....................Sympathetic root of submandibular ganglion (>1840)
....................Sympathetic root of otic ganglion (>1840)
..........Jugular nerves (>1840)
..........Laryngopharyngeal branches of superior cervical ganglion (>1840)
..........Superior cardiac nerve (Neubauer, 1772)
..........Thyroid branches of middle cervical ganglion (>1840)

....................Thyroid plexus (Portal, 1803)
..........Middle cardiac nerve (Cloquet, 1816)
..........Inferior cardiac nerve (Cloquet, 1816)
..........Subclavian plexus (>1840)
..........Vertebral nerve (Cruveilhier, 1836)
....................Vertebral plexus (Cloquet, 1816)
..........Thoracic cardiac nerves (>1840)
..........Thoracic pulmonary nerves (>1840)
....................Esophageal branches of sympathetic trunk (>1840)
..........Greater splanchnic nerve (Walter, 1783)
..........Lesser splanchnic nerve (Haller, 1762)
....................Renal branch of lesser splanchnic nerve (>1840)
..........Least splanchnic nerve (>1840)
..........Lumbar splanchnic nerves (Cruveilhier, 1836)
..........Sacral splanchnic nerves (>1840)
.....Prevertebral plexuses (Quain, 1832)
..........Thoracic aortic plexus (>1840)
..........Celiac plexus (Winslow, 1733)
....................Phrenic plexus (Loder, 1778)
....................Gastroduodenal plexus (>1840)
..............................Right gastroepiploic plexus (Wrisberg, 1800)
..............................Pancreaticoduodenal plexus (Wrisberg, 1800)
....................Left gastric plexus (>1840)
..........Superior mesenteric plexus (Rau, 1720)
....................Pancreatic branches of superior mesenteric plexus (>1840)
....................Jejunal & ileal plexuses (>1840)
....................Right colic plexus (>1840)
....................Middle colic plexus (>1840)
..........Intermesenteric plexus (>1840)
..........Inferior mesenteric plexus (Rau, 1720)
....................Left colic plexus (>1840)
....................Superior rectal plexus (>1840)
..........Superior hypogastric plexus (Tiedemann, 1822)
....................Iliac plexus (>1840)
..........Hypogastric nerve (Walter, 1783)
..........Inferior hypogastric plexus (Tiedemann, 1822)
....................Middle rectal plexus (>1840)
....................Extrinsic vesical plexus (>1840)
..............................Deferential plexus (Cruveilhier, 1840)
....................Urethral branches of inferior hypogastric plexus (>1840)
....................Prostatic plexus (>1840)
....................Uterovaginal plexus (>1840)
.....Prevertebral nerves (Swanson & Bota, 2010)
..........Renal nerves (Haase, 1781)
..........Superior ureteric nerves (Walter, 1783)
..........Middle ureteric nerves (>1840)
..........Inferior ureteric nerves (>1840)
..........Superior testicular nerves (>1840)
..........Superior ovarian nerves (>1840)
..........Middle testicular nerves (>1840)
..........Middle ovarian nerves (>1840)
..........Inferior testicular nerves (>1840)
..........Inferior ovarian nerves (>1840)
....................Tubo-uterine plexus (>1840)
....................Tubo-uterine nerve (>1840)
..........Seminal vesicle nerves (Bock, 1827)
..........Cavernous nerves of penis (>1840)

.... Vaginal nerves (Walter, 1783)
.... Cavernous nerves of clitoris (>1840)
..... Terminal plexuses (Swanson & Bota, 2010)
.... Pharyngeal plexus (Neubauer, 1772)
.... Pulmonary plexus (Winslow, 1733)
.... Anterior pulmonary plexus (Haller, 1762)
.... Posterior pulmonary plexus (Haller, 1762)
.... Cardiac plexus (Keill, 1698)
.... Preaortic plexus (Arnulf, 1939)
.... Coronary plexuses (Meckel, 1817)
.... Right coronary plexus (Scarpa, 1794)
.... Left coronary plexus (Scarpa, 1794)
.... Atrial plexuses (>1840)
.... Intrinsic cardiac plexus (>1840)
.... Hepatic plexus (Rau, 1720)
.... Cystic plexus (Wrisberg, 1808)
.... Hepatic plexus branches to bile ducts (>1840)
.... Right gastric plexus (>1840)
.... Splenic plexus (Palfijn, 1726)
.... Left gastroepiploic plexus (Wrisberg, 1800)
.... Pancreatic plexus (Cruveilhier, 1836)
.... Adrenal plexus (>1840)
.... Renal plexus (Drake, 1707)
.... Intrinsic renal nerves (>1840)
.... Intrinsic vesical plexus (>1840)
.... Ureteric plexus (>1840)
.... Ovarian plexus (Cruveilhier, 1836)
.... Testicular plexus (Cruveilhier, 1836)
.... Enteric plexuses (Hill, 1927)
..... Terminal autonomic nerves (Swanson & Bota, 2010)
.... Short ciliary nerves (>1840)
.... Communicating branch of otic ganglion with auriculotemporal nerve (>1840)
.... Glandular branches of submandibular ganglion (>1840)

Appendix 10

Human nervous system supporting structures (ventricular-subarachnoid space, meninges, and choroid plexus)

This hierarchical Nomenclature Table provides a set of ***standard terms*** for describing the ***supporting structures (Swanson & Bota, 2010)*** of the macrodissected adult human ***central nervous system (Carus, 1814)***. The scheme is based on topographic architecture (see Figure 15, left side). The overall scheme can be adapted for all vertebrates.

NERVOUS SYSTEM [HUMAN] (MONRO, 1783)

.....Nervous system topographic architecture (Swanson & Bota, 2010)
..........Nervous system supporting structures (Swanson & Bota, 2010)
...............Ventricular-subarachnoid space (Swanson & Bota, 2010)
....................Cerebrospinal fluid (Magendie, 1827)
....................Subarachnoid space (Magendie, 1827)
.........................Septal fissure (Burdach, 1822)
....................Ventricles (Hippocrates)
.........................Ependyma (>1840)
.........................Subependymal zone (>1840)
.........................Lateral ventricle (Vesalius, 1543a)
..............................Anterior horn of lateral ventricle (Bell, 1803b)
...................................Olfactory ventricle (>1840)
..............................Body of lateral ventricle (Bell, 1803b)
...................................Lamina affixa (>1840)
..............................Atrium of lateral ventricle (>1840)
...................................Collateral triangle (>1840)
..............................Posterior horn of lateral ventricle (Haller, 1747)
...................................Calcarine spur (Morand, 1748)
...................................Bulb of posterior horn (>1840)
..............................Inferior horn of lateral ventricle (Bell, 1802)
...................................Collateral eminence (Meckel, 1767)
..............................Choroid epithelium of lateral ventricle (>1840)
..............................Choroid line of lateral ventricle (>1840)
..............................Fimbrial line of lateral ventricle (>1840)
.........................Interventricular foramen (>1840)
.........................Third ventricle (>1840)
..............................Hypothalamic part of third ventricle (Swanson, 2004)
...................................Preoptic recess (>1840)
...................................Infundibular recess (>1840)
...................................Mammillary recess (>1840)
..............................Hypothalamic sulcus (>1840)
..............................Thalamic part of third ventricle (Swanson, 2004)
...................................Interthalamic adhesion (>1840)
...................................Roof of third ventricle (>1840)
....Choroid epithelium of third ventricle (>1840)
....Suprapineal recess (>1840)
....Choroid line of third ventricle (>1840)
....Pineal recess (>1840)
.........................Opening of cerebral aqueduct (>1840)

................Cerebral aqueduct (>1840)
................Opening of fourth ventricle (>1840)
................Fourth ventricle (Galen, c192)
....................Floor of fourth ventricle (Reil, 1807–1808a)
........................Median sulcus of fourth ventricle (>1840)
........................Medial eminence (>1840)
........................Facial colliculus (>1840)
........................Rostral fovea (>1840)
........................Vestibular area of fourth ventricle (>1840)
........................Auditory tubercle (>1840)
........................Caudal fovea (>1840)
........................Hypoglossal triangle (>1840)
........................Vagal triangle (>1840)
........................Funiculus separans (>1840)
........................Area postrema (1840)
........................Obex (Burdach, 1822)
........................Limiting sulcus of fourth ventricle (>1840)
....................Roof of fourth ventricle (Vesalius, 1543a)
........................Rostral medullary velum (>1840)
............................Frenulum (Vieussens, 1684)
........................Fastigium of fourth ventricle (Burdach, 1822)
........................Choroid epithelium of fourth ventricle (>1840)
........................Choroid line of fourth ventricle (>1840)
........................Lateral recess of fourth ventricle (>1840)
............................Lateral aperture of fourth ventricle (>1840)
........................Median aperture of fourth ventricle (>1840)
........................Caudal medullary velum (>1840)
................Central canal (Bellingeri, 1823)
....................Central canal of medulla (>1840)
....................Central canal of spinal cord (>1840)
........................Terminal ventricle (>1840)
........Meninges (Smith Papyrus, c1700 BC)
............Pia-arachnoid (>1840)
................Pia (Galen, c192)
....................Choroid membrane of lateral ventricle (>1840)
....................Choroid membrane of third ventricle (>1840)
....................Choroid membrane of fourth ventricle (>1840)
....................Denticulate ligament (Monro, 1783)
................Arachnoid (Blasius, 1666)
....................Epipial layer (Key & Retzius, 1875–1876)
....................Arachnoid trabeculae (>1840)
....................Arachnoid membrane (Meckel, 1817)
....................Arachnoid granulations (>1840)
............Dura (Galen, c177)
................Cerebral falx (Vesalius, 1543a)
................Sellar diaphragm (>1840)
................Cerebellar falx (Günther, 1786)
................Cerebellar tentorium (Winslow, 1733)
....................Tentorial notch (>1840)
........Choroid plexus (Galen, c177)
............Choroid plexus of lateral ventricle (Vicq d'Azyr, 1784)
................Choroid enlargement (>1840)
............Choroid plexus of third ventricle (Vicq d'Azyr, 1784)
............Choroid plexus of fourth ventricle (Vieussens, 1684)

Bibliography

Achillini, A. (1520) *Annotationes Anatomicae* (Benedictis, Bologna).

Ackermann, J.F. (1813) *De Nervei Systematis Primordiis Commintatio* (Schwan et Goetz; Mannheim, Heidelberg).

Adams, F. (1972), *see* Hippocrates, *On the Sacred Disease*.

Adelmann, H.B. (1966) *Marcello Malpighi and the Evolution of Embryology* (Cornell University Press, Ithaca NY).

Al, J., Epstein, P.N., Gozal, D., Yang, B., Wurster, R., & Cheng, Z.J. (2007) Morphology and topography of nucleus ambiguus projections to cardiac ganglia in rats and mice. *Neuroscience* **149**:845–860.

Albertus Magnus (13th century) *On Animals: A Medieval Summa Zoologica / Albertus Magnus*; translated and annotated by K.F. Kitchell, Jr. & I. M. Resnick (Johns Hopkins University Press, Baltimore), 1999.

Albertus Magnus (1490) *Philosophia Pauperum* (Farfengus, Brescia).

Albinus, B.S. (1744) *Explicatio Tabularum Anatomicarum Bartholomaei Eustachii* (Verbeek, Leiden).

Albinus, B.S. (1761) *Explicatio Tabularum Anatomicarum Bartholomaei Eustachii, Anatomici Summi. Auctor Recognovit, Castigavit, Auxit, Denuo Edidit* (Verbeek, Leiden).

Albinus, B.S. (1768) *Academicarum Annotationum*, Liber 8 (Verbeek, Leiden).

Allen, G.V. & Hopkins, D.A. (1990) Topography and synaptology of mamillary body projections to the mesencephalon and pons in the rat. *Journal of Comparative Neurology* **301**:214–231.

Allen, J.P. (2005) *The Art of Medicine in Ancient Egypt* (The Metropolitan Museum of Art, New York).

Alvarez-Bolado, G. & Swanson, L.W. (1996) *Developmental Brain Maps: Structure of the Embryonic Rat Brain* (Elsevier, Amsterdam).

Anatomia Magistri Nicolai physici (early 12th century), *see* Corner (1927).

Andersch, K.S. (1797) *Tractatio Anatomico-Physiologica de Nervis Humani Corporis Aliquibus, quam Edidit Ernst. Philipp. Andersch. Pars Prior [-Pars Altera]*, 2 Vols. (Fasch, Königsberg). Ernst Phillip Andersch found and published his uncle's thesis printed c1751–c1755 but it was not distributed and was then lost until the unusual translation in Andersch, K.S. & Soemmerrig, S.T. (1792).

Andersch, K.S. & Soemmerrig, S.T. (1792) *Anderschii Fragmentum Descriptionis Nervorum Cardiacorum (Vel Potius Arteriarum Prope Cor) Dextri Lateris iam ante Aliquot Decinnia Typis Impressum, Nunc Demum a. MDCCXCI Subjuncta Autoris Tabula Notulisque Adiectis Editum a S. Th. Soemmerring*. In: Ludwig, C.F. (1791–1795), Vol. 2, pp. 113–203. Soemmerring edited fragments of Andersch's "lost" thesis, printed c1751–c1755 but never circulated; *see* Haller (1772), Andersch (1797).

Anderson, J. (1837) *Sketch of the Comparative Anatomy of the Nervous System; with Remarks on its Development in the Human Embryo. To which is Added, an Arranged Descriptive list of the Series of Illustrative Preparations and Drawings, and an Anatomical Table of the Analogies Existing between the Brain of the Human Foetus and that of the Lower Animals* (Sherwood, Gilbert, & Piper; London).

Angevine, J.B. Jr., Mancall, E.L., & Yakovlev, P.I. (1961) *The Human Cerebellum: An Atlas of Gross Topography in Serial Sections* (Little, Brown; Boston).

Aranzi, G.C. (1587) *De Humano Foetu Liber Tertio Editus, ac Recognitus. Ejusdem Anatomicarum Observationum Liber ac De Tumoribus Secundum Locos Affectos Liber nunc Primum Editi* (Brechtanum, Venice).

Aranzi, G.C. (1595) *De Humano Foetu Liber Tertio Editus, ac Recognitus. Ejusdem Anatomicarum Observationum Liber ac De Tumoribus Secundum Locos Affectos Liber nunc Primum Editi* (Carampellum, Venice).

Ariëns Kappers, C.U., Huber, G.C., & Crosby, E.C. (1936) *The Comparative Anatomy of the Nervous System of Vertebrates, Including Man*, 2 Vols. (Macmillan, New York).

Aristotle, *Historia Animalium*. In: *The Works of Aristotle*, Translated into English under the Editorship of Sir David Ross, Volume IV, Translated by D'Arcy Wentworth Thompson (Oxford University Press, London) 1962 (reprint of original 1910 edition).

Aristotle, *De Partibus Animalium*. In: *The Works of Aristotle*, Translated into English under the Editorship of Sir David Ross, Volume V, Translated by William Ogle (Oxford University Press, London) 1958 (reprint of original 1912 edition).

Aristotle, *De Generatione Animalium*. In: *The Works of Aristotle*, Translated into English under the Editorship of Sir David Ross, Volume V, Translated by Arthur Platt (Oxford University Press, London) 1958 (reprint of original 1912 edition).

Arnold, F. (1826a) *Sistens Observationes Nonnullas Neurologicas de Parte Cephalica Nervi Sympathici in Homine* (Osswald, Heidelberg).

Arnold, F. (1826b) Beschreibung des Kipftheils des sympathischen Nerven beim Kalb, nebst einigen Beobachtungen über diesen Theil beim Menschen. *Zeitschrift für Physiologie* **2**:125–172.

Arnold, F. (1828) *Ueber den Ohrknoten; eine Anatomisch-Physiologische Abhandlung* (Winger, Heidelberg).

Arnold, F. (1834) *Icones Nervorum Capitis* (Sumtibus Auctoris, Heidelberg).

Arnold, F. (1835) Bemerkungen über einige Entdickungen und Ansichten in der Anatomie und Physiologie. *Zeitschrift für Physiologie* **5**:175–189.

Arnold, F. (1838a) *Untersuchungen im Gebiete der Anatomie und Physiologie mit besonderer Hinsicht auf seine Anatomischen Tafeln. 1. Bändchen. Bemerkungen über den Bau des Hirns und Rückenmarks* (Höhr, Zürich).

Arnold, F. (1838b) *Tabulae Anatomicae. Fasc. i. Icones Cerebri et Medullae Spinalis* (Turici, Orelli, Fuesslin; Zürich).

Arnold, F. (1839) *Tabulae Anatomicae. Fasc. ii. Icones Organorum Sensuum* (Turici, Orelli, Fuesslin; Zürich).

Arnulf, G. (1939) De la section du plexus préaortic: justification et technique. *Presse Médicale* **47**:1635–1638.

Arsaky, A. (1813) *De Piscium Cerebro et Medulla Spinali* (Hendelianis, Halle).

Asch, G.T. (1750) *Dissertatio Inauguralis de Primo Pare Nervorum Medullae Spinalis, quam Auctoritate Gratiosae Facultatis Medicae in Academia in Academia Georgia Augusta pro gradu Doctoris d. XIX Augusti MDCCL. Publice Defendet Georgius Thomas Asch Petropolitanus* (In Officina Vandenhoekiana, Göttingen).

Baer, K.E. von (1828) *Über Entwickelungsgeschichte der Thiere. Beobachtung und Reflexion.* Part 1 (Bornträger, Königsberg).

Baer, K.E. von (1837) *Über Entwickelungsgeschichte der Thiere. Beobachtung und Reflexion.* Part 2 (Bornträger, Königsberg).

Bailey, P. & von Bonin, G. (1951) *The Isocortex of Man* (University of Illinois Press, Urbana).

Baillarger, J.G.F. (1840) Researches sur la structure de la couche corticale des circonvolutions du cerveau. *Mémoires de l'Academie Royale de Medicine* **8**:149–183.

Baker, F. (1909) The two Sylviuses. An historical study. *Bulletin of the Johns Hopkins Hospital* **20**:329–339.

Bang, J. (1770) *Nervorum Cervicalium Anatome* (Möllerus, Copenhagen). Reprinted in Ludwig, C.F. (1791–1795), Vol. 1, pp. 343–348, 1791, with Tab. XI.

Bannister, J. (1578) *The Historie of Man* (Daye, London). Facsimile published by De Capo Press, New York, 1969.

Barker, L.F. (1899) *The Nervous System and its Constituent Parts. Designed for the Use of Practitioners of Medicine and of Students of Medicine and Psychology* (Appleton, New York).

Bartels, E.D.A. (1813) *Die Respiration als vom Gehirn Abhaengige Bewegung und als Chemischer Process nebst ihren Physiologischen und Pathologischen Abweichungen Untersucht* (Korn, Breslau).

Bartholin, C. (1611) *Casp. Bartholini Philosophi & Medici Anatomicae Institutiones Corporis Humani Utriusque Sexus Historiam & Declarationem Exhibentes cum Plurimis Novis Observationibus & Opinionibus nec non Illustriorum quae in Anthropologia Occurrunt, Controversiarum Decisionibus; Cum Indice Capitum & Rerum Locupletissimo* (Raabe, Wittenberg).

Bartholin, C. (1632) *Casp. Bartholini d. Phil. Medici &Theologi ac Profess. Regii, Institutiones Anatomicae, Corporis Humani Utriusque Sexus, Historiam & Declarationem Exhibentes; Cum Plurimis Novis Observationibus Opinionibus & Controversiarum Occurrentium Decisionibus Adjecto Indice Capitum & Rerum Locupletissimo* (Goslariae, no place indicated).

Bartholin, T. (1641) *Casp. Bartholini D. & Profes. Regii Institutiones Anatomicae: Novis Recentiorum Opinionibus & Observationibus, quarum Innumerae Nactenus Editae Non Sunt, Figurisque Auctae ab Auctoris Filio Thoma Bartholino Movendo* (Hack, Leiden).

Bartholin, T. (1651) *Thomae Bartholini Casp. F. Anatomia: Ex Caspari Bartholini Parentis Institutionibus, Omniumque Recentiorum & Propriis Observationibus: Tertiùm ad Sanguinis Circulationem Reformata cum Iconibus Novis Accuratissimis* (Hack, Leiden), *see* English translation, Bartholin, T. (1662).

Bartholin, T. (1654) *Thomae Bartholini Historiarum Anatomicarum: Rariorum Centuria I et II* (Henrici, Amsterdam).

Bartholin, T. (1655) *Thomae Bartholini Casp. F. Anatomia: Ex Caspari Bartholini Parentis Institutionibus, Omniumque Recentiorum & Propriis Observationibus: Tertiùm ad Sanguinis Circulationem Reformata: Cum Iconibus Novis Accuratissimis: Accessit Nuic Postremae Editioni Th. Bartholini Appendix de Lacteis Thoracicis & Vasis Lymphaticis* (Vlacq, Hague).

Bartholin, T. (1662) *Bartholinus Anatomy; Made from the Precepts of his Father, and from the Observations of All Modern Anatomists; Together with his Own: With One Hundred Fifty and Three Figures Cut in Brass, Much Larger and Better than Any Have Been Heretofore Printed in English: in Four Books and Four Manuals, Answering to the Said Books; Also Two Epistles of the Circulation of the Blood. Published by Nich. Culpeper Gent. and Abdiah Cole* (Cole, London). A more common edition with same pagination published in 1668 (Streater, London); both were from the Latin original, Bartholin, T. (1651).

Bartholin, T. (1673) *Thomae Bartholini Anatome ex Omnium Veterum Recentiorumque Observationibus Imprimis Institutionibus B. M. Parentis Caspari Batholini, ad Circulationem Harveianum, et Vasa Lymphatica Quartum Novata. Cum Inconibus Novis, & Indicibus* (Hackiana, Leiden).

Bartholin, T. (1686) *Thomae Bartholini Anatome ex Omnium Veterum Recentiorumque Observationibus Imprimis Institutionibus B. M. Parentis Caspari Batholini, ad Circulationem Harveianum, et Vasa Lymphatica Quartum Novata. Cum Inconibus Novis, & Indicibus* (Hackium, Leiden).

Bartisch, G. (1583) *Ophthalmodouleia, das ist, Augendienst. Newer und Wolgegründter Bericht von Ursachen und Erkentnüs aller Gebrechen, Schäden und Mängel der Augen und des Gesichtes, wie Mon Solchen Anfenglich mit Gebürlichen Mitteln Begegenen, Vorkommen und Wehren, auch wie Man Alle Solche Gebresten Künstlich durch Artzney, Instrument und Handgrieffe Curiren, Wircken und Vertreiben Sol; mit Schönen Herrlichen Contrafectischen Figuren der Anatomiae beyde des Heubtes und der Augen, so wol Derselbigen Vornembsten Schäden und Gebrechen, Desgleichen Aller Instrument und Gefesse, so zu Solcher Augen Cur Gehörig und Dienstlich; Desgleichen von Künstlichen Praeparationen, Purgationen, Calcinationen, Distillationen Vieler Gebreuchlicher Materialium, zur Augenartzney Nötig und Nützlich; Sambt einem Kurtzen Auszuge Etlicher Zeugnüssen derer Personen, welchen durch Gottes Hülfe und Solche Mittel an Augen und Gesicht Schäden Geholffen Worden; Allken Benötigen Ertzten,*

Trewhertzigen Hausvätern, und Sonderlichen denen Menschen, die mit Gebrechen, Schäden und Mängeln der Augen und des Geschtes behafft und Beladen sein, oder sich Dessen zu Besorgen und zu Befahren haben, zu Trost, Nutz und Gute Gestellet und Beschrieben (Stöckel, Dresden).

Basel Nomina Anatomica (1895), *see* His, W. (1895). Also spelled *Basle Nomina Anatomica.*

Bauhin, C. (1605) *Caspari Bauhini Basileenis Theatrum Anatomicum; Novis Figuris Aeneis Illustratum et in Lucem Emissum Opera & Sumptibus Theodori de Brÿ P. M. Relictae Viduae & Filiorum Joannis Theodori & Joannis Israelis de Brÿ* (Beckeri, Frankfurt).

Bauhin, C. (1616) *Caspari Bauhini Institutiones Anatomicae: Hippoc. Aristot. Galeni Auctorita. Illustratae*, 5th Edn. (Jacobi, Frankfurt).

Bauhin, C. (1620) *Vivae Imagines Partium Corporis Humani Aeneis Formis Expressae*, et ex Theatro Anatomico C. Bauhini Desumptae (de Bry, Frankfurt).

Beccari, N. (1911) La sostanza perforata anteriore e i suoi rapporti col rinencefalo nel cervello dell'uomo. *Archivio Italiano de Anatomia e di Embriologia* **10**:261–328.

Bechterew, W. (1885a) Über eine bischer unbekannte Verbindung der grossen Oliven mit dem Grosshirn. *Neurologisches Centralblatt* **4**:194–196.

Bechterew, W. (1885b) Über die Schleifenschicht. *Neurologisches Centralblatt* **4**:356–359.

Bechterew, W. (1889) *Die Leitungsbahnen im Gehirn und Rückenmark* (Georgi, Leipzig).

Beck, B. (1846) *Anatomisch-Physiologische Abhandlung über einige in Knochen Verlaufenden und an der Markhaut derselben sich Verzweigenden Nerven* (Herder, Freiburg im Breisgau).

Beevor, C.E. (1891) On the course of the fibres of the cingulum and the posterior parts of the corpus callosum and fornix in the marmoset monkey. *Proceedings of the Royal Society of London; Philosophical Transactions of the Royal Society of London, Series B* **182**:135–199.

Behrends, J.B.J. (1792) *Dissertatio Inauguralis Anatomico-Physiologica qua Demonstratur Cor Nervis Carere Addita Disquisitione de Vi Nervorum Arterias Cingentium*, Moguntia (Crass, Mainz). Reprinted in Ludwig, C.F. (1791–1795) Vol. 3, pp. 1–23, 1793.

Bell, C. (1802) *The Anatomy of the Brain, Explained in a Series of Engravings* (Longman & Rees, London). Facsimile, *Engravings of the Brain and Nerves*, published by The Classics of Medicine Library, Birmingham, 1982.

Bell, C. (1803a) *A Series of Engravings Explaining the Course of the Nerves* (Longman and Rees, and Cadell and Davies; London). Facsimile, *Engravings of the Brain and Nerves*, published by The Classics of Medicine Library, Birmingham, 1982.

Bell, C. (1803b) *The Anatomy of the Human Body, Vol. 3. Containing the Nervous System, with Plates* (Longman and Rees, and Cadell and Davies; London).

Bell, C. (1821) On the nerves; giving an account of some experiments on their structure and functions, which lead to new arrangements of the system. *Philosophical Transactions of the Royal Society of London* **111**:398–424.

Bell, C. (1822) On the nerves which associate the muscles of the chest, in the actions of breathing, speaking, and expression. Being a continuation of the paper on the structure and functions of the nerves. *Philosophical Transactions of the Royal Society of London* **112**: 284-312.

Bell, C. (1823) Second part of the paper on the nerves of the orbit. *Philosophical Transactions of the Royal Society of London* **113**:289–307.

Bell, C. (1826) On the nervous circle which connects the voluntary muscles with the brain. *Philosophical Transactions of the Royal Society of London* **116**:163–173.

Bell, C. (1829) On the nerves of the face; being a second paper on that subject. *Philosophical Transactions of the Royal Society of London* **119**:317–330.

Bell, C. (1834) On the functions of some parts of the brain, and on the relations between the brain and nerves of motion and sensation. *Philosophical Transactions of the Royal Society of London* **124**:471–483.

Bell, C. (1835) Continuation of the paper on the relations between the nerves of motion and of sensation, and the brain; more particularly on the structure of the medulla oblongata and the spinal marrow. *Philosophical Transactions of the Royal Society of London* **125**:255–262.

Bell, J. & Bell, C. (1816) *The Anatomy and Physiology of the Human Body*, 4th Edn., 3 Vols., *see* Vol. 2 for nervous system (Longmans et al., London).

Bell, J. & Bell, C. (1823) *The Anatomy and Physiology of the Human Body*, 5th Edn., 3 Vols., *see* Vol. 2 for nervous system (Longmans et al., London).

Bell, J. & Bell, C. (1826) *The Anatomy and Physiology of the Human Body*, 6th Edn., 3 Vols., *see* Vol. 2 for nervous system (Longmans et al., London).

Bell, J. & Bell, C. (1829) *The Anatomy and Physiology of the Human Body*, 7th Edn., 3 Vols., *see* Vol. 2 for nervous system (Longmans et al., London).

Bellingeri, C.F. (1818) *Dissertatio Inauguralis quam Publice Defendebat in Regio Athenaeo Anno MDCCCXVIII die IX Maji Hora IX Matutina. Data Cuique Post Sextum Argumentandi Facultate* (Favale, Turin).

Bellingeri, C.F. (1823) *De Medulla Spinali Nervisque ex ea Prodeuntibus Annotationes Anatomico-Physiologiae* (Typographia Regia, Turin).

Belon, P. (1551) *L'Histoire Naturelle des Estranges Poissons Marins* (Chaudiere, Paris).

Bendz, H.C.B. (1833) *Dissertatio de Anastomosi Jacobsonii et Ganglio Arnoldi* (ex officina typographica Quistii, Copenhagen).

Benedetti, A. (1502) *Historia Corporis Humani; Sive Anatomice* (Guerraldo, Venice).

Benedetti, A. (1539) *Omnium a Vertice ad Calcem Morborum Signa, Causae, Indicationes & Remediorum Compositiones Utendique Rationes, Generatim Libris XXX Conscripta. Praeterea, Aphorismorum Lib. I. De Pestilentiae Causis, Praeservationione, & Auxiliorum Materia Lib. I. Humani Corporis Anatome, Tractata Lib. V* (Petrum, Basel).

Benedetti, A. (1998) *Historia Corporis Humani, Sive Anatomice / Alessandro Benedetti.* Introduzione, traduzione e cura di Giovanni Ferrari (Giunti, Florence).

Bennett, M.R. & Hacker, P.M.S. (2002) The motor system in neuroscience: a history and analysis of conceptual developments. *Progress in Neurobiology* **67**:1–52.

Berengario da Carpi, J. (1521) *Commentaria cum Amplissimis Additionibus super Anatomia Mundini una cum Textu ejusdem in Pristinum et Verum Nitorem Redacto* (Benedictis, Bologna).

Berengario da Carpi, J. (1522) *A Short Introduction to Anatomy (Isagogae Breves)*, Translated with an Introduction and Historical Notes by L.R. Lind (The University of Chicago Press, Chicago) 1959.

Berengario da Carpi, J. (1523) *Isagogae Breves Perlucide ac Uberrimae in Anatomiam Humani Corporis*, 2nd Edn. (Benedictus Hectoris, Bologna).

Bergen, C.A. von (1731) *Dissertatio Inauguralis Anatomico-Medica De Nervo Intercostali, Quam Publico Eruditorum Examini Subjicit Carolum Augustus à Bergen* (Schwartii, Frankfurt an der Oder).

Bergen, C.A. von (1734) *De Ventriculis Cerebri Lateralibus* (no publisher indicated, Frankfurt an der Oder).

Bergmann, G.H. (1831) *Neue Untersuchungen über die Innere Organisation des Gehirns; als Beiträge zu einer Grundlage der Physiologie und Pathologie Desselben* (Helwing'schen Hof-Buchhandlung, Hannover).

Berman, A.L. (1968) *The Brain Stem of the Cat: A Cytoarchitectonic Atlas with Stereotaxic Coordinates* (University of Wisconsin Press, Madison).

Berrettini, P., *see* Pietro da Cortona (1741) *Tabulae Anatomicae.*

Best, A.E. (1969) Pourfour du Petit's experiments on the origin of the sympathetic nerve. *Medical History* **13**:154-174.

Bichat, X. (1801) *Anatomie Général, Appliquée à la Physiologie et à la Médecine*, 4 Vols. (Brosson, Paris). There was an English translation, Bichat, X. (1822) *General Anatomy, Applied to Physiology and Medicine*, translated by George Hayward (Richarson and Lord, Boston).

Bichat, X. (1802) *Traité d'Anatomie Descriptive*, Vol. 3 (Gabon, Paris).

Bichat, X. (1822), *see* Bichat, X. (1801).

Bichat, X., Buisson, M.F.R., & Roux, P.J. (1801–1803) *Traité d'Anatomie Descriptive*, 5 Vols. (Gabon, Paris). Vols. 1–3 completed by Bichat before he died in 1802.

Bidloo, G. (1685) *Godefridi Bidloo Medicinae Doctoris & Chirurgi, Anatomia Humani Corporis; Centum & Quinque Tabulis* (Someren, with Dyk, and the heirs to Boom; Leiden).

Bischoff, L.W.T. (1832) *Nervi Accessorii Willisii Anatomia et Physiologia* (Leske, Darmstadt).

Blackstad, T. (1956) Commissural connections of the hippocampal region in the rat, with special reference to their mode of termination. *Journal of Comparative Neurology* **105**:417–537.

Blainville, H.-M.D. (1821) Considérations générales sur le système nerveux. *Journal de Physique, de Chimie et d'Histoire Naturelle et des Arts* **93**:200–222.

Blancard, S. (1702) *The Physical Dictionary wherein The Terms of Anatomy, the Names and Causes of Diseases, Chyrurgical Instruments, and their Use are Accurately Describ'd. Also the Names and Virtues of Medicinal Plants, Minerals, Stones, Gums, Salts, Earths, Etc. And the Method of Choosing the Best Drugs; the Terms of Chemistry, and of the Apothecaries Art; and the Various Forms of Medicines, and the Ways of Compounding Them* (Crouch and Sprint, London).

Blanchard, D.L. (1996) Translation of Bartisch, G. (1583) *Ophthalmodouleia* (Wayenborogh, Ostend).

Blasius, G.L. (1666) *Gerardi Blasii Med. Doct. & Prof. Ord. Anatome Medullae Spinalis, et Nervorum Inde Provenientium* (Commelinum, Amsterdam).

Blasius, G.L. (1674) *Gerardi Blasii ab Oost-Vliet, Med. Doct & Prof. Amsteod. Observata Anatomica in Homine, Simia, Equo, Vitulo, Ove, Testudine, Echine, Glire, Serpente, Ardea, Variisque Anamalibus Aliis. Accedunt Extraordinaria in Homine Reperta Praxin Medicam Aeque ac Anatomen Illustratia* (Gaasbeeck, Leiden & Amsterdam).

Bochenek, A. (1908) Ueber die zentrale Endigung des Nervus opticus. *Bulletin International de l'Académie des Sciences de Cracovie, Classe des Sciences Mathématiques et Naturelles* [no volume number], pp. 91–96.

Bock, A.C. (1817) *Beschreibund des Fünften Nervenpaares und seiner Verbindungen mit Andern Nerven, Vorzüglich mit den Gangliensysteme* (Goedsche, Meissen).

Bock, A.C. (1820) *Die Allgemeine Anatomie und die Beschreibung des Kopfes Enthaltend* (Goedsche, Meissen). Vol. 1 of *Handbuch der Practischen Anatomie* in 2 Vols. (Goedsche, Meissen).

Bock, A.C. (1824) *Darstellung des Gehirnes, des Rückenmarkes und der Sinneswerkzeuge so wie auch des Menschlichens Körpers über haupt, Allgemeine Encyklopädie der Anatomie*, Vol. 8, Part 1 (Baumgärtner, Leipzig).

Bock, A.C. (1827) *Die Rückenmarksnerven nach ihrem Ganzen Verlaufe, Vertheilungen und Verbindungen* (Baumgärtner, Leipzig).

Boehmer, J.F.W. (1777) *De Nono Pare Nervorum Cerebri. Dissertatio Inauguralis* (Dieterich, Göttingen).

Bojanus, L.H. (1819–1821) *Anatome Testudinis Europaeae. Accedunt Tabulae XXXI. Quarum IX. Duplici Exemplo* (Impensis Auctoris, Typis Zawadzki; Vilnius/Wilno).

Bolk, L. (1906) *Das Cerebellum der Säugetiere* (Bohn, Haarlem; Fischer, Jena).

Bonhomme, J.P. (1748) *Traité de la Cephalatomie, ou Description Anatomique. Des Parties que la Tête Renferme. Ouvrage Enrichi de Figures en Taille Douee, Dessinées & Gravées d'apré Nature* (Girard, Avignon).

Bota, M., Dong, H.-W., & Swanson, L.W. (2003) From gene networks to brain networks. *Nature Neuroscience* **6**:795–799.

Bota, M. & Swanson, L.W. (2007) The neuron classification problem. *Brain Research Reviews* **56**:79–88.

Bota, M. & Swanson, L.W. (2010) Collating and curating neuroanatomical nomenclatures: principles and use of the Brain Architecture Knowledge Management System (BAMS). *Frontiers in Neuroinformatics* **4**(3):1–16.

Bourdon, A. (1683) *Nouvelles Description Anatomique de Toutes les Parties du Corps Humain, et de Leurs Usages, avec le Cours de Toutes les Humeurs; sur le Principe de la Circulation, et Conformént aux Nouvelles Découvertes; le Tout Representé au Naturel sur Plusieurs Grandes Tables, Reduit en un Tres-bel Ordre, Expliqué in peu de Mots, et d'une Maniere tres Intelligible* (Houry, Paris). An Atlas volume was published in 1678.

Bowden, D.M. & Dubach, M.F. (2002) Neuronames 2002. *Neuroinformatics* **1**:43–59.

Boyd, J.D. (1937) Observations on the human carotid sinus and its nerve supply. *Anatomischer Anzeiger* **84**:386–399.

Breasted, J.H. (1930) *The Edwin Smith Surgical Papyrus* (University of Chicago Press, Chicago).

Briggs, W. (1685) *Ophthalmo-graphia, Sive Oculi Ejusque Partium Descriptio Anatomica* (Simpson, London).

Brittain, D.B. (1988) The Efferent Connections of the Infralimbic Area in the Rat. Ph.D. Dissertation. University of California, San Diego.

Broca, P. (1876) Note sur la topographie cérébrale et sur quelques points de l'histoire des circonvolutions. *Bulletin de l'Académie de Médecine* **5**:824–834.

Broca, P. (1878a) Nomenclature cérébrale: dénomination et subdivision des hémisphères et des anfractuosités de la surface. *Revue d'Anthropologie* **1**:193–236.

Broca, P. (1878b) Anatomie comparée des circonvolutions cérébrales. Le grand lobe limbique et la scissure limbique dans la série des mammifères. *Revue d'Anthropologie* **1**:385–498.

Broca, P. (1879) Localisations cérébrales: recherches sur les centres olfactifs. *Revue d'Anthropologie* **2**:385–455.

Brodal, A. (1948) *Neurological Anatomy: In Relation to Clinical Medicine* (Oxford University Press, London).

Brodal, A. (1957a) *The Cranial Nerves: Anatomy and Anatomico-Clinical Correlations*, 2nd Edn. (Blackwell, Oxford).

Brodal, A. (1957b) *The Reticular Formation of the Brain Stem. Anatomical Aspects and Functional Correlations* (Oliver and Boyd, Edinburgh).

Brodal, P. (1992) *The Central Nervous System: Structure and Function* (Oxford University Press, New York).

Brödel, M. (1946) *Three Unpublished Drawings of The Anatomy of the Human Ear* (Saunders, Philadelphia).

Brodmann, K. (1906) Fünfte mitteilung: Ueber den allgemeinen bauplan des cortex pallii bei den mammaliern und zwei homologe rindenfelder im besonderen zugleich ein beitrag zur furchenlehre. *Journal für Psychologie und Neurologie* **6**:275–400.

Brodmann, K. (1909) *Vergleichende Lokalisationslehre der Grosshirnrinde in ihren Prinzipien Dargestellt auf Grund des Zellenbaues* (Barth, Leipzig). For English translation see Garey, L.J. (1994).

Brown, R.A. & Swanson, L.W. (2013) Neural Systems Language: a formal modeling language for the systematic description, unambiguous communication, and automated digital curation of neural connectivity. *Journal of Comparative Neurology* **521**:2889–2906.

Brunet, C. (1698) *Le progrès de la medecine, contenant un recueil de tout ce qui s'observe de singulier par rapport à sa pratique. Avec un jugement sur toute sorte d'ouvrages de physique et de nouvelles expliçations des principaux phénomenes de la nature. Pour l'année 1697* (Laurent d'Houry, Paris).

Brunn, J.H. von (1753) *Dissertatio Inauguralis Medica Sistens Experimenta quaedam circa Ligaturas Nervorum in Vivis Animalibus Instituta* (Schultzii, Göttingen).

Brunner, J.C. (1688) *Exercitatio Anatomica de Glandula Pituitaria* (Bergmanni, Heidelberg).

Brunschwig (1525) *The Noble experyence of the vertuous handy warke of surgeri practysed & compyled by the moost Experte Mayster Iherome of Bruynswyke borne ine Straesborowe in Almayne ye whiche hath it Fyrst Proved and Trewly Founde by His Awne Dayly Exerycsynge. Item there after he hath authorysed and done it to vnderstande thrugh the trewe sentences of the olde doctours and maysters very experte in the scyence of surgery, as Galienus, Ipocras, Auicenna, Gwydo, Haly abbas, Lancfransus of Mylen, Iamericus, Rogerius, Albucasis, Place[n]tinus, Brunus, Gwilhelmus de Saliceto, & by many other maysters whose names be wryten in this same boke. Here also shall ye fynde for to cure & hele all wounded me[m]bres, and other swellyges. Item yf ye fynde only names of herbes or of other thynges whereof ye haue no knowlege, yt shall ye knowe playnly by the potecarys. Item here shall you fynde also for to make salues, plasters, powders, oyles, and drynkes for woundes. Item who so desyreth of this science ye playne knowlege let hym oftentymes rede this boke, and than he shall gette perfyte vnderstandynge of the noble surgery* (Treueris, London).

Brusca, R.C. & Brusca, G.J. (1990) *Invertebrates* (Sinauer, Sunderland, MA).

Bullock, T.H. & Horridge, G.A. (1965) *Structure and Function in the Nervous Systems of Invertebrates* (Freeman, San Francisco).

Burdach, K.F. (1819, 1822, 1826) *Vom Baue und Leben des Gehirns* (Dyk'schen Buchhandlung, Leipzig).

Burdin, J. (1803) *Cours d'Études Médicales ou Exposition de la Structure de l'Homme Comparée à celle des Animaux; de l'Histoire de ses Maladies, des Connaissances Acquises sur l'Action Régulière de ses Organes, etc. etc. Ouvrage Destiné aux Jeunes Médecins, aux Vétérinaires, aux Savans, et à Toutes les Personnes qui Désirent Acquérir Facilement, sur la Science de l'Homme Physique, des Notions Assez Étendues pour en Faire des Applications Utiles*, 3 Vols. (Lupret, Paris).

Burdin, J. (1803) *Course of Medical Studies, Containing a Comparative View of the Anatomical Structure of Man and of Animals, a History of Diseases, and an Account of the Knowledge Hitherto Acquired with Regard to the Regular Action of the Different Organs; a Work Chiefly Designed for the Use of Medical Students*, 3 Vols. (Cuthell & Martin, London). Translated from the French of the same year.

Cajal, S.R. (1895) *Apuntes para el Estudio del Bulbo Raquídeo, Cerebelo y Origen de los Nervios Encefálicos* (Fortanet, Madrid).

Cajal, S.R. (1899-1904) *Textura del Sistema Nervioso del Hombre y de los Vertebrados: Estudios sobre el Plan Estructural y Composición de los Centros Serviosos Adicionados de Consideraciones Fisiológicas Fundadas en los Nuevos Descubrimientos*, 2 Vols. (Moya, Madrid).

Cajal, S.R. (1901-1902) Estructura del septum lucidum. *Trabajos del Laboratoria de Investigaciones Biologicas de la Universidad de Madrid* **1**:159–188.

Cajal, S.R. (1904), *see* Cajal, S.R. (1899-1904), Vol. 2.

Cajal, S.R. (1909–1911) *Histologie du Système Nerveux de l'Homme et des Vertébrés*, 2 Vols., Translated by L. Azoulay (Maloine, Paris). See English translation by N. Swanson & L.W. Swanson, *Histology of the Nervous System of Man and Vertebrates* by S. Rámon y Cajal, 2 Vols. (Oxford University Press, New York) 1995.

Cajal, S.R. (1999) *Advice to a Young Investigator*, Translated by Neely Swanson and Larry W. Swanson (MIT Press, Cambridge).

Caldani, L.M.A. (1813, 1814) *Icones Anatomicae, quotquot sunt Celebriores ex Optimis Neotericorum Operibus Summa Diligentia Depromptae et Collectae. Tabulas Selegerunt et Nonnullas ex Cadaveribus ad Vivum Delineatas Addere Curavunt Leopoldus Marcus Antonius et Florianus Caldani*, Atlas and Text Vol. 3, part 2 (Picotti, Venice).

Calleja, C. (1893) *La Región Olfatoria del Cerebro* (Moya, Madrid).

Camper, P. (1760) *Demonstrationum Anatomico-Pathologicarum, Liber Primus. Continens Brachii Humani Fabricam et Morbos* (Schrueder & Mortier, Amsterdam).

Camper, P. (1762) *Demonstrationum Anatomico-Pathologicarum, Liber Secundus. Continens Pelvis Humanae Fabricam et Morbos* (Schrueder & Mortier, Amsterdam).

Camper, P. & Albinus, B.S. (1767) *Epistola ad Anatomicorum Principem Magnum Albinum* (Crebas, Groningen).

Cannieu, A. (1894) Recherches sur les origins du nerf auditif. Ses rameaux et ses ganglions (Doin, Paris), reprinted from the *Revue de Laryngologie, d'Otologie et de Rhinologie.*

Canteras, N.S., Ribeiro-Barbosa, É., Goto, M., Cipolla-Neto, J., & Swanson, L.W. (2011) The retinohypothalamic tract: comparison of axonal projection patterns from four major targets. *Brain Research Reviews* **65**:150–183.

Canteras, N.S., Simerly, R.B., & Swanson, L.W. (1992) The connections of the posterior nucleus of the amygdala. *Journal of Comparative Neurology* **324**:143–179.

Carpenter, M.B. (1976) *Human Neuroanatomy*, 7th Edn. (Williams & Wilkins, Baltimore).

Carpenter, M.B. & Suttin, J. (1983) *Human Neuroanatomy*, 8th Edn. (Williams & Wilkins, Baltimore).

Carus, C.G. (1814) *Versuch einer Darstellung des Nervensystems und Insbesondere des Gehirns nach Ihrer Bedeutung, Entwickelung und Vollendung im Thierischen Organismus* (Breitkopf und Härtel, Leipzig).

Carus, C.G. (1818) *Lehrbuch der Zootomie; mit Stäter Hinsicht auf Physiologie Ausgearb, und durch Zwanzig Kupfertafeln Erläutert* (Fleischer, Leipzig).

Cassell's Concise Latin-English, English-Latin Dictionary, 3rd Edn. (1979) (Cassell, London).

Casseri, G.C. [1601] *Julii Casserii Placentini Philosophi atq[ue] Medici Patavii vtranqve Medicinam Exercentis De Vocis Auditvsq[ue] Organis Historia Anatomica Singvlari fide Methodo ac Indvstria Concinnata Tractatibvs Dvobvs Explicata ac Variis Iconibvs aere Excvsis Illustrata* (Baldinus, Ferrara).

Casseri, G.C. (1609) *Pentaestheseion, hoc est, De Quinque Sensibus Liber, Organorum Fabricam Variis Iconibus Fideliter aere Incisis Illustratam, nec non Actionem et Usum, Discursu Anatomico & Philosophico Accuratè Explicata Continens* (Misserinum, Venice).

Casseri, G.C. (1627) *Tabulae Anatomicae LXXIIX* (Bucretius, Venice). Facsimile published by Editions Medicina Rara [no place indicated], [1971?].

Castiglioni, A. (1947) *A History of Medicine*, Translated from the Italian and edited by E.B. Krumbhaar, 2nd Edn. (Knopf, New York).

Celsus (c30), *De Medicina*, with an English translation by W.G. Spencer, in 3 Vols. (Harvard University Press, Cambridge) 1935–1938.

Charpy, A. (1889) *Cours de Splanchnologie. Les Centres Nerveux* (Guillau, Montauban).

Chaussier, F. (1789) *Table Synoptique du Nerf Tri-Splanchnic.* No imprint, copy at National Library of Medicine. In: Chaussier, F. [1789–1815] [*Tables Synoptiques du Plan Général des Divisions et Sou-Divisions Principales d'Anatomie*] (Barrois, Paris). As bound into copy at National Library of Medicine.

Chaussier, F. (1807) *Exposition Sommaire de la Structure et des Différentes Parties de l'Encéphale ou Cerveau* (Barrois, Paris).

Chaussier, F. (1809) *Table synoptique des nerfs.* In: Chaussier, F. [1789–1815] [*Tables Synoptiques du Plan Général des Divisions et Sou-Divisions Principales d'Anatomie*] (Barrois, Paris). As bound into copy at National Library of Medicine.

Cheng, Z. & Powley, T.L. (2000) Nucleus ambiguus projections to cardiac ganglia of rat atria: an anterograde tracing study. *Journal of Comparative Neurology* **424**:588–606.

Cheselden, W. (1713) *The Anatomy of the Human Body* (Cliff and Jackson, London).

Cheselden, W. (1722) *The Anatomy of the Human Body*, 2nd Edn. (Collins, London).

Cheselden, W. (1726) *The Anatomy of the Human Body*, 3rd Edn. (Bowyer, London).

Cheselden, W. (1712) [i.e., 1742] *The Anatomy of the Human Body*, 6th Edn. (Bowyer, London).

Choulant, L. (1852) *Geschichte und Bibliographie der Anatomischen Abbildung nach Ihrer Beziehung auf Anatomische Wissenschaft und Bildende Kunst* (Weigel, Leipzig).

Choulant, L. (1962) *History and Bibliography of Anatomic Illustration.* Translated and Annotated by Mortimer Frank (Hafner, New York).

Christ, J.F. (1969) Derivation and boundaries of the hypothalamus, with atlas of hypothalamic grisea. In: Haymaker, W., Anderson, E., & Nauta, W.J.H. (Eds.) *The Hypothalamus* (Thomas, Springfield IL), pp. 13–60.

Clark, F. Le Gros (1836) *The Practical Anatomy and Elementary Physiology of the Nervous System; Designed for the Use of Students in the Dissecting Room* (Longman, Rees, Orme, Brown, Green, and Longmans; London).

Clark, W.E. Le Gros (1951) Central nervous system. In: Brash, J.C. (Ed.), *Cunningham's Text-Book of Anatomy*, 9th Edn. (Oxford University Press, Oxford), pp. 835–1008.

Clarke, E. (1968) The doctrine of the hollow nerve in the seventeenth and eighteenth centuries. In: Stevenson, L.G. & Multhauf, R.P. (Eds.) *Medicine, Science, and Culture: Historical Essays in Honor of Owsei Temkin* (Johns Hopkins Press, Baltimore), pp. 123–141.

Clarke, E. & Dewhurst, K. (1996) *An Illustrated History of Brain Function: Imaging the Brain from Antiquity to the Present*, 2nd Edn. (Norman, San Francisco).

Clarke, E. & Jacyna, L.S. (1987) *Nineteenth-Century Origins of Neuroscientific Concepts* (University of California Press, Berkeley).

Clarke, E. & O'Malley, C.D. (1996) *The Human Brain and Spinal Cord: A Historical Study Illustrated by Writings from Antiquity to the Twentieth Century*, 2nd Edn. (Norman, San Francisco).

Clarke, E. & Stannard, J. (1963) Aristotle on the anatomy of the brain. *Journal of the History of Medicine* **18**:130–148.

Clarke, J.A.L. (1851) Researches into the structure of the spinal cord. *Philosophical Transactions of the Philosophical Society, London* **141**:607–621.

Cloquet, H. (1815) *Dissertation sur les Odeurs, sur le Sens et les Organes de l'Olfaction Présentée et Soutenue à la Faculté de Médecine de Paris le 21 Février 1815* (Crochard, Paris).

Cloquet, H. (1816) *Traité d'Anatomie Descriptive: Rédigé d'après l'Ordre Adopté à la Faculté de Médecine de Paris* (Crochard, Paris).

Cloquet, J. (1828) *Anatomie de l'Homme, ou Description et Figures de Toutes les Parties du Corps Humain.* 3, *Néurologie* (Engelmann, Paris).

Cobb, J.L.S. (1995) The nervous systems of Echinodermata: recent results and new approaches. In: Breidbach, O. & Kutsch, W. (Eds.) *The Nervous System of Invertebrates: An Evolutionary and Comparative Approach* (Birkhäuser, Basel), pp. 407–424.

Cochet, B. (1967) Contribution à l'étude du plexus tympanique. Anatomie macroscopique et microscopique. *Archives d'Anatomie, d'Histologie et d'Embryologie Normales et Expérimentales* **50**:1–46.

Coiter, V. (1564) *Tabulae Externarum Partium Humani Corporis; in Quibus Unaquaeque Paras Varijs Nominibus & Etymologiis Breviter, & Dilucide Explicatur* (Benaccius, Bologna).

Coiter, V. (1566) *Volcheri Coeiter Frisii; De Ossibus, et Cartilaginibus Humani Corporis; Tabulae, Quae eorum Obscuras Uoces, Numerum, & Nomenclaturas tam Partium Uniuscuiusque, quàm Singulorum Complectuntur* (Rossium, Bologna).

Coiter, V. (1572) *Externarum et Internarum Principalium Humani Corporis Partium Tabulae, atque Anatomicae Exercitationes Observationesque Variae, Novis, Diversis, ac Artificiosissimis Figuris Illustratae, Philosophis, Medicis, in Primis autem Anatomico Studio Addictis Summè Utiles* (Gerlatzeni, Nuremberg). English translation by A. Schierbeek in *Opuscula Selecta Neerlandicorum de Arte Medica*, Vol. 18 (Sumptibus Societatis, Amsterdam), 1955, pp. 1–159.

Cole, F.J. (1944) *A History of Comparative Anatomy* (Macmillan, London).

Collins (1685) *A Systeme of Anatomy, Treating of the Body of Man, Beasts, Birds, Fish, Insects and Plants* (Newcomb, In the Savoy [London]).

Colombo, R. (1559) *De Re Anatomica Libri XV* (Bevilacqua, Venice). Facsimile published by Culture et Civilisation, Brussels, 1983.

Combe, G., Combe, A., & Gall, F.J. (1838) *On the Functions of the Cerebellum*, by Drs Gall, Vimont, and Broussais, Translated from the French by George Combe: Also, Answers to the Objections Urged Against Phrenology by Drs Roget, Rudolphi, Prichard, and Tiedeman; by George Combe and Dr A. Combe (Maclachlan & Stewart, Edinburgh).

Comparetti, A. (1789) *Observationes Anatomicae de Aure Interna Comparata* (Bartholomaeum, Padua).

Coopmans, G. (1754), *see* Monro, A. *primus* (1754) *Celebris Anatomici Alexandri Monro.*

Coopmans, G. (1789) *Neurologia, et Observatio de Calculo, ex Urethra Excreto, Tabulis Illustrata* (Romar, Franeker).

Copho (c1070–c1100), *see* Corner, G.W. (1927).

Corner, G.W. (1927) *Anatomical Texts of the Earlier Middle Ages: A Study in the Transmission of Culture, With a Revised Latin Text of Anatomia Cophonis and Translation of Four Texts* (Carnegie Institution of Washington, Washington DC).

Cortesi, G.B. (1625) *Ioannis Baptistae Cortesii Medici ac Philosophi Almi Collegi Bononiensis Comitis Palatini in Patrio Olim Gymnasio Medicinae, et Anatomes Professoris; nunc in Messanensi Academia Praxim Ordinariam e' Prima Sede Interpretantis Miscellaneorum Medicinalium Decades Denae in Quibus Pulcherrima ac Utilissima Quaeque ad Anatomen, Chirurgiam, et Totius Fere Medicinae Theoriam, et Praxim Spectantia Sparsim Quidem, sed Iucundissimo Ordine Continentur um ad Illustriss; Senatum Nobilis Urbis Messanae* (Breae, Reinae; Messina).

Cotugno, D. (1760) *De Aquaeductibus Auris Humanae Internae* (Neapoli). In: Sandifort, E. (1768) *Thesaurus Dissertationum, Programmatum, Aliorumque Opusculorum Selectissimorum, ad Omnem Medicinae Ambitum Pertinentium*, Vol. 1 (Beman, Rotterdam), pp. 389–450. Published in book form in 1774.

Cotugno, D. (1764) *De Ischiade Nervosa Commintarius* (Simonios, Naples).

Cowper, W. (1698) *The Anatomy of Humane Bodies* (Smith and Walford, London).

Craigie, E.H. (1910–1911) History of anatomy, section of article, *Anatomy*. In: *Encyclopaedia Britannica*, 11th Edn. (Encyclopaedia Britannica, New York), pp. 921–937. Reprinted with new footnotes from the 9th Edn. (1875–1889), where the rest of the article on anatomy was written by W. Turner.

Craigie, E.H. (1925) *An Introduction to the Finer Anatomy of the Central Nervous System Based upon that of the Albino Rat, with Twenty-eight Plates and Ten Illustrations in the Text* (Blakiston's Son & Co., Philadelphia).

Crooke, H. (1615) *Microcosmographia. A Description of the Body of Man* (Jaggard, London).

Crooke, H. (1616) *Somatographia Anthropine [Greek]; or A Description of the Body of Man. By Artificiall Figures Representing the Members, and Fit Termes Expressing the Same. Set Forth Either to Pleasure or to Profite Those Who are Addicted to this Study* (Jaggard, London). Extracted by Alexander Read from Crooke (1615).

Crooke, H. (1618) *Microcosmographia. A Description of the Body of Man* (Jaggard, London). Reissue of the 1615 first edition with identical pagination.

Crosby, E.C. & Humphrey, T. (1941) Studies of the vertebrate telencephalon. II. The nuclear pattern of the anterior olfactory nucleus, tuberculum olfactorium and the amygdaloid complex in adult man. *Journal of Comparative Neurology* **74**:309–352.

Crosby, E.C, Humphrey, T., & Lauer, E.W. (1962) *Correlative Anatomy of the Nervous System* (Macmillan, New York).

Crosby, E.C. & Schnitzlein, H.N., Eds. (1982) *Comparative Correlative Neuroanatomy of the Vertebrate Telencephalon* (Macmillan, New York).

Crosby, E.C. & Woodbourne, R.T. (1940) The comparative anatomy of the preoptic area and the hypothalamus. In: *Association for Research on Nervous and Mental Diseases, Proceedings* **20**:52–169.

Cruveilhier, J. (1836) *Anatomie Descriptive*, Vol. 4 (Béchet jeune, Paris).

Cruveilhier, J. (1844) *The Anatomy of the Human Body*; the First American, from the Last Paris Edition, edited by G.S. Pattison (Harper & Brothers, New York).

Cunningham, D.J. (1892) *Contribution to the Surface Anatomy of the Cerebral Hemispheres, with a Chapter upon Cranio-Cerebral Topography by Victor Horsley* (Academy House, Dublin).

Cunningham (1951), *see* Clark (1951), Durward (1951).

Cushing, H. (1943) *A Bio-bibliography of Andreas Vesalius* (Schuman's, New York).

Cuvier, G. (1800) *Leçons d'Anatomie Comparée* (Baudouin, Paris).

Dail, W.G. (1996) The pelvic plexus: innervation of pelvic and extrapelvic visceral tissues. *Microscopy Research and Technique* **35**:95–106.

Daniel, P.M. & Prichard, M.M. (1975) Studies of the hypothalamus and the pituitary gland: with special reference to the effects of transection of the pituitary stalk. *Acta Endocrinologica*, Suppl. 201, Vol. **80**:1–216.

Dashti, A.E., Ghandeharizadeh, S., Stone, J., Swanson, L.W., & Thompson, R.H. (1997) Database challenges and solutions in neuroscientific applications. *Neuroimage* **5**:97–115.

Davies, F., Gladstone, R.J., & Stibbe, E.P. (1931) The anatomy of the intercostal nerves. *Journal of Anatomy* **66**:323–333.

de Koning, P. (1903), *see* Razi, Abu Bakr Muhammad ibn Zakariya (1903).

De Lacy (1978, 1980, 1984), *see* Galen (c162–c166) *On the Doctrines of Hippocrates and Plato.*

De Lacy (1992), *see* Galen (c170–c172) *On Semen.*

de Laguna, A. (1535) *Anatomica Methodus, Seu de Sectione Humani Corporis Contemplatio* (Cyaneum simultaneously with Keruer, Paris).

De Schutter, E. (2005) Changes and opportunities. *Neuroinformatics* **3**:79–80.

Deiters, O. (1865) *Untersuchungen über Gehirn und Rückenmark des Menschen und der Säugethiere. Nach dem Tode des Verfassers Hrsg. von Max Schultze* (Vieweg, Braunschweig).

Dejerine, J.J. & Dejerine-Klumpke, A. (1895, 1901) *Anatomie des Centres Nerveux*, 2 Vols. (Rueff, Paris).

Demeter, S., Rosene, D.L., & van Hoesen, G.W. (1985) Interhemispheric pathways of the hippocampal formation, presubiculum, and entorhinal and posterior parahippocampal cortices in the rhesus monkey: the structure and organization of the hippocampal commissures. *Journal of Comparative Neurology* **233**:30–47.

Desmoulins, A. (1825) *Anatomie des Systèmes Nerveux des Animaux a Vertèbres: Appliquée à la Physiologie et à la Zoologie / Ouvrage dont la Partie Physiologique est faite Conjointement avec F. Magendie*, 2 Vols. & Atlas (Méquignon-Marvis, Paris). Complete list of his earlier publications on pp. xxiv–xxvi.

Dessort, H. (1820) *Wegweiser durch Henry Dessort's Ethnologisches und Anatomisches Museum, der Grössten Sammlung Künstlerischer Darstellungen aus dem Gebiete des Körperlebens der Menschen* (Dessort, Mainz).

Diemerbroeck, Y. van (1672) *Anatome Corporis Humani: Plurimis Novis Inventis Instructa, Variisque Observationibus, & Paradoxis, cúm Medicis túm Physiologicis Adornata, Conscripta Ab Isbrando de Diemerbroeck, Medicinae & Anatomes Professore* (Meinardi & Dreunen, Utrecht).

Diemerbroeck, Y. van (1689) *The Anatomy of Human Bodies, Comprehending the Most Modern Discoveries and Curiosities in that Art. To which is Added a Particular Treatise of the Small-pox and Measles. Together with Several Practical Observations and Experienc'd Cures. Written in Latin* (Brewster, London).

Dixon, A.F. (1899) The sensory distribution of the facial nerve in man. *Journal of Anatomy and Physiology* **33**:471–492.

Döllinger, I. (1814) *Beiträge zur Entwicklungsgeschichte des Menschlichen Gehirns* (Brönner, Frankfurt).

Dong, H.-W. & Allen Institute for Brain Science (2008) *Allen Reference Atlas: A Digital Color Brain Atlas of the C57Black/6J Male Mouse* (Wiley, Hoboken NJ).

Dorland's Illustrated Medical Dictionary, 30th Edn. (2003) (Saunders, Philadelphia).

Dowling, J.E. (2012) *The Retina: An Approachable Part of the Brain* (Harvard University Press, Cambridge).

Drake, J. (1707) *Anthropologia Nova; Or, a New System of Anatomy Describing the Animal Oeconomy, and a Short Rationale of many Distembers Incident to Human Bodies. In Which are Inserted Divers* Anatomical Discoveries, *and* Medicinal Observations, *with the History of the Parts. Illustrated with Above Fourscore Figures, Drawn after the Life: And to every Chapter a Syllabus of the Parts Describ'd, for the Instruction of Young* Anatomists, 2 Vols. (Smith & Walford, London).

Drelincourt, C. (1672) *Caroli Drelincurlii Medici Regii in Galliis; Nec non Leidensis Professoris Practici & Anatomici Praeludium Anatomicum, Quod Lugdunensium in Ampitheatro suam ad Primam Anatomes Encheiresin Adhibuit* (Gaasbekiana, Leiden).

Dryander, J. (1536) *Anatomia Capitis Humani* (Eucharium Ceruicoznum, Marburg).

du Laurens, A. (1589) *Historia Anatomica Humani Corporis et Singularum eius Partium, Multis Controversiis et Observationibus Novis Illustrata* (Paris). Quoted in Choulant (1962, p. 222). Undoubtedly a "ghost" due to misprint of another mistake in Choulant (1852, p. 75) where another "ghost", 1598, is cited); *see* du Laurens, A. (1599) and du Laurens, A. (1600).

du Laurens, A. (1595) *Historia Anatomica Humani Corporis et Singularum ejus Partium Multis Controversiis et Observationibus Novis Illustrata* (Becker, Frankfurt).

du Laurens, A. (1599) *Historia Anatomica Humani Corporis et Singularum ejus Partium Multis Controversiis et Observationibus Novis Illustrata* (Becker, Frankfurt).

du Laurens, A. (1600) *Historia Anatomica, Humani Corporis & Singularum ejus Partium Multis Controversiis & Observationibus Novis Illustrata* (Orry, Paris).

Du Verney, G.J. (1683) *Traité de l'Organe de l'Ouie, Contenant la Structure, les Usages & les Maladies de Toutes les Parties de l'Oreille* (Michallet, Paris). An English translation was published in 1737 by Samuel Baker, London, and a facsimile was published in 1973 by AMS Press, New York.

Du Verney, G.J. (1697), *see* Winslow, J.B. (1733) Section VI, p. 79.

Du Verney, G.J. (1761) *Oeuvers Anatomiques* (Jombert, Paris).

Du Verney, G.J. (1737), *see* Du Verney, G.J. (1683).

Du Verney, M., *see* Duverney, G.J.

Dubois, J. (1551) *Vaesani Cujusdam [sc. Vesalii] Calumniarum in Hippocratis Galeníque Rem Anatomicam Depulsio* (Barbé, Paris).

Dubois, J. (1555) *In Hippocratis et Galeni Physiologiae Partem Anatomicam Isagoge* (Hulpeau, Paris).

Dubois, J. (1556) *In Hippocratis et Galeni Physiologiae Partem Anatomicam Isagoge* (Valgrisii, Venice).

Dubois, J. (1634) *Jacobi Sylvii Ambiani Medici et Professoris Regii Parisiensis Opera Medica: Iam Demum in Sex Partes Digesta, Castigata & Indicibus Necessariis Instructa: Adjuncta est Eiusdem Vita et Icon* (Jacobum Chouët, Geneva).

Duckworth, W.L. (1962), *see* Galen (c192) *On Anatomical Procedures, The Later Books.*

Dunglison, R. (1874) *A Dictionary of Medical Science* (Lea, Philadelphia).

Durward, A. (1951) Peripheral nervous system. In: Brash, J.C. (Ed.) *Cunningham's Text-Book of Anatomy*, 9th Edn. (Oxford University Press, Oxford), pp. 1009–1150.

Dutrochet, R.J.H. (1824) *Recherches Anatomiques et Physiologiques sur la Structure Intime des Animaux et des Végétaux, et sur leur Motilité* (Baillière, Paris).

Duvernoy, H.M. (1988) *The Human Hippocampus: An Atlas of Applied Anatomy* (Bergmann, Munich).

Duvernoy, J.G. (1735) De sinibus cerebri. *Commentarii Academiae Scientiarum Imperialis Petropolitanae, ad Annum MDCCXXIX* **4**:130–135.

Ebel, J.G. (1789) *Observationes Neurologicae ex Anatome Compara.* (Apitziano, Frankfurt an der Oder).

Economo, C. (1929) *The Cytoarchitectonics of the Human Cerebral Cortex*, Translated by S. Parker (Oxford University Press, London).

Economo, C. & Koskinas, G.N. (1925) *Die Cytoarchitektonik der Hirnrinde des Erwachsenen Menschen* (Springer, Vienna).

Edgley, S.A. & Grant, G.M. (1991) Inputs to spinocerebellar tract neurones located in Stilling's nucleus in the sacral segments of the rat spinal cord. *Journal of Comparative Neurology* **305**:130–138.

Edinger, L. (1890) *Twelve Lectures on the Structure of the Central Nervous System for Physicians and Students*, 2nd Edn., translated by Willis Hall Vittum, edited by C. Eugene Riggs (Davis, Philadelphia). Second printing in 1891.

Edinger, L. (1893) *Vorlesungen über den Bau der Nervösen Centralorgane des Menschen und der Thiere* (Vogel, Leipzig).

Edwin Smith Surgical Papyrus (c1700 BC), *see* Smith Papyrus (c1700 BC), Breasted (1930), Allen (2005).

Egenhofer, M. & Franzosa, R. (1991) Point-set topological spatial relations. *International Journal of Geographical Information Systems* **5**:161–174.

Ehrenberg, C.G. (1833) Nothwendigkeit einer feineren mechanischen Zerlegung des Gehirns und der Nerven vor den chemischen, dargestellt aus Beobachtungen. *Annalen der Physik und Chemie* **28**:449–473.

Ehrenritter, J. (1790) [No title] *Medizinisch-chirurgische Zeitung* **1**(4):319–320.

Emmel, V.E. (1921) *The BNA Arranged as an Outline of Regional and Systematic Anatomy* (University of California Press, Berkeley).

Eschricht, D.F. (1826) De functionibus septimi et quinti paris nervorum in facie propriis. *Journal de Physiologie Expérimentale et Pathologique* **6**:228–259.

Estienne, C. (1545) *De Dissectione Partium Corporis Humani Libri Tres* (Colines, Paris).

Estienne, C. (1546) *La Dissection des Parties du Corps Humain Divisee en Trois Livres* (Colines, Paris).

Eustachi, B. [1552], *see* Eustachi, B. (1714). The plates were finished by 1552 but not published until 1714.

Eustachi, B. (1714) *Tabulae Anatomicae*, edited by G.M. Lancisi (Gonzaga, Rome). Also see Albinus, B.S. (1744) *Explicatio Tabularum Anatomicarum Bartholomaei Eustachii*, and the revised second edition in 1761.

Eycleshymer, A.C. (1917) *Anatomical Names, Especially the Basle Nomina Anatomica ("BNA")* (Wood, New York).

Fabricius ab Aquapendente (c1610), see Zanchin, G. & De Caro, R. (2006).

Fabricius ab Aquapendente (1613) *Tractus Anatomicus Triplex Quorum Primus De Oculo, Visus; Secundus De Aure, Auditus; Tertius De Laringe, Vocis Admirandam Tradit Historiam, Actiones, Utilitates...* (de Bry, [Frankfurt am Main]).

Falloppio, G. (1561) *Observationes Anatomicae* (Ulmo & Perchachino, Venice).

Fantoni, G. (1738) *Johannis Fantoni Medici Gegii, et in Taurinensi Academia Professoris Emeriti, Opuscula Medica et Physiologia* (Sumptibus Pellisari, & soc.; Geneva).

Fay-Lund, H. (1986) Projection from the inferior colliculus to the superior olivary complex in the albino rat. *Anatomy and Embryology* **175**:35–52.

Fernel, J. (1542) *Ioannis Fernelij Ambianatis, De Naturali Parte Medicinae Libri Septem; ad Henricum Francisci Galliae Regis Filium* (Collinaeum, Paris).

Ferrari, G. (1998), *see* Benedetti, A. (1998).

Finger, S. (1994) *Origins of Neuroscience: A History of Explorations into Brain Function* (Oxford University Press, New York).

Fischer, J.L. (1791) *Descriptio Anatomica Nervorum Lumbalium Sacralium et Extremitatum Inferiorum* (Crusius, Leipzig).

Flatau, E. & Jacobsohn, L. (1899) *Handbuch der Anatomie und Vergleichenden Anatomie des Centralnervensystems der Säugetiere. I. Makroskopischer Teil* (Karger, Berlin).

Forel, A. (1872) Beiträge zur Kentniss des Thalamus opticus und der ihn umgebenden Gebilde bei den Säugethieren. *Sitzungsberichte der Kaiserlichen Akademie der Wissenschaften. Mathematisch-Naturwissenschftliche Classe. Abt. III, Physiologie, Anatomie und theoretische Medicin* **66**:25–58. Also exists as reprint with 33 pp.

Forel, A. (1877) Untersuchingen über die Haubenregion und ihre obern Verknüpfungen im Gehirne des Menschen und einiger Säugethiere, mit Beiträgen zu den Methoden der Gehirnuntersuchung. *Archiv für Psychiatrie und Nervenkrankheiten* **7**:393–495.

Foster, F.P. (1892–1894) *An Illustrated Encyclopaedic Medical Dictionary* (Appleton, New York).

Foster, M. & Sherrington, S.C. (1897) *A Textbook of Physiology*, 7th Edn., Part 3 (Macmillan, New York).

Freer, S. (1996), *see* Wharton, T. (1656).

Fritzau, A.F. (1811) *De Tertio Ramo Paris Quinti Nervorum Cerebri s. Nervi Maxillari Inferiori* (no publisher indicated, Leipzig).

Frotcher, G.C. (1788) *Descriptio Medullae Spinalis eiusque Nervorum: Iconibus Illustrata* (Walther, Erlangen). Reprinted in Ludwig, C.F. (1791–1795), Vol. 4, pp. 70–105, 1795.

Funke, J. (1904) The carotid body: anatomy, histology, embryology, and tumors arising from it. *Proceedings of the Pathological Society of Philadelphia*, New Series **7**:209–225.

Fuse, S. (1950) On the so-called intercarotid plexus; a macroscopical study on 56 Japanese cadavers. *Folia Psychiatrica et Neurologica Japonica* **4**:1–11.

Fyfe, A. (1800) *A Compendium of the Anatomy of the Human Body; Illustrated by Upwards of One Hundred and Sixty Tables, Containing Near Seven Hundred Figures, Copied from the Most Celebrated Authors, and From Nature* (Pillans & Sons, Edinburgh).

Galen (c130–c200) *Selected Works*, Translated with an Introduction and Notes by P.N. Singer (Oxford University Press, Oxford, 1997).

Galen (c162–c166) *On the Doctrines of Hippocrates and Plato*, edition, translation and commentary by Phillip De Lacy, 3 parts (Akademie-Verlag, Berlin) 1978, 1980, 1984.

Galen (c170–c172) *On Semen*; *see* Greek text and English translation in De Lacy, P. (1992) *On Semen* (Akademie-Verlag, Berlin).

Galen (c173) *On the Usefulness of the Parts of the Body*. Translated from the Greek with an Introduction and Commentary by M.T. May (Cornell University Press, Ithaca), 1968.

Galen (c177) *On Anatomical Procedures*. Translation of the Surviving Books with Introduction and Notes by Charles Singer (Oxford University Press, Oxford, 1999; a special edition for Sandpiper Books of the 1956 edition).

Galen (c180) *On Anatomy of Nerves, see* Goss (1966).

Galen (c181) *On Bones, for Beginners; see* Galen (1821).

Galen (c192) *On Anatomical Procedures, The Later Books*. A Translation of the Later Books by the late W.L. Duckworth, edited by M.C. Lyons and B. Towers (Cambridge University Press, Cambridge) 1962.

Galen (after 192) *On the Affected Parts, see* Siegel (1976).

Galen (1528) *De Usu Partium Corporis Humani* (Colines, Paris).

Galen (1531); *see* Günther, J., of Andernach (1531).

Galen (1821) *De Ossibus ad Tirones*. In: Kühn, C.G. (Ed.) *Opera Omnia*, Vol. II (Cnobloch, Leipzig), pp. 732–778.

Gall, F.J. & Spurzheim, J.C. (1809) *Recherches sur le System Nerveux General et sur Celui du Cerveau en Particulier; Mémoire Présenté à l'Institut de France, le 14 mars 1808, Suivi d'Observations sur le Rapport qui a été Fiat à cette Compagnie par ses Commissaires* (Schoell & Nicolle, Paris).

Gall, F.J. & Spurzheim, J.C. (1810) *Anatomie et Physiologie du Système Nerveux en Général et du Cerveau in Particulier*, Vol. 1 & Atlas (Schoell, Paris). In all, 5 Vols. & Atlas were published between 1810–1819. Another edition of Vols. 1 and 2, with different pagination and different back matter, was published by Schoell (Paris; 1810, 1812).

Ganser, S. (1882) Vergleichend-anatomische Studien über das Gehirn des Maulwurfs. *Morphologisches Jahrbuch* **7**:591–725.

Garengeot, R.-J.C. (1728) *Splanchnologie, Ou l'Anatomie des Visceres* (Cavelier, Paris).

Garey, L.J. (1994) *Brodmann's 'Localization in the Cerebral Cortex'* (Smith-Gordon, London).

Garrison, F.H. (1929) *An Introduction to the History of Medicine, With Medical Chronology, Suggestions for Study and Bibliographic Data*, 4th Edn., Reprinted (Saunders, Philadelphia).

Garrison, F.H. & McHenry, L.C. (1969) *Garrison's History of Neurology, Revised and Enlarged with a Bibliography of Classical, Original and Standard Works in Neurology by Lawrence C. McHenry* (Thomas, Springfield IL).

Gaskell, W.H. (1886) On the structure, distribution and function of the nerves which innervate the visceral and vascular systems. *Journal of Physiology* **7**:1–80.

Gehuchten, A. van (1897) *Anatomie du Systéme Nerveux de l'Homme*, 2nd Edn. (Uystpruyst-Dieudonné, Louvain).

Gehuchten, A. van (1906) *Anatomie du Systéme Nerveux de l'Homme*, 4th Edn. (Uystpruyst-Dieudonné, Louvain).

Geminus, Thomas (1553) *Compendiosa Totius Anatomie Delineatio* (Hyll, London); *see* facsimile published in 1959 by Dawsons (London), with Introduction by C.D. O'Malley.

Gennari, F. (1782) *De Peculiari Structura Cerebri Nonnullisque ejus Morbis* (Regio Typographeo, Parma).

Gerdy, P.N. (1838) Récherches sur l'encephale. *Journal des Connaissances Médico-Chirurgicales*, décembre, [no volume number indicated], pp. 258–263.

Gerssdorff, Hans von (1517) *Feldtbuch der Wundtartzney* (Schott, Strasbourg). Facsimile published by Editions Medicina Rara (no date or place indicated).

Giacomini, C.H. (1884) Fascia dentata du grand hippocampe dans le cerveau de l'homme. *Archives Italiennes de Biologie* **5**:1–16, 205–219, 396–417.

[Gibson, T.] Anonomyous (1682) *The Anatomy of Humane Bodies Epitomized* (Flesher, Flesher; London).

Gibson, T. (1684) *The Anatomy of Human Bodies Epitomized: Wherein All the Parts of Man's Body, with their Actions and Uses, are Succinctly Described, According to the Newest Doctrine of the Most Accurate and Learned Modern Anatomists*, 2nd Edn. (Heptinstall, Flesher; London).

Gillispie, C.C., Ed. (1970–1980) *Dictionary of Scientific Biography*, 12 Vols. (Scribner, New York).

Girardi, M. (1791) *De Nervo Intercostali* (Tofani, Florence).

Gloor, P., Salanova, V., Olivier, A., & Quesney, L.F. (1993) The human dorsal hippocampal commissure: an anatomically identifiable and functional pathway. *Brain* **116**:1249–1273.

Goette A. (1873) Kurze Mittheilungen aus der Entwicklungsgeschichte der Unke. *Archiv für Mikroskopische Anatomie* **9**:396–412.

Goll, F. (1860) *Beiträge zur Feinern Anatomie des Menschlichen Rückenmarks* (Zürcher und Furrer, Zürich).

Gomez-Perez, A., Corcho, O., & Fernandez-Lopez, M. (2003) *Ontological Engineering: With Examples from the Areas of Knowledge Management, e-Commerce and the Semantic Web* (Springer, New York).

Gordh, G. & Headrick, D.H. (2001) *A Dictionary of Entomology* (CABI, Wallingford).

Gordon, J. (1815) *A System of Human Anatomy* (Blackwood, Edinburgh).

Gordon, J. (1817) *Observations on the Structure of the Brain, Comprising an Estimate of the Claims of Drs. Gall and Spurzheim to Discovery in the Anatomy of that Organ* (Blackwood, Edinburgh).

Goss, C.M. (1966) On Anatomy of Nerves by Galen of Pergamon. *American Journal of Anatomy* **118**:327–336.

Grainger, R.D. (1837) *Observations on the Structure and Functions of the Spinal Cord* (Highley, London).

Grant, R.E. (1834a) Lectures on comparative anatomy and animal physiology. Lecture XXXVI. On the nervous system of the radiated and helminthoid classes. *Lancet* **2**:481–487.

Grant, R.E. (1834b) Lectures on comparative anatomy and animal physiology. Lecture XXXVII. On the nervous system of the entomoid and molluscous classes. *Lancet* **2**:513–520.

Grant, R.E. (1834c) Lectures on comparative anatomy and animal physiology. Lecture XXXVIII. On the nervous system of the vertebrata. *Lancet* **2**:545–554.

Gratiolet, L.P. (1854) *Mémoire sur les Plis Cérébraux de l'Homme et des Primatès* (Bertrand, Paris).

Gratiolet, L.P. (1857); *see* Leuret, F. & Gratiolet, P. (1839–1857).

Grönberg, G. (1902) Die ontogenese eines niedern Säugergehirns nach Untersuchungen an Erinaceus europaeus. *Zoologische Jahrbücher. Abtheilung für Anatomie und Ontogenie der Thiere* **15**:261–384.

Gross, C.G. (1998) *Brain, Vision, Memory: Tales in the History of Neuroscience* (MIT Press, Cambridge).

Gruber, T.R. (1993) A translation approach to portable ontology specifications. *Knowledge Acquisition* **5**:199–220.

Gudden, B.v. (1870) Ueber einen bisher nicht beschriebenen Nervenfasernstrang im Gehirne der Säugerthiere und des Menschen. *Archiv für Psychiatrie und Nervenkrankheiten* **2**:364–366.

Gudden, B.v. (1889) Ueber das Corpus mammillare und die sogennaten Schenkel des Fornix. In: Grashley, H. (Ed.) *Bernhard von Gudden's Gesammelte und Hinterlassene Abhandlungen* (Bergmann, Wiesbaden), pp. 190–192. From a lecture in 1884.

Guidi, G. (1611) *De Anatome Corporis Humani* (Iuntas, Venice).

Guillaume de Conches (c1100–1154) Dogmaticon Philosophiae. In: Maccagnolo, E. (Ed.) *Il Divino e il Megacosmo. Testi Filosofici e Scientifici della Scuola di Chartres* (Rusconi, Milan), pp. 241–453, 1980.

Günther, D.E. (1786) *Cerebri et Nervorum Distributionis Expositio* (Typis viduae Benthonianae Acad. Typogr., Duisburg).

Günther, D.E. (1789) *Kurzer Entwurf der Anatomischen Nervenlehre* (Dänzer, Düsseldorf). Translation of Günther (1786).

Günther [Guenther], J., of Andernach (1531) *De Anatomicis Administrationibus Libri Novem. De Constitutione Artis Medicae Liber. De Theriaca, ad Pisonem Commentariolus. De Pulsibus, ad Medicinae Candidatos Liber. Per Joan. Guinterium Andernacum Latinitate jam Recens Donata* (Colinaeus, Paris).

Günther [Guenther], J., of Andernach (1536) *Anatomicarum Institutionum ex Galeni Sententia Libri IIII* (Lasium & Platterum, Basel).

Günz, J.G. (1750) *Prolusio: Observationes Anatomicae de Cerebro Continens* (Langenheim, Leipzig). Also appeared that year as Observationes anatomiques. *Mémoires de Mathématique et de Physique* **1**:283–292.

Günz, J.G. (1753) *Lapilli Glandulae Pinealis in Quinque Mente Alienatis Inventos Proponit* (Langenheim, Leipzig). Reprinted in Haller, A.v. (1757) *Disputationes ad Morborum et Curationem Facientes*, Vol. 1 (Bousquet, Lausanne), pp. 233–249.

Gurdjian, E.S. (1925) Olfactory connections in the albino rat, with special reference to the stria medullaris and the anterior commissure. *Journal of Comparative Neurology* **38**:127–163.

Gurdjian, E.S. (1927) The diencephalon of the albino rat. *Journal of Comparative Neurology* **43**:1–114.

Guy de Chauliac (1363) *Chirurgia Magna*. English translation by Leonard D. Rosenman, as *The Major Surgery of Guy de Chauliac* (Xlibris Corp., no place indicated) 2005.

Haase, J.G. (1781) *Cerebri Nervorumque Corporis Humani Anatome Repitita* (Junius, Leipzig).

Haberly, L.B. & Price, J.L. (1978) Association and commissural fiber systems of the olfactory cortex in the rat. II. Systems originating in the olfactory peduncle. *Journal of Comparative Neurology* **181**:781–808.

Hagelin, O. (1989) *Rare and Important Medical Books in the Library of the Swedish Society of Medicine* (Swedish Society of Medicine, Stockholm).

Hall, J. (1565) *A Most Excellent and Learned Woorke of Chirurgerie, Called Chirurgia Parva Lanfranci, Lanfranke of Mylayne his Briefe: Reduced from Dyvers Translations to our Vulgar or Usual Frase, and Now First Published in the Englysche Prynte by John Halle Chirurgien. Who Hath Thereunto Necessarily Annexed. A Table, as Wel of the Names of Diseases and Simples with their Vertues, as also of All Other Termes of the Arte Opened. Very Profitable for the Better Understanding of the Same, or Other Like Workes. And in the Ende A Compendious Worke of Anatomie, More Utile and Profitable, then Any Here Tofore in the Englyshe Tongue Publyshed. An Historiall Expostvlation Also Against the Beastly Abusers, Both of Chyrurgie and Phisicke in our Tyme: With a nd Goodly Doctrine, and Instruction, Necessary to be Marked and Solved of All xxx Chirurgies. All these Faithfully Gathered, and Diligently Set Forth, by the sayde John Halle* (Marshe, London).

Haller, A.v. (1743–1756) *Iconum Anatomicarum quibus Praecipuae Partes Corporis Humanae Delineatae Continentur Fasc. I [-VIII]*, 8 Fascicles (Vandenhoeck, Göttingen).

Haller, A.v. (1743) *Iconum Anatomicarum quibus Praecipuae Partes Corporis Humanae Delineatae Continentur Fasc. I* (Vandenhoeck, Göttingen).

Haller, A.v. (1747) *Primae Lineae Physiologiae in Usum Praelectionum Academicarum* (Vandenhoeck, Göttingen).

Haller, A.v. (1747–1751) *Disputationum Anatomicarum* (Vandenhoeck, Göttingen).

Haller, A.v. (1754a) *Iconum Anatomicarum quibus Praecipuae Partes Corporis Humanae Delineatae Continentur*, Fasc. VII (Vandenhoeck, Göttingen).

Haller, A.v. (1754b) *Dr. Albert Haller's Physiology; Being a Course of Lectures upon the Visceral Anatomy and Vital Oeconomy of Human Bodies: Including the Latest and Most Considerable Discoveries and Improvements, which have been Made by the Most Eminent Professors, Through All Parts of Europe, Down to the Present Year: Compiled for the Use of the University of Gottingen: Now Illustrated with Useful Remarks, with an History of Medicine, and with a Nosology, or Doctrine of Diseases* (Innys and Richardson, London). Translated by Samuel Mihles.

Haller, A.v. (1762) *Elementa Physiologiae Corporis Humani*, Vol. 4 (Grasset, Lausanne).

Haller, A.v. (1768) De cerebro avium et picium. In: *Operum Anatomici Argumenti Minorum*, Vol. 3. Last volume of *Opera Minora Emendata, Aucta, Renovata* (Grasset, Lausanne).

Haller, A.v. (1772) Alberti de Haller ad Figuram nervorum cordis lateris sinistri. Cl. Ivvenis Anderschii descipuli sui divinatio missa ad societatem regiam scientiarum d. XIV. aug. MDCCLXXI. *Novi Commentarii Societatis Regiae Scientairum Gottingensis (ad a. MDCCLXXI)* **2**:1–13. Haller described a figure his student C.S. Andersch had produced for his dissertation c1751–c1755 but never distributed; *see* Andersch (1797).

Haller, A.v. (1774–1777) *Bibliotheca Anatomica. Qua Scripta ad Anatomen et Physiologiam Facientia a Rerum Initiis Recensentur* (Tiguri, Orell, Gessner, Fuessli; no place indicated). Facsimile published by Olms (in Hildesheim) 1969.

Haller, A.v., Cullen, W., & Wrisberg, H.A. (1786) *First Lines of Physiology, by the Celebrated Baron Albertus Haller, M.D. Etc. Translated from the Correct Latin Edition Printed under the Inspection of William Cullen, M.D. and Compared with the Edition Published by H.A. Wrisberg, M.D. Professor at Gottingen. To which are Added, The Valuable Index Originally Composed for Dr Cullen's Edition; and All the Notes and Illustrations of Prof. Wrisberg, Now First Translated into English*, 2 Vols. (Elliot & Robinson, Edinburgh).

Haller, A.v. & Wrisberg, H.A. (1780) *Alberti v. Haller Primae Lineae Physiologiae in Usum Praelectionum Academicarum nunc Quarto Conscriptae Emendatae et Pluribus Animadversionibus Auctae ab Henrico Augusto Wrisberg Med. et Philos. Doct. Med. Anatomes et Art. Obst. Prof. Ord. Soc. Reg. Scient. Membro* (Vandenhoeck, Göttingen).

Haly Abbas or Ali ibn' ul-Abbas (d. 944); *see* Razi (1903), Wiberg, J. (1914).

Hamilton, W.J., Ed. (1976) *Textbook of Human Anatomy*, 2nd Edn. (Mosby, St. Louis).

Hamilton, W.J., Boyd, J.D., & Mossman, H.W. (1952) *Human Embryology: Prenatal Development of Form and Function* (Williams & Wilkins, Baltimore).

Hamilton, W.J. and Mossman, H.W. (1972) *Human Embryology: Prenatal Development of Form and Function*, 4th Edn. (Heffer & Sons, Cambridge).

Hanström, B. (1928) *Vergleichende Anatomie des Nervensystems der Wirbellosen Tiere, unter Berücksichtigung seiner Funktion* (Springer, Berlin).

Hanström, B. (1966) Gross anatomy of the hypophysis in mammals. In: Harris, G.W. & Donovan, B.T. (Eds.) *The Pituitary Gland*, Vol. 1 (University of California Press, Berkeley), pp. 1–57.

Harting, J.K. (1977) Descending pathways from the superior colliculus: an autoradiographic analysis in the rhesus monkey (*Macaca mulatta*). *Journal of Comparative Neurology* **173**:583–612.

Harvey, W. (1651) *Exercitationes de Generatione Animalium: Quibus Accedunt Quaedam de Partu: de Membranis ac Humoribus Uteri: & de Conceptione* (Pulleyn, London).

Harvey, W. (1653) *Anatomical Exercitations, Concerning the Generation of Living Creatures to which are Added Particular Discourses, of Births, and of Conceptions, Etc.* (Pulleyn, London).

Harvey, W. (1961) *Lectures on the Whole of Anatomy*, An Annotated Translation of *Prelectiones Anatomiae Universalis* by C.D. O'Malley, F.N.L. Poynter, & K.F. Russell (University of California Press, Berkeley).

Hayakawa, T. & Zyo, K. (1989) Retrograde double-labeling study of the mammillothalamic and the mammillotegmental projections in the rat. *Journal of Comparative Neurology* **284**:1–11.

Hayashi, M. (1924) Einige wichtige Tatsachen aus der ontogenetischen Entwicklung des menschlichen Kleinhirns. *Deutsche Zeitschrift für Nervenheilkunde* **81**:74–82.

Hayhow, W.R., Webb, C., & Jervie, A. (1960) The accessory optic fiber system in the rat. *Journal of Comparative Neurology* **115**:187–215.

Haymaker, W. & Woodhall, B. (1953) *Peripheral Nerve Injuries: Principles of Diagnosis* (Saunders, Philadelphia).

Heimer, L. & Wilson, R.D. (1975) The subcortical projections of the allocortex: similarities in the neural associations of the hippocampus, the piriform cortex, and the neocortex. In: Santini, M. (Ed.) *Golgi Centennial Symposium Proceedings* (Raven Press, New York), pp. 177–193.

Heinzeller, T. & Welsch, U. (2001) The echinoderm nervous system and its phylogenetic interretation. In: Roth, G. & Wullimann, M.F. (Eds.) *Brain Evolution and Cognition* (Wiley, New York), pp. 41–75.

Heister, L. (1717) *Compendium Anatomicum: Veterum Recentiorumque Observationes et Inventa Brevissime Complectens; in Usum Praecipue Auditorum Suorum Concinnatum* (Kohles, Altdorf).

Heister, L. (1721) *A Compendium of Anatomy. Containing a Short But Perfect View of All Parts of Humane Bodies. Wherein are Inserted, the Modern Discoveries: Together with a Variety of Curious Observations Never Before Made Publik.Translated from the Last Edition of D. Laurentius Heister, Professor of Anatomy, Surgery, and Physick in the University of Altorse, Etc. Adorn'd with Copper Plates* (Combes and Lacy, London).

Heister, L. (1752) *A Compendium of Anatomy. In which All the Parts of the Human Body are Succinctly and Clearly Described; and their Uses Explained. By Laurence Heister, M.D. Professor of Physick and Surgery in the University of Helmstadt, and Fellow of the Royal Societies of London and Paris. Translated from the Last Edition of the Original Latin: Greatly Augmented and Improved by the Author. To which are Added, Notes by M. Henault, and the Editor. Illustrated with Eight Large Copper Plates* (Innes & Richardson, Davis, Clarke, Manby, Whistlton & White, Rivington & Rivington, Cox; London).

Henle, J. (1871) *Handbuch der Nervenlehre des Menschen*. Part of *Handbuch der Systematischen Anatomie des Menschen*, Vol. III, Pt. II; published between 1855–1871 (Viewig, Braunschweig).

Hering, H.E. (1924) Die Aenderung des Herzschlagzahl durch Aenderung des arteriellen Blutdruckes erfolgt auf reflectorischem Wege. *Pflüger's Archiv für die Gesamte Physiologie des Menschen und der Tiere* **206**:721–723.

Herophilus (c335–c280 BC); *see* Solmsen (1961), von Staden (1969), Longrigg (1993).

Herrick, C.J. (1910) The morphology of the forebrain in amphibia and reptilia. *Journal of Comparative Neurology and Psychology* **20**:413–547.

Herrick, C.J. (1915) *An Introduction to Neurology* (Saunders, Philadelphia).

Herrick, C.J. (1917) The internal structure of the midbrain and thalamus of Necturus. *Journal of Comparative Neurology* **28**:215–348.

Heschl, R.L. (1878) *Ueber die Vordere quere Schläfenwindung des Menschlichen Grosshirns* (Braumüller, Vienna).

Hierons, R. & Meyer, A. (1962) Some priority questions arising from Thomas Willis' work on the brain. *Proceedings of the Royal Society of Medicine* **55**:287–292.

Hildebrandt, G.F. (1803) *Lehrbuch der Anatomie des Menschen*, 3rd Edn. (Schulbuchhandlung, Braunschweig).

Hill, A. (1893) The hippocampus. *Proceedings of the Royal Society of London B* **184**:389–429.

Hill, C.J. (1927) A contribution to our knowledge of the enteric plexuses. *Philosophical Transactions of the Royal Society of London B* **215**:355–387.

Hines, M. (1922) Studies in the growth and differentiation of the telencephalon in man. The fissura hippocampi. *Journal of Comparative Neurology* **34**:73–171.

Hippocrates, *Fleshes*. Edited and translated by P. Potter: *Hippocrates*, Vol. VIII (Harvard University Press, Cambridge) 1995, pp. 132–165. Hippocratic Corpus or writers is implied.

Hippocrates, *Places in Man*. Edited and translated by P. Potter: *Hippocrates*, Vol. VIII (Harvard University Press, Cambridge) 1995, pp. 18–101. Hippocratic Corpus or writers is implied.

Hippocrates, *On the Sacred Disease*. In *The Genuine Works of Hippocrates*, translated from the Greek by Francis Adams (reprinted by Krieger, Huntington NY, 1972). Hippocratic Corpus or writers is implied.

Hirsch, A.B.R. (1765) *Pars Quinti Nervorum Encephali Disquisition Anatomica* (no publisher provided, Vienna).

Hirschfeld, L. & Léveillé, J.B. (1853) *Névrologie; Ou, Description et Iconographie du Système Nerveux et des Organes des Sens de l'Homme avec leur Mode de Préparation* (Baillière, Paris).

His, W. (1889) Die Neuroblasten und deren Entstehung im embryonalen Mark. *Abhandlungen der Mathematisch-physischen Classe der Königlich Sächsischen Gesellschaft der Wissenschaften* **15**:313–372.

His, W. (1892) Zur allgemeine Morphologie des Gehirns. *Archiv für Anatomie und Entwickelungsgeschichte* (1892), [no volume indicated] pp. 346–383.

His, W. (1893a) Ueber das frontale Ende des Gehirnrohres. *Archiv für Anatomie und Entwickelungsgeschichte*, [no volume indicated] pp. 157–171.

His, W. (1893b) Vorschläge zur Eintheilung des. *Gehirns Archiv für Anatomie und Entwickelungsgeschichte*, [no volume indicated] pp. 172–179.

His, W. (1895) Die anatomische Nomenclatur. Nomina anatomica. *Archiv für Anatomie und Physiologie*, Supplement-Band, pp. 1–180.

Hitchings, H. (2005) *Defining the Word: the Extraordinary Story of Dr. Johnson's Dictionary* (Farrar, Straus and Giroux; New York).

Hoffmann, J.M. (1703) *Idea Machinae Humaae Anatomico-Physiologica ad Observationes Recentiores Conformata et ad Methodum Sectionum Solennium Accomodata: Annexa est Ejusdem Decas Programmatum Anatomicorum* (Meyeri, Altdorf).

Holmes, R.L. & Ball, J.N. (1974) *The Pituitary Gland: A Comparative Account* (Cambridge University Press, Cambridge).

Honegger, J. (1890) Vergleichend-anatomische untersuchungen über den Fornix und die zu ihm in beziehung gebrachten gebilde im Gehirn des Menschen und der Säugethiere. *Recueil Zoologique Suisse* **5**:201–434.

Hooper, R. (1797) *The Anatomist's Vade-Mecum Containing a Concise and Accurate Description of the Structure, Situation, and Use of Every Part of the Human Body, To Which is Added, an Explanation of Anatomical Terms. For the Use of Students, Etc. By Robert Hooper, of Pembroke College, Oxford. M.D. F.L.S. Etc.* (Bell, London).

Horne, J. van (1662) *Mikrokosmos; Seu, Brevis Manuductio ad Historiam Corporis Humani*, 3rd Edn. (Chouët, Leiden).

Horne, J. van (1707) *Opuscula Anatomico-Chirurgica* (Fritsch, Leipzig).

Hovelacque, A. (1927) *Anatomie des Nerfs Craniens et Rachidiens du Système Grand Sympathique chez l'Homme* (Doin, Paris).

Huard, P. & Imbault-Huart, M.-J. (1980) *André Vésale: Iconographie Anatomique* (Dacosta, Paris).

Huber, J.J. (1741) *De Medulla Spinali, Speciatim de Nervis ab ea Provenientibus Commentatio: Cum Adiunctis Icon* (Vandenhoeck, Göttingen).

Huber, J.J. (1744) *Epistola Anatomica de Nervo Intercostali, de Nervis Octavi et Noni Paris deque Accessorio; Nonnulla Tradens ad Virum Ilustrem D.D. Wolrath Wigand Potentissimi Suecorum Regis Consiliarium et Archiatrum Ioh. Iacobi Huberi D* (Vandenhoeck, Göttingen).

Huber, J.J. (1760) *Observationes Aliquot Anatomicae* (Schmiedt, Kassel).

Hundt, M. (1501) *Antropologium de Ho[min]is Dignitate, Natura, et P[ro]prietatibus: de Elementis, Partibus, et Me[m]bris Humani Corp[or]is: de Iuuamentis Nocume[n]tis, Accide[n] tib[us], Vicijs, Remedijs, et Physionomia Ipsorum: de Exceme[n]tis et Exeu[n]tib[us]: de Spiritu Hu[m]ano eiusq[ue] Natura P[ar]tib[us] et Op[er]ib[us]: de Ani[m] a Hu[m]ana et Ipsius Appendicijs* (per Baccalareu[m] Wolfgangu[m] Monacensem, Leipzig).

Huschke, E. (1854) *Schädel, Hirn und Seele des Menschen und der Thiere nach Alter, Geschlecht und Race, dargestellt nach Neuen Methoden und Untersuchungen* (Mauke, Jena).

International Anatomical Nomenclature Committee (1955), *see Nomina Anatomica* (1955).

International Anatomical Nomenclature Committee (1983), *see Nomina Anatomica* (1983).

International Commission on Zoological Nomenclature (1999) *International Code of Zoological Nomenclature* (International Trust for Zoological Nomenclature, London).

Jacobaeus, O. (1675) Anatome Psittaci. *Acta Medica & Philosophica Hafniensia, Anni 1673* (published 1675) **2**:314–318.

Jacobsohn, L. (1909) *Über die Kerne des Menschlichen Hirnstamms (Medulla Oblongata, Pons und Pedunculus cerebri.)* (Königlich Akademie der Wissenschaften, Berlin).

Jacobson, L. (1818) *De Quinto Nervorum Pari Animalium* (Hartungianis, Königsberg).

Jacobson, L.L. (1809) Description anatomique d'un organe observé dans les mammifères. *Annales du Muséum d'Histoire Naturelle* **18**:412–423.

Jacobson, L.L. (1813) Anatomisk Beskrivelse over et nyt Organ i Huusdyrenes Naese. *Veterinair-Selskabets Skrifter* **2**:209–246.

Jacobson, L.L. (1818) Supplementa ad otojatriam. Supplementum primum de anastomosi nervorum nova in aure detecta. *Acta Nova Regiae Societatis Medicae Havniensis* **5**:292–303.

Jacobson, L.L. (1948) *Ouvrages sur L'Organe Voméro-Nasal* (Munksgaard, Copenhagen).

Jacobson, M. (1993) *Foundations of Neuroscience* (Plenum, New York).

Jansen, J. & Brodal, A. (1954) *Aspects of Cerebellar Anatomy* (Tanum, Olso).

Johnson, S. (1775) *A Dictionary of the English Language in which the Words are Deduced from their Originals, and Illustrated in their Different Significations by Examples from the best Writers. To which are Prefixed, a History of the Language, and an English Grammar* (Knapton et al., London).

Johnston, J.B. (1913) The morphology of the septum, hippocampus, and pallial commissures in repl[t]iles and mammals. *Journal of Comparative Neurology* **23**:371–478.

Johnston, J.B. (1923) Further contributions to the study of the evolution of the forebrain. *Journal of Comparative Neurology* **35**:337–481.

Johnstone, J. (1765) Essay on the use of the ganglions of the nerves. *Philosophical Transactions of the Philosophical Society of London* **54**:177–187.

Johnstone, J. (1767) History of a foetus born with a very imperfect brain; to which is subjoined a supplement of the essay on the use of ganglions, published in Philos. Trans. for 1764. *Philosophical Transactions of the Philosophical Society of London* **57**:118–131.

Johnstone, J. (1795) *Medical Essays and Observations with Disquisitions Relating to the Nervous System* (Agg, Evesham).

Jones, E.G. (1985) *The Thalamus* (Plenum Press, New York).

Jördens, J.H. (1788) *Descriptio Nervi Ischiadici* (Waltheri, Erlangen).

Ju, G. & Swanson, L.W. (1989) Studies on the cellular architecture of the bed nuclei of the stria terminalis in the rat: I. Cytoarchitecture. *Journal of Comparative Neurology* **280**:587–602.

Judas, M., Sedmar, G., & Pletikos, M. (2010) Early history of subplate and interstitial neurons: from Theodor Meynert (1867) to the discovery of the subplate zone (1974). *Journal of Anatomy* **217**:344–367.

Kawai, T., Oka, Y., & Eisthen, H. (2009) The role of the terminal nerve and GnRH in olfactory system neuromodulation. *Zoological Science* **26**:669–680.

Keill, J. (1698) *The Anatomy of the Human Body Abridged, or, A Short and Full View of All the Parts of the Body Together with their Several Uses Drawn from their Compositions and Structures* (Kebelwhite, London).

Kerr, A.T. (1918) The brachial plexus of nerves in man, the variations in its formation and branches. *The American Journal of Anatomy* **23**:285–395.

Keuffel, G.G.T. (1810) *De Medulla Spinali* (In officina Batheana, Halle).

Key, A. & Retzius, G. (1875–1876) *Studien in der Anatomie des Nervensystems und des Bindegewebes*, 2 Vols. (Samson & Wallin, Stockholm).

Kilian, H.F. (1822) *Anatomische Untersuchungen über das Neunte Hirnnervenpaar oder den Nervus Glossopharyngeus: Nebst Angehängten Bemerkungen über das Anatomische Museum zu Strassburg* (Hartleben, Pesth/Budapest).

Kimmel, D.L. (1961) Innervation of spinal dura mater and dura mater of posterior cranial fossa. *Neurology* **11**:800–809.

Kingsbury, B.F. (1934) The development of the septum medullae (mammals: cat). *Journal of Comparative Neurology* **60**:81–109.

Kitchell, K.F. & Resnick, I.M. (1999), *see* Albertus Magnus (13th century) *On Animals: A Medieval Summa Zoologica.*

Klint, J.J. (1784) *Commentatio Inauguralis Anatomica de Nervis Brachii* (Vandenhoeck, Göttingen).

Knox, R. (1832) *Engravings of the Cardiac Nerves, the Nerves of the Ninth Pair, the Glossopharyngeal, and the Pharyngeal Branch of the Pneumogastric*, 3rd Edn. (MacLachlan & Stewart, Edinburgh).

Kobler, J.B., Datta, S., Goyal, R.K., & Benecchi, E.J. (1994) Innervation of the larynx, pharynx, and upper esophageal sphincter of the rat. *Journal of Comparative Neurology* **349**:129–147.

Kölliker, A. (1896) *Handbuch der Gewebelehre des Menschen*, 6th Edn., Zweiter Band: *Nervensystem des Menschen und der Thiere* (Engelmann, Leipzig).

Koning, P. de (1903); *see* Razi, Abu Bakr Muhammad ibn Zakariya (1903) *Trois Traités d'Anatomie Arabes.*

Koslow, S.H. & Huerta, M.F. (1997) *Neuroinformatics* (Erlbaum, Mahwah NJ).

Krettek, J.E. & Price, J.L. (1978) A description of the amygdaloid complex in the rat and cat with observations on intra-amygdaloid axonal connections. *Journal of Comparative Neurology* **178**:255–279.

Krüger, E. (1758) *De Nervo Phrenico* (Oficina Breitkopfia, Leipzig).

Kruger, L, Saporta, S., & Swanson, L.W. (1995) *Photographic Atlas of the Rat Brain: The Cell and Fiber Architecture Illustrated in Three Planes with Stereotaxic Coordinates* (Cambridge University Press, Cambridge).

Kuhlenbeck, H. (1927) *Vorlesungen über das Zentralnervensystem der Wirbeltiere* (Fischer, Jena).

Kuhlenbeck, H. (1928) Bemerkungen zur Morphologie des Occipitallappens des menschlichen Grosshirns. *Anatomischer Anzeiger* **65**:273–294.

Kuhlenbeck, H. (1975a) *The Central Nervous System of Vertebrates. A General Survey of its Comparative Anatomy with an Introduction to the Pertinent Fundamental Biologic and Logical Concepts; Vol. 4: Spinal Cord and Deuterencephalon* (Karger, Basel).

Kuhlenbeck, H. (1975b) *The Central Nervous System of Vertebrates. A General Survey of its Comparative Anatomy with an Introduction to the Pertinent Fundamental Biologic and Logical Concepts; Vol. 5, Pt. 2: Mammalian Telencephalon: Surface Morphology and Cerebral Cortex. The Vertebrate Neuraxis as a Whole* (Karger, Basel).

Kühn, C.G. (1821–1823) *Opera Omnia*, 20 Vols. (Cnobloch, Leipzig). Galen's complete works.

Kuntz, A. (1929) *The Autonomic Nervous System* (Lea & Fibiger, Philadelphia).

Künzle, H. (2004) The hippocampal continuation (indusium griseum): its connectivity in the hedgehog tenrec and its status within the hippocampal formation of higher vertebrates. *Anatomy and Embryology* **208**:183–213.

Kupffer, C.v. (1885) Primäre Metamerie des Neuralrohrs der Vertebraten. *Sitzungsberichte der Mathematisch-Physikalischen Classe der Königlich-Bayerische Akademie der Wissenschaften zu München* **15**:469–476.

Kwak, H.H., Ko, S.J., Jung, H.S., Park, H.D., Chung, I.H., & Kim, H.J. (2003) Topographic anatomy of the deep temporal nerves, with references to the superior head of lateral pterygoid. *Surgical and Radiological Anatomy* **25**:393–399.

La Charrière, J. de (1703) *Anatomie Nouvelle de la Tête de l'Homme, et de ses Dépendances: avec l'Usage de ses Parties, suivant leur Structure et la Physique Moderne* (Hortemels, Paris).

Lancisi, G.M. (1713) Joh. Mariae Lancisi diss. de sede cogitantis animae ad Joh. Fantonum. In: Fantoni, G.B. (1713) *Jo. Baptistae Fantoni Regiae Celsitudinis Victorii Amedei II... Medici... Observationes Anatomico-Medicae* (Poleti, Venice). Quoted by Burdach, K.F. (1822), p. 365.

Lancisi, G.M. (1714), *see* Eustachi, B. (1714).

Lancisi, G.M. (1718) *Dissertatio Altera de Sede Cogitantis Animae*. In: *Jo. Mariae Lancissi Opera quae Hactenus Prodierun Omnia Dissertationibus Nonnullis adhuc dum Ineditis Locupletata, & ab ipso Auctore, Recognita atque Emendata*, Vol. 2 (Cramer, Geneva).

Lancisi, G.M. (1719) *De Vena Sine Pari*. In: Morgagni, G. (1719) *Adversaria Anatomica Sexti* (Cominus, Padua), pp. 75–95.

Lancisi, G.M. (1728) *Joannis Mariae Lancisii: A Secretiori Cubiculo, & Archiatri Pontificii: De Motu Cordis et Aneurysmatibus Opus Posthumum in Duas Partes Divisum; Sanctissimo Patri Clementi XI. Felicis Recordationis Dicatum* (Salvioni, Rome).

Landi, B. (1542) *De Humana Historia vel Singularum Hominis Partium Cognitione Libri Duo, nunc Primùm & Scripti & in Lucem Editi: Adiectus est Rerum et Verborum in his Memorabilium Index Locupletissimus* (Oporinus, Basel).

Langenbeck, C.J.M. (1826–1830) *Icones Anatomicae, Neurologia*. Fasc. I–III (Dieterich, Göttingen).

Langley, J.N. (1878) On the physiology of the salivary secretion. Part I. The influence of the chorda tympani and sympathetic nerves upon the secretion of the sub-maxillary gland of the cat. *Journal of Physiology (London)* **1**:96–103.

Langley, J.N. (1898) On the union of cranial autonomic (visceral) fibres with the nerve cells of the superior cervical ganglion. *Journal of Physiology (London)* **23**:240–270.

Langley, J.N. (1900) The sympathetic and other related systems of nerves. In: Schäfer, E.A. (Ed.) *Textbook of Physiology*, Vol. 2 (Pentland, Edinburgh), pp. 616–696.

Langley, J.N. (1905) On the reactions of cells and of nerve endings to certain poisons, chiefly as regards the reaction of striated muscle to nicotine and to curare. *Journal of Physiology (London)* **33**:374–413.

Langley, J.N. (1921) *The Autonomic Nervous System* (Heffer & Sons, Cambridge).

Langley, J.N. & Anderson, H.K. (1895) On the innervation of the pelvic and adjoining viscera. Part I. The lower portion of the intestine. *Journal of Physiology* **18**:67–105.

Larriva-Sahd, J. (2008) The accessory olfactory bulb in the adult rat: a cytological study of its cell types, neuropil, neuronal modules, and interactions with the main olfactory system. *Journal of Comparative Neurology* **510**:309–350.

Larsell, O. (1937) The cerebellum: a review and interpretation. *Archives of Neurology & Psychiatry* **38**:580–607.

Larsell, O. (1967) *The Comparative Anatomy and Histology of the Cerebellum, from Myxinoids through Birds* (University of Minnesota Press, Minneapolis).

Larsell, O. & Jansen, J. (1972) *The Comparative Anatomy and Histology of the Cerebellum; the Human Cerebellum, Cerebellar Connections, and Cerebellar Cortex* (University of Minnesota Press, Minneapolis).

Last, R.J. & Tompsett, D.H. (1953) Casts of the cerebral ventricles. *British Journal of Surgery* **40**:525–543.

Laumonier, J.-B. (1793) Observation anatomico-physiologique, Extraite d'un ouvrage sur les sympathies nerveuses, considérées dans l'état de santé et de maladie. *Journal de Médecine, Chirurgie et Pharmacie* **93**:259–263.

Laurencet, M. (1825) *Anatomie du Cerveau dans les Quarte Classes d'Animaux Vertébres* (The Author and Croullebois, Paris).

[Guyton de Morveau, L.-B.], Lavoisier, A.L., Berthollet, C.-L., Fourcroy, A.-F. de, Hassenfratz, J.H., & Adet, P.-A. (1787) *Méthode de Nomenclature Chemique: Proposée par MM. de Morveau, Lavoisier, Bertholet et de Fourcroy. On y a Joint un Nouveau Systéme de Caractéres Chimiques Adaptés a cette Nomenclature, par MM. Hassenfratz et Adet* (Cuchet, Paris).

Lazorthes, G. (1949) *Le Système Neurovasculaire: Étude Anatomique, Physiologique, Pathologique et Chirurgicale* (Masson, Paris).

Le Boë, F. de (1663) *Disputationum Medicarum Pars Prima: Primarias Corporis Humani Functiones Natural, ex Anatomicus Practicis & Chimicis Experimentis Deductus Complectens* (van den Bergh, Amsterdam).

Le Boë, F. de (1680) *Francisci Deleboe, Sylvii Opera Medica: Tam Hactenus Inedita, quam Variis Locis & Formis Edita: Nunc Verò Certo Ordine Disposita, & in Unum Volumen Redacta: cum Duplici Indice, uno Librorum & Capitum, oeri Praemisso Altero Rerum ad Calcem Adjecto* (Elsevier, Amsterdam).

Le Boë, F. de (1695) *Francisci Deleboe, Sylvii Opera Medica, Tam Hactenus Inedita, quàm Variis Locis & Formis Edita Nunc Verò Certo Ordine Disposita, & in Unum Volumen redacta. Editio Nova cui Accedunt Casus Medicinales Annor. 1659. 60. & 61. quos ex ore cl. Sylvii Calamo Excepti Joachimus Merian* (van de Water, Utrecht & Schelte, Amsterdam).

Le Cat, C.N. (1768) *Oeuvres Physiologiques*, Vol. 3. *La Théorie de l'Ouie: Supplément a cet Article du Traité des Sens* (Vallat-la-Chapelle, Paris).

Leeuwenhoek, A. van (1684) De formatione tumoris Cristallini in variis animalibus, avibus, ac piscibus; de substantia fibrosa quae in oculo apparet; de liquore in & per tunicam corneam; de formatione exiquae arteriae; de epidermide Aethiopissae. Nobilissimo domino Francisco Aston. Regio collegio à Secretis. S.P.D. Antonius a Leeuwenhoek. April 1684. In: *Arcana Naturae Detecta* (Langerak, Leiden, 1722).

Leeuwenhoek, A. van (1685) An abstract of a letter from Mr. Anthony Leeuwenhoek, Fellow of the Royal Society, concerning the parts of the brain of several animals. *Philosophical Transactions of the Royal Society of London* **15**:883–895.

Leeuwenhoek, A. van (1722) *Arcana Naturae Detecta* (Arnold, Langenrak; Leiden).

Lekakis, G.K. (2003) Philipp Friedrich Arnold, Ludvig Levin Jacobson and their contribution to head and neck anatomy. *Journal of Laryngology and Otolaryngology* **117**:28–31.

Leonardo da Vinci, *see* O'Malley & Saunders (1982).

Leuret, F. (1839) *Anatome Comparée du Système Nerveux Considéré dans ses Rapports avec l'Intelligence* (Ballière, Paris).

Leuret, F. & Gratiolet, P. (1839–1857) *Anatomie Comparée du Système Nerveux Considéré dans ses Rapports avec l'Intelligence*, 2 Vols. & Atlas (Baillière et Fils, Paris).

Lewandowsky, M. (1903) Beiträge zur anatomie des Hirnstammes. *Journal für Psychologie und Neurologie* **2**:18–28.

Lewis, F.T. (1923) The significance of the term hippocampus. *Journal of Comparative Neurology* **35**:213–230.

Lewy, F.H. (1942) Historical introduction: the basal ganglia and their diseases. In: *The Diseases of the Basal Ganglia*, Association for Research in Nervous and Mental Disease Vol. XXI (Williams & Wilkins, Baltimore), pp. 1–20.

Lieutaud, J. (1742) *Essais Anatomiques, Contenant l'Histoire Exacte des toutes les Parties qui Composent le Corps de l'Homme*, 2 Vols. (Huart, Paris).

Lind, L.R. (1949) *The Epitome of Andreas Vesalius*, Translated from the Latin with Preface and Introduction by L.R. Lind, with Anatomical Notes by C.W. Asling, and a Foreword by the late Logan Clendening (Macmillan, New York).

Lind, L.R. (1959), *see* Berengario da Carpi (1522) *A Short Introduction to Anatomy.*

Lind, L.R. (1975) *Studies in Pre-Vesalian Anatomy: Biography, Translations, Documents* (American Philosophical Society, Philadelphia).

Linnaeus, C. (1758) *Systema Naturae: per Regna Tria Naturae Secundum Classes, Ordines, Genera, Species; cum characteribus et Differentiis*, 10th Edn. (Salvius, Holmiae).

Lissauer, H. (1886) Beitrag zum Faserverlauf im Hinterhorn des menschlichen Rückenmarks und zum Verhalten desselben bei Tabes dorsalis. *Archiv für Psychiatrie un Nervenkrankheiten* **17**:377–437.

Lloyd, G.E.R. (1975) Alcmaeon and the early history of dissection. *Sudhoff's Archiv* **59**:113–147.

Lobstein, J.F. (1760) *Dissertatio Inauguralis Anatomica de Nervo Spinali ad Par Vagum Accessorio, quam sub Divini Numinis Auspicio ex Decreto Gratiosae Facultatatis Medicae pro Licentia Summos in Arte Medica Honores et Provilegia Doctoralia Rite Consequendi; Publice Defendet Johannes Fridericus Lobstein Argentinensis.Die XVI Julii MDCCLX. H.L.Q.C.* (Pauschingerianae, Strasbourg).

Lobstein, J.F. (1823) *De Nervi Sympathetici Humani Fabrica Usu et Morbis: Commentatio Anatomico-physiologico-pathologica: Tabulis Aeneis et Lithographicis Illustrata* (Levrault, Paris).

Lobstein, J.F. (1831) *A Treatise on the Structure, Functions and Diseases of the Human Sympathetic Nerve. Illustrated with Plates* (Auner, Philadelphia).

Loder, J.C. (1778) *Primae Lineae Neurologicae Corporis Humani, Commentatio I* (Finkelscheer, Jena).

Loder, J.C. (1794–1803) *Tabulae Anatomicae*, 2 Vols. & Atlas (Landes-Industrie-Comptoir, Weimar).

Longet, F.-A. (1842) *Anatomie et Physiologie du Système Nerveux de l'Homme et des Animaux Vertébrés*, 2 Vols. (Fortin, Masson; Paris).

Longrigg, J. (1993) *Greek Rational Medicine: Philosophy and Medicine from Alcmaeon to the Alexandrians* (Routledge, New York).

Longrigg, J. (1998) *Greek Medicine: From the Heroic to the Hellenistic Age: A Source Book* (Routledge, New York).

Loo, Y.T. (1931) The forebrain of the opossum, Didelphis virginiana. *Journal of Comparative Neurology* **52**:1–148.

Lorente de Nó, R. (1934) Studies on the structure of the cerebral cortex. II. Continuation of the study of the ammonic system. *Journal für Psychologie und Neurologie (Leipzig)* **46**:113–177.

Ludwig, C.F. (1779) *De Cinerea Cerebri Substantia Consensu Gratiosi Medicorum Ordinis pro Summis in Arte Medica Honoribus* (Ex Officina Breitkopfia, Leipzig).

Ludwig, C.F. (1791–1795) *Scriptores Nevrologici Minores Selecti sive Opera Minora ad Anatomiam Physilogiam et Pathologiam Nervorum Spectantia*, 4 Vols. (Ivnivm, Leipzig).

Ludwig, C.G. (1772) *De Plexibus Nervorum Abdominalium atque Nervo Intercostali Duplici Observationes Nonnullae* (Ex Officina Langenhemia, Leipzig).

Luschka, H. von (1862) Ueber die drüsenartige natur der sogenannten ganglion intercaroticum. *Archiv für Anatomie Physiologie und Wissenschaftliche Medicin* [no volume indicated], pp. 406–414.

Lyonnet, P. (1762) *Traité Anatomique de la Chenille: Qui Ronge le Bois de Saule, Augmenté d'Une Explication Abregée des Planches, et d'Une Description de l'Instrument et des outils dont l'Auteur s'Est Servi, pour Anatomiser à la Loupe & au Microscope, & pour Déterminer la Force de ses Verres, Suivant les Règles de l'Optique, & Méchaniquement* (Gosse & Pinet et Rey, The Hague).

Mackay, A.L. (1977) *Scientific Quotations: The Harvest of a Quiet Eye* (Crane, Russak; New York).

Magendie, F. (1825) Sur un liquide qui se trouve dans le crane et le canal vertébral de l'homme et des animaux mammifères. *Journal de Physiologie Expérimentale et Pathologique* **5**:27–37.

Magendie, F. (1827) Second mémoire sur le liquide qui se trouve dans le crane et l'épine de l'homme et des animaux vertébrés. *Journal de Physiologie Expérimentale et Pathologique* **7**:1–29.

Magendie, F. (1828) Memoire physiologique sur le cerveau. *Journal de Physiologie Expérimentale et Pathologique* **8**:221–229.

Malacarne, V. (1776) *Nuova Esposizione della Vera Struttura del Cervelletto Umano* (Briolo, Turin); reprinted in Malacarne, V. (1780), Pt. 3, pp. 17–129.

Malacarne, V. (1780) *Encefalotomia Nuova Universale* (Briolo, Turin).

Malacarne, V. (1791) *Neuro-Encefalotomia* (no publisher provided, Pavia).

Malacarne, V. (1795) Encefalotomia di alcuni quadrupedi. *Memorie della Reale Accademia di Scienze, Belle Lettere ed Arti di Mantova* **1**:55–95.

Malone E. (1910) Über die Kerne des menschlichen Zwischenhirns. *Neurologisches Centralblatt* **29**:290–300.

Malpighi, M. (1665) De cerebro. In: *Tetras Anatomicarum Epistolarum de Lingua, et Cerebro* (Benati, Bologna), pp. 1–46.

Malpighi, M. (1666) *De Viscerum Structura Exercitatio Anatomica* (Montius, Bologna).

Malpighi, M. (1669) *Marcelli Malpighii Dissertatio Epistolica de Bombyce: Societati Regiae, Londini ad Scientiam Naturalem Promovendam Institutae Dicta* (Martyn & Allestry, London).

Malpighi, M. (1673) *Dissertatio Epistolica de Formatione Pulli in Ovo* (Martin, London).

Malpighi, M. (1675–1679) *Anatome Plantarum. Cui Subjungitur Appendix Iteratas et Auctas ejusdem Authoris de Ovo Incubato Observationes Continens*, 2 Vols. (Martin, London).

Manfredi, H. (1490), *see* Singer, C. (1917).

Mangili, G. (1804) *Nuove Ricerche Zootomiche sopra Alcune Specie de Conchiglie Bivalvi* (Genio, Milan).

Manzoni, T. (1998) The cerebral ventricles, the animal spirits and the dawn of brain localization of function. *Archives Italiennes de Biologie* **136**:103–152.

Marchetti, D. de (1652) *Anatomia, cui Responsiones ad Riolanum, Antomicum Parisiensem, in Ipsius Animadversionibus Contra Veslingium Additae sunt* (Bolzettam, Padua).

Martin, R. (1781) *Institutiones Neurologicae, Sive de Nervis Corporis Humani Tractatio: Praemissa est Oratio de Proprietatibus Nervorum Generalioribus, Publice Habita in Regia Academia Scientiarum Suecana. Editio Altera, Latine Reddita, Recentiorum Observationibus Aucta et Priori Emendatior*, 2 Vols. (Sumtibus Magni Swederi, Stockholm and Leipzig).

Massa, N. (1536) *Liber Introductorius Anatomiae* (Bindoni & Pasini, Venice).

Matsuda N. (1914) Über das Brückengrau des Menschen (Griseum pontis) und dessen nähere Beziehungen zum Kleinhirn und Grosshirn. *Arbeiten aus dem Hirnanatomischen Institut in Zürich* **9**:1–249.

May, M.T. (1968), *see* Galen (c173) *On the Usefulness of the Parts of the Body.*

Mayer, J.C.A. (1779) *Anatomisch-Physiologische Abhandlung vom Gehirn, Rückmark, und Ursprung der Nerven* (Decker, Berlin).

Mayer, J.C.A. (1783–1794) *Beschreibung des Ganzen Menschlichen Körpers*, 8 Vols. (Decker, Berlin).

Mayer, J.C.A. (1783–1794) *Anatomische Kupfertafeln, nebst dazu Gehörigen Erklärungen*, 6 Parts (Decker, Berlin & Leipzig for Parts 1–4; Rottmann, Berlin for Parts 5–6).

Mayer, J.C.A. (1786) *Anatomische Kupfertafeln, nebst dazu Gehörigen Erklärungen*, Part 4 (Decker, Berlin).

Mayer, J.C.A. (1794) *Anatomische Kupfertafeln, nebst dazu Gehörigen Erklärungen*, Parts 5 and 6 (Rottmann, Berlin). Also published as *Anatomische Kupfertafeln zur Erläuterung des Nervensystems, nebst dazu Gehörigen Erklärungen*, 2 Parts (Rotmann, Berlin).

Mayo, H. (1822) *Anatomical and Physiological Commentaries*, Number I (Underwood, London). Facsimile published together with Number II by The Classics of Neurology & Neurosurgery Library (Birmingham, 1985).

Mayo, H. (1823) *Anatomical and Physiological Commentaries*, Number II (Underwood, London). Provided rough translations of much of Reil's work on the brain. Facsimile published together with Number I by The Classics of Neurology & Neurosurgery Library (Birmingham, 1985).

Mayo, H. (1827) *A Series of Engravings Intended to Illustrate the Structure of the Brain and Spinal Chord in Man* (Burgess and Hill, London).

Mazzolini, R.G. (1991) Schemes and models of the thinking machine (1662–1762). In: Corsi, P. (Ed.), *The Enchanted Loom: Chapters in the History of Neuroscience* (Oxford University Press, New York), pp. 68–143, 198–200.

Meckel, J.F., the Elder (1748) *Tractus Anatomico Physiologicus de Quinto Pare Nervorum Cerebri* (Vandenhoek, Göttingen).

Meckel, J.F., the Elder (1751) Observation anatomique sur un noeud, ou ganglion, du second rameau de la cinquieme paire des nerfs du cerveau, nouvellement découvert, avec l'examen physiologique du véritable usage des noeuds, ou ganglions des nerfs. *Histoire de l'Académie Royale des Sciences et Belle-Lettres de Berlin, Année 1749* **5**:84–102.

Meckel, J.F., the Elder (1753) Dissertation anatomique sur les nerfs de la face. *Histoire de l'Académie Royale des Sciences et Belle-Lettres de Berlin, Année 1751* **9**:19–130.

Meckel, J.F., the Elder (1767) Observations anatomiques sur la glande pineale, sur la cloison transparente, et sur l'origine du nerf de la septieme paire. *Histoire de l'Académie Royale des Sciences et des Belles-Lettres de Berlin, Année 1765* **21**:91–101.

Meckel, J.F., the Younger (1815) Versuch einer Entwicklung der Centraltheile des nervensystems bei den Säugthieren. *Deutsches Archiv für die Physiologie* **1**:1–108, 334–422, 589–639.

Meckel, J.F., the Younger (1817) *Handbuch der Menschlichen Anatomie*, Vol. 3 (Buchhandlung des Hallischen Maisenhauses, Berlin).

Meckel, J.F., the Younger (1832) *Manual of General, Descriptive, and Pathological Anatomy*, 3 Vols. (Carey & Lea, Philadelphia).

Meessen, H. & Olszewski, J. (1949) *A Cytoarchitectonic Atlas of the Rhombencephalon of the Rabbit* (Karger, Basel).

Meissner, F.L. (1830) *Encyclopädie der Medicinischen Wissenschaften, nach dem Dictionnaire de Médecine Frei Bearb. und mit Nöthigen Zusätzen Versehen* (Fest, Leipzig).

Mery, J. (1698), *see* Brunet (1697)

Mettler, C.C. (1947) *History of Medicine: A Correlative Text, Arranged According to Subjects* (Blakiston, Philadelphia).

Mettler, F.A. (1948) *Neuroanatomy*, 2nd Edn. (Mosby, St. Louis).

Meyer, A. (1967) Marcello Malpighi and the dawn of neurohistology. *Journal of Neurological Sciences* **4**:185–193.

Meyer, A. (1971) *Historical Aspects of Cerebral Anatomy* (Oxford University Press, London).

Meynert, T. (1867) Der Bau der Gross-Hirnrinde und seine örtlichen Verschiedenheiten, nebst einem pathologisch-anatomischen Corollarium, I. *Vierteljahrsschrift für Psychiatrie in ihren Beziehungen zur Morphologie und Pathologie des Central-Nervensystems, der physiologischen Psychologie, Statistik und gerichtlichen Medicin* **1**:77–93, 119–124.

Meynert, T. (1872) The brain of mammals. In: Stricker, S. (Ed.) *A Manual of Histology* (Wood, New York), pp. 650–766. American translation of the first German edition (1871–1872; Engelmann, Leipzig).

Mihalkovics, V.v. (1877) *Entwicklungsgeschichte des Gehirns, nach Untersuchungen an Höheren Wirbelthieren und dem Menschen* (Engelmann, Leipzig).

Millen, J.H. & Woollam, D.H.M. (1961) Observations on the nature of the pia mater. *Brain* **84**:514–520.

Millen, J.H. & Woollam, D.H.M. (1962) *The Anatomy of the Cerebrospinal Fluid* (Oxford University Press, Oxford).

Mistichelli, D. (1709) *Tratto dell'Apoplessia* (Rossi, Rome).

Mitchell, G.A.G. (1953) *Anatomy of the Autonomic Nervous System* (Livingston, Edinburgh).

Miyazaki, T., Yoshida, Y., Hirano, M., Shin, T., & Kanaseki, T. (1981) Central location of the motoneurons supplying the thyrohyoid and the geniohyoid muscles as demonstrated by horseradish peroxidase method. *Brain Research* **219**:423–427.

Molinetti, A. (1669) *Antonio Molinetti Phil. et Medici Veneti Prima Sede* (Cadorinis, Padua).

Molinetti, A. (1675) *Dissertationes Anatomico-Pathologicae Quibus Humani Corpus Partes Accuratissimè Describuntur Morbique Singular Diuextantes Explicantur* (Balleonium, Venice).

Mondino (1316) *Anatomy*. In: *The Fasciculo di Medicina Venice, 1493, with Introduction and Translation by Charles Singer*, 2 Vols. (Lier, Florence), 1925.

Mondino dei Luzzi (1316) *Anathomia Corporis Humani, see* Mondino (1316).

Monro, A., *primus* (1732) *The Anatomy of the Human Bones, to Which are Added an Anatomical Treatise of the Nerves; an Account of the Reciprocal Motions of the Heart; and a Description of the Humane Lacteal Sac and Duct* (W. Monro, Edinburgh).

Monro, A. *primus*, translated by Coopmans, G. (1754) *Celebris Anatomici Alexandri Monro. R.S.L.S. in Acad. Edinburgensi Professoris. Nervorum Anatome Contracta. Latine Reddita. cui Subjectae sunt Ejusdem Explicatio Motus Reciproci Cordis, & Ductus Thoracici Descriptio* (Petrum Romar, Franeker).

Monro, A., *secundus* (1783) *Observations on the Structure and Functions of the Nervous System: Illustrated with Tables* (Creech & Johnson, Edinburgh).

Morand, S.F. [*sic* M.] (1748) Observations anatomiques sur quelques parties du cerveau. *Histoire de l'Académie Royale des Sciences avec les Mémoires de Mathématique et de Physique (Année 1744)* [no volume indicated], pp. 312–322.

Morand, S.F. (1768–1772) *Opuscules de Chirurgie* (Desprez, Paris).

Morgagni, G. (1719) *Adversaria Anatomica Sexti* (Cominus, Padua).

Morgagni, G. (1762) *Adversaria Anatomica Omnia: Archetypis Aereis Tabulis Cominianis ab Auctore ipso Communicatis, & Universali Accuratissimo Indice Ornata: Opus Nunc Vere Absolutum, Inventis, et Innumeris Observationibus, ac Monitis Refertum, Quibus Universa Humani Corporis Anatome, & Subinde Etiam quae ab hac Pendent, Res Medica, & Chirurgica Admodum Illustrantur* (Remondiniana, Venice).

Morton, L.T. & Norman, J.M. (1991) *Morton's Medical Bibliography: An Annotated Check-list of Texts Illustrating the History of Medicine (Garrison and Morton)*, 5th Edn. (Scolar Press, Aldershot).

Müller, J. (1828a) Über ein eigenthümlichens, dem *nervus sympathicus* analoges Nervensystem der eingeweide bei den insecten. *Nova Acta Physico-medica Academiae Caesareae Leopoldino-Carolinae Naturae Curiosorum* **14**:71–108.

Müller, J. (1828b) Über die Metamorphose des Nervensystems in der Thierwelt. *Archiv für Anatomie und Physiologie [Meckel's Archiv]* [no volume indicated], pp. 1–22.

Müller, J. (1834) *Handbüch der Physiologie des Menschen für Vorlesungen*, Vol. 1, Pt. 2 (Hölscher, Coblenz).

Müller, J. (1837) Historisch-anatomische Bemerkungen. *Archiv für Anatomie, Physiologie und Wissenschaftliche Medicin* [no volume indicated], pp. 273–296.

Müller, J. (1838) *Elements of Physiology*, Vol. 1 (Taylor and Walton, London).

Munniks, J. (1805) *Observationes Variae: quas, Favente Summo Numine, ex Auctoritate Rectoris Magnifici, Seerpiigratami, J.U.D. Jur. Nat. Publ. Gent. et Criminalis Prof. Ordinarii, ut et Amplissimi Senatue Academici Confensu, et Nobilissimae Facultatis Medicae Decreto, Pro Gradu Doctoratus Summisque in Medicina Honoribus ac Privilegiis Rite et Legitime Capessendis, Publice Eruditis ad Disceptandum Proponit Jacobus Munniks Groninganus* (Kamerling, Groningen).

Murray, A. (1780) *De Sensibilitate Ossium Morbosa* (Edman, Uppsala). Reprinted in Ludwig, C.F. (1791–1795), Vol. 4, pp. 252–265, 1795.

Nahin, R.L., Madsen, A.M., & Giesler, G.J. Jr. (1983) Anatomical and physiological studies of the gray matter surrounding the spinal cord central canal. *Journal of Comparative Neurology* **220**:321–335.

Nauta, W.J.H. & Feirtag, M. (1986) *Fundamental Neuroanatomy* (Freeman, New York).

Nauta, W.J.H. & Haymaker, W. (1969) Hypothalamic nuclei and fiber connections. In: Haymaker, W., Anderson, E., & Nauta, W.J.H. (Eds.) *The Hypothalamus* (Thomas, Springfield IL), pp. 136–209.

Nemesius (1636) *The Nature of Man. A Learned and Usefull Tract, Written in Greek by Nemesius, Surnamed the Philosopher; Sometime Bishop of a City in Phoeniecia, and One of the Most Ancient Fathers of the Church. Englished, and Divided into Sections, with Briefs of their Principall Contents: by Geo. Wither* (Taunton, London).

Neubauer, J.E. (1772) *Descripto Anatomica Nervorum Cardiacorum: Sectio 1. De Nervo Intercostali Cervicali Dextri Imprimis Lateris* (Officina Fleischeriana, Frankfurt).

Neuburger, M. (1981) *The Historical Development of Experimental Brain and Spinal Cord Physiology before Flourens* (Johns Hopkins University Press, Baltimore).

Newport, G. (1832) On the nervous system of the *Sphinx ligustri*, Linn., and on the changes which it undergoes during a part of the metamorphoses of the insect. *Philosophical Transactions of the Royal Society of London* **122**:383–398.

Newport, G. (1834) On the nervous system of the *Sphinx ligustri*, Linn., (Part II.) during the latter stages of its pupa and its imago state; and on the means by which its development is effected. *Philosophical Transactions of the Royal Society of London* **124**:389–423.

Nicolai, Th. G.I. (1812) Ueber das Rückenmark der Vögel und die Bildung desselben im bebrüteten Ey. *Archiv für die Physiologie* **11**(2):156–219. Published in thesis form one year earlier.

Nieuwenhuys, R. (2002) Deuterostome brains: synopsis and commentary. *Brain Research Bulletin* **57**:257–270.

Nieuwenhuys, R., ten Donkellar, H.J., & Nicholson, C. (1998) *The Central Nervous System of Vertebrates*, 3 Vols. (Springer, Berlin).

Nieuwenhuys, R., Voogd, J., & Huijzen, Chr. van (2008) *The Human Central Nervous System*, 4th Edn. (Springer-Verlag, Berlin).

Noguez, P. (1726) *L'Anatomie du Corps de l'Homme in Abrégé; Ou, Description Courte de Toutes ses Parties, Ou l'On Donne l'Explication de Leurs Differens Usages, Tirée de Leur Structure & des Observations les plus Modernes*, 2nd Edn. (Cavelier, Paris).

Nomina Anatomica (1955) (no publisher indicated, [London]).

Nomina Anatomica (1983) 5th Edn. (Williams & Wilkins, Baltimore).

Nunn, J.F. (2002) *Ancient Egyptian Medicine* (University of Oklahoma Press, Norman).

Nysten, P. H. (1814) *Dictionnaire de Médecine, et des Sciences Accessories de la Médecine, avec l'Étymologie de Chaque Terme; suivi de Deux Vocabulaires l'un Latin, l'autre Grec* (Brosson, Paris).

Obersteiner, H. (1888) *Anleitung beim Studium des Baues der Nervösen Centralorgane: Im Gesunden und Kranken Zustande* (Toeplitz & Deuticke, Vienna).

Obersteiner, H. & Hill, A. (1900) *The Anatomy of the Central Nervous Organs in Health and in Disease*, 2nd Edn. (Griffin, London).

Ogle, W. (1958); *see* Aristotle, *De Partibus Animalium*.

Ollivier, C.P. (1824) *De la Moelle Épinière et des ses Maladies*, Vol. 1 (Crevot, Paris).

Olszewski, J. & Baxter, D. (1954) *Cytoarchitecture of the Human Brain Stem* (Karger, New York).

O'Malley, C.D. (1964) *Andreas Vesalius of Brussels, 1514–1564* (University of California Press, Berkeley).

O'Malley, C.D. & Saunders, J.B. de C.M. (1982) *Leonardo de Vinci on the Human Body* (Crown Publishers, New York).

Oort, H. (1918) Über die verästelung des nervus octavus bei Säugetieren. *Anatomischer Anzeiger* **51**:272–280.

Ortega, F., Gascón, S., Masserdotti, G., Deshpande, A., Simon, C., Fischer, J., Dimou, L., Lie, D.C., Schroeder, T., & Berninger, B. (2013) Oligodendrogliogenic and neurogenic adult subependymal zone neural stem cells constitute distinct lineages and exhibit differential responsiveness to Wnt signalling. *Nature Cell Biology* **15**:602–613.

Osborn, H.F. (1888) A contribution to the internal structure of the amphibian brain. *Journal of Morphology* **2**:51–96.

Owen, R. (1832) *Memoir on the Pearly Nautilus (*Nautilus Pompilius, *Linn.) with Illustrations of its External Form and Internal Structure* (Wood, London).

Owen, R. (1837) On the structure of the brain in marsupial animals. *Philosophical Transactions of the Royal Society of London* **127**:87–96.

Owen, R. (1866) *On the Anatomy of Vertebrates* (Longmans, Green; London).

Oxford English Dictionary, *see* Online version.

Oxford Latin Dictionary, edited by P.G.W. Clare (Oxford University Press, Oxford, 1982).

Pacchioni, A. (1705) *Dissertatio Epistolaris De Glandulis Conglobatis Durae Meningis Humanae, Indeque Ortis Lymphaticis ad Piam Meningem Productis* (Buagni, Rome).

Pacchioni, A. (1741) *Antonii Pacchioni Regienssi Medici, & Anatomici Ramani Opera, Editio Quarta, Novis Accessionibus Auctior* (Pagliarinos, Rome).

Pagel, W. (1958) Medieval and renaissance contributions to knowledge of the brain and its structure. In: Poynter, F.L.N. (Ed.) *The History and Philosophy of Knowledge of the Brain and its Functions* (Blackwell, Oxford), pp. 95–114.

Palfijn, J. (1726) *Anatomie du Corps Humain* (Cavelier, Paris).

Palletta, G.B. (1784) *De Nervis Crotaphitico et Buccinatorio* (Typis Imperialis Monasterii, Milan).

Palmgren, A. (1921) Embryological and morphological studies on the mid-brain and cerebellum of vertebrates. *Acta Zoologica* **2**:1–94.

Papez, J.W. (1929) *Comparative Neurology: A Manual and Text for the Study of the Nervous System of Vertebrates* (Crowell, New York).

Paré, A. (1550) *Briefve Collection de l'Administration Anatomique* (Cauellat, Paris). There was also a 1549 edition or issue with the same collation and publisher; also see Solomon, C. & Trouilloud, P. (2003).

Paré, A. (1561) *Anatomie Universelle du Corps Humain, Composee par A. Paré, Chirurgien Ordinaire du Roy et Juré à Paris: Reveuë et Augmentee par Ledit Autheur, avec l. Rostaing du Bignosc Provençal, aussi Chirurgien Juré à Paris* (Le Royer, Paris).

Paré, A. (1564) *Dix Livres de la Chirurgie, avec le Magasin des Instrumens Necessaires à Icelle* (Le Royer, Paris).

Paré, A. (1634) *The Works of that Famous Chirurgion Ambrose Parey*, translated out of the Latine and compared with the French by Th. Johnson (Cotes, London). Facsimile published by Milford House, New York, 1968.

Paterson, A.M. (1887) The limb plexuses of mammals. *Journal of Anatomy and Physiology* **21**:611–634.

Pearson (1947) The roots of the facial nerve in human embryos and fetuses. *Journal of Comparative Neurology* **87**:139–159.

Pechura, C.M. & Martin, J.B., Eds. (1991) *Mapping the Brain and its Functions: Integrating Enabling Technologies into Neuroscience Research* (National Academy Press, Washington DC).

Peipers, G.F. (1793) *Dissertatio Inauguralis, Sistens Tertii et Quarti Nervorum Cervicalium Descriptionem, cui Accedit Succincta Eorundem Nervorum Quinti; Nervi Phrenici, Praesertim Ratione Originis; Nervi Accessorii Willisii; Nervi Duri, Ejusque Praecipue Rami Inferioris; Nervi Hypoglossi et Occipitalis Maximi a Secundo Cervicalium Nervo, Adumbratio; cum Tab. Aenea* (Typo Grunertiano, Halle).

[Perrault, C.] (1671–1676) *Memoires pour Servir a l'Histoire Naturelle des Animaux* (Imprimerie Royale, Paris).

[Perrault, C.] (1687) *Memoires for a Natural History of Animals. Being the Anatomical Descriptions of Several Animals Dissected by the Royal Academy at Paris* (No publisher or place provided). Originally published in French, see [Perrault, C.] (1671–1676).

[Perrault, C.] (1688) *Memoir's for a Natural History of Animals. Containing the Anatomical Descriptions of Several Creatures*

Dissected by the Royal Academy of Sciences at Paris (Streater, London).

Peters, A., Palay, S.L., & Webster, H.deF. (1991) *The Fine Structure of the Nervous System: Neurons and Their Supporting Cells*, 3rd Edn. (Oxford University Press, New York).

Petrioli, G. (1741), see Pietro da Cortona (1741) *Tabulae Anatomicae.*

Peyligk, H. (1499) *Philosophiae Naturalis Compendium* (Lother, Leipzig).

Pfeffinger, J. (1783) *Dissertatio Anatomico-Physiologica de Structura Nervorum Cujus Sectionen Primam Cujus Sectionem* (Strasbourg, thesis published in two parts, done under Johann Friedrich Lobstein; this first part published under Lobstein's name).

Phillips, E. & Kersey, J. (1706) *The New World of Words: or Universal English Dictionary*, 6th Edn. (Phillips, Rhodes, and Taylor; London).

Piccolomini, A. (1586) *Anatomicae Praelectiones, Archangeli Piccolhomini, Ferrariensis, Civisque Romani, Explicantes Mirificam Corporis Humani Fabricam: Et quae Animae Vires, quibus Corporis Partibus, Tanquàm Instrumentis, ad suas Obeundas Actiones, Utantur; Sicuti Tota Anima, Toto Corpore* (Bodfadinus, Rome).

Pietro da Cortona (c1618), see Pietro da Cortona (1741) *Tabulae Anatomicae.*

Pietro da Cortona (1741) *Tabulae Anatomicae a Celeberrimo Pictore Petro Berrettini Cortonensi Delineatae. & Egregiè Aeri Incisae Nunc Primum Prodeunt, et a Cajetano Petrioli Romano Doctore, Regis Sardiniae Chirurgo Notis Illustratae* (Fausti Amidei, Rome). Edited and expanded by G. Petrioli, based on unpublished plates finished about 1618.

Plato, *Timaeus and Critias*, translated with an introduction and an appendix on *Atlantis* by Desmond Lee (Penguin, London) 1965.

Platt, A. (1958); *see* Aristotle, *De Generatione Animalium.*

Platter, F. (1583) *De Corporis Humani Structura et Usu Felicis Plateri Bas. Medici Abtecessoris Libri III: Tabulis Methodicè Explicati, Iconibus Accuratè Illustrati* (Froben, [Basel]).

Platter, F. (1603) *De Corporis Humani Structura et Usu Libri III* (König, Basel).

Polyak, S.L. (1941) *The Retina: The Anatomy and the Histology of the Retina in Man, Ape, and Monkey, Including the Consideration of Visual Functions, the History of Physiological Optics, and the Histological Laboratory Technique* (University of Chicago Press, Chicago).

Polyak, S.L. (1957) *The Vertebrate Visual System*, edited by H. Klüver (University of Chicago Press, Chicago).

Pordage, S. (1681), *see* Willis (1664).

Pordage, S. (1683), *see* Willis (1672).

Portal, A. (1803a) Description du nerf intercostal dans l'homme. *Mémoires de l'Institut National des Sciences et Arts. Sciences Mathématiques et Physiques* **4**:151–208.

Portal, A. (1803b) *Cours d'Anatomie Médicale, ou Élémens de l'Anatomie de l'Homme*, Vol. 4 (Baudouin, Paris).

Potter, P. (1995); *see* Hippocrates, *Places in Man*, and *Fleshes.*

Poupart, F. (1712) An anatomical history of the brain. In: Le Clerc, D. & Manget, J.-J. (1711–1714) *Bibliotheca Anatomica, Medica, Chirurgica, Etc.: Containing a Description of the Several Parts of the Body: Each Done by Some One or More Eminent Physician or Chirurgeon; with their Diseases and Cures. Wherein are not only all the Tracts of Use that are in the Second Edition of the Bibliotheca Anatomica, Lately Publish'd by Daniel Clericus and Jacob Mangetus, in Two Volumes in Folio, but an addition also of Near Double the Number of Other Curious Tracts, which were either Omitted in the said Bibliotheca, or have been Publishd since, some of them Translated, Others Faithfully Abridg'd; Very Few of which were ever before in English. Illustrated with several Hundred Figures, Done by the Best Artists, and from the Truest Designs; as will Appear from the Name to Each Figure.* To be Published Monthly, Vol. 2, pp. 639–644.

Pourfour du Petit, F. (1710) *Lettres d'un Médecin des Hôpitaux du Roy à un autre Médecin des ses Amis* (Albert, Namur).

Pourfour du Petit, F. (1729) Mémoire dans lequel il est démontré que les nerfs intercostaux fournissent des rameaux qui portent des esprits dans les yeax. *Mémoires de Mathématique et de Physique, pour la même Année*, in *Histoire de l'Académie Royal des Sciences, Année MDCCXVII*, pp. 1–19 (and one plate).

Price, J.L. (1973) An autoradiographic study of complementary laminar patterns of termination of afferent fibers to the olfactory cortex. *Journal of Comparative Neurology* **150**:87–108.

Price, J.L., Russchen, F.T., & Amaral, D.G. (1987) The limbic region. II: The amygdaloid complex. In: Björklund, A., Hökfelt, T., & Swanson, L.W. (Eds.) *Handbook of Chemical Neuroanatomy*, Vol. 5, *Integrated Systems of the CNS*, Part I, (Elsevier, Amsterdam), pp. 279–388.

Privat, A. & LeBlond, C.P. (1972) The subependymal layer and neighboring region in the brain of the young rat. *Journal of Comparative Neurology* **146**:277–302.

Procháska, G. (1779) *De Structura Nervorum. Tractus Anatomicus* (Graeffer, Vienna).

Procháska, G. (1800) *Operum Minorum Anatomici, Physiologici et Pathologici Argumenti*, 2 Parts (Wappler et Beck, Vienna).

Purkinje, J.E. (1838) "Neueste Untersuchungen aus der Nerven- und Hirn-anatomie… [from first sentence]" *Bericht über die Versammlung Deutscher Naturforscher und Aertze in Prag im September 1837* (Gottlieb Haas Söhne, Prague), pp. 174–175.

Quain, J. (1828) *Elements of Descriptive and Practical Anatomy: For the Use of Students* (Simpkin and Marshall, London).

Quain, J. (1832) *The Elements of Anatomy*, 2nd Edn. (Taylor, London).

Quain, J. (1834) *The Elements of Anatomy*, 3rd Edn. (Taylor, London).

Quain, J. (1837) *The Elements of Anatomy*, 4th Edn. (Taylor & Walton, London).

Quain, J. & Wilson, W.J.E. (1839) *The Nerves of the Human Body; Including the Brain and Spinal Marrow, and Organs of Sense in a Series of Plates with References and Physiological Comments* (Taylor & Walton, London).

Racchetti, V. (1816) *Della Struttura, delle Funzioni e delle Malattie della Midolla Spinale, Opera* (Giusti, Milan).

Ramsay, A. (1813) *Anatomy of the Heart, Cranium, and Brain: Adapted to the Purposes of the Medical and Surgical Practitioner: to which is Added, in Notes, Observations*

on the Laws of Life and Sensation, 2nd Edn. (Constable, Edinburgh).
Ranson, S.W. (1920) *The Anatomy of the Nervous System, From the Standpoint of Development and Function* (Saunders, Philadelphia).
Rasmussen, A.T. (1932) *The Principal Nervous Pathways: Neurological Charts and Schemas with Explanatory Notes* (Macmillan, New York).
Rasmussen, A.T. (1933) Origin and course of the fasciculus uncinatus (Russell) in the cat, with observations on other fiber tracts arising from the cerebellar nuclei. *Journal of Comparative Neurology* **57**:165–197.
Rasmussen, A.T. (1947) *Some Trends in Neuroanatomy* (Brown, Dubuque IO).
Rau, J.J. (1694) *Disputatio Anatomico-Medica Inauguralis de Ortu et Regeneratione Dentium*. In: Haller, A. von (1747–1751) *Disputationum Anatomicarum Selectarum Volumen I [-VII]. Collegit, Edidit, Praefatus est Albertus Haller*, Vol. 6 (Vandenhoeck, Göttingen), pp. 181–207.
Rau, J.J. (1720) Neurologia Rauiana. In: Valentini, M.B., *Amphitheatrum Zootomicum*, Appendix III (Zunner, Frankfurt am Main).
Ray, J. (1671) An account of the dissection of a Porpess. *Philosophical Transactions of the Royal Society of London* **6**:2274–2279.
Razi (c910), *see* next entry.
Razi, Abu Bakr Muhammad ibn Zakariya (1903) *Trois Traités d'Anatomie Arabes par Muhammed ibn Zakariyya al-Razi, Ali ibn al-Abbas et Ali ibn Sina. Text Inédit de Deux Traités. Traduction de P. de Koning* (Brill, Leiden).
Read, A. (1638) *The Manuall of the Anatomy or Dissection of the Body of Man, Containing the Enumeration, and Description of the Parts of the Same, which Usually are Shewed in the Publike Anatomicall Exercises. Enlarged and More Methodically Digested into 6 Books* (Constable, London).
Read, A. (1650) *The Manuall of the Anatomy or Dissection of the Body of Man: Containing the Enumeration and Description of the Parts of the Same; which Usually are Shewn in the Publick Anatomicall Exercises. With Sundry Figures thereunto Belonging*, 4th Edn. (Newcomb, Thrale; London).
Reichert, K.B. (1859) *Der Bau des Menschlichens Gehirns: Durch Abbildungen mit Erläuterndem Texte* (Engelmann, Leipzig).
Reil, J.C. (1796) *Exercitationum Anatomicarum Fasciculus Primus. De Structura Nervorum* (Venalis, Halle).
Reil, J.C. (1807) Ueber die Eigenschaften des Ganglien-Systems und sein Verhältniss zum Cerebral-System. *Archiv für die Physiologie* **7**:189–254. Much of the material published by Reil in the articles between 1807–1809 was translated into English by H. Mayo (1822–1823).
Reil, J.C. (1807–1808a) Fragmente über die Bildung des kleinen Gehirns im Menschen. *Archiv für die Physiologie* **8**:1–58.
Reil, J.C. (1807–1808b) Erste Fortsetzung der Untersuchungen über den Bau des kleinen Gehirns im Menschen. *Archiv für die Physiologie* **8**:273–304.
Reil, J.C. (1807–1808c) Untersuchungen über den Bau des kleinen Gehirns im Menschen. Zweyte Fortsetzung, über die Organisation der Lappen und Läppchen. *Archiv für die Physiologie* **8**:385–426.
Reil, J.C. (1809a) Nachtrag zur Anatomie des kleinen Gehirns. *Archiv für die Physiologie* **9**:129–135.
Reil, J.C. (1809b) Untersuchungen über den Bau des grossen Gehirns im Menschen... *Archiv für die Physiologie* **9**:136–208.
Reil, J.C. (1809c) Das verlängerte Rückenmark, die hintern, seitlichen und vörderen Schenkel des kleinen Gehirns und die theils strangförmig, theils als Ganglienkette in der Axe des Rückenmarks und des Gehirns fortlausende graue Substanz, vom Prof. Reil. Fünfte Fortsetzung. *Archiv für die Physiologie* **9**:485–524.
Reil, J.C. (1812a) Die vördere Commissur im grossen Gehirn. *Archiv für die Physiologie* **11**:89–100.
Reil, J.C. (1812b) Die Scheidewand, ihre Höhle, die Zwillingsbinde und die Höhlen im Gehirn. *Archiv für die Physiologie* **11**:101–116.
Reil, J.C. (1812c) Nachträge zur Anatomie des grossen und kleinen Gehirns. *Archiv für die Physiologie* **11**:345–376.
Reisinger, E. (1925) Untersuchungen am Nervensystem der Bothrioplana. *Zeitschrift für Morphologie und Ökologie der Tiere* **5**:119–149.
Reisinger. E. (1972) Die Evolution des Orthogons der Spiralier und das Archicölomatenproblem. *Zeitschrift für Zoologische Systematik und Evolutionsforschung* **10**:1–43.
Remmelin, J. (1670) *An Exact Survey of the Microcosmus or Little World Being an Anatomie, of the Bodies of Man and Woman: Wherein the Skin, Veins, Nerves, Muscles, Bones, Sinews and Ligaments are Accurately Delineated. And Curiously Pasted Together, so as at First Sight You May Behold All the Outward Parts of Man and Woman. And by Turning Up the Several Dissections of the Paper Take a View of All Their Inwards. With Alphabetical Referrences to Every Member and Part of the Body: Usefull for all Doctors, Chirurgeons, Etc. As Also for Painters, Carvers, and All Persons that Desire to be Acquainted with the Parts, and their Names, in the Bodies of Man, or Woman* (Moxon, London).
Retzius, G. (1884) *Das Gehörorgan der Wirbeltier* (Samson & Wallin, Stockholm).
Retzius, G. (1896) *Das Menschenhirn* (Nordstedt & Söner, Stockholm).
Rexed (1952) The cytoarchitectonic organization of the spinal cord in the cat. *Journal of Comparative Neurology* **96**:415–495.
Rhazes (c910), *see* Razi, Abu Bakr Muhammad ibn Zakariya (1903).
Rhoton, A.L., Kobayashi, S., & Hollinshead, W.H. (1968) Nervus intermedius. *Journal of Neurosurgery* **29**:609–618.
Ribes, F. (1811) Recherches anatomiques et physiologiques sur quelques partes de l'oeil, à l'occasion d'une plaie de tête. *Mémoires de la Société Médicale d'Émulation* **7**:86–104.
Ribes, F. (1817) Exposé sommaire de quelques recherches anatomiques, physiologiques et pathologiques. *Mémoires de la Société Médicale d'Émulation*, **8**:604–630.
Richardson, R.F. & Carman, J.B.; *see* Vesalius, A. (2002) *On the Fabric of the Human Body*. A Translation of *De Humani Corporis Fabrica Libri Septem, Book III, The Veins and Arteries, and Book IV, The Nerves.*
Richardson, R.F. & Carman, J.B.; *see* Vesalius, A. (2009) *On the Fabric of the Human Body. A Translation of De Humani Corporis Fabrica Libri Septem, Book VI, The Heart and Associated Organs, and Book VII, The Brain.*
Ridley, H. (1695) *The Anatomy of the Brain. Containing its Mechanism and Physiology; Together with some New*

Discoveries and Corrections of Ancient and Modern Authors Upon that Subject. To which is Annex'd a Particular Account of Animal Functions and Muscular Motion. The Whole Illustrated with Elegant Sculptures After the Life (Smith & Walford, London). Facsimile published by The Classics of Neurology & Neurosurgery Library, Birmingham, 1987.

Riley, H.A. (1943) *An Atlas of the Basal Ganglia, Brain Stem and Spinal Cord: Based on Myelin-stained Material* (Williams & Wilkins, Baltimore).

Rioch, D.McK., Wislocki, G.B., & O'Leary, J.L. (1940) A précis of preoptic, hypothalamic and hypophysial terminology with atlas. In: *The Hypothalamus and Central Levels of Autonomic Function*. Research Publications: Association for Research in Nervous and Mental Disease **20**:3–30.

Riolan, J. (1610) *Joannis Riolani Ambiani, Medici Parisiensis, Viri Clarissimi Opera Omnia: Tam Hactenus Edita, quam Postuma Authoris Postrema Manu Exarata & Exornata: Quibus Universam Medicinam Fideliter & Accurate Descripsit, atque Illustrauit* (Perier, Paris).

Riolan, J. (1618) *Anthropographia* (Perier, Paris).

Riolan, J. (1628–1629) *Les Oeuvres Anatomiques* (Moreau, Paris).

Riolan, J. (1649) *Encheiridium Anatomicum et Pathologicum: in quo ex Naturali Constitutione Partium, Recessus à Naturali Statu Demonstratur ad Usum Theatri Anatomici Adornatum* (Wyngaerden, Leiden). For English translation see Riolan (1657).

Riolan, J. (1657) *A Sure Guide; Or, the Best and Nearest Way to Physick and Chyrurgery: That is to say, the Arts of Healing by Medicine and Manual Operation. Being an Anatomical Description of the Whol Body of Man and its Parts: with their Respective Diseases Demonstrated from the Fabrick and Use of the Said Parts. In Six Books. Viz. 1 Describing all, and every of the Bones of Mans Body, According to the Ancient Method. 2 Describing the Belly, and All Its Parts and Bowels, with their Respective Diseases. 3 Describing the Chest, and All Its Parts and Contents, with their Respective Diseases. 4 Describing the Head, and Face, with All their Parts Containing and Contained, and their Respective Diseases. 5. Describing the Limbs of the Body, with the Many Regiments of Muscles, and their Diseases. 6. Containing a New Description of the Bones, by a Method First Invented by our Author, Handling Al the Diseases and Symptomes of the Said Bones. At the End of the Six Books, are Added Twenty Four Tables, Cut in Brass, Containing One Hundred Eighty Four Figures, with an Explanation of Them: Which are Referred to in the Above a Thousand Places in the Books, for the Help of Yong Artists* (Cole, London). For original edition see Riolan (1649).

Risold, P.Y. & Swanson, L.W. (1997) Connections of the rat lateral septal complex. *Brain Research Reviews* **24**:115–195.

Roberts, K.B. & Tomlinson, J.D.W. (1992) *The Fabric of the Body: European Traditions of Anatomical Illustration* (Oxford University Press, Oxford).

Rocca, J. (2003) *Galen on the Brain: Anatomical Knowledge and Physiological Speculation in the Second Century A.D.* (Brill, Leiden).

Rolando, L. (1809) *Saggio sopra la Vera Struttura del Cervello dell'Uomo e degli Animali e sopra la Funzioni del Sistema Nervoso* (Nella Stamperìa da S.S.R.M. Privilegiata, Sassari).

Rolando, L. (1819) *Anatomes Physiologica* (Bianco, Turin).

Rolando, L. (1824) *Ricerche Anatomiche sulla Struttura del Midollo Spinale* (Stamperia reale, Turin). Reprinted from *Dizionario Periodice di Medicina*.

Rolando, L. (1825a) Recherches anatomiques sur la moelle alongée. *Memorie della Reale Accademia delle Scienze di Torino* **29**:1–78.

Rolando, L. (1825b) Osservazioni sul cervelletto. *Memorie della Reale Accademia delle Scienze di Torino* **29**:163–188.

Rolando, L. (1831) Della struttura degli emisferi cerebrali. *Memorie della Reale Accademia della Scienze di Torino* **35**:103–146.

Rolfinck, W. (1656) *Dissertationes Anatomicae Methodo Synthetica Exaratae, Sex Libris Comprehensae, Theoricis & Practicis Veterum, & Recentiorum Propriisque Observationibus Illustratae, & ad Circulationem Accommodatae* (Endter, Nuremberg).

Romer, A.S. (1962) *The Vertebrate Body*, 3rd Edn. (Saunders, Philadelphia).

Rose, J.E. & Woolsey, C.N. (1948) Structure and relations of limbic cortex and anterior thalamic nuclei in rabbit and cat. *Journal of Comparative Neurology* **89**:279–347.

Rosenman, L.D. (1998), *see* William of Saliceto (1275) *The Surgery of William of Saliceto.*

Rosenman, L.D. (2005), *see* Guy de Chauliac (1363) *The Major Surgery of Guy de Chauliac.*

Rosenmüller, J.C. (1819) *Handbuch der Anatomie des Meschlichen Körpers zum Gebrauch der Vorlesungen*, 3rd Edn. (Köhler, Leipzig).

Rosenthal, F.C. (1815) *Ein Beitrag zur Encephalotomie* (Landes-Industrie-Compt, Weimar).

Rufus of Ephesus (fl. c90–120), *Oeuvres*, translated with Greek and Latin texts by C.V. Daremberg (completed by C.E. Ruelle) (Impr. nationale, Paris) 1879.

Ruskell, G.L. (1970) An ocular parasympathetic nerve pathway of facial nerve origin and its influence on intraocular pressure. *Experimental Eye Research* **10**:319–330.

Ruskell, G.L. (1971) The distribution of autonomic post-ganglionic nerve fibres to the lacrimal gland in monkeys. *Journal of Anatomy* **109**:229–242.

Ruskell, G.L. (1974) Ocular fibres of the maxillary nerve in monkeys. *Journal of Anatomy* **118**:195–203.

Russell, J.S.R. (1897) The origin and destination of certain afferent and efferent tracts in the medulla oblongata. *Brain* **20**:409–440.

Ruysch, F. (1702) *Thesaurus Anatomicis Secundus* (Wolters, Amsterdam).

Ruysch, F. (1728), *see* Ruysch, F. (1737) *Opera Omnia*. Epist. XII appeared in 1728.

Ruysch, F. (1737) [*Opera Omnia Anatomico-Medico-Chirurgica*], 2 Vols. (Janssonio-Waesbergios, Amsterdam). Epist. XII appeared in 1728. Actually covers 1725–1751 in at least some copies.

Sabatier, R.B. [*sic* M] (1775) *Traité Complet d'Anatomie, ou Description de Toutes les Parties du Corps Humain*, 2 Vols. (Didot le jeune, Paris).

Sabatier, R.B. [*sic* M] (1777) *Traité Complet d'Anatomie, ou Description de Toutes les Parties du Corps Humain*, 3 Vols. (Didot le jeune, Paris).

Sabatier, R.B. [*sic* M] (1781) *Traité Complet d'Anatomie, ou Description de Toutes les Parties du Corps Humain*, Nouvelle édition, 3 Vols. (Didot le jeune, Paris).

Sabin, F.R. (1901) *An Atlas of the Medulla and Midbrain: A Laboratory Manual* (Friedenwald, Baltimore).
Saint Hilaire, de (1680) *L'Anatomie du Corps Humain; avec ses Maladies, et les Remedes pour les Guerir, selon les Auteurs Anciens & Modernes* (Couterot, Paris).
Salmon, W. (1714) *Ars Anatomica: Or, The Anatomy of Humane Bodies* (Brown, Taylor, Browne; London).
Salomon, C. & Trouilloud, P. (2003) *Le Corps & ses Mots: Présentation de la Briefve Collection de l'Administration Anatomique d'Ambroise Paré avec Translation* (L'Harmattan, Paris).
Santorini, G.D. (1724) *Observationes Anatomicae* (Recurti, Venice).
Santorini, G.D. (1775) *Septemdecim Tabulae quas nunc Primum Edit atque Explicat iisque alias addit De Structura Mammarum et De Tunica Testis Vaginali Michael Girardi* (Bodoni, Parma).
Saper, C.B., Loewy, A.D., Swanson, L.W., & Cowan, W.M. (1976) Direct hypothalamo-autonomic connections. *Brain Research* **117**:305–312.
Sapolini, G. (1883) Etudes anatomiques sur le nerf de Wrisberg et la corde du tympan ou treizième nerf cranien. *Journal de Médecine, de Chirurgie et de Pharmacologie de Bruxelles* **77**:33–344, 460–470, 570–577.
Savage-Smith, E. (1971) Galen's account of the cranial nerves and the autonomic nervous system. *Clio Medica* **6**:77–98.
Sawyer, S.E., Young, S.J., & Groves, P.M. (1989) Quantitative Golgi study of anatomically identified subdivisions of motor thalamus in the rat. *Journal of Comparative Neurology* **286**:1–27.
Scalia, F. (1972) The termination of retinal axons in the pretectal region of mammals. *Journal of Comparative Neurology* **145**:223–258.
Scarpa, A. (1772) *Antonii Scarpa in Mutinensi Archigymnasio Publici Anatomes, et Chirurgiae Professoris: De Structura Fenestrae Rotundae Auris, et de Tympano Secundario Anatomicae Observationes* (Societatem Typographicam, Modena).
Scarpa, A. (1779) *Anatomicarum Annotationum Liber Primus. De Nervorum Gangliis, et Plexubus* (no publisher indicated, Modena).
Scarpa, A. (1785) *Anatomicarum Annotationum; Liber Secundus, De Organo Olfactus Praecipuo* (Typis R. & I. Monasterii S. Salvatoris, Pavia).
Scarpa, A. (1788) De nervo spinali ad octavum cerebri accessorio commentarius. *Acta Academiae Caesareae Regiae Josephinae Medico-Chirurgicae Vindobonenis* **1**:337–374.
Scarpa, A. (1789) *Anatomicae Disquisitiones de Auditu et Olfactu* (Galeat, Pavia).
Scarpa, A. (1794) *Tabulae Nevrologicae ad Illustrandam Historiam Anatomicam Cardiacorum Nervorum, Noni Nervorum Cerebri, Glossopharygaei, et Pharyngaei ex Octavo Cerebri* (Comini, Turin).
Schaarschmidt, A. (1750) *Neurologische Tabellen* (Schutz, Berlin).
Schiller, F. (1965) The rise of the "enteroid processes" in the 19th century: some landmarks in cerebral nomenclature. *Bulletin of the History of Medicine* **39**:326–334.
Schiller, F. (1967) The vicissitudes of the basal ganglia (further landmarks in cerebral nomenclature). *Bulletin of the History of Medicine* **41**:515–538.
Schiller, F. (1969) Stilling's nuclei—turning point in basic neurology. *Bulletin of the History of Medicine* **43**:67–84.
Schiller, F. (1992) *Paul Broca: Founder of French Anthropology, Explorer of the Brain* (Oxford University Press, New York).
Schleiden, M.J. (1838) Beiträge zur phytogenesis. *Archiv für Anatomie, Physiologie und Wissenschaftliche Medicin* [no volume indicated], pp. 137–176.
Schlemm, F. (1834) *Observationes Neurologicae: Cum III. Tabulas Aeri Incisis* (Hirschwald, Berlin).
Schlosser, G. (2006) Induction and specification of cranial placodes. *Developmental Biology* **294**:303–351.
Schmidel, C.C. (1754) *Dissertatio Inauguralis Medic a qua quaedam de Nervo Intercostali* (Typis Tetzschnerianis, Erlangen).
Schmidt, J.A. (1794) *Commentarius de Nervis Lumbalibus Eorumque Plexu Anatomico-Pathologicus. Adiecta est Duorum, qui in Plexu Brachiali Major Continentur, Neperque Inveniebantur, Plexuum Minorum Descriptio & Adumbratio* (Wappler, Vienna).
Schönlein, J.L. (1816) *Von der Hirnmetamorphose. Inauguralabhandlung* (Nitribitt, Würzburg).
Schreger, C.H.T. (1803) *Synonymia Anatomica* (Bureau par Literatur, Furthi), or second title-page, *Synonymik der Anatomischen Nomenclatur* (Bureau für Literatur, Fürth).
Schroeder van der Kolk, J.L.C. (1854) *Anatomisch Physiologisch Onderzoek over het Fijnere Zamenstel en de Werking van het Ruggemerg* (Van der Post, Amsterdam). For translation see Schroeder van der Kolk, J.L.C. (1859).
Schroeder van der Kolk, J.L.C. (1859) *On the Minute Structure and Fuctions of the Spinal Cord and Medulla Oblongata, and On the Proximate Cause and Rational Treatment of Epilepsy*, Translated from the original by William Daniel Moore (New Sydenham Society, London).
Schulte, B.P.M. & Endtz, L.J. (1977) *A Short History of Neurology in the Netherlands* (no publisher indicated, Amsterdam).
Schütz, H. (1891) Anatomische Untersuchungen über den Faserverlauf im centralen Höhlengrau und den Nervenfaserschwund in demselben bei der progressiven Paralyse der Irren. *Archiv für Psychiatrie und Nervenkrankheiten* **22**:527–587.
Schwalbe, G. (1881) *Lehrbuch der Neurology* (Besold, Erlangen).
Schwann, T. (1839) *Mikroskopische Untersuchungen über die Uebereinstimmung in der Struktur und dem Wachsthum der Thiere und Pflanzen* (Sander, Berlin).
Second Salernitan Demonstration (c1070–c1100), *see* Corner, G.W. (1927) *Anatomical Texts of the Earlier Middle Ages.*
Senac, J.-B. (1749) *Traité de la Structure du Coeur, de son Action, et de ses Maladies*, 2 Vols. (Vincent, Paris).
Serres, E.R.A. (1824–1826) *Anatomie Comparée du Cerveau, dans les Quatre Classes des Animaux Vertébrés*, 2 Vols. & Atlas (Gabon, Paris).
Sharpey, W., Thomson, A., & Cleland, J. (1867) *Quain's Elements of Anatomy*, 7th Edn. (Walton, London).
Sheehan, D. (1936) Discovery of the autonomic nervous system. *Archives of Neurology and Psychiatry* **35**:1081–1115.
Shepherd, G.M. (1991) *Foundations of the Neuron Doctrine* (Oxford University Press, New York).
Sherrington, C.S. (1906) *The Integrative Action of the Nervous System* (Scribner's Sons, New York).

Sherrington, C.S. (1946) *The Endeavour of Jean Fernel, With a List of the Editions of his Writings* (Cambridge University Press, Cambridge).

Shipley, M.T., McLean, J.H., Zimmer, L.A., & Ennis, M. (1996) The olfactory system. In: Swanson, L.W., Björklund, A., & Hökfelt, T. (Eds.), *Handbook of Chemical Neuroanatomy*, Vol. 12, *Integrated Systems of the CNS, Part III* (Elsevier, Amsterdam), pp. 469–573.

Siegel, R.E. (1970) *Galen On Sense Perception* (Karger, Basel).

Siegel, R.E. (1976) *Galen On the Affected Parts* (Karger, Basel).

Sigerist, H.E. (1960) *On the History of Medicine* (MD Publications, New York).

Simmons, D.M., Voss, J.W., Ingraham, H.A., Holloway, J.M., Broide, R.S., Rosenfeld, M.G., & Swanson, L.W. (1990) Pituitary cell phenotypes involve cell-specific Pit-1 mRNA translation and synergistic interactions with other classes of transcription factors. *Genes and Development* **4**:695–711.

Simpson, G.G. (1961) *Principles of Animal Taxonomy* (Columbia University Press, New York).

Sinclair, H.M. & Robb-Smith, A.H.T. (1950) *A Short History of Anatomical Teaching in Oxford* (Oxford University Press, Oxford).

Singer, C. (1917) A study in early Renaissance anatomy, with a new text: the *Anothomia* of Hieronymo Manfredi (1490). In: Singer, C. (Ed.) *Studies in the History and Method of Science* (Oxford University Press, Oxford), pp. 79–130.

Singer, C. (1925) Anatomy of Mundinus. In: *The Fasciculo di Medicina Venice 1493 with an Introduction etc. by Charles Singer. Part I. Description of the Fasciculo, Discussion of its Editions Art Language Sources and Influence, Translation of the "Anathomia" of Mondino da Luzzi, An Account of Mediaeval Anatomy and Physiology, and An Atlas of Illustrative Figures from Manuscript and Printed Sources.* Volume II of *Monumenta Medica* under the General Editorship of Henry E. Sigerist (Lier, Florence), pp. 45–112.

Singer, C., (1952) *Vesalius on the Human Brain: Introduction, Translation of the Text, Translation of Descriptions of Figures, Notes to the Translations, Figures* (Oxford University Press, London).

Singer, C. (1957) *A Short History of Anatomy and Physiology from the Greeks to Harvey* (Dover, New York).

Singer, C. (1959) *A Short History of Scientific Ideas to 1900* (Oxford University Press, New York).

Singer, C. (1999), *see* Galen (c177) *On Anatomical Procedures.*

Singer, C. & Rabin, C. (1946) *A Prelude to Modern Science, being a Discussion of the History, Sources and Circumstances of the 'Tabulae Anatomicae Sex' of Vesalius* (Cambridge University Press, Cambridge).

Singer, P.N. (1997), *see* Galen (c130–c200) *Selected Works.*

Skinner, H.A. (1949) *The Origin of Medical Terms* (Williams & Wilkins, Baltimore).

Slevogt, J.P. (1690) *Dissertatio Medica, De Dura Matre* (Wertherus, Jena).

Smith, G.E. (1895) The morphology of the true limbic lobe, corpus callosum, septum pellucidum and fornix. *Journal of Anatomy and Physiology* **30**:157–167, 185–205.

Smith, G.E. (1897) The morphology of the indusium and striae Lancisii. *Anatomische Anzeiger* **13**:23–27.

Smith, G.E. (1898) Further observations upon the fornix, with special reference to the brain of *Nyctophilus. Journal of Anatomy and Physiology* **32**:231–246.

Smith, G.E. (1902) The primary subdivision of the mammalian cerebellum. *Journal of Anatomy and Physiology* **36**:381–385.

Smith, G.E. (1903) The morphology of the human cerebellum. *Review of Neurology and Psychiatry* **1**:629–639.

Smith, G.E. (1919): A preliminary note on the morphology of the corpus striatum and the origin of the neopallium. *Journal of Anatomy* **53**:271–291.

Smith Papyrus (c1700 BC), *see* Breasted (1930), Allen (2005).

Soemmerring, S.T. (1778) *De Basi Encephali et Originibus Nervorum Cranio Egredientium Libri Quinque* (Widow of Abraham Vandenhoeck, Göttingen).

Soemmerring, S.T. (1788) *Vom Hirn und Rückenmark* (Winkopp, Mainz).

Soemmerring, S.T. (1791) *Vom Baue des Menschlichen Körpers*, Vol. 5, *Hirnlehre und Nervenlehre* (Varrentrapp & Wenner, Frankfurt am Main).

Soemmerring, S.T. (1792) *Vom Baue des Menschlichen Körpers*, Vol. 4, *Gefasselehre* (Varrentrapp & Wenner, Frankfurt am Main).

Soemmerring, S.T. (1796) *Über das Organ der Seele* (Nicolovius, Königsberg).

Soemmerring, S.T. (1798) *De Corporis Humani Fabrica*, Vol. 4 (Varrentrapp & Wenner, Frankfurt).

Soemmerring, S.T. (1799) *Icones Embryonum Humanorum* (Moenum, Frankfurt).

Soemmerring, S.T. (1800) *Vom Baue des Menschlichen Körpers*, 2nd Edn., Vol. 5, Part 1: *Lehre vom Hirne und von den Nerven* (Varrentrapp & Wenner, Frankfurt).

Soemmerring, S.T. (1801) *Abbildungen des Menschlichen Auges* (Varrentrapp und Wenner, Frankfurt am Main).

Soemmerring, S.T. (1806) *Abbildungen des Menslischen Hoerorganes* (Varrentrapp und Wenner, Frankfurt am Main). A Latin version was published in the same year, *Icones Organi Auditus Humani* (Varrentrapp und Wenner, Frankfurt am Main).

Soemmerring, S.T. (1809) De cerebri administrationibus anatomicis, vasorumque ejus habitu. *Denkschriften der Königlichen Akademie der Wissenschaften zu München* **1**:57–80.

Soemmerring, S.T. & Lisignolo, N. (1785) *Dissertatio Inauguralis Anatomica de Lapillis vel Prope vel Intra Glandulam Pinealem Sitis sive de Acervulo Cerebri* (Moguntiae, Mainz).

Soemmerring, S.T. & Noethig, F.N. (1786) *Dissertatio Inauguralis Anatomico de Decussatione Nervorum Opticorum* (Moguntiae, Mainz).

Solly, S. (1836) *The Human Brain, Its Configuration, Structure, Development, and Physiology* (Longman, Rees, Orme, Brown, Green and Longman; London).

Solmsen, F. (1961) Greek philosophy and the discovery of the nerves. *Museum Helveticum* **18**:150–197.

Solomon, C. & Trouilloud, P. (2003) *Le Corps & ses Mots: Présentation de la Briefve Collection de l'Administration Anatomique d'Ambroise Paré avec Translation* (l'Harmattan, Paris).

Sommé, C.L. (1824) *Recherches sur l'Anatomie Comparèe du Cerveau* (Ancelle, Antwerp).

Spiegel, A. (1627) *Adriani Spiegelli Bruxellenis Equitis D. Marci etc. De Humani Corporis Fabrica Libri Decem: Tabulis XCIIX Aeri Incisis Elegantissimis, nec Ante has Visis Exornati; Opus Posthumum Daniel Bucretius Jussu Autoris in Lucem Profert* (Deuchium, Venice).

Sporns, O., Tononi, G., & Kötter, R. (2005) The human connectome: a structural description of the human brain. *PLoS Computational Biology* **1**:e42.

Sprague, J.M. & Meyer, M. (1950) An experimental study of the fornix in the rabbit. *Journal of Anatomy* **84**:354–368.

Spurzheim, J.G. (1826) *The Anatomy of the Brain, With a General View of the Nervous System* (Highley, London).

Stamm, R.H. (1932) Ludvig Levin Jacobson. In: Meisen, V. (Ed.) *Prominent Danish Scientists Through the Ages with Facsimiles from their Works* (Oxford University Press, Oxford), pp. 97–99.

Standring, S. (2008) *Gray's Anatomy: The Anatomical Basis of Clinical Practice*, 40th Edn. (Churchill Livingston/Elsevier, Edinburgh).

Starkie, C. & Stewart D. (1931) The intra-mandibular course of the inferior dental nerve. *Journal of Anatomy* **65**:319–323.

Stedman's Medical Dictionary, 22nd Edn. (1972) (Williams & Wilkins, Baltimore).

Steenbergen, J.G. (1731) *Dissertatio Anatomico-Medica Inauguralis de Cerebro* (Kerckhem, Leiden).

Stein, M.B. & Carpenter, M.B. (1967) Central projections of portions of the vestibular ganglia innervating specific parts of the labyrinth in the rhesus monkey. *American Journal of Anatomy* **120**:281–318.

Steno, N. (1669) *Discourse de Monsieur Stenon sur l'Anatomie du Cerveau* (Ninville, Paris). Facsimile published with an English translation as *Nicolaus Steno's Lecture on the Anatomy of the Brain*, introduction by G. Scherz (Busck, Copenhagen), 1965.

Stieda, I. (1869) Studien über das centrale Nervensystem der Vögel und Säugethiere. *Zeitschrift für Wissenchaftliche Zoologie* **19**:1–94.

Stilling, B. (1840) *Physiologische, Pathologische und Medicinisch-practische Untersuchungen über die Spinal-Irritation* (Wigand, Leipzig).

Stilling, B. (1859) *Neue Untersuchungen über den Feineren Bau des Rüchenmarks* (Hotop, Cassel/Kassel).

Stilling, B. & Wallach, J. (1842–1843) *Untersuchungen über den Bau des Nervensystems*, 2 Vols. & Atlas (Wigand, Leipzig). Vol. 1 titled *Untersuchungen über die Textur des Rückenmarks.*

Straus Durckheim, H. (1828) *Considerations Generales sur l'Anatomie Comparee des Animaus Articules, Auxquelles On a Joint l'Anatomie Descriptive du Melolontha Vulgaris*, Text & Plate Volumes (Levrault, Paris).

Streeter, G.L. (1907) On the development of the membranous labyrinth and the acoustic and facial nerves in the human embryo. *American Journal of Anatomy* **6**:139–165.

Stricker, J. (1860) Entwickelungsgeschichte von *Bufo cinereus* bis zum Erscheinen der äusseren Kiemen. *Sitzungsberichte der Mathematisch-Naturwissenschaftlichen Classe der Kaiserlichen Akademie der Wissenschaften* **39**:472–478.

Strong, O.S. & Elwyn, A. (1943) *Human Neuroanatomy* (Williams & Wilkins, Baltimore).

Stroud, B.B. (1895) The mammalian cerebellum. Part I: The development of the cerebellum in man and the cat. *Journal of Comparative Neurology* **5**:71–118.

Stumphius, N. (1736) *Dissertatio Anatomica Inauguralis, de Cerebro* (Wishoff, Leiden).

Styx, M.E. (1782) *Descriptio Anatomica Nervi Cruralis et Obturatorii Icone Illustrata* (Fickelscherr, Jena).

Sutin, J. (1966) The periventricular stratum of the hypothalamus. *International Review of Neurobiology* **9**:263–300.

Swammerdam, J. (1669) *Historia Insectorum Generalis, Ofte, Algemeene Verhandeling van de Bloedeloose Dierkens waar in, de Waaragtige Gronden van Haare Langsaame Aangroeingen in Leedemaaten, Klaarelijk Werden Voorgestelt: Kragtiglijk, van de Gemeene Dwalling der Vervorming, Anders Metamorphosis Genoemt, Gesuyvert: Ende Beknoptelijk, in Vier Onderscheide Orderen van Veranderingen, Ofte Natuurelijke Uytbottingen in Leeden, Begreepen* (van Dreunen, Utrecht).

Swammerdam, J. (c1675), *see* Swammerdam (1737–1738), Swammerdam (1758).

Swammerdam, J. (1737–1738 but completed c1675) *Bybel der Natuure/Biblia Naturae; sive, Historia Insectorum*, 2 Vols. (Severinus, Leiden).

Swammerdam, J. (1758) *The Book of Nature, or, The History of Insects: Reduced to Distinct Classes, Confirmed by Particular Instances, Displayed in the Anatomical Analysis of Many Species, and Illustrated with Copper-Plates: Including the Generation of the Frog, the History of the Ephemerus, the Changes of Flies, Butterflies, and Beetles: with the Original Discovery of the Milk-vessels of the Cuttle-fish, and Many Other Curious Particulars* (Seyffert, London).

Swan, J. (1830) *A Demonstration of the Nerves of the Body* (Longman, Rees, Orme, Brown and Green; London).

Swanson, L.W. (1976) An autoradiographic study of the efferent connections of the preoptic region in the rat. *Journal of Comparative Neurology* **167**:227–256.

Swanson, L.W. (1986) Organization of mammalian neuroendocrine system. In: Bloom, F.E. (Ed.) *Handbook of Physiology, The Nervous System*, Vol. IV (Waverly Press, Baltimore), pp. 317–363.

Swanson, L.W. (1987) The hypothalamus. In: Björklund, A., Hökfelt, T., & Swanson, L.W. (Eds.) *Handbook of Chemical Neuroanatomy*, Vol. 5, *Integrated Systems of the CNS*, Part I, (Elsevier, Amsterdam), pp. 1–124.

Swanson, L.W. (1991) Biochemical switching in hypothalamic circuits mediating responses to stress. *Progress in Brain Research* **87**:181–200.

Swanson, L.W. (1992) *Brain Maps: Structure of the Rat Brain* (Elsevier, Amsterdam).

Swanson, L.W. (1993) *Brain Maps: Computer Graphics Files* (Elsevier, Amsterdam).

Swanson, L.W. (1998–1999) *Brain Maps: Structure of the Rat Brain. A Laboratory Guide with Printed and Electronic Templates for Data, Models and Schematics*, 2nd Edn. (Elsevier, Amsterdam).

Swanson, L.W. (2000a) Cerebral hemisphere regulation of motivated behavior. *Brain Research* **886**:113–164.

Swanson, L.W. (2000b) What is the brain? *Trends in Neuroscience* **23**:519–527.

Swanson, L.W. (2003) *Brain Architecture: Understanding the Basic Plan* (Oxford University Press, Oxford).

Swanson, L.W. (2004) *Brain Maps: Structure of the Rat Brain. A Laboratory Guide with Printed and Electronic Templates for Data, Models and Schematics*, 3rd Edn. (Elsevier, Amsterdam).

Swanson, L.W. (2012) *Brain Architecture: Understanding the Basic Plan*, 2nd Edn. (Oxford University Press, Oxford).

Swanson, L.W. & Bota, M. (2010) Foundational model of structural connectivity in the nervous system with a schema for wiring diagrams, connectome, and basic plan architecture. *Proceeding of the National Academy of Sciences USA* **107**:20610–20617.

Swanson, L.W. & Cowan, W.M. (1977) An autoradiographic study of the organization of the efferent connections of the hippocampal formation in the rat. *Journal of Comparative Neurology* **172**:49–84.

Swanson, L.W. & Cowan, W.M. (1979) The connections of the septal region in the rat. *Journal of Comparative Neurology* **186**:621–665.

Swanson, L.W. & Hartman, B.K. (1975) The central adrenergic system. An immunofluorescence study of the location of cell bodies and their efferent connections in the rat utilizing dopamine-β-hydroxylase as a marker. *Journal of Comparative Neurology* **163**:467–506.

Swanson, L.W., Köhler, C., & Björklund, A. (1987) The limbic region. I: The septohippocampal system. In: Björklund, A., Hökfelt, T., & Swanson, L.W. (Eds.) *Handbook of Chemical Neuroanatomy*, Vol. 5, *Integrated Systems of the CNS*, Part I, (Elsevier, Amsterdam), pp. 125–277.

Swanson, L.W. & McKellar, S. (1979) The distribution of oxytocin- and neurophysin-stained fibers in the spinal cord of the rat and monkey. *Journal of Comparative Neurology* **188**:87–106.

Swanson, L.W. & Petrovich, G.D. (1998) What is the amygdala? *Trends in Neurocience* **21**:323–331.

Swanson, L.W., Sanchez-Watts, G., & Watts, A.G. (2005) Comparison of melanin-concentrating hormone and hypocretin/orexin mRNA expression patterns in a new parcelling scheme of the lateral hypothalamic zone. *Neuroscience Letters* **387**:80–84.

Swanson, L.W., Wyss, J.M., & Cowan, W.M. (1978) An autoradiographic study of the organization of intrahippocampal association pathways in the rat. *Journal of Comparative Neurology* **181**:681–716.

Swanson, N. & Swanson, L.W. (1995), *see* Cajal, S.R. (1909–1911).

Sylvius; *see* Dubois, J.

Sylvius, F.; *see* Le Boë, F. de.

Szabó, N.-E., Zhao, T., Cankaya, M., Stoykova, A., Zhou, X, & Alvarez-Bolado, G. (2011) Interaction between axons and specific populations of surrounding cells is indispensable for collateral formation in the mammillary system. *PLoS One* **6**:e20315.

Talbot, S.A. (1942) A lateral localization in the cat's visual cortex. *Federation Proceedings* **1**:84.

Tarin, P. (1750) *Adversaria Anatomica, De Omnibus Corporis Humani Partium, tum Descriptionibus, cum Picturis. Adversaria Anatomica Prima, De Omnibus Cerebri, Nervorum & Organorum Functionibus Animalibus Inferventium, Descriptionibus & Iconismis* (Moreau, Paris).

Tarin, P. (1753) *Dictionnaire Anatomique suivi d'une Bibliotheque Anatomique et Physiologique* (Briasson, Paris).

Terminologia Anatomica (1998) (Thieme, Stuttgart). The terms are defined in *Dorland's* (2003).

Theophilos Protospatharios (1540) *In Galeni de Usu Partium Libros Epitome, quam de Corporis Humani Fabrica Inscripsit. J.P. Crasso Interprete* (Neobarium, Paris).

Thomas, H.M. (1910) Decussation of the pyramids—an historical inquiry. *Johns Hopkins Hospital Bulletin* **21**:304–311.

Thompson, D.W. (1962); *see* Aristotle, *Historia Animalium*.

Tiedemann, F. (1815) Beobachtungen über das Nervensystem und die sensiblen Erscheinungen der Seesterne. *Deutsches Archiv für die Physiologie* **1**:161–175.

Tiedemann, F. (1816) *Anatomie und Bildungsgeschichte des Gehirns im Foetus des Menschen: Nebst einer Vergleichenden Darstellung des Hirnbaues in den Thieren* (Steinishchen, Nuremberg). For translation see Tiedemann, F. (1826).

Tiedemann, F. (1821) *Icones Cerebri Simiarum et Quorundam Mammalium Rariorum* (Mohr et Winter, Heidelberg).

Tiedemann, F. (1822) *Tabulae Nervorum Uteri* (Oswald, Heidelberg).

Tiedemann, F. (1826) *The Anatomy of the Foetal Brain; with a Comparative Exposition of its Structure in Animals* (Carfrae & Son, Edinburgh). For the original German edition see Tiedemann, F. (1816).

Tilney, F. (1936) The development and constituents of the human hypophysis. *Bulletin of the Neurological Institute of New York* **5**:387–436.

Tilney, F. & Riley, H.A. (1923) *The Form and Functions of the Central Nervous System: An Introduction to the Study of Nervous Diseases* (Hoeber, New York).

Tiscornia, O.M., Drieling, D.A., Yacomotti, J., Kurtzbart, R., Torre, A. de La, & Farache, S. (1987) Neural control of the exocrine pancreas: an analysis of the cholinergic, adrenergic, and peptidergic pathways and their positive and negative components. 1: neural mechanisms. *Mount Sinai Journal of Medicine* **54**:366–383.

Todd, E.M. (1983) *The Neuroanatomy of Leonardo da Vinci* (Capra Press, Santa Barbara CA).

Todd, R.B., Ed. (1836–1839) *The Cyclopaedia of Anatomy and Physiology*, Vol. 2 (Sherwood, Gilbert, and Piper; London).

Todd, R.B. (1845) *The Descriptive and Physiological Anatomy of the Brain, Spinal Cord, and Ganglions, and of their Coverings* (Sherwood, Gilbert, and Piper; London). Facsimile published by Classics of Neurology & Neurosurgery Library, Birmingham, 1987.

Torres-Reveron, J. & Friedlander, M.J. (2007) Properties of persistent postnatal cortical subplate neurons. *Journal of Neuroscience* **27**:9962–9974.

Tóth, I.E., Boldogkoi, Z., Medveczky, I., & Palkovits, M. (1999) Lacrimal preganglionic neurons form a subdivision of the superior salivatory nucleus of rat: transneuronal labelling by pseudorabies virus. *Journal of the Autonomic Nervous System* **77**:45–54.

Treviranus, G.R. (1820), *see* Treviranus, G.R. & Treviranus, L.C. (1816–1821), Vol. 3.

Treviranus, G.R. (1835–1838) *Beiträge zur Aufklärung und der Erscheinungen Gesetze des Organischen Lebens*, one Vol. in 4 Pts. (Heyse, Bremen).

Treviranus, G.R. & Treviranus, L.C. (1816–1821) *Vermischte Schriften Anatomischen und Physiologischen Inhalts*, 4 Vols. (Röwen, Göttingen). Vol. 2 was published in 1817, Vol. 3 in 1820.

Tsai, C. (1925) The optic tracts and centers of the opossum, *Didelphis virginiana*. *Journal of Comparative Neurology* **39**:173–216.

Turner, W. (1891) The convolutions of the brain. A study in comparative anatomy. *Journal of Anatomy and Physiology* **25**:105–153.

Tyson, E. (1699) *Orang-Outang, sive Homo Sylvestris: or, the Anatomy of a Pygmie Compared with that of a Monkey, an Ape, and a Man* (Bennet & Brown for Hunt, London). Facsimile published by Dawsons of Pall Mall, London, 1966.

Valentin, G.G. (1841) *Hirn- und Nervenlehre*. In: Soemmerring, S.T., et al. (Eds.), *Vom Baue des Menschlichen Körpers*, Vol. 4 (Voss, Leipzig).

Valsalva, A.M. (1704) *De Aure Humana Tractus* (Pisarii, Bologna).

Valsalva, A.M. (1740) *Opera*, 3 Vols. (Pittari, Venice).

Valverde de Amusco, J. (1556) *Historia de la Composicion del Cuerpo Humano* (Salamanca y Lafrery, Rome).

Valverde de Amusco, J. (1560) *Anatome Corporis Humani* (Salamanca et Lafreri, Rome).

Valverde de Amusco, J. (1589) *Anatome Corporis Humani, Auctore Joanne Valverdo, Nunc Primùm à Michaele Colúmbo Latine Reddita, et Additis Novis Aliquot Tabulis Exornata* (Juntarum, Venice).

Van Hoesen, G.W. (1982) The parahippocampal gyrus. New observations regarding its cortical connections in the monkey. *Trends in Neurosciences* **5**:345–350.

Varoli, C. (1573) *De Neruis Opticis Nonnullisq; Aliis Praeter Communem Opinionem in Humano Capite Obseruatis* (Meitti, Padua). Facsimile and translation published by Culture et Civilisation, Brussels, 1969. It was reprinted in Varoli (1591).

Varoli, C. (1591) *Constanti Varolii, Philosophi ac Medici Bononiensis Anatomie, sive de Resolutione Corporis Humani ad Caesarem Mediovillanum Libri IIII: a Ioan. Baptista Cortesio nunc Primum Editi* (Wechelum & Fischerum, Frankfurt).

Verheyen, P. (1693) *Corporis Humani Anatomia, in qua Omnia tam Veterum, quam Recentiorum Anatomicarum Inventa Methodo Nova & Intellectu Facillima Describuntur, ac Tabulis Aenis Repraesentantur* (Aegidium Denique, Louvain).

Vesalius, A. (1543a) *De Humani Corporis Fabrica Libri Septem* (Oporinus, Basel).

Vesalius, A. (1543b) *Suorum de Humani Corporis Fabrica Librorum Epitome* (Oporinus, Basel).

Vesalius, A. (1555) *De Humani Corporis Fabrica Libri Septem*, 2nd folio Edn. (Oporinus, Basel).

Vesalius, A. (2002) *On the Fabric of the Human Body*. A Translation of *De Humani Corporis Fabrica Libri Septem, Book III, The Veins and Arteries, and Book IV, The Nerves*. W.F. Richardson and J.B. Carman (Norman, Novato).

Vesalius, A. (2009) *On the Fabric of the Human Body. A Translation of De Humani Corporis Fabrica Libri Septem, Book VI, The Heart and Associated Organs, and Book VII, The Brain*. W.F. Richardson and J.B. Carman (Norman, Novato).

Vesling, J. (1647) *Syntagma Anatomicum: Locis Plurimis Auctum, Emendatum, Novisque Iconibus Diligenter Exornatum* (Frambotti, Padua). See translation by Nicholas Culpeper in Vesling (1653).

Vesling, J. (1653), *The Anatomy of the Body of Man: Wherein is Exactly Described Every Part Thereof, in the Same Manner as It is Commonly Shewed in Publick Anatomies. And for the Further help of Yong Physitians and Chyrurgions, there is Added Very Many Copper Cuts, Far larger than is Printed in Any Book Written in the English Tongue. Also Explanations of Every Particular Expressed in the Copper Plates*, Englished by Nich. Culpeper (Cole, London).

Vicary, T. (1548) *The Anatomie of the Bodie of Man*. The edition of 1548 as reissued by the surgeons of the St. Bartholomew's in 1577, with a life of Vicary, notes on surgeons in England, Bartholomew's Hospital, and London, in Tudor times, an appendix of documents, and illustrations edited by F.J. Furnivall and P. Furnivall, Early English Text Society, Extra Series LIII, 1888, second impression 1930 (Milford, London).

Vicq d'Azyr, F. (1784) Recherches sur la structure de cerveau, du cervelet, de la moelle alongée, de la moelle épinière, et sur l'origine des nerfs de l'homme et des animaux [in 3 Parts]. *Histoire de l'Academie Royale des Sciences. Année MDCCLXXXI. Avec les Mémoires de Mathématique & de Physique, pour la même Année, Tirés des Registres de cette Académi, année 1781*, pp. 495–622 (published 1784). A fourth part in the series was published in the *Memoirs of the Royal Academy* for the year 1783, pp. 468–504 (published in 1786).

Vicq d'Azyr, F. (1786) *Traité d'Anatomie et de Physiologie, avec des Planches Coloriées Représentant au Naturel les Divers Organes de l'Homme et des Animaux*. Tome premier (Didot, Paris). All that was published.

Vicq d'Azyr, F. (1805) *Oeuvres de Vicq-d'Azyr, Recueillies et Publiées avec ces Notes et un Discours sur sa Vie et ses Ouvrages* (Duprat-Duverge, Paris). A poor edition with some illustrations omitted and others combined.

Vieussens, R. (1684) *Neurographia Universalis* (Certe, Lyons).

Villiger, E., Ludwig, E., & Rasmussen, A.T. (1951) *Atlas of Cross Section Anatomy of the Brain; Guide to the Study of the Morphology and Fiber Tracts of the Human Brain, Fifth Section of Emil Villiger's Brain and Spinal Cord*, 14th Edn. (Blakiston, New York).

Virchow R. (1846) Über das granulierte anschen der Wandungen der Gehirnventrikel. *Allgemeine Zeitschrift für Psychiatrie* **3**:242–250.

Vogt, C. & Vogt, O. (1919) Allgemeine Ergebnisse underer Hirnforschung. Vierte Mitteilung: Die physiologische Bedeutung der architektonischen Rindenfelderung auf Grund neuer Rindenreizungen. *Journal für Psychologie und Neurologie (Leipzig)* **25**:279–462.

Volkmann, A.W. (1831) *Anatomia Animalium, Tabulis Illustrata*, Bd. 1, Liber 1–2 (Lauffer, Leipzig).

von Bonin, G. (1960) *Some Papers on The Cerebral Cortex* (Thomas, Springfield IL).

von Staden, H. (1989) *Herophilus: The Art of Medicine in Early Alexandria* (Cambridge University Press, Cambridge).

Wagner, R. (1839) *Icones Physiologicalae. Tabulae Physiologiam et Geneseos Historiam Illustrantes* (Voss, Leipzig).

Waldeyer, W. (1889) Das Gorilla-Rückenmark. *Abhandlung der Königlich Preussischen Akademie der Wissenschaften zu Berlin vom Jahre 1888*, pp. 1–147.

Waldeyer, W. (1891) Über einige neuere Forschungen im Gebiete der Anatomie des Centralnervensystems. *Deutsche Medicinische Wochenschrift* **17**:1352–1356.

Walker, E.A. (1998) *The Genesis of Neuroscience* (The American Association of Neurological Surgeons, Washington DC).

Walsh, J. (1937) Galen's writings and influences inspiring them, part IV. *Annals of Medical History*, New Series **9**:34–61.

Walter, J.G. (1783) *Tabulae Nervorum Thoracis et Abdominis* (Deckeri, Berlin).

Walther, A.F. (1733) *Facultatis Medicae in Academia Lipsiensi H.T. Pro-cancellarius D. Aug. Frid. Walther Archiat. Regius et P.P.: Paris Intercostalis et Vagi Corporis Humani Nervorum et ab Utroque Eius Latere Obviorum Anatomen Exhibet Postquam Expositionem Cl. Winslow Nuperrime cum Cadavere Contulit atque Panegyrin Medicam Indicit* (Langenheim, Leipzig).

Walther, A.F. (1735) *Facultatis Medicae in Academia Lipsiensi H.T. Pro-cancellarius D. Aug. Frid. Walther Archiat. Regius et P.P.: Paris Intercostalis et Vagi Corporis Humani Nervorum et ab Utroque Eius Latere Obviorum Anatomen Exhibet Postquam Expositionem Cl. Winslow Nuperrime cum Cadavere Contulit atque Panegyrin Medicam Indicit* (Ex Officiana Langenhemiana, Leipzig). Reprinted in Haller, A.v. (1747–1751) *Disputationum Anatomicarum*, Vol. 2.

Weber, E.H. (1817) *Dissertatio Inauguralis Medica de Anatomia Comparata Nervi Sympathici* (Reclam, Leipzig).

Weber, E.H. (1827) Ueber das Geschmacksorgan der Karpfen und den Ursprung seiner Nerven. *Archiv für Anatomie und Physiologie* [**12**]:309–315.

Wecker, J.J. (1562) *Medicae Syntaxes, Medicinam Universam Ordine Pulcherrimo Complectentes: ex Selectioribus Medicis, tam Graecis quam Latinis et Arabibus Collectae et Concinnatae* (Parcum, Basel).

Weitbrecht, J. (1751) De vera significatione processuum mamillarium cerebri. *Commentarii Academiae Scientiarum Imperialis Petropolitanae*, Vol. 14 for 1744–1746 (published in 1751), pp. 276–285.

Wenzel, J. & Wenzel, K. (1811) *Observations sur le Cervelet, et sur les Diverses Parties du Cerveau dans les Épileptiques* (Dufour, Paris).

Wenzel, J. & Wenzel, K. (1812) *De Penitiori Structura Cerebri Hominis et Brutorum* (Cotta, Tübingen).

Wharton, T. (1656) *Adenographia: sive, Glandularum Totius Corporis Descriptio* (Typis J. G. impensis Authoris, London). A facsimile and English translation by S. Freer were published by Clarendon Press (Oxford University Press, Oxford), 1996.

Wiberg, J. (1914) The anatomy of the brain in the works of Galen and 'Ali' Abbas: a comparative historical-anatomical study. *Janus* **19**:17–32.

Wilder B.G. & Gage, S.H. (1882) *Anatomical Technology as Applied to the Domestic Cat* (Barnes, New York).

William of Saliceto (1275) *The Surgery of William of Saliceto*, English translation by Leonard D. Rosenman (Xlibris Corp., Philadelphia, 1998).

Williams, P.L. (1989) *Gray's Anatomy*, 37th Edn. (Livingstone, Edinburgh).

Williams, P.L. & Warwick, R. (1975) *Fuctional Neuroanatomy of Man: Being the Neurology Section from Gray's Anatomy*, 35th British Edn. (Saunders, Philadelphia).

Williams, P.L. & Warwick, R. (1980) *Gray's Anatomy*, 36th Edn. (Saunders, Philadelphia).

Willis, T. (1664) *Cerebri Anatome: Cui Accessit Nervorum Descriptio et Usus* (Flesher, Martyn and Allestry; London), the 4to edition. English translation by Pordage, S. (1681) *The Remaining Medical Works of that Famous and Renowned Physician Dr. Thomas Willis* (Dring, Harper, Leigh, & Martyn; London). Facsimile published by The Classics of Medicine Library, Birmingham, 1978.

Willis, T. (1667) *Pathologiae Cerebri et Nervosi Generis Specimen. In quo Agitur de Morbis Convulsivis, et de Scorbuto* (Excudebat Guil. Hall, impensis Ja. Allestry; Oxford). English translation published as *An Essay of the Pathology of the Brain and Nervous Stock: In which Convulsive Diseases are Treated of / Translated out of Latine into English, by S[amuel] P[ordage]* (Dring, London), 1681.

Willis, T. (1672) *De Anima Brutorum* (Davis, London). English translation published as *Two Discourses Concerning the Soul of Brutes, which is that of the Vital and Sensitive of Man*, Englished by S. Pordage (Dring, London), 1683. Facsimile published by Scholars' Facsimiles & Reprints, Gainsville FL, 1971.

Willis, T. (1681) *Clarissimi Viri Thomae Willis, Medicinae Doctoris, Naturalis Philosophiae Professoris Oxoniensis, Necnon Inclyti Medicorum Collegii Londinensis & Societatis Regiae Socii; Opera Omnia: Cum Elenchis Rerum et Rerum et Indicibus Necessariis, ut & Multis Figuris Aneis*, 2 Vols., 1st Edn., 2nd printing (Huguetan, Lyon).

Wilson, W.J.E. (1838) *Practical and Surgical Anatomy* (Longman, Orme, Brown, Green, Longmans; London).

Winslow, J.B. (1732) *Exposition Anatomique de la Structure du Corps Humain* (Desprez, Paris).

Winslow, J.B. (1733) *An Anatomical Exposition of the Structure of the Human Body*, translated from the French Original [1732] by G. Douglas (Prevost, London).

Woollam, D.H.M. (1958) Concepts of the brain and its functions in classical antiquity. In: Poynter, F.L.N. (Ed.) *The History and Philosophy of Knowledge of the Brain and its Functions* (Blackwell, Oxford), pp. 5–18.

Wreeden, O.J. (1741) *Kurze und Gründliche Demonstration des Gehirns und derer Theile, welche Selbes Umgeben, denen Chirurgis und Anatomicis zum Besten Nach der Lage und Structur Entworffen von Otto Just Wreden* (Gsellius, Leipzig).

Wrisberg, H.A. (1777) Observationes anatomicae de quinto pare nervorum encephali et de nervis qui ex eodem duram matrem ingredi falso dicuntur (d. X. Febr. 1776. praelectae). *Novi Commentarii Societatis Regiae Scientiarum Gottingensis* **7**:41–66. This article was also published as a pamphlet by Dieterich in Göttingen (1777, pp. 28 with one plate), and reprinted in Wrisberg (1800).

Wrisberg, H.A. (1780) *Observationum Anatomicarum de Nervis Viscerum Abdominalium Particula Prima quae de Ganglio Plexuque Semilunari Agit* (Dieterich, Göttingen). Also published as: Observationes anatomico neurologicae de ganglio plexuque semilunari in abdomine ex nervis illum formantibus (Praelect. d. XVIII. Dec. 1779). *Commentationes Societatis Regiae Scientiarum Gottingensis* **2**:79–111. This article was also reprinted in Wrisberg (1800).

Wrisberg, H.A. (1786) *Sylloge Commentationum Anatomicarum. I. de Membranarum ac Involucrorum Contenuationibus II. Nervis Arterias Venasque Comitantibus Et III. de Nervis Pharyngis* (Dieterich, Göttingen). Also published as: "Observationes anatomico-physiologicae de nervis arterias venasque comitantibus", and "Observationes anatomico-medicae de nervis pharyngis (Praelectae d. 11. Apr. a. 1785)". *Commentationes Societatis Regiae Scientiarum Gottingensis* **7**:95–134 and 135–160, respectively. These articles were also reprinted in Wrisberg (1800).

Wrisberg, H.A. (1800) *Commentationum Medici, Physiologici, Anatomici et Obstetricii Argumenti*, Vol. 1, Societatis Regiae Scientiarum Goettingensi oblatarum et editarum (Dietrich, Göttingen).

Wrisberg, H.A. (1804) Observationum anatomico-neurologicarum de nervis viscerum abdominalium Partic. II. De nervis systematis coeliaci Sectio I. De nervis gastricis quae est observationum de ganglio plexuque semilunari continuatio I. (Praelecta in publico soc. reg. scient. consensus d. XVII. Nov. 1798). *Commentationes Societatis Regiae Scientiarum Gottingensis* **15**:3–17. This article also appeared in Wrisberg (1800).

Wrisberg, H.A. (1808) Observationum anatomico-neurologicarum de nervis viscerum abdominalium partic. III. De nervis systematis coeliaci sectio II. De nervis hepaticis et splenicis, quae est observationum de ganglio plexuque semilunari continuatio II. (Praelecta in consessu soc. reg. scient. d. XXVII. Decembr. 1800) *Commentationes Societatis Regiae Scientiarum Gottingensis* **16**:15–47.

Wutzer, K.W. (1817) *De Corporis Humani Gangliorum Fabrica atque Usu, Monographia* (Nicolai, Berlin).

Wyss, J.M. & Sripanidkulchai, K. (1983) The indusium griseum and anterior hippocampal continuation in the rat. *Journal of Comparative Neurology* **219**:251–272.

Yoss, R.E. (1953) Studies of the spinal cord. Part II. Topographic localization within the ventral spono-cerebellar tract in the macaque. *Journal of Comparative Neurology* **99**:613–638.

Zanchin, G. & De Caro, R. (2006) The nervous system in colours: the *tabulae pictae* of G.F. d'Acquapendente (ca. 1533–1619). *Journal of Headache Pain* **7**:360–366.

Zerbi, G. (1502) *Liber Anathomie Corporis Humani et Singulorum Membrorum Illius* (Heirs of Ottaviano Scoto of Monza, Venice).

Ziehen, T. (1897–1901) Das Centralnervensystem der Monotremen und Marsupialier. *Denkschriften der Medicinisch-naturwissenschaftlichen Gesellschaft zu Jena* **6**(1):1–187, 677–728.

Zinn, J.G. (1755) *Descriptio Anatomica Oculi Humani* (Vandenhoeck, Göttingen).

Zuckerkandl, E. (1887) *Über das Riechcentrum. Eine Vergleichend-anatomische Studie* (Enke, Stuttgart).

List of All Defined Terms

There are two kinds of defined terms. Either they are ***standard terms (Author, date)*** used in the current nomenclature hierarchy (Figure 15 and Nomenclature Tables in Appendix) or they are *nonstandard terms (Author, date)*, which are listed chronologically by type (alternate spelling, translation, earlier synonym, later synonym, partly corresponds) under ***standard terms*** in the Lexicon. The preferred language for ***standard terms*** is American English.

abdominal aortic plexus (Chaussier, 1789), see ***prevertebral plexuses (Quain, 1832)***

abdominal aortic plexus (>1840), see ***intermesenteric plexus (>1840)***

abdominal brain (Wrisberg, 1780), see ***peripheral nervous system (Meckel, 1817)***

abdominal branch of first lumbar nerve (Bock, 1827), see ***ilio-inguinal nerve (Schmidt, 1794)***

abdominal branch of intercostal branches of dorsal nerves (Cruveilhier, 1836), see ***intercostal nerves (Vesalius, 1543a)***

abdominal branch of lumbar nerves (Bock, 1827), see ***spinal nerve ventral branch (>1840)***

abdominal branch of second nerve of body (Andersch, 1797), see ***phrenico-abdominal branches of phrenic nerve (Günther, 1786)***

abdominal branch proper of greater abdominal branch of lumbar plexus (Cruveilhier, 1836), see ***anterior cutaneous branch of iliohypogastric nerve (>1840)***

abdominal branches of first lumbar pair (Cruveilhier, 1836), see ***lumbar plexus ventral branches (>1840)***

abdominal branches of lateral left vagus nerve (Haase, 1781), see ***gastric branches of anterior vagal trunk (>1840)***

abdominal branches of lumbar plexus (Cruveilhier, 1836), see ***iliohypogastric nerve (Schmidt, 1794)***

abdominal chord (Grant, 1834a), see ***ventral cord (Anderson, 1837)***

abdominal column (Grant, 1834a), see ***ventral cord (Anderson, 1837)***

abdominal cord of spinal medulla (Cloquet, 1828), see ***dorsal funiculus (>1840)***

abdominal cord of spinal medulla (Desmoulins, 1825), see ***ventral funiculus (>1840)***

abdominal ganglia (Grant, 1834a), see ***ventral ganglia (Anderson, 1837)***

abdominal ganglion (Günther, 1786), see ***celiac ganglion (Walter, 1783)***

abdominal ganglions of limiting cord (Meckel, 1817), see ***sympathetic trunk ganglia (Winslow, 1733)***

abdominal medulla (Carus, 1818), see ***ventral cord (Anderson, 1837)***

abdominal nerves (Bock, 1827), see ***lumbar nerves (Diemerbroeck, 1672)***

abdominal nerves (Lobstein, 1823), see ***paravertebral nerves (Swanson & Bota, 2010)***

abdominal nervous cord (Anderson, 1837), see ***ventral cord (Anderson, 1837)***

abdominal part of pneumogastric nerve (Arnold, 1834), see ***vagus nerve trunk (Wrisberg, 1786; Günther, 1786)***

abdominal part of tenth pair (Arnold, 1834), see ***vagus nerve trunk (Wrisberg, 1786; Günther, 1786)***

abdominal part of vagus nerve (Arnold, 1834), see ***vagus nerve trunk (Wrisberg, 1786; Günther, 1786)***

abdominal plexus (Ludwig, 1772), see ***prevertebral plexuses (Quain, 1832)***

abdominal plexus (Meckel, 1817), see ***celiac plexus (Winslow, 1733)***

abdominal root (Desmoulins, 1825), see ***ventral root (>1840)***

abducens nerve branch to sympathetic (Langenbeck, 1826–1830), see ***communicating branch from internal carotid plexus to abducens nerve (>1840)***

abducens nerve central root (>1840)

abducens nerve central rootlets (>1840)

abducens nerve root (>1840)

abducens nerve rootlets (>1840)

abducens nerve trunk (>1840)

abducens nucleus (>1840)

abducent nerve (Heister, 1752)

abducent oculo-muscular nerve (Swan, 1830), see ***abducens nerve (Heister, 1717)***

abductor nerve of eye (Gordon, 1815), see ***abducens nerve (Heister, 1717)***

accessories of cornua Ammonis (Burdin, 1803), see ***parahippocampal gyrus (>1840)***

accessories of cylindroid protuberances (Burdin, 1803), see ***parahippocampal gyrus (>1840)***

accessory branch of saphenous nerve (Cruveilhier, 1836), see ***medial cutaneous branch of femoral nerve (>1840)***

accessory crural nerve (Styx, 1782), see ***lumbar plexus dorsal divisions (Paterson, 1887)***

accessory cuneate nucleus (>1840)

accessory cutaneous branch of internal saphenous nerve (Cruveilhier, 1836), see ***medial cutaneous branch of femoral nerve (>1840)***

accessory foot of hippocampus (Cruveilhier, 1836), see ***hippocampal region (Swanson et al., 1987)***

accessory ganglia (Walter, 1783), see ***intermediate ganglia (>1840)***

accessory great sympathetic nerve (Schmidt, 1794), see ***sympathetic cord (>1840)***

accessory internal crural nerve (Schmidt, 1794), see **accessory obturator nerve (Schmidt, 1794)**
accessory internal cutaneous nerve of arm (Cruveilhier, 1826), see **medial cutaneous nerve of arm (>1840)**
accessory nerve (Vieussens, 1684)
accessory nerve of internal crural nerve (Schmidt, 1794), see **accessory obturator nerve (Schmidt, 1794)**
accessory nerve of obturator nerve (Cloquet, 1828), see **accessory obturator nerve (Schmidt, 1794)**
accessory nerve of wandring pair (Willis, 1664), see **accessory nerve (Vieussens, 1684)**
accessory nerve of Weber (Bischoff, 1832), see **accessory nerve (Vieussens, 1684)**
accessory nerve of Willis (Vieussens 1684), see **spinal accessory nerve (Willis, 1664)**
accessory nerve to vagal pair (Frotscher, 1788), see **accessory nerve (Vieussens, 1684)**
accessory nerve trunk (Frotscher, 1788), see **spinal root of accessory nerve trunk (>1840)**
accessory nerve trunk (Wrisberg, 1786)
accessory nerves to eighth pair of Lobstein (Frotscher, 1788), see **accessory nerve (Vieussens, 1684)**
accessory obturator nerve (Schmidt, 1794)
accessory olfactory bulb (>1840)
accessory phrenic nerve (>1840)
accessory roots from medulla oblongata (Scarpa, 1788), see **cranial root of accessory nerve rootlets (>1840)**
accessory splanchnic nerve (Walter, 1783), see **lesser splanchnic nerve (Haller, 1762)**
accessory splanchnic nerve roots (Walter, 1783), see **lesser splanchnic nerve (Haller, 1762)**
accessory splanchnic nerve trunk (Walter, 1783), see **lesser splanchnic nerve (Haller, 1762)**
accessory sympathetic nerve (Walter, 1783), see **lesser splanchnic nerve (Haller, 1762)**
accessory sympathetic nerve trunk (Walter, 1783), see **lesser splanchnic nerve (Haller, 1762)**
accumbens nucleus (Ziehen, 1897–1901)
acervulo cerebri (Soemmerring & Lisignolo, 1785), see **brain sand (Soemmerring & Lisignolo, 1785)**
acervulus (Soemmerring & Lisignolo, 1785), see **brain sand (Soemmerring & Lisignolo, 1785)**
acervulus of pineal gland (Bock, 1824), see **brain sand (Soemmerring & Lisignolo, 1785)**
acoustic nerve (Galen, c173), see **vestibulocochlear nerve (>1840)**
acoustic nerve (Straus Durckheim, 1828), see **invertebrate nerves (>1840)**
acoustic nerve trunk (Scarpa, 1789), see **vestibulocochlear nerve trunk (>1840)**
acromial branch of descending superficial branches of cervical plexus (Quain, 1828), see **lateral supraclavicular nerves (>1840)**
acromial branch of descending superficial branches of cervical plexus (Quain, 1834), see **lateral supraclavicular nerves (>1840)**
acromial branch of thoracic part of tracheosubcutaneous nerves (Chaussier, 1809), see **intermediate supraclavicular nerves (>1840)**
acromial nerve (Quain, 1832), see **lateral supraclavicular nerves (>1840)**
acromial nerves (Bang, 1770), see **intermediate supraclavicular nerves (>1840)**
acromial supraclavicular branch (Peipers, 1793), see **lateral supraclavicular nerves (>1840)**
acromian branch of thoracic part of trachelo-cutanean plexus (Burdin, 1803), see **intermediate supraclavicular nerves (>1840)**
adcessory pair of cerebral nerves (Soemmerring, 1798), see **accessory nerve (Vieussens, 1684)**
adductor longus femoris nerve (Jördens, 1788), see **common fibular nerve (>1840)**
aden colatorius (Hall, 1565), see **pituitary gland (>1840)**
adenohypophysis (Rioch et al., 1940)
adhesio interthalamica (>1840), see **interthalamic adhesion (>1840)**
aditus ad aquaeductum (Bartholin, 1654), see **opening of cerebral aqueduct (>1840)**
aditus ad aquaeductum Sylvii (Haase, 1781), see **opening of cerebral aqueduct (>1840)**
aditus ad infundibulum (Bock, 1824), see **ventricles (Hippocrates)**
aditus ad infundibulum (Haase, 1781), see **interventricular foramen (>1840)**
aditus ad ventriculum tertium (Haase, 1781), see **interventricular foramen (>1840)**
adrenal plexus (>1840)
afterbrain (Baer, 1837)
after-brain (Crooke, 1615), see **cerebellum (Aristotle)**
afterbrain vesicle (Baer, 1837)
agger lunatus (Meckel, 1817), see **trigeminal ganglion (>1840)**
agranular frontal area (Brodmann, 1909), see **frontal region (Vicq d'Azyr, 1786)**
agranular retrolimbic area (Brodmann, 1909), see **agranular retrosplenial area (>1840)**
agranular retrosplenial area (>1840)
ais (Smith Papyrus, c1700 BC), see **brain (Smith Papyrus, c1700 BC)**
ajaz (Avicenna or Ibn Sina, c1030), see **fornix (Vesalius, 1543a)**
ala cinerea (Arnold, 1838b), see **vagal triangle (>1840)**
ala lobulus centralis (Reil, 1807–1808a), see **central lobule (Burdach, 1822)**
alae of inferior vermiform process (Gordon, 1815), see **caudal medullary velum (>1840)**
alar plate (>1840)
albicantes prominentiae duae pone infundibulum (Vieussens, 1684), see **mammillary body (Ludwig, 1779)**
almond-like lobe (Reil, 1807–1808a), see **tonsil (Malacarne, 1776)**
alveolar branch of inferior maxillary nerve (Jacobson, 1818), see **inferior dental nerve (Meckel, 1817)**
alveolar branch of second branch of fifth pair (Haase, 1781), see **posterior superior dental nerve (Haller, 1762)**
alveolar branch of superior maxillary nerve (Cuvier, 1800), see **posterior superior dental nerve (Haller, 1762)**

alveolar fascicles proper of inferior alveolar surculus of inferior maxillary branch (Bellingeri, 1818), see **inferior dental plexus (>1840)**

alveolar plexus (>1840), see **inferior dental plexus (>1840)**

alveus (Burdach, 1822)

alveus (Haller, 1762), see **foramen cecum of medulla (>1840)**

alveus (Le Böe, 1663), see **opening of fourth ventricle (>1840)**

alveus Sylvii (Haller, 1762), see **cerebral aqueduct (>1840)**

ambient gyrus (>1840)

ambiguus nucleus (>1840)

ambulatorium (Vesling, 1647), see **cranial nerves (Soemmerring, 1791)**

amiculum of olive (>1840)

amiculum olivare (>1840), see **amiculum of olive (>1840)**

Ammonic bundle of tuber cinereum (Cajal, 1901–1902), see **medial corticohypothalamic tract (Gurdjian, 1927)**

Ammon's horn (Garengeot, 1728), see **hippocampal region (Swanson et al., 1987)**

Ammon's horn (Noguez, 1726), see **fimbria (Honegger, 1890)**

Ammon's horn (Vicq d'Azyr, 1784)

Ammon's horn commissure (Forel, 1872), see **hippocampal commissures (Johnston, 1913)**

amygdala (Arnold, 1838a), see **basolateral amygdalar complex (>1840)**

amygdala (Malacarne, 1776), see **tonsil (Malacarne, 1776)**

amygdala (>1840), see **endbrain (Kuhlenbeck, 1927)**

amygdala input from small palatine nerves (Meckel, 1817), see **tonsillar branches of lateral palatine nerve (>1840)**

amygdalar nucleus (Burdach, 1822), see **basolateral amygdalar complex (>1840)**

amygdalar region (>1840), see **endbrain (Kuhlenbeck, 1927)**

anal cutaneous nerve (Walter, 1783), see **inferior rectal nerves (>1840)**

anal nerve (Cruveilhier, 1836), see **inferior rectal nerves (>1840)**

anastomoseos cum sympathico (Martin, 1781), see **communicating branches of spinal nerves (Wutzer, 1817)**

anastomoses between ulnar and radial dorsal nerves of thumb (Caldani, 1813, 1814), see **dorsal digital nerves of radial nerve (>1840)**

anastomosing branch of great sympathetic (Knox, 1832), see **communicating branches of sympathetic trunk (>1840)**

anastomosing branches communicate with limiting ganglions of ganglionnary system (Meckel, 1817), see **communicating branches of spinal nerves (Wutzer, 1817)**

anastomosing nerve of sympathetic (Knox, 1832), see **communicating branches of spinal nerves (>1840)**

anastomosis between anterior thoracic nerve and long anterior thoracic nerve (Cloquet, 1828), see **lateral pectoral nerve (>1840)**

anastomosis between first and second cervical nerve (Cloquet, 1828), see **communicating loops of cervical plexus (>1840)**

anastomosis between fourth and fifth cervical nerve (Cloquet, 1828), see **brachial plexus (Camper, 1760)**

anastomosis between internal palmar branch and external palmar branch of index finger (Cloquet, 1828), see **proper palmar digital nerves of median nerve (>1840)**

anastomosis between supratrochlear nerve and infratrochlear (Langenbeck, 1826–1830), see **supratrochlear nerve (Schaarschmidt, 1750)**

anastomosis between supreme cervical ganglion and vagus nerve (Langenbeck, 1826–1830), see **jugular nerves (>1840)**

anastomosis between third and fourth cervical nerve (Cloquet, 1828), see **communicating loops of cervical plexus (>1840)**

anastomosis of digastric branch of facial nerve with glossopharyngeal nerve (Meckel, 1817), see **communicating branch of digastric branch of facial nerve with glossopharyngeal nerve (>1840)**

anastomosis of glossopharyngeal nerve with pharyngeal nerves of eighth pair (Scarpa, 1788), see **glossopharyngeal nerve (Huber, 1744)**

anastomosis of internal branch of accessory nerve with eighth nerve fibers (Scarpa, 1788), see **internal branch of accessory nerve trunk (Meckel, 1817)**

anastomosis of Jacobson's nerve with sympathetic nerve (Langenbeck, 1826–1830), see **caroticotympanic nerves (>1840)**

anastomosis of Jacobson's nerve with Vidian nerve (Langenbeck, 1826–1830), see **tympanic nerve (Arnold, 1834)**

anastomosis of lacrimal nerve with subcutaneous malar nerve (Martin, 1781), see **communicating branch of lacrimal nerve with zygomatic nerve (>1840)**

anastomosis of left recurrent with anterior pulmonary plexus of right pneumogastric nerve (Knox, 1832), see **recurrent laryngeal nerve (Albinus, 1744)**

anastomosis of ninth nerve with lingual nerve of fifth pair (Scarpa, 1794), see **communicating branches of lingual nerve with hypoglossal nerve (>1840)**

anastomosis of second and third cervical nerves (Cloquet, 1828), see **communicating loops of cervical plexus (>1840)**

anastomosis of sympathetic nerve with second branch of trigeminal (Langenbeck, 1826–1830), see **internal carotid plexus (>1840)**

anastomosis of third cervical nerve with recurrent nerve of Willis (Peipers, 1793), see **accessory nerve (Vieussens, 1684)**

anastomotic arcade of palmar nerves of index finger (Cloquet, 1828), see **proper palmar digital nerves of median nerve (>1840)**

anastomotic arch of dorsal nerves of hand (Mayer, 1794), see **communicating branch of radial nerve with ulnar nerve (>1840)**

anastomotic branch between anterior branch of second cervical nerve and vagus (Langenbeck, 1826–1830), see **vagus nerve trunk (Wrisberg, 1786; Günther, 1786)**

anastomotic branch between anterior branches of cervical nerve two and cervical nerve three (Langenbeck, 1826–1830), see **communicating loops of cervical plexus (>1840)** *anastomotic branch between cervical nerves three and four (Langenbeck, 1826–1830)*, see **communicating loops of cervical plexus (>1840)**

anastomotic branch between oculomotor nerve and anterior branch of sympathetic (Langenbeck, 1826–1830), see **communicating branch from internal carotid plexus to oculomotor nerve (>1840)**

anastomotic branch of accessory nerve of Willis with glossopharyngeal nerve (Günther, 1786), see **accessory nerve trunk (Wrisberg, 1786)**

anastomotic branch of accessory nerve of Willis with ninth nerve (Günther, 1786), see **accessory nerve trunk (Wrisberg, 1786)**

anastomotic branch of accessory nerve of Willis with vagus nerve (Günther, 1786), see **accessory nerve trunk (Wrisberg, 1786)**

anastomotic branch of anterior branch of first cervical nerve with supreme cervical ganglion (Arnold, 1834), see **gray communicating branch (>1840)**

anastomotic branch of anterior branch of third cervical nerve with supreme cervical ganglion (Arnold, 1834), see **gray communicating branch (>1840)**

anastomotic branch of anterior gastric plexus with branch of semilunar ganglion (Günther, 1786), see **celiac branches of anterior vagal trunk (>1840)**

anastomotic branch of external branch of carotid branch of superior cervical ganglion with sphenopalatine ganglion (Cruveilhier, 1836), see **deep petrosal nerve (Meckel, 1817)**

anastomotic branch of first cervical nerve with second cervical nerve (Arnold, 1834), see **communicating loops of cervical plexus (>1840)**

anastomotic branch of first lumbar pair (Cruveilhier, 1836), see **genitofemoral nerve (>1840)**

anastomotic branch of ganglion of pneumogastric with facial nerve (Cruveilhier, 1836), see **communicating branch of intermediofacial nerve trunk with vagus nerve (>1840)**

anastomotic branch of glossopharyngeal nerve to facial nerve (Cruveilhier, 1836), see **communicating branch of digastric branch of facial nerve with glossopharyngeal nerve (>1840)**

anastomotic branch of glossopharyngeal nerve with internal deep branch of hard nerve (Günther, 1786), see **communicating branch of digastric branch of facial nerve with glossopharyngeal nerve (>1840)**

anastomotic branch of greater frontal nerve (Mayer, 1794), see **frontal nerve (Cheselden, 1726)**

anastomotic branch of greater frontal nerve (Meckel, 1753), see **supraorbital nerve (Meckel, 1753)**

anastomotic branch of hard nerve (Günther, 1786), see **communicating branch of intermediofacial nerve with tympanic plexus (>1840)**

anastomotic branch of internal branch of superior laryngeal nerve with recurrent laryngeal nerve (Meckel, 1817), see **communicating branch of superior laryngeal nerve with inferior laryngeal nerve (Langenbeck, 1826–1830)**

anastomotic branch of median and cubital nerves (Cloquet, 1828), see **communicating branch of median nerve with ulnar nerve (Bock, 1827)**

anastomotic branch of ninth pair with branch of lingual nerve of fifth pair (Günther, 1786), see **communicating branches of lingual nerve with hypoglossal nerve (>1840)**

anastomotic branch of peroneal saphenous nerve with tibial saphenous nerve (Cruveilhier, 1836), see **sural communicating branch of common fibular nerve (>1840)**

anastomotic branch of radial nerve with cubital nerve (Klint, 1784), see **communicating branch of radial nerve with ulnar nerve (>1840)**

anastomotic branch of spinal nerve (Cruveilhier, 1836), see **internal branch of accessory nerve trunk (Meckel, 1817)**

anastomotic branch of volar deep branch of ulnar nerve with superficial nerve (Günther, 1786), see **deep branch of ulnar nerve (>1840)**

anastomotic branches of carotid branch of superior cervical ganglion to sixth pair (Cruveilhier, 1836), see **communicating branch from internal carotid plexus to abducens nerve (>1840)**

anastomotic branches of external accessory nerve with second and third cervical nerves (Scarpa, 1788), see **external branch of accessory nerve trunk (Meckel, 1817)**

anastomotic branches of superficial temporal nerve with facial nerve (Meckel, 1817), see **communicating branches of auriculotemporal nerve with facial nerve (>1840)**

anastomotic fascicles of cutaneous temporal surculus of inferior maxillary branch (Bellingeri, 1818), see **communicating branches of auriculotemporal nerve with facial nerve (>1840)**

anastomotic fibril of external subcutaneous filament of deep frontal thread of supraorbital fascicle (Bellingeri, 1818), see **supraorbital nerve (Meckel, 1753)**

anastomotic fifth nerve (Meckel, 1817), see **nerve of pterygoid canal (>1840)**

anastomotic filament of cubital nerve (Cruveilhier, 1836), see **ulnar nerve (Cheselden, 1726)**

anastomotic filament of digastric branch (Bellingeri, 1818), see **digastric nerve (Meckel, 1753)**

anastomotic filament of external branch of carotid branch of superior cervical ganglion with branch of Jacobson (Cruveilhier, 1836), see **caroticotympanic nerves (>1840)**

anastomotic filament of external dorsal branch of cubital nerve internal dorsal branch of hand (Cruveilhier, 1836), see **dorsal digital nerves of ulnar nerve (>1840)**

anastomotic filament of portio major and minor of facial nerve with accessory nerve of Willis (Bellingeri, 1818), see **intermediofacial nerve trunk (>1840)**

anastomotic filament of portio major and minor of facial nerve with intercostal branch (Bellingeri, 1818), see **external carotid plexus (>1840)**

anastomotic filament of posterior mastoid branch of facial nerve with glossopharyngeal nerve (Cruveilhier, 1836), see **communicating branch of digastric branch of facial nerve with glossopharyngeal nerve (>1840)**

anastomotic filament of stylo-hyoid branch (Bellingeri, 1818), see **stylohyoid nerve (Meckel, 1753)** *anastomotic filament of superior facial branch of pes anserinus (Bellingeri, 1818)*, see **zygomatic branches of facial nerve (>1840)**

anastomotic filament of superior laryngeal branches of pneumogastric nerve (Cruveilhier, 1836), see **communicating branch of superior laryngeal nerve with inferior laryngeal nerve (Langenbeck, 1826–1830)**

anastomotic nerve between median and cubital nerves (Caldani, 1813, 1814), see **communicating branch of median nerve with ulnar nerve (Bock, 1827)**

anastomotic nerve of great sympathetic nerve (Walter, 1783), see **communicating branches of sympathetic trunk (>1840)**

anastomotic nerve of intercostal nerve (Walter, 1783), see **communicating branches of sympathetic trunk (>1840)**

anastomotic nerve with second common digital branch of median nerve and ulnar volar nerve of fourth finger (Caldani, 1813, 1814), see **brachial plexus medial cord (Schwalbe, 1881)**

anastomotic petrosal thread of Vidian fascicle with trunk of facial nerve (Bellingeri, 1818), see **greater petrosal nerve (>1840)**

anastomotic root between ganglia and trunk of great sympathetic nerve (Walter, 1783), see **communicating branches of spinal nerves (Wutzer, 1817)**

anastomotic thread of supratrochlear fascicle (Bellingeri, 1818), see **supratrochlear nerve (Schaarschmidt, 1750)**

anastomotic threads of internal dental fascicle with anterior dental fascicle (Bellingeri, 1818), see **superior dental plexus (>1840)**

anastomotic threads of supratrochlear fascicle (Bellingeri, 1818), see **supratrochlear nerve (Schaarschmidt, 1750)**

anceformes (Hall, 1565), see **tectum (Baer, 1837)**

anchae (Massa, 1536), see **caudate nucleus (Arnold, 1838b)**

anchae (Mondino, 1316), see **vertebrate brain (Cuvier, 1800)**

anchor (Chaussier, 1807), see **hippocampal region (Swanson et al., 1987)**

anchyroïde (Morand, 1748), see **posterior horn of lateral ventricle (Haller, 1747)**

ancyroid cavity (Morand, 1748), see **posterior horn of lateral ventricle (Haller, 1747)**

ancyroïde (Morand, 1748), see **posterior horn of lateral ventricle (Haller, 1747)**

anfractuosa cerebri fissura (Tarin, 1753), see **lateral cerebral sulcus (>1840)**

anfractuosity (Perrault, 1688), see **cerebral cortex gray matter (>1840)**

anfractuosity of digital cavity (Cruveilhier, 1836), see **posterior horn of lateral ventricle (Haller, 1747)**

anfractuosity of olfactory nerves (Cruveilhier, 1836), see **olfactory sulcus (Quain, 1834)**

anfractus (Vicq d'Azyr, 1786), see **cerebral sulci (Vesalius, 1543a)**

anfractus (Zerbi, 1502), see **cerebral cortex gray matter (>1840)**

angle of mouth filament of middle facial branch of pes anserinus (Bellingeri, 1818), see **zygomatic branches of facial nerve (>1840)**

angular area (Brodmann, 1909), see **angular gyrus (>1840)**

angular branch of lower jaw of inferior facial branch of hard nerve (Meckel, 1753), see **marginal mandibular branch of facial nerve (>1840)**

angular fossette of fourth ventricle (Chaussier, 1807), see **fourth ventricle (Galen, c192)**

angular gyrus (>1840)

angular muscle branch of brachial plexus (Cruveilhier, 1836), see **dorsal scapular nerve (Bock, 1827)**

annular convolution (Gerdy, 1838), see **limbic region (>1840)**

annular prominence (Schreger, 1803), see **pons (Haller, 1747)**

annular protuberance (Cloquet, 1828), see **brainstem (Schwalbe, 1881)**

annular protuberance and its prolongations (Bichat, 1801), see **brainstem (Schwalbe, 1881)**

annular tubercle (Swan, 1830), see **pons (Haller, 1747)**

annulary process (Vieussens, 1684), see **pons (Haller, 1747)**

annulary protuberance (Willis, 1664), see **pons (Haller, 1747)**

annuli (Günther, 1786), see **cerebellar cortex (Willis, 1664)**

annulus gangliformis (Cruveilhier, 1836), see **nerves (Herophilus, c335–c280 BC)**

anococcygeal nerves (>1840)

anonymous cavity (Haller, 1747), see **septal fissure (Burdach, 1822)**

ansa carotidi communi (Neubauer, 1772), see **ansa cervicalis (>1840)**

ansa cervicalis (>1840)

ansa formed by descending branch of hypoglossal nerve and third cervical nerve (Langenbeck, 1826–1830), see **ansa cervicalis (>1840)**

ansa magna circa subclaviam arteriam (Haller, 1772), see **ansa subclavia (Neubauer, 1772)**

ansa of intercostal nerve (Krüger, 1758), see **ansa subclavia (Neubauer, 1772)**

ansa of superior cerebellar peduncle (Reil, 1809c), see **superior cerebellar peduncle (Procháska, 1800)**

ansa peduncularis (>1840), see **peduncular loop (Gratiolet, 1857)**

ansa peduncularis of Gratiolet (Dejerine & Dejerine-Klumpke, 1895), see **peduncular loop (Gratiolet, 1857)**

ansa spermaticae (Walter, 1783), see **superior ovarian nerves (>1840)**

ansa subclavia (Neubauer, 1772)

ansa Vieussenii (Camper, 1760–1762), see **ansa subclavia (Neubauer, 1772)**

ansam communicationis nervorum cervicalium cum nono pari cerebri nervorum (Neubauer, 1772), see **ansa cervicalis (>1840)**

anse du pédoncule (Gratiolet, 1857), see **peduncular loop (Gratiolet, 1857)**

ansiform lobule (Bolk, 1906)

ansiform lobule crus 1 (Bolk, 1906)

ansiform lobule crus 2 (Bolk, 1906)

ansoparamedian fissure (>1840)
ansularam subclavias (Camper, 1760–1762), see **ansa subclavia (Neubauer, 1772)**
antennal nerve (Straus Durckheim, 1828), see **invertebrate nerves (>1840)**
anterior accessory optic tract (Bochenek, 1908), see **inferior fascicle of accessory optic system (Hayhow et al., 1960)**
anterior alveolar nerve (Günther, 1786), see **infraorbital nerve (Schaarschmidt, 1750)**
anterior alveolar nerves (Soemmerring, 1798), see **anterior superior dental nerve (Haller, 1762)**
anterior alveolar nerves of superior maxillary nerve (Schaarschmidt, 1750), see **anterior superior dental nerve (Haller, 1762)**
anterior alveolo-dental nerve (Cruveilhier, 1836), see **anterior superior dental nerve (Haller, 1762)**
anterior ampullary nerve (>1840)
anterior and exterior cerebral ganglion (Gall & Spurzheim, 1810), see **cerebral nuclei (Swanson, 2000a)**
anterior and internal pyramidal bodies (Günther, 1786), see **pyramid (Willis, 1664)**
anterior and lateral pyramid of Tarin (Günther, 1786), see **inferior cerebellar peduncle (Günther, 1786)**
anterior and posterior plexus gulae (Bell & Bell, 1816), see **esophageal plexus (Haller, 1762)**
anterior and posterior roots of trigeminal nerve (Meckel, 1817), see **trigeminal nerve motor root (Bell, 1829)**
anterior and superior nasal nerves (Schaarschmidt, 1750), see **posterior superior nasal nerves (Soemmerring, 1791)**
anterior aortic plexus (Andersch, 1797), see **cardiac plexus (Keill, 1698)**
anterior aortic plexus (Andersch & Soemmerring, 1792), see **preaortic plexus (Arnulf, 1939)**
anterior aperture of aqueduct of Sylvius (Mayer, 1794), see **opening of cerebral aqueduct (>1840)**
anterior aperture of third ventricle (Haase, 1781), see **interventricular foramen (>1840)**
anterior appendix of cerebellum (Willis, 1664), see **tectum (Baer, 1837)**
anterior arms of cerebrum (Chaussier, 1807), see **cerebral peduncle (Tarin, 1753)**
anterior auricular branch of hard nerve (Bang, 1770), see **auricular branch of posterior auricular nerve (Arnold, 1834)**
anterior auricular branches of anterior auricular nerve (Arnold, 1834), see **anterior auricular nerves (>1840)**
anterior auricular branches of deep cardiac plexus (Cruveilhier, 1836), see **cardiac plexus (Keill, 1698)**
anterior auricular branches of posterior zygomatic nerve (Meckel, 1753), see **temporal branches of facial nerve (Swan, 1830)**
anterior auricular branches of superficial temporal nerve (Arnold, 1834), see **anterior auricular nerves (>1840)**
anterior auricular nerve (Bock, 1817), see **auriculotemporal nerve (Haller, 1762)**
anterior auricular nerve (Mayer, 1794), see **temporal branches of facial nerve (Swan, 1830)**

anterior auricular nerves (>1840)
anterior belly of brain (William of Saliceto, 1275), see **endbrain (Kuhlenbeck, 1927)**
anterior bigeminal bodies (Owen, 1837), see **superior colliculus (Haller, 1762)**
anterior brachial branches of musculocutaneous nerve (Cruveilhier, 1836), see **muscular branches of musculocutaneous nerve (Günther, 1786)**
anterior brachial plexus (Günther, 1786), see **brachial plexus (Camper, 1760)**
anterior brachium of quadrigeminal body (Arnold, 1838a), see **brachium of superior colliculus (>1840)**
anterior brain (Aristotle), see **vertebrate brain (Cuvier, 1800)**
anterior brain (Vesalius, 1543a), see **vertebrate brain (Cuvier, 1800)**
anterior brain cell (Baer, 1837), see **primary forebrain vesicle (Baer, 1837)**
anterior brain vesicle (Baer, 1837), see **primary forebrain vesicle (Baer, 1837)**
anterior branch of acoustic nerve (Cloquet, 1828), see **cochlear nerve (Cotugno, 1760)**
anterior branch of anterior branch of fourth pair of cervical nerves (Bang, 1770), see **medial supraclavicular nerves (>1840)**
anterior branch of anterior commissure (Reil, 1812a), see **olfactory limb of anterior commissure (>1840)**
anterior branch of auditory nerve (Soemmerring, 1791), see **cochlear nerve (Cotugno, 1760)**
anterior branch of auricular nerve of third pair of cervical nerves (Meckel, 1753), see **anterior branch of great auricular nerve (>1840)**
anterior branch of auricular portion of hard part of acoustic nerve (Frotscher, 1788), see **auricular branch of posterior auricular nerve (Arnold, 1834)**
anterior branch of cardiac ganglion (Lobstein, 1823), see **cardiac plexus (Keill, 1698)**
anterior branch of cubital nerve (Frotscher, 1788), see **dorsal branch of ulnar nerve (Günther, 1786)**
anterior branch of dorsal branch of radial nerve (Cloquet, 1828), see **superficial branch of radial nerve (Martin, 1781)**
anterior branch of dorsal branch of radial nerve (Loder, 1803), see **superficial branch of radial nerve (Martin, 1781)**
anterior branch of external cutaneous branch of lumbar plexus (Quain, 1828), see **anterior cutaneous branch of iliohypogastric nerve (>1840)**
anterior branch of external cutaneous nerve (Fischer, 1791), see **lateral cutaneous nerve of thigh (>1840)**
anterior branch of external cutaneous nerve (Quain & Wilson, 1839), see **lateral cutaneous nerve of forearm (>1840)**
anterior branch of external deep branch of hard nerve (Haase, 1781), see **auricular branch of posterior auricular nerve (Arnold, 1834)**
anterior branch of external inguinal branch of lumbar plexus (Cruveilhier, 1836), see **ilio-inguinal nerve (Schmidt, 1794)**
anterior branch of fifth pair (Rau, 1694), see **ophthalmic nerve (Winslow, 1733)**

anterior branch of first lumbar nerve (Haller, 1762), see **subcostal nerve (>1840)**

anterior branch of great auricular nerve (Bock, 1827)

anterior branch of greater posterior auricular nerve (Bang, 1770), see **anterior branch of great auricular nerve (>1840)**

anterior branch of inferior maxillary nerve (Todd, 1836–1839), see **mandibular nerve trunk (>1840)**

anterior branch of internal cutaneous nerve (Loder, 1803), see **anterior branch of medial cutaneous nerve of forearm (>1840)**

anterior branch of internal deep nerve of hard nerve (Meckel, 1753), see **stylohyoid nerve (Meckel, 1753)**

anterior branch of lateral abdominal cutaneous nerve (Bock, 1827), see **anterior branch of lateral cutaneous branch of intercostal nerves (>1840)**

anterior branch of lateral cerebral sulcus (>1840)

anterior branch of lateral cutaneous branch of intercostal nerves (>1840)

anterior branch of lateral cutaneous nerve of intercostal nerve (Bock, 1827), see **anterior branch of lateral cutaneous branch of intercostal nerves (>1840)**

anterior branch of lateral pectoral cutaneous nerve of intercostal nerve (Bock, 1827), see **anterior branch of lateral cutaneous branch of intercostal nerves (>1840)**

anterior branch of lateral pectoral nerve (Bock, 1827), see **anterior branch of lateral cutaneous branch of intercostal nerves (>1840)**

anterior branch of mandibular nerve (>1840)

anterior branch of medial cutaneous nerve of forearm (>1840)

anterior branch of medulla oblongata (Winslow, 1733), see **brainstem (Schwalbe, 1881)**

anterior branch of musculocutaneous nerve (Bock, 1827), see **lateral cutaneous nerve of forearm (>1840)**

anterior branch of musculo-spiral nerve (Quain, 1832), see **superficial branch of radial nerve (Martin, 1781)**

anterior branch of nerve from spinal medulla (Vesalius, 1543a), see **spinal nerve ventral branches (>1840)**

anterior branch of obturator nerve (Haase, 1781; Martin, 1781)

anterior branch of palatine nerve (Bang, 1770), see **greater palatine nerve (Cloquet, 1816)**

anterior branch of posterior auricular nerve (Meckel, 1817), see **auricular branch of posterior auricular nerve (Arnold, 1834)**

anterior branch of posterior branch of auricular nerve (Meckel, 1753), see **posterior branch of great auricular nerve (Bock, 1827)**

anterior branch of posterior terminal branch of internal saphenous nerve (Cruveilhier, 1836), see **saphenous nerve (Haase, 1781)**

anterior branch of principal auricular nerve (Bang, 1770), see **anterior branch of great auricular nerve (>1840)**

anterior branch of proper intercostal nerve (Monro, 1783), see **intercostal nerves (Vesalius, 1543a)**

anterior branch of radial nerve (Caldani, 1813, 1814), see **superficial branch of radial nerve (Martin, 1781)**

anterior branch of radial nerve (Cloquet, 1828), see **superficial branch of radial nerve (Martin, 1781)**

anterior branch of radial nerve (Loder, 1803), see **superficial branch of radial nerve (Martin, 1781)**

anterior branch of right superior cardiac nerve (Cruveilhier, 1836), see **superior cardiac nerve (Neubauer, 1772)**

anterior branch of superficial temporal branch (Loder, 1778), see **superficial temporal branches of auriculotemporal nerve (>1840)**

anterior branch of sympathetic nerve (Langenbeck, 1826–1830), see **internal carotid plexus (>1840)**

anterior branch of third branch of fifth cerebral pair (Albinus, 1744), see **anterior branch of mandibular nerve (>1840)**

anterior branch of trunk of maxillary nerve (Le Cat, 1768), see **anterior branch of mandibular nerve (>1840)**

anterior branch of twelfth thoracic nerve (Meckel, 1817), see **subcostal nerve (>1840)**

anterior branches of anal nerve (Cruveilhier, 1836), see **inferior rectal nerves (>1840)**

anterior branches of auricular branch of cervical plexus (Cloquet, 1816), see **anterior branch of great auricular nerve (>1840)**

anterior branches of cerebrum (Chaussier, 1807), see **cerebral peduncle (Tarin, 1753)**

anterior branches of dorsal nerves (Cruvielhier, 1836), see **intercostal nerves (Vesalius, 1543a)**

anterior branches of facial nerve (Meckel, 1817), see **buccal branch of facial nerve (>1840)**

anterior branches of lumbar ganglia of intercostal nerve (Günther, 1786), see **lumbar splanchnic nerves (Cruveilhier, 1836)**

anterior branches of nerves coming forth from lumbar vertebrae (Vesalius, 1543a), see **lumbar plexus ventral branches (>1840)**

anterior branches of spheno-palatine ganglion (Quain & Wilson, 1839), see **posterior superior nasal nerves (Soemmerring, 1791)**

anterior branches of superior dorsal and four inferior cervical nerves (Meckel, 1817), see **brachial plexus roots (Schwalbe, 1881)**

anterior branches of superior laryngeal branches of pneumogastric nerve (Cruveilhier, 1836), see **internal branch of superior laryngeal nerve (Fyfe, 1800)**

anterior branches of thoracic nerves (Bock, 1827), see **intercostal nerves (Vesalius, 1543a)**

anterior bundle (Monro, 1783), see **ventral root (>1840)**

anterior bundle of anterior funiculus (Rosenthal, 1815), see **ventral funiculus (>1840)**

anterior bundles (Swan, 1830), see **ventral rootlets (>1740)**

anterior cardiac nerves (Mayer, 1794), see **gastric branches of anterior vagal trunk (>1840)**

anterior cardiac plexus (Burdin, 1803), see **cardiac plexus (Keill, 1698)**

anterior cerebellar crus (Mayer, 1779), see **middle cerebellar peduncle (Rolando, 1819)**

anterior cerebellar fissure (Reil, 1807–1808a), see **anterior cerebellar notch (Chaussier, 1807)**

anterior cerebellar notch (Chaussier, 1807)

anterior cerebellar peduncle (Chaussier, 1807), see **middle cerebellar peduncle (Rolando, 1819)**

anterior cerebellar peduncle (Prochâska, 1800, p. 371), see **superior cerebellar peduncle (Prochâska, 1800)**

anterior cerebellar peduncle (Prochâska, 1800, p. 372), see **middle cerebellar peduncle (Rolando, 1819)**

anterior cerebellar process (Haase, 1781), see **middle cerebellar peduncle (Rolando, 1819)**

anterior cerebellar process (Willis, 1664), see **superior cerebellar peduncle (Prochâska, 1800)**

anterior cerebral artery plexus (Chaussier, 1789)

anterior cerebral cell (Wagner, 1839), see **endbrain vesicle (Kuhlenbeck, 1927)**

anterior cerebral commissure (Tarin, 1753), see **anterior commissure (Lieutaud, 1742)**

anterior cerebral ganglion (Gall & Spurzheim, 1810), see **cerebral nuclei (Swanson, 2000a)**

anterior cerebral lobe (Willis, 1664), see **frontal region (Vicq d'Azyr, 1786)**

anterior cerebral prominence (Varoli, 1573), see **frontal region (Vicq d'Azyr, 1786)**

anterior cineritious substance (Monro, 1783), see **ventral horn (>1840)**

anterior cingulate region (>1840)

anterior clinoid sinus (Vicq d'Azyr, 1786), see **anterior intercavernous sinus (>1840)**

anterior collateral fissure (Bellingeri, 1823), see **ventrolateral sulcus of spinal cord (>1840)**

anterior column descending from hemisphere (Bell, 1834), see **corticospinal tract (>1840)**

anterior column of fornix (Riolan, 1618), see **fornix (Vesalius, 1543a)**

anterior column of fornix (>1840), see **postcommissural fornix (Loo, 1931)**

anterior column of fornix column (Dejerine & Dejerine-Klumpke, 1901), see **postcommissural fornix (Loo, 1931)**

anterior column of medullary triangle (Vicq d'Azyr, 1786), see **fornix (Vesalius, 1543a)**

anterior column of spinal marrow (Bell, 1822), see **ventral funiculus (>1840)**

anterior column of trigone (Dejerine & Dejerine-Klumpke, 1901), see **postcommissural fornix (Loo, 1931)**

anterior column of true fornix (Vieussens, 1684), see **postcommissural fornix (Loo, 1931)**

anterior column of vault (Longet, 1842), see **postcommissural fornix (Loo, 1931)**

anterior column of vault with three pillars (Vicq d'Azyr, 1786), see **fornix (Vesalius, 1543a)**

anterior commissure (Lieutaud, 1742)

anterior commissure (Vicq d'Azyr, 1784), see **ventral white commissure (>1840)**

anterior commissure central part (Reil, 1809c, 1812a), see **anterior commissure (Lieutaud, 1742)**

anterior commissure of middle lobe (Knox, 1832), see **anterior commissure (Lieutaud, 1742)**

anterior cord (Rolando, 1824), see **funiculi of spinal cord (Burdach, 1822)**

anterior cord of oblong medulla (Rolando, 1825a), see **ventrolateral fascicle (>1840)**

anterior cord of spinal marrow (Monro, 1783), see **spinal cord (Galen, c162–c166)**

anterior cord of spinal medulla (Desmoulins, 1825), see **ventral funiculus (>1840)**

anterior cords of spinal medulla (Rolando, 1825a), see **funiculi of spinal cord (Burdach, 1822)**

anterior coronary plexus (Scarpa, 1794), see **right coronary plexus (Scarpa, 1794)**

anterior corticospinal tract (>1840), see **uncrossed pyramidal tract (>1840)**

anterior cranial pairs (Cruveilhier, 1836), see **cranial nerves (Soemmerring, 1791)**

anterior cribriform plate (Meckel, 1817), see **cerebral nuclei (Swanson, 2000a)**

anterior crural nerve (Vieussens, 1684), see **femoral nerve (Haller, 1762)**

anterior crus of fornix (Beevor, 1891), see **postcommissural fornix (Loo, 1931)**

anterior crus of fornix (Colombo, 1559), see **fornix (Vesalius, 1543a)**

anterior crus of fornix (Haller, 1762), see **fornix (Vesalius, 1543a)**

anterior crus of fornix (Monro, 1783), see **hypothalamic postcommissural fornix (>1840)**

anterior crus of fornix (Vesling, 1647), see **fornix (Vesalius, 1543a)**

anterior crus of gray substance (Keuffel, 1810), see **ventral horn (>1840)**

anterior crus of lateral ventricle (Günther, 1786), see **lateral ventricle (Vesalius, 1543a)**

anterior crus of spinal medulla (Arnold, 1838b), see **ventral horn (>1840)**

anterior cutaneous branch of crural nerve (Fyfe, 1800), see **anterior cutaneous branches of femoral nerve (Quain & Wilson, 1839)**

anterior cutaneous branch of iliohypogastric nerve (>1840)

anterior cutaneous branch of intercostal nerves (>1840)

anterior cutaneous branches of anterior crural nerve (Quain, 1837), see **femoral nerve (Haller, 1762)**

anterior cutaneous branches of crural nerve (Quain & Wilson, 1839), see **anterior cutaneous branches of femoral nerve (Quain & Wilson, 1839)**

anterior cutaneous branches of dorsal nerves (Cruveilhier, 1836), see **anterior cutaneous branch of intercostal nerve (>1840)**

anterior cutaneous branches of femoral nerve (Quain, 1837), see **femoral nerve (Haller, 1762)**

anterior cutaneous branches of femoral nerve (Quain & Wilson, 1839)

anterior cutaneous nerve (Bell, 1803b), see **anterior cutaneous branches of femoral nerve (Quain & Wilson, 1839)**

anterior cutaneous nerve (Cloquet, 1828), see **anterior cutaneous branches of femoral nerve (Quain & Wilson, 1839)**

anterior cutaneous nerve (Styx, 1782), see **anterior cutaneous branches of femoral nerve (Quain & Wilson, 1839)**

anterior cutaneous nerve of crural nerve (Styx, 1782), see **anterior cutaneous branches of femoral nerve (Quain & Wilson, 1839)** *anterior cutaneous nerve of foot (Soemmerring, 1791)*, see **superficial fibular nerve (Fyfe, 1800)**

anterior cutaneous nerve of thigh (Bell, 1803a), see **anterior cutaneous branches of femoral nerve (Quain & Wilson, 1839)**

anterior cutaneous nerves of temple (Meckel, 1753), see **zygomaticotemporal nerve (>1840)**

anterior cystic nerves (Mayer, 1794), see **cystic plexus (Wrisberg, 1808)**

anterior deep nerve of ductus arteriosus (Andersch, 1797), see **cardiac plexus (Keill, 1698)**

anterior deep temporal branch of inferior maxillary nerve (Todd, 1836–1839), see **anterior deep temporal nerve (>1840)**

anterior deep temporal nerve (Arnold, 1834)

anterior dental branch of infraorbital nerve (Meckel, 1748), see **anterior superior dental nerve (Haller, 1762)**

anterior dental branch of superior maxillary branch (Meckel, 1748), see **anterior superior dental nerve (Haller, 1762)**

anterior dental branch of superior maxillary nerve (Quain, 1832), see **anterior superior dental nerve (Haller, 1762)**

anterior dental fascicles of inferior alveolar surculus of inferior maxillary branch (Bellingeri, 1818), see **inferior dental plexus (>1840)**

anterior dental nerve (Günther, 1786), see **infraorbital nerve (Schaarschmidt, 1750)**

anterior dental nerve (Meckel, 1748), see **anterior superior dental nerve (Haller, 1762)**

anterior dentar nerves (Meckel, 1817), see **anterior superior dental nerve (Haller, 1762)**

anterior division of auditory nerve (Bergmann, 1831), see **medullary striae (Scarpa, 1788)**

anterior dorsal cutaneous nerve of foot (Martin, 1781), see **superficial fibular nerve (Fyfe, 1800)**

anterior eminence (Ramsay, 1813), see **superior colliculus (Haller, 1762)**

anterior end of lateral part of spinal ashen-colored substance (Vicq d'Azyr, 1784), see **ventral horn (>1840)**

anterior end of worm (Galen, c173), see **cerebellar vermis (Meckel, 1817)**

anterior epiglottal nerve (Andersch & Soemmerring, 1792), see **internal branch of superior laryngeal nerve (Fyfe, 1800)**

anterior esophageal plexus (Haller, 1762)

anterior ethmoidal nerve (>1840)

anterior external branch of internal cutaneous nerve of arm (Cruveilhier, 1836), see **medial cutaneous nerve of arm (>1840)**

anterior external femoral cutaneous nerve (Bock, 1827), see **lateral cutaneous nerve of thigh (>1840)**

anterior extremity of vault (Cloquet, 1816), see **fornix (Vesalius, 1543a)**

anterior face of cerebellar ventricle (Chaussier, 1807), see **floor of fourth ventricle (Reil, 1807–1808a)**

anterior fascicle of spinal medulla (Bellingeri, 1823), see **ventral funiculus (>1840)**

anterior fascicles of acoustic nerve (Scarpa, 1789), see **caudal part of vestibular nerve (>1840)**

anterior fasciculus (Winslow, 1733), see **ventral root (>1840)**

anterior fasciculus of acustic nerve (Bell, 1803b), see **caudal part of vestibular nerve (>1840)**

anterior fasciculus proprius (>1840), see **ventral intersegmental tract (>1840)**

anterior femoral nerve (Keill, 1698), see **femoral nerve (Haller, 1762)**

anterior fibers of vagus nerve pair (Morgagni, 1719), see **glossopharyngeal nerve (Huber, 1744)**

anterior filament of internal branch of accessory nerve (Bischoff, 1832), see **internal branch of accessory nerve trunk (Meckel, 1817)**

anterior filament of perforating branch of intercostal branches of dorsal nerves (Cruveilhier, 1836), see **anterior branch of lateral cutaneous branch of intercostal nerves (>1840)**

anterior filaments (Huber, 1741), see **ventral root (>1840)**

anterior filaments of nerves of eighth pair (Winslow, 1733), see **glossopharyngeal nerve rootlets (>1840)**

anterior fissure (Burdach, 1822), see **anterior branch of lateral cerebral sulcus (>1840)**

anterior fissure (Vicq d'Azyr, 1784), see **ventral median fissure of spinal cord (>1840)**

anterior floor of third ventricle (Cruveilhier, 1836), see **terminal lamina (Burdach, 1822)**

anterior fold of corpus callosum (Reil, 1809b), see **genu of corpus callosum (Reil, 1809b)**

anterior foramen (Tyson, 1699), see **opening of cerebral aqueduct (>1840)**

anterior foramen coecum of pons (Mayer, 1794), see **interpeduncular fossa (>1840)**

anterior forceps (Arnold, 1838a), see **frontal forceps (>1840)**

anterior fovea (Arnold, 1838a), see **rostral fovea (>1840)**

anterior frontal branch of infratrochlear nerve (Meckel, 1753), see **infratrochlear nerve (Schaarschmidt, 1750)**

anterior frontal horn of lateral ventricle (Cruveilhier, 1836), see **lateral ventricle (Vesalius, 1543a)**

anterior funiculus (Burdach, 1822), see **ventral funiculus (>1840)**

anterior funiculus (Rosenthal, 1815), see **funiculi of spinal cord (Burdach, 1822)**

anterior ganglia (Serres, 1824–1826), see **ventral ganglia (Anderson, 1837)**

anterior ganglion (Bell, 1821), see **invertebrate brain (>1840)**

anterior ganglion of spinal cord (Solly, 1836), see **cerebral nuclei (Swanson, 2000a)**

anterior gastric plexus (Günther, 1786), see **gastric branches of anterior vagal trunk (>1840)**

anterior gastric plexus (Loder, 1778), see **peripheral nervous system (Meckel, 1817)**

anterior geniculate (Gerdy, 1838), see **dorsal lateral geniculate nucleus (>1840)**

anterior geniculate tubercle (Rolando, 1831), see **anterior thalamic nuclei (>1840)**

anterior gluteal cutaneous nerve (Bock, 1827), see **subcostal nerve (>1840)**

anterior gray bodies (Arnold, 1838b), see **medulla (Winslow, 1733)** *anterior gray column (Burdach, 1819)*, see **ventral horn (>1840)**

anterior gray fascicle (Wagner, 1839), see **ventral horn (>1840)**

anterior gray substance (Rolando, 1824), see **spinal cord (Galen, c162–c166)**

anterior greater branch of palatine nerve (Loder, 1778), see **greater palatine nerve (Cloquet, 1816)**

anterior greater palatine nerve (Meckel, 1748), see **greater palatine nerve (Cloquet, 1816)**

anterior half of spinal medulla (Meckel, 1817), see **spinal cord (Galen, c162–c166)**

anterior hepatic plexus (Mayer, 1794), see **hepatic plexus (Rau, 1720)**

anterior horn of cineritious substance (Bellingeri, 1823), see **ventral horn (>1840)**

anterior horn of lateral ventricle (Bell, 1803b)

anterior horn of lateral ventricle (Haller, 1747), see **inferior horn of lateral ventricle (Bell, 1802)**

anterior horn of lateral ventricle (Vicq d'Azyr, 1786), see **lateral ventricle (Vesalius, 1543a)**

anterior horn of medulla (Quain, 1828), see **ventral horn (>1840)**

anterior horn of spinal cord (Quain, 1828), see **ventral horn (>1840)**

anterior horn of tricornate ventricle (Soemmerring, 1791), see **lateral ventricle (Vesalius, 1543a)**

anterior hypothalamic nucleus (>1840)

anterior inferior dental branch of inferior maxillary nerve proper (Günther, 1786), see **inferior dental branches of inferior dental plexus (>1840)**

anterior inner ganglia of optic tubercles (Carus, 1814), see **cerebral nuclei (Swanson, 2000a)**

anterior intercavernous sinus (>1840)

anterior intercostal nerve (Haase, 1781), see **paravertebral nerves (Swanson & Bota, 2010)**

anterior intercostal nerve (Schaarschmidt, 1750), see **greater splanchnic nerve (Walter, 1783)**

anterior internal tubercle of optic thalamus (Vicq d'Azyr, 1786), see **anterior thalamic nuclei (>1840)**

anterior interosseous deep nerve (Mayer, 1794), see **anterior interosseous nerve (Quain, 1832)**

anterior interosseous nerve (Quain, 1832)

anterior intersegmental tract (>1840), see **ventral intersegmental tract (>1840)**

anterior junction of middle lobe (Knox, 1832), see **anterior commissure (Lieutaud, 1742)**

anterior labial nerves (>1840)

anterior lateral furrow of spinal marrow (Mayo, 1827), see **ventrolateral sulcus of spinal cord (>1840)**

anterior lateral part of central fissure (Gordon, 1815), see **inferior horn of lateral ventricle (Bell, 1802)**

anterior lateral sulcus of spinal marrow (Meckel, 1817), see **ventrolateral sulcus of spinal cord (>1840)**

anterior legs of cerebrum (Chaussier, 1807), see **cerebral peduncle (Tarin, 1753)**

anterior limb of internal capsule (>1840)

anterior limbus of striate body (Willis, 1672), see **external capsule (Burdach, 1822)**

anterior lobe (Burdach, 1822), see **frontal region (Vicq d'Azyr, 1786)**

anterior lobe (Fyfe, 1800), see **orbital region (Rolando, 1831)**

anterior lobe of cerebrum (Winslow, 1733), see **cerebral cortex gray matter (>1840)**

anterior lobe of pituitary gland (Haller, 1762)

anterior lobes of cerebellum (Gordon, 1815), see **cerebellar hemisphere (Willis, 1664)**

anterior lobule of median lobe of cerebellum (Serres, 1824–1826), see **cerebellar vermis (Burdach, 1822)**

anterior lobule of pituitary gland (Arnold, 1834), see **anterior lobe of pituitary gland (Haller, 1762)**

anterior longitudinal fissure (Arnold, 1838b), see **ventral median fissure of medulla (>1840)**

anterior longitudinal groove (Tiedemann, 1816), see **ventral median fissure of spinal cord (>1840)**

anterior mastoid branch of auricular nerve (Cruveilhier, 1836), see **posterior branch of great auricular nerve (Bock, 1827)**

anterior median fissure of neural mass of spinal column (Gall & Spurzheim, 1810), see **ventral median fissure of spinal cord (>1840)**

anterior median fissure of spinal cord (Gall & Spurzheim, 1810), see **ventral median fissure of spinal cord (>1840)**

anterior median furrow (Mayo, 1823), see **ventral median fissure of spinal cord (>1840)**

anterior median furrow of medulla oblongata (Mayo, 1827), see **ventral median fissure of medulla (>1840)**

anterior median sulcus (Bellingeri, 1823), see **ventral median fissure of spinal cord (>1840)**

anterior median sulcus of medulla oblongata (Quain, 1832), see **ventral median fissure of medulla (>1840)**

anterior medullar fibers (Coiter, 1572), see **ventral rootlets (>1840)**

anterior medullar filaments (Coiter, 1572), see **ventral rootlets (>1840)**

anterior medullar threads (Coiter, 1572), see **ventral rootlets (>1840)**

anterior medullary cord (Meckel, 1817), see **ventral funiculus (>1840)**

anterior medullary nuclei of Reil (Tiedemann, 1821), see **cerebral nuclei (Swanson, 2000a)**

anterior medullary velum (Reil, 1807–1808a), see **rostral medullary velum (>1840)**

anterior middle furrowed line of spinal cord (Knox, 1832), see **ventral median fissure of spinal cord (>1840)**

anterior nerve of back of foot (Meckel, 1817), see **medial dorsal cutaneous nerve (>1840)**

anterior nerve of foot (Meckel, 1817), see **medial dorsal cutaneous nerve (>1840)**

anterior nerve of lesser curvature (>1840)

anterior nerve of sixth conjugation of nerves of brain (Bauhin, 1605), see **glossopharyngeal nerve (Huber, 1744)**

anterior nerve of sixth conjugation of nerves of brain fibers (Bauhin, 1605), see **glossopharyngeal nerve rootlets (>1840)** *anterior nervous filaments (Winslow, 1733)*, see **ventral rootlets (>1740)**

anterior occipital nerve (Meckel, 1817), see **lesser occipital nerve (Mayer, 1794)**

anterior olfactory nucleus (Herrick, 1910)

anterior opening of aqueduct of Sylvius (Mayer, 1794), see ***opening of cerebral aqueduct (>1840)***

anterior orbital gyrus (>1840)

anterior oriface of third ventricle (Haase, 1781), see ***interventricular foramen (>1840)***

anterior palatine branches of naso-palatine ganglion (Quain & Wilson, 1839), see ***nasopalatine nerve (Scarpa, 1785)***

anterior palatine fascicle of sphenopalatine ganglion (Bellingeri, 1818); see ***greater palatine nerve (Cloquet, 1816)***

anterior palatine nerve (Meckel, 1748), see ***greater palatine nerve (Cloquet, 1816)***

anterior palatine nerves (Quain & Wilson, 1839), see ***nasopalatine nerve (Scarpa, 1785)***

anterior pancreatic nerves from splenic plexus (Walter, 1783), see ***pancreatic plexus (Cruveilhier, 1836)***

anterior paracentral gyrus (>1840)

anterior parolfactory sulcus (>1840)

anterior part of anterior commissure (>1840), see ***olfactory limb of anterior commissure (>1840)***

anterior part of brain (Aristole), see ***vertebrate brain (Cuvier, 1800)***

anterior part of brain (Berengario da Carpi, 1522), see ***vertebrate brain (Cuvier, 1800)***

anterior part of inferior vermiform process (Gordon, 1815), see ***nodule (Reil, 1807–1808a)***

anterior part of olivary fasciculus (Arnold, 1838b), see ***medial lemniscus (>1840)***

anterior part of tail of medulla oblongata (Pourfour du Petit, 1710), see ***medulla (Winslow, 1733)***

anterior part of trigeminal nerve (Vicq d'Azyr, 1786; Günther, 1786), see ***trigeminal nerve motor root (Bell, 1829)***

anterior part of white substance of spinal medulla (Arnold, 1838b), see ***ventral funiculus (>1840)***

anterior partition (Pourfour du Petit, 1710), see ***ventral median fissure of spinal cord (>1840)***

anterior pectoral nerves (Bock, 1827), see ***medial pectoral nerve (>1840)***

anterior peduncle of trigone (Chaussier, 1807), see ***fornix (Vesalius, 1543a)***

anterior peduncles (Cruveilhier, 1836), see ***cerebral peduncle (Tarin, 1753)***

anterior peduncles of cerebral protuberance (Cloquet, 1816), see ***cerebral peduncle (Tarin, 1753)***

anterior peduncles of pineal gland (Serres, 1824–1826), see ***medullary stria (Wenzel & Wenzel, 1812)***

anterior perforated plate (Meckel, 1817), see ***cerebral nuclei (Swanson, 2000a)***

anterior perforated substance (Vicq d'Azyr, 1784), see ***cerebral nuclei (Swanson, 2000a)***

anterior perforating branches of dorsal nerves (Cruveilhier, 1836), see ***anterior cutaneous branch of intercostal nerves (>1840)***

anterior perforating filaments of intercostal branch of intercostal branches of dorsal nerves (Cruveilhier, 1836), see ***anterior cutaneous branch of intercostal nerves (>1840)***

anterior peroneal nerve (Meckel, 1817), see ***medial dorsal cutaneous nerve (>1840)***

anterior pillar of fornix (Dejerine & Dejerine-Klumpke, 1901), see ***postcommissural fornix (Loo, 1931)***

anterior pillar of fornix (Herrick, 1915), see ***fornix (Vesalius, 1543a)***

anterior pillar of fornix (Paré, 1564), see ***fornix (Vesalius, 1543a)***

anterior pillar of fornix (Winslow, 1733), see ***fornix (Vesalius, 1543a)***

anterior pillar of fornix column (Dejerine & Dejerine-Klumpke, 1901), see ***postcommissural fornix (Loo, 1931)***

anterior pillar of longitudinal commissure (Solly, 1836), see ***fornix (Vesalius, 1543a)***

anterior pillar of trigone (Dejerine & Dejerine-Klumpke, 1901), see ***postcommissural fornix (Loo, 1931)***

anterior plate of spinal marrow (Meckel, 1817), see ***floor plate (>1840)***

anterior plexus gulae (Bell, 1803b), see ***anterior esophageal plexus (Haller, 1762)***

anterior pontine sulcus (Günther, 1786), see ***pontine sulcus (Soemmerring, 1778)***

anterior portion of oblong marrow (Willis, 1664), see ***vertebrate brain (Cuvier, 1800)***

anterior portion of three-fold nerve (Swan, 1830), see ***trigeminal nerve motor root (Bell, 1829)***

anterior primary brain vesicle (Baer, 1837), see ***primary forebrain vesicle (Baer, 1837)***

anterior process (Fyfe, 1800), see ***orbital region (Rolando, 1831)***

anterior processes of brain (Crooke, 1615), see ***cerebral cortex (>1840)***

anterior prolongation of cerebral protuberance (Bichat et al., 1801–1803), see ***cerebral peduncle (Tarin, 1753)***

anterior pulmonary branches of pneumogastric nerve (Cruveilhier, 1836), see ***pulmonary branches of vagus nerve (Cloquet, 1828)***

anterior pulmonary plexus (Haller, 1762)

anterior pulmonary plexus of eighth nerve (Scarpa, 1794), see ***anterior pulmonary plexus (Haller, 1762)***

anterior pulmonic plexus (Bell & Bell, 1816), see ***anterior pulmonary plexus (Haller, 1762)***

anterior pyramid (Rolando, 1825a), see ***brainstem (Schwalbe, 1881)***

anterior pyramidal body (Tarin, 1750, Tab. I), see ***trigeminal tubercle (>1840)***

anterior pyramidal body (Tarin, 1750, Tab. II), see ***pyramid (Willis, 1664)***

anterior quadrangular lobule (>1840), see ***culmen (Stroud, 1895)***

anterior quadrigeminal bodies (Tiedemann, 1821), see ***superior colliculus (Haller, 1762)***

anterior renal ganglion (Tiedemann, 1822)

anterior renal nerves (Mayer, 1794), see ***intrinsic renal nerves (>1840)***

anterior renal nerves (Walter, 1783), see **intrinsic renal nerves (>1840)**
anterior rima of medulla oblongata (Monro, 1783), see **median sulcus of fourth ventricle (>1840)**
anterior root (Asch, 1750), see **ventral root (>1840)**
anterior root of fifth nerve (Bell, 1829), see **trigeminal nerve motor root (Bell, 1829)**
anterior root of sphenopalatine ganglion (Meckel, 1751), see **pterygopalatine nerves (Wrisberg, 1786)**
anterior scrotal nerves (>1840)
anterior semilunar notch (Tiedemann, 1816), see **anterior cerebellar notch (Chaussier, 1807)**
anterior set of primary divisions of brachial plexus (Quain, 1828), see **brachial plexus ventral divisions (Paterson, 1887)**
anterior sinus (de Laguna, 1535), see **lateral ventricle (Vesalius, 1543a)**
anterior sinus of lateral ventricle (Bell, 1802), see **lateral ventricle (Vesalius, 1543a)**
anterior sinus of lateral ventricle (Bell, 1803b), see **anterior horn of lateral ventricle (Bell, 1803b)**
anterior sinus of superior ventricle (Vicq d'Azyr, 1786), see **lateral ventricle (Vesalius, 1543a)**
anterior spinal branches (Cruveilhier, 1836), see **spinal nerve ventral branches (>1840)**
anterior spinal marrow (Varoli, 1573), see **brainstem (Schwalbe, 1881)**
anterior spinocerebellar tract (>1840), see **ventral spinocerebellar tract (>1840)**
anterior stomachic nerve (Winslow, 1733), see **anterior vagal trunk (Wrisberg, 1780)**
anterior striated body (Solly, 1836), see **cerebral nuclei (Swanson, 2000a)**
anterior subcutaneous branch of intercostal branch of thoracic nerve (Bock, 1827), see **anterior cutaneous branch of intercostal nerves (>1840)**
anterior subcutaneous nerves of temple (Meckel, 1753), see **zygomaticotemporal nerve (>1840)**
anterior sulcus (Vieussens, 1684), see **ventral median fissure of spinal cord (>1840)**
anterior sulcus of medulla oblongata (Vicq d'Azyr, 1786), see **ventral median fissure of medulla (>1840)**
anterior superclavicular nerves (Bell & Bell, 1816), see **medial supraclavicular nerves (>1840)**
anterior superficial branch of peroneal nerve (Mayer, 1794), see **superficial fibular nerve (Fyfe, 1800)**
anterior superficial nerve of neck (Peipers, 1793), see **inferior branch of transverse nerve of neck (>1840)**
anterior superior alveolar nerve (Henle, 1871), see **anterior superior dental nerve (Haller, 1762)**
anterior superior branches of nasal branches from fifth pair (Scarpa, 1785), see **posterior superior nasal nerves (Soemmerring, 1791)**
anterior superior dental nerve (Haller, 1762)
anterior superior internal nerves of palatine nerve (Bell & Bell, 1826), see **posterior inferior nasal nerves (>1840)**
anterior superior labial nerve (Mayer, 1794), see **superior labial branches of infraorbital nerve (Meckel, 1748)**
anterior superior nasal branches of Vidian nerve (Meckel, 1748), see **lateral posterior superior nasal nerves (>1840)**
anterior superior nasal fascicles of sphenopalatine ganglion (Bellingeri, 1818), see **posterior superior nasal nerves (Soemmerring, 1791)**
anterior superior nasal nerves (Soemmerring, 1791), see **pterygopalatine nerves (Wrisberg, 1786)**
anterior superior nucleus of thalamus of optic nerve (Arnold, 1838b), see **anterior thalamic nuclei (>1840)**
anterior superior ventricle of cerebrum (Winslow, 1733), see **lateral ventricle (Vesalius, 1543a)**
anterior supraclavicular nerves (Meckel, 1817), see **medial supraclavicular nerves (>1840)**
anterior surface of cerebellum (Vicq d'Azyr, 1784), see **cerebellum (Aristotle)**
anterior temporal nerve (Soemmerring, 1791), see **temporal branches of facial nerve (Swan, 1830)**
anterior temporal nerve of hard nerve (Meckel, 1753), see **temporal branches of facial nerve (Swan, 1830)**
anterior terminal branch of internal saphenous nerve (Cruveilhier, 1836), see **infrapatellar branch of saphenous nerve (>1840)**
anterior thalamic nuclei (>1840)
anterior thalamic tubercle (Gordon, 1815), see **anterior thalamic nuclei (>1840)**
anterior thoracic branch of brachial plexus (Cloquet, 1816), see **medial pectoral nerve (>1840)**
anterior thoracic branch of brachial plexus (Cruveilhier, 1836), see **lateral pectoral nerve (>1840)**
anterior thoracic nerve (Cloquet, 1828), see **lateral pectoral nerve (>1840)**
anterior thoracic nerves (Günther, 1786), see **spinal nerve ventral branch (>1840)**
anterior thoracic nerves (Meckel, 1817), see **brachial plexus cords (Schwalbe, 1881)**
anterior tibial branch of external popliteal nerve (Cloquet, 1816), see **deep fibular nerve (Fyfe, 1800)**
anterior tibial nerve (Haller, 1762), see **common fibular nerve (>1840)**
anterior tibial nerve (Meckel, 1817), see **deep fibular nerve (Fyfe, 1800)**
anterior trunk of eighth pair of nerves (Wrisberg, 1780), see **anterior vagal trunk (Wrisberg, 1780)**
anterior trunk of ethmoidal nerve (Meckel, 1817), see **anterior ethmoidal nerve (>1840)**
anterior trunk of gastric and hepatic nerve (Walter, 1783), see **anterior vagal trunk (Wrisberg, 1780)**
anterior trunk of gastric and hepatic plexus (Walter, 1783), see **anterior vagal trunk (Wrisberg, 1780)**
anterior trunk of sub-occipital nerve (Swan, 1830), see **suboccipital nerve (Winslow, 1733)**
anterior tubercle (Winslow, 1733), see **superior colliculus (Haller, 1762)**
anterior tubercle of optic thalamus (Vicq d'Azyr, 1786), see **anterior thalamic nuclei (>1840)**
anterior tubercle of thalamus opticus (Gordon, 1815), see **dorsal lateral geniculate nucleus (>1840)**
anterior twig of deep branch of peroneal nerve (Jördens, 1788), see **muscular branches of deep fibular nerve (>1840)**
anterior twig of great cervical auricular nerve (Soemmerring, 1791), see **anterior branch of great auricular nerve (>1840)**

anterior vagal trunk (Wrisberg, 1780)

anterior valve (Burdach, 1822), see **rostral medullary vellum (>1840)**

anterior ventricle (Galen, c173), see **lateral ventricle (Vesalius, 1543a)**

anterior ventricle (Gordon, 1815), see **third ventricle (Galen, c173)**

anterior ventricular aperture (Günther, 1786), see **interventricular foramen (>1840)**

anterior ventricular oriface (Günther, 1786), see **interventricular foramen (>1840)**

anterior vermicular eminences of cerebellum (Palfijn, 1726), see **cerebellar vermis (Meckel, 1817)**

anterior vermiform appendix (Winslow, 1733), see **cerebellar vermis (Meckel, 1817)**

anterior vermiform process (Vieussens, 1684), see **cerebellar vermis (Meckel, 1817)**

anterior vermiform process proper (Meckel, 1817), see **cerebellar vermis (Meckel, 1817)**

anterior vertical branch of Sylvian fissure (Vicq d'Azyr, 1784), see **ascending branch of lateral cerebral sulcus (>1840)**

anterior white commissure (Vicq d'Azyr, 1784), see **ventral white commissure (>1840)**

anterior worm (Massa, 1536), see **cerebellar vermis (Meckel, 1817)**

anterior zygomatic threads of temporal surculus (Bellingeri, 1818), see **temporal branches of facial nerve (Swan, 1830)**

anterioris plexus pulmonis (Haller, 1762), see **anterior pulmonary plexus (Haller, 1762)**

anterolateral column (>1840), see **lateral funiculus (Burdach, 1822)**

anterolateral cord (Rolando, 1825a), see **ventrolateral fascicle (>1840)**

anterolateral cord of oblong medulla (Rolando, 1825a), see **ventrolateral fascicle (>1840)**

anterolateral cord of spinal medulla (Rolando, 1825a), see **funiculi of spinal cord (Burdach, 1822)**

anterolateral fasciculus (>1840), see **ventrolateral fascicle (>1840)**

anterolateral funiculus (>1840), see **funiculi of spinal cord (Burdach, 1822)**

anteromedial arch (Rolando, 1831), see **uncinate fascicle (Reil, 1809b)**

antibrachial deep branch of radial nerve (Cruveilhier, 1836), see **deep branch of radial nerve (Martin, 1781)**

antibrachial muscular branch of radial nerve (Cruveilhier, 1836), see **deep branch of radial nerve (Martin, 1781)**

antilaryngeal cutaneous nerve of neck (Peipers, 1793), see **inferior branch of transverse nerve of neck (>1840)**

antrum nervorum motoriorum communium oculorum (Malacarne, 1776), see **interpeduncular fossa (>1840)**

anus (Bartholin, 1662), see **cerebral aqueduct (>1840)**

anus (Bauhin, 1605), see **opening of cerebral aqueduct (>1840)**

anus (Willis, 1664), see **opening of cerebral aqueduct (>1840)**

anus (Vesalius, 1543a), see **opening of fourth ventricle (>1840)**

aortic branch of ninth thoracic ganglion (Walter, 1783), see **paravertebral nerves (Swanson & Bota, 2010)**

aortic filaments from thoracic ganglia of great sympathetic (Cloquet, 1828), see **paravertebral nerves (Swanson & Bota, 2010)**

aortic plexus (Cloquet, 1816), see **intermesenteric plexus (>1840)**

aortic plexus (Fyfe, 1800), see **prevertebral plexuses (Quain, 1832)**

aortic plexus (Lobstein, 1823), see **thoracic aortic plexus (>1840)**

aortic plexus (Quain, 1837, p. 814), see **cardiac plexus (Keill, 1698)**

aortic plexus (Quain, 1837, p. 819), see **prevertebral plexuses (Quain, 1832)**

aorticorenal ganglion (>1840)

apertura ad ventriculum tertium (Haase, 1781), see **interventricular foramen (>1840)**

apertura anterior ventriculi tertii (Malacarne, 1780), see **interventricular foramen (>1840)**

apertura aqueductus cerebri (>1840), see **opening of cerebral aqueduct (>1840)**

apertura declivis (Willis, 1664), see **opening of cerebral aqueduct (>1840)**

apertura lateralis ventriculi quarti (>1840), see **lateral aperture of fourth ventricle (>1840)**

apertura mediana ventriculi quarti (>1840), see **median aperture of fourth ventricle (>1840)**

aperture (Galen, c177), see **interventricular foramen (>1840)**

apex of medulla oblongata (Ridley, 1695), see **cerebral nuclei (Swanson, 2000a)**

apex of spinal medulla (Tiedemann, 1821), see **medullary cone (>1840)**

apophysis (Diemerbroeck, 1689), see **spinal cord (Galen, c162–c166)**

apoplectic nerve (Berengario da Carpi, 1522), see **vagus nerve (Galen, c192)**

apparatus of formation (Gall & Spurzheim, 1810), see **central nervous system white matter tracts (>1840)**

apparatus of union (Gall & Spurzheim, 1810), see **central nervous system white matter tracts (>1840)**

apparent origin of accessory nerve of Willis (Cruveilhier, 1836), see **spinal roots of accessory nerve rootlets (>1840)**

apparent origin of common motor nerve of eye (Cruveilhier, 1836), see **oculomotor nerve rootlets (>1840)**

apparent origin of external ocular motor nerve (Cruveilhier, 1836), see **abducens nerve rootlets (>1840)**

apparent origin of olfactory nerve (Cruveilhier, 1836), see **endbrain (Kuhlenbeck, 1927)**

apparent origin of pathetic nerve (Cruveilhier, 1836), see **trochlear nerve (Molinetti, 1669)**

apparent origin of portio dura (Cruveilhier, 1836), see **facial nerve root (>1840)**

apparent origin of trigeminal nerve (Cruveilhier, 1836), see **trigeminal nerve (Winslow, 1733)**

appendices of ventricles (Burdin, 1803), see **posterior horn of lateral ventricle (Haller, 1747)**

appendicula cerebri (Ebel, 1789), see **pituitary gland (>1840)**

appendix (Morgagni, 1719), see **posterior lobe of pituitary gland (Haller, 1762)**

appendix cerebri (Haller, 1762), see **pituitary gland (>1840)**

appendix flabelli (Bergmann, 1831), see **internal capsule (Burdach, 1822)**
appendix glandulae pituitariae (Santorini, 1724), see **posterior lobe of pituitary gland (Haller, 1762)**
appendix of brain (Willis, 1664), see **central nervous system (Carus, 1814)**
appendix of cerebrum (Soemmerring, 1778), see **cerebellum (Aristotle)**
appendix of nates (Willis, 1664), see **brachium of superior colliculus (>1840)**
appendix of spinal medulla (Malpighi, 1665), see **vertebrate brain (Cuvier, 1800)**
appendix of spinal pith (Diemerbroeck, 1689), see **vertebrate brain (Cuvier, 1800)**
aqua emissarium (Vieussens, 1684), see **cerebral aqueduct (>1840)**
aqueduct (Aranzi, 1587), see **cerebral aqueduct (>1840)**
aqueduct (Brunn, 1753), see **hypothalamus (Kuhlenbeck, 1927)**
aqueduct of quadrigeminal tubercles (Cruveilhier, 1836), see **cerebral aqueduct (>1840)**
aqueductus cerebri (>1840), see **cerebral aqueduct (>1840)**
arachnoid (Blasius, 1666)
arachnoid (Rufus of Ephesus, c90–120), see **retina (Herophilus, c335–c280 BC)**
arachnoid cavity (Magendie, 1825), see **subarachnoid space (Magendie, 1827)**
arachnoid granulations (>1840)
arachnoid membrane (Günther, 1786), see **arachnoid (Blasius, 1666)**
arachnoid membrane (Meckel, 1817)
arachnoid trabeculae (>1840)
arbor medullaris (Arnold, 1838a), see **arbor vitae (Winslow, 1733)**
arbor vitae (Winslow, 1733)
arbor vitae of brain (Cruveilhier, 1836), see **cerebral cortex white matter (>1840)**
arbusculis medullaribus (Heister, 1717), see **arbor vitae (Winslow, 1733)**
arch (Galen, c173), see **fornix (Vesalius, 1543a)**
arch (Hall, 1565), see **fornix (Vesalius, 1543a)**
arch (Vesalius, 1543a), see **cerebral cortex white matter (>1840)**
arch-like body (Galen, c177), see **fornix (Vesalius, 1543a)**
arch of hyoidiam nerves (Burdin, 1803), see **ansa cervicalis (>1840)**
arch with three columns (Crooke, 1615), see **fornix (Vesalius, 1543a)**
arched anastomosis between first and second cervical nerves (Knox, 1832), see **communicating loops of cervical plexus (>1840)**
arched chamber (Willis, 1664), see **fornix (Vesalius, 1543a)**
arched roof of ventricles (Riolan, 1657), see **fornix (Vesalius, 1543a)**
arched vault (Willis, 1664), see **fornix (Vesalius, 1543a)**
arching fascicles (Serres, 1824–1826), see **ventral external arcuate fibers (>1840)**
arcuate fascicle (Burdach, 1822), see **superior longitudinal fascicle (>1840)**
arcuate fascicle (>1840), see **superior longitudinal fascicle (>1840)**
arcuate fascicle of septum pellucidum (Ganser, 1882), see **dorsal fornix (Sprague & Meyer, 1950)**
arcuate fibers (Arnold, 1838b)
arcuate fibers (Rolando, 1825a), see **ventral external arcuate fibers (>1840)**
arcuate filaments (Rolando, 1825a), see **ventral external arcuate fibers (>1840)**
arcuate nucleus of medulla (>1840)
area 1 (Brodmann, 1909), see **parietal region (>1840)**
area 2 (Brodmann, 1909), see **parietal region (>1840)**
area 3 (Brodmann, 1909), see **parietal region (>1840)**
area 4 (Brodmann, 1909), see **frontal region (Vicq d'Azyr, 1786)**
area 5 (Brodmann, 1909), see **parietal region (>1840)**
area 6 (Brodmann, 1909), see **frontal region (Vicq d'Azyr, 1786)**
area 7 (Brodmann, 1909), see **parietal region (>1840)**
area 8 (Brodmann, 1909), see **frontal region (Vicq d'Azyr, 1786)**
area 9 (Brodmann, 1909), see **frontal region (Vicq d'Azyr, 1786)**
area 10 (Brodmann, 1909), see **frontal region (Vicq d'Azyr, 1786)**
area 11 (Brodmann, 1909), see **orbital region (Rolando, 1831)**
area 12 (Brodmann, 1909), see **frontal region (Vicq d'Azyr, 1786)**
area 13 (Brodmann, 1909), see **insular region (Brodmann, 1909)**
area 14 (Brodmann, 1909), see **insular region (Brodmann, 1909)**
area 15 (Brodmann, 1909), see **insular region (Brodmann, 1909)**
area 16 (Brodmann, 1909), see **insular region (Brodmann, 1909)**
area 17 (Brodmann, 1909), see **primary visual area (>1840)**
area 18 (Brodmann, 1909), see **occipital region (Vesalius, 1543a)**
area 19 (Brodmann, 1909), see **occipital region (Vesalius, 1543a)**
area 20 (Brodmann, 1909), see **temporal region (>1840)**
area 21 (Brodmann, 1909), see **middle temporal gyrus (>1840)**
area 22 (Brodmann, 1909), see **superior temporal gyrus (>1840)**
area 23 (Brodmann, 1909), see **ventral posterior cingulate area (Brodmann, 1909)**
area 24 (Brodmann, 1909), see **ventral anterior cingulate area (Brodmann, 1909)**
area 25 (Brodmann, 1909), see **infralimbic area (Rose & Woolsey, 1948)**
area 26 (Brodmann, 1909), see **fasciola cinerea (Arnold, 1838b)**
area 27 (Brodmann, 1909), see **presubiculum (>1840)**
area 28 (Brodmann, 1909), see **entorhinal area (Brodmann, 1909)**
area 29 (Brodmann, 1909), see **granular retrosplenial area (>1840)**
area 30 (Brodmann, 1909), see **agranular retrosplenial area (>1840)**

area 31 (Brodmann, 1909), see ***dorsal posterior cingulate area (Brodmann, 1909)***

area 32 (Brodmann, 1909), see ***dorsal anterior cingulate area (Brodmann, 1909)***

area 33 (Brodmann, 1909), see ***hippocampal region (Swanson et al., 1987)***

area 34 (Brodmann, 1909), see ***entorhinal area (Brodmann, 1909)***

area 35 (Brodmann, 1909), see ***medial occipitotemporal gyrus (>1840)***

area 36 (Brodmann, 1909), see ***medial occipitotemporal gyrus (>1840)***

area 37 (Brodmann, 1909), see ***temporal region (>1840)***

area 38 (Brodmann, 1909), see ***temporal region (>1840)***

area 39 (Brodmann, 1909), see ***angular gyrus (>1840)***

area 40 (Brodmann, 1909), see ***supramarginal gyrus (>1840)***

area 41 (Brodmann, 1909), see ***transverse temporal gyri (>1840)***

area 42 (Brodmann, 1909), see ***transverse temporal gyri (>1840)***

area 43 (Brodmann, 1909), see ***cerebral cortex gray matter (>1840)***

area 44 (Brodmann, 1909), see ***opercular part of inferior frontal gyrus (>1840)***

area 45 (Brodmann, 1909), see ***triangular part of inferior frontal gyrus (>1840)***

area 46 (Brodmann, 1909), see ***inferior frontal gyrus (>1840)***

area 47 (Brodmann, 1909), see ***lateral orbital gyrus (>1840)***

area 48 (Brodmann, 1909), see ***postsubiculum (Swanson & Cowan, 1977)***

area 49 (Brodmann, 1909), see ***parasubiculum (>1909)***

area 50 (Brodmann, 1909), see ***parietal region (>1840)***

area 51 (Brodmann, 1909), see ***piriform area (Smith, 1919)***

area 52 (Brodmann, 1909), see ***transverse temporal gyri (>1840)***

area angularis (Brodmann, 1909), see ***angular gyrus (>1840)***

area cingularis anterior dorsalis (Brodmann, 1909), see ***dorsal anterior cingulate area (Brodmann, 1909)***

area cingularis anterior ventralis (Brodmann, 1909), see ***ventral anterior cingulate area (Brodmann, 1909)***

area cingularis posterior dorsalis (Brodmann, 1909), see ***dorsal posterior cingulate area (Brodmann, 1909)***

area cingularis posterior ventralis (Brodmann, 1909), see ***ventral posterior cingulate area (Brodmann, 1909)***

area ectorhinalis (Brodmann, 1909), see ***medial occipitotemporal gyrus (>1840)***

area ectosplenialis (Brodmann, 1909), see ***fasciola cinerea (Arnold, 1838b)***

area entorhinalis (Brodmann, 1909), see ***entorhinal area (Brodmann, 1909)***

area frontalis agranularis (Brodmann, 1909), see ***frontal region (Vicq d'Azyr, 1786)***

area frontalis granularis (Brodmann, 1909), see ***frontal region (Vicq d'Azyr, 1786)***

area frontalis intermedia (Brodmann, 1909), see ***frontal region (Vicq d'Azyr, 1786)***

area frontalis media (Brodmann, 1909), see ***inferior frontal gyrus (>1840)***

area frontopolaris (Brodmann, 1909, p. 137), see ***frontal region (Vicq d'Azyr, 1786)***

area frontopolaris (Brodmann, 1909, p. 156), see ***frontal region (Vicq d'Azyr, 1786)***

area gigantopyramidalis (Brodmann, 1909), see ***frontal region (Vicq d'Azyr, 1786)***

area occipitalis (Brodmann, 1909), see ***occipital region (Vesalius, 1543a)***

area occipito-temporalis (Brodmann, 1909), see ***temporal region (>1840)***

area opercularis (Brodmann, 1909), see ***opercular part of inferior frontal gyrus (>1840)***

area orbitalis (Brodmann, 1909), see ***lateral orbital gyrus (>1840)***

area parainsularis (Brodmann, 1909), see ***transverse temporal gyri (>1840)***

area parasubicularis (Brodmann, 1909), see ***parasubiculum (>1840)***

area parietalis superior (Brodmann, 1909), see ***parietal region (>1840)***

area perirhinalis (Brodmann, 1909), see ***medial occipitotemporal gyrus (>1840)***

area postcentralis caudalis (Brodmann, 1909), see ***parietal region (>1840)***

area postcentralis intermedia (Brodmann, 1909), see ***parietal region (>1840)***

area postcentralis oralis (Brodmann, 1909), see ***parietal region (>1840)***

area postrema (>1840)

area praefrontalis (Brodmann, 1909), see ***orbital region (Rolando, 1831)***

area praegenualis (Brodmann, 1909), see ***hippocampal region (Swanson et al., 1987)***

area praeoccipitalis (Brodmann, 1909), see ***occipital region (Vesalius, 1543a)***

area praeparietalis (Brodmann, 1909), see ***parietal region (>1840)***

area praepyriformis (Brodmann, 1909), see ***piriform area (Smith, 1919)***

area praesubicularis (Brodmann, 1909), see ***presubiculum (>1840)***

area praeterminalis (Brodmann, 1909), see ***infralimbic area (Rose & Woolsey, 1948)***

area retrolimbica agranularis (Brodmann, 1909), see ***agranular retrosplenial area (>1840)***

area retrolimbica granularis (Brodmann, 1909), see ***granular retrosplenial area (>1840)***

area striata (Brodmann, 1909), see ***primary visual area (>1840)***

area subcentralis (Brodmann, 1909), see ***cerebral cortex gray matter (>1840)***

area subgenualis (Brodmann, 1909), see ***infralimbic area (Rose & Woolsey, 1948)***

area supramarginalis (Brodmann, 1909), see ***supramarginal gyrus (>1840)***

area temporalis inferior (Brodmann, 1909), see ***temporal region (>1840)***

area temporalis media (Brodmann, 1909), see ***middle temporal gyrus (>1840)***

area temporalis superior (Brodmann, 1909), see ***superior temporal gyrus (>1840)***

area temporalis transversa external (posterior) (Brodmann, 1909), see ***transverse temporal gyri (>1840)***

area temporalis transversa interna (anterior) (Brodmann, 1909), see **transverse temporal gyri (>1840)**
area temporopolaris (Brodmann, 1909), see **temporal region (>1840)**
area triangularis (Brodmann, 1909), see **triangular part of inferior frontal gyrus (>1840)**
arm of fornix (Willis, 1664), see **fimbria (Honegger, 1890)**
armilla (Malacarne, 1791), see **trigeminal ganglion (>1840)**
Arnold's nerve (>1840), see **auricular branch of vagus nerve (Arnold, 1834)**
arse-hole (Riolan, 1657), see **opening of fourth ventricle (>1840)**
arse-hole (Willis, 1664), see **opening of cerebral aqueduct (>1840)**
articular and periosteal filaments of internal nerve of vastus internus (Cruveilhier, 1836), see **muscular branches of femoral nerve (Quain & Wilson, 1839)**
articular branch of anterior branch of dorsal branch of radial nerve (Bock, 1827), see **superficial branch of radial nerve (Martin, 1781)**
articular branch of biceps branches of musculocutaneous nerve (Cruveilhier, 1836), see **muscular branches of musculocutaneous nerve (Günther, 1786)**
articular branch of deep fibular nerve (>1840)
articular branch of external popliteal nerve (Bock, 1827), see **articular branches of common fibular nerve (>1840)**
articular branch of internal branch of musculocutaneous nerve (Cruveilhier, 1836), see **lateral cutaneous nerve of forearm (>1840)**
articular branch of nerve to popliteus (>1840)
articular branch of nerve to quadratus femoris (>1840)
articular branch of posterior branch of obturator nerve (>1840)
articular branch of tibial nerve to ankle joint (>1840)
articular branches of auriculotemporal nerve (>1840)
articular branches of common fibular nerve (>1840)
articular branches of nerve of quadratus femoris and gemellus inferior (Cruveilhier, 1836), see **articular branch of nerve to quadratus femoris (>1840)**
articular branches of radial nerve (>1840)
articular branches of sciatic nerve (Cruveilhier, 1836), see **articular branches of common fibular nerve (>1840)**
articular branches of tibial nerve (>1840)
articular branches of tibial nerve to knee joint (>1840)
articular circumflex nerve (Monro, 1783), see **axillary nerve (Winslow, 1733)**
articular fascicles of cutaneous temporal surculus of inferior maxillary branch (Bellingeri, 1818), see **articular branches of auriculotemporal nerve (>1840)**
articular filament of internal saphenous nerve (Cruveilhier, 1836), see **saphenous nerve (Haase, 1781)**
articular filaments of cubital nerve (Cruveilhier, 1836), see **ulnar nerve (Cheselden, 1726)**
articular filaments of deep terminal branch of external plantar nerve (Cruveilhier, 1836), see **deep branch of lateral plantar nerve (>1840)**
articular filaments of elbow from pronator teres branch of median nerve (Cruveilhier, 1836), see **muscular branches of median nerve (Martin, 1781)**
articular filaments of external branch of superficial terminal branch of external plantar nerve (Cruveilhier, 1836), see **common plantar digital nerves of lateral plantar nerve (>1840)**
articular filaments of first terminal branch of internal plantar nerve (Cruveilhier, 1836), see **common plantar digital nerves of medial plantar nerve (>1840)**
articular filaments of posterior terminal branch of internal saphenous nerve (Cruveilhier, 1836), see **saphenous nerve (Haase, 1781)**
articular filaments of radial nerve (Cruveilhier, 1836), see **posterior interosseous nerve (Quain & Wilson, 1839)**
articular nerve (Cheselden, 1726), see **axillary nerve (Winslow, 1733)**
articular nerve of knee (Cruveilhier, 1836, p. 840), see **articular branch of posterior branch of obturator nerve (>1840)**
articular nerve of knee (Cruveilhier, 1836, p. 861), see **articular branches of common fibular nerve (>1840)**
articular nerves of internal branch of superficial terminal branch of external plantar nerve (Cruveilhier, 1836), see **common plantar digital nerves of lateral plantar nerve (>1840)**
arytenoid filament of superior laryngeal branches of pneumogastric nerve (Cruveilhier, 1836), see **internal branch of superior laryngeal nerve (Fyfe, 1800)**
ascending anastomotic branch of third cervical nerve (Arnold, 1834), see **communicating loops of cervical plexus (>1840)**
ascending anastomotic branchlet of second cervical nerve with first cervical nerve (Arnold, 1834), see **communicating loops of cervical plexus (>1840)**
ascending anastomotic nerve of second cervical nerve (Meckel, 1817), see **communicating loops of cervical plexus (>1840)**
ascending and external branches of muscular branches of inferior gluteal nerve (Cruveilhier, 1836), see **inferior gluteal nerve (Martin, 1781)**
ascending branch of auriculotemporal nerve (Cruveilhier, 1836), see **superficial temporal branches of auriculotemporal nerve (>1840)**
ascending branch of crus fornicis (Meynert, 1872), see **mammillothalamic tract (>1840)**
ascending branch of fourth cervical nerve (Arnold, 1834), see **communicating loops of cervical plexus (>1840)**
ascending branch of glossopharyngeal nerve to accessory nerve of Willis (Kilian, 1822), see **glossopharyngeal nerve (Huber, 1744)**
ascending branch of hard nerve (Mayer, 1794), see **facial nerve trunk (1840)**
ascending branch of intercostal nerve (Winslow, 1733), see **internal carotid nerve (>1840)**
ascending branch of lateral cerebral sulcus (>1840)
ascending branch of left vagus nerve (Mayer, 1794), see **hepatic branches of anterior vagal trunk (>1840)**
ascending branch of portio dura (Bell & Bell, 1816), see **temporal branches of facial nerve (Swan, 1830)**

ascending branch of superficial branch of hard nerve (Günther, 1786), see **facial nerve trunk (1840)**
ascending branch of superficial cervical branch of cervical plexus (Cruveilhier, 1836), see **superior branches of transverse nerve of neck (>1840)**
ascending branch of superior branch of hard nerve (Meckel, 1753), see **facial nerve trunk (1840)**
ascending branch of superior gluteal nerve (Cruveilhier, 1836), see **superior gluteal nerve (Martin, 1781)**
ascending branches of anterior trunk of eighth pair of nerves (Walter, 1783), see **hepatic branches of anterior vagal trunk (>1840)**
ascending branches of buccal nerve (Cruveilhier, 1836), see **buccal nerve (Meckel, 1748)**
ascending branches of external frontal nerve (Cruveilhier, 1836), see **supraorbital nerve (Meckel, 1753)**
ascending branches of facial nerve (Meckel, 1817), see **facial nerve trunk (1840)**
ascending branches of inferior laryngeal nerve (Günther, 1786), see **inferior laryngeal nerve (>1840)**
ascending branches of pharyngeal nerves (Scarpa, 1794), see **pharyngeal branches of vagus nerve (>1840)**
ascending branches of recurrent nerve (Haase, 1781), see **inferior laryngeal nerve (>1840)**
ascending branches of spheno-palatine ganglion (Quain, 1828), see **pterygopalatine nerves (Wrisberg, 1786)**
ascending branches of superior cervical ganglion (Cloquet, 1816), see **internal carotid nerve (>1840)**
ascending branches of supraorbital nerve (Cruveilhier, 1836), see **supraorbital nerve (Meckel, 1753)**
ascending communicating branch part of tenth nerves of head with superior lingual nerve (Andersch & Soemmerring, 1792), see **communicating branches of lingual nerve with hypoglossal nerve (>1840)**
ascending crura of cerebellum (Palletta, 1784), see **superior cerebellar peduncle (Procháska, 1800)**
ascending crus of fornix (Volkmann, 1831), see **postcommissural fornix (Loo, 1931)**
ascending esophageal branch of fourth branch of recurrent nerves of neck (Andersch & Soemmerring, 1792), see **pharyngeal branches of vagus nerve (>1840)**
ascending filament of posterior auricular branch of facial nerve (Cruveilhier, 1836), see **auricular branch of posterior auricular nerve (Arnold, 1834)**
ascending filaments of anterior alveolo-dental nerve (Cruveilhier, 1836), see **nasal branch of anterior superior dental nerve (>1840)**
ascending filaments of anterior terminal branch of internal saphenous nerve (Cruveilhier, 1836), see **infrapatellar branch of saphenous nerve (>1840)**
ascending filaments of internal frontal nerve (Cruveilhier, 1836), see **supratrochlear nerve (Schaarschmidt, 1750)**
ascending filaments of superior maxillary nerve (Cruveilhier, 1836), see **inferior palpebral branches of infraorbital nerve (>1840)**
ascending filaments of supratrochlear nerve (Cruveilhier, 1836), see **supratrochlear nerve (Schaarschmidt, 1750)**
ascending minor branch of inferior anterior nasal nerves (Scarpa, 1785), see **posterior inferior nasal nerves (Günther, 1786)**
ascending nerve (Meckel, 1817), see **recurrent laryngeal nerve (Albinus, 1744)**
ascending part of cerebellar brachia (Malacarne, 1776), see **superior cerebellar peduncle (Procháska, 1800)**
ascending part of eleventh nerves of head (Andersch & Soemmerring, 1792), see **superior root of ansa cervicalis (>1840)**
ascending part of tenth nerves of head (Andersch & Soemmerring, 1792), see **superior root of ansa cervicalis (>1840)**
ascending root of fornix (Burdach, 1822), see **hypothalamic postcommissural fornix (>1840)**
ascending root of mammillary body (Arnold, 1838b), see **postcommissural fornix (Loo, 1931)**
ascending root of trigone (Dejerine & Dejerine-Klumpke, 1895), see **mammillothalamic tract (>1840)**
ascending spinal nerve (Swan, 1830), see **accessory nerve (Vieussens, 1684)**
ascending superficial branches of cervical plexus (Quain, 1828)
ascending suprazygomatic branch of superior branch of hard nerve (Meckel, 1753), see **facial nerve trunk (1840)**
ascending trunk of accessory spinal nerve (Willis, 1664), see **spinal root of accessory nerve (>1840)**
ascending trunk of spinal nerves (Swan, 1830), see **spinal nerve ventral branch (>1840)**
ascending uterine nerves (Cruveilhier, 1836), see **uterovaginal plexus (>1840)**
ascending vesicle plexus (Cruveilhier, 1836), see **extrinsic vesical plexus (>1840)**
ash-colored substance (Winslow, 1733), see **central nervous system gray matter regions (>1840)**
ash-coloured matter (Bell, 1803b), see **central nervous system gray matter regions (>1840)**
ashen part (Valverde de Amusco, 1556), see **central nervous system gray matter regions (>1840)**
ash-gray substance (Vesalius, 1543a), see **central nervous system gray matter regions (>1840)**
ashy orange substance of brain (Vesalius, 1543a), see **central nervous system gray matter regions (>1840)**
associate of eighth pair of nerves (Swan, 1830), see **glossopharyngeal nerve (Huber, 1744)**
association fibers of cerebral cortex (>1840)
atrial plexuses (>1840)
atrium of lateral ventricle (>1840)
auditory nerve (Galen, c192), see **vestibulocochlear nerve (>1840)**
auditory nerve (Willis, 1664), see **cranial nerves (Soemmerring, 1791)**
auditory nerve proper (Willis, 1664), see **vestibulocochlear nerve (>1840)**
auditory nerve trunk (Meckel, 1817), see **vestibulocochlear nerve trunk (>1840)**
auditory radiation (>1840)
auditory tubercle (>1840)
Augenknöchtchen (Soemmerring, 1801), see **ciliary ganglion (Loder, 1778)**

Augennervenknötchens (Soemmerring, 1801), see **ciliary ganglion (Loder, 1778)**

auricular branch of auriculotemporal nerve (Cruveilhier, 1836), see **anterior auricular nerves (>1840)**

auricular branch of cervical plexus (Cloquet, 1816), see **great auricular nerve (Haase, 1781)**

auricular branch of external deep branch of hard nerve (Meckel, 1753), see **auricular branch of posterior auricular nerve (Arnold, 1834)**

auricular branch of inferior maxillary nerve (Quain, 1832), see **auriculotemporal nerve (Haller, 1762)**

auricular branch of lesser occipital nerve (Bock, 1827), see **lesser occipital nerve (Mayer, 1794)**

auricular branch of petrosal small ganglion (Andersch, 1797), see **tympanic nerve (Arnold, 1834)**

auricular branch of pneumogastric nerve (Cruveilhier, 1836), see **auricular branch of vagus nerve (Arnold, 1834)**

auricular branch of posterior auricular nerve (Arnold, 1834)

auricular branch of superficial temporal branch of third branch of fifth pair (Meckel, 1748), see **anterior auricular nerves (>1840)**

auricular branch of third trunk of fifth pair (Haller, 1762), see **auriculotemporal nerve (Haller, 1762)**

auricular branch of vagus nerve (Arnold, 1834)

auricular branch proper of auricular nerve of third cervical pair (Meckel, 1753), see **posterior branch of great auricular nerve (Bock, 1827)**

auricular branch proper of external deep branch of hard nerve (Günther, 1786), see **auricular branch of posterior auricular nerve (Arnold, 1834)**

auricular branches of great auricular nerve (Arnold, 1834), see **posterior branch of great auricular nerve (Bock, 1827)**

auricular fascicles proper of cutaneous temporal surculus of inferior maxillary branch (Bellingeri, 1818), see **external acoustic meatus nerves (Meckel, 1817)**

auricular filament of posterior auricular branch of facial nerve (Cruveilhier, 1836), see **auricular branch of posterior auricular nerve (Arnold, 1834)**

auricular filament of posterior zygomatic threads of temporal surculus (Bellingeri, 1818), see **temporal branches of facial nerve (Swan, 1830)**

auricular ganglion (Arnold, 1828), see **otic ganglion (Arnold, 1828)**

auricular nerve (Günther, 1786), see **auriculotemporal nerve (Haller, 1762)**

auricular nerve (Meckel, 1753), see **great auricular nerve (Haase, 1781)**

auricular nerve of hard nerve (Bang, 1770), see **posterior auricular nerve (Meckel, 1753)**

auricular nerve of third cervical pair (Meckel, 1753), see **great auricular nerve (Haase, 1781)**

auricular nerves (Haase, 1781), see **anterior auricular nerves (>1840)**

auricular plexus (Cruveilhier, 1836), see **external carotid plexus (>1840)**

auricular plexus (Swan, 1830), see **atrial plexuses (>1840)**

auricular surculus of external deep branch of portio major and minor of facial nerve (Bellingeri, 1818), see **auricular branch of posterior auricular nerve (Arnold, 1834)**

auriculofacial branch of middle cutaneous nerve of neck (Peipers, 1793), see **superior branch of transverse nerve of neck (>1840)**

auriculo-occipital branch of facial nerve (Cruveilhier, 1836), see **posterior auricular nerve (Meckel, 1753)**

auriculotemporal nerve (Haller, 1762)

automatic system ganglia (Wutzer, 1817), see **autonomic ganglia (Langley, 1900)**

autonomic ganglia (Langley, 1900)

autonomic nerves (Langley, 1898)

autonomic plexuses (Strong & Elwyn, 1943), see **autonomic nerves (Langley, 1898)**

axillary circumflex nerve (Monro, 1783), see **axillary nerve (Winslow, 1733)**

axillary nerve (Cheselden, 1713), see **brachial plexus (Camper, 1760)**

axillary nerve (Cheselden, 1722), see **musculocutaneous nerve (Du Verney, 1697)**

axillary nerve (Winslow, 1733)

axillary nerves (Salmon, 1714), see **brachial plexus (Camper, 1760)**

axillary plexus (Salmon, 1714), see **brachial plexus (Camper, 1760)**

axis of nervous system (Reil, 1809c), see **central nervous system (Carus, 1814)**

azygos ganglion (Quain & Wilson, 1839), see **ganglion impar (Quain & Wilson, 1839)**

back mary (Brunschwig, 1525), see **spinal cord (Galen, c162–c166)**

back part of brain (Galen, c177), see **cerebellum (Aristotle)**

back-ward brain (Crooke, 1615), see **cerebellum (Aristotle)**

backward branches of conjugations of neck, chest, loynes, and sacral bone (Crooke, 1615), see **spinal nerve dorsal branch (Meckel, 1817)**

backward prominence of brain (Crooke, 1615), see **cerebral cortex gray matter (>1840)**

backward ventricle (Crooke, 1615), see **fourth ventricle (Gelen, c192)**

Balkensystem (Reil, 1809b), see **cerebral cortex white matter (>1840)**

band of fornix (Tiedemann, 1816), see **fimbria (Honegger, 1890)**

band of Giacomini (>1840), see **dentate gyrus (>1840)**

band of optic nerves (Cruveilhier, 1836), see **optic tract (Vicq d'Azyr, 1784)**

band of roots of spinal marrow (Riolan, 1657), see **pons (Haller, 1747)**

bandelette du grand hippocampe (Vicq d'Azyr, 1786), see **fimbria (Honegger, 1890)**

bark as it were (Bartholin, 1662), see **cerebral cortex gray matter (>1840)**

barley-shaped ganglioform enlargement of accessory nerve (Cruveilhier, 1836), see **cranial nerve ganglia (>1840)**

basal ganglia (>1840), see **cerebral nuclei (Swanson, 2000a)**

basal grayish substance of cerebrum (Vesalius, 1543a), see **cerebral nuclei (Swanson, 2000a)**

basal plate (>1840)

base of anterior pillar of fornix (Winslow, 1733), see **septal postcommissural fornix (>1840)**
base of anterior ventricle both right and left (Manfredi, 1490), see **caudate nucleus (Arnold, 1838b)**
base of brain (Benedetti, 1502), see **spinal cord (Galen, c162–c166)**
base of brain (Bidloo, 1685), see **vertebrate brain (Cuvier, 1800)**
base of brain (Galen, c173), see **brainstem (Schwalbe, 1881)**
base of brain (Herophilus, c335–c280 BC), see **fourth ventricle (Galen, c192)**
base of brain (Piccolomini, 1586), see **vertebrate brain (Cuvier, 1800)**
base of brain (Rufus of Ephesus, fl. c90–120), see **brainstem (Schwalbe, 1881)**
base of brain (Varoli, 1573), see **vertebrate brain (Cuvier, 1800)**
base of cerebellum (Galen, c173), see **rhombicbrain (His, 1893b)**
base of cerebral cortex (Willis, 1664), see **cerebral cortex white matter (>1840)**
base of cerebral peduncle (Meckel, 1817), see **cerebral peduncle (Tarin, 1753)**
base of cerebrum (Vesalius, 1543a), see **vertebrate brain (Cuvier, 1800)**
base of corona radiata (Burdach, 1822), see **internal capsule (Burdach, 1822)**
base of crus cerebri (Reil, 1809b), see **cerebral peduncle (Tarin, 1753)**
base of encephalon (Galen, c173), see **brainstem (Schwalbe, 1881)**
base of fore ventricle (Mondino, 1316), see **vertebrate brain (Cuvier, 1800)**
base of fornix (Willis, 1664), see **septal postcommissural fornix (>1840)**
base of oblong marrow (Willis, 1664), see **brainstem (Schwalbe, 1881)**
base of parencephalis (Galen, c173), see **rhombicbrain (His, 1893b)**
base of peduncle (Arnold, 1838b), see **cerebral peduncle (Tarin, 1753)**
base of striate body (Willis, 1672), see **head of caudate nucleus (>1840)**
base of third ventricle (Galen, c177), see **hypothalamus (Kuhlenbeck, 1927)**
basilar furrow of medulla oblongata (Reil, 1807–1808a), see **ventral median fissure of medulla (>1840)**
basilar furrow of pons (Gordon, 1815), see **basilar sulcus of pons (Gordon, 1815)**
basilar gland (Chaussier, 1807), see **pituitary gland (>1840)**
basilar part of pons (>1840), see **pons (Haller, 1747)**
basilar plexus (Cruveilhier, 1836), see **vertebral plexus (Cloquet, 1816)**
basilar sulcus of pons (Gordon, 1815)
basin (Rufus of Ephesus, fl. c90–120), see **hypothalamus (Kuhlenbeck, 1927)**
basin of fourth ventricle (Reil, 1809c), see **rhombicbrain (His, 1893b)**
basis crus cerebri (Reil, 1809b), see **cerebral peduncle (Tarin, 1753)**
basis of brain (Bidloo, 1685), see **vertebrate brain (Cuvier, 1800)**
basis of fornix (Willis, 1664), see **septal postcommissural fornix (>1840)**
basis of medulla of brain (Haller, 1754b), see **brainstem (Schwalbe, 1881)**
basis of oblong marrow (Willis, 1664), see **brainstem (Schwalbe, 1881)**
basis of roof of ventricles (Poupart, 1712), see **septal postcommissural fornix (>1840)**
basis of striate body (Willis, 1672), see **head of caudate nucleus (>1840)**
basis pedunculi (Arnold, 1838b), see **cerebral peduncle (Tarin, 1753)**
basis pedunculi (Henle 1871), see **tegmentum (Swanson, 2000b)**
basis septi (Burdach, 1822), see **medial septal complex (Swanson et al., 1987)**
basolateral amygdalar complex (>1840)
basyn (Geminus, 1553), see **hypothalamus (Kuhlenbeck, 1927)**
beak of corpus callosum (Reil, 1809b), see **rostrum of corpus callosum (Reil, 1809b)**
beak of infundibulum (Winslow, 1733), see **pituitary gland (>1840)**
bed nuclei of stria terminalis (Swanson et al., 1987), see **bed nuclei of terminal stria (Gurdjian, 1925)**
bed nuclei of terminal stria (Gurdjian, 1925)
bed nucleus of stria terminalis (Gurdjian, 1925), see **bed nuclei of terminal stria (Gurdjian, 1925)**
bed of ethmoidal nerve (Chaussier, 1807), see **cerebral nuclei (Swanson, 2000a)**
bed of gray substance (Reil, 1812c), see **interbrain (Baer, 1837)**
bed of ocular nerve (Chaussier, 1807), see **interbrain (Baer, 1837)**
bed of optic nerve (Riolan, 1657), see **interbrain (Baer, 1837)**
beginnings and twigs of sixth pair of cerebral nerves (Vesalius, 1543a), see **cranial nerves (Soemmerring, 1791)**
Bell's nerve (>1840), see **long thoracic nerve (Quain & Wilson, 1839)**
belly (Willis, 1664), see **ventricles (Hippocrates)**
belly of lute (Bartholin, 1662), see **fornix (Vesalius, 1543a)**
bendings (Vesalius, 1543a), see **cerebral cortex gray matter (>1840)**
biceps branches of musculocutaneous nerve (Cruveilhier, 1836), see **muscular branches of musculocutaneous nerve (Günther, 1786)**
bifid branch of main communicating branches of glossopharyngeal nerve (Kilian, 1822), see **glossopharyngeal nerve (Huber, 1744)**
bifid cutaneous digital branches of median nerve (Günther, 1786), see **common palmar digital nerves of median nerve (>1840)**
bifid digital branches of internal plantar nerve (Günther, 1786), see **common plantar digital nerves of medial plantar nerve (>1840)**
bigeminal bodies (Spurzheim, 1826), see **tectum (Baer, 1837)**
bigeminal prominences (Rolando, 1809), see **tectum (Baer, 1837)**

biventral lobe (Malacarne, 1776), see **biventral lobule (>1840)**

biventral lobule (>1840)

black matter (Reil, 1809c), see **locus ceruleus (Wenzel & Wenzel, 1812)**

black region (Vicq d'Azyr, 1784), see **substantia nigra (Soemmerring, 1791)**

black substance in peduncles of brain (Spurzheim, 1826), see **substantia nigra (Soemmerring, 1791)**

blackish body (Vicq d'Azyr, 1784), see **substantia nigra (Soemmerring, 1791)**

blackish segment (Vicq d'Azyr, 1786), see **substantia nigra (Soemmerring, 1791)**

blackish substance (Vicq d'Azyr, 1784), see **substantia nigra (Soemmerring, 1791)**

blind hole of middle ventricle (Gerdy, 1838), see **hypothalamic part of third ventricle (Swanson, 2004)**

blind nerve (Albertus Magnus, 13th century), see **intermediofacial nerve (Strong & Elwyn, 1943)**

blue place (Meckel, 1832), see **locus ceruleus (Wenzel & Wenzel, 1812)**

blueish-white body (Piccolomini, 1586), see **central nervous system gray matter regions (>1840)**

Bock's ganglion (>1840), see **carotid ganglion (Wutzer, 1817; Bock, 1817)**

body like arch (Geminus, 1553), see **fornix (Vesalius, 1543a)**

body made like vault (Geminus, 1553), see **fornix (Vesalius, 1543a)**

body of brain (Steno, 1669), see **endbrain (Kuhlenbeck, 1927)**

body of caudate nucleus (Arnold, 1838b), see **caudate nucleus (Arnold, 1838b)**

body of caudate nucleus (>1840)

body of cerebellum (Meckel, 1817), see **cerebellum (Aristotle)**

body of corona radiata (Arnold, 1838a), see **cerebral cortex white matter (>1840)**

body of corpus callosum (Arnold, 1838a)

body of fornix (Burdach, 1822), see **fimbria (Honegger, 1890)**

body of fornix (Monro, 1783), see **fornix (Vesalius, 1543a)**

body of fornix (Reil, 1812b), see **fornix (Vesalius, 1543a)**

body of fornix (Ridley, 1695), see **fornix (Vesalius, 1543a)**

body of fornix (Vesalius, 1543a), see **fimbria (Honegger, 1890)**

body of fornix (>1840), see **fimbria (Honegger, 1890)**

body of great commissure (Arnold, 1838b), see **body of corpus callosum (Arnold, 1838a)**

body of ischiatic nerve (Bell, 1803b), see **sciatic nerve (Keill, 1698)**

body of lateral part of spinal ashen-colored substance (Vicq d'Azyr, 1784), see **intermediate spinal zone (>1840)**

body of lateral ventricle (Bell, 1803b)

body of spinal medulla (Günther, 1786), see **spinal cord (Galen, c162–c166)**

body of spinal prolongation (Chaussier, 1807), see **spinal cord (Galen, c162–c166)**

body of superior cerebellar peduncle (Reil, 1809c), see **superior cerebellar peduncle (Procháska, 1800)**

body of vertebral medulla (Cloquet, 1828), see **spinal cord (Galen, c162–c166)**

bombicine appendix (Malacarne, 1780), see **hippocampal region (Swanson et al., 1987)**

bombycinus Aurantius (Ridley, 1695), see **hippocampal region (Swanson et al., 1987)**

bombyx (Marchetti, 1652), see **hippocampal region (Swanson et al., 1987)**

border of brain (Willis, 1664), see **limbic region (>1840)**

border of inferior lobe (Burdach, 1822), see **parahippocampal gyrus (>1840)**

bordered or fringed bodies (Burdin, 1803), see **fimbria (Honegger, 1890)**

bottom of cerebral cortex (Willis, 1664), see **cerebral cortex white matter (>1840)**

bourelet di Vicq-d'Azir (Rolando, 1831), see **splenium of corpus callosum (Burdach, 1822)**

bourrelet antérieur du corps calleux (Vicq d'Azyr, 1786), see **genu of corpus callosum (Reil, 1809b)**

bourrelet postérieur du corps calleux (Vicq d'Azyr, 1786), see **splenium of corpus callosum (Burdach, 1822)**

brachia cerebelli ad pontem (Arnold, 1838a), see **middle cerebellar peduncle (Rolando, 1819)**

brachia cerebri (Chaussier, 1807), see **cerebral peduncle (Tarin, 1753)**

brachia medulla oblongata (Winslow, 1733), see **cerebral peduncle (Tarin, 1753)**

brachial branch of anterior branch of second dorsal pair (Cloquet, 1815), see **intercostobrachial nerves (>1840)**

brachial branch of anterior branch of third dorsal pair (Cloquet, 1815), see **intercostobrachial nerves (>1840)**

brachial cutaneous branch (Bock, 1827), see **posterior cutaneous nerve of arm (>1840)**

brachial muscular nerve (Günther, 1786), see **radial nerve (Du Verney, 1697)**

brachial nerve (Günther, 1786), see **radial nerve (Du Verney, 1697)**

brachial nerve (Meckel, 1817), see **intercostobrachial nerves (>1840)**

brachial nerve (Vesalius, 1543a), see **brachial plexus (Camper, 1760)**

brachial nerves (Camper, 1760), see **brachial plexus roots (Schwalbe, 1881)**

brachial plexus (Camper, 1760)

brachial plexus cords (Schwalbe, 1881)

brachial plexus divisions (Paterson, 1887)

brachial plexus dorsal cord (Paterson, 1887)

brachial plexus dorsal divisions (Paterson, 1887)

brachial plexus lateral cord (Schwalbe, 1881)

brachial plexus lower trunk (>1840)

brachial plexus medial cord (Schwalbe, 1881)

brachial plexus middle trunk (>1840)

brachial plexus roots (Schwalbe, 1881)

brachial plexus trunks (Schwalbe, 1881)

brachial plexus upper trunk (>1840)

brachial plexus ventral divisions (Paterson, 1887)

brachial swelling of spinal cord (Quain & Wilson, 1839), see **cervical enlargement (Arnold, 1838b)**

brachium conjunctivum (>1840), see **superior cerebellar peduncle (Procháska, 1800)**

brachium copulativum (Burdach, 1822), see **superior cerebellar peduncle (Procháska, 1800)** *brachium of fornix (Willis, 1664)*, see **fimbria (Honegger, 1890)**

brachium of inferior colliculus (>1840)

brachium of inferior quadrigeminal body (Burdach, 1822), see **brachium of inferior colliculus (>1840)**

brachium of medulla oblongata (Reil, 1807–1808a), see **inferior cerebellar peduncle (Günther, 1786)**

brachium of pons (Reil, 1807–1808a), see **middle cerebellar peduncle (Rolando, 1819)**

brachium of superior colliculus (>1840)

brachium of tubercula quadrigemina (Reil, 1807–1808a), see **superior cerebellar peduncle (Procháska, 1800)**

brachium pontis (Burdach, 1822), see **middle cerebellar peduncle (Rolando, 1819)**

braegen (Anglo-Saxon), see **brain (Smith Papyrus, c1700 BC)**

brain (Aristotle), see **invertebrate brain (>1840)**

brain (Piccolomini, 1586, definition 1), see **central nervous system (Carus, 1814)**

brain (Piccolomini, 1586, definition 2), see **cerebral cortex gray matter (>1840)**

brain (Quain, 1828), see **vertebrate brain (Cuvier, 1800)**

brain (Smith Papyrus, c1700 BC)

brain (Solly, 1836), see **supraesophageal ganglion (Grant, 1834a)**

brain (Willis, 1664), see **endbrain (Kuhlenbeck, 1927)**

brain and its appendix (Willis, 1664), see **central nervous system (Carus, 1814)**

brain bark (Crooke, 1615), see **cerebral cortex gray matter (>1840)**

brain-caul (Aristotle), see **pia (Galen, c192)**

brain cells (Baer, 1837), see **brain vesicles (Malpighi, 1673)**

brain commonly so called (Bartholin, 1662), see **vertebrate brain (Cuvier, 1800)**

brain ganglia (Gall & Spurzheim, 1810), see **central nervous system gray matter regions (>1840)**

brain ganglia (Meckel, 1815), see **interbrain (Baer, 1837)**

brain ganglion (Carus, 1814), see **invertebrate brain (>1840)**

brain hemisphere (Tarin, 1753), see **cerebral cortex (>1840)**

brain in general (Gibson, 1682), see **vertebrate brain (Cuvier, 1800)**

brain in particular (Ridley, 1695), see **endbrain (Kuhlenbeck, 1927)**

brain itself (Aristotle), see **vertebrate brain (Cuvier, 1800)**

brain itself (Bartholin, 1662), see **cerebral cortex gray matter (>1840)**

brain itself (Galen, c173), see **vertebrate brain (Cuvier, 1800)**

brain marrow (Crooke, 1615), see **central nervous system (Carus, 1814)**

brain marrow (Galen, c173), see **vertebrate brain (Cuvier, 1800)**

brain pans (Nemesius, 1636), see **ventricles (Hippocrates)**

brain prominences (Crooke, 1615), see **cerebral cortex gray matter (>1840)**

brain proper (Bartholin, 1662), see **cerebral cortex gray matter (>1840)**

brain proper (Chaussier, 1807), see **forebrain (Goette, 1873)**

brain proper (Haller, 1747), see **vertebrate brain (Cuvier, 1800)**

brain proper (Piccolomini, 1586), see **cerebral cortex gray matter (>1840)**

brain proper (Willis, 1664), see **endbrain (Kuhlenbeck, 1927)**

brain properly so-called (Bartholin, 1662), see **cerebral cortex gray matter (>1840)**

brain properly so called (Willis, 1664), see **endbrain (Kuhlenbeck, 1927)**

brain ring (Treviranus, 1816–1821), see **central nervous system (Carus, 1814)**

brain sand (Soemmerring & Lisignolo, 1785)

brain shell (Crooke, 1615), see **cerebral cortex gray matter (>1840)**

brain stem (Coiter, 1572), see **cerebrospinal trunk (>1840)**

brain strictly so called (Bartholin, 1662), see **cerebral cortex gray matter (>1840)**

brain trunk (Coiter, 1572), see **cerebrospinal trunk (>1840)**

brain vesicles (Malpighi, 1673)

braine (archaic English), see **brain (Smith Papyrus, c1700 BC)**

brainlet (Bartholin, 1662), see **cerebellum (Aristotle)**

brainstem (Burdach, 1822), see **vertebrate brain (Cuvier, 1800)**

brainstem (Schwalbe, 1881)

brakes of pineal gland (Cruveilhier, 1836), see **medullary stria (Wenzel & Wenzel, 1812)**

branch from first cervical ganglion to pharyngeal plexus (Swan, 1830), see **laryngopharyngeal branches of superior cervical ganglion (>1840)**

branch from wandring pair [to hard part of seventh pair of nerves arising within skull] (Willis, 1664), see **communicating branch of digastric branch of facial nerve with glossopharyngeal nerve (>1840)**

branch of anterior branch of second cervical nerve to descending nerve of hypoglossal nerve (Arnold, 1834), see **inferior root of ansa cervicalis (>1840)**

branch of anterior branch of vestibular nerve to ampulla of external semicircular canal (Langenbeck, 1826–1830), see **lateral ampullary nerve (>1840)**

branch of anterior branches of obturator nerve to adductor brevis muscle (Styx, 1782), see **muscular branches of anterior branch of obturator nerve (>1840)**

branch of anterior branches of obturator nerve to gracilis muscle (Styx, 1782), see **muscular branches of anterior branch of obturator nerve (>1840)**

branch of anterior vestibular nerve to ampulla of anterior membranous semicircular canal (Langenbeck, 1826–1830), see **anterior ampullary nerve (>1840)**

branch of anterior vestibular nerve to ampulla of external membranous semicircular canal (Langenbeck, 1826–1830), see **lateral ampullary nerve (>1840)**

branch of axillary nerve partly to deltoid and partly to teres minor muscle (Caldani, 1813, 1814), see **muscular branch of axillary nerve (>1840)**

branch of axillary nerve to infraspinatus muscle (Caldani, 1813, 1814), see **muscular branch of axillary nerve (>1840)**

branch of axillary nerve to long belly of triceps (Caldani, 1813, 1814), see **muscular branch of axillary nerve (>1840)**

branch of chorda tympani to external malleus muscle (Langenbeck, 1826–1830), see **chorda tympani (Falloppio, 1561)** *branch of communication from radial nerve to external cutaneous nerve (Quain & Wilson, 1839)*, see **lateral cutaneous nerve of forearm (>1840)**

branch of communication of posterior branch of internal cutaneous nerve with radial cutaneous nerve (Quain & Wilson, 1839), see **brachial plexus cords (Schwalbe, 1881)**

branch of cubital nerve communicating with radial nerve (Cloquet, 1828), see **communicating branch of radial nerve with ulnar nerve (>1840)**

branch of deep branch of ulnar nerve to adductor muscle of little finger and last lumbrical muscle (Swan, 1830), see **deep branch of ulnar nerve (>1840)**

branch of digastric branch of facial joining glosso-pharyngeal nerve (Swan, 1830), see **communicating branch of digastric branch of facial nerve with glossopharyngeal nerve (>1840)**

branch of dorsal branch of peroneal nerve to middle peroneal muscle (Swan, 1830), see **muscular branch of superficial fibular nerve (>1840)**

branch of extensor of little finger of radial nerve (Cruveilhier, 1836), see **posterior interosseous nerve (Quain & Wilson, 1839)**

branch of extensor proper of index finger of radial nerve (Cruveilhier, 1836), see **posterior interosseous nerve (Quain & Wilson, 1839)**

branch of exterior branch of sciatic nerve to short head of biceps (Günther, 1786), see **nerve to short head of biceps femoris (>1840)**

branch of facial nerve to internal malleus muscle (Langenbeck, 1826–1830), see **nerve to tensor tympani (>1840)**

branch of first external radial muscle of radial nerve (Cruveilhier, 1836), see **muscular branches of radial nerve (>1840)**

branch of first metacarpal space of radial nerve (Quain & Wilson, 1839), see **superficial branch of radial nerve (Martin, 1781)**

branch of glossopharyngeal nerve for digastric and stylohyoid (Cruveilhier, 1836), see **communicating branch of digastric branch of facial nerve with glossopharyngeal nerve (>1840)**

branch of glossopharyngeal nerve to nodular plexus of vagus nerve of Meckel (Kilian, 1822), see **glossopharyngeal nerve (Huber, 1744)**

branch of hard nerve to Eustachian muscle (Günther, 1786), see **nerve to tensor tympani (>1840)**

branch of hard nerve to stapedial muscle (Günther, 1786), see **stapedial nerve (>1840)**

branch of hard nerve to tensor tympani muscle (Günther, 1786), see **nerve to tensor tympani (>1840)**

branch of humeral circumflex nerve to capsular ligament (Langenbeck, 1826–1830), see **axillary nerve (Winslow, 1733)**

branch of humeral circumflex nerve to teres minor muscle (Langenbeck, 1826–1830), see **muscular branch of axillary nerve (>1840)**

branch of hypoglossal nerve descending branch to hyothyreoidei muscle (Arnold, 1834), see **thyrohyoid branch of hypoglossal nerve (Meckel, 1817)**

branch of hypoglossal nerve descending branch to omohyoid muscle (Arnold, 1834), see **ansa cervicalis (>1840)**

branch of hypoglossal nerve descending branch to sternohyoid muscle (Arnold, 1834), see **ansa cervicalis (>1840)**

branch of hypoglossal nerve descending branch to sternothyroid muscle (Arnold, 1834), see **ansa cervicalis (>1840)**

branch of inferior maxillary marginal nerve to buccinator muscle (Arnold, 1834), see **marginal mandibular branch of facial nerve (>1840)**

branch of inferior maxillary marginal nerve to depressor muscle (Arnold, 1834), see **marginal mandibular branch of facial nerve (>1840)**

branch of inferior maxillary marginal nerve to levator menti muscle (Arnold, 1834), see **marginal mandibular branch of facial nerve (>1840)**

branch of inferior maxillary marginal nerve to quadrati muscle (Arnold, 1834), see **marginal mandibular branch of facial nerve (>1840)**

branch of Jacobson's nerve to sympathetic nerve (Langenbeck, 1826–1830), see **caroticotympanic nerves (>1840)**

branch of jugular fossa of pneumogastric nerve (Cruveilhier, 1836), see **communicating branch of intermediofacial nerve trunk with vagus nerve (>1840)**

branch of lateral peroneus brevis of musculocutaneous branch of external popliteal sciatic nerve (Cruveilhier, 1836), see **muscular branch of superficial fibular nerve (>1840)**

branch of long extensor proper of thumb of radial nerve (Cruveilhier, 1836), see **posterior interosseous nerve (Quain & Wilson, 1839)**

branch of long supinator of radial nerve (Cruveilhier, 1836), see **muscular branches of radial nerve (>1840)**

branch of major anterior vestibular nerve to ampulla of anterior semicircular canal (Langenbeck, 1826–1830), see **anterior ampullary nerve (>1840)**

branch of median nerve communicating with ulnar (Swan, 1830), see **communicating branch of median nerve with ulnar nerve (Bock, 1827)**

branch of median nerve to abductor and opponent muscles of thumb (Swan, 1830), see **muscular branches of median nerve (Martin, 1781)**

branch of median nerve to muscles of deep layer (Cruveilhier, 1836), see **median nerve (Du Verney, 1697)**

branch of median nerve to muscles of superficial layer (Cruveilhier, 1836), see **muscular branches of median nerve (Martin, 1781)**

branch of median nerve to origin of round pronator muscle of radius and radial flexor of wrist (Swan, 1830), see **muscular branches of median nerve (Martin, 1781)**

branch of median nerve to round pronator muscle of radius (Swan, 1830), see **muscular branches of median nerve (Martin, 1781)**

branch of median nerve to short flexor muscle of thumb (Swan, 1830), see **muscular branches of median nerve (Martin, 1781)**

branch of musculocutaneous nerve to biceps muscle (Langenbeck, 1826–1830), see **muscular branches of musculocutaneous nerve (Günther, 1786)** *branch of musculocutaneous nerve to brachialis anticus muscle (Quain & Wilson, 1839)*, see **muscular branches of musculocutaneous nerve (Günther, 1786)**

branch of musculocutaneous nerve to internal brachial muscle (Langenbeck, 1826–1830), see **muscular branches of musculocutaneous nerve (Günther, 1786)**

branch of musculocutaneous nerve to short head of biceps muscle (Quain & Wilson, 1839), see **muscular branches of musculocutaneous nerve (Günther, 1786)**

branch of musculo-spiral nerve distributed to joint (Quain & Wilson, 1839), see **articular branches of radial nerve (>1840)**

branch of nasal nerve to ophthalmic ganglion (Quain & Wilson, 1839), see **communicating branch of nasociliary nerve with ciliary ganglion (>1840)**

branch of obturator nerve to adductor longus muscle (Styx, 1782), see **muscular branches of anterior branch of obturator nerve (>1840)**

branch of obturator nerve to gracile muscle (Swan, 1830), see **muscular branch of anterior branch of obturator nerve (>1840)**

branch of obturator nerve to long head of triceps muscle (Swan, 1830), see **branch of anterior branch of obturator nerve (>1840)**

branch of obturator nerve to short head of triceps muscle (Swan, 1830), see **muscular branch of anterior branch of obturator nerve (>1840)**

branch of oculomotor nerve to ciliary ganglion (>1840)

branch of ophthalmic ganglion to inferior division of third nerve (Quain & Wilson, 1839), see **branch of oculomotor nerve to ciliary ganglion (>1840)**

branch of peroneal nerve to anterior tibial artery (Swan, 1830), see **deep fibular nerve (Fyfe, 1800)**

branch of posterior cubital muscle of radial nerve (Cruveilhier, 1836), see **posterior interosseous nerve (Quain & Wilson, 1839)**

branch of posterior tibial nerve to long flexor muscle of great toe (Swan, 1830), see **nerve to flexor hallucis longus (>1840)**

branch of posterior tibial nerve to long flexor muscle of toes (Swan, 1830), see **nerve to flexor digitorum longus (>1840)**

branch of sciatic nerve distributing to quadratus femoris (Meckel, 1817), see **nerve to quadratus femoris (>1840)**

branch of sciatic nerve to long head of biceps muscle (Swan, 1830), see **nerve to hamstring muscles (>1840)**

branch of sciatic nerve to obturator internus (Meckel, 1817), see **nerve to obturator internus (>1840)**

branch of sciatic nerve to plantar muscle (Swan, 1830), see **nerve to plantaris (>1840)**

branch of sciatic nerve to semi-membranous muscle (Swan, 1830), see **nerve to hamstring muscles (>1840)**

branch of sciatic nerve to semi-tendinous muscle (Swan, 1830), see **nerve to hamstring muscles (>1840)**

branch of sciatic nerve to short head of biceps muscle (Swan, 1830), see **nerve to short head of biceps femoris (>1840)**

branch of sciatic nerve trunk to short head of biceps (Meckel, 1817), see **nerve to short head of biceps femoris (>1840)**

branch of second external radial muscle of radial nerve (Cruveilhier, 1836), see **posterior interosseous nerve (Quain & Wilson, 1839)**

branch of second metacarpal space of radial nerve (Quain & Wilson, 1839), see **superficial branch of radial nerve (Martin, 1781)**

branch of short supinator of radial nerve (Cruveilhier, 1836), see **posterior interosseous nerve (Quain & Wilson, 1839)**

branch of sixth pair of sinews stretched to roots of ribs (Geminus, 1553), see **sympathetic trunk (Winslow, 1733)**

branch of sixth pair stretching along roots of ribs (Vesalius, 1543a), see **sympathetic trunk (Winslow, 1733)**

branch of sixth pair stretching along roots of ribs offshoots to testes (Vesalius, 1543a), see **prevertebral nerves (Swanson & Bota, 2010)**

branch of spiral nerve to internal brachial muscle (Swan, 1830), see **muscular branches of radial nerve (>1840)**

branch of spiral nerve to long supinator muscle of radius (Swan, 1830), see **muscular branches of radial nerve (>1840)**

branch of spiral nerve to long supinator muscle of radius and longer radial extensor of wrist (Swan, 1830), see **muscular branches of radial nerve (>1840)**

branch of spiral nerve to short supinator muscle of radius (Swan, 1830), see **posterior interosseous nerve (Quain & Wilson, 1839)**

branch of spiral nerve to shorter radial extensor muscle of wrist (Swan, 1830), see **posterior interosseous nerve (Quain & Wilson, 1839)**

branch of splenic plexus to pancreas and spleen (Günther, 1786), see **splenic plexus (Palfijn, 1726)**

branch of superficial branch of Vidian nerve to internal malleus muscle (Langenbeck, 1826–1830), see **greater petrosal nerve (>1840)**

branch of superficial peroneal nerve to small peroneal muscle (Günther, 1786), see **superficial fibular nerve (Fyfe, 1800)**

branch of superior laryngeal nerve to cricothyroid muscle (Langenbeck, 1826–1830), see **external branch of superior laryngeal nerve (Fyfe, 1800)**

branch of superior laryngeal nerve to lateral cricoarytenoid muscle (Langenbeck, 1826–1830), see **external branch of superior laryngeal nerve (Fyfe, 1800)**

branch of superior scapular nerve to capsular ligament of shoulder joint (Swan, 1830), see **suprascapular nerve (Bang, 1770)**

branch of superior scapular nerve to superior spinous muscle (Swan, 1830), see **suprascapular nerve (Bang, 1770)**

branch of supreme cervical ganglion to intercarotid ganglion (Arnold, 1834), see **laryngopharyngeal branches of superior cervical ganglion (>1840)**

branch of tentorium cerebelli of pathetic nerve (Cruveilhier, 1836), see **trochlear nerve (Molinetti, 1669)**

branch of tibial nerve to tibialis posterior muscle (Günther, 1786), see **nerve to tibialis posterior (>1840)**

branch of ulnar nerve to deep flexor muscle of fingers (Swan, 1830), see **muscular branches of ulnar nerve (>1840)**
branch of union with sympathetic (Bell & Bell, 1816), see **communicating branches of spinal nerves (Wutzer, 1817)**
branch of vastus externus and anconeus muscles of radial nerve (Cruveilhier, 1836), see **muscular branches of radial nerve (>1840)**
branch to ceratoglossus muscle (Andersch & Soemmerring, 1792), see **lingual branches of hypoglossal nerve (Cloquet, 1816)**
branch to gemellus and quadratus femoris muscles (Bock, 1827), see **nerve to quadratus femoris (>1840)**
branch to genioglossus muscle from hypoglossal nerve (Arnold, 1834), see **lingual branches of hypoglossal nerve (Cloquet, 1816)**
branch to inferior oblique from third pair (Haller, 1743), see **nerve to inferior oblique (>1840)**
branch to inferior rectus from third pair (Haller, 1743), see **nerve to inferior rectus (>1840)**
branch to infraspinatus muscle (Bock, 1827), see **suprascapular nerve (Bang, 1770)**
branch to internal rectus from third pair (Haller, 1743), see **nerve to medial rectus (>1840)**
branch to levator ani muscle (Bock, 1827), see **perineal branch of fourth sacral nerve (>1840)**
branch to mammary papilla from anterior branch of lateral pectoral cutaneous nerve of intercostal nerve (Bock, 1827), see **lateral mammary branches of intercostal nerves (>1840)**
branch to muscles of femoral trochlea (Bock, 1827), see **nerve to quadratus femoris (>1840)**
branch to nasal septum of ethmoidal branch of nasal nerve (Arnold, 1834), see **medial nasal branches of internal nasal branches of anterior ethmoidal nerve (>1840)**
branch to nasal septum of ethmoidal branch of nasociliary nerve (Arnold, 1834), see **medial nasal branches of internal nasal branches of anterior ethmoidal nerve (>1840)**
branch to obturator internus muscle (Bock, 1827), see **nerve to obturator internus (>1840)**
branch to plantaris muscle from internal popliteal nerve (Bock, 1827), see **nerve to plantaris (>1840)**
branch to semitendinosus muscle (Bock, 1827), see **nerve to hamstring muscles (>1840)**
branch to supraspinatus muscle (Bock, 1827), see **suprascapular nerve (Bang, 1770)**
branch to teres minor muscle (Bock, 1827), see **muscular branch of axillary nerve (>1840)**
branch to tonsil from external palatine nerve (Scarpa, 1785), see **tonsillar branches of lateral palatine nerve (>1840)**
branch to vastus internus of radial nerve (Cruveilhier, 1836), see **muscular branches of radial nerve (>1840)**
branche de communication du ganglion cervical supérieur au ganglion cervical moyen (Cruveilhier, 1836), see **communicating branch of superior and middle cervical ganglia (Cruveilhier, 1836)**
branche linguale du nerf hypoglosse (Cloquet, 1816), see **lingual branches of hypoglossal nerve (Cloquet, 1816)**
branches for three muscles of hypothenar eminence from deep terminal branch of cubital nerve (Cruveilhier, 1836), see **deep branch of ulnar nerve (>1840)**
branches from curve of recurrent nerve to pulmonary plexus (Quain & Wilson, 1839), see **tracheal branches of recurrent laryngeal nerve (>1840)**
branches from sacral nerves communicating with lateral portion of hypogastric plexus (Quain & Wilson, 1839), see **pelvic splanchnic nerves (Gaskell, 1886)**
branches in thorax to esophagus from sixth pair of nerves (Galen, c173), see **vagus nerve trunk (Wrisberg, 1786; Günther, 1786)**
branches in thorax to heart from sixth pair of nerves (Galen, c173), see **thoracic cardiac branches of vagus nerve (>1840)**
branches in thorax to lung from sixth pair of nerves (Galen, c173), see **pulmonary branches of vagus nerve (Cloquet, 1828)**
branches of anterior tibial nerve to extensor brevis digitorum muscle (Quain & Wilson, 1830), see **muscular branches of deep fibular nerve (>1840)**
branches of anterior tibial nerve to joints of foot (Quain & Wilson, 1839), see **articular branch of deep fibular nerve (>1840)**
branches of common extensor of digits of radial nerve (Cruveilhier, 1836), see **posterior interosseous nerve (Quain & Wilson, 1839)**
branches of communication of lingual nerve with gustatory nerve (Quain & Wilson, 1839), see **communicating branches of lingual nerve with hypoglossal nerve (>1840)**
branches of communication of ninth nerve with gustatory nerve (Quain & Wilson, 1839), see **communicating branches of lingual nerve with hypoglossal nerve (>1840)**
branches of communication of superior maxillary nerve from Meckel's ganglion (Quain & Wilson, 1839), see **pterygopalatine nerves (Wrisberg, 1786)**
branches of deep layer of posterior region of forearm of antibrachial deep branch of radial nerve (Cruvielhier, 1836), see **posterior interosseous nerve (Quain & Wilson, 1839)**
branches of dorsal nerve of penis to prepuce (Langenbeck, 1826–1830), see **dorsal nerve of penis (Camper, 1762)**
branches of facial nerve to stapedial muscle (Langenbeck, 1826–1830), see **stapedial nerve (>1840)**
branches of fifth pair (Rau, 1694), see **trigeminal nerve branches (Winslow, 1733)**
branches of glosso-pharyngeal nerve to pharyngeal plexus (Quain & Wilson, 1839), see **pharyngeal branches of glossopharyngeal nerve (Neubauer, 1772)**
branches of glossopharyngeal nerve to soft nerves (Kilian, 1822), see **glossopharyngeal nerve (Huber, 1744)**
branches of great hypoglossal for hyoglossal and styloglossal (Cruveilhier, 1836), see **lingual branches of hypoglossal nerve (Cloquet, 1816)**
branches of gustatory nerve to maxillary ganglion (Arnold, 1834), see **communicating branches of lingual nerve with submandibular ganglion (>1840)**

branches of humeral circumflex nerve to deltoid muscle (Langenbeck, 1826–1830), see **muscular branches of axillary nerve (>1840)**

branches of inferior laryngeal nerve to posterior and lateral cricoarytenoid muscles (Langenbeck, 1826–1830), see **inferior laryngeal nerve (>1840)**

branches of internal plantar nerve (Bock, 1827), see **common plantar digital nerves of medial plantar nerve (>1840)**

branches of internal saphenous nerve to knee-joint (Quain & Wilson, 1839), see **saphenous nerve (Haase, 1781)**

branches of interosseous nerve to extensor brevis digitorum muscle (Quain & Wilson, 1830), see **muscular branches of deep fibular nerve (>1840)**

branches of interosseous nerve to joints of foot (Quain & Wilson, 1839), see **articular branch of deep fibular nerve (>1840)**

branches of lateral peroneus longus of musculocutaneous branch of external popliteal sciatic nerve (Cruveilhier, 1836), see **muscular branches of superficial fibular nerve (>1840)**

branches of lingual nerve to maxillary ganglion (Arnold, 1834), see **communicating branches of lingual nerve with submandibular ganglion (>1840)**

branches of maxillary ganglion to sublingual gland (Langenbeck, 1826–1830), see **glandular branches of submandibular ganglion (>1840)**

branches of maxillary ganglion to submaxillary gland (Langenbeck, 1826–1830), see **glandular branches of submandibular ganglion (>1840)**

branches of maxillary ganglion to Wharton's duct (Arnold, 1834), see **submandibular ganglion (>1840)**

branches of median nerve to lumbrical muscles (Swan, 1830), see **muscular branches of median nerve (Martin, 1781)**

branches of median nerve to radial flexor muscle of wrist (Swan, 1830), see **muscular branches of median nerve (Martin, 1781)**

branches of median nerve to sublime flexor muscle of fingers (Swan, 1830), see **muscular branches of median nerve (Martin, 1781)**

branches of middle cutaneous nerve joining volar cutaneous branch of median nerve (Caldani, 1813, 1814), see **anterior branch of medial cutaneous nerve of forearm (>1840)**

branches of musculocutaneous nerve inserted into volar branch of median nerve (Caldani, 1814, 1814), see **lateral cutaneous nerve of forearm (>1840)**

branches of olfactory nerve (Swan, 1830), see **olfactory nerve (Winslow, 1733)**

branches of peroneal nerve to anterior tibial muscle (Swan, 1830), see **muscular branches of deep fibular nerve (>1840)**

branches of peroneal nerve to long peroneal muscle (Swan, 1830), see **muscular branches of superficial fibular nerve (>1840)**

branches of radial nerve to anterior brachial muscle (Cloquet, 1828), see **muscular branches of radial nerve (>1840)**

branches of sciatic nerve trunk to flexor muscles of thigh (Meckel, 1817), see **nerve to hamstring muscles (>1840)**

branches of superficial layer of posterior region of forearm of antibrachial deep branch of radial nerve (Cruvielhier, 1836), see **posterior interosseous nerve (Quain & Wilson, 1839)**

branches of superior laryngeal branch of pneumo-gastric nerve to pharyngeal plexus (Quain & Wilson, 1839), see **superior laryngeal nerve (Loder, 1778)**

branches of superior laryngeal nerve to arytenoid muscle (Langenbeck, 1826–1830), see **external branch of superior laryngeal nerve (Fyfe, 1800)**

branches of superior laryngeal nerve to epiglottis (Langenbeck, 1826–1830), see **internal branch of superior laryngeal nerve (Fyfe, 1800)**

branches of superior laryngeal nerve to mucosal tunic of larynx (Langenbeck, 1826–1830), see **internal branch of superior laryngeal nerve (Fyfe, 1800)**

branches of superior laryngeal nerve to tunica intima of trachea (Langenbeck, 1826–1830), see **internal branch of superior laryngeal nerve (Fyfe, 1800)**

branches of third pair (Marchetti, 1652), see **trigeminal nerve branches (Winslow, 1733)**

branches of ulnar nerve to ulnar flexor muscle of wrist (Swan, 1830), see **muscular branches of ulnar nerve (>1840)**

branches to cucullaris muscle from external ramus of accessory nerve of Willis (Arnold, 1834), see **muscular branches of external branch of accessory nerve trunk (>1840)**

branches to gingiva of dental nerve anastomosis (Arnold, 1834), see **inferior gingival branches of inferior dental plexus (>1840)**

branches to hyoglossus muscle from hypoglossal nerve (Arnold, 1834), see **lingual branches of hypoglossal nerve (Cloquet, 1816)**

branches to long portion of triceps of radial nerve (Cruveilhier, 1836), see **muscular branches of radial nerve (>1840)**

branches to sternocleidomastoid muscle from external ramus of accessory nerve of Willis (Arnold, 1834), see **muscular branches of external branch of accessory nerve trunk (>1840)**

branches which communicate with great sympathetic nerve (Winslow, 1733), see **communicating branches of spinal nerves (Wutzer, 1817)**

branchial nerve (Leuret, 1839), see **vagus nerve (Galen, c192)**

branchiogastric nerve (Solly, 1836), see **vagus nerve (Galen, c192)**

branchlet of auricular branch of vagus nerve to external auditory meatus (Arnold, 1834), see **auricular branch of vagus nerve (Arnold, 1834)**

branchlet of otic ganglion to anterior auricular nerve (Arnold, 1834), see **communicating branches of otic ganglion with auriculotemporal nerve (>1840)**

branchlet to geniohyoid muscle from hypoglossal nerve (Arnold, 1834), see **lingual branches of hypoglossal nerve (Cloquet, 1816)** *branchlet to styloglossus muscle from hypoglossal nerve (Arnold, 1834)*, see **lingual branches of hypoglossal nerve (Cloquet, 1816)**

branchlets from lingual nerve to maxillary ganglion (Meckel, 1748), see **communicating branches of lingual nerve with submandibular ganglion (>1840)**

branchlets of lingual nerve in sublingual gland (Meckel, 1748), see **sublingual nerve (Henle, 1871)**

brane (archaic English), see **brain (Smith Papyrus, c1700 BC)**

brawny body (Diemerbroeck, 1689), see **cerebral cortex white matter (>1840)**

brawny body (Geminus, 1553), see **corpus callosum (Galen, c177)**

brayn (archaic English), see **brain (Smith Papyrus, c1700 BC)**

brayne (archaic English), see **brain (Smith Papyrus, c1700 BC)**

braynes (archaic English), see **brain (Smith Papyrus, c1700 BC)**

breaches (Crooke, 1615), see **cerebral cortex gray matter (>1840)**

breine (archaic English), see **brain (Smith Papyrus, c1700 BC)**

bridge of cerebel (Diemerbroeck, 1689), see **pons (Haller, 1747)**

bright glass (du Laurens, 1600), see **cerebral nuclei (Swanson, 2000a)**

bright mirror (du Laurens, 1600), see **cerebral nuclei (Swanson, 2000a)**

brim of corpus callosum (Willis, 1664), see **splenium of corpus callosum (Burdach, 1822)**

bronchial branches of inferior laryngeal nerve (Arnold, 1834), see **tracheal branches of recurrent laryngeal nerve (>1840)**

bronchial branches of recurrent laryngeal nerve (Arnold, 1834), see **tracheal branches of recurrent laryngeal nerve (>1840)**

bronchial branches of vagus nerve (Quain, 1832), see **pulmonary branches of vagus nerve (Cloquet, 1828)**

bronchial plexus (Cruveilhier, 1836), see **pulmonary plexus (Winslow, 1733)**

brown region (Vicq d'Azyr, 1784), see **substantia nigra (Soemmerring, 1791)**

brown ridge on peduncle of cord (Gordon, 1815), see **cochlear nuclei (>1840)**

brown substance (Vicq d'Azyr, 1784), see **substantia nigra (Soemmerring, 1791)**

brown substance of brain (Vesalius, 1543a), see **central nervous system gray matter regions (>1840)**

Brückenkerns (Jacobsohn, 1909), see **pontine nuclei (Jacobsohn, 1909)**

buccal branch of facial nerve (>1840)

buccal branch of gustatory nerve (Arnold, 1834), see **sublingual nerve (Henle, 1871)**

buccal branch of hard nerves (Mayer, 1794), see **buccal branch of facial nerve (>1840)**

buccal branch of inferior branch of hard nerve (Meckel, 1753), see **buccal branch of facial nerve (>1840)**

buccal branch of lingual nerve (Arnold, 1834), see **sublingual nerve (Henle, 1871)**

buccal branch of portio dura of auditory nerve (Albinus, 1761), see **buccal branch of facial nerve (>1840)**

buccal branch of portio dura of seventh cerebral nerve (Albinus, 1761), see **buccal branch of facial nerve (>1840)**

buccal branch of superior primary branch of inferior maxillary nerve (Quain, 1832), see **buccal nerve (Meckel, 1748)**

buccal branch of third branch of fifth pair (Loder, 1778), see **buccal nerve (Meckel, 1748)**

buccal branches of cervicofacial branch of facial nerve (Cruveilhier, 1836), see **buccal branch of facial nerve (>1840)**

buccal branches of lower facial branches of descending branch of superficial branch of hard nerve (Günther, 1786), see **buccal branch of facial nerve (>1840)**

buccal branches of posterior alveolar nerve (Arnold, 1834), see **posterior superior dental nerve (Haller, 1762)**

buccal branches of posterior dental nerve (Arnold, 1834), see **posterior superior dental nerve (Haller, 1762)**

buccal branches of superior branch of facial nerve (Arnold, 1834), see **buccal branch of facial nerve (>1840)**

buccal branches of temporofacial branch of facial nerve (Cruveilhier, 1836), see **zygomatic branches of facial nerve (>1840)**

buccal fascicle of buccal surculus of glanglioform plexus with inferior maxillary branch (Bellingeri, 1818), see **buccal nerve (Meckel, 1748)**

buccal nerve (Meckel, 1748)

buccal nerve of inferior branch of hard nerve (Meckel, 1753), see **buccal branch of facial nerve (>1840)**

buccal nerves (Meckel, 1817), see **buccal branch of facial nerve (>1840)**

buccal plexus (Le Cat, 1768), see **buccal branch of facial nerve (>1840)**

buccal surculus of cervico-facial branch of portio major and minor of facial nerve (Bellingeri, 1818), see **buccal branches of facial nerve (>1840)**

buccal surculus of ganglioform plexus with inferior maxillary branch (Bellingeri, 1818), see **buccal nerve (Meckel, 1748)**

buccal surculus of inferior branch of portio major and minor of facial nerve (Bellingeri, 1818), see **buccal branches of facial nerve (>1840)**

buccinator nerve (Meckel, 1753), see **buccal nerve (Meckel, 1748)**

buccolabial branch of fifth nerve (Bell, 1829), see **buccal nerve (Meckel, 1748)**

bucco-labial fascicle of buccal surculus of ganglioform plexus with inferior maxillary branch (Bellingeri, 1818), see **buccal nerve (Meckel, 1748)**

bucco-labial filament of inferior facial branch of pes anserinus (Bellingeri, 1818), see **zygomatic branches of facial nerve (>1840)**

bucco-labian nerve (Burdin, 1803), see **buccal nerve (Meckel, 1748)**

bulb (Chaussier, 1807), see **medulla (Winslow, 1733)**

bulb of medulla oblongata (Serres, 1824–1826), see **medulla (Winslow, 1733)**

bulb of olfactory nerves (Soemmerring, 1798), see **olfactory bulb (Weitbrecht, 1751)**

bulb of posterior horn (>1840)
bulbi fornicis (Santorini, 1724), see **mammillary body (Ludwig, 1779)**
bulbi priorum crurum fornicis (Santorini, 1724), see **mammillary body (Ludwig, 1779)**
bulbi Santorini (Haase, 1781), see **mammillary body (Ludwig, 1779)**
bulbo-urethral branch of perineal branch of internal pudendal nerve (Cruveilhier, 1836), see **muscular branches of perineal nerve (>1840)**
bulbous extremity of olfactory nerve (Swan, 1830), see **olfactory bulb (Weitbrecht, 1751)**
bulbs of vault with three pillars (Chaussier, 1807), see **mammillary body (Ludwig, 1779)**
bulbum cinereum (Soemmerring, 1778), see **olfactory bulb (Weitbrecht, 1751)**
bulbum cinereum oblongum (Soemmerring, 1778), see **olfactory bulb (Weitbrecht, 1751)**
bulbus cornus posterioris (>1840), see **bulb of posterior horn (>1840)**
bulge (Soemmerring, 1788), see **cerebral cortex gray matter (>1840)**
bundle of lumbar and sacral nerves (Burdin, 1803), see **cauda equina (Anatomia Magistri Nicolai physici, early 12th century)**
bundle of striated bodies (Spurzheim, 1826), see **anterior limb of internal capsule (>1840)**
buttocks (Berengario da Carpi, 1522), see **interbrain (Baer, 1837)**
buttocks (Crooke, 1615), see **superior colliculus (Haller, 1762)**
buttocks (Galen, c173, definition 1), see **tectum (Baer, 1837)**
buttocks (Galen, c173, definition 2), see **inferior colliculus (Haller, 1762)**
buttocks (Massa, 1536), see **caudate nucleus (Arnold, 1838b)**
buttocks (Mondino, 1316), see **vertebrate brain (Cuvier, 1800)**
buttocks of brain (Vesalius, 1543a), see **fimbria (Honegger, 1890)**
button (Willis, 1664), see **pineal gland (Galen, c192)**
button of choroid plexus of lateral ventricle (Vicq d'Azyr, 1784), see **choroid enlargement (>1840)**
caelamina inter pedunculos corporis callosi (Burdach, 1822), see **endbrain (Kuhlenbeck, 1927)**
calamus (Mayer, 1779), see **median sulcus of fourth ventricle (>1840)**
calamus scriptorius (Haller, 1762), see **median sulcus of fourth ventricle (>1840)**
calamus scriptorius (Herophilus, c335–c280 BC), see **floor of fourth ventricle (Reil, 1807–1808a)**
calamus scriptorius (Read, 1638), see **fourth ventricle (Galen, c192)**
calamus scriptorius (Ridley, 1695), see **fourth ventricle (Galen, c192)**
calcaneal branches of peroneal saphenous nerve (Cruveilhier, 1836), see **sural communicating branch of common fibular nerve (>1840)**
calcaneal cutaneous branch of tibial nerve (Bock, 1827), see **lateral calcaneal branches of sural nerve (>1840)**
calcaneus bone cutaneous nervelet (Fischer, 1791), see **medial calcaneal nerve (>1840)**
calcar avis (Arnold, 1838a), see **calcarine spur (Morand, 1748)**
calcarine spur (Morand, 1748)
calcarine sulcus (>1840)
callosal substance (Steno, 1669), see **central nervous system white matter tracts (>1840)**
callosal sulcus (>1840), see **sulcus of corpus callosum (>1840)**
callosomarginal sulcus (>1840), see **cingulate sulcus (>1840)**
callous body (Haller, 1754b), see **corpus callosum (Galen, c177)**
camaratum (Vesalius, 1543a), see **fornix (Vesalius, 1543a)**
camarion (Hall, 1565), see **fornix (Vesalius, 1543a)**
camera (Galen, c177), see **fornix (Vesalius, 1543a)**
camera anteriorum ventriculorum (Vieussens, 1684), see **cerebral cortex white matter (>1840)**
camera medullaris (Winslow, 1733), see **cerebral cortex white matter (>1840)**
camerae (Berengario da Carpi, 1521), see **ventricles (Hippocrates)**
cameratum (Vesalius, 1543a), see **fornix (Vesalius, 1543a)**
canal (Le Böe, 1663), see **cerebral aqueduct (>1840)**
canal below corpus callosum (Pourfour du Petit, 1710), see **septal fissure (Burdach, 1822)**
canal connecting posterior ventricle with third ventricle (Spiegel, 1627), see **cerebral aqueduct (>1840)**
canal of Charles Estienne (Günther, 1786), see **central canal (Bellingeri, 1823)**
canal of medulla oblongata (Arnold, 1838b), see **central canal of medulla (>1840)**
canal of quadrigeminal eminences (Günz, 1750), see **cerebral aqueduct (>1840)**
canal of quadrigeminal tubercles (Vicq d'Azyr, 1786), see **cerebral aqueduct (>1840)**
canal of spinal cord (Spurzheim, 1826), see **central canal (Bellingeri, 1823)**
canal of spinal marrow (Carus, 1814), see **central canal (Bellingeri, 1823)**
canalis sub corporibus quadrigeminis (Wenzel & Wenzel, 1812), see **cerebral aqueduct (>1840)**
cap of cerebral peduncle (Meckel, 1817), see **tegmentum (Swanson, 2000b)**
capita medulla oblongata (Ridley, 1695), see **interbrain (Baer, 1837)**
capsula externa (Burdach, 1822), see **external capsule (Burdach, 1822)**
capsular plexus (Wrisberg, 1808), see **adrenal plexus (>1840)**
capsule (Reil, 1809b), see **central nervous system white matter tracts (>1840)**
caput rosae (Avicenna or Ibn Sina, c1030), see **hypothalamus (Kuhlenbeck, 1927)**
cardiac branch of glossopharyngeal nerve (Kilian, 1822), see **glossopharyngeal nerve (Huber, 1744)**
cardiac branch of hypoglossal nerve descending branch (Arnold, 1834), see **ansa cervicalis (>1840)**
cardiac branch of vagus nerve (Loder, 1803), see **superior cervical cardiac branches of vagus nerve (>1840)**
cardiac branch of wandring pair (Willis, 1664), see **thoracic cardiac branches of vagus nerve (>1840)**

cardiac branches of cervical part of pneumogastric nerve (Arnold, 1834), see **superior cervical cardiac branches of vagus nerve (>1840)**

cardiac branches of cervical part of tenth pair (Arnold, 1834), see **superior cervical cardiac branches of vagus nerve (>1840)**

cardiac branches of cervical part of vagus nerve (Arnold, 1834), see **superior cervical cardiac branches of vagus nerve (>1840)**

cardiac branches of descending branch of left vagus nerve (Mayer, 1794), see **gastric branches of anterior vagal trunk (>1840)**

cardiac branches of eighth pair (Walter, 1783), see **thoracic cardiac branches of vagus nerve (>1840)**

cardiac branches of pneumo-gastric nerve (Quain & Wilson, 1839), see **superior cervical cardiac branches of vagus nerve (>1840)**

cardiac branches of recurrent laryngeal nerve (>1840)

cardiac branches of superior cervical ganglion (Cruveilhier, 1836), see **superior cardiac nerve (Neubauer, 1772)**

cardiac branches of vagus nerve (Cloquet, 1828), see **thoracic cardiac branches of vagus nerve (>1840)**

cardiac communicating branch (Andersch & Soemmerring, 1792), see **superior cervical cardiac branches of vagus nerve (>1840)**

cardiac filaments of recurrent nerve (Cruveilhier, 1836), see **cardiac branches of recurrent laryngeal nerve (>1840)**

cardiac ganglion (Neubauer, 1772; Haller, 1772)

cardiac ganglion (Soemmerring, 1791), see **inferior cervical ganglion (Vieussens, 1684)**

cardiac ganglion of sympathetic (Knox, 1832), see **cardiac ganglion (Neubauer, 1772; Haller, 1772)**

cardiac ganglion of Wrisberg (Quain, 1828), see **cardiac plexus (Keill, 1698)**

cardiac ganglion of Wrisberg (Scarpa, 1794), see **cardiac ganglion (Neubauer, 1772; Haller, 1772)**

cardiac infolding (Willis, 1664), see **cardiac ganglion (Neubauer, 1772; Haller, 1772)**

cardiac nerve of eighth pair (Haase, 1781), see **superior cervical cardiac branches of vagus nerve (>1840)**

cardiac nerve of vagal pair (Haase, 1781), see **superior cervical cardiac branches of vagus nerve (>1840)**

cardiac nerves (Willis, 1664), see **nerves (Herophilus, c335–c280 BC)**

cardiac nerves from pneumogastric nerve (Meckel, 1817), see **superior cervical cardiac branches of vagus nerve (>1840)**

cardiac nerves near heart (Lobstein, 1823), see **cardiac plexus (Keill, 1698)**

cardiac nerves of anterior trunk of eighth pair of nerves (Walter, 1783), see **gastric branches of anterior vagal trunk (>1840)**

cardiac plexus (Keill, 1698)

caro glandulosa (Berengario da Carpi, 1522), see **pineal gland (Galen, c192)**

carotic plexus (Lobstein, 1831), see **internal carotid plexus (>1840)**

caroticotympanic nerves (>1840)

carotid branch of posterior branch of spheno-palatine ganglion (Quain & Wilson, 1839), see **deep petrosal nerve (Meckel, 1817)**

carotid branch of pterygoid nerve (Cloquet, 1816), see **deep petrosal nerve (Meckel, 1817)**

carotid branch of superior cervical ganglion (Cruveilhier, 1836), see **internal carotid nerve (>1840)**

carotid branch of vagus nerve (>1840)

carotid branch of Vidian nerve (Cloquet, 1816), see **deep petrosal nerve (Meckel, 1817)**

carotid branches of glossopharyngeal nerve (Todd, 1836–1839)

carotid filaments of glossopharyngeal nerve (Cruveilhier, 1836), see **carotid branches of glossopharyngeal nerve (Todd, 1836–1839)**

carotid ganglion (Wutzer, 1817; Bock, 1817)

carotid nerve (Arnold, 1834), see **paravertebral nerves (Swanson & Bota, 2010)**

carotid nerve (Lobstein, 1823), see **internal carotid nerve (>1840)**

carotid plexus (Bock, 1817), see **internal carotid plexus (>1840)**

carotid plexus of glossopharyngeal nerves (Kilian, 1822), see **external carotid plexus (>1840)**

carotid sinus branch of glossopharyngeal nerve (>1840), see **carotid branches of glossopharyngeal nerve (Todd, 1836–1839)**

carotid sinus nerve (Hering, 1924), see **carotid sinus branches of glossopharyngeal nerve (>1840)**

caruncle (Anatomia Magistri Nicolai physici, early 12th century), see **olfactory bulb (Weitbrecht, 1751)**

caruncula (Albertus Magnus, 13th century), see **choroid plexus of lateral ventricle (Vicq d'Azyr, 1784)**

caruncula mammilaris (Arnold, 1838a), see **olfactory bulb (Weitbrecht, 1751)**

carunculae (Mondino, 1316), see **cerebral cortex (>1840)**

carunculae similes capitibus mammillarum (Mondino, 1316), see **cerebral cortex (>1840)**

caruncular nerves (Leonardo da Vinci, c1504–1506), see **cerebral cortex (>1840)**

Casserian ganglion (Todd, 1836–1839), see **trigeminal ganglion (>1840)**

cauda cerebelli (Molinetti, 1669), see **cerebellar vermis (Meckel, 1817)**

cauda corporis striati (Malacarne, 1780), see **caudate nucleus (Arnold, 1838b)**

cauda equina (Anatomia Magistri Nicolai physici, early 12th century)

cauda nucleus caudatus (Arnold, 1838b), see **tail of caudate nucleus (Arnold, 1838b)**

cauda of inner portion of corpus striatum (Reil, 1809b), see **caudate nucleus (Arnold, 1838b)**

cauda of medulla oblongata (Winslow, 1733), see **medulla (Winslow, 1733)**

cauda of spinal ash-colored substance (Winslow, 1733), see **dorsal horn (>1840)**

caudal fovea (>1840)

caudal medullary velum (>1840)

caudal pairs of nerves (Burdin, 1803), see **coccygeal nerves (Camper, 1762)**

caudal part of vestibular nerve (>1840)
caudal postcentral area (Brodmann, 1909), see ***parietal region (>1840)***
caudate nucleus (Arnold, 1838b)
caudex (Collins, 1685), see ***brainstem (Schwalbe, 1881)***
caudex (Pacchioni, 1741), see ***cerebral falx (Vesalius, 1543a)***
caudex cerebri (Burdach, 1822), see ***vertebrate brain (Cuvier, 1800)***
caudex cerebri (Coiter, 1572), see ***cerebrospinal trunk (>1840)***
caudex dorsalis (Burdach, 1819), see ***spinal cord (Galen, c162–c166)***
caudex encephali (Burdach, 1822), see ***vertebrate brain (Cuvier, 1800)***
caudex medullaris (Cowper, 1698), see ***medulla (Winslow, 1733)***
caudex medullaris (Ridley, 1695), see ***brainstem (Schwalbe, 1881)***
caudex medullaris (Willis, 1664), see ***central nervous system (Carus, 1814)***
caudex of medulla oblongata (Collins, 1685), see ***brainstem (Schwalbe, 1881)***
caudicem (Willis, 1664), see ***vertebrate brain (Cuvier, 1800)***
caudici medullari (Willis, 1664), see ***central nervous system (Carus, 1814)***
caudiform expansion (Tiedemann, 1816), see ***cauda equina (Anatomia Magistri Nicolai physici, early 12th century)***
caudoputamen (Heimer & Wilson, 1975)
cavernous ganglion (Laumonier, 1793), see ***carotid ganglion (Wutzer, 1817; Bock, 1817)***
cavernous nerves of clitoris (>1840)
cavernous nerves of penis (>1840)
cavernous part of abducens nerve (Arnold, 1834), see ***abducens nerve trunk (>1840)***
cavernous part of scornful nerve (Arnold, 1834), see ***abducens nerve trunk (>1840)***
cavernous part of sixth pair (Arnold, 1834), see ***abducens nerve trunk (>1840)***
cavernous plexus (Arnold, 1834), see ***internal carotid plexus (>1840)***
cavernous plexus (Quain, 1837), see ***internal carotid plexus (>1840)***
cavernous sinus (Winslow, 1733)
caverns (Averroes, 12th century), see ***ventricles (Hippocrates)***
cavitas (Vieussens, 1684), see ***septal fissure (Burdach, 1822)***
cavitas Vieussenii (Stumphius, 1736), see ***septal fissure (Burdach, 1822)***
cavité sous-arachnoïdienne (Magendie, 1827), see ***subarachnoid space (Magendie, 1827)***
cavities (Galen, c173), see ***ventricles (Hippocrates)***
cavity of medulla dorsalis forming part of fourth ventricle (Vesalius, 1543a), see ***floor of fourth ventricle (Reil, 1807–1808a)***
cavity of septum lucidum (Sabatier, 1775), see ***septal fissure (Burdach, 1822)***
celiac branches of anterior vagal trunk (>1840)
celiac branches of posterior vagal trunk (>1840)
celiac ganglion (Walter, 1783)
celiac plexus (Winslow, 1733)
celiac plexus proper (Günther, 1786), see ***celiac plexus (Winslow, 1733)***
cell for cerebellum and medulla oblongata (Wagner, 1839), see ***primary hindbrain vesicle (Baer, 1837)***
cell for eye and optic thalamus (Wagner, 1839), see ***primary forebrain vesicle (Baer, 1837)***
cell for optic thalamus and cerebral peduncle (Wagner, 1839), see ***interbrain vesicle (Baer, 1837)***
cell for optic thalamus and third ventricle (Wagner, 1839), see ***interbrain vesicle (Baer, 1837)***
cell for quadrigeminal body (Wagner, 1839), see ***primary midbrain vesicle (Baer, 1837)***
cell for third ventricle (Wagner, 1839), see ***interbrain vesicle (Baer, 1837)***
cells (Anatomia Magistri Nicolai physici, early 12th century), see ***ventricles (Hippocrates)***
cellula fantastica (Anatomia Magistri Nicolai physici, early 12th century; Guillaume de Conches, c1100–1154), see ***lateral ventricle (Vesalius, 1543a)***
cellula logistica or rationalis (Anatomia Magistri Nicolai physici, early 12th century; Guillaume de Conches, c1100–1154), see ***third ventricle (Galen, c173)***
cellula memorialis (Anatomia Magistri Nicolai physici, early 12th century; Guillaume de Conches, c1100–1154), see ***fourth ventricle (Galen, c192)***
cendré supérieur (Gerdy, 1838), see ***cerebral nuclei (Swanson, 2000a)***
center of optic thalamus (Rolando, 1825a), see ***ventral thalamic nuclei (>1840)***
central amygdalar nucleus (Johnston, 1923)
central canal (Bellingeri, 1823)
central canal of medulla (>1840)
central canal of spinal cord (>1840)
central cervical ganglion (Meckel, 1817), see ***middle cervical ganglion (Haller, 1762)***
central cingulate gyrus (Burdach, 1822), see ***cingulate region (Brodmann, 1909)***
central column of spinal cord (Gordon, 1815), see ***cerebrospinal trunk (>1840)***
central commissure (Owen, 1832), see ***supraesophageal ganglion (Grant, 1834a)***
central end of accessory nerve of Willis (Cruveilhier, 1836), see ***white matter tracts (Bell & Bell, 1826)***
central end of auditory nerve (Cruveilhier, 1836), see ***white matter tracts (Bell & Bell, 1826)***
central end of common motor nerve of eye (Cruveilhier, 1836), see ***white matter tracts (Bell & Bell, 1826)***
central end of external ocular motor nerve (Cruveilhier, 1836), see ***white matter tracts (Bell & Bell, 1826)***
central end of facial nerve (Cruveilhier, 1836), see ***white matter tracts (Bell & Bell, 1826)***
central end of glossopharyngeal and pneumogastric nerves (Cruveilhier, 1836), see ***white matter tracts (Bell & Bell, 1826)***
central end of great hypoglossal nerve (Cruveilhier, 1836), see ***white matter tracts (Bell & Bell, 1826)***
central end of olfactory nerve (Cruveilhier, 1836), see ***endbrain (Kuhlenbeck, 1927)***
central end of optic nerves (Cruveilhier, 1836), see ***optic tract (Vicq d'Azyr, 1784)***

central end of pathetic nerve (Cruveilhier, 1836), see ***white matter tracts (Bell & Bell, 1826)***

central end of portio dura of seventh pair (Cruveilhier, 1836), see ***white matter tracts (Bell & Bell, 1826)***

central end of spinal nerve of Willis (Cruveilhier, 1836), see ***white matter tracts (Bell & Bell, 1826)***

central end of trigeminal nerves (Cruveilhier, 1836), see ***white matter tracts (Bell & Bell, 1826)***

central fissure (Meckel, 1817), see ***ventricles (Hippocrates)***

central fissure of brain proper (Gordon, 1815), see ***ventricles (Hippocrates)***

central fissure of cerebellum (Gordon, 1815), see ***fourth ventricle (Galen, c192)***

central ganglia (>1840)

central ganglion (Mangili, 1804), see ***invertebrate brain (>1840)***

central ganglions of ganglionnary nerve (Meckel, 1817), see ***prevertebral ganglia (Quain, 1832)***

central gray layer (Meckel, 1817), see ***pons (Haller, 1747)***

central gray of medulla oblongata (Arnold, 1838b), see ***medulla (Winslow, 1733)***

central gray substance of spinal medulla (Rolando, 1825a), see ***spinal cord (Galen, c162–c166)***

central lobe (Malacarne, 1776), see ***central lobule (Burdach, 1822)***

central lobule (Burdach, 1822)

central longitudinal communicating branch (>1840)

central marrow of cerebellar hemisphere (Vieussens, 1684), see ***arbor vitae (Winslow, 1733)***

central mass (Gordon, 1815), see ***central nervous system (Carus, 1814)***

central mass of cerebellum (Gordon, 1815), see ***arbor vitae (Winslow, 1733)***

central masses of nervous system (Carus, 1814), see ***central nervous system (Carus, 1814)***

central medullary nucleus (Reil, 1807–1808a), see ***arbor vitae (Winslow, 1733)***

central nerve cord (Serres, 1824–1826)

central nerve cord trunk (>1840)

central nerve mass (Carus, 1814), see ***central nervous system white matter tracts (>1840)***

central nerve of retina (Langenbeck, 1826–1830), see ***short ciliary nerves (>1840)***

central nervous system (Carus, 1814)

central nervous system gray matter (Meckel, 1817), see ***central nervous system gray matter regions (>1840)***

central nervous system gray matter regions (>1840)

central nervous system surface features (>1840)

central nervous system white matter (Meckel, 1817), see ***central nervous system white matter tracts (>1840)***

central nervous system white matter tracts (>1840)

central nucleus (Chaussier, 1807), see ***dentate nucleus (>1840)***

central nucleus of brain (Cruveilhier, 1836), see ***forebrain (Goette, 1873)***

central nucleus of olivary eminence (Chaussier, 1807), see ***amiculum of olive (>1840)***

central nucleus of peduncles (Chaussier, 1807), see ***arbor vitae (Winslow, 1733)***

central part of cerebellum (Meckel, 1817), see ***cerebellar vermis (Meckel, 1817)***

central part of great sympathetic (Cruveilhier, 1836), see ***peripheral nervous system (Meckel, 1817)***

central part of inferior vermiform process (Meckel, 1817), see ***pyramis (Malacarne, 1776)***

central part of lateral part of spinal ashen-colored substance (Vicq d'Azyr, 1784), see ***intermediate spinal zone (>1840)***

central part of lateral ventricle (Meckel, 1817), see ***body of lateral ventricle (Bell, 1803b)***

central part of nervous system (Carus, 1818), see ***central nervous system (Carus, 1814)***

central root of trigeminal nerve (Meckel, 1817), see ***trigeminal nerve sensory root (>1840)***

central sulcus (Huschke, 1854)

central sulcus of insula (>1840)

central sulcus separating four quadrigeminal tubercles (Cloquet, 1828), see ***cruciform sulcus (>1840)***

central tegmental tract (Bechterew, 1889)

central transverse communicating branch (>1840)

central white mass of convolutions (Gordon, 1815), see ***cerebral cortex white matter (>1840)***

central white nucleus of cerebellum (Cruveilhier, 1836), see ***arbor vitae (Winslow, 1733)***

central white substance (Baillarger, 1840), see ***cerebral cortex white matter (>1840)***

centralen Nervensystems (Carus, 1814), see ***central nervous system (Carus, 1814)***

Centralfurche (Huschke, 1854), see ***central sulcus (Huschke, 1854)***

centrum geminum (Haase, 1781), see ***terminal stria (Wenzel & Wenzel, 1812)***

centrum ovale (Ridley, 1695), see ***cerebral cortex white matter (>1840)***

centrum semicirculare (Günther, 1786), see ***terminal stria (Wenzel & Wenzel, 1812)***

centrum semicirculare geminum (Monro, 1783), see ***terminal stria (Wenzel & Wenzel, 1812)***

centrum semicirculare geminum (Vieussens, 1684), see ***internal capsule (Burdach, 1822)***

centrum semiovale Vieussenii (Mayer, 1779), see ***cerebral cortex white matter (>1840)***

cephalic part of medulla oblongata (Meckel, 1817), see ***medulla (Winslow, 1733)***

cephalic part of spinal marrow (Haase, 1781), see ***medulla (Winslow, 1733)***

cephalic part of spinal prolongation (Chaussier, 1807), see ***medulla (Winslow, 1733)***

cephalic part of trachelo-cutanean plexus (Burdin, 1803), see ***ascending superficial branches of cervical plexus (Quain, 1828)***

cephalic part of tracheosubcutaneous nerves (Chaussier, 1809), see ***ascending superficial branches of cervical plexus (Quain, 1828)***

cephalic part of vegetative nervous system (Arnold, 1834), see ***peripheral nervous system (Meckel, 1817)***

cephalo-rachidian nerves (Cruveilhier, 1836), see ***cerebrospinal nerves (Herrick, 1915)***

ceratobasioglossus nerve (Andersch & Soemmerring, 1792), see ***lingual branches of hypoglossal nerve (Cloquet, 1816)***

ceratobasiostyloglossus plexus (Andersch & Soemmerring, 1792), see **lingual branches of hypoglossal nerve (Cloquet, 1816)**
ceratoglossal plexus of hypoglossal (Knox, 1832), see **lingual branches of hypoglossal nerve (Cloquet, 1816)**
cerebel (Willis, 1664), see **cerebellum (Aristotle)**
cerebellar bark (Willis, 1664), see **cerebellar cortex (Willis, 1664)**
cerebellar brachia (Malacarne, 1776), see **cerebellar peduncles (Ridley, 1695)**
cerebellar choroid plexus (Desmoulins, 1825), see **choroid plexus of fourth ventricle (Vieussens, 1684)**
cerebellar cistern (Aranzi, 1587), see **fourth ventricle (Galen, c192)**
cerebellar commissure (Arnold, 1838a), see **pons (Haller, 1747)**
cerebellar commissure (Spurzheim, 1826), see **middle cerebellar peduncle (Rolando, 1819)**
cerebellar commissure (>1840)
cerebellar cortex (Willis, 1664)
cerebellar crura (Haller, 1747), see **cerebellar peduncles (Ridley, 1695)**
cerebellar eminence (Molinetti, 1669), see **cerebellar hemisphere (Willis, 1664)**
cerebellar falx (Günther, 1786)
cerebellar fascicle (Bellingeri, 1823), see **dorsal funiculus (>1840)**
cerebellar fasciculus (Tiedemann, 1816), see **inferior cerebellar peduncle (Günther, 1786)**
cerebellar fissures (>1840)
cerebellar ganglion (Gall & Spurzheim, 1810), see **dentate nucleus (>1840)**
cerebellar hemisphere (Willis, 1664)
cerebellar lobe (Winslow, 1733), see **cerebellar hemisphere (Willis, 1664)**
cerebellar nerves (Gordon, 1815), see **cranial nerves (Soemmerring, 1791)**
cerebellar nuclei (>1840)
cerebellar nucleus (Malacarne, 1776), see **arbor vitae (Winslow, 1733)**
cerebellar olive (Cruveilhier, 1836), see **dentate nucleus (1840)**
cerebellar pedestal (Willis, 1664), see **cerebellar peduncles (Ridley, 1695)**
cerebellar peduncle (Cruveilhier, 1836), see **middle cerebellar peduncle (Rolando, 1819)**
cerebellar peduncle (Willis, 1664), see **cerebellar peduncles (Ridley, 1695)**
cerebellar peduncle (Winslow, 1733), see **inferior cerebellar peduncle (Günther, 1786)**
cerebellar peduncles (Ridley, 1695)
cerebellar process (Ridley, 1695), see **cerebral peduncle (Tarin, 1753)**
cerebellar processes (Günther, 1786), see **cerebellar peduncles (Ridley, 1695)**
cerebellar prolongation of cerebral protuberance (Cloquet, 1828), see **middle cerebellar peduncle (Rolando, 1819)**
cerebellar protuberances (Winslow, 1733), see **cerebellar hemisphere (Willis, 1664)**
cerebellar roots (Lieutaud, 1742), see **cerebellar peduncles (Ridley, 1695)**
cerebellar stalks (Ridley, 1695), see **cerebellar peduncles (Ridley, 1695)**
cerebellar tentorium (Winslow, 1733)
cerebellar trunk (Willis, 1664), see **cerebellar peduncles (Ridley, 1695)**
cerebellar vermis (Meckel, 1817)
cerebellar vesicle (Malpighi, 1675), see **hindbrain (Baer, 1837)**
cerebelli anterior pars (Casseri, 1609), see **cerebral peduncle (Tarin, 1753)**
cerebellopontine angle (>1840)
cerebellopontine trigone (>1840), see **cerebellopontine angle (>1840)**
cerebellum (Aristotle)
cerebellum (Galen, c173), see **rhombicbrain (His, 1893b)**
cerebellum (Haller, 1762), see **hindbrain (Baer, 1837)**
cerebellum (Varoli, 1573), see **hindbrain (Baer, 1837)**
cerebellum (Willis, 1672), see **invertebrate brain (>1840)**
cerebral aqueduct (>1840)
cerebral brainstem (Burdach, 1822), see **vertebrate brain (Cuvier, 1800)**
cerebral cavities (Spurzheim, 1826), see **ventricles (Hipppocrates)**
cerebral ceiling (Gerdy, 1838), see **corpus callosum (Galen, c177)**
cerebral cells (Baer, 1837), see **brain vesicles (Malpighi, 1673)**
cerebral colliculi (Arnold, 1838a), see **vertebrate brain (Cuvier, 1800)**
cerebral convolutions (Smith Papyrus, c1700 BC), see **cerebral cortex gray matter (>1840)**
cerebral cortex (Bauhin, 1605), see **cerebral cortex gray matter (>1840)**
cerebral cortex (>1840)
cerebral cortex gray matter (>1840)
cerebral cortex white matter (>1840)
cerebral crus (Günther, 1786), see **cerebral peduncle (Tarin, 1753)**
cerebral epiphysis (Serres, 1824–1826), see **pineal gland (Galen, c192)**
cerebral falx (Vesalius, 1543a)
cerebral fascicle (Bellingeri, 1823), see **ventral funiculus (>1840)**
cerebral fissure (Cruveilhier, 1836), see **inner part of transverse cerebral fissure (>1840)**
cerebral ganglia (Arnold, 1838a), see **vertebrate brain (Cuvier, 1800)**
cerebral ganglia (Leuret, 1839), see **endbrain (Kuhlenbeck, 1927)**
cerebral ganglia (Newport, 1834), see **supraesophageal ganglion (Grant, 1834a)**
cerebral granulations (Bichat et al., 1801–1803), see **arachnoid granulations (>1840)**
cerebral gyri (Vesalius, 1543a), see **cerebral cortex gray matter (>1840)**
cerebral gyrus (Vesalius, 1543a), see **cerebral cortex gray matter (>1840)**
cerebral hemisphere (Willis, 1664), see **cerebral cortex (>1840)**

cerebral part of vagus nerve (Arnold, 1834), see **vagus nerve root (>1840)**
cerebral peduncle (Tarin, 1753)
cerebral peduncle (Treveranus, 1817), see **circumesophageal connective (>1840)**
cerebral peduncle (Vicq d'Azyr, 1784), see **tegmentum (Swanson, 2000b)**
cerebral peduncle (Winslow, 1733), see **brainstem (Schwalbe, 1881)**
cerebral peduncle system (Reil, 1809b), see **central nervous system white matter tracts (>1840)**
cerebral process (Mayer, 1794), see **cerebral peduncle (Tarin, 1753)**
cerebral prolongation (Burdin, 1803), see **medulla (Winslow, 1733)**
cerebral prolongation of cerebral protuberance (Bichat et al., 1801–1803), see **cerebral peduncle (Tarin, 1753)**
cerebral prominences (Varoli, 1573), see **cerebral cortex gray matter (>1840)**
cerebral proper nerves (Gordon, 1815), see **nervous system (Monro, 1783)**
cerebral protuberance (Bichat et al., 1801–1803), see **brainstem (Schwalbe, 1881)**
cerebral protuberance (Cloquet, 1816), see **brainstem (Schwalbe, 1881)**
cerebral protuberance (Quain, 1832), see **pons (Haller, 1747)**
cerebral protuberance (Rolando, 1825a), see **pons (Haller, 1747)**
cerebral ring around esophagus (Burdin, 1803), see **central nervous system (Carus, 1814)**
cerebral roots of accessory nerve of Willis (Günther, 1786), see **cranial root of accessory nerve rootlets (>1840)**
cerebral roots of great intercostal nerve (Günther, 1786), see **sympathetic trunk (Winslow, 1733)**
cerebral sphere (Willis, 1664), see **cerebral cortex (>1840)**
cerebral stem (Burdach, 1822), see **vertebrate brain (Cuvier, 1800)**
cerebral substance (Dryander, 1536), see **vertebrate brain (Cuvier, 1800)**
cerebral sulci (Vesalius, 1543a)
cerebral system (Burdin, 1803), see **central nervous system (Carus, 1814)**
cerebral system (Reil, 1807), see **craniospinal nerves (Herrick, 1915)**
cerebral system ganglia (Wutzer, 1817), see **cranial nerve ganglia (>1840)**
cerebral testicle (Vesalius, 1543a), see **superior colliculus (Haller, 1762)**
cerebral testicles (Casseri, 1609), see **mammillary body (Ludwig, 1779)**
cerebral trigone (Burdin, 1803), see **fornix (Vesalius, 1543a)**
cerebral trunk (Burdach, 1822), see **vertebrate brain (Cuvier, 1800)**
cerebral valve (Vicq d'Azyr, 1784), see **rostral medullary velum (>1840)**
cerebral ventricles (Galen, c192), see **ventricles (Hippocrates)**
cerebri medulla (Malpighi, 1665), see **cerebral cortex white matter (>1840)**
cerebri penis (Bauhin, 1605), see **pineal gland (Galen, c192)**
cerebri portionem albam qua spinali medullae principium exporrigit (Soemmerring, 1778), see **mammillary body (Ludwig, 1779)**
cerebri processus anteriores (Bauhin, 1605), see **cerebral cortex (>1840)**
cerebri vesiculae (Malpighi, 1673), see **brain vesicles (Malpighi, 1673)**
cerebrine nerves (Hooper, 1797), see **cranial nerves (Soemmerring, 1791)**
cerebrospinal axis (Meckel, 1817)
cerebrospinal fluid (Magendie, 1827)
cerebro-spinal mass (Quain, 1832), see **central nervous system (Carus, 1814)**
cerebrospinal nerve (Portal, 1803a), see **cervical nerve (Galen, c173)**
cerebro-spinal nerves (Müller, 1834), see **craniospinal nerves (Herrick, 1915)**
cerebrospinal nervous center (Cruveilhier, 1836), see **central nervous system (Carus, 1814)**
cerebrospinal nervous system (Cloquet, 1828), see **central nervous system (Carus, 1814)**
cerebrospinal system (Desmoulins, 1825), see **central nervous system (Carus, 1814)**
cerebrospinal trunk (>1840)
cerebrovertebral nerve (Portal, 1803a), see **cervical nerve (Galen, c173)**
cerebrum (Aristotle), see **vertebrate brain (Cuvier, 1800)**
cerebrum (Celsus, c30), see **brain (Smith Papyrus, c1700 BC)**
cerebrum (Cloquet, 1816), see **vertebrate brain (Cuvier, 1800)**
cerebrum (Colombo, 1559), see **forebrain (Goette, 1873)**
cerebrum (Obersteiner & Hill, 1900), see **endbrain (Kuhlenbeck, 1927)**
cerebrum (Piccolomini, 1586), see **cerebral cortex gray matter (>1840)**
cerebrum (Ramsay, 1813), see **cerebral cortex (>1840)**
cerebrum (Vesalius, 1543a), see **vertebrate brain (Cuvier, 1800)**
cerebrum (Willis, 1664), see **endbrain (Kuhlenbeck, 1927)**
cerebrum applied to frontal bone (Vesalius, 1543a), see **frontal region (Vicq d'Azyr, 1786)**
cerebrum broadly (Günther, 1786), see **central nervous system (Carus, 1814)**
cerebrum cineritium (Piccolomini, 1586), see **cerebral cortex gray matter (>1840)**
cerebrum elongatum (Bannister, 1578), see **cerebrospinal trunk (>1840)**
cerebrum elongatum (Collins, 1685), see **cerebrospinal trunk (>1840)**
cerebrum longum (Colombo, 1559), see **cerebrospinal trunk (>1840)**
cerebrum medium (Wagner, 1839), see **interbrain vesicle (Baer, 1837)**
cerebrum oblongatum (Colombo, 1559), see **cerebrospinal trunk (>1840)**
cerebrum proper (Chaussier, 1807), see **forebrain (Goette, 1873)**
cerebrum proper (Haller, 1747), see **vertebrate brain (Cuvier, 1800)**

cerebrum proper (Piccolomini, 1586), see **cerebral cortex gray matter (>1840)**
cerebrum proper (Willis, 1664), see **endbrain (Kuhlenbeck, 1927)**
cerebrum properly so called (Willis, 1664), see **endbrain (Kuhlenbeck, 1927)**
cervical auricular nerve (Meckel, 1817), see **great auricular nerve (Haase, 1781)**
cervical branch of facial nerve (>1840)
cervical branches of cervicofacial branch of facial nerve (Cruveilhier, 1836), see **cervical branch of facial nerve (>1840)**
cervical enlargement (Arnold, 1838b)
cervical fold (Diemerbroeck, 1689), see **superior cervical ganglion (Vieussens, 1684)**
cervical ganglia of intercostal nerve (Günther, 1786), see **cervical sympathetic ganglia (>1840)**
cervical ganglions of limiting cord (Meckel, 1817), see **cervical sympathetic ganglia (>1840)**
cervical infolding in trunk of intercostal nerve (Willis, 1664), see **middle cervical ganglion (Haller, 1762)**
[cervical nerves] (Colombo, 1559), see **cervical nerves (Galen, c173)**
cervical nerves (Galen, c173)
cervical nerves (William of Saliceto, 1275), see **cervical nerves (Galen, c173)**
cervical nerves (Winslow, 1733), see **cervical nerves (Galen, c173)**
cervical part of accessory nerve of Willis (Arnold, 1834), see **accessory nerve (Vieussens, 1684)**
cervical part of eleventh pair (Arnold, 1834), see **accessory nerve (Vieussens, 1684)**
cervical part of hypoglossal nerve (Arnold, 1834), see **hypoglossal nerve trunk (Günther, 1786)**
cervical part of pneumogastric nerve (Arnold, 1834), see **vagus nerve trunk (Wrisberg, 1786; Günther, 1786)**
cervical part of speaking nerve (Arnold, 1834), see **hypoglossal nerve trunk (Günther, 1786)**
cervical part of spinal cord (>1840)
cervical part of spinal medulla (Tiedemann, 1821), see **cervical part of spinal cord (>1840)**
cervical part of tenth pair (Arnold, 1834), see **vagus nerve trunk (Wrisberg, 1786; Günther, 1786)**
cervical part of twelfth pair (Arnold, 1834), see **hypoglossal nerve trunk (Günther, 1786)**
cervical part of vagus nerve (Arnold, 1834), see **vagus nerve trunk (Wrisberg, 1786; Günther, 1786)**
cervical plexus (Diemebroeck, 1672), see **peripheral nervous system (Meckel, 1817)**
cervical plexus (Keill, 1698), see **superior cervical ganglion (Vieussens, 1684)**
cervical plexus (Molinetti, 1675)
cervical portion of cord (Gordon, 1815), see **cervical part of spinal cord (>1840)**
cervical prominence (Meckel, 1817), see **cervical enlargement (Arnold, 1838b)**
cervical spinal ganglia (>1840)
cervical spinal medulla (Galen, c173), see **cervical part of spinal cord (>1840)**
cervical sympathetic ganglia (>1840)
cervico-brachial plexus (Cruveilhier, 1836), see **spinal nerve ventral branch (>1840)**
cervicobrachial plexus (Portal, 1803b), see **brachial plexus (Camper, 1760)**
cervicofacial branch of facial nerve (Meckel, 1817), see **facial nerve trunk (1840)**
cervicothoracic ganglion (>1840), see **sympathetic trunk ganglia (Winslow, 1733)**
chamber (Willis, 1664), see **cerebral cortex white matter (>1840)**
chamber built after manner of arch (Geminus, 1553), see **fornix (Vesalius, 1543a)**
chamber of brain (Willis, 1664), see **cerebral cortex white matter (>1840)**
chamber of fourth ventricle (Reil, 1809c), see **rhombicbrain (His, 1893b)**
chambered body (Willis, 1664), see **cerebral cortex white matter (>1840)**
chambers (Galen, c173), see **ventricles (Hippocrates)**
chambers of optic nerve (Willis, 1664), see **interbrain (Baer, 1837)**
chamfered body (Willis, 1664), see **cerebral nuclei (Swanson, 2000a)**
channel stretching from third to fourth ventricle (Vesalius, 1543a), see **cerebral aqueduct (>1840)**
channeled bodies (Poupart, 1712), see **cerebral nuclei (Swanson, 2000a)**
channels (Alcmaeon, c490–c430 BC), see **nerves (Herophilus, c335–c280 BC)**
chiasm (Loder, 1803), see **brachial plexus medial cord (Schwalbe, 1881)**
chiasm of Camper (Günther, 1786), see **brachial plexus medial cord (Schwalbe, 1881)**
chiasma Camperi (Günther, 1786), see **brachial plexus medial cord (Schwalbe, 1881)**
chief mesenteric infolding (Willis, 1664), see **celiac ganglion (Walter, 1783)**
chimney (Galen, c177), see **pineal recess (>1840)**
chine-marrow (Nemesius, 1636), see **spinal cord (Galen, c162–c166)**
chink (Bartholin, 1662), see **cerebral aqueduct (>1840)**
chink (Willis, 1664), see **opening of cerebral aqueduct (>1840)**
chinks (Willis, 1664), see **cerebral sulci (Vesalius, 1543a)**
choane (Galen, c177), see **hypothalamus (Kuhlenbeck, 1927)**
choane (Vesalius, 1543a), see **pituitary gland (>1840)**
chone (Galen, c177), see **hypothalamus (Kuhlenbeck, 1927)**
chord of tympanum (Swan, 1830), see **chorda tympani (Falloppio, 1561)**
chorda laminosa transversalis (Malacarne, 1776), see **folium vermis (>1840)**
chorda oblongata (Quain, 1832), see **medulla (Winslow, 1733)**
chorda spinalis (Quain, 1837), see **spinal cord (Galen, c162–c166)**
chorda tympani (Falloppio, 1561)
chorda tympani nerve (Quain & Wilson, 1839), see **chorda tympani (Falloppio, 1561)**
chorda Willisii (Santorini, 1775), see **anterior commissure (Lieutaud, 1742)**

chordae serpentinae (Bergmann, 1831), see **superior cerebellar peduncle (Procháska, 1800)**
chordae sinuosae (Bergmann, 1831), see **superior cerebellar peduncle (Procháska, 1800)**
chordae tortuosae (Bergmann, 1831), see **superior cerebellar peduncle (Procháska, 1800)**
chordae verticillatae (Bergmann, 1831), see **middle cerebellar peduncle (Rolando, 1819)**
chordae volubiles (Bergmann, 1831), see **superior cerebellar peduncle (Procháska, 1800)**
chordal process of cerebellum (Ridley, 1695), see **inferior cerebellar peduncle (Günther, 1786)**
chordis contortis (Bergmann, 1831), see **posterior limb of internal capsule (>1840)**
chorioeidê sustremmata (Galen, c177), see **choroid plexus (Galen, c177)**
chorioeides (Galen, c173), see **pia (Galen, c192)**
chorioid fissure (>1840), see **choroid fissure (>1840)**
chorioid meninx (Herophilus, c335–c280 BC), see **choroid plexus (Galen, c177)**
chorioid plexus (Galen, c177), see **choroid plexus (Galen, c177)**
chorioid tunic (Rufus of Ephesus, c90–c120), see **choroid plexus (Galen, c177)**
choroeidê plegmata (Galen, c177), see **choroid plexus (Galen, c177)**
choroid bodies (Galen, c173), see **choroid plexus (Galen, c177)**
choroid coils (Herophilus, c335–c280 BC), see **choroid plexus (Galen, c177)**
choroid concatenations (Herophilus, c335–c280 BC), see **choroid plexus (Galen, c177)**
choroid enlargement (>1840)
choroid epithelium of fourth ventricle (>1840)
choroid epithelium of lateral ventricle (>1840)
choroid epithelium of third ventricle (>1840)
choroid fissure (>1840)
choroid fold (Diemerbroeck, 1689), see **choroid plexus (Galen, c177)**
choroid lamina of fourth ventricle (Chaussier, 1807), see **choroid membrane of fourth ventricle (>1840)**
choroid line of fourth ventricle (>1840)
choroid line of lateral ventricle (>1840)
choroid line of third ventricle (>1840)
choroid membrane (Galen, c173), see **pia (Galen, c192)**
choroid membrane (Gordon, 1815), see **choroid membrane of third ventricle (>1840)**
choroid membrane (Herophilus, c335–c280 BC), see **choroid plexus (Galen, c177)**
choroid membrane of fourth ventricle (>1840)
choroid membrane of lateral ventricle (>1840)
choroid membrane of third ventricle (>1840)
choroid meninx (Herophilus, c335–c280 BC), see **choroid plexus (Galen, c177)**
choroid plexus (Galen, c177)
choroid plexus minor (Quain, 1832), see **choroid plexus of fourth ventricle (Vieussens, 1684)**
choroid plexus of brain (Cruveilhier, 1836), see **choroid plexus of lateral ventricle (Vicq d'Azyr, 1784)**
choroid plexus of fourth ventricle (Vieussens, 1684)
choroid plexus of lateral ventricle (Vicq d'Azyr, 1784)
choroid plexus of pineal gland (Vicq d'Azyr, 1786), see **choroid plexus of third ventricle (Vicq d'Azyr, 1784)**
choroid plexus of third ventricle (Vicq d'Azyr, 1784)
choroid twisted clusters (Herophilus, c335–c280 BC), see **choroid plexus (Galen, c173)**
choroidal fissure of lateral ventricle (>1840), see **choroid fissure (>1840)**
choroides minor (Quain, 1828), see **choroid plexus of fourth ventricle (Vieussens, 1684)**
ciliary body (Reil, 1807–1808a), see **dentate nucleus (>1840)**
ciliary branch of nasal nerves (Wutzer, 1817), see **communicating branch of nasociliary nerve with ciliary ganglion (>1840)**
ciliary branch of nasociliary nerve (Meckel, 1817), see **communicating branch of nasociliary nerve with ciliary ganglion (>1840)**
ciliary branches of nasal nerve (Todd, 1836–1839), see **long ciliary nerves (Soemmerring, 1801)**
ciliary branches of ophthalmic ganglion (Quain & Wilson, 1839), see **short ciliary nerves (>1840)**
ciliary fascicle of nasal surculus (Bellingeri, 1818), see **long ciliary nerves (Soemmerring, 1801)**
ciliary ganglion (Loder, 1778)
ciliary ganglion branch of communication to carotid plexus (Quain & Wilson, 1839), see **sympathetic root of ciliary ganglion (>1840)**
ciliary ganglion branch of communication to inferior branch of third nerve (Quain & Wilson, 1839), see **branch of oculomotor nerve to ciliary ganglion (>1840)**
ciliary ganglion branch of communication to nasal nerve (Quain & Wilson, 1839), see **communicating branch of nasociliary nerve with ciliary ganglion (>1840)**
ciliary nerves (Albinus,1744), see **short ciliary nerves (>1840)**
ciliary nerves (Chaussier, 1809), see **nerves (Herophilus, c335–c280 BC)**
ciliary nerves (Meckel, 1748), see **short ciliary nerves (>1840)**
ciliary nerves (Ruysch, 1702), see **short ciliary nerves (>1840)**
ciliary plexus (Meckel, 1748), see **nerves (Herophilus, c335–c280 BC)**
cinerea taenola (Wenzel & Wenzel, 1812), see **cochlear nuclei (>1840)**
cineritia substantia (Malpighi, 1665), see **central nervous system gray matter regions (>1840)**
cineritious matter (Bell & Bell, 1816), see **gray matter (Meckel, 1817)**
cineritious matter (Monro, 1783), see **central nervous system gray matter regions (>1840)**
cineritious neurine (Solly, 1836), see **gray matter (Meckel, 1817)**
cineritious part (Valverde de Amusco, 1560), see **central nervous system gray matter regions (>1840)**
cineritious root of olfactory nerve (Knox, 1832), see **tenia tecta (Swanson, 1992)**
cineritious substance (Ridley, 1695), see **central nervous system gray matter regions (>1840)**
cineritious tubercle (Spurzheim, 1826), see **hypothalamus (Kuhlenbeck, 1927)**

cingulate gyrus (Burdach, 1822), see ***cerebral cortex gray matter (>1840)***
cingulate gyrus behind splenium of corpus callosum (Burdach, 1822), see ***isthmus of cingulate region (>1840)***
cingulate region (Brodmann, 1909)
cingulate sulcus (>1840)
cingulum (Burdach, 1822)
circilli (Tyson, 1699), see ***cerebellar cortex (Willis, 1664)***
circle of Reil (Gordon, 1817), see ***central nervous system white matter tracts (>1840)***
circles (Hall, 1565), see ***cerebellar cortex (Willis, 1664)***
circular oral nervous chord (Grant, 1834a), see ***circumoral nerve ring (>1840)***
circular protuberance (Gibson, 1684), see ***pons (Haller, 1747)***
circular ruts (Bauhin, 1605), see ***cerebral sulci (Vesalius, 1543a)***
circular sinus (Ridley, 1695)
circular sulcus (Schwalbe, 1881)
circular sulcus of Reil (Schwalbe, 1881), see ***circular sulcus (Schwalbe, 1881)***
circulus tonsillaris (Andersch & Soemmerring, 1792), see ***glossopharyngeal nerve (Huber, 1744)***
circulus tonsillaris Anderschii (Cloquet, 1828), see ***glossopharyngeal nerve (Huber, 1744)***
circumenteric nerve ring (>1840)
circumesophageal connective (>1840)
circumflex glossopharyngeal branch (Scarpa, 1794), see ***pharyngeal branches of glossopharyngeal nerve (Neubauer, 1772)***
circumflex nerve (Haller, 1762), see ***axillary nerve (Winslow, 1733)***
circumflex nerve of arm (Meckel, 1817), see ***axillary nerve (Winslow, 1733)***
circumflex nerves of stylopharyngeal muscle (Andersch & Soemmerring, 1792), see ***stylopharyngeal branch of glossopharyngeal nerve (>1840)***
circumflex stylopharyngeal nerves (Andersch, 1797), see ***stylopharyngeal branch of glossopharyngeal nerve (>1840)***
circumgyrationes (Soemmerring, 1778), see ***cerebral cortex gray matter (>1840)***
circumjacent eminences (Riolan, 1649), see ***tectum (Baer, 1837)***
circumoral nerve ring (Tiedemann, 1815)
circumvolutions (Bartholin, 1662), see ***cerebellar cortex (Willis, 1664)***
cistern (Galen, c192), see ***hypothalamic part of third ventricle (Swanson, 2004)***
cistern between cerebellum and spinal cord (Aranzi, 1587), see ***fourth ventricle (Galen, c192)***
cistern of Aranzi (Tarin, 1753), see ***fourth ventricle (Galen, c192)***
cistern of fourth ventricle (Diemerbroeck, 1689), see ***roof of fourth ventricle (Vesalius, 1543a)***
cisterna spirituum (Aranzi, 1587), see ***fourth ventricle (Galen, c192)***
Clarke's column (Kölliker, 1896), see ***dorsal thoracic nucleus (>1840)***
claustral complex (Swanson, 2000a), see ***cortical subplate (>1840)***
claustrum (Burdach, 1822)
clava (Burdach, 1822), see ***gracile tubercle (>1840)***
clavicular branches of descending superficial branches of cervical plexus (Quain, 1828), see ***supraclavicular nerves (Meckel, 1817)***
clavicular branches of supraclavicular branches (Cruveilhier, 1836), see ***intermediate supraclavicular nerves (>1840)***
clavicular nerve (Quain, 1828), see ***supraclavicular nerves (Meckel, 1817)***
cliff (Malacarne, 1776), see ***anterior cerebellar notch (Chaussier, 1807)***
clitoral branch of internal pudendal nerve (Cruveilhier, 1836), see ***dorsal nerve of clitoris (>1840)***
clitoral nerve (Walter, 1783), see ***dorsal nerve of clitoris (>1840)***
clitoral pudendal nerve (Walter, 1783), see ***dorsal nerve of clitoris (>1840)***
cloison pulpeuse du troisieme ventricule (Bell, 1803b), see ***hypothalamus (Kuhlenbeck, 1927)***
Cloquet's ganglion (Quain & Wilson, 1839), see ***nasopalatine nerve (Scarpa, 1785)***
clouds (Vesalius, 1543a), see ***cerebral cortex gray matter (>1840)***
clunes (Vesalius, 1543a), see ***inferior colliculus (Haller, 1762)***
coalition of optic nerves (Willis, 1664), see ***optic chiasm (Galen, c173)***
coalitu nervorum opticorums (Bartholin, 1651), see ***optic chiasm (Galen, c173)***
coat of eye (Geminus, 1553), see ***retina (Herophilus, c335–c280 BC)***
coccygeal ganglion (Mayer, 1794), see ***coccygeal sympathetic ganglia (>1840)***
coccygeal ganglion (Walter, 1783), see ***ganglion impar (Quain & Wilson, 1839)***
coccygeal ganglion of intercostal nerve (Günther, 1786), see ***coccygeal sympathetic ganglia (>1840)***
coccygeal nerves (Camper, 1762)
coccygeal part of spinal cord (>1840)
coccygeal plexus (>1840)
coccygeal spinal ganglia (>1840)
coccygeal sympathetic ganglia (>1840)
cochlear communicating branch of vestibular nerve (>1840)
cochlear ganglion (>1840)
cochlear nerve (Arnold, 1834), see ***cochlear nerve (Cotugno, 1760)***
cochlear nerve (Cotugno, 1760)
cochlear nerve (Haase, 1781), see ***vestibulocochlear nerve (>1840)***
cochlear nerve central root (>1840)
cochlear nuclei (>1840)
cochlear root of auditory nerve (>1840), see ***cochlear nerve (Cotugno, 1760)***
cochlear root of vestibulocochlear nerve (>1840), see ***cochlear nerve (Cotugno, 1760)***
cochlear root proper of auditory nerve (>1840), see ***cochlear nerve (Cotugno, 1760)***
coeliac ganglia (Fyfe, 1800), see ***celiac plexus (Winslow, 1733)***

coils (Vesalius, 1543a), see **cerebral cortex gray matter (>1840)**
coition of optic nerves (Crooke, 1615), see **optic chiasm (Galen, c173)**
coitus nervorum opticorum (Schreger, 1803), see **optic chiasm (Galen, c173)**
colatorium (Günther, 1536), see **hypothalamus (Kuhlenbeck, 1927)**
collateral branch of intercostal nerves (Davies et al., 1931)
collateral branch of obturator nerve (Cruveilhier, 1836), see **posterior branch of obturator nerve (Haase, 1781; Martin, 1781)**
collateral branch of principal cardiac nerve (Lobstein, 1823), see **cardiac plexus (Keill, 1698)**
collateral branches of crural nerve (Cruveilhier, 1836), see **muscular branches of femoral nerve (Quain & Wilson, 1839)**
collateral branches of external plantar nerve (Cruveilhier, 1836), see **muscular branches of lateral plantar nerve (>1840)**
collateral branches of external popliteal sciatic nerve (Cruveilhier, 1836), see **common fibular nerve (>1840)**
collateral branches of facial nerve (Cruveilhier, 1836), see **intermediofacial nerve (Strong & Elwyn, 1943)**
collateral branches of inferior maxillary nerve (Cruveilhier, 1836), see **mandibular nerve (>1840)**
collateral branches of internal plantar nerve (Cruveilhier, 1836), see **medial plantar nerve (>1840)**
collateral branches of internal saphenous nerve (Cruveilhier, 1836), see **saphenous nerve (Haase, 1781)**
collateral branches of lumbar plexus (Cruveilhier, 1836), see **lumbar plexus ventral divisions (Paterson, 1887)**
collateral branches of musculocutaneous branch of external popliteal sciatic nerve (Cruveilhier, 1836), see **muscular branches of superficial fibular nerve (>1840)**
collateral branches of perineal branch of internal pudendal nerve (Cruveilhier, 1836), see **perineal nerve (Camper, 1762)**
collateral branches of recurrent nerve (Cruveilhier, 1836), see **recurrent laryngeal nerve (Albinus, 1744)**
collateral branches of sacral plexus (Cruveilhier, 1836), see **sacral plexus (Vesalius, 1543a)**
collateral branches of superior maxillary nerve (Cruveilhier, 1836), see **maxillary nerve (Meckel, 1753)**
collateral branches to thumb of median nerve (Quain & Wilson, 1839), see **proper palmar digital nerves of median nerve (>1840)**
collateral cerebral eminence (Mayer, 1779), see **collateral eminence (Meckel, 1767)**
collateral cerebral eminence of Meckel (Günther, 1786), see **collateral eminence (Meckel, 1767)**
collateral eminence (Meckel, 1767)
collateral eminence of Meckel (Meckel, 1817), see **collateral eminence (Meckel, 1767)**
collateral ganglia (Gaskell, 1886), see **prevertebral ganglia (Quain, 1832)**
collateral ganglia (Straus Durckheim, 1828), see **invertebrate peripheral ganglia (Swanson & Bota, 2010)**
collateral intercostal nerve (Günther, 1786), see **greater splanchnic nerve (Walter, 1783)**
collateral nerves of fingers (Cruveilhier, 1836), see **median nerve (Du Verney, 1697)**
collateral rope of great sympathetic nerve (Winslow, 1733), see **paravertebral nerves (Swanson & Bota, 2010)**
collateral sulcus (Chaussier, 1807), see **dorsolateral sulcus of spinal cord (>1840)**
collateral sulcus (Gall & Spurzheim, 1810), see **dorsal intermediate sulcus (>1840)**
collateral sulcus (>1840)
collateral triangle (>1840)
collateral trigone (>1840), see **collateral triangle (>1840)**
collateral trunk (Chaussier, 1789), see **greater splanchnic nerve (Walter, 1783)**
collateral trunk of great sympathetic nerve (Winslow, 1733), see **paravertebral nerves (Swanson & Bota, 2010)**
collicular ganglia (Burdach, 1822), see **central nervous system gray matter regions (>1840)**
colliculi nervorum ethmoidalium (Chaussier, 1807), see **caudate nucleus (Arnold, 1838b)**
colliculi of optic nerve (Soemmerring, 1791), see **interbrain (Baer, 1837)**
colliculus (Haller, 1754a), see **calcarine spur (Morand, 1748)**
colliculus caveae posterioris ventriculi lateralis (Vicq d'Azyr, 1786), see **calcarine spur (Morand, 1748)**
colliculus nervi ethmoïdalis (Chaussier, 1807), see **cerebral nuclei (Swanson, 2000a)**
colliculus on side of inferior vermiform eminence (Haller, 1762), see **cerebellar hemisphere (Willis, 1664)**
colliculus opticus (Wenzel & Wenzel, 1812), see **interbrain (Baer, 1837)**
colliculus striatus (Wenzel & Wenzel, 1812), see **caudate nucleus (Arnold, 1838b)**
column of cerebellar medullary velum (Vicq d'Azyr, 1786), see **superior cerebellar peduncle (Procháska, 1800)**
column of fornix (Craigie, 1925), see **postcommissural fornix (Loo, 1931)**
column of medulla oblongata (Vicq d'Azyr, 1784), see **inferior cerebellar peduncle (Günther, 1786)**
column of valve of Vieussens (Vicq d'Azyr, 1786), see **superior cerebellar peduncle (Procháska, 1800)**
column of white matter (Vicq d'Azyr, 1786), see **hypothalamic postcommissural fornix (>1840)**
columna anonyma (Haller, 1762), see **superficial medullary lamina of subiculum (Dejerine & Dejerine-Klumpke, 1895)**
columna externa anonyma (Haller, 1762), see **superficial medullary lamina of subiculum (Dejerine & Dejerine-Klumpke, 1895)**
columna medullaris (Tarin, 1750), see **medullary stria (Wenzel & Wenzel, 1812)**
columna medullaris centralis cerebri (Malacarne, 1780), see **cerebral peduncle (Tarin, 1753)**
columnae pituitariae (Tarin, 1750), see **pituitary gland (>1840)**
columnae veli medullaris cerebelli (Vicq d'Azyr, 1786), see **superior cerebellar peduncle (Procháska, 1800)**
columnas anteriores veri fornicis (Vieussens, 1684), see **postcommissural fornix (Loo, 1931)**
columnas posteriores veri fornicis (Vieussens, 1684), see **fimbria (Honegger, 1890)**

columns of spinal marrow (Heister, 1717), see **spinal cord (Galen, c162–c166)**
columns of spinal medulla (Chaussier, 1807), see **spinal cord (Galen, c162–c166)**
combinatio secunda (Molinetti, 1675), see **white matter tracts (Bell & Bell, 1826)**
combinatio tertia (Molinetti, 1675), see **oculomotor nerve (Estienne, 1545)**
combinationem primam (Molinetti, 1675), see **cerebral cortex (>1840)**
combinationibus nervorum (Molinetti, 1675), see **nervous system (Monro, 1783)**
commissura (Willis, 1664), see **anterior commissure (Lieutaud, 1742)**
commissura cerebelli (Malacarne, 1776), see **folium vermis (>1840)**
commissura cerebri (Meckel, 1817), see **pons (Haller, 1747)**
commissura cerebri maxima (Lieutaud, 1742), see **cerebral cortex white matter (>1840)**
commissura communi posterior (Bonhomme, 1748), see **interthalamic adhesion (>1840)**
commissura crassioris nervi aemula (Vieussens, 1684), see **anterior commissure (Lieutaud, 1742)**
commissura magna (Meckel, 1817), see **anterior commissure (Lieutaud, 1742)**
commissura magna cerebri (Bell, 1802), see **cerebral cortex white matter (>1840)**
commissura mediana (Gall & Spurzheim,1810), see **interthalamic adhesion (>1840)**
commissura mollis (Vicq d'Azyr, 1784), see **dorsal part of thalamus (Herrick, 1910)**
commissura processuum e testibus in cerebelli medítullia protensorum (Willis, 1664), see **rostral medullary velum (>1840)**
commissura taeniae (Haller, 1762), see **habenular commissure (>1840)**
commissural bundle of stria terminalis (Johnston, 1923), see **terminal stria commissure (>1840)**
commissure between gracile fascicles (Arnold, 1839), see **obex (Burdach, 1822)**
commissure of acoustic nerves (Gall & Spurzheim, 1810), see **trapezoid body (Treviranus, 1820)**
commissure of anterior cerebral ganglia (Combe et al., 1838), see **anterior commissure (Lieutaud, 1742)**
commissure of anterior lobe (Spurzheim, 1826), see **genu of corpus callosum (Reil, 1809b)**
commissure of anterior quadrigeminal bodies (Desmoulins, 1825), see **superior colliculus commissure (>1840)**
commissure of auditory nerves (Desmoulins, 1825), see **trapezoid body (Treviranus, 1820)**
commissure of cerebellar hemispheres (Arnold, 1838a), see **pons (Haller, 1747)**
commissure of cerebellum with cerebrum (Arnold, 1838a), see **superior cerebellar peduncle (Procháska, 1800)**
commissure of cord (Solly, 1836), see **ventral white commissure (>1840)**
commissure of corpus striatum (Combe et al., 1838), see **anterior commissure (Lieutaud, 1742)**
commissure of fimbria (Craigie, 1925), see **ventral hippocampal commissure (Craigie, 1925)**
commissure of fourth pair (Laurencet, 1825), see **trochlear nerve decussation (>1840)**
commissure of hemispheres (Carus, 1814), see **anterior commissure (Lieutaud, 1742)**
commissure of hemispheres (Owen, 1837), see **corpus callosum (Galen, c177)**
commissure of inferior quadrigeminal tubercles (Rolando, 1825a), see **inferior colliculus commissure (>1840)**
commissure of medullary process of cerebellum and testes (Tyson, 1699), see **superior cerebellar peduncle decussation (>1840)**
commissure of natiform eminences (Rolando, 1825), see **superior colliculus commissure (>1840)**
commissure of olfactory ganglion (Schönlein, 1816), see **anterior commissure (Lieutaud, 1742)**
commissure of olfactory nerve (Spurzheim, 1826), see **olfactory limb of anterior commissure (>1840)**
commissure of olfactory nerve ganglia (Carus, 1814), see **anterior commissure (Lieutaud, 1742)**
commissure of optic ganglions (Spurzheim, 1826), see **superior colliculus commissure (>1840)**
commissure of optic lobes (Serres, 1824–1826), see **superior colliculus commissure (>1840)**
commissure of optic nerve ganglia (Schönlein, 1816), see **posterior commissure (Winslow, 1733)**
commissure of optic nerves (Tarin, 1753), see **optic chiasm (Galen, c173)**
commissure of optic tracts (Reil, 1809b), see **optic chiasm (Galen, c173)**
commissure of posterior cerebral ganglia (Combe et al., 1838), see **interthalamic adhesion (>1840)**
commissure of quadrigeminal bodies (Bojanus, 1819–1821), see **tegmentum (Swanson, 2000b)**
commissure of quadrigeminal bodies (Spurzheim, 1826), see **superior colliculus commissure (>1840)**
commissure of superior posterior lobes (Malacarne, 1776), see **folium vermis (>1840)**
commissure of thalami optici (Gordon, 1815), see **interthalamic adhesion (>1840)**
commissure of two ventricles (Haly Abbas or Ali ibn' ul-Abbas, d. 994), see **interventricular foramen (>1840)**
commixtion of intercostall nerves with descending branch of sixt conjugation of brain (Crooke, 1615), see **communicating branches of spinal nerves (Wutzer, 1817)**
common anastomotic filament of superior facial branch of pes anserinus (Bellingeri, 1818), see **zygomatic branches of facial nerve (>1840)**
common branch to semitendinosus, semimembranosus, and abductor femoris magnus muscles (Bock, 1827), see **nerve to hamstring muscles (>1840)**
common canal (Winslow, 1733), see **cerebral aqueduct (>1840)**
common carotid plexus (Cloquet, 1816)
common cavity (Galen, c173), see **third ventricle (Galen, c173)**
common cavity of cerebellum and dorsal marrow (Vesalius, 1543a), see **fourth ventricle (Galen, c192)**
common coccygeal ganglion (Soemmerring, 1798), see **ganglion impar (Quain & Wilson, 1839)**
common digital branches of median nerve (Loder, 1803), see **common palmar digital nerves of median nerve (>1840)**

common fibular nerve (>1840)

common gluteal cutaneous nerve (Bock, 1827), see **lateral branch of spinal nerve dorsal branch (>1840)**

common lateral cerebellar fissure (Malacarne, 1776), see **horizontal fissure (Malacarne, 1776)**

common motor nerve (Meckel, 1817), see **oculomotor nerve (Estienne, 1545)**

common motor nerve inferior branch (Meckel, 1817), see **oculomotor nerve inferior branch (>1840)**

common motor nerve inferior terminal branch (Cruveilhier, 1836), see **oculomotor nerve inferior branch (>1840)**

common motor nerve of eye (Malacarne, 1791), see **oculomotor nerve (Estienne, 1545)**

common motor nerve superior branch (Meckel, 1817), see **oculomotor nerve superior branch (>1840)**

common motor nerve superior terminal branch (Cruveilhier, 1836), see **oculomotor nerve superior branch (>1840)**

common nerve for soleus, popliteus, and gastrocnemius muscles (Fischer, 1791), see **muscular branches of tibial nerve (>1840)**

common nerve to extensor digitorum longus and extensor pollicis longus muscles (Fischer, 1791), see **muscular branches of deep fibular nerve (>1840)**

common nerve to gastrocnemius and plantaris muscles (Fischer, 1791), see **muscular branches of tibial nerve (>1840)**

common nerve to left head of gastrocnemius muscle, soleus muscle, and tibial communicating nerve (Fischer, 1791), see **muscular branches of tibial nerve (>1840)**

common nerve to popliteus muscle and interosseous ligament (Fischer, 1791), see **muscular branches of tibial nerve (>1840)**

common nerve to soleus and flexor longus of big toe muscles (Fischer, 1791), see **muscular branches of tibial nerve (>1840)**

common nerve to tibialis anterior, extensor digitorum longus, and extensor pollicis longus muscles (Fischer, 1791), see **muscular branches of deep fibular nerve (>1840)**

common nerve to tibialis posterior, flexor digitorum longus, and flexor longus of big toe muscles and first internal inferior posterior cutaneous nerve (Fischer, 1791), see **muscular branches of tibial nerve (>1840)**

common nerves (Bell, 1829), see **spinal nerves (Camper, 1760–1762)**

common oculo-muscular pair of nerves (Burdin, 1803), see **oculomotor nerve (Estienne, 1545)**

common palmar digital nerves of median nerve (>1840)

common palmar digital nerves of ulnar nerve (>1840)

common peroneal nerve (>1840), see **common fibular nerve (>1840)**

common perpendicular cavity (Malacarne, 1776), see **posterior cerebellar notch (Chaussier, 1807)**

common plantar digital nerves of lateral plantar nerve (>1840)

common plantar digital nerves of medial plantar nerve (>1840)

common plexus (Chaussier, 1789), see **celiac plexus (Winslow, 1733)**

common pudendal nerve (Haase, 1781), see **pudendal nerve (Camper, 1762)**

common pudendal plexus (Frotscher, 1788), see **peripheral nervous system (Meckel, 1817)**

common sciatic nerve trunk (Jördens, 1788), see **sciatic nerve (Keill, 1698)**

common sensory (Willis, 1672), see **cerebral nuclei (Swanson, 2000a)**

common space (Constantine the African, c1017–1087), see **ventricles (Hippocrates)**

common station for optic nerves (Mondino, 1316), see **optic chiasm (Galen, c173)**

common trunk (Willis, 1664), see **vertebrate brain (Cuvier, 1800)**

common trunk for nerves to adductor femoris magnus, semimembranosus, biceps, and semitendinosus muscles (Fischer, 1791), see **nerve to hamstring muscles (>1840)**

common trunk for nerves to extensor pollicis longus and anterior peroneal muscles (Fischer, 1791), see **muscular branches of superficial fibular nerve (>1840)**

common trunk for nerves to gemellus superior, obturator internus, gemellus inferior, and quadratus femoris muscles (Fischer, 1791), see **nerve to obturator internus (>1840)**

common trunk for peroneal communicating and sural nerves (Fischer, 1791), see **sural communicating branch of common fibular nerve (>1840)**

common trunk formed by union of eighth cervical and first dorsal nerve (Meckel, 1817), see **brachial plexus lower trunk (>1840)**

common trunk formed by union of fifth and sixth cervical nerves (Meckel, 1817), see **brachial plexus upper trunk (>1840)**

common trunk of cerebellar peduncle (Chaussier, 1807), see **cerebellar peduncles (Ridley, 1695)**

common trunk of dorsal branch of cubital nerve for ulnar dorsal nerve of ring finger, radial dorsal nerve of auricular finger, and radial dorsal nerve of ring finger (Caldani, 1813, 1814), see **dorsal branch of ulnar nerve (Günther, 1786)**

common trunk of pterygoid and palatine nerves (Soemmerring, 1791), see **pterygopalatine nerves (Wrisberg, 1786)**

common trunk to major belly of biceps and superior internal cutaneous nerve (Jördens, 1788), see **nerve to hamstring muscles (>1840)**

common trunks of brachial plexus (Meckel, 1817), see **brachial plexus trunks (Schwalbe, 1881)**

common trunks of great plexus (Winslow, 1733), see **brachial plexus trunks (Schwalbe, 1881)**

common twig to extensor digitorum brevis muscle and superior interossei muscles (Fischer, 1791), see **muscular branches of deep fibular nerve (>1840)**

common uterine plexus (Tiedemann, 1822), see **superior hypogastric plexus (Tiedemann, 1822)**

common ventricle of marrow of back and cerebellum (Geminus, 1553), see **fourth ventricle (Galen, c192)**

common vesicle for medulla oblongata and cerebellum (Serres, 1824–1826), see **primary hindbrain vesicle (Baer, 1837)**

communicating arch between dorsal branches of radial and cubital nerves (Loder, 1803), see **brachial plexus cords (Schwalbe, 1881)**

communicating branch (Winslow, 1733)

communicating branch between fourth and fifth sacral nerves (Bock, 1827), see **coccygeal plexus (>1840)**

communicating branch between supreme cervical ganglion and second cervical nerve (Bischoff, 1832), see **communicating branch of spinal nerves (Wutzer, 1817)**

communicating branch between supreme cervical ganglion and second vagal ganglion (Bischoff, 1832), see **jugular nerves (>1840)**

communicating branch from anterior rami of first nerve of neck to inferior branches (Andersch & Soemmerring, 1792), see **communicating branches of cervical plexus (>1840)**

communicating branch from internal carotid plexus to abducens nerve (>1840)

communicating branch from internal carotid plexus to oculomotor nerve (>1840)

communicating branch from internal carotid plexus to ophthalmic nerve (>1840)

communicating branch from internal carotid plexus to trochlear nerve (>1840)

communicating branch from medial pterygoid nerve to otic ganglion (>1840), see **medial pterygoid nerve (>1840)**

communicating branch from phrenic nerve to pericardium (Krüger, 1758), see **pericardial branch of phrenic nerve (>1840)**

communicating branch from submaxillary branch of inferior submaxillary nerve to great sympathetic nerve (Andersch & Soemmerring, 1792), see **internal carotid plexus (>1840)**

communicating branch from submaxillary branches of inferior maxillary nerves to great harmonic nerve of body (Andersch, 1797), see **internal carotid plexus (>1840)**

communicating branch into forty-fourth (sympathetic) nerve of body (Andersch & Soemmerring, 1792), see **communicating branches of sympathetic trunk (>1840)**

communicating branch of anterior aortic plexus (Andersch, 1797), see **cardiac plexus (Keill, 1698)**

communicating branch of anterior rami of first nerve of neck and inferior rami (Andersch, 1797), see **communicating branches of cervical plexus (>1840)**

communicating branch of ascending part of tenth nerves of head and superior lingual nerves (Andersch & Soemmerring, 1792), see **craniospinal nerves (Herrick, 1915)**

communicating branch of digastric nerve with glossopharyngeal nerve (>1840)

communicating branch of dorsal branch of ulnar nerve with radial (Quain & Wilson, 1839), see **communicating branch of radial nerve with ulnar nerve (>1840)**

communicating branch of first lumbar nerve with second lumbar nerve (Bock, 1827), see **lumbar plexus (Vesalius, 1543a)**

communicating branch of glossopharyngeal nerve with auricular branch of vagus nerve (>1840)

communicating branch of glossopharyngeal nerve with meningeal branch of vagus nerve (>1840)

communicating branch of ilio-inguinal nerve with second lumbar nerve (Bock, 1827), see **ilio-inguinal nerve (Schmidt, 1794)**

communicating branch of inferior maxillary branch of hard nerve with medial cutaneous nerve of neck (Meckel, 1753), see **marginal mandibular branch of facial nerve (>1840)**

communicating branch of inferior maxillary branch of hard nerve with superior cutaneous nerves of neck (Meckel, 1753), see **marginal mandibular branch of facial nerve (>1840)**

communicating branch of intercostal nerve (Lobstein, 1823), see **communicating branches of sympathetic trunk (>1840)**

communicating branch of intermediofacial nerve with tympanic plexus (>1840)

communicating branch of intermediofacial nerve with vagus nerve (>1840)

communicating branch of internal laryngeal nerve and recurrent nerve (Andersch & Soemmerring, 1792), see **communicating branch of superior laryngeal nerve with inferior laryngeal nerve (Langenbeck, 1826–1830)**

communicating branch of lacrimal nerve with zygomatic nerve (>1840)

communicating branch of median nerve with ulnar nerve (Bock, 1827)

communicating branch of nasociliary nerve with ciliary ganglion (>1840)

communicating branch of ninth nerves of head and right cardiac nerves (Andersch & Soemmerring, 1792), see **superior cervical cardiac branches of vagus nerve (>1840)**

communicating branch of otic ganglion with chorda tympani (>1840)

communicating branch of otic ganglion with greater petrosal nerve (>1840), see **communicating branch of intermediofacial nerve with tympanic plexus (>1840)**

communicating branch of radial nerve with ulnar nerve (>1840)

communicating branch of recurrent nerves of neck and internal laryngeal nerves (Andersch, 1797), see **vagus nerve trunk (Wrisberg, 1786; Günther, 1786)**

communicating branch of second lumbar nerve with third lumbar nerve (Bock, 1827), see **lumbar plexus (Vesalius, 1543a)**

communicating branch of submaxillary branches of inferior maxillary nerves and lingual nerves of fifth pair of nerves of head (Andersch, 1797), see **mylohyoid nerve (Meckel, 1748)**

communicating branch of superior and middle cervical ganglia (Cruveilhier, 1836)

communicating branch of superior laryngeal nerve with inferior laryngeal nerve (Langenbeck, 1826–1830)

communicating branch of superior laryngeal nerve with recurrent laryngeal nerve (>1840), see **communicating branch of superior laryngeal nerve with inferior laryngeal nerve (Langenbeck, 1826–1830)**

communicating branch of tenth nerves of head and right nerves of heart (Andersch, 1797), see ***superior cervical cardiac branches of vagus nerve (>1840)***
communicating branch of tibial nerve (Bock, 1827), see ***tibial root of sural nerve (>1840)***
communicating branch of tympanic plexus with greater petrosal nerve (>1840)
communicating branch of ulnar nerve with median (Quain & Wilson, 1839), see ***communicating branch of median nerve with ulnar nerve (Bock, 1827)***
communicating branch of vagus nerve with glossopharyngeal nerve (>1840)
communicating branch of vagus nerve with ninth pair of cerebral nerves (Loder, 1778), see ***vagus nerve (Galen, c192)***
communicating branches between abducens nerve and great sympathetic nerve (Langenbeck, 1826–1830), see ***communicating branch from internal carotid plexus to abducens nerve (>1840)***
communicating branches between lumbar pairs and ganglia (Cruveilhier, 1836), see ***communicating branches of spinal nerves (Wutzer, 1817)***
communicating branches of anterior auricular nerve with facial nerve (Arnold, 1834), see ***communicating branches of auriculotemporal nerve with facial nerve (>1840)***
communicating branches of auriculotemporal nerve with facial nerve (>1840)
communicating branches of cervical plexus (>1840)
communicating branches of [eleventh nerves of head and] tenth nerves of head (Andersch, 1797), see ***hypoglossal nerve (Winslow, 1733)***
communicating branches of lingual nerve with hypoglossal nerve (>1840)
communicating branches of lingual nerve with submandibular ganglion (>1840)
communicating branches of lumbar ganglia (Cloquet, 1816), see ***communicating branches of sympathetic trunk (>1840)***
communicating branches of ninth nerves of head and right nerves of heart (Andersch & Soemmerring, 1792), see ***thoracic cardiac branches of vagus nerve (>1840)***
communicating branches of otic ganglion with auriculotemporal nerve (>1840)
communicating branches of recurrent and internal laryngeal nerves (Andersch & Soemmerring, 1792), see ***vagus nerve trunk (Wrisberg, 1786; Günther, 1786)***
communicating branches of spinal nerves (Wutzer, 1817)
communicating branches of spinal pairs with ganglia of great sympathetic (Cruveilhier, 1836), see ***communicating branches of spinal nerves (Wutzer, 1817)***
communicating branches of superficial aortic nerves with anterior aortic plexus (Andersch & Soemmerring, 1792), see ***cardiac plexus (Keill, 1698)***
communicating branches of superficial temporal nerve with facial nerve (Arnold, 1834), see ***communicating branches of auriculotemporal nerve with facial nerve (>1840)***
communicating branches of sympathetic nerve (Lobstein, 1823), see ***communicating branches of spinal nerves (Wutzer, 1817)***
communicating branches of sympathetic trunk (>1840)
communicating branches of [tenth nerves of head and] ninth nerves of head (Andersch & Soemmerring, 1792), see ***hypoglossal nerve (Winslow, 1733)***
communicating branches of tenth nerves of head and right nerves of heart (Andersch, 1797), see ***thoracic cardiac branches of vagus nerve (>1840)***
communicating branches of thoracic ganglia (Cloquet, 1816), see ***communicating branches of sympathetic trunk (>1840)***
communicating branches to sympathetic (Bell, 1803b), see ***communicating branches of spinal nerves (Wutzer, 1817)***
communicating branchlet of dorsal branch of cubital nerve with middle cutaneous nerve (Caldani, 1813, 1814), see ***dorsal branch of ulnar nerve (Günther, 1786)***
communicating branchlets of tenth nerves of head (Andersch, 1797), see ***communicating branch of vagus nerve with glossopharyngeal nerve (>1840)***
communicating cord (Leuret, 1839), see ***central longitudinal communicating branch (>1840)***
communicating filament between ophthalmic ganglion and superior cervical ganglion (Cruveilhier, 1836), see ***sympathetic root of ciliary ganglion (>1840)***
communicating filament between otic ganglion and nervus tympanicus (Quain & Wilson, 1839), see ***lesser petrosal nerve (>1840)***
communicating filament of cavernous plexus with ophthalmic ganglion (Cruveilhier, 1836), see ***sympathetic root of ciliary ganglion (>1840)***
communicating filaments of cavernous plexus with fifth pair (Cruveilhier, 1836), see ***communicating branch from internal carotid plexus to ophthalmic nerve (>1840)***
communicating filaments of cavernous plexus with third nerve (Cruveilhier, 1836), see ***communicating branch from internal carotid plexus to oculomotor nerve (>1840)***
communicating loops of cervical plexus (>1840)
communicating nerve (Quain, 1828), see ***lumbosacral trunk (Cruveilhier, 1836)***
communicating nerve betwixt internal laryngeal nerve and recurrent branch of par vagum (Bell & Bell, 1816), see ***communicating branch of superior laryngeal nerve with inferior laryngeal nerve (Langenbeck, 1826–1830)***
communicating nerve of great sympathetic nerve (Walter, 1783), see ***communicating branches of sympathetic trunk (>1840)***
communicating nerve of peroneal and posterior inferior cutaneous nerve (Knox, 1832), see ***sural communicating branch of common fibular nerve (>1840)***
communicating nerve of sympathetic (Knox, 1832), see ***communicating branches of sympathetic trunk (>1840)***
communicating nerves of anterior aortic plexus (Andersch, 1797), see ***cardiac plexus (Keill, 1698)***
communicating root between ganglia and trunk of great sympathetic nerve (Walter, 1783), see ***communicating branches of spinal nerves (Wutzer, 1817)***
communicating tibial branch from sciatic nerve (Swan, 1830), see ***sural communicating branch of common fibular nerve (>1840)***

communicating twigs between oculomotor nerve and abducens nerve (Langenbeck, 1826–1830), see **oculomotor nerve trunk (>1840)**
communicatio recentaculorum (Vieussens, 1684), see **circular sinus (Ridley, 1695)**
communication of facial nerve with digastric nerve (Scarpa, 1794), see **communicating branch of digastric branch of facial nerve with glossopharyngeal nerve (>1840)**
communication of glosso-pharyngeal nerve with facial nerve (Quain & Wilson, 1839), see **communicating branch of digastric branch of facial nerve with glossopharyngeal nerve (>1840)**
communication of sympathetic with second division of fifth pair of nerves (Todd, 1836–1839), see **communicating branch from internal carotid plexus to abducens nerve (>1840)**
communications between musculocutaneous nerve and middle cutaneous nerve (Caldani, 1813, 1814), see **lateral cutaneous nerve of forearm (>1840)**
communications between radial and ulnar volar nerves of thumb (Caldani, 1813, 1814), see **proper palmar digital nerves of median nerve (>1840)**
compact part of substantia nigra (>1840)
compassings (Geminus, 1553), see **cerebral cortex gray matter (>1840)**
compound nerve (Bell, 1826), see **nerve (Herophilus, c335–c280 BC)**
compound nerve (Grainger, 1837), see **spinal nerve trunk (Frotscher, 1788)**
compound spinal nerve (Grant, 1834c), see **spinal nerve trunk (Frotscher, 1788)**
conarium (Galen, c177), see **pineal gland (Galen, c192)**
concameration (Tyson, 1699), see **fornix (Vesalius, 1543a)**
concave margin of hippocampus major (Vicq d'Azyr, 1786), see **dentate gyrus (>1840)**
concave nerve (William of Saliceto, 1275), see **white matter tracts (Bell & Bell, 1826)**
concavitas conchularis (Benedetti, 1502), see **hypothalamic part of third ventricle (Swanson, 2004)**
concentric arcs (Günther, 1786), see **cerebellar cortex (Willis, 1664)**
concha (Berengario da Carpi, 1521), see **hypothalamus (Kuhlenbeck, 1927)**
concourse of optic nerves (Crooke, 1615), see **optic chiasm (Galen, c173)**
conduit of spinal medulla (Lyonnet, 1762), see **central longitudinal communicating branch (>1840)**
condyloid part of hypoglossal nerve (Arnold, 1834), see **hypoglossal nerve trunk (Günther, 1786)**
condyloid part of speaking nerve (Arnold, 1834), see **hypoglossal nerve trunk (Günther, 1786)**
condyloid part of twelfth pair (Arnold, 1834), see **hypoglossal nerve trunk (Günther, 1786)**
cone of cerebellum (Ramsay, 1813), see **cerebellum (Aristotle)**
cone of spinal medulla (Bock, 1824), see **medullary cone (>1840)**
cone of striate body (Willis, 1672), see **caudate nucleus (Arnold, 1838b)**
cone-like body (Galen, c177), see **pineal gland (Galen, c192)**
congress of optic nerves (Vesalius, 1543a), see **optic chiasm (Galen, c173)**
coniugatio (Galen, c192), see **cranial nerves (Soemmerring, 1791)**
conjoining of optic nerves (Galen, c192), see **optic chiasm (Galen, c173)**
conjugatio (Galen, c192), see **cranial nerves (Soemmerring, 1791)**
conjugations of nerves from brain (Galen, c192), see **cranial nerves (Soemmerring, 1791)**
conjunction of Jacobson's branch with superficial branch of Vidian nerve (Langenbeck, 1826–1830), see **tympanic nerve (Arnold, 1834)**
conjunction of lingual nerve with chorda tympani (Arnold, 1834), see **lingual nerve (Vesalius, 1543a)**
conjunction of nerves of vision (Vesalius, 1543a), see **optic chiasm (Galen, c173)**
conjunction of optic nerves (Vesalius, 1543a), see **optic chiasm (Galen, c173)**
conjunction of round trunks (Bartholin, 1662), see **interbrain (Baer, 1837)**
conjunctival filaments of lacrimal fascicle proper (Bellingeri, 1818), see **lacrimal nerve (Meckel, 1748; Bonhomme, 1748)**
connecting layer for gray fascicles (Desmoulins, 1825), see **spinal central gray (>1840)**
connecting plate of upper corpora bigemina (Gordon, 1815), see **superior colliculus (Haller, 1762)**
connection of anterior branch of second cervical nerve with supreme cervical ganglion (Arnold, 1834), see **gray communicating branch (>1840)**
connection of auricular branch of pneumogastric nerve with facial nerve (Arnold, 1834), see **communicating branch of intermediofacial nerve trunk with vagus nerve (>1840)**
connection of auricular branch of vagus nerve with facial nerve (Arnold, 1834), see **communicating branch of intermediofacial nerve trunk with vagus nerve (>1840)**
connection of carotid nerve with abducens nerve (Arnold, 1834), see **communicating branch from internal carotid plexus to abducens nerve (>1840)**
connection of carotid nerve with nasal ganglion (Arnold, 1834), see **deep petrosal nerve (Meckel, 1817)**
connection of carotid nerve with tympanic nerve (Arnold, 1834), see **caroticotympanic nerves (>1840)**
connection of cavernous sinus with ophthalmic ganglion (Arnold, 1834), see **sympathetic root of ciliary ganglion (>1840)**
connection of external branch of accessory nerve of Willis with third and second cervical nerves (Arnold, 1834), see **external branch of accessory nerve trunk (Meckel, 1817)**
connection of external branch of superior laryngeal nerve with filaments of superior cervical ganglion (Arnold, 1834), see **jugular nerves (>1840)**
connection of facial nerve with tympanic nerve (Arnold, 1834), see **communicating branch of intermediofacial nerve with tympanic plexus (>1840)**

copula alba cerebri (Varoli, 1573), see **corpus callosum (Galen, c177)**
coracobrachialis muscle branch of musculocutaneous nerve (Scarpa, 1794), see **muscular branches of musculocutaneous nerve (Günther, 1786)**
cord (Gerdy, 1838), see **anterior commissure (Lieutaud, 1742)**
cord (Malpighi, 1669), see **ventral cord (Anderson, 1837)**
cord of communication between ganglia (Quain & Wilson, 1839), see **communicating branches of sympathetic trunk (>1840)**
cord of tympanum (Meckel, 1832), see **chorda tympani (Falloppio, 1561)**
cordis plexum (Haase, 1781), see **cardiac plexus (Keill, 1698)**
cordon pterigoïdien (Le Cat, 1768), see **nerve of pterygoid canal (>1840)**
cords (Rufus of Ephesus (fl. c90–120), see **nerves (Herophilus, c335–c280 BC)**
cords of connexion of sympathetic nerve (Quain, 1828), see **communicating branches of sympathetic trunk (>1840)**
cords of esophageal collar (Cuvier, 1800), see **circumesophageal connectives (>1840)**
cords of spinal marrow (Monro, 1783), see **spinal cord (Galen, c162–c166)**
cornice of vault (Bonhomme, 1748), see **fimbria (Honegger, 1890)**
cornix (Valverde de Amusco, 1589), see **fornix (Vesalius, 1543a)**
cornu ammonis (Burdach, 1822), see **cerebral cortex (>1840)**
cornu ammonis (Malacarne, 1780), see **inferior horn of lateral ventricle (Bell, 1802)**
cornu arietis (Günz, 1750), see **hippocampal region (Swanson et al., 1987)**
cornua fornicis (Lancisi, 1714), see **fimbria (Honegger, 1890)**
corona radiata (Reil, 1809b), see **central nervous system white matter tracts (>1840)**
coronary nerve of posterior ventricle (Andersch, 1797), see **coronary plexuses (Meckel, 1817)**
coronary plexus (Winslow, 1733), see **prevertebral plexuses (Quain, 1832)**
coronary plexus of stomach (Cruveilhier, 1836), see **left gastric plexus (>1840)**
coronary plexuses (Meckel, 1817)
corpora albicantia (Santorini, 1775), see **mammillary body (Ludwig, 1779)**
corpora bigemina (Soemmerring, 1798), see **tectum (Baer, 1837)**
corpora duo subrotunda (Vieussens, 1684), see **superior colliculus (Haller, 1762)**
corpora glandularia (Soemmerring, 1778), see **mammillary body (Ludwig, 1779)**
corpora in turbinem acuminata (Vieussens, 1684), see **inferior colliculus (Haller, 1762)**
corpora mammillaria (Ludwig, 1779), see **mammillary body (Ludwig, 1779)**
corpora olivaria (Vieussens, 1684), see **olive (Tiedemann, 1821)**
corpora olivaria (Winslow, 1733), see **pyramid (Willis, 1664)**
corpora olivaria Fallopii (Tarin, 1753), see **peripheral ganglia (>1840)**
corpora ovalia (Soemmerring, 1791), see **olive (Tiedemann, 1821)**
corpora ovata (Soemmerring, 1791), see **olive (Tiedemann, 1821)**
corpora pyramidalia (Winslow, 1733), see **olive (Tiedemann, 1821)**
corpora pyramidalia interiora (Procháska, 1800), see **pyramid (Willis, 1664)**
corpora pyramidalia lateralia (Burdach, 1822), see **olive (Tiedemann, 1821)**
corpora pyramidalia lateralia vel anteriora Tarini (Vicq d'Azyr, 1786), see **trigeminal tubercle (>1840)**
corpora pyramidalia posteriora (Tarin, 1750), see **olive (Tiedemann, 1821)**
corpora pyramidalia superiora (Mayer, 1779), see **pyramid (Willis, 1664)**
corpora quadrigemina (Wenzel & Wenzel, 1812), see **tectum (Baer, 1837)**
corpora quadrigemina anteriora (Soemmerring, 1778), see **superior colliculus (Haller, 1762)**
corpora quadrigemina posteriora (Soemmerring, 1778), see **inferior colliculus (Haller, 1762)**
corpora striata antica inferiora (Meckel, 1817), see **caudate nucleus (Arnold, 1838b)**
corpora striata inferiora exteriora posteriora (Vieussens, 1684), see **cerebral nuclei (Swanson, 2000a)**
corpora striata interiora anteriora (Schreger, 1803), see **cerebral nuclei (Swanson, 2000a)**
corpora teretia (Arnold, 1838a), see **floor of fourth ventricle (Reil, 1807–1808a)**
corpora teretia (Willis, 1664), see **olive (Tiedemann, 1821)**
corpora vorticosa (Malpighi, 1665), see **cerebral cortex gray matter (>1840)**
corporis striati limbus anterior (Willis, 1672), see **external capsule (Burdach, 1822)**
corporis striati limbus posterior (Willis, 1672), see **internal capsule (Burdach, 1822)**
corporum striatorum propaginis (Rau, 1720), see **cerebral cortex (>1840)**
corps canelés (Lieutaud, 1742), see **cerebral nuclei (Swanson, 2000a)**
corps canelez (Bourdon, 1683), see **cerebral nuclei (Swanson, 2000a)**
corps cannellez (Pourfour du Petit, 1710), see **cerebral nuclei (Swanson, 2000a)**
corpus bigeminum (Wenzel & Wenzel, 1812), see **tectum (Baer, 1837)**
corpus callosum (Galen, c177)
corpus callosum (Malpighi, 1665), see **central nervous system white matter tracts (>1840)**
corpus callosum (Read, 1638), see **vertebrate brain (Cuvier, 1800)**
corpus callosum (Willis, 1664), see **cerebral cortex white matter (>1840)**
corpus callosum medium (Haller, 1747), see **corpus callosum (Galen, c177)**

corpus callosum of cerebellum (Cruveilhier, 1836), see **middle cerebellar peduncle (Rolando, 1819)**
corpus callosum of cerebellum (Ridley, 1695), see **arbor vitae (Winslow, 1733)**
corpus callosum system (Reil, 1809b), see **cerebral cortex white matter (>1840)**
corpus cameratum (Colombo, 1559), see **fornix (Vesalius, 1543a)**
corpus candicum (Bauhin, 1605), see **central nervous system white matter tracts (>1840)**
corpus cerebelli (Meckel, 1817), see **cerebellum (Aristotle)**
corpus cinereum (Albinus, 1744), see **hypothalamus (Kuhlenbeck, 1927)**
corpus cinereum (Volkmann, 1831), see **hypothalamus (Kuhlenbeck, 1927)**
corpus cineritium (Piccolomini, 1586), see **cerebral cortex gray matter (>1840)**
corpus communionis cerebri (Gall & Spurzheim, 1810), see **fornix (Vesalius, 1543a)**
corpus corporis callosi (Arnold, 1838a), see **body of corpus callosum (Arnold, 1838a)**
corpus dentatum olivae (Burdach, 1822), see **inferior olivary complex (>1840)**
corpus eminens oblongum album (Santorini, 1775), see **anterior thalamic nuclei (>1840)**
corpus fimbriatum (Bonhomme, 1748), see **hippocampal region (Swanson et al., 1987)**
corpus fimbriatum (Longet, 1842), see **fimbria (Honegger, 1890)**
corpus fimbriatum (Meckel, 1817), see **dentate nucleus (>1840)**
corpus fimbriatum (Winslow, 1733), see **fimbria (Honegger, 1890)**
corpus fimbriatum Sylvii (Bergen, 1734), see **fimbria (Honegger, 1890)**
corpus fornicatum (Hall, 1565), see **fornix (Vesalius, 1543a)**
corpus geniculatum (Santorini, 1724), see **medial geniculate complex (>1840)**
corpus geniculatum externum (Ramsay, 1813), see **anterior thalamic nuclei (>1840)**
corpus geniculatum internum (Ramsay, 1813), see **pulvinar (Burdach, 1822)**
corpus globosum (Ruysch, 1728), see **pons (Haller, 1747)**
corpus in toto tractu bifidum (Willis, 1664), see **spinal cord (Galen, c162–c166)**
corpus medullare crassiorem nervum referens (Vieussens, 1684), see **anterior commissure (Lieutaud, 1742)**
corpus nigrum (Bell & Bell, 1829), see **substantia nigra (Soemmerring, 1791)**
corpus olivae fimbriatum (Meckel, 1817), see **inferior olivary complex (>1840)**
corpus psalloeides (Dubois, 1556), see **fornix (Vesalius, 1543a)**
corpus psalloides (Riolan, 1649), see **fornix (Vesalius, 1543a)**
corpus psalloïdes (Vicq d'Azyr, 1786), see **dorsal hippocampal commissure (Craigie, 1925)**
corpus psalloideum (Mayer, 1779), see **dorsal hippocampal commissure (Craigie, 1925)**
corpus pyramidale anticum laterale (Gordon, 1815), see **olive (Tiedemann, 1821)**
corpus quadrilaterum (Knox, 1832), see **optic chiasm (Galen, c173)**
corpus speculare (Piccolomini, 1586), see **cerebral nuclei (Swanson, 2000a)**
corpus striatum (Willis, 1664), see **cerebral nuclei (Swanson, 2000a)**
corpus striatum superior and internal part (Vicq d'Azyr, 1786), see **caudate nucleus (Arnold, 1838b)**
corpus transversale (Tyson, 1699), see **splenium of corpus callosum (Burdach, 1822)**
corpus trapezoideum (Treviranus, 1820), see **trapezoid body (Treviranus, 1820)**
corpus trifidum (Riolan, 1649), see **fornix (Vesalius, 1543a)**
corpus truncus medullaris (Günther, 1786), see **dentate nucleus (>1840)**
corpus turbinatum (Galen, c177), see **pineal gland (Galen, c192)**
corpus vermiforme (Bell & Bell, 1816), see **cerebellar vermis (Meckel, 1817)**
corpuscula quatuor eminentia (Bauhin, 1605), see **tectum (Baer, 1837)**
corrugations (Smith Papyrus, c1700 BC), see **cerebral cortex gray matter (>1840)**
cortex (Malpighi, 1665), see **central nervous system gray matter regions (>1840)**
cortical amygdalar area (>1840)
cortical amygdalar complex (>1840)
cortical amygdalar nucleus (Johnston, 1923), see **cortical amygdalar area (Swanson, 2004)**
cortical commissure of spinal marrow (Meckel, 1817), see **spinal central gray (>1840)**
cortical layer of cerebral convolution (Baillarger, 1840), see **cerebral cortex gray matter (>1840)**
cortical mantle (>1840), see **cerebral cortex gray matter (>1840)**
cortical plate (>1840)
cortical subplate (>1840)
cortical substance (Carus, 1814), see **cerebral cortex gray matter (>1840)**
cortical substance (Willis, 1664), see **central nervous system gray matter regions (>1840)**
cortical tubercle (Weitbrecht, 1751), see **olfactory bulb (Weitbrecht, 1751)**
corticopontine fibers (>1840), see **corticospinal tract (>1840)**
corticospinal tract (>1840)
costal branch (Frotscher, 1788), see **intercostal nerves (Vesalius, 1543a)**
costal branch of sixth pair of nerves (Vesling, 1647), see **sympathetic trunk (Winslow, 1733)**
costal nerve (Paré, 1561), see **sympathetic trunk (Winslow, 1733)**
costal nerves (Camper, 1760), see **intercostal nerves (Vesalius, 1543a)**
costal nerves (Winslow, 1733), see **thoracic nerves (Diemerbroeck, 1672)**
costall branch of sixth conjugation (Paré, 1634), see **sympathetic trunk (Winslow, 1733)**
costohyoid nerve (Scarpa, 1794), see **ansa cervicalis (>1840)**
costothoracic branch of subscapular nerves (Chaussier, 1809), see **thoracodorsal nerve (>1840)**

couche optique (Saint Hilaire, 1680), see ***interbrain (Baer, 1837)***
couchette des nerf optique (Riolan, 1628–1629), see ***interbrain (Baer, 1837)***
covered bands (Reil, 1809b), see ***cingulum (Burdach, 1822)***
covered gyri (Arnold, 1838a), see ***limbic region (>1840)***
covered part of fornix column (His, 1895), see ***hypothalamic postcommissural fornix (>1840)***
covering organs (Burdach, 1822), see ***cerebral cortex (>1840)***
cranial branch of pterygoid branch of superior maxillary branch of trigeminal nerve (Bichat et al., 1801–1803), see ***greater petrosal nerve (>1840)***
cranial branch of Vidian nerve (Cloquet, 1828), see ***greater petrosal nerve (>1840)***
cranial bulb (Cruveilhier, 1836), see ***medulla (Winslow, 1733)***
cranial marrow (Plato), see ***vertebrate brain (Cuvier, 1800)***
cranial nerve ganglia (>1840)
cranial nerves (Cruveilhier, 1836), see ***nervous system (Monro, 1783)***
cranial nerves (Haller & Wrisberg, 1780), see ***nervous system (Monro, 1783)***
cranial nerves (Soemmerring, 1791)
cranial portion of spinal cord (Gordon, 1815), see ***medulla (Winslow, 1733)***
cranial root of accessory nerve (>1840)
cranial root of accessory nerve rootlets (>1840)
cranial root of accessory nerve trunks (>1840)
craniospinal ganglia (>1840)
craniospinal nerves (Herrick, 1915)
crassa (Galen, c173), see ***dura (Galen, c177)***
crassa meninx (Hall, 1565), see ***dura (Galen, c177)***
cremasteric branch of singular nerve from second and third lumbar nerves (Monro & Coopmans, 1754), see ***genital branch of genitofemoral nerve (>1840)***
crenate part of hippocampus major (Vicq d'Azyr, 1786), see ***dentate gyrus (>1840)***
crested process (Rolando, 1831), see ***limbic region (>1840)***
cribriform plate (Reil, 1809b), see ***cerebral nuclei (Swanson, 2000a)***
cribriform plate of brain (Mayo, 1827), see ***cerebral nuclei (Swanson, 2000a)***
cristate vesicle of brain (Malpighi, 1675), see ***primary midbrain vesicle (Baer, 1837)***
crooked nerve (Willis, 1664), see ***ansa cervicalis (>1840)***
crossed corticospinal tract (>1840)
crossed reticulospinal tract (>1840), see ***medial reticulospinal tract (>1840)***
crotaphitic surculus of ganglioform plexus of inferior maxillary branch (Bellingeri, 1818), see ***deep temporal nerves (Haase, 1781)***
crucial depression (Meckel, 1817), see ***cruciform sulcus (>1840)***
cruciate sulcus (Leuret, 1839), see ***central sulcus (Huschke, 1854)***
cruciform sulcus (Rolando, 1831), see ***lateral cerebral sulcus (>1840)***
cruciform sulcus (>1840)
crura ad testes (Schreger, 1803), see ***superior cerebellar peduncle (Procháska, 1800)***
crura cerebelli ad cerebrum (Burdach, 1822), see ***superior cerebellar peduncle (Procháska, 1800)***
crura cerebelli ad eminentiam quadrigeminam (Meckel, 1817), see ***superior cerebellar peduncle (Procháska, 1800)***
crura cerebelli ad pontem (Soemmerring, 1778), see ***middle cerebellar peduncle (Rolando, 1819)***
crura cerebelli adscendentia (Haller, 1762), see ***superior cerebellar peduncle (Procháska, 1800)***
crura cerebelli superiora (Mayer, 1779), see ***superior cerebellar peduncle (Procháska, 1800)***
crura cerebri posteriora (Tarin, 1750), see ***middle cerebellar peduncle (Rolando, 1819)***
crura magna cerebelli (Haller, 1762), see ***pons (Haller, 1747)***
crura medullae oblongatae (Vieussens, 1684), see ***interbrain (Baer, 1837)***
crura medullae oblongatae ad corpora quadrigemina (Langenbeck, 1826–1830), see ***medial eminence (>1840)***
crura medullae spinalis superiora (Wharton, 1656), see ***vertebrate brain (Cuvier, 1800)***
crura medullaria glandulae pinealis (Mayer, 1779), see ***medullary stria (Wenzel & Wenzel, 1812)***
crura medullarica (Mayer, 1794), see ***cerebral peduncle (Tarin, 1753)***
crura minora medullae oblongatae (Haller, 1762), see ***cerebellar peduncles (Ridley, 1695)***
crura of brain (Haller, 1754b), see ***brainstem (Schwalbe, 1881)***
crura of brain (Swan, 1830), see ***cerebral peduncle (Tarin, 1753)***
crura of cerebellum (Swan, 1830), see ***middle cerebellar peduncle (Rolando, 1819)***
crura of corpora candicantia (Knox, 1832), see ***hypothalamic postcommissural fornix (>1840)***
crura of medulla oblongata (Cruveilhier, 1836), see ***middle cerebellar peduncle (Rolando, 1819)***
crura posteriora medullae oblongatae (Winslow, 1733), see ***inferior cerebellar peduncle (Günther, 1786)***
crural branch of external pudic nerve (Quain & Wilson, 1839), see ***genital branch of genitofemoral nerve (>1840)***
crural branch of external spermatic nerve (Quain & Wilson, 1839), see ***genital branch of genitofemoral nerve (>1840)***
crural branch of genito-crural nerve (Quain & Wilson, 1839), see ***genital branch of genitofemoral nerve (>1840)***
crural branch of inferior gluteal nerve (Cloquet, 1816), see ***posterior cutaneous nerve of thigh (Günther, 1786)***
crural musculocutaneous nerve (Cruveilhier, 1836), see ***femoral nerve (Haller, 1762)***
crural nerve (Crooke, 1615), see ***lumbosacral plexus (Vesalius, 1543a)***
crural nerve (Heister, 1717), see ***femoral nerve (Haller, 1762)***
crural nerve of forelegs (Straus Durckheim, 1828), see ***invertebrate nerves (>1840)***
crural nerve proper (Salmon, 1713), see ***sciatic nerve (Keill, 1698)***
crural nerve roots (Walter, 1783), see ***femoral nerve (Haller, 1762)***

crural nerve trunk (Styx, 1782), see ***femoral nerve (Haller, 1762)***
crural plexus (Chaussier, 1809), see ***lumbosacral plexus (Vesalius, 1543a)***
crural plexus (Cruveilhier, 1836), see ***sacral plexus (Vesalius, 1543a)***
crural plexus (Reil, 1796), see ***lumbar plexus (Vesalius, 1543a)***
crural trunk (Verheyen, 1693), see ***sciatic nerve (Keill, 1698)***
cruralis magnus nervus (Pietro da Cortona, 1741), see ***sciatic nerve (Keill, 1698)***
crurum cerebelli ad medullam oblongatam (Haase, 1781), see ***inferior cerebellar peduncle (Günther, 1786)***
crurum cerebri pars ante nervos opticos locata (Soemmerring, 1778), see ***cerebral peduncle (Tarin, 1753)***
crurum medullae oblongatae cerebelli (Neubauer, 1772), see ***inferior cerebellar peduncle (Günther, 1786)***
crus ad corpora quadrigemina (Soemmerring, 1791), see ***superior cerebellar peduncle (Prochάska, 1800)***
crus ad medullam spinalem (Soemmerring, 1791), see ***inferior cerebellar peduncle (Günther, 1786)***
crus anteriora medulla oblongata (Winslow, 1733), see ***brainstem (Schwalbe, 1881)***
crus cerebelli (Bell, 1803b), see ***middle cerebellar peduncle (Rolando, 1819)***
crus cerebelli (Monro, 1783), see ***arbor vitae (Winslow, 1733)***
crus cerebelli (Vicq d'Azyr, 1786), see ***middle cerebellar peduncle (Rolando, 1819)***
crus cerebelli ad corpora quadrigemina (Arnold, 1834), see ***superior cerebellar peduncle (Procháska, 1800)***
crus cerebri (Bell, 1803b), see ***tegmentum (Swanson, 2000b)***
crus cerebri (Haller, 1747), see ***brainstem (Schwalbe, 1881)***
crus cerebri (Quain, 1832), see ***tegmentum (Swanson, 2000b)***
crus cerebri (Vicq d'Azyr, 1784), see ***tegmentum (Swanson, 2000b)***
crus cerebri anteriora (Tarin, 1750), see ***cerebral peduncle (Tarin, 1753)***
crus cerebri magna (Meckel, 1817), see ***tegmentum (Swanson, 2000b)***
crus cerebri posteriora (Tarin, 1750), see ***cerebellar peduncles (Ridley, 1695)***
crus cerebri posteriora Tarini (Soemmerring, 1778), see ***pyramid (Willis, 1664)***
crus cerebri super pontem emergentia (Soemmerring, 1778), see ***pyramid (Willis, 1664)***
crus descendens cerebri (Chaussier, 1807), see ***cerebral peduncle (Tarin, 1753)***
crus fornicis (Wreeden, 1741), see ***hippocampal region (Swanson et al., 1987)***
crus medulla oblongata (Collins, 1685), see ***cerebral peduncle (Tarin, 1753)***
crus medullae posticum ad cerebellum ascendens (Tiedemann, 1821), see ***inferior cerebellar peduncle (Günther, 1786)***
crus oblongata cerebri (Camper & Albinus, 1767), see ***cerebral peduncle (Tarin, 1753)***
crus of cerebellum (Meckel, 1817), see ***inferior cerebellar peduncle (Günther, 1786)***
crus of fornix (Burdach, 1822), see ***fimbria (Honegger, 1890)***
crus of fornix (Riolan, 1618), see ***fimbria (Honegger, 1890)***
crus of fornix (>1840a), see ***fimbria (Honegger, 1890)***
crus of fornix (>1840b), see ***fimbria (Honegger, 1890)***
crus of medulla oblongata (Willis, 1664), see ***vertebrate brain (Cuvier, 1800)***
crus of true olfactory nerve ganglia (Carus, 1814), see ***cerebral peduncle (Tarin, 1753)***
crust of crus cerebri (Reil, 1809b), see ***cerebral peduncle (Tarin, 1753)***
cubital branch of internal cutaneous nerve of arm (Cruveilhier, 1836), see ***medial cutaneous nerve of arm (>1840)***
cubital nerve (Du Verney, 1697), see ***ulnar nerve (Cheselden, 1726)***
cubital nerve branch of deep flexor muscle (Cruveilhier, 1836), see ***muscular branches of ulnar nerve (>1840)***
cubital nerve branch of palmar collateral nerves of fingers (Cruveilhier, 1836), see ***superficial branch of ulnar nerve (Fyfe, 1800)***
cubital nerve branches of anterior cubital muscle (Cruveilhier, 1836), see ***muscular branches of ulnar nerve (>1840)***
cubital nerve internal dorsal branch of hand (Cruveilhier, 1836), see ***dorsal branch of ulnar nerve (Günther, 1786)***
cubito-cutaneous nerve (Burdin, 1803), see ***brachial plexus medial cord (Schwalbe, 1881)***
cubito-digital nerve (Burdin, 1803), see ***ulnar nerve (Cheselden, 1726)***
cubito-dorsal nerve of fifth finger (Meckel, 1817), see ***dorsal digital nerves of ulnar nerve (>1840)***
cubito-dorsal nerve of fourth finger (Meckel, 1817), see ***dorsal digital nerves of ulnar nerve (>1840)***
cubito-dorsal nerve of index finger (Meckel, 1817), see ***dorsal digital nerves of radial nerve (>1840)***
cubito-dorsal nerve of middle finger (Meckel, 1817), see ***dorsal digital nerves of radial nerve (>1840)***
cubito-palmar nerve of fifth finger (Meckel, 1817), see ***proper palmar digital nerves of ulnar nerve (>1840)***
cubito-palmar nerve of fourth finger (Meckel, 1817), see ***proper palmar digital nerves of ulnar nerve (>1840)***
cubito-palmar nerve of index finger (Meckel, 1817), see ***proper palmar digital nerves of median nerve (>1840)***
cubito-palmar nerve of third finger (Meckel, 1817), see ***proper palmar digital nerves of median nerve (>1840)***
cubito-palmar nerve of thumb (Meckel, 1817), see ***proper palmar digital nerves of median nerve (>1840)***
culmen (Burdach, 1822), see ***cerebellar vermis (Meckel, 1817)***
culmen (Stroud, 1895)
cuneate fascicle (Müller, 1834)
cuneate nucleus (>1840)
cuneate tubercle (>1840)
cuneiform lobe (Meckel, 1817), see ***biventral lobule (>1840)***
cuneus (Burdach, 1822)
cupola (Galen, c192), see ***fornix (Vesalius, 1543a)***
curvatura perpendicularis communis (Malacarne, 1776), see ***cerebellar vermis (Meckel, 1817)***

custodian of brain (Benedetti, 1502), see **dura (Galen, c177)**

cutaneous branch of circumflex nerve (Swan, 1830), see **superior lateral cutaneous nerve of arm (>1840)**

cutaneous branch of cubital nerve (Mayer, 1794), see **ulnar nerve (Cheselden, 1726)**

cutaneous branch of deep branch of internal pudendal nerve (Cruveilhier, 1836), see **dorsal nerve of penis (Camper, 1762)**

cutaneous branch of dorsal branch of penis of internal pudendal nerve (Cruveilhier, 1836), see **dorsal nerve of penis (Camper, 1762)**

cutaneous branch of external cutaneous nerve (Soemmerring, 1791), see **lateral cutaneous nerve of forearm (>1840)**

cutaneous branch of external inguinal branch of lumbar plexus (Cruveilhier, 1836), see **ilio-inguinal nerve (Schmidt, 1794)**

cutaneous branch of external plantar nerve (Günther, 1786), see **superficial branch of lateral plantar nerve (>1840)**

cutaneous branch of external spermatic nerve (Bock, 1827), see **femoral branch of genitofemoral nerve (>1840)**

cutaneous branch of inferior gluteal nerve (Cruveilhier, 1836), see **posterior cutaneous nerve of thigh (Günther, 1786)**

cutaneous branch of intercostal branches of dorsal nerves (Cruveilhier, 1836), see **lateral cutaneous branch of intercostal nerves (>1840)**

cutaneous branch of musculocutaneous nerve (Camper, 1760), see **lateral cutaneous nerve of forearm (>1840)**

cutaneous branch of obturator nerve (>1840)

cutaneous branch of palmar branch of ulnar nerve (Meckel, 1817), see **superficial branch of ulnar nerve (Fyfe, 1800)**

cutaneous branch of radial nerve (Meckel, 1817), see **superficial branch of radial nerve (Martin, 1781)**

cutaneous branch of shoulder of axillary nerve (Cruveilhier, 1836), see **superior lateral cutaneous nerve of arm (>1840)**

cutaneous branch of subcostal branch of twelfth thoracic nerve (Bock, 1827), see **subcostal nerve (>1840)**

cutaneous branch of ulnar nerve (Quain & Wilson, 1839), see **ulnar nerve (Cheselden, 1726)**

cutaneous branches of axillary nerve (Bock, 1827), see **superior lateral cutaneous nerve of arm (>1840)**

cutaneous branches of cervical plexus (Cruveilhier, 1836), see **cervical plexus (Molinetti, 1675)**

cutaneous branches of crural nerve (Günther, 1786), see **femoral nerve (Haller, 1762)**

cutaneous branches of dorsal branches of intercostal nerves (Quain & Wilson, 1839), see **spinal nerve dorsal branch (Meckel, 1817)**

cutaneous branches of dorsal nerves (Cruveilhier, 1836), see **lateral cutaneous branch of intercostal nerves (>1840)**

cutaneous branches of dorsal plexus of penis (Bock, 1827), see **dorsal nerve of penis (Camper, 1762)**

cutaneous branches of lateral pectoral nerve (Bock, 1827), see **anterior branch of lateral cutaneous branch of intercostal nerves (>1840)**

cutaneous branches of muscular spiral nerve (Bell, 1803a), see **posterior cutaneous nerve of forearm (>1840)**

cutaneous branches of volar superficial nerve of ulnar nerve (Bock, 1827), see **superficial branch of ulnar nerve (Fyfe, 1800)**

cutaneous calcanean nerve (Cruveilhier, 1836), see **medial plantar nerve (>1840)**

cutaneous dorsal branch of cubital nerve (Cruveilhier, 1836), see **dorsal branch of ulnar nerve (Günther, 1786)**

cutaneus externus et radialis (Klint, 1784), see **musculocutaneous nerve (Du Verney, 1697)**

cutaneous femoral branch of internal inguinal branch of lumbar plexus (Cruveilhier, 1836), see **femoral branch of genitofemoral nerve (>1840)**

cutaneous filaments of abdominal branch of intercostal branches of dorsal nerves (Cruveilhier, 1836), see **intercostal nerves (Vesalius, 1543a)**

cutaneous filaments of first terminal branch of internal plantar nerve (Cruveilhier, 1836), see **common plantar digital nerves of medial plantar nerve (>1840)**

cutaneous filaments of obturator nerve (Quain & Wilson, 1839), see **cutaneous branch of obturator nerve (>1840)**

cutaneous long palmar branch of ulnar nerve (Bock, 1827), see **palmar branch of ulnar nerve (Soemmerring, 1791)**

cutaneous malar branch of second division of fifth pair of nerves (Todd, 1836–1839), see **zygomatic nerve (>1840)**

cutaneous nerve (Cheselden, 1726), see **medial cutaneous nerve of forearm (>1840)**

cutaneous nerve of anterior thoracic nerves (Günther, 1786), see **anterior cutaneous branch of intercostal nerves (>1840)**

cutaneous nerve of armpit (Chaussier, 1809), see **intercostal nerves (Vesalius, 1543a)**

cutaneous nerve of axilla (Burdin, 1803), see **intercostobrachial nerves (>1840)**

cutaneous nerve of cubital side of arm (Chaussier, 1809), see **intercostobrachial nerves (>1840)**

cutaneous nerve of foot (Martin, 1781), see **superficial fibular nerve (Fyfe, 1800)**

cutaneous nerve of neck (Meckel, 1753), see **transverse nerve of neck (>1840)**

cutaneous nerve of shoulder (Cruveilhier, 1836), see **superior lateral cutaneous nerve of arm (>1840)**

cutaneous nerve of shoulder (Meckel, 1817), see **superior lateral cutaneous nerve of arm (>1840)**

cutaneous nerve of Wrisberg (Bell, 1803b), see **medial cutaneous nerve of arm (>1840)**

cutaneous nerve of zygomatic bone (Meckel, 1753), see **zygomaticofacial nerve (>1840)**

cutaneous nervelet of internal plantar nerve (Fischer, 1791), see **medial plantar nerve (>1840)**

cutaneous nerves of collateral branches of internal plantar nerve (Cruveilhier, 1836), see **medial plantar nerve (>1840)**

cutaneous nerves of external branch of superficial terminal branch of external plantar nerve (Cruveilhier, 1836), see **common plantar digital nerves of lateral plantar nerve (>1840)**

cutaneous nerves of intercostal nerve (Bock, 1827), see **anterior branch of lateral cutaneous branch of intercostal nerves (>1840)**
cutaneous nerves of internal branch of superficial terminal branch of external plantar nerve (Cruveilhier, 1836), see **common plantar digital nerves of lateral plantar nerve (>1840)**
cutaneous nerves of nose (Meckel, 1753), see **external nasal branches of infraorbital nerve (>1840)**
cutaneous palmar branch of cubital nerve (Cruveilhier, 1836), see **superficial branch of ulnar nerve (Fyfe, 1800)**
cutaneous palmar branch of median nerve (Cloquet, 1816), see **palmar branch of median nerve (Bock, 1827)**
cutaneous palmar branch of middle cutaneous branch from internal cutaneous nerve (Knox, 1832), see **anterior branch of medial cutaneous nerve of forearm (>1840)**
cutaneous peroneal nerve (Bock, 1827), see **superficial fibular nerve (Fyfe, 1800)**
cutaneous peroneal nerve (Martin, 1781), see **lateral cutaneous nerve of calf (>1840)**
cutaneous peroneal nerve (Mayer, 1794), see **intermediate dorsal cutaneous nerve (>1840)**
cutaneous peroneal nerve (Meckel, 1817), see **intermediate dorsal cutaneous nerve (>1840)**
cutaneous plantar nervelet (Fischer, 1791) **common plantar digital nerves of medial plantar nerve (>1840)**
cutaneous sublaryngeal nerve (Peipers, 1793), see **inferior branch of transverse nerve of neck (>1840)**
cutaneous sub-pelvian nerve (Burdin, 1803), see **posterior cutaneous nerve of thigh (Günther, 1786)**
cutaneous temporal branches of superficial temporal nerve (Günther, 1786), see **superficial temporal branches of auriculotemporal nerve (>1840)**
cutaneous temporal nerve (Burdin, 1803), see **auriculotemporal nerve (Haller, 1762)**
cutaneous temporal surculus of inferior maxillary branch (Bellingeri, 1818), see **auriculotemporal nerve (Haller, 1762)**
cutaneous twig of internal branch of internal plantar nerve (Fischer, 1791), see **medial plantar nerve (>1840)**
cutaneous twig of middle branch of external plantar nerve (Fischer, 1791), see **superficial branch of lateral plantar nerve (>1840)**
cuticular membrane (Galen, c177), see **dura (Galen, c177)**
cuticularis (Galen, c177), see **dura (Galen, c177)**
cyathus (Vesalius, 1543a), see **hypothalamus (Kuhlenbeck, 1927)**
cyclo-ganglionic system (Solly, 1836), see **peripheral nervous system (Meckel, 1817)**
cylinder of crus cerebri (Reil, 1809b), see **vertebrate brain (Cuvier, 1800)**
cylinder of crus cerebri (Reil, 1809c), see **midbrain (Baer, 1837)**
cylindrical fascicle (Reil, 1809c), see **medial longitudinal fascicle (>1840)**
cylindrical protuberance (Cruveilhier, 1836), see **Ammon's horn (Vicq d'Azyr, 1784)**
cylindroid protuberance (Burdin, 1803), see **hippocampal region (Swanson et al., 1987)**
cystic nerves (Walter, 1783), see **cystic plexus (Wrisberg, 1808)**
cystic plexus (Wrisberg, 1808)
declive (>1840)
decussation of anterior pyramids (Spurzheim, 1826), see **pyramidal decussation (Reil, 1809c)**
decussation of optic nerves (Collins, 1685), see **optic chiasm (Galen, c173)**
decussation of posterior column (Bell, 1834), see **medial lemniscus decussation (>1840)**
decussation of posterior part (Bell, 1834), see **medial lemniscus decussation (>1840)**
decussation of posterior tract (Bell, 1834), see **medial lemniscus decussation (>1840)**
decussation of pyramidal bodies (Spurzheim, 1826), see **pyramidal decussation (Reil, 1809c)**
decussation of sensitive part (Bell, 1834), see **medial lemniscus decussation (>1840)**
deep auricular branch of auricular nerve (Cruveilhier, 1836), see **posterior branch of great auricular nerve (Bock, 1827)**
deep auricular branch of nerve to left auricle (Andersch, 1797), see **atrial plexuses (>1840)**
deep auricular nerve (Meckel, 1817), see **posterior auricular nerve (Meckel, 1753)**
deep branch of cubital nerve (Caldani, 1813, 1814), see **deep branch of ulnar nerve (Fyfe, 1800)**
deep branch of deep peroneal nerve (Fischer, 1791), see **muscular branches of deep fibular nerve (>1840)**
deep branch of external cutaneous nerve (Soemmerring, 1791), see **muscular branches of musculocutaneous nerve (Günther, 1786)**
deep branch of external plantar branch of tibial nerve (Martin, 1781), see **deep branch of lateral plantar nerve (>1840)**
deep branch of external plantar nerve (Günther, 1786), see **deep branch of lateral plantar nerve (>1840)**
deep branch of foot of deeper seated branch of fibular nerve (Bell, 1803b), see **superficial fibular nerve (Fyfe, 1800)**
deep branch of fourth pair of cervical nerves (Neubauer, 1772), see **muscular branches of cervical plexus (Cruveilhier, 1836)**
deep branch of hard nerve (Günther, 1786), see **facial nerve trunk (1840)**
deep branch of internal pudendal nerve (Cruveilhier, 1836), see **dorsal nerve of penis (Camper, 1762)**
deep branch of lateral plantar nerve (>1840)
deep branch of median nerve (Bock, 1827), see **anterior interosseous nerve (Quain, 1832)**
deep branch of muscular spiral nerve (Monro, 1783), see **deep branch of radial nerve (Martin, 1781)**
deep branch of musculocutaneous nerve (Soemmerring, 1791), see **muscular branches of musculocutaneous nerve (Günther, 1786)**
deep branch of palmar branch of cubital nerve (Cloquet, 1828), see **deep branch of ulnar nerve (Fyfe, 1800)**
deep branch of peroneal nerve (Haase, 1781), see **deep fibular nerve (Fyfe, 1800)**
deep branch of radial nerve (Martin, 1781)

deep branch of supraorbital nerve (Günther, 1786), see **lateral branch of supraorbital nerve (>1840)**

deep branch of ulnar nerve (Fyfe, 1800)

deep branch of Vidian nerve (Neubauer, 1772), see **deep petrosal nerve (Meckel, 1817)**

deep branch of volar branch of cubital nerve (Loder, 1803), see **deep branch of ulnar nerve (Fyfe, 1800)**

deep branch of volar branch of ulnar nerve (Langenbeck, 1826–1830), see **superficial branch of ulnar nerve (Fyfe, 1800)**

deep branches of cervical plexus (Quain, 1828), see **muscular branches of cervical plexus (Cruveilhier, 1836)**

deep branches of frontal branches of external frontal nerve (Todd, 1836–1839), see **medial branch of supraorbital nerve (>1840)**

deep branches of suborbital branches of temporofacial branch of facial nerve (Cruveilhier, 1836), see **zygomatic branches of facial nerve (>1840)**

deep branchlets of superior laryngeal nerve (Loder, 1778), see **internal branch of superior laryngeal nerve (Fyfe, 1800)**

deep cardiac plexus (Mayer, 1794), see **cardiac plexus (Keill, 1698)**

deep cervical branches of cervical plexus (Cloquet, 1816), see **muscular branches of cervical plexus (Cruveilhier, 1836)**

deep convolutions of great cerebral sulcus (Gall & Spurzheim, 1810), see **insular region (Brodmann, 1909)**

deep cystic nerve (Mayer, 1794), see **cystic plexus (Wrisberg, 1808)**

deep dorsal branch of foot (Bell, 1803b), see **digital branch of deep fibular nerve (>1840)**

deep dorsal branch of foot of deeper seated branch of fibular nerve (Bell & Bell, 1816), see **muscular branches of deep fibular nerve (>1840)**

deep dorsal external collateral nerve of big toe (Cruveilhier, 1836), see **dorsal digital nerves of digital branch of deep fibular nerve (>1840)**

deep dorsal twig of foot of deep branch of peroneal nerve (Jördens, 1788), see **digital branch of deep fibular nerve (>1840)**

deep femoral branch from sacral plexus (Mayer, 1794), see **sacral plexus ventral divisions (Paterson, 1887)**

deep fibular nerve (Fyfe, 1800)

deep frontal thread of supraorbital fascicle (Bellingeri, 1818), see **supraorbital nerve (Meckel, 1753)**

deep internal branch of external plantar nerve (Cloquet, 1828), see **deep branch of lateral plantar nerve (>1840)**

deep layer of cardiac nerves (Cruveilhier, 1836), see **cardiac plexus (Keill, 1698)**

deep lingual branches of glossopharyngeal nerve (Bell, 1803b), see **lingual branches of glossopharyngeal nerve (Haller, 1762)**

deep lobule of superior fissure of Vicq d'Azyr (Dejerine & Dejerine-Klumpke, 1901), see **ansiform lobule crus I (Bolk, 1906)**

deep major branch of Vidian nerve (Meckel, 1748), see **deep petrosal nerve (Meckel, 1817)**

deep median nerve (Günther, 1786), see **anterior interosseous nerve (Quain, 1832)**

deep muscular branch of hard nerve (Mayer, 1794), see **facial nerve trunk (1840)**

deep muscular branch of peroneal nerve (Soemmerring, 1791), see **deep fibular nerve (Fyfe, 1800)**

deep nerve of muscular spiral nerve (Bell & Bell, 1816), see **deep branch of radial nerve (Martin, 1781)**

deep nerve of nerve layers of septum of heart (Andersch, 1797), see **coronary plexuses (Meckel, 1817)**

deep palmar branch of ulnar nerve (Quain & Wilson, 1839), see **deep branch of ulnar nerve (>1840)**

deep palmar nerve (Fyfe, 1800), see **deep branch of ulnar nerve (Fyfe, 1800)**

deep peroneal nerve (Bell, 1803a), see **deep fibular nerve (Fyfe, 1800)**

deep peroneal nerve (Günther, 1781), see **deep fibular nerve (Fyfe, 1800)**

deep petrosal nerve (Meckel, 1817)

deep petrous nerve (Meckel, 1832), see **deep petrosal nerve (Meckel, 1817)**

deep plantar nerve (Swan, 1830), see **deep branch of lateral plantar nerve (>1840)**

deep posterior auricular nerve (Meckel, 1753), see **posterior auricular nerve (Meckel, 1753)**

deep posterior supraclavicular nerves (Bock, 1827), see **lateral supraclavicular nerves (>1840)**

deep seated branch of fibular nerve (Bell & Bell, 1829), see **deep fibular nerve (Fyfe, 1800)**

deep-seated branches of anterior crural nerve (Quain, 1832), see **femoral nerve (Haller, 1762)**

deep-seated branches of crural nerve (Quain, 1828), see **femoral nerve (Haller, 1762)**

deep seated cardiac plexus (Lobstein, 1823), see **cardiac plexus (Keill, 1698)**

deep seated nerves of heart (Lobstein, 1823), see **cardiac plexus (Keill, 1698)**

deep-seated palmar branch of ulnar nerve (Quain, 1828), see **deep branch of ulnar nerve (Fyfe, 1800)**

deep-seated Vidian nerve (Lobstein, 1823), see **greater petrosal nerve (>1840)**

deep smaller cardiac nerves (Scarpa, 1794), see **inferior cardiac nerve (Cloquet, 1816)**

deep temporal branches of inferior maxillary nerve (Todd, 1836–1839), see **deep temporal nerves (Haase, 1781)**

deep temporal branches of third branch of fifth pair (Meckel, 1748), see **deep temporal nerves (Haase, 1781)**

deep temporal nerves (Haase, 1781)

deep terminal branch of cubital nerve (Cruveilhier, 1836), see **deep branch of ulnar nerve (Fyfe, 1800)**

deep terminal branch of external plantar nerve (Cruveilhier, 1836), see **deep branch of lateral plantar nerve (>1840)**

deep thread of Vidian fascicle (Bellingeri, 1818), see **deep petrosal nerve (Meckel, 1817)**

deep trunk of external plantar nerve (Meckel, 1817), see **deep branch of lateral plantar nerve (>1840)**

deep twig of deep branch of external plantar nerve (Jördens, 1788), see **deep branch of lateral plantar nerve (>1840)** *deep twig of palmar branch of ulnar nerve (Meckel, 1817)*, see ***deep branch of ulnar nerve (Fyfe, 1800)***

deep Vidian nerve (Günther, 1786), see ***deep petrosal nerve (Meckel, 1817)***

deep volar branch of ulnar nerve (Günther, 1786), see ***superficial branch of ulnar nerve (Fyfe, 1800)***

deep white substance of quadrigeminal body (Arnold, 1838a), see ***superior colliculus (Haller, 1762)***

deeper division of fibular nerve (Bell & Bell, 1829), see ***deep fibular nerve (Fyfe, 1800)***

deeper transverse septum of pons (Bell, 1834), see ***transverse pontine fibers (>1840)***

deferential plexus (Cruveilhier, 1836)

delicate membrane (Galen, c177), see ***pia (Galen, c192)***

deltoid branch of axillary nerve (Cruveilhier, 1836), see ***muscular branch of axillary nerve (>1840)***

dental branch of maxillary branch of inferior maxillary branch of fifth pair of nerves (Bock, 1817), see ***inferior dental nerve (Meckel, 1817)***

dental branches of dental nerve (Arnold, 1834), see ***inferior dental branches of inferior dental plexus (>1840)***

dental branches of dental nerve anastomosis (Arnold, 1834), see ***inferior dental branches of inferior dental plexus (>1840)***

dental branches of greater anterior alveolar nerve (Arnold, 1834), see ***anterior superior dental nerve (Haller, 1762)***

dental branches of greater anterior dental nerve (Arnold, 1834), see ***anterior superior dental nerve (Haller, 1762)***

dental branches of inferior maxillary branch (Loder, 1778), see ***inferior dental branches of inferior dental plexus (>1840)***

dental branches of maxillodental nerve (Chaussier, 1809), see ***inferior dental branches of inferior dental plexus (>1840)***

dental branches of posterior alveolar nerve (Arnold, 1834), see ***posterior superior dental nerve (Haller, 1762)***

dental branches of posterior dental nerve (Arnold, 1834), see ***posterior superior dental nerve (Haller, 1762)***

dental nerve (Arnold, 1834), see ***inferior dental plexus (>1840)***

dental nerve (Meckel, 1817), see ***inferior dental nerve (Meckel, 1817)***

dental nerve (Quain & Wilson, 1839), see ***inferior dental nerve (Meckel, 1817)***

dental nerve anastomosis (Arnold, 1834), see ***superior dental plexus (>1840)***

dental threads of internal dental fascicles (Bellingeri, 1818), see ***superior dental branches of superior dental plexus (>1840)***

dentar nerve (Meckel, 1817), see ***inferior dental nerve (Meckel, 1817)***

dentate body of cerebellar peduncles (Desmoulins, 1825), see ***dentate nucleus (>1840)***

dentate body of cerebellum (Vicq d'Azyr, 1784), see ***dentate nucleus (>1840)***

dentate body of olivary body (Langenbeck, 1826–1830), see ***olivocerebellar tract (>1840)***

dentate body of olivary eminence (Vicq d'Azyr, 1786), see ***inferior olivary complex (>1840)***

dentate body of olives (Desmoulins, 1825), see ***amiculum of olive (>1840)***

dentate gyrus (>1840)

dentate margin of hippocampus major (Vicq d'Azyr, 1786), see ***dentate gyrus (>1840)***

dentate nucleus (>1840)

denticulate ligament (Monro, 1783)

dento-muscular fascicle of posterior dental surculus of superior maxillary branch (Bellingeri, 1818), see ***posterior superior dental nerve (Haller, 1762)***

descending anastomotic branch of second cervical nerve with third cervical nerve (Arnold, 1834), see ***communicating loops of cervical plexus (>1840)***

descending anastomotic branch of third cervical nerve (Arnold, 1834), see ***communicating loops of cervical plexus (>1840)***

descending anastomotic nerve of second cervical nerve (Meckel, 1817), see ***communicating loops of cervical plexus (>1840)***

descending and internal branches of muscular branches of inferior gluteal nerve (Cruveilhier, 1836), see ***inferior gluteal nerve (Martin, 1781)***

descending branch of anterior pillar of fornix (Meynert, 1872), see ***postcommissural fornix (Loo, 1931)***

descending branch of auriculotemporal nerve (Cruveilhier, 1836), see ***anterior auricular nerves (>1840)***

descending branch of crus fornicis (Meynert, 1872), see ***postcommissural fornix (Loo, 1931)***

descending branch of hard nerve (Mayer, 1794), see ***facial nerve trunk (1840)***

descending branch of hypoglossal nerve (Günther, 1786), see ***superior root of ansa cervicalis (>1840)***

descending branch of inferior maxillary branch of fifth pair of nerves (Bock, 1817), see ***marginal mandibular branch of facial nerve (>1840)***

descending branch of internal laryngeal nerve (Knox, 1832), see ***communicating branch of superior laryngeal nerve with inferior laryngeal nerve (Langenbeck, 1826–1830)***

descending branch of left vagus nerve (Mayer, 1794), see ***gastric branch of left vagus nerve (Mayer, 1794)***

descending branch of middle cutaneous nerve of neck (Peipers, 1793), see ***inferior branches of transverse nerve of neck (>1840)***

descending branch of ninth pair of nerves of head (Asch, 1750), see ***superior root of ansa cervicalis (>1840)***

descending branch of pharyngeal nerves (Scarpa, 1794), see ***pharyngeal branches of vagus nerve (>1840)***

descending branch of pterygopalatine nerve (Meckel, 1817), see ***palatine nerves (Schaarschmidt, 1750)***

descending branch of superficial branch of hard nerve (Günther, 1786), see ***facial nerve trunk (1840)***

descending branch of superficial cervical branch of cervical plexus (Cruveilhier, 1836), see ***inferior branches of transverse nerve of neck (>1840)***

descending branch of superior branch of hard nerve (Meckel, 1753), see ***zygomatic branches of facial nerve (>1840)***

descending branch of superior gluteal nerve (Cruveilhier, 1836), see ***superior gluteal nerve (Martin, 1781)***

descending branch of superior maxillary nerve (Meckel, 1748), see ***pterygopalatine nerves (Wrisberg, 1786)*** *descending branches of anterior trunk of eighth pair of nerves (Walter, 1783)*, see **gastric branches of anterior vagal trunk (>1840)**

descending branches of buccal nerve (Cruveilhier, 1836), see **buccal nerve (Meckel, 1748)**

descending branches of cervical plexus (Knox, 1832), see **descending superficial branches of cervical plexus (Quain, 1828)**

descending branches of external frontal nerve (Cruveilhier, 1836), see **supraorbital nerve (Meckel, 1753)**

descending branches of facial nerve (Meckel, 1817), see **facial nerve trunk (1840)**

descending branches of inferior laryngeal nerve (Günther, 1786), see **tracheal branches of recurrent laryngeal nerve (>1840)**

descending branches of recurrent nerve (Haase, 1781), see **recurrent laryngeal nerve (Albinus, 1744)**

descending branches of recurrent nerves (Scarpa, 1794), see **cardiac branches of recurrent laryngeal nerve (>1840)**

descending branches of spheno-palatine ganglion (Quain, 1828), see **lesser palatine nerves (Meckel, 1817)**

descending branches of spheno-palatine ganglion (Quain & Wilson, 1839), see **palatine nerves (Schaarschmidt, 1750)**

descending branches of supraorbital nerve (Cruveilhier, 1836), see **supraorbital nerve (Meckel, 1753)**

descending cerebellar crus (Meckel, 1817), see **inferior cerebellar peduncle (Günther, 1786)**

descending cervical branch (Neubauer, 1772), see **inferior root of ansa cervicalis (>1840)**

descending cervical nerve (Meckel, 1817), see **inferior root of ansa cervicalis (>1840)**

descending column of fornix (Sprague & Meyer, 1950), see **postcommissural fornix (Loo, 1931)**

descending cornu of fornix (Volkmann, 1831), see **postcommissural fornix (Loo, 1931)**

descending cutaneous nerve of neck (Peipers, 1793), see **inferior branch of transverse nerve of neck (>1840)**

descending esophageal branches of fourth branch of recurrent nerves of neck (Andersch & Soemmerring, 1792), see **pharyngeal branches of vagus nerve (>1840)**

descending external branches of cervical plexus (Cloquet, 1816), see **descending superficial branches of cervical plexus (Quain, 1828)**

descending fascicle of inferior maxillary nerve (Günther, 1786), see **posterior branch of mandibular nerve (>1840)**

descending fibers of calamus scriptorius (Laurencet, 1825), see **hypoglossal triangle (>1840)**

descending filament of superior laryngeal branches of pneumogastric nerve (Cruveilhier, 1836), see **communicating branch of superior laryngeal nerve with inferior laryngeal nerve (Langenbeck, 1826–1830)**

descending filaments of anterior alveolo-dental nerve (Cruveilhier, 1836), see **anterior superior dental nerve (Haller, 1762)**

descending filaments of anterior terminal branch of internal saphenous nerve (Cruveilhier, 1836), see **infrapatellar branch of saphenous nerve (>1840)**

descending filaments of internal frontal nerve (Cruveilhier, 1836), see **supratrochlear nerve (Schaarschmidt, 1750)**

descending filaments of superior maxillary nerve (Cruveilhier, 1836), see **superior labial branches of infraorbital nerve (>1840)**

descending filaments of supratrochlear nerve (Cruveilhier, 1836), see **supratrochlear nerve (Schaarschmidt, 1750)**

descending horn of lateral ventricle (Haller, 1762), see **inferior horn of lateral ventricle (Bell, 1802)**

descending laryngeal nerve (Quain, 1827), see **superior laryngeal nerve (Loder, 1778)**

descending major branch of inferior anterior nasal nerves (Scarpa, 1785), see **posterior inferior nasal nerves (Günther, 1786)**

descending neck branch of hypoglossal nerve (Soemmerring, 1791), see **superior root of ansa cervicalis (>1840)**

descending nerve (Soemmerring, 1798), see **buccal branch of facial nerve (>1840)**

descending part of cerebellar brachia (Malacarne, 1776), see **inferior cerebellar peduncle (Günther, 1786)**

descending part of fornix (Cajal, 1904), see **septal postcommissural fornix (>1840)**

descending part of lateral ventricle (Valverde de Amuso, 1556), see **inferior horn of lateral ventricle (Bell, 1802)**

descending part of medullary stria (Kölliker, 1896), see **hypothalamic medullary stria (>1840)**

descending root of fornix (Burdach, 1822), see **mammillothalamic tract (>1840)**

descending root of mammillary body (Arnold, 1838a), see **mammillothalamic tract (>1840)**

descending superficial branches of cervical plexus (Quain, 1828)

descending third branch of fifth pair (Meckel, 1748), see **posterior branch of mandibular nerve (>1840)**

descending trunk of accessory spinal nerve (Willis, 1664), see **external branch of accessory nerve trunk (Meckel, 1817)**

descending uterine nerves (Cruveilhier, 1836), see **uterovaginal plexus (>1840)**

diagonal band (Broca, 1879)

diagonal band of quadrilateral space (Broca, 1879), see **diagonal band (Broca, 1879)**

diagonal sulcus (Beccari, 1911)

diaphragm (Galen, c177), see **cerebral nuclei (Swanson, 2000a)**

diaphragm of brain (Winslow, 1733), see **cerebellar tentorium (Winslow, 1733)**

diaphragma (Galen, c177), see **cerebral nuclei (Swanson, 2000a)**

diaphragma interpositum (Bell & Bell, 1816), see **choroid membrane of third ventricle (>1840)**

diaphragma sellae (>1840), see **sellar diaphragm (>1840)**

diaphragmatic branch of cervical plexus (Cloquet, 1816), see **phrenic nerve (Galen, c173)**

diaphragmatic nerve (Diemerbroeck, 1689), see **phrenic nerve (Galen, c173)**

diaphragmatic plexus (Loder, 1778), see **phrenic plexus (Loder, 1778)**

didymia (Galen, c173, definition 1), see **tectum (Baer, 1837)**
didymia (Galen, c173, definition 2), see **superior colliculus (Haller, 1762)**
didymos (Vesalius, 1543a), see **superior colliculus (Haller, 1762)**
diencephalon (Sharpey et al., 1867), see **interbrain (Baer, 1837)**
digastric branch of communicating nerve of face (Knox, 1832), see **digastric nerve (Meckel, 1753)**
digastric branch of facial nerve (Meckel, 1817), see **digastric nerve (Meckel, 1753)**
digastric branch of glossopharyngeal nerves (Kilian, 1822), see **glossopharyngeal nerve (Huber, 1744)**
digastric branch of hard part of acoustic nerve (Scarpa, 1794), see **digastric nerve (Meckel, 1753)**
digastric branch of internal deep nerve of hard nerve (Meckel, 1753), see **digastric nerve (Meckel, 1753)**
digastric branch of submaxillary branch of inferior maxillary nerve (Andersch, 1797), see **mylohyoid nerve (Meckel, 1748)**
digastric lobe (Meckel, 1817), see **biventral lobule (>1840)**
digastric muscle nerve (Soemmerring, 1798), see **digastric nerve (Meckel, 1753)**
digastric nerve (Meckel, 1753)
digastric surculus proper of digastric branch (Bellingeri, 1818), see **digastric nerve (Meckel, 1753)**
digital branch of cubital nerve (Cloquet, 1828), see **common palmar digital nerves of ulnar nerve (>1840)**
digital branch of deep fibular nerve (>1840)
digital branch of external plantar branch of tibial nerve (Martin, 1781), see **superficial branch of lateral plantar nerve (>1840)**
digital branch of external plantar nerve (Quain & Wilson, 1839), see **common plantar digital nerves of lateral plantar nerve (>1840)**
digital branch of first finger of median nerve (Quain & Wilson, 1839), see **proper palmar digital nerves of median nerve (>1840)**
digital branch of peroneal nerve (Mayer, 1794), see **intermediate dorsal cutaneous nerve (>1840)**
digital branch of superficial peroneal nerve (Mayer, 1794), see **intermediate dorsal cutaneous nerve (>1840)**
digital branches of internal plantar branches of tibial nerve (Martin, 1781), see **common plantar digital nerves of medial plantar nerve (>1840)**
digital branches of internal plantar nerve (Quain & Wilson, 1839), see **proper plantar digital nerves of medial plantar nerve (>1840)**
digital branches of median nerve (Cloquet, 1816), see **common palmar digital nerves of median nerve (>1840)**
digital branches of superficial peroneal nerve (Günther, 1786), see **superficial fibular nerve (Fyfe, 1800)**
digital cavity (Bartholin, 1641), see **posterior horn of lateral ventricle (Haller, 1747)**
digital eminence (Meckel, 1817), see **calcarine spur (Morand, 1748)**
digital filaments of external plantar nerve to dorsal surface of toes (Quain & Wilson, 1839), see **proper plantar digital nerves of lateral plantar nerve (>1840)**
digital fovea (Meckel, 1817), see **posterior horn of lateral ventricle (Haller, 1747)**
digital median nerve (Burdin, 1803), see **median nerve (Du Verney, 1697)**
digital nerves of foot from internal plantar nerve (Soemmerring, 1798), see **common plantar digital nerves of medial plantar nerve (>1840)**
digital nerves of median nerve (Schaarschmidt, 1750), see **proper palmar digital nerves of median nerve (>1840)**
digital process (Bergen, 1734), see **posterior horn of lateral ventricle (Haller, 1747)**
digital processes of Ammon's horn (Günther, 1786), see **hippocampal region (Swanson et al., 1987)**
digital sinus of lateral ventricle (Ramsay, 1813), see **posterior horn of lateral ventricle (Haller, 1747)**
digitationes pes hippopotami major (Mayer, 1779), see **hippocampal region (Swanson et al., 1987)**
digiti pedis hippocampi (Haller, 1762), see **hippocampal region (Swanson et al., 1987)**
digiti pedis minoris hippocampi (Haase, 1781), see **calcarine spur (Morand, 1748)**
digits of small foot of seahorse (Haase, 1781), see **calcarine spur (Morand, 1748)**
direct reticulospinal tract (>1840), see **medial reticulospinal tract (>1840)**
direct terminal branch of internal saphenous nerve (Cruveilhier, 1836), see **saphenous nerve (Haase, 1781)**
discolored substance of brain (Vesalius, 1543a), see **central nervous system gray matter regions (>1840)**
distal glossopharyngeal ganglion (>1840)
distal part of neurohypophysis (Daniel & Pritchard, 1975), see **posterior lobe of pituitary gland (Haller, 1762)**
distal vagal ganglion (>1840)
ditch (Rufus of Ephesus, fl. c90–120), see **hypothalamic part of third ventricle (Swanson, 2004)**
diverging fibres (Spurzheim, 1826), see **central nervous system white matter tracts (>1840)**
diverticulum (Günz, 1753), see **posterior horn of lateral ventricle (Haller, 1747)**
divided branch of dorsal branch of radial nerve (Loder, 1803), see **superficial branch of radial nerve (Martin, 1781)**
divisions of fifth pair (Bell, 1803a), see **trigeminal nerve branches (Winslow, 1733)**
dorsal anterior cingulate area (Brodmann, 1909)
dorsal arch of hand (Meckel, 1817), see **brachial plexus cords (Schwalbe, 1881)**
dorsal branch of cubital nerve (Loder, 1803), see **dorsal branch of ulnar nerve (Günther, 1786)**
dorsal branch of cubital nerve (Martin, 1781), see **dorsal branch of ulnar nerve (Günther, 1786)**
dorsal branch of deep peroneal nerve (Bock, 1827), see **digital branch of deep fibular nerve (>1840)**
dorsal branch of deeper seated branch of fibular nerve (Bell, 1803b), see **superficial fibular nerve (Fyfe, 1800)**
dorsal branch of hand of ulnar nerve (Bock, 1827), see **dorsal branch of ulnar nerve (Günther, 1786)**
dorsal branch of median nerve external collateral branch of index finger (Cruveihier, 1836), see **proper palmar digital nerves of median nerve (>1840)**

dorsal branch of median nerve external collateral branch of thumb (Cruveilhier, 1836), see ***common palmar digital nerves of median nerve (>1840)***
dorsal branch of penis of internal pudendal nerve (Cruveilhier, 1836), see ***dorsal nerve of penis (Camper, 1762)***
dorsal branch of peroneal nerve (Swan, 1830), see ***superficial fibular nerve (Fyfe, 1800)***
dorsal branch of plantar internal collateral nerve of big toe (Cruveilhier, 1836), see ***proper plantar digital nerves of medial plantar nerve (>1840)***
dorsal branch of radial nerve (Bock, 1827), see ***superficial branch of radial nerve (Martin, 1781)***
dorsal branch of radial nerve (Cloquet, 1828), see ***superficial branch of radial nerve (Martin, 1781)***
dorsal branch of radial nerve (Loder, 1803), see ***superficial branch of radial nerve (Martin, 1781)***
dorsal branch of superficial branch of spiral nerve (Fyfe, 1800), see ***dorsal digital nerves of radial nerve (>1840)***
dorsal branch of ulnar nerve (Günther, 1786)
dorsal branches of dorsal nerves (Cloquet, 1816), see ***spinal nerve dorsal branch (Meckel, 1817)***
dorsal branches of foot (Bell, 1803b), see ***superficial fibular nerve (Fyfe, 1800)***
dorsal branches of intercostal nerves (Quain & Wilson, 1839), see ***spinal nerve dorsal branch (Meckel, 1817)***
dorsal branches of superficial branch of radial nerve (Martin, 1781), see ***dorsal digital nerves of radial nerve (>1840)***
dorsal collateral branches of cubital nerve internal dorsal branch of hand (Cruveilhier, 1836), see ***dorsal digital nerves of ulnar nerve (>1840)***
dorsal collateral branches of digital nerves of ulnar nerve (Quain & Wilson, 1839), see ***dorsal digital nerves of ulnar nerve (>1840)***
dorsal collateral nerves of musculocutaneous nerve (Cruveilhier, 1836), see ***superficial fibular nerve (Fyfe, 1800)***
dorsal column nuclei (>1840)
dorsal commissure of Ammon's horn (Kölliker, 1896), see ***dorsal hippocampal commissure (Craigie, 1925)***
dorsal cord (Galen, c170–c180), see ***spinal cord (Galen, c162–c166)***
dorsal crest of plate (Wagner, 1839), see ***neural crest (>1840)***
dorsal cutaneous branches of dorsal superficial branch of radial nerve (Günther, 1786), see ***dorsal digital nerves of radial nerve (>1840)***
dorsal cutaneous nerves of thumb (Meckel, 1817), see ***dorsal digital nerves of radial nerve (>1840)***
dorsal digital branches of dorsal branch of ulnar nerve (Günther, 1786), see ***dorsal digital nerves of ulnar nerve (>1840)***
dorsal digital nerves (Bock, 1827), see ***brachial plexus cords (Schwalbe, 1881)***
dorsal digital nerves of anterior cutaneous branch of peroneal nerve (Langenbeck, 1826–1830), see ***superficial fibular nerve (Fyfe, 1800)***
dorsal digital nerves of deep branch of peroneal nerve (Langenbeck, 1826–1830), see ***dorsal digital nerves of deep fibular nerve (>1840)***
dorsal digital nerves of deep fibular nerve (>1840)
dorsal digital nerves of dorsal branch of radial nerve (Langenbeck, 1826–1830), see ***dorsal digital nerves of radial nerve (>1840)***
dorsal digital nerves of dorsal branch of ulnar nerve (Langenbeck, 1826–1830), see ***dorsal digital nerves of ulnar nerve (>1840)***
dorsal digital nerves of foot (Bock, 1827), see ***sciatic nerve (Keill, 1698)***
dorsal digital nerves of intermediate dorsal cutaneous nerve (>1840)
dorsal digital nerves of lateral dorsal cutaneous nerve (>1840)
dorsal digital nerves of medial dorsal cutaneous nerve (>1840)
dorsal digital nerves of radial nerve (>1840)
dorsal digital nerves of ulnar nerve (>1840)
dorsal entorhinal area (Brodmann, 1909), see ***entorhinal area (Brodmann, 1909)***
dorsal external collateral nerve of thumb (Cruveilhier, 1836), see ***dorsal digital nerves of radial nerve (>1840)***
dorsal external twig of fourth digit (Jördens, 1788), see ***dorsal digital nerves of intermediate dorsal cutaneous nerve (>1840)***
dorsal external twig of second digit (Jördens, 1788), see ***dorsal digital nerves of medial dorsal cutaneous nerve (>1840)***
dorsal external twig of third digit (Jördens, 1788), see ***dorsal digital nerves of intermediate dorsal cutaneous nerve (>1840)***
dorsal fasciculus proprius (>1840), see ***dorsal intersegmental tract (>1840)***
dorsal fornix (Smith, 1898), see ***fimbria (Honegger, 1890)***
dorsal fornix (Sprague & Meyer, 1950)
dorsal funiculus (>1840)
dorsal ganglion (Mayer, 1794), see ***thoracic sympathetic ganglia (1840)***
dorsal hippocampal commissure (Craigie, 1925)
dorsal horn (>1840)
dorsal intermediate sulcus (>1840)
dorsal internal collateral nerve of second toe (Cruveilhier, 1836), see ***dorsal digital nerves of digital branch of deep fibular nerve (>1840)***
dorsal internal twig of fifth digit (Jördens, 1788), see ***dorsal digital nerves of intermediate dorsal cutaneous nerve (>1840)***
dorsal internal twig of fourth digit (Jördens, 1788), see ***dorsal digital nerves of intermediate dorsal cutaneous nerve (>1840)***
dorsal internal twig of third digit (Jördens, 1788), see ***dorsal digital nerves of medial dorsal cutaneous nerve (>1840)***
dorsal intersegmental tract (>1840)
dorsal intervertebral nerves (Schaarschmidt, 1750), see ***thoracic nerves (Diemerbroeck, 1672)***
dorsal lateral geniculate nucleus (>1840)
dorsal longitudinal fascicle (Schütz, 1891)
dorsal marrow (Bauhin, 1605), see ***cerebrospinal trunk (>1840)***
dorsal marrow (Hippocrates), see ***spinal cord (Galen, c162–c166)***

dorsal median fissure of spinal cord (Spurzheim, 1826), see **dorsal median sulcus of spinal cord (>1840)**

dorsal median septum (>1840)

dorsal median sulcus of medulla (>1840)

dorsal median sulcus of spinal cord (>1840)

dorsal medulla (Galen, c192), see **spinal cord (Galen, c162–c166)**

dorsal medulla (Hippocrates), see **spinal cord (Galen, c162–c166)**

dorsal medulla (Vesalius, 1543a), see **cerebrospinal trunk (>1840)**

dorsal midbrain sulcus (>1840)

dorsal motor nucleus of vagus nerve (>1840)

dorsal nerve (Fyfe, 1800), see **dorsal branch of ulnar nerve (Günther, 1786)**

dorsal nerve from internal cutaneous nerve (Knox, 1832), see **posterior branch of medial cutaneous nerve of forearm (>1840)**

dorsal nerve of clitoris (Mayer, 1794), see **dorsal nerve of clitoris (>1840)**

dorsal nerve of clitoris (>1840)

dorsal nerve of hand (Klint, 1784), see **dorsal branch of ulnar nerve (Günther, 1786)**

dorsal nerve of penis (Camper, 1762)

dorsal nerve of penis (Mayer, 1794), see **dorsal nerve of penis (Camper, 1762)**

dorsal nerves (Coiter, 1572), see **spinal nerves (Camper, 1760–1762)**

dorsal nerves (Haller, 1762), see **thoracic nerves (Diemerbroeck, 1762)**

dorsal nerves (Winslow, 1733), see **thoracic nerves (Diemerbroeck, 1672)**

dorsal nerves of fourth toe (Meckel, 1817), see **dorsal digital nerves of intermediate dorsal cutaneous nerve (>1840)**

dorsal nerves of index finger (Bock, 1827), see **dorsal digital nerves of radial nerve (>1840)**

dorsal nerves of thumb (Bock, 1827), see **dorsal digital nerves of radial nerve (>1840)**

dorsal nerves of two external toes and peroneal nerve of third (Meckel, 1817), see **dorsal digital nerves of medial dorsal cutaneous nerve (>1840)**

dorsal nucleus of spinal cord (>1840), see **dorsal thoracic nucleus (>1840)**

dorsal part of thalamus (Herrick, 1910)

dorsal peroneal nerve of fifth toe (Meckel, 1817), see **lateral dorsal cutaneous nerve (>1840)**

dorsal plexus of penis (Bock, 1827), see **dorsal nerve of penis (Camper, 1762)**

dorsal portion of cord (Gordon, 1815), see **spinal cord (Galen, c162–c166)**

dorsal posterior cingulate area (Brodmann, 1909)

dorsal premammillary nucleus (>1840)

dorsal radial nerve (Bock, 1824), see **superficial branch of radial nerve (Martin, 1781)**

dorsal reticulospinal tract (>1840), see **lateral reticulospinal tract (>1840)**

dorsal root (Spurzheim, 1826)

dorsal root central part (>1840)

dorsal rootlets (>1840)

dorsal scapular nerve (Bock, 1827)

dorsal spinal medulla (Galen, c173), see **thoracic part of spinal cord (>1840)**

dorsal spinocerebellar tract (>1840)

dorsal superficial branch of radial nerve (Günther, 1786), see **superficial branch of radial nerve (Martin, 1781)**

dorsal superior nasal nerves (Günther, 1786), see **external nasal branch of anterior ethmoidal nerve (>1840)**

dorsal tegmental decussation (>1840)

dorsal thoracic nucleus (>1840)

dorsal twig of foot of superficial branch of external plantar nerve (Jördens, 1788), see **superficial branch of lateral plantar nerve (>1840)**

dorsal ulnar nerve of ring-finger (Knox, 1832), see **dorsal digital nerves of ulnar nerve (>1840)**

dorsales Längsbündel (Schütz, 1891), see **dorsal longitudinal fascicle (Schütz, 1891)**

dorsi-lumbar communicating branch (Quain, 1832), see **lumbar plexus (Vesalius, 1543a)**

dorsi-lumbar nerve (Quain & Wilson, 1839), see **lumbar plexus (Vesalius, 1543a)**

dorsolateral fascicle (>1840), see **dorsolateral tract (>1840)**

dorsolateral fissure (>1840), see **dorsal midbrain sulcus (>1840)**

dorsolateral sulcus of medulla (>1840)

dorsolateral sulcus of spinal cord (>1840)

dorsolateral tract (>1840)

double anastomosis of great hypoglossal nerve with lingual branch of fifth pair (Knox, 1832), see **communicating branches of lingual nerve with hypoglossal nerve (>1840)**

double infolding within bason (Willis, 1664), see **inferior hypogastric plexus (Tiedemann, 1822)**

double origination of olfactory nerve (Collins, 1685), see **endbrain (Kuhlenbeck, 1927)**

double panniculus (Benedetti, 1502), see **meninges (Smith Papyrus, c1700 BC)**

dropping pan (Hall, 1565), see **hypothalamus (Kuhlenbeck, 1927)**

duct (Aristotle), see **white matter tracts (Bell & Bell, 1826)**

ducts (Aristotle), see **cranial nerves (Soemmerring, 1791)**

ductus ad infundibulum (Ridley, 1695), see **hypothalamic part of third ventricle (Swanson, 2004)**

ductus instrumenti olfactus (Varoli, 1573), see **cerebral cortex (>1840)**

ductus nervei olfactus (Varoli, 1573), see **cerebral cortex (>1840)**

dug-like process (Riolan, 1657), see **olfactory bulb (Weitbrecht, 1751)**

dull white nucleus inside olivary eminence (Vicq d'Azyr, 1784), see **olivocerebellar tract (>1840)**

duobus tuberculis (Haller, 1762), see **spinal cord (Galen, c162–c166)**

duodenal nerves (Walter, 1783), see **gastroduodenal plexus (>1840)**

duodenal plexus (Wrisberg, 1800), see **gastroduodenal plexus (>1840)**

dura (Galen, c177)

dura cerebri meninx (Wrisberg, 1777), see **dura (Galen, c177)**

encephalon (Galen, c173), see ***central nervous system (Carus, 1814)***

encephalon (Galen, c173, c177), see ***brain (Smith Papyrus, c1700 BC)***

encephalon (Homer, c9th century BC), see ***brain (Smith Papyrus, c1700 BC)***

encephalon (Soemmerring, 1778), see ***vertebrate brain (Cuvier, 1800)***

encephalon extension to crystalline humor (Galen, c173), see ***white matter tracts (Bell & Bell, 1826)***

encephalon itself (Galen, c173), see ***vertebrate brain (Cuvier, 1800)***

encephalos (Homer, c9th century BC), see ***brain (Smith Papyrus, c1700 BC)***

enclosing of right and left ventricles (Geminus, 1553), see ***cerebral nuclei (Swanson, 2000a)***

encranion (Galen, c173), see ***cerebellum (Aristotle)***

encranis (Galen, c173), see ***cerebellum (Aristotle)***

encranium (Galen, c173), see ***cerebellum (Aristotle)***

encranon (Galen, c173), see ***cerebellum (Aristotle)***

endbrain (Kuhlenbeck, 1927)

endbrain vesicle (Kuhlenbeck, 1927)

Endhirn (Kuhlenbeck, 1927), see ***endbrain (Kuhlenbeck, 1927)***

Endhirnblasen (Kuhlenbeck, 1927), see ***endbrain vesicle (Kuhlenbeck, 1927)***

Endplatte (Burdach, 1822), see ***terminal lamina (Burdach, 1822)***

enkar (Salmon, 1714), see ***cerebral cortex gray matter (>1840)***

enkaros (Salmon, 1714), see ***cerebral cortex gray matter (>1840)***

enkephalon (Aristotle), see ***vertebrate brain (Cuvier, 1800)***

enkephalon (Galen, c177), see ***brain (Smith Papyrus, c1700 BC)***

enkephalon (Homer, c9th century BC), see ***brain (Smith Papyrus, c1700 BC)***

enkephalos (Homer, c9th century BC), see ***brain (Smith Papyrus, c1700 BC)***

enteric nervous system (Langley, 1900), see ***terminal plexuses (Swanson & Bota, 2010)***

enteric plexuses (Hill, 1927)

enteroid processes (Soemmerring, 1778), see ***cerebral cortex gray matter (>1840)***

entire base of brain (Galen, c173), see ***brainstem (Schwalbe, 1881)***

entire base of encephalon (Galen, c173), see ***brainstem (Schwalbe, 1881)***

entire brain (Aristotle), see ***vertebrate brain (Cuvier, 1800)***

entire encephalon (Aristotle), see ***vertebrate brain (Cuvier, 1800)***

entorhinal area (Brodmann, 1909)

entrelacement transversal du gros faisceau fibreux (Gall & Spurzheim, 1810), see ***transverse peduncular tract (Gudden, 1870)***

epencephalon (Sharpey et al., 1867), see ***hindbrain (Baer, 1837)***

epencranis (Erasistratus, c310–c250 BC), see ***cerebellum (Aristotle)***

ependyma (>1840)

ependymal roof plate (>1840)

epicranis (Benedetti, 1502), see ***spinal cord (Galen, c162–c166)***

epigastric nervous center (Cruveilhier, 1836), see ***autonomic nerves (Langley, 1896)***

epigastric plexus (Cruveilhier, 1836), see ***autonomic nerves (Langley, 1896)***

epiglottal branches of superior laryngeal branches of pneumogastric nerve (Cruveilhier, 1836), see ***internal branch of superior laryngeal nerve (Fyfe, 1800)***

epipial layer (Key & Retzius, 1875)

epiploic nerves (Cloquet, 1828), see ***right gastroepiploic plexus (Wrisberg, 1800)***

epiploic plexus (Wrisberg, 1800), see ***peripheral nervous system (Meckel, 1817)***

epithalamic medullary stria (>1840)

epithalamus (His, 1893b)

epitrochlear branch of internal cutaneous nerve of arm (Cruveilhier, 1836), see ***medial cutaneous nerve of arm (>1840)***

ergot (Morand, 1748), see ***calcarine spur (Morand, 1748)***

ergot de Morand (Cruveilhier, 1836), see ***calcarine spur (Morand, 1748)***

erta della corna d' Ammone (Malacarne, 1780), see ***superficial medullary lamina of subiculum (Dejerine & Dejerine-Klumpke, 1895)***

esophageal branches of inferior laryngeal nerve (Arnold, 1834), see ***esophageal branches of recurrent laryngeal nerve (>1840)***

esophageal branches of pneumogastric nerve (Chaussier, 1809), see ***vagus nerve trunk (Wrisberg, 1786; Günther, 1786)***

esophageal branches of recurrent laryngeal nerve (Arnold, 1834)

esophageal branches of recurrent nerve (Cruveilhier, 1836), see ***esophageal branches of recurrent laryngeal nerve (>1840)***

esophageal branches of sympathetic trunk (>1840)

esophageal bridle (Lyonnet, 1762), see ***circumesophageal connective (>1840)***

esophageal cord of left side (Cloquet, 1816), see ***anterior vagal trunk (Wrisberg, 1780)***

esophageal cord of right side (Cloquet, 1816), see ***posterior vagal trunk (Wrisberg, 1780)***

esophageal ganglion (Cloquet, 1828), see ***autonomic ganglia (Langley, 1900)***

esophageal nerves (Loder, 1778) see ***upper esophageal branches of vagus nerve (Cloquet, 1828)***

esophageal plexus (Haller, 1762)

esophageal ring (Andersch & Soemmerring, 1792), see ***pharyngeal branches of vagus nerve (>1840)***

esophageal ring (Serres, 1824–1826), see ***circumesophageal connective (>1840)***

esophageal small ganglion (Walter, 1783), see ***autonomic ganglia (Langley, 1900)***

ethmoidal branch of nasal nerve (Arnold, 1834), see ***anterior ethmoidal nerve (>1840)***

ethmoidal branch of nasociliary nerve (Arnold, 1834), see ***anterior ethmoidal nerve (>1840)***

ethmoidal bulb (Quain, 1837), see ***olfactory bulb (Weitbrecht, 1751)*** *ethmoidal fascicle of nasal surculus (Bellingeri, 1818)*, see **anterior ethmoidal nerve (>1840)**

ethmoidal nerve (Burdin, 1803), see **greater palatine nerve (Cloquet, 1816)**

ethmoidal nerve (Chaussier, 1807), see **cerebral cortex (>1840)**

ethmoidal nerve (Günther, 1786), see **anterior ethmoidal nerve (>1840)**

ethmoidal pair of nerves (Burdin, 1803), see **nervous system (Monro, 1783)**

éventail de Vieussens (Cruveilhier, 1836), see **central nervous system white matter tracts (>1840)**

exortus crurum fornicis (Santorini, 1724), see **hypothalamic postcommissural fornix (>1840)**

exterior and posterior cardiac nerves (Lobstein, 1823), see **cardiac plexus (Keill, 1698)**

exterior branch of first branch of fifth pair (Haller, 1743), see **lacrimal nerve (Meckel, 1748; Bonhomme, 1748)**

exterior branch of fourth pair of cervical nerves (Neubauer, 1772), see **cervical plexus (Molinetti, 1675)**

exterior branch of nasal nerve (Scarpa, 1785), see **external nasal branch of anterior ethmoidal nerve (>1840)**

exterior branch of praetibio-digital nerve (Burdin, 1803), see **intermediate dorsal cutaneous nerve (>1840)**

exterior branch of supraorbital nerve (Günther, 1786), see **lateral branch of supraorbital nerve (>1840)**

exterior branch of tibial nerve (Burdin, 1803), see **lateral plantar nerve (>1840)**

exterior branch to tonsils of exterior palatine nerve (Günther, 1786), see **tonsillar branches of lateral palatine nerve (>1840)**

exterior branches of sympathetic nerve (Lobstein, 1823), see **communicating branches of spinal nerves (Wutzer, 1817)**

exterior dorsal nerve (Günther, 1786), see **sural nerve (Pietro da Cortona, 1741)**

exterior dorsal twig of foot of tibial communicating branch (Jördens, 1788), see **lateral calcaneal branches of sural nerve (>1840)**

exterior minor branch of major palatine nerve (Scarpa, 1785), see **greater palatine nerve (Cloquet, 1816)**

exterior minor lingual branch of glossopharyngeal nerve (Cloquet, 1828), see **lingual branches of glossopharyngeal nerve (Haller, 1762)**

exterior oculo-muscular pair of nerves (Burdin, 1803), see **abducens nerve (Heister, 1717)**

exterior palatine nerve (Günther, 1786), see **lateral palatine nerve (Henle, 1871)**

exterior palpebral branch of infraorbital nerve (Loder, 1778), see **inferior palpebral branches of infraorbital nerve (Meckel, 1748)**

exterior palpebral nerve (Haase, 1781), see **inferior palpebral branches of infraorbital nerve (Meckel, 1748)**

exterior scapular nerve (Mayer, 1794), see **suprascapular nerve (Bang, 1770)**

exterior sciatic nerve (Günther, 1786), see **common fibular nerve (>1840)**

exterior smaller medullary tract of anterior process of medulla oblongata (Vieussens, 1684), see **external capsule (Burdach, 1822)**

exterior twig of superior branch of first branch of fifth pair (Haller, 1743), see **supraorbital nerve (Meckel, 1753)**

externa membrana cerebri (Wenzel & Wenzel, 1812), see **dura (Galen, c177)**

external acoustic meatus nerves (Meckel, 1817)

external anastomotic filament of superficial frontal thread of supraorbital fascicle (Bellingeri, 1818), see **supraorbital nerve (Meckel, 1753)**

external and deep branch of back of foot of anterior tibial branch of external popliteal nerve (Cloquet, 1816), see **digital branch of deep fibular nerve (>1840)**

external and internal deep-seated branches of crural nerve (Quain, 1828), see **muscular branches of femoral nerve (Quain & Wilson, 1839)**

external and internal plantar nerves of external plantar nerve (Meckel, 1817), see **proper plantar digital nerves of lateral plantar nerve (>1840)**

external and internal plantar nerves of internal plantar nerve (Meckel, 1817), see **proper plantar digital nerves of medial plantar nerve (>1840)**

external and posterior cutaneous nerve (Bell, 1803b), see **posterior cutaneous nerve of thigh (Günther, 1786)**

external and posterior root of facial nerve (Meckel, 1817), see **intermediate nerve (>1840)**

external and superficial branch to back of foot of musculocutaneous branch of external popliteal nerve (Cloquet, 1816), see **intermediate dorsal cutaneous nerve (>1840)**

external and superior posterior femoral cutaneous nerve (Mayer, 1794), see **lateral cutaneous nerve of calf (>1840)**

external anterior branch of first pair of lumbar nerves (Winslow, 1733), see **iliohypogastric nerve (Schmidt, 1794)**

external anterior branch of small sciatic branch (Winslow, 1733), see **superficial fibular nerve (Fyfe, 1800)**

external anterior femoral cutaneous nerve (Bock, 1827), see **lateral cutaneous nerve of thigh (>1840)**

external appendix of fimbria (Volkmann, 1831), see **alveus (Burdach, 1822)**

external arcuate fibers (>1840), see **ventral external arcuate fibers (>1840)**

external arcuate fibers of septum (Cajal, 1901–1902), see **lateral arcuate fibers of septum (>1840)**

external auditory meatus branch of anterior auricular nerve (Arnold, 1834), see **external acoustic meatus nerves (Meckel, 1817)**

external auditory meatus branch of superficial temporal nerve (Arnold, 1834), see **external acoustic meatus nerves (Meckel, 1817)**

external auricular branches of superficial temporal nerve (Todd, 1836–1839), see **anterior auricular nerves (>1840)**

external branch of accessory nerve (Scarpa, 1788), see **external branch of accessory nerve trunk (Meckel, 1817)**

external branch of accessory nerve trunk (Meckel, 1817)

external branch of accessory vagal pair (Soemmerring, 1791), see **external branch of accessory nerve trunk (Meckel, 1817)** *external branch of anterior branch of obturator nerve (Cloquet, 1816)*, see **cutaneous branch of obturator nerve (>1840)**

external branch of ascending branch of external frontal nerve (Cruveilhier, 1836), see **lateral branch of supraorbital nerve (>1840)**

external branch of ascending branch of supraorbital nerve (Cruveilhier, 1836), see **lateral branch of supraorbital nerve (>1840)**

external branch of carotid nerve (Arnold, 1834), see **internal carotid plexus (>1840)**

external branch of common motor nerve inferior terminal branch (Cruveilhier, 1836), see **nerve to inferior oblique (>1840)**

external branch of conjugations of nerves from loynes and holy bone (Paré, 1561), see **spinal nerve dorsal branch (Meckel, 1817)**

external branch of crural nerve proper (Salmon, 1713), see **common fibular nerve (>1840)**

external branch of crural trunk (Diemerbroeck, 1672), see **common fibular nerve (>1840)**

external branch of cubital nerve (Haase, 1781), see **superficial branch of ulnar nerve (Fyfe, 1800)**

external branch of cutaneous nerve (Fyfe, 1800), see **anterior branch of medial cutaneous nerve of forearm (>1840)**

external branch of deep branch of internal pudendal nerve (Cruveilhier, 1836), see **dorsal nerve of penis (Camper, 1762)**

external branch of deep peroneal nerve (Bock, 1827), see **digital branch of deep fibular nerve (>1840)**

external branch of deep peroneal nerve (Fischer, 1791), see **muscular branches of deep fibular nerve (>1840)**

external branch of descending laryngeal nerve (Swan, 1830), see **external branch of superior laryngeal nerve (Fyfe, 1800)**

external branch of dorsal branch of penis of internal pudendal nerve (Cruveilhier, 1836), see **dorsal nerve of penis (Camper, 1762)**

external branch of dorsal branch of radial nerve (Bock, 1827), see **superficial branch of radial nerve (Martin, 1781)**

external branch of dorsal branch of thoracic nerve (Bock, 1827), see **lateral branch of spinal nerve dorsal branch (>1840)**

external branch of dorsal nerve (Swan, 1830), see **lateral cutaneous branch of intercostal nerves (>1840)**

external branch of dorsal radial nerve (Bock, 1824), see **dorsal digital nerves of radial nerve (>1840)**

external branch of external cutaneous nerve of arm (Cloquet, 1816), see **lateral cutaneous nerve of forearm (>1840)**

external branch of external least branch of palatine nerve (Meckel, 1748), see **tonsillar branches of lateral palatine nerve (>1840)**

external branch of external plantar nerve (Jördens, 1788), see **superficial branch of lateral plantar nerve (>1840)**

external branch of external plantar nerve (Meckel, 1817), see **common plantar digital nerves of lateral plantar nerve (>1840)**

external branch of external pudic nerve (Quain, 1828), see **femoral branch of genitofemoral nerve (>1840)**

external branch of external spermatic nerve (Walter, 1783), see **femoral branch of genitofemoral nerve (>1840)**

external branch of fibular nerve (Quain, 1828), see **intermediate dorsal cutaneous nerve (>1840)**

external branch of first division of fifth pair of nerves (Todd, 1836–1839), see **lacrimal nerve (Meckel, 1748; Bonhomme, 1748)**

external branch of frontal branch of external frontal nerve (Cruveilhier, 1836), see **lateral branch of supraorbital nerve (>1840)**

external branch of frontal branch of supraorbital nerve (Cruveilhier, 1836), see **lateral branch of supraorbital nerve (>1840)**

external branch of frontal nerve (Quain, 1828), see **supraorbital nerve (Meckel, 1753)**

external branch of genitocrural nerve (Meckel, 1817), see **femoral branch of genitofemoral nerve (>1840)**

external branch of greater frontal nerve (Meckel, 1753), see **lateral branch of supraorbital nerve (>1840)**

external branch of hypogastric nerve of second accessory lumbar ganglion (Walter, 1783), see **lumbar splanchnic nerve (Cruveilhier, 1836)**

external branch of iliohypogastric nerve (Bock, 1827), see **lateral cutaneous nerve of iliohypogastric nerve (>1840)**

external branch of iliohypogastric nerve (Cloquet, 1828), see **iliohypogastric nerve (Schmidt, 1794)**

external branch of ilio-inguinal nerve (Cloquet, 1828), see **ilio-inguinal nerve (Schmidt, 1794)**

external branch of internal cutaneous nerve of arm (Cloquet, 1816), see **medial cutaneous nerve of arm (>1840)**

external branch of internal inguinal branch of lumbar plexus (Cruveilhier, 1836), see **femoral branch of genitofemoral nerve (>1840)**

external branch of internal plantar nerve (Fischer, 1791), see **medial plantar nerve (>1840)**

external branch of internal plantar nerve (Jördens, 1788), see **common plantar digital nerves of medial plantar nerve (>1840)**

external branch of lacrimal nerve (Arnold, 1834), see **communicating branch of lacrimal nerve with zygomatic nerve (>1840)**

external branch of laryngeal nerve (Haase, 1781), see **external branch of superior laryngeal nerve (Fyfe, 1800)**

external branch of lumboinguinal nerve (Bock, 1827), see **femoral branch of genitofemoral nerve (>1840)**

external branch of musculocutaneous nerve (Cruveilhier, 1836), see **lateral cutaneous nerve of forearm (>1840)**

external branch of musculo-cutaneous nerve (Quain & Wilson, 1839), see **intermediate dorsal cutaneous nerve (>1840)**

external branch of nasal nerve (Scarpa, 1785), see **external nasal branch of anterior ethmoidal nerve (>1840)**

external branch of nasociliary nerve (Meckel, 1817), see **communicating branch of nasociliary nerve with ciliary ganglion (>1840)**

external branch of orbital nerve (Jacobson, 1818), see **ophthalmic nerve (Winslow, 1733)**
external branch of palatine nerve (Bang, 1770), see **lateral palatine nerve (Henle, 1871)**
external branch of palmar cutaneous nerve (Cruveilhier, 1836), see **palmar branch of median nerve (Bock, 1827)**
external branch of palpebro-frontal nerve (Burdin, 1803), see **lateral branch of supraorbital nerve (>1840)**
external branch of penile nerve (Bock, 1827), see **dorsal nerve of penis (Camper, 1762)**
external branch of perforating or cutaneous branch of second dorsal nerve (Cruveilhier, 1836), see **intercostobrachial nerves (>1840)**
external branch of peroneal nerve (Quain, 1828), see **intermediate dorsal cutaneous nerve (>1840)**
external branch of posterior branch of abdominal nerve (Bock, 1827), see **lateral branch of spinal nerve dorsal branch (>1840)**
external branch of posterior branch of lumbar nerve (Bock, 1827), see **lateral branch of spinal nerve dorsal branch (>1840)**
external branch of posterior crural nerve (Vieussens, 1684), see **common fibular nerve (>1840)**
external branch of radial nerve (Haase, 1781), see **superficial branch of radial nerve (Martin, 1781)**
external branch of recurrent branch of cutaneous branch of inferior gluteal nerve (Cruveilhier, 1836), see **inferior clunial nerves (>1840)**
external branch of sciatic nerve trunk (Günther, 1786), see **common fibular nerve (>1840)**
external branch of spinal nerve dorsal branch (Meckel, 1817), see **lateral branch of spinal nerve dorsal branch (>1840)**
external branch of superficial branch of radial nerve (Cruveilhier, 1836), see **dorsal digital nerves of radial nerve (>1840)**
external branch of superficial peroneal nerve (Fischer, 1791), see **intermediate dorsal cutaneous nerve (>1840)**
external branch of superficial terminal branch of cubital nerve (Cruveilhier, 1836), see **common palmar digital nerves of ulnar nerve (>1840)**
external branch of superficial terminal branch of external plantar nerve (Cruveilhier, 1836), see **common plantar digital nerves of lateral plantar nerve (>1840)**
external branch of superior laryngeal nerve (Fyfe, 1800)
external branch of third pair (Haller, 1743), see **nerve to inferior oblique (>1840)**
external branch of trunk of pharyngeal branches of vagus (Bischoff, 1832), see **pharyngeal branches of vagus nerve (>1840)**
external branches of dorsal branches of foot (Bell, 1803b), see **intermediate dorsal cutaneous nerve (>1840)**
external branches of inferior maxillary nerve (Cruveilhier, 1836), see **anterior branch of mandibular nerve (>1840)**
external branches of metatarsal nerves (Bell, 1803b), see **intermediate dorsal cutaneous nerve (>1840)**
external branches of olfactory nerves (Langenbeck, 1826–1830), see **olfactory nerve (Winslow, 1733)**
external branches of spermatic nerve (Fyfe, 1800), see **genital branch of genitofemoral nerve (>1840)**
external branches of superior cervical ganglion (Cruveilhier, 1836), see **communicating branches of spinal nerves (Wutzer, 1817)**
external branches of thoracic part of great sympathetic (Cruveilhier, 1836), see **communicating branches of spinal nerves (Wutzer, 1817)**
external calcanean nerves (Cruveilhier, 1836), see **lateral calcaneal branches of sural nerve (>1840)**
external capsule (Burdach, 1822)
external capsule (Reil, 1809b), see **central nervous system white matter tracts (>1840)**
external carotid nerve (Arnold, 1834), see **internal carotid plexus (>1840)**
external carotid plexus (>1840)
external carotid soft nerve trunk (Arnold, 1834), see **external carotid plexus (>1840)**
external carotid vascular nerve trunk (Arnold, 1834), see **external carotid plexus (>1840)**
external collateral branch of little finger of dorsal collateral branches of cubital nerve internal dorsal branch of hand (Cruveilhier, 1836), see **dorsal digital nerves of ulnar nerve (>1840)**
external collateral branch of middle finger of fifth terminal branch of median nerve (Cruveilhier, 1836), see **proper palmar digital nerves of median nerve (>1840)**
external collateral branch of ring finger of dorsal collateral branches of cubital nerve internal dorsal branch of hand (Cruveilhier, 1836), see **dorsal digital nerves of ulnar nerve (>1840)**
external collateral nerve of big toe (Cruveilhier, 1836), see **proper plantar digital nerves of medial plantar nerve (>1840)**
external collateral nerve of fourth toe (Cruveilhier, 1836), see **proper plantar digital nerves of lateral plantar nerve (>1840)**
external collateral nerve of little toe (Cruveilhier, 1836), see **proper plantar digital nerves of lateral plantar nerve (>1840)**
external collateral nerve of third toe (Cruveilhier, 1836), see **proper plantar digital nerves of medial plantar nerve (>1840)**
external common hemorrhoidal nerve (Meckel, 1817), see **pudendal nerve (Camper, 1762)**
external common pudendal nerve (Mayer, 1794), see **dorsal nerve of penis (Camper, 1762)**
external common pudendohemorrhoidal nerve (Meckel, 1817), see **pudendal nerve (Camper, 1762)**
external cutaneous branch of lumbar plexus (Quain, 1832), see **lateral cutaneous nerve of thigh (>1840)**
external cutaneous branch of peroneal nerve (Martin, 1781), see **lateral cutaneous nerve of calf (>1840)**
external cutaneous branch of peroneal nerve (Meckel, 1817), see **intermediate dorsal cutaneous nerve (>1840)**
external cutaneous branch of radial nerve (Günther, 1786), see **posterior cutaneous nerve of forearm (>1840)**
external cutaneous nerve (Du Verney, 1697), see **musculocutaneous nerve (Du Verney, 1697)**

external cutaneous nerve (Jördens, 1788), see **lateral cutaneous nerve of calf (>1840)**

external cutaneous nerve (Styx, 1782), see **lateral cutaneous nerve of thigh (>1840)**

external cutaneous nerve of arm (Cloquet, 1816), see **musculocutaneous nerve (Du Verney, 1697)**

external cutaneous nerve of arm (Mayer, 1794), see **inferior lateral cutaneous nerve of arm (>1840)**

external cutaneous nerve of back of foot (Bock, 1827), see **lateral dorsal cutaneous nerve (>1840)**

external cutaneous nerve of foot (Günther, 1786), see **sural nerve (Pietro da Cortona, 1741)**

external cutaneous nerve of foot (Mayer, 1794), see **intermediate dorsal cutaneous nerve (>1840)**

external cutaneous nerve of leg (Bock, 1827), see **lateral cutaneous nerve of calf (>1840)**

external cutaneous nerve of thigh (Bell, 1803a), see **lateral cutaneous nerve of thigh (>1840)**

external cutaneous tibial nerve of foot (Meckel, 1817), see **sural nerve (Pietro da Cortona, 1741)**

external deep branch of dorsum of foot of anterior tibial branch of external peroneal sciatic nerve (Cruveilhier, 1836), see **digital branch of deep fibular nerve (>1840)**

external deep branch of hard nerve (Meckel, 1753), see **posterior auricular nerve (Meckel, 1753)**

external deep branch of portio major and minor of facial nerve (Bellingeri, 1818), see **posterior auricular nerve (Meckel, 1753)**

external deep nerve of hard nerve (Meckel, 1753), see **posterior auricular nerve (Meckel, 1753)**

external deep temporal branch of inferior maxillary nerve (Todd, 1836–1839), see **posterior deep temporal nerve (Arnold, 1834)**

external deep temporal branch of masseteric branch (Loder, 1778), see **masseteric nerve (Meckel, 1748)**

external deep temporal branch of third branch of fifth pair (Meckel, 1748), see **posterior deep temporal nerve (Arnold, 1834)**

external descending nerve of neck (Andersch & Soemmerring, 1792), see **inferior root of ansa cervicalis (>1840)**

external descending nerve of neck of third nerves of neck (Andersch & Soemmerring, 1792), see **inferior root of ansa cervicalis (>1840)**

external division of great sciatic nerve (Quain, 1828), see **common fibular nerve (>1840)**

external dorsal branch of cubital nerve internal dorsal branch of hand (Cruveilhier, 1836), see **dorsal digital nerves of ulnar nerve (>1840)**

external dorsal branch of deep peroneal nerve (Fischer, 1791), see **muscular branches of deep fibular nerve (>1840)**

external dorsal branch of hand of radial nerve (Cruveilhier, 1836), see **superficial branch of radial nerve (Martin, 1781)**

external dorsal branch of inframalleolar nerve (Fischer, 1791), see **lateral dorsal cutaneous nerve (>1840)**

external dorsal branch of superficial peroneal nerve (Fischer, 1791), see **intermediate dorsal cutaneous nerve (>1840)**

external dorsal branch of thumb of anterior branch of radial nerve (Cloquet, 1828), see **dorsal digital nerves of radial nerve (>1840)**

external dorsal collateral branch of index finger of radial nerve (Cruveilhier, 1836), see **dorsal digital nerves of radial nerve (>1840)**

external dorsal collateral nerve of big toe (Cruveilhier, 1836), see **dorsal digital nerves of medial dorsal cutaneous nerve (>1840)**

external dorsal collateral nerve of fifth metatarsal (Cruveilhier, 1836), see **dorsal digital nerves of lateral dorsal cutaneous nerve (>1840)**

external dorsal collateral nerve of fourth toe (Cruveilhier, 1836), see **dorsal digital nerves of lateral dorsal cutaneous nerve (>1840)**

external dorsal collateral nerve of second toe (Cruveilhier, 1836), see **dorsal digital nerves of medial dorsal cutaneous nerve (>1840)**

external dorsal collateral nerve of third toe (Cruveilhier, 1836), see **dorsal digital nerves of intermediate dorsal cutaneous nerve (>1840)**

external dorsal digital nerve of big toe from external metatarsal twig (Fischer, 1791), see **dorsal digital nerves of medial dorsal cutaneous nerve (>1840)**

external dorsal digital nerve of big toe from metatarsus pollicis nerve (Fischer, 1791), see **dorsal digital nerves of digital branch of deep fibular nerve (>1840)**

external dorsal digital nerve of fifth toe from external metatarsal branch of inframalleolar nerve (Fischer, 1791), see **dorsal digital nerve of lateral dorsal cutaneous nerve (>1840)**

external dorsal digital nerve of fourth toe from external branch of superficial peroneal nerve (Fischer, 1791), see **dorsal digital nerves of intermediate dorsal cutaneous nerve (>1840)**

external dorsal digital nerve of fourth toe from internal metatarsal branch of inframalleolar nerve (Fischer, 1791), see **dorsal digital nerves of lateral dorsal cutaneous nerve (>1840)**

external dorsal digital nerve of second toe (Fischer, 1791), see **dorsal digital nerves of medial dorsal cutaneous nerve (>1840)**

external dorsal digital nerve of third toe from external branch of superficial peroneal nerve (Fischer, 1791), see **dorsal digital nerves of intermediate dorsal cutaneous nerve (>1840)**

external dorsal digital nerve of third toe from internal metatarsal branch of inframalleolar nerve (Fischer, 1791), see **dorsal digital nerves of lateral dorsal cutaneous nerve (>1840)**

external dorsal nerve of big toe (Bock, 1827), see **dorsal digital nerves of medial dorsal cutaneous nerve (>1840)**

external dorsal nerve of big toe (Mayer, 1794), see **dorsal digital nerves of digital branch of deep fibular nerve (>1840)**

external dorsal nerve of first small toe (Mayer, 1794), see **dorsal digital nerves of digital branch of deep fibular nerve (>1840)**

external dorsal nerve of foot (Bock, 1827), see **lateral dorsal cutaneous nerve (>1840)**

external dorsal nerve of fourth small toe (Mayer, 1794), see **dorsal digital nerves of intermediate dorsal cutaneous nerve (>1840)**
external dorsal nerve of fourth toe (Bock, 1827), see **dorsal digital nerves of lateral dorsal cutaneous nerve (>1840)**
external dorsal nerve of index finger (Mayer, 1794), see **dorsal digital nerves of radial nerve (>1840)**
external dorsal nerve of little finger (Mayer, 1794), see **dorsal digital nerves of ulnar nerve (>1840)**
external dorsal nerve of little toe (Bock, 1827), see **dorsal digital nerves of lateral dorsal cutaneous nerve (>1840)**
external dorsal nerve of middle finger (Mayer, 1794), see **dorsal digital nerves of radial nerve (>1840)**
external dorsal nerve of ring finger (Mayer, 1794), see **dorsal digital nerves of ulnar nerve (>1840)**
external dorsal nerve of second small toe (Mayer, 1794), see **dorsal digital nerves of intermediate dorsal cutaneous nerve (>1840)**
external dorsal nerve of second toe (Bock, 1827), see **dorsal digital nerves of medial dorsal cutaneous nerve (>1840)**
external dorsal nerve of smallest toe (Mayer, 1794), see **dorsal digital nerves of intermediate dorsal cutaneous nerve (>1840)**
external dorsal nerve of third small toe (Mayer, 1794), see **dorsal digital nerves of intermediate dorsal cutaneous nerve (>1840)**
external dorsal nerve of third toe (Bock, 1827), see **dorsal digital nerves of lateral dorsal cutaneous nerve (>1840)**
external dorsal nerve of thumb (Mayer, 1794), see **dorsal digital nerves of radial nerve (>1840)**
external dorsal twig of foot of deep branch of peroneal nerve (Jördens, 1788), see **digital branch of deep fibular nerve (>1840)**
external dorsal twig of foot of superficial branch of peroneal nerve (Jördens, 1788), see **intermediate dorsal cutaneous nerve (>1840)**
external fascicle of crotaphitic surculus of ganglioform plexus of inferior maxillary branch (Bellingeri, 1818), see **posterior deep temporal nerve (Arnold, 1834)**
external filament of ethmoidal branch of nasal nerve (Cruveilhier, 1836), see **external nasal branch of anterior ethmoidal nerve (>1840)**
external filament of internal branch of ilio-inguinal nerve (Cloquet, 1828), see **ilio-inguinal nerve (Schmidt, 1794)**
external filament of internal nasal branch of nasal nerve (Cruveilhier, 1836), see **external nasal branch of anterior ethmoidal nerve (>1840)**
external filament of superior anastomotic thread of malo-palpebral fascicle of subcutaneous malar surculus (Bellingeri, 1818), see **zygomaticofacial nerve (>1840)**
external fornix (Arnold, 1838b), see **cingulum (Burdach, 1822)**
external frontal nerve (Cruveilhier, 1836; Todd, 1836–1839), see **supraorbital nerve (Meckel, 1753)**
external frontal thread of supratrochlear fascicle (Bellingeri, 1818), see **supratrochlear nerve (Schaarschmidt, 1750)**
external ganglionnary cord (Meckel, 1817), see **sympathetic cord (>1840)**
external gastrocnemius branch of internal popliteal nerve (Bock, 1827), see **nerves to gastrocnemius (>1840)**
external geniculate body (Burdach, 1822), see **dorsal lateral geniculate nucleus (>1840)**
external geniculate tubercle (Arnold, 1838b), see **dorsal lateral geniculate nucleus (>1840)**
external gray matter mass of great superior cerebral ganglion (Gall & Spurzheim, 1810), see **cerebral nuclei (Swanson, 2000a)**
external gray nucleus (Burdach, 1822), see **dorsal part of thalamus (Herrick, 1910)**
external head of median nerve (Quain & Wilson, 1839), see **lateral root of median nerve (>1840)**
external hemorrhoidal branch of internal pudic nerve (Quain & Wilson, 1839), see **inferior rectal nerves (>1840)**
external hemorrhoidal branch of pudendal nerve (Quain & Wilson, 1839), see **inferior rectal nerves (>1840)**
external hemorrhoidal branches of fourth sacral pair (Fischer, 1791), see **perineal branch of fourth sacral nerve (>1841)**
external hemorrhoidal nerves (Bock, 1827), see **inferior rectal nerves (>1840)**
external hemorrhoidal nerves (Walter, 1783), see **inferior rectal nerves (>1840)**
external humeral cutaneous nerve (Frotscher, 1788), see **superior lateral cutaneous nerve of arm (>1840)**
external inferior cutaneous nasal nerve (Meckel, 1817), see **external nasal branches of infraorbital nerve (>1840)**
external inferior labial branch (Meckel, 1748), see **inferior labial branches of mental nerve (Meckel, 1753)**
external inferior labial nerve (Mayer, 1794), see **inferior labial branches of mental nerve (Meckel, 1753)**
external inferior palpebral nerve (Arnold, 1834), see **inferior palpebral branches of infraorbital nerve (Meckel, 1748)**
external inferior palpebral threads of outermost superior labial fascicle of infraorbital surculus (Bellingeri, 1818), see **superior labial branches of infraorbital nerve (Meckel, 1748)**
external inferior part of striated body (Pourfour du Petit, 1710), see **cerebral nuclei (Swanson, 2000a)**
external inferior posterior cutaneous nerve (Cloquet, 1828), see **sural nerve (Pietro da Cortona, 1741)**
external inferior sulcus (Meckel, 1817), see **prepyramidal fissure (Hayashi, 1924)**
external inferior superficial nasal nerve (Meckel, 1817), see **external nasal branches of infraorbital nerve (>1840)**
external inferior twig of common motor nerve (Meckel, 1817), see **nerve to inferior oblique (>1840)**
external inguinal branch of eternal spermatic branch of first lumbar nerve (Günther, 1786), see **femoral branch of genitofemoral nerve (>1840)**
external inguinal branch of lumbar plexus (Cruveilhier, 1836), see **ilio-inguinal nerve (Schmidt, 1794)**
external inguinal nerve (Fischer, 1791), see **femoral branch of genitofemoral nerve (>1840)**

external inguinal nerve (Martin, 1781), see **genitofemoral nerve (>1840)**

external interosseous nerve (Günther, 1786), see **posterior interosseous nerve (Quain & Wilson, 1839)**

external interosseous nerve of forearm (Bock, 1827), see **deep branch of radial nerve (Martin, 1781)**

external labial branch of infraorbital nerve (Bock, 1817), see **superior labial branches of infraorbital nerve (Meckel, 1748)**

external labial thread of mental fascicle of inferior alveolar surculus of inferior maxillary branch (Bellingeri, 1818), see **inferior labial branches of mental nerve (Meckel, 1753)**

external lacrimal nerve (Le Cat, 1768), see **lacrimal nerve (Meckel, 1748; Bonhomme, 1748)**

external laryngeal branch of superior laryngeal branch of pneumogastric nerve (Cruveilhier, 1836), see **external branch of superior laryngeal nerve (Fyfe, 1800)**

external laryngeal branch of vocal nerve (Bock, 1817), see **external branch of superior laryngeal nerve (Fyfe, 1800)**

external laryngeal nerve (Soemmerring, 1791), see **external branch of superior laryngeal nerve (Fyfe, 1800)**

external lateral lingual branch of eighth pair of nerves of head (Andersch & Soemmerring, 1792), see **lingual branches of glossopharyngeal nerve (Haller, 1762)**

external lateral lingual branch of ninth nerves of head (Andersch, 1797), see **lingual branches of glossopharyngeal nerve (Haller, 1762)**

external lesser frontal nerve (Meckel, 1753), see **supratrochlear nerve (Schaarschmidt, 1750)**

external maleolar filament of musculocutaneous branch of external popliteal sciatic nerve (Cruveilhier, 1836), see **muscular branches of superficial fibular nerve (>1840)**

external medullary lamina (>1840)

external medullary root of olfactory nerve (Haase, 1781), see **lateral olfactory tract (>1840)**

external metatarsal branch of inframalleolar nerve (Fischer, 1791), see **lateral dorsal cutaneous nerve (>1840)**

external metatarsal twig of external dorsal twig of foot of superficial branch of peroneal nerve (Jördens, 1788), see **intermediate dorsal cutaneous nerve (>1840)**

external metatarsal twig of internal branch of superficial peroneal nerve (Fischer, 1791), see **medial dorsal cutaneous nerve (>1840)**

external motor nerve filaments (Meckel, 1817), see **abducens nerve rootlets (>1840)**

external motor nerve roots (Günther, 1786), see **abducens nerve root (>1840)**

external motor nerve trunk (Günther, 1786), see **abducens nerve trunk (>1840)**

external musculo-cutaneous branch of lumbar plexus (Quain, 1828), see **ilio-inguinal nerve (Schmidt, 1794)**

external musculo-cutaneous nerve (Quain & Wilson, 1839), see **ilio-inguinal nerve (Schmidt, 1794)**

external nasal branch of anterior ethmoidal nerve (>1840)

external nasal branch of ethmoidal branch of nasal nerve (Arnold, 1834), see **external nasal branch of anterior ethmoidal nerve (>1840)**

external nasal branch of ethmoidal branch of nasociliary nerve (Arnold, 1834), see **external nasal branch of anterior ethmoidal nerve (>1840)**

external nasal branch of nasal nerve (Cruveilhier, 1836), see **infratrochlear nerve (Schaarschmidt, 1750)**

external nasal branches of infraorbital nerve (>1840)

external nasal nerve (Meckel, 1817), see **infratrochlear nerve (Schaarschmidt, 1750)**

external nasal nerve (>1840), see **external nasal branch of anterior ethmoidal nerve (>1840)**

external nasal threads of ethmoidal fascicle (Bellingeri, 1818), see **lateral nasal branches of internal nasal branches of anterior ethmoidal nerve (>1840)**

external nerve of back of foot (Bock, 1827), see **lateral dorsal cutaneous nerve (>1840)**

external nerve of vastus internus (Cruveilhier, 1836), see **muscular branches of femoral nerve (Quain & Wilson, 1839)**

external nervous system (Meckel, 1817), see **peripheral nervous system (Meckel, 1817)**

external nucleus of colliculus of optic nerve (Arnold, 1838b), see **dorsal part of thalamus (Herrick, 1910)**

external nucleus of thalamus of optic nerve (Arnold, 1838b), see **dorsal part of thalamus (Herrick, 1910)**

external occipital branch of cervical plexus (Cruveilhier, 1836), see **lesser occipital nerve (Mayer, 1794)**

external olfactory convolution (Gerdy, 1838), see **medial orbital gyrus (>1840)**

external palatine fascicle of sphenopalatine ganglion (Bellingeri, 1818), see **lateral palatine nerve (Henle, 1871)**

external palatine nerve (Scarpa, 1785), see **lateral palatine nerve (Henle, 1871)**

external palatine thread of anterior palatine fascicle (Bellingeri, 1818), see **greater palatine nerve (Cloquet, 1816)**

external palmar branch of index finger of first common digital branch of median nerve (Cloquet, 1828), see **proper palmar digital nerves of median nerve (>1840)**

external palmar branch of middle finger of second common digital branch of median nerve (Cloquet, 1828), see **proper palmar digital nerves of median nerve (>1840)**

external palmar branch of ring finger of third common digital branch of median nerve (Cloquet, 1828), see **proper palmar digital nerves of median nerve (>1840)**

external palmar branch of thumb of median nerve (Cloquet, 1828), see **common palmar digital nerves of median nerve (>1840)**

external palmar nerve of little finger (Cloquet, 1828), see **proper palmar digital nerves of ulnar nerve (>1840)**

external part of brain (Bartholin, 1662), see **cerebral cortex gray matter (>1840)**

external part of corpus striatum (Vicq d'Azyr, 1786), see **cerebral nuclei (Swanson, 2000a)**

external part of lemniscus (Reil, 1809c), see **medial lemniscus (>1840)**

external part of medullary capsule (Reil, 1809b), see **central nervous system white matter tracts (>1840)**

external part of superior great cerebral ganglion (Gall & Spurzheim, 1810), see **putamen (Burdach, 1822)**

external pectoral subcutaneous supraclavicular branch (Peipers, 1793), see **intermediate supraclavicular nerves (>1840)**
external perineal branch of perineal branch of internal pudendal nerve (Cruveilhier, 1836), see **perineal nerve (Camper, 1762)**
external peroneal branch of external popliteal sciatic nerve (Cruveilhier, 1836), see **superficial fibular nerve (Fyfe, 1800)**
external pia mater (Meckel, 1817), see **pia (Galen, c192)**
external plantar branch of tibial nerve (Martin, 1781), see **lateral plantar nerve (>1840)**
external plantar collateral nerve of second toe (Cruveilhier, 1836), see **proper plantar digital nerves of medial plantar nerve (>1840)**
external plantar digital twig of big toe (Fischer, 1791), see **proper plantar digital nerves of medial plantar nerve (>1840)**
external plantar digital twig of fourth toe (Fischer, 1791), see **proper plantar digital nerves of medial plantar nerve (>1840)**
external plantar digital twig of second toe (Fischer, 1791), see **proper plantar digital nerves of medial plantar nerve (>1840)**
external plantar digital twig of third toe (Fischer, 1791), see **proper plantar digital nerves of medial plantar nerve (>1840)**
external plantar nerve (Winslow, 1733), see **lateral plantar nerve (>1840)**
external plantar nerve of big toe (Mayer, 1794), see **proper plantar digital nerves of medial plantar nerve (>1840)**
external plantar nerve of first small toe (Mayer, 1794), see **proper plantar digital nerves of medial plantar nerve (>1840)**
external plantar nerve of fourth small toe (Mayer, 1794), see **proper plantar digital nerves of lateral plantar nerve (>1840)**
external plantar nerve of fourth toe (Bock, 1827), see **proper plantar digital nerves of lateral plantar nerve (>1840)**
external plantar nerve of little toe (Mayer, 1794), see **proper plantar digital nerves of lateral plantar nerve (>1840)**
external plantar nerve of second small toe (Mayer, 1794), see **proper plantar digital nerves of medial plantar nerve (>1840)**
external plantar nerve of second toe (Meckel, 1817), see **proper plantar digital nerve of medial plantar nerve (>1840)**
external plantar nerve of third toe (Meckel, 1817), see **proper plantar digital nerve of medial plantar nerve (>1840)**
external plantar twig of big toe (Jördens, 1788), see **proper plantar digital nerves of medial plantar nerve (>1840)**
external plantar twig of fifth digit (Jördens, 1788), see **proper plantar digital nerves of lateral plantar nerve (>1840)**
external plantar twig of fourth digit (Jördens, 1788), see **proper plantar digital nerves of medial plantar nerve (>1840)**
external plantar twig of second digit (Jördens, 1788), see **proper plantar digital nerves of medial plantar nerve (>1840)**
external plantar twig of third digit (Jördens, 1788), see **proper plantar digital nerves of medial plantar nerve (>1840)**
external popliteal nerve (Winslow, 1733), see **common fibular nerve (>1840)**
external popliteal sciatic nerve (Sabatier, 1775), see **common fibular nerve (>1840)**
external portion of fifth pair of nerves (Todd, 1836–1839), see **trigeminal nerve branches (Winslow, 1733)**
external posterior cord of spinal marrow (Meckel, 1817), see **cuneate fascicle (Müller, 1834)**
external pterygoid branch of buccal nerve (Arnold, 1834), see **lateral pterygoid nerve (>1840)**
external pterygoid branch of inferior maxillary nerve (Quain & Wilson, 1839), see **lateral pterygoid nerve (>1840)**
external pterygoid nerve (Quain & Wilson, 1839), see **lateral pterygoid nerve (>1840)**
external pudendal nerve (Mayer, 1794), see **pudendal nerve (Camper, 1762)**
external pudendal plexus (Bock, 1827), see **sacral plexus (Vesalius, 1543a)**
external pudic nerve (Bell, 1803), see **perineal nerve (Camper, 1762)**
external pudic nerve (Meckel, 1817), see **genitofemoral nerve (>1840)**
external radial cutaneous branch of radial nerve (Cruveilhier, 1836), see **posterior cutaneous nerve of forearm (>1840)**
external ramus of ophthalmic nerve (Winslow, 1733), see **lacrimal nerve (Meckel, 1748; Bonhomme, 1748)**
external respiratory nerve (Bell, 1821), see **long thoracic nerve (Quain & Wilson, 1839)**
external root of external ocular motor nerve (Cruveilhier, 1836), see **abducens nerve rootlets (>1840)**
external root of olfactory nerve (Swan, 1830), see **lateral olfactory tract (>1840)**
external saphenous branch of internal popliteal nerve (Cloquet, 1816), see **tibial root of sural nerve (>1840)**
external saphenous nerve (Cloquet, 1816), see **sural nerve (Pietro da Cortona, 1741)**
external saphenous nerve branch of communication with external branch of musculo-cutaneous (Quain & Wilson, 1839), see **sural nerve (Pietro da Cortona, 1741)**
external scapular nerve (Günther, 1786), see **suprascapular nerve (Bang, 1770)**
external sciatic nerve (Winslow, 1733), see **common fibular nerve (>1840)**
external spermatic branch of first lumbar nerve (Günther, 1786), see **genitofemoral nerve (>1840)**
external spermatic nerve (Walter, 1783), see **genitofemoral nerve (>1840)**
external sphenopalatine nerves (Cruveilhier, 1836), see **lateral posterior superior nasal nerves (>1840)**
external striated body (Rolando, 1831), see **cerebral nuclei (Swanson, 2000a)**

external subcutaneous branch of radial nerve (Klint, 1784), see **posterior cutaneous nerve of forearm (>1840)**

external subcutaneous branch of radial nerve (Loder, 1803), see **inferior lateral cutaneous nerve of arm (>1840)**

external subcutaneous filament of deep frontal thread of supraorbital fascicle (Bellingeri, 1818), see **supraorbital nerve (Meckel, 1753)**

external subcutaneous nerve of radial nerve (Loder, 1803), see **inferior lateral cutaneous nerve of arm (>1840)**

external superior carotid nerve (Arnold, 1834), see **internal carotid plexus (>1840)**

external superior labial fascicle of infraorbital surculus (Bellingeri, 1818), see **superior labial branches of infraorbital nerve (Meckel, 1748)**

external superior labial nerve (Mayer, 1794), see **superior labial branches of infraorbital nerve (Meckel, 1748)**

external superior nasal nerves (Günther, 1786), see **external nasal branch of anterior ethmoidal nerve (>1840)**

external superior palpebral nerve (Meckel, 1753), see **supraorbital nerve (Meckel, 1753)**

external superior subsural cutaneous nerve (Knox, 1832), see **sural nerve (Pietro da Cortona, 1741)**

external supraorbital branch of greater frontal nerve (Meckel, 1753), see **lateral branch of supraorbital nerve (>1840)**

external suture of corpus callosum (Bock, 1824), see **longitudinal striae (>1840)**

external suture of corpus callosum (Meckel, 1817), see **corpus callosum (Galen, c177)**

external temporal branch of inferior maxillary nerve (Le Cat, 1768), see **auriculotemporal nerve (Haller, 1762)**

external temporal branch of temporo-malar branch of second division of fifth pair of nerves (Todd, 1836–1839), see **zygomaticotemporal nerve (>1840)**

external temporal branch of zygomatic branch of hard nerve (Meckel, 1753), see **temporal branches of facial nerve (Swan, 1830)**

external temporal nerve (Le Cat, 1768), see **auriculotemporal nerve (Haller, 1762)**

external terminal branch of obturator nerve (Cruveilhier, 1836), see **muscular branch of anterior branch of obturator nerve (>1840)**

external thoracic nerve (Bell, 1821), see **long thoracic nerve (Quain & Wilson, 1839)**

external thoracic nerves (Meckel, 1817), see **lateral cutaneous branch of intercostal nerves (>1840)**

external thoracic nerves (Monro, 1783), see **brachial plexus (Camper, 1760)**

external thumb nerve (Mayer, 1794), see **proper palmar digital nerves of median nerve (>1840)**

external tibial nerve (Haller, 1762), see **common fibular nerve (>1840)**

external tibial nerve (Meckel, 1817), see **medial calcaneal nerve (>1840)**

external trunk (Schmidel, 1754), see **paravertebral nerves (Swanson & Bota, 2010)**

external trunk of vagus nerve (Drake, 1707), see **anterior vagal trunk (Wrisberg, 1780)**

external twig from superficial dorsal twig of foot of deep branch of peroneal nerve (Jördens, 1788), see **dorsal digital nerves of digital branch of deep fibular nerve (>1840)**

external volar nerve of index finger (Mayer, 1794), see **proper palmar digital nerves of median nerve (>1840)**

external volar nerve of little finger (Mayer, 1794), see **proper palmar digital nerves of ulnar nerve (>1840)**

external volar nerve of middle finger (Mayer, 1794), see **proper palmar digital nerves of median nerve (>1840)**

external volar nerve of ring finger (Mayer, 1794), see **proper palmar digital nerves of median nerve (>1840)**

external volar nerve of thumb (Mayer, 1794), see **proper palmar digital nerves of median nerve (>1840)**

extremitas vaccinis papillis similis (Casseri, 1609), see **olfactory bulb (Weitbrecht, 1751)**

extremitates septi (Massa, 1536), see **fornix (Vesalius, 1543a)**

extremities of spinal ash-colored substance (Winslow, 1733), see **dorsal horn (>1840)**

extremity of genu of corpus callosum (Reil, 1809b), see **rostrum of corpus callosum (Reil, 1809b)**

extremity of medulla oblongata (Winslow, 1733), see **medulla (Winslow, 1733)**

extremity of septum (Massa, 1536), see **fornix (Vesalius, 1543a)**

extrinsic vesical plexus (>1840)

eye-mover pair of nerves from brain (Bartholin, 1662), see **oculomotor nerve (Estienne, 1545)**

facial branch of great auricular nerve (Arnold, 1834), see **anterior branch of great auricular nerve (>1840)**

facial branch of hard nerve (Meckel, 1753), see **zygomatic branches of facial nerve (>1840)**

facial branch of superior branch of hard nerve (Meckel, 1753), see **zygomatic branches of facial nerve (>1840)**

facial branches of ascending branch of superficial branch of hard nerve (Günther, 1786), see **zygomatic branches of facial nerve (>1840)**

facial branches of second division of fifth pair of nerves (Todd, 1836–1839), see **infraorbital nerve (Schaarschmidt, 1750)**

facial branches of superior branch of hard part of seventh pair (Haller, 1762), see **buccal branch of facial nerve (>1840)**

facial branches proper of superior branch of hard nerve (Meckel, 1753), see **zygomatic branches of facial nerve (>1840)**

facial branchlets of auricular nerve (Cruveilhier, 1836), see **anterior branch of great auricular nerve (>1840)**

facial colliculus (>1840)

facial communicating branch (Mayer, 1794), see **buccal branch of facial nerve (>1840)**

facial communicating nerve (Wrisberg, 1786), see **greater petrosal nerve (>1840)**

facial ganglion (Lazorthes, 1949)

facial ganglion (>1840), see **geniculate ganglion (Bischoff, 1832)** *facial nerve (Meckel, 1753)*, see **zygomatic branches of facial nerve (>1840)**

facial nerve (Meckel, 1817), see **intermediofacial nerve (Strong & Elwyn, 1943)**

facial nerve (Vicq d'Azyr, 1784), see **intermediofacial nerve (>1840)**

facial nerve central root (>1840)

facial nerve proper (Kölliker, 1896), see **intermediofacial nerve (Strong & Elwyn, 1943)**

facial nerve root (>1840)

facial nerve trunk (Meckel, 1817), see **intermediofacial nerve (Strong & Ewlyn, 1943)**

facial nerve trunk (>1840)

facial nucleus (>1840)

facial plexus (Cruveilhier, 1836), see **external carotid plexus (>1840)**

facial plexus (Mayer, 1794), see **facial nerve trunk (1840)**

facial surculus of superior branch of portio major and minor of facial nerve (Bellingeri, 1818), see **zygomatic branches of facial nerve (>1840)**

facial surculus of temporo-facial branch of portio major and minor of facial nerve (Bellingeri, 1818), see **zygomatic branches of facial nerve (>1840)**

faisceau primitif du cervelet (Gall & Spurzheim, 1810), see **inferior cerebellar peduncle (Günther, 1786)**

falciform fold (Chaussier, 1807), see **cerebral falx (Vesalius, 1543a)**

falx (Fyfe, 1800), see **cerebral falx (Vesalius, 1543a)**

falx cerebelli (Günther, 1786), see **cerebellar falx (Günther, 1786)**

falx cerebri (Vesalius, 1543a), see **cerebral falx (Vesalius, 1543a)**

falx durae matris (Vesalius, 1543a), see **cerebral falx (Vesalius, 1543a)**

falx major (Meckel, 1817), see **cerebral falx (Vesalius, 1543a)**

falx minor (Mayer, 1779), see **cerebellar falx (Günther, 1786)**

falx of brain (Burdin, 1803), see **cerebral falx (Vesalius, 1543a)**

falx of cerebellum (Bell, 1803b; Burdin, 1803), see **cerebellar falx (Günther, 1786)**

falx of cerebrum (Meckel, 1832), see **cerebral falx (Vesalius, 1543a)**

falx of dura mater (Winslow, 1733), see **cerebral falx (Vesalius, 1543a)**

falx transversalis (Ruysch, 1702), see **cerebellar tentorium (Winslow, 1733)**

fascia (Molinetti, 1675), see **fimbria (Honegger, 1890)**

fascia communicans memorabilis (Wrisberg, 1800), see **celiac branch of posterior vagal trunk (>1840)**

fascia communicans of Wrisberg (Lobstein, 1823), see **celiac branch of posterior vagal trunk (>1840)**

fascia dentata (Arnold, 1838b), see **fasciola cinerea (Arnold, 1838b)**

fascia dentata (Döllinger, 1814), see **dentate gyrus (>1840)**

fasciae medullares (Malacarne, 1776), see **pyramid (Willis, 1664)**

fascicle from olivary ganglion (Gall & Spurzheim, 1810), see **central nervous system white matter tracts (>1840)**

fascicle of great superior cerebral ganglion (Gall & Spurzheim, 1810), see **internal capsule (Burdach, 1822)**

fascicles of cerebellum (Chaussier, 1807), see **cerebellar hemisphere (Willis, 1664)**

fasciculi mesenterici posterioris (Winslow, 1733), see **intermesenteric plexus (>1840)**

fasciculi unciformes (Burdach, 1822), see **uncinate fascicle (Reil, 1809b)**

fasciculus (Bergmann, 1831), see **thalamic medial lemniscus (>1840)**

fasciculus baseosis interni (Burdach, 1822), see **occipital forceps (>1840)**

fasciculus cuneatus (Müller, 1834), see **cuneate fascicle (Müller, 1834)**

fasciculus gracilis (Müller, 1834), see **gracile fascicle (Müller, 1834)**

fasciculus longitudinalis inferior (Burdach, 1822), see **inferior longitudinal fascicle (Burdach, 1822)**

fasciculus mammillaris princeps (Kölliker, 1896), see **principal mammillary tract (Kölliker, 1896)**

fasciculus of external root of facial nerve (Meckel, 1817), see **intermediate nerve trunk (>1840)**

fasciculus olivarum (Burdach, 1822), see **ventral funiculus (>1840)**

fasciculus retroflexus (>1840), see **habenulo-interpeduncular tract (>1840)**

fasciculus siliqualis externus (Wagner, 1839), see **uncrossed pyramidal tract (>1840)**

fasciculus siliqualis internus (Wagner, 1839), see **spinal medial longitudinal fascicle (>1840)**

fasciculus tegmento-mammillaris (Kölliker, 1896), see **mammillotegmental tract (Kölliker, 1896)**

fasciculus teres (Arnold, 1838b), see **floor of fourth ventricle (Reil, 1807–1808a)**

fasciculus teres (Wagner, 1839), see **hypoglossal triangle (>1840)**

fasciculus thalamo-mammillaris (Kölliker, 1896), see **mammillotegmental tract (Kölliker, 1896)**

fasciculus uncinatus (>1840), see **uncinate fascicle (Reil, 1809b)**

fasciculus uncinatus cerebelli (>1840), see **superior cerebellar peduncle (Procháska, 1800)**

fasciola cinerea (Arnold, 1838b)

fasciola cinerea (Procháska, 1779), see **cochlear nuclei (>1840)**

fasciola cinerea cinguli (>1840), see **fasciola cinerea (Arnold, 1838b)**

fasciola dentata (Arnold, 1838a), see **fasciola cinerea (Arnold, 1838b)**

fasciolar gyrus (>1840), see **fasciola cinerea (Arnold, 1838b)**

fastigial nucleus (>1840)

fastigium of fourth ventricle (Burdach, 1822)

fastigium ventriculi quarti (Burdach, 1822), see **fastigium of fourth ventricle (Burdach, 1822)**

femora medulla oblongata (Winslow, 1733), see **brainstem (Schwalbe, 1881)**

femoral anterior cutaneous nerve (Fischer, 1791), see **femoral branch of genitofemoral nerve (>1840)**

femoral branch of genitofemoral nerve (>1840)

femoral cutaneous branch of internal saphenous nerve (Cruveilhier, 1836), see **saphenous nerve (Haase, 1781)**

femoral nerve (Haller, 1762)

femoral plexus (Meckel, 1817), see **lumbosacral plexus (Vesalius, 1543a)**

femoro-praetibial nerve (Burdin, 1803), see **femoral nerve (Haller, 1762)**

fence (Bartholin, 1662), see **pons (Haller, 1747)**

fessiers nerve (Burdin, 1803), see **sacral plexus ventral divisions (Paterson, 1887)**

fibrae ad facialem accessoriae (Soemmerring, 1778), see **intermediate nerve rootlets (>1840)**

fibrae arcuatae (Arnold, 1838b), see **arcuate fibers (Arnold, 1838b)**

fibrae arcuatae cerebri (>1840), see **arcuate fibers (Arnold, 1838b)**

fibrae arcuatae externae ventrales (>1840), see **ventral external arcuate fibers (>1840)**

fibrae longitudinales pontis (Arnold, 1838b), see **longitudinal pontine fibers (Arnold, 1838b)**

fibrae primitivae pyramidalis (Arnold, 1838b), see **uncrossed pyramidal tract (>1840)**

fibres of nerves (Grainger, 1837), see **peripheral nervous system white matter tracts (>1840)**

fibres of union (Spurzheim, 1826), see **central nervous system white matter tracts (>1840)**

fibrillae nervaeae ad par communicans faciei accessoriae (Vicq d'Azyr, 1786), see **intermediate nerve rootlets (>1840)**

fibrillae nerveae ad par communicans faciei accessoriae Wrisbergii (Soemmerring, 1778), see **intermediate nerve (>1840)**

fibrils of nerve of Wrisberg (Scarpa, 1789), see **intermediate nerve rootlets (>1840)**

fibrous cone (Reil, 1809b), see **central nervous system white matter tracts (>1840)**

fibrous envelope of cornu ammonis (Meckel, 1817), see **alveus (Burdach, 1822)**

fibrous matter of central organs of nervous system (Grainger, 1837), see **central nervous system white matter tracts (>1840)**

fibrous nerve (Salmon, 1714), see **sympathetic trunk (Winslow, 1733)**

fibrous protuberance (Diemerbroeck, 1689), see **brachium of superior colliculus (>1840)**

fibrous protuberance (Salmon, 1714), see **cerebral nuclei (Swanson, 2000a)**

fibrous substance of central organs of nervous system (Grainger, 1837), see **central nervous system white matter tracts (>1840)**

fibular communicating branch (Bock, 1827), see **sural communicating branch of common fibular nerve (>1840)**

fibular nerve (Coopmans, 1789), see **common fibular nerve (>1840)**

fibular nerve (Quain, 1828), see **common fibular nerve (>1840)**

field CA1 (Lorente de Nó, 1934)

field CA2 (Lorente de Nó, 1934)

field CA3 (Lorente de Nó, 1934)

fifteenth pair (Malacarne, 1791), see **accessory nerve (Vieussens, 1684)**

fifth and sixth pairs of nerves from brain (Bartholin, 1641), see **trigeminal nerve (Winslow, 1733)**

fifth brachial nerve (Vieussens, 1684), see **radial nerve (Du Verney, 1697)**

fifth branch of fifth pair (Desmoulins, 1825), see **trigeminal nerve (Winslow, 1733)**

fifth branch of glossopharyngeal nerve (Wrisberg, 1786), see **lingual branches of glossopharyngeal nerve (Haller, 1762)**

fifth internal lateral twig of deep branch of peroneal nerve (Jördens, 1788), see **muscular branches of deep fibular nerve (>1840)**

fifth nerve entering arm (Vesalius, 1543a), see **ulnar nerve (Cheselden, 1726)**

fifth nerve from spine to upper arm (Galen, c177), see **median nerve (Du Verney, 1697)**

fifth nerve of hand (Bauhin, 1605), see **ulnar nerve (Cheselden, 1726)**

fifth nerve of third pair of nerves arising from brain (Falloppio, 1561), see **lingual nerve (Vesalius, 1543a)**

fifth nerve to soleus muscle (Fischer, 1791), see **nerve to soleus (>1840)**

fifth pair (Estienne, 1545), see **cranial nerves (Soemmerring, 1791)**

fifth pair of cerebral nerves (Soemmerring, 1791), see **trigeminal nerve (Winslow, 1733)**

fifth pair of cranial nerves (Soemmerring, 1791), see **trigeminal nerve (Winslow, 1733)**

fifth pair of nerves (Malacarne, 1791), see **trochlear nerve (Molinetti, 1669)**

fifth pair of nerves arising within skull (Willis, 1664), see **trigeminal nerve (Winslow, 1733)**

fifth pair of nerves from brain (Benedetti, 1502), see **mandibular nerve (>1840)**

fifth pair of nerves from brain (Galen, c192), see **cranial nerves (Soemmerring, 1791)**

fifth pair of sinews of brain (Geminus, 1553), see **cranial nerves (Soemmerring, 1791)**

fifth plantar nerve of toes (Meckel, 1817), see **common plantar digital nerves of lateral plantar nerve (>1840)**

fifth sinew going into arm (Geminus, 1553), see **ulnar nerve (Cheselden, 1726)**

fifth temporal branch of hard nerve (Meckel, 1753), see **zygomatic branches of facial nerve (>1840)**

fifth terminal branch of median nerve (Cruveilhier, 1836), see **common palmar digital nerves of median nerve (>1840)**

fifth toe of foot of hippocampus (Malacarne, 1780), see **cerebral cortex (>1840)**

fifth toe of pes hippocampi (Malacarne, 1780), see **cerebral cortex (>1840)**

fifth ventricle (Aranzi, 1587), see **third ventricle (Galen, c173)**

fifth ventricle (Meckel, 1817), see **fourth ventricle (Galen, c192)**

fifth ventricle (Soemmerring, 1791), see **septal fissure (Burdach, 1822)** *fifth ventricle (Wenzel & Wenzel, 1812)*, see **fourth ventricle (Galen, c192)**

filament from carotid plexus to ciliary ganglion (Todd, 1836–1839), see **sympathetic root of ciliary ganglion (>1840)**

filament from cavernous ganglion to ciliary ganglion (Todd, 1836–1839), see **sympathetic root of ciliary ganglion (>1840)**

filament from spheno-palatine ganglion to ciliary ganglion (Todd, 1836–1839), see **ciliary ganglion (Loder, 1778)**

filament from sympathetic to third division of fifth pair of nerves (Todd, 1836–1839), see **internal carotid plexus (>1840)**

filament of arytenoid muscle (Cruveilhier, 1836), see **internal branch of superior laryngeal nerve (Fyfe, 1800)**

filament of communication with superior cervical ganglion (Meckel, 1817), see **internal carotid nerve (>1840)**

filament of cubital nerve to cubital artery (Cruveilhier, 1836), see **ulnar nerve (Cheselden, 1726)**

filament of first lumbrical of first terminal branch of internal plantar nerve (Cruveilhier, 1836), see **common plantar digital nerves of medial plantar nerve (>1840)**

filament of third lumbrical of deep terminal branch of external plantar nerve (Cruveilhier, 1836), see **deep branch of lateral plantar nerve (>1840)**

filament of transverse abductor of deep terminal branch of external plantar nerve (Cruveilhier, 1836), see **deep branch of lateral plantar nerve (>1840)**

filament to tensor tympani muscle (Quain & Wilson, 1839), see **nerve to tensor tympani (>1840)**

filaments forming external and posterior root of facial nerve (Meckel, 1817), see **intermediate nerve rootlets (>1840)**

filaments from superior mesenteric plexus to large intestine (Meckel, 1817), see **superior mesenteric plexus (Rau, 1720)**

filaments from superior mesenteric plexus to small intestine (Meckel, 1817), see **jejunal and ileal plexuses (>1840)**

filaments into nose from anterior dentar nerves (Meckel, 1817), see **nasal branch of anterior superior dental nerve (>1840)**

filaments of cavernous plexus joining first branch of fifth pair (Arnold, 1834), see **communicating branch from internal carotid plexus to ophthalmic nerve (>1840)**

filaments of cavernous plexus joining Gasserian ganglion (Arnold, 1834), see **communicating branch from internal carotid plexus to ophthalmic nerve (>1840)**

filaments of communication of internal cutaneous nerve with external cutaneous nerve (Quain & Wilson, 1839), see **lateral cutaneous nerve of forearm (>1840)**

filaments of communication of otic ganglion with auricular nerve (Quain & Wilson, 1839), see **communicating branches of otic ganglion with auriculotemporal nerve (>1840)**

filaments of communication with anterior cords of spinal nerves (Meckel, 1817), see **communicating branches of spinal nerves (Wutzer, 1817)**

filaments of interosseous muscles of deep terminal branch of external plantar nerve (Cruveilhier, 1836), see **deep branch of lateral plantar nerve (>1840)**

filaments of lingual nerve to maxillary ganglion (Meckel, 1817), see **communicating branches of lingual nerve with submandibular ganglion (>1840)**

filaments of medulla oblongata roots of accessory nerve (Meckel, 1817), see **cranial root of accessory nerve rootlets (>1840)**

filaments of nervi accessorii of eighth pair (Winslow, 1733), see **spinal roots of accessory nerve rootlets (>1840)**

filaments of par linguale (Winslow, 1733), see **hypoglossal nerve rootlets (>1840)**

filaments of union of limiting ganglia (Meckel, 1817), see **communicating branches of sympathetic trunk (>1840)**

filaments to cardiac nerves from pneumogastric nerve (Meckel, 1817), see **cardiac branches of recurrent laryngeal nerve (>1840)**

filamentum terminale (Arnold, 1838b), see **terminal filament (Tiedemann, 1821)**

fillet (Reil, 1809b), see **central nervous system white matter tracts (>1840)**

fillet of great commissure (Mayo, 1827), see **cingulum (Burdach, 1822)**

fillet of medulla oblongata (Mayo, 1827), see **central nervous system white matter tracts (>1840)**

films (Willis, 1664), see **meninges (Smith Papyrus, c1700 BC)**

filum terminale (Tiedemann, 1821), see **terminal filament (Tiedemann, 1821)**

fimbria (Günz, 1750), see **fimbria (Honegger, 1890)**

fimbria (Honegger, 1890)

fimbria fornicis (Vieussens, 1684), see **fornix (Vesalius, 1543a)**

fimbria hippocampi (Wenzel & Wenzel, 1812), see **fimbria (Honegger, 1890)**

fimbria medullaria transparente (Malacarne, 1780), see **cerebral cortex (>1840)**

fimbria medullosa (Wenzel & Wenzel, 1812), see **fimbria (Honegger, 1890)**

fimbria of fornix (Vieussens, 1684), see **fornix (Vesalius, 1543a)**

fimbria of fornix (>1840), see **fimbria (Honegger, 1890)**

fimbria of hippocampus (Henle, 1871), see **fimbria (Honegger, 1890)**

fimbrial appendix of true fornix (Vieussens, 1684), see **fornix (Vesalius, 1543a)**

fimbrial line of lateral ventricle (>1840)

fimbrial part of fornix (Cajal, 1904), see **septal postcommissural fornix (>1840)**

fimbriatae veri fornicis appendix (Vieussens, 1684), see **fornix (Vesalius, 1543a)**

fimbriodentate sulcus (>1840)

fine membrane (Hippocrates), see **pia (Galen, c192)**

first accessory lumbar ganglion (Walter, 1783), see **intermediate ganglia (>1840)**

first anastomotic ansa of cervical nerves (Cloquet, 1828), see **communicating loops of cervical plexus (>1840)**

first and superior branch of third pair (Marchetti, 1652), see **ophthalmic nerve (Winslow, 1733)**

first ansa cervicalis (Bock, 1827), see **communicating loops of cervical plexus (>1840)** *first auricular branch of superficial temporal nerve* (Bock, 1817), see **anterior auricular nerves (>1840)**

first brachial nerve (Vieussens, 1684), see **axillary nerve (Winslow, 1733)**

first branch of anterior crural nerve to straight muscle of thigh (Swan, 1830), see **muscular branches of femoral nerve (Quain & Wilson, 1839)**

first branch of eighth pair (Winslow, 1733), see **glossopharyngeal nerve (Huber, 1744)**

first branch of fifth pair of nerves (Meckel, 1753), see **ophthalmic nerve (Winslow, 1733)**

first branch of fourth branch of second division of fifth pair of nerves arising within skull (Willis, 1664), see **superior gingival branches of superior dental plexus (>1840)**

first branch of fourth conjugation of nerves of brain (Crooke, 1615), see **anterior branch of mandibular nerve (>1840)**

first branch of glossopharyngeal nerve (Wrisberg, 1786), see **glossopharyngeal nerve trunk (Wrisberg, 1786; Günther, 1786)**

first branch of lower branch of second division of fifth pair of nerves arising within skull (Willis, 1664), see **superior gingival branches of superior dental plexus (>1840)**

first branch of second nerve entering upper arm from spine (Galen, c177), see **inferior lateral cutaneous nerve of arm (>1840)**

first branch of superior palpebral nerve (Meckel, 1753), see **frontal nerve (Cheselden, 1726)**

first branch of third conjugation of nerves of brain (Crooke, 1615), see **supraorbital nerve (Meckel, 1753)**

first branch of tibial nerve to flexor digitorum longus muscle (Jördens, 1788), see **nerve to flexor digitorum longus (>1840)**

first branchlet of major branch of fifth pair (Rau, 1694), see **zygomatic nerve (>1840)**

first cardiac branch of recurrent nerves (Mayer, 1794), see **cardiac branches of recurrent laryngeal nerve (>1840)**

first cerebellar peduncle (Procháska, 1800), see **superior cerebellar peduncle (Procháska, 1800)**

first cerebral mass (Anderson, 1837), see **cerebral cortex (>1840)**

first cervical ganglion (Winslow, 1733), see **superior cervical ganglion (Vieussens, 1684)**

first cervical nervous plexus (Meckel, 1817), see **cervical plexus (Molinetti, 1675)**

first common digital branch of median nerve (Caldani, 1813, 1814), see **common palmar digital nerves of median nerve (>1840)**

first communicating branch of glossopharyngeal nerve (Wrisberg, 1786), see **glossopharyngeal nerve trunk (Wrisberg, 1786; Günther, 1786)**

first cutaneous nerve of thigh (Galen, c177), see **lateral cutaneous nerve of thigh (>1840)**

first deep nerve of thigh (Galen, c177), see **femoral nerve (Haller, 1762)**

first dental nerve of second trunk of fifth nerve (Swan, 1830), see **posterior superior dental nerve (Haller, 1762)**

first division of fifth pair (Bell, 1803a), see **ophthalmic nerve (Winslow, 1733)**

first division of fifth pair of nerves arising within skull (Willis, 1664), see **mandibular nerve (>1840)**

first dorsal ganglion (Neubauer, 1772), see **inferior cervical ganglion (Vieussens, 1684)**

first dorsal ganglion (Winslow, 1733), see **superior thoracic ganglion (Lieutaud, 1742)**

first epiglottal branch of posterior epiglottal nerve (Andersch & Soemmerring, 1792), see **internal branch of superior laryngeal nerve (Fyfe, 1800)**

first exterior supraclavicular branch (Peipers, 1793), see **lateral supraclavicular nerves (>1840)**

first external inferior posterior cutaneous nerve (Fischer, 1791), see **sural nerve (Pietro da Cortona, 1741)**

first external lateral twig of deep branch of peroneal nerve (Jördens, 1788), see **muscular branches of deep fibular nerve (>1840)**

first external posterior inferior cutaneous nerve (Knox, 1832), see **sural nerve (Pietro da Cortona, 1741)**

first ganglion of neck (Andersch & Soemmerring, 1792), see **superior cervical ganglion (Vieussens, 1684)**

first ganglion of neck (Lyonnet, 1762), see **ventral ganglia (Anderson, 1837)**

first great brachial nerve (Albinus, 1744), see **musculocutaneous nerve (Du Verney, 1697)**

first inferior internal spermatic nerve (Walter, 1783), see **superior ovarian nerves (>1840)**

first intermediate white layer of cortical layer (Baillarger, 1840), see **cerebral cortex gray matter (>1840)**

first internal inferior posterior cutaneous nerve (Fischer, 1791), see **tibial nerve (Haase, 1781)**

first internal lateral twig of deep branch of peroneal nerve (Jördens, 1788), see **muscular branches of deep fibular nerve (>1840)**

first internal posterior inferior cutaneous nerve (Knox, 1832), see **tibial nerve (Haase, 1781)**

first labial branch of infraorbital nerve (Bock, 1817), see **superior labial branches of infraorbital nerve (Meckel, 1748)**

first lateral ganglion (Soemmerring, 1798), see **intermediate ganglia (>1840)**

first medullary process of cerebellum (Cowper, 1698), see **middle cerebellar peduncle (Rolando, 1819)**

first nerve entering arm (Vesalius, 1543a), see **suprascapular nerve (Bang, 1770)**

first nerve entering leg (Vesalius, 1543a), see **lumbar plexus dorsal divisions (Paterson, 1887)**

first nerve entering thigh (Vesalius, 1543a), see **lumbar plexus dorsal divisions (Paterson, 1887)**

first nerve for vastus externus muscle (Fischer, 1791), see **muscular branches of femoral nerve (Quain & Wilson, 1839)**

first nerve from spine to upper arm (Galen, c177), see **musculocutaneous nerve (Du Verney, 1697)**

first nerve of body (Andersch, 1797), see **sympathetic trunk (Winslow, 1733)**

first nerve of hand (Bauhin, 1605), see **suprascapular nerve (Bang, 1770)**

first nerve of seventh pair (Vicq d'Azyr, 1784), see **intermediofacial nerve (Strong & Elwyn, 1943)**

first nerve of trunk (Andersch, 1797), see **sympathetic trunk (Winslow, 1733)**
first nerve sulcus (Soemmerring, 1778), see **olfactory sulcus (Quain, 1834)**
first nerve to extensor digitorum longus muscle (Fischer, 1791), see **muscular branches of deep fibular nerve (>1840)**
first nerve to flexor digitorum longus muscle (Fischer, 1791), see **nerve to flexor digitorum longus (>1840)**
first nerve to flexor longus of big toe muscle (Fischer, 1791), see **nerve to flexor hallucis longus (>1840)**
first nerve to left head of gastrocnemius muscle (Fischer, 1791), see **nerves to gastrocnemius (>1840)**
first nerve to long head of crural biceps muscle (Fischer, 1791), see **nerve to hamstring muscles (>1840)**
first nerve to plantaris muscle (Fischer, 1791), see **nerve to plantaris (>1840)**
first nerve to popliteus muscle (Fischer, 1791), see **nerve to popliteus (>1840)**
first nerve to popliteus muscle from tibial nerve trunk (Jördens, 1788), see **nerve to popliteus (>1840)**
first nerve to posterior tibial muscle (Fischer, 1791), see **muscular branches of deep fibular nerve (>1840)**
first nerve to right head of gastrocnemius muscle (Fischer, 1791), see **nerves to gastrocnemius (>1840)**
first nerve to short head of biceps muscle (Fischer, 1791), see **nerve to hamstring muscles (>1840)**
first nerve to soleus muscle (Fischer, 1791), see **nerve to soleus (>1840)**
first nerve to tibialis anterior muscle (Fischer, 1791), see **muscular branches of deep fibular nerve (>1840)**
first nerve to tibialis posterior muscle (Fischer, 1791), see **nerve to tibialis posterior (>1840)**
first of three anterior branches of first lumbar pair (Sabatier, 1775), see **genitofemoral nerve (>1840)**
first offshoot of thinner root of third pair (Vesalius, 1543a), see **supraorbital nerve (Meckel, 1753)**
first or second medullary process of cerebellum (Cowper, 1698), see **superior cerebellar peduncle (Procháska, 1800)**
first pair of cerebral nerves (Arnold, 1834), see **nervous system (Monro, 1783)**
first pair of neck (Fyfe, 1800), see **suboccipital nerve (Winslow, 1733)**
first pair of nerves (Theophilus Protospatharius, fl. 610–641), see **cerebral cortex (>1840)**
first pair of nerves arising within skull (Willis, 1664), see **nervous system (Monro, 1783)**
first pair of nerves from brain (Benedetti, 1502), see **white matter tracts (Bell & Bell, 1826)**
first pair of nerves from brain (Galen, c173), see **white matter tracts (Bell & Bell, 1826)**
first pair of nerves from brain (Massa, 1536), see **nervous system (Monro, 1783)**
first pair of nerves of medulla oblongata (Haller & Wrisberg, 1780), see **glossopharyngeal nerve (Huber, 1744)**
first pair of sinews of hand (Colombo, 1559), see **cervical nerves (Galen, c173)**
first pair of thoracic nerves (Vesalius, 1543a), see **cervical nerves (Galen, c173)**
first pair of tubercles (Steno, 1669), see **cerebral nuclei (Swanson, 2000a)**
first part of optic nerve (Perrault, 1688), see **optic tract (Vicq d'Azyr, 1784)**
first part of spinal marrow (Vesalius, 1543a), see **rhombicbrain (His, 1893b)**
first pectoral ganglion (Schreger, 1803), see **superior thoracic ganglion (Lieutaud, 1742)**
first pharyngeal branch of main communicating branch of glossopharyngeal nerve (Kilian, 1822), see **pharyngeal branches of glossopharyngeal nerve (Neubauer, 1772)**
first pharyngeal nerve (Andersch & Soemmerring, 1792), see **pharyngeal branches of vagus nerve (>1840)**
first posterior inferior external cutaneous nerve (Knox, 1832), see **sural nerve (Pietro da Cortona, 1741)**
first posterior inferior internal cutaneous nerve (Knox, 1832), see **tibial nerve (Haase, 1781)**
first process of cerebellum (Ridley, 1695), see **superior cerebellar peduncle (Procháska, 1800)**
first ramification of trunk of portio dura (Du Verney, 1683), see **posterior auricular nerve (Meckel, 1753)**
first root of intercostal nerve (Bang, 1770), see **communicating branch from internal carotid plexus to abducens nerve (>1840)**
first root of sciatic nerves (Mayer, 1794), see **sciatic nerve (Keill, 1698)**
first shoot of uppermost branch of second division of fifth pair of nerves arising within skull (Willis, 1664), see **nasociliary nerve (Meckel, 1817; Wutzer, 1817)**
first sinew coming to arm (Geminus, 1553), see **suprascapular nerve (Bang, 1770)**
first sinew going under thigh (Geminus, 1553), see **lumbar plexus dorsal divisions (Paterson, 1887)**
first sinew of leg (Geminus, 1553), see **lumbar plexus dorsal divisions (Paterson, 1887)**
first spinal nerve (Soemmerring, 1778), see **glossopharyngeal nerve (Huber, 1744)**
first subscapular branch of brachial plexus (Cloquet, 1816), see **thoracodorsal nerve (>1840)**
first superior labial nerve (Mayer, 1794), see **superior labial branches of infraorbital nerve (Meckel, 1748)**
first terminal branch of median nerve (Cruveilhier, 1836), see **median nerve (Du Verney, 1697)**
first thoracic ganglion (Winslow, 1733), see **superior thoracic ganglion (Lieutaud, 1742)**
first trunk of fifth nerve (Swan, 1830), see **ophthalmic nerve (Winslow, 1733)**
first trunk of fifth pair (Swan, 1830), see **ophthalmic nerve (Winslow, 1733)**
first trunk of third pair (Falloppio, 1561), see **ophthalmic nerve (Winslow, 1733)**
first trunk of three-fold nerve (Swan, 1830), see **ophthalmic nerve (Winslow, 1733)**
first twig of deep twig of deep branch of external plantar nerve to flexor digiti minimi brevis (Jördens, 1788), see **deep branch of lateral plantar nerve (>1840)**
first ventricle (Galen, c192), see **fourth ventricle (Galen, c192)**

first ventricle (Geminus, 1553), see **anterior horn of lateral ventricle (Bell, 1803b)**
first ventricle (Wenzel & Wenzel, 1812), see **septal fissure (Burdach, 1822)**
first visual area (Talbot, 1942), see **primary visual area (>1840)**
fissura cerebralis magna (Bichat, 1802), see **inner part of transverse cerebral fissure (>1840)**
fissura cerebri (Winslow, 1733), see **lateral cerebral sulcus (>1840)**
fissura cerebri transversa cerebelli (Burdach, 1822), see **transverse cerebellar fissure (Burdach, 1822)**
fissura cerebri transversa magna (Meckel, 1817), see **inner part of transverse cerebral fissure (>1840)**
fissura cerebri transversa parva (Meckel, 1817), see **transverse cerebellar fissure (Burdach, 1822)**
fissura choroidea (>1840), see **choroid fissure (>1840)**
fissura inter lobulos (Rosenthal, 1815), see **third ventricle (Galen, c173)**
fissura magna anterior (Ramsay, 1813), see **lateral cerebral sulcus (>1840)**
fissura magna Silvii (Winslow, 1733), see **lateral cerebral sulcus (>1840)**
fissura major Sylvii (Tarin, 1753), see **lateral cerebral sulcus (>1840)**
fissura posterior (Ramsay, 1813), see **inner part of transverse cerebral fissure (>1840)**
fissure (Le Böe, 1663), see **lateral cerebral sulcus (>1840)**
fissure dividing external root of olfactory nerve from superincumbent hemisphere (Owen, 1837), see **rhinal sulcus (>1840)**
fissure of Bichât (Quain, 1828), see **inner part of transverse cerebral fissure (>1840)**
fissure of cerebellar peduncles (Vicq d'Azyr, 1784), see **posterolateral fissure (Larsell, 1937)**
fissure of Monro (Quain, 1828), see **interventricular foramen (>1840)**
fissure of Rolando (Leuret, 1839), see **central sulcus (Huschke, 1854)**
fissure of Sylvius (Fyfe, 1800), see **septal fissure (Burdach, 1822)**
fissure upon which hippocampus is folded (Owen, 1837), see **hippocampal sulcus (Gratiolet, 1854)**
fistula sacra (Schreger, 1803), see **spinal cord (Galen, c162–c166)**
five cerebral vesicles (Malpighi, 1673), see **secondary brain vesicles (>1840)**
five morphological elements of brain (Baer, 1837), see **secondary brain vesicles (>1840)**
five vesicles (Baer, 1837), see **secondary brain vesicles (>1840)**
flabellum (Bergmann, 1831), see **internal capsule (Burdach, 1822)**
flegmaticke glandule (Crooke, 1615), see **pituitary gland (>1840)**
flexor digitorum brevis nerve from external plantar nerve (Jördens, 1788), see **muscular branches of lateral plantar nerve (>1840)**
flexus (Soemmerring, 1778), see **cerebral cortex gray matter (>1840)**
floccular peduncle (Burdach, 1822)
flocculus (Meckel, 1817)
flock (Reil, 1807–1808a), see **flocculus (Meckel, 1817)**
floor of cerebrum (Winslow, 1733), see **cerebellar tentorium (Winslow, 1733)**
floor of fourth ventricle (Reil, 1807–1808a)
floor of third ventricle (Langenbeck, 1826–1830), see **hypothalamus (Kuhlenbeck, 1927)**
floor plate (>1840)
flossi laminosi (Malacarne, 1776), see **flocculus (Meckel, 1817)**
foldings together of brain (Geminus, 1553), see **cerebral cortex gray matter (>1840)**
folds (Erasistratus, c310–c250 BC, definition 1), see **cerebral cortex gray matter (>1840)**
folds (Erasistratus, c310–c250 BC, definition 2), see **cerebellar cortex (Willis, 1664)**
folia (Malacarne, 1776), see **cerebellar cortex (Willis, 1664)**
foliatus arbori (Tiedemann, 1821), see **arbor vitae (Winslow, 1733)**
folium cacuminis (Burdach, 1822), see **folium vermis (>1840)**
folium vermis (>1840)
foot of larger hippocampus (Haase, 1781), see **hippocampal region (Swanson et al., 1987)**
foot of larger hippopotamus (Mayer, 1779), see **hippocampal region (Swanson et al., 1987)**
foot of larger seahorse (Haase, 1781), see **hippocampal region (Swanson et al., 1987)**
foot of seahorse (Riolan, 1618), see **hippocampal region (Swanson et al., 1987)**
foot-stalk of hippocampus (Haller, 1747), see **hippocampal region (Swanson et al., 1987)**
foramen ani (Salmon, 1714), see **opening of cerebral aqueduct (>1840)**
foramen caecum anterius (Soemmerring, 1778), see **interpeduncular fossa (>1840)**
foramen cecum of medulla (>1840)
foramen coecum (Vicq d'Azyr, 1784), see **foramen cecum of medulla (>1840)**
foramen commune anterius (Ramsay, 1813), see **ventricles (Hippocrates)**
foramen commune anterius (Winslow, 1733), see **interventricular foramen (>1840)**
foramen commune posterius (Winslow, 1733), see **opening of cerebral aqueduct (>1840)**
foramen of Bichat (Solly, 1836), see **inner part of transverse cerebral fissure (>1840)**
foramen of Monro (Ramsay, 1813), see **interventricular foramen (>1840)**
foramen pontis coecum anterius (Günther, 1786), see **interpeduncular nucleus (>1840)**
foramen profundum (Lieutaud, 1742), see **interventricular foramen (>1840)**
forceps (Arnold, 1838a), see **occipital forceps (>1840)**
forceps frontalis (>1840), see **frontal forceps (>1840)**
forceps major (Arnold, 1838a), see **occipital forceps (>1840)**
forceps minor (Arnold, 1838a), see **frontal forceps (>1840)**
forceps occipitalis (>1840), see **occipital forceps (>1840)**
forceps of corpus callosum (Reil, 1809b), see **corpus callosum (Galen, c177)**

fore lobe of brain (Gibson, 1682), see ***frontal region (Vicq d'Azyr, 1786)***

fore nerves of pairs of nerves of medulla spinalis (Salmon, 1714), see ***spinal nerve ventral branches (>1840)***

fore part of brain (Mondino, 1316), see ***endbrain (Kuhlenbeck, 1927)***

fore part of medulla oblongata (Gibson, 1684), see ***vertebrate brain (Cuvier, 1800)***

forebrain (Baer, 1837), see ***endbrain (Kuhlenbeck, 1927)***

fore-brain (Galen, c177), see ***vertebrate brain (Cuvier, 1800)***

forebrain (Goette, 1873)

forebrain vesicle (Baer, 1837), see ***endbrain vesicle (Kuhlenbeck, 1927)***

foremore and uppermore ventricle (Bartholin, 1662), see ***lateral ventricle (Vesalius, 1543a)***

foremore nerves of pairs of nerves of medulla spinalis (Salmon, 1714), see ***spinal nerve ventral branches (>1840)***

foremost border of streaked body (Willis, 1672), see ***external capsule (Burdach, 1822)***

foremost branch of pairs of sinews or nerves from neck, back, loins, and os sacrum (Read, 1638), see ***spinal nerve ventral branch (>1840)***

foremost figure of brain (Geminus, 1553), see ***anterior horn of lateral ventricle (Bell, 1803b)***

foremost leg of vault (Riolan, 1657), see ***fornix (Vesalius, 1543a)***

foremost lobe of brain (Cowper, 1698), see ***frontal region (Vicq d'Azyr, 1786)***

foremost portion of basis of brain (Riolan, 1657), see ***hypothalamus (Kuhlenbeck, 1927)***

foremost thigh of arch (Diemerbroeck, 1689), see ***fornix (Vesalius, 1543a)***

foremost ventricle (Salmon, 1714), see ***lateral ventricle (Vesalius, 1543a)***

foremost ventricles (Galen, c177), see ***anterior horn of lateral ventricle (Bell, 1803b)***

forepart of brain (Crooke, 1615), see ***frontal region (Vicq d'Azyr, 1786)***

forepart of brain commonly so called (Bartholin, 1662), see ***cerebral cortex gray matter (>1840)***

forepart of whole brain (Crooke, 1615), see ***cerebral cortex gray matter (>1840)***

foreward ventricle (Galen, c173), see ***lateral ventricle (Vesalius, 1543a)***

former lobe of brain (Ridley, 1695), see ***frontal region (Vicq d'Azyr, 1786)***

former pans of braine (Nemesius, 1636), see ***lateral ventricle (Vesalius, 1543a)***

former ventricle (Hall, 1565), see ***lateral ventricle (Vesalius, 1543a)***

fornicate body (Hall, 1565), see ***fornix (Vesalius, 1543a)***

fornicate gyrus (Arnold, 1838a), see ***limbic region (>1840)***

fornicem (Hall, 1565), see ***fornix (Vesalius, 1543a)***

fornicis crurum anteriorum ad tubercula mammillaria descensus (Haase, 1781), see ***hypothalamic postcommissural fornix (>1840)***

fornix (Colombo, 1559), see ***fimbria (Honegger, 1890)***

fornix (Demeter et al., 1985), see ***fornix (Vesalius, 1543a)***

fornix (Galen, c177), see ***fornix (Vesalius, 1543a)***

fornix (Meynert, 1867), see ***postcommissural fornix (Loo, 1931)***

fornix (Ridley, 1695), see ***fornix (Vesalius, 1543a)***

fornix (Vesalius, 1543a)

fornix (Willis, 1664), see ***fornix (Vesalius, 1543a)***

fornix callosus (Winslow, 1733), see ***fornix (Vesalius, 1543a)***

fornix column (Burdach, 1822), see ***septal postcommissural fornix (>1840)***

fornix column (Herrick, 1915), see ***fornix (Vesalius, 1543a)***

fornix column (Honegger, 1890), see ***postcommissural fornix (Loo, 1931)***

fornix commissure (Smith, 1895), see ***hippocampal commissures (Johnston, 1913)***

fornix itself (Willis, 1664), see ***fornix (Vesalius, 1543a)***

fornix longus (Forel, 1876), see ***fimbria (Honegger, 1890)***

fornix obliquus (Honegger, 1890), see ***precommissural fornix (Loo, 1931)***

fornix superior (Kölliker, 1896), see ***fimbria (Honegger, 1890)***

fornix transversus (Forel, 1872), see ***hippocampal commissures (Johnston, 1913)***

fornix trilaterus (Chaussier, 1807), see ***fornix (Vesalius, 1543a)***

fornix vera (Vieussens, 1684), see ***cerebral cortex white matter (>1840)***

fortieth pair of nerves (Fyfe, 1800), see ***terminal filament (Tiedemann, 1821)***

forty-fifth nerve of body (Andersch, 1797), see ***sympathetic trunk (Winslow, 1733)***

forty-fourth nerve (Soemmerring, 1791), see ***sympathetic trunk (Winslow, 1733)***

forty-fourth nerve of body (Andersch & Soemmerring, 1792), see ***sympathetic trunk (Winslow, 1733)***

forty-third nerve of body (Andersch & Soemmerring, 1792), see ***phrenic nerve (Galen, c173)***

forty-third pair of nerves (Cloquet, 1828), see ***sympathetic trunk (Winslow, 1733)***

forward branches of conjugations of neck, chest, loynes, and sacral bone (Crooke, 1615), see ***spinal nerve ventral branches (>1840)***

forward prominence of brain (Crooke, 1615), see ***frontal region (Vicq d'Azyr, 1786)***

fossa eminentiae olivaris (Burdach, 1822), see ***medullopontine sulcus (>1840)***

fossa of base of septum lucidum (Vicq d'Azyr, 1786), see ***septal fissure (Burdach, 1822)***

fossa of fourth ventricle (Meckel, 1817), see ***fourth ventricle (Galen, c192)***

fossa of oculo-muscular nerves (Vicq d'Azyr, 1786), see ***interpeduncular fossa (>1840)***

fossa of olivary body (Vicq d'Azyr, 1786), see ***medullopontine sulcus (>1840)***

fossae (Gordon, 1815), see ***cerebral sulci (Vesalius, 1543a)***

fossette of fourth ventricle (Chaussier, 1807), see ***fourth ventricle (Galen, c192)***

fossulas (Soemmerring, 1778), see ***cerebral sulci (Vesalius, 1543a)***

foundation of brain (Bannister, 1578), see ***vertebrate brain (Cuvier, 1800)***

foundation of brain (Brunschwig, 1525), see **brainstem (Schwalbe, 1881)**
foundation of brain (Geminus, 1553), see **vertebrate brain (Cuvier, 1800)**
four bellies (Willis, 1664), see **fourth ventricle (Galen, c192)**
four-horned medullary tracts (Haller, 1747), see **fornix (Vesalius, 1543a)**
four mole hills (Willis, 1664), see **tectum (Baer, 1837)**
four protuberances of oblong marrow (Willis, 1664), see **tectum (Baer, 1837)**
fourteenth pair, intermediate sympathetic (Malacarne, 1791), see **vagus nerve (Galen, c192)**
fourteenth pair of nerves (Malacarne, 1791), see **cranial nerves (Soemmerring, 1791)**
fourth and fifth pairs of nerves from brain (Theophilos Protospatharios, fl. 610-641), see **trigeminal nerve (Winslow, 1733)**
fourth ansa lumbalis (Bock, 1827), see **lumbar plexus (Vesalius, 1543a)**
fourth branch of anterior crural nerve to sartorius muscle (Swan, 1830), see **muscular branches of femoral nerve (Quain & Wilson, 1839)**
fourth branch of fifth pair (Desmoulins, 1825), see **trigeminal nerve (Winslow, 1733)**
fourth branch of glossopharyngeal nerve (Wrisberg, 1786), see **tonsillar branches of glossopharyngeal nerve (Wrisberg, 1786)**
fourth branch of second division of fifth pair of nerves arising within skull (Willis, 1664), see **maxillary nerve (Meckel, 1753)**
fourth branch of third conjugation of nerves of brain (Crooke, 1615), see **zygomaticotemporal nerve (>1840)**
fourth choroid plexus (Haller, 1754a), see **choroid plexus of fourth ventricle (Vieussens, 1684)**
fourth choroid plexus of Haller (Soemmerring, 1778), see **choroid plexus of fourth ventricle (Vieussens, 1684)**
fourth conjugation of nerves of brain (Bauhin, 1605), see **trigeminal nerve (Winslow, 1733)**
fourth crural nerve (Crooke, 1615), see **sciatic nerve (Keill, 1698)**
fourth cutaneous nerve of thigh (Galen, c177), see **genitofemoral nerve (>1840)**
fourth deep nerve of thigh (Galen, c177), see **sciatic nerve (Keill, 1698)**
fourth facial nerve (Mayer, 1794), see **zygomatic branches of facial nerve (>1840)**
fourth great brachial nerve (Albinus, 1744), see **ulnar nerve (Cheselden, 1726)**
fourth internal lateral twig of deep branch of peroneal nerve (Jördens, 1788), see **muscular branches of deep fibular nerve (>1840)**
fourth nerve entering arm (Vesalius, 1543a), see **radial nerve (Du Verney, 1697)**
fourth nerve entering leg (Vesalius, 1543a), see **sciatic nerve (Keill, 1698)**
fourth nerve for vastus externus muscle (Fischer, 1791), see **muscular branches of femoral nerve (Quain & Wilson, 1839)**
fourth nerve from spine to upper arm (Galen, c177), see **ulnar nerve (Cheselden, 1726)**
fourth nerve of hand (Bauhin, 1605), see **radial nerve (Du Verney, 1697)**
fourth nerve of third pair of nerves arising from brain (Falloppio, 1561), see **inferior dental nerve (Meckel, 1817)**
fourth nerve to short head of biceps muscle (Fischer, 1791), see **nerve to hamstring muscles (>1840)**
fourth nerve to soleus muscle (Fischer, 1791), see **nerve to soleus (>1840)**
fourth nerve traveling to thigh (Vesalius, 1543a), see **sciatic nerve (Keill, 1698)**
fourth offshoot of thinner root of third nerve (Vesalius, 1543a), see **zygomaticotemporal nerve (>1840)**
fourth pair of cerebral nerves (Soemmerring, 1791), see **trochlear nerve (Molinetti, 1669)**
fourth pair of cerebral nerves (Vesalius, 1543a), see **trigeminal nerve motor root (Bell, 1829)**
fourth pair of cranial nerves (Soemmerring, 1791), see **trochlear nerve (Molinetti, 1669)**
fourth pair of nerves (Bartholin, 1632), see **trochlear nerve (Molinetti, 1669)**
fourth pair of nerves (Malacarne, 1791), see **oculomotor nerve (Estienne, 1545)**
fourth pair of nerves from brain (Benedetti, 1502), see **maxillary nerve (Meckel, 1753)**
fourth pair of nerves from brain (Estienne, 1545), see **vestibulocochlear nerve (>1840)**
fourth pair of nerves from brain (Falloppio, 1561), see **abducens nerve (Heister, 1717)**
fourth pair of nerves from brain (Galen, c192), see **trigeminal nerve (Winslow, 1733)**
fourth pair of sinews of brain (Geminus, 1553), see **trigeminal nerve motor root (Bell, 1829)**
fourth pharyngeal branch of pharyngolingual branch of glossopharyngeal nerve (Kilian, 1822), see **pharyngeal branches of glossopharyngeal nerve (Neubauer, 1772)**
fourth sinew going into leg (Geminus, 1553), see **sciatic nerve (Keill, 1698)**
fourth sinew going into thigh (Geminus, 1553), see **sciatic nerve (Keill, 1698)**
fourth sinew going under arm (Geminus, 1553), see **radial nerve (Du Verney, 1697)**
fourth sinus (du Laurens, 1600), see **fourth ventricle (Galen, c192)**
fourth supraclavicular branch (Peipers, 1793), see **medial supraclavicular nerves (>1840)**
fourth temporal branch of hard nerve (Meckel, 1753), see **temporal branches of facial nerve (Swan, 1830)**
fourth terminal branch of median nerve (Cruveilhier, 1836), see **common palmar digital nerves of median nerve (>1840)**
fourth terminal branch of obturator nerve (Cruveilhier, 1836), see **muscular branch of anterior branch of obturator nerve (>1840)**
fourth trunk of fifth nerve (Swan, 1830), see **buccal nerve (Meckel, 1748)**
fourth ventricle (Galen, c173), see **third ventricle (Galen, c173)**
fourth ventricle (Galen, c192)

fourth ventricle (Meckel, 1817), see **fourth ventricle (Galen, c192)**
fourth ventricle (Molinetti, 1675), see **floor of fourth ventricle (Reil, 1807–1808a)**
fourth ventricle (Willis, 1664), see **cerebral aqueduct (>1840)**
fourth ventricle fovea (Arnold, 1838a), see **floor of fourth ventricle (Reil, 1807–1808a)**
fourth ventrycle (Geminus, 1553), see **fourth ventricle (Galen, c192)**
fovea of Tarin (Günther, 1786), see **subarachnoid space (Magendie, 1827)**
fovea triangularis infra septi lucidi partem inferiorem obvia (Tarin, 1750), see **septal fissure (Burdach, 1822)**
foveae inter corpora orbicularia & protuberantiam annularem (Tarin, 1750), see **interpeduncular fossa (>1840)**
foveola ante nervorum opticorum confluxum (Soemmerring, 1778), see **preoptic recess (>1840)**
foveola ventriculi quarti (Chaussier, 1807), see **fourth ventricle (Galen, c192)**
free part of fornix column (His, 1895), see **septal postcommissural fornix (>1840)**
frenulum (Vieussens, 1684)
frenulum novum (Tarin, 1750), see **terminal stria (Wenzel & Wenzel, 1812)**
frenulum veli anterioris (Arnold, 1838a), see **frenulum (Vieussens, 1684)**
frondosae arbori (Tiedemann, 1821), see **arbor vitae (Winslow, 1733)**
front cavities (Galen, c177), see **anterior horn of lateral ventricle (Bell, 1803b)**
front part of brain (Galen, c177), see **vertebrate brain (Cuvier, 1800)**
front part of middle part of cerebellum (Vesalius, 1543a), see **cerebellar vermis (Meckel, 1817)**
frontal branch of first branch of fifth pair of nerves (Meckel, 1753), see **frontal nerve (Cheselden, 1726)**
frontal branch of ophthalmic nerve (Knox, 1832), see **frontal nerve (Cheselden, 1726)**
frontal branch of supraorbital nerve (>1840), see **medial branch of supraorbital nerve (>1840)**
frontal branch of supratrochlear nerve (Meckel, 1753), see **supratrochlear nerve (Schaarschmidt, 1750)**
frontal branches of external frontal nerve (Cruveilhier, 1836), see **supraorbital nerve (Meckel, 1753)**
frontal branches of supraorbital nerve (Cruveilhier, 1836), see **supraorbital nerve (Meckel, 1753)**
frontal cerebral lobule (Chaussier, 1807), see **frontal region (Vicq d'Azyr, 1786)**
frontal cutaneous branch of infratrochlear nerve (Meckel, 1753), see **infratrochlear nerve (Schaarschmidt, 1750)**
frontal filaments of external nasal branch of nasal nerve (Cruveilhier, 1836), see **infratrochlear nerve (Schaarschmidt, 1750)**
frontal filaments of internal frontal nerve (Cruveilhier, 1836), see **supratrochlear nerve (Schaarschmidt, 1750)**
frontal filaments of supratrochlear nerve (Cruveilhier, 1836), see **supratrochlear nerve (Schaarschmidt, 1750)**
frontal forceps (>1840)
frontal horn (Cruveilhier, 1836), see **frontal pole (>1840)**
frontal lobe (Arnold, 1838a), see **frontal region (Vicq d'Azyr, 1786)**
frontal lobe (Rolando, 1831), see **frontal region (Vicq d'Azyr, 1786)**
frontal nerve (Cheselden, 1726)
frontal nerve (>1840), see **medial branch of supraorbital nerve (>1840)**
frontal nerve proper (Meckel, 1817), see **supraorbital nerve (Meckel, 1753)**
frontal operculum (>1840)
frontal pole (>1840)
frontal ramus of ophthalmic nerve (Winslow, 1733), see **frontal nerve (Cheselden, 1726)**
frontal region (Vicq d'Azyr, 1786)
frontalis nervus (Haase, 1781), see **frontal nerve (Cheselden, 1726)**
frontonasal branch of frontal nerve (Cruveilhier, 1836), see **frontal nerve (Cheselden, 1726)**
frontopolar area (Brodmann, 1909, p. 137), see **frontal region (Vicq d'Azyr, 1786)**
frontopolar area (Brodmann, 1909, p. 156), see **frontal region (Vicq d'Azyr, 1786)**
fundament (Vesalius, 1543a), see **opening of fourth ventricle (>1840)**
fundamental part of cerebellum (Gall & Spurzheim, 1810), see **cerebellar vermis (Meckel, 1817)**
fundus of third ventricle (Günther, 1786), see **hypothalamus (Kuhlenbeck, 1927)**
funiculi inter pedunculos corporis callosi (Burdach, 1822), see **endbrain (Kuhlenbeck, 1927)**
funiculi nervei (Le Boë, 1663), see **central nervous system (Carus, 1814)**
funiculi of spinal cord (Burdach, 1822)
funiculi pyramidum (Burdach, 1822), see **pyramid (Willis, 1664)**
funiculus cuneatus (Burdach, 1822), see **cuneate fascicle (Müller, 1834)**
funiculus gracilis (Burdach, 1822), see **gracile fascicle (Müller, 1834)**
funiculus medullaris transversus (Haller, 1762), see **pineal stalk (Burdach, 1822)**
funiculus nuclei olivae (Burdach, 1822), see **olivocerebellar tract (>1840)**
funiculus olivae (Burdach, 1822), see **olivocerebellar tract (>1840)**
funiculus separans (>1840)
funiculus siliquae externus (Burdach, 1822), see **amiculum of olive (>1840)**
funiculus siliquae internus (Burdach, 1822), see **olive (Tiedemann, 1821)**
funiculus teres (Arnold, 1828a), see **floor of fourth ventricle (Reil, 1807–1808a)**
funiculus terete (Burdach, 1822), see **medial longitudinal fascicle (>1840)**
funnel (Galen, c173), see **hypothalamus (Kuhlenbeck, 1927)**
funyil (Geminus, 1553), see **hypothalamus (Kuhlenbeck, 1927)**
furrowed hillock (Diemerbroeck, 1689), see **cerebral nuclei (Swanson, 2000a)**

furrows (Heister, 1722), see **cerebellar fissures (>1840)**
furrows (Winslow, 1733), see **cerebral sulci (Vesalius, 1543a)**
fusiform ganglion (Portal, 1803a), see **superior cervical ganglion (Vieussens, 1684)**
fusiform gyrus (>1840), see **temporal region (>1840)**
gadroonate margin of hippocampus major (Vicq d'Azyr, 1786), see **dentate gyrus (>1840)**
gamberuolo (Malacarne, 1780), see **collateral eminence (Meckel, 1767)**
ganglia (Galen, c173)
ganglia cerebri magna antica (Meckel, 1817), see **cerebral nuclei (Swanson, 2000a)**
Ganglia der Rückenmarknerven (Burdach, 1819), see **spinal nerve ganglia (Burdach, 1819)**
ganglia for optic nerves (Carus, 1814), see **superior colliculus (Haller, 1762)**
ganglia hepatica (Walter, 1783), see **hepatic ganglia (Walter, 1783)**
ganglia lumbalia (Soemmerring, 1791), see **lumbar sympathetic ganglia (>1840)**
ganglia of brain (Carus, 1814), see **invertebrate brain (>1840)**
ganglia of cord (Solly, 1836), see **forebrain (Goette, 1873)**
ganglia of lower nerve cord (Carus, 1814), see **ventral ganglia (Anderson, 1837)**
ganglia of oculomuscular nerves (Carus, 1814), see **oculomotor nucleus (>1840)**
ganglia of pneumogastric nerve (Leuret, 1839), see **nucleus of solitary tract (>1840)**
ganglia of spinal medulla (Lyonnet, 1762), see **ventral ganglia (Anderson, 1837)**
ganglia of sympathetic nervous system (Wutzer, 1817), see **autonomic ganglia (Langley, 1900)**
ganglia of third nerves (Carus, 1814), see **oculomotor nucleus (>1840)**
ganglia ovalia intumescentiae magnae (Gall & Spurzheim, 1810), see **inferior olivary complex (>1840)**
ganglia renalia (Walther, 1735), see **renal ganglia (Walther, 1735)**
gangliaform tubercles (Winslow, 1733), see **peripheral ganglia (>1840)**
gangliated cord (Newport, 1834), see **central nerve cord (Serres, 1824–1826)**
gangliformis intumescentia (Scarpa, 1789), see **vestibular ganglion (>1840)**
ganglio dorsali magno (Camper, 1760–1762), see **superior thoracic ganglion (Lieutaud, 1742)**
ganglio plexuque semilunari (Wrisberg, 1780), see **peripheral nervous system (Meckel, 1817)**
ganglioform branches (Neubauer, 1772), see **jugular nerves (>1840)**
ganglioform infoldings (Willis, 1664), see **peripheral ganglia (>1840)**
ganglioform intumescence at origin of optic nerve (Arnold, 1834), see **dorsal lateral geniculate nucleus (>1840)**
ganglioform intumescence of genu of facial nerve (Arnold,1834), see **geniculate ganglion (Bischoff, 1832)**
ganglioform plexus (Vieussens, 1684), see **trigeminal ganglion (>1840)**
ganglioform plexus of par vagum (Collins, 1685), see **distal vagal ganglion (>1840)**
ganglioform plexus of pharyngeal nerve (Knox, 1832), see **terminal ganglia (Gaskell, 1886)**
ganglioform plexus of pharyngeal nerves (Scarpa, 1794), see **pharyngeal plexus (Neubauer, 1772)**
ganglioform plexus of vagus nerve (Arnold, 1834), see **vagus nerve (Galen, c192)**
ganglioform plexuses (Tarin, 1750), see **peripheral nervous system (Meckel, 1817)**
ganglioform trunk of pneumogastric (Knox, 1832), see **distal vagal ganglion (>1840)**
ganglioform tumor (Rau, 1694), see **trigeminal ganglion (>1840)**
ganglion (Reil, 1809c), see **central nervous system gray matter regions (>1840)**
ganglion (Swammerdam, c1675), see **central ganglia (>1840)**
ganglion after esophagus (Serres, 1824–1826), see **ventral ganglia (Anderson, 1837)**
ganglion annulare (Cruveilhier, 1836), see **nerves (Herophilus, c335–c280 BC)**
ganglion before esophagus (Serres, 1824–1826), see **supraesophageal ganglion (Grant, 1834a)**
ganglion caroticum (Bock, 1817), see **carotid ganglion (Wutzer, 1817; Bock, 1817)**
ganglion celiacum (Walter, 1783), see **celiac ganglion (Walter, 1783)**
ganglion cervicale imum (Haller, 1762), see **inferior cervical ganglion (Vieussens, 1684)**
ganglion cervicale imum (Neubauer, 1772), see **cardiac ganglion (Neubauer, 1772; Haller, 1772)**
ganglion cervicale infimum (Winslow, 1733), see **inferior cervical ganglion (Vieussens, 1684)**
ganglion cervicale medium (Haller, 1762), see **middle cervical ganglion (Haller, 1762)**
ganglion cervicale supremum (Haller, 1762), see **superior cervical ganglion (Vieussens, 1684)**
ganglion chain (Carus, 1814), see **ventral cord (Anderson, 1837)**
ganglion ciliare (Loder, 1778), see **ciliary ganglion (Loder, 1778)**
ganglion dorsale superius (Camper, 1760–1762), see **superior thoracic ganglion (Lieutaud, 1742)**
ganglion hordeiforme (Günther, 1786), see **lumbar sympathetic ganglia (>1840)**
ganglion impar (Quain & Wilson, 1839)
ganglion in posterior fasciculus of spinal nerves (Monro, 1783), see **spinal nerve ganglia (Burdach, 1819)**
ganglion in trunk of fifth pair of nerves (Monro, 1783), see **trigeminal ganglion (>1840)**
ganglion intervertebrale capitis anticum (Arnold, 1834), see **trigeminal ganglion (>1840)**
ganglion magnum cervicale imum (Haller, 1772), see **inferior cervical ganglion (Vieussens, 1684)**
ganglion molle and pellucidum of Scarpa (Bell, 1803b), see **cardiac ganglion (Neubauer, 1772; Haller, 1772)**
ganglion of acoustic nerve (Gall & Spurzheim, 1810), see **cochlear nuclei (>1840)**
ganglion of Andersch (Todd, 1836–1839), see **distal glossopharyngeal ganglion (>1840)**

ganglion of anterior columns (Solly, 1836), see **cerebral nuclei (Swanson, 2000a)**

ganglion of Arnold (Bendz, 1833), see **otic ganglion (Arnold, 1828)**

ganglion of auditory nerve (Tiedemann, 1816), see **cochlear nuclei (>1840)**

ganglion of cardiac nerves (Soemmerring, 1798), see **cardiac ganglion (Neubauer, 1772; Haller, 1772)**

ganglion of coccygeal nerve (Arnold, 1838b), see **coccygeal spinal ganglia (>1840)**

ganglion of fifth nerve (Ridley, 1695), see **trigeminal ganglion (>1840)**

ganglion of increase to cerebellum (Quain, 1832), see **dentate nucleus (1840)**

ganglion of intellectual faculties (Spurzheim, 1826), see **cerebral nuclei (Swanson, 2000a)**

ganglion of Laumonier (Lobstein, 1831), see **carotid ganglion (Wutzer, 1817; Bock, 1817)**

ganglion of Miekel (Bell & Bell, 1803a), see **pterygopalatine ganglion (>1840)**

ganglion of motory columns (Solly, 1836), see **cerebral nuclei (Swanson, 2000a)**

ganglion of olfactory nerve (Gall & Spurzheim, 1810), see **olfactory bulb (Weitbrecht, 1751)**

ganglion of optic nerve (Gall & Spurzheim, 1810), see **superior colliculus (Haller, 1762)**

ganglion of pituitary (Carus, 1814), see **hypothalamus (Kuhlenbeck, 1927)**

ganglion of pneumogastric (Cruveilhier, 1836), see **distal vagal ganglion (>1840)**

ganglion of radiation to ceiling of great ventricles (Carus, 1814), see **cerebral nuclei (Swanson, 2000a)**

ganglion of temporal nervi molles (Knox, 1832), see **temporal ganglion (Andersch & Soemmerring, 1792)**

ganglion of trifacial nerve (Leuret, 1839), see **spinal nucleus of trigeminal nerve (>1840)**

ganglion of uterine plexus (Tiedemann, 1822), see **uterine cervical ganglion (>1840)**

ganglion of Walter (Hovelacque, 1927), see **ganglion impar (Quain & Wilson, 1839)**

ganglion parvum cervicale imum (Neubauer, 1772), see **cardiac ganglion (Neubauer, 1772; Haller, 1772)**

ganglion renale anterius (Tiedemann, 1822), see **anterior renal ganglion (Tiedemann, 1822)**

ganglion sine pare (Bell & Bell, 1826), see **ganglion impar (Quain & Wilson, 1839)**

ganglion substance (Carus, 1814), see **central nervous system gray matter regions (>1840)**

ganglion system (Carus, 1814), see **central nervous system (Carus, 1814)**

ganglion system (Reil, 1807), see **peripheral nervous system (Meckel, 1817)**

ganglion thoracicum supernum (Haller, 1772), see **inferior cervical ganglion (Vieussens, 1684)**

ganglion thoracicum supremum (Meckel, 1817), see **superior thoracic ganglion (Lieutaud, 1742)**

ganglion ultimum cervicis (Neubauer, 1772), see **inferior cervical ganglion (Vieussens, 1684)**

ganglion ultimum thyreoideum (Soemmerring, 1791), see **inferior cervical ganglion (Vieussens, 1684)**

ganglionated circle around oesophagus (Grant, 1834a), see **central nervous system (Carus, 1814)**

ganglionated nerve (Bock, 1827), see **sympathetic cord (>1840)**

ganglionated nervous cord (Müller, 1834), see **ventral cord (Anderson, 1837)**

ganglionated oesophageal ring (Grant, 1834a), see **central nervous system (Carus, 1814)**

ganglionated part of nervous system (Blainville, 1821), see **craniospinal ganglia (>1840)**

ganglionated spinal cord (Grainger, 1837), see **ventral cord (Anderson, 1837)**

ganglionated trunk (Burdach, 1819), see **sympathetic trunk (Winslow, 1733)**

ganglionic abdominal cord (Anderson, 1837), see **ventral cord (Anderson, 1837)**

ganglionic branch of nasociliary nerve (Meckel, 1817), see **communicating branch of nasociliary nerve with ciliary ganglion (>1840)**

ganglionic branches to maxillary nerve (>1840), see **pterygopalatine nerves (Wrisberg, 1786)**

ganglionic branches to submandibular ganglion (>1840), see **communicating branches of lingual nerve with submandibular ganglion (>1840)**

ganglionic chain (Leuret, 1839), see **central nervous system (Carus, 1814)**

ganglionic fascicles of lingual surculus with chorda tympani (Bellingeri, 1818), see **communicating branches of lingual nerve with submandibular ganglion (>1840)**

ganglionic nerves (Cruveilhier, 1836), see **paravertebral nerves (Swanson & Bota, 2010)**

ganglionic nervous system (Bichat et al., 1801–1803), see **peripheral nervous system (Meckel, 1817)**

ganglionic portion of fifth pair of nerves (Todd, 1836–1839), see **trigeminal nerve sensory root (>1840)**

ganglionic root (Cruveilhier, 1836), see **dorsal root (Spurzheim, 1826)**

ganglionic root of nasal surculus (Bellingeri, 1818), see **communicating branch of nasociliary nerve with ciliary ganglion (>1840)**

ganglionic root of ophthalmic ganglion (Cruveilhier, 1836), see **sympathetic root of ciliary ganglion (>1840)**

ganglionic root of trigeminal nerve (Cruveilhier, 1836), see **trigeminal nerve sensory root (>1840)**

ganglionic spinal branches (Cruveilhier, 1836), see **communicating branches of spinal nerves (Wutzer, 1817)**

Ganglionmasse (Carus, 1814), see **central nervous system gray matter regions (>1840)**

ganglionnary nerve (Meckel, 1817), see **peripheral nervous system (Meckel, 1817)**

ganglionnary nerve anastomosis with external motor nerve (Meckel, 1817), see **communicating branch from internal carotid plexus to abducens nerve (>1840)**

ganglionnary nerve anastomosis with sixth pair (Meckel, 1817), see **communicating branch from internal carotid plexus to abducens nerve (>1840)**

ganglionnary plexuses (Meckel, 1817), see **peripheral nervous system (Meckel, 1817)**

ganglionnary system (Meckel, 1817), see **peripheral nervous system (Meckel, 1817)**

ganglions (Winslow, 1733), see **peripheral ganglia (>1840)**

ganglions communicate by short branches with vertebral nerves (Winslow, 1733), see **communicating branches of spinal nerves (Wutzer, 1817)**

ganglions of medulla spinalis (Winslow, 1733), see **spinal nerve ganglia (Burdach, 1819)**

ganglions of trunk (Winslow, 1733), see **sympathetic trunk ganglia (Winslow, 1733)**

ganglioso-abdominal centre (Lobstein, 1832), see **celiac ganglion (Walter, 1783)**

ganglium temporale (Andersch & Soemmerring, 1792), see **temporal ganglion (Andersch & Soemmerring, 1792)**

Gasserian ganglion (Hirsch, 1765), see **trigeminal ganglion (>1840)**

gastric branch of left vagus nerve (Mayer, 1794), see **gastric branches of anterior vagal trunk (>1840)**

gastric branch of right vagus nerve (Mayer, 1794), see **gastric branches of posterior vagal trunk (>1840)**

gastric branches of anterior trunk of eighth pair of nerves (Walter, 1783), see **gastric branches of anterior vagal trunk (>1840)**

gastric branches of anterior vagal trunk (>1840)

gastric branches of posterior trunk of gastric and hepatic plexus (Walter, 1783), see **gastric branches of posterior vagal trunk (>1840)**

gastric branches of posterior vagal trunk (>1840)

gastric plexus (Günther, 1786), see **prevertebral plexuses (Quain, 1832)**

gastric plexus (Walter, 1783), see **left gastric plexus (>1840)**

gastroduodenal plexus (>1840)

gastrohepatic plexus (Wrisberg, 1800), see **peripheral nervous system (Meckel, 1817)**

gastropulmonary nerve (Gordon, 1815), see **vagus nerve (Galen, c192)**

Gefässblatt (Meckel, 1817), see **choroid membrane of third ventricle (>1840)**

Gefässvorhang (Meckel, 1817), see **choroid membrane of third ventricle (>1840)**

gelatinous gray substance (Gall & Spurzheim, 1810), see **central nervous system gray matter regions (>1840)**

gelatinous substance (Gall & Spurzheim, 1809), see **central nervous system gray matter regions (>1840)**

gelatinous substance of spinal medulla (Stilling & Wallach, 1842–1843), see **dorsal horn (>1840)**

gemelli (Vesalius, 1543a), see **superior colliculus (Haller, 1762)**

gemellus inferior branch of nerve of quadratus femoris and gemellus inferior (Cruveilhier, 1836), see **nerve to quadratus femoris (>1840)**

geminum centrum semicirculare (Meckel, 1817), see **terminal stria (Wenzel & Wenzel, 1812)**

general commissure (Owen, 1832), see **supraesophageal ganglion (Grant, 1834a)**

general commissure of cerebellum (Reil, 1807–1808a), see **cerebellar vermis (Meckel, 1817)**

geniculate body (Santorini, 1724), see **medial geniculate complex (>1840)**

geniculate ganglion (Bischoff, 1832)

geniculate gyrus of Zuckerkandl (Dejerine & Dejerine-Klumpke, 1895), see **endbrain (Kuhlenbeck, 1927)**

geniculate tubercle (Rolando, 1825a), see **dorsal lateral geniculate nucleus (>1840)**

genioglossus nerves (Andersch & Soemmerring, 1792), see **lingual branches of hypoglossal nerve (Cloquet, 1816)**

genital branch of genitofemoral nerve (>1840)

genitocrural branch of lumbar plexus (Cloquet, 1816), see **genitofemoral nerve (>1840)**

genitocrural nerve (Meckel, 1817), see **genitofemoral nerve (>1840)**

genitofemoral nerve (>1840)

genu of corpus callosum (Reil, 1809b)

genu of facial nerve (Langenbeck, 1826–1830), see **intermediofacial nerve trunk (1840)**

genu of great commissure (Arnold, 1838b), see **genu of corpus callosum (Reil, 1809b)**

genu of internal capsule (>1840)

genus nervosum (Willis, 1667), see **central nervous system (Carus, 1814)**

gerollte Wulst (Soemmerring, 1788), see **Ammon's horn (Vicq d'Azyr, 1784)**

giant pyramidal area (Brodmann, 1909), see **frontal region (Vicq d'Azyr, 1786)**

gibber inferius (Soemmerring, 1778), see **dorsal lateral geniculate nucleus (>1840)**

gingival fascicles of lingual surculus with chorda tympani (Bellingeri, 1818), see **lingual nerve (Vesalius, 1543a)**

gland (Galen, c173), see **pituitary gland (>1840)**

gland at infundibulum (Galen, c173), see **pituitary gland (>1840)**

gland below extreme end of funnel (Vesalius, 1543a), see **pituitary gland (>1840)**

gland like a penis (Vesalius, 1543a), see **pineal gland (Galen, c192)**

gland resembling spinning top (Vesalius, 1543a), see **pineal gland (Galen, c192)**

glands of Pacchioni (Fantoni, 1738), see **arachnoid granulations (>1840)**

glandula behind tunnel (Willis, 1664), see **mammillary body (Ludwig, 1779)**

glandula cunearis (Wharton, 1656), see **pituitary gland (>1840)**

glandula in sphenoïdis sella posita (Colombo, 1559), see **pituitary gland (>1840)**

glandula pituitaria potior (Santorini, 1724), see **anterior lobe of pituitary gland (Haller, 1762)**

glandula turbinata (Galen, c177), see **pineal gland (Galen, c192)**

glandulae candicantes (Willis, 1664), see **mammillary body (Ludwig, 1779)**

glandulae duae albae ponè infundibulum (Willis, 1664), see **mammillary body (Ludwig, 1779)**

glandulae duae candidae (Bartholin, 1651), see **mammillary body (Ludwig, 1779)**

glandulae durae matris (Mayer, 1794), see **arachnoid granulations (>1840)**

glandulae pinealis frena (Tarin, 1750), see **habenular commissure (>1840)**

glandulae sub infundibulo (Marchetti, 1652), see **mammillary body (Ludwig, 1779)**

glandular branches of submandibular ganglion (>1840)
glandular fascicles of buccal surculus of ganglioform plexus with inferior maxillary branch (Bellingeri, 1818), see ***buccal nerve (Meckel, 1748)***
glandular lobe of hypophysis (Tilney, 1936), see ***adenohypophysis (Rioch et al., 1940)***
glandulas albas (Soemmerring, 1778), see ***mammillary body (Ludwig, 1779)***
glandulis conglobatis durae meningis (Pacchioni, 1705), see ***arachnoid granulations (>1840)***
glandulocutaneous nerve (Jacobson, 1818), see ***auriculotemporal nerve (Haller, 1762)***
glandulous flesh (Berengario da Carpi, 1522), see ***pineal gland (Galen, c192)***
glans branch of deep branch of internal pudendal nerve (Cruveilhier, 1836), see ***dorsal nerve of penis (Camper, 1762)***
glans branch of dorsal branch of penis of internal pudendal nerve (Cruveilhier, 1836), see ***dorsal nerve of penis (Camper, 1762)***
glans pituitaria (du Laurens, 1600), see ***pituitary gland (>1840)***
globes (Bartholin, 1662), see ***cerebellar cortex (Willis, 1664)***
globes (Vesalius, 1543a), see ***cerebellar hemisphere (Willis, 1664)***
globosa cerebri medulla (Piccolomini, 1586), see ***vertebrate brain (Cuvier, 1800)***
globose marrow (Crooke, 1615), see ***vertebrate brain (Cuvier, 1800)***
globose part of marrow (Bartholin, 1662), see ***vertebrate brain (Cuvier, 1800)***
globose tubercles (Günther, 1786), see ***tectum (Baer, 1837)***
globous marrow (Crooke, 1615), see ***vertebrate brain (Cuvier, 1800)***
globular part of thalamus (Reil, 1809c), see ***dorsal part of thalamus (Herrick, 1910)***
globules (Malpighi, 1669), see ***central ganglia (>1840)***
globuli (Burdach, 1822), see ***mammillary body (Ludwig, 1779)***
globuli albicantia (Santorini, 1775), see ***mammillary body (Ludwig, 1779)***
globus pallidus (Burdach, 1822)
glomus choroideum (>1840), see ***choroid enlargement (>1840)***
glossopalatine nerve (>1840), see ***intermediate nerve (>1840)***
glosso-pharyngeal anastomotic surculus of digastric branch (Bellingeri, 1818), see ***communicating branch of digastric branch of facial nerve with glossopharyngeal nerve (>1840)***
glossopharyngeal branch of eighth pair (Haller, 1762), see ***glossopharyngeal nerve (Huber, 1744)***
glossopharyngeal branches to stylopharyngeal muscle (Scarpa, 1788), see ***stylopharyngeal branch of glossopharyngeal nerve (>1840)***
glossopharyngeal eighth pair of nerves (Haller, 1772), see ***glossopharyngeal nerve (Huber, 1744)***
glossopharyngeal nerve (Huber, 1744)
glossopharyngeal nerve branches of plexus of soft nerves (Langenbeck, 1826–1830), see ***paravertebral nerves (Swanson & Bota, 2010)***
glossopharyngeal nerve central root (>1840)
glossopharyngeal nerve central rootlets (>1840)
glossopharyngeal nerve filaments (Meckel, 1817), see ***glossopharyngeal nerve rootlets (>1840)***
glossopharyngeal nerve ganglion (Huber, 1744), see ***distal glossopharyngeal ganglion (>1840)***
glossopharyngeal nerve root (>1840)
glossopharyngeal nerve rootlets (>1840)
glossopharyngeal nerve trunk (Wrisberg, 1786; Günther, 1786)
glossopharyngeal roots (Bischoff, 1832), see ***glossopharyngeal nerve rootlets (>1840)***
glottic ganglion (Arnold, 1834), see ***submandibular ganglion (>1840)***
gloutia (Galen, c173, definition 1), see ***tectum (Baer, 1837)***
gloutia (Galen, c173, definition 2), see ***inferior colliculus (Haller, 1762)***
gloution (Vesalius, 1543a), see ***inferior colliculus (Haller, 1762)***
glove of corpus callosum (Reil, 1809b), see ***splenium of corpus callosum (Burdach, 1822)***
gluteal branch of external inguinal branch of lumbar plexus (Cruveilhier, 1836), see ***ilio-inguinal nerve (Schmidt, 1794)***
gluteal branches proper of inferior gluteal nerve (Cloquet, 1816), see ***inferior gluteal nerve (Martin, 1781)***
gluteal cutaneous branch of greater abdominal branch of lumbar plexus (Cruveilhier, 1836), see ***iliohypogastric nerve (Schmidt, 1794)***
gluteal nerve (Cloquet, 1816), see ***superior gluteal nerve (Martin, 1781)***
gluteal nerves (Fyfe, 1800), see ***sacral plexus dorsal divisions (Paterson, 1887)***
going together of sinews of sight (Geminus, 1553), see ***optic chiasm (Galen, c173)***
Goll's fasciculus (>1840), see ***gracile fascicle (Müller, 1834)***
goodliest and safest root of fifth pair of sinews of brain (Geminus, 1553), see ***cranial nerves (Soemmerring, 1791)***
gracile bundle (Reil, 1809c), see ***gracile fascicle (Müller, 1834)***
gracile fascicle (Müller, 1834)
gracile lobe (Malacarne, 1776), see ***gracile lobule (>1840)***
gracile lobule (>1840)
gracile nucleus (>1840)
gracile tubercle (>1840)
grand nerf palatin (Cloquet, 1816), see ***greater palatine nerve (Cloquet, 1816)***
grand renflement au dessus des nerfs cervicaux (Gall & Spurzheim, 1810), see ***medulla (Winslow, 1733)***
grand soleil (Cruveilhier, 1836), see ***central nervous system white matter tracts (>1840)***
granular frontal area (Brodmann, 1909), see ***frontal region (Vicq d'Azyr, 1786)***
granular retrolimbic area (Brodmann, 1909), see ***granular retrosplenial area (>1840)***
granular retrosplenial area (>1840)
grapes (Albertus Magnus, 13th century), see ***cerebellar vermis (Meckel, 1817)***
graue Schleier (Valentin, 1841), see ***indusium griseum (Valentin, 1841)***

gravel (Winslow, 1733), see **brain sand (Soemmerring & Lisignolo, 1785)**
gray band (Procháska, 1779), see **cochlear nuclei (>1840)**
gray body of medulla oblongata (Arnold, 1838a), see **spinal nucleus of trigeminal nerve (>1840)**
gray bulb of olfactory nerve (Langenbeck, 1826–1830), see **olfactory bulb (Weitbrecht, 1751)**
gray colliculus (Wenzel & Wenzel, 1812), see **auditory tubercle (>1840)**
gray commissure (Cruveilhier, 1836), see **spinal central gray (>1840)**
gray commissure of thalamus (Rolando, 1831), see **dorsal part of thalamus (Herrick, 1910)**
gray communicating branch (>1840)
gray cortical substance of convolutions of brain (Baillarger, 1840), see **cerebral cortex gray matter (>1840)**
gray cribriform plate (Meckel, 1817), see **interpeduncular nucleus (>1840)**
gray equally rounded spaces (Vicq d'Azyr, 1786), see **midbrain reticular nucleus (>1840)**
gray lamina of optic chiasm (Vicq d'Azyr, 1784), see **terminal lamina (Burdach, 1822)**
gray lanceolate leaves (Desmoulins, 1825), see **nucleus of solitary tract (>1840)**
gray layer of insula (Rolando, 1831), see **claustrum (Burdach, 1822)**
gray layer of taenia striata (Vicq d'Azyr, 1786), see **bed nuclei of terminal stria (Gurdjian, 1825)**
gray mass of infundibulum (Carus, 1814), see **hypothalamus (Kuhlenbeck, 1927)**
gray matter (Meckel, 1817)
gray matter regions (Swanson & Bota, 2010)
gray-medullary appendix of acoustic nerve (Rolando, 1831), see **vestibular nuclei (>1840)**
gray nucleus (Ludwig, 1779), see **central nervous system gray matter regions (>1840)**
gray nucleus (Reil, 1812c), see **inferior colliculus (Haller, 1762)**
gray nucleus of globular portions of cerebral nucleus (Reil, 1812c), see **inferior colliculus (Haller, 1762)**
gray nucleus of medulla oblongata (Arnold, 1838a), see **spinal nucleus of trigeminal nerve (>1840)**
gray optic thalamus (Sommé, 1824), see **hypothalamus (Kuhlenbeck, 1927)**
gray perforated space (Cloquet, 1816), see **interpeduncular nucleus (>1840)**
gray plate (Meckel, 1817), see **hypothalamus (Kuhlenbeck, 1927)**
gray pyramid (Cruveilhier, 1836), see **olfactory tubercle (Calleja, 1893)**
gray root of olfactory nerve (Cruveilhier, 1836), see **olfactory tubercle (Calleja, 1893)**
gray rounded spaces (Vicq d'Azyr, 1786), see **tectum (Baer, 1837)**
gray stria (Soemmerring, 1791), see **indusium griseum (Valentin, 1841)**
gray stria of Lancisi (>1840), see **indusium griseum (Valentin, 1841)**
gray substance (Vesalius, 1543a), see **central nervous system gray matter regions (>1840)**
gray substance leaves (Rolando, 1825a), see **vagal triangle (>1840)**
gray substance of restiform body (Arnold, 1838b), see **medulla (Winslow, 1733)**
gray terminal lamina (Burdach, 1822), see **terminal lamina (Burdach, 1822)**
gray transverse lamina (Keuffel, 1810), see **spinal central gray (>1840)**
gray transverse lamina of Morgagni (Tarin, 1753), see **dorsal part of thalamus (Herrick, 1910)**
gray tubercle (Cloquet, 1828), see **spinal nucleus of trigeminal nerve (>1840)**
gray tubercle (Rolando, 1825a), see **trigeminal tubercle (>1840)**
gray tubercle of first pair (Vicq d'Azyr, 1784), see **olfactory tubercle (Calleja, 1893)**
great abdominal ganglion (Wrisberg, 1780), see **celiac ganglion (Walter, 1783)**
great abdomino-cephalic anastomotic branch (Lobstein, 1823), see **celiac branch of posterior vagal trunk (>1840)**
great anastomotic branch between median and cubital nerves (Loder, 1803), see **brachial plexus medial cord (Schwalbe, 1881)**
great anterior and superior cerebral ganglion (Arnold, 1838a), see **cerebral nuclei (Swanson, 2000a)**
great anterior plexus of heart (Senac, 1749), see **cardiac plexus (Keill, 1698)**
great auricular branch of auricular nerve of third cervical pair (Meckel, 1753), see **posterior branch of great auricular nerve (Bock, 1827)**
great auricular nerve (Haase, 1781)
great branch of medulla oblongata (Winslow, 1733), see **brainstem (Schwalbe, 1881)**
great buccal nerve (Meckel, 1753), see **buccal nerve (Meckel, 1748)**
great cardiac plexus (Lobstein, 1823), see **cardiac plexus (Keill, 1698)**
great cardiac plexus (Neubauer, 1772), see **cardiac plexus (Keill, 1698)**
great celiac ganglion (Günther, 1786), see **celiac ganglion (Walter, 1783)**
great cerebellar commissure (Gall & Spurzheim, 1810), see **middle cerebellar peduncle (Rolando, 1819)**
great cerebellar fissure (Vicq d'Azyr, 1784), see **horizontal fissure (Malacarne, 1776)**
great cerebellic commissure (Grant, 1834c), see **middle cerebellar peduncle (Rolando, 1819)**
great cerebral commissure (Arnold, 1838a), see **corpus callosum (Galen, c177)**
great cerebral commissure (Lieutaud, 1742), see **cerebral cortex white matter (>1840)**
great cerebral fissure (Bartholin, 1641), see **lateral cerebral sulcus (>1840)**
great cerebral fissure (Bichat, 1802), see **inner part of transverse cerebral fissure (>1840)**
great cerebral ganglion (Reil, 1809b), see **cerebral nuclei (Swanson, 2000a)**
great cervical ganglion (Neubauer, 1772), see **superior cervical ganglion (Vieussens, 1684)**

great chink of brain (Bartholin, 1662), see ***lateral cerebral sulcus (>1840)***

great cleft of brain (Bartholin, 1662), see ***lateral cerebral sulcus (>1840)***

great commissure (Bell & Bell, 1823), see ***corpus callosum (Galen, c177)***

great commissure (Meckel, 1817), see ***anterior commissure (Lieutaud, 1742)***

great commissure of brain (Mayo, 1827), see ***cerebral cortex white matter (>1840)***

great commissure of cerebrum (Mayo, 1827), see ***cerebral cortex white matter (>1840)***

great common uterine plexus (Tiedemann, 1822), see ***superior hypogastric plexus (Tiedemann, 1822)***

great cornu of optic nerve (Winslow, 1733), see ***optic tract (Vicq d'Azyr, 1784)***

great crural nerve trunk (Pietro da Cortona, 1741), see ***femoral nerve (Haller, 1762)***

great curvature of optic nerve (Winslow, 1733), see ***optic tract (Vicq d'Azyr, 1784)***

great cutaneous palmar branch of median nerve (Cloquet, 1828), see ***palmar branch of median nerve (Bock, 1827)***

great deep cardiac plexus (Scarpa, 1794), see ***cardiac plexus (Keill, 1698)***

great dentate branch of brachial plexus (Cruveilhier, 1836), see ***long thoracic nerve (Quain & Wilson, 1839)***

great dorsal ganglion (Neubauer, 1772), see ***inferior cervical ganglion (Vieussens, 1684)***

great double plexus of arteries of heart (Andersch, 1797), see ***coronary plexuses (Meckel, 1817)***

great esophageal plexus of eighth pair (Scarpa, 1794), see ***esophageal plexus (Haller, 1762)***

great facial branch of hard nerve (Meckel, 1753), see ***zygomatic branches of facial nerve (>1840)***

great facial branch of superior branch of anterior branch of hard nerve (Loder, 1778), see ***zygomatic branches of facial nerve (>1840)***

great facial nerve (Meckel, 1753), see ***zygomatic branches of facial nerve (>1840)***

great femoral nerve (Haller, 1762), see ***femoral nerve (Haller, 1762)***

great femoro-poplitean nerve (Burdin, 1803), see ***sciatic nerve (Keill, 1698)***

great fiber tract of hemisphere (Gall & Spurzheim, 1810), see ***cerebral peduncle (Tarin, 1753)***

great fissure of Bichat (Broca, 1878b), see ***inner part of transverse cerebral fissure (>1840)***

great fore ventricle (Mondino, 1316), see ***lateral ventricle (Vesalius, 1543a)***

great ganglion of middle and posterior lobes (Combe et al., 1838), see ***interbrain (Baer, 1837)***

great ganglions of affective powers (Spurzheim, 1826), see ***interbrain (Baer, 1837)***

great gastric plexus (Langenbeck, 1826–1830), see ***right gastric plexus (>1840)***

great harmonic ganglion (Andersch, 1797), see ***celiac ganglion (Walter, 1783)***

great harmonic nerve of body (Andersch, 1797), see ***sympathetic trunk (Winslow, 1733)***

great hole of third ventricle (Bauhin, 1605), see ***cerebral aqueduct (>1840)***

great horizontal sulcus (Arnold, 1834), see ***horizontal fissure (Malacarne, 1776)***

great hypoglossal nerve (Cuvier, 1800), see ***hypoglossal nerve (Winslow, 1733)***

great inferior cerebral ganglion (Gall & Spurzheim, 1810), see ***interbrain (Baer, 1837)***

great inferior ganglion (Arnold, 1838a), see ***interbrain (Baer, 1837)***

great intercostal nerve (Cuvier, 1800), see ***sympathetic trunk (Winslow, 1733)***

great interlobar fissure (Chaussier, 1807), see ***lateral cerebral sulcus (>1840)***

great internal cutaneous nerve (Bell, 1803b), see ***medial cutaneous nerve of forearm (>1840)***

great internal cutaneous nerve (Mayer, 1794), see ***saphenous nerve (Haase, 1781)***

great internal cutaneous nerve of leg (Mayer, 1794), see ***saphenous nerve (Haase, 1781)***

great internal respiratory nerve (Bell, 1821), see ***phrenic nerve (Galen, c173)***

great internal saphenous nerve (Bock, 1827), see ***saphenous nerve (Haase, 1781)***

great ischiatic nerve (Bell, 1803a), see ***sciatic nerve (Keill, 1698)***

great kernel (Hippocrates), see ***vertebrate brain (Cuvier, 1800)***

great king (Galen, c173), see ***vertebrate brain (Cuvier, 1800)***

great limbic lobe (Broca, 1878), see ***limbic region (>1840)***

great lobe of brain (Winslow, 1733), see ***cerebral cortex (>1840)***

great longitudinal septum (Winslow, 1733), see ***cerebral falx (Vesalius, 1543a)***

great median fissure of cerebellum (Cruveilhier, 1836), see ***vallecula of cerebellum (Haller, 1762)***

great median fissure of cerebrum (Cruveilhier, 1836), see ***longitudinal cerebral fissure (Gordon, 1815)***

great medullary nucleus (Tiedemann, 1816), see ***dentate nucleus (>1840)***

great mesenteric plexus (Winslow, 1733), see ***prevertebral plexuses (Quain, 1832)***

great nerve (Galen, c192), see ***vagus nerve (Galen, c192)***

great nerve of body (Andersch, 1797), see ***sympathetic trunk (Winslow, 1733)***

great occipital nerve (Winslow, 1733), see ***greater occipital nerve (Haase, 1781)***

great oesophageal plexus (Fyfe, 1800), see ***esophageal plexus (Haller, 1762)***

great oval notch (Winslow, 1733), see ***tentorial notch (>1840)***

great palatine nerve (Meckel, 1832), see ***greater palatine nerve (Cloquet, 1816)***

great pectoral ganglion (Schreger, 1803), see ***superior thoracic ganglion (Lieutaud, 1742)***

great plexus (Winslow, 1733), see ***brachial plexus (Camper, 1760)***

great posterior auricular nerve (Neubauer, 1772), see ***posterior branch of great auricular nerve (Bock, 1827)***

great posterior ganglion (Arnold, 1838a), see **interbrain (Baer, 1837)**
great posterior plexus of heart (Senac, 1749), see **cardiac plexus (Keill, 1698)**
great root of fifth nerve (Cruveilhier, 1836), see **trigeminal nerve central sensory root (>1840)**
great saphenous nerve (Bell, 1803a), see **saphenous nerve (Haase, 1781)**
great sciatic nerve (Knox, 1832), see **sciatic nerve (Keill, 1698)**
great semilunar ganglion (Haller, 1762), see **celiac ganglion (Walter, 1783)**
great splanchnic nerve (Burdin, 1803), see **paravertebral nerves (Swanson & Bota, 2010)**
great splanchnic nerve (Knox, 1832), see **greater splanchnic nerve (Walter, 1783)**
great striated cerebral ganglion (Reil, 1809b), see **cerebral nuclei (Swanson, 2000a)**
great sublingual nerve (Winslow, 1732), see **hypoglossal nerve (Winslow, 1733)**
great superficial division of fibular nerve (Bell & Bell, 1816), see **superficial fibular nerve (Fyfe, 1800)**
great superficial division of muscular spiral nerve (Bell & Bell, 1816), see **superficial branch of radial nerve (Martin, 1781)**
great superior cerebral ganglion (Gall & Spurzheim, 1810), see **cerebral nuclei (Swanson, 2000a)**
great superior commissure of cerebral hemispheres (Grant, 1834c), see **corpus callosum (Galen, c177)**
great suprarenal nerve (Chaussier, 1789), see **greater splanchnic nerve (Walter, 1783)**
great suprarenal nerve (Chaussier, 1807), see **paravertebral nerves (Swanson & Bota, 2010)**
great Sylvian fissure (Winslow, 1733), see **lateral cerebral sulcus (>1840)**
great sympathetic (Cruveilhier, 1836), see **peripheral nervous system (Meckel, 1817)**
great sympathetic nerve (Winslow, 1733), see **sympathetic trunk (Winslow, 1733)**
great sympathetic nerves (Cruveilhier, 1836), see **paravertebral nerves (Swanson & Bota, 2010)**
great sympathetic part of nervous system (Blainville, 1821), see **paravertebral ganglia (Durward, 1951)**
great thoracic ganglion (Lobstein, 1823), see **superior thoracic ganglion (Lieutaud, 1742)**
great thoracic ganglion (Neubauer, 1772), see **inferior cervical ganglion (Vieussens, 1684)**
great thoracic nerve (Bang, 1770), see **long thoracic nerve (Quain & Wilson, 1839)**
great toe of foot of hippocampus (Malacarne, 1780), see **cerebral cortex (>1840)**
great toe of pes hippocampi (Malacarne,1780), see **cerebral cortex (>1840)**
great transverse commissure (Solly, 1836), see **cerebral cortex white matter (>1840)**
great transverse commissure of hemispheres (Combe et al., 1838), see **cerebral cortex white matter (>1840)**
great transverse protuberance (Winslow, 1733), see **pons (Haller, 1747)**
great trunk of great sympathetic nerve (Winslow, 1733), see **paravertebral nerves (Swanson & Bota, 2010)**
great ventricles (Varoli, 1573), see **lateral ventricle (Vesalius, 1543a)**
great zygomatic branch of hard nerve (Meckel, 1753), see **facial nerve trunk (1840)**
greater abdominal branch of lumbar plexus (Cruveilhier, 1836), see **iliohypogastric nerve (Schmidt, 1794)**
greater and grosser root of third pair of sinews of brain (Geminus, 1553), see **mandibular nerve sensory root (>1840)**
greater and superior ganglion of brain (Knox, 1832), see **cerebral nuclei (Swanson, 2000a)**
greater anterior alveolar nerve (Arnold, 1834), see **anterior superior dental nerve (Haller, 1762)**
greater anterior dental nerve (Arnold, 1834), see **anterior superior dental nerve (Haller, 1762)**
greater anterior gastric nerve (>1840), see **gastric branches of anterior vagal trunk (>1840)**
greater anterior thoracic nerve (Günther, 1786), see **lateral pectoral nerve (>1840)**
greater branch of fifth pair of nerves arising within skull (Willis, 1664), see **trigeminal nerve (Winslow, 1733)**
greater branches of conjugations of neck, chest, loynes, and sacral bone (Crooke, 1615), see **spinal nerve ventral branches (>1840)**
greater cardiac infolding (Willis, 1664), see **cardiac ganglion (Neubauer, 1772; Haller, 1772)**
greater cerebellar commissure (Knox, 1832), see **middle cerebellar peduncle (Rolando, 1819)**
greater cutaneous branch of musculocutaneous nerve (Loder, 1803), see **lateral cutaneous nerve of forearm (>1840)**
greater deep branch of middle subcutaneous nerve of neck (Peipers, 1793), see **transverse nerve of neck (>1840)**
greater external branch of accessory eighth nerve (Scarpa, 1794), see **external branch of accessory nerve trunk (Meckel, 1817)**
greater external branch of spinal accessory nerve (Knox, 1832), see **external branch of accessory nerve trunk (Meckel, 1817)**
greater frontal nerve (Meckel, 1753), see **supraorbital nerve (Meckel, 1753)**
greater geniculate body (Solly, 1836), see **dorsal lateral geniculate nucleus (>1840)**
greater inferior branch of third branch of fifth pair (Meckel, 1748), see **posterior branch of mandibular nerve (>1840)**
greater occipital nerve (Haase, 1781)
greater or thicker root of third pair of nerves (Vesalius, 1543a), see **mandibular nerve sensory root (>1840)**
greater orbicular prominences (Palfijn, 1726), see **superior colliculus (Haller, 1762)**
greater palatine nerve (Cloquet, 1816)
greater petrosal nerve (>1840)
greater pons (Serres, 1824–1826), see **middle cerebellar peduncle (Rolando, 1819)**
greater posterior auricular nerve (Meckel, 1753), see **great auricular nerve (Haase, 1781)**
greater posterior thoracic nerve (Günther, 1786), see **thoracodorsal nerve (>1840)**
greater protuberance (Willis, 1664), see **pons (Haller, 1747)**

greater ring (Willis, 1664), see **pons (Haller, 1747)**

greater root of fifth pair of sinews of brain (Geminus, 1553), see **cranial nerves (Soemmerring, 1791)**

greater root of posterior pectoral nerve (Bock, 1827), see **lateral pectoral nerve (>1840)**

greater sciatic nerve (Chaussier, 1809), see **sciatic nerve (Keill, 1698)**

greater splanchnic nerve (Walter, 1783)

greater superficial petrosal nerve (Arnold, 1834), see **greater petrosal nerve (>1840)**

greater superior branch of middle cutaneous nerve of neck (Peipers, 1793), see **superior branch of transverse nerve of neck (>1840)**

greater thoracic nerve (Haase, 1781), see **long thoracic nerve (Quain & Wilson, 1839)**

greater trunk of fourth nerve of thigh (Vesalius, 1543a), see **tibial nerve (Haase, 1781)**

greater trunk or stock of fourth sinew of thigh (Geminus, 1553), see **tibial nerve (Haase, 1781)**

greater volar branch of cubital nerve (Loder, 1803), see **superficial branch of ulnar nerve (Fyfe, 1800)**

greater volar branch of dorsal nerve from internal cutaneous nerve (Knox, 1832), see **posterior branch of medial cutaneous nerve of forearm (>1840)**

greatest infolding of mesentery (Willis, 1664), see **peripheral nervous system (Meckel, 1817)**

greatest mesenteric infolding (Willis, 1664), see **peripheral nervous system (Meckel, 1817)**

grey band of Wenzels (Tiedemann, 1816), see **cochlear nuclei (>1840)**

grey matter of ganglions (Grainger, 1837), see **peripheral nervous system gray matter regions (>1840)**

grey tubercle (Solly, 1836), see **hypothalamus (Kuhlenbeck, 1927)**

greyish-brown matter (Gordon, 1815), see **gray matter (Meckel, 1817)**

grooves (Massa, 1536), see **cerebral sulci (Vesalius, 1543a)**

grooves (Vesalius, 1543a), see **cerebellar fissures (>1840)**

grossa mininga (Zerbi, 1502), see **dura (Galen, c177)**

ground of brain (Geminus, 1553), see **vertebrate brain (Cuvier, 1800)**

gustatory nerve (Galen, c180), see **lingual nerve (Vesalius, 1543a)**

gustatory nerve (Soemmerring, 1791), see **mandibular nerve (>1840)**

gustatory nerve (Winslow, 1733), see **hypoglossal nerve (Winslow, 1733)**

gustatory pair of nerves (Heister, 1717), see **trigeminal nerve (Winslow, 1733)**

gutturo-palatine nerve (Burdin, 1803), see **lesser palatine nerves (Meckel, 1817)**

gutturo-palatine nerves (Chaussier, 1809), see **nerves (Herophilus, c335–c280 BC)**

gyres (Collins, 1685), see **cerebral cortex gray matter (>1840)**

gyri (Vesalius, 1543a), see **cerebellar cortex (Willis, 1664)**

gyrus ambiens (>1840), see **ambient gyrus (>1840)**

gyrus rectus (Valentin, 1841), see **straight gyrus (Valentin, 1841)**

gyrus semilunaris (>1840), see **semilunar gyrus (>1840)**

haakenförmige Markbundel (Reil, 1809b), see **uncinate fascicle (Reil, 1809b)**

habenae (Cruveilhier, 1836), see **medullary stria (Wenzel & Wenzel, 1812)**

habenular commissure (>1840)

habenular ganglion (Meynert, 1872), see **habenular nuclei (>1840)**

habenular nuclei (>1840)

habenular sulcus (>1840)

habenular triangle (>1840)

habenulo-interpeduncular tract (>1840)

halves of cerebrum (Diemerbroeck, 1672), see **cerebral cortex (>1840)**

hamular fasciculus (Mayo, 1823), see **uncinate fascicle (Reil, 1809b)**

hard body (Geminus, 1553), see **corpus callosum (Galen, c177)**

hard cerebral membrane (Vesalius, 1543a), see **dura (Galen, c177)**

hard membrane (Galen, c177), see **dura (Galen, c177)**

hard mother (Diemerbroeck, 1689), see **dura (Galen, c177)**

hard nerve (Willis, 1664), see **intermediofacial nerve (Strong & Elwyn, 1943)**

hard nerve anastomosis with eighth pair (Meckel, 1753), see **communicating branch of digastric branch of facial nerve with glossopharyngeal nerve (>1840)**

hard nerve trunk (Günther, 1786), see **intermediofacial nerve (Strong & Elwyn, 1943)**

hard pannicle (Geminus, 1553), see **dura (Galen, c177)**

hard part of seventh pair of nerves arising within skull (Willis, 1664), see **intermediofacial nerve (Strong & Elwyn, 1943)**

harmonic nerve (Burdach, 1819), see **sympathetic trunk (Winslow, 1733)**

harp fashioned body (Riolan, 1657), see **fornix (Vesalius, 1543a)**

Hauben-Bündel (Gudden, 1889), see **mammillotegmental tract (>1840)**

haunches (Mondino, 1316), see **vertebrate brain (Cuvier, 1800)**

head cells (Baer, 1837), see **brain vesicles (Malpighi, 1673)**

head ganglion (Lyonnet, 1762), see **invertebrate brain (>1840)**

head of anterior cerebellar process (Willis, 1664), see **inferior colliculus (Haller, 1762)**

head of caudate nucleus (>1840)

head of former ventricle (Willis, 1664), see **lateral ventricle (Vesalius, 1543a)**

head of hippocampus (Duvernoy, 1735), see **cerebral cortex (>1840)**

head of inferior vermiform process (Gordon, 1815), see **nodule (Reil, 1807–1808a)**

head of marrow (Bartholin, 1662), see **vertebrate brain (Cuvier, 1800)**

head of oblong marrow (Willis, 1672), see **invertebrate brain (>1840)**

head of olfactory nerve (Vicq d'Azyr, 1786), see **olfactory bulb (Weitbrecht, 1751)**

head of rose (Avicenna or Ibn Sina, c1030), see **hypothalamus (Kuhlenbeck, 1927)**

head of spinal marrow (Gibson, 1684), see ***vertebrate brain (Cuvier, 1800)***

head of striated body (Willis, 1664), see ***head of caudate nucleus (>1840)***

heads of instruments of smell (Berengario da Carpi, 1522), see ***olfactory bulb (Weitbrecht, 1751)***

hearing nerve (Falloppio, 1561), see ***vestibulocochlear nerve (>1840)***

hearing nerve (Willis, 1664), see ***cranial nerves (Soemmerring, 1791)***

hedge of right and left ventricles (Geminus, 1553), see ***cerebral nuclei (Swanson, 2000a)***

hemiglobi cerebelli (Molinetti, 1669), see ***cerebellar hemisphere (Willis, 1664)***

hemisphaericorum tuberculorum (Soemmerring, 1778), see ***mammillary body (Ludwig, 1779)***

hemisphere (Willis, 1664), see ***cerebral cortex (>1840)***

hemispheres (Swammerdam, c1675), see ***invertebrate brain (>1840)***

hemispheric commissure (Arnold, 1838a), see ***pons (Haller, 1747)***

hemispheric crus (Rolando, 1819), see ***cerebral peduncle (Tarin, 1753)***

hemispheric ganglia (Solly, 1836), see ***forebrain (Goette, 1873)***

hemispheric ganglion (Carus, 1814), see ***interbrain (Baer, 1837)***

hemispheric lobes (Serres, 1824–1826), see ***endbrain (Kuhlenbeck, 1927)***

hemispheric sulcus (Grönberg, 1902)

hemispheric tubercle (Serres, 1824–1826), see ***cerebral nuclei (Swanson, 2000a)***

hemispherical ganglia (Solly, 1836), see ***cerebral cortex gray matter (>1840)***

hemorrhoidal branch of fifth sacral nerve (Cloquet, 1828), see ***pelvic splanchnic nerves (Gaskell, 1886)***

hemorrhoidal branches of third and fourth sacral nerves (Cloquet, 1828), see ***pelvic splanchnic nerves (Gaskell, 1886)***

hemorrhoidal nerve (Günther, 1786), see ***perineal nerve (Camper, 1762)***

hemorrhoidal nerves (Bock, 1827), see ***middle rectal plexus (>1840)***

hemorrhoidal nerves (Martin, 1781), see ***inferior rectal nerves (>1840)***

hemorrhoidal plexus (Cruveilhier, 1836), see ***superior rectal plexus (>1840)***

hemorrhoidal plexus (Mayer, 1794), see ***middle rectal plexus (>1840)***

hepatic branch of left vagus nerve (Mayer, 1794), see ***hepatic branches of anterior vagal trunk (>1840)***

hepatic branches of anterior trunk of eighth pair of nerves (Walter, 1783), see ***hepatic branches of anterior vagal trunk (>1840)***

hepatic branches of anterior vagal trunk (>1840)

hepatic branches of posterior vagal trunk (>1840)

hepatic ganglia (Walter, 1783)

hepatic nerves (Walter, 1783), see ***hepatic plexus (Rau, 1720)***

hepatic plexus (Keill, 1698), see ***celiac plexus (Winslow, 1733)***

hepatic plexus (Rau, 1720)

hepatic plexus (Walter, 1783), see ***hepatic plexus (Rau, 1720)***

hepatic plexus branches to bile ducts (>1840)

hepatick infolding (Willis, 1664), see ***celiac ganglion (Walter, 1783)***

hepatico-gastric branch of posterior trunk of gastric and hepatic plexus (Walter, 1783), see ***hepatic branch of posterior vagal trunk (>1840)***

hepaticogastric nerve (Walter, 1783), see ***hepatic plexus (Rau, 1720)***

hepaticogastric plexus (Mayer, 1794), see ***hepatic plexus (Rau, 1720)***

heterocrania (Benedetti, 1502), see ***meninges (Smith Papyrus, c1700 BC)***

hiatus ad canalem natibus et testibus substratum ducens (Vieussens, 1684), see ***opening of cerebral aqueduct (>1840)***

hiatus ad infundibulum (Vieussens, 1684), see ***ventricles (Hippocrates)***

hidden lobe (Arnold, 1838a), see ***cerebral cortex gray matter (>1840)***

high road (Willis, 1664), see ***vertebrate brain (Cuvier, 1800)***

higher branch of fourth nerve entering arm (Vesalius, 1543a), see ***superficial branch of radial nerve (Martin, 1781)***

higher part of third deep nerve of thigh (Galen, c177), see ***anterior branch of obturator nerve (Haase, 1781; Martin, 1781)***

highest cardiac nerve (Neubauer, 1772; Haller, 1772), see ***superior cardiac nerve (Neubauer, 1772)***

highest ganglioform infolding of intercostal nerve (Willis, 1664), see ***superior cervical ganglion (Vieussens, 1684)***

highest ganglion of vagus nerve (Bischoff, 1832), see ***proximal vagal ganglion (>1840)***

highest knot of intercostal nerve (Willis, 1664), see ***superior cervical ganglion (Vieussens, 1684)***

highest lateral plexus of neck (Andersch & Soemmerring, 1792), see ***nerves (Herophilus, c335–c280 BC)***

highest soft nerve (Andersch & Soemmerring, 1792), see ***jugular nerves (>1840)***

highest superficial cardiac nerve (Soemmerring, 1791), see ***superior cardiac nerve (Neubauer, 1772)***

highest superficial nerve of anterior ventricle of heart (Andersch, 1797), see ***cardiac plexus (Keill, 1698)***

highest trunk of nerves of superficial layer of septum of heart (Andersch, 1797), see ***coronary plexuses (Meckel, 1817)***

hillock (Vesalius, 1555), see ***cerebral cortex (>1840)***

hind brain (Galen, c192), see ***cerebellum (Aristotle)***

hind brain (Mondino, 1316), see ***rhombicbrain (His, 1893b)***

hind part of middle part of cerebellum (Vesalius, 1543a), see ***cerebellar vermis (Meckel, 1817)***

hind passage of third ventricle (Vesalius, 1543a), see ***cerebral aqueduct (>1840)***

hind recess of ventricle (Vesalius, 1543a), see ***body of lateral ventricle (Bell, 1803b)***

hind shank of fornix (Bartholin, 1662), see ***fimbria (Honegger, 1890)***

hind ventricle (Mondino, 1316), see ***fourth ventricle (Galen, c192)***
hindbrain (Baer, 1837)
hindbrain vesicle (Baer, 1837)
hinder border of streaked body (Willis, 1672), see ***internal capsule (Burdach, 1822)***
hinder braine-pan (Nemesius, 1636), see ***fourth ventricle (Galen, c192)***
hinder cell of brain (Geminus, 1553), see ***cerebellum (Aristotle)***
hinder leg of vault (Vesling, 1647), see ***fimbria (Honegger, 1890)***
hinder lobe of brain (Gibson, 1682), see ***cerebral cortex gray matter (>1840)***
hinder nerves of pairs of nerves of medulla spinalis (Salmon, 1714), see ***spinal nerve dorsal branch (Meckel, 1817)***
hinder part of medulla oblongata (Gibson, 1684), see ***rhombicbrain (His, 1893b)***
hinder part of trunk of long marrow (Diemerbroeck, 1689), see ***pons (Haller, 1747)***
hinder region of oblong marrow (Willis, 1664), see ***rhombicbrain (His, 1893b)***
hinder roots of oblongata medulla (Ridley, 1695), see ***cerebellar peduncles (Ridley, 1695)***
hinder thigh of fornix (Bartholin, 1662), see ***fimbria (Honegger, 1890)***
hindermore nerves of pairs of nerves of medulla spinalis (Salmon, 1714), see ***spinal nerve dorsal branch (Meckel, 1817)***
hindermost branch of pairs of sinews or nerves from neck, back, loins, and os sacrum (Read, 1638), see ***spinal nerve dorsal branch (Meckel, 1817)***
hindmost lobe of brain (Cowper, 1698), see ***cerebral cortex gray matter (>1840)***
hindmost ventricle (Avicenna, c1030), see ***fourth ventricle (Galen, c192)***
hindpart of brain (Crooke, 1615), see ***cerebral cortex gray matter (>1840)***
hinter oder beutelförmiger Ausschnitt (Reil, 1807–1808a), see ***cerebellar vermis (Meckel, 1817)***
hinteres primären Hirnbläschen (Baer, 1837), see ***primary hindbrain vesicle (Baer, 1837)***
Hinterhirn (Baer, 1837), see ***hindbrain (Baer, 1837)***
hintre oder kleine Wulst (Tiedemann, 1816), see ***calcarine spur (Morand, 1748)***
hippocampal commissure (Owen, 1837), see ***fornix (Vesalius, 1543a)***
hippocampal commissures (Johnston, 1913)
hippocampal decussation (Demeter et al., 1985), see ***intermediate hippocampal commissure (>1840)***
hippocampal fissure (Gratiolet, 1854), see ***hippocampal sulcus (Gratiolet, 1854)***
hippocampal formation (Swanson & Cowan, 1977)
hippocampal gyrus (>1840), see ***parahippocampal gyrus (>1840)***
hippocampal lobe (Serres, 1824–1826), see ***parahippocampal gyrus (>1840)***
hippocampal lobule (Serres, 1824–1826), see ***parahippocampal gyrus (>1840)***
hippocampal region (Swanson et al., 1987)
hippocampal sulcus (Gratiolet, 1854)
hippocampal ventricle (Aranzi, 1587), see ***inferior horn of lateral ventricle (Bell, 1802)***
hippocampus (Aranzi, 1587), see ***hippocampal region (Swanson et al., 1987)***
hippocampus (Vicq d'Azyr, 1784), see ***Ammon's horn (Vicq d'Azyr, 1784)***
hippocampus Aurantius (Ridley, 1695), see ***hippocampal region (Swanson et al., 1987)***
hippocampus major (Vicq d'Azyr, 1786), see ***Ammon's horn (Vicq d'Azyr, 1784)***
hippocampus minor (Vicq d'Azyr, 1786), see ***calcarine spur (Morand, 1748)***
hippocampus proper (Vicq d'Azyr, 1786), see ***Ammon's horn (Vicq d'Azyr, 1784)***
Hirnschenkelsystem (Reil, 1809b), see ***central nervous system white matter tracts (>1840)***
Hirnstamm (Schwalbe, 1881), see ***brainstem (Schwalbe, 1881)***
Hirschfeld's ganglion (>1840), see ***posterior renal ganglion (>1840)***
hole (Galen, c177), see ***interventricular foramen (>1840)***
hollow (Aristotle), see ***ventricles (Hippocrates)***
hollow (Rufus of Ephesus, fl. c90–120), see ***hypothalamic part of third ventricle (Swanson, 2004)***
hollow medullary prominences (Willis, 1664), see ***tectum (Baer, 1837)***
hollowness common to cerebellum and marrow of back (Geminus, 1553), see ***fourth ventricle (Galen, c192)***
hollowness common to right and left ventricles (Geminus, 1553), see ***third ventricle (Galen, c173)***
holy mother (Diemerbroeck, 1689), see ***pia (Galen, c192)***
hordeiforme ganglia (Portal, 1803a), see ***thoracic sympathetic ganglia (1840)***
horizontal fibers (Burdach, 1822), see ***ventrolateral fascicle (>1840)***
horizontal filament of posterior auricular branch of facial nerve (Cruveilhier, 1836), see ***occipital branch of posterior auricular nerve (Arnold, 1834)***
horizontal fissure (Malacarne, 1776)
horizontal portion of nucleus of cerebrum (Reil, 1809b), see ***cerebral cortex white matter (>1840)***
horizontal vesicle plexus (Cruveilhier, 1836), see ***extrinsic vesical plexus (>1840)***
horn of right and left ventricle (Vesalius, 1543a), see ***inferior horn of lateral ventricle (Bell, 1802)***
horny layer of taenia striata (Vicq d'Azyr, 1786), see ***bed nuclei of terminal stria (Gurdjian, 1925)***
horse's tail (Anatomia Magistri Nicolai physici, early 12th century), see ***cauda equina (Anatomia Magistri Nicolai physici, early 12th century)***
Hügel (Vesalius, 1555), see ***cerebral cortex (>1840)***
humeral circumflex nerve (Mayer, 1794), see ***axillary nerve (Winslow, 1733)***
humeral subcutaneous supraclavicular branch (Peipers, 1793), see ***lateral supraclavicular nerves (>1840)***
hyo-glossian pair of nerves (Burdin, 1803), see ***hypoglossal nerve (Winslow, 1733)***
hyothyroid nerves (Scarpa, 1794), see ***thyrohyoid branch of hypoglossal nerve (Meckel, 1817)***

hyo-thyroidian branch of hyoglossal nerve (Burdin, 1803), see **thyrohyoid branch of hypoglossal nerve (Meckel, 1817)**

hypogastric branch of first accessory lumbar ganglion (Walter, 1783), see **lumbar splanchnic nerves (Cruveilhier, 1836)**

hypogastric branch of fourth sacral pair (Walter, 1783), see **pelvic splanchnic nerves (Gaskell, 1886)**

hypogastric branch of second accessory lumbar ganglion (Walter, 1783), see **lumbar splanchnic nerves (Cruveilhier, 1836)**

hypogastric branch of third lumbar ganglion (Walter, 1783), see **lumbar splanchnic nerves (Cruveilhier, 1836)**

hypogastric branches of great sympathetic (Cloquet, 1828), see **lumbar splanchnic nerves (Cruveilhier, 1836)**

hypogastric branches of great sympathetic forming hypogastric plexus (Cloquet, 1828), see **lumbar splanchnic nerves (Cruveilhier, 1836)**

hypogastric branches of sacral nerves (Cloquet, 1828), see **pelvic splanchnic nerves (Gaskell, 1886)**

hypogastric branches of third sacral nerve (Walter, 1783), see **pelvic splanchnic nerves (Gaskell, 1886)**

hypogastric nerve (Walter, 1783)

hypogastric nerves (Chaussier, 1809), see **inferior hypogastric plexus (Tiedemann, 1822)**

hypogastric plexus (Haller, 1762), see **prevertebral plexuses (Quain, 1832)**

hypogastric plexus (Mitchell, 1953), see **superior hypogastric plexus (Tiedemann, 1822)**

hypogastric plexus (Winslow, 1733), see **inferior hypogastric plexus (Tiedemann, 1822)**

hypoglossal nerve (Winslow, 1733)

hypoglossal nerve central root (>1840)

hypoglossal nerve central rootlets (>1840)

hypoglossal nerve fasciculi (Soemmerring, 1791), see **hypoglossal nerve rootlets (>1840)**

hypoglossal nerve fibers (Günther, 1786), see **hypoglossal nerve rootlets (>1840)**

hypoglossal nerve root (>1840)

hypoglossal nerve rootlets (>1840)

hypoglossal nerve trunk (Günther, 1786)

hypoglossal nucleus (>1840)

hypoglossal triangle (>1840)

hypophysial plexus (>1840)

hypophysial stalk (Rioch et al., 1940), see **infundibulum (Rioch et al., 1940)**

hypophysis (Soemmerring, 1791), see **pituitary gland (>1840)**

hypophysis cerebri (Arnold, 1834), see **pituitary gland (>1840)**

hypophysis cerebri lobulus anterior (Arnold, 1834), see **anterior lobe of pituitary gland (Haller, 1762)**

hypophysis cerebri lobulus posterior (Arnold, 1834), see **posterior lobe of pituitary gland (Haller, 1762)**

hypothalamic mammillotegmental tract (>1840)

hypothalamic mammillothalamic tract (>1840)

hypothalamic medial forebrain bundle (>1840)

hypothalamic medullary stria (>1840)

hypothalamic optic tract (>1840)

hypothalamic part of fornix (Cajal, 1904), see **hypothalamic postcommissural fornix (>1840)**

hypothalamic part of third ventricle (Swanson, 2004)

hypothalamic postcommissural fornix (>1840)

hypothalamic sulcus (>1840)

hypothalamohypophysial tract (>1840)

hypothalamus (His, 1893a), see **hypothalamus (Kuhlenbeck, 1927)**

hypothalamus (His, 1893b), see **hypothalamus (Kuhlenbeck, 1927)**

hypothalamus (Kuhlenbeck, 1927)

hyppocampum (Cortesi, 1625), see **hippocampal region (Swanson et al., 1987)**

ilamide (Benedetti, 1502), see **pia (Galen, c192)**

iliac plexus (Fischer, 1791), see **muscular branches of femoral nerve (Quain & Wilson, 1839)**

iliac plexus (>1840)

iliacus branches of crural nerve (Cruveilhier, 1836), see **muscular branches of femoral nerve (Quain & Wilson, 1839)**

iliohypogastric nerve (Schmidt, 1794)

iliohypogastric plexus (Bock, 1827), see **superior hypogastric plexus (Tiedemann, 1822)**

ilio-inguinal nerve (Schmidt, 1794)

iliosacral nerve (Cloquet, 1828), see **lumbosacral trunk (Cruveilhier, 1836)**

ilioscrotal branch of lumbar plexus (Cruveilhier, 1836), see **iliohypogastric nerve (Schmidt, 1794)**

ilio-scrotal branches of first lumbar pair (Cruveilhier, 1836), see **lumbar plexus ventral branches (>1840)**

ilioscrotal nerve (Chaussier, 1807), see **ilio-inguinal nerve (Schmidt, 1794)**

implexus (Vesalius, 1543a), see **cerebral cortex gray matter (>1840)**

incile (Haller, 1762), see **cerebral aqueduct (>1840)**

incisor dental branch of inferior dental nerve (Cruveilhier, 1836), see **incisor nerve (>1840)**

incisor nerve (>1840)

incisura anterior cerebelli (Burdach, 1822), see **anterior cerebellar notch (Chaussier, 1807)**

incisura cerebelli anterior (Burdach, 1822), see **anterior cerebellar notch (Chaussier, 1807)**

incisura cerebelli posterior (Burdach, 1822), see **posterior cerebellar notch (Chaussier, 1807)**

incisura pallii (Burdach, 1822), see **longitudinal cerebral fissure (Gordon, 1815)**

incisura posterior cerebelli (Burdach, 1822), see **posterior cerebellar notch (Chaussier, 1807)**

incisura septi (Burdach, 1822), see **septal fissure (Burdach, 1822)**

incisura tentorii (>1840), see **tentorial notch (>1840)**

incrementa fibrosa (Drelincourt, 1672), see **rostral medullary velum (>1840)**

incrementa fibrosa a cerebro ad cerebellum obliqua (Drelincourt, 1672), see **superior cerebellar peduncle (Procháska, 1800)**

incruciatio (Berengario da Carpi, 1521), see **optic chiasm (Galen, c173)**

indented band (Gordon, 1815), see **dentate gyrus (>1840)**

indented border (Reil, 1812c), see **dentate gyrus (>1840)**

indented margin of pedes hippocampi (Fyfe, 1800), see **dentate gyrus (>1840)**

induseum griseum (>1840), see **indusium griseum (Valentin, 1841)**

indusium griseum (Valentin, 1841)
indusium griseum corporis callosi (Valentin, 1841), see **indusium griseum (Valentin, 1841)**
inferior acoustic fovea (Bergmann, 1831), see **foramen cecum of medulla (>1840)**
inferior alveolar branch of inferior maxillary branch of fifth pair of nerves (Bock, 1817), see **inferior dental nerve (Meckel, 1817)**
inferior alveolar nerve (Arnold, 1834), see **inferior dental nerve (Meckel, 1817)**
inferior alveolar surculus of inferior maxillary branch (Bellingeri, 1818), see **inferior dental nerve (Meckel, 1817)**
inferior anastomotic thread of malo-palpebral fascicle of subcutaneous malar surculus with external palpebral thread of infraorbital surculus (Bellingeri, 1818), see **zygomaticofacial nerve (>1840)**
inferior anastomotic thread of malo-palpebral fascicle of subcutaneous malar surculus with inferior orbital thread of seventh pair (Bellingeri, 1818), see **zygomaticofacial nerve (>1840)**
inferior anastomotic thread of malo-palpebral fascicle of subcutaneous malar surculus with subcutaneous temporal fascicle (Bellingeri, 1818), see **zygomaticofacial nerve (>1840)**
inferior anastomotic thread of malo-palpebral fascicle of subcutaneous malar surculus with superior facial branch of seventh pair (Bellingeri, 1818), see **zygomaticofacial nerve (>1840)**
inferior anastomotic threads of malo-palpebral fascicle of subcutaneous malar surculus (Bellingeri, 1818), see **zygomaticofacial nerve (>1840)**
inferior and internal cutaneous nerve (Bell, 1803b), see **medial cutaneous nerve of thigh (>1840)**
inferior and internal cutaneous nerve (Cloquet, 1828), see **medial cutaneous nerve of calf (>1840)**
inferior and internal cutaneous nerve (Jördens, 1788), see **nerve to hamstring muscles (>1840)**
inferior and middle subcutaneous nerve of neck (Arnold, 1834), see **transverse nerve of neck (>1840)**
inferior and superior floor of hippocampus major (Vicq d'Azyr, 1786), see **parahippocampal gyrus (>1840)**
inferior and superior level of annular protuberance (Desmoulins, 1825), see **transverse pontine fibers (>1840)**
inferior anterior branch of auditory nerve proper (Günther, 1786), see **cochlear nerve (Cotugno, 1760)**
inferior anterior branches of muscular nerve (Martin, 1781), see **dorsal digital nerves of deep fibular nerve (>1840)**
inferior anterior lobe (Meckel, 1817), see **biventral lobule (>1840)**
inferior anterior nasal nerves (Scarpa, 1785), see **posterior inferior nasal nerves (>1840)**
inferior anterior tubercle of Tarin (Günther, 1786), see **cerebellar hemisphere (Willis, 1664)**
inferior aortic plexus (Bock, 1827), see **inferior mesenteric plexus (Rau, 1720)**
inferior auricular fascicle of cutaneous temporal surculus of inferior maxillary branch (Bellingeri, 1818), see **parotid branches of auriculotemporal nerve (>1840)**
inferior auricular nerve (Meckel, 1817), see **posterior auricular nerve (Meckel, 1753)**
inferior bigeminal prominences (Rolando, 1831), see **inferior colliculus (Haller, 1762)**
inferior brachial plexus (Günther, 1786), see **brachial plexus dorsal cord (Peterson, 1887)**
inferior branch of auriculotemporal nerve (Cruveilhier, 1836), see **anterior auricular nerves (>1840)**
inferior branch of buccal nerve (Meckel, 1753), see **buccal branch of facial nerve (>1840)**
inferior branch of crural plexus (Meckel, 1817), see **lateral cutaneous nerve of thigh (>1840)**
inferior branch of external branch of inferior maxillary nerve (Meckel, 1753), see **marginal mandibular branch of facial nerve (>1840)**
inferior branch of facial nerve (Arnold, 1834), see **facial nerve trunk (1840)**
inferior branch of facial nerve (Meckel, 1753), see **zygomatic branches of facial nerve (>1840)**
inferior branch of fifth pair (Winslow, 1733), see **mandibular nerve (>1840)**
inferior branch of first and superior branch of third pair (Marchetti, 1652), see **nasociliary nerve (Meckel, 1817; Wutzer, 1817)**
inferior branch of first branch of fifth pair (Haller, 1743), see **nasociliary nerve (Meckel, 1817; Wutzer, 1817)**
inferior branch of first division of fifth pair of nerves (Todd, 1836–1839), see **nasociliary nerve (Meckel, 1817; Wutzer, 1817)**
inferior branch of great facial nerve (Meckel, 1753), see **zygomatic branches of facial nerve (>1840)**
inferior branch of hard nerve (Meckel, 1753), see **facial nerve trunk (1840)**
inferior branch of hard part of nerve of seventh pair (Bonhomme, 1748), see **facial nerve trunk (1840)**
inferior branch of internal pudendal nerve (Cruveilhier, 1836), see **perineal nerve (Camper, 1762)**
inferior branch of middle cutaneous nerve of neck (Peipers, 1793), see **inferior branches of transverse nerve of neck (>1840)**
inferior branch of middle subcutaneous nerve of neck (Bock, 1827), see **superior branches of transverse nerve of neck (>1840)**
inferior branch of obturator nerve (Soemmerring, 1798), see **posterior branch of obturator nerve (Haase, 1781; Martin, 1781)**
inferior branch of perineal branch of internal pudendal nerve (Cruveilhier, 1836), see **perineal nerve (Camper, 1762)**
inferior branch of portio dura (Du Verney, 1683), see **facial nerve trunk (1840)**
inferior branch of portio major and minor of facial nerve (Bellingeri, 1818), see **facial nerve trunk (1840)**
inferior branch of pterygoid nerve (Cloquet, 1816), see **deep petrosal nerve (Meckel, 1817)**
inferior branch of right vagus nerve (Mayer, 1794), see **gastric branches of posterior vagal trunk (>1840)**

inferior branch of subcutaneous malar nerve (Arnold, 1834), see ***zygomaticofacial nerve (>1840)***

inferior branch of subcutaneous nerve of neck (Meckel, 1753), see ***inferior branches of transverse nerve of neck (>1840)***

inferior branch of superior cervical ganglion (Cloquet, 1816), see ***communicating branch of superior and middle cervical ganglia (>1840)***

inferior branch of superior maxillary branch of nerve of fifth pair (Bonhomme, 1748), see ***maxillary nerve (Meckel, 1753)***

inferior branch of trigeminal nerve (Winslow, 1733), see ***mandibular nerve (>1840)***

inferior branch of vestibular nerve (Arnold, 1839), see ***posterior ampullary nerve (>1840)***

inferior branch of Vidian nerve (Burdin, 1803), see ***deep petrosal nerve (Meckel, 1817)***

inferior branches of inferior maxillary nerve (Cruveilhier, 1836), see ***mandibular nerve (>1840)***

inferior branches of pudendal nerve (Bock, 1827), see ***perineal nerve (Camper, 1762)***

inferior branches of spermatic nerve (Fyfe, 1800), see ***genital branch of genitofemoral nerve (>1840)***

inferior branches of transverse nerve of neck (>1840)

inferior cardiac nerve (Cloquet, 1816)

inferior cardiac plexus (Cuvier, 1800), see ***cardiac plexus (Keill, 1698)***

inferior caroticotympanic nerve (>1840)

inferior cavity of foremost ventricle (Vesling, 1647), see ***inferior horn of lateral ventricle (Bell, 1802)***

inferior cerebellar fissure (Vic d'Azyr, 1784), see ***posterior superior fissure (>1840)***

inferior cerebellar peduncle (Günther, 1786)

inferior cerebellar peduncle (Santorini, 1775), see ***middle cerebellar peduncle (Rolando, 1819)***

inferior cerebellar process (Günther, 1786), see ***inferior cerebellar peduncle (Günther, 1786)***

inferior cerebellar vermis (Tiedemann, 1821), see ***cerebellar vermis (Meckel, 1817)***

inferior cerebral ganglion (Quain, 1828), see ***interbrain (Baer, 1837)***

inferior cervical cardiac branches of vagus nerve (>1840)

inferior cervical ganglion (Neubauer, 1772), see ***middle cervical ganglion (Haller, 1762)***

inferior cervical ganglion (Vieussens, 1684)

inferior ciliary filaments (Todd, 1836–1839), see ***short ciliary nerves (>1840)***

inferior circumflex nerve of arteries of heart (Andersch, 1797), see ***coronary plexuses (Meckel, 1817)***

inferior clunial nerves (>1840)

inferior coccygeal nerve (Schlemm, 1834), see ***coccygeal nerves (Camper, 1762)***

inferior colliculus (Haller, 1762)

inferior colliculus commissure (>1840)

inferior column of cerebellum (Chaussier, 1807), see ***inferior cerebellar peduncle (Günther, 1786)***

inferior cord (Desmoulins, 1825), see ***ventral funiculus (>1840)***

inferior cornu of lateral ventricle (Fyfe, 1800), see ***inferior horn of lateral ventricle (Bell, 1802)***

inferior coronary plexus (Meckel, 1817), see ***autonomic nerves (Langley, 1896)***

inferior corpora olivaria (Schroeder van der Kolk, 1858), see ***inferior olivary complex (>1840)***

inferior cubital nerve (Cheselden, 1713), see ***ulnar nerve (Cheselden, 1726)***

inferior cutaneous branch of crural nerve (Martin, 1781), see ***saphenous nerve (Haase, 1781)***

inferior cutaneous nerve (Fischer, 1791), see ***saphenous nerve (Haase, 1781)***

inferior cutaneous nerve of face (Mayer, 1794), see ***branches of transverse nerve of neck (>1840)***

inferior cutaneous nerve of foot (Günther, 1786), see ***saphenous nerve (Haase, 1781)***

inferior cutaneous nerve of haunches (Knox, 1832), see ***perforating cutaneous nerve (>1840)***

inferior cutaneous nerve of neck (Meckel, 1753), see ***inferior branches of transverse nerve of neck (>1840)***

inferior cutaneous nerves of buttocks (Walter, 1783), see ***perforating cutaneous nerve (>1840)***

inferior cutaneous nerves of neck (Peipers, 1793), see ***inferior branches of transverse nerve of neck (>1840)***

inferior cutaneous perforant branch of crural musculocutaneous nerve (Cruveilhier, 1836), see ***medial cutaneous branches of femoral nerve (>1840)***

inferior cystic nerves (Mayer, 1794), see ***cystic plexus (Wrisberg, 1808)***

inferior dental branch of inferior maxillary nerve (Cloquet, 1816), see ***inferior dental nerve (Meckel, 1817)***

inferior dental branches of inferior dental plexus (>1840)

inferior dental branches of inferior maxillary nerve proper (Günther, 1786), see ***inferior dental branches of inferior dental plexus (>1840)***

inferior dental nerve (Meckel, 1817)

inferior dental plexus (>1840)

inferior dentar nerve (Meckel, 1832), see ***inferior dental nerve (Meckel, 1817)***

inferior descending prolongation of cerebellum (Meckel, 1817), see ***inferior cerebellar peduncle (Günther, 1786)***

inferior division of facial nerve (Swan, 1830), see ***facial nerve trunk (1840)***

inferior division of fifth cervical nerve (Bell & Bell, 1816), see ***cervical nerve (Galen, c173)***

inferior enlargement (Serres, 1824–1826), see ***lumbosacral enlargement (>1840)***

inferior external cutaneous nerve of arm (Mayer, 1794), see ***lateral cutaneous nerve of forearm (>1840)***

inferior external cutaneous nerve of leg (Mayer, 1794), see ***femoral nerve (Haller, 1762)***

inferior external femoral cutaneous nerve (Mayer, 1794), see ***femoral nerve (Haller, 1762)***

inferior external palpebral nerve (Mayer, 1794), see ***inferior palpebral branches of infraorbital nerve (Meckel, 1748)***

inferior external pudendal nerve (Mayer, 1794), see ***inferior pudendal nerve (Camper, 1762)***

inferior external respiratory nerve (Bell & Bell, 1826), see ***long thoracic nerve (Quain & Wilson, 1839)*** *inferior external subsural cutaneous nerve (Knox, 1832)*, see **tibial nerve (Haase, 1781)**

inferior external subsural nerve (Fischer, 1791), see **tibial nerve (Haase, 1781)**

inferior extremity of spinal prolongation (Chaussier, 1807), see **medullary cone (Bock, 1827)**

inferior facial branch of facial nerve (Cloquet, 1828), see **buccal branch of facial nerve (>1840)**

inferior facial branch of hard nerve (Haller, 1762), see **facial nerve trunk (1840)**

inferior facial branch of hard nerve (Meckel, 1753), see **facial nerve trunk (1840)**

inferior facial branch of hard nerve (Peipers, 1793), see **buccal branch of facial nerve (>1840)**

inferior facial branch of inferior branch of anterior branch of hard nerve (Loder, 1778), see **marginal mandibular branch of facial nerve (>1840)**

inferior facial branch of pes anserinus (Bellingeri, 1818), see **zygomatic branches of facial nerve (>1840)**

inferior facial branch of portio dura (Knox, 1832), see **buccal branch of facial nerve (>1840)**

inferior facial nerve (Bell & Bell, 1816), see **zygomatic branches of facial nerve (>1840)**

inferior facial nerve (Mayer, 1794), see **zygomatic branches of facial nerve (>1840)**

inferior fascicle of accessory optic system (Hayhow et al., 1960)

inferior fascicle of buccal surculus of cervico-facial branch of portio major and minor of facial nerve (Bellingeri, 1818), see **buccal branch of facial nerve (>1840)**

inferior fascicle of buccal surculus of inferior branch of portio major and minor of facial nerve (Bellingeri, 1818), see **buccal branch of facial nerve (>1840)**

inferior fascicle of inferior maxillary nerve (Günther, 1786), see **posterior branch of mandibular nerve (>1840)**

inferior filaments of sympathetic labial threads of mental fascicle of inferior alveolar surculus of inferior maxillary branch (Bellingeri, 1818), see **mental branches of mental nerve (>1840)**

inferior fissure (Burdach, 1822), see **lateral cerebral sulcus (>1840)**

inferior floor of fourth ventricle (Vicq d'Azyr, 1786), see **floor of fourth ventricle (Reil, 1807–1808a)**

inferior foramen (Tyson, 1699), see **opening of fourth ventricle (>1840)**

inferior fornix (Cajal, 1904), see **postcommissural fornix (Loo, 1931)**

inferior frontal gyrus (>1840)

inferior frontal nerve (Martin, 1781), see **infratrochlear nerve (Schaarschmidt, 1750)**

inferior frontal sulcus (>1840)

inferior ganglion (Leuret, 1839), see **hypothalamus (Kuhlenbeck, 1927)**

inferior ganglion of glossopharyngeal nerve (Todd, 1836–1839), see **distal glossopharyngeal ganglion (>1840)**

inferior ganglionic plexus (Tiedemann, 1822), see **inferior hypogastric plexus (Tiedemann, 1822)**

inferior gastric nerves (Wrisberg, 1800), see **autonomic nerves (Langley, 1896)**

inferior gastric plexus (Portal, 1803a), see **autonomic nerves (Langley, 1896)**

inferior gingival branches of inferior dental plexus (>1840)

inferior gland (Steno, 1669), see **pituitary gland (>1840)**

inferior gluteal branches of lesser sciatic nerve (Quain, 1828), see **inferior clunial nerves (>1840)**

inferior gluteal branches of small sciatic nerve (Quain, 1832), see **inferior gluteal nerve (Martin, 1781)**

inferior gluteal cutaneous nerve (Fischer, 1791), see **inferior clunial nerves (>1840)**

inferior gluteal cutaneous nerve (Walter, 1783), see **perforating cutaneous nerve (>1840)**

inferior gluteal nerve (Cloquet, 1816), see **sacral plexus (Vesalius, 1543a)**

inferior gluteal nerve (Martin, 1781)

inferior gluteal nerve (Quain, 1832), see **sacral plexus (Vesalius, 1543a)**

inferior gray fascicles of central medulla (Desmoulins, 1825), see **ventral horn (>1840)**

inferior hemorrhoidal nerve (Meckel, 1817), see **inferior rectal nerves (>1840)**

inferior hemorrhoidal plexus (Cruveilhier, 1836), see **middle rectal plexus (>1840)**

inferior horn of lateral ventricle (Bell, 1802)

inferior horn of tricornate ventricle (Soemmerring, 1791), see **inferior horn of lateral ventricle (Bell, 1802)**

inferior hypogastric plexus (Tiedemann, 1822)

inferior intercosto-humeral nerve (Knox, 1832), see **anterior branch of lateral cutaneous branch of intercostal nerves (>1840)**

inferior intermediate cerebellar lobule (Mayer, 1794), see **cerebellar vermis (Meckel, 1817)**

inferior internal cutaneous nerve (Cloquet, 1828), see **medial cutaneous nerve of calf (>1840)**

inferior internal cutaneous nerve (Fischer, 1791), see **sciatic nerve (Keill, 1698)**

inferior internal cutaneous nerve (Fyfe, 1800), see **posterior cutaneous nerve of thigh (Günther, 1786)**

inferior internal cutaneous nerve (Meckel, 1817), see **medial cutaneous nerve of forearm (>1840)**

inferior internal cutaneous nerve of foot (Mayer, 1794), see **saphenous nerve (Haase, 1781)**

inferior internal lobe (Meckel, 1817), see **tonsil (Malacarne, 1776)**

inferior internal nerves of nose (Bell & Bell, 1826), see **posterior inferior nasal nerves (>1840)**

inferior internal palpebral nerve (Mayer, 1794), see **inferior palpebral branches of infraorbital nerve (Meckel, 1748)**

inferior internal subsural cutaneous nerve (Fischer, 1791), see **tibial nerve (Haase, 1781)**

inferior internal subsural nerve (Fischer, 1791), see **tibial nerve (Haase, 1781)**

inferior labial branches of inferior maxillary nerve (Todd, 1836–1839), see **inferior labial branches of mental nerve (Meckel, 1753)**

inferior labial branches of inferior maxillary nerve proper (Günther, 1786), see **inferior labial branches of mental nerve (Meckel, 1753)**

inferior labial branches of mental nerve (Meckel, 1753)
inferior labial nerves (Schaarschmidt, 1750), see **inferior labial branches of mental nerve (Meckel, 1753)**
inferior laryngeal branch of pneumogastric nerve (Cloquet, 1816), see **recurrent laryngeal nerve (Albinus, 1744)**
inferior laryngeal nerve (Albinus, 1744), see **recurrent laryngeal nerve (Albinus, 1744)**
inferior laryngeal nerve (>1840)
inferior lateral cutaneous nerve of arm (>1840)
inferior lateral plexus of neck (Andersch, 1797), see **paravertebral nerves (Swanson & Bota, 2010)**
inferior lingual branch of glossopharyngeal nerve (Kilian, 1822), see **glossopharyngeal nerve (Huber, 1744)**
inferior lobe (Burdach, 1822), see **temporal region (>1840)**
inferior lobe (Gordon, 1815), see **cerebellar hemisphere (Willis, 1664)**
inferior lobes of cerebellum (Ramsay, 1813), see **cerebellum (Aristotle)**
inferior lobule of cerebellum (Chaussier, 1807), see **cerebellar hemisphere (Willis, 1664)**
inferior longitudinal commissure (Solly, 1836), see **fornix (Vesalius, 1543a)**
inferior longitudinal fascicle (Burdach, 1822)
inferior masticatory nerve (Malacarne, 1791), see **mandibular nerve (>1840)**
inferior maxillary angle branch of inferior facial branch of inferior branch of anterior branch of hard nerve (Loder, 1778), see **marginal mandibular branch of facial nerve (>1840)**
inferior maxillary angular branch (Soemmerring, 1791), see **marginal mandibular branch of facial nerve (>1840)**
inferior maxillary angular branch of lower facial branches of descending branch of superficial branch of hard nerve (Günther, 1786), see **marginal mandibular branch of facial nerve (>1840)**
inferior maxillary branch (Meckel, 1748), see **inferior dental nerve (Meckel, 1817)**
inferior maxillary branch of fifth nerve (La Charrère, 1703), see **mandibular nerve (>1840)**
inferior maxillary branch of hard nerve (Meckel, 1753), see **marginal mandibular branch of facial nerve (>1840)**
inferior maxillary marginal branch (Soemmerring, 1791), see **marginal mandibular branch of facial nerve (>1840)**
inferior maxillary nerve (Heister, 1717), see **mandibular nerve (>1840)**
inferior maxillary nerve (Meckel, 1748), see **inferior dental nerve (Meckel, 1817)**
inferior maxillary nerve (Meckel, 1753), see **marginal mandibular branch of facial nerve (>1840)**
inferior maxillary nerve proper (Schaarschmidt, 1750), see **inferior dental nerve (Meckel, 1817)**
inferior maxillary nerve trunk (Meckel, 1817), see **mandibular nerve trunk (>1840)**
inferior medullary velum (Arnold, 1838b), see **caudal medullary vellum (>1840)**
inferior mesenteric ganglion (>1840)
inferior mesenteric plexus (Cruveilhier, 1836), see **prevertebral plexuses (Quain, 1832)**
inferior mesenteric plexus (Haller, 1762), see **prevertebral plexuses (Quain, 1832)**
inferior mesenteric plexus (Rau, 1720)
inferior mesenteric plexus proper (Meckel, 1817), see **inferior mesenteric plexus (Rau, 1720)**
inferior midbrain tubercles (Chaussier, 1807), see **inferior colliculus (Haller, 1762)**
inferior musculocutaneous branch of lumbar plexus (Cloquet, 1816), see **iliohypogastric nerve (Schmidt, 1794)**
inferior musculocutaneous branch of lumbar plexus (Cruveilhier, 1836), see **ilio-inguinal nerve (Schmidt, 1794)**
inferior musculo-cutaneous nerve (Quain & Wilson, 1839), see **iliohypogastric nerve (Schmidt, 1794)**
inferior nasal branch of anterior palatine nerve (Meckel, 1748), see **posterior inferior nasal nerves (>1840)**
inferior nasal branch of greater palatine nerve (Cruveilhier, 1836), see **posterior inferior nasal nerves (>1840)**
inferior nasal cutaneous nerve (Mayer, 1794), see **external nasal branch of infraorbital nerve (>1840)**
inferior nasal filament of middle facial branch of pes anserinus (Bellingeri, 1818), see **zygomatic branches of facial nerve (>1840)**
inferior nasal nerves (Schaarschmidt, 1750), see **greater palatine nerve (Cloquet, 1816)**
inferior nasal nerves (Soemmerring, 1791), see **posterior inferior nasal nerves (>1840)**
inferior nasal subcutaneous branch of infraorbital nerve (Bock, 1817), see **external nasal branches of infraorbital nerve (>1840)**
inferior nasal subcutaneous fasciculi of infraorbital surculus (Bellingeri, 1818), see **external nasal branch of infraorbital nerve (>1840)**
inferior nerve (Jacobson, 1818), see **anterior ethmoidal nerve (>1840)**
inferior nerve (Soemmerring, 1798), see **buccal branch of facial nerve (>1840)**
inferior nerve for crural muscle (Fischer, 1791), see **muscular branches of femoral nerve (Quain & Wilson, 1839)**
inferior nerve for sartorius muscle (Fischer, 1791), see **muscular branches of femoral nerve (Quain & Wilson, 1839)**
inferior nerve for vastus externus muscle (Fischer, 1791), see **muscular branches of femoral nerve (Quain & Wilson, 1839)**
inferior nerve of foot (Mayer, 1794), see **saphenous nerve (Haase, 1781)**
inferior nerve of penis (Soemmerring, 1798), see **perineal nerve (Camper, 1762)**
inferior nerve to flexor longus of big toe muscle (Fischer, 1791), see **nerve to flexor hallucis longus (>1840)**
inferior nerve to soleus muscle (Jördens, 1788), see **nerve to soleus (>1840)**
inferior nerve to vastus internus muscle (Fischer, 1791), see **muscular branches of femoral nerve (Quain & Wilson, 1839)**
inferior oblique nerve of ductus arteriosus (Andersch, 1797), see **cardiac plexus (Keill, 1698)**
inferior occipital gyri (>1840)

inferior olfactory tubercle (Haller, 1768), see **hypothalamus (Kuhlenbeck, 1927)**

inferior olivary body (Günther, 1786), see **cuneate tubercle (>1840)**

inferior olivary complex (>1840)

inferior olivary eminence (>1840), see **olive (Tiedemann, 1821)**

inferior opening (Galen, c173), see **interventricular foramen (>1840)**

inferior orbital nerve of hard nerve (Meckel, 1753), see **zygomatic branches of facial nerve (>1840)**

inferior orbital thread of temporal surculus (Bellingeri, 1818), see **temporal branches of facial nerve (Swan, 1830)**

inferior oriface of fourth ventricle (Cruveilhier, 1836), see **median aperture of fourth ventricle (>1840)**

inferior ovarian nerves (>1840)

inferior palatine nerve (Cloquet, 1816), see **greater palatine nerve (Cloquet, 1816)**

inferior palpebral branches of infraorbital nerve (Meckel, 1748)

inferior palpebral branches of orbital branches of temporofacial branch of facial nerve (Cruveilhier, 1836), see **zygomatic branches of facial nerve (>1840)**

inferior palpebral nerves (Schaarschmidt, 1750), see **inferior palpebral branches of infraorbital nerve (>1840)**

inferior parietal lobule (>1840)

inferior part of gluteal plexus (Swan, 1830), see **inferior gluteal nerve (Martin, 1781)**

inferior part of medullary crura (Pourfour du Petit, 1710), see **cerebral peduncle (Tarin, 1753)**

inferior part of vestibular nerve (>1840), see **caudal part of vestibular nerve (>1840)**

inferior pedicle of cerebellum (Mayo, 1827), see **inferior cerebellar peduncle (Günther, 1786)**

inferior peduncles of conarium (Cruveilhier, 1836), see **habenulo-interpeduncular tract (>1840)**

inferior peduncles of pineal body (Cruveilhier, 1836), see **habenulo-interpeduncular tract (>1840)**

inferior petrosal nerve (Meckel, 1817), see **deep petrosal nerve (Meckel, 1817)**

inferior pharyngeal branch of pharyngolingual branch of glossopharyngeal nerve (Kilian, 1822), see **pharyngeal branches of glossopharyngeal nerve (Neubauer, 1772)**

inferior pharyngeal nerve (Meckel, 1817), see **pharyngeal branches of vagus nerve (>1840)**

inferior pharyngeal plexus (Bock, 1817), see **nerves (Herophilus, c335–c280 BC)**

inferior pontine sulcus (>1840), see **medullopontine sulcus (>1840)**

inferior popliteal nerve (Günther, 1786), see **nerve to popliteus (>1840)**

inferior portion of choroid plexus (Cruveilhier, 1836), see **choroid plexus of lateral ventricle (Vicq d'Azyr, 1784)**

inferior portion of lateral ventricle (Chaussier, 1807), see **lateral ventricle (Vesalius, 1543a)**

inferior portion of lateral ventricle (Cruveilhier, 1836), see **inferior horn of lateral ventricle (Bell, 1802)**

inferior portion of oblong marrow (Willis, 1664), see **medulla (Winslow, 1733)**

inferior posterior cutaneous branch of exterior branch of sciatic nerve (Günther, 1786), see **lateral cutaneous nerve of calf (>1840)**

inferior posterior cutaneous nerve (Jördens, 1788), see **tibial nerve (Haase, 1781)**

inferior posterior cutaneous nerve (Martin, 1781), see **posterior cutaneous nerve of thigh (Günther, 1786)**

inferior posterior cutaneous nerve (Meckel, 1817), see **articular branches of common fibular nerve (>1840)**

inferior posterior lobe (Burdach, 1822), see **cerebellar hemisphere (Willis, 1664)**

inferior posterior lobe (Malacarne, 1776), see **ansiform lobule crus 2 (Bolk, 1906)**

inferior posterior renal nerve (Walter, 1783), see **least splanchnic nerve (>1840)**

inferior process of vermis (Haller, 1762), see **cerebellar vermis (Meckel, 1817)**

inferior prolongation of cerebellum (Burdin, 1803), see **inferior cerebellar peduncle (Günther, 1786)**

inferior pudendal nerve (Camper, 1762), see **perineal nerve (Camper, 1762)**

inferior pudendal nerve (Walter, 1783), see **posterior labial nerves (>1840)**

inferior pudic nerve (Knox, 1832), see **pudendal nerve (Camper, 1762)**

inferior pudic nerve (Meckel, 1817), see **inferior rectal nerves (>1840)**

inferior pyramidal body (Mayer, 1794), see **pyramid (Willis, 1664)**

inferior pyramids (Desmoulins, 1825), see **pyramid (Willis, 1664)**

inferior quadrigeminal body (Wenzel & Wenzel, 1812), see **inferior colliculus (Haller, 1762)**

inferior quadrigeminal eminences (Günther, 1786), see **inferior colliculus (Haller, 1762)**

inferior quadrigeminal tubercle (Vicq d'Azyr, 1786), see **inferior colliculus (Haller, 1762)**

inferior raphe of corpus callosum (Reil, 1809b), see **corpus callosum (Galen, c177)**

inferior rectal nerves (>1840)

inferior region of anterior lobe (Rolando, 1831), see **orbital region (Rolando, 1831)**

inferior root (Desmoulins, 1825), see **ventral root (>1840)**

inferior root of ansa cervicalis (>1840)

inferior root of posterior thoracic nerve (Bock, 1827), see **long thoracic nerve (Quain & Wilson, 1839)**

inferior rope of intercostal nerve (Winslow, 1733), see **sympathetic trunk (Winslow, 1733)**

inferior salivatory nucleus (>1840)

inferior segment of fornix (Cajal, 1904), see **hypothalamic postcommissural fornix (>1840)**

inferior semilunar lobe (Meckel, 1817), see **cerebellar hemisphere (Willis, 1664)**

inferior smaller branch of fifth pair (Ridley, 1695), see **maxillary nerve (Meckel, 1753)**

inferior sphenoidal horn of lateral ventricle (Cruveilhier, 1836), see **inferior horn of lateral ventricle (Bell, 1802)**

inferior splanchnic nerve (Haller, 1762), see **paravertebral nerves (Swanson & Bota, 2010)**
inferior splanchnic nerve (Mayer, 1794), see **lesser splanchnic nerve (Haller, 1762)**
inferior splanchnic nerves (Tiedemann, 1822), see **least splanchnic nerve (>1840)**
inferior splenic nerves (Mayer, 1794), see **splenic plexus (Palfijn, 1726)**
inferior stomachical branch of wandring pair (Willis, 1664), see **posterior vagal trunk (Wrisberg, 1780)**
inferior subcutaneous malar nerve (Mayer, 1794), see **zygomaticofacial nerve (>1840)**
inferior subcutaneous nerves of neck (Meckel, 1753), see **inferior branches of transverse nerve of neck (>1840)**
inferior subcutaneous surculus of cervico-facial branch of portio major and minor of facial nerve (Bellingeri, 1818), see **cervical branch of facial nerve (>1840)**
inferior subcutaneous surculus of inferior branch of portio major and minor of facial nerve (Bellingeri, 1818), see **cervical branch of facial nerve (>1840)**
inferior subscapular nerve (Bock, 1827), see **thoracodorsal nerve (>1840)**
inferior subscapular nerve (Cruveilhier, 1836), see **lower subscapular nerve (>1840)**
inferior subsural external cutaneous nerve (Knox, 1832), see **tibial nerve (Haase, 1781)**
inferior sulcus of spinal medulla (Bojanus, 1819–1821), see **ventral median fissure of spinal cord (>1840)**
inferior superficial branch of hard nerves (Mayer, 1794), see **zygomatic branches of facial nerve (>1840)**
inferior superficial nerve to pulmonary arteries (Andersch, 1797), see **pulmonary plexus (Winslow, 1733)**
inferior surface of cerebellum (Malacarne, 1776), see **cerebellum (Aristotle)**
inferior temporal area (Brodmann, 1909), see **temporal region (>1840)**
inferior temporal gyrus (>1840)
inferior temporal sulcus (>1840)
inferior testicular nerves (>1840)
inferior thalamic commissure (Günz, 1753), see **interthalamic adhesion (>1840)**
inferior thalamic radiation peduncular loop (>1840)
inferior third branch of fifth pair (Meckel, 1748), see **posterior branch of mandibular nerve (>1840)**
inferior tonsillar nerve (Andersch & Soemmerring, 1792), see **tonsillar branches of glossopharyngeal nerve (Wrisberg, 1786)**
inferior tracheal nerves (Meckel, 1817), see **pulmonary branches of vagus nerve (Cloquet, 1828)**
inferior tracheal nerves proceeding before trachea (Meckel, 1817), see **pulmonary branches of vagus nerve (Cloquet, 1828)**
inferior tracheal nerves proceeding behind trachea (Meckel, 1817), see **pulmonary branches of vagus nerve (Cloquet, 1828)**
inferior ureteric nerves (>1840)
inferior uterine plexus (Teidemann, 1822), see **inferior hypogastric plexus (Tiedemann, 1822)**
inferior ventricle (Gerdy, 1838), see **lateral ventricle (Vesalius, 1543a)**
inferior vermicular eminence of cerebellum (Burdin, 1803), see **cerebellar vermis (Meckel, 1817)**
inferior vermiform appendix (Winslow, 1733), see **cerebellar vermis (Meckel, 1817)**
inferior vermiform process (Reil, 1807–1808a), see **cerebellar vermis (Meckel, 1817)**
inferior vermis (>1840), see **cerebellar vermis (Meckel, 1817)**
inferior wall of middle ventricle (Gerdy, 1838), see **hypothalamic part of third ventricle (Swanson, 2004)**
inferior worm of cerebellum (Chaussier, 1807), see **cerebellar vermis (Meckel, 1817)**
inflexus (Vesalius, 1543a), see **cerebral cortex gray matter (>1840)**
infolding of brain (Willis, 1664), see **lateral ventricle (Vesalius, 1543a)**
infolding of third pair (Willis, 1664), see **ciliary ganglion (Loder, 1778)**
infoldings (Willis, 1664), see **peripheral ganglia (>1840)**
infra orbitar nerve (Monro, 1783), see **infraorbital nerve (Schaarschmidt, 1750)**
infralimbic area (Rose & Woolsey, 1948)
inframalleolar nerve (Fischer, 1791), see **lateral dorsal cutaneous nerve (>1840)**
inframaxillary branch of trigeminal nerve (Bojanus, 1819–1821), see **mandibular nerve (>1840)**
inframaxillary nerve (Quain & Wilson, 1839), see **mandibular nerve (>1840)**
inframesenteric plexus (Winslow, 1733), see **inferior hypogastric plexus (Tiedemann, 1822)**
infraoccipital nerve (Schaarschmidt, 1750), see **suboccipital nerve (Winslow, 1733)**
infraoesophageal ganglia (Anderson, 1837), see **ventral ganglia (Anderson, 1837)**
infra-oesophageal ganglia (Müller, 1834), see **ventral ganglia (Anderson, 1837)**
infraorbital branch of superior branch of anterior branch of hard nerve (Loder, 1778), see **buccal branch of facial nerve (>1840)**
infraorbital branch of superior facial branch (Meckel, 1753), see **zygomatic branches of facial nerve (>1840)**
infraorbital branch of superior maxillary nerve (Jacobson, 1818), see **infraorbital nerve (Schaarschmidt, 1750)**
infraorbital cutaneous branch of great facial nerve (Meckel, 1753), see **zygomatic branches of facial nerve (>1840)**
infraorbital nerve (Bang, 1770), see **suboccipital nerve (Winslow, 1733)**
infraorbital nerve (Meckel, 1748), see **maxillary nerve (Meckel, 1753)**
infraorbital nerve (Schaarschmidt, 1750)
infraorbital plexus (Meckel, 1753), see **cranial nerves (Soemmerring, 1791)**
infraorbitar nerve (Meckel, 1832), see **maxillary nerve (Meckel, 1753)**
infrapatellar branch of saphenous nerve (>1840)
infrascapular nerve (Mayer, 1794), see **brachial plexus dorsal cord (Peterson, 1887)**
infraspinal nerve (Bang, 1770), see **suboccipital nerve (Winslow, 1733)**

infratrochlear branch of nasal branch of first branch of fifth pair (Meckel, 1748), see **infratrochlear nerve (Schaarschmidt, 1750)**

infratrochlear branch of nasal nerve (Arnold, 1834), see **infratrochlear nerve (Schaarschmidt, 1750)**

infratrochlear branch of nasociliary nerve (Arnold, 1834), see **infratrochlear nerve (Schaarschmidt, 1750)**

infratrochlear nerve (Schaarschmidt, 1750)

infundibular process (Tilney, 1936), see **posterior lobe of pituitary (Haller, 1762)**

infundibular recess (>1840)

infundibular stem (Hanström, 1966)

infundibular stem (Tilney, 1936), see **infundibular stem (Hanström, 1966)**

infundibulum (Galen, c173), see **hypothalamus (Kuhlenbeck, 1927)**

infundibulum (Rioch et al., 1940)

infundibulum (Rufus of Ephesis, fl. c90–120), see **hypothalamic part of third ventricle (Swanson, 2004)**

infundibulum (Tilney, 1936), see **infundibular stem (Hanström, 1966)**

infundibulum (Vesalius, 1543a), see **pituitary gland (>1840)**

infundibulum (>1840)

infusorium (Avicenna or Ibn Sina, c1030), see **hypothalamus (Kuhlenbeck, 1927)**

inguinal branch of singular nerve from second and third lumbar nerves (Monro & Coopmans, 1754), see **femoral branch of genitofemoral nerve (>1840)**

inguinal branches of lumbar plexus (Cruveilhier, 1836), see **lumbar plexus ventral divisions (Paterson, 1887)**

inguinal nerve (Burdin, 1803), see **ilio-inguinal nerve (Schmidt, 1794)**

inguinal nerve (Camper, 1762), see **genitofemoral nerve (>1840)**

inguino-cutaneous branch of lumbar plexus (Cruveilhier, 1836), see **ilio-inguinal nerve (Schmidt, 1794)**

inguino-cutaneous nerve (Burdin, 1803), see **iliohypogastric nerve (Schmidt, 1794)**

inguino-cutaneous nerve (Quain & Wilson, 1839), see **lateral cutaneous nerve of thigh (>1840)**

initial part of fornix (Cajal, 1904), see **septal postcommissural fornix (>1840)**

inner and thicker trunk or stock of great division of fourth sinew (Geminus, 1553), see **tibial nerve (Haase, 1781)**

inner branch of portio mollis (Monro, 1783), see **cochlear nerve (Cotugno, 1760)**

inner branch of sixth pair of nerves (Crooke, 1615), see **sympathetic trunk (Winslow, 1733)**

inner bundle of posterior funiculus (Rosenthal, 1815), see **gracile fascicle (Müller, 1834)**

inner cutaneous branch of anterior femoral nerve (Soemmerring, 1791), see **medial cutaneous nerve of thigh (>1840)**

inner gray fascicle (Wagner, 1839), see **spinal central gray (>1840)**

inner intermediate white layer of cortical layer (Baillarger, 1840), see **cerebral cortex gray matter (>1840)**

inner laryngeal nerve (Günther, 1786), see **internal branch of superior laryngeal nerve (Fyfe, 1800)**

inner lesser frontal nerve (Meckel, 1753), see **infratrochlear nerve (Schaarschmidt, 1750)**

inner lobule of middle lobe (Gordon, 1815), see **cerebral cortex (>1840)**

inner margin of middle lobe (Gordon, 1815), see **parahippocampal gyrus (>1840)**

inner membrane (Aristotle), see **pia (Galen, c192)**

inner oculo-muscular nerve (Solly, 1836), see **trochlear nerve (Molinetti, 1669)**

inner part of transverse cerebral fissure (>1840)

inner plantar nerve (Swan, 1830), see **medial plantar nerve (>1840)**

inner portion of cerebral ganglion (Reil, 1809b), see **caudate nucleus (Arnold, 1838b)**

inner portion of corpus striatum (Vicq d'Azyr, 1786), see **caudate nucleus (Arnold, 1838b)**

inner ramus of ophthalmic nerve (Winslow, 1733), see **nasociliary nerve (Meckel, 1817; Wutzer, 1817)**

inner toe of foot of hippocampus (Malacarne, 1780), see **cerebral cortex (>1840)**

inner toe of pes hippocampi (Malacarne, 1780), see **cerebral cortex (>1840)**

inner trunk of fourth nerve entering leg (Vesalius, 1543a), see **tibial nerve (Haase, 1781)**

inner wall of capsule (Reil, 1809b), see **internal capsule (Burdach, 1822)**

innermost arcade of striate body (Vicq d'Azyr, 1786), see **medial globus pallidus (>1840)**

innermost supraclavicular branch (Peipers, 1793), see **medial supraclavicular nerves (>1840)**

innern gespaltnen Hügel (Reil, 1812b), see **cerebral cortex (>1840)**

innervation apparatus (Cruveilhier, 1836), see **nervous system (Monro, 1783)**

innervation organs (Cloquet, 1828), see **nervous system (Monro, 1783)**

instrument of smelling (Geminus, 1553), see **cerebral cortex (>1840)**

instruments of communication (Spurzheim, 1826), see **central nervous system white matter tracts (>1840)**

instruments of union (Spurzheim, 1826), see **central nervous system white matter tracts (>1840)**

insula (Reil, 1809b), see **insular region (Brodmann, 1909)**

insular region (Brodmann, 1909)

insular threshold (Schwalbe, 1881), see **ambient gyrus (>1840)**

insulas (Meckel, 1753), see **nerves (Herophilus, c335–c280 BC)**

integumentum (Arnold, 1838a), see **tegmentum (Swanson, 2000b)**

interarterial superficial plexus (Andersch, 1797), see **cardiac plexus (Keill, 1698)**

interbrain (Baer, 1837)

interbrain corticospinal tract (>1840)

interbrain vesicle (Baer, 1837)

intercerebral commissure (Solly, 1836), see **superior cerebellar peduncle (Procháska, 1800)**

intercostal axillary nerves (Bell & Bell, 1826), see **intercostobrachial nerves (>1840)**

intercostal branch of costal nerve (Bock, 1827), see **intercostal nerves (Vesalius, 1543a)**

intercostal branch of intercostal branches of dorsal nerves (Cruveilhier, 1836), see **intercostal nerves (Vesalius, 1543a)**

intercostal branches of dorsal nerves (Cruveilhier, 1836), see **intercostal nerves (Vesalius, 1543a)**

intercostal branches of intercostal nerves (Quain & Wilson, 1839), see **intercostal nerves (Vesalius, 1543a)**

intercostal branches proper (Günther, 1786), see **intercostal nerves (Vesalius, 1543a)**

intercostal infolding (Willis, 1664), see **sympathetic trunk ganglia (Winslow, 1733)**

intercostal nerve (Bauhin, 1605), see **sympathetic trunk (Winslow, 1733)**

intercostal nerve (Lobstein, 1823), see **sympathetic cord (>1840)**

intercostal nerve (Willis, 1664), see **sympathetic trunk (Winslow, 1733)**

intercostal nerve ganglia (Günther, 1786), see **sympathetic trunk ganglia (Winslow, 1733)**

intercostal nerve properly so called (Bell & Bell, 1826), see **intercostal nerves (Vesalius, 1543a)**

intercostal nerves (Bell, 1803b), see **thoracic nerves (Diemerbroeck, 1672)**

intercostal nerves (Vesalius, 1543a)

intercostal pharyngeal nerves (Wrisberg, 1786), see **laryngopharyngeal branches of superior cervical ganglion (>1840)**

intercostal plexus (Drake, 1707), see **superior thoracic ganglion (Lieutaud, 1742)**

intercostal sinewes (Crooke, 1615), see **intercostal nerves (Vesalius, 1543a)**

intercostal thread of Vidian fascicle (Bellingeri, 1818), see **deep petrosal nerve (Meckel, 1817)**

intercostal trunk (Neubauer, 1772), see **communicating branches of sympathetic trunk (>1840)**

intercostal trunk (Willis, 1664), see **sympathetic trunk (Winslow, 1733)**

intercostobrachial nerves (>1840)

intercosto-humeral nerve from third dorsal nerve (Quain & Wilson, 1839), see **intercostobrachial nerves (>1840)**

intercosto-humeral nerves (Fyfe, 1800), see **intercostobrachial nerves (>1840)**

intercrossing (Meckel, 1817), see **optic chiasm (Galen, c173)**

interganglionic branches of sympathetic trunk (>1840), see **communicating branches of sympathetic trunk (>1840)**

interganglionic cord (Serres, 1824–1826), see **central longitudinal communicating branch (>1840)**

interior and anterior cardiac nerves (Lobstein, 1823), see **cardiac plexus (Keill, 1698)**

interior and superior nasal nerve (Arnold, 1834), see **internal nasal branches of infraorbital nerve (>1840)**

interior branch of nasal nerve (Scarpa, 1785), see **internal nasal branches of anterior ethmoidal nerve (>1840)**

interior branch of praetibio-digital nerve (Burdin, 1803), see **medial dorsal cutaneous nerve (>1840)**

interior branch of superficial nerve of neck (Bang, 1770), see **inferior branches of transverse nerve of neck (>1840)**

interior branch of supraorbital nerve (Günther, 1786), see **medial branch of supraorbital nerve (>1840)**

interior branch of tibial nerve (Burdin, 1803), see **medial plantar nerve (>1840)**

interior branch of trunk of pharyngeal branches of vagus (Bischoff, 1832), see **pharyngeal branches of vagus nerve (>1840)**

interior branches of sympathetic nerve (Lobstein, 1823), see **paravertebral nerves (Swanson & Bota, 2010)**

interior deep branch of hard nerve (Mayer, 1794), see **facial nerve trunk (1840)**

interior dorsal twig of foot from tibial communicating branch (Jördens, 1788), see **medial calcaneal nerve (>1840)**

interior inferior palpebral nerve (Günther, 1786), see **inferior palpebral branches of infraorbital nerve (Meckel, 1748)**

interior oculo-muscular pair of nerves (Burdin, 1803), see **trochlear nerve (Molinetti, 1669)**

interior palpebral branch of infraorbital nerve (Loder, 1778), see **inferior palpebral branches of infraorbital nerve (Meckel, 1748)**

interior superclavicular branches (Soemmerring, 1798), see **medial supraclavicular nerves (>1840)**

interior superior spermatic plexus (Soemmerring, 1798), see **superior testicular nerves (>1840)**

interior twig of superior branch of first branch of fifth pair (Haller, 1743), see **supratrochlear nerve (Schaarschmidt, 1750)**

interiorem ramum credo esse splanchnicum (Lancisi, 1719), see **paravertebral nerves (Swanson & Bota, 2010)**

interlobar fissure (Cloquet, 1816), see **longitudinal cerebral fissure (Gordon, 1815)**

inter-lobar scissure (Burdin, 1803), see **lateral cerebral sulcus (>1840)**

intermediate branches of supraclavicular branches (Cruveilhier, 1836), see **intermediate supraclavicular nerves (>1840)**

intermediate canal of ventricles (Burdin, 1803), see **cerebral aqueduct (>1840)**

intermediate commissure (Bergmann, 1831), see **interthalamic adhesion (>1840)**

intermediate dorsal cutaneous nerve (>1840)

intermediate frontal area (Brodmann, 1909), see **frontal region (Vicq d'Azyr, 1786)**

intermediate ganglia (>1840)

intermediate ganglion (>1840), see **geniculate ganglion (Bischoff, 1832)**

intermediate hippocampal commissure (>1840)

intermediate lobe (Arnold, 1838a), see **cerebral cortex gray matter (>1840)**

intermediate lobe (Mayer, 1779), see **cerebellar vermis (Meckel, 1817)**

intermediate nerve (Huber, 1744), see **accessory nerve (Vieussens, 1684)**

intermediate nerve (>1840)

intermediate nerve root (>1840)

intermediate nerve rootlets (>1840)

intermediate nerve trunk (>1840)

intermediate nervous filaments (Vicq d'Azyr, 1786), see ***intermediate nerve (>1840)***

intermediate nervous system (Blainville, 1821), see ***paravertebral ganglia (Durward, 1951)***

intermediate olfactory stria (>1840), see ***lateral olfactory tract (>1840)***

intermediate part of facial nerve (Arnold, 1834), see ***intermediate nerve (>1840)***

intermediate portio of seventh pair of nerves (Haller & Wrisberg, 1780), see ***intermediate nerve (>1840)***

intermediate postcentral area (Brodmann, 1909), see ***parietal region (>1840)***

intermediate spinal zone (>1840)

intermediate supraclavicular nerves (>1840)

intermediate sympathetic nerve (Malacarne, 1791), see ***cranial nerves (Soemmerring, 1791)***

intermediate trunk (Arnold, 1834), see ***communicating branches of sympathetic trunk (>1840)***

intermediate trunk between supreme and middle cervical ganglia (Arnold, 1834), see ***communicating branch of superior and middle cervical ganglia (>1840)***

intermediate white matter (Reil, 1809b), see ***superior longitudinal fascicle (>1840)***

intermediofacial nerve (Strong & Elwyn, 1943)

intermediofacial nerve roots (>1840)

intermediofacial nerve trunk (>1840)

intermediolateral column (>1840), see ***intermediolateral nucleus (>1840)***

intermediolateral nucleus (>1840)

intermesenteric plexus (>1840)

intermuscular branch to genioglossus muscle (Andersch & Soemmerring, 1792), see ***lingual branches of hypoglossal nerve (Cloquet, 1816)***

internal anastomotic filament of superficial frontal thread of supraorbital fascicle (Bellingeri, 1818), see ***supraorbital nerve (Meckel, 1753)***

internal and anterior root of facial nerve (Meckel, 1817), see ***facial nerve root (>1840)***

internal and deep branch of back of foot of anterior tibial branch of external popliteal nerve (Cloquet, 1816), see ***digital branch of deep fibular nerve (>1840)***

internal and superficial branch to back of foot of musculocutaneous branch of external popliteal nerve (Cloquet, 1816), see ***medial dorsal cutaneous nerve (>1840)***

internal and superior posterior femoral cutaneous nerve (Mayer, 1794), see ***medial cutaneous nerve of thigh (>1840)***

internal anterior branch of first pair of lumbar nerves (Winslow, 1733), see ***ilio-inguinal nerve (Schmidt, 1794)***

internal anterior branches of muscular branch of peroneal nerve (Martin, 1781), see ***dorsal digital nerves of deep fibular nerve (>1840)***

internal anterior femoral cutaneous nerve (Bock, 1827), see ***medial cutaneous nerve of thigh (>1840)***

internal anterior superior nasal nerves (Günther, 1786), see ***posterior superior nasal nerves (Soemmerring, 1791)***

internal appendix of fimbria (Volkmann, 1831), see ***alveus (Burdach, 1822)***

internal arcuate fibers (>1840)

internal arcuate fibers of septum (Cajal, 1901–1902), see ***diagonal band (Broca, 1879)***

internal articular branch of internal popliteal nerve (Bock, 1827), see ***articular branches of tibial nerve (>1840)***

internal ascending superficial branch of cervical plexus (Quain, 1828), see ***transverse nerve of neck (>1840)***

internal auricular branches of superficial temporal nerve (Todd, 1836–1839), see ***external acoustic meatus nerves (Meckel, 1817)***

internal branch of accessory nerve (Scarpa, 1788), see ***internal branch of accessory nerve trunk (Meckel, 1817)***

internal branch of accessory nerve trunk (Meckel, 1817)

internal branch of accessory vagal pair (Soemmerring, 1791), see ***internal branch of accessory nerve trunk (Meckel, 1817)***

internal branch of anterior branch of obturator nerve (Cloquet, 1816), see ***muscular branches of anterior branch of obturator nerve (>1840)***

internal branch of ascending branch of external frontal nerve (Cruveilhier, 1836), see ***medial branch of supraorbital nerve (>1840)***

internal branch of ascending branch of supraorbital nerve (Cruveilhier, 1836), see ***medial branch of supraorbital nerve (>1840)***

internal branch of carotid nerve (Arnold, 1834), see ***internal carotid plexus (>1840)***

internal branch of cervical plexus (Quain & Wilson, 1839), see ***transverse nerve of neck (>1840)***

internal branch of common motor nerve inferior terminal branch (Cruveilhier, 1836), see ***nerve to medial rectus (>1840)***

internal branch of conjugations of nerves from loynes and holy bone (Paré, 1561), see ***spinal nerve ventral branch (>1840)***

internal branch of crural nerve (Winslow, 1733), see ***medial cutaneous nerve of thigh (>1840)***

internal branch of crural nerve proper (Salmon, 1713), see ***tibial nerve (Haase, 1781)***

internal branch of crural trunk (Diemerbroeck, 1672), see ***tibial nerve (Haase, 1781)***

internal branch of cubital nerve (Haase, 1781), see ***deep branch of ulnar nerve (Fyfe, 1800)***

internal branch of cutaneous nerve (Fyfe, 1800), see ***posterior branch of medial cutaneous nerve of forearm (>1840)***

internal branch of deep branch of internal pudendal nerve (Cruveilhier, 1836), see ***dorsal nerve of penis (Camper, 1762)***

internal branch of deep peroneal nerve (Bock, 1827), see ***digital branch of deep fibular nerve (>1840)***

internal branch of deep peroneal nerve (Fischer, 1791), see ***deep fibular nerve (Fyfe, 1800)***

internal branch of descending laryngeal nerve (Swan, 1830), see ***internal branch of superior laryngeal nerve (Fyfe, 1800)*** *internal branch of dorsal branch of penis of internal pudendal nerve (Cruveilhier, 1836)*, see **dorsal nerve of penis (Camper, 1762)**

internal branch of dorsal branch of thoracic nerve (Bock, 1827), see **medial branch of spinal nerve dorsal branch (>1840)**

internal branch of dorsal branches of foot (Bell, 1803b), see **medial dorsal cutaneous nerve (>1840)**

internal branch of dorsal nerve (Swan, 1830), see **anterior cutaneous branch of intercostal nerves (>1840)**

internal branch of external cutaneous nerve of arm (Cloquet, 1816), see **muscular branches of musculocutaneous nerve (Günther, 1786)**

internal branch of external dorsal nerve of foot (Bock, 1827), see **lateral dorsal cutaneous nerve (>1840)**

internal branch of external plantar nerve (Jördens, 1788), see **deep branch of lateral plantar nerve (>1840)**

internal branch of external plantar nerve (Meckel, 1817), see **common plantar digital nerves of lateral plantar nerve (>1840)**

internal branch of external spermatic nerve (Walter, 1783), see **genital branch of genitofemoral nerve (>1840)**

internal branch of fibular nerve (Quain, 1828), see **medial dorsal cutaneous nerve (>1840)**

internal branch of first division of fifth pair of nerves (Todd, 1836–1839), see **nasociliary nerve (Meckel, 1817; Wutzer, 1817)**

internal branch of frontal branch of external frontal nerve (Cruveilhier, 1836), see **medial branch of supraorbital nerve (>1840)**

internal branch of frontal branch of supraorbital nerve (Cruveilhier, 1836), see **medial branch of supraorbital nerve (>1840)**

internal branch of frontal nerve (Quain, 1828), see **supratrochlear nerve (Schaarschmidt, 1750)**

internal branch of greater frontal nerve (Meckel, 1753), see **medial branch of supraorbital nerve (>1840)**

internal branch of hypogastric nerve of second accessory lumbar ganglion (Walter, 1783), see **lumbar splanchnic nerves (Cruveilhier, 1836)**

internal branch of iliohypogastric nerve (Bock, 1827), see **anterior cutaneous branch of iliohypogastric nerve (>1840)**

internal branch of iliohypogastric nerve (Cloquet, 1828), see **iliohypogastric nerve (Schmidt, 1794)**

internal branch of ilio-inguinal nerve (Cloquet, 1828), see **ilio-inguinal nerve (Schmidt, 1794)**

internal branch of inferior maxillary nerve (Cruveilhier, 1836), see **medial pterygoid nerve (>1840)**

internal branch of internal cutaneous nerve of arm (Cloquet, 1816), see **medial cutaneous nerve of forearm (>1840)**

internal branch of internal inguinal branch of lumbar plexus (Cruveilhier, 1836), see **genital branch of genitofemoral nerve (>1840)**

internal branch of internal plantar nerve (Fischer, 1791), see **medial plantar nerve (>1840)**

internal branch of internal plantar nerve (Jördens, 1788), see **common plantar digital nerves of medial plantar nerve (>1840)**

internal branch of lacrimal nerve (Arnold, 1834), see **lacrimal nerve (Meckel, 1748; Bonhomme, 1748)**

internal branch of laryngeal nerve (Haase, 1781), see **internal branch of superior laryngeal nerve (Fyfe, 1800)**

internal branch of lumbo-inguinal nerve (Cloquet, 1828), see **femoral branch of genitofemoral nerve (>1840)**

internal branch of metatarsal nerves (Bell, 1803b), see **medial dorsal cutaneous nerve (>1840)**

internal branch of musculocutaneous nerve (Cruveilhier, 1836), see **lateral cutaneous nerve of forearm (>1840)**

internal branch of musculo-cutaneous nerve (Quain & Wilson, 1839), see **medial dorsal cutaneous nerve (>1840)**

internal branch of nasal nerve (Scarpa, 1785), see **internal nasal branches of anterior ethmoidal nerve (>1840)**

internal branch of nervi motores oculorum communes (Winslow, 1733), see **nerve to medial rectus (>1840)**

internal branch of palmar cutaneous nerve (Cruveilhier, 1836), see **palmar branch of median nerve (Bock, 1827)**

internal branch of palpebro-frontal nerve (Burdin, 1803), see **medial branch of supraorbital nerve (>1840)**

internal branch of penile nerve (Bock, 1827), see **dorsal nerve of penis (Camper, 1762)**

internal branch of perforating or cutaneous branch of second dorsal nerve (Cruveilhier, 1836), see **intercostobrachial nerves (>1840)**

internal branch of peroneal nerve (Quain, 1828), see **medial dorsal cutaneous nerve (>1840)**

internal branch of posterior branch of lumbar nerve (Bock, 1827), see **medial branch of spinal nerve dorsal branch (>1840)**

internal branch of posterior crural nerve (Vieussens, 1684), see **tibial nerve (Haase, 1781)**

internal branch of radial nerve (Haase, 1781), see **deep branch of radial nerve (Martin, 1781)**

internal branch of recurrent branch of cutaneous branch of inferior gluteal nerve (Cruveilhier, 1836), see **perineal branches of posterior cutaneous nerve of thigh (>1840)**

internal branch of sciatic nerve trunk (Günther, 1786), see **tibial nerve (Haase, 1781)**

internal branch of spinal nerve (Cruveilhier, 1836), see **internal branch of accessory nerve trunk (Meckel, 1817)**

internal branch of spinal nerve dorsal branch (Meckel, 1817), see **medial branch of spinal nerve dorsal branch (>1840)**

internal branch of superficial branch of radial nerve (Cruveilhier, 1836), see **dorsal digital nerves of radial nerve (>1840)**

internal branch of superficial peroneal nerve (Fischer, 1791), see **medial dorsal cutaneous nerve (>1840)**

internal branch of superficial terminal branch of cubital nerve (Cruveilhier, 1836), see **palmar digital nerves of ulnar nerve (>1840)**

internal branch of superficial terminal branch of external plantar nerve (Cruveilhier, 1836), see **common**

internal descending neck branch of ninth nerve (Scarpa, 1794), see **superior root of ansa cervicalis (>1840)**

internal descending nerve of neck (Andersch & Soemmerring, 1792), see **superior root of ansa cervicalis (>1840)**

internal descending nerve of neck of third nerves of neck (Andersch, 1797), see **inferior root of ansa cervicalis (>1840)**

internal dorsal branch of cubital nerve internal dorsal branch of hand (Cruveilhier, 1836), see **dorsal digital nerves of ulnar nerve (>1840)**

internal dorsal branch of deep peroneal nerve (Cloquet, 1828), see **digital branch of deep fibular nerve (>1840)**

internal dorsal branch of deep peroneal nerve (Fischer, 1791), see **digital branch of deep fibular nerve (>1840)**

internal dorsal branch of inframalleolar nerve (Fischer, 1791), see **lateral dorsal cutaneous nerve (>1840)**

internal dorsal branch of superficial peroneal nerve (Fischer, 1791), see **medial dorsal cutaneous nerve (>1840)**

internal dorsal branch of thumb of anterior branch of radial nerve (Cloquet, 1828), see **dorsal digital nerves of radial nerve (>1840)**

internal dorsal branch of thumb of palmar branch of radial nerve (Coquet, 1828), see **dorsal digital nerves of radial nerve (>1840)**

internal dorsal collateral branch of cubital nerve internal dorsal branch of hand (Cruveilhier, 1836), see **dorsal digital nerves of ulnar nerve (>1840)**

internal dorsal collateral branch of index finger of radial nerve (Cruveilhier, 1836), see **dorsal digital nerves of radial nerve (>1840)**

internal dorsal collateral branch of thumb of radial nerve (Cruveilhier, 1836), see **dorsal digital nerves of radial nerve (>1840)**

internal dorsal collateral nerve of big toe (Cruveilhier, 1836), see **dorsal digital nerves of medial dorsal cutaneous nerve (>1840)**

internal dorsal collateral nerve of fourth toe (Cruveilhier, 1836), see **dorsal digital nerves of intermediate dorsal cutaneous nerve (>1840)**

internal dorsal collateral nerve of little toe (Cruveilhier, 1836), see **dorsal digital nerves of lateral dorsal cutaneous nerve (>1840)**

internal dorsal collateral nerve of second toe (Cruveilhier, 1836), see **dorsal digital nerves of medial dorsal cutaneous nerve (>1840)**

internal dorsal collateral nerve of third toe (Cruveilhier, 1836), see **dorsal digital nerves of medial dorsal cutaneous nerve (>1840)**

internal dorsal digital nerve of big toe (Fischer, 1791), see **dorsal digital nerves of medial dorsal cutaneous nerve (>1840)**

internal dorsal digital nerve of fifth toe from external branch of superficial peroneal nerve (Fischer, 1791), see **dorsal digital nerves of intermediate dorsal cutaneous nerve (>1840)**

internal dorsal digital nerve of fourth toe from external branch of superficial peroneal nerve (Fischer, 1791), see **dorsal digital nerves of intermediate dorsal cutaneous nerve (>1840)**

internal dorsal digital nerve of fourth toe from internal metatarsal branch of inframalleolar nerve (Fischer, 1791), see **dorsal digital nerves of lateral dorsal cutaneous nerve (>1840)**

internal dorsal digital nerve of little toe from internal metatarsal branch of inframalleolar nerve (Fischer, 1791), see **dorsal digital nerves of lateral dorsal cutaneous nerve (>1840)**

internal dorsal digital nerve of second toe from external metatarsal twig (Fischer, 1791), see **dorsal digital nerves of medial dorsal cutaneous nerve (>1840)**

internal dorsal digital nerve of second toe from metatarsus pollicis nerve (Fischer, 1791), see **dorsal digital nerves of medial dorsal cutaneous nerve (>1840)**

internal dorsal digital nerve of third toe (Fischer, 1791), see **dorsal digital nerves of medial dorsal cutaneous nerve (>1840)**

internal dorsal nerve of auricular finger (Mayer, 1794), see **dorsal digital nerves of ulnar nerve (>1840)**

internal dorsal nerve of big toe (Mayer, 1794, p. 26), see **saphenous nerve (Haase, 1781)**

internal dorsal nerve of big toe (Mayer, 1794, p. 27), see **dorsal digital nerves of medial dorsal cutaneous nerve (>1840)**

internal dorsal nerve of first small toe (Mayer, 1794), see **dorsal digital nerves of digital branch of deep fibular nerve (>1840)**

internal dorsal nerve of foot (Bock, 1827), see **medial dorsal cutaneous nerve (>1840)**

internal dorsal nerve of fourth small toe (Mayer, 1794), see **dorsal digital nerves of intermediate dorsal cutaneous nerve (>1840)**

internal dorsal nerve of fourth toe (Bock, 1827), see **dorsal digital nerves of lateral dorsal cutaneous nerve (>1840)**

internal dorsal nerve of index finger (Mayer, 1794), see **dorsal digital nerves of radial nerve (>1840)**

internal dorsal nerve of little toe (Bock, 1827), see **dorsal digital nerves of lateral dorsal cutaneous nerve (>1840)**

internal dorsal nerve of middle finger (Mayer, 1794), see **dorsal digital nerves of ulnar nerve (>1840)**

internal dorsal nerve of ring finger (Mayer, 1794), see **dorsal digital nerves of ulnar nerve (>1840)**

internal dorsal nerve of second small toe (Mayer, 1794), see **dorsal digital nerves of intermediate dorsal cutaneous nerve (>1840)**

internal dorsal nerve of second toe (Bock, 1827), see **dorsal digital nerves of medial dorsal cutaneous nerve (>1840)**

internal dorsal nerve of smallest toe (Mayer, 1794), see **dorsal digital nerves of intermediate dorsal cutaneous nerve (>1840)**

internal dorsal nerve of third small toe (Mayer, 1794), see **dorsal digital nerves of intermediate dorsal cutaneous nerve (>1840)**

internal dorsal nerve of third toe (Bock, 1827), see **dorsal digital nerves of medial dorsal cutaneous nerve (>1840)**

internal dorsal nerve of thumb (Mayer, 1794), see **dorsal digital nerves of radial nerve (>1840)**

internal dorsal twig of big toe (Jördens, 1788), see **dorsal digital nerves of medial dorsal cutaneous nerve (>1840)**

internal dorsal twig of foot of superficial branch of peroneal nerve (Jördens, 1788), see **medial dorsal cutaneous nerve (>1840)**

internal fascicle of crotaphitic surculus of ganglioform plexus of inferior maxillary branch (Bellingeri, 1818), see **deep temporal nerves (Haase, 1781)**

internal filament of ethmoidal branch of nasal nerve (Cruveilhier, 1836), see **internal nasal branches of anterior ethmoidal nerve (>1840)**

internal filament of internal branch of ilio-inguinal nerve (Cloquet, 1828), see **ilio-inguinal nerve (Schmidt, 1794)**

internal filament of internal nasal branch of nasal nerve (Cruveilhier, 1836), see **internal nasal branches of anterior ethmoidal nerve (>1840)**

internal filament of superior anastomotic thread of malo-palpebral fascicle of subcutaneous malar surculus (Bellingeri, 1818), see **zygomaticofacial nerve (>1840)**

internal filaments of superior maxillary nerve (Cruveilhier, 1836), see **external nasal branches of infraorbital nerve (>1840)**

internal fornix (Arnold, 1838b), see **fornix (Vesalius, 1543a)**

internal frontal nerve (Meckel, 1753), see **supratrochlear nerve (Schaarschmidt, 1750)**

internal frontal thread of supratrochlear fascicle (Bellingeri, 1818), see **supratrochlear nerve (Schaarschmidt, 1750)**

internal ganglions of ganglionnary nerve (Meckel, 1817), see **prevertebral ganglia (Quain, 1832)**

internal gastrocnemius branch of internal popliteal nerve (Bock, 1827), see **nerves to gastrocnemius (>1840)**

internal geniculate body (Reil, 1809b), see **medial geniculate complex (>1840)**

internal geniculate tubercle (Arnold, 1838b), see **medial geniculate complex (>1840)**

internal gray nucleus (Burdach, 1822), see **medial thalamic nuclei (>1840)**

internal head of median nerve (Quain & Wilson, 1839), see **medial root of median nerve (>1840)**

internal hemorrhoidal nerve (Walter, 1783), see **inferior rectal nerves (>1840)**

internal hemorrhoidal nerve of third sacral nerve (Cloquet, 1828), see **pelvic splanchnic nerves (Gaskell, 1886)**

internal hemorrhoidal plexus (Mayer, 1794), see **middle rectal plexus (>1840)**

internal inferior carotid nerve (Arnold, 1834), see **internal carotid plexus (>1840)**

internal inferior cutaneous nerve (Cloquet, 1828), see **medial cutaneous nerve of calf (>1840)**

internal inferior cutaneous nerve (Knox, 1832), see **sciatic nerve (Keill, 1698)**

internal inferior labial branch (Meckel, 1753), see **inferior labial branches of mental nerve (Meckel, 1753)**

internal inferior labial nerve (Mayer, 1794), see **inferior labial branches of mental nerve (Meckel, 1753)**

internal inferior lobe (Meckel, 1817), see **biventral lobule (>1840)**

internal inferior palpebral fascicle of infraorbital surculus (Bellingeri, 1818), see **inferior palpebral branches of infraorbital nerve (>1840)**

internal inferior palpebral nerve (Arnold, 1834), see **inferior palpebral branches of infraorbital nerve (Meckel, 1748)**

internal inferior subsural cutaneous nerve (Knox, 1832), see **tibial nerve (Haase, 1781)**

internal inguinal branch of external spermatic branch of first lumbar nerve (Günther, 1786), see **genital branch of genitofemoral nerve (>1840)**

internal inguinal branch of lumbar plexus (Cruveilhier, 1836), see **genitofemoral nerve (>1840)**

internal inguinal branch of second lumbar pair (Cruveilhier, 1836), see **genitofemoral nerve (>1840)**

internal inguinal nerve (Martin, 1781), see **genital branch of genitofemoral nerve (>1840)**

internal interosseous nerve (Günther, 1786), see **anterior interosseous nerve (Quain, 1832)**

internal interosseous plexus (Caldani, 1813, 1814), see **muscular branches of median nerve (Martin, 1781)**

internal labial branch of infraorbital nerve (Bock, 1817), see **superior labial branches of infraorbital nerve (Meckel, 1748)**

internal labial thread of mental fascicle of inferior alveolar surculus of inferior maxillary branch (Bellingeri, 1818), see **inferior labial branches of mental nerve (Meckel, 1753)**

internal laryngeal branch of vocal nerve (Bock, 1817), see **internal branch of superior laryngeal nerve (Fyfe, 1800)**

internal laryngeal nerve (Soemmerring, 1791), see **internal branch of superior laryngeal nerve (Fyfe, 1800)**

internal laryngeal nerve of pneumogastric (Knox, 1832), see **internal branch of superior laryngeal nerve (Fyfe, 1800)**

internal lateral cutaneous nerve (Fischer, 1791), see **medial cutaneous nerve of thigh (>1840)**

internal lateral lingual branch of eighth pair of nerves of head (Andersch & Soemmerring, 1792), see **lingual branches of glossopharyngeal nerve (Haller, 1762)**

internal lateral lingual branch of ninth nerves of head (Andersch, 1797), see **lingual branches of glossopharyngeal nerve (Haller, 1762)**

internal lateral twig to abductor pollicis muscle from internal branch of internal plantar nerve (Jördens, 1788), see **common plantar digital nerves of medial plantar nerve (>1840)**

internal lingual nerve (Schaarschmidt, 1750), see **lingual nerve (Vesalius, 1543a)**

internal major branch of sciatic nerve trunk (Soemmerring, 1791), see **tibial nerve (Haase, 1781)**

internal margin of hippocampus major (Vicq d'Azyr, 1786), see **dentate gyrus (>1840)**

internal maxillary plexus (Le Cat, 1768), see **buccal branch of facial nerve (>1840)**

internal medullary circumvolution (Winslow, 1733), see **cerebral cortex white matter (>1840)**
internal medullary lamina (>1840)
internal medullary root of olfactory nerve (Haase, 1781), see **lateral olfactory tract (>1840)**
internal metatarsal branch of inframalleolar nerve (Fischer, 1791), see **lateral dorsal cutaneous nerve (>1840)**
internal metatarsal nerve (Knox, 1832), see **dorsal digital nerves of medial dorsal cutaneous nerve (>1840)**
internal metatarsal twig of external dorsal twig of foot of superficial branch of peroneal nerve (Jördens, 1788), see **intermediate dorsal cutaneous nerve (>1840)**
internal metatarsal twig of internal branch of superficial peroneal nerve (Fischer, 1791), see **medial dorsal cutaneous nerve (>1840)**
internal minor cutaneous nerve (Klint, 1784), see **medial cutaneous nerve of arm (>1840)**
internal motor nerve (Meckel, 1817), see **trochlear nerve (Molinetti, 1669)**
internal muscular branch of hard nerve (Meckel, 1753), see **facial nerve trunk (1840)**
internal musculo-cutaneous branch of lumbar plexus (Quain, 1828), see **ilio-inguinal nerve (Schmidt, 1794)**
internal musculo-cutaneous branch of lumbar plexus (Quain, 1837), see **iliohypogastric nerve (Schmidt, 1794)**
internal musculo-cutaneous nerve (Quain & Wilson, 1839), see **iliohypogastric nerve (Schmidt, 1794)**
internal nasal branch of nasal branch of ophthalmic nerve (Quain, 1837), see **anterior ethmoidal nerve (>1840)**
internal nasal branch of nasal nerve (Cruveilhier, 1836), see **anterior ethmoidal nerve (>1840)**
internal nasal branch of nasociliary nerve (>1840), see **anterior ethmoidal nerve (>1840)**
internal nasal branches of anterior ethmoidal nerve (>1840)
internal nasal branches of infraorbital nerve (>1840)
internal nasal nerve (Willis, 1664), see **anterior ethmoidal nerve (>1840)**
internal nasal threads of ethmoidal fascicle (Bellingeri, 1818), see **medial nasal branches of internal nasal branches of anterior ethmoidal nerve (>1840)**
internal nerve of great toe (Meckel, 1817), see **proper plantar digital nerves of medial plantar nerve (>1840)**
internal nerve of vastus internus (Cruveilhier, 1836), see **muscular branches of femoral nerve (Quain & Wilson, 1839)**
internal nervous system (Meckel, 1817), see **central nervous system (Carus, 1814)**
internal nucleus of colliculus of optic nerve (Arnold, 1838b), see **medial thalamic nuclei (>1840)**
internal nucleus of thalamus of optic nerve (Arnold, 1838b), see **medial thalamic nuclei (>1840)**
internal olfactory convolution (Gerdy, 1838), see **straight gyrus (Valentin, 1841)**
internal or larger division of sciatic nerve (Quain, 1828), see **tibial nerve (Haase, 1781)**
internal palatine nerve (Bock, 1817), see **posterior palatine nerve (Günther, 1786)**
internal palatine thread of anterior palatine fascicle (Bellingeri, 1818), see **greater palatine nerve (Cloquet, 1816)**
internal palmar branch furnished by cubital nerve (Cloquet, 1828), see **common palmar digital nerves of ulnar nerve (>1840)**
internal palmar branch of index finger of second common digital branch of median nerve (Cloquet, 1828), see **proper palmar digital nerves of median nerve (>1840)**
internal palmar branch of middle finger of third common digital branch of median nerve (Cloquet, 1828), see **proper palmar digital nerves of median nerve (>1840)**
internal palmar branch of thumb of first common digital branch of median nerve (Cloquet, 1828), see **proper palmar digital nerves of median nerve (>1840)**
internal palmar nerve of little finger (Cloquet, 1828), see **proper palmar digital nerves of ulnar nerve (>1840)**
internal palmar nerve of ring finger (Cloquet, 1828), see **proper palmar digital nerves of ulnar nerve (>1840)**
internal palpebral branch (Meckel, 1753), see **lacrimal nerve (Meckel, 1748; Bonhomme, 1748)**
internal part of brain (Bartholin, 1662), see **vertebrate brain (Cuvier, 1800)**
internal part of lemniscus (Reil, 1809c), see **lateral lemniscus (Bechterew, 1885b)**
internal part of superior great cerebral ganglion (Gall & Spurzheim, 1810), see **caudate nucleus (Arnold, 1838b)**
internal pectoral subcutaneous supraclavicular branch (Peipers, 1793), see **medial supraclavicular nerves (>1840)**
internal pia mater (Meckel, 1817), see **pia (Galen, c192)**
internal plantar branch of posterior tibial nerve (Quain, 1828), see **medial plantar nerve (>1840)**
internal plantar branch of tibial nerve (Martin, 1781), see **medial plantar nerve (>1840)**
internal plantar collateral nerve of third toe (Cruveilhier, 1836), see **proper plantar digital nerves of medial plantar nerve (>1840)**
internal plantar digital twig of big toe (Fischer, 1791), see **proper plantar digital nerves of medial plantar nerve (>1840)**
internal plantar digital twig of fifth toe (Fischer, 1791), see **proper plantar digital nerves of medial plantar nerve (>1840)**
internal plantar digital twig of fourth toe (Fischer, 1791), see **proper plantar digital nerves of medial plantar nerve (>1840)**
internal plantar digital twig of second toe (Fischer, 1791), see **proper plantar digital nerves of medial plantar nerve (>1840)**
internal plantar digital twig of third toe (Fischer, 1791), see **proper plantar digital nerves of medial plantar nerve (>1840)**
internal plantar nerve (Winslow, 1733), see **medial plantar nerve (>1840)**
internal plantar nerve of big toe (Mayer, 1794), see **proper plantar digital nerves of medial plantar nerve (>1840)**

internal plantar nerve of first small toe (Mayer, 1794), see **proper plantar digital nerves of medial plantar nerve (>1840)**
internal plantar nerve of fourth toe (Meckel, 1817), see **proper plantar digital nerve of medial plantar nerve (>1840)**
internal plantar nerve of little toe (Mayer, 1794), see **proper plantar digital nerves of lateral plantar nerve (>1840)**
internal plantar nerve of second small toe (Mayer, 1794), see **proper plantar digital nerves of medial plantar nerve (>1840)**
internal plantar nerve of second toe (Bock, 1827), see **proper plantar digital nerve of medial plantar nerve (>1840)**
internal plantar nerve of third small toe (Mayer, 1794), see **proper plantar digital nerves of medial plantar nerve (>1840)**
internal plantar nerve of third toe (Meckel, 1817), see **proper plantar digital nerve of medial plantar nerve (>1840)**
internal plantar twig of big toe (Jördens, 1788), see **proper plantar digital nerves of medial plantar nerve (>1840)**
internal plantar twig of fifth digit (Jördens, 1788), see **proper plantar digital nerves of medial plantar nerve (>1840)**
internal plantar twig of fourth digit (Jördens, 1788), see **proper plantar digital nerves of medial plantar nerve (>1840)**
internal plantar twig of second digit (Jördens, 1788), see **proper plantar digital nerves of medial plantar nerve (>1840)**
internal plantar twig of third digit (Jördens, 1788), see **proper plantar digital nerves of medial plantar nerve (>1840)**
internal popliteal nerve (Winslow, 1733), see **tibial nerve (Haase, 1781)**
internal popliteal sciatic nerve (Sabatier, 1775), see **tibial nerve (Haase, 1781)**
internal portion of fifth pair of nerves (Todd, 1836–1839), see **nervous system (Monro, 1783)**
internal posterior cord of mammillary bodies (Spurzheim, 1826), see **mammillothalamic tract (>1840)**
internal posterior cord of spinal marrow (Meckel, 1817), see **gracile fascicle (Müller, 1834)**
internal posterior cutaneous nerve (Bock, 1827), see **posterior cutaneous nerve of arm (>1840)**
internal pterygoid nerve (Arnold, 1834), see **medial pterygoid nerve (>1840)**
internal pudendal nerve (Cruveilhier, 1836), see **pudendal nerve (Camper, 1762)**
internal pudendal nerve (Mayer, 1794), see **pelvic splanchnic nerves (Gaskell, 1886)**
internal pudic nerve (Quain & Wilson, 1839), see **pudendal nerve (Camper, 1762)**
internal radial cutaneous branch of radial nerve (Cruveilhier, 1836), see **posterior cutaneous nerve of arm (>1840)**
internal ramus of orbitary nerve (Winslow, 1733), see **nasociliary nerve (Meckel, 1817; Wutzer, 1817)**
internal ramusculus of external pudic nerve (Quain, 1828), see **genital branch of genitofemoral nerve (>1840)**
internal root of external ocular motor nerve (Cruveilhier, 1836), see **abducens nerve rootlets (>1840)**
internal root of olfactory nerve (Knox, 1832), see **lateral olfactory tract (>1840)**
internal root of olfactory nerve (Swan, 1830), see **tenia tecta (Swanson, 1992)**
internal saphenous nerve (Cloquet, 1816), see **saphenous nerve (Haase, 1781)**
internal scapular nerve (Günther, 1786), see **lower subscapular nerve (>1840)**
internal sciatic nerve (Winslow, 1733), see **tibial nerve (Haase, 1781)**
internal spermatic nerve (Mayer, 1794), see **superior testicular nerves (>1840)**
internal sphenopalatine nerve (Cruveilhier, 1836), see **medial posterior superior nasal nerves (>1840)**
internal striated body (Rolando, 1831), see **cerebral nuclei (Swanson, 2000a)**
internal subcutaneous branch of radial nerve (Loder, 1803), see **posterior cutaneous nerve of arm (>1840)**
internal subcutaneous branch of third subcostal nerve (Bock, 1827), see **anterior cutaneous branch of intercostal nerves (>1840)**
internal subcutaneous nerve (Klint, 1784), see **posterior cutaneous nerve of arm (>1840)**
internal subsural cutaneous nerve (Knox, 1832), see **tibial nerve (Haase, 1781)**
internal superior cutaneous nasal nerve (Meckel, 1817), see **internal nasal branches of infraorbital nerve (>1840)**
internal superior cutaneous nerve (Knox, 1832), see **nerve to hamstring muscles (>1840)**
internal superior labial fascicle of infraorbital surculus (Bellingeri, 1818), see **superior labial branches of infraorbital nerve (Meckel, 1748)**
internal superior labial nerve (Mayer, 1794), see **superior labial branches of infraorbital nerve (Meckel, 1748)**
internal superior nasal nerves (Günther, 1786), see **internal branches of anterior ethmoidal nerve (>1840)**
internal superior oculomuscular nerve (Cruveilhier, 1836), see **trochlear nerve (Molinetti, 1669)**
internal superior palpebral nerve (Meckel, 1753), see **lacrimal nerve (Meckel, 1748; Bonhomme, 1748)**
internal superior palpebral thread of supratrochlear fascicle (Bellingeri, 1818), see **supratrochlear nerve (Schaarschmidt, 1750)**
internal superior part of striated body (Pourfour du Petit, 1710), see **caudate nucleus (Arnold, 1838b)**
internal superior subsural cutaneous nerve (Knox, 1832), see **tibial nerve (Haase, 1781)**
internal superior superficial nasal nerve (Meckel, 1817), see **internal nasal branches of infraorbital nerve (>1840)**
internal supraclavicular branches (Soemmerring, 1791), see **medial supraclavicular nerves (>1840)**

internal terminal branch of obturator nerve (Cruveilhier, 1836), see **muscular branch of anterior branch of obturator nerve (>1840)**

internal trunk of vagus nerve (Drake, 1707), see **posterior vagal trunk (Wrisberg, 1780)**

internal tuberosity of temporal lobe (Gerdy, 1838), see **parahippocampal gyrus (>1840)**

internal twig from superficial dorsal twig of foot of deep branch of peroneal nerve (Jördens, 1788), see **dorsal digital nerves of digital branch of deep fibular nerve (>1840)**

internal twig of common motor nerve (Meckel, 1817), see **nerve to medial rectus (>1840)**

internal volar nerve of index finger (Mayer, 1794), see **proper palmar digital nerves of median nerve (>1840)**

internal volar nerve of little finger (Mayer, 1794), see **proper palmar digital nerves of ulnar nerve (>1840)**

internal volar nerve of middle finger (Mayer, 1794), see **proper palmar digital nerves of median nerve (>1840)**

internal volar nerve of ring finger (Mayer, 1794), see **proper palmar digital nerves of ulnar nerve (>1840)**

internal volar nerve of thumb (Mayer, 1794), see **proper palmar digital nerves of median nerve (>1840)**

interosseal branch of external popliteal sciatic nerve (Cruveilhier, 1836), see **deep fibular nerve (Fyfe, 1800)**

interosseal branch of median nerve (Cloquet, 1816), see **anterior interosseous nerve (Quain, 1832)**

interosseal nerve (Mayer, 1794), see **deep fibular nerve (Fyfe, 1800)**

interosseal nerve (Soemmerring, 1791), see **deep fibular nerve (Fyfe, 1800)**

interosseal nerve of leg (>1840)

interosseal twigs of metatarsal nerves (Fischer, 1791), see **common plantar digital nerves of medial plantar nerve (>1840)**

interosseous branches of anterior tibial nerve (Quain & Wilson, 1839), see **muscular branches of deep fibular nerve (>1840)**

interosseous branches of interosseous nerve (Quain & Wilson, 1839), see **muscular branches of deep fibular nerve (>1840)**

interosseous nerve (Fyfe, 1800), see **posterior interosseous nerve (Quain & Wilson, 1839)**

interosseous nerve (Quain, 1828), see **anterior interosseous nerve (Quain, 1832)**

interpeduncular fascicle (Cruveilhier, 1836), see **habenulo-interpeduncular tract (>1840)**

interpeduncular fossa (>1840)

interpeduncular nucleus (>1840)

interpeduncular space (Cruveilhier, 1836), see **interpeduncular fossa (>1840)**

interposed nucleus (>1840)

interstitium between hemispheres (Willis, 1664), see **longitudinal cerebral fissure (Gordon, 1815)**

intertexture of nervi sacri (Winslow, 1733), see **sacral plexus (Vesalius, 1543a)**

interthalamic adhesion (>1840)

intervallum inter ganglia magna inferiora (Gall & Spurzheim, 1810), see **third ventricle (Galen, c173)**

intervening medullary tract (Ridley, 1695), see **transverse pontine fibers (>1840)**

interventricular foramen (>1840)

intervertebral ganglia (Serres, 1824–1826), see **spinal nerve ganglia (Burdach, 1819)**

intervertebral nerves (Schaarschmidt, 1750), see **spinal nerves (Camper, 1760–1762)**

intervertebral nerves of neck (Schaarschmidt, 1750), see **cervical nerves (Galen, c173)**

intestine flexures of brain (Collins, 1685), see **cerebral cortex gray matter (>1840)**

intestinorum simulacra (Soemmerring, 1778), see **cerebral cortex gray matter (>1840)**

intracranial medulla oblongata (Piccolomini, 1586), see **medulla (Winslow, 1733)**

intralaminar thalamic nuclei (>1840)

intraparietal sulcus (>1840)

intrinsic cardiac plexus (>1840)

intrinsic renal nerves (>1840)

intrinsic vesical plexus (>1840)

intumescentia cervicalis (Arnold, 1838b), see **cervical enlargement (Arnold, 1838b)**

intumescentia lumbosacralis (>1840), see **lumbosacral enlargement (>1840)**

intumescentiam ganglio affinem (Scarpa, 1779), see **trigeminal ganglion (>1840)**

invertebrate brain (>1840)

invertebrate nerves (>1840)

invertebrate peripheral ganglia (Swanson & Bota, 2010)

involuntary nerves (Willis, 1664), see **nerves (Herophilus, c335–c280 BC)**

involutiones (Vesalius, 1543a), see **cerebral cortex gray matter (>1840)**

involutiones intestiniformes (Soemmerring, 1778), see **cerebral cortex gray matter (>1840)**

irian nerves (Burdin, 1803), see **short ciliary nerves (>1840)**

iridic nerves (Chaussier, 1809), see **nerves (Herophilus, c335–c280 BC)**

irregular nerves (Bell & Bell, 1829), see **craniospinal nerves (Herrick, 1915)**

irregular system of nerves (Bell & Bell, 1826), see **craniospinal nerves (Herrick, 1915)**

ischiatic nerve (Cheselden, 1726), see **sciatic nerve (Keill, 1698)**

ischioclitoral nerve (Chaussier, 1809), see **dorsal nerve of clitoris (>1840)**

ischio-clitorian nerve (Burdin, 1803), see **pudendal nerve (Camper, 1762)**

ischio-penian nerve (Burdin, 1803), see **pudendal nerve (Camper, 1762)**

ischio-trochanterian branches of small femoro-poplitean nerve (Burdin, 1803), see **sacral plexus (Vesalius, 1543a)**

island (Reil, 1809b), see **insular region (Brodmann, 1909)**

island of Reil (Cruveilhier, 1836), see **insular region (Brodmann, 1909)**

island of Sylvian fissure (Meckel, 1817), see **insular region (Brodmann, 1909)**

isthmus (Reil, 1807–1808a), see **paramedian fissure (>1840)**

isthmus (Ridley, 1695), see **tectum (Baer, 1837)**

lacuna cerebri (Mondino, 1316), see **hypothalamic part of third ventricle (Swanson, 2004)**

lacunar (Vieussens, 1684), see **dorsal part of thalamus (Herrick, 1910)**

lacunar ventriculi quarti (Soemmerring, 1778), see **rostral medullary velum (>1840)**

laqueus (Burdach, 1822), see **lateral lemniscus (Bechterew, 1885b)**

lamellae (Willis, 1664), see **cerebellar cortex (Willis, 1664)**

lamina affixa (>1840)

lamina chorioidea inferior (Burdach, 1822), see **choroid membrane of fourth ventricle (>1840)**

lamina conjunctiva (Burdach, 1822), see **Ammon's horn (Vicq d'Azyr, 1784)**

lamina connectens (Gordon, 1815), see **posterior commissure (Winslow, 1733)**

lamina cornea (Meckel, 1817), see **lamina affixa (>1840)**

lamina cornea (Vicq d'Azyr, 1786), see **reticular thalamic nucleus (>1840)**

lamina cribrosa (Reil, 1809b), see **cerebral nuclei (Swanson, 2000a)**

lamina genu corpus callosi (Burdach, 1822), see **rostrum of corpus callosum (Reil, 1809b)**

lamina medullaris (Burdach, 1822), see **superficial medullary lamina of subiculum (Dejerine & Dejerine-Klumpke, 1895)**

lamina medullaris triangularis (Günz, 1750), see **dorsal hippocampal commissure (Craigie, 1925)**

lamina rostralis (>1840), see **rostrum of corpus callosum (Reil, 1809b)**

lamina septi medullaris triangularis intermedii interventriculos laterales (Soemmerring, 1778), see **cerebral nuclei (Swanson, 2000a)**

lamina terminalis (Burdach, 1822), see **terminal lamina (Burdach, 1822)**

laminated flakes (Malacarne, 1776), see **flocculus (Meckel, 1817)**

laminated leaflets (Malacarne, 1776), see **cerebellar cortex (Willis, 1664)**

laminated lingula (Malacarne, 1776), see **lingula (Malacarne, 1776)**

laminated pyramid (Cruveilhier, 1836), see **cerebellar vermis (Meckel, 1817)**

laminated pyramid (Malacarne, 1776), see **pyramis (Malacarne, 1776)**

laminated tubercle (Malacarne, 1776), see **nodule (Reil, 1807–1808a)**

laminated tubercle of fourth ventricle (Chaussier, 1807), see **nodule (Reil, 1807–1808a)**

lang Ciliarnerven (Soemmerring, 1801), see **long ciliary nerves (Soemmerring, 1801)**

Langley's ganglion (>1840), see **submandibular ganglion (>1840)**

lapis specularis (du Laurens, 1600), see **cerebral nuclei (Swanson, 2000a)**

lappets (Willis, 1664), see **cerebellar cortex (Willis, 1664)**

laquei subclavici (Andersch & Soemmerring, 1792), see **ansa subclavia (Neubauer, 1772)**

laqueus ordinarius arteriae subclaviae (Andersch & Soemmerring, 1792), see **ansa subclavia (Neubauer, 1772)**

laqueus subclavicus (Andersch, 1797), see **ansa subclavia (Neubauer, 1772)**

large brain (Aristotle), see **vertebrate brain (Cuvier, 1800)**

large branch of medulla oblongata (Winslow, 1733), see **brainstem (Schwalbe, 1881)**

large branch of oblong medulla (Tarin, 1753), see **cerebral peduncle (Tarin, 1753)**

large cord formed by all five undermost cervical nerves (Monro, 1783), see **brachial plexus lateral cord (Schwalbe, 1887)**

large cord formed by great part of fourth and fifth cervicals (Monro, 1783), see **brachial plexus dorsal cord (Peterson, 1887)**

large falx (Chaussier, 1807), see **cerebral falx (Vesalius, 1543a)**

large root of trigeminal nerve (Cruveilhier, 1836), see **trigeminal nerve sensory root (>1840)**

large round eminences (Manfredi, 1490), see **hypothalamus (Kuhlenbeck, 1927)**

large round eminences (Mondino, 1316), see **hypothalamus (Kuhlenbeck, 1927)**

large round tubercle (Vicq d'Azyr, 1786), see **dorsal lateral geniculate nucleus (>1840)**

large sciatic branch (Winslow, 1733), see **tibial nerve (Haase, 1781)**

large transverse cerebral fissure (Meckel, 1817), see **inner part of transverse cerebral fissure (>1840)**

large transverse fissure (Bichat, 1802), see **inner part of transverse cerebral fissure (>1840)**

larger portion of fifth pair of nerves (Todd, 1836–1839), see **trigeminal nerve sensory root (>1840)**

larger root of fifth pair of cerebral nerves (Vesalius, 1543a), see **cranial nerves (Soemmerring, 1791)**

largest nerve of arm (Paré, 1550), see **median nerve (Du Verney, 1697)**

largest pharyngeal branch of pharyngolingual branch of glossopharyngeal nerve (Kilian, 1822), see **pharyngeal branches of glossopharyngeal nerve (Neubauer, 1772)**

laryngeal anastomotic surculus of digastric branch (Bellingeri, 1818), see **digastric nerve (Meckel, 1753)**

laryngeal branch of cervical intercostal trunk (Neubauer, 1772), see **laryngopharyngeal branches of superior cervical ganglion (>1840)**

laryngeal branch of pneumogastric nerve (Chaussier, 1809), see **superior laryngeal nerve (Loder, 1778)**

laryngeal branch of vagus nerve (Mayer, 1794), see **superior laryngeal nerve (Loder, 1778)**

laryngeal branches of inferior laryngeal nerve (Arnold, 1834), see **inferior laryngeal nerve (>1840)**

laryngeal branches of recurrent laryngeal nerve (Arnold, 1834), see **inferior laryngeal nerve (>1840)**

laryngeal branches of superior cervical ganglion (Cruveilhier, 1836), see **laryngopharyngeal branches of superior cervical ganglion (>1840)**

lateral hypothalamic zone (Nauta & Haymaker, 1969)

lateral intersegmental tract (>1840)

lateral left vagus nerve (Haase, 1781), see ***anterior vagal trunk (Wrisberg, 1780)***

lateral lemniscus (Bechterew, 1885b)

lateral line nerve (Desmoulins, 1825), see ***vagus nerve (Galen, c192)***

lateral lingual branches of eighth nerves of head (Andersch & Soemmerring, 1792), see ***lingual branches of glossopharyngeal nerve (Haller, 1762)***

lateral lingual branches of glossopharyngeal (Knox, 1832), see ***lingual branches of glossopharyngeal nerve (Haller, 1762)***

lateral lingual branches of glossopharyngeal nerve (Bell, 1803b), see ***lingual branches of glossopharyngeal nerve (Haller, 1762)***

lateral lingual branches of ninth nerves of head (Andersch, 1797), see ***lingual branches of glossopharyngeal nerve (Haller, 1762)***

lateral lingual nerve (Fyfe, 1800), see ***glossopharyngeal nerve (Huber, 1744)***

lateral lobe (Fyfe, 1800), see ***temporal region (>1840)***

lateral lobes of cerebrum (Gerdy, 1838), see ***cerebral cortex (>1840)***

lateral lobule of inferior vermiform process (Vicq d'Azyr, 1784), see ***biventral lobule (>1840)***

lateral longitudinal cord (Lancisi, 1713), see ***lateral longitudinal stria (Arnold, 1838a)***

lateral longitudinal stria (Arnold, 1838a)

lateral longitudinal striae (Meckel, 1817), see ***cingulum (Burdach, 1822)***

lateral longitudinal striae (Rolando, 1831), see ***superior longitudinal fascicle (>1840)***

lateral mammary branches of intercostal nerves (>1840)

lateral medullary lamina (>1840)

lateral midbrain sulcus (>1840)

lateral nasal branch of ethmoidal branch of nasal nerve (Arnold, 1834), see ***lateral nasal branches of internal nasal branches of anterior ethmoidal nerve (>1840)***

lateral nasal branch of ethmoidal branch of nasociliary nerve (Arnold, 1834), see ***lateral nasal branches of internal nasal branches of anterior ethmoidal nerve (>1840)***

lateral nasal branches of internal nasal branches of anterior ethmoidal nerve (>1840)

lateral nervous system (Desmoulins, 1825), see ***peripheral nervous system (Meckel, 1817)***

lateral occipital sulcus (>1840)

lateral occipitotemporal gyrus (>1840)

lateral olfacto-habenular tract (Gurdjian, 1925), see ***hypothalamic medullary stria (>1840)***

lateral olfactory gyrus (Craigie, 1925), see ***piriform area (Smith, 1919)***

lateral olfactory gyrus (>1840a), see ***ambient gyrus (>1840)***

lateral olfactory gyrus (>1840b), see ***ambient gyrus (>1840)***

lateral olfactory stria (>1840), see ***lateral olfactory tract (>1840)***

lateral olfactory tract (>1840)

lateral orbital gyrus (>1840)

lateral oval center (Vicq d'Azyr, 1786), see ***cerebral cortex white matter (>1840)***

lateral palatine nerve (Henle, 1871)

lateral part of cerebellum (Meckel, 1817), see ***cerebellar hemisphere (Willis, 1664)***

lateral part of white substance of spinal medulla (Arnold, 1838b), see ***lateral funiculus (Burdach, 1822)***

lateral pectoral cutaneous nerve (Bock, 1827), see ***lateral cutaneous branch of intercostal nerves (>1840)***

lateral pectoral nerve (>1840)

lateral pectoral nerves (Bock, 1827), see ***lateral cutaneous branch of intercostal nerves (>1840)***

lateral pedicles of laminated tubercles (Chaussier, 1807), see ***caudal medullary velum (>1840)***

lateral perforated substance (Arnold, 1834), see ***cerebral nuclei (Swanson, 2000a)***

lateral plantar nerve (>1840)

lateral popliteal nerve (>1840), see ***common fibular nerve (>1840)***

lateral portions of spinal marrow (Fyfe, 1800), see ***spinal cord (Galen, c162–c166)***

lateral posterior superior nasal nerves (>1840)

lateral (posterior) transverse temporal area (Brodmann, 1909), see ***transverse temporal gyri (>1840)***

lateral process (Fyfe, 1800), see ***temporal region (>1840)***

lateral process of dura mater (Fyfe, 1800), see ***cerebellar tentorium (Winslow, 1733)***

lateral pterygoid nerve (>1840)

lateral pyramid (Vicq d'Azyr, 1786), see ***trigeminal tubercle (>1840)***

lateral pyramidal body (Tarin, 1750), see ***trigeminal tubercle (>1840)***

lateral recess of fourth ventricle (>1840)

lateral reticulospinal tract (>1840)

lateral retinohypothalamic tract (>1840)

lateral ridge of lower corpus bigeminum (Gordon, 1815), see ***brachium of inferior colliculus (>1840)***

lateral ridge of upper corpus bigeminum (Gordon, 1815), see ***brachium of superior colliculus (>1840)***

lateral root of median nerve (>1840)

lateral septal arcuate fibers (>1840)

lateral septal complex (Risold & Swanson, 1997)

lateral small ganglion of neck (Andersch, 1797), see ***cervical spinal ganglia (>1840)***

lateral spinoreticular tract (>1840), see ***medullary reticulospinal tract (>1840)***

lateral spinothalamic tract (>1840)

lateral stria (Arnold, 1838b), see ***lateral longitudinal stria (Arnold, 1838a)***

lateral subcutaneous branch of intercostal branch of thoracic nerve (Bock, 1827), see ***lateral cutaneous branch of intercostal nerves (>1840)***

lateral sulcus of isthmus (Cruveilhier, 1836), see ***pontine sulcus (Soemmerring, 1778)***

lateral superficial nerves of ductus arteriosus (Andersch, 1797), see ***cardiac plexus (Keill, 1698)***

lateral supraclavicular nerves (>1840)

lateral terminal branch of deep peroneal nerve (>1840), see ***digital branch of deep fibular nerve (>1840)***

lateral thalamic nuclei (>1840)

lateral tract of medulla oblongata (Vicq d'Azyr, 1784), see ***trigeminal tubercle (>1840)***

lateral triangular fascicle of isthmus (Cruveilhier, 1836), see **lateral lemniscus (Bechterew, 1885b)**
lateral trunks of central lobule (Malacarne, 1776), see **central lobule (Burdach, 1822)**
lateral twig of tibial nerve to interosseal ligament (Jördens, 1788), see **tibial nerve (Haase, 1781)**
lateral ventricle (Vesalius, 1543a)
lateral vermiform process (Winslow, 1733), see **cerebellar hemisphere (Willis, 1664)**
lateral vestibulospinal tract (>1840)
lateral walls of cerebellar ventricle (Chaussier, 1807), see **floor of fourth ventricle (Reil, 1807–1808a)**
latter border of streaked body (Willis, 1672), see **internal capsule (Burdach, 1822)**
layer of peduncle of hemisphere (Rolando, 1831), see **internal capsule (Burdach, 1822)**
layers of ocular nerves (Burdin, 1803), see **interbrain (Baer, 1837)**
layers of optic nerves (Burdin, 1803), see **interbrain (Baer, 1837)**
least external branch of palatine nerve (Meckel, 1748), see **lateral palatine nerve (Henle, 1871)**
least infolding of abdomen (Willis, 1664), see **inferior mesenteric ganglion (>1840)**
least infolding of mesentery (Willis, 1664), see **inferior mesenteric ganglion (>1840)**
least palatine nerve (Bock, 1817), see **lateral palatine nerve (Henle, 1871)**
least splanchnic nerve (>1840)
left anterior and superior gastric nerves (Mayer, 1794), see **gastric branches of anterior vagal trunk (>1840)**
left colic plexus (Chaussier, 1789), see **inferior mesenteric plexus (Rau, 1720)**
left colic plexus (Meckel, 1817)
left cord of pneumogastric nerve (Meckel, 1817), see **anterior vagal trunk (Wrisberg, 1780)**
left coronary artery nerve (Behrends, 1792), see **left coronary plexus (Scarpa, 1794)**
left coronary plexus (Scarpa, 1794)
left gastric nerves (Wrisberg, 1800), see **gastric branches of anterior vagal trunk (>1840)**
left gastric plexus (>1840)
left gastro-epiploic nerve (Albinus, 1744), see **anterior nerve of lesser curvature (>1840)**
left gastroepiploic nerve (Mayer, 1794), see **left gastroepiploic plexus (Wrisberg, 1800)**
left gastroepiploic plexus (Wrisberg, 1800)
left hepatic nerves (Mayer, 1794), see **hepatic plexus (Rau, 1720)**
left hepatic plexus (Wrisberg, 1780), see **hepatic branches of anterior vagal trunk (>1840)**
left lateral cardiac plexus (Swan, 1830), see **cardiac plexus (Keill, 1698)**
left omental nerves (Mayer, 1794), see **left gastroepiploic plexus (Wrisberg, 1800)**
left pancreatic nerves (Mayer, 1794), see **pancreatic plexus (Cruveilhier, 1836)**
left posterior and superior gastric nerves (Mayer, 1794), see **gastric branches of posterior vagal trunk (>1840)**
left stomach nerve (Crooke, 1615), see **anterior vagal trunk (Wrisberg, 1780)**
left thoracic plexus (Swan, 1830), see **paravertebral nerves (Swanson & Bota, 2010)**
left vagus nerve (Mayer, 1794), see **vagus nerve (Galen, c192)**
leg of vault (Vesling, 1647), see **fimbria (Honegger, 1890)**
leg of vaulted body (Paré, 1550), see **fornix (Vesalius, 1543a)**
lemniscus (Reil, 1809b), see **central nervous system white matter tracts (>1840)**
lemniscus of lamina cribrosa (Reil, 1812a,b), see **diagonal band (Broca, 1879)**
lenticular branch of nasal nerve (Todd, 1836–1839), see **communicating branch of nasociliary nerve with ciliary ganglion (>1840)**
lenticular ganglion (Winslow, 1733), see **ciliary ganglion (Loder, 1778)**
lenticular ganglion branch of communication to carotid plexus (Quain & Wilson, 1839), see **sympathetic root of ciliary ganglion (>1840)**
lenticular ganglion branch of communication to inferior branch of third nerve (Quain & Wilson, 1839), see **branch of oculomotor nerve to ciliary ganglion (>1840)**
lenticular ganglion branch of communication to nasal nerve (Quain & Wilson, 1839), see **communicating branch of nasociliary nerve with ciliary ganglion (>1840)**
lenticular nucleus (Burdach, 1822), see **cerebral nuclei (Swanson, 2000a)**
lentiform nucleus (Burdach, 1822), see **cerebral nuclei (Swanson, 2000a)**
lentiform process (Willis, 1664), see **cerebral nuclei (Swanson, 2000a)**
lentiform prominence (Willis, 1664), see **cerebral nuclei (Swanson, 2000a)**
leptomeninges (>1840), see **pia-arachnoid (>1840)**
less trunk of fourth sinew of thigh (Geminus, 1553), see **common fibular nerve (>1840)**
lesser abdominal branch of lumbar plexus (Cruveilhier, 1836), see **iliohypogastric nerve (Schmidt, 1794)**
lesser annulary process (Willis, 1664), see **trapezoid body (Treviranus, 1820)**
lesser annulary protuberance (Willis, 1664), see **trapezoid body (Treviranus, 1820)**
lesser anterior dental nerve (Arnold, 1834), see **middle superior dental nerve (Henle, 1871)**
lesser anterior thoracic nerve (Günther, 1786), see **medial pectoral nerve (>1840)**
lesser apartments of cerebellum (Collins, 1685), see **cerebellar hemisphere (Willis, 1664)**
lesser auricular nerves (Günther, 1786), see **auriculotemporal nerve (Haller, 1762)**
lesser brain (Geminus, 1553), see **cerebellum (Aristotle)**
lesser branches of conjugations of neck, chest, loynes, and sacral bone (Crooke, 1615), see **spinal nerve dorsal branch (Meckel, 1817)**
lesser cardiac infolding (Willis, 1664), see **cardiac ganglion (Neubauer, 1772; Haller, 1772)**
lesser cardiack plex of par vagum (Collins, 1685), see **cardiac plexus (Keill, 1698)**

lesser circuits of cerebellum (Collins, 1685), see **cerebellar hemisphere (Willis, 1664)**
lesser cutaneous branch of musculocutaneous nerve (Loder, 1803), see **lateral cutaneous nerve of forearm (>1840)**
lesser deep petrosal nerve (Arnold, 1834), see **deep petrosal nerve (Meckel, 1817)**
lesser external palatine nerve (Mayer, 1794), see **lateral palatine nerve (Henle, 1871)**
lesser frontal nerve (Meckel, 1753), see **supratrochlear nerve (Schaarschmidt, 1750)**
lesser hippocampus (Bell & Bell, 1816), see **calcarine spur (Morand, 1748)**
lesser ilioscrotal branch of lumbar plexus (Cruveilhier, 1836), see **iliohypogastric nerve (Schmidt, 1794)**
lesser internal branch of accessory eighth cranial nerve (Scarpa, 1794), see **internal branch of accessory nerve trunk (Meckel, 1817)**
lesser nerves out of infolding of third pair (Willis, 1664), see **short ciliary nerves (>1840)**
lesser occipital branch of cervical plexus (Quain, 1832), see **lesser occipital nerve (Mayer, 1794)**
lesser occipital nerve (Mayer, 1794)
lesser occipital nerve (Meckel, 1753), see **lesser occipital nerve (Mayer, 1794)**
lesser orbicular protuberances (Willis, 1664), see **inferior colliculus (Haller, 1762)**
lesser palatine nerve (Bock, 1817), see **posterior palatine nerve (Günther, 1786)**
lesser palatine nerves (Meckel, 1817)
lesser petrosal nerve (>1840)
lesser pons (Serres, 1824–1826), see **trapezoid body (Treviranus, 1820)**
lesser posterior auricular nerve (Neubauer, 1772), see **anterior branch of great auricular nerve (>1840)**
lesser posterior palatine nerve (Meckel, 1748), see **posterior palatine nerve (Günther, 1786)**
lesser posterior thoracic nerve (Günther, 1786), see **long thoracic nerve (Quain & Wilson, 1839)**
lesser protuberance of auditory nerve (Willis, 1664), see **trapezoid body (Treviranus, 1820)**
lesser protuberances (Willis, 1664), see **inferior colliculus (Haller, 1762)**
lesser ring (Willis, 1664), see **trapezoid body (Treviranus, 1820)**
lesser root of fifth pair of sinews of brain (Geminus, 1553), see **trigeminal nerve motor root (Bell, 1829)**
lesser saphenous nerve (Fischer, 1791), see **saphenous nerve (Haase, 1781)**
lesser sciatic nerve (Chaussier, 1809), see **sacral plexus (Vesalius, 1543a)**
lesser splanchnic nerve (Haller, 1762)
lesser stories of cerebellum (Collins, 1685), see **cerebellar hemisphere (Willis, 1664)**
lesser superficial branch of middle subcutaneous nerve of neck (Peipers, 1793), see **transverse nerve of neck (>1840)**
lesser superficial petrosal nerve (Arnold, 1828), see **lesser petrosal nerve (>1840)**
lesser superficial petrosal nerve (Quain & Wilson, 1839), see **caroticotympanic nerves (>1840)**
lesser superior branch of third branch of fifth pair (Meckel, 1748), see **mandibular nerve trunk (>1840)**
lesser, thinner, harder root of third pair of nerves (Vesalius, 1543a), see **trigeminal nerve (Winslow, 1733)**
lesser, thinner, harder root of third pair of sinews (Geminus, 1553), see **trigeminal nerve (Winslow, 1733)**
lesser thoracic nerve (Bang, 1770), see **lateral pectoral nerve (>1840)**
lesser thoracic nerve (Haase, 1781), see **long thoracic nerve (Quain & Wilson, 1839)**
lesser trunk of nerve of thigh (Vesalius, 1543a), see **common fibular nerve (>1840)**
lesser volar branch of cubital nerve (Loder, 1803), see **superficial branch of ulnar nerve (Fyfe, 1800)**
lesser volar branch of dorsal nerve from internal cutaneous nerve (Knox, 1832), see **posterior branch of medial cutaneous nerve of forearm (>1840)**
ligamentous twig of internal branch of internal plantar nerve (Fischer, 1791), see **medial plantar nerve (>1840)**
ligamentum piae matris (Fyfe, 1800), see **terminal filament (Tiedemann, 1821)**
ligula (Arnold, 1838b), see **choroid line of fourth ventricle (>1840)**
ligula (Bergmann, 1831), see **choroid membrane of fourth ventricle (>1840)**
limbi medullares (Lancisi, 1718), see **lateral longitudinal stria (Arnold, 1838a)**
limbic convolution (Foville, 1844), see **limbic region (>1840)**
limbic lobe (Broca, 1878), see **limbic region (>1840)**
limbic region (>1840)
limbus (Molinetti, 1669), see **central nervous system gray matter regions (>1840)**
limbus cerebri (Willis, 1664), see **limbic region (>1840)**
limbus of Ammon's horn (Soemmerring, 1791), see **fimbria (Honegger, 1890)**
limbus of brain (Bartholin, 1662), see **limbic region (>1840)**
limbus of brain (Gibson, 1682), see **limbic region (>1840)**
limbus posterior (Vieussens, 1684), see **limbic region (>1840)**
limbus Sylvii (Haller, 1762), see **fimbria (Honegger, 1890)**
limen fissura Sylvii (Reil, 1809b), see **ambient gyrus (>1840)**
limen insulae (>1840), see **ambient gyrus (>1840)**
limiting cord (Meckel, 1817), see **sympathetic cord (>1840)**
limiting cord trunk (Meckel, 1817), see **sympathetic trunk (Winslow, 1733)**
limiting ganglions of ganglionnary nerve (Meckel, 1817), see **paravertebral ganglia (Durward, 1951)**
limiting sulcus (>1840)
limiting sulcus of fourth ventricle (>1840)
linea alba (Haller, 1754a), see **medullary stria (Wenzel & Wenzel, 1812)**
linea Lancisii (Reil, 1812c), see **longitudinal striae (>1840)**
linea media mesolobii (Chaussier, 1807), see **longitudinal striae (>1840)**
lineae transversae of calamus scriptorius (Quain, 1837), see **medullary striae (Scarpa, 1788)**

lobule of medulla oblongata (Vicq d'Azyr, 1784), see **tonsil (Malacarne, 1776)**
lobule of striate body (Cruveilhier, 1836), see **insular region (Brodmann, 1909)**
lobule of Sylvian fissure (Cruveilhier, 1836), see **insular region (Brodmann, 1909)**
lobule of vagus nerve (Vicq d'Azyr, 1786), see **flocculus (Meckel, 1817)**
lobules of cerebellum (Haller, 1762), see **cerebellar hemisphere (Willis, 1664)**
lobules of cerebellum (Heister, 1717), see **cerebellar hemisphere (Willis, 1664)**
lobuli minima (Günther, 1786), see **flocculus (Meckel, 1817)**
lobuli parvi cerebelli, que communiter septimo et octavo pari interjacent (Prochàska, 1800), see **flocculus (Meckel, 1817)**
lobus caudicis (Burdach, 1822), see **insular region (Brodmann, 1909)**
lobus posterior (Leuret, 1839), see **spinal nucleus of trigeminal nerve (>1840)**
lobus striatus (Leuret, 1839), see **nucleus of solitary tract (>1840)**
lobus subtilus (Malacarne, 1776), see **gracile lobe (Malacarne, 1776)**
localis membrana (Ramsay, 1813), see **pia (Galen, c192)**
locality where olfactory apparatus originates (Varoli, 1573), see **cerebral nuclei (Swanson, 2000a)**
loculos caeruleos (Wenzel & Wenzel, 1812), see **locus ceruleus (Wenzel & Wenzel, 1812)**
locus caeruleus (Burdach, 1822), see **locus ceruleus (Wenzel & Wenzel, 1812)**
locus ceruleus (Wenzel & Wenzel, 1812)
locus coeruleus (Arnold, 1838a), see **locus ceruleus (Wenzel & Wenzel, 1812)**
locus niger crurum cerebri (Vicq d'Azyr, 1784), see **substantia nigra (Soemmerring, 1791)**
locus perforatus (Quain, 1828), see **interpeduncular nucleus (>1840)**
long anterior thoracic nerve (Loder, 1803), see **lateral pectoral nerve (>1840)**
long arch of neck (Andersch & Soemmerring, 1792), see **ansa cervicalis (>1840)**
long brain (Benedetti, 1502), see **spinal cord (Galen, c162–c166)**
long brain (Crooke, 1615), see **cerebrospinal trunk (>1840)**
long branches of frontal branches of external frontal nerve (Todd, 1836–1839), see **lateral branch of supraorbital nerve (>1840)**
long cervical ganglion of intercostal nerve (Meckel, 1751), see **superior cervical ganglion (Vieussens, 1684)**
long chink (Bartholin, 1662), see **third ventricle (Galen, c173)**
long ciliary nerves (Soemmerring, 1801)
long convolution (Reil, 1809b), see **cingulate region (Brodmann, 1909)**
long crus of lateral ventricle (Günther, 1786), see **inferior horn of lateral ventricle (Bell, 1802)**
long cutaneous branch of internal interosseous nerve (Caldani, 1813, 1814), see **anterior interosseous nerve (Quain, 1832)**
long cutaneous branch of leg (Bock, 1827), see **sural nerve (Pietro da Cortona, 1741)**
long cutaneous branch of median nerve (Knox, 1832), see **palmar branch of median nerve (Bock, 1827)**
long cutaneous branch of peroneal nerve (Swan, 1830), see **lateral cutaneous nerve of calf (>1840)**
long cutaneous nerve (Bell, 1803a), see **saphenous nerve (Haase, 1781)**
long cutaneous nerve (Günther, 1786), see **sural nerve (Pietro da Cortona, 1741)**
long cutaneous nerve of foot (Günther, 1786), see **saphenous nerve (Haase, 1781)**
long cutaneous nerve of leg (Bock, 1827), see **sural nerve (Pietro da Cortona, 1741)**
long descending branch of obturator nerve communicating with internal saphenous nerve (Quain & Wilson, 1839), see **obturator nerve (Cheselden, 1726)**
long external branch of external plantar nerve (Bock, 1827), see **common plantar digital nerves of lateral plantar nerve (>1840)**
long external root of olfactory nerve (Soemmerring, 1778), see **lateral olfactory tract (>1840)**
long gyrus of insula (Valentin, 1841)
long hidden commissure of cerebellum (Reil, 1807–1808a), see **tuber vermis (>1840)**
long inferior branch of nervi motores oculorum communes (Winslow, 1733), see **nerve to inferior oblique (>1840)**
long inferior branch of third pair of nerves (Winslow, 1733), see **nerve to inferior oblique (>1840)**
long inferior pudendal nerve (Walter, 1783), see **posterior labial nerves (>1840)**
long internal convolution (Reil, 1812b), see **parahippocampal gyrus (>1840)**
long internal root of olfactory nerve (Vicq d'Azyr, 1786), see **lateral olfactory tract (>1840)**
long marrow (Crooke, 1615), see **cerebrospinal trunk (>1840)**
long marrow (Willis, 1664), see **vertebrate brain (Cuvier, 1800)**
long marrow of brain (Crooke, 1615), see **cerebrospinal trunk (>1840)**
long nerve (Bell, 1803b), see **muscular branches of femoral nerve (Quain & Wilson, 1839)**
long nerve to crural muscle (Styx, 1782), see **muscular branches of femoral nerve (Quain & Wilson, 1839)**
long nerve to sartorius muscle (Styx, 1782), see **muscular branches of femoral nerve (Quain & Wilson, 1839)**
long nerve to vastus externus muscle (Styx, 1782), see **muscular branches of femoral nerve (Quain & Wilson, 1839)**
long nerve to vastus internus muscle (Styx, 1782), see **muscular branches of femoral nerve (Quain & Wilson, 1839)**
long palmar branch of median nerve (Bock, 1827), see **palmar branch of median nerve (Bock, 1827)**
long palmar branch of ulnar nerve (Bock, 1827), see **palmar branch of ulnar nerve (Soemmerring, 1791)**
long palmar cutaneous branch of median nerve (Loder, 1803), see **palmar branch of median nerve (Bock, 1827)**

looking glass (du Laurens, 1600), see **cerebral nuclei (Swanson, 2000a)**

lower and internal part of auditory nerve (Meckel, 1817), see **vestibular nerve central root (>1840)**

lower branch of fifth pair of nerves arising within skull (Willis, 1664), see **mandibular nerve (>1840)**

lower branch of fourth nerve entering arm (Vesalius, 1543a), see **deep branch of radial nerve (Martin, 1781)**

lower branch of second division of fifth pair of nerves arising within skull (Willis, 1664), see **maxillary nerve (Meckel, 1753)**

lower bundle of trigeminal nerve (Gordon, 1815), see **trigeminal nerve sensory root (>1840)**

lower cervical ganglion (Bell, 1803b), see **inferior cervical ganglion (Vieussens, 1684)**

lower commissure of cerebellum (Carus, 1814), see **middle cerebellar peduncle (Rolando, 1819)**

lower corpora bigeminum (Gordon, 1815), see **inferior colliculus (Haller, 1762)**

lower esophageal branches of vagus nerve (>1840), see **esophageal plexus (>1840)**

lower facial branches of descending branch of superficial branch of hard nerve (Günther, 1786), see **facial nerve trunk (1840)**

lower filament of inferior orbital thread of temporal surculus (Bellingeri, 1818), see **temporal branches of facial nerve (Swan, 1830)**

lower ganglia (Carus, 1814), see **ventral ganglia (Anderson, 1837)**

lower ganglion of nerve ring (Carus, 1818), see **ventral ganglia (Anderson, 1837)**

lower hinder seat of ventricle (Geminus, 1553), see **lateral ventricle (Vesalius, 1543a)**

lower infolding of intercostal nerve (Willis, 1664), see **sympathetic trunk ganglia (Winslow, 1733)**

lower infolding of wandring pair (Willis, 1664), see **vagus nerve (Galen, c192)**

lower internal cutaneous nerve (Bell, 1803a), see **sciatic nerve (Keill, 1698)**

lower maxillary nerve (Bell, 1809b), see **mandibular nerve (>1840)**

lower mesenteric plexus (Bell & Bell, 1816), see **inferior mesenteric plexus (Rau, 1720)**

lower-middle-white portion of brain (Haller, 1747), see **rhombicbrain (His, 1893b)**

lower nerve chain (Carus, 1814), see **ventral cord (Anderson, 1837)**

lower nerve cord (Cuvier, 1800), see **ventral cord (Anderson, 1837)**

lower part of third deep nerve of thigh (Galen, c177), see **posterior branch of obturator nerve (Haase, 1781; Martin, 1781)**

lower recess of ventricle (Vesalius, 1543a), see **inferior horn of lateral ventricle (Bell, 1802)**

lower ring (Willis, 1664), see **trapezoid body (Treviranus, 1820)**

lower stomachical branch of wandring pair (Willis, 1664), see **posterior vagal trunk (Wrisberg, 1780)**

lower subscapular nerve (>1840)

lower substance of brain (Dryander, 1536), see **temporal region (>1840)**

lower tract of cerebellum (Vesalius, 1543a), see **inferior cerebellar peduncle (Günther, 1786)**

lowest brain substance (Dryander, 1536), see **frontal region (Vicq d'Azyr, 1786)**

lowest cardiac nerve (Günther, 1786), see **inferior cardiac nerve (Cloquet, 1816)**

lowest cervical ganglion (Winslow, 1733), see **inferior cervical ganglion (Vieussens, 1684)**

lowest coccygeal ganglion (Bock, 1827), see **ganglion impar (Quain & Wilson, 1839)**

lowest facial nerve of superior branch of hard nerve (Meckel, 1753), see **zygomatic branches of facial nerve (>1840)**

lowest filament of inferior orbital thread of temporal surculus (Bellingeri, 1818), see **temporal branches of facial nerve (Swan, 1830)**

lowest foot of oblong marrow (Willis, 1664), see **medulla (Winslow, 1733)**

lowest infolding of abdomen (Willis, 1664), see **superior hypogastric plexus (Tiedemann, 1822)**

lowest infolding of mesentery (Willis, 1664), see **superior hypogastric plexus (Tiedemann, 1822)**

lowest nerve of posterior ventricle of heart (Andersch, 1797), see **coronary plexuses (Meckel, 1817)**

lowest soft branch (Andersch, 1797), see **jugular nerves (>1840)**

lowest soft nerve (Andersch & Soemmerring, 1792), see **jugular nerves (>1840)**

lowest superficial branch of anterior ventricle of heart (Andersch, 1797), see **cardiac plexus (Keill, 1698)**

lowest superficial branch of superficial nerve of neck (Bang, 1770), see **inferior branches of transverse nerve of neck (>1840)**

lowest trunk of superficial nerve of nerve layers of septum of heart (Andersch, 1797), see **coronary plexuses (Meckel, 1817)**

lozenge (Reil, 1809c), see **floor of fourth ventricle (Reil, 1807–1808a)**

lozenge-shaped field (Reil, 1809c), see **floor of fourth ventricle (Reil, 1807–1808a)**

lucid enclosure (Diemerbroeck, 1689), see **cerebral nuclei (Swanson, 2000a)**

lucid fence (Diemerbroeck, 1689), see **cerebral nuclei (Swanson, 2000a)**

lumbal branch of abdominal nerve (Bock, 1827), see **spinal nerve dorsal branch (Meckel, 1817)**

lumbal branch of lumbar nerve (Bock, 1827), see **spinal nerve dorsal branch (Meckel, 1817)**

lumbal nerve of lumbar nerve (Bock, 1827), see **spinal nerve dorsal branch (Meckel, 1817)**

lumbar aortic and splanchnic branches (Cruveilhier, 1836), see **lumbar splanchnic nerves (Cruveilhier, 1836)**

lumbar branches of lumbar nerves (Meckel, 1817), see **spinal nerve dorsal branch (Meckel, 1817)**

lumbar extremity of spinal prolongation (Chaussier, 1807), see **medullary cone (>1840)**

lumbar ganglia of intercostal nerve (Günther, 1786), see **lumbar sympathetic ganglia (>1840)**

lumbar ganglion (Walter, 1783), see **lumbar sympathetic ganglia (>1840)**
lumbar ganglion of great sympathetic nerve (Walter, 1783), see **lumbar sympathetic ganglia (>1840)**
lumbar ganglions of limiting cord (Meckel, 1817), see **lumbar sympathetic ganglia (>1840)**
lumbar intervertebral nerves (Schaarschmidt, 1750), see **lumbar nerves (Diemerbroeck, 1672)**
lumbar nerves (Diemerbroek, 1672)
lumbar nerves (Haller, 1762), see **spinal nerves (Camper, 1760–1762)**
lumbar nerves (Vesalius, 1543a), see **spinal nerves (Camper, 1760–1762)**
lumbar part of crural plexus (Chaussier, 1809), see **lumbar plexus (Vesalius, 1543a)**
lumbar part of spinal cord (>1840)
lumbar part of spinal medulla (Tiedemann, 1821), see **lumbar part of spinal cord (>1840)**
lumbar plexus (Vesalius, 1543a)
lumbar plexus abdominal branches (Meckel, 1817), see **lumbar plexus ventral branches (>1840)**
lumbar plexus anterior branches (Meckel, 1817), see **lumbar plexus ventral branches (>1840)**
lumbar plexus dorsal divisions (Paterson, 1887)
lumbar plexus ventral branches (>1840)
lumbar plexus ventral divisions (Paterson, 1887)
lumbar prominence (Meckel, 1817), see **lumbosacral enlargement (>1840)**
lumbar spinal ganglia (>1840)
lumbar spinal medulla (Galen, c173), see **lumbar part of spinal cord (>1840)**
lumbar splanchnic nerves (Cruveilhier, 1836)
lumbar swelling of spinal cord (Quain & Wilson, 1839), see **lumbosacral enlargement (>1840)**
lumbar sympathetic ganglia (>1840)
lumbar trunk (Bell, 1803b), see **femoral nerve (Haller, 1762)**
lumbo-abdominal plexus (Schmidt, 1794), see **lumbar plexus (Vesalius, 1543a)**
lumboaortic plexus (Cruveilhier, 1836), see **intermesenteric plexus (>1840)**
lumbo-dorsal communicating branch (Quain, 1828), see **lumbar plexus (Vesalius, 1543a)**
lumboinguinal nerve (Schmidt, 1794), see **femoral branch of genitofemoral nerve (>1840)**
lumbo-intercostal ganglia (Schmidt, 1794), see **lumbar sympathetic ganglia (>1840)**
lumbo-sacral communicating branch (Quain, 1828), see **lumbosacral trunk (Cruveilhier, 1836)**
lumbosacral cord (Bichat et al., 1801–1803), see **lumbosacral trunk (Cruveilhier, 1836)**
lumbosacral enlargement (>1840)
lumbosacral nerve (Cruveilhier, 1836), see **lumbosacral trunk (Cruveilhier, 1836)**
lumbosacral plexus (Vesalius, 1543a)
lumbosacral trunk (Cruveilhier, 1836)
lunate sulcus (>1840)
lupine-bean-shaped spongy flesh (Galen, c192), see **pituitary gland (>1840)**
lyra Davidis (Mayer, 1779), see **dorsal hippocampal commissure (Craigie, 1925)**
lyra minima (Bergmann, 1831), see **ventral hippocampal commissure (Craigie, 1925)**
lyra veli anterioris (Bergmann, 1831), see **rostral medullary vellum (>1840)**
lyre (Winslow, 1733), see **dorsal hippocampal commissure (Craigie, 1925)**
maeandros (Soemmerring, 1778), see **cerebral cortex gray matter (>1840)**
magna reunio cerebri (Gall & Spurzheim, 1810), see **cerebral cortex white matter (>1840)**
magno nervo cardiaco (Wrisberg, 1786), see **cardiac plexus (Keill, 1698)**
main body of filaments of nerves of eighth pair (Winslow, 1733), see **vagus nerve rootlets (>1840)**
main communicating branch of glossopharyngeal nerve (Kilian, 1822), see **glossopharyngeal nerve (Huber, 1744)**
main nerve cord of body (Carus, 1814), see **central nerve cord (Serres, 1824–1826)**
main olfactory bulb (>1840)
major anterior branches of auricular nerve (Soemmerring, 1791), see **superficial temporal branches of auriculotemporal nerve (>1840)**
major anterior vestibular nerve (Langenbeck, 1826–1830), see **rostral part of vestibular nerve (>1840)**
major brachial plexus (Günther, 1786), see **brachial plexus (Camper, 1760)**
major branch of anterior fascicles of acoustic nerve (Scarpa, 1789), see **rostral part of vestibular nerve (>1840)**
major branch of cubital nerve trunk (Loder, 1803), see **superficial branch of ulnar nerve (Fyfe, 1800)**
major branch of fifth pair (Rau, 1694), see **maxillary nerve (Meckel, 1753)**
major branch of interior nasal nerve (Scarpa, 1785), see **internal nasal branches of anterior ethmoidal nerve (>1840)**
major branch of posterior branch of acoustic nerve (Cloquet, 1828), see **rostral part of vestibular nerve (>1840)**
major branch of sciatic nerve trunk (Günther, 1786), see **tibial nerve (Haase, 1781)**
major branches of inferior maxillary nerve (Loder, 1778), see **posterior branch of mandibular nerve (>1840)**
major cardiac nerve (Neubauer, 1772), see **inferior cardiac nerve (Cloquet, 1816)**
major cerebellar lobes (Günther, 1786), see **cerebellar hemisphere (Willis, 1664)**
major crura of ventricle (Bergen, 1734), see **lateral ventricle (Vesalius, 1543a)**
major inferior branch of inferior maxillary branch of fifth pair of nerves (Bock, 1817), see **marginal mandibular branch of facial nerve (>1840)**
major inferior cutaneous branch of anterior femoral nerve (Soemmerring, 1798), see **saphenous nerve (Haase, 1781)**
major internal cutaneous nerve (Klint, 1784), see **medial cutaneous nerve of forearm (>1840)**
major internal musculo-cutaneous nerve (Frotscher, 1788), see **medial cutaneous nerve of forearm (>1840)**
major part of facial nerve (Arnold, 1834), see **intermediofacial nerve (Strong & Elwyn, 1943)**

major pharyngeal branch of pharyngolingual branch of glossopharyngeal nerve (Kilian, 1822), see **pharyngeal branches of glossopharyngeal nerve (Neubauer, 1772)**

major pharyngeal nerve (Soemmerring, 1791), see **pharyngeal branch of vagus nerve (>1840)**

major posterior fissure (Blasius, 1666), see **dorsal median septum (>1840)**

major pudendal nerve (Günther, 1786), see **sacral plexus (Vesalius, 1543a)**

major subcutaneous branch of radial nerve (Haase, 1781), see **posterior cutaneous nerve of forearm (>1840)**

major twig of posterior branch of auditory nerve (Soemmerring, 1791), see **rostral part of vestibular nerve (>1840)**

malar branch of lacrimal nerve (Cruveilhier, 1836), see **lacrimal nerve (Meckel, 1748; Bonhomme, 1748)**

malar branch of malar nerve (Swan, 1830), see **zygomaticofacial nerve (>1840)**

malar branch of temporo-malar branch of second division of fifth pair of nerves (Todd, 1836–1839), see **zygomaticofacial nerve (>1840)**

malar branches of facial nerve (Quain, 1837), see **zygomatic branches of facial nerve (>1840)**

malar branches of orbital branches of temporofacial branch of facial nerve (Cruveilhier, 1836), see **zygomatic branches of facial nerve (>1840)**

malar branches of superior branch of facial nerve (Arnold, 1834), see **zygomatic branches of facial nerve (>1840)**

malar filament of middle facial branch of pes anserinus (Bellingeri, 1818), see **zygomatic branches of facial nerve (>1840)**

malar filament of temporo-malar branch of orbital branch of superior maxillary nerve (Cruveilhier, 1836), see **orbital branches of pterygopalatine ganglion (>1840)**

malar nerve of hard nerve (Meckel, 1753), see **zygomatic branches of facial nerve (>1840)**

malar nerve of second trunk of fifth (Swan, 1830), see **zygomatic nerve (>1840)**

malar nerves (Meckel, 1817), see **zygomatic branches of facial nerve (>1840)**

maleolar branch of peroneal saphenous nerve (Cruveilhier, 1836), see **sural communicating branch of common fibular nerve (>1840)**

malleal filament of portio major and minor of facial nerve (Bellingeri, 1818), see **intermediofacial nerve trunk (1840)**

malo-palpebral fascicle of subcutaneous malar surculus (Bellingeri, 1818), see **zygomaticofacial nerve (>1840)**

malo-temporal fascicle of lacrimal surculus (Bellingeri, 1818), see **lacrimal nerve (Meckel, 1748; Bonhomme, 1748)**

mamillares cerebri (Brunschwig, 1525), see **cerebral cortex (>1840)**

mamillaris processus cerebri (Geminus, 1553), see **frontal pole (>1840)**

mamillary body (His, 1895), see **mammillary body (Ludwig, 1779)**

mamillary body peduncle (Honegger, 1890), see **mammillary peduncle (>1840)**

mamillary eminence of inferior vermis (Cloquet, 1828), see **uvula (Malacarne, 1776)**

mamillary eminences (Haller, 1754a), see **mammillary body (Ludwig, 1779)**

mamillary process (Soemmerring, 1778), see **mammillary body (Ludwig, 1779)**

mamillary process (Vesalius, 1543a), see **frontal pole (>1840)**

mamillary swelling of posterior median çolumn (Cruveilhier, 1836), see **gracile nucleus (>1840)**

mammary nerves (Horne, 1707), see **medial mammary branches of intercostal nerves (>1840)**

mammelon (Morand, 1748), see **cerebral cortex (>1840)**

mammillares (Bartholin, 1662), see **olfactory bulb (Weitbrecht, 1751)**

mammillary bodies of Willis (Günther, 1786), see **mammillary body (Ludwig, 1779)**

mammillary body (Ludwig, 1779)

mammillary caruncle (Arnold, 1838b), see **frontal pole (>1840)**

mammillary carunculae (Benedetti, 1502), see **cerebral cortex (>1840)**

mammillary carunculae (Berengario da Carpi, 1522), see **olfactory bulb (Weitbrecht, 1751)**

mammillary eminence of inferior vermis (Vicq d'Azyr, 1784), see **cerebellar vermis (Meckel, 1817)**

mammillary peduncle (>1840)

mammillary process (Willis, 1664), see **olfactory bulb (Weitbrecht, 1751)**

mammillary process (Willis, 1672, Tab. III), see **invertebrate nerves (>1840)**

mammillary process (Willis, 1672, Tab. VI), see **cerebral cortex (>1840)**

mammillary processes (Guy de Chauliac, 1363), see **cerebral cortex (>1840)**

mammillary prominence (Vesalius, 1543a), see **frontal pole (>1840)**

mammillary protuberances (Lieutaud, 1742), see **mammillary body (Ludwig, 1779)**

mammillary recess (>1840)

mammillary sulcus (>1840)

mammillary tubercles (Winslow, 1733), see **mammillary body (Ludwig, 1779)**

mammillotegmental tract (Kölliker, 1896)

mammillothalamic tract (Kölliker, 1896)

mandibular branch of inferior maxillary branch of fifth pair of nerves (Bock, 1817), see **inferior dental nerve (Meckel, 1817)**

mandibular nerve (Straus Durckheim, 1828), see **invertebrate nerves (>1840)**

mandibular nerve (>1840)

mandibular nerve sensory root (>1840)

mandibular nerve trunk (>1840)

mandibulolabial branch of fifth nerve (Bell, 1829), see **inferior dental nerve (Meckel, 1817)**

mandibulo-labial nerve (Soemmerring, 1798), see **inferior dental nerve (Meckel, 1817)**

manducatory nerve (Bell, 1829), see **trigeminal nerve (Winslow, 1733)**

manducatory portion of fifth nerve (Bell, 1829), see **trigeminal nerve motor root (Bell, 1829)**

mantle (Rosenthal, 1815), see **cerebral cortex gray matter (>1840)**
marginal body (Vicq d'Azyr, 1786), see **fimbria (Honegger, 1890)**
marginal branch of hard nerve (Peipers, 1793), see **marginal mandibular branch of facial nerve (>1840)**
marginal branch of inferior facial branch of inferior branch of anterior branch of hard nerve (Loder, 1778), see **marginal mandibular branch of facial nerve (>1840)**
marginal branch of lower facial branches of descending branch of superficial branch of hard nerve (Günther, 1786), see **marginal mandibular branch of facial nerve (>1840)**
marginal branch of lower jaw of inferior facial branch of hard nerve (Meckel, 1753), see **marginal mandibular branch of facial nerve (>1840)**
marginal bulge (Burdach, 1822), see **cerebral cortex gray matter (>1840)**
marginal ganglia (>1840)
marginal inferior maxillary nerve (Soemmerring, 1798), see **marginal mandibular branch of facial nerve (>1840)**
marginal mandibular branch of facial nerve (>1840)
marginal nerve (Mayer, 1794), see **marginal mandibular branch of facial nerve (>1840)**
marginal sulcus (>1840)
marginal surculus of cervico-facial branch of portio major and minor of facial nerve (Bellingeri, 1818), see **marginal mandibular branch of facial nerve (>1840)**
marginal surculus of inferior branch of portio major and minor of facial nerve (Bellingeri, 1818), see **marginal mandibular branch of facial nerve (>1840)**
markigen Leistchen der Zirbel (Soemmerring, 1791), see **medullary stria (Wenzel & Wenzel, 1812)**
markiger Saum (Bock, 1820), see **fimbria (Honegger, 1890)**
markiger Streisen (Soemmerring, 1791), see **medullary stria (Wenzel & Wenzel, 1812)**
marrow (Collins, 1685), see **vertebrate brain (Cuvier, 1800)**
marrow (Crooke, 1615), see **central nervous system (Carus, 1814)**
marrow collar (Carus, 1814), see **central nervous system (Carus, 1814)**
marrow in neck and back (Plato), see **spinal cord (Galen, c162–c166)**
marrow itself (Bartholin, 1662), see **vertebrate brain (Cuvier, 1800)**
marrow of back (Geminus, 1553), see **cerebrospinal trunk (>1840)**
marrow of brain (Plato), see **vertebrate brain (Cuvier, 1800)**
marrow of chine (Nemesius, 1636), see **spinal cord (Galen, c162–c166)**
marrow of head (Plato), see **vertebrate brain (Cuvier, 1800)**
marrow of skull (Smith Papyrus, c1700 BC), see **brain (Smith Papyrus, c1700 BC)**
marrow of spondles (Vicary, 1548), see **spinal cord (Galen, c162–c166)**
marrow ring (Carus, 1814), see **central nervous system (Carus, 1814)**
marrowy appendix (Willis, 1664), see **central nervous system (Carus, 1814)**
marrowy substance (Willis, 1664), see **central nervous system white matter tracts (>1840)**
massa intermedia (>1840), see **interthalamic adhesion (>1840)**
masseteric branch of inferior maxillary nerve (Loder, 1778), see **masseteric nerve (Meckel, 1748)**
masseteric branch of superior primary branch of inferior maxillary nerve (Quain, 1832), see **masseteric nerve (Meckel, 1748)**
masseteric nerve (Meckel, 1748)
masseteric surculus of ganglioform plexus with inferior maxillary branch (Bellingeri, 1818), see **masseteric nerve (Meckel, 1748)**
masticatory nerve (Eschricht, 1826), see **trigeminal nerve motor root (Bell, 1829)**
masticatory nerve (>1840), see **mandibular nerve trunk (>1840)**
mastoid branch of cervical plexus (Cloquet, 1816), see **lesser occipital nerve (Mayer, 1794)**
mastoid process (Vesalius, 1543a), see **frontal pole (>1840)**
mastoid swelling (Vesalius, 1543a), see **frontal pole (>1840)**
matres (Stephen of Antioch, 1127), see **meninges (Smith Papyrus, c1700 BC)**
maxillary branch of inferior maxillary branch of fifth pair of nerves (Bock, 1817), see **inferior dental nerve (Meckel, 1817)**
maxillary branch of second division of fifth pair of nerves arising within skull (Willis, 1664), see **cranial nerves (Soemmerring, 1791)**
maxillary eminences (Desmoulins, 1825), see **mammillary body (Ludwig, 1779)**
maxillary fasciculi of infraorbital surculus (Bellingeri, 1818), see **anterior superior dental nerve (Haller, 1762)**
maxillary ganglion (Meckel, 1748), see **submandibular ganglion (>1840)**
maxillary ganglion of Meckel (Wutzer, 1817; Bock, 1817), see **submandibular ganglion (>1840)**
maxillary nerve (Burdin, 1803), see **mandibular nerve (>1840)**
maxillary nerve (Meckel, 1753)
maxillary nerve (Straus Durckheim, 1828), see **invertebrate nerves (>1840)**
maxillo-dentary nerve (Burdin, 1803), see **inferior dental nerve (Meckel, 1817)**
maxillo-pterygoid plexus (Le Cat, 1768), see **pterygopalatine ganglion (>1840)**
maxillo-Vidian plexus (Le Cat, 1768), see **pterygopalatine ganglion (>1840)**
maximus medullae orbis (Tiedemann, 1821), see **cerebral cortex white matter (>1840)**
meatus (Vicary, 1548), see **interventricular foramen (>1840)**
meatus inter ventriculos anteriores et posteriorem (Benedetti, 1539), see **ventricles (Hippocrates)**
Meckel's ganglion (Portal, 1803a), see **pterygopalatine ganglion (>1840)**
medial amygdalar nucleus (Johnston, 1923)
medial and internal branch of third branch of fifth pair (Comparetti, 1789), see **lingual nerve (Vesalius, 1543a)**

medial (anterior) transverse temporal area (Brodmann, 1909), see ***transverse temporal gyri (>1840)***
medial branch of external plantar nerve (Bock, 1827), see ***common plantar digital nerves of lateral plantar nerve (>1840)***
medial branch of musculocutaneous nerve (>1840), see ***medial dorsal cutaneous nerve (>1840)***
medial branch of spinal nerve dorsal branch (>1840)
medial branch of supraorbital nerve (>1840)
medial calcaneal branches of tibial nerve (>1840), see ***medial calcaneal nerve (>1840)***
medial calcaneal nerve (>1840)
medial calcanean nerve (>1840), see ***medial calcaneal nerve (>1840)***
medial clunial nerves (>1840)
medial corticohypothalamic tract (Gurdjian, 1927)
medial cutaneous nerve of arm (>1840)
medial cutaneous nerve of calf (>1840)
medial cutaneous nerve of forearm (>1840)
medial cutaneous nerve of leg (Bock, 1827), see ***medial cutaneous nerve of calf (>1840)***
medial cutaneous nerve of thigh (>1840)
medial dorsal cutaneous nerve (>1840)
medial eminence (>1840)
medial fascicles (Rolando, 1825a), see ***interpeduncular nucleus (>1840)***
medial forebrain bundle (Edinger, 1893)
medial frontal gyrus (>1840)
medial geniculate complex (>1840)
medial globus pallidus (>1840)
medial hypothalamic zone (Nauta & Haymaker, 1969)
medial lemniscus (>1840)
medial lemniscus decussation (>1840)
medial longitudinal cord (Lancisi, 1713), see ***medial longitudinal stria (>1840)***
medial longitudinal fascicle (>1840)
medial longitudinal stria (>1840)
medial longitudinal sulcus of annular protuberance (Vicq d'Azyr, 1786), see ***basilar sulcus of pons (Gordon, 1815)***
medial mammary branches of intercostal nerves (>1840)
medial medullary lamina (>1840)
medial midbrain sulcus (>1840)
medial nasal branches of internal nasal branches of anterior ethmoidal nerve (>1840)
medial occipitotemporal gyrus (>1840)
medial olfactory stria (>1840), see ***tenia tecta (Swanson, 1992)***
medial orbital gyrus (>1840)
medial pectoral nerve (>1840)
medial plantar nerve (>1840)
medial popliteal nerve (>1840), see ***tibial nerve (Haase, 1781)***
medial posterior superior nasal nerves (>1840)
medial preoptic nucleus (>1840)
medial pterygoid nerve (>1840)
medial reticulospinal tract (>1840)
medial retinohypothalamic tract (>1840)
medial root of median nerve (>1840)
medial septal complex (Swanson et al., 1987)
medial supraclavicular nerves (>1840)
medial sural cutaneous nerve (>1840), see ***medial cutaneous nerve of calf (>1840)***
medial tectospinal tract (>1840), see ***tectospinal tract (>1840)***
medial thalamic nuclei (>1840)
median aperture of fourth ventricle (>1840)
median commissure of spinal marrow (Meckel, 1817), see ***spinal central gray (>1840)***
median eminence (Tilney, 1936)
median eminence of tuber cinereum (Tilney, 1936), see ***median eminence (Tilney, 1936)***
median eminences of spinal bulb (Chaussier, 1807), see ***pyramid (Willis, 1664)***
median fossa (Gordon, 1815), see ***vallecula of cerebellum (Haller, 1762)***
median furrow of lozenge (Reil, 1809c), see ***median sulcus of fourth ventricle (>1840)***
median line of mesolobe (Chaussier, 1807), see ***corpus callosum (Galen, c177)***
median line of midbrain (Chaussier, 1807), see ***pontine raphe nucleus (>1840)***
median lobe of cerebellum (Serres, 1824–1826), see ***cerebellar vermis (Meckel, 1817)***
median lobule (Burdin, 1803), see ***cerebellar vermis (Meckel, 1817)***
median lobule of median lobe of cerebellum (Serres, 1824–1826), see ***cerebellar vermis (Meckel, 1817)***
median nerve (Du Verney, 1697)
median nerve common trunk for internal collateral branch of index finger and external collateral branch of middle finger (Cruveilhier, 1836), see ***common palmar digital nerves of median nerve (>1840)***
median nerve common trunk for internal collateral branch of middle finger and external collateral branch of ring finger (Cruveilhier, 1836), see ***common palmar digital nerves of median nerve (>1840)***
median nerve external collateral branch of index finger (Cruveihier, 1836), see ***common palmar digital nerves of median nerve (>1840)***
median nerve external collateral branch of thumb (Cruveilhier, 1836), see ***common palmar digital nerves of median nerve (>1840)***
median nerve internal collateral branch of thumb (Cruveilhier, 1836), see ***common palmar digital nerves of median nerve (>1840)***
median nerve terminal branch to thenar muscles (Cruveilhier, 1836), see ***median nerve (Du Verney, 1697)***
median part of great sympathetic (Cruveilhier, 1836), see ***peripheral nervous system (Meckel, 1817)***
median plexus (Chaussier, 1789), see ***celiac plexus (Winslow, 1733)***
median protuberance of cerebellum (Burdin, 1803), see ***cerebellar vermis (Meckel, 1817)***
median septum of brain (Burdin, 1803), see ***cerebral falx (Vesalius, 1543a)***
median septum of cerebellum (Burdin, 1803), see ***cerebellar falx (Günther, 1786)***
median septum of ventricles (Burdin, 1803), see ***cerebral nuclei (Swanson, 2000a)***

median sulcus of bulb (Cruveilhier, 1836), see **ventral median fissure of medulla (>1840)**

median sulcus of fourth ventricle (>1840)

median volar nerve (Knox, 1832), see **palmar branch of median nerve (Bock, 1827)**

mediastinum cerebri (Winslow, 1733), see **cerebral falx (Vesalius, 1543a)**

meditulli albi pars anterior (Arnold, 1838b), see **anterior limb of internal capsule (>1840)**

meditulli albi pars posterior (Arnold, 1838b), see **retrolentiform limb of internal capsule (>1840)**

meditullium (Willis, 1664), see **arbor vitae (Winslow, 1733)**

meditullium album (Arnold, 1838b), see **internal capsule (Burdach, 1822)**

meditullium of cerebellar hemisphere (Arnold, 1838a), see **arbor vitae (Winslow, 1733)**

meditullium palii (Burdach, 1822), see **cerebral cortex gray matter (>1840)**

medulla (Berengario da Carpi, 1523), see **vertebrate brain (Cuvier, 1800)**

medulla (Piccolomini, 1586), see **central nervous system (Carus, 1814)**

medulla (Winslow, 1733)

medulla cauda (Bartholin, 1651), see **brainstem (Schwalbe, 1881)**

medulla cerebrales (Plato), see **vertebrate brain (Cuvier, 1800)**

medulla dorsalis (Hippocrates), see **spinal cord (Galen, c162–c166)**

medulla elongata (Bartholin, 1651), see **central nervous system (Carus, 1814)**

medulla elongata (Meckel, 1817), see **rhombicbrain (His, 1893b)**

medulla globosa (Piccolomini, 1586), see **vertebrate brain (Cuvier, 1800)**

medulla incognita (Reil, 1809b), see **substantia innominata (Meynert, 1872)**

medulla oblongata (Bartholin, 1651), see **central nervous system (Carus, 1814)**

medulla oblongata (Collins, 1685), see **medulla (Winslow, 1733)**

medulla oblongata (Meckel, 1817), see **rhombicbrain (His, 1893b)**

medulla oblongata (Piccolomini, 1586), see **cerebrospinal trunk (>1840)**

medulla oblongata (Vicq d'Azyr, 1786), see **brainstem (Schwalbe, 1881)**

medulla oblongata (Willis, 1664), see **vertebrate brain (Cuvier, 1800)**

medulla oblongata brainstem (Burdach, 1822), see **medulla (Winslow, 1733)**

medulla oblongata intra calvariam (Bartholin, 1651), see **medulla (Winslow, 1733)**

medulla oblongata properly so-called (Soemmerring, 1778), see **medulla (Winslow, 1733)**

medulla oblongata roots of accessory nerve (Meckel, 1817), see **cranial root of accessory nerve (>1840)**

medulla oblongata vesicle (Serres, 1824–1826), see **afterbrain vesicle (Baer, 1837)**

medulla of alhosis (Achillini, 1520), see **coccygeal part of spinal cord (>1840)**

medulla of alhovius (Achillini, 1520), see **sacral part of spinal cord (>1840)**

medulla of chest (Achillini, 1520), see **thoracic part of spinal cord (>1840)**

medulla of encephalon (Galen, c173), see **vertebrate brain (Cuvier, 1800)**

medulla of head (Plato), see **vertebrate brain (Cuvier, 1800)**

medulla of kidney (Achillini, 1520), see **lumbar part of spinal cord (>1840)**

medulla rotunda (Piccolomini, 1586), see **vertebrate brain (Cuvier, 1800)**

medulla spinalis (Bauhin, 1605, p. 625), see **central nervous system (Carus, 1814)**

medulla spinalis (Bauhin, 1605, p. 628), see **cerebrospinal trunk (>1840)**

medulla spinalis (Hippocrates), see **spinal cord (Galen, c162–c166)**

medulla vero (Bauhin, 1605), see **central nervous system (Carus, 1814)**

medulla vero cerebri oblongata (Bauhin, 1605), see **cerebrospinal trunk (>1840)**

medulla vero spinalis proprie dicta (Bauhin, 1605), see **spinal cord (Galen, c162–c166)**

medullae oblongatae caudex (Willis, 1664), see **vertebrate brain (Cuvier, 1800)**

medullar substance (Coiter, 1572), see **white matter tracts (Bell & Bell, 1826)**

medullares striae (Scarpa, 1788), see **medullary striae (Scarpa, 1788)**

medullary appendix (Willis, 1664), see **central nervous system (Carus, 1814)**

medullary arch (Winslow, 1733), see **cerebral cortex white matter (>1840)**

medullary body of cerebellar hemisphere (Arnold, 1838b), see **arbor vitae (Winslow, 1733)**

medullary body of cerebellum (Arnold, 1838b), see **arbor vitae (Winslow, 1733)**

medullary branch of nerve to popliteus (>1840)

medullary canal (Bojanus, 1819–1821), see **central canal (Bellingeri, 1823)**

medullary capsule (Reil, 1809b), see **central nervous system white matter tracts (>1840)**

medullary capsule of lentiform nucleus (Arnold, 1838b), see **external capsule (Burdach, 1822)**

medullary cavity (Winslow, 1733), see **septal fissure (Burdach, 1822)**

medullary center of cerebrum (Vicq d'Azyr, 1786), see **cerebral cortex white matter (>1840)**

medullary central tegmental tract (>1840)

medullary cerebral matter (Blainville, 1821), see **white matter (Meckel, 1817)**

medullary cerebral radiation with cortex (Arnold, 1838b), see **cerebral cortex white matter (>1840)**

medullary columns (Vicq d'Azyr, 1784), see **funiculi of spinal cord (Burdach, 1822)**

medullary cone (Bock, 1827)

medullary cord (Cuvier, 1800), see **central nerve cord (Serres, 1824–1826)**
medullary cord (Rolando, 1825a), see **mammillothalamic tract (>1840)**
medullary cord (Willis, 1664), see **central nervous system (Carus, 1814)**
medullary cord of laminated flakes (Malacarne, 1776), see **floccular peduncle (Burdach, 1822)**
medullary cuneate fascicle (>1840)
medullary curtain of cerebellum (Knox, 1832), see **rostral medullary vellum (>1840)**
medullary dorsal spinocerebellar tract (>1840)
medullary eminences (Meckel, 1817), see **mammillary body (Ludwig, 1779)**
medullary fascicle of crested process (Rolando, 1831), see **cerebral cortex white matter (>1840)**
medullary gracile fascicle (>1840)
medullary lamina (Winslow, 1733), see **cerebral cortex white matter (>1840)**
medullary lamina of cerebellum (Burdin, 1803), see **rostral medullary velum (>1840)**
medullary lateral reticulospinal tract (>1840)
medullary lateral vestibulospinal tract (>1840)
medullary layer of cornu Ammonis (Meckel, 1817), see **alveus (Burdach, 1822)**
medullary matter (Monro, 1783), see **central nervous system white matter regions (>1840)**
medullary medial forebrain bundle (>1840)
medullary medial lemniscus (>1840)
medullary medial longitudinal fascicle (>1840)
medullary medial reticulospinal tract (>1840)
medullary nerves (Bock, 1827), see **spinal nerves (Camper, 1760–1762)**
medullary neurine (Solly, 1836), see **white matter (Meckel, 1817)**
medullary nucleus (Reil, 1807–1808b), see **arbor vitae (Winslow, 1733)**
medullary nucleus of cerebrum (Winslow, 1733), see **cerebral cortex white matter (>1840)**
medullary nucleus of hemisphere (Reil, 1807–1808a), see **arbor vitae (Winslow, 1733)**
medullary part (Willis, 1664), see **central nervous system white matter tracts (>1840)**
medullary part of brain (Ridley, 1695), see **cerebral cortex white matter (>1840)**
medullary part of cerebral peduncle (Vicq d'Azyr, 1786), see **cerebral peduncle (Tarin, 1753)**
medullary part of crus medulla oblongata (Ridley, 1695), see **cerebral peduncle (Tarin, 1753)**
medullary plate (Reil, 1809b), see **cerebral cortex white matter (>1840)**
medullary plates (Baer, 1837), see **neural folds (>1840)**
medullary plates (Malacarne, 1795), see **trapezoid body (Treviranus, 1820)**
medullary processes of brain (Knox, 1832), see **cerebral peduncle (Tarin, 1753)**
medullary processes of cerebellum (Arnold, 1838a), see **cerebellar peduncles (Ridley, 1695)**
medullary rays (Vieussens, 1684), see **cerebral cortex white matter (>1840)**
medullary reticular nucleus
medullary reticulospinal tract (>1840), see **lateral reticulospinal tract (>1840)**
medullary root of olfactory nerve (Owen, 1837), see **lateral olfactory tract (>1840)**
medullary rope (Willis, 1664), see **central nervous system (Carus, 1814)**
medullary rope (Winslow, 1733), see **olfactory peduncle (Solly, 1836)**
medullary rubrospinal tract (>1840)
medullary segment of spinal tract of trigeminal nerve (>1840)
medullary semicircular band (Meckel, 1817), see **terminal stria (Wenzel & Wenzel, 1812)**
medullary septum of third ventricle (Vicq d'Azyr, 1786), see **terminal lamina (Burdach, 1822)**
medullary spinothalamic tract (>1840)
medullary stem of laminated flakes (Malacarne, 1776), see **floccular peduncle (Burdach, 1822)**
medullary stria (Wenzel & Wenzel, 1812)
medullary stria of colliculus of optic nerve (Arnold, 1838a), see **medullary stria (Wenzel & Wenzel, 1812)**
medullary striae (Scarpa, 1788)
medullary substance (Berengario da Carpi, 1523), see **vertebrate brain (Cuvier, 1800)**
medullary substance (Coiter, 1572), see **white matter tracts (Bell & Bell, 1826)**
medullary substance (Colombo, 1559), see **central nervous system white matter tracts (>1840)**
medullary tectospinal tract (>1840)
medullary tract (Ridley, 1695), see **medullary stria (Wenzel & Wenzel, 1812)**
medullary tract of fourth ventricle (Drake, 1707), see **medullary striae (Scarpa, 1788)**
medullary triangle (Lieutaud, 1742), see **fornix (Vesalius, 1543a)**
medullary trunk (Willis, 1664), see **central nervous system (Carus, 1814)**
medullary tube (Baer, 1837), see **neural tube (Baer, 1837)**
medullary vault (Tarin, 1753), see **fornix (Vesalius, 1543a)**
medullary vault (Winslow, 1733), see **cerebral cortex white matter (>1840)**
medullary velum (Malacarne, 1776), see **rostral medullary velum (>1840)**
medullary ventral spinocerebellar tract (>1840)
medullary ventrolateral fascicle (>1840)
medullopontine sulcus (>1840)
meek mother (Geminus, 1553), see **pia (Galen, c192)**
meeting of optic nerves (Galen, c173), see **optic chiasm (Galen, c173)**
membrana cornea (Tarin, 1750), see **lamina affixa (>1840)**
membrana interna cerebri (Wenzel & Wenzel, 1812), see **pia (Galen, c192)**
membrana media cerebri (Wenzel & Wenzel, 1812), see **arachnoid (Blasius, 1666)**
membrana medullaris (Haase, 1781), see **pineal stalk (Burdach, 1822)**
membrana medullaris inter crura posteriora fornicis (Haase, 1781), see **dorsal hippocampal commissure (Craigie, 1925)**

membrana mucosa (Meckel, 1817), see **arachnoid (Blasius, 1666)**
membrana vasculosa (Soemmerring, 1791), see **meninges (Smith Papyrus, c1700 BC)**
membrane (Hippocrates), see **meninges (Smith Papyrus, c1700 BC)**
membrane partitioning ventricles (Galen, c177), see **cerebral nuclei (Swanson, 2000a)**
membranes (Smith Papyrus, c1700 BC), see **meninges (Smith Papyrus, c1700 BC)**
membranous membrane (Galen, c177), see **pia (Galen, c192)**
meningeal branch of mandibular nerve (>1840), see **nervus spinosus (>1840)**
meningeal branch of maxillary nerve (>1840)
meningeal branch of spinal nerve trunk (>1840)
meningeal branch of vagus nerve (>1840)
meningeal layer (Meckel, 1817), see **pia-arachnoid (>1840)**
meningeal nerve (>1840), see **meningeal branch of maxillary nerve (>1840)**
meninges (Smith Papyrus, c1700 BC)
meningina (Meckel, 1817), see **pia-arachnoid (>1840)**
meningine (Burdin, 1803), see **pia-arachnoid (>1840)**
meninx (Chaussier, 1807), see **dura (Galen, c177)**
meninx (Hippocrates), see **meninges (Smith Papyrus, c1700 BC)**
meninx exterior (Soemmerring, 1798), see **dura (Galen, c177)**
meninx fibrosa (Burdach, 1822), see **dura (Galen, c177)**
meninx interior (Soemmerring, 1798), see **meninges (Smith Papyrus, c1700 BC)**
meninx media (Bidloo, 1685), see **arachnoid (Blasius, 1666)**
meninx pachéia (Chaussier, 1807), see **dura (Galen, c177)**
meninx scléra (Chaussier, 1807), see **dura (Galen, c177)**
meninx vasculosa (Ruysch, 1737), see **meninges (Smith Papyrus, c1700 BC)**
mental branch of inferior dental nerve (Cruveilhier, 1836), see **mental nerve (Cheselden, 1726)**
mental branch of maxillary branch of inferior maxillary branch of fifth pair of nerves (Bock, 1817), see **mental nerve (Cheselden, 1726)**
mental branch of submaxillary branch of inferior maxillary nerve (Andersch, 1797), see **mylohyoid nerve (Meckel, 1748)**
mental branches of cervicofacial branch of facial nerve (Cruveilhier, 1836), see **marginal mandibular branch of facial nerve (>1840)**
mental branches of facial nerve (Chaussier, 1809), see **marginal mandibular branch of facial nerve (>1840)**
mental branches of mental nerve (Arnold, 1834)
mental fascicle of inferior alveolar surculus of inferior maxillary branch (Bellingeri, 1818), see **mental nerve (Cheselden, 1726)**
mental nerve (Cheselden, 1726)
mental plexus (Cruveilhier, 1836), see **cranial nerves (Soemmerring, 1791)**
mental subcutaneous branch of mental branch of maxillary branch of third branch of fifth pair of nerves (Bock, 1817), see **mental branches of mental nerve (>1840)**
mental subcutaneous nerve (Peipers, 1793), see **superior branch of transverse nerve of neck (>1840)**
mentonniar branches of facial nerve (Burdin, 1803), see **marginal mandibular branch of facial nerve (>1840)**
mesencephalic tract of trigeminal nerve (>1840), see **midbrain tract of trigeminal nerve (>1840)**
mesencephalon (Sharpey et al., 1867), see **midbrain (Baer, 1837)**
mesenteric branch of intercostal nerve (Willis, 1664), see **greater splanchinc nerve (Walter, 1783)**
mesenteric infolding (Willis, 1664), see **celiac ganglion (Walter, 1783)**
mesenteric infoldings (Willis, 1664), see **peripheral nervous system (Meckel, 1817)**
mesenteric nerve (Willis, 1664), see **greater splanchinc nerve (Walter, 1783)**
mesenteric plexus (Chaussier, 1789), see **superior mesenteric plexus (Rau, 1720)**
mesenteric plexus (Keill, 1698), see **prevertebral plexuses (Quain, 1832)**
mesenteric plexus (Meckel, 1817), see **inferior mesenteric plexus (Rau, 1720)**
mesenteric plexus (Vieussens, 1684), see **prevertebral plexuses (Quain, 1832)**
mesenterical plexure (Vesling, 1647), see **superior mesenteric plexus (Rau, 1720)**
mesial abdominal fissure (Spurzheim, 1826), see **ventral median fissure of spinal cord (>1840)**
mesocephalon (Burdach, 1822), see **brainstem (Schwalbe, 1881)**
mesocolic plexus (Soemmerring, 1791), see **inferior mesenteric plexus (Rau, 1720)**
mesolobe (Burdin, 1803), see **corpus callosum (Galen, c177)**
metatarsal branch of external dorsal branch of superficial peroneal nerve (Cloquet, 1828), see **superficial fibular nerve (Fyfe, 1800)**
metatarsal branch of internal dorsal branch of superficial peroneal nerve (Cloquet, 1828), see **dorsal digital nerves of medial dorsal cutaneous nerve (>1840)**
metatarsal nerves (Bell, 1803b), see **superficial fibular nerve (Fyfe, 1800)**
metatarsal nerves (Fischer, 1791), see **common plantar digital nerves of medial plantar nerve (>1840)**
metatarsal nerves (Soemmerring, 1798), see **dorsal digital nerves of intermediate dorsal cutaneous nerve (>1840)**
metatarsus pollicis nerve (Fischer, 1791), see **digital branch of deep fibular nerve (>1840)**
metencephalon (Nomina Anatomica, 1983), see **pons (Haller, 1747)**
metencephalon (Sharpey et al., 1867), see **afterbrain (Baer, 1837)**
Meynert's bundle (>1840), see **habenulo-interpeduncular tract (>1840)**
mid part of brain (Mondino, 1316), see **brainstem (Schwalbe, 1881)**
mid ventricle (Mondino, 1316), see **ventricles (Hippocrates)**
midbrain (Baer, 1837)
midbrain (Burdin, 1803), see **brainstem (Schwalbe, 1881)**
midbrain reticular nucleus (>1840)

midbrain tract of trigeminal nerve (>1840)

midbrain vesicle (Baer, 1837)

middle and anterior most inferior fascicle of soft nerve (Cotugno, 1760), see ***cochlear nerve (Cotugno, 1760)***

middle and inferior cerebral prominence (Varoli, 1573), see ***temporal region (>1840)***

middle and inferior cutaneous nerves of neck (Neubauer, 1772), see ***inferior branches of transverse nerve of neck (>1840)***

middle and inferior subcutaneous cervical nerves (Meckel, 1817), see ***inferior branches of transverse nerve of neck (>1840)***

middle anterior and superior gastric nerves (Mayer, 1794), see ***gastric branches of anterior vagal trunk (>1840)***

middle anterior femoral cutaneous nerve (Bock, 1827), see ***anterior cutaneous branches of femoral nerve (Quain & Wilson, 1839)***

middle ascending superficial branch of cervical plexus (Quain, 1828), see ***great auricular nerve (Haase, 1781)***

middle belly of brain (William of Saliceto, 1275), see ***brainstem (Schwalbe, 1881)***

middle brain cell (Baer, 1837), see ***primary midbrain vesicle (Baer, 1837)***

middle brain vesicle (Baer, 1837), see ***primary midbrain vesicle (Baer, 1837)***

middle branch of anterior branch of fourth pair of cervical nerves (Bang, 1770), see ***intermediate supraclavicular nerves (>1840)***

middle branch of cardiac ganglion (Lobstein, 1823), see ***cardiac plexus (Keill, 1698)***

middle branch of cervical plexus (Quain & Wilson, 1839), see ***great auricular nerve (Haase, 1781)***

middle branch of common motor nerve inferior terminal branch (Cruveilhier, 1836), see ***nerve to inferior rectus (>1840)***

middle branch of external plantar nerve (Fischer, 1791), see ***superficial branch of lateral plantar nerve (>1840)***

middle branch of external plantar nerve (Meckel, 1817), see ***deep branch of lateral plantar nerve (>1840)***

middle branch of fifth pair (Rau, 1694), see ***maxillary nerve (Meckel, 1753)***

middle branch of first division of fifth pair of nerves (Todd, 1836–1839), see ***frontal nerve (Cheselden, 1726)***

middle branch of orbital nerve (Jacobson, 1818), see ***ophthalmic nerve (Winslow, 1733)***

middle branch of posterior branch of acoustic nerve (Cloquet, 1828), see ***saccular nerve (>1840)***

middle branch of posterior branch of auricular nerve (Meckel, 1753), see ***posterior branch of great auricular nerve (Bock, 1827)***

middle branch of third pair (Haller, 1743), see ***nerve to inferior rectus (>1840)***

middle branch of trigeminal nerve (Winslow, 1733), see ***maxillary nerve (Meckel, 1753)***

middle branch of vestibular nerve (Arnold, 1839), see ***saccular nerve (>1840)***

middle branch of vestibular nerve to common utricle (Langenbeck, 1826–1830), see ***utricular nerve (>1840)***

middle branches of anal nerve (Cruveilhier, 1836), see ***inferior rectal nerves (>1840)***

middle branches of buccal nerve (Cruveilhier, 1836), see ***buccal nerve (Meckel, 1748)***

middle branches of dorsal nerves (Cruveilhier, 1836), see ***lateral cutaneous branches of intercostal nerves (>1840)***

middle branches of third cervical pair (Winslow, 1733), see ***cervical plexus (Molinetti, 1675)***

middle bundle (Rosenthal, 1815), see ***central nervous system white matter tracts (>1840)***

middle canal (Winslow, 1733), see ***cerebral aqueduct (>1840)***

middle cardiac nerves (Lobstein, 1823), see ***cardiac plexus (Keill, 1698)***

middle cell (Geminus, 1553), see ***third ventricle (Galen, c173)***

middle cerebellar crus (Günther, 1786), see ***middle cerebellar peduncle (Rolando, 1819)***

middle cerebellar medullary process (Soemmerring, 1778), see ***middle cerebellar peduncle (Rolando, 1819)***

middle cerebellar peduncle (Procháska, 1800), see ***middle cerebellar peduncle (Rolando, 1819)***

middle cerebellar peduncle (Rolando, 1819)

middle cerebellar process (Günther, 1786), see ***middle cerebellar peduncle (Rolando, 1819)***

middle cerebellar process (Willis, 1664), see ***middle cerebellar peduncle (Rolando, 1819)***

middle cerebral artery plexus (>1840)

middle cerebral canal (Tiedemann, 1821), see ***cerebral aqueduct (>1840)***

middle cerebral commissure (Tiedemann, 1821), see ***interthalamic adhesion (>1840)***

middle cerebral prominence (Varoli, 1573), see ***temporal region (>1840)***

middle cerebral septum (Günther, 1786), see ***cerebral nuclei (Swanson, 2000a)***

middle cervical ganglion (Haller, 1762)

middle cervical plexus (Burdin, 1803), see ***middle cervical ganglion (Haller, 1762)***

middle choroid plexus (Günther, 1786), see ***choroid plexus of third ventricle (Vicq d'Azyr, 1784)***

middle cingulate gyrus (Burdach, 1822), see ***cingulate region (Brodmann, 1909)***

middle colic plexus (>1840)

middle commissure (>1840)

middle commissure of optic chambers (Tiedemann, 1816), see ***interthalamic adhesion (>1840)***

middle commissure of quadrigeminal bodies (Bojanus, 1819–1821), see ***tectum (Baer, 1837)***

middle commissure of third ventricle (Quain, 1838), see ***interthalamic adhesion (>1840)***

middle cord (Tiedemann, 1816), see ***middle cerebellar peduncle (Rolando, 1819)***

middle crural nerve (Lieutaud, 1742), see ***femoral nerve (Haller, 1762)***

middle crural nerve (Straus Durckheim, 1828), see ***invertebrate nerves (>1840)***

middle cutaneous branch of internal cutaneous nerve (Caldani, 1813, 1814), see ***anterior branch of medial cutaneous nerve of forearm (>1840)***

middle cutaneous branch of small sciatic nerve (Quain, 1832), see **posterior cutaneous nerve of thigh (Günther, 1786)**
middle cutaneous nerve (Caldani, 1813, 1814), see **anterior branch of medial cutaneous nerve of forearm (>1840)**
middle cutaneous nerve (Fyfe, 1800), see **anterior cutaneous branches of femoral nerve (Quain & Wilson, 1839)**
middle cutaneous nerve (Klint, 1784), see **medial cutaneous nerve of forearm (>1840)**
middle cutaneous nerve of arm (Soemmerring, 1791), see **medial cutaneous nerve of forearm (>1840)**
middle cutaneous nerve of back of foot (Meckel, 1817), see **intermediate dorsal cutaneous nerve (>1840)**
middle cutaneous nerve of crural nerve (Styx, 1782), see **anterior cutaneous branches of femoral nerve (Quain & Wilson, 1839)**
middle cutaneous nerve of haunches (Knox, 1832), see **perforating cutaneous nerve (>1840)**
middle cutaneous nerve of neck (Meckel, 1754), see **superior branches of transverse nerve of neck (>1840)**
middle cutaneous nerve of temple (Meckel, 1753), see **zygomaticotemporal nerve (>1840)**
middle cutaneous nerve of thigh (Bell, 1803a), see **anterior cutaneous branches of femoral nerve (Quain & Wilson, 1839)**
middle cutaneous nerve of Wrisberg (Klint, 1784), see **medial cutaneous nerve of forearm (>1840)**
middle cutaneous nerves of anterior crural nerve (Quain & Wilson, 1839), see **anterior cutaneous branches of femoral nerve (Quain & Wilson, 1839)**
middle cutaneous nerves of buttocks (Walter, 1783), see **perforating cutaneous nerve (>1840)**
middle deep temporal nerve (>1840)
middle dental nerve (Le Cat, 1768), see **middle superior dental nerve (Henle, 1871)**
middle dorsal nerve of foot (Bock, 1827), see **intermediate dorsal cutaneous nerve (>1840)**
middle facial branch of facial nerve (Cloquet, 1828), see **zygomatic branches of facial nerve (>1840)**
middle facial branch of hard nerve (Meckel, 1753), see **zygomatic branches of facial nerve (>1840)**
middle facial branch of pes anserinus (Bellingeri, 1818), see **zygomatic branches of facial nerve (>1840)**
middle facial branch of portio dura (Knox, 1832), see **zygomatic branches of facial nerve (>1840)**
middle facial branch of superior branch of anterior branch of hard nerve (Loder, 1778), see **zygomatic branches of facial nerve (>1840)**
middle facial nerve (Bell & Bell, 1816), see **zygomatic branches of facial nerve (>1840)**
middle facial nerve (Meckel, 1753), see **zygomatic branches of facial nerve (>1840)**
middle fascicle of buccal surculus of cervico-facial branch of portio major and minor of facial nerve (Bellingeri, 1818), see **buccal branch of facial nerve (>1840)**
middle fascicle of buccal surculus of inferior branch of portio major and minor of facial nerve (Bellingeri, 1818), see **buccal branch of facial nerve (>1840)**
middle fasciculus of medulla oblongata (Rosenthal, 1815), see **central nervous system white matter tracts (>1840)**
middle filament of inferior orbital thread of temporal surculus (Bellingeri, 1818), see **temporal branches of facial nerve (Swan, 1830)**
middle filaments of anterior terminal branch of internal saphenous nerve (Cruveilhier, 1836), see **infrapatellar branch of saphenous nerve (>1840)**
middle fissure (Bichat, 1802), see **inner part of transverse cerebral fissure (>1840)**
middle fluted body (Pourfour du Petit, 1710), see **internal capsule (Burdach, 1822)**
middle frontal area (Brodmann, 1909), see **inferior frontal gyrus (>1840)**
middle frontal gyrus (>1840)
middle hemorrhoidal nerves (Meckel, 1817), see **pelvic splanchnic nerves (Gaskell, 1886)**
middle hepatic nerves (Mayer, 1794), see **hepatic plexus (Rau, 1720)**
middle hepatic plexus (Wrisberg, 1808), see **cystic plexus (Wrisberg, 1808)**
middle horn of lateral ventricle (Tiedemann, 1816), see **inferior horn of lateral ventricle (Bell, 1802)**
middle inferior palpebral thread of internal superior labial fascicle of infraorbital surculus (Bellingeri, 1818), see **superior labial branches of infraorbital nerve (Meckel, 1748)**
middle infolding in trunk of intercostal nerve (Willis, 1664), see **middle cervical ganglion (Haller, 1762)**
middle labial branch of infraorbital nerve (Bock, 1817), see **superior labial branches of infraorbital nerve (Meckel, 1748)**
middle lateral cord (Tiedemann, 1816), see **middle cerebellar peduncle (Rolando, 1819)**
middle layer of cardiac nerves (Cruveilhier, 1836), see **cardiac plexus (Keill, 1698)**
middle lingual nerve (Haller, 1762), see **hypoglossal nerve (Winslow, 1733)**
middle lingual pair (Haller, 1762), see **hypoglossal nerve (Winslow, 1733)**
middle lobe (Fyfe, 1800), see **temporal region (>1840)**
middle lobe of cerebrum (Winslow, 1733), see **temporal region (>1840)**
middle marrow of brain proper (Willis, 1664), see **cerebral cortex white matter (>1840)**
middle marrow of cerebellum (Willis, 1664), see **arbor vitae (Winslow, 1733)**
middle marrow of cerebrum (Willis, 1664), see **cerebral cortex white matter (>1840)**
middle medullary lamina of cerebellum (Vicq d'Azyr, 1784), see **rostral medullary velum (>1840)**
middle medullary tract (Ridley, 1695), see **transverse pontine fibers (>1840)**
middle meningeal nerve (>1840), see **meningeal branch of maxillary nerve (>1840)**
middle mesenteric plexus (Soemmerring, 1791), see **inferior mesenteric plexus (Rau, 1720)**
middle mesenteric plexus (Vieussens, 1684), see **prevertebral plexuses (Quain, 1832)**

middle musculocutaneous branch of lumbar plexus (Cloquet, 1816), see **lumbar plexus ventral divisions (Paterson, 1887)**
middle musculocutaneous branch of lumbar plexus (Cruveilhier, 1836), see **iliohypogastric nerve (Schmidt, 1794)**
middle musculo-cutaneous nerve (Frotscher, 1788), see **medial cutaneous nerve of forearm (>1840)**
middle nasal cutaneous nerve (Mayer, 1794), see **external nasal branch of infraorbital nerve (>1840)**
middle nerve for vastus externus muscle (Fischer, 1791), see **muscular branches of femoral nerve (Quain & Wilson, 1839)**
middle nerve of nerve layers of septum of heart (Andersch, 1797), see **coronary plexuses (Meckel, 1817)**
middle nerve to sartorius muscle (Fischer, 1791), see **muscular branches of femoral nerve (Quain & Wilson, 1839)**
middle nerves of cardiac plexus (Lobstein, 1823), see **cardiac plexus (Keill, 1698)**
middle of brain (Willis, 1664), see **cerebral cortex white matter (>1840)**
middle of cerebrum (Willis, 1664), see **cerebral cortex white matter (>1840)**
middle ovarian nerves (>1840)
middle palatine nerve (Cloquet, 1816), see **posterior palatine nerve (Günther, 1786)**
middle palatine nerve (Todd, 1836–1839), see **lateral palatine nerve (Henle, 1871)**
middle palatine threads of posterior palatine fascicle (Bellingeri, 1818), see **posterior palatine nerve (Günther, 1786)**
middle palpebral branches of orbital branches of temporofacial branch of facial nerve (Cruveilhier, 1836), see **zygomatic branches of facial nerve (>1840)**
middle pan of braine (Nemesius, 1636), see **third ventricle (Galen, c173)**
middle pancreatic nerves (Mayer, 1794), see **pancreatic plexus (Cruveilhier, 1836)**
middle part of base of corona radiata (Arnold, 1838b), see **posterior limb of internal capsule (>1840)**
middle part of brain (Crooke, 1615), see **temporal region (>1840)**
middle part of central fissure (Gordon, 1815), see **lateral ventricle (Vesalius, 1543a)**
middle part of cerebellum (Vesalius, 1543a), see **cerebellar vermis (Meckel, 1817)**
middle part of corpus callosum (Spurzheim, 1826), see **body of corpus callosum (Arnold, 1838a)**
middle part of inferior vermal process (Gordon, 1815), see **uvula (Malacarne, 1776)**
middle part of lateral ventricle (Meckel, 1817), see **body of lateral ventricle (Bell, 1803b)**
middle part of nervous system (Cuvier, 1800), see **central nervous system (Carus, 1814)**
middle part of spinal cord ashen-colored substance (Vicq d'Azyr, 1784), see **spinal central gray (>1840)**
middle pedicle of cerebellum (Mayo, 1827), see **middle cerebellar peduncle (Rolando, 1819)**
middle perforated substance (Vicq d'Azyr, 1784), see **interpeduncular nucleus (>1840)**
middle pharyngeal branch of pharyngolingual branch of glossopharyngeal nerve (Kilian, 1822), see **pharyngeal branches of glossopharyngeal nerve (Neubauer, 1772)**
middle plexus of neck (Andersch & Soemmerring, 1792), see **ansa cervicalis (>1840)**
middle plexus of semilunar ganglia (Winslow, 1773), see **celiac plexus (Winslow, 1733)**
middle posterior and superior gastric nerves (Mayer, 1794), see **gastric branches of posterior vagal trunk (>1840)**
middle posterior branch of auditory nerve proper (Günther, 1786), see **caudal part of vestibular nerve (>1840)**
middle posterior cutaneous nerve (Meckel, 1817), see **lateral cutaneous nerve of calf (>1840)**
middle posterior cutaneous nerve (Quain & Wilson, 1839), see **perineal branches of posterior cutaneous nerve of thigh (>1840)**
middle posterior cutaneous nerve (Soemmerring, 1791), see **posterior cutaneous nerve of thigh (Günther, 1786)**
middle primary brain vesicle (Baer, 1837), see **primary midbrain vesicle (Baer, 1837)**
middle primary part of spinal prolongation (Chaussier, 1807), see **spinal cord (Galen, c162–c166)**
middle process (Fyfe, 1800), see **temporal region (>1840)**
middle projection of central lobe (Malacarne, 1776), see **central lobule (Burdach, 1822)**
middle prolongation of cerebellum (Burdin, 1803), see **middle cerebellar peduncle (Rolando, 1819)**
middle prominence of brain (Crooke, 1615), see **temporal region (>1840)**
middle protuberance of cerebellum (Chaussier, 1807), see **cerebellar vermis (Meckel, 1817)**
middle rectal plexus (>1840)
middle root of ciliary ganglion (Arnold, 1834), see **sympathetic root of ciliary ganglion (>1840)**
middle root of olfactory nerve (Swan, 1830), see **lateral olfactory tract (>1840)**
middle root of ophthalmic ganglion (Arnold, 1834), see **sympathetic root of ciliary ganglion (>1840)**
middle root of trigeminal nerve (Meckel, 1817), see **trigeminal nerve sensory root (>1840)**
middle sinus (Landi, 1542), see **ventricles (Hippocrates)**
middle splenic nerves (Mayer, 1794), see **splenic plexus (Palfijn, 1726)**
middle striated body (Pourfour du Petit, 1710), see **internal capsule (Burdach, 1822)**
middle subcutaneous nerve of neck (Bock, 1817), see **superior branches of transverse nerve of neck (>1840)**
middle subcutaneous nerve of neck (Mayer, 1794), see **transverse nerve of neck (>1840)**
middle subcutaneous nerve of neck (Meckel, 1817), see **transverse nerve of neck (>1840)**
middle subcutaneous surculus of cervico-facial branch of portio major and minor of facial nerve (Bellingeri, 1818), see **cervical branch of facial nerve (>1840)**

minor twig of posterior branch of auditory nerve (Soemmerring, 1791), see **posterior ampullary nerve (>1840)**

minuca (Vicary, 1548), see **spinal cord (Galen, c162–c166)**

mirabilis plexus reticularis (Vesalius, 1543a), see **rete mirabile (Herophilus, c335–c280 BC)**

Mittelhirn (Baer, 1837), see **midbrain (Baer, 1837)**

mixed nerve (Gall & Spurzheim, 1810), see **trigeminal nerve (Winslow, 1733)**

mixed nerves (Haase, 1781), see **nerves (Herophilus, c335–280 BC)**

mixed pair (Gall & Spurzheim, 1810), see **trigeminal nerve (Winslow, 1733)**

mole (Willis, 1664), see **cerebral cortex (>1840)**

mons cerebelli (Gordon, 1815), see **cerebellar vermis (Meckel, 1817)**

monticule of inferior vermiform process (Vicq d'Azyr, 1784), see **biventral lobule (>1840)**

monticuli (Schreger, 1803), see **tectum (Baer, 1837)**

monticuli of cerebellum (Fyfe, 1800), see **cerebellar hemisphere (Willis, 1664)**

monticulus (Vesalius, 1555), see **cerebral cortex (>1840)**

monticulus (Vicq d'Azyr, 1784), see **tonsil (Malacarne, 1776)**

monticulus (Vicq d'Azyr, 1786), see **temporal pole (Broca, 1878a)**

monticulus cerebelli (Meckel, 1817), see **cerebellar vermis (Meckel, 1817)**

moriform body (Tiedemann, 1816), see **dentate nucleus (>1840)**

most anterior branch of crural nerve forming cutaneous nerves (Winslow, 1733), see **anterior cutaneous branches of femoral nerve (Quain & Wilson, 1839)**

most anterior fasciculi of second–fourth lumbar nerves (Meckel, 1817), see **lumbar plexus ventral divisions (Paterson, 1887)**

most noble bowel (Diemerbroeck, 1689), see **vertebrate brain (Cuvier, 1800)**

most principal ventricle (Herophilus, c335–c280 BC), see **fourth ventricle (Galen, c192)**

most superficial of cardiac nerves (Chaussier, 1789), see **superior cardiac nerve (Neubauer, 1772)**

motor cervical nerve (Hoffmann, 1703), see **suboccipital nerve (Winslow, 1733)**

motor nerve for tongue (Galen, c173), see **hypoglossal nerve (Winslow, 1733)**

motor nerve of eye (Spurzheim, 1826), see **oculomotor nerve (Estienne, 1545)**

motor nucleus of trigeminal nerve (>1840)

motor occipital nerve (Hoffmann, 1703), see **suboccipital nerve (Winslow, 1733)**

motor part of facial nerve (Kölliker, 1896), see **facial nerve root (>1840)**

motor portion of fifth nerve (Bell, 1829), see **trigeminal nerve motor root (Bell, 1829)**

motor root (Bell, 1829), see **ventral root (>1840)**

motor root of facial nerve (>1840), see **facial nerve root (>1840)**

motor tract (Bell, 1834), see **corticospinal tract (>1840)**

motory ganglion of spinal cord (Solly, 1836), see **cerebral nuclei (Swanson, 2000a)**

mouth of ventricles (Gerdy, 1838), see **inner part of transverse cerebral fissure (>1840)**

mucous filaments of superior laryngeal branches of pneumogastric nerve (Cruveilhier, 1836), see **internal branch of superior laryngeal nerve (Fyfe, 1800)**

mundöffnung umgebenden Nervenringe (Tiedemann, 1815), see **circumoral nerve ring (Tiedemann, 1815)**

muscular branch of accessory nerve (Cruveilhier, 1836), see **external branch of accessory nerve trunk (Meckel, 1817)**

muscular branch of external cutaneous nerve (Soemmerring, 1791), see **muscular branches of musculocutaneous nerve (Günther, 1786)**

muscular branch of external musculo-cutaneous nerve (Quain & Wilson, 1839), see **ilio-inguinal nerve (Schmidt, 1794)**

muscular branch of external plantar nerve (Günther, 1786), see **deep branch of lateral plantar nerve (>1840)**

muscular branch of glossopharyngeal nerve (Wrisberg, 1786), see **stylopharyngeal branch of glossopharyngeal nerve (>1840)**

muscular branch of hand of cubital nerve (Cruveilhier, 1836), see **deep branch of ulnar nerve (>1840)**

muscular branch of ilio-inguinal nerve (Quain & Wilson, 1839), see **ilio-inguinal nerve (Schmidt, 1794)**

muscular branch of ilio-scrotal nerve (Quain & Wilson, 1839), see **ilio-inguinal nerve (Schmidt, 1794)**

muscular branch of inferior maxillary nerve (Jacobson, 1818), see **anterior branch of mandibular nerve (>1840)**

muscular branch of mental nerve (Meckel, 1753), see **mental nerve (Cheselden, 1726)**

muscular branch of musculo-spiral nerve (Quain, 1832), see **deep branch of radial nerve (Martin, 1781)**

muscular branch of peroneal nerve (Martin, 1781), see **deep fibular nerve (Fyfe, 1800)**

muscular branch of radial nerve (Meckel, 1817), see **deep branch of radial nerve (Martin, 1781)**

muscular branch of spinal nerve (Cruveilhier, 1836), see **external branch of accessory nerve trunk (Meckel, 1817)**

muscular branch of superior musculo-cutaneous nerve (Quain & Wilson, 1839), see **ilio-inguinal nerve (Schmidt, 1794)**

muscular branch of third cervical nerve (Haller, 1762), see **muscular branches of cervical plexus (Cruveilhier, 1836)**

muscular branch of volar deep branch of ulnar nerve (Günther, 1786), see **deep branch of ulnar nerve (>1840)**

muscular branches of anterior branch of obturator nerve (>1840)

muscular branches of anterior tibial nerve (Quain & Wilson, 1839), see **muscular branches of deep fibular nerve (>1840)**

muscular branches of axillary nerve (>1840)

muscular branches of brachial plexus roots (>1840)

muscular branches of cervical plexus (Cruveilhier, 1836)

muscular branches of crural musculocutaneous nerve (Cruveilhier, 1836), see **muscular branches of femoral nerve (Quain & Wilson, 1839)** *muscular branches of crural nerve (Günther, 1786)*, see **muscular branches of femoral nerve (Quain & Wilson, 1839)**

muscular branches of cubital nerve (Cruveilhier, 1836), see **muscular branches of ulnar nerve (>1840)**

muscular branches of deep fibular nerve (>1840)

muscular branches of dorsal nerves (Cruveilhier, 1836), see **muscular branches of intercostal nerves (Quain & Wilson, 1839)**

muscular branches of external branch of accessory nerve trunk (>1840)

muscular branches of external plantar nerve (Quain & Wilson, 1839), see **muscular branches of lateral plantar nerve (>1840)**

muscular branches of femoral nerve (Quain & Wilson, 1839)

muscular branches of hypoglossal nerve (Günther, 1786), see **lingual branches of hypoglossal nerve (Cloquet, 1816)**

muscular branches of inferior gluteal nerve (Cruveilhier, 1836), see **inferior gluteal nerve (Martin, 1781)**

muscular branches of intercostal nerves (Quain & Wilson, 1839)

muscular branches of internal plantar nerve (Quain & Wilson, 1839), see **muscular branches of medial plantar nerve (>1840)**

muscular branches of interosseous nerve (Quain & Wilson, 1839), see **muscular branches of deep fibular nerve (>1840)**

muscular branches of lateral plantar nerve (>1840)

muscular branches of lumbar plexus ventral branches (>1840)

muscular branches of medial plantar nerve (>1840)

muscular branches of median nerve (Martin, 1781)

muscular branches of musculocutaneous nerve (Günther, 1786)

muscular branches of musculo-cutaneous nerve (Quain & Wilson, 1839), see **muscular branches of superficial fibular nerve (>1840)**

muscular branches of ninth pair (Günther, 1786), see **lingual branches of hypoglossal nerve (Cloquet, 1816)**

muscular branches of perineal nerve (>1840)

muscular branches of popliteal nerve (Quain & Wilson, 1839), see **muscular branches of tibial nerve (>1840)**

muscular branches of posterior branch of obturator nerve (>1840)

muscular branches of posterior tibial nerve (Quain & Wilson, 1839), see **muscular branches of tibial nerve (>1840)**

muscular branches of radial nerve (>1840)

muscular branches of sciatic nerve (Cruveilhier, 1836), see **sciatic nerve (Keill, 1698)**

muscular branches of spiral nerve (Quain & Wilson, 1839), see **muscular branches of radial nerve (>1840)**

muscular branches of superficial fibular nerve (>1840)

muscular branches of tibial nerve (>1840)

muscular branches of ulnar nerve (Quain & Wilson, 1839)

muscular branches of ulnar nerve to triceps muscle (Quain & Wilson, 1839), see **muscular branches of ulnar nerve (>1840)**

muscular cutaneous nerve (Meckel, 1817), see **superficial fibular nerve (Fyfe, 1800)**

muscular division of inferior maxillary nerve (Quain & Wilson, 1839), see **anterior branch of mandibular nerve (>1840)**

muscular fascicles of buccal surculus of ganglioform plexus with inferior maxillary branch (Bellingeri, 1818), see **buccal nerve (Meckel, 1748)**

muscular fascicles of lingual surculus with chorda tympani (Bellingeri, 1818), see **lingual nerve (Vesalius, 1543a)**

muscular filaments of abdominal branch of intercostal branches of dorsal nerves (Cruveilhier, 1836), see **intercostal nerves (Vesalius, 1543a)**

muscular nerve of fifth pair (Bell, 1826), see **trigeminal nerve motor root (Bell, 1829)**

muscular nerves of collateral branches of internal plantar nerve (Cruveilhier, 1836), see **muscular branches of medial plantar nerve (>1840)**

muscular nerves of crural nerve (Bock, 1827), see **muscular branches of femoral nerve (Quain & Wilson, 1839)**

muscular spiral nerve (Monro, 1783), see **radial nerve (Du Verney, 1697)**

muscular thread of supratrochlear fascicle (Bellingeri, 1818), see **supratrochlear nerve (Schaarschmidt, 1750)**

muscular trunk of external plantar nerve (Meckel, 1817), see **deep branch of lateral plantar nerve (>1840)**

muscular twig of palmar branch of ulnar nerve (Meckel, 1817), see **deep branch of ulnar nerve (Fyfe, 1800)**

muscularis nerve (Cheselden, 1713), see **median nerve (Du Verney, 1697)**

muscularis nerve (Cheselden, 1726), see **radial nerve (Du Verney, 1697)**

musculocutaneous branch of external popliteal nerve (Cloquet, 1816), see **superficial fibular nerve (Fyfe, 1800)**

musculo-cutaneous branch of fibular nerve (Quain, 1832), see **superficial fibular nerve (Fyfe, 1800)**

musculo-cutaneous branch of peroneal nerve (Quain, 1832), see **superficial fibular nerve (Fyfe, 1800)**

musculo-cutaneous branches of lumbar plexus (Quain, 1828), see **lumbar plexus ventral divisions (Paterson, 1887)**

musculocutaneous nerve (Du Verney, 1697)

musculo-cutaneous nerve (Quain & Wilson, 1839), see **superficial fibular nerve (Fyfe, 1800)**

musculocutaneous nerve branches for pectoral muscle (Caldani, 1813, 1814), see **muscular branches of musculocutaneous nerve (Günther, 1786)**

musculocutaneous nerve of arm (Mayer, 1794), see **musculocutaneous nerve (Du Verney, 1697)**

musculocutaneous nerve of crural nerve (Cloquet, 1828), see **femoral nerve (Haller, 1762)**

musculo-cutaneous nerve of external plantar nerve (Meckel, 1817), see **common plantar digital nerves of lateral plantar nerve (>1840)**

musculocutaneous nerve twigs for subscapularis muscle (Caldani, 1813, 1814), see **muscular branches of musculocutaneous nerve (Günther, 1786)**

musculocutaneous trunk of crural nerve (Cloquet, 1828), see **femoral nerve (Haller, 1762)**

musculus triventer & quadritendineus (Pacchioni, 1741), see **dura (Galen, c177)**

mylohyoid branch of inferior dental nerve (Quain, 1828), see **mylohyoid nerve (Meckel, 1748)**

mylohyoid branch of inferior maxillary branch (Loder, 1778), see **mylohyoid nerve (Meckel, 1748)**

mylohyoid branch of inferior maxillary nerve proper (Haase, 1781), see **mylohyoid nerve (Meckel, 1748)**

mylohyoid fascicle of inferior alveolar surculus of inferior maxillary branch (Bellingeri, 1818), see **mylohyoid nerve (Meckel, 1748)**

mylohyoid nerve (Meckel, 1748)

mylo-hyoid surculus of stylo-hyoid branch (Bellingeri 1818), see **stylohyoid nerve (Meckel, 1753)**

mynuca (Vicary, 1548), see **spinal cord (Galen, c162–c166)**

myo-glossal nerve (Swan, 1830), see **hypoglossal nerve (Winslow, 1733)**

Nachhirn (Baer, 1837), see **afterbrain (Baer, 1837)**

nape (Berengario da Carpi, 1523), see **spinal cord (Galen, c162–c166)**

nape alhosis (Berengario da Carpi, 1523), see **coccygeal part of spinal cord (>1840)**

nape alhovius (Berengario da Carpi, 1523), see **sacral part of spinal cord (>1840)**

nape of back (Berengario da Carpi, 1523), see **thoracic part of spinal cord (>1840)**

nape of kidney (Berengario da Carpi, 1523), see **lumbar part of spinal cord (>1840)**

nape of neck (Berengario da Carpi, 1523), see **cervical part of spinal cord (>1840)**

nape of ribs (Berengario da Carpi, 1523), see **thoracic part of spinal cord (>1840)**

narrow den (Willis, 1664), see **cerebral aqueduct (>1840)**

narrow plate arising from margin of spinal marrow (Tiedemann, 1816), see **rhombic lip (>1840)**

nasal branch of anterior superior dental nerve (>1840)

nasal branch of first branch of fifth pair (Meckel, 1748), see **nasociliary nerve (Meckel, 1817; Wutzer, 1817)**

nasal branch of first branch of fifth pair (Monro, 1783), see **nasal branches of anterior ethmoidal nerve (>1840)**

nasal branch of first trunk of fifth nerve (Swan, 1830), see **nasociliary nerve (Meckel, 1817; Wutzer, 1817)**

nasal branch of greater anterior alveolar nerve (Arnold, 1834), see **nasal branch of anterior superior dental nerve (>1840)**

nasal branch of greater anterior dental nerve (Arnold, 1834), see **nasal branch of anterior superior dental nerve (>1840)**

nasal branch of ophthalmic branch of nerve of fifth pair (Bonhomme, 1748), see **nasociliary nerve (Meckel, 1817; Wutzer, 1817)**

nasal branch of second branch of fifth pair (Monro, 1783), see **posterior superior nasal nerves (Soemmerring, 1791)**

nasal branch of supraorbital branch of first branch of fifth pair of nerves (Bock, 1817), see **nasociliary nerve (Meckel, 1817; Wutzer, 1817)**

nasal branch to septum from Vidian nerve (Scarpa, 1785), see **nerve of pterygoid canal (>1840)**

nasal branches of anterior ethmoidal nerve (>1840)

nasal branches of Meckel's ganglion (Quain & Wilson, 1839), see **posterior superior nasal nerves (Soemmerring, 1791)**

nasal filaments of external nasal branch of nasal nerve (Cruveilhier, 1836), see **infratrochlear nerve (Schaarschmidt, 1750)**

nasal filaments of superior maxillary nerve (Cruveilhier, 1836), see **external nasal branches of infraorbital nerve (>1840)**

nasal ganglion (Arnold, 1834), see **pterygopalatine ganglion (>1840)**

nasal ganglion (Blainville, 1821), see **nasopalatine nerve (Scarpa, 1785)**

nasal infratrochlear nerve (Günther, 1786), see **nasociliary nerve (Meckel, 1817; Wutzer, 1817)**

nasal nerve (Meckel, 1753), see **nasociliary nerve (Meckel, 1817; Wutzer, 1817)**

nasal nerve from ophthalmic nerve of fifth pair (Scarpa, 1785), see **nasal branches of anterior ethmoidal nerve (>1840)**

nasal nerves (Meckel, 1748), see **posterior superior nasal nerves (Soemmerring, 1791)**

nasal ramus of orbitary nerve (Winslow, 1733), see **nasociliary nerve (Meckel, 1817; Wutzer, 1817)**

nasociliary branch of supraorbital branch of first branch of fifth pair of nerves (Bock, 1817), see **nasociliary nerve (Meckel, 1817; Wutzer, 1817)**

nasociliary nerve (Meckel, 1817; Wutzer, 1817)

nasociliary root of ciliary ganglion (>1840), see **communicating branch of nasociliary nerve with ciliary ganglion (>1840)**

naso-frontalis filament of superior facial branch of pes anserinus (Bellingeri, 1818), see **zygomatic branches of facial nerve (>1840)**

naso-labial filament of superior facial branch of pes anserinus (Bellingeri, 1818), see **zygomatic branches of facial nerve (>1840)**

nasolacrymal nerve (Le Cat, 1768), see **nasociliary nerve (Meckel, 1817; Wutzer, 1817)**

naso-lobar nerve (Todd, 1836–1839), see **external nasal branch of anterior ethmoidal nerve (>1840)**

naso-ocular nerve (Soemmerring, 1791), see **nasociliary nerve (Meckel, 1817; Wutzer, 1817)**

nasopalatine branch of Scarpa (Wrisberg, 1786), see **nasopalatine nerve (Scarpa, 1785)**

nasopalatine branch of sphenopalatine nerves (Cloquet, 1816), see **nasopalatine nerve (Scarpa, 1785)**

nasopalatine fascicle of sphenopalatine ganglion (Bellingeri, 1818), see **nasopalatine nerve (Scarpa, 1785)**

nasopalatine ganglion (Cloquet, 1815), see **nasopalatine nerve (Scarpa, 1785)**

naso-palatine ganglion filament of communication with Meckel's ganglion (Quain & Wilson, 1839), see **nasopalatine nerve (Scarpa, 1785)**

nasopalatine nerve (Meckel, 1817), see **nasopalatine nerve (Scarpa, 1785)**

nasopalatine nerve (Scarpa, 1785)

naso-palatine nerve (Todd, 1836–1839), see **pterygopalatine nerves (Wrisberg, 1786)**

nasopalatine nerve of Scarpa (Bock, 1817), see **nasopalatine nerve (Scarpa, 1785)** *naso-palpebral nerve (Burdin, 1803)*, see **nasociliary nerve (Meckel, 1817; Wutzer, 1817)**

nates (Galen, c173, definition 1), see **tectum (Baer, 1837)**

nates (Galen, c173, definition 2), see **inferior colliculus (Haller, 1762)**

nates (Massa, 1536), see **caudate nucleus (Arnold, 1838b)**

nates (Read, 1638), see **superior colliculus (Haller, 1762)**

naticulae (Hall, 1565), see **tectum (Baer, 1837)**

natiform eminences (Cruveilhier, 1836), see **superior colliculus (Haller, 1762)**

natiform eminences (Rolando, 1825a), see **inferior colliculus (Haller, 1762)**

natiform processes (Willis, 1664), see **superior colliculus (Haller, 1762)**

natiform protuberance (Malacarne, 1780), see **limbic region (>1840)**

natulae (Vesalius, 1543a), see **inferior colliculus (Haller, 1762)**

neck of medulla spinalis (Collins, 1685), see **brainstem (Schwalbe, 1881)**

nerf auriculaire postérieur (Meckel, 1753), see **posterior auricular nerve (Meckel, 1753)**

nerf cardiaque inférieur (Cloquet, 1816), see **inferior cardiac nerve (Cloquet, 1816)**

nerf digastrique (Meckel, 1753), see **digastric nerve (Meckel, 1753)**

nerf du jambier postérieur (Cruveilhier, 1836), see **nerve to tibialis posterior (Cruveilhier, 1836)**

nerf honteux (Cloquet, 1816), see **dorsal nerve of penis (Camper, 1762)**

nerf honteux chez la femme (Cloquet, 1816), see **dorsal nerve of clitoris (>1840)**

nerf infra-trochléaire (Meckel, 1753), see **infratrochlear nerve (Schaarschmidt, 1750)**

nerf lachrymal (Bonhomme, 1748), see **lacrimal nerve (Meckel, 1748; Bonhomme, 1748)**

nerf maxillaire (Meckel, 1753), see **maxillary nerve (Meckel, 1753)**

nerf stylohyoïde (Meckel, 1753), see **stylohyoid nerve (Meckel, 1753)**

nerf sus-trochleaire (Meckel, 1753), see **infratrochlear nerve (Schaarschmidt, 1750)**

nerf vertébral (Cruveilhier, 1836), see **vertebral nerve (Cruveilhier, 1836)**

nerfs spino-crânio-trapèziens (Portal, 1803b), see **accessory nerve (Vieussens, 1684)**

nerfs splanchniques lombaires (Cruveilhier, 1836), see **lumbar splanchnic nerves (Cruveilhier, 1836)**

nerve between right auricle and ventricle of heart (Andersch, 1797), see **coronary plexuses (Meckel, 1817)**

nerve branch to kidney (Galen, c192), see **renal nerves (Haase, 1781)**

nerve branch to liver (Galen, c192), see **hepatic plexus (Rau, 1720)**

nerve branch to spleen (Galen, c192), see **splenic plexus (Palfijn, 1726)**

nerve branches to esophagus (Galen, c192), see **upper esophageal branches of vagus nerve (Cloquet, 1828)**

nerve branches to trachea (Galen, c192), see **tracheal branches of recurrent laryngeal nerve (>1840)**

nerve collar (Carus, 1818), see **central nervous system (Carus, 1814)**

nerve conferred on bladder called container of bile (Galen, c173), see **cystic plexus (Wrisberg, 1808)**

nerve conferred on kidney (Galen, c173), see **renal nerves (Haase, 1781)**

nerve conferred on liver (Galen, c173), see **hepatic plexus (Rau, 1720)**

nerve conferred on spleen (Galen, c173), see **splenic plexus (Palfijn, 1726)**

nerve cord (Cuvier, 1800), see **central nerve cord (Serres, 1824–1826)**

nerve cord (Serres, 1824–1826)

nerve cord trunk (>1840)

nerve cords (Le Boë, 1663), see **central nervous system (Carus, 1814)**

nerve emerging from petrosal bone (Galen, c192), see **sympathetic trunk (Winslow, 1733)**

nerve entering phrenes (Galen, c177), see **phrenic nerve (Galen, c173)**

nerve extending along roots of ribs (Galen, c173), see **sympathetic trunk (Winslow, 1733)**

nerve filaments of first pair (Scarpa, 1785), see **olfactory nerve (Winslow, 1733)**

nerve for popliteus muscle (Fischer, 1791), see **nerve to popliteus (>1840)**

nerve for radial side of little finger (Knox, 1832), see **dorsal digital nerves of ulnar nerve (>1840)**

nerve for soleus muscle and flexor pollicis pedis longus (Fischer, 1791), see **muscular branches of tibial nerve (>1840)**

nerve for urinary bladder (Galen, c173), see **pelvic splanchnic nerves (Gaskell, 1886)**

nerve from auricular ganglion to tensor tympani (Arnold, 1834), see **communicating branch of otic ganglion with chorda tympani (>1840)**

nerve from otic ganglion to tensor tympani (Arnold, 1834), see **communicating branch of otic ganglion with chorda tympani (>1840)**

nerve from supreme cervical ganglion joining with external branch of superior laryngeal nerve (Arnold, 1834), see **laryngopharyngeal branches of superior cervical ganglion (>1840)**

nerve implanted in liver (Galen, c173), see **hepatic plexus (Rau, 1720)**

nerve inserted into kidney (Galen, c173), see **renal nerves (Haase, 1781)**

nerve inserted into liver (Galen, c173), see **hepatic plexus (Rau, 1720)**

nerve into glandules prostatae (Willis, 1664), see **prostatic plexus (>1840)**

nerve issuing from blind perforation (Galen, c173), see **intermediofacial nerve (Strong & Elwyn, 1943)**

nerve joining together corpus striatum (Ridley, 1695), see **terminal stria (Wenzel & Wenzel, 1812)**

nerve knots (Carus, 1814), see **central ganglia (>1840)**

nerve layers of septum of heart (Andersch, 1797), see **coronary plexuses (Meckel, 1817)**

nerve net (Behrends, 1792), see **plexus (Galen, c192)**

nerve net (>1840)

nerve of adductor magnus (Cruveilhier, 1836), see **nerve to hamstring muscles (>1840)**
nerve of arytenoid (Cruveilhier, 1836), see **inferior laryngeal nerve (>1840)**
nerve of carapace (Straus Durckheim, 1828), see **invertebrate nerves (>1840)**
nerve of clitoris (Meckel, 1817), see **dorsal nerve of clitoris (>1840)**
nerve of common flexor (Cruveilhier, 1836), see **nerve to flexor digitorum longus (>1840)**
nerve of common flexor digitorum brevis muscle (Cruveilhier, 1836), see **muscular branches of medial plantar nerve (>1840)**
nerve of Cotunnius (Todd, 1836–1839, p. 282), see **external nasal branch of anterior ethmoidal nerve (>1840)**
nerve of Cotunnius (Todd, 1836–1839, p. 287), see **nasopalatine nerve (Scarpa, 1785)**
nerve of coxofemoral joint (Cruveilhier, 1836), see **accessory obturator nerve (Schmidt, 1794)**
nerve of cricoarytenoid and thyroarytenoid together (Cruveilhier, 1836), see **inferior laryngeal nerve (>1840)**
nerve of crural artery proper (Schmidt, 1794), see **femoral branch of genitofemoral nerve (>1840)**
nerve of diaphragma (Willis, 1664), see **phrenic nerve (Galen, c173)**
nerve of external gastrocnemius (Cruveilhier, 1836), see **nerves to gastrocnemius (>1840)**
nerve of external wall of nasal fossa (Cruveilhier, 1836); see **external nasal branch of anterior ethmoidal nerve (>1840)**
nerve of flexor hallucis brevis muscle (Cruveilhier, 1836), see **muscular branches of medial plantar nerve (>1840)**
nerve of flexor hallucis longus proper (Cruveilhier, 1836), see **nerve to flexor hallucis longus (>1840)**
nerve of gemellus superior (Cruveilhier, 1836), see **nerve to obturator internus (>1840)**
nerve of great dorsal muscle (Cruveilhier, 1836), see **thoracodorsal nerve (>1840)**
nerve of internal gastrocnemius (Cruveilhier, 1836), see **nerves to gastrocnemius (>1840)**
nerve of internal pterygoid muscle (Cruveilhier, 1836), see **medial pterygoid nerve (>1840)**
nerve of long portion of biceps (Cruveilhier, 1836), see **nerve to hamstring muscles (>1840)**
nerve of midriffe (Crooke, 1615), see **phrenic nerve (Galen, c173)**
nerve of nasal septum (Cruveilhier, 1836, p. 916), see **internal nasal branches of anterior ethmoidal nerve (>1840)**
nerve of nasal septum (Cruveilhier, 1836, p. 923), see **medial posterior superior nasal nerves (>1840)**
nerve of obturator externus (Cruveilhier, 1836), see **muscular branch of posterior branch of obturator nerve (>1840)**
nerve of obturator internus muscle (Cruveilhier, 1836), see **nerve to obturator internus (>1840)**
nerve of plantaris longus (Cruveilhier, 1836), see **nerve to plantaris (>1840)**
nerve of posterior cricoarytenoid muscle (Cruveilhier, 1836), see **inferior laryngeal nerve (>1840)**
nerve of pterygoid canal (>1840)
nerve of quadratus femoris and gemellus inferior (Cruveilhier, 1836), see **nerve to quadratus femoris (>1840)**
nerve of right pulmonary artery branches (Andersch, 1797), see **pulmonary plexus (Winslow, 1733)**
nerve of right pulmonary branches (Andersch & Soemmerring, 1792), see **pulmonary plexus (Winslow, 1733)**
nerve of semitendinosus (Cruveilhier, 1836), see **nerve to hamstring muscles (>1840)**
nerve of septum of nose (Meckel, 1817), see **nasopalatine nerve (Scarpa, 1785)**
nerve of short portion of biceps (Cruveilhier, 1836), see **nerve to short head of biceps femoris (>1840)**
nerve of soleus (Cruveilhier, 1836), see **nerve to soleus (>1840)**
nerve of soleus muscle and flexor longus pollicis pedis (Knox, 1832), see **muscular branches of tibial nerve (>1840)**
nerve of spinal marrow anterior branch (Meckel, 1817), see **spinal nerve ventral branch (>1840)**
nerve of spinal marrow dorsal branch (Meckel, 1817), see **spinal nerve dorsal branch (Meckel, 1817)**
nerve of spinal marrow posterior branch (Meckel, 1817), see **spinal nerve dorsal branch (Meckel, 1817)**
nerve of subseptum (Cruveilhier, 1836), see **internal nasal branches of infraorbital nerve (>1840)**
nerve of superior oblique muscle of eye (Gall & Spurzheim, 1810), see **trochlear nerve (Molinetti, 1669)**
nerve of supraspinatus and infraspinatus muscles (Cruveilhier, 1836), see **suprascapular nerve (Bang, 1770)**
nerve of taste (Galen, c173), see **lingual nerve (Vesalius, 1543a)**
nerve of tensoris palati mollis (Arnold, 1834), see **nerve to tensor veli palatini (>1840)**
nerve of tenth pair (Willis, 1664), see **cervical nerves (Galen, c173)**
nerve of teres major (Cruveilhier, 1836), see **lower subscapular nerve (>1840)**
nerve of teres minor (Cruveilhier, 1836), see **muscular branches of axillary nerve (>1840)**
nerve of transverse septum (Vesalius, 1543a), see **phrenic nerve (Galen, c173)**
nerve of vastus externus (Cruveilhier, 1836), see **muscular branches of femoral nerve (Quain & Wilson, 1839)**
nerve of wing (Straus Durckheim, 1828), see **invertebrate nerves (>1840)**
nerve of Wrisberg (Bell & Bell, 1816), see **medial cutaneous nerve of arm (>1840)**
nerve of Wrisberg (Quain & Wilson, 1839), see **intercostobrachial nerves (>1840)**
nerve of Wrisberg (Scarpa, 1788), see **intermediate nerve (>1840)**
nerve outgrowths from skull (Vesalius, 1543a), see **cranial nerves (Soemmerring, 1791)**
nerve plexus of abdomen (Wharton, 1656), see **superior mesenteric plexus (Rau, 1720)**
nerve plexus of hepatic artery (Walter, 1783), see **hepatic plexus (Rau, 1720)**

nerve plexus to coronary arteries (Walter, 1783), see **gastric branches of anterior vagal trunk (>1840)**
nerve ring (Lyonnet, 1762), see **invertebrate nerves (>1840)**
nerve ring (Tiedemann, 1815)
nerve ring around esophagus (Carus, 1814), see **central nervous system (Carus, 1814)**
nerve ring around mouth (Carus, 1818), see **central nervous system (Carus, 1814)**
nerve to abductor brevis muscle of Albinus (Fischer, 1791), see **muscular branches of femoral nerve (Quain & Wilson, 1839)**
nerve to abductor digiti minimi and flexor digiti minimi brevis muscles (Jördens, 1788), see **lateral plantar nerve (>1840)**
nerve to abductor pollicis muscle (Jördens, 1788), see **muscular branches of medial plantar nerve (>1840)**
nerve to abductor pollicis muscle from deep branch of external plantar nerve (Fischer, 1791), see **deep branch of lateral plantar nerve (>1840)**
nerve to adductor femoris magnus muscle (Fischer, 1791), see **nerve to hamstring muscles (>1840)**
nerve to anterior peroneal muscle (Fischer, 1791), see **muscular branches of superficial fibular nerve (>1840)**
nerve to calcaneal periosteum (Jördens, 1788), see **lateral plantar nerve (>1840)**
nerve to caruncle of nose (Anatomia Magistri Nicolai physici, early 12th century), see **cerebral cortex (>1840)**
nerve to coracohyoid muscle (Andersch & Soemmerring, 1792), see **ansa cervicalis (>1840)**
nerve to extensor pollicis longus muscle (Fischer, 1791), see **muscular branches of superficial fibular nerve (>1840)**
nerve to fascial muscle (Fischer, 1791), see **superior gluteal nerve (Martin, 1781)**
nerve to flexor digiti minimi brevis muscle from deep branch of external plantar nerve (Fischer, 1791), see **deep branch of lateral plantar nerve (>1840)**
nerve to flexor digitorum longus (>1840)
nerve to flexor hallucis longus (>1840)
nerve to flexor pollicis proper (Jördens, 1788), see **nerve to flexor hallucis longus (>1840)**
nerve to gastrocnemius muscle from tibial nerve trunk (Jördens, 1788), see **nerves to gastrocnemius (>1840)**
nerve to gemellus and internal obturator muscles (Jördens, 1788), see **nerve to obturator internus (>1840)**
nerve to genioglossus muscle (Andersch & Soemmerring, 1792), see **lingual branches of hypoglossal nerve (Cloquet, 1816)**
nerve to geniohyoid muscle (Andersch & Soemmerring, 1792), see **lingual branches of hypoglossal nerve (Cloquet, 1816)**
nerve to genital organs (Galen, c192), see **perineal nerve (Camper, 1762)**
nerve to gluteus maximus muscle (Jördens, 1788), see **inferior gluteal nerve (Martin, 1781)**
nerve to gracilis antici muscle (Fischer, 1791), see **muscular branches of femoral nerve (Quain & Wilson, 1839)**
nerve to gracilis muscle (Fischer, 1791), see **muscular branches of anterior branch of obturator nerve (>1840)**
nerve to hamstring muscles (>1840)
nerve to heart (Vesalius, 1543a), see **thoracic cardiac branches of vagus nerve (>1840)**
nerve to inferior oblique (>1840)
nerve to inferior rectus (>1840)
nerve to latissimus dorsi muscle (Langenbeck, 1826–1830), see **thoracodorsal nerve (>1840)**
nerve to left auricle of heart (Andersch, 1797), see **atrial plexuses (>1840)**
nerve to left pulmonary sinus (Andersch, 1797), see **pulmonary plexus (Winslow, 1733)**
nerve to left pulmonary sinus of heart (Andersch, 1797), see **pulmonary plexus (Winslow, 1733)**
nerve to liver (Galen, c173), see **hepatic plexus (Rau, 1720)**
nerve to livid muscle (Styx, 1782), see **muscular branches of femoral nerve (Quain & Wilson, 1839)**
nerve to longissimi tibiae muscle (Fischer, 1791), see **muscular branches of femoral nerve (Quain & Wilson, 1839)**
nerve to medial rectus (>1840)
nerve to obturator internus (>1840)
nerve to pectineus muscle (Styx, 1782), see **muscular branches of femoral nerve (Quain & Wilson, 1839)**
nerve to pectoral muscle (Camper, 1760), see **lateral pectoral nerve (>1840)**
nerve to penis (Galen, c192), see **dorsal nerve of penis (Camper, 1762)**
nerve to plantaris (>1840)
nerve to popliteus (>1840)
nerve to quadratus femoris (>1840)
nerve to quadratus femoris muscle (Fischer, 1791), see **nerve to quadratus femoris (>1840)**
nerve to recti cruris muscle (Styx, 1782), see **muscular branches of femoral nerve (Quain & Wilson, 1839)**
nerve to rectum (Galen, c192), see **inferior rectal nerves (>1840)**
nerve to rectus femoris muscle (Frotscher, 1788), see **muscular branches of femoral nerve (Quain & Wilson, 1839)**
nerve to rectus muscle (Styx, 1782), see **muscular branches of femoral nerve (Quain & Wilson, 1839)**
nerve to right auricle of heart (Andersch & Soemmerring, 1792), see **atrial plexuses (>1840)**
nerve to right pulmonary sinus (Andersch & Soemmerring, 1792), see **pulmonary plexus (Winslow, 1733)**
nerve to right pulmonary sinus of heart (Andersch, 1797), see **pulmonary plexus (Winslow, 1733)**
nerve to semimembranosus muscle (Fischer, 1791), see **nerve to hamstring muscles (>1840)**
nerve to seminervosi muscle (Fischer, 1791), see **nerve to hamstring muscles (>1840)**
nerve to semitendinosus muscle (Fischer, 1791), see **nerve to hamstring muscles (>1840)**
nerve to short head of biceps femoris (>1840)
nerve to soleus (>1840)
nerve to soleus muscle (Fischer, 1791), see **nerve to soleus (>1840)**
nerve to sternothyroid muscle (Andersch & Soemmerring, 1792), see **ansa cervicalis (>1840)**
nerve to stylohyoid muscle (Peipers, 1793), see **stylohyoid nerve (Meckel, 1753)**

nerve to stylopharyngeal muscle (Andersch & Soemmerring, 1792), see **stylopharyngeal branch of glossopharyngeal nerve (>1840)**
nerve to superior and inferior gemellus muscles (Fischer, 1791), see **sacral plexus ventral divisions (Paterson, 1887)**
nerve to tensor tympani (Arnold, 1834)
nerve to tensor veli palatini (>1840)
nerve to teres major muscle (Langenbeck, 1826–1830), see **lower subscapular nerve (>1840)**
nerve to tibialis posterior (Cruveilhier, 1836)
nerve to triceps muscle (Fischer, 1791), see **obturator nerve (Cheselden, 1726)**
nerve traversing canal in petrosal bone (Galen, c192), see **sympathetic trunk (Winslow, 1733)**
nerve trunk to soleus and popliteus muscles and right head of gastrocnemius muscle (Fischer, 1791), see **muscular branches of tibial nerve (>1840)**
Nervenring (Tiedemann, 1815), see **nerve ring (Tiedemann, 1815)**
nerveo plexu stomachico (Vieussens, 1684), see **left gastric plexus (>1840)**
nerveo plexui cardiaco superiorem (Vieussens, 1684), see **cardiac plexus (Keill, 1698)**
nerveo plexui renali (Vieussens, 1684), see **renal plexus (Drake, 1707)**
nerveos funiculos (Le Boë, 1663), see **trochlear nerve (Molinetti, 1669)**
nerveos plexus mesentericos (Vieussens, 1684), see **prevertebral plexuses (Quain, 1832)**
nerveos plexus pneumonicos (Vieussens, 1684), see **pulmonary plexus (Winslow, 1733)**
nerves (Herophilus, c335–c280 BC)
nerves (Hippocrates), see **nerves (Herophilus, c335–c280 BC)**
nerves (Malpighi, 1669), see **invertebrate nerves (>1840)**
nerves disappearing in hepatic duct (Walter, 1783), see **hepatic plexus (Rau, 1720)**
nerves ending in cystic duct (Walter, 1783), see **hepatic plexus branches to bile ducts (>1840)**
nerves for all intestines (Galen, c173), see **prevertebral plexuses (Quain, 1832)**
nerves from brain and spinal cord (Galen, c192), see **craniospinal nerves (Herrick, 1915)**
nerves from marrow of thorax or chest (Crooke, 1615), see **spinal nerves (Camper, 1760–1762)**
nerves from medulla of alhosis (Achillini, 1520), see **coccygeal nerves (Camper, 1762)**
nerves from medulla of alhovius (Achillini, 1520), see **sacral nerves (Camper, 1760)**
nerves from medulla of chest (Achillini, 1520), see **thoracic nerves (Diemerbroeck, 1672)**
nerves from medulla of kidney (Achillini, 1520), see **lumbar nerves (Diemerbroek, 1672)**
nerves from medulla of neck (Achillini 1520), see **cervical nerves (Galen, c173)**
nerves from spinal marrow of neck (Crooke, 1615), see **cervical nerves (Galen, c173)**
nerves from tuber annulare and its extensions (Bichat, 1801), see **cranial nerves (Soemmerring, 1791)**
nerves in intercostal muscles (Galen, c173), see **intercostal nerves (Vesalius, 1543a)**
nerves into womb (Willis, 1664), see **uterovaginal plexus (>1840)**
nerves of accessory muscle of common long flexor (Cruveilhier, 1836), see **muscular branches of lateral plantar nerve (>1840)**
nerves of animal life (Bichat, 1801), see **craniospinal nerves (Herrick, 1915)**
nerves of animal life (Bichat et al., 1801–1803), see **craniospinal nerves (Herrick, 1915)**
nerves of back (Diemerbroeck, 1689), see **thoracic nerves (Diemerbroeck, 1672)**
nerves of breast (Diemerbroeck, 1689), see **thoracic nerves (Diemerbroeck, 1672)**
nerves of cerebral protuberance (Bichat et al., 1801–1803), see **cranial nerves (Soemmerring, 1791)**
nerves of chest (Crooke, 1615), see **spinal nerves (Camper, 1760–1762)**
nerves of chest or back (Bartholin, 1662), see **spinal nerves (Camper, 1760–1762)**
nerves of collar (Cuvier, 1800), see *circumesophageal connective (>1840)*
nerves of encephalon (Bell, 1834), see **nervous system (Monro, 1783)**
nerves of flexor digiti minimi brevis (Cruveilhier, 1836), see **common plantar digital nerves of lateral plantar nerve (>1840)**
nerves of head (Bell, 1823), see **nervous system (Monro, 1783)**
nerves of head (Gall & Spurzheim, 1810), see **nervous system (Monro, 1783)**
nerves of holy bone (Crooke, 1615), see **spinal nerves (Camper, 1760–1762)**
nerves of intercostal spaces (Galen, c177), see **intercostal nerves (Vesalius, 1543a)**
nerves of interosseous muscles of fourth space (Cruveilhier, 1836), see **common plantar digital nerves of lateral plantar nerve (>1840)**
nerves of loins (Diemerbroeck, 1689), see **lumbar nerves (Diemerbroeck, 1672)**
nerves of love (Drake, 1707), see **trochlear nerve (Molinetti, 1669)**
nerves of loynes (Crooke, 1615), see **spinal nerves (Camper, 1760–1762)**
nerves of loyns (Bartholin, 1662), see **spinal nerves (Camper, 1760–1762)**
nerves of medulla oblongata (Le Cat, 1768), see **nervous system (Monro, 1783)**
nerves of medulla spinalis (Winslow, 1733), see **spinal nerves (Camper, 1760–1762)**
nerves of nape alhosos (Berengario da Carpi, 1523), see **coccygeal nerves (Camper, 1762)**
nerves of nape alhovius (Berengario da Carpi, 1523), see **sacral nerves (Camper, 1760)**
nerves of nape of back (Berengario da Carpi, 1523), see **thoracic nerves (Diemerbroeck, 1672)**
nerves of nape of kidney (Berengario da Carpi, 1523), see **lumbar nerves (Diemerbroek, 1672)**
nerves of nape of neck (Berengario da Carpi, 1523), see **cervical nerves (Galen, c173)**

nerves of nape of ribs (Berengario da Carpi, 1523), see **thoracic nerves (Diemerbroeck, 1672)**

nerves of neck (Diemerbroeck, 1689), see **cervical nerves (Galen, c173)**

nerves of organic life (Bichat et al., 1801–1803), see **peripheral nervous system (Meckel, 1817)**

nerves of origin of vertebral medulla (Bichat et al., 1801–1803), see **craniospinal nerves (Herrick, 1915)**

nerves of os sacrum (Crooke, 1615), see **spinal nerves (Camper, 1760–1762)**

nerves of semimembranosus (Cruveilhier, 1836), see **nerve to hamstring muscles (>1840)**

nerves of smelling (Piccolomni, 1586), see **cerebral cortex (>1840)**

nerves of spinal marrow (Heister, 1717), see **spinal nerves (Camper, 1760–1762)**

nerves of spinal marrow of os sacrum (Heister, 1717), see **sacral nerves (Camper, 1760)**

nerves of spinal marrow sections (Meckel, 1817), see **spinal nerve groups (Durward, 1951)**

nerves of spinal medulla (Lieutaud, 1742), see **spinal nerves (Camper, 1760–1762)**

nerves of spinall marey of brest (Bannister, 1578), see **spinal nerves (Camper, 1760–1762)**

nerves of spinall marey of loynes (Bannister, 1578), see **spinal nerves (Camper, 1760–1762)**

nerves of stylopharyngeal muscle proper (Scarpa, 1794), see **stylopharyngeal branch of glossopharyngeal nerve (>1840)**

nerves of thigh (Bartholin, 1651), see **lumbosacral plexus (Vesalius, 1543a)**

nerves of vastus internus (Cruveilhier, 1836), see **muscular branches of femoral nerve (Quain & Wilson, 1839)**

nerves of vegetative life (Meckel, 1817), see **peripheral nervous system (Meckel, 1817)**

nerves originating from spinal marrow (Bichat, 1801), see **craniospinal nerves (Herrick, 1915)**

nerves proceeding from pith of os sacrum (Diemerbroeck, 1689), see **sacral nerves (Camper, 1760)**

nerves proceeding from pith within skull (Diemerbroeck, 1689), see **cranial nerves (Soemmerring, 1791)**

nerves properly so-called (Galen, c173), see **nerves (Herophilus, c335–c280 BC)**

nerves that move muscles of eyes (Galen, c173), see **oculomotor nerve (Estienne, 1545)**

nerves to arm (Vesalius, 1543), see **brachial plexus (Camper, 1760)**

nerves to foot (Bauhin, 1605), see **lumbosacral plexus (Vesalius, 1543a)**

nerves to gastrocnemius (>1840)

nerves to hand (Bauhin, 1605), see **brachial plexus (Camper, 1760)**

nerves to leg (Galen, c177), see **lumbosacral plexus (Vesalius, 1543a)**

nerves to sheaths of lungs (Galen, c192), see **pulmonary plexus (Winslow, 1733)**

nerves to spongy flesh (Galen, c192), see **autonomic nerves (Langley, 1898)**

nerveum plexum cardiacum inferiorem (Vieussens, 1684), see **cardiac plexus (Keill, 1698)**

nerveum plexum cardiacum superiorem (Vieussens, 1684), see **cardiac plexus (Keill, 1698)**

nerveum plexum hepaticum (Vieussens, 1684), see **hepatic plexus (Rau, 1720)**

nerveum plexum lienarem (Vieussens, 1684), see **splenic plexus (Palfijn, 1726)**

nerveum plexum renalem (Vieussens, 1684), see **renal plexus (Drake, 1707)**

nerveum plexum stomachium (Vieussens, 1684), see **left gastric plexus (>1840)**

nerveus plexus cardiacus superior (Vieussens, 1684), see **cardiac plexus (Keill, 1698)**

nerveus plexus hepaticum (Vieussens, 1684), see **hepatic plexus (Rau, 1720)**

nerveus plexus renalis (Vieussens, 1684), see **renal plexus (Drake, 1707)**

nerveus plexus stomachius (Vieussens, 1684), see **left gastric plexus (>1840)**

nervi à parte spinalis medulae anteriore procedents (Blasius, 1666), see **ventral rootlets (>1840)**

nervi à parte spinalis medulae posteriore procedents (Blasius, 1666), see **dorsal rootlets (>1840)**

nervi accessorii de' Motori comuni (Malacarne, 1791), see **transverse peduncular tract (Gudden, 1870)**

nervi amatorii (Drake, 1707), see **trochlear nerve (Molinetti, 1669)**

nervi audibiles (Hall, 1565), see **vestibulocochlear nerve (>1840)**

nervi coccygei (Camper, 1762), see **coccygeal nerves (Camper, 1762)**

nervi colli (Haase, 1781), see **cervical nerves (Galen, c173)**

nervi erigentes (>1840), see **pelvic splanchnic nerves (Gaskell, 1886)**

nervi extremitatis superioris (Meckel, 1817), see **brachial plexus (Camper, 1760)**

nervi gastrici (Walter, 1783), see **peripheral nervous system (Meckel, 1817)**

nervi glandulae pinealis (Wharton, 1656), see **central nervous system (Carus, 1814)**

nervi glossopharyngei (Huber, 1744), see **glossopharyngeal nerve (Huber, 1744)**

nervi gustatorii (Winslow, 1733), see **hypoglossal nerve (Winslow, 1733)**

nervi hypoglossi (Winslow, 1733), see **hypoglossal nerve (Winslow, 1733)**

nervi hypoglossi externi (Winslow, 1733), see **hypoglossal nerve (Winslow, 1733)**

nervi hypoglossi majores (Winslow, 1733), see **hypoglossal nerve (Winslow, 1733)**

nervi ileo-hypogastrici (Bock, 1827), see **iliohypogastric nerve (Schmidt, 1794)**

nervi indeterminati (Salmon, 1714), see **hypoglossal nerve (Winslow, 1733)**

nervi innominati (Winslow, 1733), see **trigeminal nerve (Winslow, 1733)**

nervi linguales (Winslow, 1733), see **hypoglossal nerve (Winslow, 1733)**

nervi mamillares (Molinetti, 1675), see **cerebral cortex (>1840)**

nervi meatus auditorii externi (Meckel, 1817), see **external acoustic meatus nerves (Meckel, 1817)**

nervi molles (Haller, 1762), see **paravertebral nerves (Swanson & Bota, 2010)**

nervi motivi (Copho, c1070–1100), see **recurrent laryngeal nerve (Albinus, 1744)**

nervi motores externi (Winslow, 1733), see **abducens nerve (Heister, 1717)**

nervi motores oculi (Winslow, 1733), see **oculomotor nerve (Estienne, 1545)**

nervi motores oculorum externi (Winslow, 1733), see **abducens nerve (Heister, 1717)**

nervi musculares communes (Winslow, 1733), see **oculomotor nerve (Estienne, 1545)**

nervi musculares externi (Winslow, 1733), see **abducens nerve (Heister, 1717)**

nervi musculares obliqui superiores (Winslow, 1733), see **trochlear nerve (Molinetti, 1669)**

nervi nasales inferiores posteriores (Günther, 1786), see **posterior inferior nasal nerves (Günther, 1786)**

nervi nasales posteriores medii et inferiores (Meckel, 1817), see **posterior inferior nasal nerves (>1840)**

nervi oculares communes (Winslow, 1733), see **oculomotor nerve (Estienne, 1545)**

nervi oculares externi (Winslow, 1733), see **abducens nerve (Heister, 1717)**

nervi oculo-musculares (Winslow, 1733), see **oculomotor nerve (Estienne, 1545)**

nervi oculo-musculares externi (Winslow, 1733), see **abducens nerve (Heister, 1717)**

nervi oculorum motorii (Estienne, 1545), see **oculomotor nerve (Estienne, 1545)**

nervi odoratorii (Piccolomini, 1586), see **cerebral cortex (>1840)**

nervi olfactorii (Winslow, 1733), see **olfactory nerve (Winslow, 1733)**

nervi opthalmici externi (Winslow, 1733), see **abducens nerve (Heister, 1717)**

nervi postici (Anatomia Magistri Nicolai physici, early 12th century), see **vestibulocochlear nerve (>1840)**

nervi pudici (Fyfe, 1800), see **pudendal nerve (Camper, 1762)**

nervi recurrentis portio in musculum aperientem (Fabricius ab Aquapendente, 1613), see **recurrent laryngeal nerve (Albinus, 1744)**

nervi renali (Haase, 1781), see **renal nerves (Haase, 1781)**

nervi sacrales (Galen, c173), see **sacral nerves (Galen, c173)**

nervi sacri (Galen, c173), see **sacral nerves (Galen, c173)**

nervi sciatico-tibiales (Winslow, 1733), see **sciatic nerve (Keill, 1698)**

nervi scrotales posteriores (Mayer, 1794), see **posterior scrotal nerves (Mayer, 1794)**

nervi stomachici (Walter, 1783), see **peripheral nervous system (Meckel, 1817)**

nervi summi humeri (Neubauer, 1772), see **supraclavicular nerves (Meckel, 1817)**

nervi supraclaviculares intermedii (>1840), see **intermediate supraclavicular nerves (>1840)**

nervi supraclaviculares laterales (>1840), see **lateral supraclavicular nerves (>1840)**

nervi supraclaviculares mediales (>1840), see **medial supraclavicular nerves (>1840)**

nervi sympathetici majores (Winslow, 1733), see **sympathetic trunk (Winslow, 1733)**

nervi sympathetici maximi (Winslow, 1733), see **sympathetic trunk (Winslow, 1733)**

nervi sympathetici medii (Wrisberg, 1777), see **trigeminal nerve (Winslow, 1733)**

nervi trigemini (Winslow, 1733), see **trigeminal nerve (Winslow, 1733)**

nervi vaginae (Walter, 1783), see **vaginal nerves (Walter, 1783)**

nervi vasorum (Bell, 1803b), see **paravertebral nerves (Swanson & Bota, 2010)**

nervi ventriculi (Walter, 1783), see **peripheral nervous system (Meckel, 1817)**

nervi vesiculae seminalis (Bock, 1827), see **seminal vesicle nerves (Bock, 1827)**

nervo harmonico magno capitis (Andersch, 1797), see **vagus nerve (Galen, c192)**

nervo linguae (Haase, 1781), see **lingual nerve (Vesalius, 1543a)**

nervo musculos colli movente externo (Andersch, 1797), see **inferior root of ansa cervicalis (>1840)**

nervo musculos colli movente interno (Andersch, 1797), see **superior root of ansa cervicalis (>1840)**

nervorum cerebralium maximum (Günther, 1786), see **trigeminal nerve (Winslow, 1733)**

nervorum motorium opticum (Pietro da Cortona, 1741), see **oculomotor nerve (Estienne, 1545)**

nervorum nodum (Neubauer, 1772), see **peripheral ganglion (>1840)**

nervorum oculosmoventium (Casseri, 1627), see **oculomotor nerve (Estienne, 1545)**

nervorum per ossa capitis egredientium (Soemmerring, 1778), see **nervous system (Monro, 1783)**

nervos cervicales imos cardiacos (Haller, 1772), see **inferior cardiac nerve (Cloquet, 1816)**

nervos mesaraicos posteriores (Schaarschmidt, 1750), see **intermesenteric plexus (>1840)**

nervos nasales priores (Soemmerring, 1798), see **pterygopalatine nerves (Wrisberg, 1786)**

nervos nasales superiores posteriores (Soemmerring, 1791), see **posterior superior nasal nerves (Soemmerring, 1791)**

nervos odoratorios (Rolfinck, 1656), see **olfactory peduncle (Solly, 1836)**

nervos olfactibiles (Hall, 1565), see **cerebral cortex (>1840)**

nervos spinali (Camper, 1760–1762), see **spinal nerves (Camper, 1760)**

nervos temporales auricularem (Haller, 1762), see **auriculotemporal nerve (Haller, 1762)**

nervos uretiricos superiores (Walter, 1783), see **superior ureteric nerves (Walter, 1783)**

nervos ventriculi sinisteriores (Soemmerring, 1798), see **left gastric plexus (>1840)**

nervous brown matter (Gordon, 1815), see **gray matter (Meckel, 1817)**

nervous cords (Spurzheim, 1826), see **nerves (Herophilus, c335–c280 BC)**

nervous filament quitting gustatory nerve to communicate with submaxillary ganglion (Quain & Wilson, 1839),

see **communicating branch of lingual nerve with submandibular ganglion (>1840)**
nervous folds (Diemerbroeck, 1689), see **peripheral ganglia (>1840)**
nervous ganglia (Cloquet, 1828), see **peripheral ganglia (>1840)**
nervous little string (Bartholin, 1662), see **pineal stalk (Burdach, 1822)**
nervous masses of phrenic life (Spurzheim, 1826), see **nervous system (Monro, 1783)**
nervous masses of vegetative life (Spurzheim, 1826), see **peripheral nervous system (Meckel, 1817)**
nervous matter (Gordon, 1815), see **nervous system (Monro, 1783)**
nervous plexure (Vesling, 1647), see **superior mesenteric plexus (Rau, 1720)**
nervous plexure of mesenterium (Vesling, 1647), see **superior mesenteric plexus (Rau, 1720)**
nervous ring of invertebrata (Müller, 1834), see **central nervous system (Carus, 1814)**
nervous ropes (Winslow, 1733), see **nerves (Herophilus, c335–c280 BC)**
nervous stock (Willis, 1664), see **central nervous system (Carus, 1814)**
nervous system (Monro, 1783)
nervous system (Willis, 1664), see **peripheral nervous system (Meckel, 1817)**
nervous system fibrous substance (Spurzheim, 1826), see **white matter (Meckel, 1817)**
nervous system gelatinous substance (Spurzheim, 1826), see **gray matter (Meckel, 1817)**
nervous system gray matter (Meckel, 1817), see **gray matter (Meckel, 1817)**
nervous system grey substance (Grainger, 1837), see **gray matter (Meckel, 1817)**
nervous system of animal life (Bichat, 1801), see **nervous system (Monro, 1783)**
nervous system of animal life (Bichat et al., 1801–1803), see **craniospinal nerves (Herrick, 1915)**
nervous system of ganglions (Bichat, 1801), see **peripheral nervous system (Meckel, 1817)**
nervous system of organic life (Bichat, 1801), see **peripheral nervous system (Meckel, 1817)**
nervous system pulpy substance (Spurzheim, 1826), see **gray matter (Meckel, 1817)**
nervous system white matter (Meckel, 1817), see **white matter (Meckel, 1817)**
nervous ungual arch of index finger (Caldani, 1813, 1814), see **brachial plexus cords (Schwalbe, 1881)**
nervous ungual arch of thumb (Caldani, 1813, 1814), see **brachial plexus cords (Schwalbe, 1881)**
nervous white matter (Gordon, 1815), see **white matter (Meckel, 1817)**
nervum axillarem (Pietro da Cortona, 1741), see **median nerve (Du Verney, 1697)**
nervum balneare (Günther, 1786), see **trigeminal nerve (Winslow, 1733)**
nervum brachialem medium (Pietro da Cortona, 1741), see **median nerve (Du Verney, 1697)**
nervum cardiacum superiorem (Neubauer, 1772), **superior cardiac nerve (Neubauer, 1772)**
nervum conjuge carentem (Bauhin, 1605), see **terminal filament (Tiedemann, 1821)**
nervum divisum (Günther, 1786), see **trigeminal nerve (Winslow, 1733)**
nervum laryngeum superiorem (Loder, 1778), see **superior laryngeal nerve (Loder, 1778)**
nervum sine conjuge (Crooke, 1615), see **terminal filament (Tiedemann, 1821)**
nervum sympatheticum medium Wrisbergii (Günther, 1786), see **trigeminal nerve (Winslow, 1733)**
nervum trium funiculorum (Günther, 1786), see **trigeminal nerve (Winslow, 1733)**
nervus abscissus (Vieussens, 1684), see **long thoracic nerve (Quain & Wilson, 1839)**
nervus accessorius (Vieussens, 1684), see **accessory nerve (Vieussens, 1684)**
nervus accessorius ad patheticum (Palletta, 1784), see **trochlear nerve (Molinetti, 1669)**
nervus accessorius motorum communium (Palletta, 1784), see **oculomotor nerve (Estienne, 1545)**
nervus accessorius octavi paris (Winslow, 1733), see **accessory nerve (Vieussens, 1684)**
nervus accessorius to cruralis (Winslow, 1733), see **lumbar plexus dorsal divisions (Paterson, 1887)**
nervus acusticus mollis (Haller, 1762), see **vestibulocochlear nerve (>1840)**
nervus ad tensorem tympani (Arnold, 1834), see **nerve to tensor tympani (Arnold, 1834)**
nervus alveolaris maxillae inferioris (Meckel, 1817), see **inferior dental nerve (Meckel, 1817)**
nervus ampullarum externarum canalis semicircularis superioris atque externi (Arnold, 1834), see **rostral part of vestibular nerve (>1840)**
nervus anterior facialis infimus (Soemmerring, 1791), see **buccal branch of facial nerve (>1840)**
nervus auricularis maximus (Haase, 1781), see **great auricular nerve (Haase, 1781)**
nervus auricularis posterior rami musculorum retrahentium (Arnold,1834), see **auricular branch of posterior auricular nerve (Arnold, 1834)**
nervus auricularis posterior ramus auricularis (Arnold, 1834), see **auricular branch of posterior auricular nerve (Arnold, 1834)**
nervus auricularis posterior ramus occipitalis (Arnold, 1834), see **occipital branch of posterior auricular nerve (Arnold, 1834)**
nervus auriculo-temporalis (Henle, 1871), see **auriculotemporal nerve (Haller, 1762)**
nervus axillaris (Winslow, 1733), see **axillary nerve (Winslow, 1733)**
nervus biventricus (Neubauer, 1772), see **digastric nerve (Meckel, 1753)**
nervus buccinatorius (Schaarschmidt, 1750), see **buccal nerve (Meckel, 1748)**
nervus cardiacus inferior (Meckel, 1817), see **inferior cardiac nerve (Cloquet, 1816)**
nervus cardiacus superior (Meckel, 1817), see **superior cardiac nerve (Neubauer, 1772)**
nervus communicans faciei (Soemmerring, 1778), see **intermediofacial nerve (Strong & Elwyn, 1943)**

nervus communicans faciei pars cerebralis (Arnold, 1834), see **intermediofacial nerve roots (>1840)**

nervus communicans faciei pars petrosa (Arnold, 1834), see **intermediofacial nerve (Strong & Elwyn, 1943)**

nervus communicans faciei portio intermedia (Arnold, 1834), see **intermediate nerve (>1840)**

nervus communicans faciei portio major (Arnold, 1834), see **intermediofacial nerve (Strong & Elwyn, 1943)**

nervus communicans faciei ramos profundos (Günther, 1786), see **facial nerve trunk (1840)**

nervus communicans faciei ramos superficiales (Günther, 1786), see **facial nerve trunk (1840)**

nervus communicans faciei ramus ad musculo Eustachii (Günther, 1786), see **nerve to tensor tympani (>1840)**

nervus communicans faciei ramus ad musculus stapedis (Günther, 1786), see **stapedial nerve (>1840)**

nervus communicans faciei ramus ad musculus tensorem tympani (Günther, 1786), see **nerve to tensor tympani (>1840)**

nervus communicans faciei ramus anastomoticus (Günther, 1786), see **communicating branch of intermediofacial nerve with tympanic plexus (>1840)**

nervus communis facili (Meckel, 1817), see **intermediofacial nerve (Strong & Elwyn, 1943)**

nervus consensorius medius capitis (Andersch, 1797), see **trigeminal nerve (Winslow, 1733)**

nervus consensorius parvus capitis (Andersch, 1797), see **intermediofacial nerve (Strong & Elwyn, 1943)**

nervus consentiens magnus capitis (Andersch, 1797), see **vagus nerve (Galen, c192)**

nervus crotaphiticus-nervus buccinatorius (Palletta, 1784), see **trigeminal nerve (Winslow, 1733)**

nervus crotaphito-buccinatorius (Meckel, 1817), see **trigeminal nerve (Winslow, 1733)**

nervus cutaneus antebrachii lateralis (>1840), see **lateral cutaneous nerve of forearm (>1840)**

nervus cutaneus antebrachii medialis (>1840), see **medial cutaneous nerve of forearm (>1840)**

nervus cutaneus brachii medialis (>1840), see **medial cutaneous nerve of arm (>1840)**

nervus cutaneus femoris lateralis (>1840), see **lateral cutaneous nerve of thigh (>1840)**

nervus cutaneus femoris posterior (Günther, 1786), see **posterior cutaneous nerve of thigh (Günther, 1786)**

nervus cutaneus longus volae (Günther, 1786), see **palmar branch of median nerve (Bock, 1827)**

nervus cutaneus minor internus vel ulnaris Wrisbergii (Klint, 1784), see **medial cutaneous nerve of arm (>1840)**

nervus cutaneus surae lateralis (>1840), see **lateral cutaneous nerve of calf (>1840)**

nervus cutaneus surae medialis (>1840), see **medial cutaneous nerve of calf (>1840)**

nervus dentalis anterior superior (Haller, 1762), see **anterior superior dental nerve (Haller, 1762)**

nervus dentalis posterior superior (Haller, 1762), see **posterior superior dental nerve (Haller, 1762)**

nervus dentalis superiores medialis (Henle, 1871), see **middle superior dental nerve (Henle, 1871)**

nervus dorsalis scapulae (Bock, 1827), see **dorsal scapular nerve (Bock, 1827)**

nervus dura portio nervi acustici (Haase, 1781), see **intermediofacial nerve (Strong & Elwyn, 1943)**

nervus facialis quinti (Cheselden, 1726), see **zygomatic nerve (>1840)**

nervus fibularis communis (>1840), see **common fibular nerve (>1840)**

nervus frontalis (Cheselden, 1726), see **frontal nerve (Cheselden, 1726)**

nervus glossopharyngeus (Haller, 1762), see **glossopharyngeal nerve (Huber, 1744)**

nervus glossopharyngeus ramus sinus carotici (>1840), see **carotid branches of glossopharyngeal nerve (Todd, 1836–1839)**

nervus gluteus inferior (Martin, 1781), see **inferior gluteal nerve (Martin, 1781)**

nervus gluteus superior (Martin, 1781), see **superior gluteal nerve (Martin, 1781)**

nervus hypogastricus (Walter, 1783), see **hypogastric nerve (Walter, 1783)**

nervus hypoglossus minor (Winslow, 1733), see **lingual nerve (Vesalius, 1543a)**

nervus ileo-inguinalis (Bock, 1827), see **ilio-inguinal nerve (Schmidt, 1794)**

nervus ilio-hypogastricus (Schmidt, 1794), see **iliohypogastric nerve (Schmidt, 1794)**

nervus ilio-inguinalis (Schmidt, 1794), see **ilio-inguinal nerve (Schmidt, 1794)**

nervus impar (Haller, 1762), see **terminal filament (Tiedemann, 1821)**

nervus imparus sacrus (Fyfe, 1800), see **terminal filament (Tiedemann, 1821)**

nervus infraorbitalis (Meckel, 1817), see **maxillary nerve (Meckel, 1753)**

nervus infraorbitalis (Schaarschmidt, 1750), see **infraorbital nerve (Schaarschmidt, 1750)**

nervus infratrochlearis (Schaarschmidt, 1750), see **infratrochlear nerve (Schaarschmidt, 1750)**

nervus innominatus (Todd, 1836–1839), see **greater petrosal nerve (>1840)**

nervus internus oculi (Andersch, 1797), see **trochlear nerve (Molinetti, 1669)**

nervus interosseus antebrachii anterior (>1840), see **anterior interosseous nerve (Quain, 1832)**

nervus inter-osseus anticus (Quain, 1832), see **anterior interosseous nerve (Quain, 1832)**

nervus ischiadicum (Heister, 1717), see **sciatic nerve (Keill, 1698)**

nervus ischiadicus (Heister, 1721), see **sciatic nerve (Keill, 1698)**

nervus jugalis posterior (Mayer, 1794), see **temporal branches of facial nerve (Swan, 1830)**

nervus jugalis primus (Soemmerring, 1791), see **temporal branches of facial nerve (Swan, 1830)**

nervus jugalis quartus (Soemmerring, 1791), see **temporal branches of facial nerve (Swan, 1830)**

nervus jugalis quintus (Soemmerring, 1791), see **zygomatic branches of facial nerve (>1840)**

nervus jugalis secundus (Soemmerring, 1791), see **temporal branches of facial nerve (Swan, 1830)**

nervus jugalis tertius (Soemmerring, 1791), see **temporal branches of facial nerve (Swan, 1830)**

nervus lingualis (Vesalius, 1543a), see **lingual nerve (Vesalius, 1543a)**
nervus lingualis rami isthmi faucium (>1840), see **isthmus of fauces branches of lingual nerve (>1840)**
nervus lingualis rami linguales (Arnold, 1834), see **lingual branches of lingual nerve (Arnold, 1834)**
nervus massetericus (Meckel, 1748), see **masseteric nerve (Meckel, 1748)**
nervus medianus (Du Verney, 1697), see **median nerve (Du Verney, 1697)**
nervus medianus nervi digitales palmares communes (>1840), see **common palmar digital nerves of median nerve (>1840)**
nervus medianus nervi digitales palmares proprii (>1840), see **proper palmar digital nerves of median nerve (>1840)**
nervus mentalis (Cheselden, 1726), see **mental nerve (Cheselden, 1726)**
nervus mentalis rami mentales (Arnold, 1834), see **mental branches of mental nerve (Arnold, 1834)**
nervus mollis (Haller, 1762), see **vestibulocochlear nerve (>1840)**
nervus motorius medius oculi (Andersch, 1797), see **oculomotor nerve (Estienne, 1545)**
nervus musculo-cutaneus (Du Verney, 1697), see **musculocutaneous nerve (Du Verney, 1697)**
nervus musculo-cutaneus ramus musculoris (Soemmerring, 1798), see **muscular branches of musculocutaneous nerve (Günther, 1786)**
nervus nasociliaris (Meckel, 1817), see **nasociliary nerve (Meckel, 1817; Wutzer, 1817)**
nervus naso-palatinus (Scarpa, 1785), see **nasopalatine nerve (Scarpa, 1785)**
nervus obturator (Cheselden, 1726), see **obturator nerve (Cheselden, 1726)**
nervus obturatorius (Meckel, 1817), see **obturator nerve (Cheselden, 1726)**
nervus obturatorius ramus anterior (Haase, 1781), see **anterior branch of obturator nerve (Haase, 1781; Martin, 1781)**
nervus obturatorius ramus posterior (Haase, 1781), see **posterior branch of obturator nerve (Haase, 1781; Martin, 1781)**
nervus occipitalis magnus (Haase, 1781), see **greater occipital nerve (Haase, 1781)**
nervus oculomuscularis communis (Burdach, 1822), see **oculomotor nerve (Estienne, 1545)**
nervus oculomuscularis inferior (Meckel, 1817), see **oculomotor nerve (Estienne, 1545)**
nervus oculomuscularis medius (Meckel, 1817), see **oculomotor nerve (Estienne, 1545)**
nervus oculomuscularis minimus (Meckel, 1817), see **trochlear nerve (Molinetti, 1669)**
nervus oculomuscularis posterior (Meckel, 1817), see **abducens nerve (Heister, 1717)**
nervus oculomuscularis superior (Meckel, 1817), see **trochlear nerve (Molinetti, 1669)**
nervus palatini major (Meckel, 1817), see **greater palatine nerve (Cloquet, 1816)**
nervus palatinus posteriorem (Günther, 1786), see **posterior palatine nerve (Günther, 1786)**
nervus perforans (Cheselden, 1713), see **muscular branches of musculocutaneous nerve (Günther, 1786)**
nervus perforans Casserii (Cheselden, 1726), see **musculocutaneous nerve (Du Verney, 1697)**
nervus plantaris internus (Meckel, 1817), see **common plantar digital nerves of medial plantar nerve (>1840)**
nervus popliteus (Winslow, 1733), see **sciatic nerve (Keill, 1698)**
nervus portio inter communicantem faciei et auditorium media (Haase, 1781), see **intermediate nerve (>1840)**
nervus pudendus (Camper, 1762), see **pudendal nerve (Camper, 1762)**
nervus quintus portio major (Soemmerring, 1778), see **trigeminal nerve sensory root (>1840)**
nervus quintus portio minor of Wrisberg (Soemmerring, 1778), see **trigeminal nerve motor root (Bell, 1829)**
nervus radialis (Du Verney, 1697), see **radial nerve (Du Verney, 1697)**
nervus radialis ramus profundus (Martin, 1781), see **deep branch of radial nerve (Martin, 1781)**
nervus radialis ramus superficialis (Martin, 1781), see **superficial branch of radial nerve (Martin, 1781)**
nervus saphenus (Haase, 1781), see **saphenous nerve (Haase, 1781)**
nervus sciatico-cruralis (Winslow, 1733), see **sciatic nerve (Keill, 1698)**
nervus sciaticus (Keill, 1698), see **sciatic nerve (Keill, 1698)**
nervus sine pari (Hall, 1565), see **terminal filament (Tiedemann, 1821)**
nervus spinalis (Winslow, 1733), see **accessory nerve (Vieussens, 1684)**
nervus spinalis ad par vagum accessorius (Vieussens, 1684), see **spinal root of accessory nerve trunk (>1840)**
nervus spinosus (>1840)
nervus splanchnicum minorem (Haller, 1762), see **lesser splanchnic nerve (Haller, 1762)**
nervus splanchnicus imus (>1840), see **least splanchnic nerve (>1840)**
nervus splanchnicus major (Walter, 1783), see **greater splanchnic nerve (Walter, 1783)**
nervus sub-occipitalis (Winslow, 1733), see **suboccipital nerve (Winslow, 1733)**
nervus suprascapularem (Bang, 1770), see **suprascapular nerve (Bang, 1770)**
nervus supraspinatus scapulae (Scarpa, 1794), see **suprascapular nerve (Bang, 1770)**
nervus supratrochlearis (Schaarschmidt, 1750), see **supratrochlear nerve (Schaarschmidt, 1750)**
nervus sympatheticus medius (Winslow, 1733), see **cranial nerves (Soemmerring, 1791)**
nervus sympathicus parvus (Haase, 1781), see **intermediofacial nerve (Strong & Elwyn, 1943)**
nervus temporalis profundus (Haase, 1781), see **deep temporal nerves (Haase, 1781)**
nervus temporalis profundus anterior (Arnold, 1834), see **anterior deep temporal nerve (Arnold, 1834)**

nervus temporalis profundus posterior (Arnold, 1834), see **posterior deep temporal nerve (Arnold, 1834)**
nervus tentorii (Arnold, 1838a), see **tentorial nerve (Arnold, 1838a)**
nervus thalamos conjugens (Burdach, 1822), see **posterior commissure (Winslow, 1733)**
nervus tibialis (Haase, 1781), see **tibial nerve (Haase, 1781)**
nervus tibialis hallucis (Meckel, 1817), see **common plantar digital nerves of medial plantar nerve (>1840)**
nervus timidus (Bidloo, 1685), see **abducens nerve (Heister, 1717)**
nervus tornabilis (Second Salernitan Demonstration, c1070–1100), see **vagus nerve (Galen, c192)**
nervus transversus colli (>1840), see **transverse nerve of neck (>1840)**
nervus trochlearis (Molinetti, 1669), see **trochlear nerve (Molinetti, 1669)**
nervus tympanicus (Arnold, 1834), see **tympanic nerve (Arnold, 1834)**
nervus ulnaris (Cheselden, 1726), see **ulnar nerve (Cheselden, 1726)**
nervus ulnaris nervi digitales palmares communes (>1840), see **common palmar digital nerves of ulnar nerve (>1840)**
nervus ulnaris ramus dorsalis (Günther, 1786), see **dorsal branch of ulnar nerve (Günther, 1786)**
netlike body (Galen, c173), see **retina (Herophilus, c335–c280 BC)**
netlike plexus (Vesalius, 1543a), see **rete mirabile (Herophilus, c335–c280 BC)**
netnet (Smith Papyrus, c1700 BC), see **meninges (Smith Papyrus, c1700 BC)**
net-resembling fold for thighs and feet (Diemerbroeck, 1689), see **lumbosacral plexus (Vesalius, 1543a)**
net-resembling fold under clavicle (Diemerbroeck, 1689), see **brachial plexus (Camper, 1760)**
network of soft nerves (Mayer, 1794), see **nerves (Herophilus, c335–c280 BC)**
neura (Herophilus, c335–c280 BC), see **nerves (Herophilus, c335–c280 BC)**
neural crest (>1840)
neural folds (>1840)
neural groove (>1840)
neural lobe of hypophysis (Tilney, 1936), see **neurohypophysis (Rioch et al., 1940)**
neural lobe of pituitary gland (Rioch et al., 1940), see **posterior lobe of pituitary gland (Haller, 1762)**
neural mass of vertebral column (Gall & Spurzheim, 1810), see **spinal cord (Galen, c162–c166)**
neural placodes (>1840)
neural plate (Stricker, 1860)
neural stalk (Rioch et al., 1940), see **infundibulum (Rioch et al., 1940)**
neural tube (Baer, 1837)
neuris (Herophilus, c335–c280 BC), see **nerve (Herophilus, c335–c280 BC)**
neurohypophysis (Rioch et al., 1940)
neuron (Herophilus, c335–c280 BC), see **nerve (Herophilus, c335–c280 BC)**
neuron (Hippocrates), see **nerve (Herophilus, c335–c280 BC)**
neuronode (Kilian, 1822), see **ganglion (Galen, c173)**
nexus thalamorum nervorum opticorum (Santorini, 1775), see **interthalamic adhesion (>1840)**
nib of calamus scriptorius (Vicq d'Azyr, 1786), see **obex (Burdach, 1822)**
nidus (Reil, 1809c)
nidus avis (>1840), see **nidus (Reil, 1809c)**
nidus hirundinus (Reil, 1807–1808c), see **nidus (Reil, 1809c)**
ninth branch of anterior crural nerve to pectineal muscle (Swan, 1830), see **muscular branches of femoral nerve (Quain & Wilson, 1839)**
ninth nerve proper of nerves of head (Andersch & Soemmerring, 1792), see **vagus nerve (Galen, c192)**
ninth nerves of head (Andersch, 1797), see **glossopharyngeal nerve (Huber, 1744)**
ninth pair of cerebral nerves (Haase, 1781), see **hypoglossal nerve (Winslow, 1733)**
ninth pair of cerebral nerves (Soemmerring, 1791), see **glossopharyngeal nerve (Huber, 1744)**
ninth pair of cranial nerves (Soemmerring, 1791), see **glossopharyngeal nerve (Huber, 1744)**
ninth pair of nerves (Malacarne, 1791), see **mandibular nerve (>1840)**
ninth pair of nerves arising within skull (Gibson, 1682), see **sympathetic trunk (Winslow, 1733)**
ninth pair of nerves arising within skull (Willis, 1664), see **hypoglossal nerve (Winslow, 1733)**
ninth pair of nerves from brain (Bartholin, 1641), see **cranial nerves (Soemmerring, 1791)**
ninth pair of nerves from brain (Colombo, 1559), see **trochlear nerve (Molinetti, 1669)**
ninth pair of nerves leaving skull (Burdach, 1822), see **glossopharyngeal nerve (Huber, 1744)**
ninth pair of nerves of head (Andersch & Soemmerring, 1792), see **vagus nerve (Galen, c192)**
nipple (Haly Abbas or Ali ibn' ul-Abbas, d. 994), see **cerebral cortex (>1840)**
noble ventricle (Herophilus, c335–c280 BC), see **fourth ventricle (Galen, c192)**
node of brain (Cruveilhier, 1836), see **brainstem (Schwalbe, 1881)**
node of nerve (Neubauer, 1772), see **peripheral ganglion (>1840)**
nodes (Gall & Spurzheim, 1810), see **central ganglia (>1840)**
nodose ganglion (>1840), see **distal vagal ganglion (>1840)**
nodose tubercle (Rolando, 1831), see **medial geniculate complex (>1840)**
nodular plexus of vagus nerves of Meckel (Kilian, 1822), see **vagus nerve (Galen, c192)**
nodule (Reil, 1807–1808a)
nodule of anterior root of crus of fornix (Reil, 1812c), see **mammillary body (Ludwig, 1779)**
nodules (Malpighi, 1669), see **central ganglia (>1840)**
nodus cerebri (Wenzel & Wenzel, 1812), see **pons (Haller, 1747)**
nodus encephali (Quain, 1828), see **brainstem (Schwalbe, 1881)**

nodus encephali (Soemmerring, 1778), see **pons (Haller, 1747)**
non-ganglionic portion of fifth pair of nerves (Todd, 1836–1839), see **trigeminal nerve motor root (Bell, 1829)**
nonganglionic root of trigeminal nerve (Cruveilhier, 1836), see **trigeminal nerve motor root (Bell, 1829)**
nonus descendens nerve (Quain & Wilson, 1839), see **superior root of ansa cervicalis (>1840)**
novo nervo cardiaco (Wrisberg, 1786), see **cardiac plexus (Keill, 1698)**
nuca (Berengario da Carpi, 1523), see **spinal cord (Galen, c162–c166)**
nucha (Constantine the African, c1017–1087), see **spinal cord (Galen, c162–c166)**
nuclear ganglia (Burdach, 1822), see **central nervous system gray matter regions (>1840)**
nucleus (Rosenthal, 1815), see **central nervous system white matter tracts (>1840)**
nucleus (Soemmerring, 1791), see **dentate nucleus (>1840)**
nucleus (Vicq d'Azyr, 1784), see **central nervous system gray matter regions (>1840)**
nucleus accumbens (Ziehen, 1897–1901), see **accumbens nucleus (Ziehen, 1897–1901)**
nucleus amygdalae (Burdach, 1822), see **basolateral amygdalar complex (>1840)**
nucleus caudatus (Arnold, 1838b), see **caudate nucleus (Arnold, 1838b)**
nucleus cinereus (Ludwig, 1779), see **central nervous system gray matter regions (>1840)**
nucleus lentiformis (Burdach, 1822), see **cerebral nuclei (Swanson, 2000a)**
nucleus of brain (Reil, 1811c), see **vertebrate brain (Cuvier, 1800)**
nucleus of cerebellum (Arnold, 1838a), see **arbor vitae (Winslow, 1733)**
nucleus of cerebellum (Reil, 1809b), see **arbor vitae (Winslow, 1733)**
nucleus of cerebrum (Reil, 1809b), see **vertebrate brain (Cuvier, 1800)**
nucleus of cerebrum (Winslow, 1733), see **cerebral cortex white matter (>1840)**
nucleus of hemisphere (Reil, 1809b), see **vertebrate brain (Cuvier, 1800)**
nucleus of hemisphere (Reil, 1812c), see **arbor vitae (Winslow, 1733)**
nucleus of olivary fasciculus (Arnold, 1838b), see **inferior olivary complex (>1840)**
nucleus of optic thalamus (Rolando, 1825a), see **ventral thalamic nuclei (>1840)**
nucleus of solitary tract (>1840)
nucleus of spinal cord (Meckel, 1817), see **spinal cord (Galen, c162–c166)**
nucleus raphes pontis (>1840), see **pontine raphe nucleus (>1840)**
nucleus teniaformis (Reil, 1809b), see **claustrum (Burdach, 1822)**
nuptual chambers of optic nerves (Diemerbroeck, 1689), see **interbrain (Baer, 1837)**
obex (Burdach, 1822)
oblique commissure (Solly, 1836), see **superior cerebellar peduncle (Procháska, 1800)**
oblique medullary striae from calamus scriptorius (Bell, 1802), see **medullary striae (Scarpa, 1788)**
oblong eminence (Gordon, 1815), see **pyramid (Willis, 1664)**
oblong flat surface (Gordon, 1815), see **cerebral nuclei (Swanson, 2000a)**
oblong inferior eminences (Winslow, 1733), see **medulla (Winslow, 1733)**
oblong marrow (Willis, 1664), see **vertebrate brain (Cuvier, 1800)**
oblong medulla (Willis, 1664), see **vertebrate brain (Cuvier, 1800)**
oblong passage (Gordon, 1815), see **choroid membrane of third ventricle (>1840)**
oblong stock (Willis, 1664), see **central nervous system (Carus, 1814)**
obturator nerve (Cheselden, 1726)
occipital area (Brodmann, 1909), see **occipital region (Vesalius, 1543a)**
occipital brain (Galen, c192), see **cerebellum (Aristotle)**
occipital branch of external deep branch of hard nerve (Meckel, 1753), see **occipital branch of posterior auricular nerve (Arnold, 1834)**
occipital branch of hard nerve (Mayer, 1794), see **posterior auricular nerve (Meckel, 1753)**
occipital branch of hard nerve (Meckel, 1753), see **occipital branch of posterior auricular nerve (Arnold, 1834)**
occipital branch of lesser occipital nerve (Peipers, 1793), see **lesser occipital nerve (Mayer, 1794)**
occipital branch of lesser posterior auricular nerve (Meckel, 1753), see **lesser occipital nerve (Mayer, 1794)**
occipital branch of occipitoauricular nerve (Peipers, 1793), see **lesser occipital nerve (Mayer, 1794)**
occipital branch of posterior auricular nerve (Arnold, 1834)
occipital cerebral lobule (Chaussier, 1807), see **occipital region (Vesalius, 1543a)**
occipital falx (Malacarne, 1776), see **cerebellar falx (Günther, 1786)**
occipital filament of posterior auricular branch of facial nerve (Cruveilhier, 1836), see **occipital branch of posterior auricular nerve (Arnold, 1834)**
occipital forceps (>1840)
occipital horn (Cruveilhier, 1836), see **occipital pole (>1840)**
occipital lobe (Arnold, 1838a), see **occipital region (Vesalius, 1543a)**
occipital nerve (Bidloo, 1685), see **suboccipital nerve (Winslow, 1733)**
occipital nerve (Meckel, 1753), see **posterior auricular nerve (Meckel, 1753)**
occipital nerve (Winslow, 1733), see **lesser occipital nerve (Mayer, 1794)**
occipital plexus (Cruveilhier, 1836), see **external carotid plexus (>1840)**
occipital pole (Broca, 1878a)
occipital region (Vesalius, 1543a)
occipital septum (Winslow, 1733), see **cerebellar falx (Günther, 1786)**

occipital surculus of external deep branch of portio major and minor of facial nerve (Bellingeri, 1818), see **occipital branch of posterior auricular nerve (Arnold, 1834)**

occipital surface of cerebellum (Vicq d'Azyr, 1784), see **cerebellum (Aristotle)**

occipitij regionis (Vesalius, 1543a), see **occipital region (Vesalius, 1543a)**

occipito-auricular branch of cephalic part of trachelo-cutanean plexus (Burdin, 1803), see **lesser occipital nerve (Mayer, 1794)**

occipitoauricular branch of cephalic part of tracheosubcutaneous nerves (Chaussier, 1809), see **lesser occipital nerve (Mayer, 1794)**

occipitotemporal area (Brodmann, 1909), see **temporal region (>1840)**

occipitotemporal sulcus (>1840)

ocrea (Günther, 1786), see **calcarine spur (Morand, 1748)**

octavi nervorum cerebri truncus gangliformis (Scarpa, 1794), see **distal vagal ganglion (>1840)**

ocular branch of fifth pair (Monro, 1783), see **ophthalmic nerve (Winslow, 1733)**

ocular fat fascicle (Bellingeri, 1818), see **frontal nerve (Cheselden, 1726)**

ocular nerve colliculus (Burdach, 1822), see **interbrain (Baer, 1837)**

ocular nerves (Zinn, 1755), see **cranial nerves (Soemmerring, 1791)**

ocular pair of nerves (Burdin, 1803), see **white matter tracts (Bell & Bell, 1826)**

oculomotor nerve (Estienne, 1545)

oculomotor nerve central root (>1840)

oculomotor nerve central rootlets (>1840)

oculomotor nerve inferior branch (Haase, 1781)

oculomotor nerve root (>1840)

oculomotor nerve rootlets (>1840)

oculomotor nerve superior branch (Winslow, 1733)

oculomotor nerve trunk (>1840)

oculomotor nucleus (>1840)

oculomotor root of ciliary ganglion (>1840), see **branch of oculomotor nerve to ciliary ganglion (>1840)**

oculo-nasal threads of infratrochlear fascicle (Bellingeri, 1818), see **infratrochlear nerve (Schaarschmidt, 1750)**

odonto-palatino-nasal nerve (Le Cat, 1768), see **palatine nerves (Schaarschmidt, 1750)**

oesophageal branches of vagus nerve (Quain, 1832), see **esophageal plexus (Haller, 1762)**

oesophageal ring (Müller, 1834), see **central nervous system (Carus, 1814)**

Ohrknoten (Arnold, 1828), see **otic ganglion (Arnold, 1828)**

olfactory arch (Rolando, 1831), see **uncinate fascicle (Reil, 1809b)**

olfactory bulb (Weitbrecht, 1751)

olfactory commissure (Solly, 1836), see **olfactory peduncle (Solly, 1836)**

olfactory fascicle of Ammon's horn of Zuckerkandl (Dejerine & Dejerine-Klumpke, 1901), see **dorsal fornix (Sprague & Meyer, 1950)**

olfactory fascicle of trigone (Dejerine & Dejerine-Klumpke, 1901), see **dorsal fornix (Sprague & Meyer, 1950)**

olfactory fasciculus of fornix (Tilney & Riley, 1923), see **dorsal fornix (Sprague & Meyer, 1950)**

olfactory field (Serres, 1824–1826), see **cerebral nuclei (Swanson, 2000a)**

olfactory ganglion (Meckel, 1817), see **olfactory bulb (Weitbrecht, 1751)**

olfactory instrument (Galen, c173), see **cerebral cortex (>1840)**

olfactory limb of anterior commissure (>1840)

olfactory lobe (Serres, 1824–1826), see **olfactory bulb (Weitbrecht, 1751)**

olfactory lobe (Vesalius, 1543a), see **cerebral cortex (>1840)**

olfactory lobes (Cruveilhier, 1836), see **cerebral nuclei (Swanson, 2000a)**

olfactory lobule (Serres, 1824–1826), see **olfactory bulb (Weitbrecht, 1751)**

olfactory nerve (Bartholin, 1611), see **olfactory peduncle (Solly, 1836)**

olfactory nerve (Cowper, 1698), see **nervous system (Monro, 1783)**

olfactory nerve (Soemmerring, 1778), see **cerebral cortex (>1840)**

olfactory nerve (Winslow, 1733)

olfactory nerve central root (>1840), see **olfactory nerve layer of main olfactory bulb (>1840)**

olfactory nerve fibers (Carus, 1814), see **olfactory nerve (Winslow, 1733)**

olfactory nerve ganglia (Carus, 1814), see **endbrain (Kuhlenbeck, 1927)**

olfactory nerve layer of main olfactory bulb (>1840)

olfactory nerve sulcus (Vicq d'Azyr, 1786), see **olfactory sulcus (Quain, 1834)**

olfactory nerves proper (Cruveilhier, 1836), see **olfactory nerve (Winslow, 1733)**

olfactory organ (Vesalius, 1543a), see **cerebral cortex (>1840)**

olfactory pair of cerebral nerves (Soemmerring, 1791), see **nervous system (Monro, 1783)**

olfactory pair of cranial nerves (Soemmerring, 1791), see **nervous system (Monro, 1783)**

olfactory peduncle (Brodmann, 1909), see **anterior olfactory nucleus (Herrick, 1910)**

olfactory peduncle (Solly, 1836)

olfactory projection from brain (Wiliam of Saliceto, 1275), see **cerebral cortex (>1840)**

olfactory region (>1840)

olfactory sense instrument (Galen, c173), see **cerebral cortex (>1840)**

olfactory stalk (Burdach, 1822), see **olfactory peduncle (Solly, 1836)**

olfactory sulcus (Quain, 1834)

olfactory tract (Burdach, 1822), see **olfactory peduncle (Solly, 1836)**

olfactory trigone (Soemmerring, 1778), see **olfactory tubercle (Calleja, 1893)**

olfactory trunk (Burdach, 1822), see **olfactory peduncle (Solly, 1836)**

olfactory tubercle (Arsaky, 1813), see ***endbrain (Kuhlenbeck, 1927)***
olfactory tubercle (Calleja, 1893)
olfactory tubercle (Grant, 1834c), see ***olfactory bulb (Weitbrecht, 1751)***
olfactory tubercle (Meckel, 1817), see ***olfactory tubercle (Calleja, 1893)***
olfactory ventricle (>1840)
oliva (Tiedemann, 1821), see ***olive (Tiedemann, 1821)***
olivaria (Du Verney, 1683), see ***pyramid (Willis, 1664)***
olivary body (Günther, 1786), see ***inferior olivary complex (>1840)***
olivary body (Vieussens, 1684), see ***olive (Tiedemann, 1821)***
olivary body gray substance (Santorini, 1775), see ***inferior olivary complex (>1840)***
olivary body yellow substance (Malacarne, 1776), see ***inferior olivary complex (>1840)***
olivary bundle (Burdach, 1822), see ***ventral funiculus (>1840)***
olivary bundle (Rosenthal, 1815), see ***central nervous system white matter tracts (>1840)***
olivary eminences (Palfijn, 1726), see ***olive (Tiedemann, 1821)***
olivary fasciculus (Tiedemann, 1816), see ***central nervous system white matter tracts (>1840)***
olivary ganglion (Cloquet, 1828), see ***cardiac ganglion (Neubauer, 1772; Haller, 1772)***
olivary ganglion (Knox, 1832), see ***inferior olivary complex (>1840)***
olivary ganglion (Mayer, 1794), see ***superior cervical ganglion (Vieussens, 1684)***
olivary nucleus (Burdach, 1822), see ***inferior olivary complex (>1840)***
olivary tubercle (Günther, 1786), see ***inferior olivary complex (>1840)***
olive (Tiedemann, 1821)
olive body (Falloppio, 1561), see ***distal vagal ganglion (>1840)***
olivi-formia nervorum (Tarin, 1753), see ***peripheral ganglia (>1840)***
olivocerebellar tract (>1840)
omenta (Macrobius, 5th century), see ***meninges (Smith Papyrus, c1700 BC)***
omental nerve (Walter, 1783), see ***right gastroepiploic plexus (>1840)***
omental plexus (Wrisberg, 1800), see ***peripheral nervous system (Meckel, 1817)***
one-eyed nerve (Albertus Magnus, 13th century), see ***intermediofacial nerve (Strong & Elwyn, 1943)***
onions of vault with three pillars (Chaussier, 1807), see ***mammillary body (Ludwig, 1779)***
opening of cerebral aqueduct (>1840)
opening of fourth ventricle (>1840)
opercula of insula (>1840), see ***central nervous system surface features (>1840)***
opercular area (Brodmann, 1909), see ***opercular part of inferior frontal gyrus (>1840)***
opercular part of inferior frontal gyrus (>1840)
operculum (Arnold, 1838a), see ***central nervous system surface features (>1840)***
operculum (Burdach, 1822), see ***central nervous system surface features (>1840)***
operculum of superior lobe (Arnold, 1838b), see ***parietal operculum (>1840)***
ophthalmic branch of fifth pair (Bell, 1803a), see ***ophthalmic nerve (Winslow, 1733)***
ophthalmic branch of fifth pair communicates with third and fourth nerves (Bell & Bell, 1829), see ***ophthalmic nerve (Winslow, 1733)***
ophthalmic branch of Willis (Cruveilhier, 1836), see ***ophthalmic nerve (Winslow, 1733)***
ophthalmic branches of second division of fifth pair of nerves arising within skull (Willis, 1664), see ***ophthalmic nerve (Winslow, 1733)***
ophthalmic ganglion (Pourfour du Petit, 1729), see ***ciliary ganglion (Loder, 1778)***
ophthalmic nerve (Winslow, 1733)
ophthalmic nerve of Willis (Winslow, 1733), see ***ophthalmic nerve (Winslow, 1733)***
ophthalmic plexus (Keill, 1698), see ***ciliary ganglion (Loder, 1778)***
ophthalmic plexus (>1840)
ophthalmico-frontal branch of first branch of fifth pair of nerves (Meckel, 1753), see ***frontal nerve (Cheselden, 1726)***
ophthalmicofrontal branch of trigeminal nerve (Günther, 1786), see ***ophthalmic nerve (Winslow, 1733)***
ophthalmicofrontal nerve (Le Cat, 1768), see ***frontal nerve (Cheselden, 1726)***
opisto-gastric plexus (Chaussier, 1789), see ***celiac plexus (Winslow, 1733)***
optic band (Meckel, 1832), see ***optic tract (Vicq d'Azyr, 1784)***
optic bed (Poupart, 1712), see ***interbrain (Baer, 1837)***
optic channel (Herophilus, c335–c280 BC), see ***white matter tracts (Bell & Bell, 1826)***
optic chiasm (Galen, c173)
optic colliculus (Soemmerring, 1809), see ***interbrain (Baer, 1837)***
optic colliculus (Wenzel & Wenzel, 1812), see ***thalamus (His, 1893a)***
optic colliculus commissure (Wenzel & Wenzel, 1812), see ***interthalamic adhesion (>1840)***
optic commissure (Vicq d'Azyr, 1786), see ***optic chiasm (Galen, c173)***
optic eminence (Poupart, 1712), see ***interbrain (Baer, 1837)***
optic ganglion (Leuret, 1839), see ***interbrain (Baer, 1837)***
optic ganglions (Spurzheim, 1826), see ***tectum (Baer, 1837)***
optic lobes (Serres, 1824–1826), see ***tectum (Baer, 1837)***
optic lobes vesicle (Serres, 1824–1826), see ***primary midbrain vesicle (Baer, 1837)***
optic lobule (Serres, 1824–1826), see ***mammillary body (Ludwig, 1779)***
optic nerve (Galen, c173), see ***white matter tracts (Bell & Bell, 1826)***
optic nerve (Malpighi, 1669), see ***invertebrate nerve (>1840)***
optic nerve (Vicq d'Azyr, 1786)
optic nerve colliculus (Arnold, 1838b), see ***interbrain (Baer, 1837)***

optic nerve colliculus (Wenzel & Wenzel, 1812), see ***thalamus (His, 1893a)***

optic pair of cerebral nerves (Soemmerring, 1791), see ***white matter tracts (Bell & Bell, 1826)***

optic pair of cranial nerves (Soemmerring, 1791), see ***white matter tracts (Bell & Bell, 1826)***

optic radiation (>1840)

optic thalamus (Bell, 1802), see ***interbrain (Baer, 1837)***

optic thalamus (Galen, c173), see ***inferior horn of lateral ventricle (Bell, 1802)***

optic thalamus (Pourfour du Petit, 1710), see ***brainstem (Schwalbe, 1881)***

optic thalamus vesicles (Serres, 1824–1826), see ***interbrain vesicle (Baer, 1837)***

optic tract (Vicq d'Azyr, 1784)

optic tubercle (Carus, 1814, p. 139), see ***vertebrate brain (Cuvier, 1800)***

optic tubercle (Carus, 1814, p. 176), see ***interbrain (Baer, 1837)***

optic tubercle (Carus, 1814, p. 268), see ***superior colliculus (Haller, 1762)***

optic tubercle (Carus, 1818), see ***superior colliculus (Haller, 1762)***

optic tubercle (Serres, 1824–1826), see ***mammillary body (Ludwig, 1779)***

optic tubercles (Solly, 1836), see ***tectum (Baer, 1837)***

opticos (Gerdy, 1838), see ***interbrain (Baer, 1837)***

ora lobi inferioris (Burdach, 1822), see ***parahippocampal gyrus (>1840)***

orange-white matter (Gordon, 1815), see ***white matter (Meckel, 1817)***

orbicular body (Tarin, 1750), see ***mammillary body (Ludwig, 1779)***

orbicular circumvolutions (Bauhin, 1605), see ***cerebral cortex gray matter (>1840)***

orbicular eminence (Tarin, 1750), see ***mammillary body (Ludwig, 1779)***

orbicular eminence (Tiedemann, 1816), see ***olfactory bulb (Weitbrecht, 1751)***

orbicular fibril of external subcutaneous filament of deep frontal thread of supraorbital fascicle (Bellingeri, 1818), see ***supraorbital nerve (Meckel, 1753)***

orbicular processes of cerebellum (Collins, 1685), see ***inferior colliculus (Haller, 1762)***

orbicular prominence (Willis, 1664), see ***superior colliculus (Haller, 1762)***

orbicular prominences (Willis, 1664), see ***tectum (Baer, 1837)***

orbicular protuberances (Heister, 1717), see ***mammillary body (Ludwig, 1779)***

orbital area (Brodmann, 1909), see ***lateral orbital gyrus (>1840)***

orbital branch of submaxillary nerve (Chaussier, 1809), see ***zygomatic nerve (>1840)***

orbital branch of superior maxillary nerve (Cruveilhier, 1836), see ***orbital branches of pterygopalatine ganglion (>1840)***

orbital branch of superior maxillary nerve (Quain & Wilson, 1839), see ***zygomatic nerve (>1840)***

orbital branches of pterygopalatine ganglion (>1840)

orbital branches of suprajugal branches of ascending branch of superficial branch of hard nerve (Günther, 1786), see ***temporal branches of facial nerve (Swan, 1830)***

orbital branches of temporofacial branch of facial nerve (Cruveilhier, 1836), see ***zygomatic branches of facial nerve (>1840)***

orbital branches of zygomatic branches of ascending branch of superficial branch of hard nerve (Günther, 1786), see ***temporal branches of facial nerve (Swan, 1830)***

orbital gyri (>1840)

orbital nerve (Cruveilhier, 1836), see ***orbital branches of pterygopalatine ganglion (>1840)***

orbital nerve (Quain, 1828), see ***zygomatic nerve (>1840)***

orbital nerve (Soemmerring, 1809), see ***infraorbital nerve (Schaarschmidt, 1750)***

orbital part of abducens nerve (Arnold, 1834), see ***abducens nerve trunk (>1840)***

orbital part of fourth pair (Arnold, 1834), see ***trochlear nerve (Molinetti, 1669)***

orbital part of inferior frontal gyrus (>1840)

orbital part of oculomotor nerve (Arnold, 1834), see ***oculomotor nerve (Estienne, 1545)***

orbital part of optic nerve (Arnold, 1834), see ***optic nerve (Vicq d'Azyr, 1786)***

orbital part of optic nerve chiasm (Arnold, 1838b), see ***optic nerve (Vicq d'Azyr, 1786)***

orbital part of scornful nerve (Arnold, 1834), see ***abducens nerve trunk (>1840)***

orbital part of second pair (Arnold, 1834), see ***optic nerve (Vicq d'Azyr, 1786)***

orbital part of sixth pair (Arnold, 1834), see ***abducens nerve trunk (>1840)***

orbital part of third pair (Arnold, 1834), see ***oculomotor nerve (Estienne, 1545)***

orbital part of trochlear or pathetic nerve (Arnold, 1834), see ***trochlear nerve (Molinetti, 1669)***

orbital region (Rolando, 1831)

orbital sulci (>1840)

orbitar branch of second division of fifth pair of nerves (Todd, 1836–1839), see ***zygomatic nerve (>1840)***

orbitar ganglion (Burdin, 1803), see ***ciliary ganglion (Loder, 1778)***

orbitary nerve (Winslow, 1733), see ***ophthalmic nerve (Winslow, 1733)***

orbito-frontal nerve (Burdin, 1803), see ***ophthalmic nerve (Winslow, 1733)***

orcheis (Galen, c177), see ***superior colliculus (Haller, 1762)***

organ of organs (Winslow, 1733), see ***vertebrate brain (Cuvier, 1800)***

organ of smell (Hippocrates), see ***cerebral cortex (>1840)***

organ of smell (Willis, 1664), see ***nervous system (Monro, 1783)***

organ of smelling (du Laurens, 1599), see ***olfactory ventricle (>1840)***

organa olfaciendi (Falloppio, 1561), see ***mammillary body (Ludwig, 1779)***

organic nerves (Ackermann, 1813), see ***peripheral nervous system (Meckel, 1817)***

oriface of third ventricle (Bartholin, 1662), see ***interventricular foramen (>1840)***

pairs of nerves of medulla oblongata (Winslow, 1733), see **nervous system (Monro, 1783)**

pairs of sinews of brain (Geminus, 1553), see **cranial nerves (Soemmerring, 1791)**

palatine gland threads of anterior palatine fascicle (Bellingeri, 1818), see **greater palatine nerve (Cloquet, 1816)**

palatine muscle threads of posterior palatine fascicle (Bellingeri, 1818), see **posterior palatine nerve (Günther, 1786)**

palatine nerve (Bonhomme, 1748), see **maxillary nerve (Meckel, 1753)**

palatine nerve (Burdin, 1803), see **lesser palatine nerves (Meckel, 1817)**

palatine nerves (Schaarschmidt, 1750)

palatine ramus of superior maxillary nerve (Winslow, 1733), see **trigeminal nerve (Winslow, 1733)**

palatino-pharyngeal nerve (Wrisberg, 1786), see **pharyngeal nerve (Bock, 1817)**

palato-pharyngeal surculus of inferior maxillary branch (Bellingeri, 1818), see **nerve to tensor veli palatini (>1840)**

palato-pharyngeal thread of posterior palatine fascicle (Bellingeri, 1818), see **posterior palatine nerve (Günther, 1786)**

palato-pharyngeal threads of external palatine fascicle (Bellingeri, 1818), see **lateral palatine nerve (Henle, 1871)**

palato-tonsillar threads of external palatine fascicle (Bellingeri, 1818), see **lateral palatine nerve (Henle, 1871)**

pallidum (Swanson, 2000a)

pallium (Burdach, 1822), see **cerebral cortex gray matter (>1840)**

pallium (>1840), see **cerebral cortex gray matter (>1840)**

palmar branch of cubital nerve (Cloquet, 1828), see **superficial branch of ulnar nerve (Fyfe, 1800)**

palmar branch of cubital nerve (Soemmerring, 1791), see **ulnar nerve (Cheselden, 1726)**

palmar branch of major internal cutaneous nerve (Bock, 1827), see **anterior branch of medial cutaneous nerve of forearm (>1840)**

palmar branch of medial cutaneous nerve (Bock, 1827), see **anterior branch of medial cutaneous nerve of forearm (>1840)**

palmar branch of median nerve (Bock, 1827)

palmar branch of median nerve external collateral branch of index finger (Cruveihier, 1836), see **proper palmar digital nerves of median nerve (>1840)**

palmar branch of median nerve external collateral branch of thumb (Cruveilhier, 1836), see **common palmar digital nerves of median nerve (>1840)**

palmar branch of radial nerve (Cloquet, 1828), see **superficial branch of radial nerve (Martin, 1781)**

palmar branch of ulnar nerve (Meckel, 1817), see **ulnar nerve (Cheselden, 1726)**

palmar branch of ulnar nerve (Soemmerring, 1791)

palmar cutaneous branch of medial cutaneous nerve trunk (Loder, 1803), see **medial cutaneous nerve of forearm (>1840)**

palmar cutaneous branch of middle cutaneous branch of internal cutaneous nerve (Caldani, 1813, 1814), see **anterior branch of medial cutaneous nerve of forearm (>1840)**

palmar cutaneous nerve (Klint, 1784), see **anterior branch of medial cutaneous nerve of forearm (>1840)**

palmar cutaneous nerve (Quain & Wilson, 1839), see **palmar branch of median nerve (Bock, 1827)**

palmar cutaneous nerve of Wrisberg (Frotscher, 1788), see **anterior branch of medial cutaneous nerve of forearm (>1840)**

palmar external collateral branch of little finger of external branch of superficial terminal branch of cubital nerve (Cruveilhier, 1836), see **proper palmar digital nerves of ulnar nerve (>1840)**

palmar internal collateral branch of internal branch of superficial terminal branch of cubital nerve (Cruveilhier, 1836), see **proper palmar digital nerves of ulnar nerve (>1840)**

palmar internal collateral branch of ring finger of external branch of superficial terminal branch of cubital nerve (Cruveilhier, 1836), see **proper palmar digital nerves of ulnar nerve (>1840)**

palpebral and nasal filaments of internal frontal nerve (Cruveilhier, 1836), see **supratrochlear nerve (Schaarschmidt, 1750)**

palpebral and nasal filaments of supratrochlear nerve (Cruveilhier, 1836), see **supratrochlear nerve (Schaarschmidt, 1750)**

palpebral branch of lacrimal nerve (Cruveilhier, 1836), see **lacrimal nerve (Meckel, 1748; Bonhomme, 1748)**

palpebral branch of supra-trochlear nerve (Todd, 1836–1839), see **supratrochlear nerve (Schaarschmidt, 1750)**

palpebral branches of external frontal nerve (Cruveilhier, 1836; Todd, 1836–1839), see **supraorbital nerve (Meckel, 1753)**

palpebral branches of infratrochlear nerve (>1840)

palpebral branches of naso-palpebral nerve (Burdin, 1803), see **palpebral branches of infratrochlear nerve (>1840)**

palpebral branches of supraorbital nerve (Cruveilhier, 1836), see **supraorbital nerve (Meckel, 1753)**

palpebral filaments of external nasal branch of nasal nerve (Cruveilhier, 1836), see **palpebral branches of infratrochlear nerve (>1840)**

palpebral filaments of lacrimal fascicle proper (Bellingeri, 1818), see **lacrimal nerve (Meckel, 1748; Bonhomme, 1748)**

palpebral filaments of superior maxillary nerve (Cruveilhier, 1836), see **inferior palpebral branches of infraorbital nerve (>1840)**

palpebral nerve (Cruveilhier, 1836), see **infratrochlear nerve (Schaarschmidt, 1750)**

palpebral threads proper of outermost superior labial fascicle of infraorbital surculus (Bellingeri, 1818), see **superior labial branches of infraorbital nerve (Meckel, 1748)**

palpebro-frontal filament of superficial frontal thread of supraorbital fascicle (Bellingeri, 1818), see **supraorbital nerve (Meckel, 1753)**

parotid plexus (Meckel, 1817)
pars anterior cerebelli (Casseri, 1609), see **vertebrate brain (Cuvier, 1800)**
pars anterior corporis cerebralis adscendentis (Gall & Spurzheim, 1810), see **middle cerebellar peduncle (Rolando, 1819)**
pars cerebri subcinerea (Tarin, 1750), see **cerebral nuclei (Swanson, 2000a)**
pars crurum cerebri ante nervos opticos locata (Soemmerring, 1778), see **cerebral nuclei (Swanson, 2000a)**
pars distalis (Daniel & Pritchard, 1975), see **posterior lobe of pituitary gland (Haller, 1762)**
pars dorsalis thalami (Herrick, 1910), see **dorsal part of thalamus (Herrick, 1910)**
pars infundibuli anterior (Tarin, 1750), see **hypothalamus (Kuhlenbeck, 1927)**
pars infundibuli anterior, pars pellucida (Tarin, 1750), see **terminal lamina (Burdach, 1822)**
pars media et anterior trunci medullaris (Haller, 1762), see **pons (Haller, 1747)**
pars nervosa (Tilney, 1936), see **neurohypophysis (Rioch et al., 1940)**
pars posterior medullae spinalis (Varoli, 1591), see **interbrain (Baer, 1837)**
pars subthalamica of forebrain (His, 1892), see **hypothalamus (Kuhlenbeck, 1927)**
pars suprema medullae spinalis (Soemmerring, 1778), see **medulla (Winslow, 1733)**
pars vaga of eighth pair (Fyfe, 1800), see **vagus nerve (Galen, c192)**
pars ventralis thalami (Herrick, 1910), see **ventral part of thalamus (Herrick, 1910)**
part within backbone of medulla oblongata (Bartholin, 1662), see **spinal cord (Galen, c162–c166)**
part within skull of medulla oblongata (Bartholin, 1662), see **vertebrate brain (Cuvier, 1800)**
partes cerebri divisae (Varoli, 1573), see **cerebral cortex gray matter (>1840)**
partes truncorum medullae cerebelli quae pertinent ad partem posteriorem medullae oblongatae (Albinus, 1744), see **inferior cerebellar peduncle (Günther, 1786)**
particulae segregatae cerebelli mediae (Soemmerring, 1778), see **flocculus (Meckel, 1817)**
particulae segregatae cerebelli posteriores (Soemmerring, 1778), see **tonsil (Malacarne, 1776)**
partis anterioris superioris cerebelli portio quaedam sulcis notata (Soemmerring, 1778), see **cerebellar hemisphere (Willis, 1664)**
partition (Galen, c177), see **cerebral nuclei (Swanson, 2000a)**
partition-skin (Bartholin, 1662), see **cerebral nuclei (Swanson, 2000a)**
parva particula septimae conjugationis (Galen, c180), see **superior root of ansa cervicalis (>1840)**
parvus ac brevis tractus medullaris (Vieussens, 1684), see **frenulum (Vieussens, 1684)**
passage by which lateral ventricles communicate with each other and with third ventricle (Monro, 1783), see **interventricular foramen (>1840)**
passage from third to fourth ventricle (Vesalius, 1543a), see **cerebral aqueduct (>1840)**
passage or canal extending from middle to posterior ventricle (Galen, c173, c177), see **cerebral aqueduct (>1840)**
passages (Herophilus, c335–c280 BC), see **nerves (Herophilus, c335–c280 BC)**
patellar plexus (>1840)
patellar terminal branch of internal saphenous nerve (Cruveilhier, 1836), see **infrapatellar branch of saphenous nerve (>1840)**
pathetic nerve (Willis, 1664), see **trochlear nerve (Molinetti, 1669)**
pectoral anterior cutaneous branch of intercostal nerves (Bock, 1827), see **anterior cutaneous branch of intercostal nerves (>1840)**
pectoral anterior subcutaneous branch of intercostal branch of thoracic nerve (Bock, 1827), see **anterior cutaneous branch of intercostal nerves (>1840)**
pectoral nerves (Camper, 1760), see **lateral pectoral nerve (>1840)**
pectoral nerves (Haase, 1781), see **thoracic nerves (Diemerbroeck, 1672)**
pectoralis major branch of brachial plexus (Cruveilhier, 1836), see **lateral pectoral nerve (>1840)**
pectoralis minor branch of brachial plexus (Cruveilhier, 1836), see **medial pectoral nerve (>1840)**
pectunculi (Arnold, 1838a), see **cerebral aqueduct (>1840)**
pede hippocampi majore (Haase, 1781), see **hippocampal region (Swanson et al., 1987)**
pedem anserinum (Haller, 1762), see **parotid plexus (Meckel, 1817)**
pedes hippocampi (Riolan, 1618), see **hippocampal region (Swanson et al., 1987)**
pedes hippocampi Arantii (Tarin, 1753), see **hippocampal region (Swanson et al., 1987)**
pedes major hippoocampi (Haase, 1781), see **hippocampal region (Swanson et al., 1987)**
pedestal of oblong marrow (Willis, 1664), see **brainstem (Schwalbe, 1881)**
pedibus hippocampi (Haller, 1747), see **hippocampal region (Swanson et al., 1987)**
pedicelli glandulae pinealis (Haller, 1762), see **medullary stria (Wenzel & Wenzel, 1812)**
pedicle of pituitary gland (Cloquet, 1828), see **hypothalamus (Kuhlenbeck, 1927)**
pedis minoris hippocampi (Haase, 1781), see **calcarine spur (Morand, 1748)**
pedum hippocampi (Haller, 1747), see **hippocampal region (Swanson et al., 1987)**
peduncle of annular protuberance (Reil, 1809b), see **middle cerebellar peduncle (Rolando, 1819)**
peduncle of brain proper (Gordon, 1815), see **cerebral peduncle (Tarin, 1753)**
peduncle of cerebellar medullary velum (Vicq d'Azyr, 1786), see **superior cerebellar peduncle (Procháska, 1800)**
peduncle of cerebellum (Gordon, 1815), see **middle cerebellar peduncle (Rolando, 1819)**
peduncle of conarium (Arnold, 1838b), see **pineal stalk (Burdach, 1822)**

peduncle of corpus callosum (Vicq d'Azyr, 1784), see **endbrain (Kuhlenbeck, 1927)**
peduncle of medulla oblongata (Vicq d'Azyr, 1784), see **inferior cerebellar peduncle (Günther, 1786)**
peduncle of olfactory lobule (Serres, 1824–1826), see **olfactory peduncle (Solly, 1836)**
peduncle of pineal body (Tiedemann, 1821), see **pineal stalk (Burdach, 1822)**
peduncle of pituitary gland (Desmoulins, 1825), see **pituitary gland (>1840)**
peduncle of septum (Burdach, 1822), see **endbrain (Kuhlenbeck, 1927)**
peduncle of septum lucidum (Arnold, 1838a), see **endbrain (Kuhlenbeck, 1927)**
peduncle of spinal cord (Gordon, 1815), see **medulla (Winslow, 1733)**
peduncle of spinal marrow (Meckel, 1832), see **inferior cerebellar peduncle (Günther, 1786)**
peduncles of brain (Spurzheim, 1826), see **cerebral peduncle (Tarin, 1753)**
peduncles of conarium (Burdin, 1803), see **medullary stria (Wenzel & Wenzel, 1812)**
peduncles of hemispheres (Rolando, 1825a), see **cerebral peduncle (Tarin, 1753)**
peduncular loop (Gratiolet, 1857)
peduncular tegmentum (Arnold, 1838b), see **tegmentum (Swanson, 2000b)**
pedunculi cerebelli in superiora producti (Santorini, 1775), see **superior cerebellar peduncle (Prochåska, 1800)**
pedunculi cerebelli inferiores (Günther, 1786), see **inferior cerebellar peduncle (Günther, 1786)**
pedunculi cerebelli rami posteriores medullae oblongatae (Winslow, 1732), see **inferior cerebellar peduncle (Günther, 1786)**
pedunculi cerebelli valvula magna cerebri (Procháska, 1800), see **superior cerebellar peduncle (Procháska, 1800)**
pedunculi chordae spinalis (Gordon, 1815), see **inferior cerebellar peduncle (Günther, 1786)**
pedunculi glandulae pinealis (Soemmerring, 1778), see **medullary stria (Wenzel & Wenzel, 1812)**
pedunculos a cerebello ad nates & testes (Zinn, 1755), see **superior cerebellar peduncle (Procháska, 1800)**
pedunculus ad corpora quadrigemina (Soemmerring, 1791), see **superior cerebellar peduncle (Procháska, 1800)**
pedunculus ad medullam spinalem (Soemmerring, 1791), see **inferior cerebellar peduncle (Günther, 1786)**
pedunculus flocci (Burdach, 1822), see **floccular peduncle (Burdach, 1822)**
pellicula subtilis (Zerbi, 1502), see **pia (Galen, c192)**
pelvian nerves (Burdin, 1803), see **inferior hypogastric plexus (Tiedemann, 1822)**
pelvian pairs of nerves (Burdin, 1803), see **sacral nerves (Diemerbroeck, 1672)**
pelvic aortic and splanchnic branches (Cruveilhier, 1836), see **lumbar splanchnic nerves (Cruveilhier, 1836)**
pelvic ganglia (>1840)
pelvic ganglions of limiting cord (Meckel, 1817), see **sympathetic trunk ganglia (Winslow, 1733)**
pelvic nerves (Andersch, 1797), see **spinal nerves (Camper, 1760–1762)**
pelvic plexus (Beck, 1846), see **prevertebral plexuses (Quain, 1832)**
pelvic plexus (Chaussier, 1789), see **inferior hypogastric plexus (Tiedemann, 1822)**
pelvic splanchnic nerves (Cruveilhier, 1836), see **paravertebral nerves (Swanson & Bota, 2010)**
pelvic splanchnic nerves (Gaskell, 1886)
pelvic visceral nerves (Cruveilhier, 1836), see **paravertebral nerves (Swanson & Bota, 2010)**
pelvis (Rufus of Ephesus, fl. c90–120), see **hypothalamus (Kuhlenbeck, 1927)**
penicillus (Bergmann, 1831), see **terminal stria (Wenzel & Wenzel, 1812)**
penile branch of internal pudendal nerve (Cruveilhier, 1836), see **dorsal nerve of penis (Camper, 1762)**
penile nerves (Mayer, 1794), see **dorsal nerve of penis (Camper, 1762)**
penile pudendal nerve (Bock, 1827), see **dorsal nerve of penis (Camper, 1762)**
penis of brain (Bauhin, 1605), see **pineal gland (Galen, c192)**
pennatula (Bergmann, 1831), see **hypothalamohypophysial tract (>1840)**
perforans nerve (Cheselden, 1722), see **muscular branches of musculocutaneous nerve (Günther, 1786)**
perforans of Casser (Knox, 1832), see **musculocutaneous nerve (Du Verney, 1697)**
perforated lamina (Rolando, 1831), see **cerebral nuclei (Swanson, 2000a)**
perforated lamina of Meckel (Rolando, 1831), see **cerebral nuclei (Swanson, 2000a)**
perforated substance (Vicq d'Azyr, 1786), see **cerebral nuclei (Swanson, 2000a)**
perforated substance of Vicq d'Azyr (Bell, 1803b), see **interpeduncular nucleus (>1840)**
perforated white substance (Vicq d'Azyr, 1786), see **cerebral nuclei (Swanson, 2000a)**
perforating branch of intercostal branches of dorsal nerves (Cruveilhier, 1836), see **lateral cutaneous branch of intercostal nerves (>1840)**
perforating branches of dorsal nerves (Cruveilhier, 1836), see **lateral cutaneous branch of intercostal nerves (>1840)**
perforating cutaneous nerve (>1840)
perforating fibers of fornix longus (Kölliker, 1896), see **fimbria (Honegger, 1890)**
perforating nerves (Walter, 1783), see **inferior rectal nerves (>1840)**
periaqueductal gray (>1840)
pericardial branch of phrenic nerve (>1840)
pericardial twigs of diaphragmatic nerve (Vieussens, 1684), see **pericardial branch of phrenic nerve (>1840)**
perineal branch of fourth sacral nerve (>1840)
perineal branch of internal pudendal nerve (Cruveilhier, 1836), see **perineal nerve (Camper, 1762)**
perineal branches of posterior cutaneous nerve of thigh (>1840)
perineal cutaneous nerve (Walter, 1783), see **inferior rectal nerves (>1840)**
perineal nerve (Camper, 1762)

periosteal and articular filaments of external nerve of vastus internus (Cruveilhier, 1836), see **muscular branches of femoral nerve (Quain & Wilson, 1839)**
periosteal and osseous external branches of nerve of quadratus femoris and gemellus inferior (Cruveilhier, 1836), see **nerve to quadratus femoris (>1840)**
peripheral cingulate gyrus (Burdach, 1822), see **medial frontal gyrus (1840)**
peripheral fornix (Arnold, 1838b), see **cingulum (Burdach, 1822)**
peripheral ganglia (>1840)
peripheral longitudinal communicating branch (Swanson & Bota, 2010)
peripheral nerve cord (Swanson & Bota, 2010)
peripheral nerve cord trunk (Swanson & Bota, 2010)
peripheral nerve mass (Carus, 1814), see **peripheral nervous system white matter tracts (>1840)**
peripheral nervous system (Meckel, 1817)
peripheral nervous system gray matter regions (>1840)
peripheral nervous system white matter tracts (>1840)
peripheral part of corona radiata (Arnold, 1838a), see **cerebral cortex white matter (>1840)**
peripheral part of fornix (Arnold, 1838b), see **cingulum (Burdach, 1822)**
peripheric portion of fifth pair of nerves (Todd, 1836–1839), see **trigeminal nerve branches (Winslow, 1733)**
perirhinal area (Brodmann, 1909), see **medial occipitotemporal gyrus (>1840)**
periventricular bundle of hypothalamus (>1840)
periventricular bundle of thalamus (>1840)
periventricular hypothalamic zone (Nauta & Haymaker, 1969)
peroneal branch of femoro-popliteal nerve (Quain, 1837), see **common fibular nerve (>1840)**
peroneal branch of great femoro-popliteal nerve (Quain, 1828), see **common fibular nerve (>1840)**
peroneal branch of large sciatic nerve (Chaussier, 1809), see **common fibular nerve (>1840)**
peroneal communicating branch (Jördens, 1788), see **sural communicating branch of common fibular nerve (>1840)**
peroneal communicating nerve (Fischer, 1791), see **sural communicating branch of common fibular nerve (>1840)**
peroneal cutaneous branch of external popliteal sciatic nerve (Cruveilhier, 1836), see **lateral cutaneous nerve of calf (>1840)**
peroneal cutaneous nerve (Soemmerring, 1791), see **common fibular nerve (>1840)**
peroneal nerve (Quain, 1828), see **common fibular nerve (>1840)**
peroneal nerve (Schaarschmidt, 1750), see **common fibular nerve (>1840)**
peroneal nerve of third toe (Meckel, 1817), see **dorsal digital nerves of intermediate dorsal cutaneous nerve (>1840)**
peroneal saphenous nerve (Cruveilhier, 1836), see **sural communicating branch of common fibular nerve (>1840)**
peroneo-cutaneous nerve (Burdin, 1803), see **lateral cutaneous nerve of calf (>1840)**
peroneo-digital nerve (Burdin, 1803), see **medial cutaneous nerve of calf (>1840)**
peroniar nerve (Burdin, 1803), see **common fibular nerve (>1840)**
perpendicular fossa (Meckel, 1817), see **horizontal fissure (Malacarne, 1776)**
pes anserinus (Mayer, 1794), see **parotid plexus (Meckel, 1817)**
pes hippocampi (Bergen, 1734), see **calcarine spur (Morand, 1748)**
pes hippocampi (Diemerbroeck, 1672), see **fimbria (Honegger, 1890)**
pes hippocampi (Malacarne, 1780), see **cerebral cortex (>1840)**
pes hippocampi (Riolan, 1618), see **hippocampal region (Swanson et al., 1987)**
pes hippopotami major (Mayer, 1779), see **hippocampal region (Swanson et al., 1987)**
pes hippopotami major & anterior (Günther, 1786), see **hippocampal region (Swanson et al., 1987)**
pes hippopotami minor (Mayer, 1779), see **calcarine spur (Morand, 1748)**
petioli glandulae pinealis (Haller, 1762), see **medullary stria (Wenzel & Wenzel, 1812)**
petrosal branch of glossopharyngeal nerves (Kilian, 1822), see **tympanic nerve (Arnold, 1834)**
petrosal ganglion (Wrisberg, 1786), see **distal glossopharyngeal ganglion (>1840)**
petrosal ganglion of eighth nerve of head (Andersch & Soemmerring, 1792), see **distal glossopharyngeal ganglion (>1840)**
petrosal nerve (Schaarschmidt, 1750), see **greater petrosal nerve (>1840)**
petrosal neuronode (Kilian, 1822), see **distal glossopharyngeal ganglion (>1840)**
petrosal small ganglion (Andersch, 1797), see **distal glossopharyngeal ganglion (>1840)**
petrous branch of posterior branch of spheno-palatine ganglion (Quain & Wilson, 1839), see **greater petrosal nerve (>1840)**
petrous branch of Vidian nerve (Quain & Wilson, 1839), see **greater petrosal nerve (>1840)**
petrous nerve (Günther, 1786), see **greater petrosal nerve (>1840)**
petrous part of acoustic nerve (Arnold, 1834), see **vestibulocochlear nerve trunk (>1840)**
petrous part of auditory nerve (Arnold, 1834), see **vestibulocochlear nerve trunk (>1840)**
petrous part of eighth pair (Arnold, 1834), see **vestibulocochlear nerve trunk (>1840)**
petrous part of facial nerve (Arnold, 1834), see **intermediofacial nerve (Strong & Elwyn, 1943)**
petrous part of glossopharyngeal nerve (Arnold, 1834), see **glossopharyngeal nerve trunk (Wrisberg, 1786; Günther, 1786)**
petrous part of hard part of acoustic nerve (Arnold, 1834), see **intermediofacial nerve (Strong & Elwyn, 1943)**
petrous part of middle sympathetic nerve (Arnold, 1834), see **intermediofacial nerve (Strong & Elwyn, 1943)**

petrous part of ninth pair (Arnold, 1834), see ***glossopharyngeal nerve trunk (Wrisberg, 1786; Günther, 1786)***
petrous part of pneumogastric nerve (Arnold, 1834), see ***vagus nerve trunk (Wrisberg, 1786; Günther, 1786)***
petrous part of seventh pair (Arnold, 1834), see ***intermediofacial nerve (Strong & Elwyn, 1943)***
petrous part of soft part of seventh pair (Arnold, 1834), see ***vestibulocochlear nerve trunk (>1840)***
petrous part of tenth pair (Arnold, 1834), see ***vagus nerve trunk (Wrisberg, 1786; Günther, 1786)***
petrous part of vagus nerve (Arnold, 1834), see ***vagus nerve trunk (Wrisberg, 1786; Günther, 1786)***
petty brain (Riolan, 1657), see ***cerebellum (Aristotle)***
pharyngeal and laryngeal part of glossopharyngeal nerve (Arnold, 1834), see ***glossopharyngeal nerve (Huber, 1744)***
pharyngeal and laryngeal part of ninth pair (Arnold, 1834), see ***glossopharyngeal nerve (Huber, 1744)***
pharyngeal branch of pneumo-gastric nerve (Quain & Wilson, 1839), see ***pharyngeal branches of vagus nerve (>1840)***
pharyngeal branch of Vidian nerve (Bock, 1817), see ***pharyngeal nerve (Bock, 1817)***
pharyngeal branch of vocal nerve (Bock, 1817), see ***pharyngeal branches of vagus nerve (>1840)***
pharyngeal branches of glossopharyngeal nerve (Neubauer, 1772)
pharyngeal branches of ninth pair trunk (Arnold, 1834), see ***pharyngeal branches of glossopharyngeal nerve (Neubauer, 1772)***
pharyngeal branches of recurrent laryngeal nerve (>1840)
pharyngeal branches of recurrent nerve (Meckel, 1817), see ***pharyngeal branches of recurrent laryngeal nerve (>1840)***
pharyngeal branches of superior cervical ganglion (Cruveilhier, 1836), see ***laryngopharyngeal branches of superior cervical ganglion (>1840)***
pharyngeal branches of superior ganglion (Chaussier, 1789), see ***laryngopharyngeal branches of superior cervical ganglion (>1840)***
pharyngeal branches of vagus nerve (Wrisberg, 1786)
pharyngeal filaments of recurrent nerve (Cruveilhier, 1836), see ***pharyngeal branches of recurrent laryngeal nerve (>1840)***
pharyngeal ganglion (Wrisberg, 1786), see ***terminal ganglia (Gaskell, 1886)***
pharyngeal nerve (Bock, 1817)
pharyngeal nerve (Meckel, 1817), see ***pharyngeal branches of vagus nerve (>1840)***
pharyngeal nerve from ninth pair (Kilian, 1822), see ***pharyngeal branches of glossopharyngeal nerve (Neubauer, 1772)***
pharyngeal nerve itself (Bischoff, 1832), see ***pharyngeal branches of vagus nerve (>1840)***
pharyngeal nerve of pneumogastric (Knox, 1832), see ***pharyngeal branches of vagus nerve (>1840)***
pharyngeal nerve of vagal pair (Haase, 1781), see ***pharyngeal branches of vagus nerve (>1840)***
pharyngeal nerve proper (Günther, 1786), see ***pharyngeal branches of vagus nerve (>1840)***
pharyngeal nerves (Chaussier, 1809), see ***nerves (Herophilus, c335–c280 BC)***
pharyngeal nerves (Kilian, 1822), see ***pharyngeal branches of glossopharyngeal nerve (Neubauer, 1772)***
pharyngeal nerves from eighth pair (Asch, 1750), see ***pharyngeal branches of vagus nerve (>1840)***
pharyngeal nerves from Vidian nerve (Wrisberg, 1786), see ***nerve of pterygoid canal (>1840)***
pharyngeal plexus (Cruveilhier, 1836), see ***pharyngeal plexus (Neubauer, 1772)***
pharyngeal plexus (Neubauer, 1772)
pharyngeal plexus of nerves (Todd, 1836–1839), see ***pharyngeal plexus (Neubauer, 1772)***
pharyngeal soft nerve (Andersch, 1797), see ***laryngopharyngeal branches of superior cervical ganglion (>1840)***
pharyngeal surculus of inferior maxillary branch (Bellingeri, 1818), see ***medial pterygoid nerve (>1840)***
pharyngocarotid plexus of vagus nerves (Kilian, 1822), see ***pharyngeal plexus (Neubauer, 1772)***
pharyngo-glossian pair of nerves (Burdin, 1803), see ***glossopharyngeal nerve (Huber, 1744)***
pharyngolaryngeal nerve (Bell, 1803b), see ***external branch of superior laryngeal nerve (Fyfe, 1800)***
pharyngolingual branch of glossopharyngeal nerve (Kilian, 1822), see ***pharyngeal branches of glossopharyngeal nerve (Neubauer, 1772)***
phrenic branch of cervical plexus (Cloquet, 1816), see ***phrenic nerve (Galen, c173)***
phrenic ganglia (Walter, 1783)
phrenic nerve (Galen, c173)
phrenic nerve cerebral roots (Günther, 1786), see ***phrenic nerve (Galen, c173)***
phrenic nerve spinal roots (Günther, 1786), see ***phrenic nerve (Galen, c173)***
phrenic nerve trunk (Neubauer, 1772), see ***phrenic nerve (Galen, c173)***
phrenic plexus (Loder, 1778)
phrenico-abdominal branches of phrenic nerve (Günther, 1786)
phrenico-hepatic ganglion (Walter, 1783), see ***phrenic ganglia (Walter, 1783)***
phrenico-hepatic plexus (Günther, 1786), see ***prevertebral plexuses (Quain, 1832)***
pia (Galen, c192)
pia-arachnoid (>1840)
pia mater (Haly Abbas or Ali ibn' ul-Abbas, d. 994), see ***pia (Galen, c192)***
pia mater (Lieutaud, 1742), see ***pia-arachnoid (>1840)***
pillar of fornix (Pourfour du Petit, 1710), see ***postcommissural fornix (Loo, 1931)***
pillar of vault (Luys, 1865), see ***postcommissural fornix (Loo, 1931)***
pillar of Vieussenian valve (Reil, 1807–1808a), see ***superior cerebellar peduncle (Procháska, 1800)***
pillars of medullary velum of cerebellum (Knox, 1832), see ***superior cerebellar peduncle (Procháska, 1800)***

pine cone-like body (Galen, c177), see **pineal gland (Galen, c192)**

pine nut (Galen, c177), see **pineal gland (Galen, c192)**

pineal body (Galen, c177), see **pineal gland (Galen, c192)**

pineal commissure (Combe et al., 1838), see **habenular commissure (>1840)**

pineal commissure (Solly, 1836), see **central nervous system white matter tracts (>1840)**

pineal gland (Galen, c192)

pineal kernel (Willis, 1664), see **pineal gland (Galen, c192)**

pineal recess (>1840)

pineal stalk (Burdach, 1822)

pineapple (Berengario da Carpi, 1522), see **pineal gland (Galen, c192)**

pine-apple kernel (Riolan, 1657), see **pineal gland (Galen, c192)**

pine-glandule (Crooke, 1615), see **pineal gland (Galen, c192)**

pine-kernel-shaped glandule (Bartholin, 1662), see **pineal gland (Galen, c192)**

pipe (Wharton, 1656), see **hypothalamus (Kuhlenbeck, 1927)**

pipe of infundibulum (Vesalius, 1543a), see **pituitary gland (>1840)**

piriform area (Smith, 1919)

piriform cortex (>1840), see **piriform area (Smith, 1919)**

piriform eminence (Laurencet, 1825), see **limbic region (>1840)**

piriform protuberance (Treviranus, 1820), see **limbic region (>1840)**

piriformis nerve (>1840)

pisiform tubercles (Burdin, 1803), see **mammillary body (Ludwig, 1779)**

pith (Crooke, 1615), see **cerebrospinal trunk (>1840)**

pith (Willis, 1664), see **central nervous system (Carus, 1814)**

pith of back (Hall, 1565), see **spinal cord (Galen, c162–c166)**

pith of back-bone (Salmon, 1714), see **spinal cord (Galen, c162–c166)**

pith of spine (Diemerbroeck, 1689), see **spinal cord (Galen, c162–c166)**

pith passing through vertebres of neck (Diemerbroeck, 1689), see **cervical part of spinal cord (>1840)**

pituitary (Galen, c192), see **pituitary gland (>1840)**

pituitary body (Quain, 1834), see **pituitary gland (>1840)**

pituitary cerebral gland (Günther, 1786), see **pituitary gland (>1840)**

pituitary flask (Vesalius, 1555), see **hypothalamus (Kuhlenbeck, 1927)**

pituitary gland (Galen, c192), see **pituitary gland (>1840)**

pituitary gland (>1840)

pituitary glandule (Crooke, 1615), see **pituitary gland (>1840)**

pituitary kernel (Willis, 1664), see **pituitary gland (>1840)**

pituitary peduncle (Burdin, 1803), see **hypothalamus (Kuhlenbeck, 1927)**

pituitary stalk (Lieutaud, 1742), see **pituitary gland (>1840)**

plaited margin of pedes hippocampi (Fyfe, 1800), see **dentate gyrus (>1840)**

plantar branch of plantar internal collateral nerve of big toe (Cruveilhier, 1836), see **proper plantar digital nerves of medial plantar nerve (>1840)**

plantar cutaneous nerve (Cruveilhier, 1836), see **medial plantar nerve (>1840)**

plantar cutaneous nerves (Günther, 1786), see **tibial nerve (Haase, 1781)**

plantar digital nerves (Bock, 1827), see **tibial nerve (Haase, 1781)**

plantar internal collateral nerve of big toe (Cruveilhier, 1836), see **proper plantar digital nerves of medial plantar nerve (>1840)**

plantar nerve (Haase, 1781), see **tibial nerve (Haase, 1781)**

plantar nerves of external plantar nerve (Meckel, 1817), see **common plantar digital nerves of lateral plantar nerve (>1840)**

plantar nerves of internal plantar nerve (Meckel, 1817), see **common plantar digital nerves of medial plantar nerve (>1840)**

planum temporale (>1840), see **temporal plane (>1840)**

plates (Perrault, 1688), see **cerebellar cortex (Willis, 1664)**

pleated capsule of olivary eminence (Cloquet, 1828), see **amiculum of olive (>1840)**

plexiform filaments surround carotid artery (Winslow, 1733), see **internal carotid plexus (>1840)**

plexu coeliaco (Haller, 1762), see **celiac plexus (Winslow, 1733)**

plexu pancreatico-duodenali (Wrisberg, 1800), see **pancreaticoduodenal plexus (Wrisberg, 1800)**

plexum circa oesophagum (Ludwig, 1772), see **esophageal plexus (Haller, 1762)**

plexum coeliacum (Haase, 1781), see **celiac plexus (Winslow, 1733)**

plexum coronariostomachicum posteriorem (Haase, 1781), see **left gastric plexus (>1840)**

plexum gulae (Soemmerring, 1798), see **esophageal plexus (Haller, 1762)**

plexum gulae priorem (Soemmerring, 1798), see **anterior esophageal plexus (Haller, 1762)**

plexum hypogastricum inferiorem (Tiedemann, 1822), see **inferior hypogastric plexus (Tiedemann, 1822)**

plexum hypogastricum superiorem (Tiedemann, 1822), see **superior hypogastric plexus (Tiedemann, 1822)**

plexum ischiadicum (Camper, 1762), see **sacral plexus (Vesalius, 1543a)**

plexum mesaraicum inferiorem (Ludwig, 1772), see **inferior mesenteric plexus (Rau, 1720)**

plexum mesenterico inferiore (Haase, 1781), see **inferior mesenteric plexus (Rau, 1720)**

plexum phrenicum (Loder, 1778), see **phrenic plexus (Loder, 1778)**

plexum pulmonalem anteriorem (Haase, 1781), see **anterior pulmonary plexus (Haller, 1762)**

plexum pulmonalem anteriorem minorem octavi (Scarpa, 1794), see **anterior pulmonary plexus (Haller, 1762)**

plexum pulmonalem posteriorem (Haase, 1781), see **posterior pulmonary plexus (Haller, 1762)**

plexum spermaticum inferiorem interiorem (Soemmerring, 1798), see **superior testicular nerves (>1840)**

plexure of costals (Vesling, 1647), see **superior mesenteric plexus (Rau, 1720)**

plexure of nerves between two kidneys (Diemerbroeck, 1672), see **peripheral nervous system (Meckel, 1817)** *plexus (Falloppio, 1561)*, see ***peripheral ganglia (>1840)***

plexus (Galen, c192)

plexus anserinus (Arnold, 1834), see ***parotid plexus (Meckel, 1817)***

plexus around vertebral artery (Wrisberg, 1786), see ***vertebral plexus (Cloquet, 1816)***

plexus brachialis (Camper, 1760), see ***brachial plexus (Camper, 1760)***

plexus caeliacus (Winslow, 1733), see ***celiac plexus (Winslow, 1733)***

plexus cardiacus (Keill, 1698), see ***cardiac plexus (Keill, 1698)***

plexus carotidien primitif (Cloquet, 1816), see ***common carotid plexus (Cloquet, 1816)***

plexus choreformes (Bauhin, 1605), see ***choroid plexus (Galen, c177)***

plexus choriformis (Günther, 1531), see ***choroid plexus of lateral ventricle (Vicq d'Azyr, 1784)***

plexus chorioïdei ventriculi quarti (Burdach, 1822), see ***choroid plexus of fourth ventricle (Vieussens, 1684)***

plexus choroidei medii pars, thalamus incumbens (Soemmerring, 1778), see ***choroid plexus of third ventricle (Vicq d'Azyr, 1784)***

plexus choroides (Galen, c177), see ***choroid plexus (Galen, c177)***

plexus choroïdes quartus ventriculus (Vieussens, 1684), see ***choroid plexus of fourth ventricle (Vieussens, 1684)***

plexus choroideus (Galen, c177), see ***choroid plexus (Galen, c177)***

plexus choroideus impar (Haase, 1781), see ***choroid membrane of third ventricle (>1840)***

plexus choroideus medius (Haase, 1781), see ***choroid membrane of third ventricle (>1840)***

plexus choroideus tertius (Haase, 1781), see ***choroid membrane of third ventricle (>1840)***

plexus choroideus ventriculi quarti (>1840), see ***choroid plexus of fourth ventricle (Vieussens, 1684)***

plexus communis (Meckel, 1817), see ***celiac plexus (Winslow, 1733)***

plexus coriformes (Bauhin, 1605), see ***choroid plexus (Galen, c177)***

plexus coronarii (Meckel, 1817), see ***coronary plexuses (Meckel, 1817)***

plexus coronarii sinistri (Scarpa, 1794), see ***left coronary plexus (Scarpa, 1794)***

plexus coronarius dexter (Scarpa, 1794), see ***right coronary plexus (Scarpa, 1794)***

plexus coronarius stomachicus (Winslow, 1733), see ***prevertebral plexuses (Quain, 1832)***

plexus cysticus (Wrisberg, 1808), see ***cystic plexus (Wrisberg, 1808)***

plexus déférentiel (Cruveilhier, 1836), see ***deferential plexus (Cruveilhier, 1836)***

plexus ganglioformes nervorum cervicalium (Vieussens, 1684), see ***cervical spinal ganglia (>1840)***

plexus ganglioformes nervorum dorsalium (Vieussens, 1684), see ***spinal nerve ganglia (Burdach, 1819)***

plexus ganglioformes nervorum lumbarium (Vieussens, 1684), see ***spinal nerve ganglia (Burdach, 1819)***

plexus ganglioformes nervorum ossis sacri (Vieussens, 1684), see ***spinal nerve ganglia (Burdach, 1819)***

plexus ganglioformes nervorum spinalem (Vieussens, 1684), see ***spinal nerve ganglia (Burdach, 1819)***

plexus ganglioformis cervicalis inferior nervis intercostalis (Vieussens, 1684), see ***inferior cervical ganglion (Vieussens, 1684)***

plexus ganglioformis cervicalis nervi octavis paris (Vieussens, 1684), see ***distal vagal ganglion (>1840)***

plexus ganglioformis hordeiformes (Vieussens, 1684), see ***sympathetic trunk ganglia (Winslow, 1733)***

plexus ganglioformis semilunaris nervi intercostalis (Vieussens, 1684), see ***celiac ganglion (Walter, 1783)***

plexus ganglioformis thoracicus nervi intercostalis (Vieussens, 1684), see ***superior thoracic ganglion (Lieutaud, 1742)***

plexus gastro-epiploicus dexter (Wrisberg, 1800), see ***right gastroepiploic plexus (Wrisberg, 1800)***

plexus gastro-epiploicus sinister (Wrisberg, 1800), see ***left gastroepiploic plexus (Wrisberg, 1800)***

plexus gemini intra pelvim (Willis, 1664), see ***inferior hypogastric plexus (Tiedemann, 1822)***

plexus glandulosi (Varoli, 1573), see ***choroid plexus (Galen, c177)***

plexus hepaticus (Rau, 1720), see ***hepatic plexus (Rau, 1720)***

plexus iliacus (>1840), see ***iliac plexus (>1840)***

plexus in neck (Vesalius, 1543a), see ***brachial plexus (Camper, 1760)***

plexus intraparotideus (>1840), see ***parotid plexus (Meckel, 1817)***

plexus medius (Meckel, 1817), see ***inferior mesenteric plexus (Rau, 1720)***

plexus mesaraicus inferior (Schaarsschmidt, 1750), see ***inferior mesenteric plexus (Rau, 1720)***

plexus mesaraicus superior (Schaarsschmidt, 1750), see ***superior mesenteric plexus (Rau, 1720)***

plexus mesenterici (Willis, 1664), see ***peripheral nervous system (Meckel, 1817)***

plexus mesentericos infimus (Vieussens, 1684), see ***inferior hypogastric plexus (Tiedemann, 1822)***

plexus mesentericus infimum (Haller, 1762), see ***inferior hypogastric plexus (Tiedemann, 1822)***

plexus mesentericus magnus (Drake, 1707), see ***peripheral nervous system (Meckel, 1817)***

plexus mesentericus medius (Haller, 1762), see ***prevertebral plexuses (Quain, 1832)***

plexus mesentericus superior (Rau, 1720), see ***superior mesenteric plexus (Rau, 1720)***

plexus mesocolicus (Haller, 1762), see ***prevertebral plexuses (Quain, 1832)***

plexus nervorum gulae posterior (Soemmerring, 1798), see ***posterior esophageal plexus (Haller, 1762)***

plexus nervorum gulae prior (Soemmerring, 1798), see ***anterior esophageal plexus (Haller, 1762)***

plexus nervorum iecoris dexter (Soemmerring, 1798), see ***right gastroepiploic nerves (Walter, 1783)***

plexus nervorum renum ganglioformis dexter (Soemmerring, 1798), see ***renal plexus (Drake, 1707)***

plexus nervorum renum ganglioformis sinister (Soemmerring, 1798), see **renal plexus (Drake, 1707)**
plexus nervoso-arteriosus of Walter (Cruveilhier, 1836), see **internal carotid plexus (>1840)**
plexus oesophageus (Haller, 1762), see **esophageal plexus (Haller, 1762)**
plexus oesophageus anterior (Haller, 1762), see **anterior esophageal plexus (Haller, 1762)**
plexus oesophageus posterior (Haller, 1762), see **posterior esophageal plexus (Haller, 1762)**
plexus of all nervi sacri (Winslow, 1733), see **sacral plexus (Vesalius, 1543a)**
plexus of lateral ventricles (Bell, 1803b), see **choroid plexus of lateral ventricle (Vicq d'Azyr, 1784)**
plexus of nerve pairs (Galen, c192), see **brachial plexus (Camper, 1760)**
plexus of nerves that enter arm (Vesalius, 1543a), see **brachial plexus (Camper, 1760)**
plexus of nerves traveling to leg (Vesalius, 1543a), see **lumbosacral plexus (Vesalius, 1543a)**
plexus of sixth pair (Falloppio, 1561), see **peripheral nervous system (Meckel, 1817)**
plexus of soft nerves (Bock, 1817), see **paravertebral nerves (Swanson & Bota, 2010)**
plexus of suprarenal capsule (Cruveilhier, 1836), see **adrenal plexus (>1840)**
plexus of third ventricle (Bell, 1803b), see **choroid plexus of third ventricle (Vicq d'Azyr, 1784)**
plexus on inferior thyroidal artery (Swan, 1830), see **thyroid branches of middle cervical ganglion (>1840)**
plexus on third nerve (Swan, 1830), see **peripheral nervous system white matter tracts (>1840)**
plexus ovarique (Cruveilhier, 1836), see **ovarian plexus (Cruveilhier, 1836)**
plexus pancréatique (Cruveilhier, 1836), see **pancreatic plexus (Cruveilhier, 1836)**
plexus parotideus (Meckel, 1817), see **parotid plexus (Meckel, 1817)**
plexus pharyngeus (Neubauer, 1772), see **pharyngeal plexus (Neubauer, 1772)**
plexus pneumonicus (Drake, 1707), see **pulmonary plexus (Winslow, 1733)**
plexus préaortique (Arnulf, 1939), see **preaortic plexus (Arnulf, 1939)**
plexus pulmonaris (Winslow, 1733), see **pulmonary plexus (Winslow, 1733)**
plexus renalis (Drake, 1707), see **renal plexus (Drake, 1707)**
plexus reteformis (Geminus, 1553), see **choroid plexus (Galen, c177)**
plexus reticulares (Colombo, 1559), see **choroid plexus (Galen, c177)**
plexus retiformis (Guidi, 1611), see **choroid plexus (Galen, c177)**
plexus retiformis (Read, 1638), see **superior mesenteric plexus (Rau, 1720)**
plexus semilunaris et ganglii (Wrisberg, 1780), see **peripheral nervous system (Meckel, 1817)**
plexus splenicus (Winslow, 1733), see **splenic plexus (Palfijn, 1726)**
plexus splenique (Palfijn, 1726), see **splenic plexus (Palfijn, 1726)**
plexus stomachicus posterior (Haase, 1781), see **left gastric plexus (>1840)**
plexus stomachus (Winslow, 1733), see **prevertebral plexuses (Quain, 1832)**
plexus surrounding subclavian artery (Swan, 1830), see **subclavian plexus (>1840)**
plexus testiculaire (Cruveilhier, 1836), see **testicular plexus (Cruveilhier, 1836)**
plexus thyroïdien (Portal, 1803a), see **thyroid plexus (Portal, 1803a)**
plexus vasorum et fibrarum usus incogniti (Heister, 1717), see **rete mirabile (Herophilus, c335–c280 BC)**
plexus vertébral (Cloquet, 1816), see **vertebral plexus (Cloquet, 1816)**
plexus which resembles a goose's foot (Winslow, 1733), see **parotid plexus (Meckel, 1817)**
plicae (Willis, 1664), see **cerebral cortex gray matter (>1840)**
ploughland (Plato), see **vertebrate brain (Cuvier, 1800)**
plumula (Arnold, 1838a), see **cerebral aqueduct (>1840)**
plumula (Bergmann, 1831), see **hypothalamohypophysial tract (>1840)**
pneumogastric ganglia (Solly, 1836), see **inferior olivary complex (>1840)**
pneumo-gastric nerve (Chaussier, 1807), see **vagus nerve (Galen, c192)**
pneumogastric nerve filaments (Meckel, 1817), see **vagus nerve rootlets (>1840)**
pneumogastric nerve trunk (Meckel, 1817), see **vagus nerve trunk (Wrisberg, 1786; Günther, 1786)**
pneumo-gastric pair of nerves (Burdin, 1803), see **vagus nerve (Galen, c192)**
pneumonic branches of wandring pair (Willis, 1664), see **pulmonary branches of vagus nerve (Cloquet, 1828)**
pneumonic nerves arising from eighth pair of cerebral nerves (Albinus, 1744), see **pulmonary branches of vagus nerve (Cloquet, 1828)**
point of a pen with which we write (Geminus, 1553), see **floor of fourth ventricle (Reil, 1807–1808a)**
pointed part of scribe's quill (Vesalius, 1543a), see **floor of fourth ventricle (Reil, 1807–1808a)**
pons (Casseri, 1609), see **medulla (Winslow, 1733)**
pons (Haller, 1747)
pons (Varoli, 1573), see **pons (Haller, 1747)**
pons cerebri (Wenzel & Wenzel, 1812), see **middle cerebellar peduncle (Rolando, 1819)**
pons mammillaris (Haller, 1762), see **spinal nucleus of trigeminal nerve (>1840)**
pons of cerebellum (Varoli, 1573), see **pons (Haller, 1747)**
pons of Sylvius (Bock, 1824), see **tectum (Baer, 1837)**
pons Tarini (Solly, 1836), see **hypothalamus (Kuhlenbeck, 1927)**
pons Tarini (Vicq d'Azyr, 1786), see **interpeduncular nucleus (>1840)**
pons testibut et natibus (in quatuor ipsius extremis eminentibus) ornatus (Le Böe, 1663), see **tectum (Baer, 1837)**
pons Varolii (Bell, 1802), see **pons (Haller, 1747)**
pons Varolii (Cowper, 1698), see **brainstem (Schwalbe, 1881)**

pons Varolii (Steno, 1669), see ***pons (Haller, 1747)***
ponticulus (Arnold, 1828a), see ***trapezoid body (Treviranus, 1820)***
ponticulus (Riolan, 1649), see ***pons (Haller, 1747)***
pontine central gray (>1840)
pontine central tegmental tract (>1840)
pontine dorsal longitudinal fascicle (>1840)
pontine gray (Reil, 1809b), see ***pontine nuclei (Jacobsohn, 1909)***
pontine medial forebrain bundle (>1840)
pontine medial lemniscus (>1840)
pontine medial longitudinal fascicle (>1840)
pontine medial reticulospinal tract (>1840)
pontine nuclei (Jacobsohn, 1909)
pontine raphe nucleus (>1840)
pontine reticular nucleus (>1840)
pontine reticulospinal tract (>1840), see ***medial reticulospinal tract (>1840)***
pontine rubrospinal tract (>1840)
pontine segment of midbrain tract of trigeminal nerve (>1840)
pontine segment of spinal tract of trigeminal nerve (>1840)
pontine spinothalamic tract (>1840)
pontine sulcus (Soemmerring, 1778)
pontine superior cerebellar peduncle (>1840)
pontine tectospinal tract (>1840)
pontine ventral spinocerebellar tract (>1840)
pontine ventrolateral fascicle (>1840)
pontocerebellar bundles (>1840), see ***transverse pontine fibers (>1840)***
pontocerebellar fibers (>1840), see ***transverse pontine fibers (>1840)***
pool (Galen, c192), see ***hypothalamic part of third ventricle (Swanson, 2004)***
poop (Constantine the African, c1017–1087), see ***rhombicbrain (His, 1893b)***
poop of brain (Zerbi, 1502), see ***cerebellum (Aristotle)***
popliteal nerve (Quain, 1828), see ***tibial nerve (Haase, 1781)***
popliteal nerve (Quain & Wilson, 1839), see ***tibial nerve (Haase, 1781)***
popliteaus nerve (Monro, 1732), see ***tibial nerve (Haase, 1781)***
poroi optikoi (Herophilus, c335–c280 BC), see ***white matter tracts (Bell & Bell, 1826)***
portal plexus (Wrisberg, 1800), see ***hepatic plexus (Rau, 1720)***
portal plexus (Wrisberg, 1808), see ***hepatic plexus (Rau, 1720)***
portio dura nervi auditorii (Winslow, 1733), see ***intermediofacial nerve (Strong & Elwyn, 1943)***
portio dura paris quinti (Falloppio, 1561), see ***intermediofacial nerve (Strong & Elwyn, 1943)***
portio media inter communicantem faciei et auditivum nervum (Vicq d'Azyr, 1784), see ***intermediate nerve (>1840)***
portio mollis nervi auditorii (Winslow, 1733), see ***vestibulocochlear nerve (>1840)***
portio mollis of seventh pair of nerves arising within skull (Willis, 1664), see ***vestibulocochlear nerve (>1840)***
portio transversa, qua radices fornicis conjunctae sunt (Albinus, 1744), see ***anterior commissure (Lieutaud, 1742)***
portione inter par communicans faciei et auditorium media Wrisbergii (Soemmerring, 1778), see ***intermediate nerve (>1840)***
portiones cerebelli processus vermiformes aemulantes (Ruysch, 1728), see ***tonsil (Malacarne, 1776)***
portiones mammillares (Cortisi, 1625), see ***cerebral cortex (>1840)***
portionis durae nervi acustici ramulus stylohyoideus (Neubauer, 1772), see ***stylohyoid nerve (Meckel, 1753)***
postcentral gyrus (>1840)
postcentral sulcus (>1840)
postcingulate subregion (Brodmann, 1909), see ***posterior cingulate region (>1840)***
postclival fissure (>1840), see ***posterior superior fissure (>1840)***
postcommissural fornix (Loo, 1931)
posterior alveolar branch of superior maxillary branch (Meckel, 1748), see ***posterior superior dental nerve (Haller, 1762)***
posterior alveolar nerve (Schaarschmidt, 1750), see ***posterior superior dental nerve (Haller, 1762)***
posterior alveolo-dental nerves (Cruveilhier, 1836), see ***posterior superior dental nerve (Haller, 1762)***
posterior ampullary nerve (>1840)
posterior and external cutaneous branches of great sciatic nerve (Quain, 1832), see ***posterior cutaneous nerve of thigh (Günther, 1786)***
posterior and external tubercle of optic bed (Meckel, 1832), see ***dorsal lateral geniculate nucleus (>1840)***
posterior and inferior branch of inferior maxillary nerve (Meckel, 1817), see ***posterior branch of mandibular nerve (>1840)***
posterior and inferior dental nerve (Cruveilhier, 1836), see ***posterior superior dental nerve (Haller, 1762)***
posterior and interior cerebral ganglion (Gall & Spurzheim, 1810), see ***interbrain (Baer, 1837)***
posterior and internal cutaneous branch of small sciatic nerve (Quain, 1832), see ***posterior cutaneous nerve of thigh (Günther, 1786)***
posterior and internal cutaneous nerve (Quain & Wilson, 1839), see ***inferior clunial nerves (>1840)***
posterior and lateral part of medullary triangle (Vicq d'Azyr, 1786), see ***fimbria (Honegger, 1890)***
posterior and lateral part of vault with three pillars (Vicq d'Azyr, 1786), see ***fimbria (Honegger, 1890)***
posterior and superior cutaneous nerve (Cloquet, 1828), see ***posterior cutaneous nerve of thigh (Günther, 1786)***
posterior and superior dental nerve (Cruveilhier, 1836), see ***posterior superior dental nerve (Haller, 1762)***
posterior and superior nasal nerves (Schaarschmidt, 1750), see ***posterior superior nasal nerves (Soemmerring, 1791)***
posterior angles of cerebral trigone (Chaussier, 1807), see ***fimbria (Honegger, 1890)***
posterior angles of cerebral trigone (Cloquet, 1816), see ***fimbria (Honegger, 1890)***

posterior aortic plexus (Andersch & Soemmerring, 1792), see **preaortic plexus (Arnulf, 1939)**
posterior aperture of third ventricle (Haase, 1781), see **opening of cerebral aqueduct (>1840)**
posterior appendix of cerebellum (Willis, 1664), see **middle cerebellar peduncle (Rolando, 1819)**
posterior arches of vault (Chaussier, 1807), see **fimbria (Honegger, 1890)**
posterior articular nerve of knee (Cruveilhier, 1836), see **articular branch of tibial nerve to knee joint (>1840)**
posterior ascending superficial branch of cervical plexus (Quain, 1828), see **lesser occipital nerve (Mayer, 1794)**
posterior auricular branch of facial nerve (Cruveilhier, 1836), see **posterior auricular nerve (Meckel, 1753)**
posterior auricular branch of hard nerve (Bang, 1770), see **occipital branch of posterior auricular nerve (Arnold, 1834)**
posterior auricular branch of hard nerve (Mayer, 1794), see **posterior auricular nerve (Meckel, 1753)**
posterior auricular branchlets of facial nerve (Chaussier, 1809), see **posterior auricular nerve (Meckel, 1753)**
posterior auricular nerve (Meckel, 1753)
posterior auricular nerve (Neubauer, 1772), see **great auricular nerve (Haase, 1781)**
posterior band of cerebral protuberance (Rolando, 1825a), see **trapezoid body (Treviranus, 1820)**
posterior belly of brain (William of Saliceto, 1275), see **rhombicbrain (His, 1893b)**
posterior bigeminal bodies (Owen, 1837), see **inferior colliculus (Haller, 1762)**
posterior brachial nerve (Pietro da Cortona, 1741), see **radial nerve (Du Verney, 1697)**
posterior brachial plexus (Günther, 1786), see **brachial plexus dorsal cord (Paterson, 1887)**
posterior brachium of quadrigeminal body (Arnold, 1838a), see **brachium of inferior colliculus (>1840)**
posterior brain (Aristotle), see **cerebellum (Aristotle)**
posterior brain cell (Baer, 1837), see **primary hindbrain vesicle (Baer, 1837)**
posterior brain vesicle (Baer, 1837), see **primary hindbrain vesicle (Baer, 1837)**
posterior branch of acoustic nerve (Cloquet, 1828), see **caudal part of vestibular nerve (>1840)**
posterior branch of anterior branch of fourth pair of cervical nerves (Bang, 1770), see **lateral supraclavicular nerves (>1840)**
posterior branch of anterior commissure (Reil, 1812a), see **temporal limb of anterior commissure (>1840)**
posterior branch of auditory nerve (Soemmerring, 1791), see **caudal part of vestibular nerve (>1840)**
posterior branch of auricular nerve of third pair of cervical nerves (Meckel, 1753), see **posterior branch of great auricular nerve (Bock, 1827)**
posterior branch of auricular portion of hard part of acoustic nerve (Frotscher, 1788), see **occipital branch of posterior auricular nerve (Arnold, 1834)**
posterior branch of cardiac ganglion (Lobstein, 1823), see **cardiac plexus (Keill, 1698)**
posterior branch of cervical plexus (Quain & Wilson, 1839), see **lesser occipital nerve (Mayer, 1794)**
posterior branch of cubital nerve (Frotscher, 1788), see **ulnar nerve (Cheselden, 1726)**
posterior branch of dorsal branch of radial nerve (Cloquet, 1828), see **superficial branch of radial nerve (Martin, 1781)**
posterior branch of external cutaneous nerve (Fischer, 1791), see **lateral cutaneous nerve of thigh (>1840)**
posterior branch of external cutaneous nerve (Quain & Wilson, 1839), see **lateral cutaneous nerve of forearm (>1840)**
posterior branch of external deep branch of hard nerve (Haase, 1781), see **occipital branch of posterior auricular nerve (Arnold, 1834)**
posterior branch of external inguinal branch of lumbar plexus (Cruveilhier, 1836), see **ilio-inguinal nerve (Schmidt, 1794)**
posterior branch of fifth pair (Rau, 1694), see **mandibular nerve (>1840)**
posterior branch of great auricular nerve (Bock, 1827)
posterior branch of greater posterior auricular nerve (Bang, 1770), see **posterior branch of great auricular nerve (Bock, 1827)**
posterior branch of inferior branch of hard nerve (Meckel, 1753), see **cervical branch of facial nerve (>1840)**
posterior branch of inferior maxillary nerve (Le Cat, 1768), see **auriculotemporal nerve (Haller, 1762)**
posterior branch of internal cutaneous nerve (Loder, 1803), see **posterior branch of medial cutaneous nerve of forearm (>1840)**
posterior branch of internal deep nerve of hard nerve (Meckel, 1753), see **digastric nerve (Meckel, 1753)**
posterior branch of lachrymal nerve (Todd, 1836–1839), see **communicating branch of lacrimal nerve with zygomatic nerve (>1840)**
posterior branch of lateral cerebral sulcus (>1840)
posterior branch of lateral cutaneous branch of intercostal nerves (>1840)
posterior branch of lateral cutaneous nerve of intercostal nerve (Bock, 1827), see **posterior branch of lateral cutaneous branch of intercostal nerves (>1840)**
posterior branch of lateral pectoral cutaneous nerve (Bock, 1827), see **posterior branch of lateral cutaneous branch of intercostal nerves (>1840)**
posterior branch of lateral pectoral cutaneous nerve of intercostal nerve (Bock, 1827), see **posterior branch of lateral cutaneous branch of intercostal nerves (>1840)**
posterior branch of mandibular nerve (>1840)
posterior branch of Meckel's ganglion (Quain, 1828), see **nerve of pterygoid canal (>1840)**
posterior branch of medial cutaneous nerve (Bock, 1827), see **posterior branch of medial cutaneous nerve of forearm (>1840)**
posterior branch of medial cutaneous nerve of forearm (>1840)
posterior branch of musculo-spiral nerve (Quain & Wilson, 1839), see **deep branch of radial nerve (Martin, 1781)**
posterior branch of nerve from spinal medulla (Vesalius, 1543a), see **spinal nerve dorsal branch (Meckel, 1817)**

posterior branch of obturator nerve (Haase, 1781; Martin, 1781)

posterior branch of palatine nerve (Bang, 1770), see ***posterior palatine nerve (Günther, 1786)***

posterior branch of posterior auricular nerve (Meckel, 1817), see ***occipital branch of posterior auricular nerve (Arnold, 1834)***

posterior branch of posterior branch of auricular nerve (Meckel, 1753), see ***posterior branch of great auricular nerve (Bock, 1827)***

posterior branch of posterior terminal branch of internal saphenous nerve (Cruveilhier, 1836), see ***saphenous nerve (Haase, 1781)***

posterior branch of principal auricular nerve (Bang, 1770), see ***posterior branch of great auricular nerve (Bock, 1827)***

posterior branch of radial nerve (Cloquet, 1816), see ***deep branch of radial nerve (Martin, 1781)***

posterior branch of radial nerve (Cloquet, 1828), see ***superficial branch of radial nerve (Martin, 1781)***

posterior branch of radial nerve (Loder, 1803), see ***superficial branch of radial nerve (Martin, 1781)***

posterior branch of right superior cardiac nerve (Cruveilhier, 1836), see ***superior cardiac nerve (Neubauer, 1772)***

posterior branch of spheno-palatine ganglion (Quain & Wilson, 1839), see ***nerve of pterygoid canal (>1840)***

posterior branch of superficial branches of cervical plexus (Quain, 1832), see ***lesser occipital nerve (Mayer, 1794)***

posterior branch of superficial temporal branch of third branch of fifth pair (Meckel, 1748), see ***anterior auricular nerves (>1840)***

posterior branch of sympathetic nerve (Langenbeck, 1826–1830), see ***internal carotid plexus (>1840)***

posterior branch of third branch of fifth pair of cerebral nerves (Albinus, 1744), see ***posterior branch of mandibular nerve (>1840)***

posterior branch of vestibular nerve to ampulla of posterior semicircular canal (Langenbeck, 1826–1830), see ***posterior ampullary nerve (>1840)***

posterior branches of anal nerve (Cruveilhier, 1836), see ***inferior rectal nerves (>1840)***

posterior branches of auricular branch of cervical plexus (Cloquet, 1816), see ***posterior branch of great auricular nerve (Bock, 1827)***

posterior branches of digital nerves of median nerve (Quain & Wilson, 1839), see ***proper palmar digital nerves of median nerve (>1840)***

posterior branches of external anterior femoral cutaneous nerve (Bock, 1827), see ***lateral cutaneous nerve of thigh (>1840)***

posterior branches of third cervical pair (Winslow, 1733), see ***muscular branches of cervical plexus (Cruveilhier, 1836)***

posterior branchlets from lingual nerve to maxillary ganglion (Meckel, 1748), see ***communicating branches of lingual nerve with submandibular ganglion (>1840)***

posterior bronchial branches of pneumogastric nerve (Cruveilhier, 1836), see ***pulmonary branches of vagus nerve (Cloquet, 1828)***

posterior bundle (Monro, 1783), see ***dorsal root (Spurzheim, 1826)***

posterior bundle ganglia (Monro, 1783), see ***spinal nerve ganglia (Burdach, 1819)***

posterior bundle of anterior funiculus (Rosenthal, 1815), see ***lateral funiculus (Burdach, 1822)***

posterior bundles of spinal nerves (Swan, 1830), see ***dorsal rootlets (>1840)***

posterior cardiac nerves (Mayer, 1794), see ***gastric branches of posterior vagal trunk (>1840)***

posterior cardiac plexus (Burdin, 1803), see ***cardiac plexus (Keill, 1698)***

posterior carotid artery nerve (Andersch & Soemmerring, 1792), see ***carotid branch of vagus nerve (>1840)***

posterior cavity of lateral ventricle (Haller, 1754), see ***posterior horn of lateral ventricle (Haller, 1747)***

posterior cerebellar crus (Mayer, 1779), see ***inferior cerebellar peduncle (Günther, 1786)***

posterior cerebellar notch (Chaussier, 1807)

posterior cerebellar peduncle (Günther, 1786), see ***inferior cerebellar peduncle (Günther, 1786)***

posterior cerebellar process (Willis, 1664), see ***inferior cerebellar peduncle (Günther, 1786)***

posterior cerebral artery plexus (Chaussier, 1789)

posterior cerebral commissure (Haller, 1762), see ***posterior commissure (Winslow, 1733)***

posterior cerebral fissure (Reil, 1809b), see ***calcarine sulcus (>1840)***

posterior cerebral ganglion (Gall & Spurzheim, 1810), see ***interbrain (Baer, 1837)***

posterior cerebral lobe (Willis, 1664), see ***cerebral cortex gray matter (>1840)***

posterior cerebral prominence (Varolio, 1573), see ***cerebral cortex gray matter (>1840)***

posterior cervical ganglia (Neubauer, 1772), see ***sympathetic trunk ganglia (Winslow, 1733)***

posterior cervical plexus (Cruveilhier, 1836), see ***spinal nerve dorsal branches (Meckel, 1817)***

posterior channel of third ventricle (Vesalius, 1543a), see ***cerebral aqueduct (>1840)***

posterior choroid plexus (Desmoulins, 1825), see ***choroid plexus of fourth ventricle (Vieussens, 1684)***

posterior cineritious substance (Monro, 1783), see ***dorsal horn (>1840)***

posterior cingulate region (>1840)

posterior clinoid sinus (Vicq d'Azyr, 1786), see ***posterior intercavernous sinus (>1840)***

posterior collateral branch to thumb of radial nerve (Quain & Wilson, 1839), see ***dorsal digital nerves of radial nerve (>1840)***

posterior collateral sulcus (Bellingeri, 1823), see ***dorsolateral sulcus of spinal cord (>1840)***

posterior column descending from hemisphere (Bell, 1834), see ***central nervous system white matter tracts (>1840)***

posterior column of fornix (Demeter et al., 1985), see ***fimbria (Honegger, 1890)***

posterior column of fornix (Riolan, 1618), see ***fimbria (Honegger, 1890)***

posterior column of medullary triangle (Vicq d'Azyr, 1786), see ***fimbria (Honegger, 1890)*** *posterior column of spinal marrow (Bell, 1822)*, see **dorsal funiculus (>1840)**

posterior column of true fornix (Vieussens, 1684), see **fimbria (Honegger, 1890)**

posterior columns of vault (Chaussier, 1807), see **fimbria (Honegger, 1890)**

posterior commissure (Winslow, 1733)

posterior commissure of brain proper (Gordon, 1815), see **posterior commissure (Winslow, 1733)**

posterior common cutaneous nerve of thigh (Bock, 1827), see **posterior cutaneous nerve of thigh (Günther, 1786)**

posterior cord (Vicq d'Azyr, 1784), see **dorsal funiculus (>1840)**

posterior cord of spinal marrow (Monro, 1783), see **spinal cord (Galen, c162–c166)**

posterior cord of spinal medulla (Rolando, 1825a), see **inferior cerebellar peduncle (Günther, 1786)**

posterior coronary plexus (Scarpa, 1794), see **left coronary plexus (Scarpa, 1794)**

posterior cranial pairs (Cruveilhier, 1836), see **cranial nerves (Soemmerring, 1791)**

posterior crural nerve (Monro, 1732), see **obturator nerve (Cheselden, 1726)**

posterior crural nerve (Straus Durckheim, 1828), see **invertebrate nerves (>1840)**

posterior crural nerve (Vieussens, 1684), see **sciatic nerve (Keill, 1698)**

posterior crus of fornix (Colombo, 1559), see **fimbria (Honegger, 1890)**

posterior crus of fornix (Haller, 1762), see **fimbria (Honegger, 1890)**

posterior crus of fornix (Reil, 1812b), see **fimbria (Honegger, 1890)**

posterior crus of fornix (Vesling, 1647), see **fimbria (Honegger, 1890)**

posterior crus of gray substance (Keuffel, 1810), see **dorsal horn (>1840)**

posterior crus of lateral ventricle (Günther, 1786), see **posterior horn of lateral ventricle (Haller, 1747)**

posterior crus of spinal medulla (Arnold, 1838b), see **dorsal horn (>1840)**

posterior cutaneous branch of posterior branches of third cervical nerve (Bock, 1827), see **third occipital nerve (>1840)**

posterior cutaneous branch of sciatic nerve (Soemmerring, 1791), see **perineal branches of posterior cutaneous nerve of thigh (>1840)**

posterior cutaneous branch of spiral nerve (Swan, 1830), see **posterior cutaneous nerve of forearm (>1840)**

posterior cutaneous branches of thigh (Bock, 1827), see **perineal branches of posterior cutaneous nerve of thigh (>1840)**

posterior cutaneous nerve (Jördens, 1788), see **posterior cutaneous nerve of thigh (Günther, 1786)**

posterior cutaneous nerve of arm (>1840)

posterior cutaneous nerve of forearm (>1840)

posterior cutaneous nerve of thigh (Chaussier, 1809), see **posterior cutaneous nerve of thigh (Günther, 1786)**

posterior cutaneous nerve of thigh (Günther, 1786)

posterior cutaneous temporal branches of zygomatic nerve (Meckel, 1753), see **temporal branches of facial nerve (Swan, 1830)**

posterior cystic nerve (Mayer, 1794), see **cystic plexus (Wrisberg, 1808)**

posterior deep branch of hard nerve (Mayer, 1794), see **posterior auricular nerve (Meckel, 1753)**

posterior deep temporal branch of inferior maxillary nerve (Todd, 1836–1839), see **posterior deep temporal nerve (Arnold, 1834)**

posterior deep temporal nerve (Arnold, 1834)

posterior dental branch of superior maxillary branch (Meckel, 1748), see **posterior superior dental nerve (Haller, 1762)**

posterior dental branches of superior maxillary nerve (Quain, 1832), see **maxillary nerve (Meckel, 1753)**

posterior dental branches of superior maxillary nerve (Quain & Wilson, 1839), see **posterior superior dental nerve (Haller, 1762)**

posterior dental nerve (Meckel, 1751), see **posterior superior dental nerve (Haller, 1762)**

posterior dentar nerves (Meckel, 1832), see **posterior superior dental nerve (Haller, 1762)**

posterior descending branchlet to sphenopalatine ganglion (Meckel, 1751), see **pterygopalatine nerves (Wrisberg, 1786)**

posterior eminence (Ramsay, 1813), see **inferior colliculus (Haller, 1762)**

posterior end of lateral part of spinal ash-colored substance (Vicq d'Azyr, 1784), see **dorsal horn (>1840)**

posterior end of worm (Galen, c173), see **cerebellar vermis (Meckel, 1817)**

posterior epiglottal nerve (Andersch & Soemmerring, 1792), see **internal branch of superior laryngeal nerve (Fyfe, 1800)**

posterior esophageal plexus (Haller, 1762)

posterior ethmoidal nerve (>1840)

posterior face of cerebellar ventricle (Chaussier, 1807), see **roof of fourth ventricle (Vesalius, 1543a)**

posterior fascicle of soft nerve (Cotugno, 1760), see **caudal part of vestibular nerve (>1840)**

posterior fascicle of spinal medulla (Bellingeri, 1823), see **dorsal funiculus (>1840)**

posterior fascicles of acoustic nerve trunk (Scarpa, 1789), see **cochlear nerve (Cotugno, 1760)**

posterior fasciculus (Winslow, 1733), see **dorsal root (Spurzheim, 1826)**

posterior fasciculus of acustic nerve (Bell, 1803b), see **cochlear nerve (Cotugno, 1760)**

posterior fasciculus proprius (>1840), see **dorsal intersegmental tract (>1840)**

posterior femoral cutaneous branch of second lumbar nerve (Günther, 1786), see **lateral cutaneous nerve of thigh (>1840)**

posterior femoral cutaneous nerve (Günther, 1786), see **posterior cutaneous nerve of thigh (Günther, 1786)**

posterior femoral nerve (Fischer, 1791), see **sciatic nerve (Keill, 1698)**

posterior fibers of vagus nerve pair (Morgagni, 1719), see **vagus nerve (Galen, c192)**

posterior ligament of cerebral hemispheres (Serres, 1824–1826), see **terminal stria (Wenzel & Wenzel, 1812)**

posterior limb of corpus striatum (Willis, 1672), see **terminal stria (Wenzel & Wenzel, 1812)**

posterior limb of internal capsule (>1840)

posterior limbus of corpus striatum (Willis, 1672), see **internal capsule (Burdach, 1822)**

posterior lobe (Burdach, 1822), see **occipital region (Vesalius, 1543a)**

posterior lobe (Fyfe, 1800), see **occipital region (Vesalius, 1543a)**

posterior lobe of cerebrum (Winslow, 1733), see **cerebral cortex gray matter (>1840)**

posterior lobe of pituitary gland (Haller, 1762)

posterior lobes of cerebellum (Gordon, 1815), see **cerebellar hemisphere (Willis, 1664)**

posterior lobule of cerebellum (Chaussier, 1807), see **ansiform lobule crus I (Bolk, 1906)**

posterior lobule of median lobe of cerebellum (Serres, 1824–1826), see **cerebellar vermis (Burdach, 1822)**

posterior lobule of pituitary gland (Arnold, 1834), see **posterior lobe of pituitary gland (Haller, 1762)**

posterior long cutaneous nerve (Quain, 1828), see **sural nerve (Pietro da Cortona, 1741)**

posterior long cutaneous nerve of leg (Mayer, 1794), see **sural nerve (Pietro da Cortona, 1741)**

posterior long cutaneous nerve of tibia (Martin, 1781), see **sural nerve (Pietro da Cortona, 1741)**

posterior longitudinal fasciculus (>1840), see **dorsal longitudinal fascicle (Schütz, 1891)**

posterior longitudinal fissure (Arnold, 1838b), see **dorsal median fissure of medulla (>1840)**

posterior longitudinal groove (Tiedemann, 1816), see **dorsal median septum (>1840)**

posterior longitudinal sulcus (Arnold, 1838a), see **dorsal median sulcus of spinal cord (>1840)**

posterior mastoid branch of facial nerve (Cruveilhier, 1836), see **digastric nerve (Meckel, 1753)**

posterior median column (Cruveilhier, 1836), see **gracile fascicle (Müller, 1834)**

posterior median fissure (Gordon, 1815), see **dorsal median sulcus of medulla (>1840)**

posterior median fissure (Morgagni, 1719), see **dorsal median septum (>1840)**

posterior median furrow of spinal marrow (Mayo, 1827), see **dorsal median sulcus of spinal cord (>1840)**

posterior median sulcus (Bellingeri, 1823), see **dorsal median septum (>1840)**

posterior median sulcus of medulla oblongata (Quain, 1832), see **dorsal median sulcus of medulla (>1840)**

posterior median sulcus of spinal medulla (Rolando, 1824), see **dorsal median sulcus of spinal cord (>1840)**

posterior medullar fibers (Coiter, 1572), see **dorsal rootlets (>1840)**

posterior medullar filaments (Coiter, 1572), see **dorsal rootlets (>1840)**

posterior medullar threads (Coiter, 1572), see **dorsal rootlets (>1840)**

posterior medullary cord (Meckel, 1817), see **dorsal funiculus (>1840)**

posterior medullary nucleus of Reil (Tiedemann, 1821), see **interbrain (Baer, 1837)**

posterior medullary velum (Reil 1807–1808a), see **caudal medullary velum (>1840)**

posterior middle nasal nerve (Meckel, 1817), see **posterior inferior nasal nerves (>1840)**

posterior nasal nerves (Cruveilhier, 1836), see **posterior superior nasal nerves (Soemmerring, 1791)**

posterior nerve of lesser curvature (>1840)

posterior nerve of sixth conjugation of nerves of brain (Bauhin, 1605), see **cranial nerves (Soemmerring, 1791)**

posterior nerve of vertebral artery (Andersch & Soemmerring, 1792), see **vertebral nerve (Cruveilhier, 1836)**

posterior nervous filaments (Winslow, 1733), see **dorsal rootlets (>1840)**

posterior notch in body of cerebellum (Winslow, 1733), see **posterior cerebellar notch (Chaussier, 1807)**

posterior notch of Reil (Tiedemann, 1816), see **posterior cerebellar notch (Chaussier, 1807)**

posterior occipital horn of lateral ventricle (Cruveilhier, 1836), see **posterior horn of lateral ventricle (Haller, 1747)**

posterior occipital nerve (Quain & Wilson, 1839), see **greater occipital nerve (Haase, 1781)**

posterior olivary body (Ruysch, 1737), see **cuneate tubercle (>1840)**

posterior olive (Huber 1741), see **cuneate tubercle (>1840)**

posterior orbital gyrus (>1840)

posterior oriface of third ventricle (Schreger, 1803), see **ventricles (Hippocrates)**

posterior palatine fascicle of sphenopalatine ganglion (Bellingeri, 1818), see **posterior palatine nerve (Günther, 1786)**

posterior palatine nerve (Günther, 1786)

posterior palatine nerve (Soemmerring, 1809), see **lesser palatine nerves (Meckel, 1817)**

posterior palatine nerves (Quain & Wilson, 1839), see **palatine nerves (Schaarschmidt, 1750)**

posterior palatine nerves from Meckel's ganglion (Quain & Wilson, 1839), see **palatine nerves (Schaarschmidt, 1750)**

posterior paracentral gyrus (>1840)

posterior parolfactory sulcus (>1840)

posterior part of anterior commissure (Rolando, 1831), see **temporal limb of anterior commissure (>1840)**

posterior part of base of corona radiata (Arnold, 1838b), see **retrolentiform limb of internal capsule (>1840)**

posterior part of brain (Aristotle), see **cerebellum (Aristotle)**

posterior part of cerebral peduncle (Arnold, 1838b), see **tegmentum (Swanson, 2000b)**

posterior part of cerebrum (Galen, c177), see **occipital region (Vesalius, 1543a)**

posterior part of eighth pair (Haase, 1781), see **vagus nerve (Galen, c192)**

posterior part of inferior vermal process (Gordon, 1815), see **pyramis (Malacarne, 1776)**

posterior part of olivary fasciculus (Arnold, 1838b), see **lateral lemniscus (Bechterew, 1885b)** *posterior part of tail of medulla oblongata (Pourfour du Petit, 1710)*, see **spinal cord (Galen, c162–c166)**

posterior part of trigeminal nerve (Vicq d'Azyr, 1786; Günther, 1786), see **trigeminal nerve sensory root (>1840)**

posterior part of white substance of spinal medulla (Arnold, 1838b), see **dorsal funiculus (>1840)**

posterior partition (Pourfour du Petit, 1710), see **dorsal median septum (>1840)**

posterior pectoral nerve (Bock, 1827), see **lateral pectoral nerve (>1840)**

posterior peduncle (Cruveilhier, 1836), see **middle cerebellar peduncle (Rolando, 1819)**

posterior peduncles of trigone (Chaussier, 1807), see **fimbria (Honegger, 1890)**

posterior perforated substance (>1840), see **interpeduncular nucleus (>1840)**

posterior pillar of fornix (Paré, 1564), see **fimbria (Honegger, 1890)**

posterior pillar of fornix (Pourfour du Petit, 1710), see **fornix (Vesalius, 1543a)**

posterior pillar of fornix (Vicq d'Azyr, 1786), see **fimbria (Honegger, 1890)**

posterior pillar of fornix (Winslow, 1733), see **fimbria (Honegger, 1890)**

posterior pillar of trigone (Dejerine & Dejerine-Klumpke, 1895), see **fimbria (Honegger, 1890)**

posterior pillar of vault (Lieutaud, 1742), see **hippocampal region (Swanson et al., 1987)**

posterior pillar of vault (Longet, 1842), see **fimbria (Honegger, 1890)**

posterior pillar of vault with three pillars (Vicq d'Azyr, 1786), see **fimbria (Honegger, 1890)**

posterior pillar proper of trigone (Dejerine & Dejerine-Klumpke, 1895), see **fimbria (Honegger, 1890)**

posterior plantar cutaneous branch of tibial nerve (Bock, 1827), see **lateral calcaneal branches of sural nerve (>1840)**

posterior plexus gulae (Bell, 1803b), see **posterior esophageal plexus (Haller, 1762)**

posterior plexus of heart (Haller, 1772), see **cardiac plexus (Keill, 1698)**

posterior pontine sulcus (Günther, 1786), see **medullopontine sulcus (>1840)**

posterior portion of lateral ventricle (Cruveilhier, 1836), see **posterior horn of lateral ventricle (Haller, 1747)**

posterior portion of three-fold nerve (Swan, 1830), see **trigeminal nerve sensory root (>1840)**

posterior primary brain vesicle (Baer, 1837), see **primary hindbrain vesicle (Baer, 1837)**

posterior process (Fyfe, 1800), see **occipital region (Vesalius, 1543a)**

posterior process of ventricle (Bergen, 1734), see **posterior horn of lateral ventricle (Haller, 1747)**

posterior prolongation of cerebral protuberance (Cloquet, 1828), see **middle cerebellar peduncle (Rolando, 1819)**

posterior prolongation of lateral ventricle (Vicq d'Azyr, 1786), see **posterior horn of lateral ventricle (Haller, 1747)**

posterior prolongations of cerebellum (Meckel, 1817), see **inferior cerebellar peduncle (Günther, 1786)**

posterior pulmonary branches of pneumogastric nerve (Cruveilhier, 1836), see **pulmonary branches of vagus nerve (Cloquet, 1828)**

posterior pulmonary plexus (Haller, 1762)

posterior pulmonic plexus (Bell & Bell, 1816), see **posterior pulmonary plexus (Haller, 1762)**

posterior pulmonoaortic plexus (Andersch, 1797), see **terminal plexuses (Swanson & Bota, 2010)**

posterior pyramid (Haller, 1762), see **gracile tubercle (>1840)**

posterior pyramidal bodies (Bell, 1834), see **inferior cerebellar peduncle (Günther, 1786)**

posterior pyramidal body (Ruysch, 1737), see **gracile tubercle (>1840)**

posterior pyramidal body (Tarin, 1750), see **pyramid (Willis, 1664)**

posterior pyramidal body of medulla oblongata (Procháska, 1800), see **inferior cerebellar peduncle (Günther, 1786)**

posterior pyramidal body of Tarin (Vicq d'Azyr, 1786), see **pyramid (Willis, 1664)**

posterior quadrigeminal bodies (Tiedemann, 1821), see **inferior colliculus (Haller, 1762)**

posterior ramus of small sciatic branch (Winslow, 1733), see **lateral cutaneous nerve of calf (>1840)**

posterior ramus of Sylvian fissure (Vicq d'Azyr, 1784), see **posterior branch of lateral cerebral sulcus (>1840)**

posterior renal ganglion (>1840)

posterior renal nerve (Walter, 1783), see **least splanchnic nerve (>1840)**

posterior renal nerves (Mayer, 1794), see **intrinsic renal nerves (>1840)**

posterior root (Asch, 1750), see **dorsal root (Spurzheim, 1826)**

posterior root of fifth pair (Bell, 1829), see **trigeminal nerve sensory root (>1840)**

posterior rope of eighth pair (Winslow, 1733), see **posterior vagal trunk (Wrisberg, 1780)**

posterior scapular nerve (Mayer, 1794), see **lateral supraclavicular nerves (>1840)**

posterior scapular nerve (Monro, 1783), see **suprascapular nerve (Bang, 1770)**

posterior scrotal nerves (Mayer, 1794)

posterior semilunar notch (Tiedemann, 1816), see **posterior cerebellar notch (Chaussier, 1807)**

posterior set of primary divisions of brachial plexus (Quain, 1828), see **brachial plexus dorsal divisions (Paterson, 1887)**

posterior sinus (de Laguna, 1535), see **fourth ventricle (Galen, c192)**

posterior sinus of lateral ventricle (Tarin, 1750), see **posterior horn of lateral ventricle (Haller, 1747)**

posterior small cerebral commissure (Meckel, 1817), see **posterior commissure (Winslow, 1733)**

posterior spinal branches (Cruveilhier, 1836), see **spinal nerve dorsal branches (Meckel, 1817)**

posterior spinocerebellar tract (>1840), see **dorsal spinocerebellar tract (>1840)**

posterior stomachic nerve (Winslow, 1733), see **posterior vagal trunk (Wrisberg, 1780)**
posterior striate body of Vieussens (Günther, 1786), see **interbrain (Baer, 1837)**
posterior striated body (Solly, 1836), see **interbrain (Baer, 1837)**
posterior subclavicular branches (Soemmerring, 1791), see **lateral supraclavicular nerves (>1840)**
posterior subcutaneous branch of hard nerve (Meckel, 1753), see **cervical branch of facial nerve (>1840)**
posterior subcutaneous branch of intercostal branch of thoracic nerve (Bock, 1827), see **lateral cutaneous branch of intercostal nerves (>1840)**
posterior subcutaneous temporal nerve of third branch of fifth pair (Meckel, 1753), see **auriculotemporal nerve (Haller, 1762)**
posterior subthalamic decussation (Honegger, 1890), see **supramammillary decussation (>1840)**
posterior sulcus (Soemmerring, 1778), see **parieto-occipital sulcus (>1840)**
posterior superclavicular branches (Bell, 1803b), see **lateral supraclavicular nerves (>1840)**
posterior superclavicular nerves (Bell & Bell, 1816), see **lateral supraclavicular nerves (>1840)**
posterior superficial nerve of ductus arteriosus (Andersch, 1797), see **cardiac plexus (Keill, 1698)**
posterior superficial temporal nerve (Mayer, 1794), see **auriculotemporal nerve (Haller, 1762)**
posterior superior alveolar nerve (Meckel, 1817), see **posterior superior dental nerve (Haller, 1762)**
posterior superior cutaneous nerve (Knox, 1832), see **inferior clunial nerves (>1840)**
posterior superior dental branches of superior maxillary nerve (Todd, 1836–1839), see **maxillary nerve (Meckel, 1753)**
posterior superior dental nerve (Haller, 1762)
posterior superior fissure (>1840)
posterior superior lateral nasal branches of pterygopalatine ganglion (>1840), see **lateral posterior superior nasal nerves (>1840)**
posterior superior medial nasal branches of pterygopalatine ganglion (>1840), see **medial posterior superior nasal nerves (>1840)**
posterior superior nasal branches (Loder, 1778), see **posterior superior nasal nerves (Soemmerring, 1791)**
posterior superior nasal branches of Vidian nerve (Meckel, 1748), see **nerve of pterygoid canal (>1840)**
posterior superior nasal nerves (Günther, 1786), see **nerve of pterygoid canal (>1840)**
posterior superior nasal nerves (Soemmerring, 1791)
posterior supraclavicular nerves (Meckel, 1817), see **lateral supraclavicular nerves (>1840)**
posterior surface of cerebellum (Vicq d'Azyr, 1784), see **cerebellum (Aristotle)**
posterior temporal nerve of hard nerve (Meckel, 1753), see **temporal branches of facial nerve (Swan, 1830)**
posterior terminal branch of internal saphenous nerve (Cruveilhier, 1836), see **saphenous nerve (Haase, 1781)**
posterior thalamic nuclei (>1840)
posterior thalamic tubercle (Vicq d'Azyr, 1786), see **pulvinar (Burdach, 1822)**
posterior thoracic branch of brachial plexus (Cloquet, 1816), see **long thoracic nerve (Quain & Wilson, 1839)**
posterior thoracic branch of brachial plexus (Cruveilhier, 1836), see **medial pectoral nerve (>1840)**
posterior thoracic nerve (Meckel, 1817), see **long thoracic nerve (Quain & Wilson, 1839)**
posterior thoracic nerves (Günther, 1786), see **brachial plexus (Camper, 1760)**
posterior thoracic nucleus (>1840), see **dorsal thoracic nucleus (>1840)**
posterior tibial nerve (Haller, 1762), see **tibial nerve (Haase, 1781)**
posterior tibial nerve (Quain, 1828), see **tibial nerve (Haase, 1781)**
posterior tract (Bell, 1834), see **central nervous system white matter tracts (>1840)**
posterior transverse band (Rolando, 1825a), see **trapezoid body (Treviranus, 1820)**
posterior trunk of eighth pair of nerves (Wrisberg, 1780), see **posterior vagal trunk (Wrisberg, 1780)**
posterior trunk of ethmoidal nerve (Meckel, 1817), see **posterior ethmoidal nerve (>1840)**
posterior trunk of gastric and hepatic plexus (Walter, 1783), see **posterior vagal trunk (Wrisberg, 1780)**
posterior trunk of spinal nerves (Swan, 1830), see **spinal nerve dorsal branch (Meckel, 1817)**
posterior trunk of sub-occipital nerve (Swan, 1830), see **suboccipital nerve (Winslow, 1733)**
posterior tubercle (Winslow, 1733), see **inferior colliculus (Haller, 1762)**
posterior twig of deep branch of peroneal nerve (Jördens, 1788), see **muscular branches of deep fibular nerve (>1840)**
posterior twig of great cervical auricular nerve (Soemmerring, 1791), see **posterior branch of great auricular nerve (Bock, 1827)**
posterior twig of posterior branch of auditory nerve (Soemmerring, 1791), see **rostral part of vestibular nerve (>1840)**
posterior vagal trunk (Wrisberg, 1780)
posterior valve (Burdach, 1822), see **caudal medullary vellum (>1840)**
posterior ventricle (Galen, c177), see **fourth ventricle (Galen, c192)**
posterior ventricular aperture (Günther, 1786), see **opening of cerebral aqueduct (>1840)**
posterior ventricular oriface (Günther, 1786), see **opening of cerebral aqueduct (>1840)**
posterior vermiform appendix (Winslow, 1733), see **cerebellar vermis (Meckel, 1817)**
posterior vermiform process (Vieussens, 1684), see **cerebellar vermis (Meckel, 1817)**
posterior vesicular column (Clarke, 1851), see **dorsal thoracic nucleus (>1840)**
posterior worm (Massa, 1536), see **cerebellar vermis (Meckel, 1817)**
posterior zygomatic nerve of superior branch of hard nerve (Meckel, 1753), see **temporal branches of facial nerve (Swan, 1830)**

posterior zygomatic threads of temporal surculus (Bellingeri, 1818), see **temporal branches of facial nerve (Swan, 1830)**
posterioris plexus pulmonis (Haller, 1762), see **posterior pulmonary plexus (Haller, 1762)**
posterolateral fissure (Larsell, 1937)
posterolateral sulcus of medulla (>1840), see **dorsolateral sulcus of medulla (>1840)**
posterolateral tract (>1840), see **dorsolateral tract (>1840)**
postsubicular area (Rose & Woolsey, 1948), see **postsubiculum (Swanson & Cowan, 1977)**
postsubiculum (Swanson & Cowan, 1977)
praetibio-digital nerve (Burdin, 1803), see **superficial fibular nerve (Fyfe, 1800)**
praetibio-super-plantaris nerve (Burdin, 1803), see **deep fibular nerve (Fyfe, 1800)**
prae-vertebral part of tri-splanchnic nervous system (Quain & Wilson, 1839), see **peripheral nervous system (Meckel, 1817)**
preaortic plexus (Arnulf, 1939)
precentral fissure (>1840)
precentral gyrus (>1840)
precentral sulcus (>1840)
precingulate subregion (Brodmann, 1909), see **limbic region (>1840)**
precommissural fornix (Loo, 1931)
preculminate fissure (Smith, 1903)
precuneus (Burdach, 1822)
predorsal bundle (>1840); see **tectospinal tract (>1840)**
prefrontal area (Brodmann, 1909), see **orbital region (Rolando, 1831)**
pregenual area (Brodmann, 1909), see **hippocampal region (Swanson et al., 1987)**
prehippocampal rudiment (>1840), see **tenia tecta (Swanson, 1992)**
prelumbar ganglia (Cloquet, 1816), see **lumbar sympathetic ganglia (>1840)**
preoccipital area (Brodmann, 1909), see **occipital region (Vesalius, 1543a)**
preoccipital notch (>1840)
preolivary sulcus (>1840), see **ventrolateral sulcus of medulla (>1840)**
preoptic recess (>1840)
preparietal area (Brodmann, 1909), see **parietal region (>1840)**
prepiriform cortex (>1840), see **piriform area (Smith, 1919)**
prepyramidal fissure (Hayashi, 1924)
prepyriform area (Brodmann, 1909), see **piriform area (Smith, 1919)**
presubicular area (Brodmann, 1909), see **presubiculum (>1840)**
presubiculum (>1840)
pretectal brachium of superior colliculus (>1840)
pretectal region (>1840)
preterminal area (Brodmann, 1909), see **infralimbic area (Rose & Woolsey, 1948)**
prevertebral ganglia (Quain, 1832)
prevertebral nerves (Swanson & Bota, 2010)
prevertebral plexuses (Quain, 1832)
prima ac interior propago rami majoris posterioris (Vieussens, 1684), see **lingual nerve (Vesalius, 1543a)**
primären Hirnbläschen (Baer, 1837), see **primary brain vesicles (Baer, 1837)**
primary auditory area (>1840), see **transverse temporal gyri (Heschl, 1878)**
primary brain vesicles (Baer, 1837)
primary branch of sixth pair (Portal, 1803a), see **abducens nerve trunk (>1840)**
primary divisions of axillary plexus (Quain, 1828), see **brachial plexus divisions (Paterson, 1887)**
primary divisions of brachial plexus (Quain, 1828), see **brachial plexus divisions (Paterson, 1887)**
primary fissure (Smith, 1902)
primary forebrain vesicle (Baer, 1837)
primary ganglion of vagus nerves (Wutzer, 1817), see **distal vagal ganglion (>1840)**
primary hindbrain vesicle (Baer, 1837)
primary midbrain vesicle (Baer, 1837)
primary nerves (Gordon, 1815), see **nerves (Herophilus, c335–c280 BC)**
primary nervous ring (Anderson, 1837), see **circumoral nerve ring (Tiedemann, 1815)**
primary nervous system (Willis, 1664), see **peripheral nervous system (Meckel, 1817)**
primary origin of spinal marrow (Varoli, 1573), see **brainstem (Schwalbe, 1881)**
primary substance (Wutzer, 1817), see **white matter (Meckel, 1817)**
primary visual area (>1840)
primitive part of cerebellum (Gall & Spurzheim, 1810), see **cerebellar vermis (Meckel, 1817)**
primum nervorum par (Theophilos Protospatharios, fl. 610–641), see **cerebral cortex (>1840)**
principal anterior nerve of lesser curve (>1840), see **anterior nerve of lesser curvature (>1840)**
principal auricular nerve (Bang, 1770), see **great auricular nerve (Haase, 1781)**
principal branches of fifth pair (Meckel, 1817), see **trigeminal nerve branches (Winslow, 1733)**
principal cardiac nerve (Lobstein, 1823), see **cardiac plexus (Keill, 1698)**
principal cavity (Ridley, 1695), see **forebrain (Goette, 1873)**
principal mammillary tract (Kölliker, 1896)
principal palatine nerve (Swan, 1830), see **greater palatine nerve (Cloquet, 1816)**
principal root of facial nerve (Meckel, 1817), see **facial nerve root (>1840)**
principal root of flock (Reil, 1809c), see **floccular peduncle (Burdach, 1822)**
principal root of trigeminal nerve (Meckel, 1817), see **trigeminal nerve sensory root (>1840)**
principal sensory nucleus of trigeminal nerve (>1840)
principal splanchnic nerve (Walter, 1783), see **greater splanchnic nerve (Walter, 1783)**
principium medullae spinalis (Spiegel, 1627), see **medulla (Winslow, 1733)**
priori plexui nervorum pulmonum (Soemmerring, 1798), see **anterior pulmonary plexus (Haller, 1762)**

process from cerebellum to testes (Haller, 1762), see **superior cerebellar peduncle (Prochâska, 1800)**
process of brain (Coiter, 1572), see **spinal cord (Galen, c162–c166)**
process of greater and superior ganglion of brain (Knox, 1832), see **internal capsule (Burdach, 1822)**
process of marrow (Bartholin, 1662), see **cerebral cortex gray matter (>1840)**
processes of longitudinal striae of Reil (Rolando, 1831), see **cerebral cortex gray matter (>1840)**
processo cristato (Rolando, 1831), see **limbic region (>1840)**
processo enteriodeo cristato (Rolando, 1831), see **limbic region (>1840)**
processus á cerebello ad medullam oblongatum (Vicq d'Azyr, 1786), see **inferior cerebellar peduncle (Günther, 1786)**
processus a cerebello ad nates (Haller, 1754a), see **superior cerebellar peduncle (Prochâska, 1800)**
processus à cerebello ad testes (Vieussens, 1684), see **superior cerebellar peduncle (Prochâska, 1800)**
processus a testibus in cerebellum adscendentes (Willis, 1664), see **superior cerebellar peduncle (Prochâska, 1800)**
processus ad medullam oblongatam (Haase, 1781), see **brainstem (Schwalbe, 1881)**
processus ad medullam oblongatam (Pourfour du Petit, 1710), see **middle cerebellar peduncle (Rolando, 1819)**
processus ad medullam spinalem (Pourfour du Petit, 1710), see **inferior cerebellar peduncle (Günther, 1786)**
processus ad pontem Varolii (Günther, 1786), see **cerebral peduncle (Tarin, 1753)**
processus ad pontem Varolii (Haase, 1781), see **middle cerebellar peduncle (Rolando, 1819)**
processus ad testes (Pourfour du Petit, 1710), see **superior cerebellar peduncle (Prochâska, 1800)**
processus anceformes (Soemmerring, 1778), see **tectum (Baer, 1837)**
processus anteriores medullae oblongatae (Vieussens, 1684), see **caudate nucleus (Arnold, 1838b)**
processus arciformis (Santorini, 1724), see **ventral external arcuate fibers (>1840)**
processus cerebellares protuberantiae cerebralis (Bichat et al., 1801–1803), see **middle cerebellar peduncle (Rolando, 1819)**
processus cerebelli ad corpora quadrigemina (Soemmerring, 1778), see **superior cerebellar peduncle (Prochâska, 1800)**
processus cerebelli ad medullam (Cruveilhier, 1836), see **inferior cerebellar peduncle (Günther, 1786)**
processus cerebelli ad testes (Bell & Bell, 1816), see **rostral medullary velum (>1840)**
processus cerebelli interiores (Günther, 1786), see **superior cerebellar peduncle (Prochâska, 1800)**
processus cerebri ad medullam oblongatam (Chaussier, 1807), see **cerebral peduncle (Tarin, 1753)**
processus cerebri ad nares (Günther, 1536), see **cerebral cortex (>1840)**
processus cerebri ad pontem varolii (Chaussier, 1807), see **cerebral peduncle (Tarin, 1753)**
processus cerebri ad pontem Varolii (Haase, 1781), see **brainstem (Schwalbe, 1881)**
processus cerebri lateralis (Wenzel & Wenzel, 1812), see **Ammon's horn (Vicq d'Azyr, 1784)**
processus durae matris longitudinalem (Slevogt, 1690), see **cerebral falx (Vesalius, 1543a)**
processus durae matris posticus (Vieussens, 1684), see **cerebellar tentorium (Winslow, 1733)**
processus durae matris secundus (Vieussens, 1684), see **cerebellar tentorium (Winslow, 1733)**
processus durae matris transversus (Slevogt, 1690), see **cerebellar tentorium (Winslow, 1733)**
processus e testibus in cerebelli meditullia protensi (Willis, 1664), see **superior cerebellar peduncle (Prochâska, 1800)**
processus enteroideos (Soemmerring, 1778), see **cerebral cortex gray matter (>1840)**
processus falciformis (Mayer, 1783–1794), see **cerebral falx (Vesalius, 1543a)**
processus falciformis cerebelli (Mayer, 1783–1794), see **cerebellar falx (Günther, 1786)**
processus falciformis cerebri (Meckel, 1817), see **cerebral falx (Vesalius, 1543a)**
processus falciformis inferior (Schreger, 1803), see **cerebellar falx (Günther, 1786)**
processus falciformis major (Haller, 1762), see **cerebral falx (Vesalius, 1543a)**
processus falciformis minor (Arnold, 1834), see **cerebellar falx (Günther, 1786)**
processus falciformis superior (Haller, 1762), see **cerebral falx (Vesalius, 1543a)**
processus glandulae pinealis (Mayer, 1779), see **medullary stria (Wenzel & Wenzel, 1812)**
processus glandulosos (Soemmerring, 1778), see **mammillary body (Ludwig, 1779)**
processus lentiformes (Ridley, 1695), see **cerebral nuclei (Swanson, 2000b)**
processus longitudinalis (Mayer, 1783–1794), see **cerebral falx (Vesalius, 1543a)**
processus mamillares (Soemmerring, 1778), see **mammillary body (Ludwig, 1779)**
processus mamillares (Vesalius, 1543a), see **frontal pole (>1840)**
processus mammarum ritu protuberantes (du Laurens, 1599), see **cerebral cortex (>1840)**
processus mammillares (Bartholin, 1611), see **olfactory bulb (Weitbrecht, 1751)**
processus medullae oblongatae ad cerebrum (Cruveilhier, 1836), see **cerebral peduncle (Tarin, 1753)**
processus medullares (Casseri, 1609), see **cerebral cortex (>1840)**
processus medullares (Lancisi, 1718), see **medullary stria (Wenzel & Wenzel, 1812)**
processus medullares à cerebello ad medullam oblongatam (Vieussens, 1684), see **middle cerebellar peduncle (Rolando, 1819)**
processus medullares à cerebello ad medullam spinalem (Vieussens, 1684), see **inferior cerebellar peduncle (Günther, 1786)**

processus medullares a cerebello recta descendentes (Willis, 1664), see **middle cerebellar peduncle (Rolando, 1819)**
processus medullares è cerebello ad testes (Vieussens, 1684), see **superior cerebellar peduncle (Procháska, 1800)**
processus medullaris (Willis, 1664), see **terminal stria (Wenzel & Wenzel, 1812)**
processus natibus antepositus (Ridley, 1695), see **posterior commissure (Winslow, 1733)**
processus papillares (Bartholin, 1611), see **olfactory bulb (Weitbrecht, 1751)**
processus papillares (Soemmerring, 1778), see **mammillary body (Ludwig, 1779)**
processus perpendicularis fissurae medianae (Meckel, 1817), see **third ventricle (Galen, c173)**
processus posteriores (Bichat et al., 1801–1803), see **middle cerebellar peduncle (Rolando, 1819)**
processus transversus corpora striata conjugens (Bartholin, 1686), see **anterior commissure (Lieutaud, 1742)**
processus transversus durae matris (Haller, 1762), see **cerebellar tentorium (Winslow, 1733)**
processus versus principia nervorum opticorum (Santorini, 1775), see **brachium of inferior colliculus (>1840)**
processuum mammillarium principia (Bauhin, 1620), see **cerebral cortex (>1840)**
production of infundibulum (Winslow, 1733), see **pituitary gland (>1840)**
productiones procerae (Coiter, 1572), see **cerebral cortex (>1840)**
profound branch of exterior branch of tibial nerve (Burdin, 1803), see **deep branch of lateral plantar nerve (>1840)**
prolongations of cerebellum (Meckel, 1817), see **cerebellar peduncles (Ridley, 1695)**
prominentia lobus inferior (Burdach, 1822), see **cerebral cortex (>1840)**
prominentiae semiovales (Soemmerring, 1778), see **olive (Tiedemann, 1821)**
pronator teres branch of median nerve (Cruveilhier, 1836), see **muscular branches of median nerve (Martin, 1781)**
proper branch for soleus and flexor longus of big toe muscles (Fischer, 1791), see **muscular branches of tibial nerve (>1840)**
proper cutaneous plantar nerve (Meckel, 1817), see **medial calcaneal nerve (>1840)**
proper dorsal nerves (Monro, 1783), see **thoracic nerves (Diemerbroeck, 1672)**
proper intercostal nerve (Bell & Bell, 1816), see **intercostal nerves (Vesalius, 1543a)**
proper intercostal nerves (Monro, 1783), see **thoracic nerves (Diemerbroeck, 1672)**
proper lower maxillary nerve (Bell & Bell, 1816), see **inferior dental nerve (Meckel, 1817)**
proper palmar digital nerves of median nerve (>1840)
proper palmar digital nerves of ulnar nerve (>1840)
proper pia mater (Bell, 1803b), see **meninges (Smith Papyrus, c1700 BC)**
proper plantar digital nerves of lateral plantar nerve (>1840)
proper plantar digital nerves of medial plantar nerve (>1840)
prosencephalon (Mihalkovics, 1877), see **forebrain (Goete, 1873)**
prostatic filaments of horizontal vesical plexus (Cruveilhier, 1836), see **prostatic plexus (>1840)**
prostatic plexus (>1840)
protensiones glandulares (Soemmerring, 1778), see **mammillary body (Ludwig, 1779)**
protubérances collatérales (Meckel, 1767), see **collateral eminence (Meckel, 1767)**
protuberantia annularis Willisii (Tarin, 1753), see **pons (Haller, 1747)**
protuberantia cinereae substantiae similis (Santorini, 1724), see **olfactory bulb (Weitbrecht, 1751)**
protuberantia mammillares Santorini (Tarin, 1753), see **mammillary body (Ludwig, 1779)**
protuberantiae crurum medullae oblongatae (Ruysch, 1728), see **mammillary body (Ludwig, 1779)**
protuberantiae orbiculares (Willis, 1664), see **tectum (Baer, 1837)**
protuberantias glandulosas (Soemmerring, 1778), see **mammillary body (Ludwig, 1779)**
prow of brain (Constantine the African, c1017–1087), see **vertebrate brain (Cuvier, 1800)**
prow of brain (Willis, 1664), see **frontal region (Vicq d'Azyr, 1786)**
proximal glossopharyngeal ganglion (>1840)
proximal vagal ganglion (>1840)
proxy of brain (Massa, 1536), see **spinal cord (Galen, c162–c166)**
psalidoeides (Galen, c177), see **fornix (Vesalius, 1543a)**
psalidoeides (Massa, 1536), see **fimbria (Honegger, 1890)**
psalidoeides (Vesalius, 1543a), see **cerebral cortex white matter (>1840)**
psalloid body (Aranzi, 1587), see **fimbria (Honegger, 1890)**
psalloides (Galen, c177), see **fornix (Vesalius, 1543a)**
psalloidique corpori (Aranzi, 1587), see **fimbria (Honegger, 1890)**
psaloides (Winslow, 1733), see **dorsal hippocampal commissure (Craigie, 1925)**
psalterium (Ganser, 1882), see **hippocampal commissures (Johnston, 1913)**
psalterium (Tarin, 1750), see **dorsal hippocampal commissure (Craigie, 1925)**
pseudoganglion (>1840), see **nerve (Herophilus, c335–c280 BC)**
pterygodorsal nerve (Desmoulins, 1825), see **trigeminal nerve (Winslow, 1733)**
pterygoid branch of facial nerve (Chaussier, 1809), see **greater petrosal nerve (>1840)**
pterygoid branch of superior branch of inferior maxillary nerve (Meckel, 1748), see **medial pterygoid nerve (>1840)**
pterygoid branch of superior maxillary branch of fifth pair (Haller, 1762), see **nerve of pterygoid canal (>1840)**
pterygoid branch of third branch of fifth pair (Loder, 1778), see **lateral pterygoid nerve (>1840)**
pterygoid filament (Cloquet, 1816), see **internal carotid plexus (>1840)**

pterygoid muscle nerve (Soemmerring, 1798), see **medial pterygoid nerve (>1840)**

pterygoid nerve (Andersch & Soemmerring, 1792), see **deep petrosal nerve (Meckel, 1817)**

pterygoid nerve (Haase, 1781), see **medial pterygoid nerve (>1840)**

pterygoid nerve (Schaarschmidt, 1750), see **lateral pterygoid nerve (>1840)**

pterygoid nerve (Soemmerring, 1791), see **nerve of pterygoid canal (>1840)**

pterygoid surculus of ganglioform plexus with inferior maxillary branch (Bellingeri, 1818), see **mandibular nerve trunk (>1840)**

pterygopalatine ganglion (>1840)

pterygopalatine nerve (Bock, 1817), see **palatine nerves (Schaarschmidt, 1750)**

pterygopalatine nerves (Wrisberg, 1786)

pubic branch of greater abdominal branch of lumbar plexus (Cruveilhier, 1836), see **lateral cutaneous nerve of iliohypogastric nerve (>1840)**

pudendal nerve (Camper, 1762)

pudendal nerves (Walter, 1783), see **posterior labial nerves (>1840)**

pudendal plexus (Bock, 1827), see **sacral plexus (Vesalius, 1543a)**

pudendal scrotal nerve (Günther, 1786), see **posterior scrotal nerves (Mayer, 1794)**

pudic nerve (Bell & Bell, 1816), see **pudendal nerve (Camper, 1762)**

pulmonary branches of left superior superficial nerve (Andersch, 1797), see **pulmonary plexus (Winslow, 1733)**

pulmonary branches of vagus nerve (Cloquet, 1828)

pulmonary nerve (Andersch, 1797), see **phrenic nerve (Galen, c173)**

pulmonary nerve (Bartels, 1813), see **vagus nerve (Galen, c192)**

pulmonary nerves (Chaussier, 1809), see **pulmonary plexus (Winslow, 1733)**

pulmonary nerves (Horne, 1707), see **nerves (Herophilus, c335–c280 BC)**

pulmonary nerves (Walter, 1783), see **pulmonary branches of vagus nerve (Cloquet, 1828)**

pulmonary plexus (Winslow, 1733)

pulpous nucleus (Dutrochet, 1824), see **invertebrate brain (>1840)**

pulpy septum of third ventricle (Vicq d'Azyr, 1784), see **terminal lamina (Burdach, 1822)**

pulpy substance (Gall & Spurzheim, 1809), see **central nervous system gray matter regions (>1840)**

pulvinar (Burdach, 1822)

pupillary nerves (Pourfour du Petit, 1729), see **peripheral nervous system (Meckel, 1817)**

purse-like fissure of cerebellum (Reil 1807–1808a), see **posterior cerebellar notch (Chaussier, 1807)**

putamen (Burdach, 1822)

pyelos (Galen, c177), see **hypothalamic part of third ventricle (Swanson, 2004)**

pyelos (Vesalius, 1543a), see **hypothalamus (Kuhlenbeck, 1927)**

pyloric branches of anterior vagal trunk (>1840)

pyloric nerves (Walter, 1783), see **right gastric plexus (>1840)**

pyramid (Willis, 1664)

pyramidal body (Willis, 1664), see **pyramid (Willis, 1664)**

pyramidal body (Winslow, 1733), see **olive (Tiedemann, 1821)**

pyramidal bundle (Rolando, 1825a), see **brainstem (Schwalbe, 1881)**

pyramidal bundles (>1840), see **longitudinal pontine fibers (>1840)**

pyramidal columns (Rolando, 1824), see **gracile tubercle (>1840)**

pyramidal commissure (Arnold, 1838a), see **ventral external arcuate fibers (>1840)**

pyramidal commissure (Arnold, 1838b), see **pyramidal decussation (Reil, 1809c)**

pyramidal decussation (Reil, 1809c)

pyramidal eminence (Garengeot, 1728), see **pyramid (Willis, 1664)**

pyramidal eminence (Gordon, 1815), see **olfactory tubercle (Calleja, 1893)**

pyramidal eminence (Malacarne, 1776), see **gracile tubercle (>1840)**

pyramidal eminences (Burdin, 1803), see **medulla (Winslow, 1733)**

pyramidal fascicle (Rolando, 1825a), see **brainstem (Schwalbe, 1881)**

pyramidal fasciculus (Tiedemann, 1816), see **pyramid (Willis, 1664)**

pyramidal fibers in pons Varolii (Langenbeck, 1826–1830), see **longitudinal pontine fibers (>1840)**

pyramidal process (Collins, 1685), see **ambient gyrus (>1840)**

pyramidal process of corpus callosum (Günther, 1786), see **longitudinal striae (>1840)**

pyramidal tracts (>1840), see **longitudinal pontine fibers (>1840)**

pyramis (Malacarne, 1776)

pyramis laminosa (Malacarne, 1776), see **pyramis (Malacarne, 1776)**

pyriform (Collins, 1685), see **ambient gyrus (>1840)**

pyriform cortex (Johnston, 1923), see **piriform area (Smith, 1919)**

pyriform eminences (Burdin, 1803), see **caudate nucleus (Arnold, 1838b)**

pyriform lobe (Johnston, 1923), see **piriform area (Smith, 1919)**

pyriform lobe (>1840), see **limbic region (>1840)**

pyriform protuberance (Owen, 1837), see **cerebral nuclei (Swanson, 2000a)**

pyriform tubercles (Burdin, 1803), see **mammillary body (Ludwig, 1779)**

pyriformes prominentiae (Rolando, 1819), see **caudate nucleus (Arnold, 1838b)**

quadrangular lobe (Meckel, 1817), see **cerebellar hemisphere (Willis, 1664)**

quadrangular lobule (>1840), see **culmen (Stroud, 1895)**

quadrangular space (Zinn, 1755), see **optic chiasm (Galen, c173)** *quadrate area (Rolando, 1825a)*, see **optic chiasm (Galen, c173)**

quadrate flesh nerve from external plantar nerve (Jördens, 1788), see **muscular branches of medial plantar nerve (>1840)**

quadrigeminal bodies (Wenzel & Wenzel, 1812), see **tectum (Baer, 1837)**

quadrigeminal colliculi (Arnold, 1838a), see **tectum (Baer, 1837)**

quadrigeminal eminences (Haller, 1762), see **tectum (Baer, 1837)**

quadrigeminal protuberances (Soemmerring, 1778), see **tectum (Baer, 1837)**

quadrigeminal tubercles (Winslow, 1733), see **tectum (Baer, 1837)**

quadrilateral fovea (Malacarne, 1791), see **medullopontine sulcus (>1840)**

quadrilateral lobe (Malacarne, 1776), see **cerebellar hemisphere (Willis, 1664)**

quarter of oblong sphere of brain (Tarin, 1753), see **cerebral cortex (>1840)**

quartus brachium ingrediens nervus (Casseri, 1627), see **radial nerve (Du Verney, 1697)**

quartus crassisimus nervus (Diemerbroeck, 1672), see **radial nerve (Du Verney, 1697)**

quatuor moleculas (Willis, 1664), see **tectum (Baer, 1837)**

queren Schläfenwindungen (Heschl, 1878), see **transverse temporal gyri (Heschl, 1878)**

qui ad musculos linguae et faucium tendit (Falloppio, 1561), see **glossopharyngeal nerve (Huber, 1744)**

quintus brachium invadens nervus (Casseri, 1627), see **ulnar nerve (Cheselden, 1726)**

rachidian bulb (Meckel, 1832), see **medulla (Winslow, 1733)**

rachidian nerves (Cruveilhier, 1836), see **nervous system (Monro, 1783)**

rachidian prolongation (Burdin, 1803), see **medulla (Winslow, 1733)**

rachidian prolongation of cerebellum (Meckel, 1817), see **inferior cerebellar peduncle (Günther, 1786)**

radial branch of median nerve (Bock, 1827), see **common palmar digital nerves of median nerve (>1840)**

radial branch of muscular spiral nerve (Bell & Bell, 1816), see **superficial branch of radial nerve (Martin, 1781)**

radial branch of spinal nerve (Swan, 1830), see **superficial branch of radial nerve (Martin, 1781)**

radial cutaneous nerve (Quain & Wilson, 1839), see **posterior cutaneous nerve of forearm (>1840)**

radial dorsal nerve of auricular finger (Loder, 1803), see **dorsal digital nerves of ulnar nerve (>1840)**

radial dorsal nerve of index finger (Loder, 1803), see **dorsal digital nerves of radial nerve (>1840)**

radial dorsal nerve of middle finger (Loder, 1803), see **dorsal digital nerves of radial nerve (>1840)**

radial dorsal nerve of ring finger (Loder, 1803), see **dorsal digital nerves of radial nerve (>1840)**

radial dorsal nerve of thumb (Loder, 1803), see **dorsal digital nerves of radial nerve (>1840)**

radial nerve (Cheselden, 1726), see **median nerve (Du Verney, 1697)**

radial nerve (Du Verney, 1697)

radial nerve (Swan, 1830), see **superficial branch of radial nerve (Martin, 1781)**

radial nerve cord (>1840)

radial volar branch of thumb of median nerve (Caldani, 1813, 1814), see **proper palmar digital nerves of median nerve (>1840)**

radial volar nerve (Knox, 1832), see **superficial branch of radial nerve (Martin, 1781)**

radial volar nerve of auricular finger (Loder, 1803), see **proper palmar digital nerves of ulnar nerve (>1840)**

radial volar nerve of index finger (Loder, 1803), see **proper palmar digital nerves of median nerve (>1840)**

radial volar nerve of little finger (Caldani, 1813, 1814), see **proper palmar digital nerves of ulnar nerve (>1840)**

radial volar nerve of middle finger (Loder, 1803), see **proper palmar digital nerves of median nerve (>1840)**

radial volar nerve of ring finger (Loder, 1803), see **proper palmar digital nerves of median nerve (>1840)**

radial volar nerve of third finger (Caldani, 1813, 1814), see **proper palmar digital nerves of median nerve (>1840)**

radial volar nerve of thumb (Loder, 1803), see **proper palmar digital nerves of median nerve (>1840)**

radiant concretion (Willis, 1664), see **peripheral nervous system (Meckel, 1817)**

radiant texture (Willis, 1664), see **peripheral nervous system (Meckel, 1817)**

radiating commissure of optic lobes (Serres, 1824–1826), see **superior colliculus commissure (>1840)**

radiating nerve (Tiedemann, 1815), see **radial nerve cord (>1840)**

radiatio caudicea (Burdach, 1822), see **central nervous system white matter tracts (>1840)**

radiation of corpus callosum (Dejerine & Dejerine-Klumpke, 1895)

radiation of posterior fold of corpus callosum (Reil, 1812c), see **occipital forceps (>1840)**

radiation to ceiling of great ventricles (Carus, 1814), see **central nervous system white matter tracts (>1840)**

radical filaments of third pair (Knox, 1832), see **oculomotor nerve rootlets (>1840)**

radicles of medulla oblongata roots of accessory nerve (Meckel, 1817), see **cranial root of accessory nerve trunks (>1840)**

radio-cutaneous nerve (Burdin, 1803), see **musculocutaneous nerve (Du Verney, 1697)**

radio-digital nerve (Burdin, 1803), see **radial nerve (Du Verney, 1697)**

radio-dorsal nerve of fifth finger (Meckel, 1817), see **dorsal digital nerves of ulnar nerve (>1840)**

radio-dorsal nerve of fourth finger (Meckel, 1817), see **dorsal digital nerves of ulnar nerve (>1840)**

radio-dorsal nerve of index finger (Meckel, 1817), see **dorsal digital nerves of radial nerve (>1840)**

radio-dorsal nerve of middle finger (Meckel, 1817), see **dorsal digital nerves of radial nerve (>1840)**

radio-palmar nerve of fifth finger (Meckel, 1817), see **proper palmar digital nerves of ulnar nerve (>1840)**

radio-palmar nerve of fourth finger (Meckel, 1817), see **proper palmar digital nerves of median nerve (>1840)**

ramus meningeus recurrens nervi ophthalmici (>1840), see **tentorial nerve (Arnold, 1838a)**
ramus minor inferior nervus quintae conjugationis (Vieussens, 1684), see **maxillary nerve (Meckel, 1753)**
ramus minor superior nervus quintae conjugationis (Vieussens, 1684), see **ophthalmic nerve (Winslow, 1733)**
ramus oculo-nasalis of ophthalmic nerve (Quain, 1832), see **nasociliary nerve (Meckel, 1817; Wutzer, 1817)**
ramus phrenicus abdominalis nervus phrenicus (Günther, 1786), see **phrenico-abdominal branches of phrenic nerve (Günther, 1786)**
ramus posterior nervi auricularis magni (Bock, 1827), see **posterior branch of great auricular nerve (Bock, 1827)**
ramus profundus volaris ramus volaris nervus cubitalis (Martin, 1781), see **deep branch of ulnar nerve (Fyfe, 1800)**
ramus subcutaneous malae proprius (Günther, 1786), see **zygomatic nerve (>1840)**
ramus superficialis volaris ramus volaris nervus cubitalis (Martin, 1781), see **superficial branch of ulnar nerve (Fyfe, 1800)**
ramus tertius quinti paris fortissimus (Meckel, 1748), see **mandibular nerve trunk (>1840)**
Randwülst (Burdach, 1822), see **cerebral cortex gray matter (>1840)**
Randwülste des innern Grundbündls (Burdach, 1822), see **lingual gyrus (>1840)**
raphe (Malacarne, 1776), see **cerebellar vermis (Meckel, 1817)**
raphe (Mayer, 1779), see **longitudinal striae (>1840)**
raphe externa (Reil, 1809b), see **corpus callosum (Galen, c177)**
raphe interna (Reil, 1809b), see **corpus callosum (Galen, c177)**
raphe of annular protuberance (Vicq d'Azyr, 1784), see **pontine raphe nucleus (>1840)**
raphe of corpus callosum (Arnold, 1838b), see **medial longitudinal stria (>1840)**
raphe of corpus callosum (Winslow, 1733), see **corpus callosum (Galen, c177)**
raphe pontis (Gordon, 1815), see **pontine raphe nucleus (>1840)**
Rautenhirn (His, 1893b), see **rhombicbrain (His, 1893b)**
real origin of common motor nerve of eye (Cruveilhier, 1836), see **oculomotor nerve central rootlets (>1840)**
real origin of external ocular motor nerve (Cruveilhier, 1836), see **abducens nerve central root (>1840)**
real origin of great hypoglossal nerve (Cruveilhier, 1836), see **hypoglossal nerve central root (>1840)**
real origin of olfactory nerve (Cruveilhier, 1836), see **olfactory limb of anterior commissure (>1840)**
real origin of pathetic nerve (Cruveilhier, 1836), see **trochlear nerve central root (>1840)**
real origin of portio dura (Cruveilhier, 1836), see **facial nerve central root (>1840)**
real origin of trigeminal nerve (Cruveilhier, 1836), see **central nervous system white matter tracts (>1840)**
rear ventricle (Berengario da Carpi, 1522), see **fourth ventricle (Galen, c192)**
receptacula sellae equinae lateribus apposita (Vieussens, 1684), see **cavernous sinus (Winslow, 1733)**
recesses (Vesalius, 1543a), see **cerebral sulci (Vesalius, 1543a)**
recurrent acoustic nerve (Le Cat, 1768), see **chorda tympani (Falloppio, 1561)**
recurrent acoustico-laryngeal nerve (Le Cat, 1768), see **chorda tympani (Falloppio, 1561)**
recurrent branch of cutaneous branch of inferior gluteal nerve (Cruveilhier, 1836), see **posterior cutaneous nerve of thigh (Günther, 1786)**
recurrent branch of glossopharyngeal nerves (Kilian, 1822), see **tympanic nerve (Arnold, 1834)**
recurrent branch of sixth conjugation (Paré, 1634), see **recurrent laryngeal nerve (Albinus, 1744)**
recurrent branches of external popliteal sciatic nerve (Cruveilhier, 1836), see **muscular branches of deep fibular nerve (>1840)**
recurrent fifth nerve (Meckel, 1817), see **nerve of pterygoid canal (>1840)**
recurrent laryngeal nerve (Albinus, 1744)
recurrent lingual nerve (Le Cat, 1768), see **chorda tympani (Falloppio, 1561)**
recurrent nerve (Arnold, 1834), see **tentorial nerve (Arnold, 1838a)**
recurrent nerve (Galen, c173), see **recurrent laryngeal nerve (Albinus, 1744)**
recurrent nerve of Galen (Günther, 1786), see **recurrent laryngeal nerve (Albinus, 1744)**
recurrent nerve of psoas magnus muscle (Fischer, 1791), see **muscular branches of lumbar plexus ventral branches (>1840)**
recurrent nerves (Swammerdam, c1675), see **invertebrate nerves (>1840)**
recurrent nerves of neck (Andersch & Soemmerring, 1792), see **pharyngeal branches of vagus nerve (>1840)**
recurrent nerves of Willis (Frotscher, 1788), see **accessory nerve (Vieussens, 1684)**
recurrent occipitoauricular nerve (Peipers, 1793), see **lesser occipital nerve (Mayer, 1794)**
recurrent pterygoid nerve (Schaarschmidt, 1750), see **nerve of pterygoid canal (>1840)**
recurrent spinal nerve (Albinus, 1744), see **accessory nerve (Vieussens, 1684)**
recurrent spinal nerve of Willis (Coopmans, 1789), see **accessory nerve (Vieussens, 1684)**
recurrent Vidian nerve (Meckel, 1748), see **nerve of pterygoid canal (>1840)**
recursive nerve (Massa, 1536), see **recurrent laryngeal nerve (Albinus, 1744)**
red nucleus (Burdach, 1822)
red worm (Haly Abbas or Ali ibn' ul-Abbas, d. 994), see **choroid plexus (Galen, c177)**
reddish spot (Vicq d'Azyr, 1786), see **red nucleus (Burdach, 1822)**
reflected filament of perforating branch of intercostal branches of dorsal nerves (Cruveilhier, 1836), see

posterior branch of lateral cutaneous branch of intercostal nerves (>1840)
reflected portion of choroid plexus (Cruveilhier, 1836), see ***choroid plexus of lateral ventricle (Vicq d'Azyr, 1784)***
reflected portion of corpus callosum (Cruveilhier, 1836), see ***endbrain (Kuhlenbeck, 1927)***
reflected terminal branch of internal saphenous nerve (Cruveilhier, 1836), see ***infrapatellar branch of saphenous nerve (>1840)***
regio cingularis (Brodmann, 1909), see ***cingulate region (Brodmann, 1909)***
regio insularis (Brodmann, 1909), see ***insular region (Brodmann, 1909)***
regio occipitalis (Brodmann, 1909), see ***occipital region (Vesalius, 1543a)***
regione orbitale (Rolando, 1831), see ***orbital region (Rolando, 1831)***
reinforcing fascicle of bulb (Cruveilhier, 1836), see ***brainstem (Schwalbe, 1881)***
reins (Cruveilhier, 1836), see ***medullary stria (Wenzel & Wenzel, 1812)***
remaining hepatic nerves (Wrisberg, 1808), see ***hepatic plexus (Rau, 1720)***
renal branch of lesser splanchnic nerve (>1840)
renal ganglia (Walther, 1735)
renal infolding (Willis, 1664), see ***aorticorenal ganglion (>1840)***
renal mesenteric infolding (Willis, 1664), see ***aorticorenal ganglion (>1840)***
renal nerve (Lobstein, 1823), see ***least splanchnic nerve (>1840)***
renal nerves (Haase, 1781)
renal plexus (Drake, 1707)
respiratory nerve of face (Bell, 1821), see ***intermediofacial nerve (Strong & Elwyn, 1943)***
respiratory nerves (Bell, 1821), see ***craniospinal nerves (Herrick, 1915)***
respiratory tract (Quain, 1832), see ***central nervous system white matter tracts (>1840)***
restiform body (Günther, 1786), see ***inferior cerebellar peduncle (Günther, 1786)***
restiform eminence (Arnold, 1838a), see ***inferior cerebellar peduncle (Günther, 1786)***
restiform fascicle (Bellingeri, 1823), see ***lateral funiculus (Burdach, 1822)***
restiform fasciculus (Tiedemann, 1816), see ***inferior cerebellar peduncle (Günther, 1786)***
restiform process (Tarin, 1750), see ***inferior cerebellar peduncle (Günther, 1786)***
restraining membrane (Willis, 1664), see ***rostral medullary velum (>1840)***
rete choroïdeum (Vicq d'Azyr, 1786), see ***choroid membrane of third ventricle (>1840)***
rete mirabile (du Laurens, 1599), see ***choroid plexus of lateral ventricle (Vicq d'Azyr, 1784)***
rete mirabile (Herophilus, c335–c280 BC)
rete nervorum mollium (Haller, 1772), see ***paravertebral nerves (Swanson & Bota, 2010)***
rete nervorum mollium (Mayer, 1794), see ***nerves (Herophilus, c335–c280 BC)***
reticular broad expansion (Ridley, 1695), see ***choroid plexus of third ventricle (Vicq d'Azyr, 1784)***
reticular layer of Arnold (>1840), see ***superficial medullary lamina of subiculum (Dejerine & Dejerine-Klumpke, 1895)***
reticular part of substantia nigra (>1840)
reticular thalamic nucleus (>1840)
reticular white substance (Arnold, 1838a), see ***superficial medullary lamina of subiculum (Dejerine & Dejerine-Klumpke, 1895)***
retiform plexus (Arnold, 1834), see ***internal carotid plexus (>1840)***
retiform plexus (Galen, c173), see ***rete mirabile (Herophilus, c335–c280 BC)***
retiform plexus (Santorini, 1775), see ***trigeminal ganglion (>1840)***
retiform plexus (Varoli, 1573), see ***choroid plexus of lateral ventricle (Vicq d'Azyr, 1784)***
retiform tunic (Galen, c173), see ***retina (Herophilus, c335–c280 BC)***
retiformis (Geminus, 1553), see ***rete mirabile (Herophilus, c335–c280 BC)***
retina (Herophilus, c335–c280 BC)
retracted lobe (Arnold, 1838a), see ***cerebral cortex gray matter (>1840)***
retrograde anterior branchlet from lingual nerve to maxillary ganglion (Meckel, 1748), see ***communicating branches of lingual nerve with submandibular ganglion (>1840)***
retrograde Vidian nerve (Meckel, 1751), see ***nerve of pterygoid canal (>1840)***
retrohippocampal region (Swanson et al., 1987)
retrolentiform part of internal capsule (>1840)
retrosplenial region (Brodmann, 1909), see ***limbic region (>1840)***
retrosplenial region (>1840)
retrosubicular area (Brodmann, 1909), see ***postsubiculum (Swanson & Cowan, 1977)***
returning nerve (Willis, 1664), see ***recurrent laryngeal nerve (Albinus, 1744)***
returning or converging nervous system (Gall & Spurzheim, 1809), see ***central nervous system white matter tracts (>1840)***
returning sinew (Geminus, 1553), see ***recurrent laryngeal nerve (Albinus, 1744)***
reunion of optic nerves (Winslow, 1733), see ***optic chiasm (Galen, c173)***
reverse nerve of aorta (Andersch, 1797), see ***preaortic plexus (Arnulf, 1939)***
reverse nerve of occipital artery (Andersch & Soemmerring, 1792), see ***external carotid plexus (>1840)***
reverse nerve of superior thyroid artery (Andersch & Soemmerring, 1792), see ***external carotid plexus (>1840)***
reverse soft nerve of occipital artery (Andersch, 1797), see ***external carotid plexus (>1840)***
reverse soft nerve of superior thyroid artery (Andersch, 1797), see ***external carotid plexus (>1840)***

revolutiones (Vesalius, 1543a), see **cerebral cortex gray matter (>1840)**

rheum-kernel (Bartholin, 1662), see **pituitary gland (>1840)**

rhinal ganglion (Arnold, 1834), see **pterygopalatine ganglion (>1840)**

rhinal sulcus (>1840)

rhinocele (>1840), see **olfactory ventricle (>1840)**

rhombencephalon (His, 1893b), see **rhombicbrain (His, 1893b)**

rhombic lip (>1840)

rhombicbrain (His, 1893b)

rhomboid body (Vieussens, 1684), see **dentate nucleus (>1840)**

rhomboid body of olivary eminence (Vicq d'Azyr, 1786), see **inferior olivary complex (>1840)**

rhomboid branch of brachial plexus (Cruveilhier, 1836), see **dorsal scapular nerve (Bock, 1827)**

rhomboid cavity (Haller, 1762), see **fourth ventricle (Galen, c192)**

rhomboid cavity (Malacarne, 1776), see **floor of fourth ventricle (Reil, 1807–1808a)**

rhomboid fossa (Burdach, 1822), see **floor of fourth ventricle (Reil, 1807–1808a)**

rhomboid sinus (Jacobaeus, 1675), see **central canal (Bellingeri, 1823)**

rhomboid substance (Vieussens, 1684), see **dentate nucleus (>1840)**

rhomboid ventricle (Albinus, 1744), see **floor of fourth ventricle (Reil, 1807–1808a)**

rhomboidaea caveae (Haller, 1762), see **fourth ventricle (Galen, c192)**

rhomboidal sinus (Meckel, 1817), see **fourth ventricle (Galen, c192)**

rib nerve (Crooke, 1615), see **sympathetic trunk (Winslow, 1733)**

ribbon of Reil (Cruveilhier, 1836), see **lateral lemniscus (Bechterew, 1885b)**

ridge bone mary (Brunschwig, 1525), see **spinal cord (Galen, c162–c166)**

ridge of anterior lobe near longitudinal fissure (Gordon, 1815), see **cerebral cortex gray matter (>1840)**

Riechkolben (Carus, 1814), see **olfactory bulb (Weitbrecht, 1751)**

right and left ventricles (Vesalius, 1543a), see **lateral ventricle (Vesalius, 1543a)**

right colic plexus (>1840)

right cord of pneumogastric nerve (Meckel, 1817), see **posterior vagal trunk (Wrisberg, 1780)**

right coronary plexus (Scarpa, 1794)

right gastric nerves (Wrisberg, 1780), see **gastric branches of posterior vagal trunk (>1840)**

right gastric plexus (>1840)

right gastro-epiploic nerve (Albinus, 1744), see **posterior nerve of lesser curvature (>1840)**

right gastroepiploic nerve (Mayer, 1794), see **right gastroepiploic plexus (Wrisberg, 1800)**

right gastroepiploic nerves (Walter, 1783), see **right gastroepiploic plexus (Wrisberg, 1800)**

right gastroepiploic plexus (Wrisberg, 1800)

right genioglossus nerves (Andersch, 1797), see **lingual branches of hypoglossal nerve (Cloquet, 1816)**

right genioglossus nerves of tenth pair of nerves of head (Andersch & Soemmerring, 1792), see **lingual branches of hypoglossal nerve (Cloquet, 1816)**

right hepatic nerves (Mayer, 1794), see **hepatic plexus (Rau, 1720)**

right inferior gastric nerves (Mayer, 1794), see **right gastroepiploic plexus (Wrisberg, 1800)**

right lateral cardiac plexus (Swan, 1830), see **cardiac plexus (Keill, 1698)**

right major posterior hepatic plexus (Soemmerring, 1791), see **hepatic plexus (Rau, 1720)**

right nerve to geniohyoid muscle (Andersch & Soemmerring, 1792), see **lingual branches of hypoglossal nerve (Cloquet, 1816)**

right omental nerves (Mayer, 1794), see **right gastroepiploic plexus (Wrisberg, 1800)**

right stomach nerve (Crooke, 1615), see **posterior vagal trunk (Wrisberg, 1780)**

right superior gastric nerves (Mayer, 1794), see **right gastric plexus (>1840)**

right thoracic plexus (Swan, 1830), see **paravertebral nerves (Swanson & Bota, 2010)**

right vagus nerve (Haase, 1781), see **posterior vagal trunk (Wrisberg, 1780)**

right vagus nerve (Mayer, 1794), see **vagus nerve (Galen, c192)**

rim of mouth of ventricles (Gerdy, 1838), see **isthmus of cingulate region (>1840)**

rima (Ridley, 1695), see **hypothalamic part of third ventricle (Swanson, 2004)**

rima (Willis, 1664), see **ventricles (Hippocrates)**

rima ad infundibulum (Ridley, 1695), see **hypothalamic part of third ventricle (Swanson, 2004)**

rima transversa cerebelli (Burdach, 1822), see **transverse cerebellar fissure (Burdach, 1822)**

rima transversa cerebri (Burdach, 1822), see **inner part of transverse cerebral fissure (>1840)**

rimae (Varoli, 1573), see **vertebrate brain (Cuvier, 1800)**

rimula Tarini (Günther, 1786), see **ventral median fissure of medulla (>1840)**

rind (Bartholin, 1662), see **cerebral cortex gray matter (>1840)**

ring of gray substance (Rolando, 1825), see **periaqueductal gray (>1840)**

roof of fourth ventricle (Vesalius, 1543a)

roof of lateral ventricle (Arnold, 1838b), see **lateral ventricle (Vesalius, 1543a)**

roof of Sylvian fissure (Meckel, 1817), see **frontal operculum (>1840)**

roof of Sylvian fissure (Reil, 1809b), see **cerebral cortex (>1840)**

roof of third ventricle (>1840)

roof plate (>1840)

root fibers of third nerve (Soemmerring, 1778), see **oculomotor nerve rootlets (>1840)**

root foundation of brain (Geminus, 1553), see **vertebrate brain (Cuvier, 1800)**

root of anterior pillar of fornix (Tiedemann, 1816), see **mammillothalamic tract (>1840)**

root of anterior pillar of fornix (Winslow, 1733), see **hypothalamic postcommissural fornix (>1840)**
root of auditory nerve (Willis, 1664), see **medullary striae (Scarpa, 1788)**
root of brain (Cruveilhier, 1836), see **forebrain (Goette, 1873)**
root of fifth nerve (Bell, 1834), see **trigeminal nerve (Winslow, 1733)**
root of fifth pair of cerebral nerves (Vesalius, 1543a), see **cranial nerves (Soemmerring, 1791)**
root of fifth pair of nerves (Monro, 1783), see **trigeminal nerve (Winslow, 1733)**
root of fifth pair of nerves (Rolando, 1825a), see **spinal tract of trigeminal nerve (>1840)**
root of fifth pair of sinews of brain (Geminus, 1553), see **cranial nerves (Soemmerring, 1791)**
root of fornix (Reil, 1809b), see **mammillothalamic tract (>1840)**
root of fornix (Willis, 1664), see **hypothalamic postcommissural fornix (>1840)**
root of fourth pair of cerebral nerves (Vesalius, 1543a), see **trigeminal nerve motor root (Bell, 1829)**
root of fourth pair of sinews of brain (Geminus, 1553), see **trigeminal nerve motor root (Bell, 1829)**
root of great arch of optic nerve (Winslow, 1733), see **optic tract (Vicq d'Azyr, 1784)**
root of great body of optic nerve (Winslow, 1733), see **optic tract (Vicq d'Azyr, 1784)**
root of intercostal nerve (Meckel, 1751), see **deep petrosal nerve (Meckel, 1817)**
root of intercostal nerve (Willis, 1664), see **internal carotid nerve (>1840)**
root of nerves (Galen, c173), see **brachial plexus roots (Schwalbe, 1881)**
root of optic nerve (Galen, c192), see **optic tract (Vicq d'Azyr, 1784)**
root of peduncle (Pourfour du Petit, 1710), see **arbor vitae (Winslow, 1733)**
root of pituitary (Chaussier, 1807), see **pituitary gland (>1840)**
root of seventh pair of cerebral nerves (Vesalius, 1543a), see **hypoglossal nerve root (>1840)**
root of seventh pair of sinews of brain (Geminus, 1553), see **hypoglossal nerve root (>1840)**
root of sixth pair of cerebral nerves (Vesalius, 1543a), see **cranial nerves (Soemmerring, 1791)**
root of sixth pair of sinews of brain (Geminus, 1553), see **cranial nerves (Soemmerring, 1791)**
root of spinal marrow (Bartholin, 1662), see **vertebrate brain (Cuvier, 1800)**
root of spinal marrow (Varoli, 1573), see **vertebrate brain (Cuvier, 1800)**
root of third pair of cerebral nerves (Vesalius, 1543a), see **trigeminal nerve (Winslow, 1733)**
root of third pair of sinews of brain (Geminus, 1553), see **trigeminal nerve (Winslow, 1733)**
roots (Galen, c192), see **nerves (Herophilus, c335–c280 BC)**
roots from brain (Bartholin, 1662), see **vertebrate brain (Cuvier, 1800)**
roots from brainlet (Bartholin, 1662), see **brainstem (Schwalbe, 1881)**
roots [of accessory nerve] from medulla oblongata (Frotscher, 1788), see **cranial root of accessory nerve rootlets (>1840)**
roots of accessory nerve from spinal medulla (Frotscher, 1788), see **spinal roots of accessory nerve rootlets (>1840)**
roots of accessory nerve of Willis (Malacarne, 1791), see **accessory nerve (Vieussens, 1684)**
roots of acoustic nerve (Malacarne, 1791), see **vestibulocochlear nerve (>1840)**
roots of acoustic nerve (Rolando, 1831), see **medullary striae (Scarpa, 1788)**
roots of common motor nerve of eye (Malacarne, 1791), see **oculomotor nerve rootlets (>1840)**
roots of external motor nerve of eyes (Malacarne, 1791), see **abducens nerve rootlets (>1840)**
roots of gustatory nerve (Malacarne, 1791), see **hypoglossal nerve rootlets (>1840)**
roots of inferior masticatory nerve (Malacarne, 1791), see **mandibular nerve (>1840)**
roots of intermediate sympathetic nerve (Malacarne, 1791), see **cranial nerves (Soemmerring, 1791)**
roots of motor nerve of eye (Vicq d'Azyr, 1786), see **oculomotor nerve central root (>1840)**
roots of nerves from spinal marrow (Vesalius, 1543a), see **spinal nerve roots (Tiedemann, 1816)**
roots of obturator nerve (Walter, 1783), see **obturator nerve (Cheselden, 1726)**
roots of ophthalmic nerve (Malacarne, 1791), see **ophthalmic nerve (Winslow, 1733)**
roots of pathetic nerve (Malacarne, 1791), see **trochlear nerve (Molinetti, 1669)**
roots of portio dura of acoustic nerve (Malacarne, 1791), see **facial nerve root (>1840)**
roots of proper intercostal nerves (Monro, 1783), see **communicating branches of spinal nerves (Wutzer, 1817)**
roots of seventh conjugation (Bauhin, 1605), see **hypoglossal nerve rootlets (>1840)**
roots of sinews of marrow of back (Geminus, 1553), see **spinal nerve roots (Tiedemann, 1816)**
roots of sixth pair of nerves from brain (Galen, c192), see **cranial nerves (Soemmerring, 1791)**
roots of spinal marrow (Bartholin, 1662), see **vertebrate brain (Cuvier, 1800)**
roots of splanchnic nerve (Haase, 1781), see **paravertebral nerves (Swanson & Bota, 2010)**
roots of subocciptial nerve (Malacarne, 1791), see **suboccipital nerve (Winslow, 1733)**
roots of superior masticatory nerve (Malacarne, 1791), see **maxillary nerve (Meckel, 1753)**
roots of third pair of nerves from brain (Galen, c192), see **trigeminal nerve (Winslow, 1733)**
rostral commissure (>1840), see **anterior commissure (Lieutaud, 1742)**
***rostral fovea* (>1840)**
rostral medullary velum (>1840)
***rostral part of vestibular nerve* (>1840)**

rostral postcentral area (Brodmann, 1909), see **parietal region (>1840)**

rostrum of corpus callosum (Reil, 1809b)

rothen Kern (Burdach, 1822), see **red nucleus (Burdach, 1822)**

round attachment (Vesalius, 1543a), see **cerebellar peduncles (Ridley, 1695)**

round bundle (Burdach, 1822), see **medial longitudinal fascicle (>1840)**

round infolding (Willis, 1664, p. 285), see **ciliary ganglion (Loder, 1778)**

round infolding (Willis, 1664, p. 348), see **ganglion impar (Quain & Wilson, 1839)**

round part of marrow (Bartholin, 1662), see **vertebrate brain (Cuvier, 1800)**

round trunk (Bartholin, 1662), see **vertebrate brain (Cuvier, 1800)**

round tubercles of optic thalamus (Tarin, 1750), see **anterior thalamic nuclei (>1840)**

rubrospinal tract (>1840)

ruling principle (Galen, c173), see **vertebrate brain (Cuvier, 1800)**

Rumpfnerve (Burdach, 1819), see **sympathetic trunk (Winslow, 1733)**

Rumpfnervensystem (Burdach, 1819), see **peripheral nervous system (Meckel, 1817)**

saccular nerve (>1840)

sacral ganglia of intercostal nerve (Günther, 1786), see **sacral sympathetic ganglia (>1840)**

sacral ganglion (Walter, 1783), see **sacral sympathetic ganglia (>1840)**

sacral nerves (Benedetti, 1502), see **spinal nerves (Camper, 1760–1762)**

sacral nerves (Camper, 1760)

sacral nerves (Galen, c173), see **sacral nerves (Camper, 1760)**

sacral nerves (Vesalius, 1543a), see **spinal nerves (Camper, 1760–1762)**

sacral nerves (Winslow, 1733), see **spinal nerves (Camper, 1760–1762)**

sacral or lumbar plexus (Molinetti, 1675), see **lumbosacral plexus (Vesalius, 1543a)**

sacral part of crural plexus (Chaussier, 1809), see **sacral plexus (Vesalius, 1543a)**

sacral part of spinal cord (>1840)

sacral plexus (Vesalius, 1543a)

sacral plexus anterior branches (Meckel, 1817), see **sacral plexus ventral branches (>1840)**

sacral plexus dorsal divisions (Paterson, 1887)

sacral plexus ventral branches (>1840)

sacral plexus ventral divisions (Paterson, 1887)

sacral spinal ganglia (>1840)

sacral splanchnic nerves (>1840)

sacral sympathetic ganglia (>1840)

sagittal part of fornix (Cajal, 1904), see **hypothalamic postcommissural fornix (>1840)**

salpingo-pharyngeal threads of Vidian fascicle (Bellingeri, 1818), see **nerve of pterygoid canal (>1840)**

saphene nerve (Burdin, 1803), see **saphenous nerve (Haase, 1781)**

saphenous nerve (Haase, 1781)

satellite branch of femoral artery of accessory cutaneous branch of internal saphenous nerve (Cruveilhier, 1836), see **medial cutaneous branch of femoral nerve (>1840)**

satellite branch of saphenous vein of accessory cutaneous branch of internal saphenous nerve (Cruveilhier, 1836), see **medial cutaneous branch of femoral nerve (>1840)**

Saum des Wulstes (Soemmerring, 1791), see **fimbria (Honegger, 1890)**

scala rhythmica (Bergmann, 1831), see **medial eminence (>1840)**

scapular branch of thoracic part of tracheosubcutaneous nerves (Chaussier, 1809), see **lateral supraclavicular nerves (>1840)**

scapular nerve (Du Verney, 1697), see **brachial plexus dorsal cord (Peterson, 1887)**

scapular nerve (Monro, 1732), see **suprascapular nerve (Bang, 1770)**

scapular nerves (Günther, 1786), see **brachial plexus (Camper, 1760)**

scapulary branch of thoracic part of trachelo-cutanean plexus (Burdin, 1803), see **lateral supraclavicular nerves (>1840)**

scapulo-humeral nerve (Burdin, 1803), see **axillary nerve (Winslow, 1733)**

Scarpa's ganglion (>1840), see **vestibular ganglion (>1840)**

Scarpa's nerve (>1840), see **nasopalatine nerve (Scarpa, 1785)**

Schedelnerven (Soemmerring, 1791), see **cranial nerves (Soemmerring, 1791)**

Schläfenfläche (Heschl, 1878), see **temporal plane (Heschl, 1878)**

Schläfenfurche quer (Heschl, 1878), see **transverse temporal sulcus (Heschl, 1878)**

Schlemm's ganglion (Müller, 1837), see **coccygeal spinal ganglia (>1840)**

sciatic branch of inferior gluteal nerve (Cloquet, 1816), see **posterior cutaneous nerve of thigh (Günther, 1786)**

sciatic nerve (Keill, 1698)

sciatic nerve trunk (Günther, 1786), see **sciatic nerve (Keill, 1698)**

sciatic plexus (Cloquet, 1816), see **sacral plexus (Vesalius, 1543a)**

sciatic plexus anterior branches (Cloquet, 1816), see **sacral plexus ventral divisions (Paterson, 1887)**

sciatic plexus posterior branches (Cloquet, 1816), see **sacral plexus (Vesalius, 1543a)**

sciatic trunk (Fischer, 1791), see **sciatic nerve (Keill, 1698)**

sciatico-peroneal nerve (Winslow, 1733), see **common fibular nerve (>1840)**

sciatico-tibialis nerve (Winslow, 1733), see **tibial nerve (Haase, 1781)**

scissure des hippocampes (Gratiolet, 1854), see **hippocampal sulcus (Gratiolet, 1854)**

scolicoides (Hall, 1565), see **cerebellar vermis (Meckel, 1817)**

sconce (Bartholin, 1662), see **pons (Haller, 1747)**

scornful nerve (Burdach, 1822), see **adbucens nerve (Heister, 1717)** *scrobs ventriculi quarti (Santorini, 1775)*, see **floor of fourth ventricle (Reil, 1807–1808a)**

scrotal branch of external musculo-cutaneous nerve (Quain & Wilson, 1839), see **ilio-inguinal nerve (Schmidt, 1794)**

scrotal branch of ilio-inguinal nerve (Quain & Wilson, 1839), see **ilio-inguinal nerve (Schmidt, 1794)**

scrotal branch of ilio-scrotal nerve (Quain & Wilson, 1839), see **ilio-inguinal nerve (Schmidt, 1794)**

scrotal branch of inferior musculo-cutaneous nerve (Quain & Wilson, 1839), see **ilio-inguinal nerve (Schmidt, 1794)**

scrotal branch of internal inguinal branch of lumbar plexus (Cruveilhier, 1836), see **genital branch of genitofemoral nerve (>1840)**

scrotal branch of recurrent branch of cutaneous branch of inferior gluteal nerve (Cruveilhier, 1836), see **perineal branches of posterior cutaneous nerve of thigh (>1840)**

scrotal nerve (Martin, 1781), see **pudendal nerve (Camper, 1762)**

scyphum (Soemmerring, 1778), see **hypothalamus (Kuhlenbeck, 1927)**

scythe (Diemerbroeck, 1689), see **cerebral falx (Vesalius, 1543a)**

seahorse (Aranzi, 1587), see **hippocampal region (Swanson et al., 1987)**

seat of brain (Bannister, 1578), see **vertebrate brain (Cuvier, 1800)**

second accessory lumbar ganglion (Walter, 1783), see **intermediate ganglia (>1840)**

second anastomotic ansa of cervical nerves (Cloquet, 1828), see **communicating loops of cervical plexus (>1840)**

second and third superior labial nerves (Mayer, 1794), see **superior labial branches of infraorbital nerve (Meckel, 1748)**

second ansa cervicalis (Bock, 1827), see **communicating loops of cervical plexus (>1840)**

second ansa lumbalis (Bock, 1827), see **lumbar plexus (Vesalius, 1543a)**

second auricular branch of superficial temporal nerve (Bock, 1817), see **auriculotemporal nerve (Haller, 1762)**

second branch of anterior crural nerve to external vast and crural muscles (Swan, 1830), see **muscular branches of femoral nerve (Quain & Wilson, 1839)**

second branch of fifth pair of nerves (Meckel, 1753), see **maxillary nerve (Meckel, 1753)**

second branch of first lumbar pair (Sabatier, 1775), see **ilio-inguinal nerve (Schmidt, 1794)**

second branch of fourth branch of second division of fifth pair of nerves arising within skull (Willis, 1664), see **palatine nerves (Schaarschmidt, 1750)**

second branch of fourth conjugation of nerves of brain (Crooke, 1615), see **maxillary nerve (Meckel, 1753)**

second branch of glossopharyngeal nerve (Wrisberg, 1786), see **stylopharyngeal branch of glossopharyngeal nerve (>1840)**

second branch of lower branch of second division of fifth pair of nerves arising within skull (Willis, 1664), see **palatine nerves (Schaarschmidt, 1750)**

second branch of second division of fifth pair of nerves arising within skull (Willis, 1664), see **lacrimal nerve (Meckel, 1748; Bonhomme, 1748)**

second branch of third conjugation of nerves of brain (Crooke, 1615), see **maxillary nerve (Meckel, 1753)**

second branch of third pair (Marchetti 1652), see **maxillary nerve (Meckel, 1753)**

second branch to flexor digitorum longus muscle (Jördens, 1788), see **nerve to flexor digitorum longus (>1840)**

second cardiac branch of recurrent nerves (Mayer, 1794), see **cardiac branches of recurrent laryngeal nerve (>1840)**

second cell (Brunschwig, 1525), see **ventricles (Hippocrates)**

second cerebellar crus (Günther, 1789), see **middle cerebellar peduncle (Rolando, 1819)**

second cerebellar peduncle (Procháska, 1800), see **middle cerebellar peduncle (Rolando, 1819)**

second cerebellar process (Günther, 1789), see **middle cerebellar peduncle (Rolando, 1819)**

second cerebral cell (Wagner, 1839), see **interbrain vesicle (Baer, 1837)**

second cerebral mass (Anderson, 1837), see **tectum (Baer, 1837)**

second cervical ganglion of sympathetic nerve (Swan, 1830), see **middle cervical ganglion (Haller, 1762)**

second cervical nervous plexus (Meckel, 1817), see **cervical plexus (Molinetti, 1675)**

second common digital branch of median nerve (Caldani, 1813, 1814), see **common palmar digital nerves of median nerve (>1840)**

second communicating branch of glossopharyngeal nerve (Wrisberg, 1786), see **glossopharyngeal nerve trunk (Wrisberg, 1786; Günther, 1786)**

second cutaneous nerve at beginning of thigh (Galen, c177), see **anterior cutaneous branches of femoral nerve (Quain & Wilson, 1839)**

second cutaneous nerve of thigh (Galen, c177), see **femoral nerve (Haller, 1762)**

second deep nerve of thigh (Galen, c177), see **muscular branches of femoral nerve (Quain & Wilson, 1839)**

second dental nerve of second trunk of fifth nerve (Swan, 1830), see **middle superior dental nerve (Henle, 1871)**

second division of fifth pair (Bell, 1803a), see **maxillary nerve (Meckel, 1753)**

second division of fifth pair of nerves arising within skull (Willis, 1664), see **trigeminal nerve (Winslow, 1733)**

second dorsal ganglion (Neubauer, 1772), see **superior thoracic ganglion (Lieutaud, 1742)**

second encephalon (Galen, c173), see **spinal cord (Galen, c162–c166)**

second epiglottal branch of posterior epiglottal nerve (Andersch & Soemmerring, 1792), see **internal branch of superior laryngeal nerve (Fyfe, 1800)**

second external inferior posterior cutaneous nerve (Fischer, 1791), see **tibial nerve (Haase, 1781)**

second external lateral twig of deep branch of peroneal nerve (Jördens, 1788), see **muscular branches of deep fibular nerve (>1840)**

second–fourth shoots of uppermost branch of second division of fifth pair of nerves arising within skull (Willis, 1664), see **frontal nerve (Cheselden, 1726)**

second glossopharyngeal branch (Neubauer, 1772), see **carotid branches of glossopharyngeal nerve (Todd, 1836–1839)**
second great brachial nerve (Albinus, 1744), see **median nerve (Du Verney, 1697)**
second hippocampus (Vicq d'Azyr, 1786), see **calcarine spur (Morand, 1748)**
second inferior internal spermatic nerve (Walter, 1783), see **superior ovarian nerves (>1840)**
second internal inferior posterior cutaneous nerve (Fischer, 1791), see **tibial nerve (Haase, 1781)**
second internal lateral twig of deep branch of peroneal nerve (Jördens, 1788), see **muscular branches of deep fibular nerve (>1840)**
second internal posterior inferior cutaneous nerve (Knox, 1832), see **tibial nerve (Haase, 1781)**
second labial branch of infraorbital nerve (Bock, 1817), see **superior labial branches of infraorbital nerve (Meckel, 1748)**
second nerve entering arm (Vesalius, 1543a), see **musculocutaneous nerve (Du Verney, 1697)**
second nerve entering leg (Vesalius, 1543a), see **femoral nerve (Haller, 1762)**
second nerve entering upper arm from spine (Galen, c177), see **radial nerve (Du Verney, 1697)**
second nerve for vastus externus muscle (Fischer, 1791), see **muscular branches of femoral nerve (Quain & Wilson, 1839)**
second nerve from spine to upper arm (Galen, c177), see **axillary nerve (Winslow, 1733)**
second nerve of body (Andersch, 1797), see **phrenic nerve (Galen, c173)**
second nerve of hand (Bauhin, 1605), see **musculocutaneous nerve (Du Verney, 1697)**
second nerve of seventh pair (Vicq d'Azyr, 1784), see **vestibulocochlear nerve (>1840)**
second nerve of trunk (Andersch, 1797), see **phrenic nerve (Galen, c173)**
second nerve to extensor digitorum longus muscle (Fischer, 1791), see **muscular branches of deep fibular nerve (>1840)**
second nerve to extensor pollicis longus muscle (Fischer, 1791), see **muscular branches of deep fibular nerve (>1840)**
second nerve to flexor digitorum longus muscle (Fischer, 1791), see **nerve to flexor digitorum longus (>1840)**
second nerve to flexor longus of big toe muscle (Fischer, 1791), see **nerve to flexor hallucis longus (>1840)**
second nerve to peroneus longus muscle (Fischer, 1791), see **muscular branches of deep fibular nerve (>1840)**
second nerve to popliteus muscle (Jördens, 1788), see **nerve to popliteus (>1840)**
second nerve to right head of gastrocnemius muscle (Fischer, 1791), see **nerves to gastrocnemius (>1840)**
second nerve to short head of biceps muscle (Fischer, 1791), see **nerve to hamstring muscles (>1840)**
second nerve to soleus muscle (Fischer, 1791), see **nerve to soleus (>1840)**
second nerve to tibialis anterior muscle (Fischer, 1791), see **muscular branches of deep fibular nerve (>1840)**
second nerve to tibialis posterior muscle (Fischer, 1791), see **nerve to tibialis posterior (>1840)**
second nerve traveling to thigh (Vesalius, 1543a), see **femoral nerve (Haller, 1762)**
second of four branches of first lumbar pair (Haase, 1781), see **ilio-inguinal nerve (Schmidt, 1794)**
second offshoot of thinner root of third pair (Vesalius, 1543a), see **maxillary nerve (Meckel, 1753)**
second pair of cerebral nerves (Arnold, 1843), see **white matter tracts (Bell & Bell, 1826)**
second pair of nerves arising within skull (Willis, 1664), see **white matter tracts (Bell & Bell, 1826)**
second pair of nerves from brain (Benedetti, 1502), see **vestibulocochlear nerve (>1840)**
second pair of nerves from brain (Galen, c173), see **oculomotor nerve (Estienne, 1545)**
second pair of nerves from brain (Piccolomini, 1586), see **cerebral cortex (>1840)**
second pair of nerves from brain (Theophilos Protospatharios, fl. 610–641), see **white matter tracts (Bell & Bell, 1826)**
second pair of nerves of medulla oblongata (Haller & Wrisberg, 1780), see **vagus nerve (Galen, c192)**
second pair of sinews of brain (Geminus, 1553), see **oculomotor nerve (Estienne, 1545)**
second pair of tubercles (Steno, 1669), see **interbrain (Baer, 1837)**
second pharyngeal branch of main communicating branch of glossopharyngeal nerve (Kilian, 1822), see **pharyngeal branches of glossopharyngeal nerve (Neubauer, 1772)**
second pharyngeal nerve (Andersch & Soemmerring, 1792), see **pharyngeal branches of vagus nerve (>1840)**
second posterior inferior external cutaneous nerve (Knox, 1832), see **tibial nerve (Haase, 1781)**
second posterior inferior internal cutaneous nerve (Knox, 1832), see **tibial nerve (Haase, 1781)**
second principal branch of fifth pair (Meckel, 1817), see **maxillary nerve (Meckel, 1753)**
second process of cerebellum (Ridley, 1695), see **middle cerebellar peduncle (Rolando, 1819)**
second process of middle lobe (Rolando, 1831), see **middle temporal gyrus (>1840)**
second root of crural nerve (Günther, 1786), see **femoral nerve (Haller, 1762)**
second root of intercostal nerve (Bang, 1770), see **communicating branch from internal carotid plexus to abducens nerve (>1840)**
second root of intercostal nerves (Mayer, 1794), see **deep petrosal nerve (Meckel, 1817)**
second saphenous nerve (Fischer, 1791), see **saphenous nerve (Haase, 1781)**
second section of oblong marrow (Willis, 1664), see **interbrain (Baer, 1837)**
second sinew going to arm (Geminus, 1553), see **musculocutaneous nerve (Du Verney, 1697)**
second sinew going to thigh (Geminus, 1553), see **femoral nerve (Haller, 1762)**
second sinew of leg (Geminus, 1553), see **femoral nerve (Haller, 1762)**

second soft nerve (Andersch & Soemmerring, 1792), see **jugular nerves (>1840)**

second spinal nerve (Soemmerring, 1778), see **vagus nerve (Galen, c192)**

second subscapular branch of brachial plexus (Cloquet, 1816), see **upper subscapular nerve (>1840)**

second supraclavicular branch (Peipers, 1793), see **lateral supraclavicular nerves (>1840)**

second temporal branch of hard nerve (Meckel, 1753), see **temporal branches of facial nerve (Swan, 1830)**

second temporal nerve (Soemmerring, 1798), see **temporal branches of facial nerve (Swan, 1830)**

second terminal branch of median nerve (Cruveilhier, 1836), see **common palmar digital nerves of median nerve (>1840)**

second to sixth soft nerves from lowest (Andersch & Soemmerring, 1792), see **jugular nerves (>1840)**

second trunk of fifth nerve (Swan, 1830), see **maxillary nerve (Meckel, 1753)**

second trunk of fifth pair (Swan, 1830), see **maxillary nerve (Meckel, 1753)**

second trunk of third pair (Falloppio, 1561), see **maxillary nerve (Meckel, 1753)**

second trunk of three-fold nerve (Swan, 1830), see **maxillary nerve (Meckel, 1753)**

second twig of deep twig of deep branch of external plantar nerve to abductor pollicis (Jördens, 1788), see **deep branch of lateral plantar nerve (>1840)**

second zygomatic branch of superior branch of hard nerve (Meckel, 1753), see **temporal branches of facial nerve (Swan, 1830)**

secondary brain vesicles (>1840)

secondary branch of sixth pair (Portal, 1803a), see **abducens nerve trunk (>1840)**

secondary fissure (Bolk, 1906)

secondary ganglion of vagus nerves (Wutzer, 1817), see **vagus nerve (Galen, c192)**

secondary hindbrain (Sharpey et al., 1867), see **hindbrain (Baer, 1837)**

secondary nerves (Gordon, 1815), see **nerves (Herophilus, c335–c280 BC)**

secondary nervous system (Willis, 1664), see **peripheral nervous system (Meckel, 1817)**

secondary plexiform cord of lumboaortic plexus (Cruveilhier, 1836), see **hypogastric nerve (Walter, 1783)**

secondary splanchnic nerve (Haller, 1762), see **lesser splanchnic nerve (Haller, 1762)**

secondary substance (Wutzer, 1817), see **gray matter (Meckel, 1817)**

secondary sympathetic nerve (Walter, 1783), see **lesser splanchnic nerve (Haller, 1762)**

secondary sympathetic nerve trunk (Walter, 1783), see **lesser splanchnic nerve (Haller, 1762)**

secondary trunk (Schmidel, 1754), see **lesser splanchnic nerve (Haller, 1762)**

secondary vagal ganglion (Bischoff, 1832), see **distal vagal ganglion (>1840)**

sectors of spinal marrow (Huber, 1741), see **spinal cord (Galen, c162–c166)**

secunda ac media propago rami majoris posterioris (Vieussens, 1684), see **inferior dental nerve (Meckel, 1817)**

secundina (Berengario da Carpi, 1522), see **pia (Galen, c192)**

secundina cerebri (Bauhin, 1605), see **pia (Galen, c192)**

secundine plexus (Vesalius, 1543a), see **choroid plexus (Galen, c177)**

secundine plexus of lateral ventricle (Vesalius, 1543a), see **choroid plexus of lateral ventricle (Vicq d'Azyr, 1784)**

secundines (Vesalius, 1543a), see **choroid plexus (Galen, c177)**

seeing nerve (Bartholin, 1662), see **white matter tracts (Bell & Bell, 1826)**

Seitenstrang (Burdach, 1822), see **lateral funiculus (Burdach, 1822)**

sellar diaphragm (>1840)

semi-annular protuberance (Winslow, 1733), see **pons (Haller, 1747)**

semicircular commissure (Serres, 1824–1826), see **terminal stria commissure (>1840)**

semicircular tape-worm of Haller (Spurzheim, 1826), see **terminal stria (Wenzel & Wenzel, 1812)**

semicircular valves of mammillary eminence of inferior vermis (Vicq d'Azyr, 1784), see **caudal medullary velum (>1840)**

semicirculare centrum (Vieussens, 1684), see **internal capsule (Burdach, 1822)**

semicircularis centri pars superior (Vieussens, 1684), see **terminal stria (Wenzel & Wenzel, 1812)**

semilunar abdominal ganglion (Wrisberg, 1808), see **celiac ganglion (Walter, 1783)**

semilunar border (Reil, 1812c), see **cerebral cortex white matter (>1840)**

semilunar cerebellar fissure (Reil, 1807–1808a), see **anterior cerebellar notch (Chaussier, 1807)**

semilunar fissure (Dejerine & Dejerine-Klumpke, 1901), see **ansoparamedian fissure (>1840)**

semilunar fossa (Gordon, 1815), see **cerebellar vermis (Meckel, 1817)**

semilunar ganglioform plexus (Tarin, 1753), see **celiac plexus (Winslow, 1733)**

semilunar ganglion (Neubauer, 1772), see **trigeminal ganglion (>1840)**

semilunar ganglion (Winslow, 1733), see **celiac ganglion (Walter, 1783)**

semilunar gyrus (>1840)

semilunar intumescence (Wrisberg, 1777), see **trigeminal ganglion (>1840)**

semilunar lobules (>1840), see **ansiform lobule (Bolk, 1906)**

semilunar notch (Ranson, 1920), see **anterior cerebellar notch (Chaussier, 1807)**

semilunar plexus (Palfijn, 1726), see **celiac plexus (Winslow, 1733)**

semilunar plexus (Winslow, 1733), see **celiac ganglion (Walter, 1783)**

semilunar valves (Malacarne, 1776), see **caudal medullary velum (>1840)**

seminal vesicle nerves (Bock, 1827)

seminal vesicle plexus (Cruveilhier, 1836), see **seminal vesicle nerves (Bock, 1827)**
sensible nerve of fifth pair (Bell, 1826), see **trigeminal nerve sensory root (>1840)**
sensible tract (Bell, 1834), see **central nervous system white matter tracts (>1840)**
sensitive column (Bell, 1835), see **lateral funiculus (Burdach, 1822)**
sensitive root (Bell, 1829), see **dorsal root (Spurzheim, 1826)**
sensitive root of fifth pair (Bell, 1829), see **trigeminal nerve sensory root (>1840)**
sensory ganglion of spinal cord (Solly, 1836), see **interbrain (Baer, 1837)**
sensory nerve for tongue (Galen, c173), see **lingual nerve (Vesalius, 1543a)**
sensory root of ciliary ganglion (>1840), see **communicating branch of nasociliary nerve with ciliary ganglion (>1840)**
sensory root of facial nerve (>1840), see **intermediate nerve (>1840)**
sensory root of otic ganglion (>1840), see **medial pterygoid nerve (>1840)**
sensory root of pterygopalatine ganglion (>1840), see **pterygopalatine nerves (Wrisberg, 1786)**
sensory root of submandibular ganglion (>1840), see **communicating branches of lingual nerve with submandibular ganglion (>1840)**
sentient portion of fifth pair of nerves (Todd, 1836–1839), see **trigeminal nerve sensory root (>1840)**
septal arcuate fibers (Burdach, 1822), see **diagonal band (Broca, 1879)**
septal branch of nasal branch of ophthalmic nerve (Quain, 1837), see **medial nasal branches of internal nasal branches of anterior ethmoidal nerve (>1840)**
septal fissure (Burdach, 1822)
septal peduncle (Burdach, 1822), see **endbrain (Kuhlenbeck, 1927)**
septal postcommissural fornix (>1840)
septal region (Swanson & Cowan, 1979), see **cerebral nuclei (Swanson, 2000a)**
septal segment of fornix (Cajal, 1904), see **septal postcommissural fornix (>1840)**
septum (Galen, c177), see **cerebral nuclei (Swanson, 2000a)**
septum cerebelli (Winslow, 1733), see **cerebellar falx (Günther, 1786)**
septum cerebri (Fyfe, 1800), see **cerebral falx (Vesalius, 1543a)**
septum encephali (Soemmerring, 1791), see **cerebellar tentorium (Winslow, 1733)**
septum inter ventriculos (Quain, 1834), see **cerebral nuclei (Swanson, 2000a)**
septum lucidum (Galen, c177), see **cerebral nuclei (Swanson, 2000a)**
septum nervosum vestibuli (Cotugno, 1760), see **vestibular nerve (Cotugno, 1760)**
septum occipitale majus (Winslow, 1733), see **cerebellar tentorium (Winslow, 1733)**
septum of lateral ventricles (Cruveilhier, 1836), see **cerebral nuclei (Swanson, 2000a)**
septum of pons (Bell, 1834), see **transverse pontine fibers (>1840)**
septum pellucidum (Galen, c177), see **cerebral nuclei (Swanson, 2000a)**
septum sagittale (Winslow, 1733), see **cerebral falx (Vesalius, 1543a)**
septum tenue (Bartholin, 1662), see **cerebral nuclei (Swanson, 2000a)**
septum verticale (Winslow, 1733), see **cerebral falx (Vesalius, 1543a)**
serrated body of cerebellum (Vicq d'Azyr, 1784), see **dentate nucleus (>1840)**
serrated body of olivary eminence (Vicq d'Azyr, 1786), see **inferior olivary complex (>1840)**
serrated margin of pedes hippocampi (Fyfe, 1800), see **dentate gyrus (>1840)**
serrated membrane (Gordon, 1815), see **denticulate ligament (Monro, 1783)**
seven pair of sensitive sinews from brain (Geminus, 1553), see **cranial nerves (Soemmerring, 1791)**
seventeenth pair of nerves (Malacarne, 1791), see **suboccipital nerve (Winslow, 1733)**
seventh, eighth, and ninth pairs (Malacarne, 1791), see **trigeminal nerve (Winslow, 1733)**
seventh nerve (Soemmerring, 1778), see **intermediofacial nerve (Strong & Elwyn, 1943)**
seventh pair of cerebral nerves (Soemmerring, 1791), see **intermediofacial nerve (Strong & Elwyn, 1943)**
seventh pair of cranial nerves (Soemmerring, 1791), see **intermediofacial nerve (Strong & Elwyn, 1943)**
seventh pair of nerves arising within skull (Willis, 1664), see **cranial nerves (Soemmerring, 1791)**
seventh pair of nerves from brain (Bartholin, 1641), see **abducens nerve (Heister, 1717)**
seventh pair of nerves from brain (Galen, c192), see **hypoglossal nerve (Winslow, 1733)**
seventh pair of nerves from brain (Theophilos Protospatharios, fl. 610–641), see **cranial nerves (Soemmerring, 1791)**
seventh pair of sinews of brain (Geminus, 1553), see **hypoglossal nerve (Winslow, 1733)**
shank of oblong marrow (Willis, 1664), see **vertebrate brain (Cuvier, 1800)**
shanks of oblong marrow (Willis, 1672), see **circumesophageal connectives (>1840)**
sheaths (Galen, c192), see **meninges (Smith Papyrus, c1700 BC)**
sheaths (Hippocrates), see **meninges (Smith Papyrus, c1700 BC)**
shoots to rough artery [from returning nerve] (Willis, 1664), see **tracheal branches of recurrent laryngeal nerve (>1840)**
short branch of oculomotor nerve (Winslow, 1733), see **branch of oculomotor nerve to ciliary ganglion (>1840)**
short branches of frontal branches of external frontal nerve (Todd, 1836–1839), see **medial branch of supraorbital nerve (>1840)**
short ciliary nerves (>1840)

short crus of lateral ventricle (Günther, 1786), see **posterior horn of lateral ventricle (Haller, 1747)**
short cutaneous nerve (Günther, 1786), see **medial cutaneous nerve of thigh (>1840)**
short cutaneous nerves (Quain & Wilson, 1839), see **lateral cutaneous branch of intercostal nerves (>1840)**
short exposed commissure of cerebellum (Reil, 1807–1808a), see **folium vermis (>1840)**
short gastric nerves (Mayer, 1794), see **splenic plexus (Palfijn, 1726)**
short gyri of insula (Gall & Spurzheim, 1810)
short inferior branch of nervi motores oculorum communes (Winslow, 1733), see **nerve to inferior rectus (>1840)**
short inferior branch of third pair of nerves (Winslow, 1733), see **nerve to inferior rectus (>1840)**
short internal root of olfactory nerve (Soemmerring, 1778), see **lateral olfactory tract (>1840)**
short internal root of olfactory nerve (Vicq d'Azyr, 1786), see **tenia tecta (Swanson, 1992)**
short nerve to crural muscle (Styx, 1782), see **muscular branches of femoral nerve (Quain & Wilson, 1839)**
short nerve to sartorius muscle (Styx, 1782), see **muscular branches of femoral nerve (Quain & Wilson, 1839)**
short nerve to vastus externus muscle (Styx, 1782), see **muscular branches of femoral nerve (Quain & Wilson, 1839)**
short nerve to vastus internus muscle (Styx, 1782), see **muscular branches of femoral nerve (Quain & Wilson, 1839)**
short root of auricular ganglion (Arnold, 1834), see **medial pterygoid nerve (>1840)**
short root of ciliary ganglion (Langenbeck, 1826–1830), see **branch of oculomotor nerve to ciliary ganglion (>1840)**
short root of glottic ganglion (Arnold, 1834), see **communicating branches of lingual nerve with submandibular ganglion (>1840)**
short root of lenticular ganglion (Todd, 1836–1839), see **branch of oculomotor nerve to ciliary ganglion (>1840)**
short root of lingual ganglion (Arnold, 1834), see **communicating branches of lingual nerve with submandibular ganglion (>1840)**
short root of maxillary ganglion (Arnold, 1834), see **communicating branches of lingual nerve with submandibular ganglion (>1840)**
short root of Meckel's ganglion (Arnold, 1834), see **communicating branches of lingual nerve with submandibular ganglion (>1840)**
short root of ophthalmic ganglion (Zinn, 1755), see **branch of oculomotor nerve to ciliary ganglion (>1840)**
short root of otic ganglion (Arnold, 1834), see **medial pterygoid nerve (>1840)**
short saphenous nerve (Quain & Wilson, 1839), see **anterior cutaneous branches of femoral nerve (Quain & Wilson, 1839)**
shorter circumvolutions of island of Sylvian fissure (Meckel, 1817), see **short gyri of insula (Gall & Spurzheim, 1810)**
silkworm (Aranzi, 1587), see **hippocampal region (Swanson et al., 1987)**
silkworm (Malacarne, 1780), see **fimbria (Honegger, 1890)**
silkworm (Vesalius, 1543a), see **cerebellar vermis (Meckel, 1817)**
silkworm ventricle (Aranzi, 1587), see **inferior horn of lateral ventricle (Bell, 1802)**
silver cord (Ecclesiastes, 3rd century BC?), see **spinal cord (Galen, c162–c166)**
simple lobule (Jansen & Brodal, 1954)
simple nerve (Bell, 1826), see **nerve (Herophilus, c335–c280 BC)**
sinew of hearing (Crooke, 1615), see **vestibulocochlear nerve (>1840)**
sinew of midriff (Geminus, 1553), see **phrenic nerve (Galen, c173)**
sinew of sight (Geminus, 1553), see **white matter tracts (Bell & Bell, 1826)**
sinew of voice (Geminus, 1553), see **recurrent laryngeal nerve (Albinus, 1744)**
sinew returning back (Geminus, 1553), see **recurrent laryngeal nerve (Albinus, 1744)**
sinew to heart (Geminus, 1553), see **thoracic cardiac branches of vagus nerve (>1840)**
sinews (Brunschwig, 1525), see **nerves (Herophilus, c335–c280 BC)**
sinews between ribs (Geminus, 1553), see **intercostal nerves (Vesalius, 1543a)**
sinews proceeding from brain (Read, 1650), see **nervous system (Monro, 1783)**
single commissure of cerebellum (Reil, 1807–1808a), see **cerebellar vermis (Meckel, 1817)**
sinowe optico (Brunschwig, 1525), see **white matter tracts (Bell & Bell, 1826)**
sinuosos cerebri flexus (Soemmerring, 1778), see **cerebral cortex gray matter (>1840)**
sinus bulbi rachidici (Meckel, 1817), see **fourth ventricle (Galen, c192)**
sinus cavernosus (Winslow, 1733), see **cavernous sinus (Winslow, 1733)**
sinus circularis Ridleyi (Tarin, 1750), see **circular sinus (Ridley, 1695)**
sinus circularis sellae equinae (Burdach, 1822), see **circular sinus (Ridley, 1695)**
sinus clinoïdeus (Malacarne, 1780), see **circular sinus (Ridley, 1695)**
sinus clinoïdeus anterior (Vicq d'Azyr, 1786), see **anterior intercavernous sinus (>1840)**
sinus clinoïdeus posterior (Vicq d'Azyr, 1786), see **posterior intercavernous sinus (>1840)**
sinus coronoïdeus (Meckel, 1817), see **circular sinus (Ridley, 1695)**
sinus ellipticus (Malacarne, 1780), see **circular sinus (Ridley, 1695)**
sinus inferiores hippocampi (Aranzi, 1587), see **inferior horn of lateral ventricle (Bell, 1802)**
sinus medius (Landi, 1542), see **third ventricle (Galen, c173)**
sinus medius (Lieutaud, 1742), see **circular sinus (Ridley, 1695)**

sinus of cerebellum (Benedetti, 1502), see **fourth ventricle (Galen, c192)**
sinus of median system (Cruveilhier, 1836), see **septal fissure (Burdach, 1822)**
sinus of medulla oblongata (Meckel, 1817), see **fourth ventricle (Galen, c192)**
sinus of septum lucidum (Vicq d'Azyr, 1784), see **septal fissure (Burdach, 1822)**
sinus ovalis (Santorini, 1724), see **circular sinus (Ridley, 1695)**
sinus polymorphi (Schreger, 1803), see **cavernous sinus (Winslow, 1733)**
sinus protuberantiae annularis (Santorini, 1775), see **basilar sulcus of pons (Gordon, 1815)**
sinus sphenoïdales (Malacarne, 1780), see **cavernous sinus (Winslow, 1733)**
sinuses (Averroes, 12th century), see **ventricles (Hippocrates)**
sinuses (Vesalius, 1543a), see **cerebral sulci (Vesalius, 1543a)**
sixteenth pair (Malacarne, 1791), see **hypoglossal nerve (Winslow, 1733)**
sixth nerve entering arm (Vesalius, 1543a), see **brachial plexus medial cord (Schwalbe, 1881)**
sixth nerve of fifth pair (Desmoulins, 1825), see **trigeminal nerve (Winslow, 1733)**
sixth nerve of hand (Bauhin, 1605), see **brachial plexus medial cord (Schwalbe, 1881)**
sixth pair (Molinetti, 1669), see **trochlear nerve (Molinetti, 1669)**
sixth pair of cerebral nerves (Soemmerring, 1791), see **abducens nerve (Heister, 1717)**
sixth pair of cranial nerves (Soemmerring, 1791), see **abducens nerve (Heister, 1717)**
sixth pair of nerves arising within skull (Willis, 1664), see **abducens nerve (Heister, 1717)**
sixth pair of nerves from brain (Benedetti, 1502), see **spinal cord (Galen, c162–c166)**
sixth pair of nerves from brain (Galen, c192), see **cranial nerves (Soemmerring, 1791)**
sixth pair of nerves from brain (Theophilos Protospatharios, fl. 610–641), see **cranial nerves (Soemmerring, 1791)**
sixth pair of nerves trunk (Vieussens, 1684), see **abducens nerve trunk (>1840)**
sixth pair of sacral nerves (Benedetti, 1502), see **coccygeal nerves (Camper, 1762)**
sixth pair of sinews of brain (Geminus, 1553), see **cranial nerves (Soemmerring, 1791)**
sixth plantar nerve of toes (Meckel, 1817), see **common plantar digital nerves of lateral plantar nerve (>1840)**
sixth sacral nerve (Camper, 1762), see **coccygeal nerve (Camper, 1762)**
sixth sinew pertaining to arm (Geminus, 1553), see **brachial plexus medial cord (Schwalbe, 1881)**
sixth terminal branch of median nerve (Cruveilhier, 1836), see **common palmar digital nerves of median nerve (>1840)**
skin-like membrane (Aristotle), see **pia (Galen, c192)**
slenderer root of third pair of sinews (Geminus, 1553), see **trigeminal nerve (Winslow, 1733)**
small bands of pyriform eminences (Burdin, 1803), see **terminal stria (Wenzel & Wenzel, 1812)**
small brain (Aristotle), see **cerebellum (Aristotle)**
small branch of eighth pair of nerves of medulla oblongata (Winslow, 1733), see **glossopharyngeal nerve (Huber, 1744)**
small branch of sheath of femoral vessels of crural nerve (Cruveilhier, 1836), see **femoral nerve (Haller, 1762)**
small branches of oblong medulla (Tarin, 1753), see **cerebellar peduncles (Ridley, 1695)**
small branches of sixth pair of sinews of brain (Geminus, 1553), see **cranial nerves (Soemmerring, 1791)**
small cerebral fissure (Meckel, 1817), see **transverse cerebellar fissure (Burdach, 1822)**
small column of fornix (Soemmerring, 1791), see **septal postcommissural fornix (>1840)**
small coronary plexus (Portal, 1803a), see **autonomic nerves (Langley, 1896)**
small eminence at superior and anterior part of optic thalamus (Pourfour du Petit, 1710), see **anterior thalamic nuclei (>1840)**
small femoro-poplitean nerve (Burdin, 1803), see **sacral plexus (Vesalius, 1543a)**
small foot of hippopotamus (Mayer, 1779), see **calcarine spur (Morand, 1748)**
small foot of seahorse (Haase, 1781), see **calcarine spur (Morand, 1748)**
small foramen (Bellingeri, 1823), see **central canal (Bellingeri, 1823)**
small ganglia of head (Lyonnet, 1762), see **invertebrate peripheral ganglion (Swanson & Bota, 2010)**
small ganglion (Neubauer, 1772), see **facial ganglion (Lazorthes, 1949)**
small ganglion of fifth nerves of neck (Andersch, 1797), see **cervical spinal ganglia (>1840)**
small ganglion of ninth nerves of head (Andersch, 1797), see **distal glossopharyngeal ganglion (>1840)**
small ganglion of second nerve of body (Andersch, 1797), see **phrenic ganglion (Walter, 1783)**
small harmonic nerve of body (Andersch, 1797), see **phrenic nerve (Galen, c173)**
small inferior plexus of stomach (Meckel, 1817), see **splenic plexus (Palfijn, 1726)**
small internal cutaneous nerve (Swan, 1830), see **medial cutaneous nerve of arm (>1840)**
small intestines (Erasistratus, c310–c250 BC), see **cerebral cortex gray matter (>1840)**
small maxillary ganglion (Meckel, 1748), see **submandibular ganglion (>1840)**
small maxillary ganglion of superior lingual nerve (Andersch, 1797), see **submandibular ganglion (>1840)**
small medullary cords (Winslow, 1733), see **longitudinal striae (>1840)**
small muscular branch of infrahyoid region from hypoglossal nerve (Cruveilhier, 1836), see **superior root of ansa cervicalis (>1840)**
small nerve of body (Andersch, 1797), see **phrenic nerve (Galen, c173)**

small occipital branch of third cervical nerve (Haase, 1781), see **lesser occipital nerve (Mayer, 1794)**

small occipital nerve (Bang, 1770), see **lesser occipital nerve (Mayer, 1794)**

small occipital septum (Winslow, 1733), see **cerebellar falx (Günther, 1786)**

small oesophageal plexus (Fyfe, 1800), see **esophageal branches of recurrent laryngeal nerve (>1840)**

small oval center (Vicq d'Azyr, 1786), see **cerebral cortex white matter (>1840)**

small palatine nerve (Cloquet, 1816), see **lateral palatine nerve (Henle, 1871)**

small petrosal nerve from tympanic branch of glosso-pharyngeal nerve (Quain, 1837), see **lesser petrosal nerve (>1840)**

small pharyngeal branch of pharyngolingual branch of glossopharyngeal nerve (Kilian, 1822), see **pharyngeal branches of glossopharyngeal nerve (Neubauer, 1772)**

small pharyngeal nerves (Soemmerring, 1791), see **pharyngeal branches of vagus nerve (>1840)**

small posterior auricular nerve (Meckel, 1753), see **lesser occipital nerve (Mayer, 1794)**

small posterior esophageal plexus of pneumogastric (Cloquet, 1828), see **upper esophageal branches of vagus nerve (Cloquet, 1828)**

small root of fifth pair (Cruveilhier, 1836), see **trigeminal nerve central motor root (>1840)**

small root of trigeminal nerve (Cruveilhier, 1836), see **trigeminal nerve motor root (Bell, 1829)**

small saphena nerve (Meckel, 1817), see **femoral nerve (Haller, 1762)**

small sciatic nerve (Quain, 1832), see **sacral plexus (Vesalius, 1543a)**

small sciatic ramus (Winslow, 1733), see **common fibular nerve (>1840)**

small semicircular bands (Burdin, 1803), see **terminal stria (Wenzel & Wenzel, 1812)**

small splanchnic nerve (Meckel, 1817), see **lesser splanchnic nerve (Haller, 1762)**

small splanchnic nerve (Portal, 1803a; Burdin, 1803), see **least splanchnic nerve (>1840)**

small suprarenal nerve (Chaussier, 1789, definition 1), see **lesser splanchnic nerve (Haller, 1762)**

small suprarenal nerve (Chaussier, 1789, defintion 2), see **least splanchnic nerve (>1840)**

small sympathetic nerve (Winslow, 1733), see **intermediofacial nerve (Strong & Elwyn, 1943)**

small transverse fissure (Meckel, 1817), see **transverse cerebellar fissure (Burdach, 1822)**

small white bodies near infundibulum (Pourfour du Petit, 1710), see **mammillary body (Ludwig, 1779)**

smaller anterior pulmonary plexus of pneumogastric (Knox, 1832), see **anterior pulmonary plexus (Haller, 1762)**

smaller cardiac nerve (Scarpa, 1794), see **inferior cardiac nerve (Cloquet, 1816)**

smaller external lingual branch of glossopharyngeal (Knox, 1832), see **glossopharyngeal nerve (Huber, 1744)**

smaller internal branch of spinal accessory (Knox, 1832), see **internal branch of accessory nerve trunk (Meckel, 1817)**

smaller nerve bundles of glossopharyngeal nerve (Wrisberg, 1786), see **glossopharyngeal nerve rootlets (>1840)**

smaller portion of fifth pair of nerves (Todd, 1836–1839), see **trigeminal nerve motor root (Bell, 1829)**

smaller posterior esophageal plexus (Scarpa, 1794), see **posterior esophageal plexus (Haller, 1762)**

smaller root of fifth pair of cerebral nerves (Vesalius, 1543a), see **trigeminal nerve motor root (Bell, 1829)**

smaller splanchnic nerve (Knox, 1832), see **lesser splanchnic nerve (Haller, 1762)**

smallest cardiac nerve (Chaussier, 1789), see **inferior cardiac nerve (Cloquet, 1816)**

smallest exterior palatine nerve (Mayer, 1794), see **lateral palatine nerve (Henle, 1871)**

smallest pharyngeal branch of pharyngolingual branch of glossopharyngeal nerve (Kilian, 1822), see **pharyngeal branches of glossopharyngeal nerve (Neubauer, 1772)**

smelling nerve (Bartholin, 1662), see **olfactory peduncle (Solly, 1836)**

smooth medulla (Benedetti, 1502), see **spinal cord (Galen, c162–c166)**

snotty kernel (Willis, 1664), see **pituitary gland (>1840)**

so-called brain of invertebrate animals (Carus, 1814), see **invertebrate brain (>1840)**

soft and pellucid ganglion of deep cardiac nerve (Knox, 1832), see **cardiac ganglion (Neubauer, 1772; Haller, 1772)**

soft branch of superior cervical ganglion (Lobstein, 1823), see **laryngopharyngeal branches of superior cervical ganglion (>1840)**

soft commissure of optic thalamus (Vicq d'Azyr, 1784), see **dorsal part of thalamus (Herrick, 1910)**

soft intercostal nerve (Neubauer, 1772), see **paravertebral nerves (Swanson & Bota, 2010)**

soft medullary branches of second branch of fifth pair (Meckel, 1748), see **maxillary nerve (Meckel, 1753)**

soft membrane (Galen, c177), see **pia (Galen, c192)**

soft mother (Hall, 1565), see **pia (Galen, c192)**

soft nerve net accompanying trunk of external carotid artery (Arnold, 1834), see **external carotid plexus (>1840)**

soft nerve of labial artery (Andersch & Soemmerring, 1792), see **external carotid plexus (>1840)**

soft nerves (Cloquet, 1816), see **superior cardiac nerve (Neubauer, 1772)**

soft nerves (Haller, 1762), see **paravertebral nerves (Swanson & Bota, 2010)**

soft nerves of anterior carotid artery (Andersch & Soemmerring, 1792), see **external carotid plexus (>1840)**

soft nerves of facial artery (Arnold, 1834), see **external carotid plexus (>1840)**

soft nerves of Haller (Günther, 1786), see **paravertebral nerves (Swanson & Bota, 2010)**

soft nerves of internal maxillary artery (Arnold, 1834), see **external carotid plexus (>1840)**

soft nerves of occipital artery (Arnold, 1834), see **external carotid plexus (>1840)**

soft nerves of temporal artery (Arnold, 1834), see **external carotid plexus (>1840)**
soft nerves of vertebral and basilar arteries (Arnold, 1834), see **vertebral plexus (Cloquet, 1816)**
soft nerves to otic ganglion from superior cervical ganglion (Quain & Wilson, 1839), see **sympathetic root of otic ganglion (>1840)**
soft pair of nerves (Galen, c192), see **trigeminal nerve (Winslow, 1733)**
soft pannicle (Hall, 1565), see **pia (Galen, c192)**
soft part of fifth pair (Falloppio, 1561), see **vestibulocochlear nerve (>1840)**
soft part of seventh pair of nerves arising within skull (Willis, 1664), see **vestibulocochlear nerve (>1840)**
soft root of auricular ganglion (Arnold, 1834), see **sympathetic root of otic ganglion (>1840)**
soft root of glottic ganglion (Arnold, 1834), see **sympathetic root of submandibular ganglion (>1840)**
soft root of lingual ganglion (Arnold, 1834), see **sympathetic root of submandibular ganglion (>1840)**
soft root of maxillary ganglion (Arnold, 1834), see **sympathetic root of submandibular ganglion (>1840)**
soft root of Meckel's ganglion (Arnold, 1834), see **sympathetic root of submandibular ganglion (>1840)**
soft root of ophthalmic ganglion (Cruveilhier, 1836), see **sympathetic root of ciliary ganglion (>1840)**
soft root of otic ganglion (Arnold, 1834), see **sympathetic root of otic ganglion (>1840)**
soft veil (Hall, 1565), see **pia (Galen, c192)**
solar ganglia (Cruveilhier, 1836), see **celiac plexus (Winslow, 1733)**
solar ganglioform plexus (Tarin, 1753), see **prevertebral plexuses (Quain, 1832)**
solar ganglion (Günther, 1786), see **celiac ganglion (Walter, 1783)**
solar plexus (Cloquet, 1816), see **autonomic nerves (Langley, 1896)**
solar plexus (Cruveilhier, 1836), see **autonomic nerves (Langley, 1896)**
solar plexus (Willis, 1664), see **peripheral nervous system (Meckel, 1817)**
solar plexus (Winslow, 1733), see **prevertebral plexuses (Quain, 1832)**
soleus branch of internal popliteal nerve (Bock, 1827), see **nerve to soleus (>1840)**
space within hemisphere (Gall & Spurzheim, 1810), see **lateral ventricle (Vesalius, 1543a)**
spatium triangulare inter crura (Tarin, 1750), see **subarachnoid space (Magendie, 1827)**
speaking nerve (Arnold, 1834), see **hypoglossal nerve (Winslow, 1733)**
special pharyngeal nerve (Galen, c192), see **glossopharyngeal nerve (Huber, 1744)**
speculum (Vesalius, 1543a), see **cerebral nuclei (Swanson, 2000a)**
speculum lucidum (du Laurens, 1600), see **cerebral nuclei (Swanson, 2000a)**
spermatic branch of external pudic nerve (Quain & Wilson, 1839), see **genital branch of genitofemoral nerve (>1840)**
spermatic branch of external spermatic nerve (Quain & Wilson, 1839), see **genital branch of genitofemoral nerve (>1840)**
spermatic branch of genito-crural nerve (Quain & Wilson, 1839), see **genital branch of genitofemoral nerve (>1840)**
spermatic ganglia (Walter, 1783)
spermatic nerve (Mayer, 1794), see **femoral branch of genitofemoral nerve (>1840)**
spermatic nerves (Walter, 1783), see **superior ovarian nerves (>1840)**
spermatic plexus (Günther, 1786), see **prevertebral nerves (Swanson & Bota, 2010)**
spermatic plexus (Haller, 1762), see **testicular plexus (>1840)**
spermatic plexus (Mayer, 1794), see **renal plexus (Drake, 1707)**
spermatic plexus (Meckel, 1817), see **peripheral nervous system (Meckel, 1817)**
spermatic plexus (Soemmerring, 1791), see **superior testicular nerves (>1840)**
sphaericas prominentias (Soemmerring, 1778), see **cerebral cortex gray matter (>1840)**
sphenoidal ganglion (Burdin, 1803), see **pterygopalatine ganglion (>1840)**
sphenoidal horn (Cruveilhier, 1836), see **temporal pole (>1840)**
sphenoidal lobe (Arnold, 1838a), see **temporal region (>1840)**
sphenoidal lobe (Serres, 1824–1826), see **inferior temporal gyrus (>1840)**
sphenoidal lobule (Serres, 1824–1826), see **temporal region (>1840)**
spheno-maxillary branch of lachrymal nerve (Todd, 1836–1839), see **communicating branch of lacrimal nerve with zygomatic nerve (>1840)**
spheno-maxillary fascicle of lacrimal surculus (Bellingeri, 1818), see **communicating branch of lacrimal nerve with zygomatic nerve (>1840)**
sphenomaxillary ganglion (Wrisberg, 1786), see **pterygopalatine ganglion (>1840)**
spheno-palatin ganglion (Bell, 1803b), see **pterygopalatine ganglion (>1840)**
sphenopalatine branch of superior maxillary branch of fifth pair of nerves (Bock, 1817), see **pterygopalatine nerves (Wrisberg, 1786)**
spheno-palatine branches of Meckel's ganglion (Quain & Wilson, 1839), see **greater palatine nerve (Cloquet, 1816)**
spheno-palatine branches of spheno-palatine ganglion (Quain, 1828), see **greater palatine nerve (Cloquet, 1816)**
sphenopalatine ganglion (Meckel, 1751), see **pterygopalatine ganglion (>1840)**
spheno-palatine ganglion ascending branches of communication with superior maxillary nerve (Quain & Wilson, 1839), see **pterygopalatine nerves (Wrisberg, 1786)**
sphenopalatine ganglion branches from superior maxillary nerve (Langenbeck, 1826–1830), see **pterygopalatine nerves (Wrisberg, 1786)**
sphenopalatine ganglion of Meckel (Bock, 1817), see **pterygopalatine ganglion (>1840)**

spinal nucleus of trigeminal nerve (>1840)
spinal part of accessory nerve (Arnold, 1838b), see ***spinal root of accessory nerve (>1840)***
spinal pith (Diemerbroeck, 1689), see ***spinal cord (Galen, c162–c166)***
spinal prolongation of brain (Chaussier, 1807), see ***central nervous system (Carus, 1814)***
spinal prolongation of cerebellum (Meckel, 1817), see ***inferior cerebellar peduncle (Günther, 1786)***
spinal root of accessory nerve (>1840)
spinal root of accessory nerve rootlets (>1840)
spinal root of accessory nerve trunk (>1840)
spinal roots of accessory nerve of Willis (Günther, 1786), see ***spinal roots of accessory nerve rootlets (>1840)***
spinal roots of great sympathetic nerve (Güther, 1786), see ***communicating branches of spinal nerves (Wutzer, 1817)***
spinal rope (Willis, 1672), see ***ventral cord (Anderson, 1837)***
spinal rubrospinal tract (>1840)
spinal segment of spinal tract of trigeminal nerve (>1840)
spinal system ganglia (Wutzer, 1817), see ***spinal nerve ganglia (Burdach, 1819)***
spinal tectospinal tract (>1840)
spinal tract of trigeminal nerve (>1840)
spinal ventral spinocerebellar tract (>1840)
spinalis medullae (Hippocrates), see ***spinal cord (Galen, c162–c166)***
spino-cerebellar ventricle (Gordon, 1815), see ***fourth ventricle (Galen, c192)***
spino-cerebral axis (Grant, 1834a), see ***central nervous system (Carus, 1814)***
spinocortical tract (>1840), see ***spinothalamic tract (>1840)***
spinohypothalamic fibers (>1840), see ***spinothalamic tract (>1840)***
spino-olivary tract (>1840), see ***spinothalamic tract (>1840)***
spinopontine fibers (>1840), see ***spinothalamic tract (>1840)***
spinoreticular fibers (>1840), see ***spinothalamic tract (>1840)***
spinotectal tract (>1840), see ***spinothalamic tract (>1840)***
spinothalamic tract (>1840)
spirae (Piccolomini, 1586), see ***cerebral cortex gray matter (>1840)***
spiraglis (Malacarne, 1780), see ***choroid fissure (>1840)***
spiral ganglion (>1840), see ***cochlear ganglion (>1840)***
spiral muscular nerve (Monro, 1783), see ***radial nerve (Du Verney, 1697)***
spiral nerve (Fyfe, 1800), see ***radial nerve (Du Verney, 1697)***
spirale intervallum nervi cochleae (Cotugno, 1760), see ***cochlear nerve (Cotugno, 1760)***
spittle kernel (Diemerbroeck, 1689), see ***pituitary gland (>1840)***
spity kernel (Diemerbroeck, 1689), see ***pituitary gland (>1840)***
splanchnic ganglia of sympathetic (Grant, 1834c), see ***prevertebral ganglia (Quain, 1832)***
splanchnic ganglion (Günther, 1786), see ***celiac ganglion (Walter, 1783)***
splanchnic ganglion (>1840)
splanchnic nerve (Günther, 1786), see ***greater splanchnic nerve (Walter, 1783)***
splanchnic nerve (Haller, 1762), see ***paravertebral nerves (Swanson & Bota, 2010)***
splanchnic nerve (Meckel, 1817), see ***paravertebral nerves (Swanson & Bota, 2010)***
splanchnic nerve roots (Wrisberg, 1780), see ***greater splanchnic nerve (Walter, 1783)***
splanchnic nerve trunk (Wrisberg, 1780), see ***greater splanchnic nerve (Walter, 1783)***
splanchnic nerves (Cruveilhier, 1836), see ***paravertebral nerves (Swanson & Bota, 2010)***
splanchnic nerves of lumbar ganglia (Cruveilhier, 1836), see ***lumbar splanchnic nerves (Cruveilhier, 1836)***
splenetick nerves (Willis, 1664), see ***splenic plexus (Palfijn, 1726)***
splenial gyrus (>1840), see ***fasciola cinerea (Arnold, 1838b)***
splenic ganglia (Wutzer, 1817), see ***splenic plexus (Palfijn, 1726)***
splenic infolding (Willis, 1664), see ***splenic plexus (Palfijn, 1726)***
splenic nerve plexus (Walter, 1783), see ***splenic plexus (Palfijn, 1726)***
splenic nerves (Walter, 1783), see ***splenic plexus (Palfijn, 1726)***
splenic plexus (Keill, 1698), see ***celiac plexus (Winslow, 1733)***
splenic plexus (Palfijn, 1726)
splenic plexus (Walter, 1783), see ***splenic plexus (Palfijn, 1726)***
splenic plexus roots (Walter, 1783), see ***splenic plexus (Palfijn, 1726)***
splenium of corpus callosum (Burdach, 1822)
splenium of great commissure (Arnold, 1838b), see ***splenium of corpus callosum (Burdach, 1822)***
spongy substance (Paré, 1550), see ***central nervous system gray matter regions (>1840)***
square lobe (Reil, 1807–1808a), see ***cerebellar hemisphere (Willis, 1664)***
staff (Crooke, 1615), see ***cerebrospinal trunk (>1840)***
stalk of oblong marrow (Willis, 1664), see ***vertebrate brain (Cuvier, 1800)***
stapedial filament of portio major and minor of facial nerve (Bellingeri, 1818), see ***stapedial nerve (>1840)***
stapedial nerve (>1840)
staphyline branch of anterior palatine nerve (Cruveilhier, 1836), see ***greater palatine nerve (Cloquet, 1816)***
stato-acoustic nerve (>1840), see ***vestibulocochlear nerve (>1840)***
stellate ganglion (Bock, 1817), see ***inferior cervical ganglion (Vieussens, 1684)***
stellate ganglion (>1840), see ***sympathetic trunk ganglia (Winslow, 1733)***
stem (du Laurens, 1600), see ***cerebrospinal trunk (>1840)***
stem lobe (Burdach, 1822), see ***insular region (Brodmann, 1909)***
stem of brain (Coiter, 1572), see ***spinal cord (Galen, c162–c166)***
stem of lateral cerebral sulcus (>1840)
stem of oblong marrow (Willis, 1664), see ***vertebrate brain (Cuvier, 1800)***

stem of sixth pair of cerebral nerves (Vesalius, 1543a), see **vagus nerve trunk (Wrisberg, 1786; Günther, 1786)**
stem of Sylvian fissure (Vicq d'Azyr, 1784), see **stem of lateral cerebral sulcus (>1840)**
stem system (Burdach, 1822), see **central nervous system white matter tracts (>1840)**
sternal branch of supraclavicular branches (Cruveilhier, 1836), see **medial supraclavicular nerves (>1840)**
sternal branch of thoracic part of trachelo-cutanean plexus (Burdin, 1803), see **medial supraclavicular nerves (>1840)**
sternal branch of thoracic part of tracheosubcutaneous nerves (Chaussier, 1809), see **medial supraclavicular nerves (>1840)**
sterno-thoracic nerve (Burdin, 1803), see **long thoracic nerve (Quain & Wilson, 1839)**
sternothyrohyoid nerves (Andersch & Soemmerring, 1792), see **cervical plexus (Molinetti, 1675)**
Stilling's nucleus (>1840), see **dorsal thoracic nucleus (>1840)**
stock of long marrow (Willis, 1664), see **vertebrate brain (Cuvier, 1800)**
stock of oblong marrow (Willis, 1664), see **vertebrate brain (Cuvier, 1800)**
stock of sixth pair of nerves of brain (Geminus, 1553), see **vagus nerve trunk (Wrisberg, 1786; Günther, 1786)**
stomach nerve (Paré, 1561), see **vagus nerve (Galen, c192)**
stomachical and splenetick infolding (Willis, 1664), see **celiac ganglion (Walter, 1783)**
stomachical branches of wandring pair (Willis, 1664), see **esophageal plexus (>1840)**
stomachical nerves (Willis, 1664), see **esophageal plexus (>1840)**
stomacke branch of sixth conjugation (Paré, 1634), see **vagus nerve (Galen, c192)**
stomogastric plexus (Chaussier, 1789), see **prevertebral plexuses (Quain, 1832)**
stones of brain (Willis, 1664), see **inferior colliculus (Haller, 1762)**
straight den (Willis, 1664), see **cerebral aqueduct (>1840)**
straight gyrus (Valentin, 1841)
straight roots of fornix (Willis, 1664), see **hypothalamic postcommissural fornix (>1840)**
straight sulcus (Santorini, 1724), see **olfactory sulcus (Quain, 1834)**
straining gland (Estienne, 1545), see **pituitary gland (>1840)**
strata (Winslow, 1733), see **cerebellar cortex (Willis, 1664)**
stratum horizontale (Burdach, 1822), see **ventrolateral fascicle (>1840)**
stratum nigrum (Burdach, 1822), see **substantia nigra (Soemmerring, 1791)**
stratum zonale thalami (Burdach, 1822), see **zonal layer of thalamus (Burdach, 1822)**
streaked body (Willis, 1664), see **cerebral nuclei (Swanson, 2000a)**
streaked membrane (Willis, 1664), see **cerebral nuclei (Swanson, 2000a)**
streaks (Winslow, 1733), see **cerebral sulci (Vesalius, 1543a)**
stria alba accedens radici brevi (Scarpa, 1785), see **lateral olfactory tract (>1840)**
stria cornea (Soemmerring, 1798), see **terminal stria (Wenzel & Wenzel, 1812)**
stria lateralis longitudinalis (Arnold, 1838a), see **lateral longitudinal stria (Arnold, 1838a)**
stria medullaris (Wenzel & Wenzel, 1812), see **medullary stria (Wenzel & Wenzel, 1812)**
stria medullaris line (>1840), see **choroid line of third ventricle (>1840)**
stria of Gennari (Obersteiner, 1888), see **primary visual area (>1840)**
stria terminalis (Wenzel & Wenzel, 1812), see **terminal stria (Wenzel & Wenzel, 1812)**
striae medullares (>1840), see **medullary striae (Scarpa, 1788)**
striae medullares of third ventricle (Arnold, 1838b), see **hypothalamic part of third ventricle (Swanson, 2004)**
striae medullares pectiniformes (Lancisi, 1718), see **corpus callosum (Galen, c177)**
striae medullares ventriculi quarti (>1840), see **medullary striae (Scarpa, 1788)**
striae medullosae (Wenzel & Wenzel, 1812), see **medullary striae (Scarpa, 1788)**
striae of Lancisi (Reil, 1812c), see **longitudinal striae (>1840)**
striae transversa corporis callosi in medio decussatae (Tarin, 1753), see **corpus callosum (Galen, c177)**
strias medullares (Procháska, 1800), see **medullary striae (Scarpa, 1788)**
striata corpora posteriora et superna (Vieussens, 1684), see **interbrain (Baer, 1837)**
striata corpora posteriora interna (Vieussens, 1684), see **interbrain (Baer, 1837)**
striata corpora superna anteriora (Vieussens, 1684), see **caudate nucleus (Arnold, 1838b)**
striata corpora superna et posteriora (Vieussens, 1684), see **interbrain (Baer, 1837)**
striatal protuberances (Diemerbroeck, 1672), see **interbrain (Baer, 1837)**
striate area (Brodmann, 1909), see **primary visual area (>1840)**
striated band (Vicq d'Azyr, 1786), see **terminal stria (Wenzel & Wenzel, 1812)**
striated body (Willis, 1664), see **cerebral nuclei (Swanson, 2000a)**
striated colliculus (Wenzel & Wenzel, 1812), see **cerebral nuclei (Swanson, 2000a)**
striated eminence (Arnold, 1838a), see **cerebral nuclei (Swanson, 2000a)**
striatum (Swanson, 2000a)
stringy protuberance (Diemerbroeck, 1689), see **dorsal lateral geniculate nucleus (>1840)**
stringy protuberance (Salmon, 1714), see **interbrain (Baer, 1837)**
strong mother (Hall, 1565), see **dura (Galen, c177)**
stronger membrane (Aristotle), see **dura (Galen, c177)**
structures under thalamus (Burdach, 1822), see **hypothalamus (Kuhlenbeck, 1927)**
styloglossus nerve (Loder, 1778), see **stylohyoid nerve (Meckel, 1753)**

stylohyoid and digastric nerve (Arnold, 1834), see ***facial nerve trunk (1840)***
stylohyoid branch of facial nerve (Chaussier, 1809), see ***stylohyoid nerve (Meckel, 1753)***
stylohyoid branch of glossopharyngeal nerves (Kilian, 1822), see ***glossopharyngeal nerve (Huber, 1744)***
stylohyoid nerve (Meckel, 1753)
stylo-hyoid surculus proper of stylo-hyoid branch (Belligeri, 1818), see ***stylohyoid nerve (Meckel, 1753)***
styloid nerve (Mayer, 1794), see ***stylohyoid nerve (Meckel, 1753)***
stylopharyngeal branch of glossopharyngeal nerve (>1840)
stylopharyngeal muscle branch of glossopharyngeal nerve (Wutzer, 1817), see ***stylopharyngeal branch of glossopharyngeal nerve (>1840)***
stylopharyngeal muscle branches of glossopharyngeal nerve (Arnold, 1837), see ***stylopharyngeal branch of glossopharyngeal nerve (>1840)***
stylus scriptorius (Ramsay, 1813), see ***fourth ventricle (Galen, c192)***
subarachnoid space (Magendie, 1827)
subatloidien nerve (Chaussier, 1809), see ***cervical nerves (Galen, c173)***
subaxoidien nerve (Chaussier, 1809), see ***cervical nerves (Galen, c173)***
subcallosal area (>1840), see ***endbrain (Kuhlenbeck, 1927)***
subcallosal gyrus (Zuckerkandl, 1887), see ***endbrain (Kuhlenbeck, 1927)***
subcallosal gyrus (>1840), see ***endbrain (Kuhlenbeck, 1927)***
subcentral area (Brodmann, 1909), see ***cerebral cortex gray matter (>1840)***
subcervical nerves (Monro, 1783), see ***spinal nerve ventral branches (>1840)***
subclavian ansa (>1840), see ***ansa subclavia (Neubauer, 1772)***
subclavian branch of brachial plexus (Cruveilhier, 1836), see ***subclavian nerve (>1840)***
subclavian nerve (Andersch, 1797), see ***subclavian plexus (>1840)***
subclavian nerve (>1840)
subclavian nerves (Cheselden, 1713), see ***brachial plexus (Camper, 1760)***
subclavian plexus (>1840)
subclavicular branches of cervical plexus (Cloquet, 1816), see ***muscular branches of cervical plexus (Cruveilhier, 1836)***
sub-costal branch of dorsal pairs (Burdin, 1803), see ***intercostal nerves (Vesalius, 1543a)***
subcostal branch of twelfth thoracic nerve (Bock, 1827), see ***subcostal nerve (>1840)***
subcostal nerve (>1840)
subcostal nerves (Chaussier, 1809), see ***intercostal nerves (Vesalius, 1543a)***
subcutaneous basilic nerves (Monro, 1783), see ***medial cutaneous nerve of forearm (>1840)***
subcutaneous branch of cubital nerve (Frotscher, 1788), see ***ulnar nerve (Cheselden, 1726)***
subcutaneous branch of dorsal branch of thoracic nerve (Bock, 1827), see ***lateral branch of spinal nerve dorsal branch (>1840)***
subcutaneous branch of lower jaw of facial nerve (Cloquet, 1828), see ***marginal mandibular branch of facial nerve (>1840)***
subcutaneous branch of neck of hard nerve (Cloquet, 1828), see ***cervical branch of facial nerve (>1840)***
subcutaneous branch of neck of inferior branch of anterior branch of hard nerve (Loder, 1778), see ***cervical branch of facial nerve (>1840)***
subcutaneous branch of ulnar nerve (Günther, 1786), see ***ulnar nerve (Cheselden, 1726)***
subcutaneous cervical branch of portio dura (Knox, 1832), see ***cervical branch of facial nerve (>1840)***
subcutaneous deltoid supraclavicular branch (Peipers, 1793), see ***lateral supraclavicular nerves (>1840)***
subcutaneous fibrils of external subcutaneous filament of deep frontal thread of supraorbital fascicle (Bellingeri, 1818), see ***supraorbital nerve (Meckel, 1753)***
subcutaneous malar branch of second branch of fifth pair (Meckel, 1748), see ***zygomatic nerve (>1840)***
subcutaneous malar nerve (Meckel, 1748), see ***zygomatic nerve (>1840)***
subcutaneous nerve (Vesling, 1647), see ***brachial plexus medial cord (Schwalbe, 1881)***
subcutaneous nerve of neck (Meckel, 1753), see ***transverse nerve of neck (>1840)***
subcutaneous nerve of zygomatic bone (Meckel, 1753), see ***zygomaticofacial nerve (>1840)***
subcutaneous temporalis nerve (Bell & Bell, 1826), see ***zygomaticotemporal nerve (>1840)***
subcutaneous thoracic nerves (Neubauer, 1772), see ***supraclavicular nerves (Meckel, 1817)***
subcutaneous twig of external plantar nerve (Fischer, 1791), see ***lateral plantar nerve (>1840)***
subdiaphragmatic plexus (Chaussier, 1789), see ***phrenic plexus (Loder, 1778)***
subdorsal nerves (Monro, 1783), see ***spinal nerve ventral branches (>1840)***
subependymal zone (>1840)
subgenual area (Brodmann, 1909), see ***infralimbic area (Rose & Woolsey, 1948)***
subicular complex (Swanson & Cowan, 1977)
subiculothalamic tract (Swanson et al., 1987)
subiculum (>1840)
subiculum of Ammon's horn (Burdach, 1822), see ***parahippocampal gyrus (>1840)***
sublentiform part of internal capsule (>1840)
sublingual fascicles of lingual surculus with chorda tympani (Bellingeri, 1818), see ***sublingual nerve (Henle, 1871)***
sublingual ganglion (>1840), see ***submandibular ganglion (>1840)***
sublingual ganglion of Mayer (>1840), see ***sublingual nerve (Henle, 1871)***
sublingual nerve (Henle, 1871)
submandibular ganglion (>1840)
sub-mastoidian branch of facial nerve (Burdin, 1803), see ***digastric nerve (Meckel, 1753)***
submaxillary branch of inferior maxillary nerve (Andersch, 1797), see ***mylohyoid nerve (Meckel, 1748)***
sub-maxillary ganglion (Burdin, 1803), see ***submandibular ganglion (>1840)***

sub-maxillary nerve (Burdin, 1803), see **maxillary nerve (Meckel, 1753)**

submaxillary nerves (Chaussier, 1809), see **lingual nerve (Vesalius, 1543a)**

submental branch of cephalic part of tracheosubcutaneous nerves (Chaussier, 1809), see **transverse nerve of neck (>1840)**

submental branch of facial nerve (Burdin, 1803), see **cervical branch of facial nerve (>1840)**

submental nerve (Loder, 1778), see **cervical branch of facial nerve (>1840)**

sub-mentonnair branch of cephalic part of trachelo-cutanean plexus (Burdin, 1803), see **transverse nerve of neck (>1840)**

sub-mentonniar branches of facial nerve (Burdin, 1803), see **cervical branch of facial nerve (>1840)**

submesenteric plexus (Winslow, 1733), see **inferior hypogastric plexus (Tiedemann, 1822)**

suboccipital nerve (Winslow, 1733)

suboccipital nerve (>1840), see **suboccipital nerve (Winslow, 1733)**

suboesophageal ganglia (Newport, 1834), see **ventral ganglia (Anderson, 1837)**

suboesophageal ganglia (Straus Durckheim, 1828), see **ventral ganglia (Anderson, 1837)**

suborbital branches of temporofacial branch of facial nerve (Cruveilhier, 1836), see **zygomatic branches of facial nerve (>1840)**

suborbital nerve (Bell, 1829), see **infraorbital nerve (Schaarschmidt, 1750)**

sub-orbitar branches of facial nerve (Burdin, 1803), see **zygomatic branches of facial nerve (>1840)**

sub-orbitary ramus of superior maxillary nerve (Winslow, 1733), see **maxillary nerve (Meckel, 1753)**

subparietal sulcus (>1840)

subpeduncular lobule (Gordon, 1815), see **flocculus (Meckel, 1817)**

subpubial nerve (Cuvier, 1800), see **obturator nerve (Cheselden, 1726)**

sub-pubio-femoral nerve (Burdin, 1803), see **obturator nerve (Cheselden, 1726)**

subrotunda corpora alba (Vieussens, 1684), see **anterior thalamic nuclei (>1840)**

subsartorial plexus (>1840)

subscapular nerve (Günther, 1786), see **lower subscapular nerve (>1840)**

subscapular nerve (Mayer, 1794), see **brachial plexus dorsal cord (Peterson, 1887)**

subscapular nerves (Bell, 1803a), see **brachial plexus dorsal cord (Peterson, 1887)**

subscapular nerves (Bock, 1817), see **upper subscapular nerve (>1840)**

sub-scapular nerves (Quain, 1832), see **brachial plexus dorsal cord (Peterson, 1887)**

sub-scapulary nerves (Burdin, 1803), see **brachial plexus dorsal cord (Peterson, 1887)**

substantia cinerea (Tarin, 1750), see **dentate gyrus (>1840)**

substantia cornea (Wenzel & Wenzel, 1812), see **lamina affixa (>1840)**

substantia ferruginea (Arnold, 1838a), see **locus ceruleus (Wenzel & Wenzel, 1812)**

substantia flavescens (Günther, 1786), see **cerebellar cortex (Willis, 1664)**

substantia glandulosa (Vieussens, 1684), see **central nervous system gray matter regions (>1840)**

substantia innominata (Meynert, 1872)

substantia innominata of Reil (Meynert, 1872), see **substantia innominata (Meynert, 1872)**

substantia medullaris (Santorini, 1775), see **cerebral cortex white matter (>1840)**

substantia nigra (Soemmerring, 1791)

substantia nigra of Soemmerring (Kölliker, 1896), see **substantia nigra (Soemmerring, 1791)**

substantia ochracea (Bergmann, 1831), see **vagal triangle (>1840)**

substantia perforata (Solly, 1836), see **interpeduncular nucleus (>1840)**

substantia succosa (Langenbeck, 1826–1830), see **central nervous system gray matter regions (>1840)**

substantia vitrea (Leeuwenhoek, 1685), see **central nervous system gray matter regions (>1840)**

subtle veil (Hall, 1565), see **pia (Galen, c192)**

subvertebral nerves (Monro, 1783), see **spinal nerve ventral branches (>1840)**

sub-zygomatic nerve (Burdin, 1803), see **masseteric nerve (Meckel, 1748)**

sulci (Heister, 1717), see **cerebellar fissures (>1840)**

sulci of posterior pyramids (Rolando, 1824), see **dorsal intermediate sulcus (>1840)**

sulcum pontem (Soemmerring, 1778), see **pontine sulcus (Soemmerring, 1778)**

sulcus ante nervorum opticorum confluxum (Günther, 1786), see **preoptic recess (>1840)**

sulcus corpora pyramidalia profunde dividens (Soemmerring, 1778), see **ventral median fissure of medulla (>1840)**

sulcus insculptus basi lobi cerebri anterioris (Scarpa, 1785), see **olfactory sulcus (Quain, 1834)**

sulcus limitans (>1840), see **limiting sulcus (>1840)**

sulcus longitudinalis (Günther, 1786), see **olfactory sulcus (Quain, 1834)**

sulcus of cerebellar ventricle (Vicq d'Azyr, 1786), see **median sulcus of fourth ventricle (>1840)**

sulcus of corpus callosum (>1840)

sulcus of posterior roots (Cruveilhier, 1836), see **dorsolateral sulcus of spinal cord (>1840)**

sulcus olfactorius (Quain, 1834), see **olfactory sulcus (Quain, 1834)**

sulcus pontis basilaris (>1840), see **basilar sulcus of pons (Gordon, 1815)**

sulcus under cuneus (Burdach, 1822), see **calcarine sulcus (>1840)**

summitates medullae oblongatae (Steenbergen, 1731), see **interbrain (Baer, 1837)**

summus corporis humani nervus (Chaussier, 1807), see **central nervous system (Carus, 1814)**

super trochlearis (Bell & Bell, 1816), see **supratrochlear nerve (Schaarschmidt, 1750)** *superadded nerves (Bell, 1821)*, see **craniospinal nerves (Herrick, 1915)**

superadded system of nerves (Bell, 1822), see **craniospinal nerves (Herrick, 1915)**

superciliary nerve (Winslow, 1733), see **frontal nerve (Cheselden, 1726)**

superclavicular nerves (Bell & Bell, 1816), see **supraclavicular nerves (Meckel, 1817)**

superficial aortic cardiac nerve (Fyfe, 1800), see **inferior cardiac nerve (Cloquet, 1816)**

superficial auricular branch of auricular nerve (Cruveilhier, 1836), see **posterior branch of great auricular nerve (Bock, 1827)**

superficial auricular branches of nerve to left auricle (Andersch, 1797), see **atrial plexuses (>1840)**

superficial branch of accessory cutaneous branch of internal saphenous nerve (Cruveilhier, 1836), see **medial cutaneous branch of femoral nerve (>1840)**

superficial branch of cubital nerve (Cloquet, 1816), see **superficial branch of ulnar nerve (Fyfe, 1800)**

superficial branch of deep peroneal nerve (Fischer, 1791), see **digital branch of deep fibular nerve (>1840)**

superficial branch of exterior branch of tibial nerve (Burdin, 1803), see **superficial branch of lateral plantar nerve (>1840)**

superficial branch of external cutaneous nerve (Soemmerring, 1791), see **lateral cutaneous nerve of forearm (>1840)**

superficial branch of external plantar branch of tibial nerve (Martin, 1781), see **superficial branch of lateral plantar nerve (>1840)**

superficial branch of external plantar nerve (Günther, 1786), see **superficial branch of lateral plantar nerve (>1840)**

superficial branch of first nerve of trunk (Andersch, 1797), see **paravertebral nerves (Swanson & Bota, 2010)**

superficial branch of hard nerve (Günther, 1786), see **facial nerve trunk (1840)**

superficial branch of lateral plantar nerve (>1840)

superficial branch of median nerve (Langenbeck, 1826–1830), see **median nerve (Du Verney, 1697)**

superficial branch of musculocutaneous nerve (Soemmerring, 1791), see **lateral cutaneous nerve of forearm (>1840)**

superficial branch of neck of superficial branches of cervical plexus (Quain, 1832), see **transverse nerve of neck (>1840)**

superficial branch of obturator nerve (Meckel, 1817), see **anterior branch of obturator nerve (Haase, 1781; Martin, 1781)**

superficial branch of palmar branch of ulnar nerve (Meckel, 1817), see **superficial branch of ulnar nerve (Fyfe, 1800)**

superficial branch of peroneal nerve (Haase, 1781), see **superficial fibular nerve (Fyfe, 1800)**

superficial branch of radial nerve (Martin, 1781)

superficial branch of supraorbital nerve (Günther, 1786), see **medial branch of supraorbital nerve (>1840)**

superficial branch of ulnar nerve (Fyfe, 1800)

superficial branch of Vidian nerve (Scarpa, 1785), see **greater petrosal nerve (>1840)**

superficial branches of anterior crural nerve (Quain, 1832), see **femoral nerve (Haller, 1762)**

superficial branches of crural nerve (Quain, 1828), see **lateral cutaneous nerve of thigh (>1840)**

superficial branches of frontal branches of external frontal nerve (Todd, 1836–1839), see **lateral branch of supraorbital nerve (>1840)**

superficial branches of suborbital branches of temporofacial branch of facial nerve (Cruveilhier, 1836), see **zygomatic branches of facial nerve (>1840)**

superficial branchlets of superior laryngeal nerve (Loder, 1778), see **external branch of superior laryngeal nerve (Fyfe, 1800)**

superficial cardiac branch of eight (Scarpa, 1794), see **superior cervical cardiac branches of vagus nerve (>1840)**

superficial cardiac branch of pneumogastric (Knox, 1832), see **superior cervical cardiac branches of vagus nerve (>1840)**

superficial cardiac branch of vagus (Scarpa, 1794), see **superior cervical cardiac branches of vagus nerve (>1840)**

superficial cardiac nerve (Neubauer, 1772), see **superior cardiac nerve (Neubauer, 1772)**

superficial cardiac plexus (Mayer, 1794), see **cardiac plexus (Keill, 1698)**

superficial cervical branches of cervical plexus (Cloquet, 1816), see **transverse nerve of neck (>1840)**

superficial cervical nerve (Meckel, 1817), see **transverse nerve of neck (>1840)**

superficial cervical plexus (Bell & Bell, 1826), see **ansa cervicalis (>1840)**

superficial communicating branch of first nerves of trunk and second nerves of trunk (Andersch, 1797), see **paravertebral nerves (Swanson & Bota, 2010)**

superficial cutaneous branch of peroneal nerve (Mayer, 1794), see **medial dorsal cutaneous nerve (>1840)**

superficial digital branch of external plantar nerve (Soemmerring, 1798), see **superficial branch of lateral plantar nerve (>1840)**

superficial dorsal branch of foot (Bell, 1803b), see **digital branch of deep fibular nerve (>1840)**

superficial dorsal branch of foot of deeper seated branch of fibular nerve (Bell & Bell, 1816), see **digital branch of deep fibular nerve (>1840)**

superficial dorsal branch of radial nerve (Caldani, 1813, 1814), see **posterior cutaneous nerve of forearm (>1840)**

superficial dorsal branch of radial nerve (Meckel, 1817), see **superficial branch of radial nerve (Martin, 1781)**

superficial dorsal twig of foot of deep branch of peroneal nerve (Jördens, 1788), see **dorsal digital nerves of deep fibular nerve (>1840)**

superficial fiber plexus of subiculum (Cajal, 1904), see **superficial medullary lamina of subiculum (Dejerine & Dejerine-Klumpke, 1895)**

superficial fibular nerve (Fyfe, 1800)

superficial frontal thread of supraorbital fascicle (Bellingeri, 1818), see **supraorbital nerve (>1840)**

superficial layer of cardiac nerves (Cruveilhier, 1836), see **cardiac plexus (Keill, 1698)**

superficial maxillary branch of inferior branch of anterior branch of hard nerve (Loder, 1778), see **marginal mandibular branch of facial nerve (>1840)**

superficial medullary lamina of subiculum (Dejerine & Dejerine-Klumpke, 1895)

superficial minor branch of Vidian nerve (Meckel, 1748), see **greater petrosal nerve (>1840)**

superficial nasal branches of infraorbital nerve (Meckel, 1748), see **external nasal branches of infraorbital nerve (>1840)**

superficial nasal nerves (Schaarschmidt, 1750), see **external nasal branches of infraorbital nerve (>1840)**

superficial nerve of deep peroneal nerve (Knox, 1832), see **digital branch of deep fibular nerve (>1840)**

superficial nerve of heart (Scarpa, 1794), see **superior cardiac nerve (Neubauer, 1772)**

superficial nerve of left artery of septum of heart (Andersch, 1797), see **left coronary plexus (Scarpa, 1794)**

superficial nerve of muscular spiral nerve (Bell & Bell, 1816), see **superficial branch of radial nerve (Martin, 1781)**

superficial nerve of neck (Bang, 1770), see **transverse nerve of neck (>1840)**

superficial nerve of nerve layers of septum of heart (Andersch, 1797), see **coronary plexuses (Meckel, 1817)**

superficial nerve of posterior ventricle of heart (Andersch, 1797), see **coronary plexuses (Meckel, 1817)**

superficial nerve of right artery of septum of heart (Andersch, 1797), see **right coronary plexus (Scarpa, 1794)**

superficial palmar arch (Meckel, 1817), see **brachial plexus medial cord (Schwalbe, 1881)**

superficial palmar branch of ulnar nerve (Quain & Wilson, 1839), see **superficial branch of ulnar nerve (Fyfe, 1800)**

superficial palmar nerve (Fyfe, 1800), see **superficial branch of ulnar nerve (Fyfe, 1800)**

superficial palmar nerve (Quain & Wilson, 1839), see **palmar branch of median nerve (Bock, 1827)**

superficial perineal branch of perineal branch of internal pudendal nerve (Cruveilhier, 1836), see **perineal nerve (Camper, 1762)**

superficial peroneal nerve (Günther, 1786), see **superficial fibular nerve (Fyfe, 1800)**

superficial petrous branch of Vidian nerve (Todd, 1836–1839), see **greater petrosal nerve (>1840)**

superficial petrous nerve (Meckel, 1817), see **greater petrosal nerve (>1840)**

superficial plexus of heart (Haller, 1772), see **cardiac plexus (Keill, 1698)**

superficial plexus of posterior carotid arteries (Andersch & Soemmerring, 1792), see **internal carotid plexus (>1840)**

superficial pudendal nerve (Bock, 1827), see **perineal nerve (Camper, 1762)**

superficial pulmonary plexus (Scarpa, 1794), see **posterior pulmonary plexus (Haller, 1762)**

superficial scapular branch of anterior branch of fourth pair of cervical nerves (Bang, 1770), see **lateral supraclavicular nerves (>1840)**

superficial scapular nerve (Mayer, 1794), see **lateral supraclavicular nerves (>1840)**

superficial stratum of crus cerebri (Mayo, 1827), see **cerebral peduncle (Tarin, 1753)**

superficial temporal branch of inferior maxillary nerve (Le Cat, 1768), see **auriculotemporal nerve (Haller, 1762)**

superficial temporal branch of superior maxillary branch of fifth pair (Haller, 1762), see **zygomatic nerve (>1840)**

superficial temporal branch of third branch of fifth pair (Meckel, 1748), see **auriculotemporal nerve (Haller, 1762)**

superficial temporal branches of anterior auricular nerve (Arnold, 1834), see **superficial temporal branches of auriculotemporal nerve (>1840)**

superficial temporal branches of auriculotemporal nerve (>1840)

superficial temporal branches of superficial temporal nerve (Arnold, 1834), see **superficial temporal branches of auriculotemporal nerve (>1840)**

superficial temporal nerve (Meckel, 1748), see **auriculotemporal nerve (Haller, 1762)**

superficial temporal nerve of third trunk of fifth (Swan, 1830), see **auriculotemporal nerve (Haller, 1762)**

superficial terminal branch of cubital nerve (Cruveilhier, 1836), see **superficial branch of ulnar nerve (Fyfe, 1800)**

superficial terminal branch of external plantar nerve (Cruveilhier, 1836), see **superficial branch of lateral plantar nerve (>1840)**

superficial transverse fibres of pons (Bell, 1834), see **transverse pontine fibers (>1840)**

superficial twig of deep branch of external plantar nerve (Jördens, 1788), see **deep branch of lateral plantar nerve (>1840)**

superficial Vidian nerve (Günther, 1786), see **greater petrosal nerve (>1840)**

superficial volar arch (Mayer, 1794), see **brachial plexus medial cord (Schwalbe, 1881)**

superficial volar branch of ulnar nerve (Bock, 1827), see **common palmar digital nerves of ulnar nerve (>1840)**

superficial white substance of quadrigeminal body (Arnold, 1838a), see **superior colliculus (Haller, 1762)**

superimposed bulge (Reil, 1809b), see **splenium of corpus callosum (Burdach, 1822)**

superior anastomotic thread of malo-palpebral fascicle of subcutaneous malar surculus with inferior orbital thread of seventh pair (Bellingeri, 1818), see **zygomaticofacial nerve (>1840)**

superior anastomotic threads of malo-palpebral fascicle of subcutaneous malar surculus (Bellingeri, 1818), see **zygomaticofacial nerve (>1840)**

superior and anterior external femoral cutaneous nerve (Mayer, 1794), see **lateral cutaneous nerve of thigh (>1840)**

superior and anterior fascicle of soft nerve (Cotugno, 1760), see **rostral part of vestibular nerve (>1840)**

superior and external inferior femoral cutaneous nerve (Mayer, 1794), see **lateral cutaneous nerve of thigh (>1840)**

superior and inferior branches of infratrochlear nerve (Haase, 1781), see **palpebral branches of infratrochlear nerve (>1840)**

superior and lesser posterior auricular nerve (Mayer, 1794), see **lesser occipital nerve (Mayer, 1794)**

superior and posterior cutaneous nerve (Jördens, 1788), see **posterior cutaneous nerve of thigh (Günther, 1786)**

superior and posterior fascicle of soft nerve (Cotugno, 1760), see **caudal part of vestibular nerve (>1840)**

superior anterior branch of auditory nerve proper (Günther, 1786), see **rostral part of vestibular nerve (>1840)**

superior anterior branch of small sciatic branch (Winslow, 1733), see **deep fibular nerve (Fyfe, 1800)**

superior anterior branches of muscular branch of peroneal nerve (Martin, 1781), see **muscular branches of deep fibular nerve (>1840)**

superior anterior gastric plexus (Langenbeck, 1826–1830), see **left gastric plexus (>1840)**

superior anterior lobe (Malacarne, 1776), see **cerebellar hemisphere (Willis, 1664)**

superior anterior tubercle (Günther, 1786), see **tonsil (Malacarne, 1776)**

superior ascending prolongation of cerebellum (Meckel, 1817), see **superior cerebellar peduncle (Procháska, 1800)**

superior auricular branch of lesser occipital nerve (Peipers, 1793), see **lesser occipital nerve (Mayer, 1794)**

superior auricular branch of occipitoauricular nerve (Peipers, 1793), see **lesser occipital nerve (Mayer, 1794)**

superior auricular fascicle of cutaneous temporal surculus of inferior maxillary branch (Bellingeri, 1818), see **anterior auricular nerves (>1840)**

superior brachial plexus (Günther, 1786), see **brachial plexus (Camper, 1760)**

superior branch of auriculotemporal nerve (Cruveilhier, 1836), see **superficial temporal branches of auriculotemporal nerve (>1840)**

superior branch of buccal nerve (Meckel, 1753), see **buccal branch of facial nerve (>1840)**

superior branch of eighth pair of nerves arising within skull (Willis, 1664), see **glossopharyngeal nerve (Huber, 1744)**

superior branch of facial nerve (Knox, 1832), see **facial nerve trunk (1840)**

superior branch of facial nerve (Meckel, 1753), see **zygomatic branches of facial nerve (>1840)**

superior branch of fifth pair (Rau, 1694), see **ophthalmic nerve (Winslow, 1733)**

superior branch of fifth pair of nerves arising within skull (Willis, 1664), see **trigeminal nerve (Winslow, 1733)**

superior branch of first and superior branch of third pair (Marchetti, 1652), see **frontal nerve (Cheselden, 1726)**

superior branch of first division of fifth pair of nerves (Todd, 1836–1839), see **frontal nerve (Cheselden, 1726)**

superior branch of great facial nerve (Meckel, 1753), see **zygomatic branches of facial nerve (>1840)**

superior branch of hard nerve (Meckel, 1753), see **facial nerve trunk (1840)**

superior branch of hard part of nerve of seventh pair (Bonhomme, 1748), see **facial nerve trunk (1840)**

superior branch of inferior facial branch of inferior branch of anterior branch of hard nerve (Loder, 1778), see **marginal mandibular branch of facial nerve (>1840)**

superior branch of inferior maxillary nerve (Schaarschmidt, 1750), see **anterior branch of mandibular nerve (>1840)**

superior branch of internal pudendal nerve (Cruveilhier, 1836), see **dorsal nerve of penis (Camper, 1762)**

superior branch of middle cervical ganglion (Meckel, 1817), see **communicating branch of superior and middle cervical ganglia (>1840)**

superior branch of middle cutaneous nerve of neck (Peipers, 1793), see **superior branches of transverse nerve of neck (>1840)**

superior branch of middle facial nerve (Meckel, 1753), see **zygomatic branches of facial nerve (>1840)**

superior branch of middle subcutaneous nerve of neck (Bock, 1827), see **superior branches of transverse nerve of neck (>1840)**

superior branch of obturator nerve (Günther, 1786), see **anterior branch of obturator nerve (Haase, 1781; Martin, 1781)**

superior branch of perineal branch of internal pudendal nerve (Cruveilhier, 1836), see **muscular branches of perineal nerve (>1840)**

superior branch of portio dura (Du Verney, 1683), see **facial nerve trunk (1840)**

superior branch of portio major and minor of facial nerve (Bellingeri, 1818), see **facial nerve trunk (1840)**

superior branch of pterygoid nerve (Cloquet, 1816), see **greater petrosal nerve (>1840)**

superior branch of right vagus nerves (Mayer, 1794), see **hepatic branch of posterior vagal trunk (>1840)**

superior branch of second cervical nerve (Bell, 1803b), see **spinal nerve ventral branch (>1840)**

superior branch of second cervical nerve (Bell & Bell, 1816), see **communicating loops of cervical plexus (>1840)**

superior branch of sixth pair of nerves (Lobstein, 1823), see **communicating branch from internal carotid plexus to abducens nerve (>1840)**

superior branch of subcutaneous malar nerve (Arnold, 1834), see **zygomaticotemporal nerve (>1840)**

superior branch of subcutaneous nerve of neck (Meckel, 1753), see **superior branches of transverse nerve of neck (>1840)**

superior branch of superficial nerve of neck (Bang, 1770), see **superior branches of transverse nerve of neck (>1840)**

superior branch of superior maxillary branch of nerve of fifth pair (Bonhomme, 1748), see **maxillary nerve (Meckel, 1753)**

superior branch of trigeminal nerve (Winslow, 1733), see **ophthalmic nerve (Winslow, 1733)**

superior branch of vestibular nerve (Arnold, 1839), see **utricular nerve (>1840)**

superior branch of Vidian nerve (Burdin, 1803), see **greater petrosal nerve (>1840)** *superior branches of external popliteal sciatic nerve (Cruveilhier, 1836)*, see ***muscular branches of deep fibular nerve (>1840)***

superior branches of spermatic nerve (Fyfe, 1800), see ***superior testicular nerves (>1840)***

superior branches of spheno-palatine ganglion (Quain, 1837), see ***pterygopalatine nerves (Wrisberg, 1786)***

superior branches of superior cervical ganglion (Cloquet, 1816), see ***internal carotid nerve (>1840)***

superior branches of third branch of fifth pair (Meckel, 1748), see ***mandibular nerve trunk (>1840)***

superior branches of transverse nerve of neck (>1840)

superior branches of vagus supply larynx (Cheselden, 1726), see ***superior laryngeal nerve (Loder, 1778)***

superior bulb of spinal prolongation (Chaussier, 1807), see ***medulla (Winslow, 1733)***

superior cardiac branch (Haller, 1762), see ***superior cardiac nerve (Neubauer, 1772)***

superior cardiac branch of vagus nerves (Mayer, 1794), see ***superior cervical cardiac branches of vagus nerve (>1840)***

superior cardiac nerve (Neubauer, 1772)

superior cardiac nerves (Haase, 1781), see ***superior cardiac nerve (Neubauer, 1772)***

superior cardiac plexus (Drake, 1707), see ***cardiac plexus (Keill, 1698)***

superior caroticotympanic nerve (>1840)

superior cerebellar commissure (Tiedemann, 1821), see ***cerebellar vermis (Meckel, 1817)***

superior cerebellar fissure (Vicq d'Azyr, 1784), see ***posterior superior fissure (>1840)***

superior cerebellar peduncle (Procháska, 1800)

superior cerebellar peduncle decussation (>1840)

superior cerebellar process (Vieussens, 1684), see ***superior cerebellar peduncle (Procháska, 1800)***

superior cerebellar vermis (Tiedemann, 1821), see ***cerebellar vermis (Meckel, 1817)***

superior cerebral commissure (Gerdy, 1838), see ***corpus callosum (Galen, c177)***

superior cerebral ganglion (Quain, 1828), see ***cerebral nuclei (Swanson, 2000a)***

superior cervical cardiac branches of vagus nerve (>1840)

superior cervical ganglion (Vieussens, 1684)

superior ciliary filaments (Todd, 1836–1839), see ***short ciliary nerves (>1840)***

superior circular sinus (Winslow, 1733), see ***circular sinus (Ridley, 1695)***

superior circumflex nerves of arteries of heart (Andersch, 1797), see ***coronary plexuses (Meckel, 1817)***

superior clunial nerves (>1840)

superior coccygeal ganglion (Bock, 1827), see ***coccygeal sympathetic ganglia (>1840)***

superior coccygeal nerve (Schlemm, 1834), see ***coccygeal nerves (Camper, 1762)***

superior colliculus (Haller, 1762)

superior colliculus commissure (>1840)

superior commissure of quadrigeminal tubercles (Serres, 1824–1826), see ***superior colliculus commissure (>1840)***

superior coronary plexus of stomach (Meckel, 1817), see ***autonomic nerves (Langley, 1896)***

superior corpora bigemina (Gordon, 1815), see ***superior colliculus (Haller, 1762)***

superior cubital nerve (Cheselden, 1713), see ***median nerve (Du Verney, 1697)***

superior cutaneous branch of crural nerve (Martin, 1781), see ***medial cutaneous nerve of thigh (>1840)***

superior cutaneous branches of neck of inferior branch of hard nerve (Meckel, 1753), see ***marginal mandibular branch of facial nerve (>1840)***

superior cutaneous cervical branches of inferior branch of hard nerve (Meckel, 1753), see ***cervical branch of facial nerve (>1840)***

superior cutaneous cervical nerves (Meckel, 1753), see ***cervical branch of facial nerve (>1840)***

superior cutaneous nerve (Günther, 1786), see ***medial cutaneous nerve of thigh (>1840)***

superior cutaneous nerve of arm (Cloquet, 1828), see ***superior lateral cutaneous nerve of arm (>1840)***

superior cutaneous nerve of hips (Knox, 1832), see ***perforating cutaneous nerve (>1840)***

superior cutaneous nerve of neck (Neubauer, 1772), see ***superior branches of transverse nerve of neck (>1840)***

superior cutaneous nerves of buttocks (Walter, 1783), see ***perforating cutaneous nerve (>1840)***

superior cutaneous perforant branch of crural musculocutaneous nerve (Cruveilhier, 1836), see ***anterior cutaneous branches of femoral nerve (Quain & Wilson, 1839)***

superior cutaneous submaxillary nerves (Meckel, 1817), see ***cervical branch of facial nerve (>1840)***

superior dental branches of superior dental plexus (>1840)

superior dental nerves (Haller, 1762), see ***maxillary nerve (Meckel, 1753)***

superior dental plexus (>1840)

superior division of facial nerve (Swan, 1830), see ***facial nerve trunk (1840)***

superior division of fifth cervical nerve (Bell & Bell, 1816), see ***cervical nerve (Galen, c173)***

superior dorsal branch of external volar nerve of index finger (Bock, 1827), see ***proper palmar digital nerves of median nerve (>1840)***

superior duodenal nerves (Mayer, 1794), see ***gastroduodenal plexus (>1840)***

superior enlargement (Serres, 1824–1826), see ***cervical enlargement (Arnold, 1838b)***

superior enteroid processes of middle lobe (Rolando, 1831), see ***superior temporal gyrus (>1840)***

superior external cutaneous nerve (Günther, 1786), see ***superior lateral cutaneous nerve of arm (>1840)***

superior external cutaneous nerve (Meckel, 1817), see ***posterior cutaneous nerve of forearm (>1840)***

superior external cutaneous nerve (Quain, 1828), see ***posterior cutaneous nerve of arm (>1840)***

superior external cutaneous nerve of infraorbital nerve (Meckel, 1753), see ***infraorbital nerve (Schaarschmidt, 1750)***

superior part of gluteal plexus (Swan, 1830), see **superior gluteal nerve (Martin, 1781)**
superior part of medullary crura (Pourfour du Petit, 1710), see **brainstem (Schwalbe, 1881)**
superior part of spinal marrow (Haase, 1781), see **vertebrate brain (Cuvier, 1800)**
superior part of vestibular nerve (>1840), see **rostral part of vestibular nerve (>1840)**
superior pectoral ganglion (Schreger, 1803), see **superior thoracic ganglion (Lieutaud, 1742)**
superior pedicle of cerebellum (Mayo, 1827), see **superior cerebellar peduncle (Procháska, 1800)**
superior peduncles of conarium (Cruveilhier, 1836), see **medullary stria (Wenzel & Wenzel, 1812)**
superior peduncles of pineal body (Cruveilhier, 1836), see **medullary stria (Wenzel & Wenzel, 1812)**
superior petrous nerve (Meckel, 1817), see **greater petrosal nerve (>1840)**
superior pharyngeal branch of pharyngolingual branch of glossopharyngeal nerve (Kilian, 1822), see **pharyngeal branches of glossopharyngeal nerve (Neubauer, 1772)**
superior pharyngeal nerve (Meckel, 1817), see **pharyngeal branches of vagus nerve (>1840)**
superior pharyngeal plexus (Bock, 1817), see **pharyngeal plexus (Neubauer, 1772)**
superior poplital nerve (Günther, 1786), see **articular branches of common fibular nerve (>1840)**
superior portion of lateral ventricle (Chaussier, 1807), see **lateral ventricle (Vesalius, 1543a)**
superior portion of spinal cord (Anderson, 1837), see **medulla (Winslow, 1733)**
superior posterior cutaneous nerve (Bock, 1827), see **posterior cutaneous nerve of forearm (>1840)**
superior posterior cutaneous nerve (Fischer, 1791), see **inferior clunial nerves (>1840)**
superior posterior gastric plexus (Langenbeck, 1826–1830), see **right gastric plexus (>1840)**
superior posterior lobe (Malacarne, 1776), see **ansiform lobule crus 1 (Bolk, 1906)**
superior posterior renal nerve (Walter, 1783), see **least splanchnic nerve (>1840)**
superior posterior renal nerve roots (Walter, 1783), see **least splanchnic nerve (>1840)**
superior posterior renal nerve trunk (Walter, 1783), see **least splanchnic nerve (>1840)**
superior posterior scapular nerve (Monro, 1783), see **suprascapular nerve (Bang, 1770)**
superior primary branch of inferior maxillary nerve (Quain, 1832), see **anterior branch of mandibular nerve (>1840)**
superior process of vermis (Haller, 1762), see **cerebellar vermis (Meckel, 1817)**
superior prolongation of cerebellum (Burdin, 1803), see **superior cerebellar peduncle (Procháska, 1800)**
superior prominences (Willis, 1664), see **tectum (Baer, 1837)**
superior protuberances (Willis, 1664), see **tectum (Baer, 1837)**
superior pudendal nerve in female (Camper, 1762), see **dorsal nerve of clitoris (>1840)**
superior pudendal nerve in male (Camper, 1762), see **dorsal nerve of penis (Camper, 1762)**
superior pudic nerve (Knox, 1832), see **dorsal nerve of clitoris (>1840)**
superior pudic nerve (Meckel, 1817), see **perineal nerve (Camper, 1762)**
superior pyramid (Desmoulins, 1825), see **gracile tubercle (>1840)**
superior pyramidal body (Mayer, 1794), see **pyramid (Willis, 1664)**
superior quadrigeminal body (Wenzel & Wenzel, 1812), see **superior colliculus (Haller, 1762)**
superior quadrigeminal eminence (Günther, 1786), see **superior colliculus (Haller, 1762)**
superior quadrigeminal tubercle (Vicq d'Azyr, 1786), see **superior colliculus (Haller, 1762)**
superior rachidian bulb (Meckel, 1817), see **medulla (Winslow, 1733)**
superior ramus of ophthalmic nerve (Winslow, 1733), see **frontal nerve (Cheselden, 1726)**
superior ramus of trunk of nerve of portio dura (Winslow, 1733), see **posterior auricular nerve (Meckel, 1753)**
superior raphe of corpus callosum (Reil, 1809b), see **corpus callosum (Galen, c177)**
superior rectal plexus (>1840)
superior recurrent nerve of eighth pair (Neubauer, 1772), see **accessory nerve (Vieussens, 1684)**
superior respiratory nerve of trunk (Bell, 1821), see **accessory nerve (Vieussens, 1684)**
superior root of ansa cervicalis (>1840)
superior root of intercostal nerve (Mayer, 1794), see **internal carotid nerve (>1840)**
superior root of olfactory nerve (Knox, 1832), see **tenia tecta (Swanson, 1992)**
superior root of posterior thoracic nerve (Bock, 1827), see **long thoracic nerve (Quain & Wilson, 1839)**
superior salivatory nucleus (>1840)
superior saphena nerve (Meckel, 1817), see **femoral nerve (Haller, 1762)**
superior scapular nerve (Swan, 1830), see **suprascapular nerve (Bang, 1770)**
superior semilunar lobe (Meckel, 1817), see **ansiform lobule crus I (Bolk, 1906)**
superior small branch of fifth pair (Ridley, 1695), see **ophthalmic nerve (Winslow, 1733)**
superior soft nerve (Neubauer, 1772), see **laryngopharyngeal branches of superior cervical ganglion (>1840)**
superior spermatic nerves (Walter, 1783), see **superior ovarian nerves (>1840)**
superior splanchnic nerve (Haase, 1781), see **greater splanchnic nerve (Walter, 1783)**
superior splenic nerves (Mayer, 1794), see **splenic plexus (Palfijn, 1726)**
superior stomachical branch of wandring pair (Willis, 1664), see **anterior vagal trunk (Wrisberg, 1780)**
superior striae of corpus striatum (Vicq d'Azyr, 1786), see **cerebral cortex white matter (>1840)**
superior subcutaneous branch of neck of descending branch of superficial branch of hard nerve (Günther, 1786), see **cervical branch of facial nerve (>1840)**

superior subcutaneous cervical nerves (Meckel, 1753), see **cervical branch of facial nerve (>1840)**
superior subcutaneous cervical nerves (Meckel, 1817), see **superior branches of transverse nerve of neck (>1840)**
superior subcutaneous malar nerve (Mayer, 1794), see **zygomaticofacial nerve (>1840)**
superior subcutaneous nerve of neck (Arnold, 1834), see **cervical branch of facial nerve (>1840)**
superior subcutaneous surculus of cervico-facial branch of portio major and minor of facial nerve (Bellingeri, 1818), see **cervical branch of facial nerve (>1840)**
superior subcutaneous surculus of inferior branch of portio major and minor of facial nerve (Bellingeri, 1818), see **cervical branch of facial nerve (>1840)**
superior subscapular branch of brachial plexus (Cruveilhier, 1836), see **upper subscapular nerve (>1840)**
superior sulcus (Burdach, 1822), see **circular sulcus (Schwalbe, 1881)**
superior sulcus of spinal medulla (Bojanus, 1819–1821), see **dorsal median sulcus of spinal cord (>1840)**
superior superficial branch of hard nerve (Mayer, 1794), see **facial nerve trunk (1840)**
superior superficial nasal branches of infraorbital nerve (Loder, 1778), see **external nasal branches of infraorbital nerve (>1840)**
superior superficial nerve to pulmonary arteries (Andersch, 1797), see **pulmonary plexus (Winslow, 1733)**
superior surface of cerebellum (Malacarne, 1776), see **cerebellum (Aristotle)**
superior swelling of spinal cord (Quain & Wilson, 1839), see **spinal cord (Galen, c162–c166)**
superior temporal area (Brodmann, 1909), see **superior temporal gyrus (>1840)**
superior temporal gyrus (>1840)
superior temporal sulcus (>1840)
superior testicular nerves (>1840)
superior thoracic ganglion (Lieutaud, 1742)
superior thoracic ganglion (Neubauer, 1772), see **inferior cervical ganglion (Vieussens, 1684)**
superior tracheal nerves (Meckel, 1817), see **tracheal branches of recurrent laryngeal nerve (>1840)**
superior twig of Vidian nerve (Todd, 1836–1839), see **greater petrosal nerve (>1840)**
superior ureteric nerves (Walter, 1783)
superior uterine plexus (Tiedemann, 1822), see **uterovaginal plexus (>1840)**
superior vagal ganglion (>1840), see **proximal vagal ganglion (>1840)**
superior ventricle (Berengario da Carpi, 1521), see **lateral ventricle (Vesalius, 1543a)**
superior ventricles (Gerdy, 1838), see **lateral ventricle (Vesalius, 1543a)**
superior vermicular eminence (Burdin, 1803), see **cerebellar vermis (Meckel, 1817)**
superior vermiform appendix (Winslow, 1733), see **cerebellar vermis (Meckel, 1817)**
superior vermiform process (Gordon, 1815), see **central lobule (Burdach, 1822)**
superior vermiform process (Reil, 1807–1808a), see **cerebellar vermis (Meckel, 1817)**
superior vermis (Massa, 1536), see **cerebellar vermis (Meckel, 1817)**
superior vermis (>1840), see **cerebellar vermis (Meckel, 1817)**
superior vesicle nerves (Walter, 1783), see **extrinsic vesical plexus (>1840)**
superior Vidian nerve (Günther, 1786), see **greater petrosal nerve (>1840)**
superior wall of middle ventricle (Gerdy, 1838), see **thalamic part of third ventricle (Swanson, 2004)**
superior worm (Massa, 1536), see **cerebellar vermis (Meckel, 1817)**
superior worm of cerebellum (Chaussier, 1807), see **cerebellar vermis (Meckel, 1817)**
super-orbitar branches of facial nerve (Burdin, 1803), see **temporal branches of facial nerve (Swan, 1830)**
super-pubian nerve (Burdin, 1803), see **genitofemoral nerve (>1840)**
superscapular nerve (Haller, 1747), see **suprascapular nerve (Bang, 1770)**
supersphenoidal peduncle (Burdin, 1803), see **hypothalamus (Kuhlenbeck, 1927)**
supertrochlear branch of frontal nerve (Quain, 1828), see **supratrochlear nerve (Schaarschmidt, 1750)**
supinator longus muscle branch of radial nerve (Bock, 1827), see **muscular branches of radial nerve (>1840)**
supposed anterior lateral sulcus (Rolando, 1824), see **ventrolateral sulcus of spinal cord (>1840)**
supra-acromial branch of supraclavicular branches (Cruveilhier, 1836), see **lateral supraclavicular nerves (>1840)**
supra-acromial branches of cervical plexus (Cloquet, 1816), see **lateral supraclavicular nerves (>1840)**
supra-acromial nerves (Cruveilhier, 1836), see **lateral supraclavicular nerves (>1840)**
supracallosal gyrus (>1840), see **indusium griseum (Valentin, 1841)**
supraclavicular branch proper of cervical plexus (Cruveilhier, 1836), see **supraclavicular nerves (Meckel, 1817)**
supraclavicular branches of cervical plexus (Cloquet, 1816), see **supraclavicular nerves (Meckel, 1817)**
supraclavicular branches of cervical plexus (Cruveilhier, 1836), see **supraclavicular nerves (Meckel, 1817)**
supraclavicular nerves (Cruveilhier, 1836), see **supraclavicular nerves (Meckel, 1817)**
supraclavicular nerves (Meckel, 1817)
supraesophageal brain (Cuvier, 1800), see **supraesophageal ganglion (Grant, 1834a)**
supraesophageal ganglion (Grant, 1834a)
suprajugal branches of ascending branch of superficial branch of hard nerve (Günther, 1786), see **temporal branches of facial nerve (Swan, 1830)**
supramalleolar nerve (Fischer, 1791), see **lateral calcaneal branches of sural nerve (>1840)**
supramalleolar twig of tibial communicating branch (Jördens, 1788), see **lateral calcaneal branches of sural nerve (>1840)**
supramammillary decussation (>1840)
supramarginal area (Brodmann, 1909), see **supramarginal gyrus (>1840)**

supramarginal gyrus (>1840)
supraoesophageal ganglia (Newport, 1834), see ***nervous system (Monro, 1783)***
supraoptic commissures (>1840), see ***supraoptic decussations (>1840)***
supraoptic decussations (>1840)
supraoptic layer (Gerdy, 1838), see ***endbrain (Kuhlenbeck, 1927)***
supraorbital branch of first branch of fifth pair of nerves (Meckel, 1753), see ***supraorbital nerve (Meckel, 1753)***
supra-orbital branch of first trunk of fifth nerve (Swan, 1830), see ***supraorbital nerve (Meckel, 1753)***
supraorbital branch of fourth temporal branch of hard nerve (Meckel, 1753), see ***temporal branches of facial nerve (Swan, 1830)***
supraorbital branch of frontal nerve (Arnold, 1834), see ***supraorbital nerve (Meckel, 1753)***
supraorbital branch of temporal branches (Meckel, 1753), see ***temporal branches of facial nerve (Swan, 1830)***
supraorbital convolution (Gerdy, 1838), see ***orbital gyri (>1840)***
supraorbital nerve (Meckel, 1753)
suprapineal recess (>1840)
suprapubic nerve (Chaussier, 1809), see ***genitofemoral nerve (>1840)***
suprarenal ganglion (Meckel, 1817), see ***celiac ganglion (Walter, 1783)***
suprarenal nerves (Cloquet, 1828), see ***adrenal plexus (>1840)***
suprarenal plexus (Haase, 1781), see ***adrenal plexus (>1840)***
suprascapular branch of brachial plexus (Cloquet, 1816), see ***suprascapular nerve (Bang, 1770)***
suprascapular nerve (Bang, 1770)
suprascapular nerve (Haase, 1781), see ***dorsal scapular nerve (>1840)***
suprasphenoidal appendix of cerebrum (Chaussier, 1807), see ***pituitary gland (>1840)***
suprasphenoidal filament (Cloquet, 1816), see ***hypophysial plexus (>1840)***
suprasphenoidal stalk (Chaussier, 1807), see ***pituitary gland (>1840)***
supratrochlear branch of frontal nerve (Meckel, 1748), see ***supratrochlear nerve (Schaarschmidt, 1750)***
supratrochlear nerve (Schaarschmidt, 1750)
suprazygomatic branch of superior branch of anterior branch of hard nerve (Loder, 1778), see ***temporal branches of facial nerve (Swan, 1830)***
supreme mesenteric branch (Willis, 1664), see ***greater splanchnic nerve (Walter, 1783)***
sural communicating branch of common fibular nerve (>1840)
sural nerve (Pietro da Cortona, 1741)
suralem nervum (Pietro da Cortona, 1741), see ***sural nerve (Pietro da Cortona, 1741)***
surculi rami majoris posterioris crassam meningem penetrantes (Vieussens, 1684), see ***nervus spinosus (>1840)***
surculus quartus crassioris ac interioris propaginis K (Vieussens, 1684), see ***infratrochlear nerve (Schaarschmidt, 1750)***
surculus secundus crassioris ac interioris propaginis K (Vieussens, 1684), see ***anterior ethmoidal nerve (>1840)***
surculus tertius crassioris ac interioris propaginis K (Vieussens, 1684), see ***nasal branches of anterior ethmoidal nerve (>1840)***
suture of corpus callosum (Günther, 1786), see ***longitudinal striae (>1840)***
sutures of cerebellum (Malacarne, 1776), see ***cerebellar vermis (Meckel, 1817)***
swallow's nest (Reil, 1807–1808a), see ***nidus (Reil, 1809c)***
swellings (Swammerdam, c1675), see ***central ganglia (>1840)***
Sylvian fissure (Vicq d'Azyr, 1784), see ***lateral cerebral sulcus (>1840)***
Sylvian fossa (Tarin, 1753), see ***lateral cerebral sulcus (>1840)***
Sylvian fossa (Vicq d'Azyr, 1784), see ***lateral cerebral fossa (>1840)***
Sylvian fossa (Vicq d'Azyr, 1786), see ***septal fissure (Burdach, 1822)***
Sylvius's aqueduct (Heister, 1721), see ***cerebral aqueduct (>1840)***
symmetrical system of nerves (Bell, 1821), see ***craniospinal nerves (Herrick, 1915)***
sympathetic branch of mental nerve (Meckel, 1753), see ***mental nerve (Cheselden, 1726)***
sympathetic branch of Vidian nerve (Arnold, 1834), see ***deep petrosal nerve (Meckel, 1817)***
sympathetic branches to esophagus (Bischoff, 1832), see ***esophageal branches of sympathetic trunk (>1840)***
sympathetic carotid ganglion (Langenbeck, 1826–1830), see ***carotid ganglion (Wutzer, 1817; Bock, 1817)***
sympathetic chain (Gaskell, 1886), see ***sympathetic cord (>1840)***
sympathetic cord (>1840)
sympathetic labial threads of mental fascicle of inferior alveolar surculus of inferior maxillary branch (Bellingeri, 1818), see ***mental branches of mental nerve (>1840)***
sympathetic nerve (Lobstein, 1823), see ***sympathetic cord (>1840)***
sympathetic nerve (Soemmerring, 1791), see ***sympathetic trunk (Winslow, 1733)***
sympathetic nerve branches to oculomotor nerve (Langenbeck, 1826–1830), see ***communicating branch from internal carotid plexus to oculomotor nerve (>1840)***
sympathetic nerve ganglia (Carus, 1814), see ***sympathetic trunk ganglia (Winslow, 1733)***
sympathetic nerves (Quain, 1828), see ***peripheral nervous system (Meckel, 1817)***
sympathetic nerves (Sharpey et al., 1867), see ***autonomic nerves (Langley, 1898)***
sympathetic nervous system (Blainville, 1821), see ***paravertebral ganglia (Durward, 1951)***
sympathetic nervous system (Wutzer, 1817), see ***peripheral nervous system (Meckel, 1817)***
sympathetic root of ciliary ganglion (>1840)
sympathetic root of otic ganglion (>1840)

sympathetic root of sphenopalatine ganglion (>1840), see **deep petrosal nerve (Meckel, 1817)**
sympathetic root of submandibular ganglion (>1840)
sympathetic system (Cruveilhier, 1844), see **peripheral nervous system (Meckel, 1817)**
sympathetic system of nerves (Bell & Bell, 1816), see **peripheral nervous system (Meckel, 1817)**
sympathetic trunk (Winslow, 1733)
sympathetic trunk ganglia (Winslow, 1733)
sympathicus minor par decimum tertium (Malacarne, 1791), see **intermediofacial nerve (Strong & Elwyn, 1943)**
systema caudiceum (Burdach, 1822), see **central nervous system white matter tracts (>1840)**
systema copulativum (Burdach, 1822), see **vertebrate brain (Cuvier, 1800)**
tactile nerves (Anatomia Magistri Nicolai physici, early 12th century), see **nerves (Herophilus, c335–c280 BC)**
taenia (Burdach, 1822), see **fimbria (Honegger, 1890)**
taenia (Fyfe, 1800), see **terminal stria (Wenzel & Wenzel, 1812)**
taenia cerebri (Haller, 1762), see **fimbria (Honegger, 1890)**
taenia cinerea foveae rhomboidalis (Burdach, 1822), see **cochlear nuclei (>1840)**
taenia corporis striati (Chaussier, 1807), see **terminal stria (Wenzel & Wenzel, 1812)**
taenia fibrosa corporis striati (Vicq d'Azyr, 1786), see **terminal stria (Wenzel & Wenzel, 1812)**
taenia fornicis (>1840), see **fimbria (Honegger, 1890)**
taenia grisea (Wenzel & Wenzel, 1812), see **cochlear nuclei (>1840)**
taenia hippocampi (Vicq d'Azyr, 1786), see **fimbria (Honegger, 1890)**
taenia nervosa (Meckel, 1748), see **trigeminal ganglion (>1840)**
taenia plexus choroidei ventriculi quarti (Burdach, 1822), see **choroid line of fourth ventricle (>1840)**
taenia semicircularis (Haller, 1754a), see **terminal stria (Wenzel & Wenzel, 1812)**
taenia striata (Vicq d'Azyr, 1786), see **terminal stria (Wenzel & Wenzel, 1812)**
taeniae foveae rhomboidalis (Burdach, 1822), see **medullary striae (Scarpa, 1788)**
taeniae medullares (Arnold, 1838a), see **medullary striae (Scarpa, 1788)**
taeniam cornu Ammonis cineream (Volkmann, 1831), see **dentate gyrus (>1840)**
taeniola conarii (Wenzel & Wenzel, 1812), see **pineal stalk (Burdach, 1822)**
taeniolae corporis callosi (Reil, 1812c), see **rostrum of corpus callosum (Reil, 1809b)**
tail of caudate nucleus (Arnold, 1838b)
tail of fascia dentata (Arnold, 1838b), see **dentate gyrus (>1840)**
tail of marrow (Bartholin, 1662), see **brainstem (Schwalbe, 1881)**
tail of oblong marrow (Willis, 1664), see **rhombicbrain (His, 1893b)**
tailed structure (Avicenna, c1030), see **caudate nucleus (Arnold, 1838b)**
Tapete (Reil, 1809b), see **tapetum (Reil, 1809b)**
tapetum (Reil, 1809b)
tapetum of thalamus (Reil, 1809b), see **zonal layer of thalamus (Burdach 1822)**
tarsal nerves (Fischer, 1791), see **medial plantar nerve (>1840)**
teat (Crooke, 1615), see **frontal pole (>1840)**
tectal stria (Arnold, 1838b), see **lateral longitudinal stria (Arnold, 1838a)**
tectospinal tract (>1840)
tectum (Baer, 1837)
tectum of white substance at anterior end of olivary nucleus (Arnold, 1838b), see **amiculum of olive (>1840)**
tectum ventriculi quarti (Burdach, 1822), see **roof of fourth ventricle (Vesalius, 1543a)**
tegimen secundinale (Zerbi, 1502), see **pia (Galen, c192)**
tegmen ventriculi quarti (>1840), see **roof of fourth ventricle (Vesalius, 1543a)**
tegmental bundle from ganglion of pineal peduncles (Meynert, 1871–1872), see **habenulo-interpeduncular tract (>1840)**
tegmental central tegmental tract (>1840)
tegmental dorsal longitudinal fascicle (>1840)
tegmental habenulo-interpeduncular tract (>1840)
tegmental mammillotegmental tract (>1840)
tegmental medial forebrain bundle (>1840)
tegmental medial lemniscus (>1840)
tegmental medial longitudinal fascicle (>1840)
tegmental rubrospinal tract (>1840)
tegmental segment of midbrain tract of trigeminal nerve (>1840)
tegmental spinothalamic tract (>1840)
tegmental superior cerebellar peduncle (>1840)
tegmental tectospinal tract (>1840)
tegmental ventrolateral fascicle (>1840)
tegmentum (Arnold, 1838b), see **tegmentum (Swanson, 2000b)**
tegmentum (Meckel, 1817), see **tegmentum (Swanson, 2000b)**
tegmentum (Reil, 1809b), see **vertebrate brain (Cuvier, 1800)**
tegmentum (Reil, 1809c), see **midbrain (Baer, 1837)**
tegmentum (Swanson, 2000b)
tegmentum caudicis cerebri (Burdach, 1822), see **tegmentum (Swanson, 2000b)**
tegmentum cruris (Arnold, 1838a), see **tegmentum (Swanson, 2000b)**
tegmentum of cerebral peduncle (Arnold, 1838b), see **tegmentum (Swanson, 2000b)**
tegmentum of cerebral peduncle (Meckel, 1817), see **tegmentum (Swanson, 2000b)**
tegmentum of third ventricle (Günther, 1786), see **fornix (Vesalius, 1543a)**
tegmentum ventriculorum (Mayer, 1779), see **cerebral cortex white matter (>1840)**
tela chorioidea (Arnold, 1838a), see **choroid membrane of fourth ventricle (>1840)**
tela choroidea (Bock, 1824), see **choroid plexus of third ventricle (Vicq d'Azyr, 1784)**
tela choroïdea (Vicq d'Azyr, 1786), see **choroid membrane of third ventricle (>1840)**

tela choroidea ventriculi lateralis (>1840), see **choroid membrane of lateral ventricle (>1840)**

tela choroidea ventriculi quarti (>1840), see **choroid membrane of fourth ventricle (>1840)**

tela choroidea ventriculi tertii (>1840), see **choroid membrane of third ventricle (>1840)**

tela choroides (Burdach, 1822), see **choroid membrane of third ventricle (>1840)**

tela choroides superior (Burdach, 1822), see **choroid membrane of third ventricle (>1840)**

telencephalon (His, 1893a), see **forebrain (Goette, 1873)**

telencephalon (His, 1893b), see **forebrain (Goette, 1873)**

telencephalon (Kuhlenbeck, 1927), see **endbrain (Kuhlenbeck, 1927)**

temporal branch of auriculotemporal nerve (Cruveilhier, 1836), see **superficial temporal branches of auriculotemporal nerve (>1840)**

temporal branch of facial nerve (Swan, 1830), see **temporal branches of facial nerve (Swan, 1830)**

temporal branch of lachrymal nerve (Todd, 1836–1839), see **communicating branch of lacrimal nerve with zygomatic nerve (>1840)**

temporal branch of lacrimal nerve (Cruveilhier, 1836), see **lacrimal nerve (Meckel, 1748; Bonhomme, 1748)**

temporal branch of malar nerve (Swan, 1830), see **zygomaticotemporal nerve (>1840)**

temporal branch of portio dura (Knox, 1832), see **temporal branches of facial nerve (Swan, 1830)**

temporal branch of subcutaneous malar nerve (Bock, 1817), see **zygomaticofacial nerve (>1840)**

temporal branch of superior branch of anterior branch of hard nerve (Loder, 1778), see **temporal branches of facial nerve (Swan, 1830)**

temporal branch of superior branch of hard nerve (Meckel, 1753), see **facial nerve trunk (1840)**

temporal branch of superior facial branch of hard part of seventh nerve (Haller, 1762), see **facial nerve trunk (1840)**

temporal branches of facial nerve (Swan, 1830)

temporal branches of hard nerve (Meckel, 1753), see **facial nerve trunk (1840)**

temporal branches of superior branch of facial nerve (Arnold, 1834), see **temporal branches of facial nerve (Swan, 1830)**

temporal branches of suprajugal branches of ascending branch of superficial branch of hard nerve (Günther, 1786), see **temporal branches of facial nerve (Swan, 1830)**

temporal branches of temporofacial branch of facial nerve (Cruveilhier, 1836), see **temporal branches of facial nerve (Swan, 1830)**

temporal branches of zygomatic branches of ascending branch of superficial branch of hard nerve (Günther, 1786), see **temporal branches of facial nerve (Swan, 1830)**

temporal cerebral lobule (Chaussier, 1807), see **temporal region (>1840)**

temporal fascicles proper of cutaneous temporal surculus of inferior maxillary branch (Bellingeri, 1818), see **superficial temporal branches of auriculotemporal nerve (>1840)**

temporal filament of temporo-malar branch of orbital branch of superior maxillary nerve (Cruveilhier, 1836), see **orbital branches of pterygopalatine ganglion (>1840)**

temporal filaments of posterior zygomatic threads of temporal surculus (Bellingeri, 1818), see **temporal branches of facial nerve (Swan, 1830)**

temporal fissure (Gerdy, 1838), see **lateral cerebral sulcus (>1840)**

temporal ganglion (Andersch & Soemmerring, 1792)

temporal limb of anterior commissure (>1840)

temporal lobe (Arnold, 1838a), see **temporal region (>1840)**

temporal lobe (Rolando, 1831), see **temporal region (>1840)**

temporal nerve (Schaarschmidt, 1750), see **deep temporal nerves (Haase, 1781)**

temporal nerves (Meckel, 1817), see **temporal branches of facial nerve (Swan, 1830)**

temporal operculum (>1840)

temporal plane (Heschl, 1878)

temporal pole (Broca, 1878a)

temporal region (>1840)

temporal small ganglion (Andersch & Soemmerring, 1792), see **temporal ganglion (Andersch & Soemmerring, 1792)**

temporal soft nerve (Andersch & Soemmerring, 1792), see **jugular nerves (>1840)**

temporal soft small ganglion (Andersch & Soemmerring, 1792), see **temporal ganglion (Andersch & Soemmerring, 1792)**

temporal surculus of superior branch of portio major and minor of facial nerve (Bellingeri, 1818), see **temporal branches of facial nerve (Swan, 1830)**

temporal surculus of temporo-facial branch of portio major and minor of facial nerve (Bellingeri, 1818), see **temporal branches of facial nerve (Swan, 1830)**

temporal surface of cerebellum (Vicq d'Azyr, 1784), see **cerebellum (Aristotle)**

temporo-buccal nerve (Meckel, 1832), see **trigeminal nerve (Winslow, 1733)**

temporofacial branch of facial nerve (Meckel, 1817), see **facial nerve trunk (1840)**

temporo-malar branch of orbital branch of superior maxillary nerve (Cruveilhier, 1836), see **orbital branches of pterygopalatine ganglion (>1840)**

temporo-malar branch of second division of fifth pair of nerves (Todd, 1836–1839), see **zygomatic nerve (>1840)**

temporo-muscular nerves (Burdin, 1803), see **deep temporal nerves (Haase, 1781)**

temporopolar area (Brodmann, 1909), see **temporal region (>1840)**

tender pannicle (Hall, 1565), see **pia (Galen, c192)**

tendril-like offshoot of thicker root of third pair (Vesalius, 1543a), see **anterior branch of mandibular nerve (>1840)**

tenia choroidea ventriculi lateralis (>1840), see **choroid line of lateral ventricle (>1840)**

tenia choroidea ventriculi quarti (>1840), see **choroid line of fourth ventricle (>1840)**

tenia fimbria ventriculi lateralis (>1840), see **fimbrial line of lateral ventricle (>1840)**

tenia of third ventricle (>1840), see **choroid line of third ventricle (>1840)**
tenia stria medullaris (>1840), see **choroid line of third ventricle (>1840)**
tenia tecta (Reil, 1809b), see **cingulum (Burdach, 1822)**
tenia tecta (Swanson, 1992)
tenia thalami (Wenzel & Wenzel, 1812), see **epithalamic medullary stria (>1840)**
tenia thalami (>1840), see **choroid line of third ventricle (>1840)**
tenōn (Hippocrates), see **nerves (Herophilus, c335–c280 BC)**
tensor fasciae latae nerve (Fischer, 1791), see **superior gluteal nerve (Martin, 1781)**
tent (Reil, 1807–1808a), see **roof of fourth ventricle (Vesalius, 1543a)**
tent of cerebellum (Winslow, 1733), see **cerebellar tentorium (Winslow, 1733)**
tenth cerebral pair of Willis (Bang, 1770), see **suboccipital nerve (Winslow, 1733)**
tenth nerve of head (Andersch & Soemmerring, 1792), see **hypoglossal nerve (Winslow, 1733)**
tenth nerve proper of nerves of head (Andersch, 1797), see **vagus nerve (Galen, c192)**
tenth nerves of head (Andersch, 1797), see **vagus nerve (Galen, c192)**
tenth pair of cerebral nerves (Soemmerring, 1791), see **vagus nerve (Galen, c192)**
tenth pair of cranial nerves (Soemmerring, 1791), see **vagus nerve (Galen, c192)**
tenth pair of head (Fyfe, 1800), see **suboccipital nerve (Winslow, 1733)**
tenth pair of nerves (Malacarne, 1791), see **abducens nerve (Heister, 1717)**
tenth pair of nerves arising within skull (Willis, 1664), see **cervical nerves (Galen, c173)**
tenth pair of nerves from brain (Bartholin, 1641), see **hypoglossal nerve (Winslow, 1733)**
tenth pair of nerves of head (Andersch, 1797), see **vagus nerve (Galen, c192)**
tenth pair of nerves of head (Andersch & Soemmerring, 1792), see **hypoglossal nerve (Winslow, 1733)**
tenth pair of nerves of medulla oblongata (Winslow, 1733), see **suboccipital nerve (Winslow, 1733)**
tenth pair of scull (Bell, 1803b), see **suboccipital nerve (Winslow, 1733)**
tenth pair of Willis (Portal, 1803a), see **cervical nerves (Galen, c173)**
tentorial nerve (Arnold, 1838a)
tentorial notch (>1840)
tentorium (Bell, 1803b), see **cerebellar tentorium (Winslow, 1733)**
tentorium cerebelli (Winslow, 1733), see **cerebellar tentorium (Winslow, 1733)**
tentorium of cerebellum (Burdin, 1803), see **cerebellar tentorium (Winslow, 1733)**
tenuis membrana cerebrum involvens (Chaussier, 1807), see **pia (Galen, c192)**
tenuis meninx (Aristotle), see **pia (Galen, c192)**
terminal autonomic nerves (Swanson & Bota, 2010)
terminal branch of axillary nerve (Cruveilhier, 1836), see **muscular branches of axillary nerve (>1840)**
terminal branch of sacral plexus (Cruveilhier, 1836), see **sciatic nerve (Keill, 1698)**
terminal branches of crural nerve (Cruveilhier, 1836), see **femoral nerve (Haller, 1762)**
terminal branches of external plantar nerve (Cruveilhier, 1836), see **lateral plantar nerve (>1840)**
terminal branches of facial nerve (Cruveilhier, 1836), see **facial nerve trunk (1840)**
terminal branches of inferior maxillary nerve (Cruveilhier, 1836), see **mandibular nerve (>1840)**
terminal branches of internal plantar nerve (Cruveilhier, 1836), see **common plantar digital nerves of medial plantar nerve (>1840)**
terminal branches of internal saphenous nerve (Cruveilhier, 1836), see **saphenous nerve (Haase, 1781)**
terminal branches of lumbar plexus (Cruveilhier, 1836), see **lumbosacral plexus (Vesalius, 1543a)**
terminal branches of median nerve (Cruveilhier, 1836), see **median nerve (Du Verney, 1697)**
terminal branches of musculocutaneous nerve (Cruveilhier, 1836), see **superficial fibular nerve (Fyfe, 1800)**
terminal branches of obturator nerve (Cruveilhier, 1836), see **muscular branches of anterior branch of obturator nerve (>1840)**
terminal branches of perineal branch of internal pudendal nerve (Cruveilhier, 1836), see **perineal nerve (Camper, 1762)**
terminal branches of radial nerve (Cruveilhier, 1836), see **radial nerve (Du Verney, 1697)**
terminal branches of recurrent nerve (Cruveilhier, 1836), see **inferior laryngeal nerve (>1840)**
terminal branches of superior maxillary nerve (Cruveilhier, 1836), see **infraorbital nerve (Schaarschmidt, 1750)**
terminal filament (Tiedemann, 1821)
terminal ganglia (Gaskell, 1886)
terminal ganglion (Quain & Wilson, 1839), see **ganglion impar (Quain & Wilson, 1839)**
terminal ganglion (>1840)
terminal lamina (Burdach, 1822)
terminal nerve (>1840)
terminal plexuses (Swanson & Bota, 2010)
terminal stria (Wenzel & Wenzel, 1812)
terminal stria commissure (>1840)
terminal sulcus (>1840)
terminal ventricle (>1840)
tertia ac exterior propago rami majoris posterioris (Viesssens, 1684), see **parotid branches of auriculotemporal nerve (>1840)**
tertium involucrum (Vieussens, 1684), see **arachnoid (Blasius, 1666)**
testes (Galen, c173, definition 1), see **tectum (Baer, 1837)**
testes (Galen, c173, definition 2), see **superior colliculus (Haller, 1762)**
testes (Willis, 1664), see **inferior colliculus (Haller, 1762)**
testes and nates (Vesalius, 1543a), see **tectum (Baer, 1837)**
testicles (Crooke, 1615), see **inferior colliculus (Haller, 1762)**
testicles (Galen, c173, definition 1), see **tectum (Baer, 1837)**

testicles (Galen, c173, definition 2), see **superior colliculus (Haller, 1762)**

testicular nerves (Horne, 1707), see **inferior testicular nerves (>1840)**

testicular plexus (Cruveilhier, 1836)

testicular plexuses (Chaussier, 1789), see **prevertebral nerves (Swanson & Bota, 2010)**

testiculi cerebri (Casseri, 1609), see **mammillary body (Ludwig, 1779)**

testiform eminences (Cruveilhier, 1836), see **inferior colliculus (Haller, 1762)**

testiforme process (Ridley, 1695), see **inferior colliculus (Haller, 1762)**

testudo (Achillini, 1520), see **fornix (Vesalius, 1543a)**

texturae radiosae (Willis, 1664), see **peripheral nervous system (Meckel, 1817)**

thalami (Berengario da Carpi, 1521), see **ventricles (Hippocrates)**

thalami nervorum opticorum (Riolan, 1618), see **interbrain (Baer, 1837)**

thalamic brachium of superior colliculus (>1840)

thalamic commissure (Chaussier, 1807), see **interthalamic adhesion (>1840)**

thalamic habenulo-interpeduncular tract (>1840)

thalamic line (>1840), see **choroid line of third ventricle (>1840)**

thalamic mammillothalamic tract (>1840)

thalamic medial lemniscus (>1840)

thalamic medullary lamina (Burdach, 1822), see **internal medullary lamina (>1840)**

thalamic optic tract (>1840)

thalamic part of third ventricle (Swanson, 2004)

thalamic radiations (Reil, 1809b)

thalamic region (Galen, c192), see **inferior horn of lateral ventricle (Bell, 1802)**

thalamic spinothalamic tract (>1840)

thalamic ventrolateral fascicle (>1840), see **thalamic spinothalamic tract (>1840)**

thalamos (Haller, 1747), see **interbrain (Baer, 1837)**

thalamus (Galen, c173), see **inferior horn of lateral ventricle (Bell, 1802)**

thalamus (His, 1893a)

thalamus (Malpighi, 1673), see **interbrain (Baer, 1837)**

thalamus (Reil, 1809b), see **interbrain (Baer, 1837)**

thalamus nervi optici (Riolan, 1618), see **interbrain (Baer, 1837)**

thalamus ophthalmicis (Haase, 1781), see **interbrain (Baer, 1837)**

thalamus opticus (Poupart, 1712), see **interbrain (Baer, 1837)**

thick membrane (Hippocrates), see **dura (Galen, c177)**

thick part of inferior vermis (Vicq d'Azyr, 1786), see **pyramis (Malacarne, 1776)**

thicker and greater root of third pair of sinews of brain (Geminus, 1553), see **mandibular nerve sensory root (>1840)**

thicker root of third pair of cerebral nerves (Vesalius, 1543a), see **mandibular nerve (>1840)**

thigh of fornix (Bartholin, 1662), see **fimbria (Honegger, 1890)**

thighs of arch (Diemerbroeck, 1689), see **hippocampal region (Swanson et al., 1987)**

thin cerebral membrane (Vesalius, 1543a), see **pia (Galen, c192)**

thin membrane (Hippocrates), see **pia (Galen, c192)**

thin pannicle (Geminus, 1553), see **pia (Galen, c192)**

thin part of dorsal hippocampal commissure (Craigie, 1925), see **intermediate hippocampal commissure (>1840)**

thinner root of fifth pair of cerebral nerves (Vesalius, 1543a), see **trigeminal nerve motor root (>1840)**

thinner root of fifth pair of sinews of brain (Geminus, 1553), see **trigeminal nerve (Winslow, 1733)**

thinner root of third pair of cerebral nerves (Vesalius, 1543a), see **trigeminal nerve (Winslow, 1733)**

third and fourth branches of second division of fifth pair of nerves arising within skull (Willis, 1664), see **maxillary nerve (Meckel, 1753)**

third and fourth pairs of nerves from brain (Galen, c192), see **trigeminal nerve (Winslow, 1733)**

third ansa cervicalis (Bock, 1827), see **communicating loop of cervical plexus (>1840)**

third ansa lumbalis (Bock, 1827), see **lumbar plexus (Vesalius, 1543a)**

third arcade of striate body (Vicq d'Azyr, 1786), see **lateral globus pallidus (>1840)**

third branch of anterior crural nerve to crural and internal vast muscles (Swan, 1830), see **muscular branches of femoral nerve (Quain & Wilson, 1839)**

third branch of anterior fascicles of acoustic nerve (Scarpa, 1789), see **saccular nerve (>1840)**

third branch of external plantar nerve (Fischer, 1791), see **muscular branches of lateral plantar nerve (>1840)**

third branch of fifth pair of nerves (Meckel, 1753), see **mandibular nerve (>1840)**

third branch of first lumbar pair (Sabatier, 1775), see **iliohypogastric nerve (Schmidt, 1794)**

third branch of fourth conjugation of nerves of brain (Crooke, 1615), see **inferior dental nerve (Meckel, 1817)**

third branch of glossopharyngeal nerve (Wrisberg, 1786), see **glossopharyngeal nerve trunk (Wrisberg, 1786; Günther, 1786)**

third branch of second division of fifth pair of nerves arising within skull (Willis, 1664), see **cranial nerves (Soemmerring, 1791)**

third branch of third conjugation of nerves of brain (Crooke, 1615), see **anterior ethmoidal nerve (>1840)**

third branch of third pair (Marchetti, 1652), see **mandibular nerve (>1840)**

third cardiac ganglion (Bock, 1817), see **inferior cervical ganglion (Vieussens, 1684)**

third cardiac nerve (Chaussier, 1789), see **inferior cardiac nerve (Cloquet, 1816)**

third cerebellar peduncle (Procháska, 1800), see **inferior cerebellar peduncle (Günther, 1786)**

third cerebral mass (Anderson, 1837), see **cerebellum (Aristotle)**

third cerebral ventricle (Vesalius, 1543a), see **ventricles (Hippocrates)**

third cervical ganglion (Günther, 1786), see **inferior cervical ganglion (Vieussens, 1684)**
third cervical nervous plexus (Meckel, 1817), see **cervical plexus (Molinetti, 1675)**
third choroid plexus (Günther, 1786), see **choroid plexus of third ventricle (Vicq d'Azyr, 1784)**
third common digital branch of median nerve (Caldani, 1813, 1814), see **common palmar digital nerves of median nerve (>1840)**
third conjugation of nerves of brain (Bauhin, 1605), see **trigeminal nerve (Winslow, 1733)**
third cutaneous nerve of thigh (Galen, c177), see **posterior cutaneous nerve of thigh (Günther, 1786)**
third deep nerve of thigh (Galen, c177), see **obturator nerve (Cheselden, 1726)**
third dental nerve of second trunk of fifth nerve (Swan, 1830), see **anterior superior dental nerve (Haller, 1762)**
third division of eighth pair of nerves (Bell, 1803b), see **accessory nerve (Vieussens, 1684)**
third division of fifth nerve (Bell, 1803a), see **mandibular nerve (>1840)**
third division of nerve of sixth pair (Galen, c192), see **accessory nerve (Vieussens, 1684)**
third facial nerve of superior branch of hard nerve (Meckel, 1753), see **zygomatic branches of facial nerve (>1840)**
third great brachial nerve (Albinus, 1744), see **radial nerve (Monro, 1732)**
third gustatory nerve (Soemmerring, 1778), see **hypoglossal nerve (Winslow, 1733)**
third inferior facial nerve (Soemmerring, 1791), see **zygomatic branches of facial nerve (>1840)**
third internal lateral twig of deep branch of peroneal nerve (Jördens, 1788), see **muscular branches of deep fibular nerve (>1840)**
third labial branch of infraorbital nerve (Bock, 1817), see **superior labial branches of infraorbital nerve (Meckel, 1748)**
third nerve entering arm (Vesalius, 1543a), see **median nerve (Du Verney, 1697)**
third nerve entering leg (Vesalius, 1543a), see **obturator nerve (Cheselden, 1726)**
third nerve for vastus externus muscle (Fischer, 1791), see **muscular branches of femoral nerve (Quain & Wilson, 1839)**
third nerve from spine to upper arm (Galen, c177), see **radial nerve (Du Verney, 1697)**
third nerve of fifth pair (Meckel, 1753), see **mandibular nerve (>1840)**
third nerve of hand (Bauhin, 1605), see **median nerve (Du Verney, 1697)**
third nerve root (Soemmerring, 1778), see **oculomotor nerve root (>1840)**
third nerve to extensor pollicis longus muscle (Fischer, 1791), see **muscular branches of deep fibular nerve (>1840)**
third nerve to flexor digitorum longus of foot muscle (Fischer, 1791), see **nerve to flexor digitorum longus (>1840)**
third nerve to long head of biceps muscle (Fischer, 1791), see **nerve to hamstring muscles (>1840)**
third nerve to short head of biceps muscle (Fischer, 1791), see **nerve to short head of biceps femoris (>1840)**
third nerve to soleus muscle (Fischer, 1791), see **nerve to soleus (>1840)**
third nerve to tibialis anterior muscle (Fischer, 1791), see **muscular branches of deep fibular nerve (>1840)**
third nerve traveling to thigh (Vesalius, 1543a), see **obturator nerve (Cheselden, 1726)**
third occipital nerve (>1840)
third of four branches of first lumbar pair (Haase, 1781), see **iliohypogastric nerve (Schmidt, 1794)**
third offshoot of thinner root of third pair (Vesalius, 1543a), see **anterior ethmoidal nerve (>1840)**
third pair of cerebral nerves (Soemmerring, 1791), see **oculomotor nerve (Estienne, 1545)**
third pair of cerebral nerves (Vesalius, 1543a), see **trigeminal nerve (Winslow, 1733)**
third pair of cranial nerves (Soemmerring, 1791), see **oculomotor nerve (Estienne, 1545)**
third pair of nerves (Bauhin, 1605), see **trochlear nerve (Molinetti, 1669)**
third pair of nerves from brain (Benedetti, 1502), see **cerebral cortex (>1840)**
third pair of nerves from brain (Falloppio, 1561), see **trigeminal nerve (Winslow, 1733)**
third pair of nerves from brain (Galen, c192), see **trigeminal nerve (Winslow, 1733)**
third pair of nerves from brain (Theophilos Protospatharios, fl. 610–641), see **oculomotor nerve (Estienne, 1545)**
third pair of nerves from medulla oblongata (Winslow, 1733), see **oculomotor nerve (Estienne, 1545)**
third pair of nerves of medulla oblongata (Haller & Wrisberg, 1780), see **hypoglossal nerve (Winslow, 1733)**
third pair of sinews of brain (Geminus, 1553), see **trigeminal nerve (Winslow, 1733)**
third pair of tubercles (Steno, 1669), see **tectum (Baer, 1837)**
third pharyngeal nerve (Andersch & Soemmerring, 1792), see **pharyngeal branches of vagus nerve (>1840)**
third principal branch of fifth pair (Meckel, 1817), see **mandibular nerve (>1840)**
third process of cerebellum (Ridley, 1695), see **inferior cerebellar peduncle (Günther, 1786)**
third process of middle lobe (Rolando, 1831), see **inferior temporal gyrus (>1840)**
third root of intercostal nerve (Bang, 1770), see **deep petrosal nerve (Meckel, 1817)**
third root of maxillary ganglion (Arnold, 1834), see **sympathetic root of submandibular ganglion (>1840)**
third sinew coming to arm (Geminus, 1553), see **median nerve (Du Verney, 1697)**
third sinew going to leg (Geminus, 1553), see **obturator nerve (Cheselden, 1726)**
third sinew pertaining to thigh (Geminus, 1553), see **obturator nerve (Cheselden, 1726)**
third spinal nerve (Soemmerring, 1778), see **hypoglossal nerve (Winslow, 1733)**

third subscapular branch of brachial plexus (Cloquet, 1816), see **lower subscapular nerve (>1840)**

third supraclavicular branch (Peipers, 1793), see **intermediate supraclavicular nerves (>1840)**

third temporal branch of hard nerve (Meckel, 1753), see **temporal branches of facial nerve (Swan, 1830)**

third terminal branch of median nerve (Cruveilhier, 1836), see **common palmar digital nerves of median nerve (>1840)**

third trunk of fifth nerve (Swan, 1830), see **mandibular nerve (>1840)**

third trunk of fifth pair (Rau, 1694), see **mandibular nerve (>1840)**

third trunk of third pair (Falloppio, 1561), see **mandibular nerve (>1840)**

third trunk of three-fold nerve (Swan, 1830), see **mandibular nerve (>1840)**

third ventricle (Avicenna, c1030), see **fourth ventricle (Galen, c192)**

third ventricle (Bell, 1802), see **hypothalamic part of third ventricle (Swanson, 2004)**

[third ventricle] (Erasistratus, c310–250 BC), see **ventricles (Hippocrates)**

third ventricle (Galen, c173)

thirteenth pair of nerves (Malacarne, 1791), see **vestibulocochlear nerve (>1840)**

thirty pair of motive sinews from spinal marrow (Geminus, 1553), see **spinal nerves (Camper, 1760–1762)**

thoracic aortic plexus (>1840)

thoracic branches of brachial plexus (Cruveilhier, 1836), see **brachial plexus cords (Schwalbe, 1881)**

thoracic cardiac branches of pneumogastric nerve (Cruveilhier, 1836), see **thoracic cardiac branches of vagus nerve (>1840)**

thoracic cardiac branches of vagus nerve (>1840)

thoracic cardiac branches proper of pneumogastric nerve (Cruveilhier, 1836), see **thoracic cardiac branches of vagus nerve (>1840)**

thoracic cardiac nerves (>1840)

thoracic ganglia of intercostal nerve (Günther, 1786), see **thoracic spinal ganglia (>1840)**

thoracic ganglioform plexus of eighth pair of nerves (Vieussens, 1684), see **vagus nerve (Galen, c192)**

thoracic ganglion (Walter, 1783), see **thoracic sympathetic ganglia (>1840)**

thoracic ganglion of great sympathetic nerve (Walter, 1783), see **thoracic sympathetic ganglia (>1840)**

thoracic ganglion of greatest sympathetic nerve (Wrisberg, 1780), see **thoracic sympathetic ganglia (>1840)**

thoracic ganglion of intercostal nerve proper (Walter, 1783), see **thoracic sympathetic ganglia (>1840)**

thoracic ganglions of limiting cord (Meckel, 1817), see **thoracic sympathetic ganglia (>1840)**

thoracic nerve (Burdin, 1803), see **long thoracic nerve (Quain & Wilson, 1839)**

thoracic nerves (Diemerbroeck, 1672)

thoracic nerves (Günther, 1786), see **spinal nerve ventral branch (>1840)**

thoracic nerves (Quain, 1828), see **brachial plexus (Camper, 1760)**

thoracic nerves (Soemmerring, 1791), see **brachial plexus (Camper, 1760)**

thoracic nerves (Vesalius, 1543a), see **spinal nerves (Camper, 1760–1762)**

thoracic nerves of axillary plexus (Bell, 1803b), see **brachial plexus cords (Schwalbe, 1881)**

thoracic nucleus (>1840), see **dorsal thoracic nucleus (>1840)**

thoracic part of pneumogastric nerve (Arnold, 1834), see **vagus nerve trunk (Wrisberg, 1786; Günther, 1786)**

thoracic part of spinal cord (>1840)

thoracic part of spinal medulla (Tiedemann, 1821), see **thoracic part of spinal cord (>1840)**

thoracic part of tenth pair (Arnold, 1834), see **vagus nerve trunk (Wrisberg, 1786; Günther, 1786)**

thoracic part of trachelo-cutanean plexus (Burdin, 1803), see **descending superficial branches of cervical plexus (Quain, 1828)**

thoracic part of tracheosubcutaneous nerves (Chaussier, 1809), see **descending superficial branches of cervical plexus (Quain, 1828).**

thoracic part of vagus nerve (Arnold, 1834), see **vagus nerve trunk (Wrisberg, 1786; Günther, 1786)**

thoracic pericardial branches of pneumogastric nerve (Cruveilhier, 1836), see **thoracic cardiac branches of vagus nerve (>1840)**

thoracic plexus (Günther, 1786), see **spinal nerve ventral branch (>1840)**

thoracic pulmonary nerves (>1840)

thoracic spinal ganglia (>1840)

thoracic spinal medulla (Galen, c173), see **thoracic part of spinal cord (>1840)**

thoracic sympathetic ganglia (>1840)

thoracical infolding (Willis, 1664), see **sympathetic trunk ganglia (Winslow, 1733)**

thoracodorsal nerve (>1840)

three conjugations proceeding out of coccyx (Crooke, 1615), see **coccygeal nerves (Camper, 1762)**

three vesicles (Malpighi, 1673), see **primary brain vesicles (Baer, 1837)**

three-fold nerve (Swan, 1830), see **trigeminal nerve (Winslow, 1733)**

threshold of Sylvian fissure (Reil, 1809b), see **ambient gyrus (>1840)**

thumb branch of median nerve (Mayer, 1794), see **common palmar digital nerve of median nerve (>1840)**

thyrde ventricle (Geminus, 1553), see **third ventricle (Galen, c173)**

thyrohyoid branch of hypoglossal nerve (Meckel, 1817)

thyrohyoid muscle twigs from hypoglossal nerve (Soemmerring, 1791), see **thyrohyoid branch of hypoglossal nerve (Meckel, 1817)**

thyroid branch of vagus nerve trunk (Neubauer, 1772), see **vagus nerve trunk (Wrisberg, 1786; Günther, 1786)**

thyroid branches of middle cervical ganglion (>1840)

thyroid cervical ganglion (Haller, 1772), see **middle cervical ganglion (Haller, 1762)**

thyroid ganglion (Haase, 1781), see **inferior cervical ganglion (Vieussens, 1684)**

thyroid ganglion (Neubauer, 1772; Haller, 1772), see **middle cervical ganglion (Haller, 1762)**

tractus medullaris nervorum opticorum thalamus interjectus (Vieussens, 1684), see **medullary stria (Wenzel & Wenzel, 1812)**
tractus medullaris nervorum opticorum thalamus intermedius (Vieussens, 1684), see **medullary stria (Wenzel & Wenzel, 1812)**
tractus medullaris striatis ex corporibus mediis emergentes (Vieussens, 1684), see **cerebral peduncle (Tarin, 1753)**
tractus medullaris transversus (Vieussens, 1684), see **rostral medullary velum (>1840)**
tractus medullaris transversus et nonnihil obliquus (Schreger, 1803), see **terminal stria (Wenzel & Wenzel, 1812)**
tractus medullaris transversus et nonnihil obliquus (Vieussens, 1684), see **anterior commissure (Lieutaud, 1742)**
tractus medullaris transversus natibus antipositus (Vieussens, 1684), see **posterior commissure (Winslow, 1733)**
tractus peduncularis transversus (Gudden, 1870), see **transverse peduncular tract (Gudden, 1870)**
transparent globules (Coiter, 1572), see **brain vesicles (Malpighi, 1673)**
transparent septum (Chaussier, 1807), see **cerebral nuclei (Swanson, 2000a)**
transversa cinerea thalamorum (Schreger, 1803), see **dorsal part of thalamus (Herrick, 1910)**
transverse arch of eleventh pair of nerves of head (Andersch, 1797), see **hypoglossal nerve (Winslow, 1733)**
transverse arch of tenth pair of nerves of head (Andersch & Soemmerring, 1792), see **hypoglossal nerve (Winslow, 1733)**
transverse band behind olivary ganglion (Gall & Spurzheim, 1810), see **ventral external arcuate fibers (>1840)**
transverse band of great superior ganglion (Spurzheim, 1826), see **posterior limb of internal capsule (>1840)**
transverse band under optic nerve (Spurzheim, 1826), see **supraoptic decussations (>1840)**
transverse branch of abductor digiti minimi muscle of external plantar nerve (Cruveilhier, 1836), see **muscular branches of lateral plantar nerve (>1840)**
transverse branch of superior branch of anterior branch of hard nerve (Loder, 1778), see **zygomatic branches of facial nerve (>1840)**
transverse bundles of medullary fibers (Monro, 1783), see **ventral external arcuate fibers (>1840)**
transverse cerebellar fissure (Burdach, 1822)
transverse cerebral fissure (>1840)
transverse cerebral fissure (>1840), see **inner part of transverse cerebral fissure (>1840)**
transverse cerebral fissure (Todd, 1845), see **outer part of transverse cerebral fissure (>1840)**
transverse cerebral septum (Günther, 1786), see **cerebellar tentorium (Winslow, 1733)**
transverse cerebral stria (Günther, 1786), see **rostral medullary vellum (>1840)**
transverse cervical nerve (>1840), see **transverse nerve of neck (>1840)**
transverse commissure (Solly, 1836), see **cerebral cortex white matter (>1840)**
transverse commissure of conarium (Cruveilhier, 1836), see **habenular commissure (>1840)**
transverse commissure of pineal body (Cruveilhier, 1836), see **habenular commissure (>1840)**
transverse commissure uniting optic thalami (Cloquet, 1828), see **interthalamic adhesion (>1840)**
transverse cord (Riolan, 1649), see **anterior commissure (Lieutaud, 1742)**
transverse eminence (Leuret, 1839), see **vestibular area of fourth ventricle (>1840)**
transverse fibers of medulla oblongata (Arnold, 1838a), see **olivocerebellar tract (>1840)**
transverse filament (Serres, 1824–1826), see **central transverse communicating branch (>1840)**
transverse furrow of corpora bigemina (Gordon, 1815), see **transverse tectal sulcus (>1840)**
transverse ganglion (Günther, 1786), see **celiac ganglion (Walter, 1783)**
transverse interweaving (Gall & Spurzheim, 1810), see **ventral external arcuate fibers (>1840)**
transverse lamina of gray substance (Keuffel, 1810), see **spinal central gray (>1840)**
transverse laminated commissures of cerebellum (Malacarne, 1776), see **tuber vermis (>1840)**
transverse laminated cords of cerebellum (Malacarne, 1776), see **tuber vermis (>1840)**
transverse medullary bundles (Monro, 1783), see **ventral external arcuate fibers (>1840)**
transverse medullary fibers of calamus scriptorius (Reil, 1809c), see **medullary striae (Scarpa, 1788)**
transverse medullary lamina (Arnold, 1838b), see **rostral medullary vellum (>1840)**
transverse medullary process (Wenzel & Wenzel, 1812), see **pons (Haller, 1747)**
transverse medullary process (Willis, 1664, p. 61), see **terminal stria (Wenzel & Wenzel, 1812)**
transverse medullary process (Willis, 1664, p. 65), see **rostral medullary velum (>1840)**
transverse medullary process of fourth ventricle (Ridley, 1695), see **medullary striae (Scarpa, 1788)**
transverse medullary striae (Meckel, 1817), see **medullary striae (Scarpa, 1788)**
transverse medullary tracts of pons Varolii (Ridley, 1695), see **transverse pontine fibers (>1840)**
transverse nerve of anterior carotid artery (Andersch & Soemmerring, 1792), see **external carotid plexus (>1840)**
transverse nerve of neck (>1840)
transverse occipital branch of hard nerve (Peipers, 1793), see **posterior auricular nerve (Meckel, 1753)**
transverse occipital sulcus (>1840)
transverse part of spinal cord ashen-colored substance (Vicq d'Azyr, 1784), see **spinal central gray (>1840)**
transverse peduncular tract (Gudden, 1870)
transverse plexus (Chaussier, 1789), see **celiac plexus (Winslow, 1733)**
transverse plexus (Portal, 1803a), see **superior mesenteric plexus (Rau, 1720)**
transverse pontine fibers (>1840)
transverse process of cerebellum (Varoli, 1573), see **pons (Haller, 1747)**

transverse prolongation of cerebellum (Meckel, 1817), see **pons (Haller, 1747)**
transverse protuberance (Winslow, 1733), see **pons (Haller, 1747)**
transverse septum (Winslow, 1733), see **cerebellar tentorium (Winslow, 1733)**
transverse striae of pons Varolii (Ridley, 1695), see **transverse pontine fibers (>1840)**
transverse striae of Willis (Günther, 1786), see **corpus callosum (Galen, c177)**
transverse sulcus (Chaussier, 1807), see **horizontal fissure (Malacarne, 1776)**
transverse sulcus of quadrigeminal tubercles (Serres, 1824–1826), see **transverse tectal sulcus (>1840)**
transverse sulcus separating annular protuberance from superior end of medulla oblongata (Cloquet, 1828), see **medullopontine sulcus (>1840)**
transverse tectal sulcus (>1840)
transverse temporal gyri (Heschl, 1878)
transverse temporal sulcus (Heschl, 1878)
transverse tract of third ventricle (Santorini, 1724), see **middle commissure (>1840)**
transversus medullaris (Willis, 1664), see **terminal stria (Wenzel & Wenzel, 1812)**
trapezium (Tiedemann, 1821), see **trapezoid body (Treviranus, 1820)**
trapezium of medulla oblongata (Serres, 1824–1826), see **trapezoid body (Treviranus, 1820)**
trapezoid body (Treviranus, 1820)
triangular area (Brodmann, 1909), see **triangular part of inferior frontal gyrus (>1840)**
triangular cavity of septum lucidum (Vicq d'Azyr, 1784), see **septal fissure (Burdach, 1822)**
triangular fascicle (Cruveilhier, 1836), see **lateral lemniscus (Bechterew, 1885b)**
triangular fossa (Gordon, 1815), see **fourth ventricle (Galen, c192)**
triangular furrow (Gordon, 1815), see **interpeduncular fossa (>1840)**
triangular leaflet (Solly, 1836), see **cerebellum (Aristotle)**
triangular part of inferior frontal gyrus (>1840)
triangular pit (Gordon, 1815), see **medullopontine sulcus (>1840)**
triangular space (Tiedemann, 1816), see **interpeduncular fossa (>1840)**
triangular surface (Laurencet, 1825), see **interpeduncular nucleus (>1840)**
triangular ventricle (Haller, 1747), see **lateral ventricle (Vesalius, 1543a)**
tricornate ventricle (Bergen, 1734), see **lateral ventricle (Vesalius, 1543a)**
trifacial pair of nerves (Burdin, 1803), see **trigeminal nerve (Winslow, 1733)**
trigeminal ganglion (>1840)
trigeminal nerve (Winslow, 1733)
trigeminal nerve branches (Winslow, 1733)
trigeminal nerve central motor root (>1840)
trigeminal nerve central sensory root (>1840)
trigeminal nerve motor root (Bell, 1829)
trigeminal nerve sensory root (>1840)
trigeminal nerve trunk (Winslow, 1733), see **trigeminal nerve (Winslow, 1733)**
trigeminal tubercle (>1840)
trigonon durum (Bergmann, 1831), see **pretectal region (>1840)**
trigonon fluctuans (Bergmann, 1831), see **pretectal region (>1840)**
trigonon molle (Bergmann, 1831), see **pretectal region (>1840)**
trigonon pensile (Bergmann, 1831), see **pretectal region (>1840)**
trigonum collaterale (>1840), see **collateral triangle (>1840)**
trigonum habenulare (>1840), see **habenular triangle (>1840)**
trigonum vagale (>1840), see **vagal triangle (>1840)**
tripartite body (Riolan, 1657), see **fornix (Vesalius, 1543a)**
tri-splanchnic nerve (Chaussier, 1789), see **sympathetic cord (>1840)**
tri-splanchnic nervous system (Quain & Wilson, 1839), see **peripheral nervous system (Meckel, 1817)**
trochlear nerve (Molinetti, 1669)
trochlear nerve central root (>1840)
trochlear nerve decussation (>1840)
tronc lombo-sacré (Cruveilhier, 1836), see **lumbosacral trunk (Cruveilhier, 1836)**
trough (Galen, c177), see **hypothalamic part of third ventricle (Swanson, 2004)**
true intercostal nerves (Winslow, 1733), see **thoracic nerves (Diemerbroeck, 1672)**
true marrow (Crooke, 1615), see **central nervous system (Carus, 1814)**
true optic tubercle (Carus, 1814), see **superior colliculus (Haller, 1762)**
true spinal marrow proper (Bauhin, 1605), see **spinal cord (Galen, c162–c166)**
trunci noni paris nervorum cerebri finis (Albinus, 1744), see **lingual branches of hypoglossal nerve (Cloquet, 1816)**
truncorum medullae cerebelli partes, quae pertinent ad medullae oblongatae partem priorem (Albinus, 1744), see **superior cerebellar peduncle (Procháska, 1800)**
truncum octavi tumidulum (Pfeffinger, 1783), see **distal vagal ganglion (>1840)**
truncus nervi glossopharyngaei (Wrisberg, 1786), see **glossopharyngeal nerve trunk (Wrisberg, 1786; Günther, 1786)**
truncus nervi vagi (Wrisberg, 1786), see **vagus nerve trunk (Wrisberg, 1786; Günther, 1786)**
trunk (Cuvier, 1800), see **central nerve cord (Serres, 1824–1826)**
trunk (Galen, c173), see **spinal cord (Galen, c162–c166)**
trunk (Varoli, 1573), see **cerebrospinal trunk (>1840)**
trunk for nerves to soleus muscle, popliteal muscle and gastrocnemius muscle (Fischer, 1791), see **muscular branches of tibial nerve (>1840)**
trunk formed by fourth and fifth subcervicals (Monro, 1783), see **brachial plexus upper trunk (>1840)**
trunk formed by union of fifth and sixth cervical nerves (Meckel, 1817), see **brachial plexus upper trunk (>1840)**
trunk itself of fourth conjugation of nerves of brain (Crooke, 1615), see **lingual nerve (Vesalius, 1543a)**
trunk nerve (Burdach, 1819), see **sympathetic trunk (Winslow, 1733)**

trunk nerve of intercostal nerve (Walter, 1783), see **communicating branches of sympathetic trunk (>1840)**

trunk nervous system (Burdach, 1819), see **peripheral nervous system (Meckel, 1817)**

trunk of anterior renal nerves (Walter, 1783), see **intrinsic renal nerves (>1840)**

trunk of arbor vitae (Langenbeck, 1826–1830), see **arbor vitae (Winslow, 1733)**

trunk of brain (Willis, 1664), see **vertebrate brain (Cuvier, 1800)**

trunk of cerebellar commissure (Arnold, 1838b), see **pons (Haller, 1747)**

trunk of cerebellum (Arnold, 1838a), see **arbor vitae (Winslow, 1733)**

trunk of corpus callosum (Burdach, 1822), see **body of corpus callosum (Arnold, 1838a)**

trunk of eighth pair of nerves (Vieussens, 1684), see **vagus nerve trunk (Wrisberg, 1786; Günther, 1786)**

trunk of fifth pair (Arnold, 1834), see **trigeminal nerve (Winslow, 1733)**

trunk of fifth pair of cerebral nerves (Procháska, 1779), see **trigeminal nerve (Winslow, 1733)**

trunk of fifth pair of nerves arising within skull (Willis, 1664), see **trigeminal nerve (Winslow, 1733)**

trunk of first division of fifth pair of nerves arising within skull (Willis, 1664), see **lingual nerve (Vesalius, 1543a)**

trunk of fornix (Willis, 1664), see **fimbria (Honegger, 1890)**

trunk of ganglionated nerves (Bock, 1827), see **sympathetic trunk (Winslow, 1733)**

trunk of gastro-hepatic nerve (Walter, 1783), see **left gastric plexus (>1840)**

trunk of great deep cardiac nerve of left side (Fyfe, 1800), see **cardiac plexus (Keill, 1698)**

trunk of great hypoglossal nerve (Knox, 1832), see **hypoglossal nerve trunk (Günther, 1786)**

trunk of great sympathetic nerve (Walter, 1783, Tab. 1), see **sympathetic trunk (Winslow, 1733)**

trunk of great sympathetic nerve (Walter, 1783, Tab. 2), see **communicating branches of sympathetic trunk (>1840)**

trunk of hard part of seventh pair of nerves arising within skull (Willis, 1664), see **intermediofacial nerve (Strong & Elwyn, 1943)**

trunk of inferior cutaneous nerves of buttocks (Walter, 1783), see **perforating cutaneous nerve (>1840)**

trunk of intercostal nerve (Willis, 1664), see **sympathetic trunk (Winslow, 1733)**

trunk of internal dorsal twig of foot of superficial peroneal nerve (Jördens, 1788), see **medial dorsal cutaneous nerve (>1840)**

trunk of internal superior spermatic nerve (Walter, 1783), see **superior ovarian nerves (>1840)**

trunk of nerve for soleus, popliteal and gastrocnemii muscles (Knox, 1832), see **muscular branches of tibial nerve (>1840)**

trunk of ninth cerebral nerve (Scarpa, 1794), see **hypoglossal nerve trunk (Günther, 1786)**

trunk of ninth pair (Haase, 1781), see **hypoglossal nerve trunk (Günther, 1786)**

trunk of oblong marrow (Willis, 1664), see **vertebrate brain (Cuvier, 1800)**

trunk of olfactory nerve (Scarpa, 1785), see **olfactory peduncle (Solly, 1836)**

trunk of par lingulae (Winslow, 1733), see **hypoglossal nerve trunk (Günther, 1786)**

trunk of pharyngeal branches of vagus (Bischoff, 1832), see **pharyngeal branches of vagus nerve (>1840)**

trunk of proper intercostal nerve (Monro, 1783), see **intercostal nerves (Vesalius, 1543a)**

trunk of pterygopalatine nerve (Meckel, 1817), see **pterygopalatine nerves (Wrisberg, 1786)**

trunk of recurrent spinal nerve (Albinus, 1744), see **accessory nerve trunk (Wrisberg, 1786)**

trunk of sixth pair (Vesalius, 1543a), see **vagus nerve trunk (Wrisberg, 1786; Günther, 1786)**

trunk of spinal marrow (Bartholin, 1662), see **vertebrate brain (Cuvier, 1800)**

trunk of superficial cardiac nerve (Scarpa, 1794), see **superior cardiac nerve (Neubauer, 1772)**

trunk of superior internal cutaneous nerve and nerve to long head of crural biceps muscle (Fischer, 1791), see **nerve to hamstring muscles (>1840)**

trunk of supraclavicular nerves (Peipers, 1793), see **supraclavicular nerves (Meckel, 1817)**

trunk of sympathetic nerve (Soemmerring, 1791), see **sympathetic trunk (Winslow, 1733)**

trunk of temporo-buccal nerve (Meckel, 1817), see **trigeminal nerve (Winslow, 1733)**

trunk of third pair of nerves (Haller, 1743), see **oculomotor nerve trunk (>1840)**

trunk of wandring pair (Willis, 1664), see **vagus nerve trunk (Wrisberg, 1786; Günther, 1786)**

trunks of medulla oblongata (Bartholin, 1662), see **vertebrate brain (Cuvier, 1800)**

trunks of spinal marrow (Bartholin, 1662), see **vertebrate brain (Cuvier, 1800)**

trunks of third pair (Falloppio, 1561), see **trigeminal nerve branches (Winslow, 1733)**

tub (Vesalius, 1543a), see **hypothalamus (Kuhlenbeck, 1927)**

tubal branch of tympanic plexus (>1840)

tubal nerves (Cruveilhier, 1836), see **tubo-uterine nerve (>1840)**

tube of infundibulum (Vesalius, 1543a), see **pituitary gland (>1840)**

tuber annulare (Bell, 1802), see **pons (Haller, 1747)**

tuber annulare (Monro, 1783), see **pons (Haller, 1747)**

tuber cinereum (Soemmerring, 1778), see **hypothalamus (Kuhlenbeck, 1927)**

tuber exterius (Günz, 1750), see **collateral eminence (Meckel, 1767)**

tuber of corpus callosum (Arnold, 1834), see **splenium of corpus callosum (Burdach, 1822)**

tuber valvulae (Burdach, 1822), see **tuber vermis (>1840)**

tuber vermis (>1840)

tubercle generating first pair (Vicq d'Azyr, 1784), see **olfactory tubercle (Calleja, 1893)**

tubercle of gray substance of medulla oblongata (Rolando, 1825a), see **trigeminal tubercle (>1840)**

tubercle of Rolando (>1840), see **trigeminal tubercle (>1840)**
tubercle of semicircular commissure (Serres, 1824–1826), see **bed nuclei of terminal stria (Gurdjian, 1825)**
tubercles (Benedetti, 1502), see **cerebral cortex (>1840)**
tubercles of mesencephalon (Burdin, 1803), see **tectum (Baer, 1837)**
tubercula anteriora inferiora Tarini (Haase, 1781), see **cerebellar hemisphere (Willis, 1664)**
tubercula lateralia anteriora inferiora cerebelli (Tarin, 1750), see **cerebellar hemisphere (Willis, 1664)**
tubercula mammillaria (Winslow, 1733), see **mammillary body (Ludwig, 1779)**
tubercula mammillarum papillis simillima (du Laurens, 1599), see **cerebral cortex (>1840)**
tubercula minima cerebelli (Tarin, 1750), see **flocculus (Meckel, 1817)**
tubercula olivaria (Soemmerring, 1778), see **olive (Tiedemann, 1821)**
tubercula ovalia (Soemmerring, 1799), see **olive (Tiedemann, 1821)**
tubercula papillaria (Benedetti, 1502), see **cerebral cortex (>1840)**
tubercula quadrigemina (Winslow, 1733), see **tectum (Baer, 1837)**
tubercula striata (Haller, 1762), see **nucleus of solitary tract (>1840)**
tubercula subrotunda Vieussenii (Tarin, 1750), see **anterior thalamic nuclei (>1840)**
tuberculum cinereum (Arnold, 1838a), see **trigeminal tubercle (>1840)**
tuberculum ganglii postici posterius (Meckel, 1817), see **pulvinar (Burdach, 1822)**
tuberculum ganglii postici posterius superius (Meckel, 1817), see **pulvinar (Burdach, 1822)**
tuberculum laminosum (Malacarne, 1776), see **nodule (Reil, 1807–1808a)**
tuberculum pedunculi cerebri (Treviranus, 1820), see **dorsal lateral geniculate nucleus (>1840)**
tuberculum thalami inferius (Soemmerring, 1778), see **medial geniculate complex (>1840)**
tuberculum thalami posticum externus (Meckel, 1817), see **dorsal lateral geniculate nucleus (>1840)**
tuberculum thalami posticum inferius (Meckel, 1817), see **dorsal lateral geniculate nucleus (>1840)**
tuberculum thalami posticum medium (Meckel, 1817), see **medial geniculate complex (>1840)**
tuberculum trigeminale (>1840), see **trigeminal tubercle (>1840)**
tubo-uterine nerve (1840)
tubo-uterine plexus (>1840)
tumors (Diemerbroeck, 1689), see **peripheral ganglia (>1840)**
tunic (Hippocrates), see **meninges (Smith Papyrus, c1700 BC)**
tunic of eye (Vesalius, 1543a), see **retina (Herophilus, c335–c280 BC)**
tunica altera (Rufus of Ephesus, c90–120), see **pia (Galen, c192)**
tunica arachnoidea (Bell, 1803b), see **arachnoid (Blasius, 1666)**
tunica cerebri propria (Meckel, 1817), see **pia (Galen, c192)**
tunica prima (Rufus of Ephesus, c90–120), see **dura (Galen, c177)**
tunica telae arachnoidis similiis (Molinetti, 1669), see **arachnoid (Blasius, 1666)**
tunica vasculosa (Bell, 1803b), see **meninges (Smith Papyrus, c1700 BC)**
tunicles (Diemerbroeck, 1689), see **meninges (Smith Papyrus, c1700 BC)**
tunnel (Crooke, 1615), see **hypothalamus (Kuhlenbeck, 1927)**
turbo (Galen, c177), see **pineal gland (Galen, c192)**
turn-again nerve (Diemerbroeck, 1689), see **recurrent laryngeal nerve (Albinus, 1744)**
turnings (Bartholin, 1662), see **cerebellar cortex (Willis, 1664)**
turnings (Geminus, 1553), see **cerebral cortex gray matter (>1840)**
twelfth pair of cerebral nerves (Soemmerring, 1791), see **hypoglossal nerve (Winslow, 1733)**
twelfth pair of cranial nerves (Soemmerring, 1791), see **hypoglossal nerve (Winslow, 1733)**
twelfth pair of encephalic nerves (Burdin, 1803), see **accessory nerve (Vieussens, 1684)**
twelfth pair of nerves (Malacarne, 1791), see **intermediofacial nerve (Strong & Elwyn, 1943)**
twig connecting inferior laryngeal nerve with superior laryngeal nerve (Arnold, 1834), see **communicating branch of superior laryngeal nerve with inferior laryngeal nerve (Langenbeck, 1826–1830)**
twig to abductor digiti minimi muscle from third branch of external plantar nerve (Fischer, 1791), see **muscular branches of lateral plantar nerve (>1840)**
twig to carne quadrata Sylvii (Fischer, 1791), see **muscular branches of lateral plantar nerve (>1840)**
twig to flexor brevis and interosseus digiti quinti (Fischer, 1791), see **muscular branches of lateral plantar nerve (>1840)**
twig to flexor digitorum brevis muscle (Jördens, 1788), see **muscular branches of medial plantar nerve (>1840)**
twig to gall bladder (Vesalius, 1543a), see **cystic plexus (Wrisberg, 1808)**
twigs from Vidian nerve to sphenoid sinus membrane (Scarpa, 1785), see **nerve of pterygoid canal (>1840)**
twigs of deep branch of volar branch of ulnar nerve to adductor pollicis muscle (Langenbeck, 1826–1830), see **superficial branch of ulnar nerve (Fyfe, 1800)**
twigs of deep branch of volar branch of ulnar nerve to interosseous muscles (Langenbeck, 1826–1830), see **superficial branch of ulnar nerve (Fyfe, 1800)**
twigs of superior subcutaneous nerve of neck to platysma muscle (Arnold, 1834), see **cervical branch of facial nerve (>1840)**
twin column of beam (Reil, 1809b), see **fornix (Vesalius, 1543a)**
twins (Galen, c173, definition 1), see **tectum (Baer, 1837)**
twins (Galen, c173, definition 2), see **superior colliculus (Haller, 1762)**
two glandular pieces of flesh (Mondino, 1316), see **mammillary body (Ludwig, 1779)**

two infoldings in pelvis (Willis, 1664), see ***inferior hypogastric plexus (Tiedemann, 1822)***

two lateral longitudinal nerves of corpus callosum (Tarin, 1753), see ***lateral longitudinal stria (Arnold, 1838a)***

two long hook-like processes from brain (Galen, c192), see ***cerebral cortex (>1840)***

two medullary protuberances behind infundibulum (Tyson, 1699), see ***mammillary body (Ludwig, 1779)***

two posterior pairs of tubercles (Steno, 1669), see ***tectum (Baer, 1837)***

two semilunar ventricles (Günther, 1786), see ***lateral ventricle (Vesalius, 1543a)***

two small roots of trigeminal nerve (Meckel, 1817), see ***trigeminal nerve motor root (Bell, 1829)***

two soft pillows (Collins, 1685), see ***mammillary body (Ludwig, 1779)***

two white glands behind tunnel (Willis, 1664), see ***mammillary body (Ludwig, 1779)***

two white kernels (Bartholin, 1662), see ***mammillary body (Ludwig, 1779)***

two white protuberances behind infundibulum (Ridley, 1695), see ***mammillary body (Ludwig, 1779)***

twofold root of fornix (Willis, 1664), see ***hypothalamic postcommissural fornix (>1840)***

tympanic branch of facial nerve (Burdin, 1803), see ***chorda tympani (Falloppio, 1561)***

tympanic branch of glosso-pharyngeal nerve (Todd, 1836–1839), see ***tympanic nerve (Arnold, 1834)***

tympanic membrane branch of external acoustic meatus nerves (>1840)

tympanic nerve (Arnold, 1834)

tympanic nerve (Bock, 1817), see ***tympanic membrane branch of external acoustic meatus nerves (>1840)***

tympanic nerve branchlet to Eustachian tube (Arnold, 1834), see ***tubal branch of tympanic plexus (>1840)***

tympanic plexus (Müller, 1834)

tympanine nerve (Swan, 1830), see ***tympanic nerve (Arnold, 1834)***

tympanum (Duvernoy, 1735), see ***cerebral nuclei (Swanson, 2000a)***

ugola (Malacarne, 1776), see ***uvula (Malacarne, 1776)***

ulnar branch of major internal cutaneous nerve (Bock, 1827), see ***posterior branch of medial cutaneous nerve of forearm (>1840)***

ulnar branch of medial cutaneous nerve (Bock, 1827), see ***posterior branch of medial cutaneous nerve of forearm (>1840)***

ulnar branch of median nerve (Bock, 1827), see ***common palmar digital nerves of median nerve (>1840)***

ulnar cutaneous nerve (Soemmerring, 1791), see ***posterior branch of medial cutaneous nerve of forearm (>1840)***

ulnar cutaneous nerve of Wrisberg (Frotscher, 1788), see ***posterior branch of medial cutaneous nerve of forearm (>1840)***

ulnar dorsal nerve of auricular finger (Loder, 1803), see ***dorsal digital nerves of ulnar nerve (>1840)***

ulnar dorsal nerve of index finger (Loder, 1803), see ***dorsal digital nerves of radial nerve (>1840)***

ulnar dorsal nerve of middle finger (Loder, 1803), see ***dorsal digital nerves of radial nerve (>1840)***

ulnar dorsal nerve of ring finger (Loder, 1803), see ***dorsal digital nerves of ulnar nerve (>1840)***

ulnar dorsal nerve of thumb (Loder, 1803), see ***dorsal digital nerves of radial nerve (>1840)***

ulnar nerve (Cheselden, 1726)

ulnar nerve of little finger of cubital nerve (Caldani, 1813, 1814), see ***dorsal digital nerves of ulnar nerve (>1840)***

ulnar nerve of Wrisberg (Klint, 1784), see ***medial cutaneous nerve of arm (>1840)***

ulnar volar branch of auricular finger (Loder, 1803), see ***proper palmar digital nerves of ulnar nerve (>1840)***

ulnar volar nerve of auricular finger (Loder, 1803), see ***proper palmar digital nerves of ulnar nerve (>1840)***

ulnar volar nerve of fourth finger (Caldani, 1813, 1814), see ***proper palmar digital nerves of ulnar nerve (>1840)***

ulnar volar nerve of index finger (Loder, 1803), see ***proper palmar digital nerves of median nerve (>1840)***

ulnar volar nerve of little finger (Caldani, 1813, 1814), see ***proper palmar digital nerves of ulnar nerve (>1840)***

ulnar volar nerve of middle finger (Loder, 1803), see ***proper palmar digital nerves of median nerve (>1840)***

ulnar volar nerve of ring finger (Loder, 1803), see ***proper palmar digital nerves of ulnar nerve (>1840)***

ulnar volar nerve of thumb (Loder, 1803), see ***proper palmar digital nerves of median nerve (>1840)***

umbilical nerves (Wrisberg, 1808), see ***hepatic plexus (Rau, 1720)***

umbilical nervous plexuses (Wrisberg, 1808), see ***hepatic plexus (Rau, 1720)***

umbilical plexuses (Wrisberg, 1808), see ***hepatic plexus (Rau, 1720)***

umm (Haly Abbas or Ali ibn' ul-Abbas, d. 994), see ***meninges (Smith Papyrus, c1700 BC)***

unciform eminence (Chaussier, 1807), see ***calcarine spur (Morand, 1748)***

unciform fascicle (Reil, 1809b), see ***uncinate fascicle (Reil, 1809b)***

unciform gyri (Arnold, 1838a), see ***limbic region (>1840)***

uncinate fascicle (Reil, 1809b)

uncinate fasciculus of cerebellum (Lewandowsky, 1903), see ***superior cerebellar peduncle (Procháska, 1800)***

uncinate fasciculus of Russell (>1840), see ***superior cerebellar peduncle (Procháska, 1800)***

uncrossed corticospinal tract (>1840)

uncus (Vicq d'Azyr, 1786), see ***cerebral cortex (>1840)***

uncus of fornicate gyrus (Arnold, 1838a), see ***cerebral cortex (>1840)***

unguinal branch of median nerve external collateral branch of thumb (Cruveilhier, 1836), see ***common palmar digital nerves of median nerve (>1840)***

unguinal branch of plantar internal collateral nerve of big toe (Cruveilhier, 1836), see ***proper plantar digital nerves of medial plantar nerve (>1840)***

unguis (Haller, 1754a), see ***calcarine spur (Morand, 1748)***

union of first and second cervical nerves (Swan, 1830), see ***communicating loops of cervical plexus (>1840)***

union of optic nerves (Galen, c173), see ***optic chiasm (Galen, c173)***

union of second and third cervical nerves (Swan, 1830), see ***communicating loops of cervical plexus (>1840)***

united caudex of optic nerves (Collins, 1685), see **optic chiasm (Galen, c173)**

unnamed fascicle of bulb (Cruveilhier, 1836), see **brainstem (Schwalbe, 1881)**

unnamed medullary substance (Reil, 1809b), see **substantia innominata (Meynert, 1872)**

unpaired nerve (Haly Abbas or Ali ibn' ul-Abbas, d. 994), see **terminal filament (Tiedemann, 1821)**

unpaired spinal marrow ganglion (Carus, 1814), see **cerebellum (Aristotle)**

upper and external part of auditory nerve (Meckel, 1817), see **cochlear nerve central root (>1840)**

upper and internal cutaneous nerve (Bell, 1803b), see **intercostobrachial nerves (>1840)**

upper and posterior dentar nerve (Meckel, 1832), see **posterior superior dental nerve (Haller, 1762)**

upper anterior branch of inferior maxillary nerve (Meckel, 1817), see **anterior branch of mandibular nerve (>1840)**

upper bundle of trigeminal nerve (Gordon, 1815), see **trigeminal nerve motor root (Bell, 1829)**

upper cervical ganglion (Lobstein, 1831), see **superior cervical ganglion (Vieussens, 1684)**

upper commissure of optic tubercles (Carus, 1814), see **posterior commissure (Winslow, 1733)**

upper corpora bigemina (Gordon, 1815), see **superior colliculus (Haller, 1762)**

upper esophageal branches of eighth pair (Walter, 1783), see **upper esophageal branches of vagus nerve (Cloquet, 1828)**

upper esophageal branches of vagus nerve (Cloquet, 1828)

upper filament of inferior orbital thread of temporal surculus (Bellingeri, 1818), see **temporal branches of facial nerve (Swan, 1830)**

upper ganglioform infolding of intercostal nerve (Willis, 1664), see **superior cervical ganglion (Vieussens, 1684)**

upper ganglioform infolding of wandring pair (Willis, 1664), see **proximal vagal ganglion (>1840)**

upper mesenteric plexus (Haller, 1762), see **superior mesenteric plexus (Rau, 1720)**

upper part of trunk of fifth pair of nerves arising within skull (Willis, 1664), see **trigeminal nerve (Winslow, 1733)**

upper pedicle of cerebellum (Mayo, 1827), see **superior cerebellar peduncle (Procháska, 1800)**

upper plexure of abdomen (Diemerbroeck, 1672), see **peripheral nervous system (Meckel, 1817)**

upper posterior nasal nerves (Meckel, 1832), see **posterior superior nasal nerves (Soemmerring, 1791)**

upper stomachical branch of wandring pair (Willis, 1664), see **anterior vagal trunk (Wrisberg, 1780)**

upper subscapular nerve (>1840)

upper ventricle (Avicenna, c1030), see **lateral ventricle (Vesalius, 1543a)**

uppermost and second branches of second division of fifth pair of nerves arising within skull (Willis, 1664), see **ophthalmic nerve (Winslow, 1733)**

uppermost branch of second division of fifth pair of nerves arising within skull (Willis, 1664), see **ophthalmic nerve (Winslow, 1733)**

uppermost cervical ganglion (Monro, 1783), see **superior cervical ganglion (Vieussens, 1684)**

upwardly recurrent nerve (Galen, c192), see **recurrent laryngeal nerve (Albinus, 1744)**

ureteric nerve to urethra (Walter, 1783), see **urethral branch of inferior hypogastric plexus (>1840)**

ureteric nerves (Tiedemann, 1822), see **superior ureteric nerves (Walter, 1783)**

ureteric plexus (>1840)

urethral branches of inferior hypogastric plexus (>1840)

urethral branchlets from hypogastric plexus (Walter, 1783), see **urethral branches of inferior hypogastric plexus (>1840)**

urinary vesicle branch of primary hypogastric plexus (Walter, 1783), see **extrinsic vesical plexus (>1840)**

uterine and vaginal nerves (Cloquet, 1816), see **sacral plexus ventral divisions (Paterson, 1887)**

uterine cervical ganglion (>1840)

uterine nerve (Cloquet, 1828), see **pelvic splanchnic nerves (Gaskell, 1886)**

uterine nerve (Fischer, 1791), see **sacral plexus ventral divisions (Paterson, 1887)**

uterine nerves (Galen, c173), see **uterovaginal plexus (>1840)**

uterovaginal nerves (Cruveilhier, 1836), see **uterovaginal plexus (>1840)**

uterovaginal plexus (>1840)

utricular nerve (>1840)

utriculoampullary nerve (>1840)

uvae (Albertus Magnus, 13th century), see **cerebellar vermis (Meckel, 1817)**

uvula (Malacarne, 1776)

uvular thread of external palatine fascicle (Bellingeri, 1818), see **lateral palatine nerve (Henle, 1871)**

vaccarum mammis (Spiegel, 1627), see **olfactory bulb (Weitbrecht, 1751)**

vaccinae papillae (Casseri, 1609), see **cerebral cortex (>1840)**

vacuities (Averroes, 12th century), see **ventricles (Hippocrates)**

vagal ganglia (Carus, 1814), see **nucleus of solitary tract (>1840)**

vagal lobes (Leuret, 1839), see **nucleus of solitary tract (>1840)**

vagal triangle (>1840)

vagal trigone (>1840), see **vagal triangle (>1840)**

vaginal branches of small plexus from first hypogastric plexus (Cloquet, 1828), see **vaginal nerves (Walter, 1783)**

vaginal nerves (Walter, 1783)

vagous nerve (Diemerbroeck, 1689), see **vagus nerve (Galen, c192)**

vague nerve (Haller, 1754b), see **vagus nerve (Galen, c192)**

vagus nerve (Galen, c192)

vagus nerve (Willis, 1664), see **cranial nerves (Soemmerring, 1791)**

vagus nerve central root (>1840)

vagus nerve central rootlets (>1840)

vagus nerve ganglion (Arnold, 1834), see **distal vagal ganglion (>1840)**

vagus nerve root (>1840)

vagus nerve rootlets (>1840)

vagus nerve roots (Günther, 1786), see **vagus nerve rootlets (>1840)**
vagus nerve trunk (Wrisberg, 1786; Günther, 1786)
vagus or pneumogastric nerve (Newport, 1834), see **invertebrate nerves (>1840)**
vallecula cerebelli (Haller, 1762), see **vallecula of cerebellum (Haller, 1762)**
vallecula inter lobos cerebri (Soemmerring, 1778), see **vallecula of cerebellum (Haller, 1762)**
vallecula of cerebellum (Haller, 1762)
valleculam (Soemmerring, 1778), see **vallecula of cerebellum (Haller, 1762)**
valley (Reil, 1809b), see **lateral cerebral sulcus (>1840)**
valley of cerebellum (Reil, 1807–1808a), see **vallecula of cerebellum (Haller, 1762)**
valve of Aqueduct of Sylvius (Gordon, 1817), see **rostral medullary vellum (>1840)**
valve of Galen (Günther, 1786), see **rostral medullary velum (>1840)**
valve of Vieussens (Lieutaud, 1742), see **rostral medullary velum (>1840)**
valviform expansion (Winslow, 1733), see **rostral medullary velum (>1840)**
valvula magna cerebelli (Günther, 1786), see **rostral medullary velum (>1840)**
valvula magna cerebri (Günther, 1786), see **rostral medullary velum (>1840)**
valvula major cerebri (Vieussens, 1684), see **rostral medullary velum (>1840)**
valvula major cerebri Vieussenii (Tarin, 1753), see **rostral medullary velum (>1840)**
valvula ovalis (Günther, 1786), see **rostral medullary velum (>1840)**
valvulae semicirculares, inferiores & posteriores (Tarin, 1750), see **caudal medullary velum (>1840)**
valvulam magnam cerebri (Haller, 1762), see **rostral medullary velum (>1840)**
valvular lamina (Winslow, 1733), see **rostral medullary velum (>1840)**
varicose part of cerebrum (du Laurens, 1600), see **cerebral cortex gray matter (>1840)**
varicosities (Rufus of Ephesus, fl. c90–c120), see **cerebral cortex gray matter (>1840)**
various filaments of portio major and minor of facial nerve (Bellingeri, 1818), see **intermediofacial nerve trunk (>1840)**
vascular commissure of optic thalamus (Cruveilhier, 1836), see **interthalamic adhesion (>1840)**
vascular nerve (Lobstein, 1823), see **sympathetic trunk (Winslow, 1733)**
vasculosa cerebri membrana (Haase, 1781), see **meninges (Smith Papyrus, c1700 BC)**
vasculosae membranae (Haller & Wrisberg, 1780), see **meninges (Smith Papyrus, c1700 BC)**
vasomotor nerve (Stilling, 1840), see **sympathetic trunk (Winslow, 1733)**
vault (Galen, c173), see **fornix (Vesalius, 1543a)**
vault (Geminus, 1553), see **fornix (Vesalius, 1543a)**
vault (Willis, 1664), see **cerebral cortex white matter (>1840)**
vault itself (Willis, 1664), see **fornix (Vesalius, 1543a)**
vault of fourth ventricle (Tiedemann, 1816), see **roof of fourth ventricle (Vesalius, 1543a)**
vault of ventricles (Riolan, 1657), see **fornix (Vesalius, 1543a)**
vault proper (Longet, 1842), see **fimbria (Honegger, 1890)**
vault-shaped body (Galen, c173), see **fornix (Vesalius, 1543a)**
vaulted arch of ventricles (Riolan, 1657), see **fornix (Vesalius, 1543a)**
vaulted body (Galen, c173), see **fornix (Vesalius, 1543a)**
vaulted body (Paré, 1550), see **fimbria (Honegger, 1890)**
vaulted body with three legs (Paré, 1550), see **fornix (Vesalius, 1543a)**
vaulted body with three pillars (Paré, 1561), see **fornix (Vesalius, 1543a)**
vegetative nerves (Reil, 1807), see **peripheral nervous system (Meckel, 1817)**
vegetative nervous system (Reil, 1807), see **peripheral nervous system (Meckel, 1817)**
vegetative system ganglia (Wutzer, 1817), see **autonomic ganglia (Langley, 1900)**
veil-like membrane (William of Saliceto, 1275), see **pia (Galen, c192)**
veils (Hall, 1565), see **meninges (Smith Papyrus, c1700 BC)**
vellum (Bell, 1803b), see **choroid membrane of third ventricle (>1840)**
velum apophysi vermiformi obtentum (Drelincourt, 1672), see **rostral medullary velum (>1840)**
velum cerebri vasculosum (Burdach, 1822), see **choroid membrane of third ventricle (>1840)**
velum choroïdes (Vicq d'Azyr, 1786), see **choroid membrane of third ventricle (>1840)**
velum commissurae anterioris (Bergmann, 1831), see **terminal lamina (Burdach, 1822)**
velum interjectum (Haller, 1762), see **rostral medullary velum (>1840)**
velum interpositum (Haller, 1754a), see **choroid membrane of third ventricle (>1840)**
velum medullare rostralis (>1840), see **rostral medullary velum (>1840)**
velum of Haller (Bell, 1802), see **choroid membrane of third ventricle (>1840)**
velum triangulare (Haller, 1762), see **choroid membrane of third ventricle (>1840)**
velum vasculosum (Bell, 1802), see **choroid membrane of third ventricle (>1840)**
velum vasculosum (Haller, 1754a), see **choroid plexus of third ventricle (Vicq d'Azyr, 1784)**
velum Vieussenii (Gordon, 1817), see **rostral medullary vellum (>1840)**
venae emissariae Santorini (Bell & Bell, 1816), see **emissary veins (Santorini, 1724)**
venter anterior (Berengario da Carpi, 1521), see **lateral ventricle (Vesalius, 1543a)**
venter medius (Berengario da Carpi, 1521), see **third ventricle (Galen, c173)**
venter posterior (Berengario da Carpi, 1522), see **fourth ventricle (Galen, c192)**
ventral anterior cingulate area (Brodmann, 1909)

ventral commissure of Ammon's horn (Kölliker, 1896), see **ventral hippocampal commissure (Craigie, 1925)**
ventral cord (Anderson, 1837)
ventral cord trunk (>1840)
ventral corticospinal tract (>1840), see **uncrossed pyramidal tract (>1840)**
ventral external arcuate fibers (>1840)
ventral fasciculus proprius (>1840), see **ventral intersegmental tract (>1840)**
ventral funiculus (>1840)
ventral ganglia (Anderson, 1837)
ventral hippocampal commissure (Craigie, 1925)
ventral horn (>1840)
ventral intersegmental tract (>1840)
ventral lateral geniculate nucleus (>1840)
ventral median fissure of medulla (>1840)
ventral median fissure of spinal cord (>1840)
ventral nervous cord (Anderson, 1837), see **ventral cord (Anderson, 1837)**
ventral part of pons (>1840), see **pons (Haller, 1747)**
ventral part of thalamus (Herrick, 1910)
ventral posterior cingulate area (Brodmann, 1909)
ventral premammillary nucleus (>1840)
ventral reticulospinal tract (>1840a), see **medial reticulospinal tract (>1840)**
ventral reticulospinal tract (>1840b), see **medial forebrain bundle (Edinger, 1893)**
ventral root (>1840)
ventral root central part (>1840)
ventral rootlets (>1840)
ventral rootlets central part (>1840)
ventral spinocerebellar tract (>1840)
ventral spinothalamic tract (>1840)
ventral tegmental decussation (>1840)
ventral thalamic nuclei (>1840)
ventral white commissure (>1840)
ventricle common to medulla dorsalis and cerebellum (Vesalius, 1543a), see **fourth ventricle (Galen, c192)**
ventricle lying under orbicular protuberances (Willis, 1664), see **cerebral aqueduct (>1840)**
ventricle of Aranzi (Mayer 1779), see **fourth ventricle (Galen, c192)**
ventricle of Aranzi (Meckel, 1817), see **fourth ventricle (Galen, c192)**
ventricle of brain (Willis, 1664), see **lateral ventricle (Vesalius, 1543a)**
ventricle of cerebellum (Herophilus, c335–c280 BC), see **fourth ventricle (Galen, c192)**
ventricle of cerebellum (Meckel, 1817), see **fourth ventricle (Galen, c192)**
ventricle of corpus callosum (Cruveilhier, 1836), see **sulcus of corpus callosum (>1840)**
ventricle of optic thalamus (Vicq d'Azyr, 1786), see **third ventricle (Galen, c173)**
ventricle of septum (Burdin, 1803), see **septal fissure (Burdach, 1822)**
ventricle of septum lucidum (Meckel, 1767), see **septal fissure (Burdach, 1822)**
ventricle of spinal marrow (Carus, 1814), see **central canal (Bellingeri, 1823)**
ventricle of Sylvius (Gall & Spurzheim, 1810), see **septal fissure (Burdach, 1822)**
ventricle of Sylvius (Müller, 1834), see **cerebral aqueduct (>1840)**
ventricle of thalamus (Rolando, 1831), see **third ventricle (Galen, c173)**
ventricles (Hippocrates)
ventricles one and two (Galen, c173, c177), see **lateral ventricle (Vesalius, 1543a)**
ventricular fluid (Cruveilhier, 1836), see **cerebrospinal fluid (Magendie, 1827)**
ventricular membrane (Cruveilhier, 1836), see **pia (Galen, c192)**
ventricular plexus (Swan, 1830), see **cardiac plexus (Keill, 1698)**
ventricular-subarachnoid space (Swanson & Bota, 2010)
ventriculum nobilem (Collins, 1685), see **fourth ventricle (Galen, c192)**
ventriculus cerebello et medullae dorsali communis (Vesalius, 1543a), see **fourth ventricle (Galen, c192)**
ventriculus medius anterior (Haller, 1762), see **third ventricle (Galen, c173)**
ventriculus nobilis (Herophilus, c335–c280 BC), see **fourth ventricle (Galen, c192)**
ventriculus septi cerebri medii (Wenzel & Wenzel, 1812), see **septal fissure (Burdach, 1822)**
ventrolateral fascicle (>1840)
ventrolateral fissure (>1840), see **lateral midbrain sulcus (>1840)**
ventrolateral sulcus of medulla (>1840)
ventrolateral sulcus of spinal cord (>1840)
ventromedial hypothalamic nucleus (>1840)
Verbindungszweig (Ram. communicans) zwischen dem Median- und dem Ulnarnerven (Bock, 1827), see **communicating branch of median nerve with ulnar nerve (Bock, 1827)**
vermiform eminence of cerebellum (Tarin, 1753), see **cerebellar vermis (Meckel, 1817)**
vermiform epiphysis (Galen, c173), see **cerebellar vermis (Meckel, 1817)**
vermiform excrescence (Galen, c177), see **cerebellar vermis (Meckel, 1817)**
vermiform process (Galen, c177), see **cerebellar vermis (Meckel, 1817)**
vermiformes (Winslow, 1733), see **flocculus (Meckel, 1817)**
vermiformis (Geminus, 1553), see **choroid plexus (Galen, c177)**
vermis (Avicenna or Ibn Sina, c1030), see **choroid plexus of lateral ventricle (Vicq d'Azyr, 1784)**
vermis (Galen, 1531), see **cerebellar vermis (Meckel, 1817)**
vermis bombycinus (Aranzi, 1587), see **hippocampal region (Swanson et al., 1987)**
vertebral branch (Willis, 1664), see **communicating branches of spinal nerves (Wutzer, 1817)**
vertebral ganglia (Bichat, 1801), see **spinal nerve ganglia (Burdach, 1819)**
vertebral ganglia (Gaskell, 1886), see **paravertebral ganglia (Durward, 1951)**
vertebral ganglion (>1840)
vertebral marrow (Cloquet, 1816), see **cerebrospinal trunk (>1840)**

wormlike epifysis (Galen, c177), see **cerebellar vermis (Meckel, 1817)**
Wulst (Burdach, 1822), see **splenium of corpus callosum (Burdach, 1822)**
Wulst (Soemmerring, 1788), see **cerebral cortex gray matter (>1840)**
yard of brain (Crooke, 1615), see **pineal gland (Galen, c192)**
yellow substance of posterior lobe (Arnold, 1838b), see **primary visual area (>1840)**
yellowish substance (Vesalius, 1543a), see **central nervous system gray matter regions (>1840)**
yellowish substance between gray and white matter of cerebellum (Soemmerring, 1778), see **cerebellar cortex (Willis, 1664)**
zac (Vesalius, 1543a), see **fornix (Vesalius, 1543a)**
zachd (Vesalius, 1543a), see **fornix (Vesalius, 1543a)**
zona (Palletta, 1784), see **trigeminal ganglion (>1840)**
zona incerta (>1840)
zonal layer of thalamus (Burdach, 1822)
zone of Lissauer (>1840), see **dorsolateral tract (>1840)**
Züngelchen (Burdach, 1822), see **lingula (Malacarne, 1776)**
Zwischenhirn (Baer, 1837), see **interbrain (Baer, 1837)**
zygomatic branch of hard nerve (Meckel, 1753), see **facial nerve trunk (1840)**
zygomatic branch of portio dura of auditory nerve (Albinus, 1744), see **zygomatic branches of facial nerve (>1840)**
zygomatic branch of portio dura of seventh pair of cerebral nerves (Albinus, 1761), see **zygomatic branches of facial nerve (>1840)**
zygomatic branches of ascending branch of superficial branch of hard nerve (Günther, 1786), see **temporal branches of facial nerve (Swan, 1830)**
zygomatic branches of facial nerve (>1840)
zygomatic branches of superior branch of facial nerve (Arnold, 1834), see **zygomatic branches of facial nerve (>1840)**
zygomatic nerve (Soemmerring, 1791), see **temporal branches of facial nerve (Swan, 1830)**
zygomatic nerve (>1840)
zygomatic orbital nerve (Le Cat, 1768), see **zygomatic nerve (>1840)**
zygomatico-auricular branch of cephalic part of trachelo-cutanean plexus (Burdin, 1803), see **great auricular nerve (Haase, 1781)**
zygomatico-auricular branch of cephalic part of tracheosubcutaneous nerves (Chaussier, 1809), see **great auricular nerve (Haase, 1781)**
zygomaticofacial nerve (>1840)
zygomaticotemporal nerve (>1840)

Index